Hematopathology of the Skin

Clinical & Pathological Approach

SECOND EDITION

Hematopathology of the Skin

Clinical & Pathological Approach

SECOND EDITION

Editors

Alejandro A. Gru, MD
Tenured Professor of Pathology & Dermatology
Departments of Pathology & Dermatology
Co-Director Cutaneous Lymphoma Program
Emily Couric Clinical Cancer Center
University of Virginia
Charlottesville, Virginia

András Schaffer, MD, PhD
Associate Professor
Division of Dermatology
University of Central Florida College of Medicine
Orlando, Florida and
Dermatology Associates of Tallahassee
Tallahassee, Florida

Alistair M. Robson, FRCPath, DipRCPath
Consultant Dermatopathologist
Departamento de Diagnóstico Laboratorial
Serviço de Anatomia Patológica
Instituto Português de Oncologia de Lisboa Francisco Gentil
Lisbon, Portugal and
Source LDPath London, UK

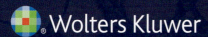

Philadelphia • Baltimore • New York • London
Buenos Aires • Hong Kong • Sydney • Tokyo

Acquisitions Editor: Nicole Dernoski
Senior Product Development Editor: Ariel S. Winter
Editorial Coordinator: Anju Radhakrishnan
Production Project Manager: Justin Wright
Manager, Graphic Arts & Design: Stephen Druding
Manufacturing Coordinator: Beth Welsh
Prepress Vendor: TNQ

2nd edition

Copyright © 2023 Wolters Kluwer

All rights reserved. This book is protected by copyright. No part of this book may be reproduced or transmitted in any form or by any means, including as photocopies or scanned-in or other electronic copies, or utilized by any information storage and retrieval system without written permission from the copyright owner, except for brief quotations embodied in critical articles and reviews. Materials appearing in this book prepared by individuals as part of their official duties as U.S. government employees are not covered by the above-mentioned copyright. To request permission, please contact Wolters Kluwer at Two Commerce Square, 2001 Market Street, Philadelphia, PA 19103, via email at permissions@lww.com, or via our website at lww.com (products and services).

9 8 7 6 5 4 3 2 1

Printed in Singapore

Library of Congress Cataloging-in-Publication Data
ISBN-13: 978-1-975158-55-2
Cataloging in Publication data available on request from publisher.

This work is provided "as is," and the publisher disclaims any and all warranties, express or implied, including any warranties as to accuracy, comprehensiveness, or currency of the content of this work.

This work is no substitute for individual patient assessment based upon healthcare professionals' examination of each patient and consideration of, among other things, age, weight, gender, current or prior medical conditions, medication history, laboratory data, and other factors unique to the patient. The publisher does not provide medical advice or guidance and this work is merely a reference tool. Healthcare professionals, and not the publisher, are solely responsible for the use of this work including all medical judgments and for any resulting diagnosis and treatments.

Given continuous, rapid advances in medical science and health information, independent professional verification of medical diagnoses, indications, appropriate pharmaceutical selections and dosages, and treatment options should be made and healthcare professionals should consult a variety of sources. When prescribing medication, healthcare professionals are advised to consult the product information sheet (the manufacturer's package insert) accompanying each drug to verify, among other things, conditions of use, warnings and side effects and identify any changes in dosage schedule or contraindications, particularly if the medication to be administered is new, infrequently used or has a narrow therapeutic range. To the maximum extent permitted under applicable law, no responsibility is assumed by the publisher for any injury and/or damage to persons or property, as a matter of products liability, negligence law or otherwise, or from any reference to or use by any person of this work.

LWW.com

To the love of my life, my wife, Lorena, my five beautiful children, Camila, Sofia, Santiago, Valentin, Nicolas, and my granddaughter, Amara.

Alejandro A. Gru

To my family, Sena, Daniel, Andrew Bence, Katalin, and Imre for their love and relentless support.

András Schaffer

For my family,

Alistair M. Robson

CONTRIBUTORS

Faizan Alawi, DDS
Associate Dean for Academic Affairs
Director, Penn Oral Pathology Services
Professor of Pathology
School of Dental Medicine
University of Pennsylvania
Philadelphia, Pennsylvania

Ali Al-Haseni
Department of Dermatology
Boston Medical center
Boston, Massachusetts

Liaqat Ali, MD
Assistant Professor
Department of Dermatology
Wayne State University
Detroit, Michigan
Pinkus Dermatopathology
Monroe, Michigan

Julia Almeida, MD, PhD
Department Medicine and IBMCC
  (USAL-CISC)
University of Salamanca
Salamanca, Spain

Martine Bagot, MD, PhD
Professor of Dermatology and Head of
  Dermatology Department
Department of Dermatology
Université de Paris and Inserm U976
Hôpital Saint Louis
Paris, France

Farrah Bakr, MBBS, MRCP
Academic Clinical Fellow
Division of Genetics and Molecular
  Medicine
St John's Institute of Dermatology
Guy's Hospital
King's College London
London, United Kingdom

Carlos Barrionuevo-Cornejo, MD, MSc
Executive Director
Department of Pathology
Instituto Nacional de Enfermedades
  Neoplásicas
Lima, Peru

Maxime Battistella, MD, PhD
Professor
Department of Pathology
Université de Paris
Paris, France

Helmut Beltraminelli, MD
Vice Chief
Dermatology and Pathology
Ente Ospedaliero Cantonale (EOC)
Bellinzona and Locarno, Switzerland

Jacob R. Bledsoe, MD
Assistant Professor of Pathology
Boston Children's Hospital
Boston, Massachusetts

Zoe O. Brown-Joel, MD
Department of Dermatology
Medical College of Wisconsin
Milwaukee, Wisconsin

Caitlin M. Brumfiel, MD
Georgetown University School of
  Medicine
Washington, DC

José Cabeçadas, MD
Director do Departamento de
  Diagnóstico Laboratorial
Instituto Português de Oncologia de
  Lisboa, Francisco Gentil
Lisboa, Portugal

Casey A. Carlos, MD, PhD
Consultant Dermatologist
Dermatology Arts
Bellevue, Washington

Yann Charlie-Joseph
Dermatologist/Dermatopathologist,
  Co-director & Founder: Cutaneous
  Hematopathology Clinic
  INCMNSZ. Secretary AMD
Mexico City, Mexico
Professor in Dermatopathology and
  Skin Lymphomas, Dermatology
  Residency, INCMNSZ, UNAM

Milda Chmieliauskaite, DMD, MPH
Assistant Professor of Oral Medicine
  and Director
Oral Medicine Graduate Program
University of Washington
Seattle, Washington

Emily Y. Chu, MD, PhD
Associate Professor
Department of Dermatology
Perelman School of Medicine
University of Pennsylvania
Philadelphia, Pennsylvania

Catherine G. Chung, MD
Associate Professor
Department of Dermatology and
  Pathology
Penn State Milton S. Hershey Medical
  Center
Hershey, Pennsylvania

Mariana Cravo, MD
Senior Consultant Dermatologist
Department of Dermatology
Portuguese Institute of Oncology
Lisbon, Portugal

Richard Danialan, DO
Dermatopathology Fellow
Department of Pathology and
  Laboratory Medicine
The University of Texas
MD Anderson Cancer Center
Houston, Texas

Louis P. Dehner, MD
Professor
Department of Pathology and
  Immunology
Washington University School of
  Medicine
St. Louis, Missouri

Martin Dittmer, MD
Dermatopathology Fellow
Division of Dermatology
University of Washington
Seattle, Washington

Jacques J. M. van Dongen, MD, PhD
Professor of Medical Immunology
Dept of Immunology
Leiden University Medical Center
Leiden, The Netherlands

Brittany O. Dulmage, MD
Assistant Professor
Dermatology
Ohio State University Wexner Medical Center
Columbus, Ohio

Juanita Duran, MD
Dermatopathology Fellow
Department of Pathology, Dermatopathology Division
University of Virginia
Charlottesville, Virginia

Benjamin H. Durham, MD
Assistant Attending Pathologist
Department of Pathology
Memorial Sloan Kettering Cancer Center
New York, New York

Andrew L. Feldman, MD
Professor
Department of Laboratory Medicine and Pathology
Mayo Clinic College of Medicine
Rochester, Minnesota

Katalin Ferenczi, MD
Associate Professor
Department of Dermatology and Dermatopathology
University of Connecticut
Farmington, Connecticut

Katherine France, DMD, MBE
Assistant Professor of Oral Medicine
University of Pennsylvania School of Dental Medicine
Philadelphia, Pennsylvania

John L. Frater, MD
Professor
Department of Pathology and Immunology
Washington University School of Medicine
St. Louis, Missouri

Aharon G. Freud, MD, PhD
Associate Professor
Department of Pathology
The Ohio State University
Wexner Medical Center
Columbus, Ohio

Crystal Gao, MBBS (Hons), BMedSc (Hons)
Doctor
Peter McCallum Cancer Centre / The Alfred Hospital
Melbourne, Victoria, Australia

Carolina M. Gentile, MD
Chief
Department of Ophthalmology
Unit of Ocular Oncology
Hospital Italiano de Buenos Aires
Buenos Aires, Argentina

Lynne J. Goldberg, MD
Professor
Department of Dermatology and Pathology and Laboratory Medicine
Boston University School of Medicine
Boston, Massachusetts

Clive E. Grattan, MA, MD, FRCP
Consultant Dermatologist
St Johns Institute of Dermatology
Guys Hospital
London, United Kingdom

Alejandro A. Gru, MD
Tenured Professor of Pathology & Dermatology
Departments of Pathology & Dermatology
Co-Director Cutaneous Lymphoma Program
Emily Couric Clinical Cancer Center
University of Virginia
Charlottesville, Virginia

Emmanuella Guenova
Professor in Dermatology
Faculty of Biology and Medicine
University of Lausanne
Lausanne, Switzerland

Ian S. Hagemann, MD, PhD
Associate Professor
Department of Pathology and Immunology
Washington University School of Medicine
St. Louis, Missouri

Yasmin Hambaroush, MD
Hematopathology Fellow
Departrment of Pathology
University of Virginia
Charlottesville, Virginia

Paul Haun
Assistant Professor
Departments of Dermatology and Anatomic Pathology and Laboratory Medicine
University of Pennsylvania
Philadelphia, Pennsylvania

Gillian Heinecke, MD
Assistant Professor
Department of Dermatology
Saint Louis University
Saint Louis, Missouri

Emmilia Hodak
Professor of Dermatology
Rabin Medical Center
Cancer Biology Research Center
Tel Aviv University
Petah Tikva, Israel

Hans-Peter Horny, MD
Professor of Pathology
Institue of Pathology
University of Munich
Munich, Germany

Andy C. Hsi, MD
Consultant Dermatopathologist
West Dermatology
Placentia, California

M. Yadira Hurley, MD
Professor
Department of Dermatology and Pathology
Director
Division of Dermatopathology
Director
Dermatopathology Fellowship
Department of Dermatology
Saint Louis University
St. Louis, Missouri

Paola de la Iglesia Niveyro, MD
Staff Pathologist
Pathology
Hospital Italiano de Buenos Aires
Buenos Aires, Argentina

Elaine S. Jaffe, MD
Chief
Hematopathology Section
Laboratory of Pathology
Center for Cancer Research
National Cancer Institute
National Institutes of Health
Bethesda, Maryland

Melinda Jen, MD
Associate Professor of Clinical Pediatrics
Perelman School of Medicine
University of Pennsylvania
The Children's Hospital of Philadelphia
Philadelphia, Pennsylvania

Jacqueline M. Junkins-Hopkins, MD
Dermatopathologist
Geisinger Medical Laboratories
Geisinger Commonwealth School of Medicine
Danville, Pennsylvania

Benjamin H. Kaffenberger, MD
Associate Professor
Department of Dermatology
The Ohio State University
Wexner Medical Center
Columbus, Ohio

Viktoryia Kazlouskaya, MD, PhD
Assistant Professor of Dermatology
Department of Dermatology
University of Pittsburgh Medical Center
Pittsburgh, Pennsylvania

Werner Kempf, MD
Co-Director Cutaneous Lymphoma Unit
Kempf und Pfaltz Histologische Diagnostik
Zurich, Switzerland

Shadi Khalil, MD, PhD
Department of Dermatology
University of California, San Diego
San Diego, California

Joseph D. Khoury, MD
Stokes-Shackleford Professor and Chairman
Department of Pathology
University of Nebraska Medical Center
Omaha, Nebraska

Ellen J. Kim, MD
Sandra J. Lazarus Professor of Dermatology
Perelman School of Medicine at the University of Pennsylvania
Philadelphia, Pennsylvania

Rebecca L. King, MD
Associate Professor
Division of Hematopathology
Mayo Clinic
Rochester, Minnesota

Eynav Klechevsky
Assistant Professor
Pathology and Immunology
Washington University School of Medicine
St. Louis, Missouri

Abraham Korman, MD
Assistant Professor
Department of Dermatology
The Ohio State University Wexner Medical Center
Columbus, Ohio

Stephen Lade, MBBS
Pathologist
University of Melbourne
Peter Maccallum Cancer Centre
Melbourne, Victoria, Australia

Jason B. Lee, MD
Professor
Department of Dermatology and Cutaneous Biology
Thomas Jefferson University
Philadelphia, Pennsylvania

Sena J. Lee, MD, PhD
Medical Reviewer
Division of Dermatology and Dentistry
Center for Drug Evaluation and Research
Food and Drug Administration
Silver Spring, Maryland

Sanam Loghavi, MD
Assistant Professor
Department of Hematopathology
The University of Texas
MD Anderson Cancer Center
Houston, Texas

Jozef Malysz, MD
Associate Professor
Department of Pathology
Penn State Milton S. Hershey Medical Center
Hershey, Pennsylvania

Kristin K. McNamara, DDS, MS
Associate Professor
Oral and Maxillofacial Pathology and Radiology
College of Dentistry
The Ohio State University
Columbus, Ohio

Christina Mitteldorff, MD
Head of Dermapathology and Cutaneous
Department of Dermatology
University of Göttingen
Göttingen, Lower Saxony, Germany

Andrea P. Moy, MD
Dermatopathologist
Memorial Sloan-Kettering Cancer Center
New York, New York

Amy C. Musiek, MD
Professor of Medicine (Dermatology)
Washington University School of Medicine
St. Louis, Missouri

Priyadharsini Nagarajan, MD, PhD
Associate Professor
Department of Pathology
The University of Texas
MD Anderson Cancer Center
Houston, Texas

Safa Najidh, MD
Dermatology
Leiden University Medical Center
Leiden, South Holland,
 The Netherlands

Rosalynn M. Nazarian, MD
Associate Professor
Department of Pathology
Harvard Medical School
Dermatopathologist
Pathology Service
Massachusetts General
 Hospital
Boston, Massachusetts

Jacob Nosewicz
Clinical Research Fellow
Department of Dematology
Ohio State University Wexner Medical
 Center
Columbus, Ohio

Roberto Novoa, MD
Clinical Associate Professor
Departments of Pathology and
 Dermatology
Stanford University
Stanford, California

Kelsey Nusbaum, MD
Clinical Instructor
Department of Dermatology
The Ohio State University
Columbus, Ohio

Pablo L. Ortiz-Romero, MD, PhD
Jefe de Servicio de Dermatologia
Hospital Universitario 12 de
 Octubre
Facultad de Medicina
Universidad Complutense
Madrid, Spain

Nicolas Ortonne
Professor
Paris Est Creteil University (UPEC),
 and Mondor
Institute of Biomédical Research
 (IMRB)
Paris, Creteil

Meera H. Patel, BS
Medical Student
Creighton University School of
 Medicine Phoenix Regional
 Campus
Phoenix, Arizona

Yvonne Perner, MBBS, MMED
Division of Anatomical Pathology
Faculty of Health Sciences
University of the Witwatersrand
Johannesburg, Gauteng, South Africa

Tony Petrella, MD
Associate Professor
Pathology
University of Montreal
Montreal, Quebec, Canada

Jennifer Picarsic, MD
Associate Professor
Cincinnati Children's Hospital
University of Cincinnati College of
 Medicine
Department of Pathology and
 Laboratory Medicine
Cincinnati, Ohio

Laura Beth Pincus, MD
Professor
Department of Dermatology and
 Pathology
University of California, San Francisco
San Francisco, California

Jose A. Plaza, MD
Professor of Pathology & Dermatology
Department of Pathology
The Ohio State University Wexner
 Medical Center
Columbus, Ohio

Pierluigi Porcu, MD
Professor
Department of Internal Medicine
Division of Hematology
Comprehensive Cancer Center
Cutaneous Lymphoma Program
The Ohio State University
Columbus, Ohio

H. Miles Prince, MD
Professor
Sir Peter MacCallum
Department of Oncology
University of Melbourne
Melbourne, Victoria, Australia

Melissa Pulitzer, MD
Associate Attending Pathologist
Memorial Sloan Kettering Cancer Center
Assistant Professor
Department of Pathology and
 Laboratory Medicine
Weill Medical College of Cornell
 University
New York, New York

Pietro Quaglino, MD
Professor of Dermatology
Director of Cutaneous Lymphoma
 Program
Medical Sciences
University of Turin
Italy, Turin

Leticia Quintanilla-Martinez, MD
Prof Dr. Med, Professor In Pathology
Institute of Pathology
University Hospital Tuebingen
Tuebingen, Germany

Egle Ramelyte, MD, PhD
Attending physician
Skin Cancer Center, Department of
 Dermatology
University Hospital Zurich
Zurich, Switzerland

Alistair M. Robson, FRCPath, DipRCPath
Consultant Dermatopathologist
Departamento de Diagnóstico
 Laboratorial
Serviço de Anatomia Patológica
Instituto Português de Oncologia de
 Lisboa Francisco Gentil
Lisbon, Portugal and
Source LDPath London,
 United Kingdom

Andrea Roggo, PhD
Department of Dermatology
University Hospital Zürich
Zürich, Switzerland

Kate Roussak, MS, MD
Postdoctoral Research Associate
Department of Pathology &
 Immunology
Washington University in Saint Louis
Saint Louis, Missouri

Adam I. Rubin, MD
Professor of Dermatology
Department of Dermatology,
 Pediatrics, and Pathology and
 Laboratory Medicine
Hospital of the University of
 Pennsylvania
The Children's Hospital of
 Philadelphia
Perelman School of Medicine
University of Pennsylvania
Philadelphia, Pennsylvania

Joya Sahu, MD
Consultant Dermatologist and Dermatopathologist
Dermatology Specialists
Madison, Alabama

Andrea L. Salavaggione, MD
Anatomic Pathology
University of Virginia
Charlottesville, Virginia

J. Martin Sangueza
Professor
Department of Pathology and Dermatology
Hospital Obrero
La Paz, Bolivia

Julia Scarisbrick, MB (Hons), ChB, FRCP, MD
Consultant Dermatologist & Lead Cutaneous Lymphoma Service
University Hospitals Birmingham NHS Foundation Trust
Birmingham, United Kingdom

András Schaffer, MD, PhD
Associate Professor
Division of Dermatology
University of Central Florida College of Medicine
Orlando, Florida and
Dermatology Associates of Tallahassee
Tallahassee, Florida

Madelie Sellers, MD, MBA
Fellow
Department of Pathology
Ohio State University Hospital
Columbus, Ohio

Sara C. Shalin, MD, PhD
Chairman, Department of Dermatology
Associate Professor, Department of Dermatology and Pathology
University of Arkansas for Medical Sciences
Little Rock, Arkansas

Archana Shenoy, MD
Clinical Assistant Professor
Nationwide Children's Hospital
The Ohio State University College of Medicine
Columbus, Ohio

Allen F. Shih, MD, MBA, MA
Instructor in Dermatology
Harvard Medical School
Beth Israel Deaconess Medical Center
Boston, Massachusetts

Michi M. Shinohara, MD
Associate Professor
Director of Dermatopathology
Division of Dermatology, Department of Medicine; Division of Dermatopathology, Department of Laboratory Medicine and Pathology
University of Washington
Seattle, Washington

Kristin C. Smith, MD
Dermatopathologist; Assistant Professor of Dermatology
Saint Louis University
St. Louis, Missouri

Bruce R. Smoller, MD
Professor and Chair
Department of Pathology and Laboratory Medicine
University of Rochester School of Medicine and Dentistry
Rochester, New York

Campbell L. Stewart, MD
Assistant Professor
Department of Dermatology
University of Connecticut
Farmington, Connecticut

Antonio Subtil, MD, MBA
Dermatopathologist and Hematopathologist
Laboratory Medicine, Pathology and Genetics
Royal Jubilee Hospital
Victoria, British Columbia, Canada

Kari E. Sufficool, MD
Dermatopathologist
United Skin Specialists
1001 Chesterfield Pkwy E, Suite 101
Chesterfield, Missouri

Tina L. Sumpter
Research Assistant Professor
Department of Dermatology
University of Pittsburgh
Pittsburgh, Pennsylvania

Michael T. Tetzlaff, MD, PhD
Professor of Pathology and Dermatology
Dermatopathology and Oral Pathology Service
University of San Francisco
San Francisco, California

Carlos A. Torres-Cabala, MD
Professor
Department of Pathology and Dermatology
The University of Texas
MD Anderson Cancer Center
Houston, Texas

Maarten H. Vermeer, MD, PhD
Head of Department
Department of Dermatology
Leiden University Medical Center
Leiden, The Netherlands

Karolyn A. Wanat, MD
Vice Chair and Clinical Associate Professor
Department of Dermatology
University of Iowa
Iowa City, Iowa

Sean Whittaker, MB, MD, FRCP
Professor of Cutaneous Oncology
School of Basic and Medical Biosciences
Faculty of Life Sciences and Medicine
Kings College
London, United Kingdom

Rein Willemze, MD, PhD
Professor Emeritus of Dermatology
Department of Dermatology
Leiden University Medical Center
Leiden, The Netherlands

Matthew J. Zirwas, MD
Director
Ohio Contact Dermatitis Center
Columbus, Ohio

PREFACE

Diagnosing hematologic neoplasms in the skin requires interdisciplinary collaboration between hematologists, dermatologists, hematopathologists, and dermatopathologists. Most dermatopathologists, especially those with a dermatology background, confess their limited knowledge of hematopathology. Conversely, hematopathologists rarely encounter skin biopsies and lack appreciation for the clinical findings and of the plethora of inflammatory mimickers, which are pertinent in consideration to reach an accurate diagnosis. It is critically important that dermatologists and cutaneous oncologists are knowledgeable about hematopathologic principles, which are increasingly salient in personalized therapeutic regimens for cancer patients. It is equally vital that pathologists understand clinical correlates, including latest treatment modalities. They must characterize each neoplasm using appropriate molecular markers, which can then facilitate proper selection of antitumor agents for patients.

Our goal was to compile a concise yet comprehensive compendium for clinicians and pathologists who care for those with cutaneous hematologic neoplasms. It was clear from the conception of the book that the experience from a single author or single institution will not be sufficient to cover the breadth of knowledge that spans four disciplines. To achieve our mission, more than 40 leading dermatopathologists, hematopathologists, dermatologists, and oncologists from more than 15 major academic centers in the United States and abroad came together to share their expertise and personal experiences.

Appropriate structuring of the book was indispensable to clarity. The authors followed the classification guidelines of the World Health Organization and European Organization for Research and Treatment of Cancer (EORTC). Most of the chapters address individual disease entities or a group of related diseases. Each chapter starts with disease definition, followed by clinical, histologic, immunophenotypic, and genetic findings. Molecular and immune pathogenesis are also emphasized at great length. Furthermore, the chapters are accompanied by many clinical and pathologic images and conclude with detailed differential diagnoses and a capsule summary. Numerous tables and figures are also included for an enhanced illustration of concepts.

Cutaneous immune cells give rise to the many neoplasms discussed in this book. It thus made sense to begin by describing the functional and phenotypic heterogeneity of these cells, as this information is the foundation for later chapters, especially in understanding pathogenesis and classification. The next chapters detail the molecular biology of T- and B-cell lymphomas, which are followed by a brief review of contemporary and emerging diagnostic techniques such as flow cytometry, cytogenetics, PCR-based gene rearrangement studies, and next-generation sequencing.

Most of the book discusses hematologic malignancies that emerge from skin-resident or skin-homing immune cells, including various T- and B-cell subsets, monocytes, dendritic cells, macrophages, and mast cells. Also, several chapters have been devoted to the cutaneous metastasis of and paraneoplastic reactions to systemic hematologic malignancies. A single chapter is dedicated to summarize the recent advances in diagnosing cutaneous lymphoproliferations in acquired immunodeficiency, such as in posttransplant patients, patients on immunosuppression for autoimmune disorders, or in acquired immunodeficiency syndrome.

The book also places a major emphasis on cutaneous inflammatory conditions and reactive lymphoproliferations that resemble hematologic malignancies and often cause diagnostic dilemmas. The reader will find thorough discussions about inflammatory mimickers of early cutaneous lymphomas, such as pityriasis lichenoides, follicular mucinosis, cutaneous lymphoid hyperplasia, and relatively new entities such as annular lichenoid dermatosis of the youth. Additionally, detailed chapters are devoted to pseudolymphomas stemming from drugs, infection, vaccination, tattoo, and epithelial neoplasia.

The last few chapters cover hematologic malignancies in special anatomical regions or patient populations: ocular and oral lymphoproliferative diseases, alopecia-associated lymphomas, and pediatric hematolymphoid neoplasias. The book ends with a chapter dedicated to adverse cutaneous reactions secondary to chemotherapy and newer targeted anticancer agents.

It is a testament to the ongoing interest and research in the field that in updating the first edition of this work after only 4 years there have had to be revisions to reflect changes in classification and nomenclature, expansion to the sections on pathogenetic mechanisms and greater attention paid to the consequences of wider therapeutic choices. In addition, two chapters outlining the approach to the treatment strategies employed in cutaneous T- and B-cell lymphomas have been introduced.

We believe this revision has succeeded in maintaining a work that is unprecedented in depth and breadth for its field and is satisfactory in achieving our goal to produce a comprehensive textbook of cutaneous hematopathology. We are delighted that the collaborative network of contributing authors, whose devotion and hard work remain very much appreciated, has only grown in number and scope. We sincerely hope that this book will serve as an interdisciplinary knowledge portal for clinicians and pathologists and, most importantly, that it will ultimately help to improve our care of patients.

Alejandro A. Gru, MD
András Schaffer, MD, PhD
Alistair M. Robson, FRCPath, DipRCPath

CONTENTS

Contributors vii
Preface xiii

Part I
Immunobiology and Molecular Pathogenesis   1

1. Cutaneous T-cell immunobiology 1
   Emmanuella Guenova, Andy C. Hsi, and András Schaffer

2. Cutaneous B-cell immunobiology 12
   Alejandro A. Gru and José Cabeçadas

3. NK cell immunobiology 21
   Aharon G. Freud and Madelie Sellers

4. Mononuclear phagocytic system of the skin–guide to pathologists 26
   Kate Roussak and Eynav Klechevsky

5. Mast cells in the skin 34
   Tina L. Sumpter

6. Molecular pathogenesis of primary cutaneous T-cell lymphomas 40
   Sean Whittaker

7. Molecular pathogenesis of primary cutaneous B-cell lymphomas 50
   Alejandro A. Gru and Pierluigi Porcu

Part II
Laboratory Techniques   59

8. Flow cytometric analysis in hematopathology diagnosis 59
   Safa Najidh, Julia Almeida, Jacques J. M. van Dongen, and Maarten H. Vermeer

9. PCR-based gene rearrangement studies 73
   Ian S. Hagemann

10. FISH and cytogenetic techniques 81
    Andrea L. Salavaggione and Alejandro A. Gru

11. Next-generation sequencing 97
    Ian S. Hagemann

Part III
Primary Cutaneous T-Cell Lymphomas   103

12. Approach to the diagnosis of primary cutaneous T-cell lymphomas 103
    Alistair M. Robson, Alejandro A. Gru, and András Schaffer

13. Mycosis fungoides 109
    Alistair M. Robson, Rein Willemze, Julia Scarisbrick, Amy C. Musiek, Emmilia Hodak, Alejandro A. Gru, and András Schaffer

14. Sézary syndrome 143
    Ellen J. Kim, Paul Haun, Martine Bagot, Maxime Battistella, and András Schaffer

15. Primary cutaneous CD30-positive T-cell lymphoproliferative disorders 158
    Rebecca L. King, Werner Kempf, Amy C. Musiek, and Andrew L. Feldman

16. Subcutaneous panniculitis-like T-cell lymphoma 178
    Alejandro A. Gru, Laura Beth Pincus, and Yann Charlie-Joseph

17. Cutaneous CD4+ small to medium lymphoproliferative disorder and other proliferations with TFH phenotype 193
    Sanam Loghavi, Farrah Bakr, Helmut Beltraminelli, Alistair M. Robson, and Michael T. Tetzlaff

18. Aggressive cytotoxic primary cutaneous T-cell lymphomas 203
    Jacqueline M. Junkins-Hopkins and Ellen J. Kim

19. Primary cutaneous peripheral T-cell lymphoma, not otherwise specified 220
    Alistair M. Robson, Andy C. Hsi, Amy C. Musiek, and András Schaffer

20. Primary cutaneous CD8+ acral lymphoproliferative disorder 225
    Alistair M. Robson, Farrah Bakr, Melissa Pulitzer, and Werner Kempf

21. Granulomatous CD8-positive lymphoproliferative disorder associated with immunodeficiency 233
    Werner Kempf and Christina Mitteldorf

22. An approach to the treatment of mycosis fungoides/Sézary syndrome and CD30 positive lymphoproliferative disorders 238
    Pietro Quaglino, Egle Ramelyte, Andrea Roggo, Crystal Gao, Rein Willemze, Stephen Lade, and H. Miles Prince

Part IV
Primary Cutaneous NK/T-Cell Malignancies   256

23. Extranodal natural killer/T-cell lymphoma, nasal type 256
    Carlos Barrionuevo-Cornejo and Leticia Quintanilla-Martinez

24. Hydroa vacciniforme lymphoproliferative disorder 262
    Jose A. Plaza and J. Martin Sangueza

25. Natural killer–cell leukemias/lymphomas 270
    Aharon G. Freud and Madelie Sellers

xv

Part V
Systemic T- and NK-Cell Lymphomas With Cutaneous Dissemination — 280

26 Systemic anaplastic large cell lymphoma 280
   Alejandro A. Gru and Werner Kempf

27 T-cell prolymphocytic leukemia 291
   Alejandro A. Gru

28 Skin manifestations of angioimmunoblastic T-cell lymphoma 298
   Nicolas Ortonne

29 Adult T-cell leukemia/lymphoma 311
   Melissa Pulitzer

Part VI
Primary Cutaneous B-Cell Lymphoproliferative Disorders — 322

30 Approach to the diagnosis of cutaneous B-cell lymphomas 322
   Alejandro A. Gru and Elaine S. Jaffe

31 Primary cutaneous follicle center B-cell lymphoma 336
   Antonio Subtil and Michi M. Shinohara

32 Primary cutaneous marginal zone B-cell lymphoma 347
   Katalin Ferenczi, Farrah Bakr, and Alistair M. Robson

33 Primary cutaneous diffuse large B-cell lymphoma 360
   Christina Mitteldorf, Alejandro A. Gru, and José Cabeçadas

34 Lymphomatoid granulomatosis 378
   Yasmin Hambaroush and Alejandro A. Gru

35 Mucocutaneous EBV- and HHV-8 associated lymphoproliferative disorders in acquired immunodeficiency 388
   Alejandro A. Gru, Melissa Pulitzer, and András Schaffer

36 An approach to the treatment of primary cutaneous B-Cell lymphomas 405
   Pablo L. Ortiz-Romero and Mariana Cravo

Part VII
Systemic B-Cell Lymphomas With Cutaneous Dissemination — 413

37 Systemic follicular lymphoma, marginal zone lymphomas, and lymphoplasmacytic lymphoma 413
   Alejandro A. Gru and Antonio Subtil

38 Intravascular large B-cell lymphoma 423
   Alejandro A. Gru and Maxime Battistella

39 Cutaneous involvement in systemic diffuse large B-cell lymphomas 431
   Alejandro A. Gru and Yvonne Perner

40 Cutaneous mantle cell lymphoma 455
   José Cabeçadas and Alejandro A. Gru

41 Cutaneous manifestations of chronic lymphocytic leukemia/small lymphocytic lymphoma 463
   Alejandro A. Gru and Maxime Battistella

42 Cutaneous plasma-cell neoplasms 474
   Liaqat Ali, Jozef Malysz, and José Cabeçadas

43 Cutaneous involvement by Hodgkin's lymphoma 480
   Alejandro A. Gru, András Schaffer, and Maxime Battistella

Part VIII
Cutaneous Reactive Infiltrates — 492

44 Pityriasis lichenoides chronica 492
   Emily Y. Chu and Werner Kempf

45 Jessner lymphocytic infiltrate and tumid lupus erythematosus 498
   Juanita Duran and Jose A. Plaza

46 Pigmented purpuric dermatoses 503
   Casey A. Carlos

47 Chronic actinic dermatitis—actinic reticuloid 506
   Sena J. Lee and András Schaffer

48 CD30 pseudolymphomas 510
   Jacqueline M. Junkins-Hopkins and Werner Kempf

49 Pseudolymphomatous reactions with associated cutaneous neoplastic proliferations 525
   Sara C. Shalin and Bruce R. Smoller

50 Cutaneous lymphoid hyperplasia and related entities 542
   Alejandro A. Gru

51 Pseudolymphomas at sites of vaccination and in tattoos 562
   Priyadharsini Nagarajan

52 Lymphoid proliferations in association with viral and bacterial infections 567
   Priyadharsini Nagarajan

53 Cutaneous plasmacytosis 572
   M. Yadira Hurley and Gillian Heinecke

54 Cutaneous IgG4-related disease 577
   Alejandro A. Gru

55 Lymphomatoid contact dermatitis 582
   Caitlin M. Brumfiel, Meera H. Patel, Alejandro A. Gru, and Matthew J. Zirwas

56 Annular lichenoid dermatosis of youth 588
   Alejandro A. Gru

57 Eosinophilic dermatosis of hematologic malignancy 592
   Joya Sahu and Jason B. Lee

Part IX
Precursor Lymphoid and Myeloid Neoplasms — 598

58 Precursor B- and T-cell neoplasms 598
   Alejandro A. Gru and Maxime Battistella

59 Leukemia cutis/aleukemic leukemia cutis/myeloid sarcoma 608
   Kari E. Sufficool and John L. Frater

60 Cutaneous manifestations of myeloproliferative neoplasms 621
   Richard Danialan and Carlos A. Torres-Cabala

61 Cutaneous extramedullary hematopoiesis 635
Shadi Khalil and András Schaffer

62 Blastic plasmacytoid dendritic cell neoplasm 638
M. Yadira Hurley, Joseph D. Khoury, Alejandro A. Gru,
Tony Petrella, and Martin Dittmer

Part X
Cutaneous Mast Cell Proliferations   650

63 Mast cell neoplasms 650
Clive E. Grattan and Hans-Peter Horny

Part XI
Benign and Malignant Histiocytic Disorders   664

64 Molecular classification of histiocytoses 664
Jennifer Picarsic and Benjamin H. Durham

65 Langerhans cell proliferations and related
disorders ("L" group) 674
Jacob R. Bledsoe, Jennifer Picarsic, Louis P. Dehner,
and Rosalynn M. Nazarian

66 Rosai–Dorfman disease 684
Kristin C. Smith and M. Yadira Hurley

67 Non-Langerhans cell histiocytoses (C and H groups) 690
Andrea P. Moy, Jacob R. Bledsoe, Louis P. Dehner,
and Rosalynn M. Nazarian

68 Histiocytic and dendritic cell sarcomas 702
Archana Shenoy and Louis P. Dehner

69 Intralymphatic histiocytosis and Melkersson–Rosenthal
syndrome 708
Andrea P. Moy, Louis P. Dehner, and Rosalynn M. Nazarian

Part XII
**Lymphoid Proliferations of Special Sites/Special
Populations**   717

70 Oral lymphoproliferative disorders 717
Kristin K. McNamara

71 Ocular lymphoproliferative disorders 751
Carolina M. Gentile and Paola de la Iglesia Niveyro

72 Cutaneous hematolymphoid proliferations in children 770
Julia Scarisbrick, Louis P. Dehner, and Alejandro A. Gru

73 Alopecia in lymphoproliferative disorders 820
Allen F. Shih, Ali Al-Haseni, and Lynne J. Goldberg

74 Cutaneous adverse reactions to chemotherapeutic
agents 834
Jacob Nosewicz, Brittany O. Dulmage, Jose A. Plaza,
and Benjamin H. Kaffenberger

75 Cutaneous adverse reactions to immunotherapy 867
Kelsey Nusbaum, Abraham Korman, Catherine G. Chung,
Benjamin H. Kaffenberger, and Brittany O. Dulmage

Part XIII
**Cutaneous Manifestations Associated With
Hematologic Malignancy**   872

76 Sweet and histiocytoid sweet syndrome 872
Jacqueline M. Junkins-Hopkins and Viktoryia Kazlouskaya

77 Wells syndrome (eosinophilic cellulitis) 883
Melinda Jen and Adam I. Rubin

78 Vasculitis 887
Alejandro A. Gru

79 Paraneoplastic pemphigus 897
Katherine France, Milda Chmieliauskaite,
and Faizan Alawi

80 Cryoglobulinemia 903
Alejandro A. Gru

81 Granulomatous reactions 910
Zoe O. Brown-Joel and Karolyn A. Wanat

82 Pyoderma gangrenosum 914
Campbell L. Stewart and Roberto Novoa

83 Schnitzler syndrome 917
Viktoryia Kazlouskaya and Jacqueline M. Junkins-Hopkins

Index 921

PART I IMMUNOBIOLOGY AND MOLECULAR PATHOGENESIS

CHAPTER 1

Cutaneous T-cell immunobiology

Emmanuella Guenova, Andy C. Hsi, and András Schaffer

INTRODUCTION

The skin is the largest organ of the human body and functions as a physical and immunologic barrier against external pathogens and chemical and physical assaults. The presence of billions of antigen-experienced memory T lymphocytes further renders the skin one of the largest tissue reservoirs for T cells.[1-3] Classically, memory T cells comprise the L-selectin+/CCR7+ central memory T cells (T_{CM}), recirculating and patrolling between the blood and the secondary lymphoid organs and the CCR7- effector memory T cells (T_{EM}), migrating into nonlymphoid peripheral tissues as sentinels for tissue immune surveillance.[4-6] The third subset, the resident memory T lymphocytes (T_{RM}), are phenotypically distinct, do not recirculate and reside permanently in peripheral tissues such as the skin, where they are indispensable for long-term immunity.[7,8] Adaptive immune responses against microorganisms and autoantigens in various inflammatory dermatoses and skin cancer are largely mediated by circulating T_{CM} and skin-resident T_{RM} cells.[9,10] However, skin T_{EM} and T_{RM} may also mediate harmful proinflammatory responses in autoimmune skin diseases or be the cells of origin of cutaneous T-cell lymphoma.[9,11]

In this chapter, we will discuss the various T-cell effector subtypes, their distinct transcriptional regulatory programs, cytokine expression patterns, and roles in cutaneous inflammatory and infectious processes. In addition, we will highlight their potential contribution to the pathobiology of cutaneous lymphoma (Figs. 1-1 and 1-2).

T-CELL RECEPTORS AND CORECEPTORS

T cells recognize their specific antigens through interaction between the membrane-bound T-cell receptors (TCRs) and the antigen-major histocompatibility complex (MHC) presented by the antigen-presenting cells (APCs). A TCR consists of a heterodimer composed of either α and β or γ and δ chains. The TCR chains undergo random genetic recombination steps to encode unique antigen receptors that recognize an infinitely diverse group of antigens present on bacteria, viruses, parasites, and tumor cells.[12,13] The αβ- or γδ-lineage commitment occurs very early during T-cell differentiation. Expression of the transcription factor SOX13 by triple-negative (TN2) (CD3−CD4−CD8−) thymocytes inhibits the Wnt/T-cell factor (TCF) pathway and promotes γδ T-cell development, while unopposed Wnt/TCF activity leads to αβ T-cell differentiation.[14] The TCR is closely associated with the pan–T-cell marker CD3, which is essential in signal transduction initiated by TCR-antigen interaction.[15] In skin T-cell lymphoma, identical TCR gene rearrangements delineate a monoclonal population of tumor cells and clonality assessment is a helpful diagnostic tool.[16] Advanced methods for clonality detection go beyond the current PCR standard and offer the advantage of higher accuracy as well as the potential of prognostic stratification of disease.[17-19]

Based on their expression of CD4 or CD8 membrane coreceptors, T cells can be divided into two subgroups.[20] CD4+ T cells recognize protein antigen bound to class II MHC molecules on APCs and mainly function as helper cells, whereas CD8+ T cells recognize protein antigen bound to class I MHC on target cells and mainly function as cytotoxic cells.[21]

RECRUITMENT OF T CELLS TO THE SKIN

Antigens encountered through the skin initiate the generation of skin-homing T cells.[22,23] APCs, including Langerhans cells (LCs) in the epidermis and myeloid-derived dendritic cells (DCs) in the dermis, phagocytose invading pathogens and migrate to skin-draining secondary lymphoid organs (SLOs). Within the SLO (ie, lymph node and lymphoid follicles), APCs migrate into the T-cell-rich paracortex through CCR7-CCL19/21-dependent chemotaxis, allowing for MHC-TCR conjugation and antigen-specific activation of naïve and memory CD4+ helper and CD8+ cytotoxic T cells.[24-28] Activated T cells upregulate skin-homing chemokine receptors CCR4 and CCR10, which promote their exit

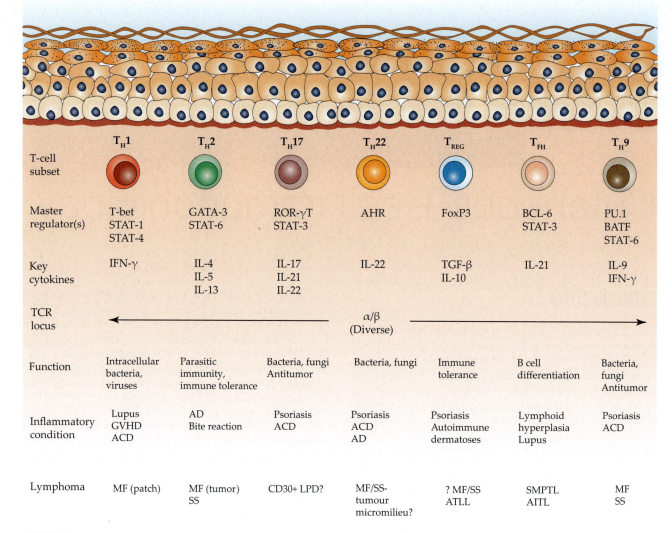

FIGURE 1-1. CD4+ T helper cell subtypes in the skin. Transcriptional master regulators, signature cytokines, postulated functions, and associated cutaneous disorders are illustrated. ACD, allergic contact dermatitis; AD, atopic dermatitis; AHR, aryl hydrocarbon receptor; AITL, angioimmunoblastic T-cell lymphoma; ATLL, adult T-cell leukemia/lymphoma; BATF, B-cell activation transcription factor-like; CD30+ LPD, CD30+ lymphoproliferative disorders; GVHD, graft-versus-host disease; MF, mycosis fungoides; SS, Sézary syndrome; SMPTLD, primary cutaneous CD4+ small/medium-sized pleomorphic T-cell lymphoproliferative disorder; STAT, signal transducer and activator of transcription; TCR, T-cell receptor; T_H, T helper; T_{reg}, regulatory T cells.

into the circulation.[29-32] Especially CCR4 is preferentially expressed on skin-homing T cells in patients with cutaneous T-cell lymphoma.[33] In addition, the same chemokine receptors upregulate T-cell cutaneous lymphocyte antigen (CLA), which targets T-cell adhesion and extravasation into the skin by binding to E- and P-selectins on cutaneous endothelial cells.[27,31-37]

The final extravasation of T cells to the skin requires firm attachment to the endothelium through interactions between T-cell integrin leukocyte function antigen (LFA-1) and intercellular/vascular cell adhesion molecules (ICAM/VCAM) expressed on the endothelium. The expression of ICAM and VCAM can be induced by proinflammatory cytokines such as TNF-α, IFN-γ, and interleukin (IL)-1 secreted at the site of infection.[36,38] Once extravasated, T cells utilize additional integrins to transmigrate through the dermal extracellular matrix.

A minority of T cells further migrate to the epidermis, a phenomenon known as epidermotropism. Epidermal hair follicles harbor large numbers of CD4+ and CD8+ T_{RM}s. In healthy skin, and especially in models of cutaneous T-cell lymphoma, hair follicle expression of IL-7 and/or IL-15 has been shown to be a major driver of epidermotropism.[39] Integrin-activated TGFβ creates selective pressure on CD8+ T cells and promotes the retention of antigen-specific resident memory T cells within the epidermal niche.[40] However, the detailed mechanisms of T cell localizing to particular layers of the epidermis have not been fully elucidated.

DIVERSE CUTANEOUS CD4+ T-CELL SUBSETS

Differentiation of CD4+ T cells into specific T helper phenotypes is highly dependent on the antigen presented by APCs as well as the cytokine/chemokine microenvironment at the time of activation.[41] In the steady-state skin, approximately 80% of T cells have an αβ+, CD4+ phenotype. Following infection, naive CD4+ T cells have the potential to

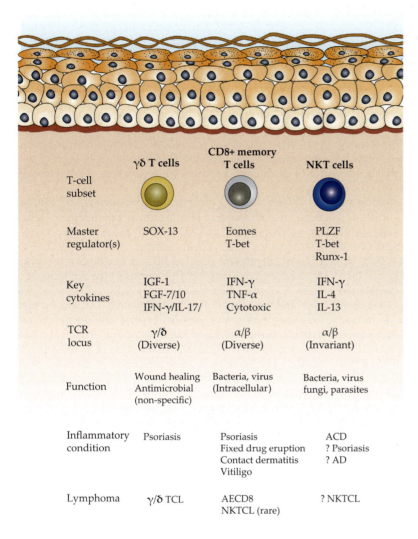

FIGURE 1-2. Innate-like T-cell subtypes in the skin. Transcriptional master regulators, signature cytokines, and postulated function and associated cutaneous disorders are illustrated. ACD, allergic contact dermatitis; AD, atopic dermatitis; AECD8, primary cutaneous aggressive epidermotropic CD8+ cytotoxic T-cell lymphoma; FGF, fibroblast growth factor; IGF, insulin-like growth factor; NKT, natural killer T cells; NKTCL, extranodal NK/T-cell lymphoma, nasal type; PLZF, promyelocytic leukemia zinc finger; γ/δ TCL, gamma/delta T-cell lymphoma.

differentiate into at least seven functionally distinct T helper (T_H) subsets with unique effector functions within the circulation, SLO, and infected tissues.[42]

Most (>85%) of these cells are T helper 1 (T_H1) cells as defined by their capability to secrete cytokines such as IFN-γ and IL-2.[43] A minority of skin-resident T cells have an IL-4-producing T helper 2 (T_H2) or IL-10/TGF-β-producing immunosuppressive regulatory T (T_{reg}) cell phenotype.[44,45]

The original distinction of type T_H1 and T_H2 cells was based on the cytokines they produced.[43,46] Later, on the basis of the preferential expression of further cytokines, such as IL-17, IL-22, IL-9, and CXCL-13, novel subtypes of T helper cells, including T_H17, T_H22, T_H9, and follicular T helper (T_{FH}) cells, have been identified.[47,48] These T cells are generally not present in steady-state skin but may be recruited during inflammation. The relevance of these CD4+ T-cell subsets in pathogen eradication, skin homeostasis, inflammatory dermatoses, and cutaneous T-cell lymphomas (CTCLs) will be discussed in more detail in the following sections.

T Helper 1 and T Helper 2 Cells

Early studies discovered that naïve T helper cells differentiate into two distinct subsets, T_H1 and T_H2, based on their cytokine profiles.[43,44] T_H1 cells mainly activate macrophages and cytotoxic T cells to eradicate intracellular pathogens, as well as act as mediators in autoimmunity.[49] As a lesser role, they may also stimulate B cells to produce IgG antibodies specific for certain extracellular pathogens. T_H2 cells, in contrast, mainly help the host in its defense against extracellular pathogens, including parasites and helminths, by interacting with eosinophils and mast cells, as well as stimulating B cells to produce most classes of antibodies. T_H1 cells secrete signature proinflammatory cytokines IFN-γ, TNF-α, and IL-2, among others. T_H2 cells are characterized by the secretion of IL-4, IL-5, IL-6, IL-9, IL-10, and IL-13.[21,44,50-53] Differentiation into the T_H1 and T_H2 pathways is highly dependent on the reciprocal expression of lineage-determining transcription factors T-bet and GATA-3, respectively.[50,52,54] T-bet is a T-box transcription factor that controls IFN-γ expression and is capable of redirecting effector T_H2 cells into the T_H1 pathway, characterized by the induction of IFN-γ and loss of IL-4 and IL-5 expressions.[52,55] T-bet expression is upregulated via activation of the signal transducer and activator of transcription 1 and 4 (STAT-1 and STAT-4) pathways after stimulation by IL-12 from APCs.[56,57]

In T_H2 differentiation, IL-4 from activated T cells, eosinophils, mast cells, and basophils triggers the STAT-6 signaling pathway that upregulates GATA-binding protein 3 (GATA-3) expression. GATA-3 is responsible for IL-4, IL-5, and IL-13 production, which may in turn stimulate more naïve T cells to undergo T_H2 differentiation through a positive feedback loop or autoactivation. In addition to its indispensable role in the T_H2 pathway, GATA-3 suppresses T_H1 development through downregulating IL-12 receptor and STAT-4 expressions in lymphocytes. Thus, the counter-regulatory roles of T-bet and GATA-3 are critical in achieving an optimal T_H1/T_H2 ratio in healthy individuals.

T_H1/T_H2 imbalance has long been the paradigm for many inflammatory dermatoses. T_H1-polarized diseases include allergic contact dermatitis (ACD) to metals, psoriasis, discoid lupus, and acute graft-versus-host disease (GVHD). In both animal models and human studies, these entities are associated with high levels of T_H1 cytokines.[58-67]

In contrast, a genetically determined predominance of T_H2-associated cytokines that are involved in the regulation of IgE synthesis and recruitment of eosinophils (IL-4, IL-5, IL-13) has been implicated in atopic dermatitis (AD), in which exposure to environmental triggers results in downregulation of IL-12 and thus shifting a primarily normal T_H1-polarized response to a pathologic T_H2-dominant response. In human keratinocyte–derived models, IL-4 and IL-13 induce spongiosis and keratinocyte apoptosis, as well as a strong increase in the expression of AD-associated genes *CAII* and *NELL2* that are positively correlated with cytokine concentration.

Furthermore, IL-4 initiates and supports T_H2 cell differentiation, when acting directly on T cells, but can also drive a negative regulatory feedback loop resulting in strong T_H1 driving phenotype in antigen-presenting innate immune cells,[68] a regulatory mechanism important for the transition from T_H2- to T_H1-dominated milieu in the chronic phase of atopic dermatitis skin lesion.[69]

T_H1 and T_H2 cells are the postulated cells of origin in mycosis fungoides (MF), Sézary syndrome (SS), and (primary cutaneous) peripheral T-cell lymphoma, not otherwise specified (PTCL-NOS). In early-stage CTCL, the Th1 phenotype is maintained by the expression of signal transducer and activator of transcription 4 (STAT-4) and IL-12 signaling via JAK2/TYK2.[70] This supports establishment of cell-mediated antitumor responses and secretion of cytotoxic molecules, including the proinflammatory cytokines IFN-α and IFN-γ.[71-75] The escape from immune recognition can lead to tumor progression as observed in advanced-stage CTCL. During disease progression, the expression of Th2 markers (eg, GATA-3) and cytokines (for example, IL-4, IL-5, and IL-10) increases, whereas the expression of Th1 transcription factors, such as T-cell-specific T box transcription factor (T-bet), interferon gamma (IFN-γ), STAT4, and IL-12 decreases.[76,77] Furthermore, T_H2 cytokines from malignant cells suppress T_H1 responses and enforce a global T_H2 bias in leukemic CTCL.[78]

Expression of the transcription factor GATA 3 had been also identified in a high-risk subset of PTCL-NOS with L-10 and Th2-associated cytokine production, alternative macrophage activation, and worse prognosis.[79]

T Helper 17 Cells

When APCs recognize extracellular bacterial and fungal organisms through their pattern recognition receptors (ie, TLR2 and TLR4 in *Candida albicans* recognition and TLR4 in nickel), they secrete cytokines, including TGF-β, IL-1β, IL-23, and IL-6.[80-83] The combination of these cytokines, especially IL-1β and IL-6 and Il-23 in humans, promotes differentiation and maintenance of activated CD4+ T cells into the T_H17 lineage through upregulation of the transcription factor RORγT.[84,85] Activated T_H17 in turn expresses cytokines including IL-17, IL-21, and IL-22.[86] IL-17 interacts with the IL-17 receptor (IL-17R) on keratinocytes to induce the expression of neutrophil-attracting chemokines (CXCL8), growth factors such as granulocyte-colony stimulating factor, and antimicrobial peptides. IL-22 functions in synergy with IL-17 to enhance keratinocyte production of antimicrobial peptides.[87]

Dysregulated T_H17 cells, along with a T_H1/T_H2 imbalance, mediate a variety of inflammatory dermatoses, including psoriasis, ACD, and AD.[84,88-90] In patients with psoriasis, keratinocytes under environmental stress activate dermal DCs, which produce IL-23 and IL-12, as well as other proinflammatory cytokines.[64,91] This results in the recruitment of T_H17, T_H1, and other inflammatory cells including neutrophils and mast cells.[91] IL-17, along with IL-22, acts on keratinocytes, leading to epidermal hyperplasia, acanthosis, and hyperkeratosis. Increased numbers of T_H17 cells have been observed in ACD[92] and AD, more often in infants than in adults.[93] This increase is more prominent in the acute phase of disease, and the amount of T_H17 recruitment appears to correlate with the degree of severity.[88,89] However, in general, T_H17 cells causing psoriasis remain mutually antagonistic to the T_H2 cell, major driver of atopic dermatitis.[94]

T_H17 cells also promote immune-related skin damage.[95] Increased T_H17 population, along with T_H1 cells, is observed in patients with acute and active chronic GVHD and epidermolysis bullosa as well.[96] The proportion of T_H17 cells in GVHD-affected skin is inversely correlated with the proportion of T_{reg} cells, and the disease severity can be significantly reduced by inhibiting T_H17 differentiation, suggesting the critical role of T_H17 in cutaneous GVHD.[59,95,97,98]

The proinflammatory nature of T_H17 is further implicated in its antitumor activity.[99-101] Tumor-specific T_H17 cells have strong tumor rejection abilities against advanced melanoma that are significantly more efficient than those exhibited by T_H1 cells.[99,102]

Regarding cutaneous lymphoma, enhanced T_H17- and reduced T_H1-related gene expression is observed in 91.7% of all lymphomatoid papulosis and 38.1% of all primary cutaneous anaplastic large-cell lymphoma cases.[103] This results from upregulated special AT-rich sequence binding protein 1 (SATB1), a thymocyte-specific chromatin organizer that promotes malignant T-cell proliferation in some CD30+ lymphoproliferative disorders (LPDs).[103,104]

While evolving T_H17 cytokine expression has been occasionally observed in some cases of CTCL progression,[105] the level of T_H17 cytokines in T_H2-biased CTCL is low.[106] The relatively low expression of IL-17 may further explain the lack of relative neutrophils during bacterial infections in CTCL skin lesions.[107]

T Helper 22 Cells

T Helper 22 (T_H22) is a recently described skin-resident T helper cell subset. Similar to T_H17 cells, T_H22 cells produce IL-22; however, T_H22 cells do not secrete IL-17 and as such are positioned as a separate T_H subset.[108,109] T_H22 differentiation depends on the master transcription factor aryl hydrocarbon receptor upon stimulation by LCs from the epidermis.[59,109] T_H22 cells express skin-homing chemokine receptors CCR4 and CCR10 and are enriched in inflammatory dermatoses, such as psoriasis, AD, and ACD.[110,111] IL-22 is a cytokine that acts mainly on epithelial cells and is essential in the host's defense against bacterial and fungal organisms as well as in epidermal homeostasis.[110,112] Increased IL-22 expression alone, without IL-17 or IFN-γ expression, can lead to classic psoriatic changes, including acanthosis with hypogranulosis and parakeratosis, along with disruption of keratinocyte terminal differentiation.[113,114] Similarly, in patients with AD and ACD to nickel, elevated IL-22 levels are also observed, along with other T_H2- and T_H1-related cytokines, respectively.[108,115-117] In the prospective population-based cohort study (Generation R Study), genotyping in 523 school-aged children with AD clearly linked higher T_H22 cell numbers to mutation in the filaggrin gene compared with children in the general and non-AD population without filaggrin mutation.[118] The role of T_H22 cells in cutaneous lymphomagenesis is currently unclear. Yet a role for T_H22 in shaping the CTCL tumor microenvironment has been proposed.[107]

Follicular T Helper Cells

T_{FH} cells are a recently discovered subset of CD4+ T cells expressing high levels of CXCR5, which promotes their homing to B-cell follicles and germinal centers (GCs).[119] Within the GC, T_{FH} cells primarily secrete IL-21 to induce the differentiation and survival of activated, antigen-specific B cells into memory B cells and long-lived plasma cells.[120,121] T_{FH} cells express high levels of transcription factor BCL-6, which serves as the master regulator for differentiation.[119] T_{FH} has been implicated in several autoimmune conditions with potential cutaneous manifestations, including juvenile dermatomyositis, systemic lupus erythematosus, systemic sclerosis, pemphigus, and rheumatoid arthritis.[122-124] These entities are characterized by dysregulation of T_{FH} cells, which are poised to promote B-cell responses within the inflamed skin lesions.[125] Several primary and secondary CTCLs have been hypothesized to originate from T_{FH} cells. Primary cutaneous CD4+ small/medium-sized pleomorphic T-cell lymphoproliferative disorder and angioimmunoblastic T-cell lymphoma are well-described primary and secondary cutaneous lymphoproliferations that express T_{FH} markers BCL-6, CD10, PD-1, and CXCL-13.[126-130]

T Helper 9 Cells

T Helper 9 (T_H9) cells are a subtype of T helper cells, closely related to the T_H2 subtype.[131] In fact, the signature T_H2 cytokine IL-4, together with TGF-β, is a major factor for the reprogramming of T_H2 cells, cytokine secretion, and promotion of IL-9-producing T_H subset.[132,133]

T_H9 cells are characterized by high expression of cytokine IL-9 and transcription factors, including PU.1, STAT-6, IRF-4, and BATF.[134-136] Of these transcription factors, BATF appears to be the master regulator of the T_H9 phenotype,[134] while the epidermal growth factor receptor seems to be supportive for IL-9 induction.[137]

Th9 is distinct from other T helper phenotypes by the lack of T-bet, GATA-3, RORγt, or FoxP3 expression.[135] Most T_H9 cells express skin-homing receptor CLA and are therefore largely skin-tropic.[136] IL-9 and TNF-α production by T_H9 cells augments cytokine production by other T_H subsets and are important in the eradication of *C. albicans*.[138] Elevation of T_H9 cells and IL-9 levels is also observed in patients with AD.[135]

T_H9 cells have also been implicated in antitumor immunity, in that loss-of-function mutations in the *IL-9* gene are associated with a higher incidence of melanoma development.[139,140] This antitumor activity is thought to be indirect and is achieved by T_H9 cells recruiting other T cells, DCs, and mast cells.[141,142]

Patients with CTCL have a higher frequency of "skin-homing" T_H9 cells in their blood,[143] and both malignant and reactive T cells produce IL-9 in MF skin lesions.[144] In MF, enhanced expression of IL-9 parallels decreased expression of SATB1, the same factor that promotes T-cell proliferation and T_H17 phenotype in CD30+ LPD (see above).[103,104,145]

Regulatory T Cells

Approximately 5% to 10% of the T cells in the skin under normal conditions are CD25+ FoxP3+ T_{reg} cells.[1,146] T_{reg} cells serve as a brake for cutaneous inflammation, as well as mediate tolerance to normal skin flora and self-antigens.[147] Differentiation of T cells into T_{reg} cells requires TCR activation, along with signals from cytokines IL-2, IL-7, and IL-15. These stimulations result in the upregulation of CD25 and FoxP3, a transcriptional master regulator for T_{reg} cells. FoxP3 induces production of immunosuppressive cytokines IL-10 and TGF-β and prevents activated T-cell precursors from differentiating into effector T-cell lineages.[148,149]

Dysfunctional T_{reg} cells may play a significant role in autoimmune/inflammatory dermatoses.[45,150-153] In psoriasis, increased percentages and absolute numbers of FoxP3+ T_{reg} cells are present in lesional skin. However, these T_{reg} cells are qualitatively defective, with decreased anti-inflammatory activity and enhanced propensity to differentiate into IL-17- and IFN-γ-producing effector T cells that are the hallmarks of psoriasis pathogenesis.[45,151,153] Dysregulation in T_{reg} cells is also observed in AD, bullous pemphigoid, pemphigus vulgaris, vitiligo, and halo nevi.[150,154,155] T_{reg}-mediated suppression of tumor-specific T-cell immunity has been postulated in cutaneous malignancies, such as basal cell carcinoma, squamous cell carcinoma, as well as primary and metastatic melanoma.[146,147,156-158]

It has been suggested that T_{reg} cells are the postulated cells of origin in adult T-cell leukemia/lymphoma (ATLL), an HTLV-1-associated aggressive PTCL that phenotypically shares the CD4+CD25+ expression profile. However, controversy remains about whether ATLL cells have similar immune inhibition functions compared with normal T_{reg} cells.[159-162] In Sézary syndrome, staphylococcal enterotoxins (SEs) induce FoxP3 expression, shaping the phenotype of both malignant and nonmalignant T cells. However, given a lack of direct response to SE, the induction of FoxP3 expression in malignant T cells seems to be indirectly mediated by signals derived from nonmalignant counterparts.[163]

CD8+ RESIDENT MEMORY T CELLS

Tissue-resident, nonrecirculating CD8+ resident memory T (T_{RM}) cells provide superior protection from infection at barrier sites such as the skin. They develop from mature cytotoxic T cells that are in the epidermis during the initial inflammation. T_{RM} cells differ from their CD8+ cytotoxic T-cell precursors by the downregulation of cytotoxic gene transcription. After the inflammation is resolved, T_{RM} cells assume an immunosurveillance mode. They reside near the dermal-epidermal junction, in contact with the basement membrane, where they proactively search for antigens by interacting with local LCs and keratinocytes.[164] T_{RM} cells can persist in an immunosurveillance mode for many months; however, upon re-exposure to the antigen, they rapidly resume cytotoxic activities and secrete IFN-γ and TNF-α without stimulation from CD4+ T helper.[164-166] This accelerated reactivation requires transcription factors T-bet and eomesodermin.[167,168]

A role for human skin-resident CD8+ memory T cells has been demonstrated in psoriasis and fixed drug eruption. Both entities are characterized by recurrent bouts of inflammatory pathology at sites of previously affected skin.[166] T_{RM} cells are also partially responsible in autoimmune dermatoses such as psoriasis, AD, and vitiligo.[169] Neoplastic proliferation of skin-homing CD8+ T_{RM} cells are the postulated cells of origin in a subset of MF, primary cutaneous aggressive epidermotropic CD8+ cytotoxic T-cell lymphoma, and, occasionally, extranodal NK/T-cell lymphoma, nasal type.[170,171]

γδ T CELLS

Contrary to the peripheral blood T-cell population, γδ T cells constitute a major T-cell component in the skin.[172-174] As a part of the innate immune response, γδ T cells produce a wide variety of cytokines, growth factors, and chemokines and have potential autocrine and paracrine functions following stimulation.[175] These include insulin-like growth factor 1 (IGF-1), IL-2, IFN-γ, and fibroblast growth factors 7 and 10 (FGF-7 and FGF-10). Both FGF-7 and FGF-10 bind to the FGFR2-IIIb receptor on the keratinocyte and are implicated in keratinocyte proliferation during wound healing. IGF-1 is required to prevent the epidermal γδ T cells from undergoing apoptosis in addition to stimulating wound closure.[175,176] Decreased IGF-1 production is observed in nonhealing chronic wounds, suggesting the critical roles of skin-resident γδ T cells in wound healing.[176,177] In animal models, TCRδ knockout mice showed a significantly slower rate of re-epithelialization and keratinocyte proliferation.[174] In addition, γδ T cells promote the activation of natural killer (NK), natural killer T (NKT), and T cells and play a nonspecific but important role in antimicrobial immunosurveillance.[178-181] A subset of γδ T cells found in patients with psoriasis are capable of producing IL-17, which is traditionally considered a T_H17-specific cytokine in the first steps of disease pathogenesis. This discovery has led to a new hypothesis that γδ T cells may provide a more rapid IL-17 production and early keratinocyte hyperproliferation that is then followed by similar activities by T_H17 cells.[182,183] Mature and activated γδ cytotoxic T cells are the postulated cells of origin in primary cutaneous γ/δ T-cell lymphoma.[171]

NATURAL KILLER T CELLS

NKT cells belong to a distinct subset of T cells that possess phenotypic features of both NK cells and T cells (CD3+ CD161+ CD56+). CD4 and CD8 expressions can be variable. Although NKT cells are TCRαβ+, they are uniquely characterized by the expression of only one type (invariant) of TCRα chain and a limited number of TCRβ chains.[184] NKT cells recognize glycolipids, rather than protein antigens, that are presented by a nonclassic, class I MHC-like molecule CD1d.[184-186]

Differentiation of T cells toward the NKT phenotype is highly dependent upon the expression of the transcription factor promyelocytic leukemia zinc finger protein.[187,188] In addition, Runx1 and T-bet are necessary regulators for early NKT cell development and terminal maturation, respectively.[189-191] Depending on the specific types of antigen presented, NKT cells are capable of producing large quantities of either T_H1 or T_H2 cytokines. The release of cytokines by NKT cells is rapid, occurring within minutes after activation, and has been shown to provide beneficial, and sometimes critical, support in clearing bacterial, viral, fungal, and parasitic infections.[186,192] Recent data have suggested that NKT cells are capable of suppressing ACD reactions independently of T_{reg} cells.[193,194] Although still controversial, NKT cells may participate in the formation and maintenance of psoriatic lesions, as well as in the pathogenesis of AD.[192,195-197]

References

1. Clark RA, Chong B, Mirchandani N, et al. The vast majority of CLA+ T cells are resident in normal skin. *J Immunol*. 2006;176(7):4431-4439.
2. Sathaliyawala T, Kubota M, Yudanin N, et al. Distribution and compartmentalization of human circulating and tissue-resident memory T cell subsets. *Immunity*. 2013;38(1):187-197.
3. Watanabe R, Gehad A, Yang C, et al. Human skin is protected by four functionally and phenotypically discrete populations of resident and recirculating memory T cells. *Sci Transl Med*. 2015;7(279):279ra39.
4. Sallusto F, Lenig D, Forster R, Lipp M, Lanzavecchia A. Two subsets of memory T lymphocytes with distinct homing potentials and effector functions. *Nature*. 1999;401(6754):708-712.
5. Sallusto F, Geginat J, Lanzavecchia A. Central memory and effector memory T cell subsets: function, generation, and maintenance. *Annu Rev Immunol*. 2004;22:745-763.
6. Mueller SN, Gebhardt T, Carbone FR, Heath WR. Memory T cell subsets, migration patterns, and tissue residence. *Annu Rev Immunol*. 2013;31:137-161.
7. Sasson SC, Gordon CL, Christo SN, Klenerman P, Mackay LK. Local heroes or villains: tissue-resident memory T cells in human health and disease. *Cell Mol Immunol*. 2020;17(2):113-122.
8. Chen L, Shen Z. Tissue-resident memory T cells and their biological characteristics in the recurrence of inflammatory skin disorders. *Cell Mol Immunol* 2020;17(1):64-75.
9. Ho AW, Kupper TS. T cells and the skin: from protective immunity to inflammatory skin disorders. *Nat Rev Immunol*. 2019;19(8):490-502.
10. Malik BT, Byrne KT, Vella JL, et al. Resident memory T cells in the skin mediate durable immunity to melanoma. *Sci Immunol*. 2017;2(10):eaam6346.

11. Campbell JJ, Clark RA, Watanabe R, Kupper TS. Sezary syndrome and mycosis fungoides arise from distinct T-cell subsets: a biologic rationale for their distinct clinical behaviors. *Blood*. 2010;116(5):767-771.
12. Qi Q, Liu Y, Cheng Y, et al. Diversity and clonal selection in the human T-cell repertoire. *Proc Natl Acad Sci USA*. 2014;111(36):13139-13144.
13. Arstila TP, Casrouge A, Baron V, Even J, Kanellopoulos J, Kourilsky P. A direct estimate of the human alphabeta T cell receptor diversity. *Science*. 1999;286(5441):958-961.
14. Melichar HJ, Narayan K, Der SD, et al. Regulation of gammadelta versus alphabeta T lymphocyte differentiation by the transcription factor SOX13. *Science*. 2007;315(5809):230-233.
15. Call ME, Pyrdol J, Wiedmann M, Wucherpfennig KW. The organizing principle in the formation of the T cell receptor-CD3 complex. *Cell*. 2002;111(7):967-979.
16. Moczko A, Dimitriou F, Kresbach H, et al. Sensitivity and specificity of T-cell receptor PCR BIOMED-2 clonality analysis for the diagnosis of cutaneous T-cell lymphoma. *Eur J Dermatol*. 2020;30(1):12-15.
17. de Masson A, O'Malley JT, Elco CP, et al. High-throughput sequencing of the T cell receptor beta gene identifies aggressive early-stage mycosis fungoides. *Sci Transl Med*. 2018;10(440):eaar5894.
18. Weng WK, Armstrong R, Arai S, Desmarais C, Hoppe R, Kim YH. Minimal residual disease monitoring with high-throughput sequencing of T cell receptors in cutaneous T cell lymphoma. *Sci Transl Med*. 2013;5(214):214ra171.
19. Wang J, Rea B, Haun P, Emerson R, Kirsch I, Bagg A. High-throughput sequencing of the T-cell receptor beta chain gene distinguishes 2 subgroups of cutaneous T-cell lymphoma. *J Am Acad Dermatol*. 2019;80(4):1148-1150.e1.
20. Bosselut R. CD4/CD8-lineage differentiation in the thymus: from nuclear effectors to membrane signals. *Nat Rev Immunol*. 2004;4(7):529-540.
21. Davis SJ, Ikemizu S, Evans EJ, Fugger L, Bakker TR, van der Merwe PA. The nature of molecular recognition by T cells. *Nat Immunol*. 2003;4(3):217-224.
22. Mackay CR, Marston WL, Dudler L, Spertini O, Tedder TF, Hein WR. Tissue-specific migration pathways by phenotypically distinct Subpopulations of memory T-cells. *Eur J Immunol*. 1992;22(4):887-895.
23. Masopust D, Vezys V, Marzo AL, Lefrancois L. Preferential localization of effector memory cells in nonlymphoid tissue. *Science*. 2001;291(5512):2413-2417.
24. Bousso P. T-cell activation by dendritic cells in the lymph node: lessons from the movies. *Nat Rev Immunol*. 2008;8(9):675-684.
25. Eisenbarth SC. Dendritic cell subsets in T cell programming: location dictates function. *Nat Rev Immunol*. 2019;19(2):89-103.
26. Bousso P, Robey E. Dynamics of CD8+ T cell priming by dendritic cells in intact lymph nodes. *Nat Immunol*. 2003;4(6):579-585.
27. Forster R, Braun A, Worbs T. Lymph node homing of T cells and dendritic cells via afferent lymphatics. *Trends Immunol*. 2012;33(6):271-280.
28. Randolph GJ, Angeli V, Swartz MA. Dendritic-cell trafficking to lymph nodes through lymphatic vessels. *Nat Rev Immunol*. 2005;5(8):617-628.
29. Campbell DJ, Butcher EC. Rapid acquisition of tissue-specific homing phenotypes by CD4(+) T cells activated in cutaneous or mucosal lymphoid tissues. *J Exp Med*. 2002;195(1):135-141.
30. Campbell JJ, O'Connell DJ, Wurbel MA. Cutting edge: chemokine receptor CCR4 is necessary for antigen-driven cutaneous accumulation of CD4 T cells under physiological conditions. *J Immunol*. 2007;178(6):3358-3362.
31. Picker LJ, Treer JR, Fergusondarnell B, Collins PA, Buck D, Terstappen LWMM. Control of lymphocyte recirculation in man. 1. Differential regulation of the peripheral lymph-node homing receptor L-selectin on T-cells during the Virgin to memory cell transition. *J Immunol*. 1993;150(3):1105-1121.
32. Soler D, Humphreys TL, Spinola SM, Campbell JJ. CCR4 versus CCR10 in human cutaneous T-H lymphocyte trafficking. *Blood* 2003;101(5):1677-1682.
33. Ferenczi K, Fuhlbrigge RC, Pinkus JL, Pinkus GS, Kupper TS. Increased CCR4 expression in cutaneous T cell lymphoma. *J Invest Dermatol* 2002;119(6):1405-1410.
34. Fuhlbrigge RC, Kieffer JD, Armerding D, Kupper TS. Cutaneous lymphocyte antigen is a specialized form of PSGL-1 expressed on skin-homing T cells. *Nature*. 1997;389(6654):978-981.
35. Kunstfeld R, Lechleitner S, Groger M, Wolff K, Petzelbauer P. HECA-452+ T cells migrate through superficial vascular plexus but not through deep vascular plexus endothelium. *J Invest Dermatol*. 1997;108(3):343-348.
36. Schon MP, Zollner TM, Boehncke WH. The molecular basis of lymphocyte recruitment to the skin: clues for pathogenesis and selective therapies of inflammatory disorders. *J Invest Dermatol*. 2003;121(5):951-962.
37. Sheridan BS, Lefrancois L. Regional and mucosal memory T cells. *Nat Immunol*. 2011;12(6):485-491.
38. Griffiths CE, Voorhees JJ, Nickoloff BJ. Characterization of intercellular adhesion molecule-1 and HLA-DR expression in normal and inflamed skin: modulation by recombinant gamma interferon and tumor necrosis factor. *J Am Acad Dermatol*. 1989;20(4):617-629.
39. Adachi T, Kobayashi T, Sugihara E, et al. Hair follicle-derived IL-7 and IL-15 mediate skin-resident memory T cell homeostasis and lymphoma. *Nat Med*. 2015;21(11):1272-1279.
40. Hirai T, Yang Y, Zenke Y, et al. Competition for active TGF beta cytokine allows for selective retention of antigen-specific tissue-resident memory T cells in the epidermal niche. *Immunity* 2021;54(1):84-98.e5.
41. Kapsenberg ML. Dendritic-cell control of pathogen-driven T-cell polarization. *Nat Rev Immunol*. 2003;3(12):984-993.
42. Bluestone JA, Mackay CR, O'Shea JJ, Stockinger B. The functional plasticity of T cell subsets. *Nat Rev Immunol*. 2009;9(11):811-816.
43. Bradley LM, Yoshimoto K, Swain SL. The cytokines IL-4, IFN-gamma, and IL-12 regulate the development of subsets of memory effector helper T cells in vitro. *J Immunol*. 1995;155(4):1713-1724.
44. Mosmann TR, Coffman RL. TH1 and TH2 cells: different patterns of lymphokine secretion lead to different functional properties. *Annu Rev Immunol*. 1989;7:145-173.
45. Sanchez Rodriguez R, Pauli ML, Neuhaus IM, et al. Memory regulatory T cells reside in human skin. *J Clin Invest*. 2014;124(3):1027-1036.
46. Mosmann TR, Cherwinski H, Bond MW, Giedlin MA, Coffman RL. Pillars article: two types of murine helper T cell clone. I. Definition according to profiles of lymphokine activities and secreted proteins. *J Immunol*. 2005;175:5-14.

47. van Beek JJP, Rescigno M, Lugli E. A fresh look at the T helper subset dogma. *Nat Immunol*. 2021;22(2):104-105.
48. Sallusto F. Heterogeneity of human CD4(+) T cells against microbes. *Annu Rev Immunol*. 2016;34:317-334.
49. Jankovic D, Liu Z, Gause WC. Th1- and Th2-cell commitment during infectious disease: asymmetry in divergent pathways. *Trends Immunol*. 2001;22(8):450-457.
50. Ho IC, Tai TS, Pai SY. GATA3 and the T-cell lineage: essential functions before and after T-helper-2-cell differentiation. *Nat Rev Immunol* 2009;9(2):125-135.
51. Romagnani S. Type 1 T helper and type 2 T helper cells: functions, regulation and role in protection and disease. *Int J Clin Lab Res* 1991;21(2):152-158.
52. Szabo SJ, Kim ST, Costa GL, Zhang X, Fathman CG, Glimcher LH. A novel transcription factor, T-bet, directs Th1 lineage commitment. *Cell*. 2000;100(6):655-669.
53. Walker JA, McKenzie ANJ. T_H2 cell development and function. *Nat Rev Immunol*. 2018;18(2):121-133.
54. Ting CN, Olson MC, Barton KP, Leiden JM. Transcription factor GATA-3 is required for development of the T-cell lineage. *Nature*. 1996;384(6608):474-478.
55. Lametschwandtner G, Biedermann T, Schwarzler C, et al. Sustained T-bet expression confers polarized human TH2 cells with TH1-like cytokine production and migratory capacities. *J Allergy Clin Immunol*. 2004;113(5):987-994.
56. Usui T, Nishikomori R, Kitani A, Strober W. GATA-3 suppresses Th1 development by downregulation of Stat4 and not through effects on IL-12Rbeta2 chain or T-bet. *Immunity*. 2003;18(3):415-428.
57. Ylikoski E, Lund R, Kylaniemi M, et al. IL-12 up-regulates T-bet independently of IFN-gamma in human CD4+ T cells. *Eur J Immunol*. 2005;35(11):3297-3306.
58. Broady R, Yu J, Chow V, et al. Cutaneous GVHD is associated with the expansion of tissue-localized Th1 and not Th17 cells. *Blood*. 2010;116(25):5748-5751.
59. Coghill JM, Sarantopoulos S, Moran TP, Murphy WJ, Blazar BR, Serody JS. Effector CD4+ T cells, the cytokines they generate, and GVHD: something old and something new. *Blood*. 2011;117(12):3268-3276.
60. Dhingra N, Shemer A, Correa da Rosa J, et al. Molecular profiling of contact dermatitis skin identifies allergen-dependent differences in immune response. *J Allergy Clin Immunol*. 2014;134(2):362-372.
61. Gambichler T, Genc Z, Skrygan M, et al. Cytokine and chemokine ligand expression in cutaneous lupus erythematosus. *Eur J Dermatol*. 2012;22(3):319-323.
62. Jabbari A, Suarez-Farinas M, Fuentes-Duculan J, et al. Dominant Th1 and minimal Th17 skewing in discoid lupus revealed by transcriptomic comparison with psoriasis. *J Invest Dermatol*. 2014;134(1):87-95.
63. Lew W, Bowcock AM, Krueger JG. Psoriasis vulgaris: cutaneous lymphoid tissue supports T-cell activation and "Type 1" inflammatory gene expression. *Trends Immunol*. 2004;25(6):295-305.
64. Lowes MA, Kikuchi T, Fuentes-Duculan J, et al. Psoriasis vulgaris lesions contain discrete populations of Th1 and Th17 T cells. *J Invest Dermatol*. 2008;128(5):1207-1211.
65. Lu Y, Sakamaki S, Kuroda H, et al. Prevention of lethal acute graft-versus-host disease in mice by oral administration of T helper 1 inhibitor, TAK-603. *Blood*. 2001;97(4):1123-1130.
66. Schlaak JF, Buslau M, Jochum W, et al. T cells involved in psoriasis vulgaris belong to the Th1 subset. *J Invest Dermatol*. 1994;102(2):145-149.
67. Uyemura K, Yamamura M, Fivenson DF, Modlin RL, Nickoloff BJ. The cytokine network in lesional and lesion-free psoriatic skin is characterized by a T-helper type 1 cell-mediated response. *J Invest Dermatol*. 1993;101(5):701-705.
68. Guenova E, Volz T, Sauer K, et al. IL-4-mediated fine tuning of IL-12p70 production by human DC. *Eur J Immunol*. 2008;38(11):3138-3149.
69. Hamid Q, Boguniewicz M, Leung DY. Differential in situ cytokine gene expression in acute versus chronic atopic dermatitis. *J Clin Invest*. 1994;94(2):870-876.
70. Showe LC, Fox FE, Williams D, Au K, Niu Z, Rook AH. Depressed IL-12-mediated signal transduction in T cells from patients with Sezary syndrome is associated with the absence of IL-12 receptor beta 2 mRNA and highly reduced levels of STAT4. *J Immunol*. 1999;163(7):4073-4079.
71. Wood GS, Edinger A, Hoppe RT, Warnke RA. Mycosis fungoides skin lesions contain CD8+ tumor-infiltrating lymphocytes expressing an activated, MHC-restricted cytotoxic T-lymphocyte phenotype. *J Cutan Pathol*. 1994;21(2):151-156.
72. Asadullah K, Friedrich M, Döcke W-D, Jahn S, Volk H-D, Sterry W. Enhanced expression of T-cell activation and natural killer cell antigens Indicates systemic anti-tumor response in early primary cutaneous T-cell lymphoma. *J Invest Dermatol*. 1997;108(5):743-747.
73. Bagot M, Echchakir H, Mami-Chouaib F, et al. Isolation of tumor-specific cytotoxic CD4+ and CD4+CD8dim+ T-cell clones infiltrating a cutaneous T-cell lymphoma. *Blood*. 1998;91(11):4331-4341.
74. Echchakir H, Bagot M, Dorothee G, et al. Cutaneous T cell lymphoma reactive CD4+ cytotoxic T lymphocyte clones display a Th1 cytokine profile and use a fas-independent pathway for specific tumor cell lysis. *J Invest Dermatol*. 2000;115(1):74-80.
75. Hsi AC, Lee SJ, Rosman IS, et al. Expression of helper T cell master regulators in inflammatory dermatoses and primary cutaneous T-cell lymphomas: diagnostic implications. *J Am Acad Dermatol*. 2015;72(1):159-167.
76. Vowels BR, Lessin SR, Cassin M, et al. Th2 cytokine mRNA expression in skin in cutaneous T-cell lymphoma. *J Invest Dermatol*. 1994;103(5):669-673.
77. Netchiporouk ELI, Moreau L, Gilbert M, Sasseville D, Duvic M. Deregulation in STAT signaling is important for cutaneous T-cell lymphoma (CTCL) pathogenesis and cancer progression. *Cell Cycle* 2014;13(21):3331-3335. doi:10.4161/15384 101.2014.965061
78. Guenova E, Watanabe R, Teague JE, et al. TH2 cytokines from malignant cells suppress TH1 responses and enforce a global TH2 bias in leukemic cutaneous T-cell lymphoma. *Clin Cancer Res*. 2013;19(14):3755-3763.
79. Wang T, Feldman AL, Wada DA, et al. GATA-3 expression identifies a high-risk subset of PTCL, NOS with distinct molecular and clinical features. *Blood*. 2014;123(19):3007-3015.
80. Hernandez-Santos N, Gaffen SL. Th17 cells in immunity to Candida albicans. *Cell Host Microbe* 2012;11(5):425-435.
81. Netea MG, Van Der Graaf CA, Vonk AG, Verschueren I, Van Der Meer JW, Kullberg BJ. The role of toll-like receptor (TLR) 2 and TLR4 in the host defense against disseminated candidiasis. *J Infect Dis*. 2002;185(10):1483-1489.
82. Romani L. Immunity to fungal infections. *Nat Rev Immunol*. 2011;11(4):275-288.
83. Schmidt M, Raghavan B, Muller V, et al. Crucial role for human Toll-like receptor 4 in the development of contact allergy to nickel. *Nat Immunol*. 2010;11:814-819.

84. Di Cesare A, Di Meglio P, Nestle FO. The IL-23/Th17 axis in the immunopathogenesis of psoriasis. *J Invest Dermatol.* 2009;129(6):1339-1350.
85. Manel N, Unutmaz D, Littman DR. The differentiation of human T(H)-17 cells requires transforming growth factor-beta and induction of the nuclear receptor RORgammat. *Nat Immunol.* 2008;9(6):641-649.
86. Conti HR, Gaffen SL. Host responses to Candida albicans: Th17 cells and mucosal candidiasis. *Microbes Infect.* 2010;12(7):518-527.
87. Liang SC, Tan XY, Luxenberg DP, et al. Interleukin (IL)-22 and IL-17 are coexpressed by Th17 cells and cooperatively enhance expression of antimicrobial peptides. *J Exp Med.* 2006;203(10):2271-2279.
88. Koga C, Kabashima K, Shiraishi N, Kobayashi M, Tokura Y. Possible pathogenic role of Th17 cells for atopic dermatitis. *J Invest Dermatol.* 2008;128(11):2625-2630.
89. Peiser M. Role of Th17 cells in skin inflammation of allergic contact dermatitis. *Clin Dev Immunol* 2013;2013:261037.
90. Guenova E, Skabytska Y, Hoetzenecker W, et al. IL-4 abrogates T(H)17 cell-mediated inflammation by selective silencing of IL-23 in antigen-presenting cells. *Proc Natl Acad Sci USA.* 2015;112(7):2163-2168.
91. Di Meglio P, Perera GK, Nestle FO. The multitasking organ: recent insights into skin immune function. *Immunity.* 2011;35(6):857-869.
92. Garzorz-Stark N, Lauffer F, Krause L, et al. Toll-like receptor 7/8 agonists stimulate plasmacytoid dendritic cells to initiate T(H)17-deviated acute contact dermatitis in human subjects. *J Allergy Clin Immun.* 2018;141(4):1320-1333.e11.
93. Renert-Yuval Y, Del Duca E, Pavel AB, et al. The molecular features of normal and atopic dermatitis skin in infants, children, adolescents, and adults. *J Allergy Clin Immunol.* 2021;148(1):148-163.
94. Eyerich S, Onken AT, Weidinger S, et al. Mutual antagonism of T cells causing psoriasis and atopic eczema. *N Engl J Med.* 2011;365(3):231-238.
95. Cheng H, Tian J, Li Z, et al. TH17 cells are critical for skin-specific pathological injury in acute graft-versus-host disease. *Transplant Proc.* 2012;44(5):1412-1418.
96. Castela E, Tulic MK, Rozieres A, et al. Epidermolysis bullosa simplex generalized severe induces a T helper 17 response and is improved by apremilast treatment. *Br J Dermatol.* 2019;180(2):357-364.
97. Dander E, Balduzzi A, Zappa G, et al. Interleukin-17-producing T-helper cells as new potential player mediating graft-versus-host disease in patients undergoing allogeneic stem-cell transplantation. *Transplantation.* 2009;88(11):1261-1272.
98. Fulton LM, Carlson MJ, Coghill JM, et al. Attenuation of acute graft-versus-host disease in the absence of the transcription factor RORgammat. *J Immunol.* 2012;189(4):1765-1772.
99. Martin-Orozco N, Muranski P, Chung Y, et al. T helper 17 cells promote cytotoxic T cell activation in tumor immunity. *Immunity.* 2009;31(5):787-798.
100. Numasaki M, Fukushi J, Ono M, et al. Interleukin-17 promotes angiogenesis and tumor growth. *Blood.* 2003;101(7):2620-2627.
101. Stockinger B, Omenetti S. The dichotomous nature of T helper 17 cells. *Nat Rev Immunol.* 2017;17:535-544.
102. Muranski P, Boni A, Antony PA, et al. Tumor-specific Th17-polarized cells eradicate large established melanoma. *Blood.* 2008;112:362-373.
103. Sun J, Yi S, Qiu L, et al. SATB1 defines a subtype of cutaneous CD30(+) lymphoproliferative disorders associated with a T-helper 17 cytokine profile. *J Invest Dermatol.* 2018;138:1795-1804.
104. Wang Y, Gu X, Zhang G, et al. SATB1 overexpression promotes malignant T-cell proliferation in cutaneous CD30+ lymphoproliferative disease by repressing p21. *Blood.* 2014;123:3452-3461.
105. Ehrentraut S, Schneider B, Nagel S, et al. Th17 cytokine differentiation and loss of plasticity after SOCS1 inactivation in a cutaneous T-cell lymphoma. *Oncotarget.* 2016;7:34201-34216.
106. Wolk K, Mitsui H, Witte K, et al. Deficient cutaneous antibacterial competence in cutaneous T-cell lymphomas: role of Th2-mediated biased Th17 function. *Clin Cancer Res.* 2014;20:5507-5516.
107. Miyagaki T, Sugaya M, Suga H, et al. IL-22, but not IL-17, dominant environment in cutaneous T-cell lymphoma. *Clin Cancer Res.* 2011;17:7529-7538.
108. Eyerich S, Eyerich K, Pennino D, et al. Th22 cells represent a distinct human T cell subset involved in epidermal immunity and remodeling. *J Clin Invest.* 2009;119:3573-3585.
109. Fujita H, Nograles KE, Kikuchi T, Gonzalez J, Carucci JA, Krueger JG. Human Langerhans cells induce distinct IL-22-producing CD4+ T cells lacking IL-17 production. *Proc Natl Acad Sci USA.* 2009;106:21795-21800.
110. Fujita H. The role of IL-22 and Th22 cells in human skin diseases. *J Dermatol Sci.* 2013;72:3-8.
111. Trifari S, Kaplan CD, Tran EH, Crellin NK, Spits H. Identification of a human helper T cell population that has abundant production of interleukin 22 and is distinct from T(H)-17, T(H)1 and T(H)2 cells. *Nat Immunol.* 2009;10:864-871.
112. Sonnenberg GF, Fouser LA, Artis D. Border patrol: regulation of immunity, inflammation and tissue homeostasis at barrier surfaces by IL-22. *Nat Immunol.* 2011;12:383-390.
113. Nograles KE, Zaba LC, Guttman-Yassky E, et al. Th17 cytokines interleukin (IL)-17 and IL-22 modulate distinct inflammatory and keratinocyte-response pathways. *Br J Dermatol.* 2008;159:1092-1102.
114. Wolk K, Haugen HS, Xu W, et al. IL-22 and IL-20 are key mediators of the epidermal alterations in psoriasis while IL-17 and IFN-gamma are not. *J Mol Med (Berl).* 2009;87:523-536.
115. Nograles KE, Zaba LC, Shemer A, et al. IL-22-producing "T22" T cells account for upregulated IL-22 in atopic dermatitis despite reduced IL-17-producing TH17 T cells. *J Allergy Clin Immunol.* 2009;123:1244-1252.e2.
116. Ricciardi L, Minciullo PL, Saitta S, Trombetta D, Saija A, Gangemi S. Increased serum levels of IL-22 in patients with nickel contact dermatitis. *Contact Dermatitis.* 2009;60:57-58.
117. Rojahn TB, Vorstandlechner V, Krausgruber T, et al. Single-cell transcriptomics combined with interstitial fluid proteomics defines cell type-specific immune regulation in atopic dermatitis. *J Allergy Clin Immunol.* 2020;146:1056-1069.
118. Looman KIM, van Mierlo MMF, van Zelm MC, et al. Increased Th22 cell numbers in a general pediatric population with filaggrin haploinsufficiency: the generation R study. *Pediatr Allergy Immunol.* 2021;32(6):1360-1368.
119. Crotty S. Follicular helper CD4 T cells (TFH). *Annu Rev Immunol.* 2011;29:621-663.
120. Ballesteros-Tato A, Randall TD. Priming of T follicular helper cells by dendritic cells. *Immunol Cell Biol.* 2014;92:22-27.

121. Morita R, Schmitt N, Bentebibel SE, et al. Human blood CXCR5(+)CD4(+) T cells are counterparts of T follicular cells and contain specific subsets that differentially support antibody secretion. *Immunity*. 2011;34:108-121.
122. Ma CS, Deenick EK. Human T follicular helper (Tfh) cells and disease. *Immunol Cell Biol*. 2014;92:64-71.
123. Zou Y, Yuan H, Zhou S, et al. The pathogenic role of CD4+ tissue-resident memory T cells bearing T follicular helper-like phenotype in pemphigus lesions. *J Invest Dermatol*. 2021;141(9):2141-2150.
124. Yang M, Cao PP, Zhao ZD, et al. An enhanced expression level of CXCR3 on Tfh-like cells from lupus skin lesions rather than lupus peripheral blood. *Clin Immunol*. 2021;226:108717.
125. Gaydosik AM, Tabib T, Domsic R, Khanna D, Lafyatis R, Fuschiotti P. Single-cell transcriptome analysis identifies skin-specific T-cell responses in systemic sclerosis. *Ann Rheum Dis*. 2021;80(11):1453-1460.
126. Dorfman DM, Brown JA, Shahsafaei A, Freeman GJ. Programmed death-1 (PD-1) is a marker of germinal center-associated T cells and angioimmunoblastic T-cell lymphoma. *Am J Surg Pathol*. 2006;30:802-810.
127. Dupuis J, Boye K, Martin N, et al. Expression of CXCL13 by neoplastic cells in angioimmunoblastic T-cell lymphoma (AITL): a new diagnostic marker providing evidence that AITL derives from follicular helper T cells. *Am J Surg Pathol*. 2006;30:490-494.
128. Gaulard P, de Leval L. Follicular helper T cells: implications in neoplastic hematopathology. *Semin Diagn Pathol*. 2011;28:202-213.
129. Krenacs L, Schaerli P, Kis G, Bagdi E. Phenotype of neoplastic cells in angioimmunoblastic T-cell lymphoma is consistent with activated follicular B helper T cells. *Blood*. 2006;108:1110-1111.
130. Rodriguez Pinilla SM, Roncador G, Rodriguez-Peralto JL, et al. Primary cutaneous CD4+ small/medium-sized pleomorphic T-cell lymphoma expresses follicular T-cell markers. *Am J Surg Pathol*. 2009;33:81-90.
131. Micosse C, von Meyenn L, Steck O, et al. Human "T_H9" cells are a subpopulation of PPAR-γ^+ T_H2 cells. *Sci Immunol*. 2019;4:eaat5943.
132. Dardalhon V, Awasthi A, Kwon H, et al. IL-4 inhibits TGF-beta-induced Foxp3+ T cells and, together with TGF-beta, generates IL-9+ IL-10+ Foxp3(−) effector T cells. *Nat Immunol*. 2008;9:1347-1355.
133. Veldhoen M, Uyttenhove C, van Snick J, et al. Transforming growth factor-beta 'reprograms' the differentiation of T helper 2 cells and promotes an interleukin 9-producing subset. *Nat Immunol*. 2008;9:1341-1346.
134. Jabeen R, Goswami R, Awe O, et al. Th9 cell development requires a BATF-regulated transcriptional network. *J Clin Invest*. 2013;123:4641-4653.
135. Ma L, Xue HB, Guan XH, Shu CM, Zhang JH, Yu J. Possible pathogenic role of T helper type 9 cells and interleukin (IL)-9 in atopic dermatitis. *Clin Exp Immunol*. 2014;175:25-31.
136. Schlapbach C, Gehad A, Yang C, et al. Human TH9 cells are skin-tropic and have autocrine and paracrine proinflammatory capacity. *Sci Transl Med*. 2014;6:219ra8.
137. Roy S, Rizvi ZA, Clarke AJ, et al. EGFR-HIF1alpha signaling positively regulates the differentiation of IL-9 producing T helper cells. *Nat Commun*. 2021;12:3182.
138. Singh TP, Schon MP, Wallbrecht K, Gruber-Wackernagel A, Wang XJ, Wolf P. Involvement of IL-9 in Th17-associated inflammation and angiogenesis of psoriasis. *PLoS One*. 2013;8:e51752.
139. Schmitt E, Bopp T. Amazing IL-9: revealing a new function for an "old" cytokine. *J Clin Invest*. 2012;122:3857-3859.
140. Yang XR, Pfeiffer RM, Wheeler W, et al. Identification of modifier genes for cutaneous malignant melanoma in melanoma-prone families with and without CDKN2A mutations. *Int J Cancer*. 2009;125:2912-2917.
141. Lu Y, Hong S, Li H, et al. Th9 cells promote antitumor immune responses in vivo. *J Clin Invest*. 2012;122:4160-4171.
142. Purwar R, Schlapbach C, Xiao S, et al. Robust tumor immunity to melanoma mediated by interleukin-9-producing T cells. *Nat Med*. 2012;18:1248-1253.
143. Kumar S, Dhamija B, Marathe S, et al. The Th9 axis reduces the oxidative stress and promotes the survival of malignant T cells in cutaneous T-cell lymphoma patients. *Mol Cancer Res*. 2020;18:657-668.
144. Vieyra-Garcia PA, Wei T, Naym DG, et al. STAT3/5-Dependent IL9 overexpression contributes to neoplastic cell survival in mycosis fungoides. *Clin Cancer Res*. 2016;22:3328-3339.
145. Fredholm S, Willerslev-Olsen A, Met O, et al. SATB1 in malignant T cells. *J Invest Dermatol*. 2018;138:1805-1815.
146. Clark RA. Skin-resident T cells: the ups and downs of on site immunity. *J Invest Dermatol*. 2010;130:362-370.
147. Beyer M, Schultze JL. Regulatory T cells in cancer. *Blood*. 2006;108:804-811.
148. Josefowicz SZ, Lu LF, Rudensky AY. Regulatory T cells: mechanisms of differentiation and function. *Annu Rev Immunol*. 2012;30:531-564.
149. Shevach EM. Mechanisms of foxp3+ T regulatory cell-mediated suppression. *Immunity*. 2009;30:636-645.
150. Antiga E, Quaglino P, Volpi W, et al. Regulatory T cells in skin lesions and blood of patients with bullous pemphigoid. *J Eur Acad Dermatol Venereol*. 2013;28(2):222-230.
151. Bovenschen HJ, van de Kerkhof PC, van Erp PE, Woestenenk R, Joosten I, Koenen HJ. Foxp3+ regulatory T cells of psoriasis patients easily differentiate into IL-17A-producing cells and are found in lesional skin. *J Invest Dermatol*. 2011;131:1853-1860.
152. de Boer OJ, van der Loos CM, Teeling P, van der Wal AC, Teunissen MB. Immunohistochemical analysis of regulatory T cell markers FOXP3 and GITR on CD4+CD25+ T cells in normal skin and inflammatory dermatoses. *J Histochem Cytochem*. 2007;55:891-898.
153. Yun WJ, Lee DW, Chang SE, et al. Role of CD4CD25FOXP3 regulatory T cells in psoriasis. *Ann Dermatol*. 2010;22:397-403.
154. Terras S, Gambichler T, Moritz RK, Altmeyer P, Lambert J. Immunohistochemical analysis of FOXP3+ regulatory T cells in healthy human skin and autoimmune dermatoses. *Int J Dermatol*. 2014;53:294-299.
155. Verhagen J, Akdis M, Traidl-Hoffmann C, et al. Absence of T-regulatory cell expression and function in atopic dermatitis skin. *J Allergy Clin Immunol*. 2006;117:176-183.
156. Clark RA, Huang SJ, Murphy GF, et al. Human squamous cell carcinomas evade the immune response by down-regulation of vascular E-selectin and recruitment of regulatory T cells. *J Exp Med*. 2008;205:2221-2234.
157. Kaporis HG, Guttman-Yassky E, Lowes MA, et al. Human basal cell carcinoma is associated with Foxp3+ T cells in a Th2 dominant microenvironment. *J Invest Dermatol*. 2007;127:2391-2398.

158. Mourmouras V, Fimiani M, Rubegni P, et al. Evaluation of tumour-infiltrating CD4+CD25+FOXP3+ regulatory T cells in human cutaneous benign and atypical naevi, melanomas and melanoma metastases. *Br J Dermatol.* 2007;157:531-539.
159. Chen S, Ishii N, Ine S, et al. Regulatory T cell-like activity of Foxp3+ adult T cell leukemia cells. *Int Immunol.* 2006;18:269-277.
160. Roncador G, Garcia JF, Garcia JF, et al. FOXP3, a selective marker for a subset of adult T-cell leukaemia/lymphoma. *Leukemia.* 2005;19:2247-2253.
161. Shimauchi T, Kabashima K, Tokura Y. Adult T-cell leukemia/lymphoma cells from blood and skin tumors express cytotoxic T lymphocyte-associated antigen-4 and Foxp3 but lack suppressor activity toward autologous CD8+ T cells. *Cancer Sci.* 2008;99:98-106.
162. Toulza F, Nosaka K, Takiguchi M, et al. FoxP3+ regulatory T cells are distinct from leukemia cells in HTLV-1-associated adult T-cell leukemia. *Int J Cancer.* 2009;125:2375-2382.
163. Willerslev-Olsen A, Buus TB, Nastasi C, et al. *Staphylococcus aureus* enterotoxins induce FOXP3 in neoplastic T cells in Sezary syndrome. *Blood Cancer J.* 2020;10(5):57.
164. Ariotti S, Beltman JB, Chodaczek G, et al. Tissue-resident memory CD8+ T cells continuously patrol skin epithelia to quickly recognize local antigen. *Proc Natl Acad Sci USA.* 2012;109:19739-19744.
165. Masopust D, Schenkel JM. The integration of T cell migration, differentiation and function. *Nat Rev Immunol.* 2013;13:309-320.
166. Mbitikon-Kobo FM, Vocanson M, Michallet MC, et al. Characterization of a CD44/CD122int memory CD8 T cell subset generated under sterile inflammatory conditions. *J Immunol.* 2009;182:3846-3854.
167. Lazarevic V, Glimcher LH, Lord GM. T-bet: a bridge between innate and adaptive immunity. *Nat Rev Immunol.* 2013;13:777-789.
168. McLane LM, Banerjee PP, Cosma GL, et al. Differential localization of T-bet and Eomes in CD8 T cell memory populations. *J Immunol.* 2013;190:3207-3215.
169. Clark RA. Resident memory T cells in human health and disease. *Sci Transl Med.* 2015;7:269rv1.
170. Gill H, Liang RH, Tse E. Extranodal natural-killer/t-cell lymphoma, nasal type. *Adv Hematol.* 2010;2010:627401.
171. Swerdlow SH; International Agency for Research on Cancer; World Health Organization. *WHO Classification of Tumours of Haematopoietic and Lymphoid Tissues.* 4th ed. International Agency for Research on Cancer; 2008.
172. Allison JP, Havran WL. The immunobiology of T cells with invariant gamma delta antigen receptors. *Annu Rev Immunol.* 1991;9:679-705.
173. Ebert LM, Meuter S, Moser B. Homing and function of human skin gammadelta T cells and NK cells: relevance for tumor surveillance. *J Immunol.* 2006;176:4331-4336.
174. Jameson J, Ugarte K, Chen N, et al. A role for skin gammadelta T cells in wound repair. *Science.* 2002;296:747-749.
175. Jameson J, Havran WL. Skin gammadelta T-cell functions in homeostasis and wound healing. *Immunol Rev.* 2007;215:114-122.
176. Toulon A, Breton L, Taylor KR, et al. A role for human skin-resident T cells in wound healing. *J Exp Med.* 2009;206:743-750.
177. Havran WL, Jameson JM. Epidermal T cells and wound healing. *J Immunol.* 2010;184:5423-5428.
178. Fink DR, Holm D, Schlosser A, et al. Elevated numbers of SCART1+ gammadelta T cells in skin inflammation and inflammatory bowel disease. *Mol Immunol.* 2010;47:1710-1718.
179. Girardi M. Immunosurveillance and immunoregulation by gammadelta T cells. *J Invest Dermatol.* 2006;126:25-31.
180. Hoq MM, Suzutani T, Toyoda T, Horiike G, Yoshida I, Azuma M. Role of gamma delta TCR+ lymphocytes in the augmented resistance of trehalose 6,6'-dimycolate-treated mice to influenza virus infection. *J Gen Virol.* 1997;78(Pt 7):1597-1603.
181. Wang T, Welte T. Role of natural killer and Gamma-delta T cells in West Nile virus infection. *Viruses.* 2013;5:2298-2310.
182. Becher B, Pantelyushin S. Hiding under the skin: interleukin-17-producing gammadelta T cells go under the skin? *Nat Med.* 2012;18:1748-1750.
183. Cai Y, Shen X, Ding C, et al. Pivotal role of dermal IL-17-producing gammadelta T cells in skin inflammation. *Immunity.* 2011;35:596-610.
184. Gapin L. The making of NKT cells. *Nat Immunol.* 2008;9:1009-1011.
185. Kawano T, Cui J, Koezuka Y, et al. CD1d-restricted and TCR-mediated activation of valpha14 NKT cells by glycosylceramides. *Science.* 1997;278:1626-1629.
186. Skold M, Behar SM. Role of CD1d-restricted NKT cells in microbial immunity. *Infect Immun.* 2003;71:5447-5455.
187. Kovalovsky D, Uche OU, Eladad S, et al. The BTB-zinc finger transcriptional regulator PLZF controls the development of invariant natural killer T cell effector functions. *Nat Immunol.* 2008;9:1055-1064.
188. Savage AK, Constantinides MG, Han J, et al. The transcription factor PLZF directs the effector program of the NKT cell lineage. *Immunity.* 2008;29:391-403.
189. Egawa T, Eberl G, Taniuchi I, et al. Genetic evidence supporting selection of the Valpha14i NKT cell lineage from double-positive thymocyte precursors. *Immunity.* 2005;22:705-716.
190. Tachibana M, Tenno M, Tezuka C, Sugiyama M, Yoshida H, Taniuchi I. Runx1/Cbfbeta2 complexes are required for lymphoid tissue inducer cell differentiation at two developmental stages. *J Immunol.* 2011;186:1450-1457.
191. Townsend MJ, Weinmann AS, Matsuda JL, et al. T-bet regulates the terminal maturation and homeostasis of NK and Valpha14i NKT cells. *Immunity.* 2004;20:477-494.
192. Bendelac A, Savage PB, Teyton L. The biology of NKT cells. *Annu Rev Immunol.* 2007;25:297-336.
193. Askenase PW, Szczepanik M, Itakura A, Kiener C, Campos RA. Extravascular T-cell recruitment requires initiation begun by Valpha14+ NKT cells and B-1 B cells. *Trends Immunol.* 2004;25:441-449.
194. Goubier A, Vocanson M, Macari C, et al. Invariant NKT cells suppress CD8(+) T-cell-mediated allergic contact dermatitis independently of regulatory CD4(+) T cells. *J Invest Dermatol.* 2013;133:980-987.
195. Ilhan F, Kandi B, Akbulut H, Turgut D, Cicek D. Atopic dermatitis and Valpha24+ natural killer T cells. *Skinmed.* 2007;6:218-220.
196. Peternel S, Kastelan M. Immunopathogenesis of psoriasis: focus on natural killer T cells. *J Eur Acad Dermatol Venereol.* 2009;23:1123-1127.
197. Prell C, Konstantopoulos N, Heinzelmann B, et al. Frequency of Valpha24+CD161+ natural killer T cells and invariant TCRAV24-AJ18 transcripts in atopic and non-atopic individuals. *Immunobiology.* 2003;208:367-380.

CHAPTER 2

Cutaneous B-cell immunobiology

Alejandro A. Gru and José Cabeçadas

INTRODUCTION

Originally termed skin-associated lymphoid tissue, the "skin immune system" is comprised of specialized skin-resident immune cells, as well as immunocompetent skin-trophic lymphocytes constantly recirculating between the skin, skin-draining lymph nodes, and the peripheral circulation.[1-5] Emerging evidence indicates that B-cells play important roles in steady-state cutaneous immune homeostasis as well as in the pathogenesis of cutaneous inflammatory and neoplastic diseases.[6,7]

In this chapter, we will review the different stages of B-cell maturation in keeping with the concept that B-cell lymphomas tend to recapitulate the stages of normal B-cell differentiation and show resemblance to the different stages of B-cell development.[8]

B-CELL DIFFERENTIATION

B-cell differentiation occurs in both an antigen-independent and -dependent fashion. We will summarize both pathways of differentiation (Fig. 2-1). The antigen-independent pathway starts with the development of precursor B-cells (Pre-B) and naïve B-cells.

Precursor B Cells

These cells develop from hematopoietic stem cells and differentiate in the bone marrow.[9] Later, they migrate into the blood as naïve mature B-cells.[10] The pre-B can develop in the liver, bone marrow, and spleen during fetal development, but in adults, their growth is restricted to the bone marrow.[11] During B-cell development, there is a rearrangement of the different parts of the immunoglobulin genes (V-D-J). The earliest type of pre-B cell is called a progenitor B-cell (pro-B), which lacks surface and cytoplasmic immunoglobulins. The pre-B cells acquire cytoplasmic light chain expression, and later express surface μ heavy chain. When the rearrangement of the gene is complete, there is surface expression of immunoglobulin M (IgM) in the immature B-cells. Mature cells express both IgM and IgD when they leave the bone marrow as naïve B-cells.[12,13]

The pre-B cells are characterized by the expression of markers of immaturity (TdT and CD34), HLA-DR, and CD10. As the cells progress in the maturation cycle, they lose CD34, TdT, and CD10. PAX-5, a B-cell transcription factor, is expressed early on the pre-B cells, as is CD19. CD20 is only acquired[10,14] later. The leukocyte common antigen (CD45) does not appear until CD20 is expressed. Pre- and pro-B cells are linked to immature blastic types of lymphomas (B-lymphoblastic leukemias and lymphomas).[8] It is important to note that the more mature stages of B-ALL might not express CD34 or TdT, but typically show a blastic morphology (Fig. 2-2) and can potentially have surface immunoglobulin expression.

Naïve B-Cells

Naïve B-cells are circulating cells expressing both surface IgM and IgD while lacking the immature markers CD10, CD34, and TdT. They are cells capable of responding to antigen stimulation that have rearranged but unmutated immunoglobulin genes.[9] The naïve B-cells and their progeny are committed to a single light chain, kappa, or lambda. These B-cells show expression of the pan B-cell markers (CD19, CD20, CD22, CD40, CD79a), Human leukocyte antigen(s) (HLA) class II molecules, the complement receptors (CD21 and CD35), CD44, and CD23. Some of these B-cells coexpress CD5 and are typically designated as activated B1a cells.[15-17] They typically represent a minute reservoir of the normal population of cells. Some of these naïve cells show expression of BCL-2, which promotes survival in the resting stage. The main functions of these cells involve "homing" or adhesion to vascular endothelium, interaction with antigen-presenting cells, and signal transduction.[17] During fetal development, naïve B-cells are confined to the spleen. In children and adults, they are the main type of circulating resting B-cells, and the more prominent population in the lymphoid follicles and mantle zones (so-called recirculating B-cells). Mantle cell lymphoma (MCL) is thought to derive from naïve B-cells and shows a characteristic rearrangement of the cyclin *D1* gene[18] (Fig. 2-2).

In antigen-dependent B-cell differentiation, the formation of mature plasma cells and the secretion of entirely specific immunoglobulins against a specific antigen occur.

T-Cell–Independent B-Cell Differentiation

Certain antigens (eg, those with repeat structures) can elicit a B-cell reaction without the direct cooperation of T-cells.

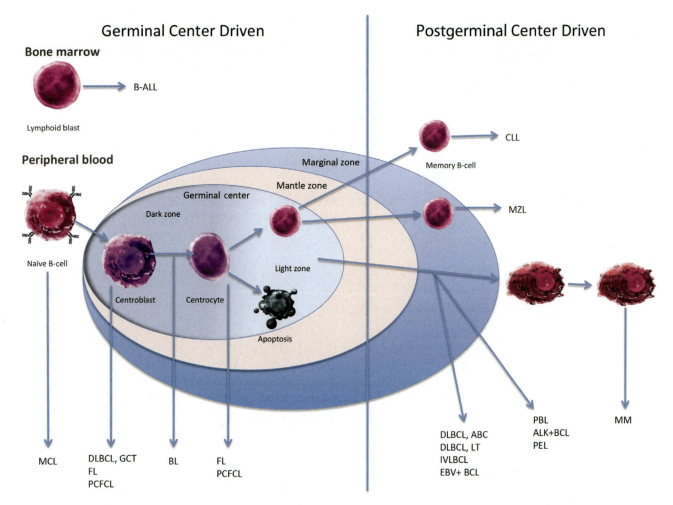

FIGURE 2-1. **B-cell differentiation in the lymph node includes multiple steps fbeginning in the bone marrow and continuing within the follicles and germinal centers, subsequently eventuating, after contact with the antigenic exposure, in plasma cell differentiation.** Lymphoid blasts are contained within the bone marrow, and as they acquire surface IgM expression, and lose immature markers, they exit into the peripheral blood circulation as naïve B-cells. B-lymphoblastic leukemias and lymphomas (B-ALL) and MCLs are derived from lymphoid blasts and naïve B-cells, respectively. Once naïve B-cells enter into contact with the specific antigens, they subsequently develop into centroblasts and centrocytes with the activation of the GC program and somatic hypermutation. B-cell lymphomas of GC origin include DLBCL, FL, PCFCL, and BL. Centrocytes with poor affinity for the specific antigen undergo the programmed cell death process, apoptosis. Those with high affinity are rescued, and some develop into memory B-cells and marginal zone B-cells. CLL derives from memory cells and marginal zone lymphomas (MZLs) from the marginal B-cells. Under plasma cell differentiation, immunoblasts, plasmablasts, and mature plasma cells later develop in the bone marrow and other organs. Many B-cell lymphomas develop from immunoblastic B-cells: DLBCL, including its primary cutaneous leg-type variant (DLBCL-LT), intravascular large B-cell lymphoma (IVLBCL), EBV[+] large B-cell lymphoma (EBV-BCL). Lymphomas with plasmablastic differentiation include plasmablastic lymphoma (PBL), ALK[+] diffuse large B-cell lymphoma (ALK[+]-DLBCL), and primary effusion lymphoma (PEL). Multiple myeloma (MM) derives from the most mature stage of differentiation.

The antigens can interact directly or indirectly (via antigen-presenting cells) with the B-cells and activate them.[19] The activated B-cells (immunoblasts) can also develop in daughter plasma cells, which are able to secrete IgM, typical of a primary immune response. However, no memory cells are generated during this process. The antibodies produced with such reaction are of low affinity to the antigens, since somatic hypermutation does not typically occur at this stage.[13] Recently, mucosal epithelial cells lining the crypts of human tonsils were shown to have the ability to support class switching through the production of B-cell activating factor (BAFF) and IL-10 upon toll-like receptor stimulation. These cells also secrete thymic stromal lymphopoietin, which stimulates production of BAFF by dendritic cells (DCs).[20]

T-Cell-Dependent Germinal Center Reaction

Antigenic stimulation is essential for this phase of the B-cell development. The germinal centers (GCs) are composed of 3 to 10 naïve B-cells and approximately 10,000 to 15,000 B-cells.[13,21] The IgM[+] B-cells are formed by naïve B-cells that have encountered an antigen in the T-cell zone (paracortex) and migrated into the center of a primary follicle, subsequently filling the follicular DC networks 3 days after antigenic stimulation, forming the GCs. The GCs are the most efficient way to generate expanded B-cell clones of a highly selected antigen receptor. Two types of effector B-cells will later emerge: memory B-cells and plasma cells. Such a process involves a series of steps, which

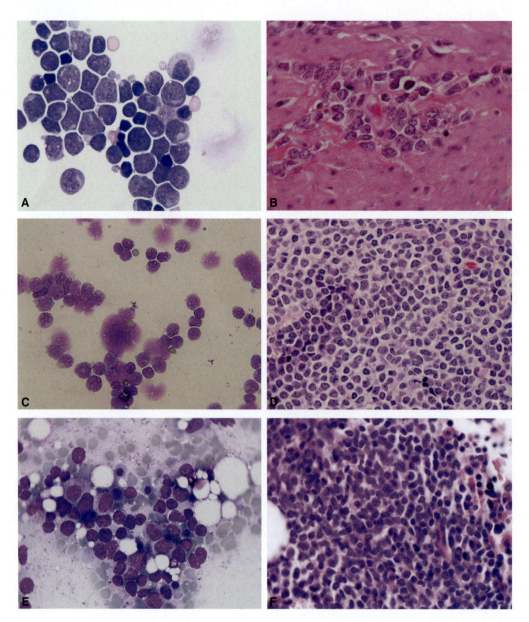

FIGURE 2-2. **B-cells at different stages of differentiation. A** and **B.** Lymphoblasts; **C** and **D.** Mantle cell lymphoma (naïve B-cells); **E** and **F.** Chronic lymphocytic leukemia (memory B-cells).

include proliferation, induction of immunoglobulins, somatic hypermutation, and class switch, selection, and differentiation.[13]

During the GC development, the B-cells acquire expression of BCL6, a nuclear zinc-finger transcription factor.[22] This protein is expressed by centrocytes, centroblasts, and follicular T-helper cells, but not by naïve B-cells, memory B-cells, mantle cells, or plasma cells. The BCL6 protein generates downregulation of genes involved in negative feedback loops of the cell cycle regulation and the genotoxic response.[22,23] As such, one of the most important targets of BCL6 is the interaction with p53.[24] Such interaction leads to the inhibition of p21, another cell cycle inhibitor, and therefore stimulates the proliferation of cells. The negative interaction with p53 also facilitates the individual cell tolerance to the DNA breaks and rearrangements that occur during somatic hypermutation and class switch. BCL6 also inhibits the differentiation of centrocytes to plasma cells and memory cells.

The B-cells that have undergone antigenic stimulation differentiate into centroblasts and accumulate in the dark zone of the GCs. Centroblasts have a short and fast cell cycle and a high proliferation.[21] They activate telomerase and prevent shortening of telomeres in each cycle.[25] Centroblasts downregulate the antiapoptotic gene *BCL2* and upregulate the proapoptotic molecule CD95 (Fas).[26] The purpose of such a program is to select cells capable of generating highly specific receptors to the antigen present in the GC. The centroblasts undergo somatic hypermutation of the variable (V) region of the immunoglobulin gene, increasing the affinity of the antibody produced by the cell. The somatic hypermutation can produce a marked intraclonal diversity of antibody-combining sites, in a population of cells which is derived from few precursors.[21]

Later, the centroblasts mature into centrocytes, which accumulate in the light zones of the GC. The mature centrocytes have surface Ig expression, with the same variable diversity joining rearrangement as the parent naïve B-cell and centroblast. Centrocytes also have a heavy-chain switch that alters the IgM constant region to IgG, IgA, or IgE. The centrocytes that do not have a high affinity for a specific antigen die by apoptosis. The "starry sky" pattern seen in GCs is the product of phagocytic macrophages and apoptotic centrocytes. The centrocytes with high affinity for a specific antigen, via a cell–cell-mediated T-cell interaction, are rescued from apoptosis.

The posterior termination of the GC program and post-GC differentiation require the inactivation of BCL6. In addition to the ubiquitination of the BCL6 protein, the B- and T-cell interaction induces expression of the transcription factor IRF4, which represses BCL6.[27] The exact mechanisms governing the formation of memory B-cells are unclear. Plasma cell differentiation involves the upregulation of IRF4 and BLIMP1 and the subsequent inactivation of the B-cell transcription factor PAX5.[28,29] Some of the most common subtypes of systemic and cutaneous B-cell lymphomas derive from the GC B-cell (Fig. 2-3). Follicular lymphomas (FLs) and a subset of primary cutaneous follicle center lymphomas are associated with the t(14; 18) translocation, which produces upregulation of the BCL2 protein.[30] Burkitt lymphoma is also derived from the GC and is associated with the t(8; 14) translocation, which activates the *MYC* gene.[31] Subsets of diffuse large B-cell lymphoma (DLBCL)

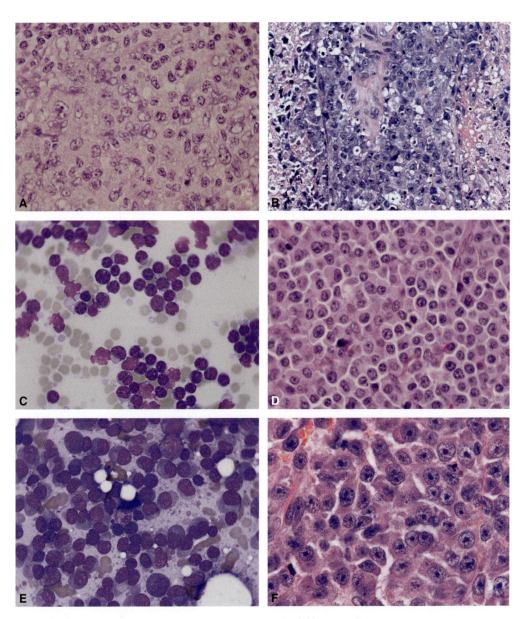

FIGURE 2-3. B-cells at different stages of differentiation. A. Centroblasts in high-grade follicular lymphoma; **B.** Immunoblasts in primary CNS lymphoma; **C** and **D.** Marginal zone lymphoma cells; **E.** Mature plasma cells (multiple myeloma); and **F.** Plasmablasts (plasmablastic lymphoma).

with GC differentiation tend to recapitulate the centroblastic morphology, and may be associated with mutations in the *BCL6* gene.[32] Many of the common DLBCLs do not recapitulate centroblasts, have an immunoblastic nature (with a vague resemblance to plasmacytoid cells), and are thought to reflect a non-GC (activated B) cell origin.

Memory B-Cells

The antigen-specific memory B-cells leave the follicles and are found in the peripheral blood and different tissue compartments, mainly in the marginal zones. Memory B-cells can have class-switched Igs (IgG, IgA, or IgE) and represent approximately 15% of all peripheral blood B-cells. Some memory B-cells arise from GC-independent activated B-cells, are IgM+, and represent 10% of all memory B-cells.[20] Many IgM+ memory cells are present in tissues, including splenic and mucosa-associated lymphoid tissues (MALT) marginal zones, tonsils, and lymph nodes.[33,34] When splenic marginal zone B-cells are reexposed to an antigen, they rapidly migrate into the GC and appear in the T-cell zone as immunoblasts, giving rise to antigen-specific plasma cells.[35] Monocytoid B-cells are cells resembling marginal zone B-cells that have an abundance of cytoplasm and irregular nuclear contours. They are typically seen in the subcapsular areas of cortical sinuses of reactive lymph nodes. The lack of or paucity of mutated V regions suggests a lack of selection by antigen. The marginal zone B-cells can migrate into the GC where they can present the antigen to the GC B-cells. If the follicular center cells have surface immunoglobulin that binds to the presented antigen, they proliferate and form the GC reaction, thus expanding the pool of B-cells responding to the antigen and differentiating into plasma cells and new memory B-cells.[36] Secondly, antigen, in association with cytokines elaborated by T-cells (but not requiring antigen-primed T-cells), can rapidly induce the differentiation of the marginal zone B-cells into plasma cells and induce synthesis and secretion of antigen-specific immunoglobulin. The B-cells residing in the mantle zone are resting lymphocytes.

Most of the nodal, splenic, and extranodal B-cell lymphomas resembling marginal zone and monocytoid B-cells show somatic hypermutations suggestive of antigen selection.[13] Chronic lymphocytic leukemia/small lymphocytic lymphoma shows somatic hypermutation in 50% of cases and appears to correspond to a subset of memory B-cells with CD5 coexpression.[31,32,37,38]

Plasma Cells

The precursors of plasma cells, plasmablasts, retain proliferating activity. Plasmablasts express MHC molecules but lose B-cell markers (PAX5, CD20, CD19) and have cytoplasmic Igs.[28,39] The mature plasma cells are divided into the short-lived, IgM secreting forms, generated in the T-cell–independent immune response, and the long-lived class-switched secreting cells. IgG-producing plasma cells accumulate in the lymph node medulla and splenic cords. Plasmablasts leave the lymph node and migrate into the bone marrow.[29,39] Mature plasma cells lack surface Igs, HLA-DR, CD40, and CD45, but keep cytoplasmic Igs. Both plasma cells and plasmablasts express CD38, CD138, and CD79a. The plasma cells also express BLIMP1, XBP1, and IRF4/MUM1. The tumors derived from the bone marrow–homing plasma cells include most of the plasmacytomas and plasma cell myelomas. There are aggressive lymphomas that have the morphology and proliferation activity of immunoblasts, yet have the immunophenotype of plasma cells (eg, lack of mature B-cell markers such as CD20 and express CD138) representing a rare subset of B-cell malignancies with plasmablastic differentiation: these include plasmablastic lymphoma, primary effusion lymphoma, and B-cell lymphomas arising in association with Castleman disease.[40]

THE ROLE OF B-CELLS IN NORMAL SKIN HOMEOSTASIS

B-cells do not represent a significant proportion of cells in the normal skin, but their presence has been well documented.[41] More importantly, these cells also display a clonally restricted pattern, a feature indicative of their capability to recognize a restricted antigenic repertoire, alluding to the possibility of a skin-resident memory B-cell population. However, it is currently unknown whether the B-cells present in normal skin are part of a specific skin-resident population or whether they are derived from circulating populations of B-cells1 (Fig. 2-4).

Recruitment of B-Cells to the Skin

The Role of B-Cells in Skin Disease
In humans, dermal B-cell infiltrates have been observed in chronic inflammatory skin conditions including cutaneous leishmaniasis, diffuse cutaneous sclerosis, and atopic dermatitis (AD).[38-40] CD19-deficient (CD19−/−) mice sensitized with ovalbumin via the epicutaneous route were found to display a less-severe histologic AD phenotype (assessed by skin thickening) compared to wild-type mice.[41] Treatment with rituximab in AD has been reported to improve skin lesions as assessed by cutaneous symptoms and histopathologic parameters.[40] Treatment of immunobullous disorders including pemphigus and bullous pemphigoid with rituximab also resulted in improvement of skin lesions and has been reported to be associated with a reduction in titers of circulating autoantibodies in some patients, and this was attributed to the systemic depletion of mature CD20+ B-cells. Recent data have also shown an association between the use of rituximab and the development of psoriasis, suggesting a possible suppressive role for the B-cells in the development of T-cell–mediated cutaneous inflammatory skin conditions.

B-cells are present in tumor-infiltrating lymphocyte populations in several cutaneous malignancies including squamous cell carcinomas and melanomas. In mouse models of melanoma, B-cells may promote tumor growth by supporting angiogenesis and lymphangiogenesis. Emerging evidence also points to systemic as well as tumor-resident B-cell responses in human cutaneous melanomas; B-cell infiltrates are detected in melanoma lesions, and lymphoid-like structures rich in B-cells are observed in some primary and

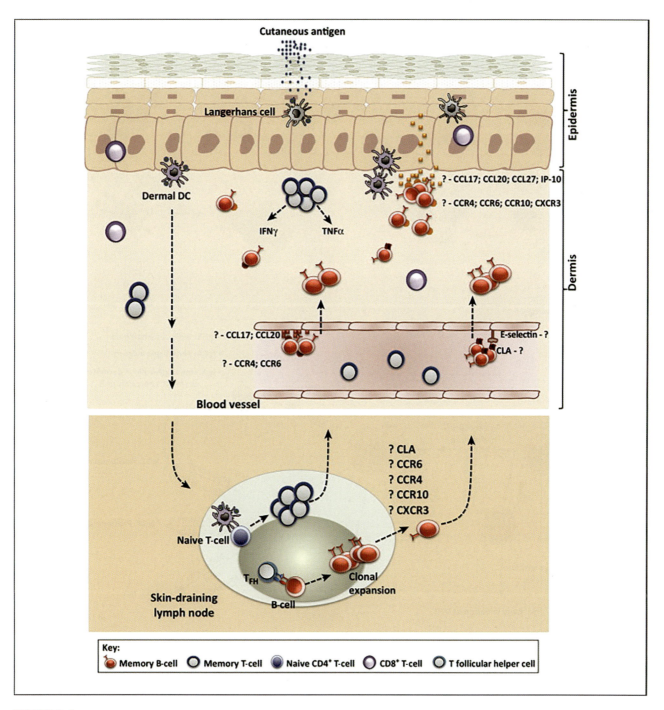

FIGURE 2-4. **Model of B-cell migration to cutaneous sites.** A diverse array of immune cells is present within the skin including Langerhans cells, dermal dendritic cells (DCs), B-cells, and T-cell subsets. Naïve T-cells are primed via presentation of cutaneous antigens by dermal DCs within skin-draining lymph nodes. Activated T-cells subsequently migrate back to the skin and can produce proinflammatory cytokines (eg, IFNγ and TNFα) as part of a cutaneous immune response. Similarly, possible interactions between cutaneous antigen-specific B-cells and appropriately primed follicular helper T-cells (TFH) within skin-draining lymph nodes may result in generation of a memory B-cell population which expresses/upregulates skin-homing chemokine receptors (such as CLA, CCR4, CCR6, CCR10, and CXCR3) and subsequently traffics into the skin. At the same time, receptor interaction with cognate ligands including E-selectin and CCL17 (from dermal blood vessels) or CCL27 (from epidermal keratinocytes), which are constitutively expressed or induced within the skin in response to proinflammatory signals, may additionally serve to direct the trafficking of activated B-cells through cutaneous vascular endothelia and into the dermis. (Reprinted from Egbuniwe IU, Karagiannis SN, Nestle FO, et al. Revisiting the role of B cells in skin immune surveillance. *Trends Immunol.* 2015;36:102-111, with permission from Elsevier.)

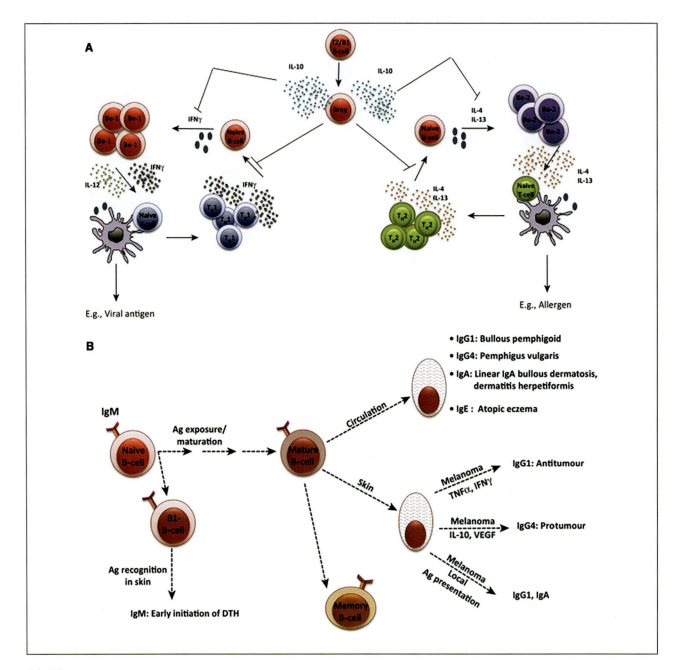

FIGURE 2-5. B-cell roles in skin immunity. A. B-cells may modulate skin immune responses through their production of pro- and antiinflammatory cytokines. Naïve B-cells primed in the presence of specific antigens (Ag) and T_H1 or T_H2 cytokines are able to adopt the same "effector phenotype" as T-cells. Be-1 (B-cells primed in a T_H1 environment) and Be-2 (B-cells primed in a T_H2 environment) cells act as a source of positive feedback by producing cytokines that maintain ongoing inflammation. Splenic transitional zone (TZ) and B1-B cells are thought to differentiate into regulatory B-cells (Bregs). **B.** Modulation of cutaneous pathology by B-cells can take place in the context of systemic (eg, immunobullous disease) or local (eg, tumor microenvironment) antibody production. Early production of low-affinity IgM antibodies also occurs in delayed-type hypersensitivity responses. (Reprinted from Egbuniwe IU, Karagiannis SN, Nestle FO, et al. Revisiting the role of B cells in skin immune surveillance. *Trends Immunol.* 2015; 36:102-111, with permission from Elsevie.)

metastatic melanomas. Ladányi et al[42] have reported correlations between the densities of tumor-infiltrating B-cells and more favorable clinical outcomes in patients with cutaneous melanomas. All these findings suggest a relevance of local B-cells to the pathogenesis, progression, and prognosis of skin cancers (Fig. 2-5).

CAPSULE SUMMARY

- The classification of cutaneous B-cell lymphomas requires an understanding of physiologic B-cell maturation.
- B-cell differentiation occurs in both an *antigen-independent* and *-dependent* fashion.

- The antigen-independent stages of B-cell differentiation include the formation of lymphoblasts and naïve B-cells. Lymphoblasts lack surface immunoglobulin expression, a feature that is acquired by naïve B-cells as they exit the bone marrow, into the circulation, and represent the largest pool of B-cells in the blood.
- The antigen-dependent stages of maturation occur as the B-cells mature into centroblasts and subsequently centrocytes. Such cells undergo somatic hypermutation to achieve high-affinity B-cell receptors. Later, the B-cells mature into memory B-cells or mature plasma cells.
- Under normal circumstances, a small population of B-cells can reside in the skin.

References

1. Streilein JW. Skin-associated lymphoid tissues (SALT): origins and functions. *J Invest Dermatol*. 1983;80(suppl l):12s-16s. doi:10.1111/1523-1747.ep12536743
2. Bos JD, Kapsenberg ML. The skin immune system its cellular constituents and their interactions. *Immunol Today*. 1986;7(7-8):235-240. doi:10.1016/0167-5699(86)90111-8
3. Egbuniwe IU, Karagiannis SN, Nestle FO, Lacy KE. Revisiting the role of B cells in skin immune surveillance. *Trends Immunol*. 2015;36(2):102-111. doi:10.1016/j.it.2014.12.006
4. Egawa G, Kabashima K. Skin as a peripheral lymphoid organ: revisiting the concept of skin-associated lymphoid tissues. *J Invest Dermatol*. 2011;131(11):2178-2185. doi:10.1038/jid.2011.198
5. Kogame T, Kabashima K, Egawa G. Putative immunological functions of inducible skin-associated lymphoid tissue in the context of mucosa-associated lymphoid tissue. *Front Immunol*. 2021;12:3387. doi:10.3389/fimmu.2021.733484
6. Karagiannis P, Gilbert AE, Nestle FO, Karagiannis SN. IgG4 antibodies and cancer-associated inflammation: insights into a novel mechanism of immune escape. *OncoImmunology*. 2013;2(7):e24889. doi:10.4161/onci.24889
7. Karagiannis P, Gilbert AE, Josephs DH, et al. IgG4 subclass Antibodies impair antitumor immunity in melanoma. *J Clin Invest*. 2013;123(4):1457-1474. doi:10.1172/JCI65579
8. Swerdlow S, Campo E, Harris N, et al, eds. *WHO Classification of Tumours of Haematopoietic and Lymphoid Tissues*. Revised 4th ed. IARC; 2017.
9. Akashi K, Reya T, Dalma-Weiszhausz D, Weissman IL. Lymphoid precursors. *Curr Opin Immunol*. 2000;12(2):144-150. doi:10.1016/S0952-7915(99)00064-3.
10. Bonnet D. Biology of human bone marrow stem cells. *Clin Exp Med*. 2003;3(3):140-149. doi:10.1007/s10238-003-0017-9
11. Kucia M, Ratajczak J, Ratajczak MZ. Are bone marrow stem cells plastic or heterogenous - that is the question. *Exp Hematol*. 2005;33(6):613-623. doi:10.1016/j.exphem.2005.01.016
12. Hirose J, Kouro T, Igarashi H, Yokota T, Sakaguchi N, Kincade PW. A developing picture of lymphopoiesis in bone marrow. *Immunol Rev*. 2002;189:28-40. doi:10.1034/j.1600-065X.2002.18904.x
13. Hardy RR, Hayakawa KB. Cell development pathways. *Annu Rev Immunol*. 2001;19:595-621. doi:10.1146/annurev.immunol.19.1.595
14. Maillard I, Fang T, Pear WS. Regulation of lymphoid development, differentiation, and function by the notch pathway. *Annu Rev Immunol*. 2005;23:945-974. doi:10.1146/annurev.immunol.23.021704.115747
15. Chen HC, Byrd JC, Muthusamy N. Differential role for cyclic AMP response element binding protein-1 in multiple stages of B cell development, differentiation, and survival. *J Immunol*. 2006;176(4):2208-2218. doi:10.4049/jimmunol.176.4.2208
16. Ishida D, Su L, Tamura A, et al. Rap1 signal controls B cell receptor repertoire and generation of self-reactive B1a cells. *Immunity*. 2006;24(4):417-427. doi:10.1016/j.immuni.2006.02.007
17. Sanz I, Wei C, Jenks SA, et al. Challenges and opportunities for consistent classification of human b cell and plasma cell populations. *Front Immunol*. 2019;10(OCT):2458. doi:10.3389/fimmu.2019.02458
18. Raffeld M, Jaffe ES. Bcl-1, t(11;14), and mantle cell-derived lymphomas. *Blood*. 1991:78(2):259-263. doi:10.1182/blood.v78.2.259.259
19. Zeng Y, Yi J, Wan Z, et al. Substrate stiffness regulates B-cell activation, proliferation, class switch, and T-cell-independent antibody responses in vivo. *Eur J Immunol*. 2015;45(6):1621-1634. doi:10.1002/eji.201444777
20. Viant C, Wirthmiller T, ElTanbouly MA, et al. Germinal center-dependent and -independent memory B cells produced throughout the immune response. *J Exp Med*. 2021;218(8):e20202489. doi:10.1084/jem.20202489
21. Gars E, Butzmann A, Ohgami R, Balakrishna JP, O'Malley DP. The life and death of the germinal center. *Ann Diagn Pathol*. 2020;44:151421. doi:10.1016/j.anndiagpath.2019.151421
22. Phan RT, Saito M, Basso K, Niu H, Dalla-Favera R. BCL6 interacts with the transcription factor miz-1 to suppress the cyclin-dependent kinase inhibitor P21 and cell cycle arrest in germinal center B cells. *Nat Immunol*. 2005:6(10):1054-1060. doi:10.1038/ni1245
23. Good-Jacobson KL, Chen Y, Voss AK, Smyth GK, Thomas T, Tarlinton D. Regulation of germinal center responses and B-cell memory by the chromatin modifier MOZ. *Proc Natl Acad Sci USA*. 2014;111(26):9585-9590. doi:10.1073/pnas.1402485111
24. Rui L, Goodnow C. Lymphoma and the control of B cell growth and differentiation. *Curr Mol Med*. 2006;6(3):291-308. doi:10.2174/156652406776894563
25. Norrback KF, Hultdin M, Dahlenborg K, Osterman P, Carlsson R, Roos G. Telomerase regulation and telomere dynamics in germinal centers. *Eur J Haematol*. 2001;67(5-6):309-317. doi:10.1034/j.1600-0609.2001.00588.x
26. Martinez-Valdez H, Guret C, De Bouteiller O, Fugier I, Banchereau J, Liu YJ. Human germinal center B cells express the apoptosis-inducing genes Fas, c-myc, P53, and Bax but not the survival gene bcl-2. *J Exp Med* 1996;183(3):971-977. doi:10.1084/jem.183.3.971
27. Lu R Interferon regulatory factor 4 and 8 in B-cell development. *Trends Immunol*. 2008;29(10):487-492. doi:10.1016/j.it.2008.07.006.
28. Nutt SL, Taubenheim N, Hasbold J, Corcoran LM, Hodgkin PD. The genetic network controlling plasma cell differentiation. *Semin Immunol*. 2011;23(5):341-349. doi:10.1016/j.smim.2011.08.010
29. Nutt SL, Hodgkin PD, Tarlinton DM, Corcoran LM. The generation of antibody-secreting plasma cells. *Nat Rev Immunol*. 2015;15(3):160-171. doi:10.1038/nri3795
30. Streubel B, Scheucher B, Valencak J, et al. Molecular cytogenetic evidence of t(14;18)(IGH;BCL2) in a substantial proportion of primary cutaneous follicle center lymphomas. *Am J Surg Pathol*. 2006;30(4):529-536. doi:10.1097/00000478-200604000-00015

31. Dalla-Favera R, Bregni M, Erikson J, Patterson D, Gallo RC, Croce CM. Human C-myc onc gene is located on the region of chromosome 8 that is translocated in burkitt lymphoma cells. *Proc Natl Acad Sci USA*. 1982;79(24 I):7824-7827. doi:10.1073/pnas.79.24.7824
32. Niu H. The proto-oncogene BCL-6 in normal and malignant B cell development. *Hematol Oncol*. 2002;155-166. doi:10.1002/hon.689
33. Klein U, Rajewsky K, Küppers R. Human immunoglobulin (Ig)M+IgD+ peripheral blood B cells expressing the CD27 cell surface antigen carry somatically mutated variable region genes: CD27 as a general marker for somatically mutated (memory) B cells. *J Exp Med*. 1998;188(9):1679-1689. doi:10.1084/jem.188.9.1679
34. Takemori T, Kaji T, Takahashi Y, Shimoda M, Rajewsky K. Generation of memory B cells inside and outside germinal centers. *Eur J Immunol*. 2014;44(5):1258-1264. doi:10.1002/eji.201343716
35. Helpap B, Grouls V, Yamashita K. Histological and autoradiographical findings in the immunologically stimulated spleen. *Virchows Arch B Cell Pathol*. 1975;19(1):269-279. doi:10.1007/BF02889373
36. Kurtin PJ. Marginal zone B cells, monocytoid B cells, and the follicular microenvironment: determinants of morphologic features in a subset of low-grade B-cell lymphomas. *Am J Clin Pathol*. 2000;114(4):505-508. doi:10.1309/L69G-F64H-4F3J-L2R5
37. Blachly JS, Ruppert AS, Zhao W, et al. Immunoglobulin transcript sequence and somatic hypermutation computation from unselected RNA-seq reads in chronic lymphocytic leukemia. *Proc Natl Acad Sci USA*. 2015:112(14):4322-4327. doi:10.1073/pnas.1503587112
38. Oscier DG, Thompsett A, Zhu D, Stevenson FK Differential rates of somatic hypermutation in V(H) genes among subsets of chronic lymphocytic leukemia defined by chromosomal abnormalities. *Blood*. 1997;89(11):4153-4160. doi:10.1182/blood.v89.11.4153
39. Baba Y, Matsumoto M, Kurosaki T. Signals controlling the development and activity of regulatory B-lineage cells. *Int Immunol*. 2015;27(10):487-493. doi:10.1093/intimm/dxv027
40. Castillo JJ, Bibas M, Miranda RN. The biology and treatment of plasmablastic lymphoma. *Blood*. 2015;125(15):2323-2330. doi:10.1182/blood-2014-10-567479
41. Nihal M, Mikkola D, Wood GS. Detection of clonally restricted immunoglobulin heavy chain gene rearrangements in normal and lesional skin: analysis of the B cell component of the skin-associated lymphoid tissue and implications for the molecular diagnosis of cutaneous B cell lymphomas. *J Mol Diagnostics*. 2000;2(1):5-10. doi:10.1016/S1525-1578(10)60609-5
42. Ladányi A, Kiss J, Mohos A, et al. Prognostic impact of B-cell density in cutaneous melanoma. *Cancer Immunol Immunother*. 2011;60(12):1729-1738.

CHAPTER 3

NK cell immunobiology

Aharon G. Freud and Madelie Sellers

INTRODUCTION

Natural killer (NK) cells are innate lymphoid cells (ILCs) that have a characteristic large granular lymphocyte morphology and that are able to recognize and kill tumor- and virus-infected cells without prior stimulation.[1] NK cells share many functional and immunophenotypic features with cytolytic T cells, yet NK cells do not rearrange their T-cell receptor genes and lack surface expression of CD3. As such, they are traditionally considered to be part of the innate immune system.[2] Nonetheless, recent data indicate that NK cells are also capable of immunologic memory.[3,4] In addition to cytotoxic function, NK cells possess the ability to produce large amounts of chemokines and cytokines, including interferon gamma (IFN-γ). NK cells play key roles in the settings of tumor surveillance,[5] antiviral immunity,[5-8] immune modulation,[5] pregnancy,[9] and solid organ[5] and stem cell transplantation.[10]

ORIGINS, BIOLOGY, AND FUNCTIONS OF NK CELLS

NK Cell Development

Similar to other leukocyte populations, NK cells ultimately derive from hematopoietic stem cells (HSCs) that reside in the bone marrow (BM). BM-derived HSCs give rise to more committed lymphoid progenitor cells that in turn are capable of differentiating into T and B lymphocytes as well as NK cells and other non-NK ILCs.[11-13] The terminal aspects of human NK cell development can be divided into five stages based on the differential surface expression of CD34, CD117, CD94, CD16, and CD56 in the absence of other lineage (Lin)-specific surface markers.[14] Stages 1 to 3 cells, which are lymphoid populations downstream of the HSC, do not possess cytotoxic function or the ability to produce IFN-γ, and are therefore considered immature, whereas stages 4 and 5 cells possess the aforementioned functions. Although the BM seems to be required for the development of NK cells or at least the HSC and potentially other early progenitor cells from which NK cells derive, cells belonging to stages 1 to 4 of NK cell development are enriched in locations other than the BM, such as secondary lymphoid tissue (SLT), the liver, and the uterus, suggesting that NK cell maturation occurs in extramedullary tissues. In the peripheral blood (PB), most NK cells are stage 5 cells and show a Lin$^-$CD34$^-$CD117$^-$CD94$^{+/-}$CD16$^+$CD56^{dim} immunophenotype. Fewer Lin$^-$CD34$^-$CD117$^{+/-}$CD94$^+$CD16$^-$CD56^{bright} NK cells, which correspond to stage 4 of NK cell development, are also detected in the circulation, but these are relatively much more abundant in other tissues, including SLTs.[15]

New in vitro research is indicative that NK cell heterogeneity may be the result of precursors not limited to common lymphoid precursors, as well as receptor expression, and maturational state.[16]

NK Function

NK cells possess two primary effector functions: cytotoxicity and cytokine production. These functional parameters are heavily dependent on competing signals derived from activating and inhibitory receptors. There are a multitude of functional surface receptors expressed by NK cells, and these include cytokine and chemokine receptors; C-type lectin receptors such as CD94/NKG2 heterodimers, NKG2D, NKp30, NKp44, NKp46, and NKp80; killer immunoglobulin-like receptors (KIRs); and CD16 (Fc-γ receptor IIIa).[5,17] Unlike T cells, NK cells are not major histocompatibility complex (MHC)–restricted per se, yet NK cells do sense MHC class I molecule expression on other cells via NK cell expression of CD94/NKG2 and KIR molecules. MHC binding of these receptors usually results in inhibition of NK cell activity, and as such, healthy cells that express MHC class I molecules are protected from NK cell killing. In contrast, cells that have become infected or malignantly transformed may downregulate MHC class I molecules and then become susceptible to NK cell killing, especially if these cells also display pathogen-derived or stress-induced ligands on their surface that can trigger activating NK cell receptors.[1]

Cytotoxicity

NK cells kill their targets via two main mechanisms: (1) through the release of constitutively expressed cytolytic granules (perforin and granzymes) that perforate and destroy target cells and (2) through receptor-ligand–mediated cytotoxicity, including tumor necrosis factor (TNF)–related apoptosis–inducing ligand (TRAIL) and Fas ligand–dependent killing; this results in target-induced apoptosis. PB CD56^{dim} NK cells show higher constitutive levels of perforin and granzyme B expression than CD56^{bright} NK cells, and thus CD56^{dim} NK cells kill MHC class I–negative targets more effectively.

Cytokine Production

Both CD56^{bright} and CD56^{dim} NK cells are capable of producing a variety of cytokines, including IFN-γ, TNF-α, macrophage inflammatory protein 1α, granulocyte-macrophage colony-stimulating factor, and interleukin (IL) 10.[1] However, they are induced to release these cytokines in response to different stimuli. For example, CD56^{bright} NK cells secrete large amounts of IFN-γ in response to other cytokines (ie, IL-12, IL-15, and IL-18), whereas CD56^{dim} NK cells release more cytokines in response to cell–cell interactions that result in receptor-mediated activation such as through NKG2D or CD16.[18]

Dendritic cells (DCs), monocytes, and macrophages are thought to be the likely source of IL-12, IL-15, and IL-18, which induce NK cell cytokine production.[1,19] Therefore, these factors are often referred to as "monokines." Monokine stimulation may occur in vivo within SLT during the process of early immune activation, and this can serve to promote CD56^{bright} NK cell production of IFN-γ, which can feed back on the antigen-presenting cells, instructing them to upregulate MHC class I molecules. IFN-γ also promotes helper CD4$^+$ T-cell differentiation toward a type 1 (T$_H$1) phenotype.[20] Therefore, CD56^{bright} NK cells in SLT likely function as a bridge between the innate and adaptive immune responses.[1,15]

Tissue Distribution and Frequency of NK Cells

NK cells are widely distributed throughout the body and can be found in a variety of tissues, including PB, BM, spleen, lymph nodes (LNs), liver, salivary gland, mucosa-associated lymphoid tissue (MALT), uterus, and skin.[21-23] NK cells play a number of different roles, and specific tissues often have distinct resident NK cell phenotypes. For example, a distinct subset of CXCR6$^+$ NK cell is found in the liver where they likely have specialized functions.[24] As we learn more about tumor-associated NK cells these phenotypes may become more important in order to differentiate tissue-resident NK cells from NK cells circulating in blood. Furthermore, NK cells are early responders to sites of inflammation.[23] Therefore, the vascular system plays an important role in facilitating NK cells transit to the sites of the body where they are needed.

Peripheral Blood and Bone Marrow

NK cells constitute approximately 10% to 20% of total PB and BM lymphocytes, and most of these (typically >90%) are CD56^{dim}CD16$^+$ NK cells. However, after BM transplantation, the CD56^{bright} NK cell subset, which is among the first leukocyte populations to engraft, can comprise up to 70% to 90% of total NK cells and 40% of circulating lymphocytes in about a third of patients.[25]

Skin

CD3$^-$CD56$^+$CD16$^-$ cells comprise ~10% of leukocytes in normal, noninflamed skin.[26] Interestingly, in contrast to circulating NK cells, most CD3$^-$CD56$^+$CD16$^-$ cells in the skin lack NKG2D and perforin.[26] Therefore, it is possible that some represent non-NK ILC.[13] CCR8 expression in the absence of CCR7 is associated with trafficking to the skin, which occurs in the steady-state and inflammatory conditions. NK cells may then return to the PB via draining lymphatics.[3] Most NK cells (~85%) found in skin-draining lymph express cutaneous lymphocyte–associated antigen (CLA), whereas only ~15% of PB NK cells express CLA.[27]

NK cells have been associated with a number of dermatologic conditions, including psoriasis,[26,28,29] atopic dermatitis,[30] alopecia areata, pemphigus vulgaris,[31] and melanoma.[32] In psoriasis, NK cells constitute 5% to 8% of the cellular infiltrate by immunohistochemistry (IHC) and flow cytometry and are found mostly in the mid and papillary dermis. Psoriatic NK cells express CD161, but only 15% express CLA. Moreover, they have high expression of CXCR3 and CCR5, which allow them to migrate toward the respective ligands, CXCL10 and CCL5, produced by keratinocytes.[28] NK cells isolated from psoriatic lesions have lower expression of CD57 than NK cells from normal tissue.[29] CD94/NKG2A expression appears to be variable in this disease, whereas high expression of KIR2DS1 has been associated with psoriasis.[30,31]

Allergic contact dermatitis is associated with an influx of CD56^{bright}CD16$^-$ NK cells, which comprise 10% of infiltrating lymphocytes and are found in the superficial dermis near areas of spongiosis.[33] In the context of melanoma, expression of MHC class I molecules on melanoma cells regulates the NK cell response.[22] Melanoma cell lines that express little to no HLA class I molecules are lysed by PB NK cells.[32] However, when melanoma cells overexpress MHC class I molecules, NK cells downregulate activation receptors including NKG2D, NKp30, and NKp44 and are unable to lyse tumor cells.[34,35]

Spleen

The spleen is an important reservoir of NK cells. However, unlike the PB, where NK cells comprise a consistent percentage of lymphocytes, the percentage of NK cells among mononuclear cells (MNCs) in the uninflamed spleen is widely variable with observations ranging from 7% to 50%.[36] NK subsets in the spleen do mirror the PB and BM; CD56^{dim} NK cells constitute about 85% of splenic NK cells, with the remaining 15% being CD56^{bright} NK cells.[36] The majority of splenic NK cells reside in the red pulp, with fewer in the marginal zone. Only a minority of NK cells are found in the white pulp follicles, and there they are predominately CD16$^-$.[37]

Lymph Nodes

NK cells are relatively rare in SLT and comprise ≤5% of MNCs in uninflamed LNs, where they primarily localize to the parafollicular T-cell zones and predominantly display a CD56^{bright}CD16$^-$ phenotype.[15,36] Given the large number of LNs present throughout the body, collectively these tissues contain approximately 2 to 10 times more NK cells than are present in the circulation. Moreover, because ~90% of NK cells in the LN are CD56^{bright}, these cells are estimated to outnumber the total CD56^{dim} population, which is primarily found in the PB, BM, and spleen.[15,36,38-40]

Liver

The liver is greatly enriched for NK cells; 30% to 50% of hepatic lymphocytes are CD3−CD56+CD16−.[23,41] Moreover, NK cells constitute a similar proportion of normal liver MNCs compared with CD8+ T cells (38% vs 42%) and considerably outnumber CD4+ T cells (14%). NK cells reside primarily within the portal tract and perisinusoidal areas, but not around the centrolobular vein.[42] Hepatic NK cells have been shown to play several different roles, including promotion of immune tolerance and antiviral immunity. In addition, a unique subset of memory NK cells have also been recently described in mouse liver.[3,43-46]

Salivary Gland

NK cells are normally found in salivary gland tissue and may play a role in regulating inflammation in pathologic states.[47] For instance, in primary Sjögren syndrome, NK cells accumulate near inflammatory loci and show aberrantly high expression of the activating receptor NKp30 that recognizes the ligand, B7-H6, expressed on salivary epithelial cells.[48] Stimulation of NK cells through NKp30:B7-H6 induces production and release of IFN-γ, which is hypothesized, in turn, to promote DC activation and subsequent T- and B-cell recruitment, ultimately resulting in tissue damage in patients with Sjögren syndrome.[48]

Mucosa-Associated Lymphoid Tissue

NK cells in human tonsils are generally similar in phenotype to LN NK cells. The predominant NK cell population is the CD56^{bright} cell, but the frequency of NK cells among total MNCs is reportedly even lower than that in the LN (≤1% vs ≤5%).[36] This is likely due to the large number of reactive B cells in secondary follicles that make up the majority of tonsil tissue.

It is now well established that other forms of MALT, including intestinal Peyer patches and crypto patches, in the gastrointestinal tract also contain NK cells as well as other non-NK ILC subsets.[49] In particular, group 3 ILC cells (ILC3) support and help to maintain homeostasis of the mucosal epithelium through the production of IL-22.[13,50] These ILC populations are present in the submucosa, lamina propria, and also to some extent within the surface mucosal epithelium. Of note, there is considerable phenotypic overlap between ILC3 and NK cells; both may express CD56 as well as other surface antigens including NKp46. Therefore, definitively distinguishing among ILC populations in MALT tissue sections would require employment of additional stains, such as those directed at lineage-defining transcription factors including eomesodermin and retinoic acid receptor–related orphan receptor gamma t (RORγt).[13]

IMMUNOPHENOTYPIC IDENTIFICATION OF NK CELLS IN TISSUES

Several NK cell–associated surface markers, including CD56, CD16, CD2, and CD7, can be used to identify NK cells in human tissue samples. However, it is important to note that these markers are not exclusive to NK cells. For example, CD2 and CD7 are also pan–T-cell antigens; CD56 can be found on other MNCs, including some T-cell subsets and monocytes; and CD16 can be expressed by T-cell subsets as well as neutrophils, monocytes, and macrophages. Thus, identification of NK cells by flow cytometry (see Chapter 8) relies also on gating strategies to include lymphocytes by forward- and side-scatter characteristics and yet exclude lineage-committed T and B lymphocytes (CD3+, CD19+) as well as few monocytes (CD14+) that may overlap with the lymphocyte gate. Selective identification of NK cells has been further complicated by the recent discovery of other non-T, -B, and -NK lymphocyte populations, which, like NK cells, are also Lin− (CD3−CD19−CD14−). Indeed, these other ILC populations share many immunophenotypic features with NK cells.[13] Despite the aforementioned caveats, NK cells are traditionally and routinely identified in clinical samples as Lin−CD56+CD16+/− cells, and the bulk of the current literature on NK cells uses this definition. See Table 3-1 for common NK cell–associated markers for IHC and flow cytometry.

Given the lack of an NK cell–specific marker, it is also challenging to specifically identify NK cells in tissue sections, because typically only one stain is applied per section. Moreover, NK cells express intracellular CD3ε and CD3ζ subunits and will therefore be labeled by polyclonal anti-CD3 antibodies.[53,54] In general, although CD56 is not specific for NK cells and can be expressed in a variety of hematologic as well as nonhematologic malignancies, its expression on NK cells is higher than on other leukocyte populations, and it can suffice to selectively identify NK cells in most cases.

NKp46 has been recently identified as a highly specific marker that can be used to identify NK cells by IHC and flow cytometry.[55-57] NKp46 is an activating C-type lectin receptor that shows ligand-binding specificity for viral hemagglutinin.[5] NKp46 is expressed on virtually all NK cells in healthy donor PB samples, and it is essentially not expressed by other leukocyte populations except rare T cells (<1%) and some ILC populations in SLT and MALT.[56] In clinical samples, staining for NKp46 labels fewer T-cell populations than CD56 and demonstrates a high level of specificity (98%) and positive predictive value (98%) for labeling NK cells in nonneoplastic human tissues. It should be noted that NKp46 expression may be significantly downregulated on CD56^{dim} NK cells in some clinical settings.[55]

As we learn more about the diverse roles of NK cells and other ILCs in human disease, it may be clinically important to be able to selectively identify and enumerate these populations by immunophenotypic analysis. Currently, non-NK ILCs are defined by characteristic expression of transcription factors and cytokines. Identification of these non-NK ILCs therefore requires the use of intracellular staining among Lin− lymphocytes for corresponding cytokines and transcription factors. Of note, non-NK ILCs are by definition noncytolytic; therefore, assessment of perforin and/or granzyme expression may become useful in future clinical settings.

TABLE 3-1 Expression of Common NK Cell–Associated Markers

Marker	Immunohistochemistry[a]	Flow Cytometry	Other Cell Types Expressing the Marker
CD56	Positive	Positive	Some T cells, monocytes, and ILCs
CD16	N/A	Positive[b]	Neutrophils, monocytes, macrophages, and some T cells
CD2	Positive	Positive	T cells and ILCs
CD7	Positive	Positive	T cells and ILCs
Surface CD3	Negative[c]	Negative	T cells
Cytoplasmic CD3	Positive[c]	Positive	T cells
NKp46	Positive	Positive	Rare T cells; some ILCs
CD94/NKG2A	N/A	Positive[d]	Some T cells
KIR	N/A	Positive[b,d]	Some T cells

[a]Refers to analysis of formalin-fixed, paraffin-embedded tissue sections. "N/A" indicates that a reliable antibody for immunohistochemistry is not currently available.
[b]A large proportion of NK cells lack this marker at a specific developmental stage or in certain tissue types.
[c]If polyclonal anti-CD3 antibodies are employed for immunohistochemical analysis, NK cells will appear CD3+ owing to the expression of intracellular CD3+ and CD3ε subunits.
[d]CD94/NKG2A and KIR expression can be assessed by flow cytometry as a surrogate for clonality testing when evaluating an NK cell population. Normal NK cell populations show variegated CD94/NKG2A and KIR surface expression, whereas the complete absence or restricted expression of these markers is characteristic of NK cell lymphoproliferative disorders.[51,52]

References

1. Caligiuri MA. Human natural killer cells. *Blood*. 2008;112(3):461-469.
2. Trinchieri G. Biology of natural killer cells. *Adv Immunol*. 1989;47:187-376.
3. Paust S, von Andrian UH. Natural killer cell memory. *Nat Immunol*. 2011;12(6):500-508.
4. Min-Oo G, Kamimura Y, Hendricks DW, et al. Natural killer cells: walking three paths down memory lane. *Trends Immunol*. 2013;34(6):251-258.
5. Vivier E, Tomasello E, Baratin M, et al. Functions of natural killer cells. *Nat Immunol*. 2008;9(5):503-510.
6. Orange JS. Human natural killer cell deficiencies. *Curr Opin Allergy Clin Immunol*. 2006;6(6):399-409.
7. Orange JS. Unraveling human natural killer cell deficiency. *J Clin Invest*. 2012;122(3):798-801.
8. Orange JS. Natural killer cell deficiency. *J Allergy Clin Immunol*. 2013;132(3):515-525.
9. Acar N, Ustunel I, Demir R. Uterine natural killer cells and their mission during pregnancy: a review. *Acta Histochem*. 2011;113(2):82-91.
10. Yu J, Venstrom JM, Liu XR, et al. Breaking tolerance to self, circulating natural killer cells expressing inhibitory KIR for non-self HLA exhibit effector function after T cell-depleted allogeneic hematopoietic cell transplantation. *Blood*. 2009;113(16):3875-3884.
11. Galy A, Travis M, Cen D, et al. Human T, B, natural killer, and dendritic cells arise from a common bone marrow progenitor cell subset. *Immunity*. 1995;3(4):459-473.
12. Miller JS, Alley KA, McGlave P. Differentiation of natural killer (NK) cells from human primitive marrow progenitors in a stroma-based long-term culture system: identification of a CD34+7+ NK progenitor. *Blood*. 1994;83(9):2594-2601.
13. Hazenberg MD, Spits H. Human innate lymphoid cells. *Blood*. 2014;124(5):700-709.
14. Freud A, Caligiuri MA. Human natural killer cell development. *Immunol Rev*. 2006;214:56-72.
15. Fehniger TA, Cooper MA, Nuovo GJ, et al. CD56bright natural killer cells are present in human lymph nodes and are activated by T cell-derived IL-2: a potential new link between adaptive and innate immunity. *Blood*. 2003;101(8):3052-3057.
16. Cichocki F, Grywacz B, Miller J. Human NK cell development: one road or many? *Front Immunol*. 2019;10:2078.
17. Long EO, Kim HS, Liu D, et al. Controlling natural killer cell responses: integration of signals for activation and inhibition. *Ann Rev Immunol*. 2013;31:227-258.
18. Fauriat C, Long EO, Ljunggren HG, et al. Regulation of human NK-cell cytokine and chemokine production by target cell recognition. *Blood*. 2010;115(11):2167-2176.
19. Moretta L, Ferlazzo G, Bottino C, et al. Effector and regulatory events during natural killer-dendritic cells interactions. *Immunol Rev*. 2006;214(1):219-228.
20. Zhou L, Chong MMW, Littman DR. Plasticity of CD4+ T cells lineage differentiation. *Immunity*. 2009;30(5):646-655.
21. Sojka DK, Tian Z, Yokoyama WM. Tissue-resident natural killer cells and their potential diversity. *Semin Immunol*. 2014;26(2):127-131.
22. Sharma R, Das A. Organ-specific phenotypic and functional features of NK cells in humans. *Immunol Res*. 2014;58(1):125-131.
23. Shi FD, Ljunggren HG, La Cava A, et al. Organ-specific features of natural killer cells. *Nat Rev Immunol*. 2011;11(10):658-671.
24. Peng H, Zhigang T. Diversity of tissue-resident NK cells. *Semin Immunol*. 2017;31:3-10.

25. Jacobs R, Stoll M, Stratmann G, et al. CD16⁻ CD56⁺ natural killer cells after bone marrow transplantation. *Blood*. 1992;79(12):3239-3244.
26. Ebert LM, Meuter S, Moser B. Homing and function of human skin gammadelta T cells and NK cells: relevance for tumor surveillence. *J Immunol*. 2006;176(7):4331-4336.
27. Hunger RE, Yawalkar N, Braathen LR, et al. The HECA-452 epitope is highly expressed on lymph cells derived from human skin. *Br J Derm*. 1999;141(3):565-569.
28. Ottaviani C, Nasorri F, Bedini C, et al. CD56brightCD16(−) NK cells accumulate in psoriatic skin in response to CXCL10 and CCL5 and exacerbate skin inflammation. *Eur J Immunol*. 2006;36(1):118-128.
29. Batista MD, Ho EL, Kuebler PJ, et al. Skewed distribution of natural killer cells in psoriasis skin lesions. *Exp Dermatol*. 2013;22(1):64-66.
30. Matusiak Ł, Białynicki-Birula R, Szepietowski JC. Emerging role for the killer-cell immunoglobulin-like receptors genotype, in the susceptibility of skin diseases. *J Dermatol Sci*. 2013;71(1):3-11.
31. Dunphy S, Gardiner CM. NK cells and psoriasis. *J Biomed Biotechnol*. 2011;2011:248317.
32. Carrega P, Pezzino G, Queirolo P, et al. Susceptibility of human melanoma cells to autologous natural killer (NK) cell killing: HLA-related effector mechanisms and role of unlicensed NK cells. *PLoS One*. 2009;4(12):e8132.
33. Carbone T, Nasorri F, Pennino D, et al. CD56highCD16-CD62L- NK cells accumulate in allergic contact dermatitis and contribute to the expression of allergic responses. *J Immunol*. 2010;184(2):1102-1110.
34. Balsamo M, Vermi W, Parodi M, et al. Melanoma cells become resistant to NK-cell-mediated killing when exposed to NK-cell numbers compatible with NK-cell infiltration in the tumor. *Eur J Immunol*. 2012;42(7):1833-1842.
35. Pietra G, Manzini C, Rivara S, et al. Melanoma cells inhibit natural killer cell function by modulating the expression of activating receptors and cytolytic activity. *Cancer Res*. 2012;72(6):1407-1415.
36. Ferlazzo G, Thomas D, Lin SL, et al. The abundant NK cells in human secondary lymphoid tissues require activation to express killer cell Ig-like receptors and become cytolytic. *J Immunol*. 2004;172(3):1455-1462.
37. Witte T, Wordelmann K, Schmidt RE. Heterogeneity of human natural killer cells in the spleen. *Immunology*. 1990;69(1):166-170.
38. Poli A, Michel T, Thérésine M, et al. CD56bright natural killer (NK) cells: an important NK cell subset. *Immunology*. 2009;126(4):458-465.
39. Westermann J, Pabst R. Distribution of lymphocyte subsets and natural killer cells in the human body. *Clin Investig*. 1992;70(7):539-544.
40. Trepel F. Number and distributions of lymphocytes in man: a critical analysis. *Klin Wochenschr*. 1974;52(11):511-515.
41. Hata K, Zhang XR, Iwatsuki S, et al. Isolation, phenotyping, and functional analysis of lymphocytes from human liver. *Clin Immunol Immunopathol*. 1990;56(3):401-419.
42. Pruvot FR, Navarro F, Janin A, et al. Characterization, qualification and localization of passenger T lymphocytes and NK cells in human liver before transplantation. *Transpl Int*. 1995;8(4):273-279.
43. Sun JC, Beilke JN, Lanier LL. Adaptive immune features of natural killer cells. *Nature*. 2009;457(7229):557-561.
44. O'Leary JG, Goodarzi M, Drayton DL, et al. T cell- and B cell-independent adaptive immunity mediated by natural killer cells. *Nat Immunol*. 2006;7(5):507-516.
45. Paust S, Gill HS, Wang BZ, et al. Critical role for the chemokine receptor CXCR6 in NK cell-mediated antigen-specific memory of haptens and viruses. *Nat Immunol*. 2010;11(12):1127-1135.
46. Paust S, Senman B, von Andrian UH. Adaptive immune responses mediated by natural killer cells. *Immunol Rev*. 2010;235(1):286-296.
47. Tessmer MS, Reilly EC, Brossay L. Salivary gland NK cells are phenotypically and functionally unique. *PLoS Pathog*. 2011;7(1):e1001254.
48. Rusakiewicz S, Nocturne G, Lazure T, et al. NCR3/NKp30 contributes to pathogenesis in primary Sjogren's syndrome. *Sci Transl Med*. 2013;5(195):195ra96.
49. Lindgren A, Pavlovic V, Flach CF, et al. Interferon-gamma secretion is induced in IL-12 stimulated human NK cells by recognition of Helicobacter pylori or TLR2 ligands. *Innate Immun*. 2011;17(2):191-203.
50. Cella M, Fuchs A, Vermi W, et al. A human natural killer cell subset provides an innate source of IL-22 for muscosal immunity. *Nature*. 2009;457(7230):722-725.
51. Morice WG, Kurtin PJ, Leibson PJ, et al. Demonstration of aberrant T-cell and natural killer-cell antigen expression in all cases of granular lymphocytic leukemia. *Br J Haematol*. 2003;120(6):1026-1036.
52. Zambello R, Teramo A, Barilà G. Activating KIRs in chronic lymphoproliferative disorder of NK cells: protection from viruses and disease induction? *Front Immunol*. 2014;5:72.
53. Moretta A, Bottino C, Vitale M, et al. Activating receptors and coreceptors involved in human natural killer cell-mediated cytolysis. *Ann Rev Immunol*. 2001;19:197-223.
54. León F, Roldán E, Sanchez L, et al. Human small-intestine epithelium contains functional natural killer lymphocytes. *Gastroenterology*. 2003;125(2):345-356.
55. Freud AG, Zhao S, Wei S, et al. Expression of the activating receptor, NKp46 (CD335), in human natural killer and T-cell neoplasia. *Am J Clin Pathol*. 2013;140(6):853-866.
56. Tomasello E, Yessaad N, Gregoire E, et al. Mapping of NKp46(+) cells in healthy human lymphoid and non-lymphoid tissues. *Front Immunol*. 2012;3:344.
57. Walzer T, Jaeger S, Chaix J, et al. Natural killer cells: from CD3(−)NKp46(+) to post-genomics meta-analyses. *Curr Opin Immunol*. 2007;19(3):365-372.

CHAPTER 4

Mononuclear phagocytic system of the skin–guide to pathologists

Kate Roussak and Eynav Klechevsky

Skin is the largest organ of the human body that provides protection from the outside world. It constantly receives immense amounts of information that must be carefully processed, evaluated, and acted upon. Importantly, a sophisticated system of immune cells referred to as the "mononuclear phagocyte system" (MPS) of the skin continually patrols and surveilles for such external signals. This system is comprised of phenotypically diverse populations of cells and is responsible for orchestrating distinct immune responses. The MPS of healthy skin is composed of Langerhans cells (LCs) situated within the epidermis, dendritic cells (DCs), macrophages, and DC progenitors that reside in the dermis. In this chapter, we will review the diverse subsets of cutaneous MPS cells including LCs, steady-state dermal DCs (DDCs), monocyte-derived inflammatory DCs (infDCs), and plasmacytoid DCs, as well as various functional macrophage subsets. We present here a helpful guide for pathologists and a summary of the skin MPS, including classifications, main functions in physiology, and contributions to cutaneous inflammatory, infectious, and neoplastic processes.

ANTIGEN-PRESENTING CELLS IN NORMAL SKIN

DCs are professional phagocytes that control most adaptive immune responses. They are superior to macrophages and monocytes in their ability to migrate to secondary lymphoid organs and exhibit enhanced naïve T-cell priming capacities in that site. In addition, they have a unique morphology and high levels of costimulatory molecules accompanying major histocompatibility complex (MHC) class II expression. Steady-state skin hosts distinct functional and phenotypic DC subsets that are microanatomically compartmentalized. LCs uniquely reside within the epidermis, while the dermis harbors three DDC lineages: heterogenous CD1c (BDCA-1)+ DDCs, CD14+ DDCs, and DCs expressing CD141 (BDCA-3) (Fig. 4-1A).

EPIDERMIS

LCs are an integral part of the antigen-presenting cell (APC) system of the skin.[1-4] LCs are localized across the epidermis and account for 3% to 5% of epidermal cells,[5] where they serve a protective role against external challenges. Though originally thought to be homogenous, LCs were recently reported to be heterogenous in human skin.[1,6] A subset of migratory LCs was shown to express CD5. More recently, two distinct epidermal steady-state subsets and two inflammatory subsets were indicated to have unique developmental requirements and differential capabilities of self-maintenance, antigen uptake and migration.[6] The relationship between CD5+ LCs and these newly defined LC subsets is yet to be determined.

Recent ontogenetic studies in mice have revealed that steady-state LCs show features of both tissue-resident macrophages and DCs.[7] They acquire DC-like phenotypes and functions upon further differentiation in the skin.[4,8] When LCs migrate from the skin to lymph nodes (LNs), they resemble the CD1c+ DDCs both in their function and phenotype.[9] LCs are derived from hematopoietic precursor cells that reside in the skin from embryonic development. Their development depends on an autocrine source of transforming growth factor beta 1 (TGF-β1) as well as on macrophage colony-stimulating factor receptor ligands.[10] Through their interaction with neighboring keratinocytes (KCs), LCs will acquire interleukin-34 (IL-34) for their survival and differentiation.[11]

LCs are characterized in situ by the presence of long, fine cytoplasmic extensions emerging from small cellular bodies. Traditional staining (H&E), used in histology, does not always effectively differentiate LCs from surrounding KCs, but the use of histochemical and histoenzymatic methods employing gold salts or enzymes such as adenosine triphosphatase or myeloperoxidase, respectively, made it possible to locate the LCs in the suprabasal layers of the epidermis. Moreover, LCs can further be identified based on the cell surface expression of CD1a, CD207/langerin, E-cadherin, and HLA-DR.[12] Additionally, a unique feature of epidermal LCs is the presence of Birbeck granules (BGs).[13] Electron microscopy reveals BGs as cytoplasmic granules that display a hemispherical bleb at one end of a linear rod-like structure, often likened to that of a tennis racquet. The formation of BGs is organized by CD207/langerin, a mannose-binding lectin. Mutations in langerin result in fewer BGs in LCs.[14] Although the function of BGs is still not completely understood, many studies suggest that they play an active role in receptor-mediated endocytosis and participate in the antigen-processing function of LCs.[15] Of note, whereas steady-state LCs that efficiently

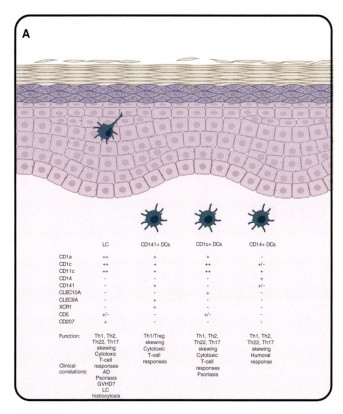 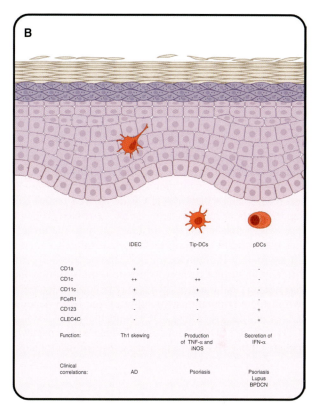

FIGURE 4-1. Dendritic cell subtypes in normal (A) and inflamed skin (B). Immunophenotype, postulated function, and associated cutaneous disorders are illustrated. AD, atopic dermatitis; DC, dendritic cell; LC, Langerhans cell; Th, helper T-cell; Treg, regulatory T-cell; Tip-DC, tumour necrosis factor alpha (TNF-α) and iNOS-producing dendritic cell; pDC, plasmacytoid dendritic cell; BPDCN, blastic plasmacytoid dendritic cell neoplasm; IDEC, inflammatory dendritic epidermal cells; IFN, interferon, GVHD, graft-versus-host disease.

internalize and process antigen exhibit high numbers of BGs, mature LCs specialized in antigen presentation are devoid of BGs.[16] In addition, the roles of BGs in directing antiviral and antimicrobial responses have also been reported. For instance, it has been suggested that the restriction factor TRIM5a, which is located in BGs, prevents HIV replication specifically in LCs (but not in DCs). This, in turn, underscores the dual function of LCs in HIV infection: virus elimination and virus transmission to CD4+ T-cells.[17] In addition, their roles in directing antiviral[18] and antimicrobial responses have also been reported.[19]

LCs that are lost during the steady-state or after minor injuries are repopulated locally and independently of circulating precursor cells throughout the individual's lifespan.[20] Furthermore, it has been well established that the bulge region of the hair follicle in the dermis serves as a niche for KCs, melanocytes, and mast cell progenitors, and there is evidence to suggest that LCs can be repopulated from the hair follicle alone following skin injury that specifically affects the epidermis but not the dermis, which contains the hair follicles.[21] Mechanistically, hair follicle KCs produce CCL2 in the infundibulum and CCL20 in the isthmus, which are signals for the CCR2- and CCR6-dependent recruitment of LC precursors to the follicle and the epidermis. Destruction of hair follicle portals for LC recruitment, such as that observed in lichen planopilaris, results in a decrease of epidermal LCs.[22] Reduction in the number of LCs has also been observed in nutritional dermatitis, likely due to zinc deficiency–induced apoptosis,[23] as well as in normal aging[24] of the skin. The latter is at least partly attributable to a decline in CXCL14-mediated recruitment of CD14+ monocytes, making CXCL14 a potential therapeutic target for the prevention of age-related LC reduction and associated infections and neoplastic consequences.[25,26] Moreover, as lower numbers and frequencies of LCs, changes in their morphological characteristics, and decreased capacities to induce a proper immune response have been reported during HPV infection, LCs may additionally play a critical role in the persistence of HPV infection.[27,28] In the mouse, under inflammatory conditions, epidermal LCs may expand by the recruitment and differentiation of circulating monocytes and circulating hematopoietic stem cells.[20] Some evidence suggests that LC repopulation may additionally require colony-stimulating factor 1 from neutrophils to attract and support monocyte entry as well as the generation of monocyte-derived LCs.[29]

LCs will continuously survey the skin and maintain homeostasis by expanding skin Treg cells. However, following a challenge, they transport antigens to the draining lymph nodes for T-cell priming,[30] induce proliferation of effector memory T-cells, and limit Treg cell activation.[31] Upon their activation, LCs were shown to be the most potent human APC subtype for the induction of primary cytotoxic CD8+ T-cell responses and share features with the mouse cross-presenting cDC1 subset.[32,33] In addition, LCs can activate T-cell responses toward Th1, Th2, Th17, and Th22 phenotypes.[34] Impaired LC function has been observed in atopic dermatitis (AD),[35] a Th2-driven disease, while defective LC migration has been demonstrated in psoriasis,[36] a Th1- and

Th17-skewed inflammatory condition. LCs were further implicated in graft-versus-host disease, and particularly, the CD5+ LCs were detected in involved patient skin[1]; however, additional studies should be performed to assess their role relative to that of long-lived macrophages.[37]

DERMIS

In contrast to the epidermis, the dermis contains a heterogenous population of immune cells that includes myeloid (conventional) DCs (cDCs), monocyte-derived cells (moDCs), and macrophages.[5] Dermal cDCs are derived from FLT3L-dependent, bone marrow-derived cDC-restricted progenitors (pre-cDCs) that terminally differentiate into mature cDCs that are found in the skin. Fully functional cDCs then distribute mainly in the upper area of the dermis.[38] Based on differential surface marker expression, transcription factor dependency, and function, cDCs may be further divided into two discrete populations (or subsets): the IRF8-dependent (CD141/CLEC9A+ DCs; cDC1) and the IRF4-dependent (CD1c+; cDC2) DCs. Monocyte-derived cells, meanwhile, include CD14+ DC-like cells and a subset of macrophages.[39]

CD141+ DCS (CDC1)

Human myeloid CD141+/CLEC9A+ DCs (cDC1) are present at a much lower frequency than CD1c+ DCs in steady-state blood and tissues.[40] Markers used to identify this population in vivo include thrombomodulin (also known as CD141), XCR1, CADM1, CLEC9A,[41,42] and CD13.[40] CD141+ DCs are detected in steady-state skin at low levels and are thought to be potentially derived from blood CD141+ DCs.[41] While their function in the skin is not clear, in the blood, they are found to possess several conserved mechanisms that make them efficient at cross-presenting cells to CD8+ T-cells. Cross-presentation of dead tumor cell–associated antigens is mediated by their selective expression of the C-type lectin CLEC9A (also known as DNGR1)—a receptor for damaged and dead cell materials[43,44] through which DCs recognize an antigen and transport it to the appropriate endosomal compartments.[45] Reductions in the CD141+ DC population, with no difference in the frequencies of CD1c+ and plasmacytoid DCs, were observed in the blood of patients with STAT3 GOF (gain-of-function) mutations.[46] Skin manifestations such as AD, alopecia, and scleroderma were documented in patients with these mutations. Hence, there might further be a connection between skin presentation and CD141+ DC reduction.[47]

CD1C+ DCS (CDC2)

The major population of myeloid cDCs in human blood, tissues, and lymphoid organs is characterized as a heterogenous population of myeloid DCs (cDC2). In the skin, this lineage can be identified by the expression of CD1c, CD1e, FcεR1 CLEC10A, LAMP3[4,48] and low levels of CD1a.[49] Intriguingly, high phenotypical diversity within this compartment was observed among different donors' skin tissues, whereas donor variance was less pronounced within the cDC1 population.[50] Similar to LCs, ex vivo human skin isolated cDC2 are potent in the activation of Th1, Th2, Th17 T-cells, suggesting their capacity to promote this range of immune responses in vivo. CD5+ DCs, a distinct population of cDC2, were shown to be potent inducers of cytotoxic T-cells and Th22 cells. The products of these T-cells, IL-22 and interferon gamma (IFN-γ), play a key role in the pathogenesis of psoriasis. Remarkably, CD5+ DCs were significantly enriched in lesional psoriatic skin compared with distal nonlesional tissues, suggesting their involvement in the disease.[1]

CD14+ DCS

Dermal CD14+ DCs are a unique population of skin immune cells that can be distinguished from macrophages by their ability to migrate out of the skin. They coexpress CD141 and IL3-Receptor/CD123 and share markers with macrophages including CD163, S100, THBS1, and MRC1. They maintain a semimature phenotype, indicated by low levels of the costimulatory molecules CD80 and CD83, but express significant levels of CD86 and MHC class I and class II molecules.[51] Functionally, they induce naïve B cell differentiation into IgM-secreting plasma cells and drive the differentiation of naïve T-cells into CXCL13+ follicular helper T-cells, which induce additional class switching and immunoglobulin production in B cells. In addition, unlike LCs, CD14+ DCs are poor activators of primary CD8+ T-cell responses[32] but are capable of reactivating memory responses. How they cooperate with other types of DCs in activating skin resident memory T-cells remains to be established.

ANTIGEN-PRESENTING CELLS IN INFLAMED SKIN

infDCs comprise a transient population that appears in response to an inflammatory stimulus and disappears when the stimulus is resolved. They share many phenotypic markers with dermal cDC2 and monocyte-derived DCs (moDCs). Their transient nature and lack of unique surface markers pose two main issues: first, how to differentiate infDCs from steady-state cDCs and moDCs; second, how best to study their mobilization kinetics and function in humans simply based on snapshot analysis during disease progression without adequate recourse to the evolution of the inflammation/disease process (Fig. 4-1B).

Interestingly, differentiation seems to take varying routes depending on the underlying cause of inflammation. In patients with psoriasis, TNF and inducible nitric oxide synthase (iNOS)–producing DCs named Tip-DCs[52,53] have been reported to produce high levels of IL-23, thereby driving Th17 activation, although more recent single cell studies imply that these two cytokines are produced by distinct cells.[54] An additional infDC subset named "slanDC" (6-sulfo LacNAc DC) was reported and was shown to additionally express CD16. These cells are now believed to be of monocytic origin and to produce large amounts of proinflammatory cytokines such as IL-12, IL-23, IL-1β, and TNF-α.[55] In contrast, in the context of AD, infDCs are called "inflammatory dendritic epidermal cells" (IDECs) and are marked by the expression of Fcε receptors. They were reported to drive Th2 responses.[56] It has also been established that IDECs tend to be present in the lower part of the epidermis (compared to resident LCs). This difference in location indicates a functional difference between IDECs and resident LCs. Due to the strategic location of LCs in the upper epidermal layer of the skin, they are able to capture antigens, which are located outside the tight junction (TJ) barrier, by extending their dendrites through the TJ barrier.[57] In contrast, IDECs residing in the lower layer of the epidermis are unable to capture antigens that are located on the surface of the skin because their dendrites extend horizontally.[58]

PLASMACYTOID DENDRITIC CELLS AND OTHER BDCA-2+ DCS

Plasmacytoid dendritic cells (pDCs), also called natural interferon (IFN) producing cells,[59] are specialized in sensing viral RNA and DNA by Toll-like receptors (TLRs)-7 and -9 and can rapidly produce massive amounts of type 1 IFNs upon viral encounter. Studies show that pDCs can also present antigens to T-cells, but they need to go through a maturation process in order to do so.[60,61] In the steady-state, pDCs circulate in the blood and lymphoid tissue, where they assume a nondendritic plasma cell–like morphology and are characterized by the expression of CD123 (IL-3Rα), CD303 (BDCA-2), and CD304 (BDCA-4). In humans, they lack the classic DC antigen CD11c.[62] An important regulator of pDC development is the E protein *TCF4*. Tcf4$^{-/-}$ mice show normal development of all immune cell types but lack pDCs, whereas Tcf4$^{+/-}$ mice and human patients with *TCF4* haplodeficiency (Pitt–Hopkins syndrome) show impaired pDC development and/or phenotype.[63] There is also murine data suggesting that a global deficiency of TCF4 or a DC-specific haplodeficiency ameliorates systemic lupus erythematosus- (SLE-) like disease, illustrating a potential role of pDCs in SLE pathogenesis.[64]

pDCs cannot be identified in healthy human skin; however, in the context of skin injury or wound repair,[65,66] as well as during certain chronic inflammatory skin disorders such as psoriasis[67] and cutaneous lupus erythematosus (LE),[68] pDCs can migrate from the blood into the skin. Histologic examination of skin lesions from individuals with cutaneous LE revealed that a subset of pDCs is localized in the dermal-epidermal junction in proximity to perforin-expressing T-cells that can secrete granzyme B and, therefore, may directly and indirectly contribute to the epithelial cell damage associated with lupus.[69] Furthermore, pDCs have been observed in skin tumors such as melanoma[70,71] and basal cell carcinoma[72] after treatment with the TLR-7 agonist imiquimod or the TLR-9 agonist PF-3512676. Hence, the effects of such antitumor treatments may be attributed, at least in part, to the activation of pDCs.

The mechanism underlying the migration of pDCs to the skin is not well understood. Human pDCs selectively express chemokine-like receptor 1, which directs pDC migration through its agonist chemerin. Chemerin is constitutively expressed as part of an inactive precursor protein by dermal endothelial cells and fibroblasts and is cleaved into the active peptide by serine proteases that are released during skin damage.[73,74]

Blastic plasmacytoid dendritic cell neoplasm (BPDCN) is a rare malignancy derived from pDCs.[75] Cutaneous lesions occur in 64% of patients with BPDCN and are often the first symptom seen in patients seeking medical care.[76] The morphology of BPDCN is heterogenous and complex. Skin biopsies often display a suffused infiltration of monomorphic medium-sized blast cells characterized by irregular, eccentrically-located nuclei; finely dispersed chromatin; and one or more small but distinctive nucleoli. The cytoplasm is dispersed and never granular.[77] Importantly, a recent report identified dual CD123 and TCF4 expression as a highly reliable and practical method for BPDCN identification in biopsy material.[78]

Recently, two novel infDC types were reported to infiltrate human skin wounds and express BDCA-2. The first type expresses lower levels of BDCA-2 and also expresses CD123, similar to pDCs. However, unlike pDCs, these cells express CD1a. The second BDCA-2–expressing population is represented by Axl+Siglec-6+ DCs. Both subsets are absent from healthy skin.[79]

In practice, some data suggest that infDCs may be a useful diagnostic tool in dermatology. Diagnostic criteria include pDC content, clustering, and distribution. Evaluation of these criteria might be useful in differentiating classes of alopecia,[80,81] LE from cutaneous lymphomas,[82] and cutaneous lymphoproliferative disorders.[83,84] Also, lesional skin samples from patients with psoriasis vulgaris, LE, and contact dermatitis were found to contain relatively high numbers of pDCs. In contrast, though, many IDECs, but very few pDCs, could be detected in AD, while LE lesions were characterized by high numbers of pDCs but low numbers of IDECs. These results demonstrate that, in addition to resident LCs, pDCs and IDECs are selectively recruited to skin lesions depending on the type of skin disease. Interestingly, a lack of pDCs in some skin diseases has been linked to a predisposition to certain secondary infections; in AD, for example, some patients may be predisposed to eczema herpeticum, a secondary infection of AD lesions with herpes simplex virus.[85]

MACROPHAGE SUBSETS AND FUNCTION IN THE SKIN

Tissue-resident macrophages comprise a heterogenous population of immune cells that perform tissue-specific and niche-specific functions. These range from dedicated homeostatic functions (such as the clearance of cellular debris) to central roles in tissue immune surveillance, response to infection, and the resolution of inflammation.[86]

Traditionally, macrophages are classified as either classically activated (M1) or alternatively activated (M2, see Fig. 4-2).[87,88] "Classical activation" occurs as a result of consistent exposure to IFN-γ or upon receptor-mediated sensing of pathogen-associated molecules (such as the sensing of lipopolysaccharide [LPS] by TLR-4). M1 macrophages play an important role in the protection against pathogens by producing high levels of iNOS and proinflammatory cytokines including TNF-α, IL-1β, IL-6, and IL-12, thereby promoting Th1-type immune responses. Canonically, M2 macrophages were thought to be alternatively activated primarily by exposure to IL-4. However, it is now believed that the M2 profile includes a number of variants, and the development of

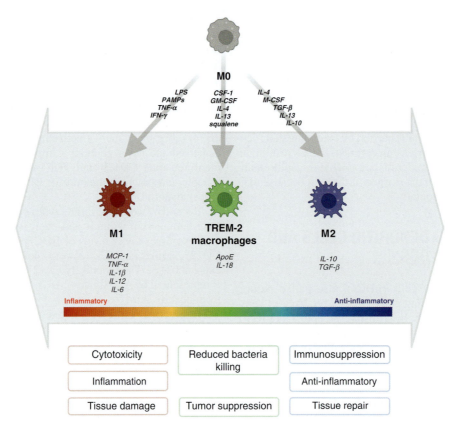

FIGURE 4-2. Macrophage subtypes in the skin. Polarization requirements, signature cytokines, and postulated functions. PAMPs, pathogen-associated molecular patterns; MCP-1, monocyte chemoattractant protein-1; MCSF, macrophage colony-stimulating factor; CSF-1, colony stimulating factor 1; GM-CSF, granulocyte-macrophage colony-stimulating factor.

such variants depends on specific stimuli. M2 macrophages exhibit antiinflammatory properties and are distinguished by a high secretion of IL-10 and the expression of arginase-1. Both M1 and M2 macrophages of the skin are characterized by the expression of CD163 and CD68; as such, their histologic discrimination requires double immunohistochemical staining. M1 and M2 macrophages can be reliably detected by double staining for CD163 and the phosphorylated forms of the transcription factors STAT1 or CMAF, respectively.[88,89]

Pathologically, the persistence of M1 macrophages has been implicated in the progression of chronic wounds,[90] and a role for M2 macrophage-driven dermal fibrosis has been linked to the pathogenesis of scleroderma.[91] CD163 has been proposed as a specific marker for macrophages with anti-inflammatory properties and was recently also described on a subset of infDCs in the skin termed "DC3". CD163 is a cell surface glycoprotein receptor that was identified as the "hemoglobin (Hb) scavenger receptor" (HbSR). When hemoglobin–haptoglobin complexes bind to CD163 on macrophages, they release anti-inflammatory mediators. CD163 expression is highly dependent on the stage of differentiation or on the activation status of macrophages. CD163-expressing macrophages are found during the healing process of acute inflammation, in chronic inflammation, and in wound healing tissues.[92]

With the introduction of new unbiased single cell technologies, the presence of distinct and diverse macrophage subsets was identified, including resident macrophages (present in the skin at steady-state) and infiltrating macrophages (only found following injury or infection).[93] Resident macrophages exist in tissue before birth and can be derived from yolk sac, fetal lever monocytes, or mature monocytes. Infiltrating macrophages are newly recruited from hematogenous precursor cells, called monocytes, which are derived from a rapidly dividing pool of cells in the bone marrow. Additionally, of note are TREM2 dermal macrophages. In the skin, they secrete oncostatin M, which inhibits hair growth by maintaining hair follicle stem cells in a quiescent state.[94] TREM2 macrophages have also been reported in tumors including melanoma and may contribute to resistance to therapy.[95,96]

A recently described population of TREM2 macrophages was found to play a role in the pathogenesis of leprosy. Specifically, TREM2 macrophages were abundant and formed large aggregates in lepromatous leprosy (L-lep) lesions- a disseminated form of the disease.[97] It was also shown that they exhibit a high level of ApoE (apolipoprotein E), an important lipid transporter that is expressed by various cells including macrophages. The potential pathogenic function of ApoE in L-lep remains to be clarified.[97] Most recently TREM2 macrophages have been shown to drive inflammation in human acne via their reduced killing of the *Cutibacterium acnes* bacteria.[98]

Cells described in this chapter play diverse, vital roles in skin health and disease. We believe that understanding their functions and regulatory pathways arms healthcare providers with invaluable tools for accurate diagnosis, rational treatment, and expanded therapeutic options.

ACKNOWLEDGMENTS

The authors would like to thank Courtney A. Iberg, PhD (Washington University in St. Louis), for expert editorial and manuscript preparation assistance, as well as Andras Schaffer, MD, PhD (Florida State University College of Medicine) for critical reading of the manuscript.

Figures were generated using Biorender.

References

1. Korenfeld D, Gorvel L, Munk A, et al. A type of human skin dendritic cell marked by CD5 is associated with the development of inflammatory skin disease. *JCI Insight*. 2017;2:(18).
2. Gorvel L, Korenfeld D, Tung T, Klechevsky E. Dendritic cell–derived IL-32α: a novel inhibitory cytokine of NK cell function. *J Immunol*. 2017;199(4):1290-1300.
3. Banchereau J, Thompson-Snipes L, Zurawski S, et al. The differential production of cytokines by human Langerhans cells and dermal CD14+ DCs controls CTL priming. *Blood*. 2012;119(24):5742-5749.
4. Artyomov MN, Munk A, Gorvel L, et al. Modular expression analysis reveals functional conservation between human langerhans cells and mouse cross-priming dendritic cells. *J Exp Med*. 2015;212:743-757.
5. Klechevsky E. Functional diversity of human dendritic cells. *Adv Exp Med Biol*. 2015;850:43-54.
6. Liu X, Zhu R, Luo Y, et al. Distinct human Langerhans cell subsets orchestrate reciprocal functions and require different developmental regulation. *Immunity*. 2021;54(10):2305-2320 e11.
7. Wu X, Briseño CG, Durai V, et al. Mafb lineage tracing to distinguish macrophages from other immune lineages reveals dual identity of Langerhans cells. *J Exp Med*. 2016;213(12):2553-2565.
8. Kabashima K, Honda T, Ginhoux F, Egawa G. *The immunological anatomy of the skin*. In: *Nature Reviews Immunology*. Springer US; 2019:19-30.
9. Klechevsky E, Morita R, Liu M, et al. Functional specializations of human epidermal Langerhans cells and CD14+ dermal dendritic cells. *Immunity*. 2008;29(3):497-510.
10. Kaplan DH, Li MO, Jenison MC, Shlomchik WD, Flavell RA, Shlomchik MJ. Autocrine/paracrine TGFbeta1 is required for the development of epidermal Langerhans cells. *J Exp Med*. 2007;204(11):2545-2552.
11. Greter M, Lelios I, Pelczar P, et al. Stroma-derived interleukin-34 controls the development and maintenance of langerhans cells and the maintenance of microglia. *Immunity*. 2012;37(6):1050-1060.
12. Collin M, Bigley V. Human dendritic cell subsets: an update. *Immunology*. 2018;154:3-20.
13. Birbeck MS, Breathnach AS, Everall JD. An Electron microscope study of basal melanocytes and high-level clear cells (langerhans cells) in Vitiligo. *J Invest Dermatol*. 1961;37(1):51-64.
14. Verdijk P, Dijkman R, Plasmeijer EI, et al. A lack of Birbeck granules in langerhans cells is associated with a naturally occurring point mutation in the human Langerin gene. *J Invest Dermatol*. 2005;124(4):714-717.
15. Valladeau J, Dezutter-Dambuyant C, Saeland S. Langerin/CD207 sheds light on formation of birbeck granules and their possible function in langerhans cells. *Immunol Res*. 2003;28:93-107.
16. Valladeau J, Ravel O, Dezutter-Dambuyant C, et al. Langerin, a novel C-type lectin specific to langerhans cells, is an endocytic receptor that induces the formation of birbeck granules cross-priming, a mechanism by which exogenous anti-gen is alternatively routed into the MHC class I pathway for presentat. *Immunity*. 2000;12:71-81.
17. Clausen BE, Romani N, Stoitzner P. Meeting report of the 16th international langerhans cell workshop: Recent developments in langerhans cell and skin dendritic cell biology and their therapeutic application. *J Invest Dermatol*. 2020;140(7):1315-1319. doi:10.1016/j.jid.2020.02.022.
18. Renn CN, Sanchez DJ, Ochoa MT, et al. TLR activation of Langerhans cell-like dendritic cells triggers an antiviral immune response. *J Immunol*. 2006;177(1):298-305.
19. Oulee A, Ma F, Teles RMB, et al. Identification of genes encoding antimicrobial proteins in langerhans cells. *Front Immunol*. 2021;12:695373.
20. Merad M, Manz MG, Karsunky H, et al. Langerhans cells renew in the skin throughout life under steady-state conditions. *Nat Immunol*. 2002;3(12):1135-1141.
21. Gilliam AC, Kremer IB, Yoshida Y, et al. The human hair follicle: a reservoir of CD40+ B7-deficient langerhans cells that repopulate epidermis after UVB exposure. *J Invest Dermatol*. 1998;110(4):422-427.
22. Nagao K, Kobayashi T, Moro K, et al. Stress-induced production of chemokines by hair follicles regulates the trafficking of dendritic cells in skin. *Nat Immunol*. 2012;13(8):744-752.
23. Kawamura T, Ogawa Y, Nakamura Y, et al. Severe dermatitis with loss of epidermal Langerhans cells in human and mouse zinc deficiency. *J Clin Invest*. 2012;122(2):722-732.
24. Zegarska B, Pietkun K, Giemza-Kucharska P, Zegarski T, Nowacki MS, Romańska-Gocka K. Changes of Langerhans cells during skin ageing. *Adv Dermatol Allergol*. 2017;3:260-267.
25. Hasegawa T, Feng Z, Yan Z, Ngo KH, Hosoi J, Demehri S. Reduction in human epidermal langerhans cells with age is associated with decline in CXCL14-mediated recruitment of CD14+ monocytes. *J Invest Dermatol*. 2020;140(7):1327-1334.
26. Schaerli P, Willimann K, Ebert LM, Walz A, Moser B. Cutaneous CXCL14 targets blood precursors to epidermal niches for langerhans cell differentiation. *Immunity*. 2005;23(3):331-342.
27. Walker F, Adle-Biassette H, Madelenat P, Hénin D, Lehy T. Increased apoptosis in cervical intraepithelial neoplasia associated with HIV infection: implication of oncogenic human papillomavirus, caspases, and langerhans cells. *Clin Cancer Res*. 2005;11(7):2451-2458.
28. Guess JC, McCance DJ. Decreased migration of langerhans precursor-like cells in response to human keratinocytes expressing human papillomavirus type 16 E6/E7 is related to reduced macrophage inflammatory protein-3α production. *J Virol*. 2005;79(23):14852-14862.
29. Wang Y, Bugatti M, Ulland TK, Vermi W, Gilfillan S, Colonna M. Nonredundant roles of keratinocyte-derived IL-34 and neutrophil-derived CSF1 in Langerhans cell renewal in the steady state and during inflammation. *Eur J Immunol*. 2016;46(3):552-559.
30. Thornton SM, Samararatne VD, Skeate JG, et al. The essential role of anxA2 in langerhans cell Birbeck granules formation. *Cells*. 2020;9(4):974.
31. Seneschal J, Clark RA, Gehad A, Baecher-Allan CM, Kupper TS. Human epidermal langerhans cells maintain immune homeostasis in skin by activating skin resident regulatory T cells. *Immunity*. 2012;36:873-884.

32. Klechevsky E, Morita R, Liu M, et al. Functional specializations of human epidermal langerhans cells and CD14+ dermal dendritic cells. *Immunity*. 2008;29:497-510.
33. Artyomov MN, Munk A, Gorvel L, et al. Modular expression analysis reveals functional conservation between human Langerhans cells and mouse cross-priming dendritic cells. *J Exp Med*. 2015;212(5):743-757.
34. Klechevsky E. Human dendritic cells - stars in the skin. *Eur J Immunol*. 2013;43:3147-3155.
35. Semper AE, Heron K, Woollard AC, et al. Surface expression of Fc epsilon RI on Langerhans' cells of clinically uninvolved skin is associated with disease activity in atopic dermatitis, allergic asthma, and rhinitis. *J Allergy Clin Immunol*. 2003;112(2):411-419.
36. Cumberbatch M, Singh M, Dearman RJ, Young HS, Kimber I, Griffiths CEM. Impaired Langerhans cell migration in psoriasis. *J Exp Med*. 2006;203:953-960.
37. Jardine L, Cytlak U, Gunawan M, et al. Donor monocyte–derived macrophages promote human acute graft-versus-host disease. *J Clin Invest*. 2020;130(9):4574-4586.
38. Wang XN, McGovern N, Gunawan M, et al. A three-dimensional atlas of human dermal Leukocytes, Lymphatics, and blood vessels. *J Invest Dermatol*. 2014;134(4):965-974.
39. McGovern N, Schlitzer A, Gunawan M, et al. Human dermal CD14+ cells are a transient population of monocyte-derived macrophages. *Immunity*: The Authors; 2014;41:465-477.
40. Granot T, Senda T, Carpenter DJ, et al. Dendritic cells display subset and tissue-specific maturation dynamics over human life. *Immunity*. 2017;46(3):504-515.
41. Haniffa M, Shin A, Bigley V, et al. Human tissues contain CD141 hi cross-presenting dendritic cells with functional homology to mouse CD103 + nonlymphoid dendritic cells. *Immunity*. 2012;37:60-73.
42. Ramos MI, Teunissen MBM, Helder B, et al. Reduced CLEC9A expression in synovial tissue of psoriatic arthritis patients after adalimumab therapy. *Rheumatology*. 2016;55(9):1575-1584.
43. Zhang J-G, Peter, Antonia, et al. The dendritic cell receptor Clec9A binds damaged cells via exposed actin filaments. *Immunity*. 2012;36(4):646-657.
44. Sancho D, Joffre OP, Keller AM, et al. Identification of a dendritic cell receptor that couples sensing of necrosis to immunity. *Nature*. 2009;458(7240):899-903.
45. Cohn L, Chatterjee B, Esselborn F, et al. Antigen delivery to early endosomes eliminates the superiority of human blood BDCA3+ dendritic cells at cross presentation. *J Exp Med*. 2013;210:1049-1063.
46. Korenfeld D, Roussak K, Dinkel S, et al. STAT3 gain-of-function mutations underlie deficiency in human nonclassical CD16 + monocytes and CD141 + dendritic cells. *J Immunol*. 2021;207:2423-2432.
47. Milner JD, Vogel TP, Forbes L, et al. Early-onset lymphoproliferation and autoimmunity caused by germline STAT3 gain-of-function mutations. *Blood*. 2015;125:591-599.
48. Villani AC, Satija R, Reynolds G, et al. Single-cell RNA-seq reveals new types of human blood dendritic cells, monocytes, and progenitors. *Science*. 2017;356(6335):eaah4573.
49. Heidkamp GF, Sander J, Lehmann CHK, et al. Human lymphoid organ dendritic cell identity is predominantly dictated by ontogeny, not tissue microenvironment. *Sci Immunol*. 2016;1:eaai7677.
50. Alcántara-Hernández M, Leylek R, Wagar LE, et al. High-dimensional phenotypic mapping of human dendritic cells reveals interindividual variation and tissue specialization. *Immunity*. 2017;47:1037-1050.e6.
51. Chu CC, Ali N, Karagiannis P, et al. Resident CD141 (BDCA3)+ dendritic cells in human skin produce IL-10 and induce regulatory T cells that suppress skin inflammation. *J Exp Med*. 2012;209:935-945.
52. Serbina NV, Salazar-Mather TP, Biron CA, Kuziel WA, Pamer EG. TNF/iNOS-Producing dendritic cells mediate innate immune defense against bacterial infection. *Immunity*. 2003;19(1):59-70.
53. Wilsmann-Theis D, Koch S, Mindnich C, et al. Generation and functional analysis of human TNF-α/iNOS-producing dendritic cells (Tip-DC). *Allergy*. 2013;68(7):890-898.
54. Hawkes JE, Yan BY, Chan TC, Krueger JG. Discovery of the IL-23/IL-17 signaling pathway and the treatment of psoriasis. *J Immunol*. 2018;201(6):1605-1613.
55. Hänsel A, Günther C, Ingwersen J, et al. Human slan (6-sulfo LacNAc) dendritic cells are inflammatory dermal dendritic cells in psoriasis and drive strong T 17/T 1 T-cell responses. *J Allergy Clin Immunol*. 2011;127(3):787-794.e9.
56. Wollenberg A, Kraft S, Hanau D, Bieber T. Immunomorphological and ultrastructural characterization of Langerhans cells and a novel, inflammatory dendritic epidermal cell (IDEC) population in lesional skin of atopic eczema. *J Invest Dermatol*. 1996;106(3):446-453.
57. Ouchi T, Kubo A, Yokouchi M, et al. Langerhans cell antigen capture through tight junctions confers preemptive immunity in experimental staphylococcal scalded skin syndrome. *J Exp Med*. 2011;208(13):2607-2613.
58. Yoshida K, Kubo A, Fujita H, et al. Distinct behavior of human Langerhans cells and inflammatory dendritic epidermal cells at tight junctions in patients with atopic dermatitis. *J Allergy Clin Immunol*. 2014;134(4):856-864.
59. Li S, Wu J, Zhu S, Liu YJ, Chen J. Disease-associated plasmacytoid dendritic cells. *Front Immunol*. 2017;8:1-12.
60. Grouard G, Rissoan MC, Filgueira L, Durand I, Banchereau J, Liu YJ. The enigmatic plasmacytoid T cells develop into dendritic cells with interleukin (IL)-3 and CD40-Ligand. *J Exp Med*. 1997;185(6):1101-1112.
61. Di Pucchio T, Chatterjee B, Smed-Sörensen A, et al. Direct proteasome-independent cross-presentation of viral antigen by plasmacytoid dendritic cells on major histocompatibility complex class I. *Nat Immunol*. 2008;9(5):551-557.
62. Kashem SW, Haniffa M, Kaplan DH. Antigen-presenting cells in the skin. *Annu Rev Immunol*. 2017;35:469-499.
63. Cisse B, Caton ML, Lehner M, et al. Transcription factor E2-2 is an essential and specific regulator of plasmacytoid dendritic cell development. *Cell*. 2008;135(1):37-48.
64. Sisirak V, Ganguly D, Lewis KL, et al. Genetic evidence for the role of plasmacytoid dendritic cells in systemic lupus erythematosus. *J Exp Med*. 2014;211(10):1969-1976.
65. Gregorio J, Meller S, Conrad C, et al. Plasmacytoid dendritic cells sense skin injury and promote wound healing through type I interferons. *J Exp Med*. 2010;207(13):2921-2930.
66. Di Domizio J, Belkhodja C, Chenuet P, et al. The commensal skin microbiota triggers type I IFN-dependent innate repair responses in injured skin. *Nat Immunol*. 2020;21(9):1034-1045.
67. Nestle FO, Conrad C, Tun-Kyi A, et al. Plasmacytoid predendritic cells initiate psoriasis through interferon-alpha production. *J Exp Med*. 2005;202(1):135-143.
68. Farkas L, Beiske K, Lund-Johansen F, Brandtzaeg P, Jahnsen FL. Plasmacytoid dendritic cells (natural interferon-α/β-producing cells) accumulate in cutaneous lupus erythematosus lesions. *Am J Pathol*. 2001;159:237-243.

69. Vermi W, Lonardi S, Morassi M, et al. Cutaneous distribution of plasmacytoid dendritic cells in lupus erythematosus. Selective tropism at the site of epithelial apoptotic damage. *Immunobiology*. 2009;214(9-10):877-886.
70. Vescovi R, Monti M, Moratto D, et al. Collapse of the plasmacytoid dendritic cell compartment in advanced cutaneous melanomas by components of the tumor cell secretome. *Cancer Immunol Res*. 2019;7:12-28.
71. Vermi W, Bonecchi R, Facchetti F, et al. Recruitment of immature plasmacytoid dendritic cells (plasmacytoid monocytes) and myeloid dendritic cells in primary cutaneous melanomas. *J Pathol*. 2003;200:255-268.
72. Hofmann MA, Kors C, Audring H, Walden P, Sterry W, Trefzer U. Phase 1 evaluation of intralesionally injected TLR9-agonist PF-3512676 in patients with basal cell carcinoma or metastatic melanoma. *J Immunother*. 2008;31(5):520-527.
73. Wittamer VR, Franssen JD, Vulcano M, et al. Specific recruitment of antigen-presenting cells by chemerin, a novel processed ligand from human inflammatory fluids. *J Exp Med*. 2003;198(7):977-985.
74. Zabel BA, Silverio AM, Butcher EC. Chemokine-like receptor 1 expression and chemerin-directed chemotaxis distinguish plasmacytoid from myeloid dendritic cells in human blood. *J Immunol*. 2005;174(1):244-251.
75. Chaperot L. Identification of a leukemic counterpart of the plasmacytoid dendritic cells. *Blood*. 2001;97(10):3210-3217.
76. Martín-Martín L, López A, Vidriales B, et al. Classification and clinical behavior of blastic plasmacytoid dendritic cell neoplasms according to their maturation-associated immunophenotypic profile. *Oncotarget*. 2015;6(22):19204-19216.
77. Cota C, Vale E, Viana I, Requena L, et al. Cutaneous manifestations of blastic plasmacytoid dendritic cell neoplasm-morphologic and phenotypic variability in a series of 33 patients. *Am J Surg Pathol*. 2010;34(1):75-87.
78. Sukswai N, Aung PP, Yin CC, et al. Dual expression of TCF4 and CD123 is highly sensitive and specific for blastic plasmacytoid dendritic cell neoplasm. *Am J Surg Pathol*. 2019;43(10):1429-1437.
79. Chen YL, Gomes T, Hardman CS, et al. Re-evaluation of human BDCA-2+ DC during acute sterile skin inflammation. *J Exp Med*. 2020;217(3):jem.20190811.
80. Fening K, Parekh V, McKay K. CD123 immunohistochemistry for plasmacytoid dendritic cells is useful in the diagnosis of scarring alopecia. *J Cutan Pathol*. 2016;43:643-648.
81. Kolivras A, Thompson C. Clusters of CD123+ plasmacytoid dendritic cells help distinguish lupus alopecia from lichen planopilaris. *J Am Acad Dermatol*. 2016;74:1267-1269.
82. Liau JY, Chuang SS, Chu CY, Ku WH, Tsai JH, Shih TF. The presence of clusters of plasmacytoid dendritic cells is a helpful feature for differentiating lupus panniculitis from subcutaneous panniculitis-like T-cell lymphoma. *Histopathology*. 2013;62:1057-1066.
83. De Souza A, Tinguely M, Burghart DR, Berisha A, Mertz KD, Kempf W. Characterization of the tumor microenvironment in primary cutaneous CD30-positive lymphoproliferative disorders: a predominance of CD163-positive M2 macrophages. *J Cutan Pathol*. 2016;43:579-588.
84. Chen SJT, Tse JY, Harms PW, Hristov AC, Chan MP. Utility of CD123 immunohistochemistry in differentiating lupus erythematosus from cutaneous T cell lymphoma. *Histopathology*. 2019;74:908-916.
85. Wollenberg A, Wagner M, Günther S, et al. Plasmacytoid dendritic cells: a new cutaneous dendritic cell subset with distinct role in inflammatory skin diseases. *J Invest Dermatol*. 2002;119:1096-1102.
86. Davies LC, Jenkins SJ, Allen JE, Taylor PR. Tissue-resident macrophages. *Nat Immunol*. 2013;14(10):986-995.
87. Tarique AA, Logan J, Thomas E, Holt PG, Sly PD, Fantino E. Phenotypic, functional, and plasticity features of classical and alternatively activated human macrophages. *Am J Respir Cell Mol Biol*. 2015;53(5):676-688.
88. Martinez FO, Gordon S. The M1 and M2 paradigm of macrophage activation: time for reassessment. *F1000Prime Reports*. 2014;6:13.
89. Barros MHM, Hauck F, Dreyer JH, Kempkes B. Macrophage polarisation: an immunohistochemical approach for identifying M1 and M2 macrophages. *PLoS One*. 2013;8(11):e80908.
90. Sindrilaru A, Peters T, Wieschalka S, et al. An unrestrained proinflammatory M1 macrophage population induced by iron impairs wound healing in humans and mice. *J Clin Invest*. 2011;121(3):985-997.
91. Higashi-Kuwata N, Makino T, Inoue Y, Takeya M, Ihn H. Alternatively activated macrophages (M2 macrophages) in the skin of patient with localized scleroderma. *Exp Dermatol*. 2009;18:727-729.
92. Ferreira DW, Ulecia-Morón C, Alvarado-Vázquez PA, et al. CD163 overexpression using a macrophage-directed gene therapy approach improves wound healing in ex vivo and in vivo human skin models. *Immunobiology*. 2020;225:151862.
93. Schulz C, Gomez Perdiguero E, Chorro L, et al. A lineage of myeloid cells independent of Myb and hematopoietic stem cells. *Science*. 2012;336(6077):86-90.
94. Wang ECE, Dai Z, Ferrante AW, Drake CG, Christiano AM. A subset of TREM2(+) dermal macrophages secretes oncostatin M to maintain hair follicle stem cell quiescence and inhibit hair growth. *Cell Stem Cell*. 2019;24(4):654-669 e6.
95. Xiong D, Wang Y, You M. A gene expression signature of TREM2(hi) macrophages and gammadelta T cells predicts immunotherapy response. *Nat Commun*. 2020;11(1):5084.
96. Molgora M, Esaulova E, Vermi W, et al. TREM2 modulation remodels the tumor myeloid Landscape enhancing anti-PD-1 immunotherapy. *Cell*. 2020;182(4):886-900 e17.
97. Ma F, Hughes TK, Teles RMB, et al. The cellular architecture of the antimicrobial response network in human leprosy granulomas. *Nat Immunol*. 2021;22(7):839-850.
98. Do TH, Ma F, Andrade PR, et al. TREM2 macrophages induced by human lipids drive inflammation in acne lesions. *Sci Immunol*. 2022;7(73):eabo2787.

CHAPTER 5

Mast cells in the skin

Tina L. Sumpter

OVERVIEW OF MAST CELLS

Mast cells (MCs) are long-lived innate immune cells that are found in the highest frequencies in barrier tissues such as the skin, the lungs, and the intestinal cells. In the skin, MCs reside in the superficial dermis proximal to blood vessels and neurons.[1-3] At these crossroads, MCs are ideally positioned to facilitate dialogue between immune and nonimmune cells to orchestrate neurogenic, innate, and adaptive immune responses (Fig. 5-1). Mast cells are host protective in the neutralization of venom, and in antihelminth, antibacterial, and antiviral immunity. However, accumulation and dysregulated activation of MCs is detrimental in cancer, autoimmunity, and allergy. In this chapter, the main pathways and outcomes of MC activation are reviewed with a focus on the roles of MCs in human disease.

LOCALIZATION, IDENTIFICATION, AND CLASSIFICATION OF MAST CELLS

In the skin of a healthy adult, MCs are unevenly distributed throughout the body with the highest density in peripheral skin sites, such as the nose, chin, and lower arms and legs. The lowest density of MCs is found in central sites, such as the abdomen.[2,4] While men and women have equivalent numbers of cutaneous MCs, MCs from females have a lower threshold of activation, in line with increased prevalence of allergy reported in women compared with men.[4,5] In healthy skin, MCs are embedded in the dermis and are not found in the epidermis.

Morphologically, MCs are either oval or spindle shaped. The MC cytoplasm is densely packed with cytoplasmic granules containing heparin or chondroitin sulfate proteoglycans complexed to inflammatory proteins including histamine, serotonin, cytokines, antimicrobial peptides, and serine proteases.[6] Mast cell granules are readily identified with basic dyes (eg, toluidine blue) or with positively charged avidin, which binds to negatively charged heparin.[6,7] On the cell surface, MCs express a myriad of receptors, including the FcεRI, c-Kit, and the receptor for IL-33, ST2.

Human MCs are classified by serine protease profiles. Mucosal MCs primarily express tryptase (MC_T). Connective tissue–type MCs, such as those found in the skin, express tryptase, chymase, carboxypeptidase A3, and cathepsin G (MC_{TC}). The relative protease composition defines the function of MC_T and MC_{TC}.[8] While MC_T are primed to respond to pathogens, MC_{TC} have a more diverse repertoire of functions, playing roles in pathogen response, as well as extracellular matrix remodeling and angiogenesis.[9]

THE HEMATOPOIETIC ORIGINS OF MAST CELLS

Mast cells are derived from $CD34^+$ hematopoietic precursors found in the bone marrow, fetal yolk sac, and fetal liver. In mice and possibly in humans, the precursors for MC_T originate from pluripotent stem cells in the bone marrow, seed the target tissue, then mature in response to tissue-specific environmental cues.[10] In contrast, MCs in the skin originate from precursor cells in the fetal yolk sac and fetal liver. From the fetal liver, MC precursors enter the blood, then the skin where MC precursors implant within the dermis. In the dermis, MCs are maintained by slow division of daughter cells.[11-13] During inflammation, established MCs proliferate and new MC precursors are recruited from the bone marrow, causing local MC accumulation.[14]

Within the skin, multiple growth factors are implicated in MC survival, including IL-3, IL-9, IL-10, IL-33, and stem cell factor (SCF).[15] Of these, SCF expressed by fibroblasts, endothelial cells, and keratinocytes is critical.[16] In vitro studies using murine mast cells demonstrate that SCF increases proteases that define connective tissue–type MCs found in the skin and inhibits apoptosis, thereby promoting survival.[17,18] The receptor for SCF, c-Kit, is constitutively expressed on the MC plasma membrane. Loss-of-function mutations in *KIT* reduce MC numbers in mice.[19] In contrast, patients with systemic mastocytosis have unchecked MC proliferation and accumulation. In 90% of these patients, dysregulated MC function is associated with a mutation that causes constitutive c-Kit activation (*KITD816V*).[20]

MAST CELL ACTIVATION

Mast cells express innate sensing receptors to integrate cues from the microenvironment (Fig. 5-2). Mast cells express Toll-like receptors (TLRs) 1 to 10, complement-binding receptors (C3aR and C5aR), cytokine receptors (notably ST2 and

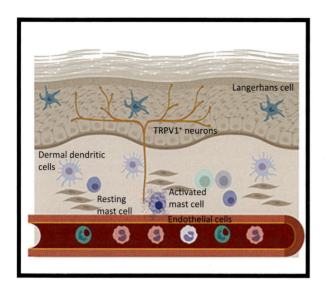

FIGURE 5-1. **Dermal mast cells interact with skin resident cells to initiate inflammation.** Mast cells in the dermis are centrally located and proximal to neurons, endothelial cells, and dendritic cells.

TSLPR), neuropeptide receptors, and receptors for IgE and IgG (FcεRI and FcγR). Mast cells also express a nonspecific cationic sensing receptor, the Mas-related G-protein-coupled receptor (MRGPR) X2, which detects diverse ligands including neuropeptides and antimicrobial peptides.[8,21-23]

Mast cell activation has three potential outcomes. First, receptor-ligand interactions increase the intracellular calcium levels, resulting in cytoskeletal rearrangement and fusion of protein-packed exocytotic vesicles with the cell membrane. Vesicle fusion liberates hundreds of granule-stabilized proteins into the extracellular space.[8,24,25] The granules directly target neighboring cells. Mast cells also extend cytoplasmic processes to reach distal cells in the skin and in the circulation to directly deliver granulated proteins to cellular targets.[26] Minimally charged proteins such as histamine rapidly dissociate from the granule core and diffuse into the microenvironment. Other positively charged proteins like TNF and some proteases remain tethered to their granule matrix and are protected from proteolytic degradation.[27] In this form, TNF can traffic through the lymphatics to affect adaptive immune responses in the skin draining lymph node and can be passed directly to neutrophils in blood vessels.[26,28] The diversity and stability of degranulation products broadly impact immune responses.

The second outcome of MC activation is the rapid synthesis and release of lipid mediators. Mast cells are equipped with high levels of arachidonic acid. Following activation, arachidonic acid is catabolized into leukotrienes, prostaglandin D_2 and prostaglandin E, and lipoxins.[27] These mediators increase vascular permeability and are chemotactic for neutrophils and T cells.

The final outcome of MC activation is de novo transcription of cytokines, occurring hours after activation.

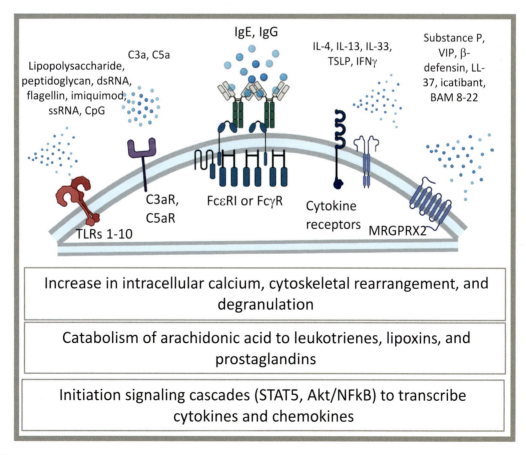

FIGURE 5-2. Mast cells respond to diverse cues in the environment causing the release of preformed proteins and lipid mediators and de novo transcription of cytokines.

Transcription is facilitated by multiple signaling pathways, including STAT5 and Akt/NFkB.[29,30] The list of cytokines in this later phase of activation is extensive and includes the classical inflammatory cytokines, TNF, IL-1β and IL-6; the type 1 cytokines, IFNγ and IL-15; the type 2 cytokines, IL-4, IL-5, IL-13, and IL-33; the type 17 cytokine, IL-17; and regulatory cytokines, IL-10 and amphiregulin, as well as IL-9 and IL-22.[8,31,32]

The outcome of MC activation is receptor dependent. For example, MC activation initiated by complement C3a or C5a primarily induces degranulation.[22] In contrast to this, MC activation initiated solely by cytokine receptors, such as the IL-33 receptor, ST2, or by TLR ligands induces de novo synthesis of leukotrienes and prostaglandins and transcription of conventional innate and Th2-skewing cytokines, but not degranulation.[21,33,34] In complex immune responses, variegated ligands are available in the microenvironment and synergistic activation of receptors may fine-tune or amplify the magnitude of MC responses.[33]

Immunoglobulin-Initiated Mast Cell Activation: FcεRI and FcγR

The best characterized pathway of MC activation is initiated by the high-affinity IgE receptor (FcεRI). All MCs constitutively express high levels of FcεRI. FcεRI comprises an extracellular IgE-binding α chain and signal-transducing β or γ chains.[35] Human MCs express FcεRI as either an $αβγ_2$ tetramer or $αγ_2$ trimer. In the skin, MCs extend processes through the junctions linking endothelial cells and acquire IgE from the circulation.[36] IgE is then displayed on FcεRIα. While monomeric IgE bound to FcεRIα can induce a modest level of mediator release, the binding of polyvalent antigen to IgE is necessary to aggregate multiple FcεRI complexes and initiate degranulation, lipid mediator synthesis, and multiple signaling cascades required for transcription.[37] Human skin MCs also express FcγRIIA, the low-affinity IgG receptor. As with IgE, signaling initiated by IgG induces degranulation, marked by the release of histamine and serotonin, synthesis and release of prostaglandins and leukotrienes, and transcription and release of cytokines.[38]

The MC response initiated by IgE is host protective. Locally, the granulated proteases directly limit bacterial and viral growth and neutralize toxins.[24,39,40] Histamine, released within 1 minute of activation, interacts with histamine receptors on endothelial cells. This interaction causes a breach in endothelial junctions and increases vascular permeability.[27] Mast cell–derived TNF initiates the leukocyte adhesion cascade promoting neutrophil egress from the bloodstream into the skin.[26]

The products of activated MCs affect neighboring dermal dendritic cells and distal Langerhans cells. Mast cell–derived histamine drives migration of Langerhans cells from the epidermis to the skin draining lymph node.[41] Notably, MCs form adhesive complexes with neighboring dermal dendritic cells following IgE-initiated activation.[42] In this complex, MCs transfer antigen to dendritic cells and release the inflammatory cytokines TNF and IL-1β. TNF and IL-1β mature dendritic cells, activate the lymphatics, and increase dermal dendritic cell migration to skin draining lymph nodes.[43] Through these pathways, MCs facilitate the migration of cutaneous dendritic cell subsets to the skin draining lymph node and initiate adaptive immune responses.

Mast Cell Activation Initiated Through the MRGPRX2

Human skin MCs uniquely express high levels of MRGPRX2, a highly promiscuous receptor that responds to a variety of environmental signals released by keratinocytes, dendritic cells, eosinophils, neutrophils, and other inflammatory cells as well as bacterial-derived toxins.[23,44,45] Ligands for MRGPRX2 are cationic and include opioids; neuropeptides such as substance P and VIP; antimicrobial peptides, including β-defensin and cathelicidin; bacterial quorum-sensing molecules; and peptidergic drugs that initiate local allergic reactions. MRGPRX2 ligation induces mast cell degranulation. When compared directly with FcεRI-initiated degranulation, MRGPRX2-initiated MC activation induces a transient and less robust increase in intracellular calcium and the release of smaller, more homogenous granulated proteins.[46] Products released following MRGPRX2 ligation include histamine and tryptase, proinflammatory cytokines, and chemokines but not prostaglandins.[47,48] Like IgE-initiated MC activation, ligation of MRGPRB2, the mouse homologue of the MRGPRX2, increases neutrophil accumulation and drives the migration of dendritic cells from the skin to the draining lymph node.[49] Neuropeptide-mediated MRGRPX2 activation perpetuates neuroinflammation and the sensations of itch and pain.[48,50] Given the pleiotropic effects of MRGPRX2 activation, understanding regulatory pathways controlling its expression may be beneficial in inflammatory diseases.

MAST CELLS IN DISEASE

Mast Cells in Allergy

Atopic dermatitis (AD) is a complex, chronic inflammatory disease involving epidermal barrier dysfunction, dysregulation of antigen-specific Th2 cells, alterations in the microbiome, and genetic factors.[51] Most patients with AD experience chronic itch, which perpetuates the cycle of barrier dysfunction.[52] In lesional skin from patients with AD, the numbers of MCs are increased, as are the density of substance P–releasing neurons and local levels of IL-33.[53,54] Systemically, circulating IgE levels are increased in patients with AD compared with healthy controls.[55,56] The combination of MC accumulation and ligand availability suggests that MC activation may be involved in the perpetuation of disease.[57] Likely, MCs promote the sensation of itch through histamine-dependent mechanisms following FcεRI aggregation and histamine-independent mechanisms following MRGPRX2 ligation.[50] IgE-activated MCs synthesize and release prostaglandin D2. Mast cell-derived prostaglandin D2 directs Th2 cells into lesional skin in AD.[58] The release of IL-4 and IL-13 from activated MCs may further perpetuate Th2-mediated barrier dysfunction. Collectively, these data suggest that targeting MC activation in AD may be a viable strategy for managing disease.

Mast Cell in Autoimmune Disease

Mast cell dysfunction has been reported in a number of autoimmune diseases, including psoriasis and bullous pemphigoid (BP). Pathogenesis in psoriasis is mediated by Th17 cells. But MCs, producing IFN and IL-17, have been documented in psoriatic lesions.[32,59] In experimental models of psoriasis, MCs degranulate in response to IL-1β and IL-23. Furthermore, in these settings MCs release extracellular traps, comprising DNA, chromatin, and histones. Mast cell–derived IL-17 embedded in these traps may be a critical player in the pathogenesis of psoriasis.[60,61]

BP is an autoimmune blistering disease in which T cells and antibodies reactive against BP180 and BP230, two components of hemidesmosomes found in the dermal-epidermal barrier, mediate disease. IgG is the predominant autoimmune isotype in patients with BP. However, anti-BP180-specific IgE has also been reported in 70% to 90% of patients.[62] Blister fluid, lesional skin, and perilesional skin are rich in MC-activating molecules, including C3a. In lesional skin, degranulating MCs accumulate at the dermal-epidermal juncture. Likely, MCs are activated through multiple pathways in lesional skin, including FcεRI, FcγR, or C3aR, and play a role in disease progression. In support of this, patients with active disease have high circulating levels of mast cell–released tryptase and tryptase levels decrease in patients who are in remission.[63] Mechanistically, the activation of MCs through multiple pathways may increase local levels of proteases such as matrix metalloproteinase-9, which has direct proteolytic activity against BP180. Local MC activation may exacerbate the symptoms of BP.

Mast Cells in Cancer

The accumulation of MCs in melanomas and other cutaneous tumors is well documented.[64-66] In patients with melanoma, circulating levels of tryptase are inversely correlated with disease progression and the accumulation of MC_{CT} in aggressive and invasive melanomas is significantly less than in benign nevi.[67] While MC activity is generally proinflammatory, the function of MCs in tumor progression and in the microenvironment may be anti-inflammatory and pro-tumor. In experimental models of UV-induced tumors, MC activation is associated with immune suppression and tumor progression.[68] Within the microenvironment, activated MCs release proangiogenic factors, such as VEGF, and proteases that remodel the tumor environment to promote metastasis. In support of this, data from mouse models of melanoma suggest that MCs are dispensable in immunity against local melanomas and promote metastasis and that MC numbers correlate with resistance to immune checkpoint inhibitors.[69-71]

References

1. Tong PL, Roediger B, Kolesnikoff N, et al. The skin immune atlas: three-dimensional analysis of cutaneous leukocyte subsets by multiphoton microscopy. *J Invest Dermatol*. 2015;135(1):84-93.
2. Janssens AS, Heide R, den Hollander JC, Mulder PG, Tank B, Oranje AP. Mast cell distribution in normal adult skin. *J Clin Pathol*. 2005;58(3):285-289.
3. Serhan N, Basso L, Sibilano R, et al. House dust mites activate nociceptor-mast cell clusters to drive type 2 skin inflammation. *Nat Immunol*. 2019;20(11):1435-1443.
4. Weber A, Knop J, Maurer M. Pattern analysis of human cutaneous mast cell populations by total body surface mapping. *Br J Dermatol*. 2003;148(2):224-228.
5. Mackey E, Ayyadurai S, Pohl CS, D'Costa S, Li Y, Moeser AJ. Sexual dimorphism in the mast cell transcriptome and the pathophysiological responses to immunological and psychological stress. *Biol Sex Differ*. 2016;7:60.
6. Metcalfe DD, Mekori YA. Pathogenesis and pathology of mastocytosis. *Annu Rev Pathol*. 2017;12:487-514.
7. Tharp MD, Seelig LL, Jr, Tigelaar RE, Bergstresser PR. Conjugated avidin binds to mast cell granules. *J Histochem Cytochem*. 1985;33(1):27-32.
8. Krystel-Whittemore M, Dileepan KN, Wood JG. Mast cell: a multi-functional master cell. *Front Immunol*. 2015;6:620.
9. McHale C, Mohammed Z, Gomez G. Human skin-derived mast cells spontaneously secrete several angiogenesis-related factors. *Front Immunol*. 2019;10:1445.
10. Nilsson G, Dahlin JS. New insights into the origin of mast cells. *Allergy*. 2019;74(4):844-845.
11. Gentek R, Ghigo C, Hoeffel G, et al. Hemogenic endothelial fate mapping reveals dual developmental origin of mast cells. *Immunity*. 2018;48(6):1160-1171 e5.
12. Li Z, Liu S, Xu J, et al. Adult connective tissue-resident mast cells originate from late erythro-myeloid progenitors. *Immunity*. 2018;49(4):640-653 e5.
13. Weitzmann A, Naumann R, Dudeck A, Zerjatke T, Gerbaulet A, Roers A. Mast cells occupy stable clonal territories in adult steady-state skin. *J Invest Dermatol*. 2020;140(12):2433-2441.
14. Weitzmann A, Naumann R, Dudeck A, Zerjatke T, Gerbaulet A, Roers A. Mast cells occupy stable clonal territories in adult steady-state skin. *J Invest Dermatol*. 2020;140(12):2433-2441 e5.
15. Elieh Ali Komi D, Wohrl S, Bielory L. Mast cell biology at molecular level: a comprehensive review. *Clin Rev Allergy Immunol*. 2020;58(3):342-365.
16. Stone KD, Prussin C, Metcalfe DD. Ige, mast cells, basophils, and eosinophils. *J Allergy Clin Immunol*. 2010;125(2 suppl 2):S73-S80.
17. Caslin HL, Kiwanuka KN, Haque TT, et al. Controlling mast cell activation and homeostasis: work influenced by bill Paul that continues today. *Front Immunol*. 2018;9:868.
18. Tsai M, Shih LS, Newlands GF, et al. The rat c-kit ligand, stem cell factor, induces the development of connective tissue-type and mucosal mast cells in vivo. Analysis by anatomical distribution, histochemistry, and protease phenotype. *J Exp Med*. 1991;174(1):125-131.
19. Galli SJ, Gaudenzio N, Tsai M. Mast cells in inflammation and disease: recent progress and ongoing concerns. *Annu Rev Immunol*. 2020;38:49-77.
20. Reiter A, George TI, Gotlib J. New developments in diagnosis, prognostication, and treatment of advanced systemic mastocytosis. *Blood*. 2020;135(16):1365-1376.
21. Sandig H, Bulfone-Paus S. TLR signaling in mast cells: common and unique features. *Front Immunol*. 2012;3:185.
22. Elieh Ali Komi D, Shafaghat F, Kovanen PT, Meri S. Mast cells and complement system: ancient interactions between components of innate immunity. *Allergy*. 2020;75(11):2818-2828.
23. Kuhn H, Kolkhir P, Babina M, et al. Mas-related g protein-coupled receptor x2 and its activators in dermatologic allergies. *J Allergy Clin Immunol*. 2021;147(2):456-469.

24. Starkl P, Watzenboeck ML, Popov LM, et al. IgE effector mechanisms, in concert with mast cells, contribute to acquired host defense against staphylococcusaureus. *Immunity*. 2020;53(4):793-804 e9.
25. Shubin NJ, Glukhova VA, Clauson M, et al. Proteome analysis of mast cell releasates reveals a role for chymase in the regulation of coagulation factor xiiia levels via proteolytic degradation. *J Allergy Clin Immunol*. 2017;139(1):323-334.
26. Dudeck J, Kotrba J, Immler R, et al. Directional mast cell degranulation of tumor necrosis factor into blood vessels primes neutrophil extravasation. *Immunity*. 2021;54(3):468-483 e5.
27. Kunder CA, St John AL, Abraham SN. Mast cell modulation of the vascular and lymphatic endothelium. *Blood*. 2011;118(20):5383-5393.
28. Kunder CA, St John AL, Li G, et al. Mast cell-derived particles deliver peripheral signals to remote lymph nodes. *J Exp Med*. 2009;206(11):2455-2467.
29. Kitaura J, Asai K, Maeda-Yamamoto M, Kawakami Y, Kikkawa U, Kawakami T. Akt-dependent cytokine production in mast cells. *J Exp Med*. 2000;192(5):729-740.
30. Barnstein BO, Li G, Wang Z, et al. Stat5 expression is required for IgE-mediated mast cell function. *J Immunol*. 2006;177(5):3421-3426.
31. Orinska Z, Maurer M, Mirghomizadeh F, et al. Il-15 constrains mast cell-dependent antibacterial defenses by suppressing chymase activities. *Nat Med*. 2007;13(8):927-934.
32. Mashiko S, Bouguermouh S, Rubio M, Baba N, Bissonnette R, Sarfati M. Human mast cells are major il-22 producers in patients with psoriasis and atopic dermatitis. *J Allergy Clin Immunol*. 2015;136(2):351-359 e1.
33. Ronnberg E, Ghaib A, Ceriol C, et al. Divergent effects of acute and prolonged interleukin 33 exposure on mast cell IgE-mediated functions. *Front Immunol*. 2019;10:1361.
34. Saluja R, Zoltowska A, Ketelaar ME, Nilsson G. IL-33 and thymic stromal lymphopoietin in mast cell functions. *Eur J Pharmacol*. 2016;778:68-76.
35. Ra C, Nunomura S, Okayama Y. Fine-tuning of mast cell activation by fcepsilonribeta chain. *Front Immunol*. 2012;3:112.
36. Cheng LE, Hartmann K, Roers A, Krummel MF, Locksley RM. Perivascular mast cells dynamically probe cutaneous blood vessels to capture immunoglobulin E. *Immunity*. 2013;38(1):166-175.
37. Kalesnikoff J, Huber M, Lam V, et al. Monomeric IgE stimulates signaling pathways in mast cells that lead to cytokine production and cell survival. *Immunity*. 2001;14(6):801-811.
38. Jonsson F, Daeron M. Mast cells and company. *Front Immunol*. 2012;3:16.
39. Marshall JS, Portales-Cervantes L, Leong E. Mast cell responses to viruses and pathogen products. *Int J Mol Sci*. 2019;20(17):4241.
40. Galli SJ, Starkl P, Marichal T, Tsai M. Mast cells and IgE in defense against venoms: possible "good side" of allergy? *Allergol Int*. 2016;65(1):3-15.
41. Jawdat DM, Albert EJ, Rowden G, Haidl ID, Marshall JS. IgE-mediated mast cell activation induces langerhans cell migration in vivo. *J Immunol*. 2004;173(8):5275-5282.
42. Carroll-Portillo A, Cannon JL, te Riet J, et al. Mast cells and dendritic cells form synapses that facilitate antigen transfer for t cell activation. *J Cell Biol*. 2015;210(5):851-864.
43. Dudeck J, Ghouse SM, Lehmann CH, et al. Mast-cell-derived TNF amplifies CD8(+) dendritic cell functionality and CD8(+) t cell priming. *Cell Rep*. 2015;13(2):399-411.
44. Azimi E, Reddy VB, Lerner EA. Brief communication: MRGPRX2, atopic dermatitis and red man syndrome. *Itch (Phila)*. 2017;2(1):e5.
45. McNeil BD, Pundir P, Meeker S, et al. Identification of a mast-cell-specific receptor crucial for pseudo-allergic drug reactions. *Nature*. 2015;519(7542):237-241.
46. Reber LL, Sibilano R, Starkl P, et al. Imaging protective mast cells in living mice during severe contact hypersensitivity. *JCI Insight*. 2017;2(9):e92900.
47. Varricchi G, Pecoraro A, Loffredo S, et al. Heterogeneity of human mast cells with respect to MRGPRX2 receptor expression and function. *Front Cell Neurosci*. 2019;13:299.
48. Green DP, Limjunyawong N, Gour N, Pundir P, Dong X. A mast-cell-specific receptor mediates neurogenic inflammation and pain. *Neuron*. 2019;101(3):412-420 e3.
49. Arifuzzaman M, Mobley YR, Choi HW, et al. MRGPR-mediated activation of local mast cells clears cutaneous bacterial infection and protects against reinfection. *Sci Adv*. 2019;5(1):eaav0216.
50. Meixiong J, Anderson M, Limjunyawong N, et al. Activation of mast-cell-expressed mas-related g-protein-coupled receptors drives non-histaminergic itch. *Immunity*. 2019;50(5):1163-1171 e5.
51. Weidinger S, Beck LA, Bieber T, Kabashima K, Irvine AD. Atopic dermatitis. *Nat Rev Dis Prim*. 2018;4(1):1.
52. Matterne U, Apfelbacher CJ, Loerbroks A, et al. Prevalence, correlates and characteristics of chronic pruritus: a population-based cross-sectional study. *Acta Derm Venereol*. 2011;91(6):674-679.
53. Tobin D, Nabarro G, Baart de la Faille H, van Vloten WA, van der Putte SC, Schuurman HJ. Increased number of immunoreactive nerve fibers in atopic dermatitis. *J Allergy Clin Immunol*. 1992;90(4 pt 1):613-622.
54. Imai Y. Interleukin-33 in atopic dermatitis. *J Dermatol Sci*. 2019;96(1):2-7.
55. Galli SJ, Tsai M. IgE and mast cells in allergic disease. *Nat Med*. 2012;18(5):693-704.
56. Bieber T. Atopic dermatitis. *Ann Dermatol*. 2010;22(2):125-137.
57. Liu FT, Goodarzi H, Chen HY. IgE, mast cells, and eosinophils in atopic dermatitis. *Clin Rev Allergy Immunol*. 2011;41(3):298-310.
58. Iwasaki M, Nagata K, Takano S, Takahashi K, Ishii N, Ikezawa Z. Association of a new-type prostaglandin D2 receptor CRTH2 with circulating T helper 2 cells in patients with atopic dermatitis. *J Invest Dermatol*. 2002;119(3):609-616.
59. Ackermann L, Harvima IT, Pelkonen J, et al. Mast cells in psoriatic skin are strongly positive for interferon-gamma. *Br J Dermatol*. 1999;140(4):624-633.
60. Lin AM, Rubin CJ, Khandpur R, et al. Mast cells and neutrophils release IL-17 through extracellular trap formation in psoriasis. *J Immunol*. 2011;187(1):490-500.
61. Hu SC, Yu HS, Yen FL, Lin CL, Chen GS, Lan CC. Neutrophil extracellular trap formation is increased in psoriasis and induces human beta-defensin-2 production in epidermal keratinocytes. *Sci Rep*. 2016;6:31119.
62. Fang H, Zhang Y, Li N, Wang G, Liu Z. The autoimmune skin disease bullous pemphigoid: the role of mast cells in autoantibody-induced tissue injury. *Front Immunol*. 2018;9:407.
63. Liu Y, Wang Y, Chen X, Jin H, Li L. Factors associated with the activity and severity of bullous pemphigoid: a review. *Ann Med*. 2020;52(3-4):55-62.

64. Toth-Jakatics R, Jimi S, Takebayashi S, Kawamoto N. Cutaneous malignant melanoma: correlation between neovascularization and peritumor accumulation of mast cells overexpressing vascular endothelial growth factor. *Hum Pathol.* 2000;31(8):955-960.
65. Ribatti D, Vacca A, Ria R, et al. Neovascularisation, expression of fibroblast growth factor-2, and mast cells with tryptase activity increase simultaneously with pathological progression in human malignant melanoma. *Eur J Cancer.* 2003;39(5):666-674.
66. Ribatti D, Ennas MG, Vacca A, et al. Tumor vascularity and tryptase-positive mast cells correlate with a poor prognosis in melanoma. *Eur J Clin Invest.* 2003;33(5):420-425.
67. Siiskonen H, Poukka M, Bykachev A, et al. Low numbers of tryptase+ and chymase+ mast cells associated with reduced survival and advanced tumor stage in melanoma. *Melanoma Res.* 2015;25(6):479-485.
68. Ch'ng S, Wallis RA, Yuan L, Davis PF, Tan ST. Mast cells and cutaneous malignancies. *Mod Pathol.* 2006;19(1):149-159.
69. Ghouse SM, Polikarpova A, Muhandes L, et al. Although abundant in tumor tissue, mast cells have no effect on immunological micro-milieu or growth of HPV-induced or transplanted tumors. *Cell Rep.* 2018;22(1):27-35.
70. Ohrvik H, Grujic M, Waern I, et al. Mast cells promote melanoma colonization of lungs. *Oncotarget.* 2016;7(42):68990-69001.
71. Somasundaram R, Connelly T, Choi R, et al. Tumor-infiltrating mast cells are associated with resistance to anti-pd-1 therapy. *Nat Commun.* 2021;12(1):346.

CHAPTER 6

Molecular pathogenesis of primary cutaneous T-cell lymphomas

Sean Whittaker

INTRODUCTION

The underlying pathogenesis of cutaneous T-cell lymphomas (CTCLs) has been enigmatic ever since the concept of primary CTCL was proposed in the late 1970s. While historically considered to be rare, recent US incidence data suggest that CTCL is one of the commonest variants of mature T-cell malignancies and it represents an accessible clinical model to study the transformation of T-cells.[1] The elegant studies of Rachel Clark and Tom Kupper provide evidence that CTCL is derived from skin-resident memory T-cells[2] and we now appreciate that different types of T-cell lymphoma are derived from specific tissue-resident T-cell populations.[3] Over the last few years, considerable insight has been gained notably through studies utilizing next-generation high-throughput sequencing (NGS) technologies supported by functional genomic studies. These reports have primarily focused on Sezary syndrome (SS) because of the ability to easily enrich for leukemic T-cells and there are now analyzes on over 186 SS cases reported, representing the largest cohort of all mature T-cell lymphomas.[4-9] These genomic findings suggest marked heterogeneity, but elegant bioinformatic and functional studies are providing clarity on both causation and dysregulation of key signaling pathways which are likely to transform mature T-cells. Importantly, there are shared genomic abnormalities between CTCL and other systemic T-cell lymphomas, but also differences (Fig. 6-1).

MYCOSIS FUNGOIDES AND SEZARY SYNDROME

A series of high-throughput NGS studies of CTCL have identified a complex genomic landscape including high rates of somatic nonsynonymous variants (SNVs) and copy number variants (CNVs).[4-11] Most studies to date have utilized whole exome sequencing (WES) of peripheral blood samples enriched for CD4+ leukemic T-cells from SS patients.[4-9] A smaller proportion ($n = 56$) of MF samples mostly from advanced stages of MF have been analyzed with either WES or whole genome sequencing (WGS) platforms using DNA extracted from whole skin biopsies ($n = 25$), while 44 samples from 31 patients have been microdissected.[4,5,7,10-12] As these studies have been based on relatively small cohorts (5-66 per study), a lack of statistical power has failed to identify all the putative driver gene mutations as small sample sizes inevitably introduce bias. However, a reanalysis of pre-2017 published genomic data from 220 CTCL cases (186 SS; 25 MF; 9 CTCL NOS) has defined at least 55 putative driver genes in CTCL which affect multiple signaling pathways (Fig. 6-2).[13] There is striking overlap between MF and SS in terms of gene mutations and pathways affected, although data on chromosomal rearrangements are limited reflecting the small WGS datasets. Overall, the most frequent recurrent gene variants affect TCR signaling pathways (*PLCG1; CARD11; CD28; RLTPR*) and selectively upregulate the NF-kB pathway (Table 6-1).[13] Other pathways often affected by driver gene mutations (>10%) include DNA damage response (DDR) pathways (*TP53; POT1; ATM; BRAC1-2*), chromatin

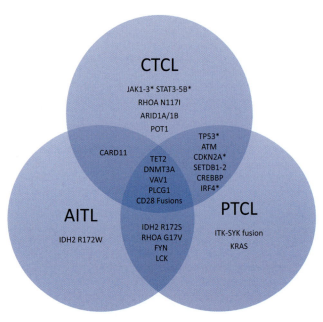

FIGURE 6-1. Most frequent gene mutations/variants in CTCL, AITL, and PTCL

modification (*ARID1A; TRRAP; DNMT3A; TET2*), and Janus tyrosine kinase (JAK)–signal transducer and activator of transcription (STAT) signaling (*STAT5B; JAK3*) (Fig. 6-3). Critically, these gene variants have been functionally validated confirming that they are bona fide driver gene mutations with either gain or loss of function (Table 6-1).[4-8,12-14]

In addition, the limited data from WGS studies mainly in advanced MF samples have shown a complex pattern of chromosomal rearrangements and translocations with no recurrent balanced translocations, although specific gains (17q, 8q) and losses (10q, 17p) are seen frequently.[15] Recurrent chromosomal translocations frequently detected in B-cell lymphomas are due to aberrant intrinsic molecular mechanisms such as V(D)J recombination, somatic hypermutation, and class switch recombination.[16] While V(D)J recombination is a feature of all lymphocytes, somatic hypermutation and class switch recombination are defining features of B-cells which may partly explain why mature T-cell lymphomas rarely have recurrent translocations with the t(2;5) in ALK + anaplastic large cell lymphomas (ALCLs) being a notable exception.

T-CELL SIGNALING AND DIFFERENTIATION

Two of the most common CTCL gene mutations, *PLCG1* and *CARD11*, including recurrent variants, appear to be mutually exclusive and occur in almost 30% of SS cases.[13] These *PLCG1* and *CARD11* gene variants are gain-of-function mutations which increase downstream T-cell signaling specifically through enhanced NF-kB transcriptional activity and also NFAT and AP1.[12,14] These transcription factors regulate the expression of genes involved in cell proliferation, survival, and differentiation. Crucially, many of these variants induce downstream signaling *without T-cell stimulation* suggesting that these mutations lead to constitutive activation of T-cell signaling.[12,14] In addition, other gene variants such CTLA4-CD28 and ICOS-CD28 gene fusions enhance CD28-dependent T-cell signaling, and *RLTPR* variants have been shown to potentiate TCR signaling and downstream activation of the NF-kB pathway.[7,13] The prevalence of these gene variants in CTCL supported by functional data indicates that there is a critical selection pressure for activation of the NF-kB pathway in the transformation of mature T-cells.

PLCG1 mutations have also been detected in other mature T-cell malignancies, notably HTLV-1-associated ATLL,[17] PTCL (NOS),[18] hepato-splenic T-cell lymphomas,[19] and AITL[20] with the *PLCG1* p.S345F and R48 W variants being two of the most frequently reported (see Table 6-1). In addition, mutations of the *JAK-STAT, CD28, VAV1, DNMT3A,* and *TET2* genes are also reported in other mature T-cell malignancies.[4-9,17-20]

Activation of T-cells via engagement with the T-cell receptor and enhanced activation of transcriptional factors such as NF-kB stimulates cytokine production which in turn activates multiple pathways including the JAK–STAT pathway, which drive proliferation and differentiation of TH cells although STAT proteins have broad functions, including gene regulation and epigenetic modification. While gain-of-function mutations of JAKs, specifically *JAK3* and *STAT5B*, only occur at low frequency in CTCL, copy number gains of both *STAT3* and *STAT5B* are common and *associated with* constitutive expression of these key transcription factors.[21,22] Specifically, overexpression of STAT3 is a consistent feature of CTCL.

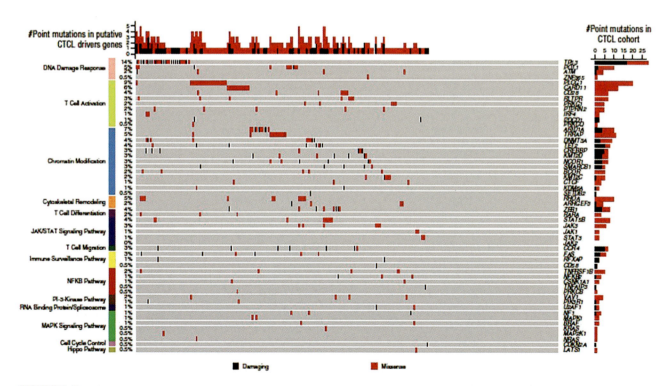

FIGURE 6-2. Putative driver genes in CTCL. (Reprinted from Park J, Yang J, Wenzel AT, et al. Genomic analysis of 220 CTCLs identifies a novel recurrent gain-of-function alteration in RLTPR (p.Q575E). *Blood.* 2017;130:1430-1440, with permission from Elsevier.)

TABLE 6-1 CTCL: Functional Impact of Putative Driver Gene Variants and Pathways

Pathway	Gene	Abnormality	Function
TCR signaling	PLCG1	SNV (RV)	GoF
	CD28	SNV (RV) and gene fusions	GoF
	CARD11	SNV (RV) and CNV	GoF
	PRKCB/Q	SNV (RV) and CNV	GoF
	RLTPR	SNV (RV)	GoF
	PTPRN2	SNV and CNV	GoF
JAK–STAT pathway	JAK1-3	SNV (RV)	GoF
	STAT3-5	SNV (RV) and copy no gain	GoF
DNA damage repair	POT1	SNV (RV)	LoF
	ATM	SNV (RV)	LoF
	BRCA1-2	SNV	LoF
Chromatin modification	TET2	SNV and CNV	LoF
	ARID1A/B	SNV and copy no loss	LoF
	DNMT3A	SNV and CNV	GoF
	SMARCB1	SNV (RV)	LoF
	SETDB2	CNV	LoF
	TRRAP	SNV (RV) and CNV	GoF
	CREBBP	SNV and CNV	LoF
	NCOR1	SNV (RV) and CNV	LoF
	BCOR	SNV	GoF
	CTCF	SNV and CNV	LoF
	KMT2C-D	SNV and CNV	LoF
Cell cycle	CDKN2A	Copy no loss	LoF
	TP53	SNV (RV) and copy no loss	LoF
NF-kB pathway	TNFRSF1B	SNV	GoF
	NFKB2	SNV	GoF
	PRKCB	CNV	GoF
	TNFAIP3	CNV	LoF
	IRF4	SNV and copy no gain	GoF
	CSNK1A1	SNV (RV) and CNV	GoF
T-cell migration	CCR4	SNV (RV)	GoF
MAPK pathway	NF1	SNV and copy no loss	LoF
	RAS	SNV	GoF
	BRAF	SNV and copy no gain	GoF
	MAP2KI	SNV	GoF
	MAPK1	SNV	GoF

TABLE 6-1 CTCL: Functional Impact of Putative Driver Gene Variants and Pathways   (Continued)

Pathway	Gene	Abnormality	Function
PI3K pathway	VAV1	SNV and fusion genes	GoF
	ARHGEF3	SNV	LoF
	RHOA	SNV (RV)	LoF

CNV, copy number variant; GoF, gain of function; LoF, loss of function; RV, recurrent gene variant; SNV, somatic non-synonymous variant.

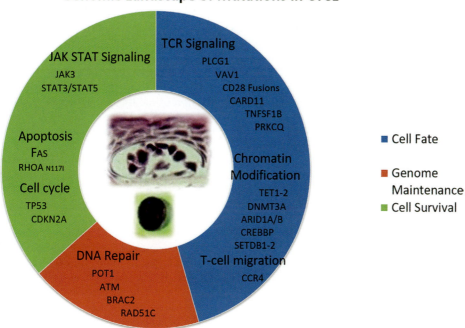

FIGURE 6-3. Genomic landscape of mutations in CTCL.

Epigenetic Modification

Epigenetics involves DNA and histone modifications which affect gene transcription and regulate cell differentiation. Global hypomethylation is a consistent feature of malignancy and contributes to genomic instability, but DNA methylation of gene promoters can lead to gene silencing. Crucially, these changes are heritable. While 7.8% of CpG sites in SS are hypomethylated, 3.2% show selection for hypermethylation of CpG sites within the proximal region of promoters.[23] Extensive studies have revealed that silencing of specific tumor suppressor genes in CTCL due to promoter hypermethylation includes genes involved in cell cycle regulation (*CDKN2A/2B*),[24] DNA repair (*MLH1* and *MGMT*),[25] apoptosis (*FAS*)[26] and JAK-STAT signaling (*SHP-1*).[27] Methylation of cytosine residues to 5-methylcytosine is mediated by DNA methyltransferases (DNMTs) and gain-of-function mutations of *DNMT3A* have been frequently identified in hematologic malignancies including MF/SS.[4,5,8,9] A second type of DNA methylation involves 5-hydroxymethylation of cytosine which is mediated by 10-11 translocation 1–3 enzymes (TET1-3) but, in contrast to 5-methylcytosine, this is associated with enhanced gene expression.[28] Loss-of-function *TET2* mutations are well documented in SS.[5,7-9,22] There is also selection in SS for mutations of other genes involved in epigenetic modifications including *IDH* encoding isocitrate dehydrogenases which inhibit TET proteins, *ARID1A/1B* which affect chromatin modeling, and *MLL* genes which mediate histone methyltransferases.[4,8,9,22] Epigenetic modification is critical for sustaining the transcriptional memory for T-cells allowing rapid transcription of inducible genes upon activation.[29,30] Large epigenomic studies in CTCL have shown that the methylation pattern of leukemic T-cells in SS can be similar to that of regulatory T-cells and that there is almost universal activation of NF-kB.[31] Recent data suggest that hypermethylation of the hTERT promoter in CTCL may be associated with telomerase activation.[32]

Micro-RNA (miR), one of a group of noncoding RNA transcripts, are key posttranscriptional regulators of messenger RNA (mRNA) contributing to the fine-tuning of protein expression. Extensive studies have implicated a functional role for dysregulation of miRs in cancer including CTCL.[33] Aberrant DNA methylation of miR promoters as well as copy number change has been reported to be associated with abnormal miR expression in CTCL.[33] In addition, constitutive activation of STAT3/5 has been shown to enhance miR-155 and miR-21 expression leading to increased apoptosis resistance and driving Th2 proliferation in CTCL.[33]

DNA Damage Response Pathways

DDR consists of numerous complex and interdependent signaling pathways which either maintain cell viability by repair of DNA or direct the damaged cell to undergo senescence or programmed cell death. Inevitably, this complex process is closely linked with pathways regulating the cell cycle, chromatin remodeling, and apoptosis.[34] Previous cytogenetic and array CGH studies in CTCL identified complex structural and numerical chromosomal abnormalities.[15] More recent WGS and WES studies have confirmed a high degree of genomic instability in CTCL[9,13] and have also identified several potential mechanisms, with one study of 101 SS samples identifying SNVs and/or CNVs affecting genes involved in DNA repair and telomere maintenance in over 50% of cases.[9] *TP53* is the most commonly mutated gene in CTCL with loss-of-function SNVs and deletions which lead to a significant detrimental effect on DDR. However, *POT1* gene mutations are also frequently detected and studies suggest that these loss-of-function variants likely contribute to telomere dysfunction considered to be a key contributor to genomic instability during cancer progression.[9] POT1 is part of the Shelterin complex and binds to single-stranded telomeric DNA, found at the ends of chromosomes, via its OB domains. Specific *POT1* variants have been shown to reduce telomere binding and induce an alternative lengthening of telomeres (ATR)-dependent DDR.[35] Germline variants of *POT1* have been detected in Li-Fraumeni-like syndromes as well as rare familial melanoma cases,[36] while somatic variants have been reported in CLL and gliomas as well as CTCL. In addition, loss-of-function *ATM* gene mutations have been identified in CTCL.[9,13] ATM is a key component of the DDR and also regulates cell cycle checkpoints and is therefore also likely to contribute to the genomic instability seen in CTCL. Notably, SNVs and CNVs affecting genes involved in homologous recombination such as *RAD51C*, *BRAC2*, and *POLD1* are also detected in CTCL.[9]

CTCL EVOLUTION

Most studies to date have been based on samples from advanced stages of MF or leukemic SS samples, which provide little insight regarding the critical early stages of CTCL development. Recent progress delineating the evolution of genomic events using mathematical models of WGS/WES data from solid malignancies has provided details of the main drivers of tumors' evolution and the impact of intratumor heterogeneity on therapeutic response.[37] Preliminary studies of paired plaques and tumors from MF patients have confirmed that subclonal evolution is a feature of CTCL linked to disease progression although these studies have not yet provided evidence of a common series of genomic events in early stages of disease.[11]

Causation

Characteristic mutational signatures have been identified in cancers and many of these signatures are linked causally to specific intrinsic and/or extrinsic mutagens.[38,39] Such mutational signatures can be identified in clonally expanded cell populations and are defined by assessment of the six substitution types and their 5′ and 3′ nucleotide context giving 96 different trinucleotide mutation types. The availability of large WES/WGS datasets of CTCL and other T-cell lymphomas has recently provided significant insight into the mutational spectrum of T-cell lymphomas and specifically the causal factors driving T-cell transformation in CTCL.[40] All mature T-cell lymphomas (403 cases) exhibited signature 1 which is related to cellular age and due to spontaneous deamination of methylated cytosine residues. Intriguingly, only MF and SS (137 cases) were associated with the UV signature 7, which contributed 52% of the mutational burden in MF and 23% in SS.[40] Overall, 41% of these patients were treatment naïve although the detection of a mutational signature is dependent on the presence of a clonal population suggesting that the malignant T-cell in CTCL accumulates UV-associated mutations before transformation and clonal expansion. The UV signature was also detected in CD4+-enriched peripheral blood leukemic cells from SS patients and represented between 7.5% and 88% of the overall SNVs. In addition, analysis of WGS data from treatment naïve patients with advanced stages of MF showed a UV signature 7 with a high frequency of CC > TT double substitutions at dipyrimidine sites and transcriptional strand bias, both of which are characteristic of UV irradiation (Fig. 6-4).[40]

CTCL exhibits a very high mutational load, as seen in other malignancies linked to exogenous mutagens such as nonmelanoma and melanoma skin cancers and smoking-associated lung cancers, and distinct from the much lower mutational burden of other types of T-cell lymphoma. It remains to be established if other CTCL variants also show a UV signature, but this would seem likely. These results confirm that environmental UV exposure contributes a significant proportion of the mutational burden in MF and SS and is a key causal factor in the transformation of T-cells that are either circulating through or are resident in the skin (Fig. 6-5). Many questions arise from these findings, notably as CTCL is a rare malignancy, why are skin resident T-cells only rarely susceptible to malignant transformation?

Primary Cutaneous CD30+ Lymphoproliferative Disorders (ALCL/LYP)

Primary cutaneous CD30+ ALCLs invariably fail to express anaplastic lymphoma kinase (ALK) but, unlike nodal ALK–ALCL, have an excellent prognosis suggesting a distinct

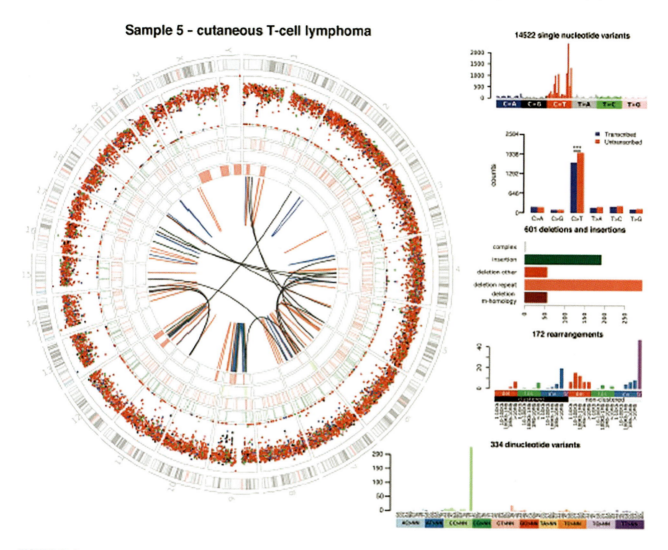

FIGURE 6-4. Characteristic features of UV-induced mutation in a tumor sample from a patient with mycosis fungoides after WGS. (Reprinted by permission from Springer: Springer Nature. Jones C, Degasperi A, Grandi V, et al. Spectrum of mutational signatures in T-cell lymphoma reveals a key role for UV radiation in cutaneous T-cell lymphoma. *Sci Rep.* 2021;11:3962-3975. doi:10.1038/s41598-021-83352-4)

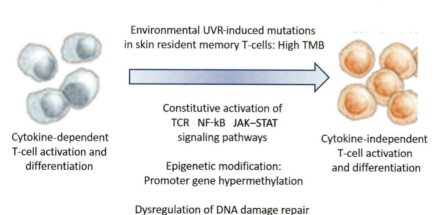

FIGURE 6-5. Malignant transformation in CTCL.

biology. In contrast nodal CD30+ ALK+ ALCL is defined by the presence of translocations producing a fusion gene involving ALK with multiple other partners, although the commonest is nucleophosphomin (NPM) associated with the t(2; 5) translocation. In ALK+ CD30+ ALCL, these fusion genes have been shown to activate the JAK STAT pathway.

In contrast, alternative mechanisms of JAK-STAT3 activation have been reported in systemic CD30+ ALK–ALCL including activating *JAK1* and/or *STAT3* mutations (37%) and in those with wild type *JAK-STAT* genes, a proportion have kinase fusions involving *ROS1*, *TYK2*, or *FRK* and diverse partners including *NF-kB* and *NPM1*, which have been shown to induce constitutive STAT expression.[41] Mutations of *JAK1* and/or *STAT3* and *NPM1-TYK2* gene fusions have only been reported rarely in pcCD30+ALCL and lymphomatoid papulosis (LYP), but the prevalence is still unclear.[41]

A subset of systemic ALK-CD30+ ALCL is characterized by chromosomal rearrangements involving the *DUSP22-IRF4* (MUM1) locus on 6p25.3 and such cases appear to have a good prognosis. This rearrangement is associated with downregulation of DUSP22 encoding dual-specificity phosphatase-22, a tumor suppressor gene, which inhibits TCR signaling and promotes apoptosis. Chromosomal rearrangements involving the same locus on 6p25.3 have also been identified in both pcCD30+ ALCL (25%) and less commonly (5%) in LYP,[42] but MUM1 expression is not specific for this rearrangement. In contrast, *TP63* rearrangements identified in aggressive variants of systemic ALK-CD30+ ALCL have not been detected in pcCD30+ lymphoproliferative disorders, which likely explain their excellent prognosis.[43]

Recent WES data suggest that a proportion of systemic and primary cutaneous ALK-ALCL, without constitutive activation of JAK-STAT, are characterized by a recurrent *MSC E116K* mutation, encoding musculin, a bHLH transcription factor, which correlates with the presence of *DUSP22* rearrangements.[44] Functional studies have demonstrated that this mutation activates the CD30-IRF4-MYC axis through a dominant negative effect and there may be dysregulation of other bHLH transcription factors in ALK-primary cutaneous ALCL. The *CDKN2A-CDKN2B* locus at 9p21 can be deleted in pcCD30+ ALCL but at a lower frequency than in advanced stages of MF, and a series of cytogenetic abnormalities have been detected using CGH techniques but comprehensive WES/WGS studies are lacking.

Subcutaneous Panniculitis-Like T-Cell Lymphoma

Recent WES studies of SPTCL have clarified the underlying pathogenesis of SPTCL, as two germline variants of *HAVCR2* were detected in a majority of cases suggesting a familial predisposition.[45] *HAVCR2* encodes T-cell immunoglobulin mucin 3 (TIM-3) which is expressed by CD8+ T-cells and NK cells and is a negative immune checkpoint involved in regulating peripheral tolerance, innate immunity, and inflammatory responses. The two homozygous *HAVCR2* variants pY82C and pIle97Met were restricted to Polynesian/East Asian and European origin, respectively.[45] Family members who were heterozygote carriers were either asymptomatic or had "lupus-like" symptoms. TIM-3 mutant SPTCL cases tend to be younger at diagnosis and to have a more severe disease course associated with hemophagocytic lymphohisticytosis and are more likely to respond to immunosuppressive therapies such as cyclosporine.[46] Both the *HAVCR2* gene variants have been shown to be pathogenic with loss of the TIM-3 immune checkpoint function. Somatic variants detected in *HAVCR2* mutant and wild type SPTCL include *TET2, ARID1B,* and other epigenetic modifiers as well as genes involved in the PI3K/AKT/mTOR pathways and the JAK–STAT pathway.[46] The association in some patients with infection or autoimmune conditions such as lupus suggests that other triggers may contribute to the development of SPTCL.

Primary Cutaneous T-Cell Lymphomas

A recent study of primary cutaneous γδ T-cell lymphomas has shown oncogenic mutations in the JAK/STAT, MAPK, MYC, and chromatin modification pathways, but interestingly, no selection for mutations in the TCR-CD28 signaling pathway as seen in MF/SS.[47] Strikingly, those γδ T-cell lymphomas which involved the subcutaneous tissues were derived from Vδ2 T-cells as opposed to those primarily involving the epidermis/dermis derived from Vδ1 T-cells. However, no differences were noted between these subtypes in terms of mutational profiles. In addition, panniculitic Vδ2 T-cell lymphomas do not show germline mutations of *HAVCR2* as seen in a majority of SPTCL patients.[47]

Other CTCL Variants

The genomic landscape of other rare primary CTCL variants has not yet been analyzed using NGS platforms, but such studies could provide important information about why these variants have such dramatically diverse clinical outcomes and might also provide clues about potential therapeutic options. Interestingly, previous CGH analysis of aggressive epidermotropic CD8+ CTCL variants showed distinct changes compared to MF/SS suggesting fundamental pathogenetic differences.[48] While we might anticipate that cutaneous lymphoma variants derived from specific T-cell subtypes such as follicular helper T-cells could share similar genomic abnormalities to those identified in AITL, it is more likely that differences may reflect their origin from skin resident T-cells.

Systemic T-Cell Lymphomas

Many of the genomic abnormalities detected in MF/SS have been detected in other systemic T-cell lymphomas, and ATLL and CTCL show a strikingly similar albeit heterogenous pattern of gene mutations.[13,17] Specifically, mature T-cell malignancies appear to be dependent on TCR and NF-kB signaling reflected in the selection for activating mutations of genes such as *PLCG1, PRKCQ, PREX2,* and *CARD11* and resistance to *TNFRSF*-mediated apoptosis with recurrent gene variants being detected in different T-cell lymphomas. Of these genes, *PLCG1* appears to be the most common TCR signaling-related gene mutation and a large number of *PLCG1* mutations have now been shown to functionally induce NFAT, AP1, and NF-kB expression in unstimulated cells.[12,14] CD28-CTLA4 and CD28-ICOS gene fusions are also detected in PTCL (NOS) and AITL and activate downstream pathways.[18] In addition, loss of epigenetic regulation, due to mutations in genes such as *TET1/2, DNMT3A,* and *ARID1A/B,* is seen in most T-cell lymphomas.[49] Abnormalities of JAK-STAT signaling are frequent in cutaneous and systemic T-cell lymphomas.[21]

However, there are exceptions, such as the recurrent *IDH2* (R172W and R172S) gene variants affecting histone methylation and the *RHOA* G17V variant that augments proximal TCR signaling via the VAV1 pathway.[49] Both appear to be restricted to AITL derived from follicular helper T-cells (TFH) and also PTCL (NOS) cases which express TFH markers.[49] Intriguingly, the recurrent *RHOA* N117I variant has only been reported in CTCL.[13] PTCL (NOS) is associated with an ITK-SYC fusion gene which has not yet been found in AITL or CTCL.[49] While IRF4 mutations are reported in CTCL, ATLL, and PTCL (NOS), a specific recurrent IRF4 K59R variant has only been described in HTLV-1-associated ATLL.[17] In contrast, rearrangements and translocations of IRF4 have been described in PTCL (NOS) and both cutaneous and systemic CD30+ ALCL.[42,49] IRF4 is a transcription factor downstream of NF-kB and has a pivotal role in differentiation of B-cells and induction of regulatory T-cells as well as a role in DNA repair via induction of PARP1 expression.[50] Specifically, IRF4 has been shown to mediate the oncogenic effects of STAT3 in ALCL.[51] In addition, DUSP22 rearrangements appear to be restricted to CD30+ ALCL, as are the tyrosine kinase gene fusions involving ROS1 or TYK2.

Finally, the tumor mutational burden in CTCL and ATLL is much higher than other mature T-cell lymphoma subtypes.[40] This may reflect the different extrinsic factors responsible for the mutational signatures, namely UVR and HTLV-1, respectively. The increasing use of NGS for T-cell lymphoma is likely to show more shared gene mutations across different subtypes, emphasizing the requirement for dysregulation of specific pathways, notably TCR signaling, to transform mature T-cells.

Prognostic Biomarkers

The prognosis for patients with MF/SS is variable even among patients with the same stage of disease. This has been partly addressed by the proposal of clinical prognostic models such as the CLIPi,[52,53] which is currently the subject of a multicenter prospective study. However, given the heterogeneity at a genomic level in CTCL, it is likely that a more accurate prognostic model will require analysis of genetic clusters which may include a combination of gene mutations including SNVs and CNVs. Recent results in systemic DLBCL suggest that a genomic classifier may be more accurate than either transcriptomic or clinical data.[54] Early studies in SS suggest that specific genomic clusters can be defined based on existing data[55] but as yet there are no data on correlation with clinical outcomes and the relative lack of genomic data in MF suggests that further NGS studies are required, especially in early stage disease.

Therapeutic Implications

While the lack of a highly prevalent recurrent mutation indicates that a targeted treatment option is not likely to be an option for MF or SS, the genomic landscape does provide insight into potential therapeutic approaches. Clearly, the selection pressure for mutations affecting specific pathways suggests that existing treatments such as ipilimumab (*CD28-CTLA4* fusion), ruxolitinib, and tofacitinib (*JAK1/3* and *JAK 1/2* mutations, respectively) and NF-kB pathway activation (bortezomib) could be reexplored in those CTCL patients who are stratified for these genomic abnormalities.[49] Patients with abnormalities of epigenetic regulation such as *DNMT3A* and *TET2* could be selected for treatment with demethylating agents such as 5-azactidine and/or HDACi, while those with *RHOA* mutations could be eligible for PI3K inhibitors. This is potentially achievable when tumor agnostic trials for refractory lymphoma become more widely available as for solid malignancies. The high mutational burden of CTCL would suggest that immunotherapies could be successful but data from phase II trials has so far shown only limited success[56] highlighting the challenges of driving a T-cell mediated immune response in a T-cell malignancy. Perhaps the most interesting option would be tumor agnostic therapies targeting the DDR pathways which show considerable promise in various solid malignancies often as maintenance therapies after platinum-based chemo regimens.[34] These approaches build on the success of PARP inhibitors inducing synthetic lethality in BRCA-mutant tumors. The DDR pathways comprise over 450 proteins and several are being targeted, including ATM and ATR inhibitors.[34] As both ATM and ATR are critically involved in identifying and directing repair of UV-induced bulky DNA adducts,[57] this would appear to be worth exploring, but the key to a successful outcome will be the identification of those genomic profiles which identify susceptible cases such as ATR inhibition in ATM-deficient CTCL cases. Several trials are currently assessing the use of drugs which inhibit DDR and sensitize cells to double strand inducing agents such as topoisomerase inhibitors or in combination with radiotherapy and liposomal doxorubicin, which are both effective in CTCL.[34]

References

1. Teras LR, DeSantis CE, Cerhan JR, Morton LM, Jemal A, Flowers CR. 2016 US lymphoid malignancy statistics by World Health Organization subtypes. *CA Cancer J. Clin.* 2016;66:443-459.
2. Campbell JJ, Clark RA, Watanabe R, Kupper TS. Sezary syndrome and mycosis fungoides arise from distinct T-cell subsets: a biologic rationale for their distinct clinical behaviors. *Blood.* 2010;116:767-771.
3. Vose J, Armitage J, Weisenburger D; International T-Cell Lymphoma Project. International peripheral T-cell and natural killer/T-cell lymphoma study: pathology findings and clinical outcomes. *J Clin Oncol Off J Am Soc Clin Oncol.* 2008;26:4124-4130.
4. Choi J, Goh G, Walradt T, et al. Genomic landscape of cutaneous T cell lymphoma. *Nat Genet.* 2015;47:1011-1019.
5. da Silva Almeida AC, Abate F, Khiabanian H, et al. The mutational landscape of cutaneous T cell lymphoma and Sézary syndrome. *Nat Genet.* 2015;47:1465-1470.
6. Prasad A, Rabionet R, Espinet B, et al. Identification of gene mutations and fusion genes in patients with Sézary syndrome. *J Invest Dermatol.* 2016;136:1490-1499.
7. Ungewickell A, Bhaduri A, Rios E, et al. Genomic analysis of mycosis fungoides and Sézary syndrome identifies recurrent alterations in TNFR2. *Nat Genet.* 2015;47:1056-1060.
8. Wang L, Ni X, Covington KR, et al. Genomic profiling of Sézary syndrome identifies alterations of key T cell signaling and differentiation genes. *Nat Genet.* 2015;47:1426-1434.
9. Woollard WJ, Pullabhatla V, Loren A, et al. Candidate driver genes involved in genome maintenance and DNA repair in Sézary syndrome. *Blood.* 2016;127:3387-3397.
10. McGirt LY, Jia P, Baerenwald DA, et al. Whole-genome sequencing reveals oncogenic mutations in mycosis fungoides. *Blood.* 2015;126:508-519.
11. Iyer A, Hennessey D, O'Keefe S, et al. Branched evolution and genomic intratumor heterogeneity in the pathogenesis of cutaneous T-cell lymphoma. *Blood Adv.* 2020;4(11):2489-2500.

12. Vaque J, Gómez-López G, Monsálvez V, et al. PLCG1 mutations in cutaneous T-cell lymphomas. *Blood*. 2014;123:2034e43.
13. Park J, Yang J, Wenzel AT, et al. Genomic analysis of 220 CTCLs identifies a novel recurrent gain-of-function alteration in RLTPR (p.Q575E). *Blood*. 2017;130:1430-1440.
14. Patel VM, Flanagan CE, Martins M, et al. Frequent and persistent PLCG1 mutations in Sézary cells directly enhance PLCγ1 activity and stimulate NFκB, AP-1, and NFAT signaling. *J Invest Dermatol*. 2020;140(2):380-389.e4.
15. Mao X, Lillington DM, Czepulkowski B, et al. Molecular cytogenetic characterization of Sezary syndrome. *Gene Chromosome Cancer*. 2003;36(3):250-260.
16. Nussenzweig A, Nussenzweig MC. Origin of chromosomal translocations in lymphoid cancer. *Cell*. 2010;141:27-38.
17. Kataoka K, Nagata Y, Kitanaka A, et al. Integrated molecular analysis of adult T cell leukemia/lymphoma. *Nat Genet*. 2015;47:1304-1315.
18. Palomero T, CouronnéL, Khiabanian H, et al. Recurrent mutations in epigenetic regulators, RHOA and FYN kinase in peripheral T cell lymphomas. *Nat Genet*. 2014;46:166-170.
19. McKinney M, Moffitt AB, Gaulard P, et al. The genetic basis of hepatosplenic T-cell lymphoma. *Cancer Discov*. 2017;7:369-379.
20. Sakata-Yanagimoto M, Enami T, Yoshida K, et al. Somatic RHOA mutation in angioimmunoblastic T cell lymphoma. *Nat Genet*. 2014;46:171-175.
21. Crescenzo R, Abate F, Lasorsa E, et al. Convergent mutations and kinase fusions lead to oncogenic STAT3 activation in anaplastic large cell lymphoma. *Cancer Cell*. 2015;27:516-532.
22. Kiel M, Sahasrabuddhe AA, Rolland DCM, et al. Genomic analyses reveal recurrent mutations in epigenetic modifiers and the JAK-STAT pathway in Sezary syndrome. *Nat Comms*. 2015;26:8470.
23. van Doorn R, Slieker RC, Boonk SE, et al. Epigenomic analysis of Sézary syndrome defines patterns of aberrant DNA methylation and identifies diagnostic markers. *J Invest Dermatol*. 2016;136:1876-1884.
24. Scarisbrick J, Woolford AJ, Calonje E, et al. Frequent abnormalities of the p15 and p16 genes in mycosis fungoides and Sezary syndrome. *J Invest Dermatol*. 2002;118(3):493-499.
25. Scarisbrick J, Woolford AJ, Russell-Jones R, Whittaker SJ. Loss of heterozygosity on 10q and microsatellite instability in advanced stages of primary cutaneous T-cell lymphoma and possible association with homozygous deletion of PTEN. *Blood*. 2000;95(9):2937-2942.
26. Jones CL, Wain EM, Chu CC, et al. Downregulation of Fas gene expression in Sézary syndrome is associated with promoter hypermethylation. *J Invest Dermatol*. 2010;130(4):1116-1125.
27. van Doorn R, Zoutman WH, Dijkman R, et al. Epigenetic silencing of cutaneous T-cell lymphoma: promoter hypermethylation of multiple tumour suppressor genes including BCL7a, PTPRG, and p73. *J Clin Oncol*. 2005;23:3886-3896.
28. Rasmussen K, Helin K. Role of TET enzymes in DNA methylation, development and cancer. *Genes Dev*. 2016;30:733e50.
29. Antigano F, Zaph C. Regulation of CD4+ T-cell differentiation and inflammation by repressive histone methylation. *Immunol Cell Biol*. 2015;93:245e52.
30. Dunn J, McCuaig R, Tu WJ, Hardy K, Rao A. Multilayered epigenetic mechanisms contribute to transcriptional memory in T lymphocytes. *BMC Immunol*. 2015;16:3e11.
31. Qu K, Zaba LC, Satpathy AT, et al. Chromatin accessibility landscape of cutaneous T-cell lymphoma and dynamic response to HDAC inhibitors. *Cancer Cell*. 2017;32(1):2741.
32. Chebly A, Ropio J, Peloponese JM, et al. Exploring *hTERT* Promoter methylation: in cutaneous T-cell lymphomas. *Mol Oncol*. Published online 2021. doi:10.1002/1878-0261.12946
33. Gluud M, Willerslev-Olsen A, Gjerdrum LMR, et al. MicroRNAs in the pathogenesis, diagnosis, prognosis and targeted treatment of cutaneous T-cell lymphomas. *Cancers*. 2020;12:1229-2247.
34. Pilie PG, Tang C, Mills GB, Yap TA. State of the art strategies for targeting the DNA damage response in cancer. *Nature Rev Clin Oncol*. 2019;16:81-104.
35. Ramsay AJ, Quesada V, Foronoda M, et al. POT1 mutations cause telomere dysfunction in chronic lymphocytic leukemia. *Nat Genet*. 2013;45(5):526-530.
36. Robles-Espinoza CD, Harland M, Ramsay AJ, et al. POT1 loss of function variants predispose to familial melanoma. *Nat Genet*. 2014;46(5):478-481.
37. McGranahan N, Swanton C. Clonal heterogeneity and tumour evolution: past, present and the future. *Cell*. 2017;168:613-624.
38. Alexandrov LB, Nik-Zainal S, Wedge DC, et al. Signatures of mutational processes in human cancer. *Nature*. 2013;500:415-421.
39. Kucab JE, Zou X, Morganella S, et al. A compendium of mutational signatures of environmental agents. *Cell*. 2019;177:1-16.
40. Jones C, Degasperi A, Grandi V, et al. Spectrum of mutational signatures in T-cell lymphoma reveals a key role for UV radiation in cutaneous T-cell lymphoma. *Sci Rep*. 2021;11:3962-3975.
41. Velusamy T, Kiel M, Sahasrabuddhe A, et al. A novel recurrent NPM1-TYK2 gene fusion in cutaneous CD30+ lymphoproliferative disoders. *Blood*. 2014;124(25):3768-3771.
42. Wada D, Law ME, Hsi ED, et al. Specificity of IRF4 translocations for primary cutaneous anaplastic large cell lymphoma: a multicenter study of 204 skin biopsies. *Mod Pathol*. 2011;24(4):596-605.
43. Schrader A, Chung Y, Jansen P, et al. No TP63 rearrangements in a selected group of primary cutaneous CD30+ lymphoproliferative disorders with aggressive clinical course. *Blood*. 2016;128(1):141-143.
44. Luchtel R, Zimmermann MT, Hu G, et al. Recurrent *MSC*^{E116K} mutations in ALK-negative anaplastic large cell lymphoma. *Blood*. 2019;133(26):2776-2789.
45. Gayden T, Sepulveda FE, Khuong-Quang DA, et al. Germline HAVCR2 mutations altering TIM-3 characterise subcutaneous panniculitis-like T-cell lymphomas with haemophagocytic lymphohistiocytic syndrome. *Nat Genet*. 2018;50:1650-1657.
46. Polprasert C, Takeuchi Y, Kakiuchi N, et al. Frequent germline mutations of HAVCR2 in sporadic subcutaneous panniculitis-like T-cell lymphoma. *Blood Adv*. 2019;3:588-595.
47. Daniels J, Doukas PG, Escala MEM, et al. Cellular origins and genetic landscape of cutaneous gamma delta T-cell lymphomas. *Nat Commun*. 2020;11:1806-1820.
48. Tomasini C, Novelli M, Fanoni D, Berti EF. Erythema multiforme like lesions in primary cutaneous aggressive cytotoxic epidermotropic CD8+ T-cell lymphoma: a diagnostic and therapeutic challenge. *J Cutan Pathol*. 2017;44(10):867-873.
49. Zhang Y, Lee D, Brimer T, et al. Genomics of peripheral T-cell lymphoma and its implications for personalized medicine. *Front Oncol*. 2020;10:898-908.

50. Alvisi G, Brummelmann J, Puccio S, et al. IRF4 instructs effector Treg differentiation and immune suppression in human cancer. *J Clin Invest*. 2020;130:3137-3150.
51. Bandini C, Pupuleku A, Spaccarotella C, et al. IRF4 mediates the oncogenic effects of STAT3 in anaplastic large cell lymphomas. *Cancers*. 2018;10:21-39.
52. Agar N, Wedgeworth E, Crichton S, et al. Survival outcomes and prognostic factors in mycosis fungoides/Sézary syndrome: validation of the revised International Society for Cutaneous Lymphomas/European Organisation for Research and Treatment of Cancer staging proposal. *J Clin Oncol*. 2010;28(31):4730.
53. Benton EC, Crichton S, Talpur R, et al. A cutaneous lymphoma international prognostic index (CLIPi) for mycosis fungoides and Sezary syndrome. *Eur J Cancer*. 2013;49(13):2859-2868.
54. Pedrosa L, Fernández-Miranda I, Pérez-Callejo D, et al. Proposal and validation of a method to classify genetic subtypes of diffuse large B-cell lymphoma. *Sci Rep*. 2021;11:1886-1990.
55. Chang LW, Patrone CC, Yang W, et al. An intergrated data resource for genomic analysis of cutaneous T-cell lymphoma. *J Invest Dermatol*. 2018;138:2681-2683.
56. Sivanand A, Surmanowicz P, Alhusayen R. Immunotherapy for cutaneous T-cell lymphoma: current landscape and future developments. *J Cutan Med Surg*. 2019;23(5):537-544.
57. Ray A, Blevins C, Wani G, Wani A. ATR- and ATM- mediated DNA damage response is dependent on excision repair assembly during G1 but not in S phase of cell cycle. *PLoS One*. 2016;21:1-20.

CHAPTER 7

Molecular pathogenesis of primary cutaneous B-cell lymphomas

Alejandro A. Gru and Pierluigi Porcu

INTRODUCTION

Cutaneous B-cell lymphomas (CBCLs) are a group of rare primary B-cell extranodal lymphomas of the skin, with an incidence of approximately 3 cases per 1,000,000 per year.[1,2] Most of them are histologically low grade and clinically indolent, but a small subset, mostly involving the lower extremities, is very aggressive. In this chapter, we will review the available data on the molecular biology of three particular subtypes of CBCL: primary cutaneous follicle center lymphoma (PCFCL), primary cutaneous marginal zone lymphoma (PCMZL), and diffuse large B-cell lymphoma, leg type (DLBCL-LT). The three subtypes of CBCL are not always easy to distinguish from systemic B-cell lymphomas. The challenging diagnostic approach to CBCL was recently reviewed by Jaffe et al.[3]

PRIMARY CUTANEOUS FOLLICLE CENTER LYMPHOMA

PCFCL is a low-grade B-cell lymphoma with a predilection for the head and neck regions. Most patients present with a solitary lesion or a small number of painless, firm, erythematous papules, plaques, nodules, or tumors.[4,5] Histologically, there is a nodular, diffuse, or mixed infiltrate of centrocytes and centroblasts.[6,7] Contrary to the systemic forms of follicular lymphoma, the number of centroblasts carries no significant prognostic information. The immunophenotype of PCFCL includes expression of the germinal center marker BCL-6 and sometimes CD10. Rearrangements of BCL-2 are typically absent, another feature that helps distinguish PCFCL from systemic FL. Reported rates of BCL-2 expression by immunohistochemistry in PCFCL vary. In a study including 47 cases of PCFCL, 25 (53%) expressed BCL-2, but only 4 (8.5%) were positive for the *IGH::BCL2* rearrangement by fluorescent in situ hybridization (FISH). Notably, the study controlled for T-cell expression of BCL-2 by comparing CD3 and BCL-2 staining on serial sections.[8] Most cases of PCFCL show a clonal rearrangement of the immunoglobulin heavy chain gene (*IGH*)[9-14] by molecular studies or monoclonality by flow cytometric analysis. Laser capture microdissection can also help improve the rates of detection of clonality.[15]

At a molecular level, gene expression profiling of PCFCL has shown significantly higher expression of the SPINK2 transcript compared with the DLBCL, leg type.[16] *SPINK2* has been recognized as one of the 43 germinal center genes that discriminate between the germinal center B-cell (GCB) and activated B-cell (ABC) types of DLBCLs with highest significance.[17] The *SPINK2* gene encodes a Kazal-type serine/threonine kinase whose role in physiologic and pathologic cellular processes remains ill defined.[18] Several genes associated with the host immune response (granzyme M, selectin P, *LCK*) were also substantially upregulated in the group of PCFCLs, which is consistent with the higher numbers of host immune cells in these tumors. Interestingly, BCL-2 mRNA levels were equivalent when comparing PCFCL and DLBCL-LT, even in the absence of BCL-2 expression. Array comparative genomic hybridization studies in PCFCL have shown recurrent 1p36 deletions.[19] A study by Dijkman et al[20] identified high-level DNA amplifications at 2p16.1 (63%) and deletion of chromosome 14q32.33 (68%). FISH analysis confirmed *c-REL* amplification in patients with gains at 2p16.1. Dijkman et al[20] demonstrated somatic hypermutation (SHM) of *BCL6* in 7 PCFCL patients (37%) and aberrant SHM in *PAX5, RhoH/TTF,* and/or *MYC* in 10 PCFCL patients (53%). The majority of mutations consisted of single base-pair substitutions with rare deletions/insertions, and displayed molecular features typical of the SHM process.[21] This shows that SHM is not restricted to DLBCL and appears to be important also in the pathogenesis of PCFCL. Perez et al[22] detected an SHM rate ranging between 1.6% and 21%, with a median rate of 9.8% among CBL (most cases of which represented PCFCL). No differences in the rates of SHM were seen according to the histologic subtypes. A more recent study by Zhou et al analyzes the key molecular differences between PCFCL and systemic FL with skin involvement: both systemic FL and skin-restricted PCFCL showed frequent *TNFRSF14* loss-of-function mutations and copy number loss at chromosome 1p36. Systemic FL showed loss-of-function *CREBBP* or *KMT2D* mutations, which were not encountered in PCFCL. Additionally, the proliferative fraction of PCFCL was higher (as measured by Ki67), compared to the one seen for sFL. *EZH2* and *EP300* mutations were rarely seen in PCFLC.[23] Another study by Barasch et al[24] showed that the most common somatic mutations in the 12-19 analyzable PCFCL were *TNFRSF14* (40%, plus 10% with 1p36 deletions), followed by *CREBBP, TNFAIP3, KMT2D, SOCS1, EP300, STAT6,* and *FOXO1* (17%-25%). *KMT2D, CREBBP,* and *BCL2* were much less frequently mutated in PCFCL compared to the systemic counterparts.

Single microRNA RT-qPCR on formalin-fixed paraffin-embedded (FFPE) tumor biopsies of cases of PCFCL and DLBCL-LT showed higher expression of miR-9-5p, miR-31-5p, miR-129-2-3p, and miR-214-3p in PCFCL as compared with DLBCL-LT. MicroRNAs that have previously shown higher levels of expression in ABC-type as compared with GCB-type nodal DLBCL were not differentially expressed between PCFCL and PCDLBCL-LT.[25]

By FISH, the *IGH::BCL2* translocation has been described in a significant subset of PCFCL[7,26-29] (approximately 10%-30%). The most recent study showed only 8% of cases with such translocation.[23] However, other studies have found a complete absence of such translocation.[28,30-33] A t(12; 21) translocation has been described in a single case of PCFCL.[34] A rare complex four-way t(2; 14; 9;3) (p11.2; q32; p13; q27) translocation involving rearrangements of *BCL-6*, immunoglobulin light chain and heavy chain genes, and an unknown gene on 9p has been described in another PCFCL.[35] In contrast to PCDLBCL, leg type, deletion of the region containing *CDKN2A* and *CDKN2B* genes on chromosome 9q21.3 has not been reported.[7]

PRIMARY CUTANEOUS MARGINAL ZONE LYMPHOMA

PCMZLs are indolent lymphomas composed of small B-cells including marginal zone (centrocyte-like), plasmacytoid, and plasma cells. The lesions most often involve the trunk and extremities, and may present as violaceous to red, papules, plaques, nodules, or more rarely tumors. Lesions are often multifocal. PCMZLs frequently recur in the skin but rarely disseminate to extracutaneous sites and have an excellent disease-specific 5-year survival of 99% to 100%.[1] The phenotype of the lymphoma cells includes expression of B-cell antigens (CD19, CD79a, CD20, PAX-5), BCL-2, and plasma cell markers (CD138, CD38) in cases with plasma cell differentiation. As opposed to other types of MZLs, the cutaneous forms are typically negative for CD43. Markers of germinal center differentiation (CD10, BCL-6) and CD5 are negative. Though all of these neoplasms are presumably monoclonal, monoclonal IgH rearrangement can only be detected in approximately 75% of cases.[36,37] Rare cases can show a rearrangement of both the B- and T-cell receptors.[38]

Because of the clinicopathologic characteristics of PCMZL, it has been suggested that the disease develops as a clonally restricted response to persistent antigenic stimulation. This finding was supported because of the specific association between PCMZL and *Borrelia burgdorferi* infection, a feature that has been noted in cases from Europe, but not in North America. This particular association has given some of these cases the name of lymphocytoma cutis (LC).[7,39-42] Colli et al[39] noted *B. burgdorferi* DNA by polymerase chain reaction analysis in 67.5% of cases of LC. As a matter of fact, several antigenic stimuli are known to eventuate into a reactive B-cell response. These reactions, variously defined as cutaneous lymphoid hyperplasia, pseudo-B-cell lymphoma, or lymphadenosis benigna cutis, may be caused by insect bites, in particular, tick bites transmitting the *B. burgdorferi* infection, acupuncture, antigen injections (drug eruptions, vaccinations, specific immune therapy), and tattoo pigments among others.[40] Indeed, many authors believe that the so-called "reactive lymphoid hyperplasias" and PCMZL represent a spectrum of cutaneous B-cell lymphoproliferative disorders with a step-wise progression from a reactive to a neoplastic state.[31,40] This may also explain why it can be so difficult to differentiate early stages of these indolent hyperplasias from frank lymphoma. Indeed, the ICC classification has proposed a change in the nomenclature from lymphma to lymphoproliferative disorder. In rare examples of localized PCMZL (T1/T2), a traumatic event such as vaccination, tattooing, or an arthropod bite could result in chronic lymphoid hyperplasia eventuating in a clonal B-cell expansion. These localized lesions may be extremely indolent and ultimately resolve with surgical excision or even antibiotics.[43] This hypothesis is supported by the fact that many PCMZLs demonstrate similar V(H) gene segments and conserved CDR3 amino acid motifs in the nontemplated areas, indicating that some of these tumors may bind the same, or similar, antigen via their surface immunoglobulin receptor.[44] SHM was also present in many of these lesions.[22,45-47] Christie et al[48] also showed frequent clusters of Langerhans cells in both lymphoid hyperplasia and PCMZL. They hypothesized that in cutaneous MALT, plasmacytoid dendritic cells are the dominant dendritic cell subtype and may act by damping the antitumor host immune response, as well as directly stimulating the growth and differentiation of the neoplastic lymphocytes.

More recently, Edinger et al[49] have established important differences between PCMZL and other MALT lymphomas. Most MALT lymphomas are IgM$^+$, but molecular studies have documented frequent heavy chain class switching in PCMZL. They found that in most cases of PCMZL, class switching occurred (IgG > IgA > IgE), and this was linked to a heavy T-cell infiltrate in the background. A small number of cases were IgM$^+$ and were characteristically composed of a predominance of B-cells. Many but not all report a predominant T_H1 T-cell microenvironment in the noncutaneous MALT lymphomas and their precursor inflammatory lesions, but the class-switched cutaneous cases reportedly have a prominent T_H2 inflammatory environment. A marked plasmacytic differentiation was also evident morphologically in their series of PCMZL. Interestingly, while most MALTs are IgM$^+$, those that typically arise in the thyroid gland in association with autoimmune disorders (such as Hashimoto thyroiditis) also reveal prominent plasmacytic differentiation and IgG class switch.[49] Furthermore, the isotype-switched PCMZLs lack CXCR3 and seem to arise in a different inflammatory environment than other extranodal MZBCLs.[50] In addition, certain translocations common in MALT lymphoma, like t(11; 18) (q21; q21) or t(1; 14) (p22; q32), have not been reported in the skin.[32,51] It also appears that nonclass-switched cases can show a propensity of dissemination and a more aggressive behavior (Figs. 7-1, 7-2).

FISH studies showed very few aberrations. Trisomy 3 has been described in two cases at levels varying from 14% to 20% of the analyzed cells.[52] Shreuder et al[51] found a t(14; 18) (q32; q21), with breakpoints in *IGH* and *MALT1*, in three

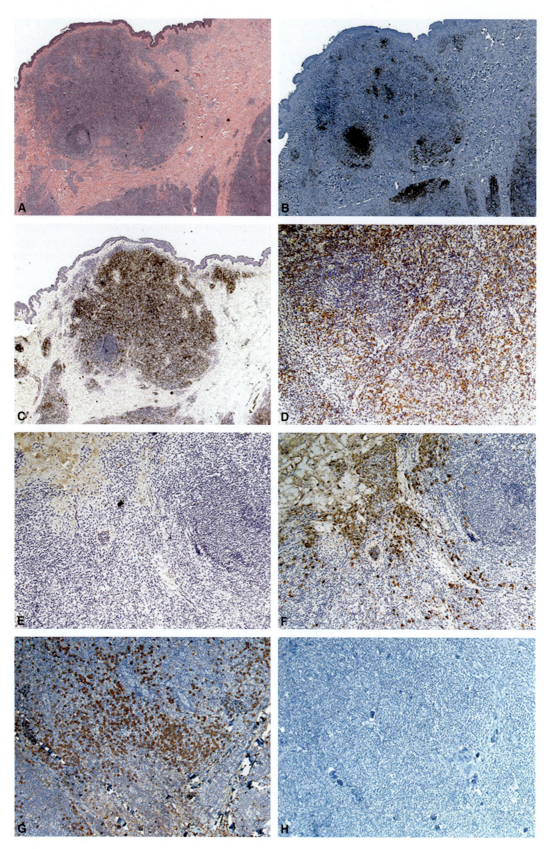

FIGURE 7-1. Class-switched PCMZL. A. Note the dense dermal nodules with predominantly small lymphoid cells and one distinct follicle with a germinal center. **B.** A CD20 stain highlights the follicle and occasional other positive aggregates but otherwise shows only scattered positive cells. **C.** There are numerous CD3⁺ cells outside of the follicle. **D.** CXCR3 is expressed on many T-cells but is negative in the B-cell aggregates. **E.** κ. **F.** λ. Note the focally marked predominance of λ light chain-restricted plasma cells. **G.** IgG. **H.** IgM. Most plasma cells are IgG⁺ and IgM⁻. (Reprinted from Edinger JT, Kant JA, Swerdlow SH. Cutaneous marginal zone lymphomas have distinctive features and include 2 subsets. *Am J Surg Pathol.* 2010;34(12):1830-1841, with permission.)

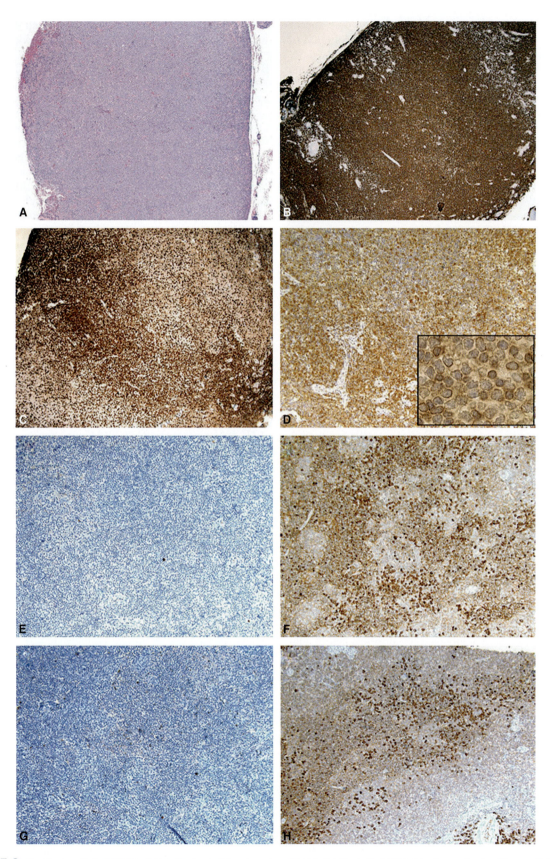

FIGURE 7-2. Nonclass-switched PCMZL. A. Note the dense diffuse dermal small lymphoid infiltrate. **B.** A CD20 stain shows extensive diffuse positivity. **C.** There are still moderately numerous admixed CD3+ T-cells. **D.** CXCR3 is diffusely positive with apparent stronger staining of T-cells and weaker staining of many B cells. **E.** κ. **F.** λ. There is a marked predominance of λ light chain-restricted plasma cells plus weak λ staining on many B cells. **G.** IgG. **H.** IgM. The IgM stain shows a similar pattern to λ, while there are only rare IgG+ cells. (Reprinted from Edinger JT, Kant JA, Swerdlow SH. Cutaneous marginal zone lymphomas have distinctive features and include 2 subsets. *Am J Surg Pathol.* 2010;34(12):1830-1841, with permission.)

cases. All three had partly monocytoid histologic appearances and lacked blastic transformation. An additional trisomy of chromosome 3 was detected in one of these cases. Trisomy 18 was present in two lymphomas without monocytoid morphology.

A comprehensive clinicopathological and molecular study[53] looking at 60 cases of PCMZL from Asia, Germany, and the United States revealed some interesting findings. Moderate to intense tissue eosinophilia was present in a significant proportion (36%) of cases from Asia, a feature not present in cases from Germany or the United States. None of the cases revealed evidence of infection by *B. burgdorferi* or of the *API2::MALT1* fusion, typical of other MALT lymphomas. Of note, tumors from the three regions were highly methylated for *DAPK* (38%-50% of the cases, mean 43%) and *p16INK4a* (42%-70%, mean 49%), and the rates of positivity were significantly higher than those of nonneoplastic skin (8%, P = .0010 and 14%, P = .0032, respectively). Methylation of these genes had no significant association with progressive features of the tumors. DAPK is a calcium/calmodulin-dependent and cytoskeletal-associated serine/threonine kinase with death-inducing functions.[54,55] *DAPK* was initially isolated as a positive mediator of apoptosis induced by interferon-γ. Overexpression of DAPK in tumor cells led to cell death in the absence of external stimuli. Recent studies showed that this molecule also participates in tumor necrosis factor-α and Fas-induced apoptosis. The *p16* gene encodes for nuclear protein that can block cell-cycle progression from the G1 to the S phase by effectively inhibiting the kinase activity of CDK4/6, thereby exerting a negative control on cell proliferation.[56-58] Loss of p16 expression gives a remarkable growth advantage in cells. Additional molecular studies have failed to reveal the *MYD88* L265 mutation in PCMZL.[59] miRNA studies show upregulation of the miR-150 in PCMZL relative to PCFCL. Low expression levels of miR-155 and miR-150 were both associated with shorter progression-free survival in PCMZLs.[60] Another study by Maurus et al[61] revealed novel molecular insights in a large proportion of PCMZLs. The most frequently detected alterations (24/38 patients, 63.2%) affected the *FAS* gene, of which 22 patients harbored alterations, which affect the functionally relevant death domain of the apoptosis-regulating FAS/CD95 protein in a dominant-negative manner. In addition, they also identified highly recurrent mutations in three other genes, namely *SLAMF1, SPEN,* and *NCOR2*.

DIFFUSE LARGE B-CELL LYMPHOMA, LEG TYPE

DLBCL-LT is an aggressive large B-cell lymphoma that typically occurs in the lower extremities of older patients. Recent SEER data on 485 US patients[62] show that the median age at diagnosis was 70 years and incidence was 0.09 case per 100,000, with male cases being about 1.6 times more common that female cases. Overall, most patients were males (52%), older than 65 years (59.4%), and Caucasians (85.6%). DLBCL-LT presents as rapidly progressive, red to bluish, often ulcerating, tumors. In approximately 10% of cases, the lesions develop in sites other than the legs. DLBCL-LT is an aggressive lymphoma with a 5-year survival of approximately 50%.[1,5,6] Histologically, tumors are composed of sheets of immunoblasts that spare the epidermis. The neoplastic cells express CD20, CD79a, and BCL-6, are strongly positive for BCL-2, IRF4/MUM1, and FOXP1,[63] and have cytoplasmic expression of IgM/IgD. p63 can help discriminate PCFCL from DLBCL-LT, being strongly expressed in the latter.[64]

Analysis of the expression of 43 genes recently described to discriminate the ABC and GCB types of DLBCLs with highest significance suggested a similarity between DLBCL-LT and ABC-like DLBCL.[16,65] The increased cellular proliferative activity in DLBCL-LT, as shown by the high expression of various genes associated with proliferation and the high percentage of Ki-67–positive tumor cells (75% in 12 of 13 cases), may be a result of the deregulated expression of several oncogenes with cell-cycle regulatory functions such as *CMYC*, *PIM1*, and *BCL6*. A correlation was found between the highest *CMYC* expression value on microarray and qPCR and the presence of a chromosomal translocation involving the *IGH* gene and *CMYC* gene (t(8; 14) (q24; q32)) detected by FISH analysis.[32] In a small CGH array study, Mao et al[66] showed gains of *CMYC* (8q24) in two of four DLBCLs-LT cases. The *CMYC* oncogene is a transcription factor involved in multiple cellular functions such as cell-cycle regulation, apoptosis, cell growth, metabolism, and differentiation. The overexpression of *CMYC* by rearrangement with the *IGH* gene is seen in Burkitt lymphoma and some cases of DLBCL. Such rearrangement has also been shown in 5 of 14 cases of DLBCL-LT.[32,67] Additionally, high expressions of *PIM1* and *PIM2* oncogenes were noted. PIM kinases are known to cooperate with *CMYC* and *NMYC* to generate T- and B-cell lymphomas. They act in multiple pathways: increasing levels of MYC-driven transcripts, inhibition of apoptosis, cell proliferation, increased protein synthesis, and others.[68] Alterations of the *BCL-6* gene pathway have also been noted in DLBCL-LT. Somatic hypermutation of the *BCL-6* gene has been detected in a small series of DLBCLs-LT, which may affect the BCL-6-negative autoregulation circuit and result in BCL-6 deregulation as described in nodal DLBCL.[69-71] Additional important genes with notable upregulation in DLBCL-LT were the B-cell transcription factors *MUM1/IRF4* and *OCT2*. *MUM1/IRF4* is strongly expressed in lymphoplasmacytoid lymphoma, multiple myeloma, and 75% of DLBCLs. *MUM1/IRF4* is transiently induced during normal lymphocyte activation and is critical for the proliferation of B lymphocytes in response to signals from the antigen receptor.[72]

More recently, Pham-Ledard et al[73] reported a very high frequency (69%) of *MYD88 L265P* mutation in DLBCL-LT. The *MYD88* mutation was significantly associated with shorter disease-specific survival in univariate (P = .03) and multivariate (odds ratio, 3.01; 95% CI, 1.03-8.78; P = .04) analyses. A separate study also showed high levels of genetic alterations in 96% of DLBCL-LT[74] in addition to *MYD88* mutations (61%). *MYD88* mutations result in the activation of the NF-κβ pathway, a previously noted molecular alteration in ABC-DLBCL[75] (Fig. 7-3). In ABC cell lines, the L265P protein was shown to promote JAK-STAT3 and NF-kB signaling and resulted in increased cell survival.[76] Targeting the MYD88 pathway using inhibitors of the Bruton tyrosine kinase (ibrutinib) has shown very promising results in these lymphomas.[77,78]

A recent exome sequencing study[79] of 37 cutaneous DLBCLs, including 31 DLBCLs, leg type (DLBCL-LT) and 6

found for BCL2 or MYC. A recent study[81] of 16 cases of DLBCL-LT and 17 cases of cutaneous DLBCL-NOS showed that 69% of DLBCL-LT and 24% of DLBCL-NOS were double expressors, whereas DH/TH cases were 15% (5/33) of all DLBCLs and mostly DLBCL-LT type.

Studies on copy number alterations described high-level amplifications for the *BCL2* gene in 67% of cases and loss of *CDKN2A* in 23% to 42% of patients. Loss of CDKN2A expression either by gene deletion or promoter methylation correlates with an adverse prognosis.[20,74,82] miRNA studies showed that miR-20a and miR-106a were overexpressed in DLBCL-LT as compared to PCFCL.[83] Multivariate Cox analysis showed that higher miR-20a and miR-20b expression levels were associated with shorter disease-free survival (DFS) and overall survival, independent of histologic type. Gene expression profiling also showed downregulation of eight candidate target genes of miR-20a, miR-20b, and miR-106a in DLBCL-LT compared with PCFCL (*PTEN*). The oncogenic miR-17-92 cluster and its paralogs were shown to be involved in CBL progression, and it was shown that the downregulation of the target gene *PTEN* was associated with shorter DFS.

CONCLUSION

Our knowledge of the molecular basis and mutational landscape of CBL remains very limited, in great part due to the rarity of these neoplasms. Novel technologies such as next-generation sequencing of tumor cell's whole genome, or whole exome, proteomics, and transcriptome profiling using RNA-seq will help define better molecular characterization of such malignancies. However, recent studies have already shown distinctive molecular alterations that will be important to direct specific therapies in these lymphomas: perhaps an example of this is the *MYD88* mutations in DLBCL-LT. Another important recent development has been the characterization of PCMZL, differentially from other types of MALT lymphomas. The current World Health Organization classification lists PCMZL together with other subtypes of MALT lymphomas. Incorporation of the knowledge and understanding of these molecular profiles will help better define some of these uncommon subtypes of cutaneous B-cell lymphoproliferative disorders.

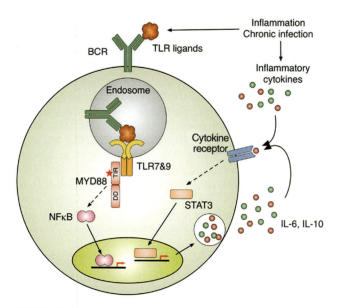

FIGURE 7-3. Inflammation induces B-cell activation. Toll-like receptor (TLR) activation by nucleic acid–protein complexes derived from inflammation and MYD88 mutation B-cell antigen receptor (BCR) delivers nucleic acid–protein complexes to TLR-containing endosomes, where MYD88 initiates the activation of intracellular signaling pathways, such as NF-κB. Intriguingly, oncogenic MYD88 mutations require intact TLR apparatuses to recognize nucleic acids. One of the potential sources for TLR ligands is nucleic acid–protein complexes derived from inflammation and chronic infection. A subset of ABC-DLBCL shows constitutive activation of JAK-STAT3 pathway, presumably due to autocrine stimulation by IL-6 and IL-10. The activation of cytokine receptor signaling can also be induced by inflammatory cytokines in the milieu of inflammation and chronic infection. (Reprinted from Wang JQ, Jeelall YS, Ferguson LL, et al. Toll-like receptors and cancer: MYD88 mutation and inflammation. *Front Immunol*. 2014;5:367, with permission.)

cutaneous DLBCLs-not otherwise specified (DLBCL-NOS), showed that 77% of DLBCL-LT harbored NF-κB-activating *MYD88* mutations and the rest had mutations in alternative NF-kB genes (*NFKBIE* or *REL*) or other canonical cancer pathways (*BRAF, MED12, PIK3R1,* and *STAT3*). Other common mutations included genes involved in immune regulation (*B2M, CIITA, HLA*) and T-cell costimulation (*CD58*). Overall, DLBCL-LT resembled other extranodal DLBCLs arising in the CNS and the testis, and nearly half-harbored *PDL1/PDL2* translocations, with overexpression of PD-L1 or PD-L2. These findings identify new treatment opportunities for these aggressive, often chemo-resistant lymphomas.

Cell of origin (COO) classification is important in the diagnosis and determination of therapeutic responses of systemic DLBCLs. Novel molecular studies in DLBCL-LT have shown that using the Hans immunohistochemical algorithm, 75% of the DLBCL-LT patients classified as non-GCB and 25% as GCB, while Lymph2C x (NanoString) classified only 18% as ABC, 43% as unclassified/intermediate, and 39% as GCB. These COO subgroups did not differ in the expression of BCL2 and IgM, mutations in *MYD88* and/or *CD79B*, loss of *CDKN2A*, or survival.[80]

Using FISH, a split of *BCL2, BCL6,* or *MYC* in 1/23, 6/23, and 3/23 of cases of DLBCL-LT has been observed, respectively.[74] *CDKN2A* deletion was detected by FISH in only 5/23 of cases. *BLIMP1* and/or 6q deletion was observed at a higher rate in 10/20 of cases. No correlation between rearrangement and immunohistochemical expression was

References

1. Vermeer MH, Willemze R. Recent advances in primary cutaneous B-cell lymphomas. *Curr Opin Oncol*. 2014;26(2):230-236.
2. Tyler KH, Haverkos BM, Hastings J, et al. The role of an integrated multidisciplinary clinic in the management of patients with cutaneous lymphoma. *Front Oncol*. 2015;5:136.
3. Jaffe ES. Navigating the cutaneous B-cell lymphomas: avoiding the rocky shoals. *Mod Pathol*. 2020;33(suppl 1):96-106.
4. Sokol L, Naghashpour M, Glass LF. Primary cutaneous B-cell lymphomas: recent advances in diagnosis and management. *Cancer Control*. 2012;19(3):236-244.
5. Willemze R. Thirty years of progress in cutaneous lymphoma research. *G Ital Dermatol Venereol*. 2012;147(6):515-521.
6. Kodama K, Massone C, Chott A, et al. Primary cutaneous large B-cell lymphomas: clinicopathologic features, classification,

and prognostic factors in a large series of patients. *Blood.* 2005;106(7):2491-2497.
7. Pileri A Jr, Patrizi A, Agostinelli C, et al. Primary cutaneous lymphomas: a reprisal. *Semin Diagn Pathol.* 2011;28(3):214-233.
8. Pham-Ledard A, Cowppli-Bony A, Doussau A, et al. Diagnostic and prognostic value of BCL2 rearrangement in 53 patients with follicular lymphoma presenting as primary skin lesions. *Am J Clin Pathol.* 2015;143(3):362-373.
9. Cerroni L, Wiesner T. Cutaneous lymphomas: from morphology to chip technology. *Actas Dermosifiliogr.* 2009;100(suppl 1):3-17.
10. Child FJ, Russell-Jones R, Calonje E, et al. Molecular genetic characterization of primary cutaneous B-cell lymphomas. *Am J Surg Pathol.* 2001;25(4):538-539.
11. Delia D, Borrello MG, Berti E, et al. Clonal immunoglobulin gene rearrangements and normal T-cell receptor, bcl-2, and c-myc genes in primary cutaneous B-cell lymphomas. *Cancer Res.* 1989;49(17):4901-4905.
12. Felcht M, Booken N, Stroebel P, et al. The value of molecular diagnostics in primary cutaneous B-cell lymphomas in the context of clinical findings, histology, and immunohistochemistry. *J Am Acad Dermatol.* 2011;64(1):135-143, e131-e134.
13. Gellrich S, Rutz S, Golembowski S, et al. Primary cutaneous follicle center cell lymphomas and large B cell lymphomas of the leg descend from germinal center cells. A single cell polymerase chain reaction analysis. *J Invest Dermatol.* 2001;117(6):1512-1520.
14. Schafernak KT, Variakojis D, Goolsby CL, et al. Clonality assessment of cutaneous B-cell lymphoid proliferations: a comparison of flow cytometry immunophenotyping, molecular studies, and immunohistochemistry/in situ hybridization and review of the literature. *Am J Dermatopathol.* 2014;36(10):781-795.
15. Cerroni L, Minkus G, Putz B, et al. Laser beam microdissection in the diagnosis of cutaneous B-cell lymphoma. *Br J Dermatol.* 1997;136(5):743-746.
16. Hoefnagel JJ, Dijkman R, Basso K, et al. Distinct types of primary cutaneous large B-cell lymphoma identified by gene expression profiling. *Blood.* 2005;105(9):3671-3678.
17. Wright G, Tan B, Rosenwald A, et al. A gene expression-based method to diagnose clinically distinct subgroups of diffuse large B cell lymphoma. *Proc Natl Acad Sci U S A.* 2003;100(17):9991-9996.
18. Chen T, Lee TR, Liang WG, et al. Identification of trypsin-inhibitory site and structure determination of human SPINK2 serine proteinase inhibitor. *Proteins.* 2009;77(1):209-219.
19. Belaud-Rotureau MA, Marietta V, Vergier B, et al. Inactivation of p16INK4a/CDKN2A gene may be a diagnostic feature of large B cell lymphoma leg type among cutaneous B cell lymphomas. *Virchows Arch.* 2008;452(6):607-620.
20. Dijkman R, Tensen CP, Jordanova ES, et al. Array-based comparative genomic hybridization analysis reveals recurrent chromosomal alterations and prognostic parameters in primary cutaneous large B-cell lymphoma. *J Clin Oncol.* 2006;24(2):296-305.
21. Dijkman R, Tensen CP, Buettner M, et al. Primary cutaneous follicle center lymphoma and primary cutaneous large B-cell lymphoma, leg type, are both targeted by aberrant somatic hypermutation but demonstrate differential expression of AID. *Blood.* 2006;107(12):4926-4929.
22. Perez M, Pacchiarotti A, Frontani M, et al. Primary cutaneous B-cell lymphoma is associated with somatically hypermutated immunoglobulin variable genes and frequent use of VH1-69 and VH4-59 segments. *Br J Dermatol.* 2010;162(3):611-618.
23. Xiaolong AZ, Yang J, Ringbloom KG, et al. Genomic landscape of cutaneous follicular lymphomas reveals 2 subgroups with clinically predictive molecular features. *Blood Adv.* 2021;5(3):649-661. doi:10.1182/bloodadvances.2020002469.
24. Barasch NJK, Liu YC, Ho J, et al. The molecular landscape and other distinctive features of primary cutaneous follicle center lymphoma. *Hum Pathol.* 2020;106:93-105.
25. Koens L, Qin Y, Leung WY, et al. MicroRNA profiling of primary cutaneous large B-cell lymphomas. *PLoS One.* 2013;8(12):e82471.
26. Abdul-Wahab A, Tang SY, Robson A, et al. Chromosomal anomalies in primary cutaneous follicle center cell lymphoma do not portend a poor prognosis. *J Am Acad Dermatol.* 2014;70(6):1010-1020.
27. Bergman R, Kurtin PJ, Gibson LE, et al. Clinicopathologic, immunophenotypic, and molecular characterization of primary cutaneous follicular B-cell lymphoma. *Arch Dermatol.* 2001;137(4):432-439.
28. Kim BK, Surti U, Pandya A, et al. Clinicopathologic, immunophenotypic, and molecular cytogenetic fluorescence in situ hybridization analysis of primary and secondary cutaneous follicular lymphomas. *Am J Surg Pathol.* 2005;29(1):69-82.
29. Mirza I, Macpherson N, Paproski S, et al. Primary cutaneous follicular lymphoma: an assessment of clinical, histopathologic, immunophenotypic, and molecular features. *J Clin Oncol.* 2002;20(3):647-655.
30. Franco R, Fernandez-Vazquez A, Rodriguez-Peralto JL, et al. Cutaneous follicular B-cell lymphoma: description of a series of 18 cases. *Am J Surg Pathol.* 2001;25(7):875-883.
31. Goodlad JR, Krajewski AS, Batstone PJ, et al. Primary cutaneous follicular lymphoma: a clinicopathologic and molecular study of 16 cases in support of a distinct entity. *Am J Surg Pathol.* 2002;26(6):733-741.
32. Hallermann C, Kaune KM, Gesk S, et al. Molecular cytogenetic analysis of chromosomal breakpoints in the IGH, MYC, BCL6, and MALT1 gene loci in primary cutaneous B-cell lymphomas. *J Invest Dermatol.* 2004;123(1):213-219.
33. Leinweber B, Colli C, Chott A, et al. Differential diagnosis of cutaneous infiltrates of B lymphocytes with follicular growth pattern. *Am J Dermatopathol.* 2004;26(1):4-13.
34. Jelic TM, Berry PK, Jubelirer SJ, et al. Primary cutaneous follicle center lymphoma of the arm with a novel chromosomal translocation t(12;21)(q13;q22): a case report. *Am J Hematol.* 2006;81(6):448-453.
35. Subramaniyam S, Magro CM, Gogineni S, et al. Primary cutaneous follicle center lymphoma associated with an extracutaneous dissemination: a cytogenetic finding of potential prognostic value. *Am J Clin Pathol.* 2015;144(5):805-810.
36. Cho-Vega JH, Vega F, Rassidakis G, et al. Primary cutaneous marginal zone B-cell lymphoma. *Am J Clin Pathol.* 2006;125(suppl):S38-S49.
37. Servitje O, Gallardo F, Estrach T, et al. Primary cutaneous marginal zone B-cell lymphoma: a clinical, histopathological, immunophenotypic and molecular genetic study of 22 cases. *Br J Dermatol.* 2002;147(6):1147-1158.
38. Gallardo F, Pujol RM, Bellosillo B, et al. Primary cutaneous B-cell lymphcoma (marginal zone) with prominent T-cell component and aberrant dual (T and B) genotype; diagnostic usefulness of laser-capture microdissection. *Br J Dermatol.* 2006;154(1):162-166.

39. Colli C, Leinweber B, Mullegger R, et al. Borrelia burgdorferi-associated lymphocytoma cutis: clinicopathologic, immunophenotypic, and molecular study of 106 cases. *J Cutan Pathol.* 2004;31(3):232-240.
40. Pimpinelli N. New aspects in the biology of cutaneous B-cell lymphomas. *J Cutan Pathol.* 2006;33(suppl 1):6-9.
41. Good DJ, Gascoyne RD. Atypical lymphoid hyperplasia mimicking lymphoma. *Hematol Oncol Clin N Am.* 2009;23(4):729-745.
42. Ponzoni M, Ferreri AJ, Mappa S, et al. Prevalence of Borrelia burgdorferi infection in a series of 98 primary cutaneous lymphomas. *Oncologist.* 2011;16(11):1582-1588.
43. Guitart J. Rethinking primary cutaneous marginal zone lymphoma: shifting the focus to the cause of the infiltrate. *J Cutan Pathol.* 2015;42(9):600-603.
44. Bahler DW, Kim BK, Gao A, et al. Analysis of immunoglobulin V genes suggests cutaneous marginal zone B-cell lymphomas recognise similar antigens. *Br J Haematol.* 2006;132(5):571-575.
45. Bortoletto G, Gerotto M, Pigozzi B, et al. Analysis of immunoglobulin variable kappa gene mutations in cutaneous B-cell lymphoma. *J Dermatol Sci.* 2007;47(3):248-252.
46. Deutsch AJ, Fruhwirth M, Aigelsreiter A, et al. Primary cutaneous marginal zone B-cell lymphomas are targeted by aberrant somatic hypermutation. *J Invest Dermatol.* 2009;129(2):476-479.
47. Ge Y, Takino H, Sato F, et al. Distinctive immunoglobulin VH gene features of cutaneous marginal zone lymphomas in Asian cases. *Br J Dermatol.* 2014;170(3):735-737.
48. Christie LJ, MacKenzie C, Palmer TJ, et al. Type and maturational status of dendritic cells in cutaneous B cell lymphoproliferative disorders. *Histopathology.* 2011;59(3):421-432.
49. Edinger JT, Kant JA, Swerdlow SH. Cutaneous marginal zone lymphomas have distinctive features and include 2 subsets. *Am J Surg Pathol.* 2010;34(12):1830-1841.
50. van Maldegem F, van Dijk R, Wormhoudt TA, et al. The majority of cutaneous marginal zone B-cell lymphomas expresses class-switched immunoglobulins and develops in a T-helper type 2 inflammatory environment. *Blood.* 2008;112(8):3355-3361.
51. Schreuder MI, Hoefnagel JJ, Jansen PM, et al. FISH analysis of MALT lymphoma-specific translocations and aneuploidy in primary cutaneous marginal zone lymphoma. *J Pathol.* 2005;205(3):302-310.
52. de la Fouchardiere A, Gazzo S, Balme B, et al. Cytogenetic and molecular analysis of 12 cases of primary cutaneous marginal zone lymphomas. *Am J Dermatopathol.* 2006;28(4):287-292.
53. Takino H, Li C, Hu S, et al. Primary cutaneous marginal zone B-cell lymphoma: a molecular and clinicopathological study of cases from Asia, Germany, and the United States. *Mod Pathol.* 2008;21(12):1517-1526.
54. Cohen O, Feinstein E, Kimchi A. DAP-kinase is a Ca2+/calmodulin-dependent, cytoskeletal-associated protein kinase, with cell death-inducing functions that depend on its catalytic activity. *EMBO J.* 1997;16(5):998-1008.
55. Deiss LP, Feinstein E, Berissi H, et al. Identification of a novel serine/threonine kinase and a novel 15-kD protein as potential mediators of the gamma interferon-induced cell death. *Genes Dev.* 1995;9(1):15-30.
56. Kamb A, Gruis NA, Weaver-Feldhaus J, et al. A cell cycle regulator potentially involved in genesis of many tumor types. *Science.* 1994;264(5157):436-440.
57. Lukas J, Parry D, Aagaard L, et al. Retinoblastoma-protein-dependent cell-cycle inhibition by the tumour suppressor p16. *Nature.* 1995;375(6531):503-506.
58. Serrano M, Hannon GJ, Beach D. A new regulatory motif in cell-cycle control causing specific inhibition of cyclin D/CDK4. *Nature.* 1993;366(6456):704-707.
59. Martinez-Lopez A, Curiel-Olmo S, Mollejo M, et al. MYD88 (L265P) somatic mutation in marginal zone B-cell lymphoma. *Am J Surg Pathol.* 2015;39(5):644-651.
60. Monsalvez V, Montes-Moreno S, Artiga MJ, et al. MicroRNAs as prognostic markers in indolent primary cutaneous B-cell lymphoma. *Mod Pathol.* 2013;26(2):171-181.
61. Maurus K, Appenzeller S, Roth S, et al. Panel sequencing shows recurrent genetic FAS alterations in primary cutaneous marginal zone lymphoma. *J Invest Dermatol.* 2018;138(7):1573-1581.
62. Arjyal L, Giri M, Uprety D, et al. Primary cutaneous diffuse large B cell lymphoma-leg type in United States: epidemiology and survival outcome. *Blood.* 2019;134(suppl 1):2202.
63. Espinet B, Garcia-Herrera A, Gallardo F, et al. FOXP1 molecular cytogenetics and protein expression analyses in primary cutaneous large B cell lymphoma, leg-type. *Histol Histopathol.* 2011;26(2):213-221.
64. Robson A, Shukur Z, Ally M, et al. Immunocytochemical p63 expression discriminates between primary cutaneous follicle centre cell and diffuse large B-cell lymphoma-leg type, and is of the TAp63 isoform. *Histopathology.* Published online September 02, 2015. doi:10.1111/his.12855
65. Hoefnagel JJ, Mulder MM, Dreef E, et al. Expression of B-cell transcription factors in primary cutaneous B-cell lymphoma. *Mod Pathol.* 2006;19(9):1270-1276.
66. Mao X, Lillington D, Child F, et al. Comparative genomic hybridization analysis of primary cutaneous B-cell lymphomas: identification of common genomic alterations in disease pathogenesis. *Genes Chromosomes Cancer.* 2002;35(2):144-155.
67. Akasaka T, Akasaka H, Ueda C, et al. Molecular and clinical features of non-Burkitt's, diffuse large-cell lymphoma of B-cell type associated with the c-MYC/immunoglobulin heavy-chain fusion gene. *J Clin Oncol.* 2000;18(3):510-518.
68. Mondello P, Cuzzocrea S, Mian M. Pim kinases in hematological malignancies: where are we now and where are we going? *J Hematol Oncol.* 2014;7:95.
69. Pasqualucci L, Migliazza A, Basso K, et al. Mutations of the BCL6 proto-oncogene disrupt its negative autoregulation in diffuse large B-cell lymphoma. *Blood.* 2003;101(8):2914-2923.
70. Paulli M, Viglio A, Vivenza D, et al. Primary cutaneous large B-cell lymphoma of the leg: histogenetic analysis of a controversial clinicopathologic entity. *Hum Pathol.* 2002;33(9):937-943.
71. Shaffer AL, Yu X, He Y, et al. BCL-6 represses genes that function in lymphocyte differentiation, inflammation, and cell cycle control. *Immunity.* 2000;13(2):199-212.
72. Mittrucker HW, Matsuyama T, Grossman A, et al. Requirement for the transcription factor LSIRF/IRF4 for mature B and T lymphocyte function. *Science.* 1997;275(5299):540-543.
73. Pham-Ledard A, Beylot-Barry M, Barbe C, et al. High frequency and clinical prognostic value of MYD88 L265P mutation in primary cutaneous diffuse large B-cell lymphoma, leg-type. *JAMA Dermatol.* 2014;150(11):1173-1179.
74. Pham-Ledard A, Prochazkova-Carlotti M, Andrique L, et al. Multiple genetic alterations in primary cutaneous large B-cell lymphoma, leg type support a common lymphomagenesis with activated B-cell-like diffuse large B-cell lymphoma. *Mod Pathol.* 2014;27(3):402-411.

75. Koens L, Zoutman WH, Ngarmlertsirichai P, et al. Nuclear factor-kappaB pathway-activating gene aberrancies in primary cutaneous large B-cell lymphoma, leg type. *J Invest Dermatol.* 2014;134(1):290-292.
76. Ngo VN, Young RM, Schmitz R, et al. Oncogenically active MYD88 mutations in human lymphoma. *Nature.* 2011;470(7332):115-119.
77. Treon SP, Tripsas CK, Meid K, et al. Ibrutinib in previously treated Waldenstrom's macroglobulinemia. *N Engl J Med.* 2015;372(15):1430-1440.
78. Wilson WH, Young RM, Schmitz R, et al. Targeting B cell receptor signaling with ibrutinib in diffuse large B cell lymphoma. *Nat Med.* 2015;21(8):922-926.
79. Zhou XA, Louissaint A Jr, Wenzel A, et al. Genomic analyses identify recurrent alterations in immune evasion genes in diffuse large B-cell lymphoma, leg type. *J Invest Dermatol.* 2018;138(11):2365-2376.
80. Schrader AMR, de Groen RAL, Willemze R, et al. Cell-of-origin classification using the Hans and Lymph2Cx algorithms in primary cutaneous large B-cell lymphomas. *Virchows Arch.* 2022;480(3):667-675.
81. Lucioni M, Pescia C, Bonometti A, et al. Double expressor and double/triple hit status among primary cutaneous diffuse large B-cell lymphoma: a comparison between leg type and not otherwise specified subtypes. *Hum Pathol.* 2021;111:1-9.
82. Senff NJ, Zoutman WH, Vermeer MH, et al. Fine-mapping chromosomal loss at 9p21: correlation with prognosis in primary cutaneous diffuse large B-cell lymphoma, leg type. *J Invest Dermatol.* 2009;129(5):1149-1155.
83. Battistella M, Romero M, Castro-Vega LJ, et al. The high expression of the microRNA 17-92 cluster and its paralogs, and the downregulation of the target gene PTEN, is associated with primary cutaneous b-cell lymphoma progression. *J Invest Dermatol.* 2015;135(6):1659-1667.

PART II LABORATORY TECHNIQUES

CHAPTER 8

Flow cytometric analysis in hematopathology diagnosis

Safa Najidh, Julia Almeida, Jacques J. M. van Dongen, and Maarten H. Vermeer

Flow cytometry (FC) is a well-established technology in clinical diagnostics of hematopathology, particularly hematological malignancies. It is a powerful tool that is used for the identification, quantitation, and characterization of normal and neoplastic hematopoietic cells in a variety of samples and, consequently, has acquired a prominent position in the current World Health Organization (WHO) classification of hematological malignancies.

This chapter will briefly describe the basic technical concept of flow cytometric analysis, explain the limitations and potential pitfalls of this method, and provide a general outline of flow cytometric markers that are currently used in the diagnosis of hematopoietic malignancies, with particular focus on cutaneous lymphoproliferative disorders.

FLOW CYTOMETRIC ANALYSIS INSTRUMENTATION

Flow cytometric analyzers are instruments that are designed to measure (metry) properties of cells (cyto) that flow suspended in liquid media (flow). Flow cytometric instruments comprise a fluidics system, optic system, signal detection system, and a computer equipped with software that controls instrument functions, data acquisition, and data analysis.

Fluidics

The fluidics system is a network of pumps, valves, tubes, and flow cell, which are all designed to deliver a single file of cells to the interrogation point in the flow chamber. The single filing of the cells is achieved by hydrodynamic focusing where a suspension of cells (sample stream) is injected into the center of a stream of sheath fluid (usually a buffered salt-based solution) flowing through a specially designed, funnel-like, flow chamber that produces laminar flow. The shape of flow cell and differences in pressures between sheet fluid (outer layer) and sample stream (centrally located) are optimized to assure that the diameter of the sample stream is no wider than the single-cell it contains, forcing cells to flow in a single file through the center of the interrogation point (Fig. 8-1). The flow of sheath fluid accelerates the particles and restricts them to the center of the sample core. This process is known as hydrodynamic focusing. Increasing the sample pressure increases the flow rate by increasing the width of the sample core. This, in turn, allows more cells to enter the stream within a given moment. With a wider sample core, some cells could pass through the laser beam off-center and intercept the laser beam at a less optimal angle. However, this might be appropriate for your application. Proper operation of fluidic components is critical for particles to properly intercept the laser beam.

Optics

The optical system comprises three major components; an excitation light source (lasers), light "handling system," and a detection system.

Light Sources

Current clinical FC instruments use low-power lasers and/or laser diodes as light sources. The light generated by these sources is monochromatic (of exact single wavelength/color) and coherent (all waves of light are parallel), allowing for the generation of a very fine light beam of desired intensity. Traditional routine flow cytometers are often equipped with three or more lasers, allowing for the generation of several different wavelength beams that can simultaneously excite a large number of different fluorochromes. The most common lasers used in traditional flow cytometers are 488 nm (blue), 405 nm (violet), 532 nm (green), 552 nm (green), 561 nm (green-yellow), 640 nm (red), and 355 nm (ultraviolet). The point at which the light beam(s) intersects with the stream of cells within the flow chamber is called the interrogation point (Fig. 8-1). As expected, the precise alignment of the laser beam with the sample stream is critical for optimal performance of a flow cytometer.

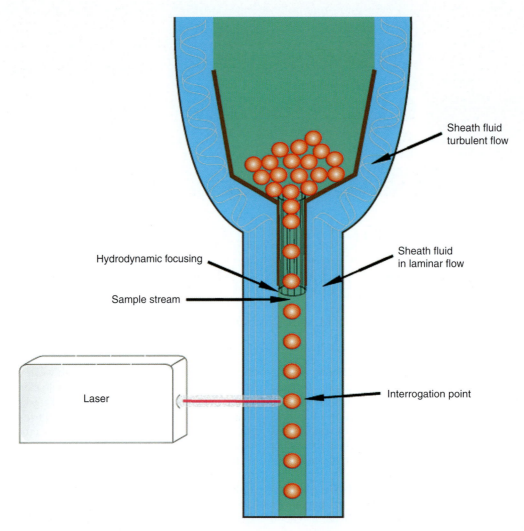

FIGURE 8-1. **Schematic representation of a flow cell.** A mixture of cells suspended in isotonic solution is injected into the stream of sheath fluid that, under conditions of hydrodynamic focusing (dictated by the shape of flow cells), forces a stream of cells to flow in a single cell file through the center of the interrogation point (the point where cells intersect a beam of laser light).

Light Handling System

The interaction of the light beam with each cell in the sample stream, at the interrogation point, results in light scatter. In addition, if a cell was stained with a fluorochrome(s), the laser beam will induce fluorescence. Both scattered light (at the wavelength of the laser) and fluorescent light (wavelength specific for fluorochrome) are emitted at 360° in a spherical fashion. To increase sensitivity and light collection efficiency, all modern flow cytometers' light handling system comprising lenses, dichroic mirrors, and band-pass filters is linked to the flow chamber at the interrogation point via a network of optic fibers. Through this system, light signals from each cell are selectively distributed to an array of photodetectors (Fig. 8-2).

Detection System

The photodetectors convert light (signal photons from scattered light or fluorescence) into electric current that is proportional to the number of photons reaching the detector and thus the intensity of the light signal for each cell. By adjusting the voltage of each photo element, their light-measuring sensitivity can be tuned up or down to assure optimal signal capture for each cell. The color of light that is delivered to a given photodetector is dictated by band-pass filters placed in the light path leading to a given detector. As a result, each detector can measure only a single color of light and is blinded to the rest of light signal generated by the analyzed cell. This combination of optic fiber, band-pass filters, and an array of detectors allows measurement of simultaneously emitted multicolored signals from each analyzed cell. The resulting pulse is transferred to the electronic system, where it is digitized and recorded for analysis. Measured light is transformed into quantifiable separate color information. As a result, depending on the FC type, commonly up to 12 different antigens (colors) can be measured on each cell at once in a highly precise and quantitative fashion. Advanced ≥20-color flow cytometers are currently becoming commercially available.

There are several fluorescence detectors that can be used on a FC, the most common types are the photomultiplier tubes (PMTs) and photodiodes (PDs). Some new-generation flow cytometers have replaced PMTs with solid-state detectors such as avalanche photodiodes (APDs) for fluorescence detection. APDs are less expensive, highly linear, and more

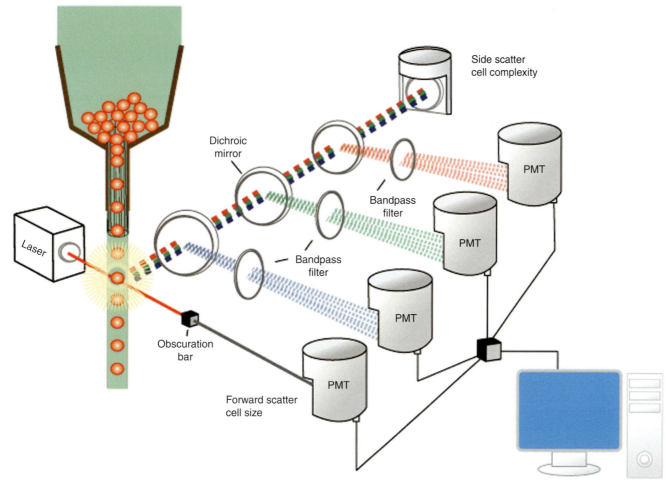

FIGURE 8-2. Schematic representation of a flow cytometer. Each cell passing through the interrogation point intersects a beam of laser light. Cells absorb, diffract, reflect, and scatter laser light according to their size and complexity. In addition, laser light induces fluorescence in colors corresponding to labeled antibodies that detect antigens expressed by a given cell subset. Strategically placed photomultiplier tubes (PMT) measure forward-scattered light (cell's size), side-scattered light (cell complexity), and fluorescence light (in colors dictated by band-pass filters). Each flow cytometry (FC) color represents a different fluorochrome label of specific antibody that is measured by just one PMT. PMTs convert photons into electric current that is proportional to each measured light signal. Data are integrated by a computer program and displayed in the form of flow plots.

sensitive, capable of detecting long-wavelength emissions (>650 nm) in the long red region. Silicon photomultipliers are another promising option as solid-state detectors.[1]

COMPUTER SYSTEM

Current FC instruments are operated via complex software packages that include instrument operation software that controls fluidics, light source, and detection systems' voltages and signal compensation. The electronic system converts scattered and emitted light signals from the detectors into electronic signals that can be read and stored by a computer system. Generally, in FC, a particle is sent to waste after it passes the laser beam. For some FC instruments with a cell sorting capacity, the electronics system is also capable of separating particles (by charging and deflecting cells) according to assigned immunophenotypic characteristics by user, thereby collecting purified samples for further analysis. Flow cytometric data are stored according to the flow cytometry standard (FCS) format, which is developed by the Society for Analytical Cytology. According to the FCS, a data storage file includes a description of the sample, the FC instrument on which the data were collected, the data set, and the results of data analysis.

All raw data from each sample are saved in a highly standardized universal format known as list mode data. Stored list mode data allow for future reanalysis with adjustments to gating strategy and certain parameters such as compensation. List mode data are also very useful for comparison between specimens from different samples for the same patient, for purposes such as detection of minimal residual disease. A separate part of the software is designed for daily instrument quality assurance (QA) monitoring that assures optimal performance of fluidics, light, and detection systems. Part of this program keeps track of daily QA activities and performance. Each instrument is also equipped with software that keeps track of sample demographics, sample acquisition, data analysis, and data reporting. In general, each major FC manufacturer provides software packages optimized for their instrument. Such packages are often Food and Drug Administration (FDA)-approved and depending on specific application may require the use of kits of reagents and flow protocol. The best examples of such kit software instrument FDA-approved combinations are T-cell subsets and stem cell quantification packages. For interpretative FC in hematopathology, the rules are less strict, and as long as proper test validation is performed, laboratories may use a combination of methods, reagents, and software of their choice.

New-Generation Advanced Flow Cytometers

FC technology is evolving rapidly. In the last decade, new-generation FCs have been launched with improved processing power while not compromising on data quality and data comparability. The most important technical breakthrough involved the incorporation of additional lasers (up to 10 lasers) and the replacement of PMTs by ADPs, having a profound impact on acquisition velocity (up to 100,000 events/second) and detection sensitivity (≥20 fluorescent parameters). Other technological advancements include the enhanced optical configurations, improved fluidics system, and more sensitive electronics. The development of new fluorochromes and, consequently, the wider selection of commercially available antibodies[2] together with the advent of spectral detectors have further attributed to the analytical potential of FC instruments.

While certain hematological malignancies are immunophenotypically well defined others are more heterogeneous and thus more complicated to comprehend with limited FC capacity. To resolve these more complex disease entities, advanced FC is being adopted by many laboratories and has established their added value in hematological research field. The implementation of such advanced technology in routine diagnostic laboratories will maximize analytic power and also facilitate rare tumor cell detection, especially in diagnostic or minimal residual disease settings.[3]

CELL CHARACTERISTICS MEASURED BY FLOW CYTOMETRIC ANALYSIS

Intrinsic Cell Properties

Several cell characteristics can be measured without the need for additional reagents. Most important are the cell size (FSC, forward scatter) and cell complexity (SSC, side scatter), which are measured by the interference in the horizontal path of visible light and associated with the refractive index in every interface of the analyzed event. These two intrinsic properties of cells are routinely measured during FC analysis.

Light scattering occurs when a particle deflects incident laser light. The extent to which this occurs depends on the physical properties of a particle, namely, its size and internal complexity. Factors that affect light scattering are the cell's membrane, nucleus, and any granular material inside the cell. Cell shape and surface topography also contribute to the total light scatter.

Forward Scatter

When a cell flows through the interrogation point and is hit by the light beam, it produces light beam absorption, reflection, diffraction, and scatter at a 360-degree angle.

A photo-element that is placed in the direct path of the laser beam is charged with a collection of light scattered along the axis of the laser beam, so-called FSC. Forward-scattered light is proportional to cell-surface area or size; a small cell produces a low FSC signal, the bigger the cell, the more the light that is scattered and the stronger the FSC signal. For example, lymphocytes that are small will produce a low FSC signal and monocytes/macrophages that are large in size will produce a strong FSC signal (Fig. 8-3).

Side Scatter

SSC is proportional to cell granularity or internal complexity. Different types of cells show differences in complexity of cell surface and internal structures. These differences are reflected by the amount of scattered light that can be measured by a photo-element that is placed at a 90-degree angle in relation to the laser beam. Light beam interaction with complex cells such as hairy cells (extensive ruffling of cell surface) or granulocytes (complex internal structures) will scatter intensely and produce a strong SSC signal. In contrast, a light beam interacting with low-complexity cells such as lymphocytes scatters less intensely and produces a low SSC signal (Fig. 8-3).

The combination of FSC and SSC parameters helps to stratify a mixed population of cells into subsets representing red blood cells, lymphocytes, monocytes, granulocytes, and platelets with good accuracy (Fig. 8-3). These parameters are also of help in distinguishing neoplastic cell populations that may show deviation from the normal ranges in FSC and SSC.

Extrinsic Cell Properties

Cell parameters that can be measured by FC with use of additional reagents such as monoclonal antibodies, DNA-binding dyes, cytoplasmic dyes, and other more specialized dyes are termed extrinsic cell properties.

Immunophenotype Characterization

Flow cytometric immunophenotyping is the most used application in FC. By adding fluorescent labeling, FC can provide information on the functional characteristics of cells. The addition of antigen-specific monoclonal antibodies (and in some cases, polyclonal antibodies) is the extrinsic property most commonly measured in clinical FC. The development of monoclonal antibodies (mAbs) that specifically recognize unique epitopes on antigens expressed on cell surface, antigens in the cell cytoplasm, and antigens in the nuclei allows for the detailed characterization of the antigenic makeup of each cell. Monoclonal antibodies are conjugated to different fluorochromes. The fluorochromes are dyes, which when excited with laser light, rapidly absorb laser light energy and emit light with lower energy that is specific for a given fluorochrome. Thus, a single laser can simultaneously induce fluorescence from a different combination of dyes that will produce several distinct fluorescence signals. These signals are then captured by designated photo-elements that recognize only a single color of fluorescent light and are "blinded" for all other colors. Photo elements transform the intensity of captured light into a digital signal that is proportional to the intensity of fluorescence emitted by each cell passing through the interrogation point. These peak emission wavelengths are far enough apart so that each signal can be detected by a separate detector.

The number of parameters than can be measured is limited by the availability of distinct fluorescent markers and the FC specifics (eg, number and types of lasers and detectors). Current (traditional) clinical FC instruments can simultaneously characterize up to 12 to 14 fluorescence signals for each cell passing through the interrogation point, allowing for high-density characterization of a cell's immunophenotype. New-generation flow cytometers enable the simultaneous measurement of ≥20 colors at a higher event rate (up to 100,000 cells per second) but are mostly used in research settings.

In its simplest form, an immunophenotyping experiment consists of cells stained with fluorochrome-conjugated mAbs that are targeted against antigens on the cell surface. Most of the antigens that are expressed on immune cells and define specific cell populations to a lineage are designated cluster of differentiation (CD) numbers by the Human Cell Differentiation Molecules organization (http://www.hcdm.org/). To date, there are currently over 400 CD molecules for which mAbs are commercially available for FC application. For example, T-helper cells express CD3 and CD4 antigens and are negative for the expression of CD8 and CD19. When these cells are stained with a combination of antibodies for CD3 APC, CD4 PB, CD8 FITC, and CD19 PECY7, they will produce a positive signal for CD3 and CD4 and will have

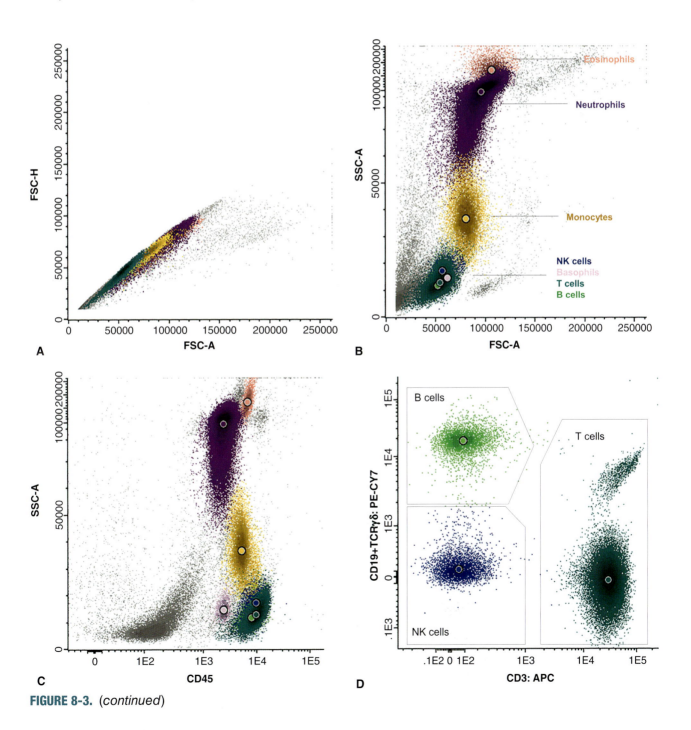

FIGURE 8-3. (*continued*)

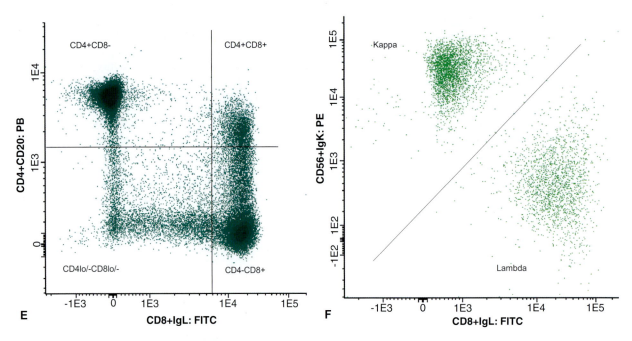

FIGURE 8-3. These graphs are based on a peripheral blood sample obtained from an adult healthy individual, stained with EuroFlow Lymphoid Screening Tube and analyzed by InfinicytTM software (Cytognos, Salamanca, Spain), and A-B represent intrinsic properties of cells by forward scatter (FSC) and side scatter (SSC) plot on a linear scale. FSC light signal is proportional to the cell size; the larger the cell the stronger the FSC signal. SSC light signal is proportional to the cell complexity; the more complex the cells (due to cytoplasmic granules, nuclear irregularities of cell membrane projections), the stronger the SSC signal. Displayed are lymphocytes (NK cells, B cells, T cells) and basophils (small cell size and low complexity cells), which show low FSC and SSC signals; monocytes (larger cell size and more complex cells), which show moderate FSC and SSC signals; granulocytes (neutrophils and eosinophils; large cell size and very complex cells), which show high FSC and SSC signals. **C.** Two-dimensional dot plot representing a combination of extrinsic properties of cells (intensity of CD45 staining) and intrinsic properties of cells (complexity) as SSC characteristics. The plot shows a population of lymphocytes and basophils characterized by strong CD45 staining and low complexity (low SSC), monocytes characterized by strong to moderate CD45 staining and moderate complexity (moderate SSC), and granulocytes (neutrophils and eosinophils) characterized by dim CD45 and high complexity (high SSC). **D.** Quadrants display double-negative cells in the left lower quadrant (NK cells; CD3-CD19-), left upper quadrant (B cells; CD3-CD19+), and right quadrant (T cells; CD3+CD19-) by extrinsic properties of cells by staining CD3 antigen (as measured by APC fluorescence) and CD19 antigen (PECy7). **E.** (Pregated) T cells are further classified depending on the expression patterns of CD4 antigen (Pacific Blue) and CD8 (FITC). Based on these plots, it can be concluded that this sample has normal CD4:CD8 ratio. **F.** (Pregated) B-cells subdivided in surface membrane IgKappa and IgLambda showing a normal polyclonal distribution. Abbreviations: APC, allophycocyanin; FITC, fluorescein isothiocyanate; PB, pacific blue; PE, phycoerythrin; PECy7, phycoerythrin-cyanin 7.

a negative signal for CD8 and CD19 (Fig. 8-3),[4] while B cells and NK cells are characterized by CD3-CD19+ and CD3-CD19- phenotypes, respectively. All circulating lymphocytes and granulocytes are positive for CD45, although with different intensities.

In addition to lineage markers that define populations of cells, other markers are used to further characterize each cell population. These markers can include activation markers, maturation markers, and chemokine receptor markers. Often, immunophenotyping experiments also include intracellular (cytoplasmic and nuclear) markers.

Other types of extrinsic properties such as the assessment of cell viability and DNA content can also be measured by FC. Of proven clinical use are exclusion dyes such as 7AAD and Propidium Iodide that are cell membrane impermeable in viable cells and used for reliable assessment of cell viability. Using DNA-binding dyes such as 4′,6-diamidino-2-phenylindole or Hoechst 33342, FC can be used for reliable determination of DNA content to assess cell cycle and ploidy. Multiple other dyes exist, useful to measure mitochondrial function, activity of enzymes involved in cell cycle regulation, cell metabolism, and apoptosis. The use of these dyes is mostly limited to research.

SAMPLE COLLECTION, PROCESSING, AND CELL PREPARATION

Sample Collection

Successful FC requires a sufficient number of viable cells. Therefore, samples submitted for FC should be delivered to the laboratory as soon as possible following procurement. It is especially important for lymph node/solid organ biopsies since "cold ischemia" results in rapid deterioration of cell viability. Samples should preferably be freshly collected on anticoagulant for blood, bone marrow aspirates of body fluids, or chilled and sterile tissue culture media can be used for FC. The FC analysis of frozen, air dried, or fixed (formalin, alcohol, etc.) is limited by progressive cell death (mainly during thawing process) and may result in the selective loss of certain proteins and/or cell populations.

In general, liquid anticoagulated blood, bone marrow aspirates, or body fluid samples, if stored/transported in ambient temperature, should preserve sufficient viability for FC analysis, and the distribution of major cell subsets remains quite stable for up to 72 hours.[5] From moment of sample collection until sample processing, samples should be preserved at room temperature. But irrespective of storage temperature, discrimination of cell population decreases as, with time, the mean fluorescence intensity (MFI) decreases on positive cell populations and unspecific staining on negative cells increases, thereby affecting cell populations unequally. This can be explained by the fact that several blood populations, mainly of myeloid origin, have half-life times equal or shorter than 24 hours and manifests as changes in immunophenotype and an increase in doublets and debris.

Freezing cellular samples facilitates the logistics of measurement but the viability of lymph node/solid tissue samples deteriorates more rapidly due to the effect of "cold ischemia." Therefore, such samples should be stored in small fragments in culture media at 4 °C and should be delivered to flow laboratory for processing within 24 hours. Concern for cell viability should be considered in the context of biopsy scheduling to prevent prolonged specimen storage (long weekends and holidays) and transport time (remote location of flow laboratory). When unavoidable, the thawing process should be active and has to be done very rapidly.

Processing of Liquid Samples

Liquid samples such as blood, body fluids, or bone marrow aspirates containing individual cells are ideally suited for FC. Following staining with an optimally titrated combination of antibodies, the red blood cells are lysed and the samples are fixed and analyzed. Sample manipulation by density gradient centrifugation or positive adhesion selection to isolate mononuclear cells is strongly discouraged due to well-known sample bias induced by such methods. Fixation of cells has no additional beneficial effect on the stability of cell surface markers and may influence the MFI values of certain marker fluorochromes.[5] Processed samples (ready for measurement on FC) should be kept at 4 °C and analyzed by FC within 4 hours.

Processing of Lymph Node and Skin Samples

Lymph nodes and solid tissue samples such as skin require processing to release a sufficient number of viable cells. With rare exceptions, fragments of lymphoid tissue within the size of a pencil eraser should produce sufficient number of cells. To extract lymphoid cells from samples with scant stromal component rich in lymphoid or lymphoma cells, the most commonly used method is mechanical tissue disruption. The tissue is sliced into very small fragments in sterile media, gently minced, and gently filtered through a metal mesh that allows passage of single cells and minimizes the presence of cell aggregates. This method can result in the loss of some of the cells of interest, especially if the cells are large and fragile. The mechanical disruption method is not well suited for stroma-rich samples such as skin or other organs where lymphoma/leukemic cells are scant. For stroma-rich samples, enzymatic digestion with collagenase (trypsin and trypsin-like digestions should be avoided to prevent destruction of antigens) can be used with subsequent cell separation by density centrifugation. This approach is gentler and may prevent preferential loss of large fragile cells; however, due to the multiple steps used in this method, it too has limitations that can result in cell or antigenic loss. Considering these limitations for samples that may be cell-poor and stroma-rich, immunohistochemical (IHC) staining of formalin-fixed paraffin-embedded tissue sections is better suited for immunophenotypic studies than for FC analysis.

INTERPRETATION OF RESULTS

The final part of an FC experiment is data analysis. Once a data file has been saved, cell populations can be displayed in several different formats. The results of FC studies are displayed in the form of different types of plots that range in complexity from single-parameter histograms through two-dimensional dot plots to multidimensional principal component displays. In clinical FC analysis, results are most commonly displayed in the form of two-dimensional dot plots where different populations of cells are represented as dots in relation to two parameters displayed on the X and Y axes. Depending on the purpose of the analysis parameter, the axes can have linear or logarithmic scales to accommodate a wide range of antigen expression levels. Based on the dot plot cell display, cells can be classified as double negative, single positive for antigen X or Y or double positive. The location of the dots on the log scale display signifies intensity of staining for antigen X or Y. The density of the dots in a given region signifies the number of cells. Further refinement of cell classification can be achieved by demarcating the subpopulations of cells of interest by so-called gates. Gates can subdivide cells according to the intensity of expressed antigens. Using gates, different subsets of cells can be tracked between different dot plots allowing integration of antigen expression patterns based on multiple plots, representing different antigens. Furthermore, logical sequential gating enables stepwise elimination of some population of cells and enrichment for cells of interest based on specific complex immunophenotypic profiles. The type and intensity of expressed antigens allow for determination of cell type (B cell, plasma cell, T cell, NK cell, myeloid cell, monocyte, etc.), their maturation status, and immunophenotypic abnormalities. The resulting multiparametric flow data (called immunophenotype) are used to diagnose specific types and subtypes of hematopoietic diseases. The process of gating (of a PB sample) is exemplified in Figure 8-3.

Recent advances in FC technology enable the simultaneous evaluation of multiple markers in a single FC measurement but is also associated with greater technical complexity, which requires novel multivariate data analysis algorithms and graphical tools for data analysis. Examples of such multidimensional analytic/visualization tools include Principal Component Analysis (PCA), Spanning-Tree Progression Analysis of Density-normalized Events (SPADE), and t-Distributed Stochastic Neighbor Embedding (tSNE) and facilitate the interpretation of complex data sets by enhancing data representation while retaining the actual measured values.[4,6]

In parallel, reference database-guided analytical algorithms of well-defined samples/cases have also been constructed for fast automated gating of the many distinct cell populations contained in an FC data file.[7-9]

Finally, despite the extensive use and widespread implementation in clinical practice, current FC protocols lack standardization both technically and in the composition of the applied antibody panels, which complicates comparability between and within laboratories. Standardization is a prerequisite for obtaining reliable and reproducible high-quality data in clinical diagnostic settings and requires the design of optimal standard operating procedures for all steps required for FC.

Immunophenotypic Profiles Used for Flow Cytometric Diagnosis of Hematopoietic Malignancies

Based on the expression of lineage-specific antigens, hematopoietic malignancies can be classified according to those of B-cell, T-cell, NK-cell, myeloid, monocytic, or histiocytic lineage. In addition, each lineage type disease can be divided into mature and immature (blastic) based on the expression of maturation antigens.[10,11]

It should be noted that certain hematological neoplasms are immunophenotypically well defined, which facilitates diagnostic routine FC. By contrast, others are more heterogeneous and require careful gating strategies. Regardless, a rational approach to differentiate neoplastic cells should be initiated with the dissection (and thereby exclusion) of normal nontransformed cell populations in specimen allowing the recognition of asynchronized and/or imbalanced representation of a particular cell population, that is, the identification of leukemia/lymphoma cells.

In difficult diagnostic cases, based on clinical and/or laboratory parameters, a suspected sample may be screened with several antibody screening panels supplemented by characterization panels for the exact classification of hematological malignancy.[12]

Flow Cytometric Analysis of B-Cell Malignancies

B-cell lineage malignancies express pan B-cell antigens, those commonly used being CD10, CD19, CD20, CD22, CD24, CD27, and CD79a.[13] CD19 is crucial as this marker is present at all stages in the life cycle of a B cell, from early progenitors through to terminally differentiated plasma cells.

Surface light chain expression is assessed by FC after the removal of circulating immunoglobulins by washing of the sample. Most mature B-cell neoplasms show restricted surface expression of immunoglobulin kappa or lambda light chain resulting in a shifted kappa:lambda ratio outside the reference range. Light chain restriction may also be observed on nonclonal reactive B-cell populations and must be interpreted with caution. B-cell malignancies with plasmacytoid differentiation, rare cases of diffuse large B-cell lymphomas, and plasma cell neoplasms are surface κ and λ negative but most often show cytoplasmic light chain restriction that can be demonstrated by staining of cells after cell membrane permeabilization.[4] The neoplastic cells in primary cutaneous follicle center lymphoma also lack expression of surface kappa and lambda light chains. In contrast, immature B-cell blasts in acute lymphoblastic lymphoma/leukemia are negative for detectable κ and λ expression for both surface and intracellular staining. In addition, immature B-cell blasts express immaturity markers including CD34 and nuclear TDT.[12]

Mature B-cell malignancies can be further subclassified based on expression of certain characteristic antigens. For example, B cells that aberrantly express T-cell antigen CD5 in the majority of cases will represent chronic lymphocytic leukemia/small lymphocytic lymphoma (CLL/SLL) or mantle cell lymphoma (MCL).[14] Therefore, detection of CD5 on B cells rapidly narrows the differential diagnosis to CLL/SLL and MCL, although atypical cases may present with weak or absent CD5 expression. Additional markers such as CD23, CD43, CD79b, and FMC7 (epitope on CD20 antigen) and careful review of intensity of staining for CD20, CD22, κ and λ light chains help to differentiate between these two entities.

CLL cases commonly present as a monoclonal accumulation of mature B lymphocytes in PB, BM, and LNs that is characterized by a homogeneous phenotypic profile with diminished expression of surface membrane Kappa or Lambda light chains, CD5 positivity, CD23 positivity, negativity or low expression of FMC7, and negativity or low expression of CD22 or CD79b (as defined by Matutes scoring system[15]). In difficult cases, additional consensus markers (CD43, CD81, CD200, CD10, and ROR1) can be used to refine the diagnosis.[16]

CLL/SLL cells are dim for CD20, CD22, CD81, CD79b, and surface immunoglobulins, but they express CD23, CD200, CD52 surface antigens while lacking FMC7. Rare IF patterns include the lack of CD23 and/or strong expression of CD20.

In contrast, MCL cells typically show bright expression of CD20, CD22, and κ or λ but are negative for CD23 and are positive for CD79b+ and FMC7+.[17] In addition, the clear absence of CD200 is a hallmark of this disease. Characteristically, CLL and MCL are almost universally negative for CD10 antigen. Detection of CD10 antigen on CD5− B cells rules out diagnosis of CLL/SLL and MCL and directs the differential diagnosis toward follicular lymphoma, diffuse large B-cell lymphoma, and Burkitt lymphoma. The expression of a unique immunophenotypic profile allows for definitive differentiation between hairy cell leukemia, which is strongly positive for CD11c+, CD25+, CD103+, CD22+, and CD123+ and shows negative staining for CD5−, CD10−, CD27−, and CD43− and very similar in terms of clinical presentation of splenic marginal zone lymphoma that is negative for CD25− and CD123− and positive for CD27+.[18]

By contrast, hairy cell leukemia neoplastic cells typically lack expression of CD43, CD5, CD10, and CD23 while remaining positive for CD11c, CD25, CD103, and CD123 and show increased surface coexpression of CD19, CD20, CD22, and FMC7.

Flow Cytometric Analysis of Plasma Cell Neoplasms

Plasma cell neoplasms (PCNs) are a group of disorders resulting from the monoclonal proliferation of neoplastic plasma cells (PCs) with indolent to aggressive disease course. PCNs include non–immunoglobulin M (IgM)-type monoclonal gammopathy of undetermined significance, myeloma, solitary plasmacytoma of bone, extraosseous plasmacytoma, monoclonal Ig deposition diseases, and PCN with associated paraneoplastic syndromes. Regardless of subtype, neoplastic PCs have distinct characteristic immunophenotypic features compared with benign (normal/reactive) PCs. Both benign and neoplastic PCs can be identified by the assessment of, at least, SSC/FSC characteristics, CD38, CD138, CD45, cytoplasmic IgKappa and/or IgLambda, CD19, CD117, and CD56 expression. Benign PCs in PB and BM are usually positive for CD19, CD27, CD45, and CD81. By contrast, neoplastic PCs are characterized by (diminished or) absent expression of CD19 (95%), CD27, CD38, CD45, and CD81 in combination with an abnormal or overexpression of CD56 (75%-80%), CD20, CD28, CD33, CD117, and CD200. Plasma cell leukemia has a less frequent expression of CD56 (negative in approximately 80%).[19]

It is important to note that plasma cells are very delicate and that many of them are lost during flow specimen processing and analysis. This often results in discrepant results of plasma cell enumeration by manual and FC methods even in liquid specimens such as blood and bone marrow aspirates with a much lower number of plasma cells detected by FCA. Loss of viable plasma cells is even more prominent in lymph nodes/solid tissue material processed by mechanical methods. For these reasons, detection and characterization of plasma cells including demonstration of light chain restriction in solid organ biopsies such as skin should be performed by IHC and in situ hybridization methods and not by FC analysis.

Flow Cytometric Analysis of Natural Killer Neoplasms

The natural killer (NK)-cell neoplasms include (nasal and extranasal) extranodal NK/T-cell lymphoma (ENKTL) and aggressive NK-cell leukemia (ANKL).[19] The most common immunophenotypic features for both types of NK-cell neoplasms include a higher FSC compared with nonneoplastic lymphocytes, in combination with consistent CD2+, membrane surface CD3−, cytoplasmic CD3ε+, and CD56+. Some cases may express CD25 or CD30. CD45 pan-leucocyte marker may be dimmer expressed on ANKL cells in half of the cases.[20] Since some T-cell neoplasms may show clinical and molecular overlapping features with NK-cell neoplasm, herein, T-cell receptors TCRαβ and TCRγδ are distinctive. Likewise, other T-cell markers CD5, CD7, CD4, and/or CD8 are negative, although CD7 and CD8 may be present in ANKL. NK cell marker CD57 is usually negative in both types, and CD16 is negative in ENKTL but positive in ANKL. The KIR (killer cell immunoglobulin-like receptor) proteins (CD158a/b/e), normally present on peripheral blood CD56dim NK cells, are mostly negative in ANKL. Overall, T-cell population can be used as an internal reference population to which neoplastic NK cells may be compared with. Nevertheless, it is important to note that the use of FC in NK-cell neoplasms is limited since neoplastic cells are usually present in low numbers especially in BM aspiration material and should therefore always be interpreted in the context of clinical and morphologic data to avoid over- or underdiagnosis based on the limited repertoire of diagnostic FC NK markers.[17] As the disease progresses, the percentage of neoplastic NK cells increases and consecutive FC analyses may be helpful when clinical suspicion remains.[20]

Flow Cytometric Diagnosis of Acute Myeloid Leukemia and Granulocytic Sarcoma

Acute myeloid leukemias (AMLs) is characterized by the clonal expansion of immature hematopoietic precursor myeloid cells. Immunophenotypic characterization of AML is typically assessed in peripheral blood and bone marrow specimens and is initiated with gating on pan-leucocyte marker CD45 in combination with SSC.[4] As opposed to lymphoblasts, myeloid blasts are commonly CD45 dim combined with a higher side scatter. AML FC antibody panel should include markers that are capable of establishing immaturity of blast population (presence of CD34 and CD117 expression and lack of maturation markers such as CD11b, CD15, CD16), accurate lineage assignment (CD13, CD15, CD33, and cytoplasmic myeloperoxidase), and delineating the aberrant antigenic expression pattern of neoplastic blasts as compared with normal progenitor cells. In this regard several precursor (CD34, CD117, CD33, CD13, HLA-DR), granulocytic (CD65, cytoplasmic MPO), monocytic (CD14, CD36, and CD64), megakaryocytic (CD41, CD61), and erythroid (CD235a, CD36, CD45neg) markers are useful.[4,21,22] Preferably, a combination of intracellular and membrane-bound markers should be combined to cover both early and late stages of maturation, respectively.

In addition, assessment of lymphoid (B- and T-cell) markers aids in the correct lineage assignment. However, it should be noted that leukemic blasts may aberrantly express antigens from another lineage including CD7, CD56, CD2, and CD19 lymphoid antigens.

Several distinct entities are recognized in AML and defined by cytogenetic or molecular genetic abnormalities that are linked to different clinical behaviors, therapy, and prognosis. Herein, FC is powerful to define these entities especially in the absence of conclusive or informative cytogenetic results.

FCA may be noncontributory for skin biopsies due to a lack of sufficient number of cells from stroma-rich tissue that shows paucity of malignant cells. For such lesions, IHC evaluation on tissue sections with use of similar antibodies may be more appropriate for the characterization of leukemic myeloid blasts. Additional helpful IHC markers used to demonstrate myeloid/monocytic lineage such as lysozyme, CD68, and CD163 may also be of use.[12,14,17]

Blastic Plasmacytoid Dendritic Cell Neoplasm

Blastic plasmacytoid dendritic cell neoplasm (BPDCN) is a rare form of hematopoietic neoplasm derived from the precursors of plasmacytoid dendritic cells. Since the 2016 revision of the WHO classification, BPDCN is now classified as a separate entity from AML. This malignancy often simultaneously involves skin and bone marrow and in advanced cases can present with a leukemic phase. The immunophenotype of skin and solid organ lesions is most often determined by a panel of IHC stains on tissue sections. However, bone marrow aspirate and blood samples are well suited for FC analysis as long as a sufficient number of malignant cells are detected. Malignant cells typically express CD4, CD43, and CD56 with bright CD123 and HLA-DR. In a subset of cases, there is expression of CD2, CD7, CD33, CD36, CD68, CD38, CD45RA, and TdT (30% of cases). The malignant cells are uniformly negative for CD3, CD5, CD13, CD14, CD15, CD16, CD19, CD20, CD34, CD45RO, CD117, and lineage-defining antigens including surface and cytoplasmic expression of CD3, CD22, CD79a, myeloperoxidase, and lysozyme.

Flow Cytometric Analysis of Mature T-Cell Lymphoma α/β Chain Type

Flow cytometric identification of mature T-cell malignancies relies on the detection of the loss of normally expressed pan T-cell antigens such as CD2, CD3, CD4,

CD5, CD7, CD8, or CD26.[23] Normal α/β mature T cells show concordant expression of all these markers with a CD4 and CD8 ratio between 1 and 4. Loss of expression of more than two pan T-cell markers (>25%) and/or massive loss of expression of single marker of more than 50% is most consistent with a T-cell lymphoproliferative disorder. T-cell clonality can be determined by FC by analysis of expression of a panel of 24 different V-β chains.[24,25] Normal/reactive T cells show variable low level of staining with all antibodies tested. In contrast, monoclonal T cells show restricted expression of a single V-β chain or are characterized by a large population of CD3+ cells that are negative for all V-β antigens tested (>50%). Only a few phenotypic findings show an association with specific subtypes of mature T-cell lymphomas. Of those, expression of CD10 antigen by CD4+ T cells is characteristic for angioimmunoblastic T-cell lymphoma, strong expression of CD25 antigen is characteristic for HTLV-induced adult T-cell lymphoma/leukemia, CD52 expression is typical of T-cell prolymphocytic leukemia, and expression of CD103 antigen is characteristic of enteropathy-associated T-cell lymphoma. Other markers that stratify abnormal T cells according to expression of CD4 (helper) or cytotoxic (CD8, CD16, CD56, and CD57) antigens aid the diagnosis but are not completely specific and should always be interpreted in the context of clinical and morphologic findings. It is also important to note that the interpretation of flow data for T-cell malignancies should always be done with caution since reactive T-cell proliferations secondary to infections and other antigenic stimulation often show abnormal loss of pan T-cell antigens and even clonally restricted T-cell receptor (TCR).

Mature T-Cell Clonality Studies by Flow Cytometric Analysis

α/β T-cell clonality can reliably be determined by FC analysis based on the expression pattern of 23 unique V-β chain (TCR-Vβ-R) antigens. A normal population of mature α/β T lymphocytes expresses a variety of Vβ segments c/w multiple different VDJ rearrangements of TCRβ chain. In contrast, monoclonal T cells will only express a single VDJ rearranged segment with a single restricted Vβ chain. FCA of V-β chain expression is performed using a set of specific monoclonal antibodies that are directed toward 23 Vβ segments that cover up to 70% of the known Vβ repertoire: Vβ1, Vβ2, Vβ3, Vβ5.1, Vβ5.2, Vβ5.3, Vβ7.1, Vβ7.2, Vβ8, Vβ9, Vβ11, Vβ12, Vβ13.1, Vβ13.2, Vβ13.6, Vβ14, Vβ16, Vβ17, Vβ18, Vβ20, Vβ21.3, Vβ22, and Vβ23. Abnormal clonal T cells will show restricted expression of one of these 23 Vβ chains and will be negative for the remaining Vβ chains or will fail to stain with any of the tested 23 Vβ chains. Normal (reactive) polytypic α/β T lymphocytes show a low and variable level of expression of each of 23 Vβ chains without evidence of restricted expression of a single Vβ chain or complete loss of Vβ chain.

TCR-β chain constant regions (TRBC) are encoded by *TRBC1* and *TRCB2* genes. Therefore, immunostaining for TRBC1 can be alternatively used to assess T-cell clonality in peripheral blood and bone marrow in most α/β peripheral T-cell lymphomas.[26,27] For both methods, T-cell population should comprise a sufficient fraction of neoplastic T cells to be detected and the admixture of normal/reactive T cells expressing the same Vβ or TRBC1 is unavoidable and should be taken into account.

Flow Cytometric Analysis of Mature T-Cell Lymphoma γ/δ Type

Mature γ/δ T-cell lymphomas are very rare and most often involve the liver and spleen in hepatosplenic γ/δ T-cell lymphoma and the skin in primary cutaneous γ/δ T-cell lymphoma. For the majority of cases, the main tumor burden involves the spleen, liver, or skin, and only a subset of patients show involvement of bone marrow or peripheral blood. Consequently, immunophenotypic characterization of this lymphoma is mostly based on IHC stains. Nonetheless, for samples with available lymphoma cells suspended in liquid such as blood, bone marrow, or tumor, fresh preparation FC can be successfully used to demonstrate characteristic diagnostic immunophenotype. γ/δ T cells are positive for CD45+, CD2+, surface CD3+, and TCR γ/δ and show characteristic negativity for CD4 and a negative or partial (diminished) expression of CD8 antigens[28] without coexpression of CD1a, CD34, and cTDT (that is diagnostic of precursor T-cell lymphoblastic lymphoma) and variable loss of CD5 and CD7 antigens. γ/δ T-cell lymphomas may acquire expression of some NK-cell markers such as CD16, CD56 (especially cutaneous form), CD57, and some KIRs with variable staining intensity.

Flow Cytometric Analysis of T-Lymphoblastic Lymphoma

The immunophenotypic profiling of immature T-cell malignancies is initiated by blast identification in the low-to-intermediate CD45 and low SSC region followed by more characteristic features including variably prominent losses of pan T-cell antigens CD2, surface CD3, CD5, CD4, and CD8 and gain of T-cell immaturity markers including CD1a, CD34, CD99, and nuclear cTDT with preserved detectable cytoplasmic cCD3. It is important to note that the cytoplasmic cCD3 must be documented by a monoclonal antibody that recognizes the CD3 ε chain and not by polyclonal antibodies that may cross-react with CD3 ζ chain, which is not specific for T lymphocytes.

Flow Cytometry in Primary Cutaneous Lymphomas

Primary cutaneous lymphomas (PCLs) are a heterogeneous group of lymphomas of mature B- or T-cell origin that present in the skin with no evidence of extracutaneous involvement at the time of diagnosis.[29,30] For most PCL types, neoplastic cells reside in the skin without extracutaneous dissemination during disease course. Consequently, diagnosis of PCL is mainly based on clinical and histopathological (determined by IHC) criteria. IHC suffers from several limitations such as low sensitivity and considerable interobserver variability. Multicolor FC overcomes some of these limitations and allows the simultaneous analysis of multiple antigens on a large number of cells and is, therefore, increasingly applied in clinic. Nevertheless, PCL skin biopsies commonly yield insufficient number of viable cells so that additional tests (FC/IHC/molecular studies) are limited. In that regard, the clinical application of FC is still challenging and subordinate as compared with IHC in terms of feasibility and applicability but provides a better alternative in PCL types with (blood) involvement other than skin. Clinical application of FC is particularly prevailing in Sézary syndrome (SS) and, to a lesser extent, mycosis fungoides (MF), both types of cutaneous T-cell lymphoma.

SS is defined by the clinical-diagnostic triad of (pruritic) erythroderma, generalized lymphadenopathy, and the presence of neoplastic, clonally related, T cells in blood and skin. Diagnosing SS is challenging and is often delayed due to nonspecific clinical and histopathological features that are also frequently seen in much more prevalent benign erythrodermic skin disorders.[31,32] Consequently, diagnosis of SS, as well as hematologic staging of SS/MF, depends on the accurate identification of circulating neoplastic cells for which FC is indispensable.

Immunophenotypic abnormalities in SS range from complete loss of pan T-cell antigen expression to quantitative changes in antigenic intensity, which are identified by comparison with the normal T cells present in each sample (Fig. 8-4).[4] The most common aberrancies include the diminished or complete loss of CD26 and/or CD7; consequently, diagnostic immunophenotypic criteria for SS are defined by the presence of ≥40% of CD4+CD26− and/or ≥40% of CD4+CD7− T cells.[31,33] Other common immunophenotypic profiles include CD3lo/-, CD4lo/-, CD2lo/-, CD5brigh/lo/-, CD45lo in combination with higher FSC and, to a lesser extent, higher SSC. It should be noted, however, that the immunophenotype of neoplastic Sézary cells is heterogeneous among and within patients and SS immunophenotype is subject to changes.[34-37] Furthermore, normal CD4+ T cells may exhibit similar phenotypes along with their physiological maturation, for instance, terminally differentiated cells are CD26lo/-. Fixed immunophenotypic criteria are therefore obsolete but improved criteria are currently lacking and international consensus guidelines have not been revised accordingly. Aiming at improving Sézary cell detection and characterization, Sézary cells were immunophenotypically profiled using highly sensitive and standardized EuroFlow-based multiparameter FC (MFC) technology and innovative software tools (Najidh et al., unpublished results). EuroFlow consortium has acquired an internationally leading role in hemato-oncology field by designing, developing, and validating standardized approaches for flow cytometric evaluation of hematological malignancies.[4,6,38] The results of this study further unraveled Sézary cell heterogeneity and established the role of standardized MFC for improved Sézary cell detection with direct consequences for clinical management of SS. Nevertheless, in some cases, accurate immunophenotypic characterization of neoplastic cells is still challenging and additional disease-specific markers are needed for FC analysis of SS. Several novel markers have been proposed for Sézary cell identification, including CD158k, CD279 (PD-1), CD194 (CCR4), and TCRCB1.[39,40] EuroFlow-based methodology as well as the addition of these novel markers are currently being investigated and validated in multicenter setting.

On the other hand, patients with MF usually present with skin patches and plaques and generally have an indolent disease course. In a minority of cases, patients develop extracutaneous disease, particularly lymph node and blood involvement, which drastically reduces survival. By FC, MF cases at different stages (and of different histologic variants) have shown abnormalities of CD2 (47%), CD3 (67%), CD4 (40%), CD5 (87%), CD7, and CD45 (67%). A study from Jokinen et al. identified abnormal T cells by FC in 14 of 18 patients (78%) with histologically and clinically confirmed MF and in zero of 14 patients whose biopsies were histologically negative or indeterminate for MF.[41] The clinical sensitivity (78%) and specificity (89%) of their FC assay seemed to be similar or superior to the sensitivity (67%) and specificity (71%) of the TCRγ-PCR assay used in the study.

The utility of FC has also been demonstrated in cutaneous B-cell lymphomas. A study from Wu et al. has shown that FC of the lesional skin detected a clonal B-cell population in 4/13 (31%) cases of atypical lymphoid hyperplasia, 8/8 (100%) cases of primary cutaneous (pcBCL) B-cell lymphoma (6 follicle center, 2 marginal zone), and 4/4 (100%) cases of secondary cutaneous B-cell lymphoma (scBCL). Molecular studies (immunoglobulin heavy chain [IGH] gene rearrangement) detected a clone in 3/14 cases of atypical lymphoid hyperplasia, 4/15 cases of pcBCL, and 6/8 cases of scBCL. Therefore, FC was significantly more sensitive than PCR for such diagnoses.[42] Similar findings were also noted by Shafernak et al.[43]

SUMMARY

Flow cytometry represents a powerful technique that provides a detailed and accurate immunophenotypic profile of malignant cells if provided access to an adequate number of viable tumor cells. Currently used clinical multicolor FC allows simultaneous determination of up to 12 to 14 stains including a combination of surface, cytoplasmic, and nuclear antigens. New-generation flow cytometers with increased detection sensitivity (≥20 fluorescent parameters) and enhanced technologies and software have established their utility in hematological research and will shape the near future in routine diagnostic laboratories. Properly performed FC analysis is unsurpassed in terms of speed and accuracy in determining hematopoietic tumor cell lineage, clonality, and maturation status. Processing fresh (viable) samples is required for FC analysis, particularly at the diagnostic stage. Specimens with poor viability that are stroma-rich or that contain few malignant cells will often fail to produce informative FC data. It is especially important for cases in which tissue necrosis or cell fragility (most prominent in large cells and in cells with plasma cell differentiation) may be present to be cognizant of the potential to produce biased results due to preferential loss of malignant cells. Therefore, while being very informative on its own, FC analysis data should always be interpreted in the context of clinical, morphologic and, if available, cytogenetic/molecular findings.

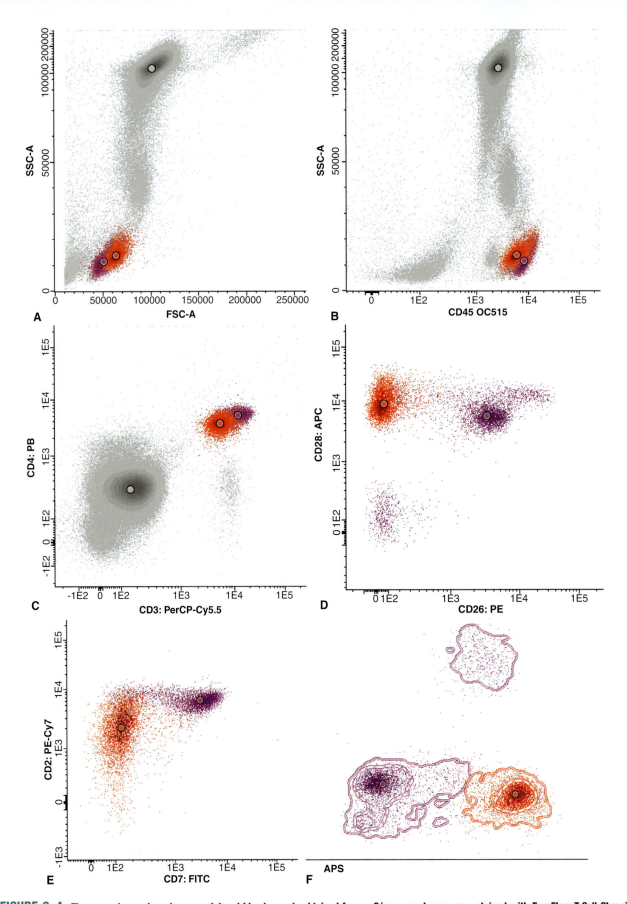

FIGURE 8–4. These graphs are based on a peripheral blood sample obtained from a Sézary syndrome case, stained with EuroFlow T-Cell Chronic Lymphoproliferative Disease (T-CLPD) Tube 1 and analyzed by InfinicytTM software (Cytognos, Salamanca, Spain) displaying the difference in immunophenotype of normal residual CD4+ T cells (depicted in purple) and neoplastic circulating Sézary cells (red) with corresponding population medians (larger dots). **A.** Compared with normal CD4+ T cells, Sézary cells are larger and more complex cells translated in higher forward scatter (FSC) and side scatter (SSC), respectively. Furthermore, Sézary cells show dimmer expression of **B.** CD45 and **C.** CD3 and CD4 and exhibit **D.** characteristic loss of CD26 while maintaining CD28 positivity and **E.** loss of CD7 and diminished expression of CD2. **F.** Automatic Population Separator (APS) plot displays a clear separation between immunophenotypically aberrant (Sézary, red) and normal residual (purple) CD4+ T-cell populations based on all parameters included in the T-CLPD antibody panel (FSC, SSC, CD45, CD3, CD4, CD8, CD2, CD7, CD26, and CD28). Given are the first (inner) and second (outer) standard deviation lines and corresponding CD4+ T-cell population medians. Abbreviations: APC, allophycocyanin; FITC, fluorescein isothiocyanate; OC515, orange cytognos 515; PB, pacific blue; PE, phycoerythrin; PECy7, phycoerythrin-cyanin 7; PerCPCy5.5, peridinin-chlorophyll protein-complex cyanin 5.5.

References

1. de Bie F, Av.d.S-G, de Bruin-Versteeg S, et al. In: *8th ESLHO Symp. Abstract Book*. Evaluation of New Generation Routine ≥20-Color Flow Cytometers. 2019;11-16.
2. Chattopadhyay PK, Roederer M. Cytometry: today's technology and tomorrow's horizons. *Methods*. 2012;57(3):251-258.
3. Bendall SC, Nolan GP, Roederer M, et al. A deep profiler's guide to cytometry. *Trends Immunol*. 2012;33(7):323-332.
4. van Dongen JJ, Lhermitte L, Böttcher S, et al. EuroFlow antibody panels for standardized n-dimensional flow cytometric immunophenotyping of normal, reactive and malignant leukocytes. *Leukemia*. 2012;26(9):1908-1975.
5. Diks AM, Bonroy C, Teodosio C, et al. Impact of blood storage and sample handling on quality of high dimensional flow cytometric data in multicenter clinical research. *J Immunol Methods*. 2019;475:112616.
6. Kalina T, Flores-Montero J, van der Velden VH, et al. EuroFlow standardization of flow cytometer instrument settings and immunophenotyping protocols. *Leukemia*. 2012;26(9):1986-2010.
7. Lhermitte L, Barreau S, Morf D, et al. Automated identification of leukocyte subsets improves standardization of database-guided expert-supervised diagnostic orientation in acute leukemia: a EuroFlow study. *Mod Pathol*. 2021;34(1):59-69.
8. Pedreira CE. Automating flow cytometry. *Cytometry*. 2012;81(2):110-111.
9. Pedreira CE, Costa ES, Lecrevisse Q, et al. Overview of clinical flow cytometry data analysis: recent advances and future challenges. *Trends Biotechnol*. 2013;31(7):415-425.
10. Braylan RC, Orfao A, Borowitz MJ, et al. Optimal number of reagents required to evaluate hematolymphoid neoplasias: results of an international consensus meeting. *Cytometry*. 2001;46(1):23-27.
11. Borowitz MJ, Bray R, Gascoyne R, et al. U.S.-Canadian Consensus recommendations on the immunophenotypic analysis of hematologic neoplasia by flow cytometry: data analysis and interpretation. *Cytometry*. 1997;30(5):236-244.
12. van Dongen JJ, Orfao A. EuroFlow: resetting leukemia and lymphoma immunophenotyping. Basis for companion diagnostics and personalized medicine. *Leukemia*. 2012;26(9):1899-1907.
13. Swerdlow SH, Campo E, Harris NL, et al. *WHO Classification of Tumour of Haematopoietic and Lymphoid Tissues*. IARC, 2008.
14. Virgo PF, Gibbs GJ. Flow cytometry in clinical pathology. *Ann Clin Biochem*. 2012;49(Pt 1):17-28.
15. Matutes E, Owusu-Ankomah K, Morilla R, et al. The immunological profile of B-cell disorders and proposal of a scoring system for the diagnosis of CLL. *Leukemia*. 1994;8(10):1640-1645.
16. Rawstron AC, Kreuzer KA, Soosapilla A, et al. Reproducible diagnosis of chronic lymphocytic leukemia by flow cytometry: an European research initiative on CLL (ERIC) & European Society for clinical cell analysis (ESCCA) Harmonisation project. *Cytometry B Clin Cytom*. 2018;94(1):121-128.
17. Heel K, Tabone T, Röhrig KJ, et al. Developments in the immunophenotypic analysis of haematological malignancies. *Blood Rev*. 2013;27(4):193-207.
18. Krause DS, Delelys ME, Preffer FI. Flow cytometry for hematopoietic cells. *Methods Mol Biol*. 2014;1109:23-46.
19. El Hussein S, Medeiros LJ, Khoury JD. Aggressive NK cell leukemia: current state of the art. *Cancers (Basel)*. 2020;12(10):2900.
20. Li C, Tian Y, Wang J, et al. Abnormal immunophenotype provides a key diagnostic marker: a report of 29 cases of de novo aggressive natural killer cell leukemia. *Transl Res*. 2014;163(6):565-577.
21. Döhner H, Estey E, Grimwade D, et al. Diagnosis and management of AML in adults: 2017 ELN recommendations from an international expert panel. *Blood*. 2017;129(4):424-447.
22. Matarraz S, Almeida J, Flores-Montero J, et al. Introduction to the diagnosis and classification of monocytic-lineage leukemias by flow cytometry. *Cytometry B Clin Cytom*. 2017;92(3):218-227.
23. Jamal S, Picker LJ, Aquino DB, et al. Immunophenotypic analysis of peripheral T-cell neoplasms. A multiparameter flow cytometric approach. *Am J Clin Pathol*. 2001;116(4):512-526.
24. Hristov AC, Vonderheid EC, Borowitz MJ. Simplified flow cytometric assessment in mycosis fungoides and Sézary syndrome. *Am J Clin Pathol*. 2011;136(6):944-953.
25. Tembhare P, Yuan CM, Xi L, et al. Flow cytometric immunophenotypic assessment of T-cell clonality by Vβ repertoire analysis: detection of T-cell clonality at diagnosis and monitoring of minimal residual disease following therapy. *Am J Clin Pathol*. 2011;135(6):890-900.
26. Maciocia PM, Wawrzyniecka PA, Philip B, et al. Targeting the T cell receptor β-chain constant region for immunotherapy of T cell malignancies. *Nat Med*. 2017;23(12):1416-1423.
27. Novikov ND, Griffin GK, Dudley G, et al. Utility of a simple and robust flow cytometry assay for rapid clonality testing in mature peripheral T-cell lymphomas. *Am J Clin Pathol*. 2019;151(5):494-503.
28. Ahmad E, Kingma DW, Jaffe ES, et al. Flow cytometric immunophenotypic profiles of mature gamma delta T-cell malignancies involving peripheral blood and bone marrow. *Cytometry B Clin Cytom*. 2005;67(1):6-12.
29. Willemze R, Jaffe ES, Burg G, et al. WHO-EORTC classification for cutaneous lymphomas. *Blood*. 2005;105(10):3768-3785.
30. Willemze R, Cerroni L, Kempf W, et al. The 2018 update of the WHO-EORTC classification for primary cutaneous lymphomas. *Blood*. 2019;133(16):1703-1714.
31. Boonk SE, Zoutman WH, Marie-Cardine A, et al. Evaluation of immunophenotypic and molecular Biomarkers for Sézary syndrome using standard operating procedures: a multicenter study of 59 patients. *J Invest Dermatol*. 2016;136(7):1364-1372.
32. Lima M, Almeida J, dos Anjos Teixeira M, et al. Utility of flow cytometry immunophenotyping and DNA ploidy studies for diagnosis and characterization of blood involvement in CD4+ Sézary's syndrome. *Haematologica*. 2003;88(8):874-887.
33. Jones D, Dang NH, Duvic M, et al. Absence of CD26 expression is a useful marker for diagnosis of T-cell lymphoma in peripheral blood. *Am J Clin Pathol*. 2001;115(6):885-892.
34. Buus TB, Willerslev-Olsen A, Fredholm S, et al. Single-cell heterogeneity in Sézary syndrome. *Blood Adv*. 2018;2(16):2115-2126.
35. Horna P, Wang SA, Wolniak KL, et al. Flow cytometric evaluation of peripheral blood for suspected Sézary syndrome or mycosis fungoides: international guidelines for assay characteristics. *Cytometry B Clin Cytom*. 2021;100(2):142-155.
36. Roelens M, Delord M, Ram-Wolff C, et al. Circulating and skin-derived Sézary cells: clonal but with phenotypic plasticity. *Blood*. 2017;130(12):1468-1471.

37. Poglio S, Prochazkova-Carlotti M, Cherrier F, et al. Xenograft and cell culture models of Sézary syndrome reveal cell of origin diversity and subclonal heterogeneity. *Leukemia.* 2020;35(6):1696-1709.
38. Botafogo V, Pérez-Andres M, Jara-Acevedo M, et al. Age distribution of multiple functionally Relevant subsets of CD4+ T cells in Human blood using a standardized and validated 14-color EuroFlow immune monitoring tube. *Front Immunol.* 2020;11:166.
39. Bagot M, Moretta A, Sivori S, et al. CD4(+) cutaneous T-cell lymphoma cells express the p140-killer cell immunoglobulin-like receptor. *Blood.* 2001;97(5):1388-1391.
40. Samimi S, Benoit B, Evans K, et al. Increased programmed death-1 expression on CD4+ T cells in cutaneous T-cell lymphoma: implications for immune suppression. *Arch Dermatol.* 2010;146(12):1382-1388.
41. Jokinen CH, Fromm JR, Argenyi ZB, et al. Flow cytometric evaluation of skin biopsies for mycosis fungoides. *Am J Dermatopathol.* 2011;33(5):483-491.
42. Wu JM, Vonderheid E, Gocke CD, et al. Flow cytometry of lesional skin enhances the evaluation of cutaneous B-cell lymphomas. *J Cutan Pathol.* 2012;39(10):918-928.
43. Schafernak KT, Variakojis D, Goolsby CL, et al. Clonality assessment of cutaneous B-cell lymphoid proliferations: a comparison of flow cytometry immunophenotyping, molecular studies, and immunohistochemistry/in situ hybridization and review of the literature. *Am J Dermatopathol.* 2014;36(10):781-795.

CHAPTER 9

PCR-based gene rearrangement studies

Ian S. Hagemann

GENE REARRANGEMENT IN LYMPHOCYTE DEVELOPMENT

Immunoglobulin Rearrangement

Human B-cell antigen receptor genes include the immunoglobulin (Ig) heavy-chain locus (*IGH*) at 14q32, the kappa light-chain locus (*IGK*) at 2p11, and the lambda light-chain locus (*IGL*) at 22q11. In the germline or nonrearranged state, antigen receptor loci are composed of separate coding segments distributed in a region of DNA estimated to be several hundred kilobases (kb) in length. The *IGH* locus consists of 38 to 46 variable (V) genes (depending on the patient's haplotype), 27 diversity (D) genes, 6 joining (J) genes, and 5 isotype-specific constant (C) genes.[1]

A similar architecture is present at the light-chain kappa (*IGK*) and lambda (*IGL*) loci. These loci include V, J, and C, but not D, genes. The combinatorial diversity available from rearranging these loci is also constrained by differences in the structure of the J and C cassettes. The *IGK* locus has a single C region. At the *IGL* locus, the J regions are interspersed between the C regions so a given J is always paired with the corresponding C.

In the pre-B cell stage of development, B cells undergo V(D)J recombination, in which they rearrange these loci to create complete Ig heavy chain open reading frames. This process provides the combinatorial diversity needed to assemble a complete immune repertoire. The cell first attempts to rearrange one *IGH* allele. An *IGH* D gene is fused to a J gene, and this DJ segment is fused with a V gene to form a functional VDJ exon that encodes the variable antigen recognition site of the IGH protein. If the result is nonfunctional, the cell will try to rearrange the other allele. Cells may therefore harbor two *IGH* rearrangements. If both alleles fail to recombine, the cell undergoes apoptotic death.

If an open reading frame has been successfully assembled at one *IGH* locus, the cell will, upon reaching the immature B stage, attempt to rearrange light chain loci, starting with *IGK* (kappa light chain). If the result at the first *IGK* allele is nonfunctional, the allele is deleted and the other allele is rearranged. If both alleles fail to rearrange productively, *IGL* (lambda light chain) rearrangement occurs at one or both loci. If a functional light chain still has not been created, the cell undergoes apoptotic death. *IGL* rearrangement is attempted only in the event that *IGK* rearrangement fails, which explains the observation that kappa B cells are more common than lambda B cells.

The main source of diversity in Ig sequences is the many available combinations of V, J, and D (for heavy chains) segments in the *IGH*, *IGK*, and *IGL* genes. A secondary source of diversity is nucleotide loss and addition at the D-J and V-D junctions by the enzyme terminal deoxynucleotidyl transferase (TdT), which is active during rearrangement. Subsequent events introduce further diversity as part of affinity maturation. V segment substitution and somatic hypermutation occur in germinal centers. Isotype switching also occurs, under the influence of T helper cells.

TCR Rearrangement

Developing thymocytes have T-cell receptor (*TCR*) α, β, γ, and δ loci, which are rearranged to form functional *TCR* open reading frames. Similarly to the Ig loci, the *TCR* loci consist of multiple cassettes. *TCRA* and *TCRG* have V, J, and C genes, while *TCRB* and *TCRD* have V, D, J, and C.

TCRB, *TCRG*, and *TCRD* undergo simultaneous rearrangement early in development. Successful *TCRB* rearrangement prompts *TCRA* rearrangement and commitment to the αβ lineage. The *TCRD* locus is entirely embedded in an intron of *TCRA*, so that *TCRA* rearrangement results in deletion of *TCRD*. The *TCRG* locus, however, is not deleted in the event of successful *TCRA*/*TCRB* rearrangement and remains present and rearranged in T cells of either αβ or γδ lineage.

CLINICAL UTILITY OF CLONALITY TESTING

Ascertainment of a Clonal Lymphoid Process

IGH and *TCR* rearrangement studies are a useful ancillary diagnostic tool in patients suspected of harboring clonal lymphoid processes. The presence of a clonal T/B-cell population is suggestive of T/B-cell malignancies, particularly when clinical or histologic suspicion is high. However, clonal populations can also be seen in nonneoplastic processes. Clinical correlation is therefore required in all cases and should be explicitly recommended in reports of clonality testing studies.

Lineage Determination

By performing *IGH* and *TCR* rearrangement studies on the same sample, it is possible to infer whether a clonal process originates from B or T lymphocytes, respectively. However, clonal lymphoid populations may show lineage infidelity. B-cell neoplasms are particularly likely to harbor *TCR* rearrangements; these have been described in half of precursor B-cell neoplasms, and as many as 5% to 10% of mature B-cell neoplasms.[2]

Monitoring for Residual/Recurrent Disease

In PCR-based clonality testing, the amplicon arising from the clonally rearranged *IGH* or *TCR* gene has a characteristic size, reported in nucleotides. Since the size resolution of capillary electrophoresis is <1 nt, an amplicon of the same size can be sought in subsequent samples. Identifying an amplicon of the same size in different samples from the same time point (eg, two different skin sites) can suggest a neoplastic process rather than a reactive one. Recovering an amplicon of the same size at a subsequent time can clarify that a biopsy shows recurrent/residual disease rather than a new neoplasm. Identification of additional amplicons can suggest clonal evolution. Any reasoning based upon amplicon size requires that the assays be performed with the same methodology and primer sets, which is often the case.

IGHV Hypermutation Testing

PCR-based *IGH* clonality testing has a role in prognostication for chronic lymphocytic leukemia/small lymphocytic lymphoma (CLL/SLL). Patients with a pre-germinal center phenotype have a significantly worse prognosis than those with a post-germinal center phenotype.[2,3] The phenotype can be ascertained by detecting features of post-germinal center B cells, including loss of ZAP-70 expression and somatic hypermutation of the rearranged *IGHV* gene.[4-6] Although ZAP-70 immunohistochemistry was previously in clinical use, this stain was technically difficult to interpret and is now deprecated.

The extent of mutation in the variable region of the *IGH* gene can also be used to differentiate pre-germinal center B cell clones from those having a post-germinal center phenotype. Hypermutation is strongly predictive of a better prognosis, while lack of hypermutation predicts a poorer prognosis. Hypermutation is defined as ≥2% difference between the clone's *IGHV* sequence and that of the germline, while <2% difference is considered lack of hypermutation.

Hypermutation is detected by amplifying, then sequencing, the clonally rearranged *IGHV* segment and comparing the patient's sequence to the reference (nonhypermutated) *IGHV* sequence. This assay only has clinical significance in the setting of a new diagnosis of CLL/SLL and is not indicated as part of disease monitoring or at any other point in the course of disease.

METHODOLOGY FOR PCR-BASED CLONALITY TESTING

Basic Principle

PCR-based clonality testing uses a forward primer located in an *IGH* or *TCR* V gene and a reverse primer located in a J gene. The method takes advantage of the fact that there is an upper limit on the size of the PCR products that can be made by *Taq* polymerase. This limit is on the order of 500 to 1000 nt, depending on the specific polymerase and other conditions. In the germline (nonrearranged) state, the primers used for clonality testing are too far from one another (hundreds of kilobases) to allow for productive PCR. In rearranged loci, however, the primer sites are brought closer together and a PCR amplicon can be made.

The test further takes advantage of the fact that all members of a clonal population can be expected to contain the same *IGH* and/or *TCR* gene rearrangements, whereas polyclonal populations of lymphocytes will contain many different gene rearrangements. In clonal populations, clonality testing will therefore reveal a restricted repertoire of gene rearrangements. Polyclonal populations will yield many different PCR products, with a Gaussian distribution of sizes, testifying to the diversity of gene rearrangements present therein.

Suitable Sample Types

The test is performed on DNA extracted from fluid or tissue containing a suspected clonal lymphoid population. The most common sample type is formalin-fixed, paraffin-embedded (FFPE) tissue, which gives acceptable performance despite DNA degradation.[7] Paraffin sections can be cut onto slides and then macrodissected with a hollow-core needle or other tool to enrich the sample in the cell population of interest, or scrolls can be collected in a microcentrifuge tube. DNA is extracted from such samples by use of an organic solvent, typically xylene or Citrasolv, to remove paraffin, followed by a standard manual or automated DNA extraction. A major advantage of FFPE specimens is that they will typically have also been examined by histopathologic methods, so that the clonality testing results can be correlated with a pathologic impression. Fresh (unfixed) tissue is suitable from a laboratory perspective, but is clinically less desirable, as there will typically be no closely associated histologic correlate (at best, there may be an FFPE specimen obtained from a nearby site). Clonality testing can be performed on fine needle aspirates, peripheral blood, or bone marrow aspirate specimens. Appropriate laboratory data such as aspirate or peripheral blood cell counts must be integrated into the eventual clinical interpretation for such specimens.

BIOMED-2/EuroClonality Consensus Primer Sets

The European BIOMED-2 network (EuroClonality consortium) developed between 2002 and 2012 a series of standardized primers and guidelines to facilitate PCR-based clonality testing.[8] This project was intended to improve interlaboratory reproducibility and make testing more widely available, including in smaller or less experienced laboratories lacking the resources to design a laboratory-developed test. Standardization also allows results of tests conducted in different laboratories to be compared. Since amplicons of the same size will be detected from the same disease with standard reagents, recurrent/residual disease can be distinguished from new disease regardless of where the testing is performed.

BIOMED-2 primer sets for rearrangement of *IGH, IGK, IGL, TCRB, TCRD,* and *TCRG* are available as analyte-specific reagents from Invivoscribe Technologies (San Diego, California). These kits are labeled for research use only, and analytical and clinical validation is required before they can be used for clinical laboratory testing. Like any ancillary method, *IGH* and *TCR* clonality studies cannot independently establish any diagnosis of malignancy and can at best be used to support a diagnosis that was already suspected on the basis of routine morphologic examination.

Assay Setup and Controls

The BIOMED-2 investigators suggest an algorithm to be used for sequential testing of suspected B-cell proliferations, T-cell proliferations, and lymphoid proliferations of unknown origin.[9] By using multiple primer sets for testing (eg, *IGH* V_H-J_H, *IGK* V_K-J_K, *IGK* Kde [kappa-deleting element], *IGH* D_H-J_H, and *IGL*), one increases the sensitivity, but this approach also increases the cost, complexity, and time of testing, with the trade-off depending in part upon whether the tests are performed simultaneously or sequentially.

Much of the benefit of testing can be obtained from using a smaller number of primer sets. In T cell lymphomas, *TCRG* Vγ-Jγ primer sets had a sensitivity (89%) comparable with *TCRB* Vβ-Jβ + Dβ-Jβ primer sets (91%) for detecting clonal rearrangements, but the combination was even more sensitive (94%).[8] Similarly, in B-cell lymphomas, using *IGH* V_H-J_H primer sets alone gave a sensitivity of 88% for detecting clonal rearrangements, while adding the results of D_H-J_H, V_K-J_K, and Kde primer sets allowed clonal peaks to be detected in 99%.[8]

In practice, a desirable cost-benefit trade-off is obtained by using a single test for TCR clonality (typically *TCRG*) and a single test for Ig clonality (typically *IGH*). The present chapter focuses on this approach, with the caveat that some laboratories may choose to implement additional assays to capture the subset of clones that will not be ascertained using a single assay.

IGH *Setup*

The BIOMED-2 *IGH* clonality assay as implemented by Invivoscribe Technologies is shown schematically in Figure 9-1. In the germline state, the primers shown in this schema are too distant from one another to yield a product. In the rearranged state, at least one combination of primers can be expected to yield a product from any given B cell. The forward primers are designed to anneal with *IGH* V_H gene sequences. Although the sequence differs from one V_H cassette to another, there are relatively conserved regions (framework regions 1, 2, and 3) such that a small number of primers, multiplexed in a single tube, cover the majority of V_H genes. The J_H genes contain a conserved region such that a single consensus reverse primer suffices to give product, regardless of the specific J_H gene that is utilized.

The *IGH* clonality assay includes three primer master mixes containing specified combinations of forward and reverse primers.[9] Several forward primers are multiplexed in each tube. It is recommended to set each tube up in two technical replicates, as spurious PCR products may be seen in one tube but not the other. For each tube, the expected size range of products is known; products falling outside of this size range are disregarded. The largest product size expected from any reaction in the assay is 360 bp, using an FR1 forward primer and the consensus reverse primer. The smallest product expected is a 100 bp band that can be produced using an FR3 forward primer and the consensus reverse primer.

Several controls are set up with the experimental tubes, including a positive control containing DNA from a known clonal B-cell population, a negative control representing a known polyclonal population, and a water blank containing no template.

A specimen control size ladder (SCSL) is also set up, using a master mix supplied by the vendor and template extracted from the specimen (Fig. 9-2). This control serves to confirm that the DNA extracted from the specimen has sufficient quality and fragment length to allow amplification of products from rearranged *IGH* loci. The SCSL consists of multiplexed PCR reactions against irrelevant genes (*VWA, FGA*), yielding products of 84, 96, 200, 300, 400, and 600 bp.[9] If the SCSL fails to show a peak of a given size, the template DNA is either absent or too degraded to support amplification of fragments of that length. For the test to be interpretable, the SCSL must show that DNA is intact up to the largest amplicon size expected as a product of the assay.

The limit of detection for the *IGH* gene clonality assay is stated by the vendor to be one clonal cell in 100 normal cells.[9] In practice, the limit of detection should be established by in-laboratory validation. The reproducibility of size determination for the clonal amplicon is 1 to 2 bp with detection by capillary electrophoresis.

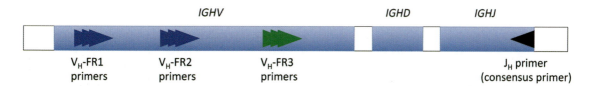

FIGURE 9-1. Schema for *IGH* clonality assay.[9] The forward primers anneal within the *IGH* V_H gene segments while the reverse primer anneals within the J_H segments. Framework regions 1, 2, and 3 are relatively conserved between V_H cassettes and allow multiple segments to be covered by a smaller number of primers, while the J_H reverse primer also represents a consensus across J segments. Fluorescent labeling of the primers allows the size and quantity of the products to be quantified by capillary electrophoresis.

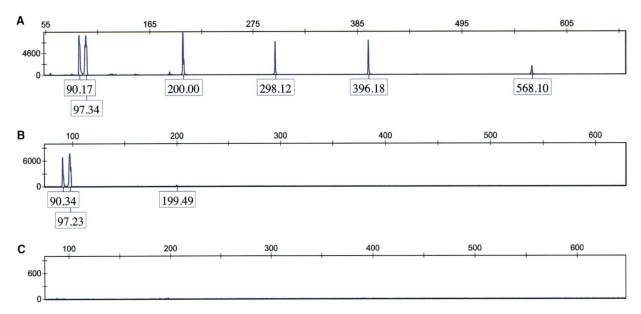

FIGURE 9-2. Specimen control size ladder. **A.** Good-quality patient DNA allows amplification of a full specimen control size ladder (SCSL). While this indicates that DNA of sufficient size and quality for testing is present, it does not prove that B lymphocytes are present within the sample. **B.** Lower-quality patient DNA still allows amplification of peaks up to 200 bp and is adequate for products only up to this size range. This factor will limit the analytical and clinical sensitivity of the assay. **C.** Degraded DNA does not support amplification of the SCSL and indicates that the specimen is not adequate for testing.

TCRG *Setup*

The Invivoscribe *TCRG* clonality assay consists of forward and reverse primer sets that support amplification of products from rearranged *TCRG* loci (Fig. 9-3). These primers are multiplexed into two master mixes, each of which contains a subset of forward primers and both blue- and green-labeled reverse primers. The largest amplicon expected to be produced from any reaction in the assay is 255 bp; the smallest is 80 bp. Similar to the *IGH* gene clonality assay, it is recommended that each tube be set up in duplicate, as spurious products will typically not occur in both technical replicates.

The limit of detection for the assay is said to be 10^6 cells, of which 10% must be from the clonal population,[10] but separate analytical and clinical validation must be performed in each laboratory implementing the test. With standard capillary electrophoresis the size resolution for detecting clonal peaks is 1 to 2 bp.

Turnaround Time

While the PCR amplification and capillary electrophoresis steps of clonality testing require only a few hours, there are other factors that contribute to a longer turnaround time for this form of testing.

Preanalytically, there may be delays in transmitting FFPE tissue to the molecular laboratory and selecting regions for analysis. Extraction of DNA from FFPE tissue requires deparaffinization followed by proteinase K digestion, which may require overnight incubation.

After PCR and electrophoresis are complete, the results must be interpreted by a molecular genetic pathologist or clinical molecular geneticist, introducing a human-factor delay.

Because of the potential for PCR inhibitors to be present in the specimen and/or for PCR reactions to fail with small amounts of input DNA, it is not uncommon for *IGH* or *TCRG* clonality testing to require troubleshooting steps and/or repeat testing.

Finally, given that most centers will perform a limited number of these tests, it is common for the test to be performed only on certain days of the week. It is prudent for users of clonality tests—both pathologists and clinicians—to be aware of the relevant turnaround time, which is similar to that of other forms of molecular testing.

INTERPRETATION OF PCR-BASED CLONALITY TESTING DATA

Reporting Categories

Monoclonal or Biclonal

Results of clonality testing are classified as monoclonal if PCR produces, in each reaction tube, no more than a single dominant amplicon, seen as a dominant well-defined peak on capillary electrophoresis (Fig. 9-4). The size of this amplicon must fall within the range expected for the PCR products in that tube. True monoclonal peaks are of an intensity comparable with that seen in the positive control reaction. The background may be polyclonal (if numerous polyclonal lymphocytes are also present) or relatively silent (if the clonal population dominates the specimen).

Some clonal populations yield two dominant peaks on gene clonality tests. This occurs because each primitive B or T cell has two *IGH* or *TCRG* loci. For both of these cell types, if one locus fails to rearrange productively, the other locus is rearranged. Clonal populations arising from such cells will contain biclonal gene rearrangements.

Biclonal results can also be obtained from a single clonal population if multiple PCR primers within a single tube compete with one another for the same template. Although this is not typically the case for *IGH* or *TCRG*, it has been reported to be more common for *IGK* and *TCRB*. In those assays, up to four peaks in a single tube are permitted within the scope of a "clonal" interpretation.[11]

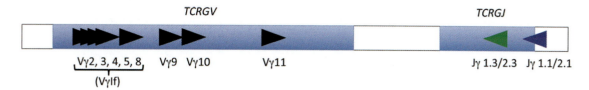

FIGURE 9-3. Schema for *TCRG* clonality assay.[10] The forward primers anneal within the TCRG Vγ gene segments. The reverse primers anneal within the Jγ gene segments. The reverse primers are fluorescently labeled, allowing the products to be sized and quantified by capillary electrophoresis.

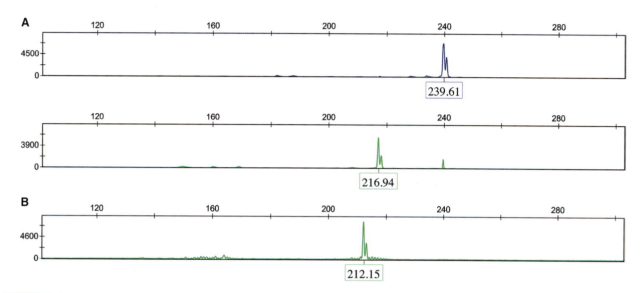

FIGURE 9-4. *TCRG* capillary electrophoresis pattern classified as monoclonal. The specimen was a punch biopsy of skin from a 55-year-old man with scaly erythematous plaques considered suspicious for cutaneous T-cell lymphoma (mycosis fungoides). The biopsy showed pan-dermal involvement by neoplastic T cells with markedly elevated CD4:CD8 ratio and CD7 loss. Focally, epidermotropism by neoplastic cells was seen. **A.** Clonal peaks were seen at 240 bp in one reaction tube and 217 bp in the other. These peaks most likely are both arising from the same clone. The peaks have an amplitude comparable with that seen in the positive control peak (**B**, from a known monoclonal T cell population). Both peaks fall within the size range expected for these reaction tubes (145-255 bp, per the package insert[10]).

Finding peaks in more than one reaction tube does not contravene a clonal interpretation, as some rearranged sequences, including those of some clonal populations, will yield a product with more than one primer pair (eg, with both FR2 and FR3 primers in the *IGH* assay). It is typically not possible to determine, without sequencing, whether peaks obtained in two different tubes arise from the same rearranged locus, from different loci within the same clonal population, or from entirely different populations.

Clonal (including monoclonal and biclonal) findings on PCR-based testing do not prove that a malignant or even neoplastic process is present. Clonality testing must be viewed as an ancillary technique in support of routine clinical, morphologic, and immunophenotypic observations. A clonal process is more likely if other observations suggest a neoplasm; if the same clone is identified at multiple anatomic sites or time points; and if there is no evidence to suggest an alternative explanation, such as a dominant immune response to a specific stimulus. Because lineage infidelity can be seen in gene rearrangement, the presence of an *IGH* or *TCRG* rearrangement does not conclusively prove that clonal process is one of B or T cells, respectively.

Monoclonal or biclonal peaks should be of an amplitude comparable with the positive control and should exceed that of the polyclonal background by a factor of 2 to 3. When these conditions are not fully met—in particular, when a peak is prominent, reproducible, but not conclusively stronger than the polyclonal background—it is acceptable to report "weak clonal" findings. The connotation of a weak clonal result is that additional evidence should be adduced before concluding that a clone is present.

Oligoclonal

An oligoclonal result is one that yields three or more dominant peaks in any given reaction tube (Fig. 9-5). To support an oligoclonal interpretation, the peaks should be significantly stronger than any polyclonal background that is present and should be of an intensity comparable with the positive control (DNA from a known clonal population).

Oligoclonal findings do not provide strong evidence of a clonal process, since a clonal population should contain at most two discrete rearranged *IGH* or *TCRG* genes. An oligoclonal result may indicate competition by multiple PCR primer pairs for a true clonal population of templates.

Oligoclonal results may also indicate an exaggerated immune response to an inflammatory or infectious stimulus, or a restricted immune repertoire in individuals who are immunocompromised or malnourished. In such patients, the repertoire of oligoclonal amplicons will typically differ if the test is repeated on material from a different anatomic site or time point.

A "pseudoclonal" pattern may be seen in specimens containing few B or T cells. The diversity of rearranged sequences within such scant specimens may be low and

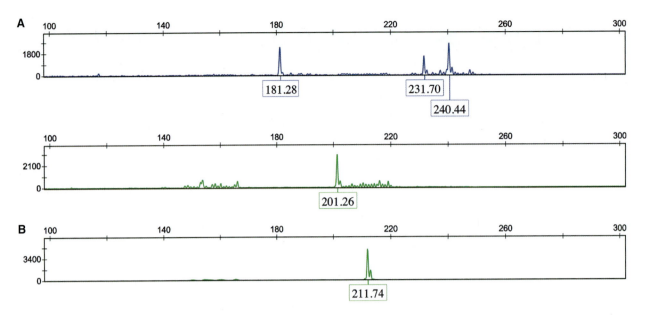

FIGURE 9-5. *TCRG* **capillary electrophoresis pattern classified as oligoclonal.** The specimen was peripheral blood from a 43-year-old man with neutropenia and a history of mature T-cell lymphocytosis with 10% large granular lymphocytes. *TCRG* rearrangement testing at an outside hospital showed a clonal T-cell population 1 year ago. The results were interpreted as an oligoclonal *TCRG* gene rearrangement pattern **(A)** with peaks not exceeding the signal intensity of the positive control **(B)**. The peaks were reproduced on technical replicates that were run in parallel (not shown). This is consistent with a small oligoclonal population of T lymphoid cells and suggests a nonneoplastic lymphocytic proliferation.

may become further restricted due to preferential amplification (PCR bias). The peaks in pseudoclonal cases may be single or multiple and are nonreproducible, including on technical replicates performed simultaneously. Such cases may be further identified by repeating DNA extraction and PCR amplification, since the sizes of the oligoclonal bands are essentially statistical artifacts and are unlikely to be reproduced upon repeat testing.

Given the variety of causes for oligoclonal results, clinical correlation is essential in interpreting such results.

Polyclonal

Polyclonal results in gene clonality testing are those that show a wide range of PCR amplicon sizes, reflecting the diverse population of rearranged *IGH* and/or *TCRG* loci contained in the specimen (Fig. 9-6). These peaks typically have a Gaussian distribution of sizes and show an intensity that is lower than that of the clonal control. A polyclonal result is generally taken as evidence of a non-neoplastic lymphocyte population. However, correlation with histopathologic findings is required to ensure that the suspicious population was contained within the specimen used for gene clonality testing. A false polyclonal result may occur if a clonal population is present below the limit of detection. A clonal postfollicular B cell process may show polyclonal *IGH* results if the neoplastic clone has undergone somatic hypermutation, abolishing the PCR primer annealing sites.

No Amplification

Other specimens failing to amplify are those that contain few to no B or T lymphocytes. In these specimens, there may be ample overall cellularity and the SCSL may show high-quality DNA, but the number of rearranged *IGH* or *TCRG* sequences is too low for detection.

No Result

Specimens that fail to yield any product (clonal or otherwise) may simply be too hypocellular or degraded to support amplification. There will usually be evidence of degradation on the SCSL, which will show poor or no amplification in the size range needed for clonality testing.

In cases classified as "no amplification" or "no result," the test does not necessarily indicate that the patient does not have a clonal hematologic process, as there may be an unsampled clone or a clone falling below the limit of detection of the assay. It behooves the laboratory to clearly indicate, in the test interpretation, whether lack of amplification is attributed to quality/quantity of the specimen or to low density of lymphocytes within the specimen.

Interobserver Reproducibility

Clonality testing data are not straightforward, and require interpretation by a molecular genetic specialist. Resources available to assist with interpretation include package inserts,[9,10] published teaching cases,[11] expert-opinion guidelines,[7] frequently asked questions,[12] and an online support form where experts will answer submitted questions.[13]

Despite the resources available, clonality test interpretation retains an element of subjectivity. Interobserver reproducibility has been reported to be higher for B cell than for T cell testing. In B-cell testing with *IGH* and *IGK* primer sets, there was 100% agreement for cases ultimately classified as clonal or nonclonal, and 60% for cases classified as indeterminate. For T-cell testing with *TCRG* and *TCRB* primer sets, agreement was reported in 67% and 98% of clonal and nonclonal cases, and 37% for indeterminate cases.[14] Thus, while the majority of raters agreed on straightforward cases, borderline cases were problematic, which is perhaps not

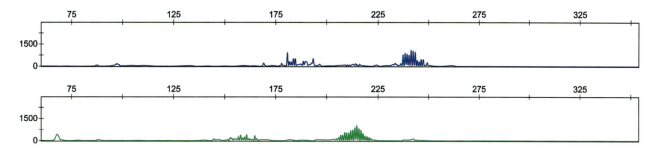

FIGURE 9-6. *TCRG* **capillary electrophoresis pattern classified as polyclonal.** The specimen was peripheral blood from a 61-year-old man with a new diagnosis of hypoplastic myelodysplastic syndrome/aplastic anemia. Peripheral blood showed a slight increase in T cells, although these appeared polyclonal with equal numbers of CD4+ and CD8+ cells. The polyclonal peaks show a Gaussian distribution of amplicon sizes, with no dominant peak. While there is no evidence for a clonal process, the findings do not exclude the presence of an unsampled clonal population or one falling below the limit of detection of the assay.

surprising. To promote consistency, it may be desirable to limit the number of individuals who review clonality testing in any given laboratory and/or to conduct periodic training inservices. A proficiency testing program is available from the College of American Pathologists.

METHODOLOGY AND INTERPRETATION OF PCR-BASED *IGHV* HYPERMUTATION TESTING

The approach to *IGH* hypermutation testing described here consists of two phases: PCR amplification and Sanger sequencing.

Amplification Phase

The amplification phase closely resembles the PCR-based *IGH* clonality test described above. Amplification is performed using FR1 forward primers and a consensus reverse primer.[15] In the presence of a clonal B-cell population, the clonally rearranged *IGH* genes will produce a dominant clonal peak, whereas nonclonal populations will not produce such a peak.

Results of this phase of testing should be specified in the clinical report. The result is "clonal rearrangement" if 1 to 2 clonal peaks are identified by PCR and capillary electrophoresis. Cases in this category are appropriate for downstream sequencing and analysis.

The result of amplification is "polyclonal rearrangements" (or, potentially, "oligoclonal rearrangements") if no specific clonal population is detected. In the absence of a predominant clonally rearranged peak, subsequent analysis cannot be performed, as the B lymphocyte population present in the sample contains a diverse population of rearranged *IGH* sequences. Sanger sequence data obtained from such a sample would represent a mixed population of cells and would therefore be meaningless and impossible to interpret.

If no clonal product is detected, but the SCSL demonstrates adequate quantity/quality of DNA, the test is reported as "no amplification." This result is typically obtained from specimens containing a very small number of B cells.

If no clonal product is detected and the SCSL does not show that the DNA is suitable for amplification, the test is reported as "no result." This result is typically obtained from specimens that are degraded and/or overall paucicellular, containing neither lymphoid elements nor other nuclei.

Sequencing Phase

If a clonal amplicon is detected, that band is purified by agarose gel electrophoresis and subjected to Sanger sequencing. If two clonal peaks are identified, both should be isolated and sequenced, although only one will represent the functional (expressed) rearranged locus. The same primer previously used for amplification is by definition suitable for use as a sequencing primer. Since the reverse (J_H) primer represents a consensus primer, it is practical to use it as the sequencing primer, rather than a mix of the forward primers. The resulting sequence describes the VDJ region of the *IGH* gene of the neoplastic clone, including the *IGHV* region, which may or may not be hypermutated.

The software must analyze the sequence to determine if the rearrangement detected is "productive" (producing a valid open reading frame) or "unproductive" (if the reading frame is disrupted at splice sites so that it no longer encodes a valid protein). It is believed that a functional *IGH* gene must be present and expressed for CLL cells to survive. In general, only productive rearrangements should be analyzed for mutation status. An unproductive rearrangement can coexist with a productive one. Rare cases may appear to lack a productive rearrangement, for which no explanation is readily available.[15]

The patient's *IGH* sequence is then aligned against reference *IGHV* sequences to determine whether hypermutation is present. This can be done using IgBLAST, a variant of the Basic Local Alignment Search Tool (BLAST).[16] A World Wide Web interface to this tool is available through the National Center for Biotechnology Information (NCBI). IgBLAST identifies the *IGHV* gene utilized by the neoplastic clone and reports the percent identity between the patient's sequence and the reference sequence. Percent identity of ≥98% is consistent with a nonhypermutated *IGHV* sequence, while <98% identity indicates hypermutation has occurred. It is appropriate to report these results as "Not hypermutated" and "Hypermutated," respectively.

Cases of CLL/SLL utilizing *IGHV*3-21 have been reported to have an adverse prognosis regardless of the state of hypermutation of the receptor.[17] If IgBLAST reports that this gene is utilized by the neoplastic clone, this result should be explicitly reported as its own sequencing result.

COMMENT

PCR-based clonality testing is a useful ancillary method in hematopathology. Performed on FFPE tissue, blood, and potentially on other specimens such as fine needle aspirates, clonality tests can provide molecular evidence for the presence of a clonal process and can provide a clue to the lineage from which the clone is derived. When sized by capillary electrophoresis, PCR amplicons derived from clonal populations have a characteristic size that can be sought in subsequent specimens to evaluate whether the same clone is present.

Formalin-fixed, paraffin-embedded skin specimens are particularly suitable for testing by these methods. The relative ease of obtaining skin biopsies makes it possible to correlate results at multiple anatomic locations and/or time points, which can help to resolve ambiguities in interpretation.

Although PCR-based clonality testing is a well-established method, next-generation sequencing (NGS)-based methods have recently been developed and are rapidly transitioning from the research setting to the clinic (see chapter on next-generation sequencing). The relative costs and benefits of these methods are changing rapidly at the present time. One notable advantage of NGS-based approaches is that they reveal the sequence of the clonally rearranged gene, providing a more specific signature than the size of the amplicon. The NGS approach may also eliminate some of the subjectivity involved in clonality test interpretation. A notable disadvantage is that the laboratory infrastructure required for NGS testing is greater than that required for PCR and capillary electrophoresis. The BIOMED-2 consortium developed standard reagents to make clonality testing more widely accessible. It remains to be seen whether it is advantageous to now concentrate this testing in the relatively small number of laboratories with NGS capabilities—or whether NGS technology will soon be as widely available as PCR is today.

References

1. Leonard DGB, ed. *Molecular Pathology in Clinical Practice*, 2nd ed. Springer International Publishing, Imprint: Springer, Cham. 2016. 10.1007/978-3-319-19674-9
2. Damle RN, Wasil T, Fais F, et al. Ig V gene mutation status and CD38 expression as novel prognostic indicators in chronic lymphocytic leukemia. *Blood*. 1999;94:1840-1847.
3. Tobin G, Rosenquist R. Prognostic usage of V(H) gene mutation status and its surrogate markers and the role of antigen selection in chronic lymphocytic leukemia. *Med Oncol Northwood Lond Engl*. 2005;22:217-228.
4. Dürig J, Nückel H, Cremer M, et al. ZAP-70 expression is a prognostic factor in chronic lymphocytic leukemia. *Leukemia*. 2003;17:2426-2434.
5. Orchard JA, Ibbotson RE, Davis Z, et al. ZAP-70 expression and prognosis in chronic lymphocytic leukaemia. *Lancet*. 2004;363:105-111.
6. Carreras J, Villamor N, Colomo L, et al. Immunohistochemical analysis of ZAP-70 expression in B-cell lymphoid neoplasms. *J Pathol*. 2005;205:507-513.
7. Langerak AW, Groenen PJTA, Brüggemann M, et al. EuroClonality/BIOMED-2 guidelines for interpretation and reporting of Ig/TCR clonality testing in suspected lymphoproliferations. *Leukemia*. 2012;26:2159-2171.
8. van Krieken JHJM, Langerak AW, Macintyre EA, et al. Improved reliability of lymphoma diagnostics via PCR-based clonality testing: report of the BIOMED-2 Concerted Action BHM4-CT98-3936. *Leukemia*. 2007;21:201-206.
9. Invivoscribe Technologies Package Insert. IGH Gene Clonality Assay. 2020.
10. Invivoscribe Technologies Package Insert. TCRG Gene Clonality Assay. 2020.
11. Groenen PJTA, Langerak AW, van Dongen JJM, van Krieken JHJM. Pitfalls in TCR gene clonality testing: teaching cases. *J Hematop*. 2008;1:97-109.
12. FAQ. Frequently Asked Questions in Clonality Testing. Accessed February 1, 2021. http://www.euroclonality.org/faq/.
13. EuroClonality Project EuroClonality Online Diagnostic Support Services. Accessed April 18, 2021. http://www.euroclonality.org/online-diagnostic-support-services/.
14. Park IJ, Bena J, Cotta CV, et al. Frequency, interobserver reproducibility and clinical significance of equivocal peaks in PCR clonality testing using Euroclonality/BIOMED-2 primers. *J Clin Pathol*. 2014;67:1093-1098.
15. Rosenquist R, Ghia P, Hadzidimitriou A, et al. Immunoglobulin gene sequence analysis in chronic lymphocytic leukemia: updated ERIC recommendations. *Leukemia*. 2017;31:1477-1481.
16. Ye J, Ma N, Madden TL, Ostell JM. IgBLAST: an immunoglobulin variable domain sequence analysis tool. *Nucleic Acids Res*. 2013;41:W34-W40.
17. Ghia EM, Jain S, Widhopf GF II, et al. Use of IGHV3-21 in chronic lymphocytic leukemia is associated with high-risk disease and reflects antigen-driven, post-germinal center leukemogenic selection. *Blood*. 2008;111:5101-5108.

CHAPTER 10

FISH and cytogenetic techniques

Andrea L. Salavaggione and Alejandro A. Gru

FLUORESCENT IN SITU HYBRIDIZATION

In situ hybridization (ISH) allows for detection and localization of a specific DNA or RNA sequence directly in tissue sections by the use of labeled complementary DNA or RNA probes. In contrast to immunohistochemistry (IHC), which analyzes surface, cytoplasmic, or nuclear expression of specific proteins, ISH is able to identify specific RNA or DNA sequences.[1,2] At the early application of ISH in the 1960s, the probes were labeled with radioactive nucleotide analogs.[3] The drawback of radiolabeling included instability of the probes, limited resolution, long exposure times, and risks associated with the handling of radioactive agents. This problem was overcome in the 1980s with the introduction of fluorochromes to make fluorescent, rather than radioactive, ISH (fluorescent in situ hybridization [FISH]).[4]

The advantages that FISH has over conventional cytogenetic methods (conventional karyotype, G-banding) are the lack of dependence on live cells and need of metaphases. FISH can be performed on interphase chromosomes of tissue samples in formalin-fixed paraffin-embedded (FFPE) tissue. Moreover, it has a much higher resolution allowing the identification and localization of short DNA or RNA fragments and the detection of numerical aberrations within single cells. One of the disadvantages is the need for probes that are at least 40 to 50 kilobase (kb) in length, as smaller probes are too difficult to identify in tissue sections. FISH has an extraordinarily high specificity. False-positive rates approximate 1% to 5% because of special colocalization in FFPE tissue.[1] One of the limiting factors in the utility of FISH is the restricted number of probes available for specific molecular diagnostic detection. One of the newer inventions in ISH is the use of chromogen-labeled probes (chromogen in situ hybridization [CISH]). CISH can be applied to FFPE allowing an easier approach with good morphologic correlation and cytogenetic findings.[5] Perhaps, the most common use of CISH techniques includes analysis of κ and λ cytoplasmic light-chain restriction, mRNA detection for Epstein-Barr virus specific sequences (Epstein–Barr–encoded RNA), human papilloma virus subtyping, and detection of HER2 amplification in biopsies of patients with breast cancer. In addition to the maturation of the technique, its applicability broadened from the detection of single nucleic acid targets to multiple targets in a single assay by the simultaneous use of multiple probes, each labeled with a spectrally distinct fluorochrome evaluated by a computer-based ratio analyses of the resulting color combinations and intensities. The discrimination of many more targets than the number of available, spectrally resolvable fluorochromes can be achieved using combinatorial labeling or ratio labeling. These different labeling strategies allow the simultaneous visualization of 24 human chromosomes in a single hybridization. The technologies using these approaches include multiplex-fluorescence in situ hybridization (M-FISH), SKY, and COBRA.[6,7]

More recently, RNA scope ultrasensitive ISH has been developed as a useful technique: Ultrasensitive bright-field RNA in situ hybridization (BRISH) technology (RNAscope, Advanced Cell Diagnostics, Newark, CA), is helpful in clonal B-cell and plasma cell proliferations because it is sensitive enough to detect single mRNA molecules in tumor cells due to simultaneous signal amplification and background suppression. This technique shows a higher level of sensitivity (with same specificity) compared to CISH studies. The cost of CISH and BRISH is very similar to the lab.[8-11] We have recently shown that BRISH was able to reduce the number of subsequent polymerase chain reaction (PCR)-based studies for molecular detection of clonality in reactive lymphoid hyperplasias and cutaneous B-cell lymphomas.[12] Additionally, in systemic B-cell lymphomas, BRISH was used successfully and shows similar clonality rates when compared to routine flow cytometric assays, which are considered the gold standard for evaluation of clonality. In fact, Tubbs et al showed that evaluation of light-chain restriction by BRISH is a reliable method of light-chain expression, with 99% concordance with results of flow cytometry, the gold standard.[10] More recently, Guo et al showed superior detection of light-chain restriction in B-cell non-Hodgkin lymphomas using BRISH compared to flow cytometry.[11] Additionally, BRISH allows for the detection of specific findings that could be missed or difficult to interpret on flow cytometric evaluation, including coexpression of kappa and lambda and biclonal/composite lymphomas. Kaseb et al also demonstrated the use of BRISH for detection of clonal B-cells in cases of nodular lymphocyte-predominant Hodgkin lymphoma.[10]

Two principal types of probes are used to detect chromosomal rearrangements: (1) "split-apart" or "break-apart" probes labeled in different colors that bind to regions on either side of a gene breakpoint and (2) "colocalizing" or "dual-fusion" probes that label each gene in a single color giving fused signals in a cell with a specific translocation.[2] Both types of probes may also reveal gene amplification, and centromeric FISH probes to allow the detection of aneuploidy are also available (Fig. 10-1). BRISH typically shows a granular staining pattern of staining in the B-cells and a cytoplasmic pattern in the plasma cells (Fig. 10-2).

COMPARATIVE GENOMIC HYBRIDIZATION AND ONCOSCAN SNP ARRAY

Chromosomal microarray analysis (CMA) enables simultaneous detection of variations in cancers at a genome-wide level, compared to detection of a limited number of genes and gene variants by fluorescence in situ hybridization (FISH), real-time PCR, and Sanger sequencing. CMA can be divided into two major categories: first is a two-color experiment also referred to as array Comparative Genomic Hybridization (aCGH), in which patient and normal samples are differentially labeled and hybridized to probes on a single microarray, and second is a one-color experiment also known as single nucleotide polymorphism (SNP)–based microarray or SNP array in which instead of including a control sample as a reference in every run, reference intensity data has been built from a population of normal samples and used as a reference for the patient sample.

Comparative genomic hybridization (CGH) is a FISH-based technology that started in the early 1990s.[13] aCGH allows for the assessment of genetic gains and losses over the whole genome. The total genomic DNA is marked with a particular fluorochrome (eg, green), and the DNA from a normal reference is labeled with a different dye (eg, red). Red and green probes are then hybridized competitively to unrelated metaphase chromosomes, which function as the reading device. The fluorescence balance between the sample and reference dyes is evaluated quantitatively. In the case of a normal genetic allocation between test and reference sample, the resulting fluorescence will be a 50/50% balance between green and red (yellow); gains (gene amplification) and losses (deletion) will be more intensive for green and red, respectively. With CGH performed on metaphase chromosomes, copy number changes at the size of several megabases can be detected. The precision to detect smaller genomic changes down to the length of kilobases (usually approximately 80-120 kb) has been achieved by exchanging the metaphase chromosomal-based reading device to a microarray platform (aCGH). With a microarray, a high number of specific and defined DNA sequences can be screened for genetic aberrations (Fig. 10-3). As CGH measurements always represent an average value over the entire cell population analyzed, copy number changes must be present in a substantial proportion of cells (approximately 30%-50%) in order to be identifiable.[14] Therefore, specific aberrations seen in a small proportion of cells will be missed by aCGH. In addition, CGH does not allow the detection of balanced chromosomal translocations, inversions, and point mutations. CGH is also cost intensive, expensive depending on the skills of a laboratory personnel, and it is hard to establish in a new laboratory. aCGH has been clinically used in the diagnosis of melanocytic lesions more extensively.[15-17]

The OncoScan assay is an accepted cancer diagnostic microarray for detection of CNVs, loss of heterozygosity (LOH), and cancer-related somatic mutations. The OncoScan array allows genomic analysis of almost all sample types regardless of source and sample age. Previously these types of samples were cumbersome with other genomic assays owing to poor quality and quantity of extracted gDNA. The OncoScan assay, however, incorporates unique ways of target generation, array hybridization, and data analysis, which make the assay significantly less dependent on gDNA quality and quantity. The OncoScan microarray has incorporated the Molecular Inversion Probe technology to generate targets, which hybridize to probes on the OncoScan microarray. gDNA is hybridized for 16 to 18 h with CNV and somatic mutation probe mixes. As low as 30 ng of DNA might be used for this assay. The OncoScan assay utilizes 335,000 probes for CNVs and allele frequencies, and 541 probes for cancer somatic mutations. Scanning takes approximately 7 min per microarray or 14 min per sample. The entire testing process is completed within 48 h. All chromosomes of a single patient can be displayed simultaneously (Fig. 10-4), and individual chromosome can also be presented with more detailed information. CNV and BAF are displayed along a chromosome where positions of cancer related genes are marked. The application also allows comparison of multiple test results to discern common and unique variations in population studies.[18]

G-BANDING—CONVENTIONAL KARYOTYPE

G-banding is a relatively straightforward and inexpensive method to screen the entire genome for numerical or structural chromosomal aberrations in viable tissues.[19] Its major restriction represents the need for viable metaphases in live cell suspensions. This requires viable tumor with a significant proliferative rate. The metaphase spreads are stained with Giemsa dye revealing a distinctive banding pattern along each chromosomal arm. As each band spans a huge part of a chromosome, subtle translocations, deletions, or insertions will produce a normal banding pattern and can therefore not be detected by this method. The addition of FISH to the conventional metaphases is routinely used in the diagnosis of specific hematologic malignancies (Fig. 10-5).

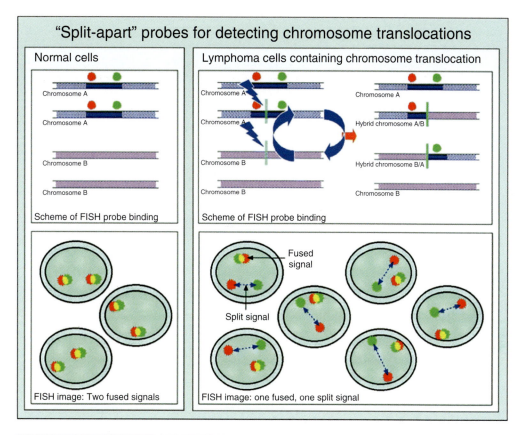
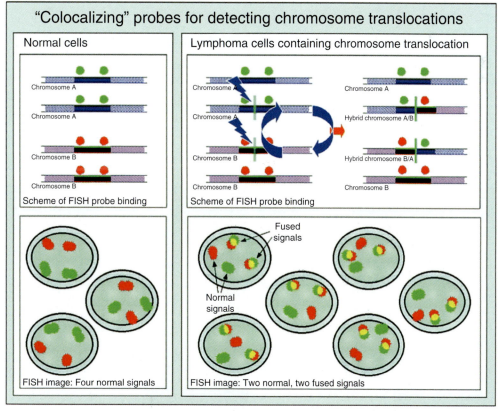

FIGURE 10-1. Probe types used for the FISH detection of chromosomal translocations. Top diagram: "split-apart" probe set, two red/green signals (often yellow) are seen in intact normal nuclei. If a gene is involved in a chromosomal translocation, one of these signals will split, generating separate red and green signals. Bottom diagram: "colocalizing" probes give four spatially separated signals (two red and two green) in normal cells. In cells carrying a reciprocal translocation, two red/green (or yellow) fused signals are seen (together with single red and green signals). It should be noted that on occasion, other combinations of FISH signals may be observed when more complex genetic rearrangements are present. Furthermore, loss of one or more signals due to tissue sectioning will be found in some nuclei. (Reprinted from Gellrich S, Ventura R, Jones M, et al. Immunofluorescent and FISH analysis of skin biopsies. *Am J Dermatopathol.* 2004;26:242-247, with permission.)

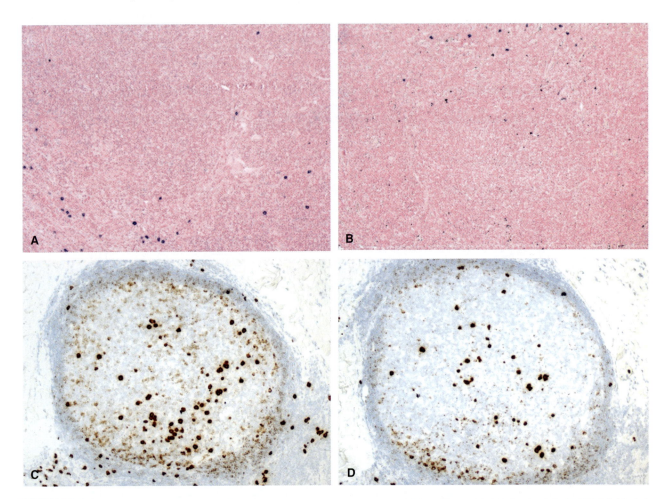

FIGURE 10-2. **A case of primary cutaneous follicle center lymphoma that showed no evidence of kappa (A, 100×) or lambda (B, 100×) light-chain expression by chromogenic in situ hybridization.** Polyclonal plasma cells serve as an internal control. On the same case, ultrasensitive bright-field RNA in situ hybridization for kappa (**C**, 100×) and lambda (**D**, 100×) light-chain RNA demonstrates kappa restriction within the small neoplastic B-cells. (Reproduced with permission from Craddock AP, Kane WJ, Raghavan SS, Williams ES, Gru AA, Gradecki SE. Use of ultrasensitive RNA in situ hybridization for determining clonality in cutaneous B-cell lymphomas and lymphoid hyperplasia decreases subsequent use of molecular testing and is cost-effective. *Am J Surg Pathol*. 2022;46(7):956-962.)

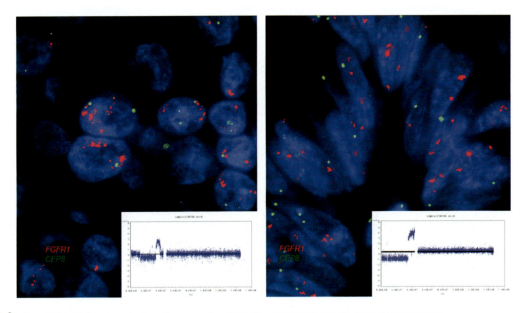

FIGURE 10-3. Array CGH (aCGH) is shown looking at two examples of *FGFR1* amplification in specific cases of breast cancer.

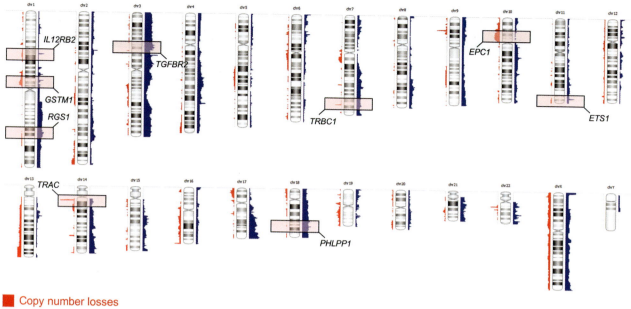

FIGURE 10-4. Multiple copy number changes are seen here displayed as a cumulative data in a cohort of patients with adult T-cell leukemia/lymphoma using OncoScan SNP array.

A comparison of FISH, aCGH, OncoScan SNP, and conventional karyotyping is summarized in Table 10-1. We will discuss the use of these techniques in the diagnosis of cutaneous lymphoproliferative disorders.

MYCOSIS FUNGOIDES AND SÉZARY SYNDROME

Chromosome abnormalities, mostly complex karyotypes, are seen in about 50% of patients with mycosis fungoides/Sézary syndrome (MF/SS), and there have only been a few instances of recurrent rearrangements.[20] Approximately 47% of cases have an abnormal karyotype. The most frequent abnormalities involve chromosome 10; followed by chromosome 6; chromosomes 3, 7, 9, 17, and 19; chromosomes 1 and 12; and chromosomes 8, 11, and 13. Most abnormalities were structural. Recurrent rearrangements included deleted chromosomes 6 and 13, and recurrent breakpoints at 1p32-36, 6q22-25, 17p11.2-13, 10q23-26, and 19p13.3. A pseudodicentric translocation between the short arms of chromosomes 8 and 17, confirmed by dual-color FISH and interpreted as psu dic (17; 8) (p11.2; p11.2), has been noted in a total of three cases. Unbalanced translocations involving chromosomes 4 and 14 have also been noted in SS.[21] Karenko et al[22] showed clonal deletions or translocations with a break point in 12q21 or 12q22 in five of seven consecutive SS patients and a clonal monosomy in the sixth patient. The translocation involved the *NAV3* gene. With locus-specific FISH, *NAV3* deletions were found in the skin lesions of

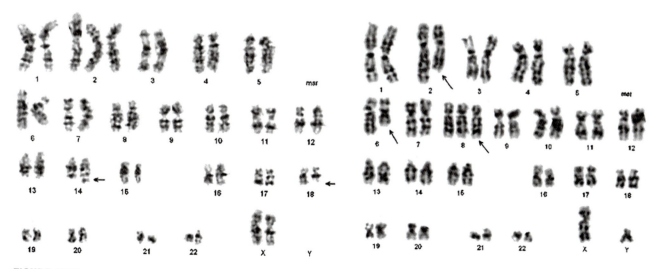

FIGURE 10-5. **Karyotyping of primary cutaneous follicle center lymphoma.** (Reprinted from Streubel B, Scheucher B, Valencak J, et al. Molecular cytogenetic evidence of t(14; 18) (*IGH::BCL2*) in a substantial proportion of primary cutaneous follicle center lymphomas. *Am J Surg Pathol*. 2006;30:529-536, with permission.)

patients were typically elderly and had localized lesions (as opposed to the typical LyP cases occurring in middle-aged adults and with more generalized lesions). A consistent histologic finding also included a typical periadnexal infiltrate and hallmark-like cells. Previously, the *IRF4* rearrangement was detected rarely in single cases of LyP.[35]

Systemic anaplastic large cell lymphoma (ALCL) and C-ALCL differ significantly in their clinical appearance, as well as immunophenotype. ALCL is divided into ALK+ and ALK− forms. The ALK+ ALCL is a disease in childhood, which can be rarely associated with cutaneous dissemination. The most typical rearrangement in ALK+ ALCL is the recurrent, reciprocal balanced translocation, t(2; 5) (p23; q35), which creates the fusion protein *NPM1::ALK*.[42] Other translocation partners of the ALK gene correlate with different patterns of ALK expression by IHC. It is important to highlight that nonhematopoietic tumors with cutaneous dissemination can also show ALK translocations, and those include inflammatory myofibroblastic tumors[43] and melanocytic spitzoid neoplasms.[44] In systemic ALK− ALCL, the t(6; 7) (p25.3; q32.3), creating a fusion between *DUSP22* and *FRA7H*, was demonstrated to be a recurrent phenomenon. Furthermore, (t6; 7) (p25.3; q32.3) was associated with downregulation of DUSP22 and upregulation of MIR29 microRNAs on 7q32.3.[45] The *DUSP22* rearrangement, present in 30% of cases, was associated with the presence of "doughnut" cells, had sheet-like growth of hallmark cells, and likely significant pleomorphic cells. Furthermore, such cases were associated with a better prognosis (similar to ALK+ ALCL), when compared to other ALK−ALCL.[46,47] *TP63* rearrangements were also shown in 8% of cases and had a worse prognosis. Rare forms of primary cutaneous ALK+ ALCL have been reported in the literature.[48] Additionally, tumors with a double hit (*DUSP22*+/*TP63*+ translocation) can occur.[49,50]

C-ALCL has shown recent specific recurrent rearrangements, similar to the systemic counterparts: an *IRF4* rearrangement has been identified in 75% of C-ALCL, and is a useful tool to distinguish them from LyP and transformed MF.[51] Pham-Ledard et al[52] found a lower frequency (26%) for such rearrangement and also identified rare cases of transformed MF with *IRF4* translocation. In the large cohort from Wada et al,[35] the translocation was present in 20% of cases. Onaindia et al[53] described three cases of C-ALCL with *IRF4–DUSP22* translocation, and found that, similar to the LyP group with 6p25.3 rearrangement, a striking biphasic pattern with an epidermotropic and diffuse dermal infiltrate was present in all cases. In addition, a spectrum of cutaneous CD30+ lymphoproliferative disorders with a prominent intralymphatic dissemination and associated *IRF4/DUSP22* rearrangement has been recently described.[54] The latter cohort includes cases that could be classified as C-ALCL or LyP (Fig. 10-8).[55]

Only limited studies have been done in other rare examples of CTCL, such as subcutaneous panniculitis-like T-cell lymphoma (SPTL). A Finnish study used CGH and showed large numbers of DNA copy number changes, the most common of which were losses of chromosomes 1pter, 2pter, 10qter, 11qter, 12qter, 16, 19, 20, and 22 and gains of chromosomes 2q and 4q. Some of the DNA copy number aberrations in SPTL, such as loss of 10q, 17p, and chromosome 19, overlap with other common forms of CTCL (MF and SS), whereas 5q and 13q gains characterize SPTL. Allelic *NAV3* aberrations (LOH or deletion by FISH), previously found in MF and SS, were identified in 44% of the SPTL samples.[56] *HAVCR-2* mutations appear to be critical in cases that develop hemophagocytosis.

A single center experience analyzing the cytogenetic karyotype of a primary cutaneous γδ T-cell lymphoma showed several chromosomal translocations involving breakpoints at 9p21, 14q11.2, 14q32.1, or 16q23.1, suggesting the involvement of *WWOX*, *TCL* gene cluster, and *BCL11B*, which are crucial for tumorigenesis in T-cell lymphomas.[57] Additionally, we have also previously identified the presence of the isochromosome i(7q) in such tumor (Fig. 10-9), a finding that is consistently present in cases of hepatosplenic T-cell lymphomas.[58,59]

A more recent study by Daniels et al revealed distinctive molecular alterations in cases of primary cutaneous gamma-delta T-cell lymphomas. They identified 20 putative driver genes, including the presence of *STAT3* and *STAT5B* mutations. They also identified 18 additional putative drivers in cutaneous gamma-delta T-cell lymphomas (CGDTLs). These mutations affect multiple, oncogenic pathways, including MAPK signaling (*KRAS*, *NRAS*, *MAPK1*), MYC pathway (*MYC*, *MYCN*, *FBXW7*), JAK/STAT signaling (*STAT3*, *STAT5B*, *JAK3*, *SOCS1*), and chromatin modification (*ARID1A*, *TRRAP*, *TET2*, *KMT2D*). Additional mutations affect consensus cancer genes (*CDKN2A*, *IDH2*, *TP53*) as well as tumor suppressors previously identified in CTCL (*TNFAIP3*, *FAS*, *PDCD1*).[60]

They also identified copy number information for 18 CGDTLs with interpretable copy number data. Analysis of SCNVs in CGDTL revealed recurrent arm level amplifications and deletions, including amplification of 1q (33%), 15q (33%), and 7q (39%) and deletions of 9p (22%) and 18q (22%). GISTIC analysis identified significantly recurrent deletions of *CDKN2A* (deleted in 61% of samples, with 45% of deletions biallelic) and *ARID1A* (deleted in 28% of samples). Significantly recurrent amplifications included *TNFRSF1B* (amplified in 33%), which encodes the NF-kB pathway activating oncogene TNFR240, and *MAP4K4* (amplified in 17%), an activator of ERK signaling associated with poor outcomes in numerous cancers. They also found focal deletions common in other T-cell cancers (*FAS and PDCD1*) in 22% of cases each, one sample each with biallelic deletion of *FAS or PDCD1*.[78]

A recent study by Lee et al revealed notorious molecular alterations in primary cutaneous aggressive epidermotropic CD8+ T-cell lymphomas (Berti lymphoma). This analysis identified *JAK2* fusions in all cases of primary cutaneous aggressive CD8+ epidermotropic T-cell lymphomas (PCAETCLs). None of the additional CTCL-not otherwise specified harbored an oncogenic fusion. Collectively, the PCAETCLs in their cohort harbored JAK2 fusions reported in other cancers (*PCM1::JAK2* and *STAT3::JAK2*), the JAK2 fusions recently reported for PCAETCL (*KHDRBS1::JAK2*), and 3 fusions not previously described in any cancer (*PICALM::JAK2*, *CAPRIN1::JAK2*, and *SELENOI::ABL1*).[61] Alterations in the JAK2 gene have also been documented in a separate large cohort of cases.[62]

PRIMARY CUTANEOUS FOLLICLE CENTER LYMPHOMA

The t(14; 18) translocation is characteristic of systemic follicular lymphomas (FLs), particularly in low-grade cases. The same translocation is present in 10% to 50% of primary cutaneous follicle center lymphoma (PCFCL) cases (Fig. 10-10).[63-66] A recent study by Zhou et al revealed the

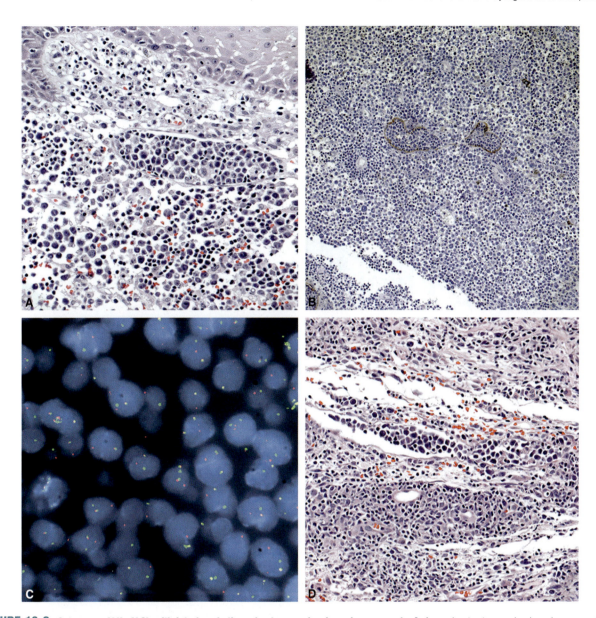

FIGURE 10-8. **Cutaneous ALK–ALCL with intralymphatic and extravascular dermal components. A.** A prominent extravascular dermal component may accompany or even mask intralymphatic CD30+large T-cell proliferations (H&E). **B.** The intralymphatic component is highlighted on D2-40 immunohistochemistry. **C.** A FISH break-apart probe reveals a translocation at the DUSP22–IRF4 locus, with aberrant separation of one pair of green and red probes per nucleus, consistent with primary cutaneous ALCL. **D.** A CD30+ cutaneous TLPD presenting as an otherwise asymptomatic papule on the nose has both an intralymphatic large cell component and a heterogenous dermal extravascular T-cell infiltrate (H&E). H&E indicates hematoxylin and eosin. (From Samols MA, Su A, Ra S, et al. Intralymphatic cutaneous anaplastic large cell lymphoma/lymphomatoid papulosis: expanding the spectrum of CD30-positive lymphoproliferative disorders. *Am J Surg Pathol*. 2014;38:1203-1211, with permission.)

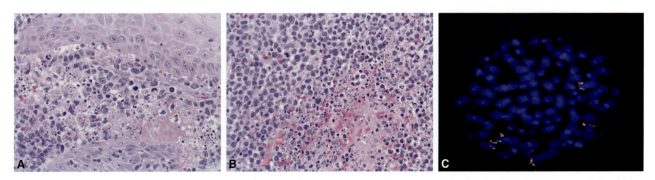

FIGURE 10-9. **FISH in primary cutaneous γδ T-cell lymphoma. A** and **B.** Malignant infiltrate in the dermis with areas of epidermotropism. **C.** Cytogenetic findings with metaphase FISH. Metaphase FISH with the ALK breakage probe, specific for 2p23.2 (Abbott Molecular), was performed. There were four normal chromosomes, two homologues, and an additional ALK signal on the derivative chromosome 19. (Courtesy of Dr. S Kawash, Nationwide Children's Hospital, Columbus, OH.)

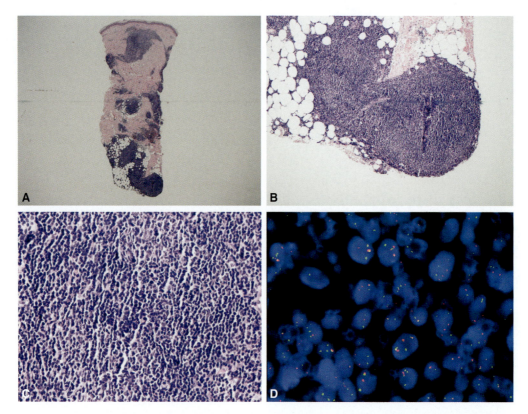

FIGURE 10-10. PCFCL with IGH-BCL2 rearrangement. A–C. Nodular infiltrate in the dermis, sparing the epidermis, and containing numerous centrocytes. **D.** Using a dual-fusion probe (*IGH-green; BCL2-red*), occasional yellow signals within the cells are noted, indicative of the translocation.

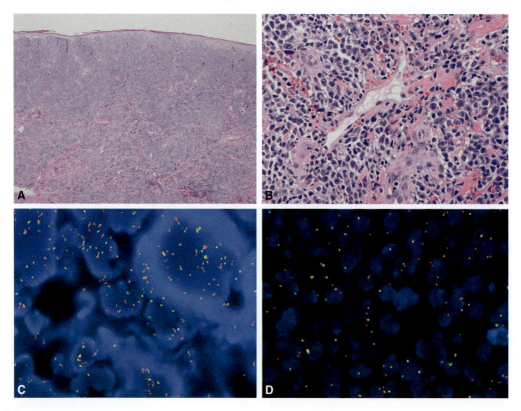

FIGURE 10-11. FISH in PCLBCL-LT. A and **B.** Dense infiltrate in the dermis composed of sheets of large malignant cells. **C.** Polysomy and copy number gains of *MYC* gene. Frequent gains of the MYC and corresponding centromeric probe are noted (CEP 8). **D.** Using a break-apart probe, splitting of the red and green signals indicates a rearrangement of the *MYC* gene.

translocation in 8% of cases, and in their algorithm, the presence of such translocation appears to be useful to distinguish between PCFLC and cutaneous involvement by systemic FL.[67] The low percentage of rearrangements has been confirmed in other studies.[68] However, the lack of this translocation is supportive of the diagnosis of PCFCL. A t(3; 14) (q27; q32) affecting *BCL6* has also been described in cases of PCFCL[66] and up to 12% can show trisomy 3.[64] Rare cases can also show more complex patterns of translocations.[69] aCGH studies in PCFCL have shown recurrent 1p36 deletions.[70] A study by Dijkman et al[71] identified high-level DNA amplifications at 2p16.1 (63%) and deletion of chromosome 14q32.33 (68%). FISH analysis confirmed *c-REL* amplification in patients with gains at 2p16.1. PCFCL showed a very different genomic profile, when compared to cases of primary cutaneous large B-cell lymphoma, leg type (PCLBCL-LT).

Copy number alterations have been observed in four of five cases of PCFCL, including copy number gains, copy number losses, and LOH. Interestingly, three of five cases of PCFCL showed loss of chromosome 1p36. Other recurrent large genomic alterations observed in at least two cases of PCFCL included gains involving chromosomes 7 and 18 and LOH of chromosomes 6p and 9/9p. Recurrent focal copy number alterations included gain of 2p16p15.1 (including *REL*) and deletions of 2p11.2 (*IGKV*), 9p21.3 (*CDKN2A*), and 14q32.33 (*IGH* locus). A high copy number gain, defined as >2 copies, was observed in only 1 case of PCFCL (2p16.1-p15 region).[72]

PRIMARY CUTANEOUS LARGE B-CELL LYMPHOMA, LEG TYPE

FISH and CGH studies have demonstrated a t(8; 14) (q24; q32) in two of six PCLBCL-LT, involving the *MYC* gene. Recurrent deletions in 9p21 (p14(ARF)/p16(INK4a) CDKN2A) were a constant finding in PCLBCL-LT (six of six).[70,73] A study of 12 cases of PCBCL-LT (using CGH and FISH) showed high-level DNA amplification of 18q21.31-q21.33 (67%), including the *BCL-2* and *MALT1* genes as confirmed by FISH, and deletions of a small region within 9p21.3 containing the *CDKN2A*, *CDKN2B*, and *NSG-x* genes.[71] *FOXP1* gene gains (three to four copies) were observed in 82% of samples of PCLBCL-LT and in 37% of PCFCL.[74] More recently, Pham-Ledard et al[75] published a large series of 23 cases of PCBCL-LT and identified a split for *BCL2*, *BCL6*, and *MYC* in 1/23, 6/23, and 3/23 of cases, respectively (Fig. 10-11). No double-hit lymphoma was observed. *CDKN2A* deletion was detected by

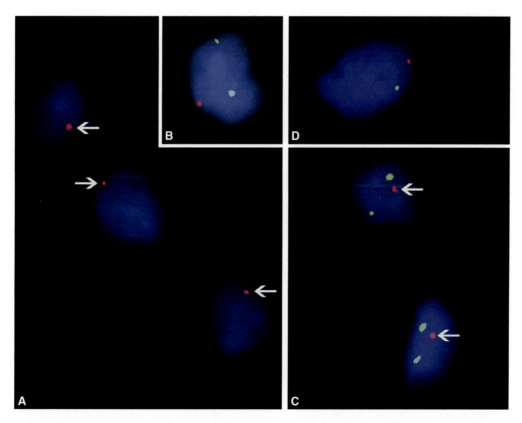

FIGURE 10-12. FISH in BPDCN. Fluorescence in situ hybridization performed on lesional tissue sections. Interphase nuclei hybridized with LSI RB1 Probe (Abbott/Vysis). The three nuclei display one orange signal indicating a loss of RB1 (13q14) (*arrows*) **(A)**. Interphase nucleus hybridized with LSI D5S23/D5S721, CEP 9, CEP15 Multicolor Probe (Abbott/Vysis). The nucleus shows one green (D5S23/D5S721), one aqua (CEP 9), and one orange (CEP15) signal pattern indicative of a loss of 5p15 (D5S23/D5S721), monosomy 9, and monosomy 15 **(B)**. Interphase nuclei hybridized with LSI p16/CEP9 Dual-Color Probe (Abbott/Vysis). The two nuclei display two green (CEP 9) and one orange (p16) signal (*arrows*), pointing to a loss of p16 (9p21) **(C)**. Interphase nuclei hybridized with LSI EGR1/D5S23, D5S721 Dual-Color Probe (Abbott/Vysis). The nucleus displays one orange (EGR1) and one green (D5S23, D5S721) signal, indicative of a loss of 5q31 (EGR1) and a loss of 5p15 (D5S23, D5S721) **(D)**. (Reprinted from Kaune KM, Baumgart M, Bertsch HP, et al. Solitary cutaneous nodule of blastic plasmacytoid dendritic cell neoplasm progressing to overt leukemia cutis after chemotherapy: immunohistology and FISH analysis confirmed the diagnosis. *Am J Dermatopathol.* 2009;31:695-701, with permission.)

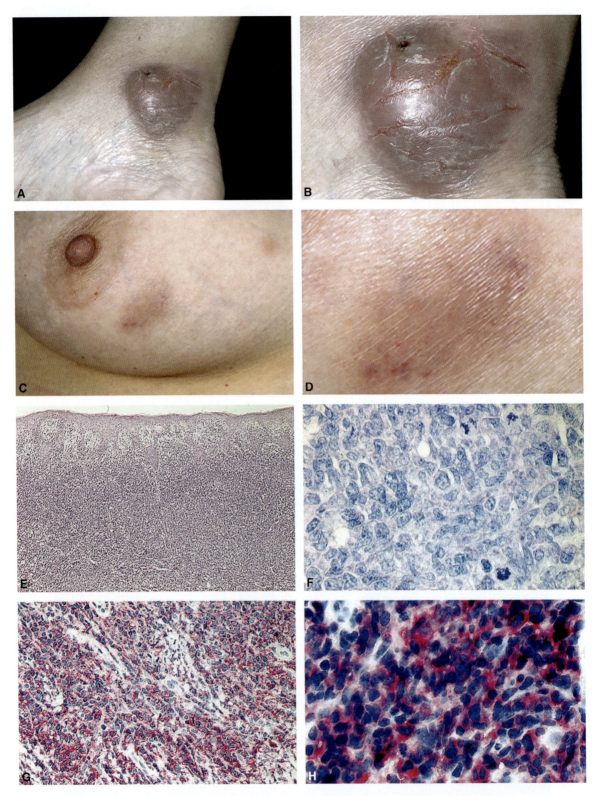

FIGURE 10-13. BPDCN. Clinical picture and histology of BPDC neoplasm. Solitary cutaneous manifestation of BPDC neoplasm as violaceous nodule on the right inner ankle (**A** and **B**). Bruise-like area on the left breast appearing as the first sign of tumor progression (**C** and **D**). Hematoxylin and eosin staining of skin sections from the skin nodule showing diffuse pandermal infiltrates (**E**). Giemsa stain reveals atypical medium-sized blastic cells with prominent nuclei and some mitotic figures (**F**). The neoplastic cells were positive for the CD56 antigen (**G**) and displayed a strong expression of CD123 (**H**). (From Kaune KM, Baumgart M, Bertsch HP, et al. Solitary cutaneous nodule of blastic plasmacytoid dendritic cell neoplasm progressing to overt leukemia cutis after chemotherapy: immunohistology and FISH analysis confirmed the diagnosis. *Am J Dermatopathol.* 2009;31:695-701, with permission.)

FISH in only 5/23 of cases. *BLIMP1* and/or 6q deletion was observed at a higher rate in 10/20 of cases. This particular study also found a high rate of *MYD88* mutations (61%) in this cohort and supported a common pathway for associated lymphomagenesis to diffuse large B-cell lymphoma—activated B-cell type.

Molecular studies looking into *BCL-2, BCL-6,* and *MYC* have been performed in PCLBCL-LT. Double hit lymphomas (*MYC* plus one of the other genes) can be seen in a substantial proportion of cases (15%).[76] *MYC* translocations can occur in as many as 32% cases of PCLBCL-LT.[77] Menguy et al have raised concerns about this disproportionate high rate of MYC translocations in PCLBCL-LT,[77] claiming the identification of such in only 1/23 cases.[78,79]

PRIMARY CUTANEOUS MARGINAL ZONE LYMPHOMA

While some extranodal marginal zone lymphomas can be associated with rearrangements of the *MALT1* gene, a study of 16 cases of primary cutaneous marginal zone lymphoma (PCMZL) failed to reveal the translocation.[80] Another study of 23 cases of PCMZL also failed to show such translocation.[81] However, Schreuder et al[82] found the translocation in 3/12 of cases.

NONLYMPHOID CUTANEOUS HEMATOLOGIC NEOPLASMS

Blastic plasmacytoid dendritic cell neoplasm (BPDCN) is a tumor that invariably has cutaneous presentations with very frequent secondary leukemic dissemination. The genetics of the disease is very poorly understood. Comprehensive aCGH studies showed complete or partial chromosomal losses that largely outnumbered the gains, with common deleted regions involving 9p21.3 (*CDKN2A/CDKN2B*), 13q13.1-q14.3 (*RB1*), 12p13.2-p13.1 (*CDKN1B*), 13q11-q12 (*LATS2*), and 7p12.2 (*IKZF1*) regions (Fig. 10-12). *CDKN2A/CDKN2B* deletion was also confirmed by FISH.[83] A study by Leroux et al[84] revealed clonal, mostly complex chromosome aberrations in 14 patients (66%). Six major recurrent chromosomal targets were defined. These were 5q, 12p, 13q, 6q, 15q, and 9, which were involved in 72% (5q), 64% (12p and 13q), 50% (6q), 43% (15q), and 28% (monosomy 9) of cases, respectively (Fig. 10-13). Subsequent studies have shown that BPDCN lacks the typical chromosomal aberrations seen in cases of acute myeloid leukemia.[85] Myeloid sarcoma (leukemia cutis) needs to be distinguished from BPDCN, given the treatment implications that both diagnoses have. In myeloid sarcoma, chromosomal aberrations were detected in about 54% of cases: monosomy 7(10.8%), trisomy 8(10.4%), and mixed lineage leukemia splitting (8.5%) (Fig. 10-14) were the commonest abnormalities, whereas t(8; 21) was rare (2.2%).[86]

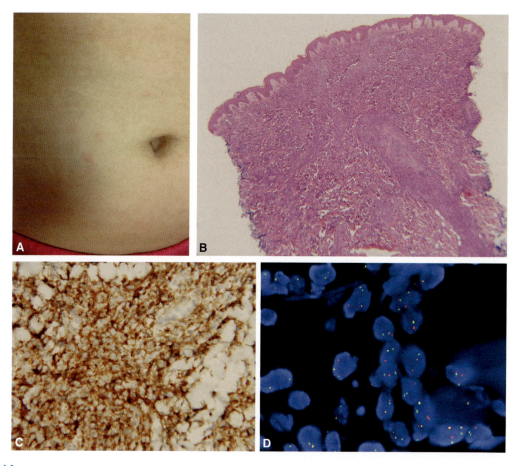

FIGURE 10-14. Leukemia cutis. Small nodular areas are seen in the abdomen of this girl **(A)**. A diffuse infiltrate in the dermis is noted **(B)**. The malignant infiltrate is positive for CD43 **(C)**. Additional FISH studies reveal a rearrangement of the *MLL* gene (splitting of green and red signals using a break-apart probe) **(D)**. In this case, the *MLL* translocation was associated with a therapy-related myeloid neoplasm.

References

1. Braun-Falco M, Schempp W, Weyers W. Molecular diagnosis in dermatopathology: what makes sense, and what doesn't. *Exp Dermatol*. 2009;18:12-23.
2. Gellrich S, Ventura R, Jones M, et al. Immunofluorescent and FISH analysis of skin biopsies. *Am J Dermatopathol*. 2004;26:242-247.
3. Gall JG, Pardue ML. Formation and detection of RNA–DNA hybrid molecules in cytological preparations. *Proc Natl Acad Sci U S A*. 1969;63:378-383.
4. Bauman JG, Wiegant J, Borst P, et al. A new method for fluorescence microscopical localization of specific DNA sequences by in situ hybridization of fluorochromelabelled RNA. *Exp Cell Res*. 1980;128:485-490.
5. Hammock L, Cohen C, Carlson G, et al. Chromogenic in situ hybridization analysis of melastatin mRNA expression in melanomas from American Joint Committee on Cancer stage I and II patients with recurrent melanoma. *J Cutan Pathol*. 2006;33:599-607.
6. Fauth C, Speicher MR. Classifying by colors: FISH-based genome analysis. *Cytogenet Cell Genet*. 2001;93:1-10.
7. Speicher MR, Carter NP. The new cytogenetics: blurring the boundaries with molecular biology. *Nat Rev Genet*. 2005;6:782-792.
8. Wang H, Su N, Wang LC, et al. Dual-color ultrasensitive brightfield RNA in situ hybridization with RNAscope. *Methods Mol Biol*. 2014;1211:139-149. doi:10.1007/978-1-4939-1459-3_12
9. Minca EC, Wang H, Wang Z, et al. Detection of immunoglobulin light-chain restriction in cutaneous B-cell lymphomas by ultrasensitive bright-field mRNA in situ hybridization. *J Cutan Pathol*. 2015;42:82-89. doi:10.1111/cup.12415
10. Tubbs RR, Wang H, Wang Z, et al. Ultrasensitive RNA in situ hybridization for detection of restricted clonal expression of low-abundance immunoglobulin light chain mRNA in B-cell lymphoproliferative disorders. *Am J Clin Pathol*. 2013;140:736-746. doi:10.1309/AJCPJTWK07FSABRJ.
11. Guo L, Wang Z, Anderson CM, et al. Ultrasensitive automated RNA in situ hybridization for kappa and lambda light chain mRNA detects B-cell clonality in tissue biopsies with performance comparable or superior to flow cytometry. *Mod Pathol*. 2018;31:385-394. doi:10.1038/modpathol.2017.142
12. Craddock AP, Kane WJ, Raghavan SS, Williams ES, Gru AA, Gradecki SE. Use of ultrasensitive RNA in situ hybridization for determining clonality in cutaneous B-cell lymphomas and lymphoid hyperplasia Decreases subsequent use of molecular testing and is cost-effective. *Am J Surg Pathol*. 2022;46(7):956-962.
13. Kallioniemi A, Kallioniemi OP, Sudar D, et al. Comparative genomic hybridization for molecular cytogenetic analysis of solid tumors. *Science*. 1992;258:818-821.
14. Bauer J, Bastian B. Genomic analysis of melanocytic neoplasia. *Adv Dermatol*. 2005;21:81-99.
15. Curtin JA, Fridlyand J, Kageshita T, et al. Distinct sets of genetic alterations in melanoma. *N Engl J Med*. 2005;353:2135-2147.
16. Moore SR, Persons DL, Sosman JA, et al. Detection of copy number alterations in metastatic melanoma by a DNA fluorescence in situ hybridization probe panel and array comparative genomic hybridization: a southwest oncology group study (S9431). *Clin Cancer Res*. 2008;14:2927-2935.
17. Shain AH, Yeh I, Kovalyshyn I, et al. The genetic evolution of melanoma from precursor lesions. *N Engl J Med*. 2015;373:1926-1936.
18. Jung HS, Lefferts JA, Tsongalis GJ. Utilization of the oncoscan microarray assay in cancer diagnostics. *Appl Cancer Res*. 2017;37:Article number: 1.
19. Sanchez O, Escobar JI, Yunis JJ. A simple G-banding technique. *Lancet*. 1973;2:269.
20. Batista DA, Vonderheid EC, Hawkins A, et al. Multicolor fluorescence in situ hybridization (SKY) in mycosis fungoides and Sézary syndrome: search for recurrent chromosome abnormalities. *Genes Chromosomes Cancer*. 2006;45:383-391.
21. Mohr B, Illmer T, Oelschlagel U, et al. Complex cytogenetic and immunophenotypic aberrations in a patient with Sézary syndrome. *Cancer Genet Cytogenet*. 1996;90:33-36.
22. Karenko L, Hahtola S, Paivinen S, et al. Primary cutaneous T-cell lymphomas show a deletion or translocation affecting NAV3, the human UNC-53 homologue. *Cancer Res*. 2005;65:8101-8110.
23. Ranki A, Vakeva L, Sipila L, et al. Molecular markers associated with clinical response to bexarotene therapy in cutaneous T-cell lymphoma. *Acta Derm Venereol*. 2011;91:568-573.
24. Caprini E, Cristofoletti C, Arcelli D, et al. Identification of key regions and genes important in the pathogenesis of sézary syndrome by combining genomic and expression microarrays. *Cancer Res*. 2009;69:8438-8446.
25. Lin WM, Lewis JM, Filler RB, et al. Characterization of the DNA copy-number genome in the blood of cutaneous T-cell lymphoma patients. *J Invest Dermatol*. 2012;132:188-197.
26. Vaque JP, Gomez-Lopez G, Monsalvez V, et al. PLCG1 mutations in cutaneous T-cell lymphomas. *Blood*. 2014;123:2034-2043.
27. Vermeer MH, van Doorn R, Dijkman R, et al. Novel and highly recurrent chromosomal alterations in Sézary syndrome. *Cancer Res*. 2008;68:2689-2698.
28. Mao X, Lillington D, Scarisbrick JJ, et al. Molecular cytogenetic analysis of cutaneous T-cell lymphomas: identification of common genetic alterations in Sézary syndrome and mycosis fungoides. *Br J Dermatol*. 2002;147:464-475.
29. Mao X, Lillington DM, Czepulkowski B, et al. Molecular cytogenetic characterization of Sézary syndrome. *Genes Chromosomes Cancer*. 2003;36:250-260.
30. Mao X, Orchard G, Lillington DM, et al. BCL2 and JUNB abnormalities in primary cutaneous lymphomas. *Br J Dermatol*. 2004;151:546-556.
31. Mao X, Orchard G, Mitchell TJ, et al. A genomic and expression study of AP-1 in primary cutaneous T-cell lymphoma: evidence for dysregulated expression of JUNB and JUND in MF and SS. *J Cutan Pathol*. 2008;35:899-910.
32. Mao X, Orchard G, Vonderheid EC, et al. Heterogeneous abnormalities of CCND1 and RB1 in primary cutaneous T-Cell lymphomas suggesting impaired cell cycle control in disease pathogenesis. *J Invest Dermatol*. 2006;126:1388-1395.
33. Salgado R, Gallardo F, Servitje O, et al. Absence of TCR loci chromosomal translocations in cutaneous T-cell lymphomas. *Cancer Genet*. 2011;204:405-409.
34. Utikal J, Poenitz N, Gratchev A, et al. Additional Her 2/neu gene copies in patients with Sézary syndrome. *Leuk Res*. 2006;30:755-760.
35. Wada DA, Law ME, Hsi ED, et al. Specificity of IRF4 translocations for primary cutaneous anaplastic large cell lymphoma: a multicenter study of 204 skin biopsies. *Mod Pathol*. 2011;24:596-605.
36. Choi J, Goh G, Walradt T, et al. Genomic landscape of cutaneous T cell lymphoma. *Nat Genet*. 2015;47:1011-1019.

37. da Silva Almeida AC, Abate F, Khiabanian H, et al. The mutational landscape of cutaneous T cell lymphoma and Sézary syndrome. *Nat Genet.* 2015;47(12):1465-1470.
38. Kiel MJ, Sahasrabuddhe AA, Rolland DC, et al. Genomic analyses reveal recurrent mutations in epigenetic modifiers and the JAK-STAT pathway in Sézary syndrome. *Nat Commun.* 2015;6:8470.
39. Ungewickell A, Bhaduri A, Rios E, et al. Genomic analysis of mycosis fungoides and Sézary syndrome identifies recurrent alterations in TNFR2. *Nat Genet.* 2015;47:1056-1060.
40. Wang L, Ni X, Covington KR, et al. Genomic profiling of Sézary syndrome identifies alterations of key T cell signaling and differentiation genes. *Nat Genet.* 2015;47(12):1426-1434.
41. Karai LJ, Kadin ME, Hsi ED, et al. Chromosomal rearrangements of 6p25.3 define a new subtype of lymphomatoid papulosis. *Am J Surg Pathol.* 2013;37:1173-1181.
42. Kadin ME, Morris SW. The t(2;5) in human lymphomas. *Leuk Lymphoma.* 1998;29:249-256.
43. Leguellec S, Tournier E, Karanian M, et al. Cutaneous inflammatory myofibroblastic tumours can be anaplastic lymphoma kinase-positive: report of the first four cases.*Histopathology.* Published online ahead of print June 23, 2015. doi:10.1111/his.12759
44. Busam KJ, Kutzner H, Cerroni L, et al. Clinical and pathologic findings of Spitz nevi and atypical Spitz tumors with ALK fusions. *Am J Surg Pathol.* 2014;38:925-933.
45. Feldman AL, Dogan A, Smith DI, et al. Discovery of recurrent t(6;7)(p25.3;q32.3) translocations in ALK-negative anaplastic large cell lymphomas by massively parallel genomic sequencing. *Blood.* 2011;117:915-919.
46. King RL, Dao LN, McPhail ED, et al. Morphologic features of ALK-negative anaplastic large cell lymphomas with DUSP22 rearrangements. *Am J Surg Pathol.* 2016;40(1):36-43.
47. Parrilla Castellar ER, Jaffe ES, Said JW, et al. ALK-negative anaplastic large cell lymphoma is a genetically heterogeneous disease with widely disparate clinical outcomes. *Blood.* 2014;124:1473-1480.
48. Melchers RC, Willemze R, van de Loo M, et al. Clinical, histologic, and molecular characteristics of anaplastic lymphoma kinase-positive primary cutaneous anaplastic large cell lymphoma. *Am J Surg Pathol.* 2020;44(6):776-781.
49. Klairmont MM, Ward N. Co-occurring rearrangements of DUSP22 and TP63 define a rare genetic subset of ALK-negative anaplastic large cell lymphoma with inferior survival outcomes. *Leuk Lymphoma.* 2022;63(2):506-508.
50. Karube K, Feldman AL. "Double-hit" of DUSP22 and TP63 rearrangements in anaplastic large cell lymphoma, ALK-negative. *Blood.* 2020;135(9):700. doi:10.1182/blood.2019004164
51. Kiran T, Demirkesen C, Eker C, et al. The significance of MUM1/IRF4 protein expression and IRF4 translocation of CD30(+) cutaneous T-cell lymphoproliferative disorders: a study of 53 cases. *Leuk Res.* 2013;37:396-400.
52. Pham-Ledard A, Prochazkova-Carlotti M, Laharanne E, et al. IRF4 gene rearrangements define a subgroup of CD30-positive cutaneous T-cell lymphoma: a study of 54 cases. *J Invest Dermatol.* 2010;130:816-825.
53. Onaindia A, Montes-Moreno S, Rodriguez-Pinilla SM, et al. Primary cutaneous anaplastic large cell lymphomas with 6p25.3 rearrangement exhibit particular histological features. *Histopathology.* 2015;66:846-855.
54. Samols MA, Su A, Ra S, et al. Intralymphatic cutaneous anaplastic large cell lymphoma/lymphomatoid papulosis: expanding the spectrum of CD30-positive lymphoproliferative disorders. *Am J Surg Pathol.* 2014;38:1203-1211.
55. Xing X, Feldman AL. Anaplastic large cell lymphomas: ALK positive, ALK negative, and primary cutaneous. *Adv Anat Pathol.* 2015;22:29-49.
56. Hahtola S, Burghart E, Jeskanen L, et al. Clinicopathological characterization and genomic aberrations in subcutaneous panniculitis-like T-cell lymphoma. *J Invest Dermatol.* 2008;128:2304-2309.
57. Yamamoto-Sugitani M, Kuroda J, Shimura Y, et al. Comprehensive cytogenetic study of primary cutaneous gamma-delta T-cell lymphoma by means of spectral karyotyping and genome-wide single nucleotide polymorphism array. *Cancer Genet.* 2012;205:459-464.
58. Hocker TL, Wada DA, McPhail ED, et al. Relapsed hepatosplenic T-cell lymphoma heralded by a solitary skin nodule. *J Cutan Pathol.* 2011;38:899-904.
59. Tripodo C, Iannitto E, Florena AM, et al. Gamma-delta T-cell lymphomas. *Nat Rev Clin Oncol.* 2009;6:707-717.
60. Daniels J, Doukas PG, Martinez Escala ME, et al. Cellular origins and genetic landscape of cutaneous gamma delta T cell lymphomas. *Nat Commun.* 2020;11(1):1806. doi:10.1038/s41467-020-15572-7
61. Lee K, Evans MG, Yang L, et al. Primary cytotoxic T-cell lymphomas harbor recurrent targetable alterations in the JAK-STAT pathway. *Blood.* 2021;138(23):2435-2440. doi:10.1182/blood.2021012536
62. Bastidas Torres AN, Cats D, Out-Luiting JJ, et al. Deregulation of JAK2 signaling underlies primary cutaneous CD8+ aggressive epidermotropic cytotoxic T-cell lymphoma. *Haematologica.* 2022;107(3):702-714.
63. Kim BK, Surti U, Pandya A, et al. Clinicopathologic, immunophenotypic, and molecular cytogenetic fluorescence in situ hybridization analysis of primary and secondary cutaneous follicular lymphomas. *Am J Surg Pathol.* 2005;29:69-82.
64. Aguilera NS, Tomaszewski MM, Moad JC, et al. Cutaneous follicle center lymphoma: a clinicopathologic study of 19 cases. *Mod Pathol.* 2001;14:828-835.
65. Pham-Ledard A, Cowppli-Bony A, Doussau A, et al. Diagnostic and prognostic value of BCL2 rearrangement in 53 patients with follicular lymphoma presenting as primary skin lesions. *Am J Clin Pathol.* 2015;143:362-373.
66. Streubel B, Scheucher B, Valencak J, et al. Molecular cytogenetic evidence of t(14;18)(IGH;BCL2) in a substantial proportion of primary cutaneous follicle center lymphomas. *Am J Surg Pathol.* 2006;30:529-536.
67. Zhou XA, Yang J, Ringbloom KG, et al. Genomic landscape of cutaneous follicular lymphomas reveals 2 subgroups with clinically predictive molecular features. *Blood Adv.* 2021;5(3):649-661. doi:10.1182/bloodadvances.2020002469
68. Barasch NJK, Liu YC, Ho J, et al. The molecular landscape and other distinctive features of primary cutaneous follicle center lymphoma. *Hum Pathol.* 2020;106:93-105. doi:10.1016/j.humpath.2020.09.014
69. Subramaniyam S, Magro CM, Gogineni S, et al. Primary cutaneous follicle center lymphoma associated with an extracutaneous dissemination: a cytogenetic finding of potential prognostic value. *Am J Clin Pathol.* 2015;144:805-810.
70. Belaud-Rotureau MA, Marietta V, Vergier B, et al. Inactivation of p16INK4a/CDKN2A gene may be a diagnostic feature of large B cell lymphoma leg type among cutaneous B cell lymphomas. *Virchows Arch.* 2008;452:607-620.

71. Dijkman R, Tensen CP, Jordanova ES, et al. Array-based comparative genomic hybridization analysis reveals recurrent chromosomal alterations and prognostic parameters in primary cutaneous large B-cell lymphoma. *J Clin Oncol.* 2006;24:296-305.
72. Zhou XA, Yang J, Ringbloom KG, et al. Genomic landscape of cutaneous follicular lymphomas reveals 2 subgroups with clinically predictive molecular features. *Blood Adv.* 2021;5(3):649-661.
73. Kaune KM, Neumann C, Hallermann C, et al. Simultaneous aberrations of single CDKN2A network components and a high Rb phosphorylation status can differentiate subgroups of primary cutaneous B-cell lymphomas. *Exp Dermatol.* 2011;20:331-335.
74. Espinet B, Garcia-Herrera A, Gallardo F, et al. FOXP1 molecular cytogenetics and protein expression analyses in primary cutaneous large B cell lymphoma, leg-type. *Histol Histopathol.* 2011;26:213-221.
75. Pham-Ledard A, Prochazkova-Carlotti M, Andrique L, et al. Multiple genetic alterations in primary cutaneous large B-cell lymphoma, leg type support a common lymphomagenesis with activated B-cell-like diffuse large B-cell lymphoma. *Mod Pathol.* 2014;27:402-411.
76. Schrader AMR, de Groen RAL, Willemze R, et al. Cell-of-origin classification using the Hans and Lymph2Cx algorithms in primary cutaneous large B-cell lymphomas. *Virchows Arch.* 2022;480(3):667-675.
77. Schrader AMR, Jansen PM, Vermeer MH, Kleiverda JK, Vermaat JSP, Willemze R. High incidence and clinical significance of MYC rearrangements in primary cutaneous diffuse large B-cell lymphoma, leg type. *Am J Surg Pathol.* 2018;42(11):1488-1494. doi:10.1097/PAS.0000000000001132
78. Menguy S, Laharanne E, Prochazkova-Carlotti M, et al. Challenges in assessing MYC rearrangement in primary cutaneous diffuse large B-cell lymphoma, leg-type. *Am J Surg Pathol.* 2020;44(3):424-427. doi:10.1097/PAS.0000000000001412
79. Menguy S, Frison E, Prochazkova-Carlotti M, et al. Double-hit or dual expression of MYC and BCL2 in primary cutaneous large B-cell lymphomas. *Mod Pathol.* 2018;31(8):1332-1342. doi:10.1038/s41379-018-0041-7
80. Wongchaowart NT, Kim B, Hsi ED, et al. t(14;18)(q32;q21) involving IGH and MALT1 is uncommon in cutaneous MALT lymphomas and primary cutaneous diffuse large B-cell lymphomas. *J Cutan Pathol.* 2006;33:286-292.
81. Espinet B, Gallardo F, Pujol RM, et al. Absence of MALT1 translocations in primary cutaneous marginal zone B-cell lymphoma. *Haematologica.* 2004;89:ELT14.
82. Schreuder MI, Hoefnagel JJ, Jansen PM, et al. FISH analysis of MALT lymphoma-specific translocations and aneuploidy in primary cutaneous marginal zone lymphoma. *J Pathol.* 2005;205:302-310.
83. Lucioni M, Novara F, Fiandrino G, et al. Twenty-one cases of blastic plasmacytoid dendritic cell neoplasm: focus on biallelic locus 9p21.3 deletion. *Blood.* 2011;118:4591-4594.
84. Leroux D, Mugneret F, Callanan M, et al. CD4(+), CD56(+) DC2 acute leukemia is characterized by recurrent clonal chromosomal changes affecting 6 major targets: a study of 21 cases by the Groupe Francais de Cytogenetique Hematologique. *Blood.* 2002;99:4154-4159.
85. Kaune KM, Baumgart M, Bertsch HP, et al. Solitary cutaneous nodule of blastic plasmacytoid dendritic cell neoplasm progressing to overt leukemia cutis after chemotherapy: immunohistology and FISH analysis confirmed the diagnosis. *Am J Dermatopathol.* 2009;31:695-701.
86. Pileri SA, Ascani S, Cox MC, et al. Myeloid sarcoma: clinicopathologic, phenotypic and cytogenetic analysis of 92 adult patients. *Leukemia.* 2007;21:340-350.

CHAPTER 11

Next-generation sequencing

Ian S. Hagemann

DNA SEQUENCING IN HISTORICAL PERSPECTIVE

Maxam–Gilbert Sequencing

Early DNA sequencing methods took advantage of chemical reactions that selectively degrade DNA at specific nucleotides. For example, treatment with dimethyl sulfate followed by hot aqueous piperazine causes cleavage at guanine nucleotides, while 60% to 80% aqueous formic acid followed by hot aqueous piperidine cleaves at both adenine and guanine.[1] One reaction tube is used for each chemical agent. If a homogeneous population of molecules is end-labeled, treated in individual tubes with nucleotide-specific cleavage agents, and separated by gel electrophoresis, the sequence can be read off the resulting gel. Maxam and Gilbert[2] described a standard set of reactions cleaving preferentially at guanine, adenine, cytosine, and equally at cytosine and thymine. While colorful (sometimes literally), these methods were cumbersome due to the variety of reagents and conditions required, including radiolabeling. They had a limited read length of ~100 nt and were poorly amenable to automation. They are now of historical interest only.

Sanger Sequencing

Sanger[3] described a method to sequence DNA by synthesis, rather than by degradation. In the dideoxynucleotide chain-terminating method as initially described, DNA is polymerized on a homogeneous population of template molecules, using four parallel reaction mixtures. Each mixture contains a 5′-radiolabeled sequencing primer and all four deoxynucleotide triphosphates (dNTPs) along with a small admixed percentage of a single dideoxynucleotide triphosphate (ddNTP). At each step of elongation, there is chance that a ddNTP will be added in place of a dNTP, in which case, in the absence of a 3′ hydroxyl group, the growing DNA chain will be terminated. The reaction produces a collection of DNA molecules of varying lengths, each terminated by a dideoxynucleotide.[4] These molecules can be separated by gel electrophoresis in four lanes, and the sequence can be read off the gel.

While Sanger sequencing originally required radiolabeling of the sequencing primer at the 5′ end, the ddNTPs today are fluorescently labeled, allowing the product to be detected by fluorimetry. A different fluorophore is attached to each ddNTP, so that the four reactions can be multiplexed together and the sequencing reaction can take place in a single tube. Sanger sequencing reactions are now read by capillary electrophoresis, yielding four-color electropherograms with subnucleotide resolution and from which the sequence can be "called" by a computer program. The time required for a typical sequencing reaction is now less than 15 minutes, with a further 60 minutes required for capillary electrophoresis. Reads of up to 1000 nt can be obtained.

These two innovations—capillary electrophoresis and fluorescent detection—have made Sanger sequencing a practical and versatile technique that is still used today. One major application is in sequencing of individual genes, where higher-throughput methods (described below) are not needed. Another application is as an adjunct to next-generation sequencing (NGS), for example, when NGS results are unclear, to "patch" regions poorly covered by NGS, or when laboratory standard operating procedures require NGS-detected variants to be confirmed by an orthogonal method.

Limitations of Sanger sequencing include relatively low sensitivity: variants must be present at ~20% allele frequency within the sample in order to be detected. In addition, Sanger sequencing cannot determine whether two variants are present in *cis* (ie, on the same DNA strand) or in *trans*, a problem referred to as "phasing." Despite these limitations, Sanger sequencing is still generally considered a gold standard and remains in common use.

Emergence of Next-Generation (Second-Generation) Methods

So-called next-generation or second-generation methods increase the throughput of DNA sequencing by making it possible to sequence multiple molecules, or a collection of molecules, at the same time. There are several platforms in current use, and the technology is changing rapidly.

Most current NGS platforms can be described as "cyclic array sequencing" platforms, as they involve fragmenting the target DNA of interest, converting these fragments into a sequencing library by adding primer-binding sites or other necessary sequences to the ends of each fragment, distributing these target sequences across a two-dimensional array, then sequencing the targets by iterative cycles of sequencing chemistry.[5] The resulting reads can be reassembled de novo or, much more commonly in clinical applications, aligned to a reference genome.

The sequence reads are on the order of 50 to 150 nucleotides, which is considerably shorter than those obtained in Sanger sequencing. If the read length is shorter than the DNA insert (fragment) length, it is often possible to sequence from both ends of the insert to obtain "paired-end" reads; the paired-end reads must align close to one another against the reference genome, which increases the confidence and speed of the alignment. To permit multiplexing of multiple samples on the same substrate, the DNA fragments derived from a single specimen are often tagged with index sequences (barcodes).

Clinical NGS-based assays can target regions ranging from a few individual genes up to the entire genome. When the region to be sequenced is less than the entire genome, target enrichment is performed to avoid wasting resources in obtaining unnecessary sequence. Two methods are in common use. In target capture methods, a library is first prepared from fragmented genomic DNA to add indexes and any adapters necessary for the sequencing chemistry. Biotinylated oligonucleotide baits corresponding to the region of interest are hybridized to this library DNA, then captured using magnetic streptavidin beads. Typically, a small number of PCR cycles are then performed to increase the mass of DNA available for sequencing.

Amplicon sequencing methods, in contrast, perform a larger number of PCR cycles on the input DNA to amplify the regions of interest and simultaneously add an index and/or other necessary adapters. Since so many cycles of PCR are performed, the quantity of input DNA required for amplicon sequencing is lower (typically on the 10-ng scale) than that required for target capture (closer to 100-ng scale). The amplification-based approach is also faster, since hybridization is typically an overnight process, but PCR takes only hours. However, the larger number of PCR cycles in amplicon sequencing has the potential to introduce polymerase errors and PCR bias, which can obscure copy number variants and assessment of variant allele fractions. For large capture spaces consisting of many exons, it can also be unwieldy to multiplex the large number of PCR reactions needed for amplicon sequencing. Thus, although both methods of target enrichment have a role, amplicon sequencing is better suited to smaller assays on smaller amounts of DNA, whereas target capture is better suited to larger capture spaces and when more input DNA is available.

Illumina Sequencing

The major platforms in current clinical use are those provided by Illumina, Inc (San Diego, California) and Ion Torrent (Thermo Fisher Scientific, Waltham, Massachusetts). In Illumina sequencing, libraries are hybridized to the two-dimensional surface of a flow cell, and each molecule is subjected to "bridge amplification" to create a cluster of about 2000 identical fragments within a diameter of ~1 μm. A single lane of a flow cell can hold >37 million individual amplified clusters. These fragments are "sequenced by synthesis" by successively incorporating fluorescently labeled, reversibly terminated nucleotides. After each elongation step, the surface of the flow cell is imaged by a charge-coupled device to query each position for the identity of the most recently incorporated nucleotide. Successive cycles of deprotection, elongation, and imaging result in a series of large image files that are then processed to determine the sequence of each cluster on the flow cell.

Illumina sequencing instruments in use today are the MiniSeq, MiSeq, and NextSeq systems. The MiSeq is framed as a smaller-scale benchtop solution and is the first NGS system cleared by the Food and Drug Administration (FDA) as an in vitro diagnostic device. These instruments vary in their run time, number of reads per run, and length of each read. Smaller instruments are less expensive to purchase but have a higher cost per base sequenced. The NovaSeq is a larger ("production-scale") instrument producing more total reads and more total data per run, with longer run times, at a lower price per sample. Clinical laboratories are advised to choose their platform on the basis of anticipated assay design, number of samples to be run at a time, frequency of runs, desired turnaround time, and tolerated error rate.

Ion Torrent Sequencing

Sanger and Illumina sequencing are based on detecting fluorescence, whereas the Ion Torrent approach measures very small changes in pH that occur as a result of H+ release when nucleotides are incorporated into an elongating sequence. Molecules of the library to be sequenced are bound to the surface of microscopic beads and amplified by emulsion PCR so that each bead becomes coated with a population of identical molecules.

The beads are distributed into wells on a chip constructed by complementary metal-oxide semiconductor technology.[6] The sequencing reaction performed on the chip is analogous to pyrosequencing, except that pH is detected instead of light. The Ion Torrent chip has the property that each well, containing an embedded field effect transistor, functions as an extremely sensitive pH meter. Sequencing reactions are accomplished by successively flooding the plate with each deoxyribonucleotide (dATP, dCTP, dGTP, dTTP). Incorporation of a nucleotide causes release of H+, causes a voltage change at the gate of the transistor, and allows current to flow across the transistor, resulting in a signal. Homopolymers cause incorporation of multiple nucleotides, with a correspondingly larger pH change.

Each method has a unique mix of advantages that may make it suitable for specific applications. Ion Torrent sequencing uses natural deoxyribonucleotides rather than synthetic derivatives, which can reduce sequencing biases related to incorporation of unnatural nucleotides. Reads are relatively long, and reaction times are relatively short (3 hours for 300 bases). Disadvantages of Ion Torrent platform include a relatively higher error rate, often attributed to difficulties in discriminating the multiplicity of longer homopolymers.[7,8] Several paired-end modes are available but require off-instrument repriming.[6]

The Ion Torrent sequencers in current use include the Ion Personal Genome Machine (PGM) Dx, a benchtop instrument, which has received FDA 510(k) clearance, and the Ion Torrent Genexus, designed as a turnkey solution with fewer manual steps.

Third-Generation Methods

Third-generation NGS platforms are those that obtain sequence from specimens closely resembling native DNA, that is, with minimal need for target amplification and library preparation. Third-generation NGS is predominantly a single-molecule approach with extremely long read lengths (greater than 10,000 nucleotides), reducing the need for assembly of short reads and improving the ability to discern the phase of detected variants. The major vendors in this area today are Pacific Biosciences (Menlo Park, California) and Oxford Nanopore Technologies (Oxford, United Kingdom).

The Pacific Biosciences approach is to perform sequencing on the surface of a SMRT cell patterned with up to 8 million wells each containing a zero-mode waveguide (ZMW). These ZMWs serve to immobilize a single template molecule and make it possible to interrogate light emission from that one molecule. As extension is carried out, fluorescent reports from each ZMW indicate the nucleotide that has been added at that position.

Oxford Nanopore sequencers contain engineered bacterial nanopores through which a molecule of DNA is fed. The electrical resistance of the pore varies in proportion to the identity of the nucleotide passing through the pore, allowing the sequence to be read off. While multiple formats have been developed, one is a portable, self-contained, disposable MinION that plugs into the universal serial bus (USB) port of a personal computer.

Third-generation technologies are at an early stage of development and have not been validated for clinical use but will undoubtedly play an important role in future diagnostics.

Analytes Other Than DNA

The methods presented above have focused on DNA sequencing. Variants of these methods have been developed to allow the detection of other analytes related to nucleic acids, including RNA sequence, epigenetic changes such as DNA methylation, and DNA-protein interactions. These methods have not yet found widespread clinical applications. DNA sequencing techniques can be readily adapted to RNA analytes by reverse transcription followed by sequencing.

BIOINFORMATIC ASPECTS

Initial Processing

The output of an NGS experiment is a collection of sequence reads annotated with quality data. Bioinformatic processing is an essential step that converts these reads into clinically meaningful data. The bioinformatics pipeline must be a validated component of any clinical NGS test and can be divided into three conceptual tiers that occur in succession.

Data analysis for NGS begins with cleaning the sequence reads, filtering them to exclude those with defects such as unacceptable quality or no recognizable index, and removing duplicates. The pipeline typically continues with alignment of the reads against the reference genome. It is at this stage that it becomes possible to determine the number of unique reads, the proportion of reads that are on target, the mean depth of coverage across the capture region, and other essential quality metrics. Regions where sequencing has failed to attain adequate coverage are flagged so that they can be retested, back-filled by Sanger sequencing, visually reviewed, and/or disclaimed.

Informatic processing continues with variant calling. The reference genome used in clinical genomics today is Genome Reference Consortium assembly GRCh38, the current human genome build. The patient's sequence is aligned against this reference, and nonreference nucleotides are analyzed by variant-calling software.

Classes of genetic variation that can potentially be detected by NGS include single-nucleotide variants, insertions and deletions (indels), structural variants such as translocations, and copy-number variants. These comprise all of the major types of genomic variants with known clinical significance. No variant caller has the ability to detect all of these, and not all formats of NGS assays permit detection of each of the variant types. For example, translocation breakpoints often occur in introns, so NGS assays that target only exons will be unable to determine the exact breakpoint. Moreover, amplicon-based methods that use PCR for library enrichment will not capture translocations between a targeted gene and an unknown partner since there will be no primers in the unknown gene. The bioinformatics pipeline for any given NGS assay must be explicitly validated for specific variant types and must be designed with attention to the types of variation that are clinically relevant in the population to be tested. Any assay designed to assess *MLL* gene status in acute myeloid leukemia, for example, must have the ability to detect translocations, which are the relevant class of variation.

Once the presence of a variant has been established, the pipeline must determine the correct nomenclature for describing it. The nomenclature established by the Human Genome Variation Society is considered standard[9] and can be reviewed on the Society's website.[10] Genomic sequence variants can be described at the genomic level ("g. nomenclature"), at the level of coding/messenger RNA sequence ("c. nomenclature"), or based on the expected effect on protein coding sequence ("p. nomenclature"). Of some note, if a gene has multiple known splice variants or isoforms, then there may be multiple valid ways to denote any given variant. In theory, most practitioners recommend focusing on the notation that corresponds to the gene's major transcript. In practice, it is not always clear which transcript is the major one, nor is it necessarily the case that the major transcript is the one that is clinically significant.

In conclusion, the initial stage of NGS bioinformatics is an automated process that pertains to sequence data but is agnostic as to the clinical significance of the sequences. The result of these steps includes quality data and a list of detected variants.

Variant Annotation

The next step in informatic processing consists of using public and proprietary databases to determine the clinical significance of variants identified in the patient's sample. The goal of this step is to assign each detected variant to one of the levels of significance in the laboratory's variant classification scheme.

The appropriate classification scheme depends directly on the type of testing at hand. In tests performed on neoplastic tissue to detect somatic variants, the variant classification system should reflect the test's goal of differentiating "actionable" variants (predictive or prognostic) from those that are not actionable. The American College of Medical Genetics has proposed an appropriate scheme for the interpretation and classification of somatic variants (Table 11-1).[11] In tests performed on germline DNA, intended to diagnose predisposition to cancer or another disease, it would be more appropriate for the variant classification scheme to separate "pathogenic" variants from those that are "likely pathogenic," "likely benign," etc.[12] Specialized tests such as lymphocyte clonality assays may not require an explicit variant classification scheme.

Numerous public databases are available to aid in determining the clinical significance of genetic variants. Internal (proprietary) databases developed by individual laboratories, containing frequency data and annotations for variants previously identified in the local population, may also be of use. Variants that have been reported in the germline of healthy individuals, as listed, for example, in Genome Aggregation Database (https://gnomad.broadinstitute.org, accessed January 1, 2021), are likely to be benign polymorphisms. At the other end of the spectrum of significance, variants with clinical-grade evidence of actionability will invariably be the subject of one or more clinical studies published in the peer-reviewed medical literature.

Reporting

The final tier of bioinformatics analysis is review by a clinical practitioner to curate the analyses performed in earlier stages. The molecular pathologist or clinical molecular geneticist will often focus on nonsynonymous variants, that is, those that alter a protein coding sequence (eg, alanine to glycine) or splice site, rather than synonymous variants (eg, alanine to alanine) or noncoding variants. Expert review is required to author clinical interpretations, although these may be based upon standardized language in the case of commonly seen variants. Expert review is also needed to appropriately report findings in light of the patient's clinical context, to take into proper consideration the ethical aspects of incidental or germline variants,[13-15] and to author a report that is comprehensive and succinct.

OPERATIONAL AND REGULATORY CONSIDERATIONS

Guidance From Professional Societies

Development and validation of NGS-based tests are generally performed by individual laboratories, as most NGS assays are currently offered as laboratory-developed tests (LDTs), subject to regulation under the Clinical Laboratory Improvement Amendments (CLIA). The MiSeqDx instrument from Illumina is FDA-approved, as are several targeted mutation detected panels run on the instrument. Individual Oncomine assays (eg, for detection of recurrent mutations in lung cancer and glioma) performed on the Ion Torrent platform have received FDA approval. The FoundationOne CDx assay (targeted sequencing of several hundred cancer-related genes) is FDA-approved for all solid tumors. NGS assays related to hematopathology of the skin are all laboratory-developed tests at the time of writing.

As clinical laboratories have begun adopting NGS technology, several organizations have issued recommendations on best practices in this area. Professional societies and regulatory bodies who have released guidelines include the College of American Pathologists,[16] the Clinical Laboratory Standards Institute,[17] the New York State Department of Health,[18] the Association for Molecular Pathology,[19] and the American College of Medical Genetics and Genomics (ACMG).[12] Many laboratories offering clinical NGS-based tests have also published their local experiences, although the relative knowledge base for oncology sequencing is much less than that for sequencing inherited disorders.[20,21]

One detailed set of guidelines for validation and quality control of clinical NGS assays was developed by the "Next-Generation Sequencing: Standardization of Clinical Testing" (Nex-StoCT) workgroup convened by the US Centers for Disease Control. An executive summary has been published, with the full document available as an extensive supplemental file.[22] The four main areas addressed in this guideline are test validation, quality control, proficiency testing or alternative

TABLE 11-1 Example of a Classification System for Somatic Variants in Cancer, Based on ACMG Recommendations[11]

Tier	Level	Significance
I		Variants of strong clinical significance
	A	FDA-approved therapy; included in professional guidelines
	B	Well-powered studies with consensus from experts
II		Variants of potential clinical significance
	C	FDA-approved therapies for different tumor types or investigational therapies; multiple small published studies with some consensus
	D	Preclinical trials or a few case reports without consensus
III		Variants of unknown clinical significance, not observed at a significant allele frequency in the general population
IV		Benign or likely benign variants, observed at significant allele frequency in the general population. Note that these are unlikely to be somatic variants and are more likely germline variants passively present in tumor tissue

assessment, and reference materials. All of these areas must be considered by laboratories implementing NGS-based testing for clinical purposes.

Assay Validation

One challenge to NGS validation is the numerous steps involved in generating NGS data that are unique to this technology. CLIA regulations dictate that laboratories assess and document the performance characteristics of LDTs, which include analytical sensitivity, analytical specificity, accuracy, precision or reproducibility, reportable range, reference range, and any other relevant test characteristics. Several validation frameworks have been proposed, including the ACMG recommendation, to separately consider three interrelated components of the test: panel design, technical performance of the assay, and reporting.[23]

Turnaround Time

The time required for NGS-based testing depends on the methodology, details of the workflow, and size of the assay space. There can also be significant preanalytic delays, related either to specimen procurement (identifying a paraffin block and transporting it to the NGS laboratory) or reimbursement (obtaining preauthorization from payors, communicating with patients regarding out-of-pocket cost).

Once the specimen reaches the laboratory, turnaround time may be as short as 5 to 10 days for amplicon-based "hotspot" testing. The time needed will be shorter if the test does not require explicit specimen review by a pathologist at the time of intake to confirm the presence of neoplastic tissue and/or estimate tumor cellularity and viability. Tests reporting on a limited range of nucleotide positions may not require laborious manual interpretation, since standardized language may be available.

At the opposite end of the spectrum, turnaround time may be on the order of 3 to 4 weeks for tests that cover dozens or hundreds of genes (potentially requiring many custom interpretations to be authored). Turnaround time may also be lengthened by capture-based methodology (requiring hybridization time) and/or by the need for orthogonal validation of certain variants, such as translocations, which may in some laboratories be confirmed by fluorescence in situ hybridization.

APPLICATIONS OF NEXT-GENERATION SEQUENCING IN CUTANEOUS HEMATOPATHOLOGY

Cancer Gene Set Testing

Cancer gene set testing uses an NGS platform to sequence multiple genes with relevance to the patient's cancer type. The analyte is DNA extracted from the patient's tumor, inevitably with an admixture of nontumor DNA. Clinically relevant (actionable) variants may be diagnostic, predictive, or prognostic. Diagnostic variants are those that assist in classifying a disease, a concept that is particularly relevant in hematopathology, where several disease entities are genetically defined. Predictive variants are those that can be used to infer the responsiveness of a tumor to a particular therapy, including targeted and nontargeted therapies. Prognostic variants are those that indicate the likely behavior of a tumor, irrespective of the use of any particular therapy.

In some tumor types, known genotype-phenotype correlations extend across numerous genes, so that it becomes desirable to assess all of them simultaneously rather than pursuing numerous single-gene tests. For acute myeloid leukemia, for example, prognostic genes specifically mentioned in the current National Comprehensive Cancer Network guideline include *FLT3*, *KIT*, *NPM1*, *DNMT3A*, *CEBPA*, *IDH1*, and *IDH2*.[24] There is emerging evidence for the importance of other genes, including *KMT2A* (*MLL*), *PHF6*, *TP53*, *U2AF1*, *ASXL1*, and *TET2*.[25,26] It would be impractical to assess such a large number of genes on an individual basis, whereas NGS testing allows all to be assessed on a single platform, and at a cost that scales less than linearly with the number of genes tested. The break-even point for NGS versus Sanger sequencing is currently three to four genes; in other words, sequencing more than this number of genes is most cost-effective using an NGS gene set approach. Several laboratories have introduced clinical tests for this purpose, either with a focus specifically on hematologic diseases, or with a pan-cancer approach.[27]

Cancer Predisposition Testing

In cancer predisposition testing, the analyte is nontumor DNA, often informally described as germline DNA. This is conveniently obtained from peripheral blood or from a buccal swab. Typically, these tests are used in cases of suspected cancer predisposition syndromes, for example, in patients with a suggestive personal or family history. The gene sets tend to be highly focused on the disease of interest in order to maximize the clinical validity of the test while minimizing incidental variants. Pre- and posttest genetic counseling is mandatory for any germline genetic test.

Clonality Testing

Lymphoid neoplasms are unique in containing clonally rearranged immunoglobulin (Ig) and/or T-cell receptor (TCR) genes. The presence of a clonal population supports a diagnosis of lymphoma, in the appropriate clinical and histologic setting; furthermore, molecular clonality detection can aid in lineage determination (although infidelity does occur) and makes it possible to differentiate recurrent lymphoma from a new clonal process.

PCR- and capillary electrophoresis–based clonality testing, described in Chapter 9 of this book, is widely available.[28] While this technique is robust, several groups have described alternative NGS-based approaches that have certain advantages[29-31] and are becoming more widely adopted: at present, clonality testing is split 50:50 between PCR and NGS methods according to survey data from the College of American Pathologists. PCR-based clonality testing can be subjective, because, while the presence of a clone is inferred from seeing a dominant peak on the electropherogram, the sequence of the sequences making up that peak is not known. NGS methods reveal the specific identity of the clonal sequence and make it possible to estimate the fraction of cells that carry that exact sequence. Cases with one or two sequences that clearly dominate the background (eg, fourfold depth of coverage compared with the polyclonal background) and make up more than a given fraction of total reads (eg, 4.5%) are classified as clonal. While these approaches are largely laboratory developed, a family of LymphoTrack assays is now available from Invivoscribe Laboratories (San Diego, California). These research-use-only reagents can be expected to speed up the validation of NGS-based clonality testing in the near future.

References

1. França LTC, Carrilho E, Kist TBL. A review of DNA sequencing techniques. *Q Rev Biophys*. 2002;35:169-200.
2. Maxam AM, Gilbert W. A new method for sequencing DNA. *Proc Natl Acad Sci U S A*. 1977;74:560-564.
3. Sanger F, Nicklen S, Coulson AR. DNA sequencing with chain-terminating inhibitors. *Proc Natl Acad Sci U S A*. 1977;74:5463-5467.
4. Slatko BE, Albright LM, Tabor S, Ju J. DNA sequencing by the dideoxy method. *Curr Protoc Mol Biol*. 2001;Chapter 7:Unit7.4A. doi:10.1002/0471142727.mb0704as47
5. Applied Biosystems, Inc (2009) *DNA Sequencing by Capillary Electrophoresis: Applied Biosystems Chemistry Guide*. [online]. http://tools.thermofisher.com/content/sfs/manuals/cms_041003.pdf Accessed April 18, 2021.
6. Shendure JA, Porreca GJ, Church GM, et al. Overview of DNA sequencing strategies. *Curr Protoc Mol Biol*. 2011; Chapter 7:Unit7.1. doi:10.1002/0471142727.mb0701s96
7. Merriman B, Rothberg JM; Ion Torrent R&D Team. Progress in ion torrent semiconductor chip based sequencing. *Electrophoresis*. 2012;33:3397-3417.
8. Loman NJ, Misra RV, Dallman TJ, et al. Performance comparison of benchtop high-throughput sequencing platforms. *Nat Biotechnol*. 2012;30:434-439.
9. Horaitis O, Cotton RGH. The challenge of documenting mutation across the genome: the Human Genome Variation Society approach. *Hum Mutat*. 2004;23:447-452.
10. *Human Genome Variation Society Sequence Variant Nomenclature*. [online]. Accessed April 18, 2021. 2020. http://varnomen.hgvs.org/
11. Li MM, Datto M, Duncavage EJ, et al. Standards and guidelines for the interpretation and reporting of sequence variants in cancer: a joint consensus recommendation of the association for molecular Pathology, American society of clinical oncology, and College of American pathologists. *J Mol Diagn*. 2017;19:4-23.
12. Richards CS, Bale S, Bellissimo DB, et al. ACMG recommendations for standards for interpretation and reporting of sequence variations: revisions 2007. *Genet Med*. 2008;10:294-300.
13. Green RC, Berg JS, Grody WW, et al. ACMG recommendations for reporting of incidental findings in clinical exome and genome sequencing. *Genet Med*. 2013;15:565-574.
14. Wolf SM, Annas GJ, Elias S. Point-counterpoint. Patient autonomy and incidental findings in clinical genomics. *Science*. 2013;340:1049-1050.
15. Kalia SS, Adelman K, Bale SJ, et al. Recommendations for reporting of secondary findings in clinical exome and genome sequencing, 2016 update (ACMG SF v2.0): a policy statement of the American College of Medical Genetics and Genomics. *Genet Med*. 2017;19:249-255.
16. College of American Pathologists. *Molecular Pathology Checklist*. 2012.
17. Clinical and Laboratory Standards Instition. *Nucleic Acid Sequencing Methods in Diagnostic Laboratory Medicine*. 2nd ed. Document MM09-A; 2014.
18. New York State Department of Health. *Oncology—Molecular and Cellular Tumor Markers: Next Generation Sequencing (NGS) Guidelines for Somatic Genetic Variant Detection*. 2018.
19. Schrijver I, Aziz N, Farkas DH, et al. Opportunities and challenges associated with clinical diagnostic genome sequencing: a report of the Association for Molecular Pathology. *J Mol Diagn*. 2012;14:525-540.
20. Hadd AG, Houghton J, Choudhary A, et al. Targeted, high-depth, next-generation sequencing of cancer genes in formalin-fixed, paraffin-embedded and fine-needle aspiration tumor specimens. *J Mol Diagn*. 2013;15:234-247.
21. Cottrell CE, Al-Kateb H, Bredemeyer AJ, et al. Validation of a next-generation sequencing assay for clinical molecular oncology. *J Mol Diagn*. 2014;16:89-105.
22. Gargis AS, Kalman L, Berry MW, et al. Assuring the quality of next-generation sequencing in clinical laboratory practice. *Nat Biotechnol*. 2012;30:1033-1036.
23. Bean LJH, Funke B, Carlston CM, et al. Diagnostic gene sequencing panels: from design to report—a technical standard of the American College of Medical Genetics and Genomics (ACMG). *Genet Med*. 2020;22:453-461.
24. National Comprehensive Cancer Network. *NCCN Clinical Practice Guidelines in Oncology: Acute Myeloid Leukemia, Version 3.2021*. [online]. https://www.nccn.org/professionals/physician_gls/pdf/aml.pdf 2021. Accessed April 18, 2021.
25. Ohgami RS, Ma L, Merker JD, et al. Next-generation sequencing of acute myeloid leukemia identifies the significance of TP53, U2AF1, ASXL1, and TET2 mutations. *Mod Pathol*. 2015;28:706-714.
26. Sanchez M, Levine RL, Rampal R. Integrating genomics into prognostic models for AML. *Semin Hematol*. 2014;51:298-305.
27. Zutter MM, Bloom KJ, Cheng L, et al. The cancer genomics resource list 2014. *Arch Pathol Lab Med*. 2015;139:989-1008.
28. Gazzola A, Mannu C, Rossi M, et al. The evolution of clonality testing in the diagnosis and monitoring of hematological malignancies. *Ther Adv Hematol*. 2014;5:35-47.
29. Schumacher JA, Duncavage EJ, Mosbruger TL, Szankasi PM, Kelley TW. A comparison of deep sequencing of TCRG rearrangements vs traditional capillary electrophoresis for assessment of clonality in T-Cell lymphoproliferative disorders. *Am J Clin Pathol*. 2014;141:348-359.
30. He J, Wu J, Jiao Y, et al. IgH gene rearrangements as plasma biomarkers in Non- Hodgkin's lymphoma patients. *Oncotarget*. 2011;2:178-185.
31. Sufficool KE, Lockwood CM, Abel HJ, et al. T-cell clonality assessment by next-generation sequencing improves detection sensitivity in mycosis fungoides. *J Am Acad Dermatol*. 2015;73:228-236.e2.

PART III PRIMARY CUTANEOUS T-CELL LYMPHOMAS

CHAPTER 12

Approach to the diagnosis of primary cutaneous T-cell lymphomas

Alistair M. Robson, Alejandro A. Gru, and András Schaffer

INTRODUCTION

The skin is the most common site of extranodal T-cell lymphomas, and mycosis fungoides (MF) is the most frequent T-cell lymphoma.[1-3] Extranodal NK-cell lymphomas are rare in the Western hemisphere but more common in Asia and some areas of central and South America, where Epstein-Barr virus (EBV) infection occurs at a young age.[4,5] The most frequent primary cutaneous and systemic T- and NK-cell lymphomas with secondary skin involvement are listed in Table 12-1.

Cutaneous T-cell lymphomas (CTCLs) encompass a range of diagnoses that include indolent and highly aggressive neoplasms, each of which may present as localized or disseminated diseases. There is considerable clinical, histological, and immunophenotypical heterogeneity, and successful diagnosis requires close attention to each of these features if misdiagnosis is to be avoided. Each of the clinical, pathological, and immunophenotypic data provides a guide to the likely differential diagnoses. For example, infiltrates that predominantly involve the epidermis generate a series of likely differential diagnoses against which the clinical presentation and subsequent immunophenotypic signature should be interpreted. Similarly, most T-cell lymphomas have well-characterized immunophenotypes; in some cases this is a defining feature of an entity. Yet, both the histological pattern and immunohistochemical signature always lie within a specific clinical context, and the appreciation of the interrelationship between these three axes is crucial to an accurate diagnosis.

SOURCES OF DIFFICULTY

Data suggest that there can be substantial disagreement among pathologists in CTCL diagnosis. The International T-cell lymphoma project reported significant diagnostic disagreement in several diagnostic categories of T-cell lymphomas, with only 66% observer concordance in cutaneous anaplastic large cell lymphoma and 75% in subcutaneous panniculitis-like T-cell lymphoma.[6] Guitart et al reported very poor (48%) consensus agreement in the diagnosis of early MF in which the initial histopathological changes may be subtle.[7] Even secondary cutaneous involvement by systemic lymphomas or leukemias, as is commonly seen in chronic lymphocytic leukemia (CLL) and angioimmunoblastic lymphoma, may have deceptively bland histology, although it does not alter the disease staging.[8-11] Furthermore, an apparent indolent subsequent clinical course in cases of cutaneous Richter transformation of CLL suggests one cannot automatically extrapolate from conclusions drawn from studies of systemic diseases to the cutaneous milieu.[12] De Souza et al confirmed the importance of synthesizing histology with clinical data in CD30+ infiltrates, in which 65% of histologically suspected benign and 72% of malignant infiltrates were confirmed. Clinical evaluation changed the preferred histological diagnosis of anaplastic large cell lymphoma (ALCL) to LyP in three patients, and one patient with a histological diagnosis of CD30+ LPD was changed to herpes virus infection.[13] Implicit to the importance of correlating histology and immunophenotype with clinical data is that the same histological pattern can be seen in several lymphomas of markedly different prognoses; similarly, a single lymphoma can have different modes of clinical presentation and, moreover, vary in its immunophenotypic signature. Accordingly, attention to these aspects in each case and the consequent likely possible diagnoses provides a starting point for making a correct diagnosis.

CLINICAL FEATURES

It cannot be overemphasized that a careful clinical history and description are essential; vastly different clinical diseases may present with an identical histology.[14,15] The location, chronology,

TABLE 12-1 Cutaneous and Systemic T- and NK-Cell Lymphomas According to the World Health Organization Classification

Cutaneous T-Cell Lymphomas

- Mycosis fungoides (MF)
- Sézary syndrome (SS)
- Subcutaneous panniculitis-like T-cell lymphoma (SPTCL)
- Primary cutaneous anaplastic large cell lymphoma (PC-ALCL)
- Lymphomatoid papulosis (LyP)
- Primary cutaneous CD8− positive aggressive epidermotropic cytotoxic T-cell lymphoma
- Primary cutaneous γδ T-cell lymphoma (PCGDTCL)
- Primary cutaneous CD4+ small to medium T-cell lymphoproliferative disorder
- Primary cutaneous acral CD8+ T-cell lymphoproliferative disorder

Systemic T-cell lymphomas with frequent cutaneous dissemination

- T-cell prolymphocytic leukemia (T-PLL)
- Peripheral T-cell lymphoma, not otherwise specified (PTCL, NOS)
- ALK+ anaplastic large cell lymphoma (ALK+ ALCL)
- ALK− anaplastic large cell lymphoma (ALK− ALCL)
- Nodal follicular T-helper cell lymphoma (including angioimmunoblastic T-cell lymphoma)
- Adult T-cell leukemia/lymphoma (ATLL)

Cutaneous and systemic NK-cell lymphomas

- Extranodal NK/T-cell lymphoma (ENKTL)
- Aggressive NK-cell leukemia
- Hydroa vacciniforme lymphoproliferative disorder

Data from Harris NL, Campo E, Jaffe ES, et al. Introduction to the Classification of Tumours of Haematopoietic and Lymphoid Tissues. International Agency for Research on Cancer; 2008.

---

areas).[16,17] In contrast, the most common sites of involvement of folliculotropic MF are the head, neck, and upper back.[18] Syringotropic MF and solitary pagetoid reticulosis have predilections for the distal extremities (acral sites).[19] Hypopigmented MF is more common in children.[20] Similarly, lymphomatoid papulosis requires the presence of multiple, often grouped, papules and/or nodules that develop and regress spontaneously over a period of several weeks or a few months; again, a solitary lesion, or a persistent tumor, excludes this diagnosis.[21] Primary cutaneous anaplastic large cell lymphoma (PC-ALCL) has the clinical appearance of ulcerated tumors or nodules in the head and neck, trunk, and extremities. Spontaneous resolution has been reported in up to 20% of cases.[22] Sézary syndrome (SS) presents as generalized erythroderma with intense and severe pruritus with diffuse scaling and very frequent nail changes. Erythroderma is not exclusive to lymphomas, as psoriasis, drug eruptions, and eczema can present similarly, whereas a significant proportion of cases are idiopathic.[23,24] Primary cutaneous CD4+ small to medium T-cell lymphoproliferative disorder usually presents in the head and neck region, as an isolated papule, plaque, or nodule, often with a recent history of rapid development. The entity is often confused with a nonmelanoma skin cancer.[25,26] Deep-seated nodules on the trunk and extremities are the frequent clinical characteristics of the lesions of subcutaneous panniculitis-like T-cell lymphoma; in contrast, knowledge of the preferred characteristic anatomic locations of the most common inflammatory panniculitides can be helpful.[27] Among the aggressive cutaneous lymphomas are aggressive epidermotropic CD8+ T-cell lymphoma and primary cutaneous γδ T-cell lymphoma; widespread acute onset of ulcerated nodules, plaques, and tumors[28-30] is the typical clinical presentation. Secondary involvement by systemic T-cell lymphomas does not show a specific clinical appearance, but patients with T-cell prolymphocytic leukemia have frequent facial involvement.[31-33] In particular, angioimmunoblastic T-cell lymphoma shows a high rate of cutaneous manifestations.

HISTOLOGICAL PATTERN

Histological infiltrates of neoplastic cells may preferentially involve the epidermis (epidermotropism), dermis, and/or subcutis; angiotropism with or without vascular destruction is an additional feature in some cases. This microanatomical distribution of neoplastic T cells is a very helpful attribute in reaching the final diagnosis (Fig. 12-2). Different CTCLs can share identical histologic findings.[14,15] For example, MF and type B lymphomatoid papulosis (LyP) present the same epidermotropic histology. Pagetoid reticulosis, LyP type D and LyP with 6p25.3 translocation, and aggressive CD8+ T-cell lymphomas (AETCLs), are each characterized by a specific florid pattern of epidermotropism, pagetoid reticulosis, usually by CD8+ lymphocytes. Epidermotropic infiltrates are typically composed of small to medium-sized cells.

Dermal infiltrates can be composed of small to medium-sized cells or large cells and may be substantial in a broad range of diagnoses. Thus, tumor-stage MF with large cell transformation, type C LyP, and PC-ALCL cannot always be reliably distinguished histologically. Angiotropic neoplastic infiltrates are a common and diagnostically useful feature of extranodal NK/T-cell and gamma-delta T-cell lymphomas, but they are also seen in aggressive epidermotropic CD8+ T-cell lymphoma and are characteristic of the angiotropic

---

and appearance of the lesions are clues to the diagnosis. The mode of presentation, whether the patient has an acute or a chronic history of lesions, is important. Furthermore, solitary or multiple skin lesions must be noted, and the nature of such lesions, for example, patches, plaques, tumors, presence of ulceration, papules, and hyopigmentation. The natural history of the cutaneous manifestations, for example, whether they persist, or undergo regression, either spontaneously or following biopsy, should be recorded. In establishing these facts an outline of possible diagnoses can then be drawn up (Fig. 12-1); for example, classical (Alibert-Bazin) MF is a clinical diagnosis dependent upon the presence of patches and plaques, and therefore an acute presentation of a solitary nodule is not consistent with this diagnosis, irrespective of the presence of histological epidermotropism. Conventional MF, of Alibert-Bazin type, typically presents on the trunk and buttocks (sun-protected

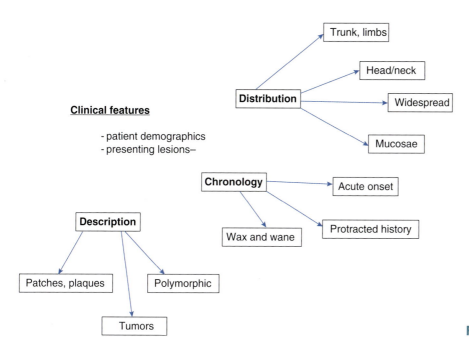

FIGURE 12-1. Clinical features.

variants of both LyP and ALCL. It follows that histology alone is often a poor predictor of either indolent or aggressive disease. For example, biopsies from patients with SS frequently show nonspecific findings, such as lack of epidermotropism and preserved CD7 expression, even though the prognosis of SS is dismal, with less than 50% survival rate at 5 years. This may also be true of cutaneous involvement by systemic lymphomas. Cases of adult T-cell leukemia/lymphoma (ATLL) are frequently associated with skin involvement and histologically resemble patches, plaques, and tumoral stages of MF, with sparse or dense infiltrates with or without a large cell component. Skin rashes occur in nearly 75% of patients with angioimmunoblastic T-cell lymphoma and may have nonspecific often granulomatous infiltrates.[9-11]

IMMUNOPHENOTYPIC PROFILE

Most CTCLs have a postthymic, that is, peripheral $CD4^+$, T-cell phenotype, with variable loss of T-cell-associated markers. However, variant phenotypes are well documented, and some diagnoses are specifically defined by a CD4 or CD8 phenotype.[3] A change in immunophenotype during disease evolution, particularly increasing loss of T-cell antigens or aberrant marker expression, is common. Rarer, but reported, is the switch from a T-helper to T-cytotoxic phenotype. The common or defining phenotypes of CTCLs are depicted in Figure 12-3. However, there are often exceptions, and in specific diseases additional more detailed immunostains are required for the diagnosis.

MOLECULAR ANALYSES IN THE DIAGNOSIS OF CTCL

The finding of a T-cell clone within the tissue pathology is supportive of a diagnosis of T-cell lymphoma but is neither a sine qua non nor proof of malignancy. It is true that in most established cases of CTCL a T-cell clone will be detected, but a polyclonal pattern may be found in the early stages of MF, and in only approximately 50% to 60% of cases of lymphomatoid papulosis. Furthermore, clonal populations of T cells are well documented in a variety of inflammatory dermatoses, such as autoimmune processes (lupus erythematosus), drug reactions, pityriasis lichenoides, and lichen planus.[34,35] The presence of *stable T-cell clones*, that is, identical T-cell clones or a restricted molecular profile from two or more anatomical sites in synchronous or sequential skin biopsies, is reported to have a specificity of >95% in discriminating MF from benign dermatoses.[36] Using the common polymerase chain reaction (PCR) approach with the BIOMED primers, the limit of detection of clonality is estimated to be 106 cells, of which approximately 10% have to be clonal. Multiple clonal peaks can sometimes be present. The use of emerging platforms, such as next-generation sequencing (NGS), has proven to be more specific and sensitive for detection of clonality and monitoring minimal residual disease in the diagnosis of T-cell lymphomas.[37,38] Interestingly, clonal T cells have recently been reported in cases of pityriasis lichenoides in children using NGS.[39]

A pathogenic role for viral infections is evident in rare subtypes of CTCL. ATLL is related to the human T-lymphotropic virus 1 (HTLV-1) while ENKTCL is linked to EBV. An association of EBV, including active lytic replication of the virus, had been observed in patients with progressive MF and systemic T-cell lymphoma.[40,41]

While the number of genetic changes underpinning CTCL is continuously growing, the diagnostic and clinical utility of this information are still in their infancy.[42,43] Recent genome-wide analyses of MF and SS revealed a broad spectrum of mutated genes that might become future therapeutic targets.[44-48] The identification of *IRF4/DUSP22* rearrangement in selected cases of LyP and PC-ALCL and systemic ALCL might have

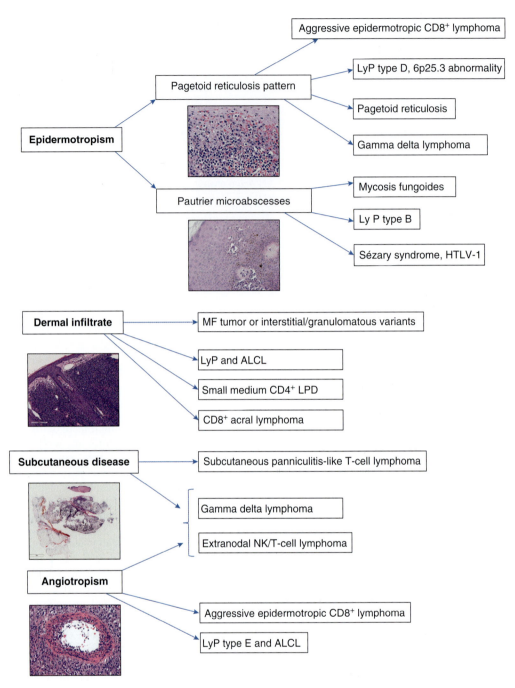

FIGURE 12-2. Histopathology.

prognostic significance. Some cases of cutaneous ALCL can also show *TP63* translocations.[49-52]

SUMMARY

Cutaneous T-cell lymphoma is a collection of disparate diseases, which differ considerably in clinical features and prognosis. There is also marked histological variation. The key patterns of the clinical, histological, and immunophenotypic features outlined in this chapter should not be considered as inviolate relationships but can nevertheless serve as a useful framework against which plausible considerations can be narrowed to the correct diagnosis, thereby guiding appropriate clinical management. The reader is directed to other chapters in the book for a detailed review of the specific disease entities, their hallmark characteristics, and less common but documented variants.

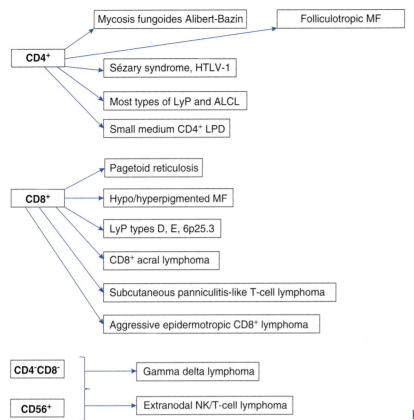

FIGURE 12-3. Immunophenotype.

References

1. Bradford PT, Devesa SS, Anderson WF, et al. Cutaneous lymphoma incidence patterns in the United States: a population-based study of 3884 cases. *Blood*. 2009;113:5064-5073.
2. Criscione VD, Weinstock MA. Incidence of cutaneous T-cell lymphoma in the United States, 1973-2002. *Arch Dermatol*. 2007;143:854-859.
3. Willemze R, Jaffe ES, Burg G, et al. WHO-EORTC classification for cutaneous lymphomas. *Blood*. 2005;105:3768-3785.
4. Liang X, Graham DK. Natural killer cell neoplasms. *Cancer*. 2008;112:1425-1436.
5. Semenzato G, Marino F, Zambello R. State of the art in natural killer cell malignancies. *Int J Lab Hematol*. 2012;34:117-128.
6. Vose J, Armitage J, Weisenburger D, et al. International peripheral T-cell and natural killer/T-cell lymphoma study: pathology findings and clinical outcomes. *J Clin Oncol*. 2008;26:4124-4130.
7. Guitart J, Kennedy J, Ronan S, et al. Histologic criteria for the diagnosis of mycosis fungoides: proposal for a grading system to standardize pathology reporting. *J Cutan Pathol*. 2001;28:174-183.
8. Robak E, Robak T. Skin lesions in chronic lymphocytic leukaemia. *Leuk Lymphoma*. 2007;48:855-865.
9. Cardoso J, Benton E, Naresh K et al. Angioimmunoblastic T-cell lymphoma: dermatopathological features in a series of 40 cases. *Mod Pathol*. 2011;24(suppl 1):p114A.
10. Balaraman B, Conley JA, Sheinbein DM. Evaluation of cutaneous angioimmunoblastic T-cell lymphoma. *J Am Acad Dermatol*. 2011;65:855-862.
11. Botros N, Cerroni L, Shawwa A, et al. Cutaneous manifestations of angioimmunoblastic T-cell lymphoma: clinical and pathological characteristics. *Am J Dermatopathol*. 2015;37:274-283.
12. Kluk J, Moonim M, Duran A, et al. Cutaneous Richter syndrome: a better place to transform? *Br J Dermatol*. 2015;172:513-521.
13. De Souza A, Carter JB, Harris NL, et al. Contribution of longitudinal follow up and clinical pathological correlation in the diagnosis CD30-positive skin infiltrates. *J Cutan Pathol*. 2015;42:452-458.
14. Subtil A. Pathology of cutaneous lymphomas. *Surg Pathol Clin*. 2014;7(2):ix.
15. Subtil A. A general approach to the diagnosis of cutaneous lymphomas and pseudolymphomas. *Surg Pathol Clin*. 2014;7:135-142.
16. Kim YH, Liu HL, Mraz-Gernhard S, et al. Long-term outcome of 525 patients with mycosis fungoides and Sézary syndrome: clinical prognostic factors and risk for disease progression. *Arch Dermatol*. 2003;139:857-866.
17. Stevens SR, Ke MS, Birol A, et al. A simple clinical scoring system to improve the sensitivity and standardization of the diagnosis of mycosis fungoides type cutaneous T-cell lymphoma: logistic regression of clinical and laboratory data. *Br J Dermatol*. 2003;149:513-522.
18. Boone SL, Guitart J, Gerami P. Follicular mycosis fungoides: a histopathologic, immunohistochemical, and genotypic review. *G Ital Dermatol Venereol*. 2008;143:409-414.

19. de Masson A, Battistella M, Vignon-Pennamen MD, et al. Syringotropic mycosis fungoides: clinical and histologic features, response to treatment, and outcome in 19 patients. *J Am Acad Dermatol.* 2014;71:926-934.
20. Hodak E, Amitay-Laish I, Feinmesser M, et al. Juvenile mycosis fungoides: cutaneous T-cell lymphoma with frequent follicular involvement. *J Am Acad Dermatol.* 2014;70:993-1001.
21. Wieser I, Oh CW, Talpur R, et al. Lymphomatoid papulosis: treatment response and associated lymphomas in a study of 180 patients. *J Am Acad Dermatol.* 2016;74:59-67.
22. Bekkenk MW, Geelen FA, van Voorst Vader PC, et al. Primary and secondary cutaneous CD30(+) lymphoproliferative disorders: a report from the Dutch Cutaneous Lymphoma Group on the long-term follow-up data of 219 patients and guidelines for diagnosis and treatment. *Blood.* 2000;95:3653-3661.
23. Olsen EA. Evaluation, diagnosis, and staging of cutaneous lymphoma. *Dermatol Clin.* 2015;33:643-654.
24. Olsen EA, Rook AH, Zic J, et al. Sézary syndrome: immunopathogenesis, literature review of therapeutic options, and recommendations for therapy by the United States Cutaneous Lymphoma Consortium (USCLC). *J Am Acad Dermatol.* 2011;64:352-404.
25. Garcia-Herrera A, Colomo L, Camos M, et al. Primary cutaneous small/medium CD4+ T-cell lymphomas: a heterogeneous group of tumors with different clinicopathologic features and outcome. *J Clin Oncol.* 2008;26:3364-3371.
26. Beltzung F, Ortonne N, Pelletier L, et al. Primary cutaneous CD4+ small/medium T-cell lymphoproliferative disorders. A clinical, pathologic, and molecular study of 60 cases presenting with a single lesion: a multicenter study of the French Cutaneous Lymphoma Study Group. *Am J Surg Pathol.* 2020;44:862-872.
27. Willemze R, Jansen PM, Cerroni L, et al. Subcutaneous panniculitis-like T-cell lymphoma definition, classification, and prognostic factors: an EORTC Cutaneous Lymphoma Group Study of 83 cases. *Blood.* 2008;111:838-845.
28. Berti E, Tomasini D, Vermeer MH, et al. Primary cutaneous CD8-positive epidermotropic cytotoxic T cell lymphomas. A distinct clinicopathological entity with an aggressive clinical behavior. *Am J Pathol.* 1999;155:483-492.
29. Guitart J, Weisenburger DD, Subtil A, et al. Cutaneous gammadelta T-cell lymphomas: a spectrum of presentations with overlap with other cytotoxic lymphomas. *Am J Surg Pathol.* 2012;36:1656-1665.
30. Robson A, Assaf C, Bagot M, et al. Aggressive epidermotropic cutaneous CD8+ lymphoma: a cutaneous lymphoma with distinct clinical and pathological features. Report of an EORTC Cutaneous Lymphoma Task Force Workshop. *Histopathology.* 2015;67:425-441.
31. De Belilovsky C, Guillaume JC, Gilles E, et al. Cutaneous manifestations of T-cell prolymphocytic leukemia [in French]. *Ann Dermatol Venereol.* 1989;116:889-891.
32. Dearden CE. T-cell prolymphocytic leukemia. *Clin Lymphoma Myeloma.* 2009;9(suppl 3):S239-S243.
33. Herling M, Valbuena JR, Jones D, et al. Skin involvement in T-cell prolymphocytic leukemia. *J Am Acad Dermatol.* 2007;57:533-534.
34. Guitart J, Magro C. Cutaneous T-cell lymphoid dyscrasia: a unifying term for idiopathic chronic dermatoses with persistent T-cell clones. *Arch Dermatol.* 2007;143:921-932.
35. Wood GS, Greenberg HL. Diagnosis, staging, and monitoring of cutaneous T-cell lymphoma. *Dermatol Ther.* 2003;16:269-275.
36. Thurber SE, Zhang B, Kim YH, et al. T-cell clonality analysis in biopsy specimens from two different skin sites shows high specificity in the diagnosis of patients with suggested mycosis fungoides. *J Am Acad Dermatol.* 2007;57:782-790.
37. Sufficool KE, Lockwood CM, Abel HJ, et al. T-cell clonality assessment by next-generation sequencing improves detection sensitivity in mycosis fungoides. *J Am Acad Dermatol.* 2015;73:228-236.e222.
38. Weng WK, Armstrong R, Arai S, et al. Minimal residual disease monitoring with high-throughput sequencing of T cell receptors in cutaneous T cell lymphoma. *Sci Transl Med.* 2013;5(214):214ra171.
39. Raghavan SS, Wang JY, Gru AA, et al. Next-generation sequencing confirms T-cell clonality in a subset of pediatric pityriasis lichenoides. *J Cutan Pathol.* 2022;49(3):252-260.
40. Haverkos BM, Gru AA, Geyer SM, et al. Increased levels of plasma Epstein Barr Virus DNA identify a poor-risk subset of patients with advanced stage cutaneous T-Cell lymphoma. *Clin Lymphoma Myeloma Leuk.* 2016;16:S181-S190.e4.
41. Haverkos BM, Gru AA, Geyer SM, et al. The Epstein-Barr Virus (EBV) in T Cell and NK Cell Lymphomas: Time for a Reassessment. *Curr Hematol Malig Rep.* 2015;10(4):456-467.
42. Gru AA, Haverkos BH, Freud AG, et al. Primary cutaneous T-cell lymphomas show a deletion or translocation affecting NAV3, the human UNC-53 homologue. *Cancer Res.* 2005;65:8101-8110.
43. Ranki A, Vakeva L, Sipila L, et al. Molecular markers associated with clinical response to bexarotene therapy in cutaneous T-cell lymphoma. *Acta Derm Venereol.* 2011;91:568-573.
44. Choi J, Goh G, Walradt T, et al. Genomic landscape of cutaneous T cell lymphoma. *Nat Genet.* 2015;47:1011-1019.
45. da Silva Almeida AC, Abate F, Khiabanian H, et al. The mutational landscape of cutaneous T cell lymphoma and Sézary syndrome. *Nat Genet.* 2015;47(12):1465-1470.
46. Kiel MJ, Sahasrabuddhe AA, Rolland DCM, et al. Genomic analyses reveal recurrent mutations in epigenetic modifiers and the JAK-STAT pathway in Sézary syndrome. *Nat Commun.* 2015;6:8470.
47. Ungewickell A, Bhaduri A, Rios E, et al. Genomic analysis of mycosis fungoides and Sézary syndrome identifies recurrent alterations in TNFR2. *Nat Genet.* 2015;47:1056-1060.
48. Wang L, Ni X, Covington KR, et al. Genomic profiling of Sézary syndrome identifies alterations of key T cell signaling and differentiation genes. *Nat Genet.* 2015;47(12):1426-1434.
49. Karai LJ, Kadin ME, Hsi ED, et al. Chromosomal rearrangements of 6p25.3 define a new subtype of lymphomatoid papulosis. *Am J Surg Pathol.* 2013;37:1173-1181.
50. Onaindia A, Montes-Moreno S, Rodriguez-Pinilla SM, et al. Primary cutaneous anaplastic large cell lymphomas with 6p25.3 rearrangement exhibit particular histological features. *Histopathology.* 2015;66:846-855.
51. Wada DA, Law ME, Hsi ED, et al. Specificity of IRF4 translocations for primary cutaneous anaplastic large cell lymphoma: a multicenter study of 204 skin biopsies. *Mod Pathol.* 2011;24:596-605.
52. Parrilla Castellar ER, Jaffe ES, Said JW, et al. ALK-negative anaplastic large cell lymphoma is a genetically heterogeneous disease with widely disparate clinical outcomes. *Blood.* 2014;124:1473-1480.

CHAPTER 13

Mycosis fungoides

Alistair M. Robson, Rein Willemze, Julia Scarisbrick, Amy C. Musiek, Emmilia Hodak, Alejandro A. Gru, and András Schaffer

DEFINITION

Mycosis fungoides (MF) is the most common form of primary cutaneous T-cell lymphoma (CTCL), characterized by epidermotropic small-to-medium–sized T lymphocytes with cerebriform nuclei. It exhibits a protracted cutaneous clinical course with slow progression from slightly scaly flat skin lesions (patches) to elevated or infiltrated lesions (plaques), both representing early stage of the disease, and eventually to tumors, representing the advanced stage of MF, which can subsequently involve lymph nodes, bone marrow, and visceral organs. Sézary syndrome (SS), ie, erythroderma with leukemic phase, was traditionally defined as a late stage of MF. However, the current prevailing concept is that it should be considered as a separate type of CTCL, since it arises from T-cell subsets that are different from those characterizing patch/plaque/tumor type of MF.[1,2] According to the current World Health Organization (WHO) and European Organization for Research and Treatment of Cancer (EORTC) classification systems, the term MF should be restricted to cases exhibiting the classical evolution of patches, plaques, and tumors.

The prototypical immunophenotype of MF is that of $CD3^+CD4^+CD8^-CD7^-$. Expression of CCR4, CLA (CD45), and lack of CCR7/L-selectin molecules suggests that MF is a malignancy of mature skin-homing effector memory T "helper" (T_H) cells. MF often shows significant clinical and histopathologic overlap with selected inflammatory dermatoses and other cutaneous lymphomas, including primary cutaneous anaplastic large cell lymphoma (PC-ALCL) and adult T-cell leukemia/lymphoma (ATLL), a mature T-cell lymphoma caused by the retrovirus human T-lymphotropic virus I (HTLV-I).

EPIDEMIOLOGY

Cutaneous lymphomas are classified as non-Hodgkin lymphomas and are a heterogeneous group of diseases with the skin as the second most common extranodal primary site after the gastrointestinal tract.[3] The specific epidemiology of MF is poorly understood. In the United States, epidemiologic data obtained from two studies examining the Surveillance, Epidemiology, and End Results Program database, which account for approximately 25% of the population, are generally concordant with one another. These studies show that the incidence of CTCL is 6.4 per million persons, with MF accounting for greater than 50% of all CTCLs.[2] The PROCLIPI (prospective international cutaneous lymphoma prognostic index) Study opened in 2015 to collect worldwide data on MF/SS, to include clinical, pathological, genotypic, treatment, and survival data, in order to develop a prognostic index for MF/SS. This cohort has found MF to occur throughout the world with a similar male predominance 1.7:1 through all stages. The median age of diagnosis is lower in those presenting with the early stages (IA-IIA) at 57 years, compared with a median age of advanced stage patients (IIB-IVAB) of 63 years.[5] This does not appear to be due to a delayed diagnosis in advanced patients as the diagnostic delay is longer in early stage patients at 3 years.[6] There are some data[7] to suggest that African American patients with MF have a poorer survival than White patients after accounting for disease characteristics, but this is not seen in the PROCLIPI data where White patients present at an older age group and more advanced stage than non-White patients; this may be due to the easier diagnosis of early stage hypopigmented MF (a specific variant of MF more common in non-White skin).[8] There are regional differences in the reported incidence of pediatric MF, defined as MF diagnosed before the age of 18 or 20 years. While pediatric MF represents only 0% to 5% of all MF cases in North America and Europe, it is much more common in Middle Eastern and Asian countries, with reported rates of 5% to 25% of all MF cases.[9] Compared to adult MF, pediatric MF is usually diagnosed at an earlier stage and has a higher rate of variant presentations, specifically the hypopigmented and folliculotropic diseases.

ETIOLOGY

The etiopathogenesis of MF is only partially understood. It has been suggested that oncogenic transformation giving rise to MF might stem from chronic antigenic stimulation by viruses or bacterial superantigens in genetically susceptible hosts. Infectious agents, such as *Staphylococcus aureus*, Epstein-Barr virus, HTLV, and human herpesvirus-8, have been implicated,[10] but this has not been proven.

Data have shown that MF and SS likely originate from two different precursors. The expression of CD3, CD4, CCR4, and cutaneous lymphocyte antigen (CLA) but not

CCR7 by MF suggests its derivation from mature skin-homing effector memory T_H cells.[1] This is in contrast to SS, in which the neoplastic cells are CCR7+, similar to those of central memory T-cells.[1] MF is a unique skin neoplasm in which the malignant T-cells are of the same lineage as the tumor infiltrating lymphocytes (Tils) fighting the tumor. The phenotype of both tumor and Tils may be important in disease progression.[11]

In MF, the malignant clone's cell surface molecules are skin homing, as CLA binds E-selectin on cutaneous vascular endothelial cells and CCR4 binds the keratinocyte-manufactured chemokines CC-chemokine ligand 17 and 22.[1] These interactions give the malignant T-cell clone access to the epidermis. The development of drugs against these molecules allows new therapeutic therapies to be used, such as mogamulizumab, an anti-CCR4 monoclonal antibody.[12] Other chemokine receptors expressed in MF include CCR10, CXCR3, and CXCR4, and additional cell surface molecules include integrin αE/β7 and LFA-1.[13-15] Basal keratinocytes, Langerhans cells, and endothelial cells all express ligands for these receptors. PD-1 expression is markedly increased on tumor T-cells compared to nontumor CD4+ T-cells in SS patients providing a potential target for new monoclonal antibodies.[16,17]

The proliferation of the malignant T-cell clone can be explained by several mechanisms. These include the expression of CD45RO, proliferating-cell nuclear antigen, and CD25 as well as the constitutive activation of the JAK/STAT pathway.[18,19] A variety of mutations in the Fas/FasL system found in MF lead to a nonfunctional Fas protein, which may confer resistance to apoptosis.[20] The expansion of the malignant T-cell clone results in the restriction of the T-cell repertoire, leading to immunodeficiency even in the early stages of the disease.[18] Identification of driver mutations will be important in understanding and hopefully preventing disease progression; a recent genomic analysis study of 220 CTCLs identified 55 gene mutations possibly involved in CTCL pathogenesis including an RLTPR (p.Q575E) mutation that potentiates T-cell receptor (TCR) signaling via selective upregulation of the NF-κB pathway.[21]

Finally, the hallmark of MF is immune dysregulation with a T_H1 skewing in patch stage,[22,23] a mixed T_H1 and T_H2 phenotype in plaques, and T_H2 skewing in tumors[22] (Fig. 13-1). The expression of T_H2 cytokines IL-4, IL-5, and IL-10 causes a decrease in T_H1 effects, cell-mediated immunity, and dendritic cells, thus propagating further immune dysregulation. The T_H2-mediated increase in IgE and eosinophilia leads to the allergic phenotype often seen in erythrodermic MF. Correcting these defects provides a proven therapeutic target.

CLINICAL PRESENTATION AND PROGNOSIS

It is essential to understand that MF is a *clinical* not a pathological diagnosis, which is predicated upon the presence of patches and plaques; in a minority of patients there will be progression to the tumor stage. A patch is defined as a palpable lesion that is not elevated; a plaque is elevated but <1 cm; a tumor is raised >1 cm. Thus, pathologists diagnose CTCL, but it is the dermatologist that determines whether it is MF. Correspondingly, while pathological changes inevitably mirror these stages of MF, as outlined below, they cannot be used to determine the clinically defined stage, and pathology reports should refrain from attempting to stage the patient from the histopathology in the biopsy. Finally, the clinical spectrum of patch, plaque, and tumor, in turn, forms the basis of the staging systems (see Tables 13-2 and 13-3) that predict likely prognosis and from which treatment strategies draw their rationalization.

Classic MF of Alibert-Bazin type typically presents on the trunk and buttocks. Characteristic sites of involvement of folliculotropic MF (FTMF) are the head, neck, and upper back. Syringotropic MF (STMF) and solitary pagetoid reticulosis (PR) have predilections for the distal extremities (Fig. 13-2). Other MF variants have widespread anatomic locations, but most often involve the typical location of classic MF around the proximal limb girdle.

Patch Stage Mycosis Fungoides

Patch stage MF typically appears as erythematous scaly patches in non–sun-exposed skin, sometimes with wrinkled-atrophic surface (Fig. 13-3A). By definition, lesions are palpable but not elevated. Patches can also appear hyperpigmented or hypopigmented. Poikilodermatous features may also be present. The clinical differential diagnosis includes both eczematous dermatitis and small plaque parapsoriasis (also known as digitate dermatosis and chronic superficial scaly dermatitis); pointers toward a clinical diagnosis of early stage MF may include asymmetrical distribution, involvement of the bathing trunk area, and failure to respond to eczema/psoriasis treatments.[24]

Patients with patches or plaques covering less than 10% of their body surface area (T1) have a 5-year disease-specific survival of 98%, while patients with patches or plaques covering greater than 10% of their body surface (T2) area have a 5-year disease-specific survival of 89%. Both have a low rate of disease progression, of 8% and 21%, respectively.[25]

Plaque Stage Mycosis Fungoides

Clinically, plaque stage denotes raised lesions <1 cm in elevation; ulceration may rarely occur (Fig. 13-3B).[24] Although the staging system does not differentiate between patches and plaques for patients with a clinical stage of T2, plaque stage disease is associated with worse disease-specific survival and a higher risk of disease progression and affected patients are more often treated with systemic therapies.[25]

Tumor Stage Mycosis Fungoides

Tumors of MF are lesions of MF that are elevated greater than 1 cm. Such tumorous lesions arise in the setting of patch/plaque disease. Historically, tumor d'emblee represented de novo presentation of tumor stage MF. Described before the advent of immunohistochemistry this is now of questionable nosological status and most authorities are skeptical of it as a bona fide entity. In practice, the acute appearance of tumorous nodules almost always represents an aggressive cutaneous lymphoma distinct from MF. Tumor stage (T3) is considered late stage disease (Fig. 13-3C).[26] IIB MF tends to have a poor prognosis with a median overall survival for patients presenting with stage IIB disease of 68 months and

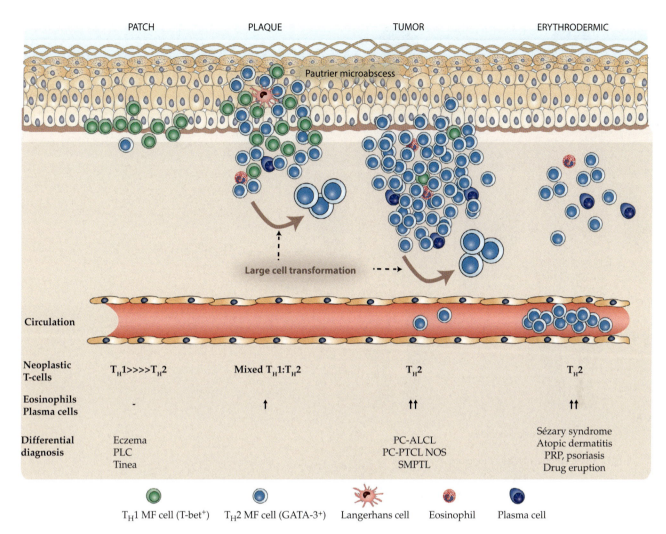

FIGURE 13-1. Histopathology, immune dysregulation, and differential diagnosis in MF progression. In patch stage, CD4+ malignant T-cells exhibit a T_H1 phenotype and home to the epidermis. In plaques, neoplastic T-cells expand in both the epidermis and dermis, have mixed T_H1 and T_H2 phenotypes, and form Pautrier microabscesses as they rosette around epidermal Langerhans cells. In tumor stage, epidermotropism is minimal; tumor cells are primarily T_H2 skewed and occupy the dermis and subcutaneous tissue. Large cell transformation occurs mostly in tumors and less frequently in plaques. Systemic spread of malignant T-cells in erythrodermic MF leads to suppressed host immune responses. The presence of plasma cells and eosinophils in plaques and tumors is likely reflective of T_H1 to T_H2 immune effector switch by neoplastic cells. PC-ALCL, primary cutaneous anaplastic large cell lymphoma; PC-PTCL-NOS, primary cutaneous peripheral T-cell lymphoma, not otherwise specified; PLC, pityriasis lichenoides chronica; PRP, pityriasis rubra pilaris; SMPTL, primary cutaneous CD4+ small/medium pleomorphic T-cell lymphoma.

is typically treated with systemic therapy; however, if disease is limited, then local site irradiation may be preferred.[5,27] Five-year disease-specific survival drops considerably to 56%, and the risk of disease progression is 48%.[25]

HISTOLOGY

Patch Stage Mycosis Fungoides

The histopathology of early MF is challenging, and distinction from inflammatory disease may not be initially possible. It is a commonplace for several biopsies to be taken before a confident diagnosis is made. To make the diagnosis of MF at an early stage, the distribution of lymphocytes, nuclear atypia of lymphocytes, and changes in the epidermis and papillary dermis have to be carefully appraised (Table 13-1).

In early patch stage, lymphocytic infiltrates in the dermis are scant and patchy and the epidermis and papillary dermis are only minimally altered. Recognition of epidermal colonization by rare single or clustered neoplastic lymphocytes, ie, epidermotropism, with minimal cytologic atypia, sometimes with surrounding lacunae, may be the only diagnostic clues at this stage of the disease (Fig. 13-4).[28,29]

In late patch stage, epidermotropism is more pronounced. Alignment of atypical lymphocytes at the dermal-epidermal junction ("tagging"), as well as pagetoid scatter within the epidermis, are characteristic (Fig. 13-5).[30,31] To clarify terminology, it should be noted that epidermotropism is used to describe neoplastic T-cell migration into the epidermis, as opposed to lymphocytic exocytosis, which is a term referring to intraepidermal lymphocytes found in inflammatory dermatoses.

Epidermal changes in early MF are usually minimal and typically exhibit three distinct patterns. (1) *Spongiosis*, or edema between keratinocytes, is usually subtle around neoplastic cells in MF compared to reactive spongiotic dermatitides. (2) *Psoriasiform* change, with thickening, and elongation of the

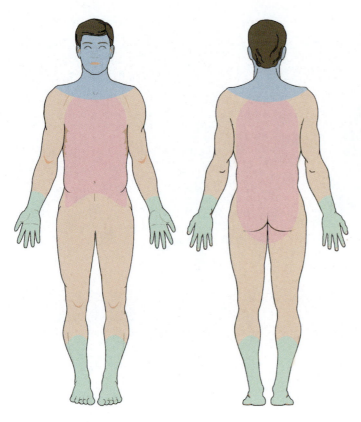

- Classical mycosis fungoides
- Folliculotropic mycosis fungoides
- Solitary pagetoid reticulosis (Woringer-Kolopp disease) Syringrotropic mycosis fungoides

FIGURE 13-2. Anatomical site predilections of MF variants.

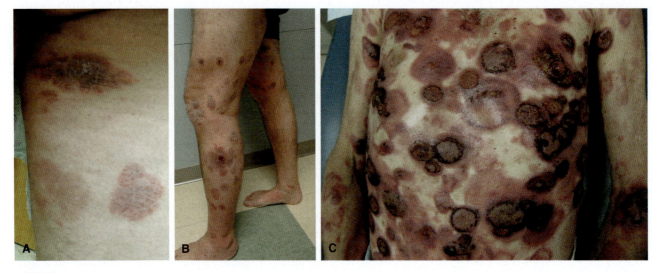

FIGURE 13-3. Classical MF. A. Erythematous scaly patches on sun-protected skin. **B.** Erythematous scaly plaques, some with ulceration. **C.** Tumor stage MF.

rete, is not uncommonly seen in MF (Fig. 13-6A). Irregular rete elongation or fusion of retes can also be observed (Fig. 13-6B). (3) *Atrophic* changes with thinning of the epidermis and effaced rete. These patterns likely reflect disturbed epidermal differentiation and/or cytotoxicity exerted by T-cells (Fig. 13-6C).

As patch stage MF progresses, neoplastic T-cells demonstrate increasing cytologic atypia including characteristic hyperchromatic nuclei with deep narrow indentations and cerebriform contours (Fig. 13-7). However, a subset of reactive T-cells with CD4+CD26− immunophenotype may also show similar "atypical" morphology with cerebriform features.[32] A clear rim around nuclei, perinuclear "halos," is a common and helpful morphological change; this should not be confused with vacuolar change seen in lichenoid

TABLE 13-1 Histologic Spectrum of Patch Stage MF

Epidermal Changes	Epidermotropism	Dermal Changes
Normal epidermis	Absence of epidermotropism	Papillary dermal fibrosis/coarse collagen bundles
Psoriasiform hyperplasia	Basilar lymphocytes	Melanophages
Epidermal atrophy	Pautrier microabscesses	Purpura
Irregular hyperplasia	"Haloed" lymphocytes	Edema of the papillary dermis
Marked spongiosis	Disproportional exocytosis	
Necrotic keratinocytes	Pagetoid epidermotropism	

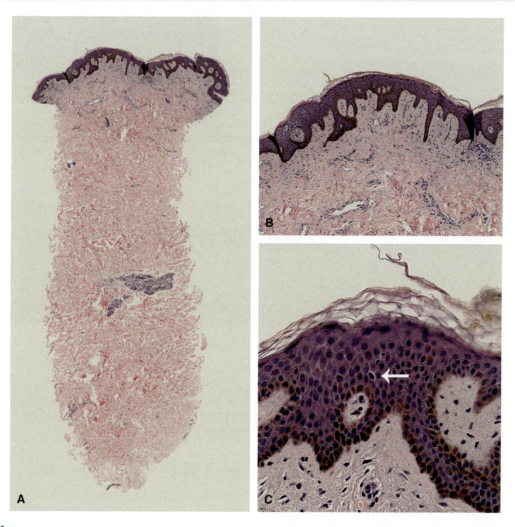

FIGURE 13-4. **Early patch stage MF. A** and **B.** Scant lymphocytic infiltrates in the papillary dermis. The epidermis shows irregular rete and hyperkeratosis. **C.** Arrow indicates a rare epidermotropic lymphocyte with nuclear hyperchromasia and perinuclear halo ("coal on a pillow"). Magnifications: A, 15×; B, 50×; C, 200×.

dermatitis, which represents a cytomorphological change in basal keratinocytes not lymphocytes. Pautrier microabscesses, a characteristic feature of the later stages of MF (see below), may start to appear in the patch stage.

Assessing the degree of solar elastosis is helpful in differentiating neoplastic from reactive lymphocytic infiltrates: classic MF lesions occur at sun-protected sites; thus, the presence of prominent solar elastosis is unusual in MF. An exception to this rule is FTMF, which typically occurs on sun-exposed sites such as the face and head. Other dermal hallmarks of patch stage MF are related to fibrotic changes elicited by chronically retained neoplastic cells in the papillary dermis ("signs of chronicity"). These changes typically occur in late rather than early patch stage MF and include (1) conversion of the papillary dermal collagen from fine fibrillary forms into wiry collagen bundles (fettuccine-like fibrosis) and (2) "halo" formation around lymphocytes

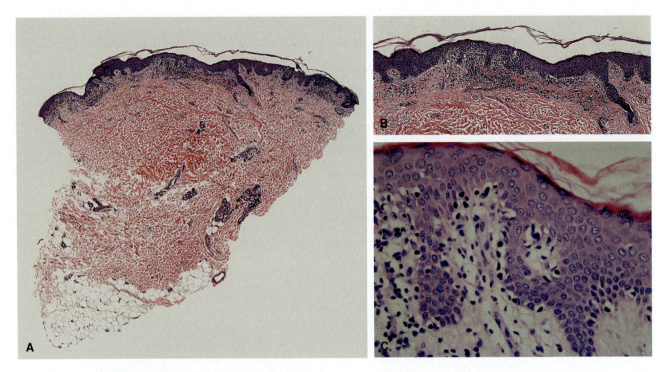

FIGURE 13-5. **Late patch stage MF. A.** Increased number of lymphoid infiltrates in the papillary dermis. **B** and **C.** Epidermal colonization by hyperchromatic neoplastic lymphocytes with perinuclear halo. Neoplastic cells lining-up along the dermoepidermal junction. Note there is no evidence of epidermal damage, eg, colloid bodies, in contrast to autoimmune lichenoid dermatides. Magnifications: A, 15×; B, 50×; C, 400×.

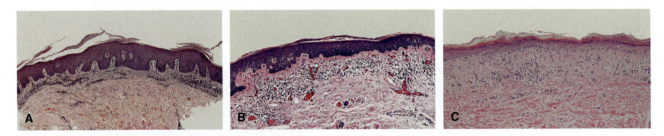

FIGURE 13-6. Epidermal changes in MF. **A.** Psoriasiform epidermal hyperplasia. **B.** Irregular rete alteration. **C.** Epidermal atrophy.

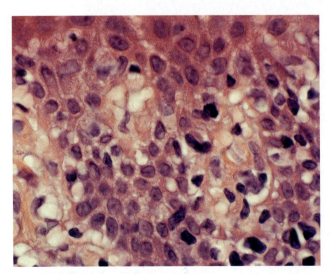

FIGURE 13-7. **Cytologic features of epidermotropic lymphocytes in MF.** Neoplastic lymphocytes are small to medium in size, and exhibit hyperchromasia and cerebriform nuclei.

(Fig. 13-8).[30,31,33,34] Nevertheless, similar collagen changes may be observed in chronic dermatitides, particularly chronic photosensitive dermatitis.

Plaque Stage Mycosis Fungoides

Progression of MF from patch stage is accompanied by the expansion of neoplastic T-cells both in the epidermis and dermis, contributing to the clinical presentation of raised, palpable plaques (see Figs. 13-1, 13-3B, and 13-9A,B). In the epidermis, expanded neoplastic T-cells may aggregate with CD1a+ Langerhans cells to form the hallmark Pautrier abscess (Fig. 13-10A,B). These neoplastic T-cell rosettes have to be distinguished from Langerhans cell microgranulomas, also known as pseudo-Pautrier abscesses, that are commonly associated with contact/eczematous dermatitides, perhaps particularly allergic/contact dermatitis (Fig. 13-11).[35] In the dermis of plaque stage MF, T-cells form broad, band-like infiltrates that extend from the papillary into the superficial reticular dermis. In both the plaque stage and much more in

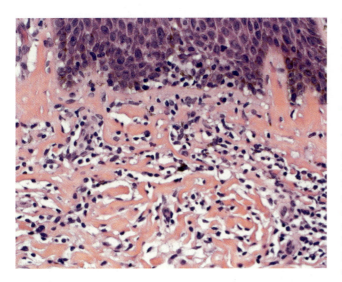

FIGURE 13-8. Papillary dermal alterations in MF: wiry collagen thickening (fettuccine-like fibrosis) and halo formation around lymphocytes and halo formation around lymphocytes ("lump of coal on a pillow").

tumor stage, it is not infrequent to observe admixed inflammatory cells, such as histiocytes, eosinophils, and plasma cells (see Fig. 13-1). This is likely a consequence of a switch in immune effector function from T_H1 to T_H2 during disease progression.

Tumor Stage Mycosis Fungoides

The clinical emergence of tumors and nodules at late disease stages correlates with frequent loss of epidermotropism and nodular or sheet-like expansion of neoplastic T-cells in the reticular dermis (see Figs. 13-1 and 13-12A–D). Cytologic atypia is readily discernible as neoplastic cells markedly outnumber admixed reactive T-cells. Neoplastic T-cells may undergo large cell transformation (LCT), which is defined histologically rather than clinically, by the occurrence of neoplastic cells four times the size of normal lymphocytes constituting more than 25% of the infiltrate (Fig. 13-12D and 13-16). LCT is not synonymous with nor restricted to tumor stage disease, as plaque and very rare instances of transformed patch stage cases have been reported.[36,37] This

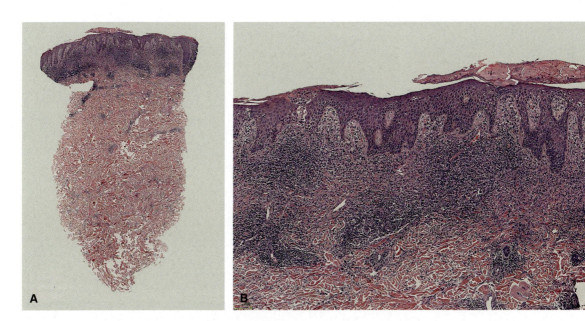

FIGURE 13-9. Histopathology of plaque stage MF. Neoplastic lymphocytes expand both in the epidermis and dermis. Magnifications: A, 15×; B, 50×.

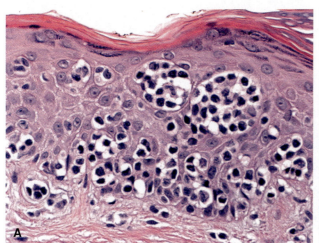
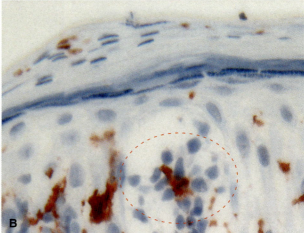

FIGURE 13-10. Pautrier microabscess. A. Neoplastic cells are grouped within the epidermis. **B.** The microabscess is centered around CD1a+ Langerhans cells.

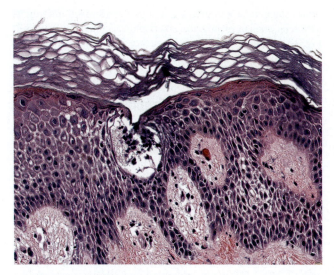

FIGURE 13-11. Vase-shaped Langerhans cell microgranuloma (pseudo-Pautrier microabscess) in spongiotic dermatitis.

transformation event portends poor prognosis[38,39] although whether it is independent of rate of stage progression is not clear. The morphology of large transformed cells varies from cells with large hyperchromatic, vesicular nuclei and scant cytoplasm to cells with large irregular nuclei, prominent nucleoli, and abundant cytoplasm, characteristic of ALCL. Differentiating MF with LCT from primary cutaneous anaplastic T-cell lymphoma is histologically unreliable, requiring both immunophenotyping and clinical correlation.[22]

Staging and Extracutaneous Spread

Clinical/prognostic stratification of MF is determined by cutaneous tumor burden, presence of lymph node involvement, visceral metastasis, and peripheral blood involvement. These parameters are recorded in the tumor-node-metastasis-blood (TNMB) classification, which stages patients from IA to IV (Tables 13-2 and 13-3).

In the updated International Society for Cutaneous Lymphomas (ISCL)/EORTC staging system for clinically

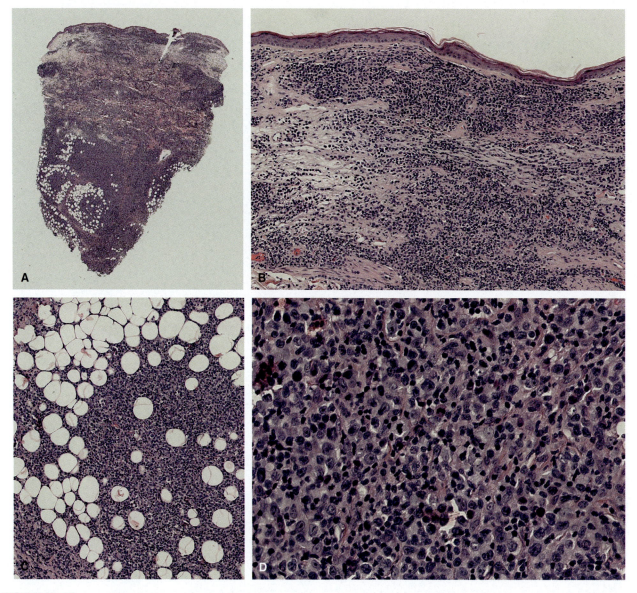

FIGURE 13-12. Histopathology of tumor stage MF. A–C. Minimal epidermotropism and diffuse dermal infiltration with subcutaneous involvement. **D.** Large cell transformation. Note admixed plasma cells and eosinophils.

abnormal peripheral lymph nodes (>1.5 cm), the following categories are recognized (Table 13-2)[40]: N1: dermatopathic lymphadenopathy (DL) without involvement by MF; N2: DL without effacement of normal lymph node architecture with early involvement by MF; N3: overt involvement with partial or complete architectural effacement. Recognition of early lymph node involvement can be difficult and can be facilitated by detection of clonal TCR gene rearrangements.[40,41]

Distinction is therefore made between stages N1a/N2a (clone negative) and N1b/N2b (clone positive) (Table 13-2).

Lungs, liver, and spleen are the most common sites of visceral involvement (M1). Rare cases involving oral mucosa, nasopharynx, orbital tissue, small bowel, and central nervous system have also been reported.[42-45] Bone marrow involvement can occur in advanced stages and is associated with a worse outcome.[46]

TABLE 13-2 MF and Sézary Syndrome TNMB Classification

Skin	
T1	Limited patches, papules, and/or plaques covering <10% of the body surface area
T2	Patches, papules, and/or plaques covering >10% of the body surface area
T2a	Patch only
T2b	Patch and plaque
T3	Tumors, one or more (≥1 cm in diameter)
T4	Erythema (≥80% of the body surface area)
Node	
N0	No abnormal lymph nodes
N1	Abnormal lymph nodes; histopathology Dutch Gr1 or NCI LN0-LN2
N1a	Clone negative
N1b	Clone positive
N2	Abnormal lymph nodes; histopathology Dutch Gr2 or NCI LN3
N2a	Clone negative
N2b	Clone positive
N3	Abnormal lymph nodes; histopathology Dutch Gr3-4 or NCI LN4
NX	Clinically abnormal node w/o histology
Visceral	
M0	No visceral organ involvement
M1	Visceral involvement (must have pathology confirmation)
MX	Abnormal visceral site; no histologic confirmation
Peripheral Blood Involvement	
B0	Absence of significant blood involvement ≤5% Sézary cells
B0a	Clone negative
B0b	Clone positive
B1	Low blood tumor burden: >5% of peripheral blood lymphocytes are >5% Sézary cells, but do not meet the criteria of B2
B1a	Clone negative
B1b	Clone positive
B2	High blood tumor burden: ≥1000/mL Sézary cells or CD4/CD8 ≥10 or ≥40% CD4$^+$/CD7$^-$ or ≥30% CD4$^+$/CD26$^-$ cells

Adapted from Olsen E, Vonderheid E, Pimpinelli N, et al. Revisions to the staging and classification of mycosis fungoides and Sézary syndrome: a proposal of the International Society for Cutaneous Lymphomas (ISCL) and the cutaneous lymphoma task force of the European Organization of Research and Treatment of Cancer (EORTC). *Blood*. 2007;110(6):1713-1722, with permission from Elsevier.

TABLE 13-3 MF and Sézary Syndrome Staging

Stage	T	N	M	Peripheral Blood Involvement
IA	T1	N0	M0	B0-1
IB	T2	N0	M0	B0-1
II	T1-2	N1-2	M0	B0-1
Late Stage				
IIB	T3	N0-2	M0	B0-1
IIIA	T4	N0-2	M0	B0
IIIB	T4	N0-2	M0	B1
IVA1	T1-4	N0-2	M0	B2
IVA2	T1-4	N3	M0	B0-2
IVB	T1-4	N0-3	M1	B0-2
Sézary Syndrome				
IVA1 or 2 or IVB	T4	N0-3	M0-1	B2

Adapted from Olsen E, Vonderheid E, Pimpinelli N, et al. Revisions to the staging and classification of mycosis fungoides and Sézary syndrome: a proposal of the International Society for Cutaneous Lymphomas (ISCL) and the cutaneous lymphoma task force of the European Organization of Research and Treatment of Cancer (EORTC). *Blood*. 2007;110(6):1713-1722, with permission from Elsevier.

Association With Other Lymphoproliferative Diseases

Contemporaneous association of MF with other hematologic neoplasms is well documented, and numerous factors have been proposed to explain the phenomenon. Immune dysregulation, therapy-related immunosuppression, and chemotherapy-induced secondary neoplastic transformation are only a few of the proposed mechanisms, although a shared biologic/genetic relationship between MF and the secondary malignancies cannot be entirely excluded. The temporal relationship between MF and secondary malignancies varies, but could be synchronous, preceding, or following the initial presentation of MF. Approximately 2% to 5% of MF cases have associated lymphomatoid papulosis (LyP).[25,47] Association with other CD30+ lymphoproliferative disorders, including ALCL and Hodgkin disease as well as various forms of T-cell lymphomas, low-grade B-cell lymphomas (ie, chronic lymphocytic leukemia), and diffuse large B-cell lymphomas, has also been observed.[48,49]

IMMUNOPHENOTYPE

In the majority of classic MF cases, neoplastic T-cells exhibit a $CD3^+\beta F1^+CD4^+CD8^-$ mature T-cell phenotype (Fig. 13-13A–D). $CD4^-CD8^+$, $CD4^-CD8^-$, and $CD4^+CD8^+$ phenotypes have also been described, although less frequently.[50-54] These variants appear to have similar clinical outcomes.[55] Rare cases of classic MF with γ/δ phenotype have also been reported.[54,56,57]

In patch stage disease, neoplastic cells preserve the expression of pan T-cell antigens, including CD2, CD3, and CD5, but they frequently lack CD7. A subset of early patch stage disease showing minimal epidermotropism can exhibit loss of CD2 and CD5 expression confirming the diagnosis (Fig.13-14A-C). The absence of CD7 expression is believed to be a result of neoplastic downregulation of CD7 expression, although some authors argue that MF cells derive from the transformation of a preexisting CD7− mature T-cell subset.[58] In the later tumor stage, partial or complete loss of CD2, CD3, and CD5 is often observed.[59]

The majority of inflammatory conditions include both CD4+ and CD8+ lymphocytes within the infiltrate. Thus, a markedly elevated CD4:CD8 ratio on immunohistochemically-stained sections may be a useful adjunct to the diagnosis, although care must be taken not to include Langerhans cells, which are also CD4+. For this reason, some authors advocate assessment of the CD3:CD8 ratio as more reliable.[60] Evaluation of immunophenotypic skewing should be performed on epidermal T-cells as dermiinfiltrates often harbor disproportionally elevated CD8 cytotoxic lymphocytes.[61] Clearly, such assessments are not useful in cases of CD8+ MF, which serve as an additional caution in overdependence on evaluation of phenotypic ratios. In practice, the diagnosis of MF is a morphological one and immunohistochemistry is often of little help in the early stages of MF in which histological distinction from a dermatitis is difficult to make, while an abnormal immunophenotypic signature is commonly seen in the later stages when the morphological diagnosis is more obvious. Nevertheless, occasionally, loss of T-cell-associated antigens can cement a tentative diagnosis of early MF despite subtle or limited histopathological changes.

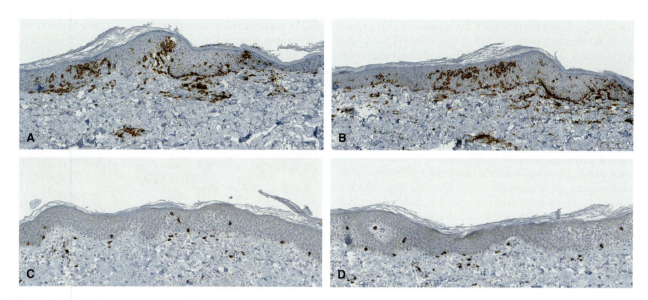

FIGURE 13-13. Classic immunophenotype of MF. **A.** CD3, **B.** CD4, **C.** CD8, and **D.** CD7.

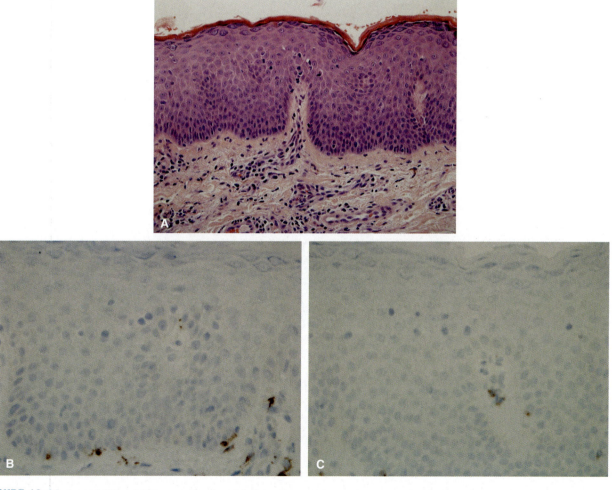

FIGURE 13-14. Loss of CD2 and CD5 expression in patch stage disease. A few atypical intraepidermal lymphocytes are present **(A)**, suspicious for T-cell lymphoma but insufficient for a firm diagnosis. However, loss of CD5 **(B)** and CD2 **(C)** expression confirms the diagnosis.

Although in most cases of MF the neoplastic cells express CD4, a CD8+ phenotype is well documented. This should not overturn a secure diagnosis of classic Alibert-Bazin MF in the correct clinical context; CD8+ variants of this disease follow the same clinical course as the more common CD4+ variant.

Progression of MF is accompanied by a switch from T_H1 and T_H2 cytokine expression: epidermal T_H1 cytokine profiles characterize patch and plaque stages, whereas T_H2 cytokine profiles dominate tumor stages.[62,63] Earlier works argued that T_H1 predominance in patch stage MF is due to the predominance of antitumoral CD8+ lymphocytes, which is followed by the outgrowth of neoplastic T_H2-skewed cells in the plaque and tumor stages.[15] A recent immunohistochemical study has found that T-cells undergo a T_H1-T_H2 effector function switch during disease progression.[22] In the early patch stage, the infiltrate expresses the T_H1-specific T-bet but not the T_H2-specific GATA-3 transcription factor. In plaques, cells exhibit a mixed T-bet: GATA-3-expression pattern. As tumors evolve, T lymphocytes become diffusely GATA-3+ with minimal T-bet expression (Fig. 13-15A-I). T-bet and GATA-3 immunohistochemistry might be helpful in differentiating MF from its benign and malignant mimics.[22]

CD30 (Ki-1 antigen) is expressed by Reed-Sternberg cells of Hodgkin lymphoma, by cells of ALCL or LyP, and by immunoblasts in certain reactive infiltrates. Additionally, CD30 expression has been observed in a subset of patch stage and tumor stage MF with LCT (Fig. 13-16).[37-39,64] Although CD30 expression correlates with better disease-specific survival in large cell–transformed MF patients, no prognostic significance for CD30 expression was found in patch stage disease.[65,66] Furthermore, therapeutic decisions are also affected

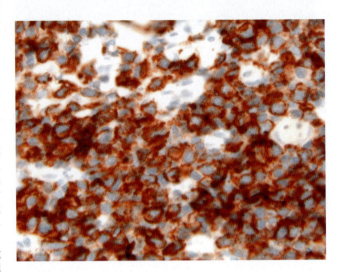

FIGURE 13-16. CD30 expression by large cell transformed MF.

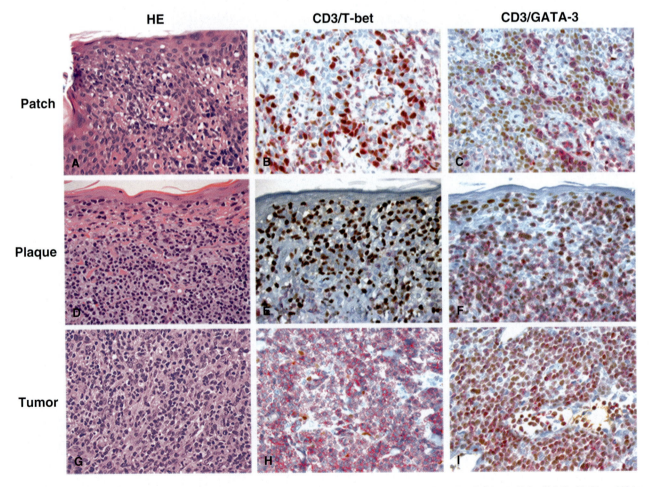

FIGURE 13-15. Immune effector phenotypes in MF progression. **A–C.** Patch: $T_H1>>T_H2$, **D–F.** plaque: $T_H1\sim T_H2$, **G–I.** tumor: $T_H2>>T_H1$. Double immunohistochemistry for CD3/T-bet and CD3/GATA-3. CD3 (red) Tbet and GATA-3 are brown.

by CD30 expression. Tumors with at least 10% CD30 expression are efficiently eradicated by CD30-targeted monoclonal antibody-immunotoxin therapy (brentuximab vedotin).[67,68]

CD25 encodes the low-affinity receptor for interleukin 2. Similar to CD30, its expression is more common in lesions from advanced MF patients.[69] Although CD25 expression is often associated with Foxp3+ regulatory T (T_{reg}) cells, and reactive Foxp3+ cells can be detected in both patch and tumor stage MF, the prognostic significance of the T_{reg} phenotype in disease progression is not fully understood.[70,71]

CD56 (neural cell adhesion molecule or NCAM), a natural killer (NK) cell marker, is very rarely expressed in MF with CD4+, CD8+, or CD4−CD8− phenotypes.[72-74] Distinction from CD56+ aggressive lymphomas including primary cutaneous NK/T-cell lymphoma, nasal type, and blastic plasmacytoid dendritic cell neoplasm is essential and requires clinical and histopathologic correlation.

Granzyme B (GrB), perforin, and T-cell-restricted intracellular antigen (TIA-1) are cytotoxic granule–associated proteins that are specifically expressed by cytotoxic CD4+ or CD8+ T-cells with either α/β or γ/δ phenotypes. They are only rarely expressed in early patch stage, but their expression increases in advanced disease.[75] Thus, a cytotoxic phenotype should not be seen as evidence against an otherwise secure diagnosis of MF.

Expression of follicular helper T-cell (T_{FH}) markers, PD-1, ICOS-1, CXCL-13, CD10, and BCL-6, has also been described in MF (Fig. 13-17).[76-79] The biologic significance of these findings is still unclear, although some authors suggest that increased expression of PD-1 and its ligand PDL-1 in tumor stage MF may be co-opted by neoplastic cells to evade antitumoral immune response.[77] Cases of MF with expression of T_{FH} markers have been associated with enriched B-cell infiltrates. More recently, Theurich et al[80] have shown that the clinical course of MF with abundant intralesional B-cells is more aggressive, and thus might be amenable to anti-CD20 therapy. The same therapy could also be exploited for rare cases of CD20+ MF (Fig. 13-18).[81,82]

GENETIC AND MOLECULAR FINDINGS

Clonal rearrangement of the TCR locus can be detected in most cases, depending on the number of neoplastic cells and the molecular technique applied. However, the early—particularly patch—stage of disease may not demonstrate a T-cell clone. Moreover, detection of monoclonality is not pathognomonic of malignancy as persistent cutaneous inflammatory infiltrates of monoclonal or oligoclonal T-cells have been documented (Table 13-4). These *clonal dermatitides* (abortive/latent lymphomas) include conditions secondary to autoimmune or iatrogenic immune dysregulation (ie, lupus profundus, lymphomatoid drug eruptions), pityriasis lichenoides et varioliformis acuta (PLEVA), actinic reticuloid (AR), lichen planus, as well as chronic idiopathic dermatoses with persistent T-cell clones

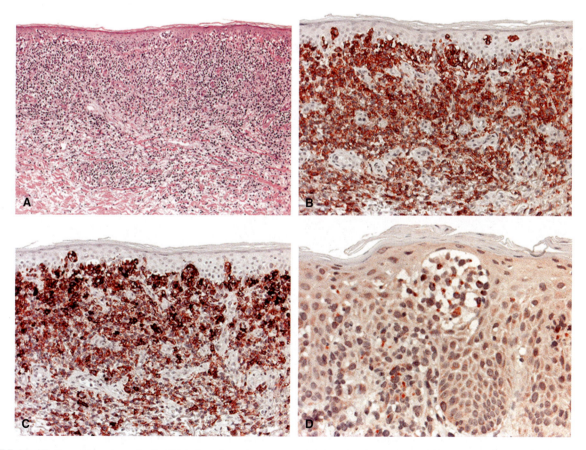

FIGURE 13-17. T_{FH} **marker expression by MF. A.** Band-like epidermotropic infiltrates of atypical lymphocytes; **B.** expression of PD-1; **C.** ICOS; and **D.** CXCL-13. (Obtained with permission from Bosisio FM, Cerroni L. Expression of T-follicular helper markers in sequential biopsies of progressive mycosis fungoides and other primary cutaneous T-cell lymphomas. *Am J Dermatopathol.* 2015;37:115-121.)

TABLE 13-4 Histological Spectrum of Clonal Dermatitides (Abortive/Latent Lymphoma)

Diagnosis	References
Eczematous/contact dermatitis	83, 84
Lymphocytic infiltrate of Jessner	83
Bullous pemphigoid	83
Lichenoid eruptions including lichen planus and lichen sclerosus et atrophicus	85
Psoriasis	85
Erythema nodosum	85
Lymphomatoid lupus profundus/discoid lupus erythematosus	86
Up to 50% of cutaneous drug-associated lymphomatoid hypersensitivity reactions (reversible)	86
Up to 30% of cases in a miscellaneous group that includes hypopigmented interface-type lesions	86, 87
Syringolymphoid hyperplasia with alopecia	87
Idiopathic follicular mucinosis	86
Pityriasis lichenoides chronica	86
Pityriasis lichenoides et varioliformis acuta (PLEVA)	86
Atypical lymphocytic lobular panniculitis	86
Idiopathic and drug-induced pigmented purpuric dermatosis	86
Morphea/scleroderma	86
HIV-associated T-cell-rich pseudolymphoma (unrelated to drug therapy)	86

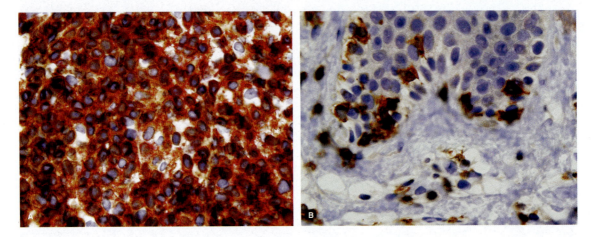

FIGURE 13-18. **CD20 expression by rare cases of MF. A** and **B.** Rust-like staining with CD3 (*red*, chromagen) and CD20 (*brown*, diaminobenzidene) indicates colocalization of CD20 expression by CD3+ T-cells. (Obtained with permission from Hagen JW, Schaefer JT, Magro CM. CD20+ mycosis fungoides: a report of three cases and review of the literature. *Am J Dermatopathol.* 2013;35(8):833-841.)

that are referred to as cutaneous T-cell lymphoid dyscrasia.[87] Although clonal dermatitides are thought to be biologically distinct from MF, 20% to 25% of these entities can progress to lymphoma within 5 years.[33,84]

Monoclonality derived from true neoplastic T-cells should be distinguished from *pseudoclonality*, which is frequently observed in small skin biopsies with sparse lymphocytic infiltrates or limited microdissected areas in the presence of inflammatory cells.[88-90] Pseudoclonality can be distinguished from true clonality by repeat PCR analyses using the same DNA template, a second independent DNA extraction from the same sample, and/or DNA from synchronous or metachronous samples. In pseudoclonality, the size of the dominant PCR amplicon varies in repeat analysis, whereas that of real clonality does not.[91]

The presence of *stable T-cell clones*, that is, identical T-cell clones or a restricted molecular profile from two or more anatomical sites in synchronous or sequential skin biopsies, is reported to be associated with a specificity of >95% in discriminating MF from most benign dermatoses.[85] However, because similar stable clones can also be found in cutaneous lymphoid dyscrasias, lymphomatoid drug reactions, as well as interstitial granulomatous dermatitis, they cannot be considered to be diagnostic of CTCL.[85,86] Therefore, lesions with nondiagnostic histopathology and stable T-cell clonal pattern should be regarded as possible precursors of early stage MF and managed as such.

Progression of MF is associated with increased cytogenomic alterations.[2,92,93] Comparative genomic hybridization studies identified highly recurrent gains in 7q36 and 7q21-7q22, and loss in 5q13 and 9p21.[2] This pattern differs markedly from chromosomal alterations observed in SS. Amplifications of chromosomal regions encompassing T-cell differentiation and activation genes, such as NOTCH1, GATA3, IL2R, FASTK1, and SKAP1, as well as chromosomal deletions affecting tumor suppressor loci such as TP53, DLEU1, and RB have been reported.[2,92] Chromosomal translocation t(3;9)(q12;p24) has been described in a case of MF with granulomatous features.[94] Patients with increased genomic instability (>5 DNA aberrations) and inactivation of loci encoding CDKN2A/p16 INK4a (9p21.3) and PTEN (10q26qter) as well as amplification of C-MYC (8q24.21) have been associated with poor clinical outcome.[92] The more recently identified genetic changes described in mycosis fungoides are summarized in Chapter 6.

POSTULATED CELL OF ORIGIN

Because classic MF cells in patch stage disease have a CD3+, CD4+, T-bet+, CD45RO, CCR4+ immunophenotype, the cells of origin are believed to be skin-homing memory T_H1-cells.

VARIANTS LISTED UNDER THE WHO/EORTC CLASSIFICATION

In addition to classic Alibert-Bazin MF numerous clinical and pathological variants are described (Table 13-5). Three of these, Folliculotropic MF, Solitary Pagetoid Reticulosis

TABLE 13-5 Histopathological Variants of MF

Diagnosis	References
Acanthosis nigricans–like	95
Anetodermic	96
Bullous	97-100
Erythrodermic	101
Folliculotropic/pilotropic	102-104
Granulomatous including granulomatous slack skin	105-107
MF with cysts and comedones	104, 108, 109
Hypopigmented	110
Hyperpigmented	54, 111
Hyperkeratotic/verrucous	112
Ichthyosis-like	113
Interstitial	114
Pagetoid reticulosis	115-117
Papular	118, 119
Pigmented purpura–like	120
Poikilodermatous	121
Pustular	122
Reticular erythematous mucinosis–like	123
Small plaque parapsoriasis	124
Syringotropic	125-130
Unilesional (other than pagetoid reticulosis)	131, 132
Zosteriform	133

FOLLICULOTROPIC MYCOSIS FUNGOIDES

FTMF, which constitutes the most common variant, has a variable clinical appearance.[102-104] The lesions tend to be indurated plaques with follicular accentuation or follicular papules coalescing into plaques. It favors the head and scalp over the bathing suit distribution of traditional MF. Infiltrated plaques in the eyebrow region with concurrent alopecia are a common and highly characteristic finding. Acneiform lesions including milia, comedones, and pustules can also occur. Rarely, there may be only a single lesion. Some patients may show keratosis pilaris–like lesions that are mainly localized on trunk and extremities. Often, the lesions have associated alopecia (Fig. 13-19A–D). Comedonal changes may be striking such that a diagnosis of MF is not initially considered (Fig. 13-21). The lesions may be accompanied by severe itching. Previous studies emphasized that FTMF has a worse prognosis compared with classic MF.[104,134] However, recent studies defined subgroups of early and advanced FTMF with a prognosis similar to early and advanced stage classic MF.[135]

Histologically, it is characterized by peri- and intra-follicular infiltrates of neoplastic T-cells (Fig. 13-20A). Infiltration of the interfollicular epidermis, characteristic of early stage classic MF, is uncommon. The sequential destruction of the follicular epithelium by neoplastic cells is reflected by a broad spectrum of histologic changes. Initially, only follicular spongiosis can be observed, which often progresses to mucinous degeneration of the follicle (follicular mucinosis) (Fig. 13-20B) with occasional involvement of the interfollicular epidermis (epidermal mucinosis). Mucin deposits can be visualized by Alcian blue or colloidal iron staining. Additional variants of FTMF include cases that lack mucin deposition or those that exhibit follicular cystic changes. Comedonal MF may be subtle

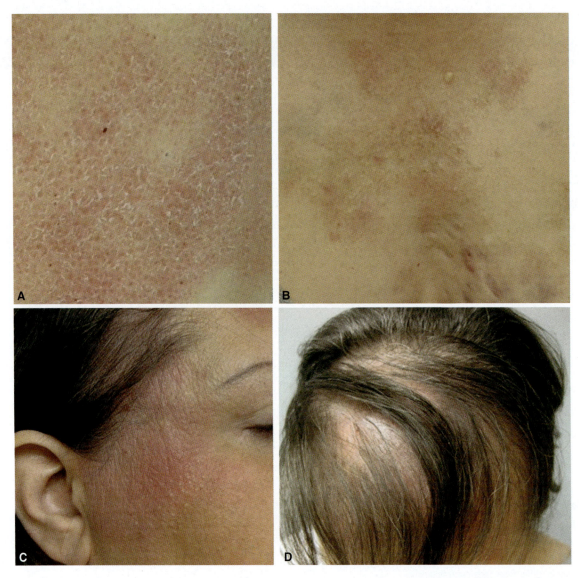

FIGURE 13-19. Folliculotropic MF. A. Erythematous plaques with follicular accentuation; **B.** acneiform lesions including milia and open comedones; **C.** facial lesion showing follicular accentuation; **D.** scalp demonstrating alopecia.

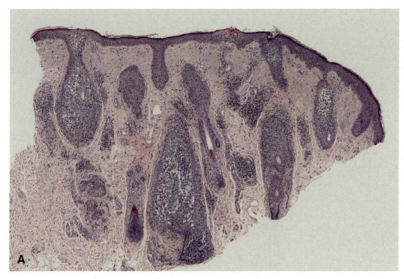 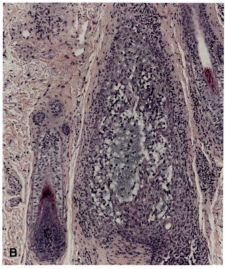

FIGURE 13-20. **Histopathology of FTMF.** Lymphocytic colonization and mucinous degeneration of the follicular epithelium. Magnifications: A, 30×; B, 100×.

with cysts having focal lymphoid epidermotropism (see Fig. 13-21).[104,108,109] In early stage lesions, clinically characterized by follicle-based patches, flat plaques, or acneiform or keratosis pilaris–like lesions, the perifollicular infiltrates are generally sparse or moderate in a lichenoid pattern and, in addition to the atypical T-cells, present variable numbers of small reactive T-cells,[136,137] histiocytes, and occasional eosinophils. The perifollicular infiltrates in more advanced plaques or tumors become more dense and more diffuse extending beyond the perifollicular dermis and may contain increasing numbers of blast cells. LCT has been reported in more than 20% of FTMF cases and is more common than in classical MF.[135] In this advanced stage there is often a considerable admixture of eosinophils and, in particular in cases with secondary bacterial infection, plasma cells. In cases with destruction of the hair follicle epithelium, a granulomatous reaction with foreign body giant cells and fibrosis can be observed. As such, one should exert caution when evaluating florid granulomatous reaction secondary to ruptured follicles, as the reactive changes can obscure the underlying neoplastic process. In virtually all cases the neoplastic T-cells have a $CD3^+$, $CD4^+$, $CD8^-$ phenotype as in classic MF. Admixture with CD30-positive blast cells is common. The follicles show abundant $CD1a^+$ cells.[137] which can be sufficiently florid to cause concern regarding Langerhans cell histiocytosis.

SYRINGOTROPIC MYCOSIS FUNGOIDES

STMF, formerly known as syringolymphoid hyperplasia with alopecia, is a rare variant of MF.[125-130] For many years, folliculotropism and syringotropism were considered closely related entities; however, a recent study serves to contrast the variants. Both are associated with alopecia and papular lesions. In contrast to folliculotropic disease, STMF often presents on the limbs, palms, and soles, but other topographical sites such as trunk, head, and neck have also been reported (see Fig. 13-22A–E).[125,126] Histologically, it is defined by the collections of perieccrine neoplastic T-cells with moderate to prominent tropism into the eccrine secretory epithelium (see Fig. 13-22F). Associated epidermotropism, folliculotropism, and syringoid hyperplasia are frequent findings.[126] Syringotropic neoplastic T-cells show similar cytologic and immunophenotypic atypia as seen in classic MF. The deep location of neoplastic cells, similar to FTMF, as well as the frequent occurrence on the palms and soles results in frequent resistance to skin-directed treatment modalities. Nonetheless, STMF appears to have a better clinical outcome than that of FTMF.[126]

SOLITARY PAGETOID RETICULOSIS OR WORINGER-KOLOPP DISEASE

Solitary pagetoid reticulosis (PR) or Woringer-Kolopp disease is a rare unilesional variant of MF named after the histologic resemblance of epidermotropic neoplastic T-cells to intraepidermal adenocarcinoma in Paget disease of the nipple. Clinical lesions are solitary, scaly patches, and plaques on distal extremities, although lesions on the trunk and even the tongue have been reported.[115] They often mimic benign dermatoses such as eczema/psoriasis (Fig. 13-23A), warts or benign or premalignant keratosis (Fig. 13-23G). Currently, PR is classified as a variant of MF with a benign, indolent clinical behavior that lacks extracutaneous dissemination. While studies are small, this variant tends to respond to skin-directed therapies.[139] Development of more disseminated skin lesions has been reported in exceptional cases.[140]

Histologically, there is prominent epidermotropism of medium-sized hyperchromatic T-cells into an acanthotic epidermis (Fig. 13-23B,C) with minimal dermal involvement. Three different phenotypes have been described, with decreasing frequency, of $CD8^+$, $CD4^+$, and $CD4^-CD8^-$ cases. Both $CD4^+$ and $CD8^+$ variants express βF1 (Fig. 13-23D–F).[115-117] Most PR cases express pan-T-cell antigens CD3, CD2, and CD5, but typically lack CD7 expression and, in some cases, CD45 (leukocyte common antigen). TIA-1 and CD30 expression by a significant proportion of $CD8^+$ PR have been described.[115,116] Because the $CD8^+CD30^+$ phenotype is also a hallmark of type D LyP,

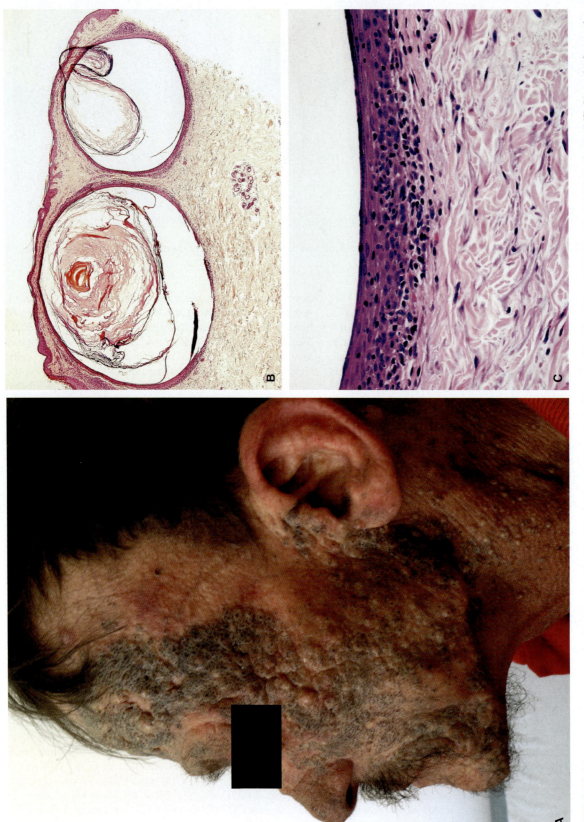

FIGURE 13-21. Florid comedonal changes in follicular MF (A). Histology demonstrates marked cystic change (B) and sparse foci of epidermotropism within the cyst wall (C). Diagnosis often requires careful clinical appraisal, with identification of a T-cell clone. (A, C/o Dr. Mariana Cravo, Department of Dermatology, Lisbon Institute of Oncology.)

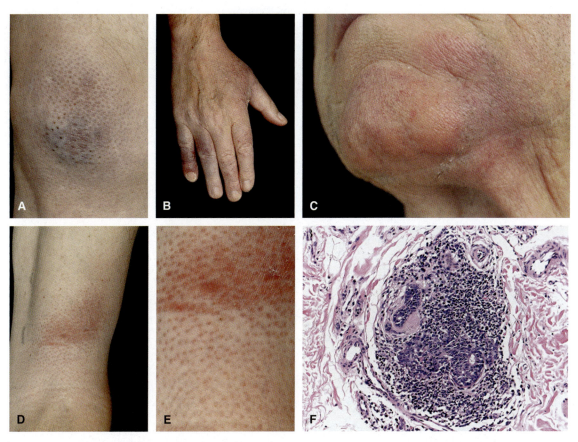

FIGURE 13-22. Clinical and histopathologic features of STMF. A. Comedones on the knee; **B.** infiltrated plaques on the fingers with follicular accentuation; **C.** alopecic plaque on the chin on a patient with a history of mycosis fungoides; **D.** confluent follicular papules on arm; **E.** note the clear follicular distribution; **F.** eccrinotropic lymphocytic infiltrates. (A, C/o Dr. Mariana Cravo, Lisbon Institute of Oncology, Portugal; Obtained with permission from Pileri A, Facchetti F, Rutten A, et al. Syringotropic mycosis fungoides: a rare variant of the disease with peculiar clinicopathologic features. *Am J Surg Pathol.* 2011;35(1):100-109.)

careful clinicopathologic interpretation is warranted as the histopathologic features can be indistinguishable.[141] Many PR lesions have monoclonal TCR rearrangements.[116,142]

Disseminated PR (Ketron-Goodman disease) is not a variant of MF and can best be considered as an archaic term for entities that we currently define as one of four disseminated primary cutaneous lymphomas.[143,144] These include conventional MF, primary aggressive epidermotropic CD8+ cytotoxic T-cell lymphoma (Berti lymphoma), cutaneous γ/δ T-cell lymphoma, and cutaneous cytotoxic NK/T-cell lymphoma.

GRANULOMATOUS SLACK SKIN

Granulomatous slack skin (GSS) is a very rare variant of MF, clinically characterized by the slow development of pendulous folds of lax skin in the major skin folds, in particular the axillae and groins[145-149] (Fig. 13-24A–H). It typically affects adolescents and adults and mostly occurs in men.[149] Extracutaneous dissemination is rare and most patients have an indolent clinical course. However, in approximately one-third of the reported patients, an association with other malignant lymphomas, particularly MF and Hodgkin lymphoma is observed.[148,149] Because of the increased risk of a second malignant lymphoma, long-term follow-up is mandatory.[145]

Histologically, GSS is characterized by the presence of dense infiltrates of small clonal CD4-positive T-cells admixed with numerous macrophages and many scattered multinucleated giant cells[147] (Fig. 13-25D–G). The presence of multinucleated giant cells containing more than 10 nuclei per cell is considered as a characteristic feature, but has also been observed in cases of granulomatous MF.[145] Loss of elastic tissue, elastophagocytosis, and emperipolesis (engulfment of lymphocytes) by multinucleated cells are commonly observed. Elastophagocytosis by giant cells (Fig. 13-25D-E) is believed to be the main mechanism of profound dermal elastolysis in GSS that leads to the characteristic pendulous skin masses. Interestingly, however, elastic van Gieson staining of sections from plaques or tumors of classic Alibert-Bazin–type MF also demonstrates elastolysis, further underlining the relationship with conventional MF. It is also found in skin lesions in other skin areas that do not develop cutis laxa-like changes.[145] The epidermis may be infiltrated by small atypical T-cells with cerebriform nuclei, as in classic MF. Most cases have a CD3+, CD4+, CD8- T-cell phenotype and show clonal TCR gene rearrangement.[145] It is common for the diagnoses of granulomatous MF and GSS to be missed, partly through dominance of the granulomatous infiltrate but also because the neoplastic lymphoid component often presents little if any atypia. Furthermore, at the end stage of the lesions in GSS there may only be residual multinucleate giant cells and only very sparse lymphoid cells (Fig. 13-25F and G).

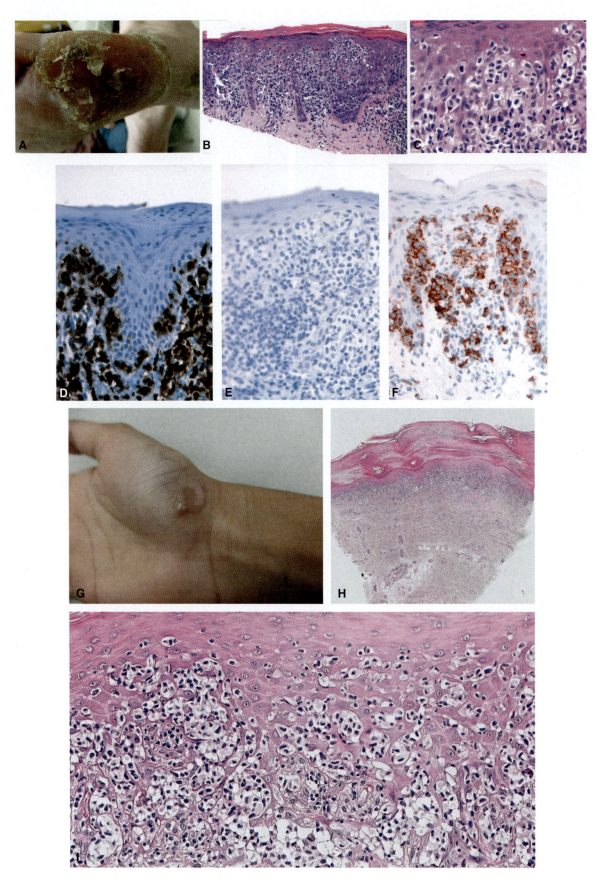

FIGURE 13-23. **Clinical and histopathologic features of pagetoid reticulosis. A.** Erythematous scaly plaque mimicking foot dermatitis (photo courtesy of Dr. Charles E. Mount III); **B** and **C.** pagetoid epidermotropism by epithelioid lymphocytes; **D.** CD3; **E.** CD4; **F.** CD8. **G.** Scaly solitary plaque mimicking benign keratosis on the hand. Histology shows hyperkeratosis **(H)** and marked pagetoid epidermotropism by epithelioid lymphocytes **(I)**.

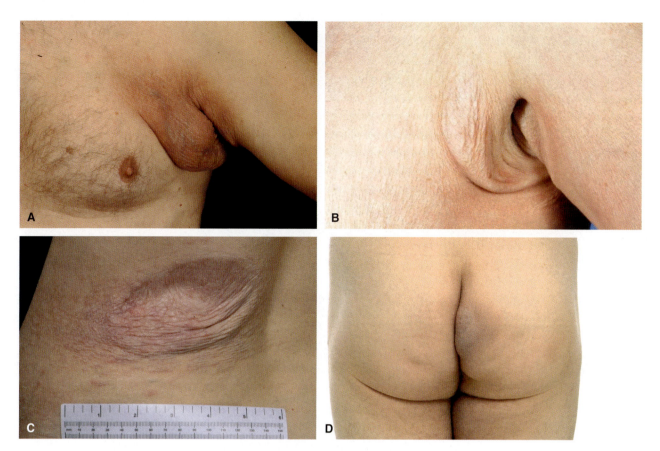

FIGURE 13-24. Typical clinical features of Granulomatous Slack Skin. **A-C.** Pendulous lax skin within axillae **D.** An area of similarly lax buttock skin.

There are overlapping histologic features between GSS and granulomatous MF, and clinicopathologic correlation is required to differentiate between these conditions. Compared with classic, nongranulomatous MF, granulomatous MF appears to have a worse prognosis, with more accelerated disease progression and a poorer response rate to skin-directed therapies, often necessitating more aggressive treatment protocols.[145,146]

VARIANTS NOT LISTED UNDER THE WHO/EORTC CLASSIFICATION

Besides the entities described above, there are additional very rare variants of MF that display distinct clinical characteristics, and, with some exceptions, exhibit a clinical course and prognosis that are similar to those of classic MF (see Table 13-5). Similar to classic MF, several of these entities exhibit histopathologic overlap with benign dermatoses.

Bullous MF is an extremely rare variant with an aggressive clinical course.[97-100] Patients present with vesicles, bullae, or erosions with negative immunofluorescence (direct and indirect) and lack of evidence for bacterial (*Staphylococcus*) or viral infections and porphyria.[97] Histopathology reveals subcorneal, intraepithelial, or subepidermal blisters, which may contain atypical T-cells. The presence of typical features of MF (eg, epidermotropism with atypical lymphocytes) is the key to the diagnosis. The pathogenesis of these lesions is not entirely clear. Direct cytotoxicity by neoplastic T-cells, decreased adhesion between basal keratinocytes and papillary dermis due to the confluence of Pautrier microabscesses, or extreme spongiosis within the epidermis are possible mechanisms. Approximately 50% of patients die within one year of diagnosis.[100]

Poikilodermatous MF presents with cigarette-paper-like thinning of the skin, reticulated red-to-brown telangiectasias, and alternating hypo- and hyperpigmentation (see Fig. 13-26A), typically with a burning sensation, predominantly located on the breast, hips, and buttocks, sometimes concomitantly with patches or plaques of classic MF. The histology demonstrates epidermal atrophy with loss of rete ridges, lichenoid interface changes with dyskeratosis, pigment incontinence, papillary dermal fibrosis, and vascular ectasia (Fig. 13-26B and C). Thus, unlike typical lichenoid MF in which lymphocytes line along the basal epidermal layer, there is often evidence of keratinocyte damage, perhaps unsurprisingly as this is thought to underlie the epidermal atrophy that characterizes this subtype (see Fig. 13-26). Immunophenotypic analysis may reveal a CD8+ or double negative signature more frequently than a CD4+ phenotype.[150]

Besides MF, prolonged lichenoid inflammation in lichen planus, lupus erythematosus, dermatomyositis, chronic radiodermatitis, and Rothmund-Thomson syndrome are associated with clinical poikiloderma. Similar features can reflect regression of nonmelanoma skin cancer or melanoma.

Papular MF is a recently recognized clinical variant of early MF characterized by papules rather than conventional patches at the onset of disease. Based on one report, this

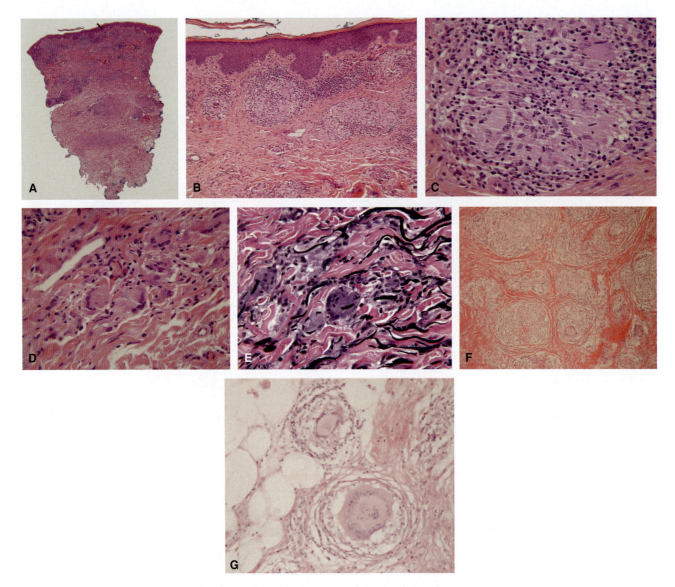

FIGURE 13-25. Histopathologic features of GMF. A–C. Superficial and deep granulomatous inflammatory infiltrates along with interstitial infiltration by neoplastic T-cells; **D.** elastophagocytosis highlighted by hematoxylin and eosin (H&E) and **E.** Verhoeff-van Gieson stains. **F** and **G.** The later stages of disease may be dominated by giant cells with a paucity of lymphocytes and the neoplastic nature of the process can be readily overlooked.

variant tends to have a less aggressive course than classic plaque- or tumor-stage MF.[118] Histology shows superficial perivascular lymphocytic infiltrates with epidermotropism, including rare Pautrier microabscesses. Neoplastic cells have a CD3+CD4+CD8−CD30− immunophenotype. The most important histologic differential diagnosis includes type B LyP, which, unlike the type A and C variants, is composed of small-to-medium–sized atypical lymphocytes without large cells.[119] The waxing and waning clinical features as well as the variable CD30 expression aid in differentiating type B LyP from papular MF.

Erythrodermic MF is characterized by generalized erythroderma, the so-called "red-man syndrome," which is often accompanied by intense pruritus (Fig. 13-27). It may develop either in patients with previously diagnosed patch/plaque disease or, more often, arise de novo. The clinical differential diagnosis includes several inflammatory erythrodermic conditions, particularly contact dermatitis, psoriasis, seborrheic dermatitis, atopic dermatitis, and pityriasis rubra pilaris. Erythrodermic MF differs from SS by the lack of the defining elevated number of circulating neoplastic cells (Sézary cells), thereby not meeting the criteria for B2 (see Table 13-2). However, in rare instances, sometimes referred to as pre-SS, these patients develop lymphadenopathy and leukemic involvement indistinguishable from classic features of SS.[151] Nonetheless, recent studies show that MF and SS are biologically and genetically distinct entities arising from distinct functional T-cell subsets with unique oncogenomic alterations.[1,2]

The histologic features of erythrodermic MF can be more subtle than the features of patch and plaque stage MF, with less pronounced epidermotropism by neoplastic T-cells. Furthermore, parakeratosis, acanthosis, and papillary dermal fibrosis, with prominent telangiectasia and increased mitotic figures, are more commonly seen in erythrodermic than in patch stage MF.[101]

Hypopigmented MF mostly presents in darkly pigmented patients and has an overrepresentation in children (Fig. 13-28).

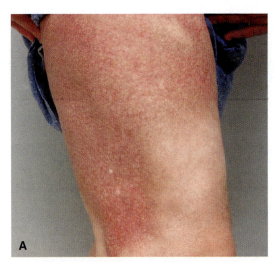
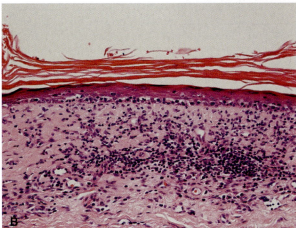
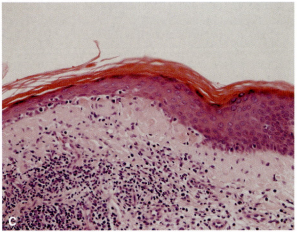

FIGURE 13-26. Clinical and histological features of poikilodermatous MF. **A.** Skin atrophy with reticulated teleangiectasia and alternating hypo- and hyperpigmentation. **B and C.** A lichenoid pattern within an atrophic epidermis. In contrast to classical MF, evidence of epidermal damage, eg, colloid bodies, and loss of stratum basalis, is often evident and underlies the clinical and pathological atrophy.

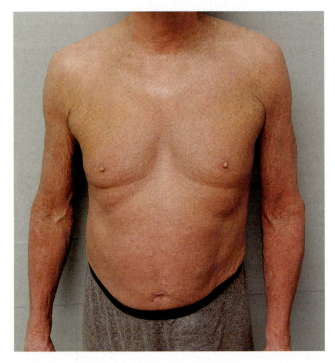

FIGURE 13-27. Erythrodermic variant of MF.

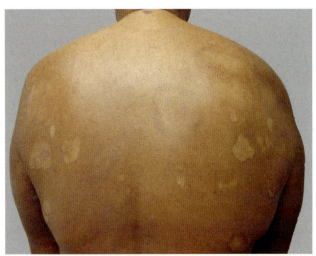

FIGURE 13-28. Hypopigmented patch stage MF.

This may account for the recent publication showing non-White skin presenting at an earlier age with an earlier stage.[9] Cases in Caucasians, including children, have also been described.[9,110] Patients demonstrate hypopigmented-to-achromic lesions, sometimes with vitiligo-like features. Similar to classic MF, patch lesions of hypopigmented MF are distributed on the trunk, proximal portions of the extremities, the buttocks, as well as the pelvic girdle and the lower limbs. However, on the arms, in contrast with classic MF, lesions show a predilection for the outer surfaces, rather than the inner sun-protected surfaces. In the pediatric age group, hypopigmented MF may be seen in combination with early folliculotropic lesions (Hodak et al).

Rare cases with involvement of the head and neck have been described. Patients may complain of pruritus. Touch-sensitivity is always preserved. The clinical differential diagnosis should include pityriasis versicolor, pityriasis alba, vitiligo, leprosy, postinflammatory hypopigmentation, pityriasis lichenoides chronica (PLC), or sarcoidosis. The histopathologic findings may be similar to classic MF, but lichenoid infiltrates are usually less striking and more focal, and fibroplasia is usually absent probably because of early patch stage presentation.[152] Parakeratosis, when present, is useful in excluding vitiligo. A CD4⁻CD8⁺ immunophenotype is more common in this variant.[153] A reduced number of epidermal melanocytes suggest a melanocyte-targeted cytotoxicity by neoplastic CD8⁺ T-cells as a possible pathomechanism.[154] The clinical course and prognosis may be more indolent than classic MF.

Hyperpigmented MF is rare and occurs almost exclusively in dark-skinned individuals (Fig. 13-29). The findings of circumscribed hyperpigmented patches or plaques raise a broad differential diagnosis, especially postinflammatory hyperpigmentation, erythema dyschromicum perstans (ashy dermatosis), drug reaction, contact dermatitis, atrophoderma of Pasini-Pierini, and idiopathic eruptive macular hyperpigmentation. Interestingly, hyperpigmented MF lesions can be associated with poikilodermatous or hypopigmented variants in the same patient.[111] By immunohistochemical studies, epidermotropic T-cells exhibit a predominantly CD8⁺ phenotype, although few CD4⁻CD8⁻ cases have also been reported. The histologic correlate of the clinical hyperpigmentation is postinflammatory melanin incontinence. Some speculate that this is caused by interface changes mediated by cytotoxic $CD8^+TIA-1^+$ or $CD4^-CD8^-TIA-1^+$ neoplastic cells.[54,111]

Ichthyosiform MF is characterized by an ichthyosis vulgaris–like eruption, or by less specific ichthyosiform lesions. Patients may present with diffuse, dry, scaling skin, or well-circumscribed scaly patches, or flat plaques affecting the trunk and extremities (Fig. 13-30).[113,155,156]

Histologically, in addition to the typical features of MF, there are findings suggestive of coexistent ichthyosis vulgaris, such as parakeratosis and focally compact orthokeratosis with thinning or absence of the granular layer. Most cases have a $CD3^+CD4^+$ phenotype, with only a few showing a predominance of CD8⁺ lymphocytes.

Hyperkeratotic, verrucous features in MF were originally recognized by Hallopeau and Bureau,[112] who noted that although hyperkeratosis of palmoplantar surfaces was a common finding in MF, similar lesions elsewhere were quite unusual. The lesions may be dormant for long periods.[157] Histology shows psoriasiform epidermal hyperplasia, confluent parakeratosis, suprapapillary thinning, spongiosis, and a dense lymphocytic infiltrate along the dermal-epidermal junction and in the superficial perivascular plexus. Atypical epidermotropic T-cells show classic cytologic and immunophenotypic features.

Interstitial MF is a rare variant that can histologically resemble granuloma annulare or inflammatory morphea.[114] Histologically, there is interstitial infiltration by single lymphocytes between collagen fibers in the reticular dermis (Fig. 13-31). Cytological atypia may be slight and the diagnosis of lymphoma not often considered without close clinical correlation.

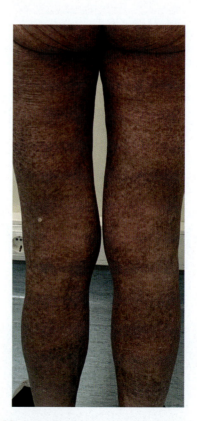

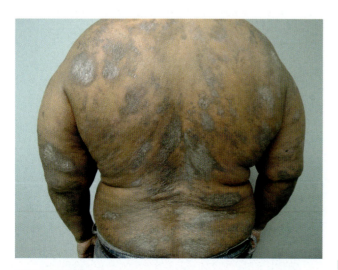

FIGURE 13-29. Hyperpigmented patch/plaque stage MF.

FIGURE 13-30. Icthyosiform MF. Dry scaly thickened skin. (C/o Dr. Mariana Cravo, Department of Dermatology, Lisbon Institute of Oncology.)

Epidermotropism is usually minimal, and subtle mucin deposition can be occasionally seen. Immunohistochemistry confirms most interstitial cells are T lymphocytes, which may have a CD4+ or CD8+ phenotype, and a variable but minority population of admixed CD68+ histiocytes.[158,159]

Solitary MF Solitary presentations of MF are documented as exceptional cases and have an uncertain relationship to classical disease.[160] The burden of proof of such a diagnosis should be high to exclude peripheral T-cell lymphoma not otherwise specified (PTCL-NOS). Patients present with a patch or plaque, or a very localized area of alopecia, with characteristic histopathology and either loss of one or more T-cell-associated antigens or detection of a T-cell clone (Fig. 13-32). The prognosis of the few cases reported is excellent. It is hypothesized that such cases simply reflect a chance occurrence of a patient presenting with such early disease, but this is speculative.

Invisible MF is an exceedingly rare form of MF.[161-163] It is characterized by neoplastic T-cell infiltrates in clinically normal-appearing skin. Pruritus without visible disease can be an associated finding, which is usually the trigger for the biopsy. The diagnostic criteria include findings of epidermotropic and superficial perivascular infiltrates of T-cells with immunophenotypic and molecular genetic evidence of clonality. Invisible MF can be seen either before or after the development of classic patches or plaques.

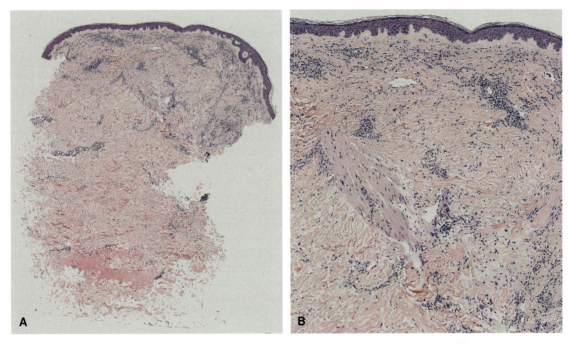

FIGURE 13-31. Histopathologic features of interstitial MF. A and **B.** Nonepidermotropic dermal interstitial infiltrates of neoplastic lymphocytes. Immunohistochemistry revealed marked elevation of CD4:CD8 ratio. Magnifications: A, 15×; B, 50×.

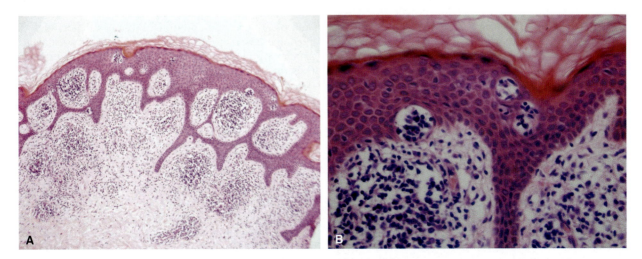

FIGURE 13-32. Solitary MF. Biopsy from an isolated plaque on the abdomen. Dermal lymphocytic infiltrate **(A)** with epidermotropism and Pautrier microabscesses **(B)**. A T-cell clone was detected.

Other very rare MF variants have been described that clinically mimic benign dermatoses. These include reticular erythematous mucinosis–like, zosteriform, and acanthosis nigricans–like MF (see Table 13-5).

HISTOLOGIC DIFFERENTIAL DIAGNOSIS

A considerable number of inflammatory dermatoses can simulate early MF. They are clinically variable, and histologically include spongiotic, lichenoid, pityriasiform, and psoriasiform reaction patterns. While most of these simulators are biologically distinct, true reactive processes, some of them might represent the earliest manifestation of patch stage MF (T-cell dyscrasia) that lack full morphologic or immunophenotypic criteria for definite diagnosis of lymphoma. Additionally, MF can be histologically and immunophenotypically indistinguishable from other types of cutaneous lymphomas.

BENIGN CONDITIONS

Spongiotic dermatitides are classically seen in eczema and contact dermatitis and can often simulate MF both clinically and histologically.[164] Spongiosis denotes increased intercellular gaps between keratinocytes in the epidermis due to intercellular edema. Lymphocytic infiltrates are mostly superficial perivascular with focal exocytosis. Lymphocyte beading along the dermoepidermal junction, characteristic of MF, is absent. The presence of perivascular eosinophils favors a spongiotic process. In patch stage MF, in which neoplastic cells are strongly T_H1-skewed, perivascular infiltrates contain only very rare, if any, eosinophils. Furthermore, intraepidermal eosinophils (eosinophilic spongiosis), as found in contact dermatitis or scabies, are almost never present in patch stage MF. Intraepidermal Langerhans cell microabscesses are classically seen in spongiotic dermatitides (typically, allergic/contact dermatitis). They are composed of CD1a+, S100+, CD4dim+ Langerhans cells, and monocytic precursors, and lack T-cells.[165] Langerhans cells have a pale, reniform/centrally indented nucleus with abundant pale cytoplasm, whereas cells within Pautrier collections in plaque stage MF are composed of neoplastic CD3+CD4+ T-cells with hyperchromatic and cerebriform nuclei.

Interface (lichenoid) dermatitides characterized by reactive lymphocytic infiltrates in the papillary dermis and epidermis can also mimic the histologic appearance of MF. Dyskeratotic cells (apoptotic keratinocytes), colloid bodies, and melanophages (pigment incontinence) are commonly associated with interface changes. Two histologic patterns can be distinguished. In the lichenoid variant of interface dermatitides, as prototypically seen in lichen planus, a band-like lymphocytic infiltrate obscures the dermoepidermal junction with exocytosis, relative paucity of dyskeratosis, and sharpening of rete ridges. In cytotoxic/vacuolar interface dermatitides, such as in lichenoid graft-versus-host disease and lupus erythematous, the dermoepidermal junction shows basovacuolar change, which is a rare finding in MF.[166] In general, evidence of epidermal keratinocyte damage is unusual in MF, in which the resident neoplastic lymphocytes colonize the epidermal compartment as bystander residents, in contrast to autoimmune lichenoid dermatitis in which immune effector T-lymphocytes attack the keratinocytes. However, the presence of lichenoid changes does not completely exclude the diagnosis of MF, since a subset of MF patients exhibit lichenoid changes; this is particularly the case in poikilodermatous and hyperpigmented subtypes. In some cases these tend to be associated with intense pruritus and may presage a poor prognosis,[167] although specifically poikilodermatous MF is associated with a more favorable prognosis.

Lymphoid infiltrates secondary to allergic or iatrogenic antigens are well-recognized simulants of MF.[168-170] Because the histologic, immunophenotypic, and even TCR genotypic features can be indistinguishable from those of lymphoma, careful clinical assessment of external causes is the cornerstone of diagnosis. Skin lesions usually resolve within months after discontinuation of the offending allergen/drug and may recur with reinitiation of the implicated agent. Lymphomatoid contact dermatitides are noneczematous allergic reactions to selected allergens such as nickel, cobalt, gold, and textile dyes (azo).[169] They are characterized by chronic accumulation of activated lymphocytes that undergo clonal selection over time.[170] Histologically, they exhibit band-like lymphocytic infiltrates and exocytosis into a nonspongiotic epidermis without significant cytologic atypia. Drug-induced pseudolymphoma syndrome is also a close imitator of MF. It is characterized by solitary or multiple plaque-like lesions or nodules such as seen following phenytoin, carbamazepine, or histamine antagonist therapies.[171,172] Digitate dermatosis–like skin changes have been described in patients taking angiotensin II inhibitors, while photo-distributed MF-like rashes have been reported after quinine intake.[173,174] In addition to medication-induced lichenoid inflammatory patterns, some drugs produce an *interstitial granulomatous reaction* with cytologic and immunophenotypic atypia and clonal restriction mimicking interstitial granulomatous MF. This reaction pattern is termed drug-associated reversible T-cell dyscrasia as most of these lesions completely regress upon cessation of the medication.[175]

Pityriasiform dermatitis is a collective term to describe chronic scaly skin conditions with small, fine, mica-like scales. The word "pityriasis" was coined by Hippocrates to describe subtle scaly skin lesions imitating the fine bran of grain called "pityron." Pityriasis lichenoides (PL) encompasses a spectrum of clinical features from acute papular eruptions with central necrosis (PLEVA or Mucha-Habermann disease) to small, scaling papules as seen in PLC (see also Chapter X). Monoclonal T-cell populations have been detected more frequently in acute and less frequently in chronic forms.[176,177] Malignant transformation in PL is controversial. Because cases of PLC evolving into MF have been described in adults and children, some authors consider PLC a form of T-cell dyscrasia with limited propensity for transformation to lymphoma.[178,179] Conversely, however, MF can present with PLC-like lesions. Histologically, PLEVA shows superficial and mid-dermal, wedge-shaped lymphocytic inflammation with exuberant exocytosis, basal vacuolar alteration, dyskeratosis, extravasation of erythrocytes, and confluent mounds of parakeratosis with serum and neutrophils. In comparison with PLEVA, the histopathology of PLC is subtle. Lymphocytic infiltrates and hemorrhage are less pronounced. Pautrier-like microabscesses may also be observed in PLC.[179] The infiltrate is predominantly composed of CD8+CD45RO+TIA-1+ cytotoxic memory T-cells, and to a lesser extent, CD4+ T-cells. Importantly, a subset of PLEVA cases have been described with a conspicuous CD30+ component, mimicking LyP.[180]

Pigmented purpuric dermatoses (PPD) encompass a broad range of clinical variants with a unifying histologic pattern composed of lymphocytic inflammation, extravasated erythrocytes, and variable hemosiderin pigment deposition. Within the PPD spectrum, the Gougerot and Blum variant and lichen aureus exhibit prominent lichenoid inflammation and could pose significant morphologic and immunophenotypic overlap with MF.[181] Cases of patients with PPD-like eruptions have been described to progress to MF.[182] In fact, one of the first cases of lichen aureus reported in the United States was eventually reclassified as MF.[183,184] The histologic differential diagnosis is further complicated by the existence of rare purpuric presentations of MF and atypical PPD-like eruptions with T-cell clonality.[120] Some of the latter have been associated with medication reaction to several drug classes, including antihistamines, β-blockers, calcium channel blockers, and lipid-lowering agents.[185] When differentiating between PPD and MF, the presence of intraepidermal lymphocytes larger than dermal lymphocytes and papillary dermal fibrosis would support a diagnosis of MF over PPD. Any pigmented and purpuric dermatitis, which appears to be atypical, either clinically or histologically, should be appraised and followed up closely for the possibility of purpuric MF.

AR is the most severe form of chronic actinic dermatitis, a photoallergic dermatitis with features of spongiotic and lichenoid changes. It can be difficult to differentiate from the eczematous form of MF. Clinically, AR shows pruritic, eczematous thickened skin on sun-exposed sites, typically on the head, neck, and upper extremities. Histologically, the papillary dermis shows brisk lymphoid infiltrates with eosinophils, plasma cells, and stellate multinucleated fibrohistiocytic cells expressing factor XIIIa.[186] Solar elastosis, a finding unusual for MF, is a common association. Features of acanthosis, reticular fibroplasia similar to lichen simplex chronicus, thickened and increased blood vessels are helpful in differentiating AR from MF.[187] Immunohistochemistry often shows an increase of CD8+ T-cells both in the epidermis and dermis, leading to a decreased CD4:CD8 ratio. Nonetheless, besides positive phototesting for ultraviolet (UV) A, UVB light, and in most cases for visible light, negative TCR gene rearrangement studies may assist in distinguishing AR from lymphoma.[186,188]

Follicular mucinosis is not a pathognomonic finding of FTMF as several benign conditions display similar features (see also Chapter X). Three clinicopathologic subgroups have been described. Benign idiopathic follicular mucinosis occurs most commonly in children and young adults (<40 years old) with two distinct clinical presentations and courses. In the first, lesions are localized to the face and clear spontaneously within a few months.[189] In the second, lesions are either confined to the face or broadly distributed with a chronic remitting relapsing course over several years.[190,191] The third group includes reactive follicular mucinosis secondary to other conditions, including lupus erythematosus, bite reactions, and lichen simplex chronicus.[192,193] In some cases, the distinction between idiopathic FM from FTMF can be challenging by morphology only, requiring clinicopathologic correlation. Clinical signs favoring FTMF over idiopathic FM include the presence of multiple versus single lesions, and the extension of lesions from the head and neck or extremities to the torso.[134] In doubtful cases, careful follow-up, with repeat biopsy and molecular analysis, is advisable. Finally, follicular mucinosis can also be seen in various types of lymphomas other than MF or SS, such as adult T-cell lymphocytic leukemia/lymphoma, cutaneous follicular center cell B-cell lymphoma, chronic lymphocytic leukemia, Hodgkin disease, and acute myeloid or lymphoblastic leukemias.[194-198]

OTHER LYMPHOMAS

ATLL, an aggressive T-cell neoplasm driven by HTLV-I (see also Chapter 29), is a rare clinical and histologic mimic of MF. While most ATLL patients initially present with widespread lymph node and peripheral blood involvement, more than 50% of patients present with skin lesions resembling either patch, plaque, or tumor stages of MF.[199-201] Histologically, Pautrier microabscesses as well as perivascular dermal infiltrates and large dermal nodules with subcutaneous extension can be observed.[200,202,203] Demonstration of HTLV-I viral integration in the tumor cells is the most reliable method for differentiating ATLL from MF.[199] Antibody serologic testing or PCR studies for HTLV-I are less reliable as these tests can be positive in patients from endemic areas such as Caribbean Islands, Southwestern Japan, or parts of Central Africa. Immunophenotyping lacks specificity as both ATLL and MF encompass CD4+CD8− and, less frequently, CD4−CD8+ or CD4+CD8+ variants.[204] Although CD25 is strongly expressed in ATLL, a subset of MF cases have a similar expression pattern.[69] A subset of ATLL express CD30, which confers a poor prognosis.[205]

PC-ALCL can show identical histopathologic features to CD30+ tumor stage MF (see Chapter 15). Clinical information is the cornerstone to accurate diagnosis. Findings of long-standing scaly patches or concomitant patch- or plaque-like lesions at sun-protected sites favor MF over C-ALCL. MF with LCT has an aggressive clinical course, often with lymph node, peripheral blood, and visceral organ involvement. Systemic treatments are often unsuccessful, with a median survival of 3 years. In contrast, C-ALCL presents as solitary or localized nodules, sometimes with ulceration. Dissemination to the lymph nodes occurs in 10% to 15% of patients, but visceral involvement almost never follows. Lack or reduction of CD3 expression by immunohistochemistry is more often observed in C-ALCL than in MF.[206] Recent data suggest a utility of GATA-3 immunostaining, as CD30+ MF with LCT exhibits strong and diffuse nuclear staining, while C-ALCL is negative for this marker (see Fig. 13-33A–C).[22]

Primary cutaneous CD4+ small/medium T-cell lymphoproliferative disease (SMPTCL) (see also Chapter 17). In contrast to classic MF, SMTCL usually presents as a single nodule, preferentially on the head and neck, and histologically as diffuse infiltrates within the dermis with minimal, if any, epidermotropism. SMPTCL is composed of a predominance of small-to-medium–sized pleomorphic T-cells

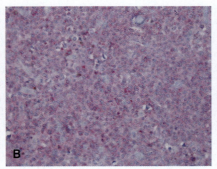

FIGURE 13-33. Lack of T-bet and GATA-3 expression by primary C-ALCL. A. H&E stain shows sheets of large anaplastic lymphocytes indistinguishable from transformed MF. **B.** Double immunohistochemistry for CD3 (*red*) and T-bet (*brown*), and **C.** CD3 (*red*) and GATA-3 (*brown*) show lack of T-bet and GATA-3 expression.

and scattered large blast cells (<30%). The proliferative rate is generally low. Almost all cases show a considerable admixture with reactive CD8-positive T-cells, CD20+ B cells, plasma cells, and histiocytes, including multinucleated giant cells. Similar to MF, SMPTCL is of CD3+CD4+CD8− phenotype. CD30 expression has been described and may rarely be widespread but is not characteristic. However, in contrast to classic MF, SMPTCL T-cells express markers of T_{FH} cells, including PD-1, CXCL-13, BCL-6, CD200, and ICOS.[207,208] Some of these B-cells display large cell morphology, express the B-cell specific transcription factor oct-2, and are surrounded by PD-1+BCL6+ neoplastic T_{FH} cells.[208,209] MF has been documented to express at least three T_{FH} markers, suggesting either T_{FH} cell derivation or capability of T_{FH} differentiation.[78,79] As such, reliance on detection of T_{FH} markers can lead to diagnostic confusion. In practice, the clinical setting of the two diseases is usually distinctive and there is rarely uncertainty.

CD8+ epidermotropic aggressive cytotoxic T-cell lymphoma (Berti lymphoma) (see Chapter 18) is a rare aggressive primary cutaneous lymphoma with a median survival of 32 months. Clinical presentation is usually more acute than MF, with generalized plaques or tumors. Metastases to the lungs, testis, oral cavity, and central nervous system, but not to the lymph nodes are typical.[210,217]

Histologically, marked pagetoid epidermotropism, in some cases with epidermal necrosis, is common and should invite consideration of this diagnosis. Neoplastic T-cells are CD3+, CD8+, βF1+, TIA-1+, GrB+, Perforin+ cells, often with preservation of CD7, but frequent loss of CD2 and CD5. Whereas rare cases are reported supervening upon CD8+ MF.[213]

PTCL-NOS rarely infiltrates the skin and mimics plaque or tumor stage MF. The overall survival rates of PTCL-NOS presenting in the skin are poor and independent of the presence or absence of extracutaneous disease, cell size, or expression of CD4 or CD8 antigens.[214] MF is a clinical diagnosis, and thorough clinical assessment to exclude the presence of patches and plaques is necessary.

CAPSULE SUMMARY

- **Clinical:** Patches, plaques, and tumors represent distinct stages of disease progression. Preferential locations are the buttocks and other sun-protected areas.
- **Morphology:** Patch and plaque stage MF: atypical lymphocytes are small to medium in size, with hyperchromatic and convoluted (cerebriform) nuclei. Epidermotropism denotes neoplastic T-cells trafficking into the epidermis and manifests as lymphocyte tagging at the dermoepidermal junction and formation of Pautrier microabscesses. Tumor stage MF: neoplastic cells expand in the dermis with concomitant loss of epidermotropism.
- **Immunophenotype:** CD3+CD4+CD8−CD7−. Early patch: T-bet+, GATA-3−. Tumor stage: T-bet−, GATA-3+. Tumor stage with large cell morphology might show CD30 positivity and/or cytotoxic markers.
- **Genetics:** Monoclonal TCR gene rearrangement might not be detected in early patch stage. Amplifications of chromosomal regions encompassing T-cell differentiation and activation genes are identified. Deletions of CDKN2A and PTEN as well as amplification of C-MYC have been associated with poor clinical outcome.
- **Differential diagnosis:** Benign mimickers include eczema, PLC, interface dermatoses, lichenoid pigmented purpura, actinic reticuloid, idiopathic alopecia mucinosa, and lichenoid drug eruptions. Neoplastic mimics include SMPTCL, Berti lymphoma, C-ALCL, ATLL and PTCL, NOS.

References

1. Campbell JJ, Clark RA, Watanabe R, et al. Sézary syndrome and mycosis fungoides arise from distinct T-cell subsets: a biologic rationale for their distinct clinical behaviors. *Blood*. 2010;116(5):767-771.
2. van Doorn R, van Kester MS, Dijkman R, et al. Oncogenomic analysis of mycosis fungoides reveals major differences with Sézary syndrome. *Blood*. 2009;113(1):127-136.
3. Willemze R, Jaffe ES, Burg G, et al. WHO-EORTC classification for cutaneous lymphomas. *Blood*. 2005;105(10): 3768-3785.
4. Criscione VD, Weinstock MA. Incidence of cutaneous T-cell lymphoma in the United States, 1973–2002. *Arch Dermatol*. 2007;143(7):854-859.
5. Quaglino P. Global patterns of care in advanced stage mycosis fungoides/Sezary syndrome: a multicenter retrospective follow-up study from the Cutaneous Lymphoma International Consortium. *Ann Oncol*. 2017;28(10):2517-2525.
6. Scarisbrick JJ, Kim YH, Whittaker SJ, et al. Prognostic factors, prognostic indices and staging in mycosis fungoides and Sézary syndrome: where are we now? *Br J Dermatol*. 2014;170(6):1226-1236.

7. Su C, Nguyen KA, Bai HX, et al. *J Am Acad Dermatol.* 2017;77(3):497-502.
8. Boulos S, Vaid R, Aladily TN, et al. Clinical presentation, immunopathology, and treatment of juvenile-onset mycosis fungoides: a case series of 34 patients. *J Am Acad Dermatol.* 2014;71(6):1117-1126.
9. Hodak E, Amitay-Laish I, Feinmesser M, et al. Juvenile mycosis fungoides: cutaneous T-cell lymphoma with frequent follicular involvement. *J Am Acad Dermatol.* 2014;70:993-1001.
10. Mirvish JJ, Pomerantz RG, Falo LD Jr, et al. Role of infectious agents in cutaneous T-cell lymphoma: facts and controversies. *Clin Dermatol.* 2013;31(4):423-431.
11. Murray D, McMurray JL, Eldershaw S, et al. Progression of mycosis fungoides occurs through divergence of tumor immunophenotype by differential expression of HLA-DR. *Blood Adv.* 2019;3(4):519-529.
12. Kim YH, Bagot M, Pinter-Brown L, et al. Mogamulizumab versus vorinostat in previously treated cutaneous T-cell lymphoma (MAVORIC): an international, open-label, randomised, controlled phase 3 trial. *Lancet Oncol.* 2018;19(9):1192-1204.
13. Lu D, Duvic M, Medeiros LJ, et al. The T-cell chemokine receptor CXCR3 is expressed highly in low-grade mycosis fungoides. *Am J Clin Pathol.* 2001;115(3):413-421.
14. Sokolowska-Wojdylo M, Wenzel J, Gaffal E, et al. Circulating clonal CLA(+) and CD4(+) T cells in Sézary syndrome express the skin-homing chemokine receptors CCR4 and CCR10 as well as the lymph node-homing chemokine receptor CCR7. *Br J Dermatol.* 2005;152(2):258-264.
15. Kim EJ, Hess S, Richardson SK, et al. Immunopathogenesis and therapy of cutaneous T cell lymphoma. *J Clin Invest.* 2005;115(4):798-812.
16. Saulite I, Ignatova D, Chang YT, et al. Blockade of programmed cell death protein 1 (PD-1) in Sézary syndrome reduces Th2 phenotype of non-tumoral T lymphocytes but may enhance tumour proliferation. *OncoImmunology.* 2020;189(1):1738797.
17. Klemke CD, Booken N, Weiss C, et al. Histopathological and immunophenotypical criteria for the diagnosis of Sézary syndrome in differentiation from other erythrodermic skin diseases: a European Organisation for Research and Treatment of Cancer (EORTC) Cutaneous Lymphoma Task Force Study of 97 cases. *Br J Dermatol.* 2015;173(1):93-105.
18. Girardi M, Heald PW, Wilson LD. The pathogenesis of mycosis fungoides. *N Engl J Med.* 2004;350(19):1978-1988.
19. Netchiporouk E, Litvinov IV, Moreau L, et al. Deregulation in STAT signaling is important for cutaneous T-cell lymphoma (CTCL) pathogenesis and cancer progression. *Cell Cycle.* 2014;13(21):3331-3335.
20. Stutz N, Johnson RD, Wood GS. The Fas apoptotic pathway in cutaneous T-cell lymphomas: frequent expression of phenotypes associated with resistance to apoptosis. *J Am Acad Dermatol.* 2012;67(6):1327.e1-e10.
21. Park J, Yang J, Wenzel AT, et al. Genomic analysis of 220 CTCLs identifies a novel recurrent gain-of-function alteration in RLTPR (p.Q575E). *Blood.* 2017;130(12):1430-1440.
22. Hsi A, Lee S, Rosman I, et al. Expression of helper T cell master regulators in inflammatory dermatoses and primary cutaneous T-cell lymphomas: diagnostic implications. *J Am Acad Dermatol.* 2015;72(1):159-167.
23. Moyal L, Gorovitz-Haris B, Yehezkel S, et al. Unilesional mycosis fungoides is associated with increased expression of microRNA-17~92 and T helper 1 skewing. *Br J Dermatol.* 2019;180(5):1123-1134.
24. Stevens SR, Ke MS, Birol A, et al. A simple clinical scoring system to improve the sensitivity and standardization of the diagnosis of mycosis fungoides type cutaneous T-cell lymphoma: logistic regression of clinical and laboratory data. *Br J Dermatol.* 2003;149(3):513-522.
25. Agar NS, Wedgeworth E, Crichton S, et al. Survival outcomes and prognostic factors in mycosis fungoides/Sézary syndrome: validation of the revised International Society for Cutaneous Lymphomas/European Organisation for Research and Treatment of Cancer staging proposal. *J Clin Oncol.* 2010;28(31):4730-4739.
26. Slater DN. The new World Health Organization-European Organization for Research and Treatment of Cancer classification for cutaneous lymphomas: a practical marriage of two giants. *Br J Dermatol.* 2005;153(5):874-880.
27. Scarisbrick JJ, Prince M, Vermeer MH, et al. Cutaneous Lymphoma International Consortium (CLIC) Study of Outcome in Advanced Stages of Mycosis Fungoides & Sézary Syndrome: effect of specific prognostic markers on survival and development of a prognostic model. *J Clin Oncol.* 2015;33(32):3766-3773.
28. Shapiro PE, Pinto FJ. The histologic spectrum of mycosis fungoides/Sézary syndrome (cutaneous T-cell lymphoma): a review of 222 biopsies, including newly described patterns and the earliest pathologic changes. *Am J Surg Pathol.* 1994;18(7):645-667.
29. Sanchez JL, Ackerman AB. The patch stage of mycosis fungoides. Criteria for histologic diagnosis. *Am J Dermatopathol.* 1979;1(1):5-26.
30. Nickoloff BJ. Light-microscopic assessment of 100 patients with patch/plaque-stage mycosis fungoides. *Am J Dermatopathol.* 1988;10(6):469-477.
31. Smoller BR, Bishop K, Glusac E, et al. Reassessment of histologic parameters in the diagnosis of mycosis fungoides. *Am J Surg Pathol.* 1995;19(12):1423-1430.
32. Bernengo MG, Novelli M, Quaglino P, et al. The relevance of the CD4+ CD26− subset in the identification of circulating Sézary cells. *Br J Dermatol.* 2001;144(1):125-135.
33. Pimpinelli N, Olsen EA, Santucci M, et al. Defining early mycosis fungoides. *J Am Acad Dermatol.* 2005;53(6):1053-1063.
34. Santucci M, Biggeri A, Feller AC, et al. Efficacy of histologic criteria for diagnosing early mycosis fungoides: an EORTC cutaneous lymphoma study group investigation. *Am J Surg Pathol.* 2000;24(1):40-50.
35. Burkert KL, Huhn K, Menezes DW, et al. Langerhans cell microgranulomas (pseudo-Pautrier abscesses): morphologic diversity, diagnostic implications and pathogenetic mechanisms. *J Cutan Pathol.* 2002;29(9):511-516.
36. Greer JP, Salhany KE, Cousar JB, et al. Clinical features associated with transformation of cerebriform T-cell lymphoma to a large cell process. *Hematol Oncol.* 1990;8(4):215-227.
37. Salhany KE, Cousar JB, Greer JP, et al. Transformation of cutaneous T cell lymphoma to large cell lymphoma: a clinicopathologic and immunologic study. *Am J Pathol.* 1988;132(2):265-277.
38. Diamandidou E, Colome-Grimmer M, Fayad L, et al. Transformation of mycosis fungoides/Sézary syndrome: clinical characteristics and prognosis. *Blood.* 1998;92(4):1150-1159.
39. Vergier B, de Muret A, Beylot-Barry M, et al. Transformation of mycosis fungoides: clinicopathological and prognostic features of 45 cases. French Study Group of Cutaneious Lymphomas. *Blood.* 2000;95(7):2212-2218.

40. Olsen E, Vonderheid E, Pimpinelli N, et al. Revisions to the staging and classification of mycosis fungoides and Sézary syndrome: a proposal of the International Society for Cutaneous Lymphomas (ISCL) and the cutaneous lymphoma task force of the European Organization of Research and Treatment of Cancer (EORTC). *Blood.* 2007;110(6):1713-1722.
41. Fraser-Andrews EA, Mitchell T, Ferreira S, et al. Molecular staging of lymph nodes from 60 patients with mycosis fungoides and Sézary syndrome: correlation with histopathology and outcome suggests prognostic relevance in mycosis fungoides. *Br J Dermatol.* 2006;155(4):756-762.
42. Barnett ML, Cole RJ. Mycosis fungoides with multiple oral mucosal lesions: a case report. *J Periodontol.* 1985;56(11):690-693.
43. Whitbeck EG, Spiers AS, Hussain M. Mycosis fungoides: subcutaneous and visceral tumors, orbital involvement, and ophthalmoplegia. *J Clin Oncol.* 1983;1(4):270-276.
44. Velagapudi P, Turagam M, Uzoaru I, et al. Small bowel obstruction due to mycosis fungoides: an unusual presentation. *Am J Med Sci.* 2011;341(6):508-509.
45. Vu BA, Duvic M. Central nervous system involvement in patients with mycosis fungoides and cutaneous large-cell transformation. *J Am Acad Dermatol.* 2008;59(2 suppl 1):S16-S22.
46. Graham SJ, Sharpe RW, Steinberg SM, et al. Prognostic implications of a bone marrow histopathologic classification system in mycosis fungoides and the Sézary syndrome. *Cancer.* 1993;72(3):726-734.
47. Zackheim HS, Jones C, LeBoit PE, et al. Lymphomatoid papulosis associated with mycosis fungoides: a study of 21 patients including analyses for clonality. *J Am Dermatol.* 2003;49(4):620-623.
48. Bekkenk MW, Geelen FA, van Voorst Vader PC, et al. Primary and secondary cutaneous CD30(+) lymphoproliferative disorders: a report from the Dutch Cutaneous Lymphoma Group on the long-term follow-up data of 219 patients and guidelines for diagnosis and treatment. *Blood.* 2000;95(12):3653-3661.
49. Barzilai A, Trau H, David M. Mycosis fungoides associated with B-cell malignancies. *Br J Dermatol.* 2006;155(2):379-386.
50. Tournier E, Laurent C, Thomas M, et al. Double-positive CD4/CD8 mycosis fungoides: a rarely reported immunohistochemical profile. *J Cutan Pathol.* 2014;41(1):58-62.
51. Knapp CF, Mathew R, Messina JL, et al. CD4/CD8 dual-positive mycosis fungoides: a previously unrecognized variant. *Am J Dermatopathol.* 2012;34(3):e37-e39.
52. Dummer R, Kamarashev J, Kempf W, et al. Junctional CD8+ cutaneous lymphomas with nonaggressive clinical behavior: a CD8+ variant of mycosis fungoides?. *Arch Dermatol.* 2002;138(2):199-203.
53. Diwan H, Ivan D. CD8-positive mycosis fungoides and primary cutaneous aggressive epidermotropic CD8-positive cytotoxic T-cell lymphoma. *J Cutan Pathol.* 2009;36(3):390-392.
54. Hodak E, David M, Maron L, et al. CD4/CD8 double-negative epidermotropic cutaneous T-cell lymphoma: an immunohistochemical variant of mycosis fungoides. *J Am Acad Dermatol.* 2006;55(2):276-284.
55. Massone C, Crisman G, Kerl H, et al. The prognosis of early mycosis fungoides is not influenced by phenotype and T-cell clonality. *Br J Dermatol.* 2008;159(4):881-886.
56. Rodriguez-Pinilla SM, Ortiz-Romero PL, Monsalvez V, et al. TCR-γ expression in primary cutaneous T-cell lymphomas. *Am J Surg Pathol.* 2013;37(3):375-384.
57. Guitart J, Weisenburger DD, Subtil A, et al. Cutaneous γδ T-cell lymphomas: a spectrum of presentations with overlap with other cytotoxic lymphomas. *Am J Surg Pathol.* 2012;36(11):1656-1665.
58. Murphy M, Fullen D, Carlson JA. Low CD7 expression in benign and malignant cutaneous lymphocytic infiltrates: experience with an antibody reactive with paraffin-embedded tissue. *Am J Dermatopathol.* 2002;24(1):6-16.
59. Washington LT, Huh YO, Powers LC, et al. A stable aberrant immunophenotype characterizes nearly all cases of cutaneous T-cell lymphoma in blood and can be used to monitor response to therapy. *BMC Clin Pathol.* 2002;2(1):5.
60. Ortonne N, Buyukbabani N, Delfau-Larue M-H, et al. Value of the CD8-CD3 ratio for the diagnosis of mycosis fungoides. *Mod Pathol.* 2003;16(9):857-862.
61. Izban KF, Hsi ED, Alkan S. Immunohistochemical analysis of mycosis fungoides on paraffin-embedded tissue sections. *Mod Pathol.* 1998;11(10):978-982.
62. Saed G, Fivenson DP, Naidu Y, et al. Mycosis fungoides exhibits a Th1-type cell-mediated cytokine profile whereas Sézary syndrome expresses a Th2-type profile. *J Invest Dermatol.* 1994;103(1):29-33.
63. Vowels BR, Cassin M, Vonderheid EC, et al. Aberrant cytokine production by Sézary syndrome patients: cytokine secretion pattern resembles murine Th2 cells. *J Invest Dermatol.* 1992;99(1):90-94.
64. Barberio E, Thomas L, Skowron F, et al. Transformed mycosis fungoides: clinicopathological features and outcome. *Br J Dermatol.* 2007;157(2):284-289.
65. Benner MF, Jansen PM, Vermeer MH, et al. Prognostic factors in transformed mycosis fungoides: a retrospective analysis of 100 cases. *Blood.* 2012;119(7):1643-1649.
66. Wu H, Telang GH, Lessin SR, et al. Mycosis fungoides with CD30-positive cells in the epidermis. *Am J Dermatopathol.* 2000;22(3):212-216.
67. Younes A, Bartlett NL, Leonard JP, et al. Brentuximab vedotin (SGN-35) for relapsed CD30-positive lymphomas. *N Engl J Med.* 2010;363(19):1812-1821.
68. Prince HM, Kim YH, Horwitz SM, et al. Brentuximab vedotin or physician's choice in CD30-positive cutaneous T-cell lymphoma (ALCANZA): an international, open-label, randomised, phase 3, multicentre trial. *Lancet.* 2017;390:555-566.
69. Talpur R, Jones DM, Alencar AJ, et al. CD25 expression is correlated with histological grade and response to denileukin diftitox in cutaneous T-cell lymphoma. *J Invest Dermatol.* 2006;126(3):575-583.
70. Krejsgaard T, Odum N, Geisler C, et al. Regulatory T cells and immunodeficiency in mycosis fungoides and Sézary syndrome. *Leukemia.* 2012;26(3):424-432.
71. Fried I, Cerroni L. FOXP3 in sequential biopsies of progressive mycosis fungoides. *Am J Dermatopathol.* 2012;34(3):263-265.
72. Wain EM, Orchard GE, Mayou S, et al. Mycosis fungoides with a CD56+ immunophenotype. *J Am Acad Dermatol.* 2005;53(1):158-163.
73. Horst BA, Kasper R, LeBoit PE. CD4+, CD56+ mycosis fungoides: case report and review of the literature. *Am J Dermatopathol.* 2009;31(1):74-76.
74. Shiomi T, Monobe Y, Kuwabara C, et al. Poikilodermatous mycosis fungoides with a CD8+ CD56+ immunophenotype: a case report and literature review. *J Cutan Pathol.* 2013;40(3):317-320.
75. Vermeer MH, Geelen FA, Kummer JA, et al. Expression of cytotoxic proteins by neoplastic T cells in mycosis fungoides increases with progression from plaque stage to tumor stage disease. *Am J Pathol.* 1999;154(4):1203-1210.

76. Wada DA, Wilcox RA, Harrington SM, et al. Programmed death 1 is expressed in cutaneous infiltrates of mycosis fungoides and Sézary syndrome. *Am J Hematol.* 2011;86(3):325-327.
77. Kantekure K, Yang Y, Raghunath P, et al. Expression patterns of the immunosuppressive proteins PD-1/CD279 and PD-L1/CD274 at different stages of cutaneous T-cell lymphoma/mycosis fungoides. *Am J Dermatopathol.* 2012;34(1):126-128.
78. Meyerson HJ, Awadallah A, Pavlidakey P, et al. Follicular center helper T-cell (TFH) marker positive mycosis fungoides/Sézary syndrome. *Mod Pathol.* 2013;26(1):32-43.
79. Bosisio FM, Cerroni L. Expression of T-follicular helper markers in sequential biopsies of progressive mycosis fungoides and other primary cutaneous T-cell lymphomas. *Am J Dermatopathol.* 2015;37:115-121.
80. Theurich S, Schlaak M, Steguweit H, et al. Targeting tumor-infiltrating B cells in cutaneous T-cell lymphoma [published online ahead of print October 27, 2014]. *J Clin Oncol.* doi:10.1200/JCO.2013.50.9471.
81. Harms KL, Harms PW, Anderson T, et al. Mycosis fungoides with CD20 expression: report of two cases and review of the literature. *J Cutan Pathol.* 2014;41(6):494-503.
82. Hagen JW, Schaefer JT, Magro CM. CD20+ mycosis fungoides: a report of three cases and review of the literature. *Am J Dermatopathol.* 2013;35(8):833-841.
83. Delfau-Larue MH, Laroche L, Wechsler J, et al. Diagnostic value of dominant T-cell clones in peripheral blood in 363 patients presenting consecutively with a clinical suspicion of cutaneous lymphoma. *Blood.* 2000;96(9):2987-2992.
84. Wood GS, Greenberg HL. Diagnosis, staging, and monitoring of cutaneous T-cell lymphoma. *Dermatol Ther.* 2003;16(4):269-275.
85. Thurber SE, Zhang B, Kim YH, et al. T-cell clonality analysis in biopsy specimens from two different skin sites shows high specificity in the diagnosis of patients with suggested mycosis fungoides. *J Am Acad Dermatol.* 2007;57(5):782-790.
86. Plaza JA, Morrison C, Magro CM. Assessment of TCR-β clonality in a diverse group of cutaneous T-cell infiltrates. *J Cutan Pathol.* 2008;35(4):358-365.
87. Guitart J, Magro C. Cutaneous T-cell lymphoid dyscrasia: a unifying term for idiopathic chronic dermatoses with persistent T-cell clones. *Arch Dermatol.* 2007;143(7):921-932.
88. Rubben A, Kempf W, Kadin ME, et al. Multilineage progression of genetically unstable tumor subclones in cutaneous T-cell lymphoma. *Exp Dermatol.* 2004;13(8):472-483.
89. Groenen PJ, Langerak AW, van Dongen JJ, et al. Pitfalls in TCR gene clonality testing: teaching cases. *J Hematop.* 2008;1(2):97-109.
90. Ponti R, Fierro MT, Quaglino P, et al. TCR gamma-chain gene rearrangement by PCR-based GeneScan: diagnostic accuracy improvement and clonal heterogeneity analysis in multiple cutaneous T-cell lymphoma samples. *J Invest Dermatol.* 2008;128(4):1030-1038.
91. Klemke C-D, Brade J, Weckesser S, et al. The diagnosis of Sézary syndrome on peripheral blood by flow cytometry requires the use of multiple markers. *Br J Dermatol.* 2008;159(4):871-880.
92. Salgado R, Servitje O, Gallardo F, et al. Oligonucleotide array-CGH identifies genomic subgroups and prognostic markers for tumor stage mycosis fungoides. *J Invest Dermatol.* 2010;130(4):1126-1135.
93. Mao X, Lillington D, Scarisbrick JJ, et al. Molecular cytogenetic analysis of cutaneous T-cell lymphomas: identification of common genetic alterations in Sézary syndrome and mycosis fungoides. *Br J Dermatol.* 2002;147(3):464-475.
94. Ikonomou IM, Aamot HV, Heim S, et al. Granulomatous slack skin with a translocation t(3;9)(q12;p24). *Am J Surg Pathol.* 2007;31(5):803-806.
95. Willemze R, Scheffer E, Van Vloten WA. Mycosis fungoides simulating acanthosis nigricans. *Am J Dermatopathol.* 1985;7(4):367-371.
96. Requena L, Gonzalez-Guerra E, Angulo J, et al. Anetodermic mycosis fungoides: a new clinicopathological variant of mycosis fungoides. *Br J Dermatol.* 2008;158(1):157-162.
97. Bowman PH, Hogan DJ, Sanusi ID. Mycosis fungoides bullosa: report of a case and review of the literature. *J Am Acad Dermatol.* 2001;45(6):934-939.
98. Kartsonis J, Brettschneider F, Weissmann A, et al. Mycosis fungoides bullosa. *Am J Dermatopathol.* 1990;12(1):76-80.
99. McBride SR, Dahl MG, Slater DN, et al. Vesicular mycosis fungoides. *Br J Dermatol.* 1998;138(1):141-144.
100. Kneitz H, Brocker EB, Becker JC. Mycosis fungoides bullosa: a case report and review of the literature. *J Med Case Rep.* 2010;4:78.
101. Kohler S, Kim YH, Smoller BR. Histologic criteria for the diagnosis of erythrodermic mycosis fungoides and Sézary syndrome: a critical reappraisal. *J Cutan Pathol.* 1997;24(5):292-297.
102. Lehman JS, Cook-Norris RH, Weed BR, et al. Folliculotropic mycosis fungoides: single-center study and systematic review. *Arch Dermatol.* 2010;146(6):607-613.
103. Gerami P, Guitart J. Folliculotropic Sézary syndrome: a new variant of cutaneous T-cell lymphoma. *Br J Dermatol.* 2007;156(4):781-783.
104. van Doorn R, Scheffer E, Willemze R. Follicular mycosis fungoides, a distinct disease entity with or without associated follicular mucinosis: a clinicopathologic and follow-up study of 51 patients. *Arch Dermatol.* 2002;138(2):191-198.
105. Scarabello A, Leinweber B, Ardigó M, et al. Cutaneous lymphomas with prominent granulomatous reaction: a potential pitfall in the histopathologic diagnosis of cutaneous T- and B-cell lymphomas. *Am J Surg Pathol.* 2002;26(10):1259-1268.
106. Gallardo F, Garcia-Muret MP, Servitje O, et al. Cutaneous lymphomas showing prominent granulomatous component: clinicopathological features in a series of 16 cases. *J Eur Acad Dermatol Venereol.* 2009;23(6):639-647.
107. LeBoit PE, Zackheim HS, White CR Jr. Granulomatous variants of cutaneous T-cell lymphoma: the histopathology of granulomatous mycosis fungoides and granulomatous slack skin. *Am J Surg Pathol.* 1988;12(2):83-95.
108. Vergier B, Beylot-Barry M, Beylot C, et al. Pilotropic cutaneous T-cell lymphoma without mucinosis: a variant of mycosis fungoides?. *Arch Dermatol.* 1996;132(6):683-687.
109. Fraser-Andrews E, Ashton R, Russell-Jones R. Pilotropic mycosis fungoides presenting with multiple cysts, comedones and alopecia. *Br J Dermatol.* 1999;140(1):141-144.
110. Ardigo M, Borroni G, Muscardin L, et al. Hypopigmented mycosis fungoides in Caucasian patients: a clinicopathologic study of 7 cases. *J Am Acad Dermatol.* 2003;49(2):264-270.
111. Pavlovsky L, Mimouni D, Amitay-Laish I, et al. Hyperpigmented mycosis fungoides: an unusual variant of cutaneous T-cell lymphoma with a frequent CD8+ phenotype. *J Am Acad Dermatol.* 2012;67(1):69-75.
112. Hallopeau H, Bureau G. Sur un cas de mycose fungoide avec localisation initiale eruptions polymorphes et vegetations axillaire et inguinales. *Bull Soc Fr Dermatol Syphiligr.* 1896;7:480-482.

113. Kutting B, Metze D, Luger TA, et al. Mycosis fungoides presenting as an acquired ichthyosis. *J Am Acad Dermatol.* 1996;34(5, pt 2):887-889.
114. Su LD, Kim YH, LeBoit PE, et al. Interstitial mycosis fungoides, a variant of mycosis fungoides resembling granuloma annulare and inflammatory morphea. *J Cutan Pathol.* 2002;29(3):135-141.
115. Haghighi B, Smoller BR, LeBoit PE, et al. Pagetoid reticulosis (Woringer–Kolopp disease): an immunophenotypic, molecular, and clinicopathologic study. *Mod Pathol.* 2000;13(5):502-510.
116. Mourtzinos N, Puri PK, Wang G, et al. CD4/CD8 double negative pagetoid reticulosis: a case report and literature review. *J Cutan Pathol.* 2010;37(4):491-496.
117. Gonzalez M, Martin-Pascual M, San Miguel J, et al. Phenotypic characterization of skin-infiltrating cells in pagetoid reticulosis by monoclonal antibodies. *Acta Derm Venereol.* 1984;64(5):421-424.
118. Kodama K, Fink-Puches R, Massone C, et al. Papular mycosis fungoides: a new clinical variant of early mycosis fungoides. *J Am Acad Dermatol.* 2005;52(4):694-698.
119. El Shabrawi-Caelen L, Kerl H, Cerroni L. Lymphomatoid papulosis: reappraisal of clinicopathologic presentation and classification into subtypes A, B, and C. *Arch Dermatol.* 2004;140(4):441-447.
120. Toro JR, Sander CA, LeBoit PE. Persistent pigmented purpuric dermatitis and mycosis fungoides: simulant, precursor, or both? A study by light microscopy and molecular methods. *Am J Dermatopathol.* 1997;19(2):108-118.
121. Samman PD. The natural history of parapsoriasis en plaques (chronic superficial dermatitis) and prereticulotic poikiloderma. *Br J Dermatol.* 1972;87(5):405-411.
122. Pabsch H, Kunze J, Schaller J. Mycosis fungoides presenting as a pustular eruption. *J Am Acad Dermatol.* 2009;61(5):908-909.
123. Twersky JM, Mutasim DF. Mycosis fungoides presenting as reticular erythematous mucinosis. *Int J Dermatol.* 2006;45(3):230-233.
124. Belousova IE, Vanecek T, Samtsov AV, et al. A patient with clinicopathologic features of small plaque parapsoriasis presenting later with plaque-stage mycosis fungoides: report of a case and comparative retrospective study of 27 cases of "nonprogressive" small plaque parapsoriasis. *J Am Acad Dermatol.* 2008;59(3):474-482.
125. Pileri A, Facchetti F, Rutten A, et al. Syringotropic mycosis fungoides: a rare variant of the disease with peculiar clinicopathologic features. *Am J Surg Pathol.* 2011;35(1):100-109.
126. de Masson A, Battistella M, Vignon-Pennamen M-D, et al. Syringotropic mycosis fungoides: clinical and histologic features, response to treatment, and outcome in 19 patients. *J Am Acad Dermatol.* 2014;7(5):926-934.
127. Dubin DB, Hurowitz JC, Brettler D, et al. Adnexotropic T-cell lymphoma presenting with generalized anhidrosis, progressive alopecia, pruritus, and Sjogren's syndrome. *J Am Acad Dermatol.* 1998;38(3):493-497.
128. Burg G, Schmockel C. Syringolymphoid hyperplasia with alopecia—a syringotropic cutaneous T-cell lymphoma? *Dermatology.* 1992;184(4):306-307.
129. Haller A, Elzubi E, Petzelbauer P. Localized syringolymphoid hyperplasia with alopecia and anhidrosis. *J Am Acad Dermatol.* 2001;45(1):127-130.
130. Hitchcock MG, Burchette JL Jr, Olsen EA, et al. Eccrine gland infiltration by mycosis fungoides. *Am J Dermatopathol.* 1996;18(5):447-453.
131. Oliver GF, Winkelmann RK, Banks PM. Unilesional mycosis fungoides: clinical, microscopic and immunophenotypic features. *Australas J Dermatol.* 1989;30(2):65-71.
132. Oliver GF, Winkelmann RK. Unilesional mycosis fungoides: a distinct entity. *J Am Acad Dermatol.* 1989;20(1):63-70.
133. Williams LR, Levine LJ, Kauh YC. Cutaneous malignancies mimicking herpes zoster. *Int J Dermatol.* 1991;30(6):432-434.
134. Gerami P, Rosen S, Kuzel T, et al. Folliculotropic mycosis fungoides: an aggressive variant of cutaneous T-cell lymphoma. *Arch Dermatol.* 2008;144(6):738-746.
135. Van Santen S., Roach RE, van Doorn R., et al. Clinical staging and prognostic factors in folliculotropic mycosis fungoides. *JAMA Dermatol.* 2016;152:992-1000.
136. Hodak E, Amitay-Laish I, Atzmony L, et al. New insights into folliculotropic mycosis fungoides (FMF): a single-center experience. *J Am Acad Dermatol.* 2016;75:347-355.
137. Atzmony L, Moyal L, Feinmesser M, et al. Stage-dependent increase in expression of miR-155 and Ki-67 and number of tumour-associated inflammatory cells in folliculotropic mycosis fungoides. *Acta DermVenereol.* 2020;100(15):adv00230.
138. Gerami P, Guitart J. The spectrum of histopathologic and immunohistochemical findings in folliculotropic mycosis fungoides. *Am J Surg Pathol.* 2007;31(9):1430-1438.
139. Lee J, Viakhireva N, Cesca C, et al. Clinicopathologic features and treatment outcomes in Woringer–Kolopp disease. *J Am Acad Dermatol.* 2008;59(4):706-712.
140. Yagi H, Hagiwara T, Shirahama S, et al. Disseminated pagetoid reticulosis: need for long-term follow-up. *J Am Acad Dermatol.* 1994;30(2, pt 2):345-349.
141. Saggini A, Gulia A, Argenyi Z, et al. A variant of lymphomatoid papulosis simulating primary cutaneous aggressive epidermotropic CD8+ cytotoxic T-cell lymphoma: description of 9 cases. *Am J Surg Pathol.* 2010;34(8):1168-1175.
142. Alaibac M, Yu R, Chu A. PCR detection of clonal TCR γ-gene rearrangements in a group of cutaneous T-cell lymphomas including a case of localized pagetoid reticulosis expressing the γ-δ TCR. *Int J Oncol.* 1995;6(6):1267-1270.
143. Nakada T, Sueki H, Iijima M. Disseminated pagetoid reticulosis (Ketron–Goodman disease): six-year follow-up. *J Am Acad Dermatol.* 2002;47(2, suppl):S183-S186.
144. Steffen C. Ketron–Goodman disease, Woringer–Kolopp disease, and pagetoid reticulosis. *Am J Dermatopathol.* 2005;27(1):68-85.
145. Kempf W, Ostheeren-Michaelis S, Paulli M, et al. Granulomatous mycosis fungoides and granulomatous slack skin: a multicenter study of the Cutaneous Lymphoma Histopathology Task Force Group of the European Organization For Research and Treatment of Cancer (EORTC). *Arch Dermatol.* 2008;144(12):1609-1617.
146. Li JY, Pulitzer MP, Myskowski PL, et al. A case-control study of clinicopathologic features, prognosis, and therapeutic responses in patients with granulomatous mycosis fungoides. *J Am Acad Dermatol.* 2013;69(3):366-374.
147. LeBoit PE. Granulomatous slack skin. *Dermatol Clin.* 1994;12:375-389.
148. van Haselen CW, Toonstra J, van der Putte SJ, van Dongen JJ, van Hees CL, van Vloten WA. Granulomatous slack skin. Report of three patients with an updated review of the literature. *Dermatology.* 1998;196:382-391.
149. Clarijs M, Poot F, Laka A, Pirard C, Bourlond A. Granulomatous slack skin: treatment with extensive surgery and review of the literature. *Dermatology.* 2003;206:393-397.

150. Abbott RA, Sahni D, Robson A, et al. Poikilodermatous mycosis fungoides: a study of its clinicopathological, immunophenotypic and prognostic features. *J Am Acad Dermatol.* 2011;65:313-319.
151. Buechner SA, Winkelmann RK. Pre-Sézary erythroderma evolving to Sézary syndrome. A report of seven cases. *Arch Dermatol.* 1983;119(4):285-291.
152. Castano E, Glick S, Wolgast L, et al. Hypopigmented mycosis fungoides in childhood and adolescence: a long-term retrospective study. *J Cutan Pathol.* 2013;40(11):924-934.
153. El-Shabrawi-Caelen L, Cerroni L, Medeiros LJ, et al. Hypopigmented mycosis fungoides: frequent expression of a CD8+ T-cell phenotype. *Am J Surg Pathol.* 2002;26(4):450-457.
154. Furlan FC, de Paula Pereira BA, da Silva LF, et al. Loss of melanocytes in hypopigmented mycosis fungoides: a study of 18 patients. *J Cutan Pathol.* 2014;41(2):101-107.
155. Hodak E, Amitay I, Feinmesser M, et al. Ichthyosiform mycosis fungoides: an atypical variant of cutaneous T-cell lymphoma. *J Am Acad Dermatol.* 2004;50:368-374.
156. Jang MS, Kang DY, Park JB, et al. Clinicopathologica lmanifestations of ichthyosiform mycosis fungoides. *Acta Derm Venereol.* 2016;96:100.
157. Price NM, Fuks ZY, Hoffman TE. Hyperkeratotic and verrucous features of mycosis fungoides. *Arch Dermatol.* 1977;113(1):57-60.
158. Reggiani C, Massone C, Fink-Puches R, et al. Interstitial mycosis fungoides. A clinicopathologic study of 21 patients. *Am J Surg Pathol.* 2016;40:1360-1367.
159. Jouary T, Beylot-Barry M, Vergier B, et al. Mycosis fungoides mimicking granuloma annulare. *Br J Dermatol.* 2002;146:1102-1104.
160. Ally MS, Pawade J, Tanaka M, et al. Solitary mycosis fungoides: a distinct clinicopathologic entity with a good prognosis. A series of 15 cases and literature review. *J Am Acad Dermatol.* 2012;67(4):736-744.
161. Pujol RM, Gallardo F, Llistosella E, et al. Invisible mycosis fungoides: a diagnostic challenge. *J Am Acad Dermatol.* 2000;42(2, pt 2):324-328.
162. Pujol RM, Gallardo F, Llistosella E, et al. Invisible mycosis fungoides: a diagnostic challenge. *J Am Acad Dermatol.* 2002;47(2 suppl):S168-S171.
163. Hwong H, Nichols T, Duvic M. "Invisible" mycosis fungoides?. *J Am Acad Dermatol.* 2001;45(2):318.
164. Ackerman AB, Breza TS, Capland L. Spongiotic simulants of mycosis fungoides. *Arch Dermatol.* 1974;109(2):218-220.
165. Candiago E, Marocolo D, Manganoni MA, et al. Nonlymphoid intraepidermal mononuclear cell collections (pseudo-Pautrier abscesses): a morphologic and immunophenotypical characterization. *Am J Dermatopathol.* 2000;22(1):1-6.
166. Friss AB, Cohen PR, Bruce S, et al. Chronic cutaneous lupus erythematosus mimicking mycosis fungoides. *J Am Acad Dermatol.* 1995;33(5, pt 2):891-895.
167. Guitart J, Peduto M, Caro WA, et al. Lichenoid changes in mycosis fungoides. *J Am Acad Dermatol.* 1997;36(3, pt 1):417-422.
168. Braun RP, French LE, Feldmann R, et al. Cutaneous pseudolymphoma, lymphomatoid contact dermatitis type, as an unusual cause of symmetrical upper eyelid nodules. *Br J Dermatol.* 2000;143(2):411-414.
169. Martinez-Moran C, Sanz-Munoz C, Morales-Callaghan AM, et al. Lymphomatoid contact dermatitis. *Contact Dermatitis.* 2009;60(1):53-55.
170. Knackstedt TJ, Zug KA. T cell lymphomatoid contact dermatitis: a challenging case and review of the literature. *Contact Dermatitis.* 2014;72(2):65-74.
171. Magro CM, Crowson AN. Drugs with antihistaminic properties as a cause of atypical cutaneous lymphoid hyperplasia. *J Am Acad Dermatol.* 1995;32(3):419-428.
172. Rijlaarsdam U, Scheffer E, Meijer CJ, et al. Mycosis fungoides-like lesions associated with phenytoin and carbamazepine therapy. *J Am Acad Dermatol.* 1991;24(2):216-220.
173. Mutasim DF. Lymphomatoid drug eruption mimicking digitate dermatosis: cross reactivity between two drugs that suppress angiotensin II function. *Am J Dermatopathol.* 2003;25(4):331-334.
174. Okun MM, Henner M, Paulson C. A quinine-induced drug reaction of photosensitive distribution with histological features mimicking mycosis fungoides. *Clin Exp Dermatol.* 1994;19(3):246-248.
175. Magro CM, Cruz-Inigo AE, Votava H, et al. Drug-associated reversible granulomatous T cell dyscrasia: a distinct subset of the interstitial granulomatous drug reaction. *J Cutan Pathol.* 2010;37(suppl 1):96-111.
176. Weinberg JM, Kristal L, Chooback L, et al. The clonal nature of pityriasis lichenoides. *Arch Dermatol.* 2002;138(8):1063-1067.
177. Weiss LM, Wood GS, Ellisen LW, et al. Clonal T-cell populations in pityriasis lichenoides et varioliformis acuta (Mucha–Habermann disease). *Am J Pathol.* 1987;126(3):417-421.
178. Magro C, Crowson AN, Kovatich A, et al. Pityriasis lichenoides: a clonal T-cell lymphoproliferative disorder. *Hum Pathol.* 2002;33(8):788-795.
179. Magro CM, Crowson AN, Morrison C, et al. Pityriasis lichenoides chronica: stratification by molecular and phenotypic profile. *Hum Pathol.* 2007;38(3):479-490.
180. Kempf W, Kazakov DV, Palmedo G, et al. Pityriasis lichenoides et varioliformis acuta with numerous CD30(+) cells – a variant mimicking lymphomatoid papulosis and other cutaneous lymphomas: a clinicopathologic, immunohistochemical, and molecular biological study of 13 cases. *Am J Surg Pathol.* 2012;36(7):1021-1029.
181. Magro CM, Schaefer JT, Crowson AN, et al. Pigmented purpuric dermatosis: classification by phenotypic and molecular profiles. *Am J Clin Pathol.* 2007;128(2):218-229.
182. Barnhill RL, Braverman IM. Progression of pigmented purpura-like eruptions to mycosis fungoides: report of three cases. *J Am Acad Dermatol.* 1988;19(1, pt 1):25-31.
183. Farrington J. Lichen aureus. *Cutis.* 1970;6:1251-1253.
184. Waisman M, Waisman M. Lichen aureus. *Arch Dermatol.* 1976;112(5):696-697.
185. Crowson AN, Magro CM, Zahorchak R. Atypical pigmentary purpura: a clinical, histopathologic, and genotypic study. *Hum Pathol.* 1999;30(9):1004-1012.
186. Sidiropoulos M, Deonizio J, Martinez-Escala ME, et al. Chronic actinic dermatitis/actinic reticuloid: a clinicopathologic and immunohistochemical analysis of 37 cases. *Am J Dermatopathol.* 2014;36(11):875-881.
187. Reddy K, Bhawan J. Histologic mimickers of mycosis fungoides: a review. *J Cutan Pathol.* 2007;34(7):519-525.
188. Bakels V, van Oostveen JW, Preesman AH, et al. Differentiation between actinic reticuloid and cutaneous T cell lymphoma by T cell receptor gamma gene rearrangement analysis and immunophenotyping. *J Clin Pathol.* 1998;51:154-158.
189. Zvulunov A, Shkalim V, Ben-Amitai D, et al. Clinical and histopathologic spectrum of alopecia mucinosa/follicular mucinosis and its natural history in children. *J Am Acad Dermatol.* 2012;67(6):1174-1181.
190. Emmerson RW. Follicular mucinosis: a study of 47 patients. *Br J Dermatol.* 1969;81(6):395-413.
191. Coskey RJ, Mehregan AH. Alopecia mucinosa: a follow-up study. *Arch Dermatol.* 1970;102(2):193-194.

192. O'Reilly K, Brauer J, Loyd A, et al. Secondary follicular mucinosis associated with systemic lupus erythematosus. *Dermatol Online J.* 2010;16(11):7.
193. Rongioletti F, De Lucchi S, Meyes D, et al. Follicular mucinosis: a clinicopathologic, histochemical, immunohistochemical and molecular study comparing the primary benign form and the mycosis fungoides-associated follicular mucinosis. *J Cutan Pathol.* 2010;37(1):15-19.
194. Benchikhi H, Wechsler J, Rethers L, et al. Cutaneous B-cell lymphoma associated with follicular mucinosis. *J Am Acad Dermatol.* 1995;33(4):673-675.
195. Thomson J, Cochran RE. Chronic lymphatic leukemia presenting as atypical rosacea with follicular mucinosis. *J Cutan Pathol.* 1978;5(2):81-87.
196. Garrido MC, Riveiro-Falkenbach E, Rodriguez-Peralto JL. Primary cutaneous follicle center lymphoma with follicular mucinosis. *JAMA Dermatol.* 2014;150(8):906-907.
197. Ishida M, Iwai M, Yoshida K, et al. Adult T-cell leukemia/lymphoma accompanying follicular mucinosis: a case report with review of the literature. *Int J Clin Exp Pathol.* 2013;6(12):3014-3018.
198. Stewart M, Smoller BR. Follicular mucinosis in Hodgkin's disease: a poor prognostic sign?. *J Am Acad Dermatol.* 1991;24(5, pt 1):784-785.
199. Tsukasaki K, Hermine O, Bazarbachi A, et al. Definition, prognostic factors, treatment, and response criteria of adult T-cell leukemia-lymphoma: a proposal from an international consensus meeting. *J Clin Oncol.* 2009;27(3):453-459.
200. Bittencourt AL, Barbosa HS, Vieira MD, et al. Adult T-cell leukemia/lymphoma (ATL) presenting in the skin: clinical, histological and immunohistochemical features of 52 cases. *Acta Oncol.* 2009;48(4):598-604.
201. Bittencourt AL, de Oliveira Mde F. Cutaneous manifestations associated with HTLV-1 infection. *Int J Dermatol.* 2010;49(10):1099-1110.
202. Yamaguchi T, Ohshima K, Karube K, et al. Clinicopathological features of cutaneous lesions of adult T-cell leukaemia/lymphoma. *Br J Dermatol.* 2005;152(1):76-81.
203. Matutes E. Adult T-cell leukaemia/lymphoma. *J Clin Pathol.* 2007;60(12):1373-1377.
204. Yokote T, Akioka T, Oka S, et al. Flow cytometric immunophenotyping of adult T-cell leukemia/lymphoma using CD3 gating. *Am J Clin Pathol.* 2005;124(2):199-204.
205. Campuzano-Zuluaga G, Cioffi-Lavina M, Lossos IS, et al. Frequency and extent of CD30 expression in diffuse large B-cell lymphoma and its relation to clinical and biologic factors: a retrospective study of 167 cases. *Leuk Lymphoma.* 2013;54(11):2405-2411.
206. Bonzheim I, Geissinger E, Roth S, et al. Anaplastic large cell lymphomas lack the expression of T-cell receptor molecules or molecules of proximal T-cell receptor signaling. *Blood.* 2004;104(10):3358-3360.
207. Ma CS, Deenick EK. Human T follicular helper (Tfh) cells and disease. *Immunol Cell Biol.* 2014;92(1):64-71.
208. Rodríguez Pinilla SM, Roncador G, Rodríguez-Peralto JL, et al. Primary cutaneous CD4+ small/medium-sized pleomorphic T-cell lymphoma expresses follicular T-cell markers. *Am J Surg Pathol.* 2009;33(1):81-90.
209. Rodriguez-Pinilla SM, Atienza L, Murillo C, et al. Peripheral T-cell lymphoma with follicular T-cell markers. *Am J Surg Pathol.* 2008;32(12):1787-1799.
210. Berti E, Tomasini D, Vermeer MH, et al. Primary cutaneous CD8-positive epidermotropic cytotoxic T cell lymphomas. A distinct clinicopathological entity with an aggressive clinical behavior. *Am J Pathol.* 1999;155:483-492.
211. Robson A, Assaf C, Bagot M, et al. Aggressive epidermotropic cutaneous CD8+ lymphoma: a cutaneous lymphoma with distinct clinical and pathological features. Report of an EORTC Cutaneous Lymphoma Task Force Workshop. *Histopathology.* 2015;67:425-441.
212. Guitart J, Martinez-Escala ME, Subtil A, et al. Primary cutaneous aggressive epidermotropic cytotoxic T-cell lymphomas: reappraisal of a provisional entity in the 2016 WHO classification of cutaneous lymphomas. *Mod Pathol.* 2017;30: 761-772.
213. Cyrenne BM, Subtil A, Girardi M, et al. Primary cutaneous aggressive epidermotropic cytotoxic CD8+ T-cell lymphoma: long-term remission after brentuximab vedotin. *Int J Dermatol.* 2017;56:1448-1450.), it is not clear whether such cases are more properly considered advanced stage MF.
214. Quintanilla-Martinez L, Jansen PM, Kinney MC, et al. Non-mycosis fungoides cutaneous T-cell lymphomas: report of the 2011 Society for Hematopathology/European Association for Haematopathology workshop. *Am J Clin Pathol.* 2013;139(4):491-514.

CHAPTER 14

Sézary syndrome

Ellen J. Kim, Paul Haun, Martine Bagot, Maxime Battistella, and András Schaffer

DEFINITION

Sézary syndrome (SS) is a rare subtype of cutaneous T-cell lymphoma (CTCL) that is closely related to, but not identical to, mycosis fungoides (MF).[1,2] These two entities are comprised of the majority of all primary CTCLs accounting for approximately 60% of all CTCLs. SS was originally described as a triad of exfoliative erythroderma, lymphadenopathy, and peripheral blood involvement by atypical T-cells (Sézary cells).[3] More recently, it has been formally defined by the International Society of Cutaneous Lymphomas (ISCL) and European Organization for the Research and Treatment of Cancer (EORTC) as erythrodermic skin involvement by atypical T-cells (covering >80% of total surface area) and significant peripheral blood involvement (Sézary count >1000 cells/mL).[4] The malignant T-cells are derived from mature skin-homing central memory T-cells that express hallmark receptors ($CD3^+CD4^+CLA^+CCR4^+CCR7^+CCR10^+$) and lack certain pan–T-cell markers (CD7, CD26 most typically). The Sézary cells are T helper cells that have T_H2 characteristics and secrete T_H2 cytokines such as IL-4, IL-5, and IL-10.[5,6]

EPIDEMIOLOGY

Similar to MF, SS is a disease of older adults with average age of onset of 50 to 60 years.[2] Recent studies examining the US Surveillance, Epidemiology, and End Results Program report the incidence of SS to be 0.01/100,000 person-years from 2005 to 2008 (MF incidence was 0.55/100,000 person-years) with a male:female incidence ratio of 1:57 and Black:Caucasian incidence ratio of 1:55 in the United States.[7] Interestingly, African American patients with MF or SS were diagnosed at a younger age and presented with a higher stage than the Caucasian patient cohort. Incidence of CTCL had increased since 1970[8,9] as have all lymphomas in general. The proportion of SS among CTCL is about 3%, homogeneous worldwide.[10]

ETIOLOGY

MF and SS are sporadic non-Hodgkin lymphomas (NHLs) derived from mature skin-derived T-cells (SALT—skin-associated lymphoid tissue) that currently have neither a confirmed driver genetic defect nor a familial pattern of inheritance (though familial MF has been rarely reported in certain populations).[11] Environmental exposures (chemical, viral) have also not been definitively shown to be oncogenic triggers of MF/SS despite extensive epidemiologic and molecular studies.[12-16]

CLINICAL PRESENTATION

The majority of SS cases have a shorter duration of onset prior to formal diagnosis than MF typically does. However, there are cases of SS that arise in patients with long-standing MF that progresses slowly over many years (erythrodermic MF) demonstrating the overlapping features of MF and SS as related entities.

Erythroderma is currently defined by the ISCL/EORTC 2007 MF/SS classification system as generalized confluent erythema >80% body surface area (BSA)[4] (Fig. 14-1) and is often accompanied by other clinical features in SS including exfoliation/scaling of skin (Fig. 14-2), alopecia (scalp and/or other body areas), ectropion (eversion of eyelids and exposure of conjunctiva), palmoplantar scaling/keratoderma (Fig. 14-3), and onychodystrophy. Erythrodermic SS patients may demonstrate sparing of the skin folds on the trunk. Secondary skin changes are common due to the intense pruritus and barrier dysfunction that is observed in majority of patients including excoriations, skin fissuring, bacterial impetiginization, and skin lichenification. Less commonly, patients can present with a generalized morbilliform eruption mimicking an allergic drug reaction or viral exanthem; these patients are often minimally scaly (Fig. 14-4). Similar to MF, SS can be the "great imitator" and at times can have clinical features identical to psoriasis or atopic dermatitis. Given this, we advise that patients with refractory "eczema" or "psoriasis" who are not improving with standard therapies should have skin biopsies (and appropriate blood studies if erythrodermic), to rule out MF/SS (especially prior to using immunosuppressive systemic agents such as TNF-α inhibitors, cyclosporine, or mycophenolate mofetil, where such treatment can potentially cause acceleration/progression of unrecognized MF/SS/CTCL).[17,18]

Erythroderma can wax and wane in severity during the day and can be exacerbated by heat, exercise, stress, or other factors that trigger vasodilation. Lower extremity edema is a commonly observed finding in older

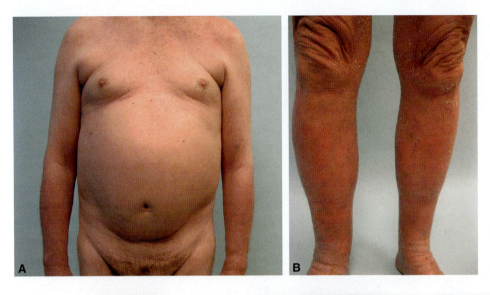

FIGURE 14-1. Sézary syndrome. A. Exfoliative erythroderma involving >80% body surface area. **B.** Concomitant lower extremity edema.

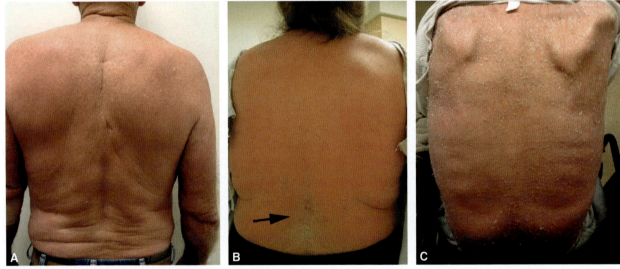

FIGURE 14-2. A–C. Spectrum of erythroderma in SS with varying degrees of exfoliation and scaling. Arrow indicates psoriasiform scale (**B**).

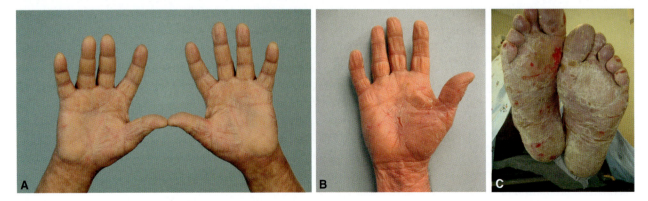

FIGURE 14-3. A–C. Palmoplantar erythema, scaling, fissuring, and/or keratoderma are common features of SS.

erythrodermic patients with underlying venous stasis (Fig. 14-1B) and or patients with significantly enlarged groin lymph nodes (LNs). With severe erythroderma, patients can rarely develop signs of high cardiac output such as pericardial or pleural effusions due to the large amount of blood flow diverted to the erythrodermic skin. Some cases of SS develop concomitant follicular papules/plaques, follicular mucinosis, or classic plaques and tumors in addition to underlying erythroderma (Fig. 14-5) and generally portend a more aggressive course. Rarely, SS can present as generalized severe skin itching and xerosis without overt erythroderma.[19]

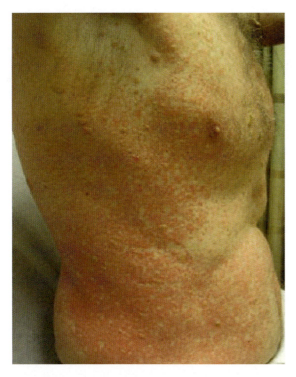

FIGURE 14-4. SS presenting as a morbilliform eruption mimicking an allergic medication reaction or viral exanthema.

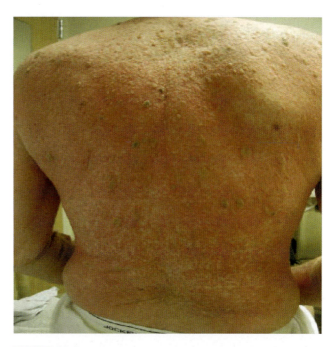

FIGURE 14-6. Multiple eruptive seborrheic keratosis (sign of Leser–Trelat) in the setting of SS erythroderma.

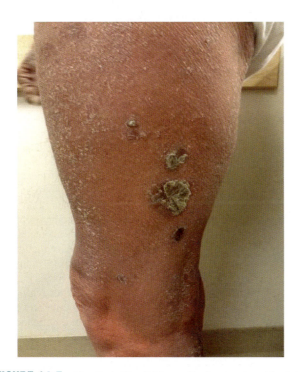

FIGURE 14-5. SS patient with exfoliative erythroderma and overlying indurated scaly plaques.

Palpable peripheral lymphadenopathy is often noted in cervical, axillary, and inguinal areas, and if >1.5 cm in diameter clinically or on imaging, generally warrant excisional or core-needle LN biopsy to distinguish between reactive dermatopathic lymphadenopathy (N1 nodal classification) and involvement by CTCL (N2, N3) for staging purposes.[4,20] Bulky lymphadenopathy (defined here as >3 cm in long axis) is unusual and should raise the possibilities of large-cell transformed disease or a second separate lymphoma (ie, Hodgkin lymphoma, systemic anaplastic large cell lymphoma, other NHL)[21]; LN biopsy is necessary to confirm diagnosis (excisional or core biopsy greatly preferred over fine needle aspirate to assess architecture).[4] Some patients will have thickening of the skin of the forehead, eyebrows, cheeks, and/or chin because of infiltration by malignant T-cells resulting in the so-called "leonine facies" described in the past. Some SS patients can also develop follicular papules/plaques, or overlying plaques/tumors, indicating a more aggressive course. Eruptive seborrheic keratoses (sign of Leser–Trelat) on the upper back/trunk/scalp (Fig. 14-6) are reported by some patients as a paraneoplastic phenomenon accompanying their SS. SS patients with darker skin types may have less prominent erythema than patients with fair skin and can present with generalized dyspigmentation (typically generalized hyperpigmentation but may be admixed with hypopigmented and depigmented areas) that masks the diffuse erythema though in body folds may see alternating bands of normal and involved skin (Fig. 14-7).[22]

Symptoms reported by SS patients often include intense pruritus, burning sensation of the skin, severe exfoliation, chills due to temperature dysregulation, impairment of sweating, fatigue, lower extremity edema (especially in older individuals with underlying venous stasis), and rarely low-grade fevers. Higher fevers (ie, "tumor fever") or drenching night sweats are uncommon in typical SS in the absence of infection or transformed disease and should prompt an infectious workup (most likely source is bacteremia from skin colonization or superinfection from skin flora bacteria such as *Staphylococcus aureus* [SA]). Infection is the leading cause of mortality in MF/SS patients.[23] SS patients can also develop herpes family viral reactivations (herpes simplex virus, varicella-zoster virus) that can disseminate because of their barrier dysfunction and their endogenous immunosuppression. The clinical differential diagnosis of SS

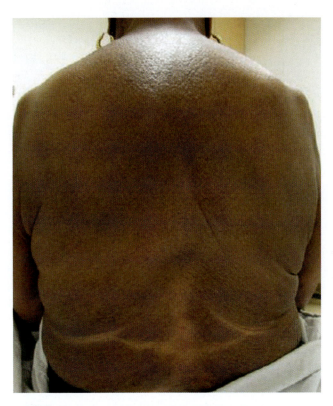

FIGURE 14-7. SS patients with darker skin types have generalized hyperpigmentation that can mask the underlying erythroderma. Note the sparing of skin folds.

erythroderma is extremely broad (see Differential Diagnosis section later) and accurate clinicopathologic diagnosis is essential. Not infrequently, the workup of the erythrodermic patient can be nondiagnostic and have to be repeated over time. In addition, interestingly, degree of erythema or exfoliation or pruritus in SS patients does not necessarily correlate with degree of peripheral blood burden by tumor cells.

Staging

The staging system for SS is identical to that used for MF–TNMB system that originated in 1978 and was revised in 2007 (see Table 12-2).[4] By current criteria, SS is defined as T4NxMxB2, which is at least stage IVA1 without taking into account nodal and visceral status.

As per current National Comprehensive Cancer Network clinical practice guidelines, the staging workup of SS patients includes (1) blood work (complete blood count with differential, comprehensive metabolic panel, lactate dehydrogenase, peripheral blood flow cytometry for CTCL panel markers, T-cell receptor gene rearrangement [TCR-GR] studies of peripheral blood, skin, and LN if applicable, Sézary prep if available) and (2) full-body scanning (computed tomography scan of neck/chest/abdomen/pelvis with IV contrast, or whole-body positron emission tomography/computed tomography scan) to evaluate for LN and/or visceral disease. If LN > 1.5 cm in long axis, excisional LN biopsy is strongly preferred over a fine needle aspirate, though in some situations, a core-needle biopsy can suffice. Any LN biopsy should be submitted for flow cytometry and histopathology (and if possible, TCR-GR). Any areas suspicious for visceral involvement should be sampled if possible—advanced, aggressive SS can involve the oropharynx, genitals,

central nervous system, lungs, liver, spleen, and colon, with less likely involvement of central LNs, bone, and kidney. Bone marrow biopsies are typically not performed unless patients demonstrate cytopenias that are unexplained.

Disease stage does predict overall prognosis. In addition, a prognostic index for MF and SS was proposed (cutaneous lymphoma international prognostic index; CLIPi) and validated with an additional external patient series. For advanced-stage patients, male gender, age > 60, blood stage B1/B2, nodal stage N2/N3, and visceral involvement M1 were significant prognostic factors and could be used to predict 10-year overall survival between low-risk (0-1 risk factors, 10-year OS 53.2%), intermediate-risk (2 risk factors, 19.8%), and high-risk (3-5 risk factors, 15.0%) patient groups.[24]

Recently, the EORTC CLTF group proposed that flow cytometry should define blood class according to absolute counts of $CD4^+7^-$ or $CD4^+26^-$ populations. This group proposed absolute counts of either $CD4^+CD7^-$ or $CD4^+CD26^-$ where B0 < 250/μL, B1 = 250/μL–<1000/μL, and B2 ≥ 1000/μL plus a T-cell blood clone with identical size to the skin.[25,26]

PROGNOSIS

SS historically has had an overall poor prognosis with infection as the leading cause of mortality. Median survival of SS patients as strictly defined (T4B2) has ranged from 2.5 to 4.6 years (26% 5-year survival, risk of disease progression in SS cohort 70% at 5 years) in several large single academic center retrospective studies with a trend toward improved survival with more recent studies, likely due to better control of infections and avoidance of indwelling central lines which are susceptible to line infection in such a population.[27-30] It is difficult to ascertain if the modest trend toward improved survival is related to newer therapies as randomized controlled data are lacking to confirm effects of current therapies on overall survival (Cochrane review). In a recent study by Agar and colleagues,[30] a multivariate analysis of their large MF/SS cohort revealed that decreased overall survival and increased risk of disease progression were associated with advanced skin (T) stage, increased LDH, B0b status, and folliculotropic MF. Approximately 30% of SS skin biopsies harbor Epstein–Barr virus (EBV)-DNA, which is thought to be related to immunosuppression. EBV infection had been linked to worse clinical outcome.[16]

MF/SS patients are at higher risk for secondary malignancies due to skin-directed therapies such as phototherapy and the use of alkylating agents. Therapy-related malignancies include nonmelanoma skin cancers, melanoma, and other lymphoproliferative disorders such as Hodgkin lymphoma and non-Hodgkin B-cell lymphomas comprising chronic lymphocytic leukemia.[21,31] In addition, 5% of MF/SS patients will develop a concomitant primary cutaneous $CD30^+$ lymphoproliferative disorder such as lymphomatoid papulosis (LyP) or primary cutaneous anaplastic large-cell lymphoma independent of their MF/SS disease activity.[32] Concomitant LyP appears to be a positive prognostic factor in MF/SS patients.[27,30]

TREATMENT

Full discussion of treatment of SS is outside the scope of this chapter, but briefly, SS treatment is stage-based and combination skin-directed (topicals, phototherapy, radiation therapy), immune-preserving biologic response modifier systemic agents (interferons, retinoids, low-dose methotrexate, extracorporeal photopheresis), targeted therapies (mogamulizumab, brentuximab vedotin, histone deacetylase inhibitors), immune checkpoint inhibitors, and single agent chemotherapy (pralatrexate, gemcitabine, liposomal doxorubicin) are utilized first prior to more immunosuppressive or multiagent cytotoxic regimens.[33-35] Durable "cure" is not routinely possible with chemotherapeutic regimens.[36] Allogeneic stem cell transplantation is a treatment option for younger patients with high-risk disease though relapses and acute and chronic graft-vs-host disease can occur.[37-39] In addition to disease stage, other factors affect treatment decisions in SS patients and they include disease tempo, comorbidities, accessibility, and cost factors. Skin-directed treatments, pruritus management, and monitoring and treating skin infection are very important measures to continue even during systemic treatment of SS.

HISTOPATHOLOGY

Similar to MF, SS can be a challenge to diagnose promptly owing to a broad clinical differential diagnosis (see Differential Diagnosis section later), but also because skin biopsies may be nonspecific/nondiagnostic in up to one-third of SS cases.[40] Because of this phenomenon, we recommend that peripheral blood studies be performed in erythrodermic patients if SS is clinically suspected.[18]

Definitive skin biopsies will demonstrate the hallmark features as described in MF: atypical small- to medium-sized hyperchromatic lymphocytes with cerebriform, hyperconvoluted nuclei demonstrating epidermotropism in a variety of patterns ("lining up") along the dermal–epidermal junction, single-cell epidermotropism without spongiosis, and discrete collections in the epidermis around Langerhans cells ("Pautrier microabscesses") (Fig. 14-8). Skin biopsies of the plaques/tumors often demonstrate large-cell morphology (Fig. 14-9). Skin "large-cell transformation" is defined, as in

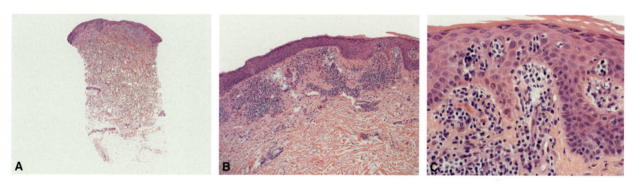

FIGURE 14-8. **Skin histopathology in SS. A** and **B.** Superficial lymphocytic infiltrates with minimal epidermotropism. **C.** Scant epidermotropic T-cells in Pautrier microabscesses. Note the subtlety of cytologic atypia.

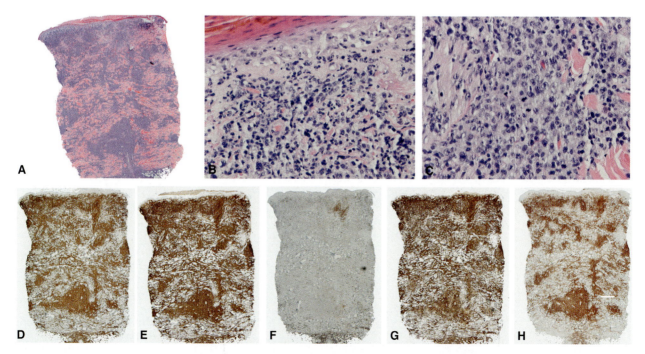

FIGURE 14-9. **SS with large-cell transformation.** Tumoral infiltrates in the dermis **(A)** show minimal epidermotropism **(B)** and large-cell morphology **(C)**. Immunohistochemistry reveals a CD3+ **(D)**, CD4+ **(E)**, CD8– **(F)**, CD7+ **(G)**, and CD30+ **(H)** phenotype. (Image courtesy of Dr. Alejandro Gru.)

MF, as >25% of the atypical infiltrate demonstrating enlarged nuclei more than four times the size of normal lymphocytes.[41-43]

However, many SS biopsies do not show marked epidermotropism and the atypical infiltrate is based in the upper dermis, with perivascular pattern.[40] Furthermore, some SS patients have nonspecific skin biopsies of spongiotic dermatitis, psoriasiform dermatitis, and lichenoid dermatitis without marked cytologic or immunophenotypic atypia. There are SS patients where the diagnosis is made only by biopsy of enlarged LNs and/or examination of the peripheral blood for Sézary cells and demonstration of consistent matching T-cell clonality in these compartments and the skin as well.[44]

IMMUNOHISTOCHEMISTRY

Immunohistochemical (IHC) stains will demonstrate a predominance of CD3+CD4+ T-cells with marked CD4:CD8 elevation (>4:1), particularly in the epidermis (Figs. 14-9 and 14-10). CD7 expression is variable and is lost by tumor T-cells in about 75% of SS cases.[45] Additionally, Sézary cells diffusely express GATA-3, a marker of T_H2 differentiation, but not T-bet, a T_H1-specific marker (Fig. 14-11).[45] SS cells will express TCRαβ receptor and will stain with IHC stain βF1. Large-cell transformed cases may express CD30 (Fig. 14-9). PD1 is often strongly expressed by Sézary cells. Its diffuse and strong expression in the context of erythroderma favors SS diagnosis over differential diagnoses (inflammatory skin disease of erythrodermic MF).[46] Increased expression of CCR4 by Sezary cells is seen both in the skin and peripheral blood.[47]

PERIPHERAL BLOOD FINDINGS

The recommended peripheral blood examination for a patient with erythroderma where SS is on the differential diagnosis includes complete blood count with differential, peripheral blood flow cytometry/fluorescence-activated cell-sorting analysis utilizing either Vβ antibodies (available in only select laboratories and relevant for only 40% of SS patients)[48] and/or T-cell markers (CD3, CD4, CD8, CD7, CD26, CD30 if available), and TCR-GR studies (either with BIOMED-2 primers or more

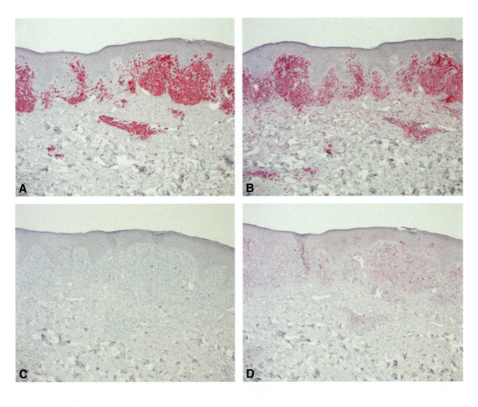

FIGURE 14-10. SS cells typically exhibit a CD3+ **(A)**, CD4+ **(B)**, CD8− **(C)**, and CD7− **(D)** immunophenotype. However, about 25% of the cases show CD7 staining.

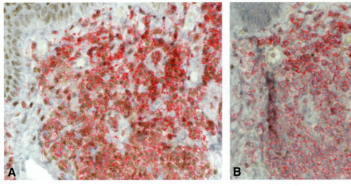

FIGURE 14-11. GATA-3 **(A)** but not T-bet **(B)** expression by CD3+ Sézary cells is indicative of T_H2 skewing. CD3+ (*red*); GATA-3 and T-bet (*brown*).

recently, next-generation deep sequencing). Sézary preps (ie, peripheral blood smears using 1-µm-thin sections) are utilized less frequently owing to operator variability (Fig. 14-12).

It is important to note that some early SS patients will have a normal white blood cell count without a lymphocytosis but have detectable Sézary cells in peripheral blood noted only on blood flow cytometry. Notably, a subset of SS patients will demonstrate CD26 loss but intact CD7 (25% of SS patients at diagnosis, in one series)[45]; thus, it is important that the flow cytometry lab utilizes the CD26 marker in addition to other pan–T-cell markers (Fig. 14-13).[18,45,49] Rarely encountered T-cell antigenic aberrancies include loss or downregulation of CD2 and a combination of decreased CD7 staining with dimmer CD2, dimmer CD3, or both.[50] Downregulated expression of CD7 can be seen in a small fraction of reactive T-cell populations. However, loss of CD7 expression in more than 40% of the CD4+ T-cells is regarded diagnostic of SS by the current ISCL recommendations.[50] CD158k (KIR3DL2) is a new reliable diagnostic marker allowing to delineate tumor cells in the blood of patients with SS.[51,52]

One important caveat is that peripheral blood flow cytometry and TCR-GR studies are not 100% specific for the diagnosis of SS/CTCL. To accurately diagnose (and avoid overdiagnosis of) SS/erythrodermic MF, one must evaluate all clinical and histologic data along with peripheral blood and molecular studies.

GENETIC AND MOLECULAR FINDINGS

Monoclonal TCR-GR can be detected in the skin and blood of SS patients. However, clonal T-cell expansions can also be observed in healthy older individuals in the absence of skin rash and also in numerous reactive skin conditions such as drug eruptions, scabies, pityriasis lichenoides et varioliformis acuta, autoimmune disease (scleroderma), and chronic graft-vs-host disease.[53,54] However, as opposed to a single neoplastic clone seen in SS, the skin and the blood in reactive dermatoses often show nonmatching clonality.[55]

Similar to advanced MF patients, chromosomal abnormalities are relatively common in SS including deletions at 6q, 10, 17p, and gains at 8q and 17q, among others.[56-58]

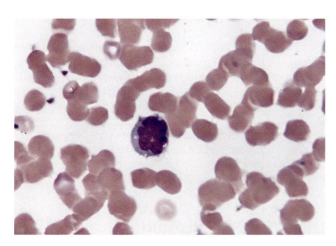

FIGURE 14-12. Sézary cell with enlarged, hyperconvoluted, cerebriform nucleus (peripheral blood smear). (Image courtesy of Dr. Alejandro A. Gru.)

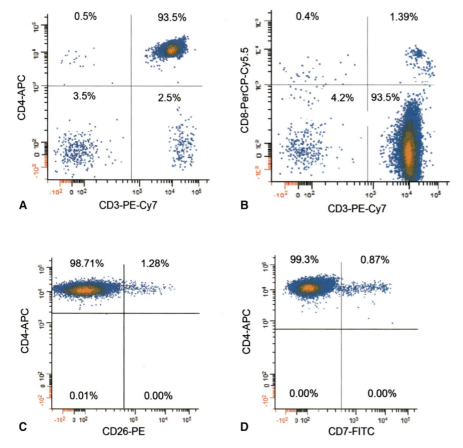

FIGURE 14-13. A–D. Flow cytometry findings in SS.

However, there is no single driver mutation observed in SS. Furthermore, results from multiple gene expression studies in MF and SS have been inconsistent, possibly attributable to differences in purity of cell populations and controls used. An early study demonstrated that SS could be distinguished from nonleukemic CTCL and from inflammatory dermatoses using a panel of five genes (*STAT4, GATA-3, PLS-3, CD1D, TRAIL*).[59] However, since then, a myriad of studies have demonstrated additional dysregulated genes some of which are observed in both MF and SS (*TWIST1, CD52, PTPRCAP, JUNB, TOX*), others which have differential expression in MF vs SS (*EPHA4, STAT4*), or are observed only in SS (*NEDD4L, STAT4*), or have conflicting results in SS (*NEDD4L, KIR3DL2*).[60] Whole exome sequencing of peripheral blood Sézary cells from a small series of 10 SS patients failed to demonstrate consistent mutations between the patients.[61] In contrast, massive parallel sequencing of TCR signaling–related genes in tumor and normal cells from 10 advanced MF/SS patients (and further validated in 42 additional patients) demonstrated activating mutations in PLCG1 in 19% of patients.[62] This study also corroborated dysregulation of genes individually highlighted previously by other groups (*JAK1, JAK3, CCR4*).

Integrated analysis of genomic studies in 121 SS patients confirmed recurrent mutations of *TP53* and of NF-κB pathway genes (*PLCG1, CARD11*), in addition to other nonrecurrent mutations.[63] Mutational signatures in SS include 25% of signature 1, indicative of age-related deamination, and 23% of signature 7, implicating UV exposure.[64]

With regards to specific signaling pathways altered in MF/SS, defects in apoptosis pathways include downregulation of SATB1,[60] Fas, FasL, and BCL2; upregulation of JUNB[65-67]; and constitutive activation of NF-κB.[68] More recently, expression of nuclear factor TOX (thymocyte selection-associated high mobility group box factor, normally expressed by T-cells only during thymic development) has been shown in both MF and SS.[69-71] In vitro, knockdown of TOX results in apoptosis of malignant T-cells.[70]

Constitutive activation of IL-2 pathways including activation of JAK-3/STAT3/STAT 5 is observed in SS[72,73] as is C-MYC depression. Tumor suppressor genes such as p16 and p53 are often inactivated especially in advanced disease.[74,75] PTEN, which is located on chromosome 10q, was recently reported to be deleted in 36% of Sézary patient samples studied, with all 44 samples demonstrating disruption of PTEN activity and subsequent upregulation of PI3/AKT pathways.[76] Activation of NOTCH1 has been recently demonstrated in both peripheral blood Sézary cells and Sézary tumor cell lines.[77] Protooncogene *TWIST* (which blocks p53 and C-MYC signaling) is expressed at higher levels in advanced MF and SS biopsies.[75]

Additionally, several studies demonstrate that MF and SS have differing gene expression signatures. MF is characterized by increased expression of *FASTK* and *SKAP1* genes and diminished expression of the *RB1* and *DLEU1* tumor suppressor genes.[78] SS is characterized by amplification of *MYC* oncogene in 75% of patients, which was detected in only a minority of MF patients.[72]

Noncoding RNA (such as long noncoding RNA and microRNA) expression is also altered in MF/SS.[12,79-81] Most notably, miR-21 is upregulated in SS and portends worse prognosis[82] and a panel of five miRNAs (miR-203, miR-205, miR-326, miR-663b, miR-711) was identified as diagnostic markers in distinguishing CTCL from inflammatory dermatoses.[81]

Skin inflammation and neoplastic progression in SS/CTCL may be enhanced by benign CD4 T-cell responses to SA on the skin.[83] Antistaphylococcal antibiotic treatment has long been reported to improve erythrodermic CTCL patients; Lindahl et al demonstrated that such treatment inhibited malignant T-cells as evidenced by decreased interleukin-2 high-affinity receptors (CD25) expression, STAT3 signaling, and cell proliferation in lesional skin.[84]

POSTULATED CELL OF ORIGIN

SS tumor cells are derived from mature skin-homing T-cells and thus express cutaneous lymphocyte antigen (CLA) on their cell surface. The malignant T-cells are derived from mature skin-homing central memory T-cells that are part of "SALT" and express hallmark receptors (CD3$^+$CD4$^+$CLA$^+$CCR4$^+$CCR7$^+$CCR10$^+$).[85]

Further studies have highlighted the great diversity of Sézary cells, in terms of naïve/memory phenotype, molecular signature, and cytokine/chemokine receptor expression. These results question the dogma of Sézary cells being exclusively derived from the T_{CM} population.[50,86]

IMMUNE DYSREGULATION

The malignant T-cells in SS are typically T-helper CD4$^+$ T-cells that are T_H2 skewed and display a T_H2 cytokine profile (IL-4, IL-5, IL-10).[5,6] T_H2 skewing is further increased by galectin-1 and -3 secreted by SS malignant T-cells that affect cross-talk with normal T-cells in the tumor environment.[87] In an organotypic model of CTCL, Thode and colleagues[88] recently demonstrated that galectins cause keratinocyte hyperproliferation, downregulation of differentiation markers, and impaired barrier function that may underlie the clinical findings in advanced CTCL of epidermal scaling and susceptibility bacterial infection.[88]

A subset of SS patients has malignant T-cells that express a regulatory T-cell phenotype (TGF-β, Foxp3, CD25).[89] With advanced disease, the higher burden of T-cells results in increased levels of T_H2 cytokines that can manifest as hypereosinophilia, elevated IgE, dampened T_H1 immune effects, and decreased number and function of dendritic cells, NK cells, and T_H1 cytokines.[90] Furthermore, CD40 ligand expression and signaling in Sézary cells is impaired resulting in decreased IL-12 and TNF-α production.[91] This results in "endogenous immunosuppression" and can explain some of the increased risk of severe skin infections and other unusual infections even in patients who have not been heavily pretreated with cytotoxic chemotherapy (progressive multifocal leukoencephalopathy, cytomegalovirus reactivation).[92] Another contributing factor potentially is the decreased normal T-cell repertoire observed by Yawalkar and colleagues in CTCL, even in early-stage disease.[93,94]

Singer and colleagues[95] demonstrated that IL-31, a T_H2 cytokine that is increased in atopic dermatitis and mastocytosis, is also elevated in CTCL patients and levels correlate with pruritus severity and disease activity. Another group reported similar elevation of serum IL-31 in SS patients, but found that IL-31 was not produced by the CTCL cells.[96]

Malek and colleagues[97] examined both MF and SS patients and could not demonstrate the association between pruritus severity and IL-31 levels in their cohort, but IL-31 IVS2+12 gene polymorphisms differentially expressed in early-stage vs late-stage disease.[97]

With CTCL disease progression, chemokine and chemokine receptor expression varies. With advanced-stage disease such as tumor MF and SS, the expression of CC chemokine receptor 4 (CCR4) increases, which results in skin homing in response to thymus and activation-regulated chemokine (also referred to as CCL17) expressed by Langerhans cells and endothelial cells. CCR10 is another chemokine receptor expressed on MF and SS cells and binds cutaneous T-cell-attracting chemokine (also referred to as CCL27).

In addition to CCR4, SS malignant T-cells also coexpress CCR7 (a chemokine receptor that homes to LN), L-selectin, and the differentiation marker CD27. In contrast, MF malignant T-cells express CLA more strongly than SS malignant T-cells, but lack CCR7/L-selectin/CD27. This differential expression of chemokine receptors raises the possibility that MF and SS arise from distinct memory T-cell subsets (SS are central memory T-cells, T_{CM}; MF originates from skin-resident effector memory T-cells, T_{EM}).[85] These observations may explain to some degree why SS malignant T-cells are less epidermotropic than MF malignant T-cells on skin histology.

Mogamulizumab, a humanized monoclonal antibody targeting CCR4, was FDA-approved in 2018 for MF/SS, with the pivotal multicenter Phase 3 randomized controlled MAVORIC trial in Stage IB-IV disease demonstrating improved progression-free survival (PFS) vs comparator vorinostat (median PFS 7.7 vs 3.1 months, $P > .0001$).[98] Overall clinical response rate was 28% but higher in SS patients (37%), reflecting that mogamulizumab is particularly effective debulking the blood compartment tumor burden. MF/SS patients treated with mogamulizumab have not as yet experienced major immunosuppression or increased infections; however, mogamulizumab-associated rash (MAR) is a frequent adverse event (23.1% mogamulizumab treated patients in the MAVORIC trial, but as high as 68% in a single center retrospective series[99]), attributed to the depletion of circulating T-reg cells, shift from Th2 to Th1 immune milieu, and may be associated with clinical response. The clinical presentation of MAR is heterogenous and may be difficult to distinguish from the patient's MF/SS but can include (1) folliculotropic–MF-like scalp plaques with alopecia, (2) psoriasiform or lichenoid papules/plaques, (3) photodistributed dermatitis, and (4) morbilliform eruption/erythroderma[100] (Fig. 14-14).

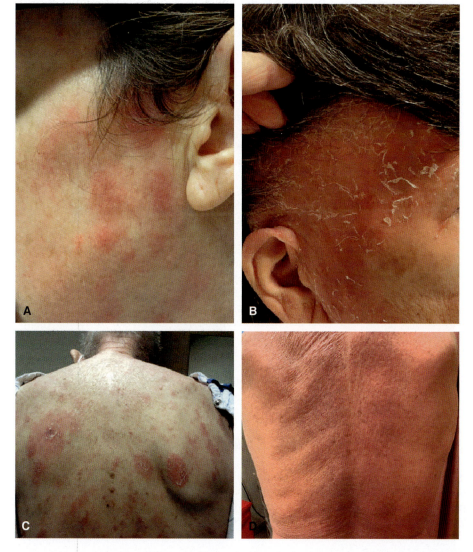

FIGURE 14-14. Clinical spectrum of mogamulizumab-induced rash includes facial rash (**A**), exfoliative rash with alopecia (**B**), psoriasiform plaques (**C**), and erythroderma (**D**).

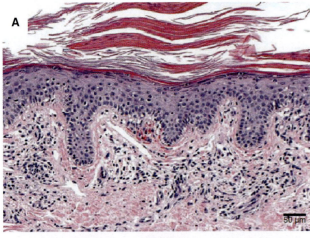
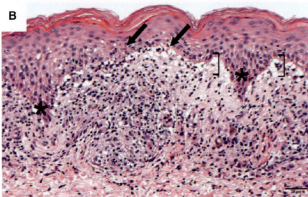
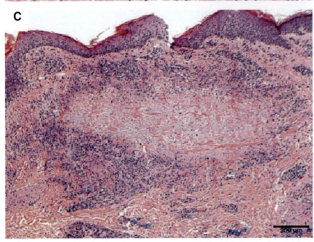

FIGURE 14-15. Histological spectrum of mogamulizumab-induced rash. Psoriasiform reaction **(A)**, lichenoid interface dermatitis **(B)** with lymphocyte exocytosis and dyskeratosis (arrows), basal vacuolar alteration (brackets) and pointed rete (asterisks). Granuloma annulare-like tissue reaction **(C)**. (Reprinted from Wang JY, Hirotsu KE, Neal TM, Raghavan SS, Kwong BY, et al. Histopathologic characterization of mogamulizumab-associated rash. *Am J Surg Pathol*. 2020;44(12):1666-1676, with permission.)

Histopathology of MAR is similarly heterogeneous with spongiotic/psoriasiform dermatitis, interface dermatitis, and granulomatous dermatitis commonly reported[101] (Fig. 14-15)[101,102] (Refs: Wang et al 2021). Immunohistochemistry (inverted CD4:CD8 ratio, retention of CD7) (Fig. 14-16) and molecular clonality studies may be helpful to distinguish MAR from MF/SS. Mild/moderate MAR that can be controlled with topical/systemic steroids/methotrexate could allow continuation of mogamulizumab treatment.[103] Other immune-related adverse events such autoimmune thyroiditis, vitiligo, alopecia areata, myositis, and myocarditis have been rarely reported with mogamulizumab.[104] In adult T-cell leukemia/lymphoma (ATLL), mogamulizumab depletion of T-regs may increase risk of severe acute graft-vs-host disease following allogeneic hematopoietic stem cell transplant though this has not been observed as yet in MF/SS patients treated with mogamulizumab who go on to transplant.[105]

CANDIDATE TUMOR MARKERS

Several candidates for a more specific SS "tumor marker" have emerged. CD158K (KIR3DL2) is a member of the killer cell Ig-like receptor family and has been reported as a specific marker for circulating malignant T-cells in SS. More recently, Ghazi and colleagues[106] have demonstrated that this receptor can mediate CpG oligodeoxynucleotide-induced malignant T-cell apoptosis.

CD164 is a sialomucin that is normally expressed on human CD34+ hematopoietic stem cells but not expressed by CD4+ T-cells in normal controls or atopic dermatitis. Wysocka and colleagues[107] have demonstrated that CD164 is expressed in SS tumor cells. The studies further showed that while CD164 is present on CD4 T-cells of SS patients with a wide range of tumor burdens, it is absent on CD4 T-cells of healthy controls and patients with atopic dermatitis. Additionally, morphologic examination of purified CD4+CD164+ T-cells demonstrates the morphology of malignant Sézary cells. Lastly, CD4+CD164+ T-cells were noted to disappear in SS patients who experienced clinical remission as a result of treatment, underscoring the potential for CD164 to serve as a marker for malignant cells in SS.

Other markers recently reported useful in flow cytometric analysis include vimentin, CD158k,[51,52,108] T-plastin (PLS3),[109] TWIST,[110] and NKp46.[111] Michel and colleagues[112] recently demonstrated that the combination of CD158k, PLS3, and TWIST gene expression profiling by quantitative PCR can be used for an efficient molecular diagnosis of SS. The authors showed that CD4+ T-cells from SS patients expressed significant PLS3, TWIST, CD158k, and NKp46 mRNA levels and that analysis of expression of these four markers accurately classified 100% patients in the study.

CD39, an ectonucleotidase involved in the process of adenosine triphosphate/adenosine diphosphate hydrolysis, has also been identified as a marker for SS tumor T-cells. This finding supports the attractive possibility of using CD39 as a specific marker for the evaluation of SS patients circulating tumor burden, but also as a promising target in the context of SS with the development of CD39-blocking antibodies that may restore efficient antitumor responses.[113]

DIFFERENTIAL DIAGNOSIS

The clinical differential diagnosis of SS is extremely broad, given the nonspecific clinical presentation of exfoliative erythroderma. MF can present with or evolve over time into exfoliative erythroderma (though by current consensus

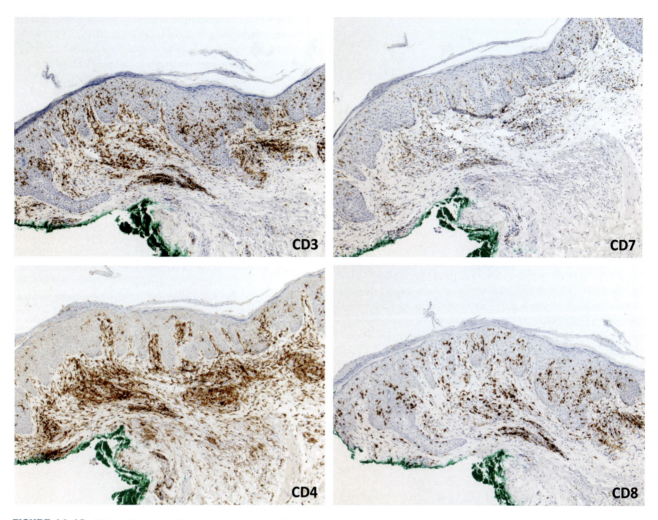

FIGURE 14-16. Lichenoid mogamulizumab-induced rash—immunophenotype. The infiltrate is positive for CD3 and has mild loss of CD7. Intraepidermal cells show a predominance of CD8+ over CD4+ T-cells.

definitions, erythrodermic MF will not have the same degree of peripheral blood involvement as SS patients) and other T-cell neoplasms can rarely present with erythroderma (ATLL associated with human T-lymphotrophic virus, T-cell prolymphocytic leukemia, large granular lymphocytic leukemia). Nonneoplastic entities that can present with erythroderma include atopic dermatitis, psoriasis, pityriasis rubra pilaris, medication reactions[114] (especially drug rash eosinophilia systemic symptoms subtype), allergic contact dermatitis, viral exanthema, erythroderma associated with HIV, severe seborrheic dermatitis, subacute cutaneous lupus, sarcoidosis, papuloerythroderma of Ofuji, paraneoplastic erythroderma, and idiopathic hypereosinophilic syndrome (lymphocytic subtype), among others. Furthermore, a large subset of erythrodermic patients will have "erythroderma not otherwise specified" without a discernible underlying etiology despite extensive investigational studies at a given time. In many of the above entities, isolated T-cell clonality can be identified in the blood or skin of unclear significance (in contrast to typical SS where matching T-cell clonality is classically observed in multiple tissue compartments—more than one skin site and blood, and often in LNs).

CAPSULE SUMMARY

- Clinical: Exfoliative erythroderma (>80% BSA) with LN and peripheral blood involvement (>1000/mL).
- Histopathology: Atypical lymphocytic infiltrates in the superficial dermis with minimal epidermotropism. About one-third of the cases show nondiagnostic skin biopsies.
- Immunophenotype: CD3+CD4+CD7−CD26−CCR4+CCR7+CD27+L-selectin+. About 25% of cases show CD7 expression.
- Cell of origin: Mature skin-homing central memory T-cells.
- Immune dysregulation: Elevated levels of T_H2 cytokines, decreased cell-mediated immunity, impaired barrier function, and symptoms of severe itching and susceptibility to infection.
- Genetics: Multiple genetic pathways are dysregulated; no single driver mutation or group of mutations has been identified.
- Differential diagnosis: Erythrodermic MF, psoriasis, atopic dermatitis, pityriasis rubra pilaris, drug reaction, and HIV-related erythrodermia.

References

1. Gaulard P, Berti E, Willemze R, et al. Primary cutaneous peripheral T-cell lymphomas, rare subtypes. In: Swerdlow SH, Campo E, Harris NL, et al., eds. *WHO Classification of Tumours of Haematopoeitic and Lymphoid Tissues*. IARC Press; 2008:302-305.
2. Willemze R, Jaffe ES, Burg G, et al. WHO-EORTC classification for cutaneous lymphomas. *Blood*. 2005;105(10):3768-3785.
3. Sézary A, Bouvrain Y. Erythrodermie avec presence de cellules monstrueuses dans le derme et le sang circulant. *Bull Soc Fr Dermatol Syph*. 1938;45:254-260.
4. Olsen E, Vonderheid E, Pimpinelli N, et al. Revisions to the staging and classification of mycosis fungoides and Sézary syndrome: a proposal of the International Society for Cutaneous Lymphomas (ISCL) and the cutaneous lymphoma task force of the European Organization of Research and Treatment of Cancer (EORTC). *Blood*. 2007;110(6):1713-1722.
5. Kim EJ, Hess S, Richardson SK, et al. Immunopathogenesis and therapy of cutaneous T cell lymphoma. *J Clin Invest*. 2005;115(4):798-812.
6. Durgin JS, Weiner DM, Wysocka M, Rook AH. The immunopathogenesis and immunotherapy of cutaneous T cell lymphoma: pathways and targets for immune restoration and tumor eradication. *J Am Acad Dermatol*. 2021;84(3):587-595. doi:10.1016/j.jaad.2020.12.027.
7. Imam MH, Shenoy PJ, Flowers CR, et al. Incidence and survival patterns of cutaneous T-cell lymphomas in the United States. *Leuk Lymphoma*. 2013;54(4):752-759.
8. Bradford PT, Devesa SS, Anderson WF, et al. Cutaneous lymphoma incidence patterns in the United States: a population-based study of 3884 cases. *Blood*. 2009;113(21):5064-5073.
9. Groves FD, Linet MS, Travis LB, et al. Cancer surveillance series: non-Hodgkin's lymphoma incidence by histologic subtype in the United States from 1978 through 1995. *J Natl Cancer Inst*. 2000;92(15):1240-1251.
10. Dobos G, Pohrt A, Ram-Wolff C, et al. Epidemiology of cutaneous T-cell lymphomas: a systematic review and meta-analysis of 16,953 patients. *Cancers (Basel)*. 2020;12(10):2921.
11. Hodak E, Klein T, Gabay B, et al. Familial mycosis fungoides: report of 6 kindreds and a study of the HLA system. *J Am Acad Dermatol*. 2005;52(3 pt 1):393-402.
12. Lee CS, Ungewickell A, Bhaduri A, et al. Transcriptome sequencing in Sézary syndrome identifies Sézary cell and mycosis fungoides-associated LncRNAs and novel transcripts. *Blood*. 2012;120(16):3288-3297.
13. Dereure O, Cheval J, Du Thanh A, et al. No evidence for viral sequences in mycosis fungoides and Sézary syndrome skin lesions: a high-throughput sequencing approach. *J Invest Dermatol*. 2013;133(3):853-855.
14. Jawed SI, Myskowski PL, Horwitz S, et al. Primary cutaneous T-cell lymphoma (mycosis fungoides and Sézary syndrome), part I—diagnosis: clinical and histopathologic features and new molecular and biologic markers. *J Am Acad Dermatol*. 2014;70(2):205.e1–e16; quiz 221-222.
15. Dulmage BO, Feng H, Mirvish E, et al. Black cat in a dark room: absence of a directly oncogenic virus does not eliminate the role of an infectious agent in CTCL pathogenesis. *Br J Dermatol*. 2015;172(5):1449-1451.
16. Novelli M, Merlino C, Ponti R, et al. Epstein-Barr virus in cutaneous T-cell lymphomas: evaluation of the viral presence and significance in skin and peripheral blood. *J Invest Dermatol*. 2009;129(6):1556-1561.
17. Dommasch E, Gelfand JM. Is there truly a risk of lymphoma from biologic therapies? *Dermatol Ther*. 2009;22(5):418-430.
18. Nagler AR, Samimi S, Schaffer A, et al. Peripheral blood findings in erythrodermic patients: importance for the differential diagnosis of Sézary syndrome. *J Am Acad Dermatol*. 2012;66(3):503-508.
19. Henn A, Michel L, Fite C, et al. Sézary syndrome without erythroderma. *J Am Acad Dermatol*. 2015;72(6):1003-1009.e1. doi:10.1016/j.jaad.2014.11.015
20. Calvani J, de Masson A, de Margerie-Mellon C, et al. Image-guided lymph node core-needle biopsy predicts survival in mycosis fungoides and Sézary syndrome. *Br J Dermatol*. 2021;185(2):419-427. doi: 10.1111/bjd.19796
21. Huang KP, Weinstock MA, Clarke CA, et al. Second lymphomas and other malignant neoplasms in patients with mycosis fungoides and Sézary syndrome: evidence from population-based and clinical cohorts. *Arch Dermatol*. 2007;143(1):45-50.
22. Hinds GA, Heald P. Cutaneous T-cell lymphoma in skin of color. *J Am Acad Dermatol*. 2009;60(3):359-375.
23. Axelrod PI, Lorber B, Vonderheid EC. Infections complicating mycosis fungoides and Sézary syndrome. *JAMA*. 1992;267(10):1354-1358.
24. Benton EC, Crichton S, Talpur R, et al. A cutaneous lymphoma international prognostic index (CLIPi) for mycosis fungoides and Sézary syndrome. *Eur J Cancer*. 2013;49(13):2859-2868.
25. Scarisbrick JJ, Hodak E, Bagot M, et al. Blood classification and blood response criteria in mycosis fungoides and Sézary syndrome using flow cytometry: recommendations from the EORTC cutaneous lymphoma task force. *Eur J Cancer*. 2018;93:47-56.
26. Scarisbrick JJ, Hodak E, Bagot M, et al. Developments in the understanding of blood involvement and stage in mycosis fungoides/Sezary syndrome. *Eur J Cancer*. 2018;101:278-280.
27. Talpur R, Singh L, Daulat S, et al. Long-term outcomes of 1,263 patients with mycosis fungoides and Sézary syndrome from 1982 to 2009. *Clin Cancer Res*. 2012;18(18):5051-5060.
28. Kim YH, Liu HL, Mraz-Gernhard S, et al. Long-term outcome of 525 patients with mycosis fungoides and Sézary syndrome: clinical prognostic factors and risk for disease progression. *Arch Dermatol*. 2003;139(7):857-866.
29. Kubica AW, Davis MD, Weaver AL, et al. Sézary syndrome: a study of 176 patients at Mayo Clinic. *J Am Acad Dermatol*. 2012;67(6):1189-1199.
30. Agar NS, Wedgeworth E, Crichton S, et al. Survival outcomes and prognostic factors in mycosis fungoides/Sézary syndrome: validation of the revised International Society for Cutaneous Lymphomas/European Organisation for Research and Treatment of Cancer staging proposal. *J Clin Oncol*. 2010;28(31):4730-4739.
31. Ai WZ, Keegan TH, Press DJ, et al. Outcomes after diagnosis of mycosis fungoides and Sézary syndrome before 30 years of age: a population-based study. *JAMA Dermatol*. 2014;150(7):709-715.
32. Liu HL, Hoppe RT, Kohler S, et al. CD30+ cutaneous lymphoproliferative disorders: the Stanford experience in lymphomatoid papulosis and primary cutaneous anaplastic large cell lymphoma. *J Am Acad Dermatol*. 2003;49(6):1049-1058.
33. Olsen EA, Rook AH, Zic J, et al. Sézary syndrome: immunopathogenesis, literature review of therapeutic options, and recommendations for therapy by the United States Cutaneous Lymphoma Consortium (USCLC). *J Am Acad Dermatol*. 2011;64(2):352-404.
34. Raphael BA, Shin DB, Suchin KR, et al. High clinical response rate of Sézary syndrome to immunomodulatory therapies: prognostic markers of response. *Arch Dermatol*. 2011;147(12):1410-1415.

35. Jawed SI, Myskowski PL, Horwitz S, et al. Primary cutaneous T-cell lymphoma (mycosis fungoides and Sézary syndrome), Part II: prognosis, management, and future directions. *J Am Acad Dermatol.* 2014;70(2):223; e1-e17; quiz 240-242.
36. Hughes CF, Khot A, McCormack C, et al. Lack of durable disease control with chemotherapy for mycosis fungoides and Sézary syndrome: a comparative study of systemic therapy. *Blood.* 2015;125(1):71-81.
37. Polansky M, Talpur R, Daulat S, et al. Long-term complete responses to combination therapies and allogeneic stem cell transplants in patients with Sézary syndrome. *Clin Lymphoma Myeloma Leuk.* 2015;15(5):e83-e93.
38. Duarte RF, Boumendil A, Onida F, et al. Long-term outcome of allogeneic hematopoietic cell transplantation for patients with mycosis fungoides and Sézary syndrome: a European society for blood and marrow transplantation lymphoma working party extended analysis. *J Clin Oncol.* 2014;32(29):3347-3348.
39. Weng WK, Armstrong R, Arai S, et al. Minimal residual disease monitoring with high-throughput sequencing of T cell receptors in cutaneous T cell lymphoma. *Sci Transl Med.* 2013;5(214):214ra171.
40. Trotter MJ, Whittaker SJ, Orchard GE, et al. Cutaneous histopathology of Sézary syndrome: a study of 41 cases with a proven circulating T-cell clone. *J Cutan Pathol.* 1997;24(5):286-291.
41. Diamandidou E, Colome-Grimmer M, Fayad L, et al. Transformation of mycosis fungoides/Sézary syndrome: clinical characteristics and prognosis. *Blood.* 1998;92(4):1150-1159.
42. Salhany KE, Cousar JB, Greer JP, et al. Transformation of cutaneous T cell lymphoma to large cell lymphoma. A clinicopathologic and immunologic study. *Am J Pathol.* 1988;132(2):265-277.
43. Benner MF, Jansen PM, Vermeer MH, et al. Prognostic factors in transformed mycosis fungoides: a retrospective analysis of 100 cases. *Blood.* 2012;119(7):1643-1649.
44. Ponti R, Quaglino P, Novelli M, et al. T-cell receptor gamma gene rearrangement by multiplex polymerase chain reaction/heteroduplex analysis in patients with cutaneous T-cell lymphoma (mycosis fungoides/Sézary syndrome) and benign inflammatory disease: correlation with clinical, histological and immunophenotypical findings. *Br J Dermatol.* 2005;153(3):565-573.
45. Novelli M, Fava P, Sarda C, et al. Blood flow cytometry in Sézary syndrome: new insights on prognostic relevance and immunophenotypic changes during follow-up. *Am J Clin Pathol.* 2015;143(1):57-69.
46. Cetinözman F, Jansen PM, Vermeer MH, Willemze R. Differential expression of programmed death-1 (PD-1) in Sézary syndrome and mycosis fungoides. *Arch Dermatol.* 2012;148(12):1379-1385.
47. Ferenczi K, Fuhlbrigge RC, Pinkus J, Pinkus GS, Kupper TS. Increased CCR4 expression in cutaneous T cell lymphoma. *J Invest Dermatol.* 2002;119:1405-1410.
48. Vonderheid EC, Boselli CM, Conroy M, et al. Evidence for restricted Vbeta usage in the leukemic phase of cutaneous T cell lymphoma. *J Invest Dermatol.* 2005;124(3):651-661.
49. Bernengo MG, Novelli M, Quaglino P, et al. The relevance of the CD4+ CD26− subset in the identification of circulating Sézary cells. *Br J Dermatol.* 2001;144(1):125-135.
50. Kelemen K, Guitart J, Kuzel TM, et al. The usefulness of CD26 in flow cytometric analysis of peripheral blood in Sézary syndrome. *Am J Clin Pathol.* 2008;129(1):146-156.
51. Moins-Teisserenc H, Daubord M, Clave E, et al. CD158k is a reliable marker for diagnosis of Sézary syndrome and reveals an unprecedented heterogeneity of circulating malignant cells. *J Invest Dermatol.* 2015;135(1):247-257.
52. Roelens M, de Masson A, Ram-Wolff C, et al. Revisiting the initial diagnosis and blood staging of mycosis fungoides and Sézary syndrome with the KIR3DL2 marker. *Br J Dermatol.* 2020;182(6):1415-1422.
53. French LE, Lessin SR, Addya K, et al. Identification of clonal T cells in the blood of patients with systemic sclerosis: positive correlation with response to photopheresis. *Arch Dermatol.* 2001;137(10):1309-1313.
54. French LE, Alcindor T, Shapiro M, et al. Identification of amplified clonal T cell populations in the blood of patients with chronic graft-versus-host disease: positive correlation with response to photopheresis. *Bone Marrow Transp.* 2002;30(8):509-515.
55. Alessi E, Coggi A, Venegoni L, et al. The usefulness of clonality for the detection of cases clinically and/or histopathologically not recognized as cutaneous T-cell lymphoma. *Br J Dermatol.* 2005;153(2):368-371.
56. Scarisbrick JJ, Woolford AJ, Russell-Jones R, et al. Loss of heterozygosity on 10q and microsatellite instability in advanced stages of primary cutaneous T-cell lymphoma and possible association with homozygous deletion of PTEN. *Blood.* 2000;95(9):2937-2942.
57. Mao X, Lillington D, Scarisbrick JJ, et al. Molecular cytogenetic analysis of cutaneous T-cell lymphomas: identification of common genetic alterations in Sézary syndrome and mycosis fungoides. *Br J Dermatol.* 2002;147(3):464-475.
58. Izykowska K, Zawada M, Nowicka K, et al. Identification of multiple complex rearrangements associated with deletions in the 6q23-27 region in Sézary syndrome. *J Invest Dermatol.* 2013;133(11):2617-2625.
59. Nebozhyn M, Loboda A, Kari L, et al. Quantitative PCR on 5 genes reliably identifies CTCL patients with 5% to 99% circulating tumor cells with 90% accuracy. *Blood.* 2006;107(8):3189-3196.
60. Dulmage BO, Geskin LJ. Lessons learned from gene expression profiling of cutaneous T-cell lymphoma. *Br J Dermatol.* 2013;169(6):1188-1197.
61. Andersson E, Eldfors S, Edgren H, et al. Novel TBL1XR1, EPHA7 and SLFN12 mutations in a Sézary syndrome patient discovered by whole exome sequencing. *Exp Dermatol.* 2014;23(5):366-368.
62. Vaque JP, Gomez-Lopez G, Monsalvez V, et al. PLCG1 mutations in cutaneous T-cell lymphomas. *Blood.* 2014;123(13):2034-2043.
63. Chang LW, Patrone CC, Yang W, et al. An integrated data resource for genomic analysis of cutaneous T-cell lymphoma. *J Invest Dermatol.* 2018;138(12):2681-2683.
64. Jones CL, Degasperi A, Grandi V, et al. Spectrum of mutational signatures in T-cell lymphoma reveals a key role for UV radiation in cutaneous T-cell lymphoma. *Sci Rep.* 2021;11(1):3962.
65. Wu J, Siddiqui J, Nihal M, et al. Structural alterations of the FAS gene in cutaneous T-cell lymphoma (CTCL). *Arch Biochem Biophys.* 2011;508(2):185-191.
66. Wu J, Wood GS. Reduction of Fas/CD95 promoter methylation, upregulation of Fas protein, and enhancement of sensitivity to apoptosis in cutaneous T-cell lymphoma. *Arch Dermatol.* 2011;147(4):443-449.
67. Wu J, Salva KA, Wood GS. c-CBL E3 ubiquitin ligase is overexpressed in cutaneous T-cell lymphoma: its inhibition promotes activation-induced cell death. *J Invest Dermatol.* 2015;135(3):861-868.

68. Sors A, Jean-Louis F, Pellet C, et al. Down-regulating constitutive activation of the NF-kappaB canonical pathway overcomes the resistance of cutaneous T-cell lymphoma to apoptosis. *Blood.* 2006;107(6):2354-2363.
69. Huang Y, Litvinov IV, Wang Y, et al. Thymocyte selection-associated high mobility group box gene (TOX) is aberrantly over-expressed in mycosis fungoides and correlates with poor prognosis. *Oncotarget.* 2014;5(12):4418-4425.
70. Huang Y, Su M, Jiang X, et al. Evidence of an oncogenic role of aberrant TOX activation in cutaneous T cell lymphoma. *Blood.* 2015;125(9):1435-1443.
71. Morimura S, Sugaya M, Suga H, et al. TOX expression in different subtypes of cutaneous lymphoma. *Arch Dermatol Res.* 2014;306(9):843-849.
72. Vermeer MH, van Doorn R, Dijkman R, et al. Novel and highly recurrent chromosomal alterations in Sézary syndrome. *Cancer Res.* 2008;68(8):2689-2698.
73. van der Fits L, Out-Luiting JJ, van Leeuwen MA, et al. Autocrine IL-21 stimulation is involved in the maintenance of constitutive STAT3 activation in Sézary syndrome. *J Invest Dermatol.* 2012;132(2):440-447.
74. Lamprecht B, Kreher S, Mobs M, et al. The tumour suppressor p53 is frequently nonfunctional in Sézary syndrome. *Br J Dermatol.* 2012;167(2):240-246.
75. Goswami M, Duvic M, Dougherty A, et al. Increased Twist expression in advanced stage of mycosis fungoides and Sézary syndrome. *J Cutan Pathol.* 2012;39(5):500-507.
76. Cristofoletti C, Picchio MC, Lazzeri C, et al. Comprehensive analysis of PTEN status in Sézary syndrome. *Blood.* 2013;122(20):3511-3520.
77. van der Fits L, Qin Y, Out-Luiting JJ, et al. NOTCH1 signaling as a therapeutic target in Sézary syndrome. *J Invest Dermatol.* 2012;132(12):2810-2817.
78. van Doorn R, van Kester MS, Dijkman R, et al. Oncogenomic analysis of mycosis fungoides reveals major differences with Sézary syndrome. *Blood.* 2009;113(1):127-136.
79. Ballabio E, Mitchell T, van Kester MS, et al. MicroRNA expression in Sézary syndrome: identification, function, and diagnostic potential. *Blood.* 2010;116(7):1105-1113.
80. Narducci MG, Arcelli D, Picchio MC, et al. MicroRNA profiling reveals that miR-21, miR486 and miR-214 are upregulated and involved in cell survival in Sézary syndrome. *Cell Death Dis.* 2011;2:e151.
81. Ralfkiaer U, Hagedorn PH, Bangsgaard N, et al. Diagnostic microRNA profiling in cutaneous T-cell lymphoma (CTCL). *Blood.* 2011;118(22):5891-5900.
82. van der Fits L, van Kester MS, Qin Y, et al. MicroRNA-21 expression in CD4+ T cells is regulated by STAT3 and is pathologically involved in Sézary syndrome. *J Invest Dermatol.* 2011;131(3):762-768.
83. Vieyra-Garcia P, Crouch JD, O'Malley JT, et al. Benign T cells drive clinical skin inflammation in cutaneous T cell lymphoma. *JCI Insight.* 2019;4(1):e124233. doi: 10.1172/jci.insight.124233
84. Lindahl LM, Willerslev-Olsen A, Gjerdrum LMR, et al. Antibiotics inhibit tumor and disease activity in cutaneous T-cell lymphoma. *Blood.* 2019;134(13):1072-1083. doi: 10.1182/blood.2018888107
85. Campbell JJ, Clark RA, Watanabe R, et al. Sézary syndrome and mycosis fungoides arise from distinct T-cell subsets: a biologic rationale for their distinct clinical behaviors. *Blood.* 2010;116(5):767-771.
86. Roelens M, Delord M, Ram-Wolff C, et al. Circulating and skin-derived Sézary cells: clonal but with phenotypic plasticity. *Blood.* 2017;130(12):1468-1471.
87. Cedeno-Laurent F, Watanabe R, Teague JE, et al. Galectin-1 inhibits the viability, proliferation, and Th1 cytokine production of nonmalignant T cells in patients with leukemic cutaneous T-cell lymphoma. *Blood.* 2012;119(15):3534-3538.
88. Thode C, Woetmann A, Wandall HH, et al. Malignant T cells secrete galectins and induce epidermal hyperproliferation and disorganized stratification in a skin model of cutaneous T-cell lymphoma. *J Invest Dermatol.* 2015;135(1):238-246.
89. Walsh PT, Benoit BM, Wysocka M, et al. A role for regulatory T cells in cutaneous T-Cell lymphoma; induction of a CD4 + CD25 + Foxp3+ T-cell phenotype associated with HTLV-1 infection. *J Invest Dermatol.* 2006;126(3):690-692.
90. Yoo EK, Cassin M, Lessin SR, et al. Complete molecular remission during biologic response modifier therapy for Sézary syndrome is associated with enhanced helper T type 1 cytokine production and natural killer cell activity. *J Am Acad Dermatol.* 2001;45(2):208-216.
91. French LE, Huard B, Wysocka M, et al. Impaired CD40L signaling is a cause of defective IL-12 and TNF-alpha production in Sézary syndrome: circumvention by hexameric soluble CD40L. *Blood.* 2005;105(1):219-225.
92. Wysocka M, Zaki MH, French LE, et al. Sézary syndrome patients demonstrate a defect in dendritic cell populations: effects of CD40 ligand and treatment with GM-CSF on dendritic cell numbers and the production of cytokines. *Blood.* 2002;100(9):3287-3294.
93. Yawalkar N, Ferenczi K, Jones DA, et al. Profound loss of T-cell receptor repertoire complexity in cutaneous T-cell lymphoma. *Blood.* 2003;102(12):4059-4066.
94. Yamanaka K, Yawalkar N, Jones DA, et al. Decreased T-cell receptor excision circles in cutaneous T-cell lymphoma. *Clin Cancer Res.* 2005;11(16):5748-5755.
95. Singer EM, Shin DB, Nattkemper LA, et al. IL-31 is produced by the malignant T-cell population in cutaneous T-Cell lymphoma and correlates with CTCL pruritus. *J Invest Dermatol.* 2013;133(12):2783-2785.
96. Möbs M, Gryzik S, Haidar A, et al. Analysis of the IL-31 pathway in mycosis fungoides and Sézary syndrome. *Arch Dermatol Res.* 2015;307(6):479-485.
97. Malek M, Glen J, Rebala K, et al. Il-31 does not correlate to pruritus related to early stage cutaneous T-cell lymphomas but is involved in pathogenesis of the disease. *Acta Derm Venereol.* 2015;95(3):283-288.
98. Kim YH, Bagot M, Pinter-Brown L, et al. Mogamulizumab versus vorinostat in previously treated cutaneous T-cell lymphoma (MAVORIC): an international, open-label, randomised, controlled phase 3 trial. *Lancet Oncol.* 2018;19(9):1192-1204. doi:10.1016/S1470-2045(18)30379-6
99. Trum NA, Zain J, Martinez XU, et al. Mogamulizumab efficacy is underscored by its associated rash that mimics cutaneous T-cell lymphoma: a retrospective single-centre case series. *Br J Dermatol.* 2022;186(1):153-166. doi:10.1111/bjd.20708
100. Hirotsu KE, Neal TM, Khodadoust MS, et al. Clinical characterization of mogamulizumab-associated rash during treatment of mycosis fungoides or sézary syndrome. *JAMA Dermatol.* 2021;157(6):700-707. doi:10.1001/jamadermatol.2021.0877
101. Wang JY, Hirotsu KE, Neal TM, et al. Histopathologic characterization of mogamulizumab-associated rash. *Am J Surg Pathol.* 2020;44(12):1666-1676.

102. Chen L, Carson KR, Staser KW, et al. Mogamulizumab-associated cutaneous granulomatous drug eruption mimicking mycosis fungoides but possibly indicating durable clinical response. *JAMA Dermatol.* 2019;155(8):968-971.
103. Musiek ACM, Rieger KE, Bagot M, et al. Dermatologic events associated with the anti-CCR4 antibody mogamulizumab: characterization and management. *Dermatol Ther.* 2022;12(1):29-40. doi:10.1007/s13555-021-00624-7
104. Bonnet P, Battistella M, Roelens M, et al. Association of autoimmunity and long-term complete remission in patients with Sézary syndrome treated with mogamulizumab. *Br J Dermatol.* 2019;180(2):419-420. doi:10.1111/bjd.17320
105. Dai J, Almazan TH, Hong EK, et al. Potential association of anti-CCR4 antibody mogamulizumab and graft-vs-host disease in patients with mycosis fungoides and sézary syndrome. *JAMA Dermatol.* 2018;154(6):728-730. doi:10.1001/jamadermatol.2018.0884
106. Ghazi B, Thonnart N, Bagot M, et al. KIR3DL2/CpG ODN interaction mediates Sézary syndrome malignant T cell apoptosis. *J Invest Dermatol.* 2015;135(1):229-237.
107. Wysocka M, Kossenkov AV, Benoit BM, et al. CD164 and FCRL3 are highly expressed on CD4+CD26− T cells in Sézary syndrome patients. *J Invest Dermatol.* 2014;134(1):229-236.
108. Bagot M, Moretta A, Sivori S, et al. CD4(+) cutaneous T-cell lymphoma cells express the p140-killer cell immunoglobulin-like receptor. *Blood.* 2001;97(5):1388-1391.
109. Begue E, Jean-Louis F, Bagot M, et al. Inducible expression and pathophysiologic functions of T-plastin in cutaneous T-cell lymphoma. *Blood.* 2012;120(1):143-154.
110. van Doorn R, Dijkman R, Vermeer MH, et al. Aberrant expression of the tyrosine kinase receptor EphA4 and the transcription factor Twist in Sézary syndrome identified by gene expression analysis. *Cancer Res.* 2004;64(16):5578-5586.
111. Bensussan A, Remtoula N, Sivori S, et al. Expression and function of the natural cytotoxicity receptor NKp46 on circulating malignant CD4+ T lymphocytes of Sézary syndrome patients. *J Invest Dermatol.* 2011;131(4):969-976.
112. Michel L, Jean-Louis F, Begue E, et al. Use of PLS3, Twist, CD158k/KIR3DL2, and NKp46 gene expression combination for reliable Sézary syndrome diagnosis. *Blood.* 2013;121(8):1477-1478.
113. Bensussan A, Janela B, Thonnart N, et al. Identification of CD39 as a marker for the circulating malignant T-cell clone of sézary syndrome patients. *J Invest Dermatol.* 2019;139(3):725-728.
114. Reeder MJ, Wood GS. Drug-induced pseudo-Sézary syndrome: a case report and literature review. *Am J Dermatopathol.* 2015;37(1):83-86.

CHAPTER 15

Primary cutaneous CD30-positive T-cell lymphoproliferative disorders

Rebecca L. King, Werner Kempf, Amy C. Musiek, and Andrew L. Feldman

INTRODUCTION

Primary cutaneous CD30-positive T-cell lymphoproliferative disorders (TLPDs) are challenging to both pathologists and clinicians due to their heterogeneous features and overlap with a multitude of reactive and neoplastic conditions. In addition to making the distinction between primary cutaneous anaplastic large cell lymphoma (pcALCL) and lymphomatoid papulosis (LyP), the two entities within this group of diseases, one must attempt to determine whether a cutaneous lesion has arisen primarily in the skin, represents secondary cutaneous involvement by a systemic lymphoma, or represents transformation of another cutaneous T-cell lymphoma (CTCL). Just as novel genetic markers emerge and bring us closer to understanding the pathogenesis of these diseases, additional pathologic subtypes are being described, further broadening the morphologic spectrum of these relatively indolent diseases. In addition, although there is evidence that pcALCL and LyP are distinct entities in many ways, there clearly are cases that show overlapping features, highlighting the pathogenic link between the two and supporting their inclusion under one subheading in current classification systems.

DEFINITION

Primary cutaneous CD30-positive TLPDs include pcALCL and LyP according to the World Health Organization (WHO) and European Organization for Research and Treatment of Cancer (EORTC) classification systems.[1,2] Together, these entities represent around 30% of CTCLs and are the second most common form of CTCL after mycosis fungoides (MF). LyP and pcALCL exist along a clinical and histopathologic spectrum of disease and "borderline" cases in which the features do not easily fit into one entity or the other exist.[3] Furthermore, both LyP and pcALCL may occur in the same patient.[4]

pcALCL is a CD30-positive T cell lymphoma that resembles systemic ALCL but arises primarily in, and is often limited to, the skin. These lesions are almost exclusively negative for anaplastic lymphoma kinase (ALK) fusion proteins and rearrangements involving the ALK gene.[2,5-8] Clinically, pcALCLs typically are localized, often solitary lesions that are large in size (>2 cm) and frequently ulcerate. Dissemination within the skin and to locoregional lymph nodes may occur; however, widespread disease is rare. The current WHO definition of pcALCL states that patients should not have concurrent MF and/or a previous history of MF[2]; however, coexisting MF and pcALCL has been reported.[9,10] The definition of pcALCL also requires distinction from secondary cutaneous involvement from systemic ALCL on clinical grounds and staging examinations.

LyP is an indolent, cutaneous TLPD characterized clinically by a recurrent papulo-nodular eruption with smaller lesions (<2 cm) that show a waxing and waning clinical course.[1,2,11,12] Six histologic subtypes (A, B, C, D, E, and DUSP22-rearranged) are recognized in the 2017 WHO classification and the 2018 WHO-EORTC classification.[1,2,13-16] A follicular variant has been proposed as type F.[17] While most show some degree of CD30-positive T-cell proliferation, the histopathologic features of the different subtypes may overlap with those of pcALCL as well as other cutaneous lymphomas and reactive entities.[4] pcALCL is considered a true malignant lymphoma, while LyP currently is not considered a malignant disorder clinically.[2] Nevertheless, both entities demonstrate an overall favorable prognosis with long-term survival rates of 90% or higher,[4,18,19] lending further support to their inclusion under the single umbrella category of primary cutaneous CD30-positive TLPDs.

EPIDEMIOLOGY

Primary Cutaneous ALCL

The median age of presentation for pcALCL is 60 years.[2] Rare cases of ALCL limited to the skin occur in the pediatric setting; ALK negativity may be helpful in recognizing the possibility of a primary cutaneous process,[2,7,20,21] although very rare ALK-positive cases limited to the skin also exist.[7] Males are affected more often than females, at a ratio of 2 to 3:1. No geographic or ethnic predilections have been reported, although poorer outcomes have been observed in Blacks in the United States with primary cutaneous CD30-positive TLPDs.[22] Possible associations with hay fever, celiac disease, and cigarette smoking have been reported.[23]

Lymphomatoid Papulosis

The incidence of LyP peaks around age 45, slightly younger than in pcALCL.[2] As with pcALCL, cases do occur in children and must be distinguished from systemic ALCL, which most often is ALK-positive in this age group.[24,25] Cases of LyP with *DUSP22* (6p25.3) rearrangements (see below) tend to occur in older individuals (67-88 years in one series).[16] As with pcALCL, LyP affects males more often than females, with a ratio of 2 to 3:1.[2] Associations between LyP and atopy have been reported, especially in young patients; however, a definitive causal link between the two conditions has not been established.[26,27] Patients with LyP are at increased risk for developing malignancies including lymphoma and non-hematolymphoid malignancies.[4,28,29] Up to 20% of patients with LyP in some series had lymphoma, most commonly MF, cutaneous or systemic ALCL, and rarely Hodgkin lymphoma.[11,28,30] Lymphoma may present before, concurrently with, or after a diagnosis of LyP in these patients, although when the lymphoma is systemic ALCL this generally follows LyP.[4,31] The association between LyP and MF appears stronger in Whites than in Blacks.[32]

ETIOLOGY

The etiology of primary cutaneous CD30-positive TLPDs is unknown. CD30 expression in lymphocytes is upregulated by viruses such as Epstein-Barr virus (EBV), human herpesviruses (HHV), and human T cell lymphotropic viruses. However, CD30 expression also is induced by various other stimuli that activate T cells, and a link to viral infection has not been confirmed in primary cutaneous CD30-positive TLPDs. Outside of rare cases occurring in the posttransplant setting, pcALCL and LyP are consistently negative for EBV.[33]

As with systemic ALK-negative ALCL, the pathogenesis of pcALCL and LyP is poorly understood. The finding of *DUSP22* rearrangements in subsets of both pcALCL and LyP (see below) provides further support for the hypothesis that these entities exist along a clinicopathologic spectrum that may include some systemic ALK-negative ALCLs as well. These rearrangements have been associated with decreased expression of the *DUSP22* gene, which encodes a dual-specificity phosphatase known to diminish mitogen-activated protein kinase activity,[34] IL-6-induced STAT3 activation,[35] and lymphocyte-specific protein tyrosine kinase phosphorylation, resulting in diminished T-cell-mediated immunity and autoimmunity.[36] *DUSP22* plays an important role in inflammatory disorders and might represent a tumor suppressor in T-cell lymphomas and lymphoproliferative disorders. *TP63* rearrangements are very rare in pcALCL. A single case of a double hit pcALCL showing both *DUSP22* and *TP63* translocations has been reported recently.

A recent study of 12 patients utilizing next-generation sequencing identified *JAK* and *STAT* alterations in cases of both LyP and pcALCL strongly implicating constitutive JAK-STAT signaling in the pathogenesis of these disorders.[37] Recurrent mutations involving *STAT3*, *STAT6*, and *STAT5B*, activating *HRAS* mutations, and fusions involving *JAK2* and *TYK2* were identified. Overall, 50% of cases showed an aberration affecting the JAK-STAT pathway, suggesting a common oncogenic mechanism between primary cutaneous CD30-positive TLPDs and systemic and breast implant–associated ALCLs that may serve as a therapeutic target.[38,39]

Differential expression of cytokines has been postulated to underlie the skin-homing properties of the neoplastic cells in primary cutaneous CD30-positive TLPDs. Gene expression studies have shown that pcALCL demonstrates higher expression of the chemokine receptor genes *CCR7*, *CCR8*, and *CCR10* than primary cutaneous peripheral T-cell lymphoma, not otherwise specified (PTCL, NOS).[40] This finding could contribute to the clinical finding that pcALCL tends to remain localized rather than disseminating to extracutaneous sites. *CCR8* expression also correlates closely with the presence of *DUSP22* rearrangements in ALCL.[31] Differential expression of chemokine receptors could direct progression or regression of primary cutaneous CD30-positive TLPDs. For example, LyP but not pcALCL may preferentially express CXCR3.[41]

The pathogenesis of pcALCL also may relate to defects in apoptotic signaling, which is known to play a critical role in cell fate of mature T cells.[40] For example, pcALCL expresses higher levels of *FAS* (CD95, TNFRSF6), *TNFRSF8* (CD30), *IRF4*, and *TRAF1* than primary cutaneous PTCL, NOS.[40] Although FAS stimulation can induce apoptosis in pcALCL cells, these cells appear resistant to tumor necrosis factor (TNF)-α- and TRAIL (TNF-related apoptosis-inducing ligand)-mediated extrinsic pro-apoptotic mechanisms.[42] TRAIL resistance might result from overexpression of cellular FLICE-like inhibitory protein (c-FLIP, CFLAR) and diminished expression of the pro-apoptotic protein, BID. Interestingly, c-FLIP has been shown to be upregulated by NF-kappa B in pcALCL cells, which in turn is activated by cross-linking of CD30. This upregulation of c-FLIP may enhance the resistance to apoptosis associated with CD95. IRF4, which is critical to the proliferation and survival of ALCL cells,[43] also increases resistance to apoptotic stimuli and activation-induced cell death in reactive CD4+ T cells.[44] TRAF1, which is involved in intracellular signal transduction from CD30 and other TNF receptor superfamily members, and the polycomb-group protein EZH2 also may contribute to resistance to apoptotic stimuli in pcALCL.[45,46]

CLINICAL PRESENTATION AND PROGNOSIS

Primary Cutaneous ALCL

pcALCL and LyP have heterogeneous and overlapping histologic features, and it is often the clinical history and presentation that distinguish these two conditions. Patients with pcALCL tend to be male more often than female and in their seventh decade of life.[4] The lesions tend to be solitary, often ulcerative tumors (Fig. 15-1), though groups of nodules also can occur (Fig. 15-2). Although spontaneous regression of

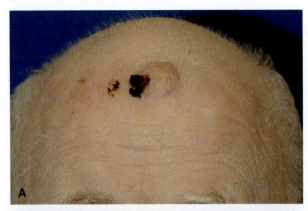

FIGURE 15-1. pcALCL presenting on the forehead, before **(A)** and after **(B)** radiation therapy. (Courtesy of Dr. Mark A. Cappel by permission of Mayo Foundation for Medical Education and Research. All rights reserved.)

pcALCL has been reported in up to 20% of cases, pcALCL is less likely to self-resolve than LyP, which can be used to help distinguish the two entities.[4] Survival rates of pcALCL are favorable, with an overall survival rate of ~75% and disease-specific survival of ~85% at both 5 and 10 years.[18,47] Despite treatment, relapse is common; the 5-year cumulative risk of developing systemic lymphoma is up to 14%.[47] Because of the favorable overall survival, it is important to not overtreat patients with this condition and patients should be staged with computed tomography or positron emission tomography scans to evaluate for systemic disease. While there are minimal data to substantiate use of one treatment modality over another, therapy should be based on tumor burden. For solitary lesions, the mainstay of treatment is excision with or without radiation. Other treatment options include radiation alone, interferon alpha, and bexarotene. In widespread disease, low-dose methotrexate, doxorubicin-based chemotherapy, and/or brentuximab vedotin can be considered.[18,48]

Lymphomatoid Papulosis

There are many histopathologic variants of LyP (see below); however, their clinical behavior and features are largely identical. In contrast to pcALCL, LyP typically occurs earlier in life, approximately the fifth decade, with a slight male predominance.[4] LyP presents as an often grouped or disseminated papular or papulonecrotic eruption (Fig. 15-3). Up to one- to two-centimeter, ulcerated nodules can occur. The lesions tend to develop as relapsing and remitting crops in different stages of evolution. When LyP occurs as papules and nodules within an erythematous, scaly plaque, it has been called persistent agmination of LyP (Fig. 15-4).[49] Generally, lesions of LyP resolve without treatment in 6 to 10 weeks (Fig. 15-5). Upon resolution, scarring, atrophy, or hyperpigmentation can result (Fig. 15-6). Overall survival rates for LyP are 100 and 92% at 5 and 10 years, respectively.[18] Staging is not required for patients

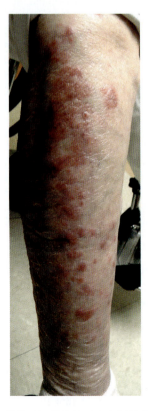

FIGURE 15-2. pcALCL presenting as a group of nodules on the lower leg.

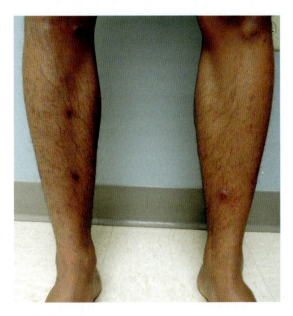

FIGURE 15-3. Lymphomatoid papulosis (LyP) showing nodules at different stages of evolution.

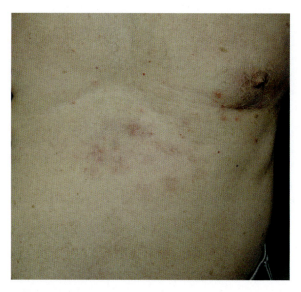

FIGURE 15-4. Persistent agmination of LyP, consisting of papules and nodules within an erythematous, scaly plaque.

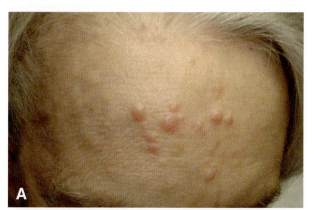

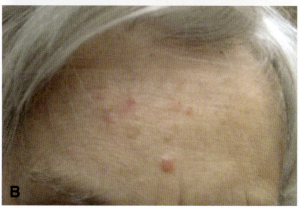

FIGURE 15-5. Lesions of LyP undergoing spontaneous resolution. A crop of lesions on the forehead is shown at presentation **(A)** and 3 weeks later without treatment **(B)**. This case had a *DUSP22* (6p25.3) rearrangement. (Reprinted from Karai LJ, Kadin ME, Hsi ED, Sluzevich JC, et al. Chromosomal rearrangements of 6p25.3 define a new subtype of lymphomatoid papulosis. *Am J Surg Pathol*. 2013;37(8):1173-1181.)

with isolated and uncomplicated (ie, no laboratory abnormalities or enlarged lymph nodes) LyP, but patients should be monitored for the development of additional malignancies including lymphoma, which has been found to be

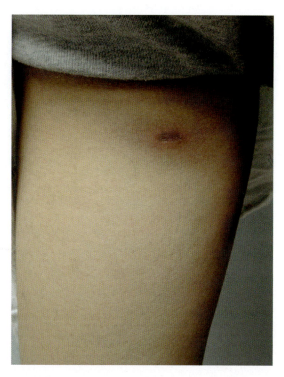

FIGURE 15-6. Resolving LyP lesion showing scarring and hyperpigmentation.

associated with LyP in 16% to 60% of cases.[4,18] Observation is an acceptable management option; low-dose methotrexate, phototherapy, antibiotics, nitrogen mustard, interferon, bexarotene, and rarely brentuximab vedotin also have been used with success.[48]

HISTOLOGY

Primary Cutaneous ALCL

Lesions of pcALCL are characterized by cohesive sheets of large, pleomorphic tumor cells growing within the dermis and occasionally extending into the subcutaneous tissue (Fig. 15-7). Epidermotropism is not characteristic; however, cases with *DUSP22* rearrangements typically show an epidermal component (see below).[50] Tumor cells of pcALCL show cytologic features similar to those of systemic ALCL including hallmark cells. A distinction between anaplastic cytology (75%-80% of cases) and nonanaplastic cytology (pleomorphic or immunoblastic, 20%-25%) has been described but is not associated with clinical presentation or outcome.[4,18,51,52]

The inflammatory background typical of LyP is less often seen in pcALCL, with the exception of a neutrophil-rich variant in which the large cells may be obscured by abundant neutrophils (Fig. 15-8).[52,53] Other histological variants including lymphohistiocytic, inflammatory, and subcutaneous have been reported but are not considered distinct morphological patterns in the WHO classification.[52] pcALCLs with spindle cell morphology may mimic mesenchymal malignancies.[54]

Cases with angiodestructive lesions, morphologically resembling LyP type E (see below), but presenting as

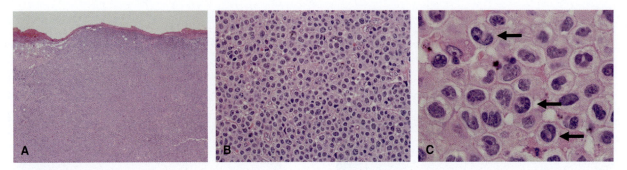

FIGURE 15-7. Typical case of pcALCL demonstrating epidermal ulceration and cohesive sheets of large, pleomorphic tumor cells in the dermis (H&E: **A**, 4×; **B**, 40×). At high magnification, the tumor cells are pleomorphic and some have the folded or reniform nuclear contours and prominent Golgi zone of so-called hallmark cells (arrows; **C**, 100×).

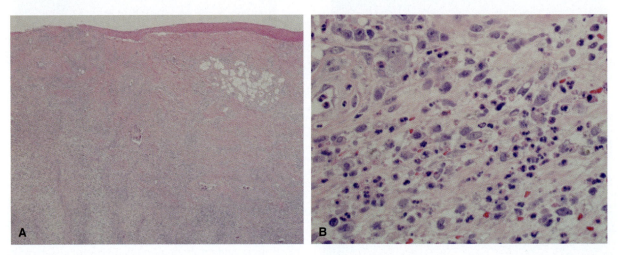

FIGURE 15-8. pcALCL with marked inflammatory background. There is an extensive infiltrate in the dermis with overlying epidermal ulceration (H&E: **A**, 2×). At higher magnification, the tumor cells are admixed with numerous neutrophils, eosinophils, and histiocytes (**B**, 50×).

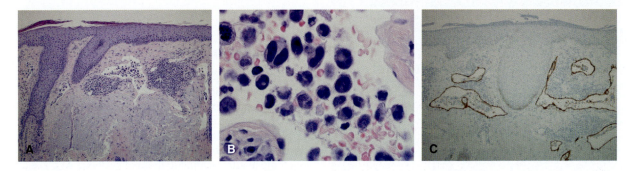

FIGURE 15-9. pcALCL with an intralymphatic pattern. The tumor cells are solely present within lymphatic spaces in the upper dermis (H&E: A, 10×; B, 100×). Immunohistochemistry for podoplanin using the D2-40 antibody highlights the lymphatic endothelium (C, 10×). (Case courtesy of Dr. Mark A. Cappel.)

solitary lesions with clinical features of pcALCL have been described.[55] These cases must be distinguished from more aggressive lymphomas such as extranodal NK/T-cell lymphoma (ENKTCL) that they may mimic pathologically. In addition, a multi-institutional case series has identified a subset of pcALCL cases with a prominent intralymphatic large cell population and lacking features of systemic disease (Fig. 15-9).[56]

pcALCLs harboring *DUSP22* rearrangements may show a unique biphasic histology with sheets of medium to large atypical cells within the dermis and a population of smaller CD30-positive cells infiltrating the epidermis in a pagetoid reticulosis–like pattern.[50]

Lymphomatoid Papulosis

Histologic features of LyP lesions vary widely depending on the histologic subtype and the age of the lesion biopsied. Early lesions show a superficial dermal and perivascular accumulation of atypical cells in an inflammatory background, while more mature lesions typically show a wedge-shaped, more diffuse infiltrate within the dermis.[11,12]

Epidermal hyperplasia is common, and ulceration, spongiosis, and focal epidermal necrosis may be seen in some cases. Neutrophils within the lumens of dermal blood vessels are common.

Six distinct subtypes (A to E and *DUSP22*-rearranged) have been recognized in the WHO classification, though there is overlap between them and lesions of different subtypes can occur in the same patient[2,11,14]; a type F has been proposed.[17]

LyP type A lesions show large, atypical cells in a robust inflammatory background (Fig. 15-10). The atypical cells often show prominent nucleoli and are sometimes reminiscent of Reed-Sternberg cells. In other cases, they resemble immunoblasts with round, eccentric nuclei, a single nucleolus, and amphophilic cytoplasm. These cells are embedded in a mixed inflammatory background characterized by variable numbers of histiocytes, small lymphocytes, neutrophils, and eosinophils, and may appear similar to the cellular background typically seen in classic Hodgkin lymphoma (CHL).

Type B lesions most closely resemble MF (patch and plaque stage), with epidermotropism and a dermal, band-like infiltrate of atypical T cells (Fig. 15-11). The lesional cells in type B are typically smaller than in types A and C (see below) and show convoluted, sometimes cerebriform nuclei without nucleoli. Background inflammation often is not prominent.

In type C lesions, the atypical cells are similar to those in type A, except they form sheets and show a less prominent inflammatory background (Fig. 15-12). Type C lesions may resemble pcALCL both morphologically and immunophenotypically, and distinction often is made on clinical grounds.

LyP type D lesions resemble pagetoid reticulosis with a markedly epidermotropic proliferation of medium-sized, pleomorphic T cells (Fig. 15-13A,B).[14] In some cases the infiltrate is limited to perivascular areas in the superficial dermis, while in others a wedge-shaped infiltrate extending into the deep dermis is seen.[14]

Type E lesions, as described by Kempf et al, are characterized by an angiocentric and angiodestructive infiltrate of medium-sized T cells within the walls of veins and small arteries in the mid-to-deep dermis (Fig. 15-13C,D).[13] Most cases contain a prominent infiltrate of eosinophils either within the dermis or clustering around blood vessels.[13] This angiodestructive growth pattern likely explains the large ulcers that occur in these cases in contrast to other subtypes of LyP.[13]

Type F, or follicular LyP, has been recently proposed by Kempf et al and represents a group of LyP lesions with prominent involvement of hair follicles.[17] These cases may show features of other subtypes, most commonly type A or C, but also demonstrate a prominent perifollicular infiltrate of CD30-positive large cells and sometimes infiltration of

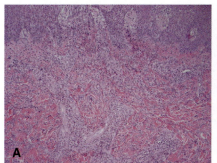
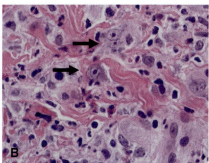
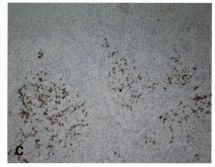

FIGURE 15-10. LyP, type A. There is a mixed inflammatory infiltrate in the upper dermis (H&E: **A**, 10×). The infiltrate contains a mixture of histiocytes, small lymphocytes, eosinophils, and neutrophils, as well as scattered large, atypical and sometimes multinucleate cells with prominent nucleoli (**B**, 100×; arrows). Immunohistochemistry for CD30 highlights the scattered and occasionally clustered distribution of the atypical cells (**C**, 10×).

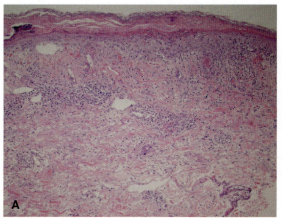
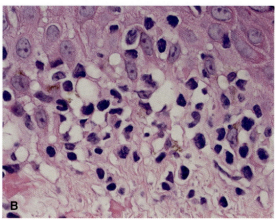

FIGURE 15-11. LyP, type B. There is a band-like lymphocytic infiltrate in the upper dermis with epidermotropism, composed of mostly small lymphocytes with convoluted, sometimes cerebriform nuclei (H&E: **A**, 10×; **B**, 100×). Correlation with clinical features is essential to distinguish this process from MF.

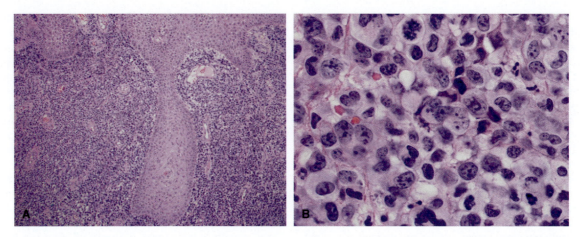

FIGURE 15-12. LyP, type C. There is sheet-like growth of large atypical lymphocytes in the dermis, with morphologic features resembling anaplastic large cell lymphoma (H&E: **A**, 10×; **B**, 100×).

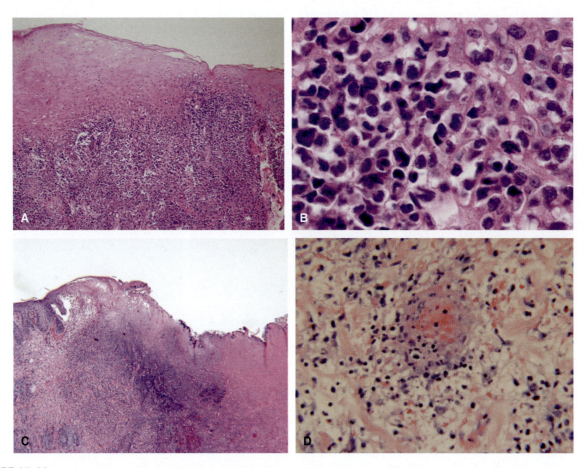

FIGURE 15-13. LyP, types D and E. **A, B.** Type D. There is hyperplastic epidermis with an epidermotropic infiltrate of mostly medium sized, pleomorphic lymphocytes (H&E: **A**, 10×; **B**, 100×). The lymphocytes had a CD8-positive, cytotoxic T-cell phenotype by immunohistochemistry (not shown). **C, D.** Type E. There is ulceration of the epidermis with an accompanying atypical lymphocytic infiltrate showing angioinvasion (H&E: **C**, 20×; **D**, 400×). (Courtesy of Dr. Alejandro Gru). The lymphocytes had a CD8-positive T-cell phenotype and co-expressed CD30 (not shown).

the follicular epithelium and/or follicular mucinosis (Fig. 15-14A,B). Thereby follicular LyP mimics folliculotropic MF with large cell transformation (MF-LCT).

LyP with *DUSP22* (6p25.3) rearrangements, as reported by Karai et al, show a biphasic growth pattern with both epidermal and dermal components, similar to the pattern seen in *DUSP22*-rearranged pcALCL (Fig. 15-15).[16] The epidermal component is composed of small to medium-sized atypical T cells, which may be cerebriform, often showing a pagetoid reticulosis–like growth pattern and occasionally accompanied by Pautrier microabscess–like collections of intraepidermal cells. The dermal component shows a nodular growth

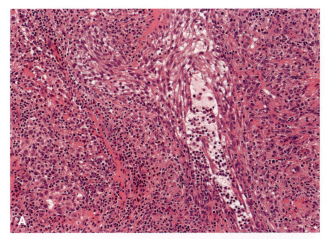

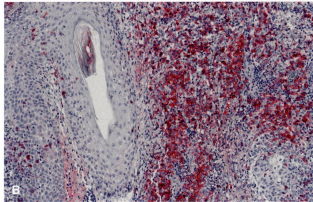

FIGURE 15-14. LyP with folliculotropism. A. Prominent folliculotropism and associated follicular mucinosis is present. **B.** Most of the cells are positive for CD30.

pattern and contains sheets of medium-sized to large transformed cells. These combined histologic features may also resemble some cases of transformed MF, from which these cases must be distinguished clinically.

IMMUNOPHENOTYPE

Primary Cutaneous ALCL

pcALCL demonstrates an immunophenotype essentially indistinguishable from systemic ALK-negative ALCL (Fig. 15-16). Although pcALCL is almost exclusively negative for the ALK protein and rearrangements involving the *ALK* gene,[5-7,57-59] rare ALK-positive ALCLs with disease limited to the skin have been reported; their relationship to ALK-negative pcALCL has not been established.[6-8] Tumor cells in pcALCL show strong, uniform expression of CD30 (>75% of tumor cells, usually 100%), typically with a membrane and Golgi pattern. Weak or partial CD30 expression on tumor cells should raise concern for cutaneous involvement by another PTCL subtype or MF-LCT.

Pan-T-cell antigens (CD2, CD3, and CD5) are variably expressed in pcALCL (Fig. 15-17), but are not lost as frequently as in systemic ALK-positive ALCL.[51,60,61] In a series of 35 pcALCLs, CD2 was expressed in 78%, CD3 in 62%, and CD5 in 48%.[62] Eleven cases (31%) showed loss of at least two pan-T-cell antigens. Although pcALCL is most commonly associated with a CD4-positive T cell phenotype, only one-third of cases showed a CD4+/CD8- phenotype, while 18% were CD4-/CD8+, 20% coexpressed these antigens, and 26% lacked both CD4 and CD8.[62] These findings suggest that the "null" phenotype, more commonly associated with systemic ALCL, may be underrecognized in the cutaneous variant. In addition, pcALCL has been shown to lack expression of transcription factors T-bet and GATA-3, which are associated with T_H1 and T_H2 cell differentiation, respectively.[63] This finding may be useful in distinguishing pcALCL from CD30-positive MF, which is typically diffusely positive for GATA-3.[63] Expression of Galectin-3 in CD30+ tumor cells is significantly lower in MF-LCT in contrast to CD30-positive TLPD, which may be an additional useful hint for the distinction.

Most pcALCLs express cytotoxic markers such as TIA-1, granzyme B, and perforin, with the CD4-/CD8- variants being more likely to lack cytotoxic protein expression.[62] *DUSP22* rearrangements also correlate with a lack of cytotoxic marker expression.[64] Cases with *DUSP22* rearrangements showed expression of LEF-1, a marker that can be used as a surrogate for the presence of the translocation. EMA is expressed less often than in systemic ALK-negative ALCL, whereas cutaneous lymphocyte antigen is expressed more commonly in pcALCL; however, both antigens lack specificity for distinguishing these entities.[57,65] Although B-cell markers (CD20, PAX5) and CD15 are typically negative, these markers can rarely be expressed in ALCL making the distinction from CHL a challenge, particularly when locoregional lymph node involvement occurs[66-68]; in practice, however, this difficulty applies more to systemic ALK-negative ALCL than to pcALCL. EBV and HHV-8 are absent. Expression of EBV should raise concern for cutaneous involvement by a systemic lymphoma such as CHL; ENKTCL, nasal type; or B-cell lymphoma with plasmablastic differentiation. HHV-8 should raise concern for cutaneous involvement by primary effusion lymphoma or plasmablastic lymphoma related to immunodeficiency. Gru et al[69] reported an unusual example of an ALCL that initially mimicked LyP clinically, was associated with immunosuppression, and displayed dissemination to lymph nodes and lung more than 6 months after the onset of skin lesions. Such tumor showed diffuse EBV expression and had a *BRAF V600E* mutation. To date, no such cases have been documented again. Another rare example of pcALCL with aberrant cytokeratins expression (OSCAR, AE1/AE3) has also been noticed (Fig. 15-18A-E). A small number of cases might show TCR-γδ expression.

Lymphomatoid Papulosis

The immunophenotype of the atypical cells in LyP types A and C is similar to that of pcALCL. The cells are CD30-positive T cells that typically express CD4 and often show loss of the pan-T cell antigens CD2, CD3, CD5, and CD7.[60] CD8 typically is negative, although occasional CD8-positive cases of LyP types A and C have been recognized; these may be more common in children.[70] Cytotoxic proteins, especially TIA-1, are commonly expressed.[60] Staining for ALK is negative. Rare cases coexpress CD56.[71,72]

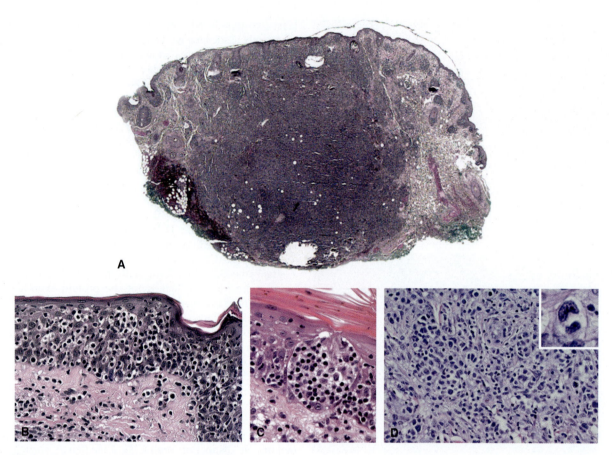

FIGURE 15-15. LyP with *DUSP22* (6p25.3) rearrangement. There is a nodular dermal infiltrate with an overlying epidermotropic component without ulceration (H&E; **A**, 2×). The epidermal component contains mostly small atypical lymphocytes with a pagetoid reticulosis–like pattern of involvement (**B**, 40×). Pautrier microabscess–like collections of intraepidermal lymphocytes occasionally may be seen (**C**, 40×). The dermis typically contains a population of medium-sized to large cells with abundant cytoplasm (**D**, 40×; inset, 100×). (Adapted from Karai LJ, Kadin ME, Hsi ED, et al. Chromosomal rearrangements of 6p25.3 define a new subtype of lymphomatoid papulosis. *Am J Surg Pathol*. 2013;37(8):1173-1181.)

LyP type B shows more variable CD30 expression in the atypical cells, but otherwise shows a similar CD4-positive T cell phenotype, commonly with loss of T-cell antigens as in types A and C. Given the predominantly epidermotropic pattern seen in this subtype, the distinction between LyP type B and MF may be impossible without clinical information.

LyP type D has a characteristic CD8-positive, cytotoxic T-cell phenotype.[14,15] Given the epidermotropic nature of this subtype, these cases may be pathologically indistinguishable from primary cutaneous CD8-positive aggressive epidermotropic cytotoxic T-cell lymphoma, as well as CD8+ MF, and clinical correlation is paramount. LyP type E also frequently is CD8-positive.[13] These cases show variable loss of pan-T cell antigens, and the majority express TIA-1.

Cases of LyP with *DUSP22* rearrangements show variable T-cell antigen expression. A common feature is biphasic expression of CD30, with weak expression in the epidermal component and strong expression in the dermal component (Fig. 15-19).[16] Sometimes a biphasic pattern can also be seen in the expression of T-cell antigens, with stronger expression in the epidermis. Rare cases also show TCR-γδ expression.[73]

GENETIC AND MOLECULAR FINDINGS

The majority of pcALCLs have clonally rearranged T-cell receptor (TCR) genes. However, the inability to detect such a rearrangement does not preclude the diagnosis, as up to 35% of cases can lack a clonal rearrangement.[74] At least 50% of LyP type C, 60% of type E, 40% of type D, and lower numbers of types A and B show clonally rearranged TCR genes, thereby limiting the diagnostic utility of this test in distinguishing LyP from pcALCL.[13,15,72,74]

pcALCL and LyP are almost exclusively negative for the t(2;5)(p23;q35) *NPM1-ALK* and other *ALK* rearrangements found in ALK-positive systemic ALCL. In general, immunohistochemistry for ALK is sufficient to screen for an *ALK* rearrangement and fluorescence in situ hybridization (FISH) is rarely necessary. ALK-positive ALCL limited to the skin had a reported incidence of 2% in a Dutch cohort of 309 pcALCLs.[6-8,59] In total, 21 cases have been reported in the literature, with clinical behavior similar to cohorts of ALK-negative pcALCL. Some cases were precipitated by arthropod bites. Given the small numbers, the relation of these cases to pcALCL has not been addressed in the current WHO classification.

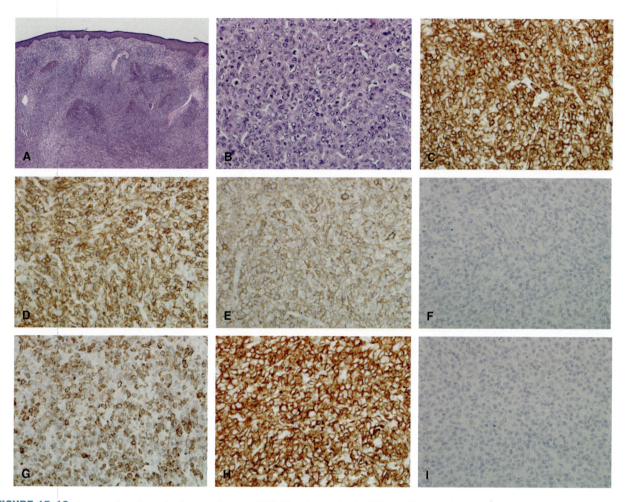

FIGURE 15-16. Immunophenotype of primary cutaneous ALCL. There is an extensive infiltrate of large, atypical lymphocytes in the dermis (H&E: **A**, 4×; **B**, 40×). The tumor cells are positive by immunohistochemistry for CD45 (**C**, 40×), CD45RO (**D**, 40×), and CD43 (**E**, 40×). They are negative for CD20 (**F**, 40×) and positive for CD3 (**G**, 40×). They show strong positivity for CD30 (**H**, 400×) and are negative for ALK (**I**, 40×).

Recurrent chromosomal rearrangements involving the *DUSP22* locus (6p25.3) have been identified in approximately 30% of systemic ALK-negative ALCLs as well as pcALCL (Fig. 15-20), LyP (Fig. 15-21), and ALK-negative ALCL limited to mucosal sites.[16,20,34,64,75-78] *DUSP22* rearrangements are present in 28% of pcALCL, making them the most common recurrent genetic abnormality in pcALCL.[34,64,75-77,79] The genomic breakpoint may be within the *DUSP22* or the neighboring *IRF4* gene, but in ALCLs the rearrangements are associated with *DUSP22* downregulation, while expression levels of *IRF4* remain constant.[34] The role of DUSP22 in the pathogenesis of CD30-positive TLPDs remains uncertain, although a tumor suppressor role has been postulated.[79] The most common partner in *DUSP22* rearrangements is a nongenic locus on 7q32.3 resulting in the t(6;7)(p25.3;q32.3) translocation; however, other partner loci of unknown significance have been described.[80] These rearrangements are distinct from t(6;14)(p25.3;q11.2) translocations, which fuse the *IRF4* gene to the TCRα (*TRA*) locus and are seen in rare cases of CD30-negative PTCL.[64,81]

Systemic ALK-negative ALCLs with *DUSP22* rearrangements have outcomes more favorable than other ALK-negative ALCLs, and similar to systemic ALK-positive ALCLs.[82] It is uncertain whether outcome within the already prognostically favorable pcALCL and LyP groups of diseases is affected by the presence of *DUSP22* rearrangements. Like LyP and pcALCL in general, distinguishing between these two entities when a *DUSP22* rearrangement is present relies on clinical correlation.[50] Rare cases of MF-LCT with *DUSP22* rearrangements have been reported, but the significance of this finding is unclear.[76]

Rearrangements involving *TP63* have been identified in systemic ALK-negative ALCL and are associated with poor prognosis.[82,83] Rare cases of pcALCL with *TP63* rearrangements have been described, both of which exhibited unusually aggressive clinical behavior (Fig. 15-22). However, there are insufficient data to know whether this represents a distinct subset of pcALCL.[83] Of note, rare cases of MF-LCT with a *TP63* rearrangement have also been described.[84] LyP with *TP63* rearrangement has not been reported.

Chromosomal copy-number analysis of pcALCL has revealed recurrent gains on chromosomes 7q and 17q and losses on 6q and 13q.[40] These cases showed higher expression levels of the skin-homing chemokine receptor genes *CCR10* and *CCR8* relative to PTCL, NOS, possibly accounting for the propensity of pcALCL to remain localized.[40] Conventional karyotyping has revealed normal cytogenetic studies in some LyP cases, while others have shown trisomy 7 and abnormalities of chromosome 10.[85] The significance of these abnormalities has not been established and no

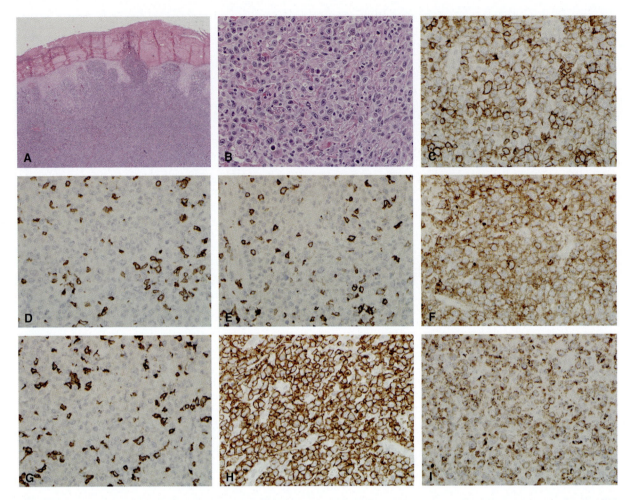

FIGURE 15-17. Primary cutaneous ALCL with loss of T-cell antigens. There is an extensive infiltrate of large, atypical lymphocytes in the dermis (H&E: **A**, 4×; **B**, 40×). The tumor cells are positive by immunohistochemistry for the pan-T-cell marker CD2 (**C**, 40×), but show aberrant loss of expression of CD3 (**D**, 40×) and CD5 (**E**, 40×). There are positive for CD4 (**F**, 40×) and negative for CD8 (**G**, 40×). The show strong and uniform expression of CD30 (**H**, 40×) and express the cytotoxic marker, TIA1 (**I**, 40×). They also were positive for the cytotoxic marker, granzyme B, and were negative for ALK (not shown).

genetic abnormality has been found to distinguish pcALCL from LyP or from cutaneous involvement by systemic ALK-negative ALCL.

Due to their rarity, there are relatively few studies looking at the mutational landscape of cutaneous CD30-positive LPDs. However, recent next-generation sequencing studies have unveiled a pattern of mutations and fusions leading to constitutive activation of the JAK-STAT pathway in cutaneous CD30-positive LPDs, a finding these lesions share with their systemic and breast implant-associated counterparts.[37,39,86]

POSTULATED CELL OF ORIGIN

Both pcALCL and LyP are believed to derive from an activated T cell, as evidenced by the CD30 expression that characterizes these lymphoproliferations.[87] CD30 is a member of the TNF receptor superfamily and is expressed on both benign and malignant activated lymphocytes.[88] However, the specific cell of origin of CD30-positive TLPDs has not been fully elucidated. While most cases have a CD4-positive T-helper phenotype, both pcALCL and LyP can show CD8 expression.[14,15,60,62] In addition, some express CD4 and CD25, consistent with a regulatory T-cell immune profile.[89] Finally, expression of the thymocyte protein SATB1 defines a group of cutaneous CD30-positive TLPDs with a T-helper 17 cytokine profile.[90]

DIFFERENTIAL DIAGNOSIS

Systemic Anaplastic Large Cell Lymphoma

Extranodal involvement of systemic ALCL occurs in up to 60% of cases, with the skin being the most common site.[91] ALK positivity by immunohistochemistry or the presence of an *ALK* gene rearrangement is associated with systemic disease in the majority of cases, but rarely may be seen in disease limited to the skin. Therefore, a diagnosis of systemic ALK-positive ALCL should not be made on the basis of a skin biopsy without careful clinical correlation and staging. The presence of EMA staining within tumor cells is more common in systemic ALCL, but also should not be used as a strict diagnostic criterion. In ALK-negative cases, histopathologic, immunophenotypic, and genetic features typically

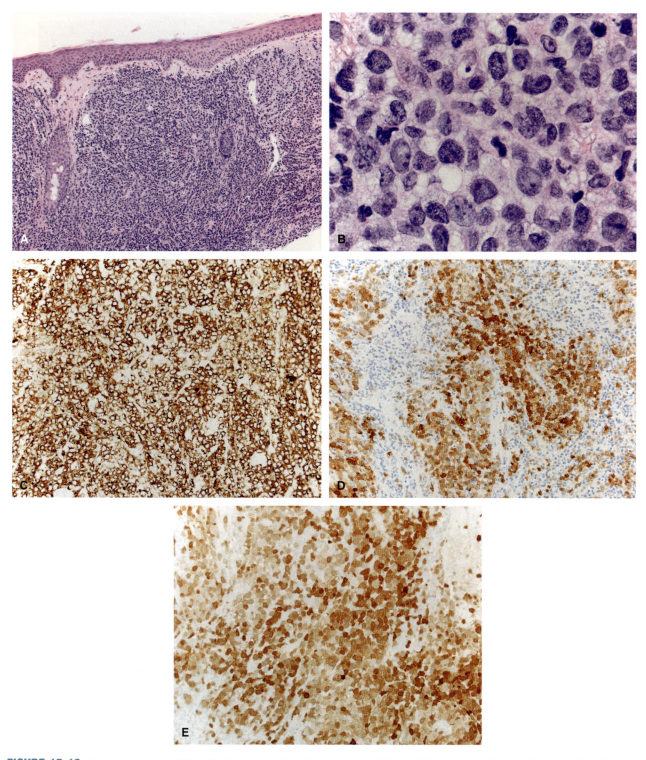

FIGURE 15-18. Primary cutaneous ALCL with aberrant cytokeratins expression. A, Dense infiltrate in the dermis, sparing the epidermis. **B**, Numerous hallmark cells are present. **C**, The cells are diffusely positive for CD30. **D**, pan-CK is positive in a significant subset of cells. **E**, OSCAR CK is also immunoreactive in the neoplastic cells. (Courtesy of Dr. Alejandro A Gru, University of Virginia).

are insufficient to distinguish between systemic ALCL and pcALCL (Fig. 15-23). Clinical features including localized lesions, lack of lymphadenopathy, and spontaneous regression favor a primary cutaneous process. Appropriate staging studies and full clinicopathologic correlation typically allow for the distinction between systemic and pcALCL. pcALCL can spread to locoregional lymph nodes without adversely affecting the generally favorable prognosis of this disease.[4] Therefore, lymph node involvement should not be taken as definitive evidence of systemic disease. When both skin and lymph node involvement are present, a careful clinical history is critical to determine the sequence of evolution of disease at the various anatomic sites to classify the disease correctly. *DUSP22* rearrangements occur with similar frequencies in

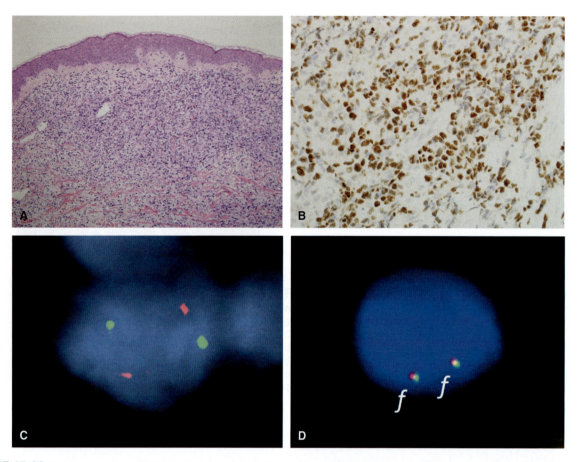

FIGURE 15-22. Primary cutaneous ALCL with *TP63* rearrangement. There is a dermal infiltrate of large atypical lymphocytes (H&E: **A**, 10×) that is positive for p63 by immunohistochemistry (**B**, 40×). The tumor cells also expressed CD30, and were negative for ALK (not shown). A break-apart FISH probe for the *TP63* locus on 3q28 shows no normal fusion signals and abnormally split red-green signals, indicating two copies of the rearranged *TP63* locus (**C**, 60×). In contrast, two fusion signals (*f*) are seen in a cell from a normal skin specimen (**D**, 60×).

these two conditions. Expression of the T_H2-associated transcription factor, GATA-3, may aid in this distinction, as pcALCL is negative for this marker, while CD30-positive MF shows diffuse positivity by IHC.[63] The possibility of true pcALCL arising in patients with a history of MF merits further study since the prognosis and management of pcALCL and MF-LCT are markedly different.[9,10]

The role of *DUSP22* rearrangements in distinguishing primary cutaneous CD30-positive TLPDs from MF-LCT remains unclear. These rearrangements are present in ~28% of pcALCLs and in at least one series were absent in cases of MF-LCT.[73] However, one study reported two cases of MF-LCT with *DUSP22* rearrangement.[76] LyP with *DUSP22* (6p25.3) rearrangements may resemble MF-LCT pathologically, with an epidermotropic infiltrate of smaller atypical T cells and a dermal nodule of larger transformed cells.[16] However, clinical data usually can differentiate these entities, as LyP with *DUSP22* rearrangement presents as localized crops of spontaneously regressing papules.

Other T-cell Lymphomas

The newly described LyP type D shows overlapping histopathologic features with the WHO provisional entity, primary cutaneous CD8-positive aggressive epidermotropic cytotoxic T-cell lymphoma.[72] This rare lymphoma shows variable clinical features, but often presents with rapidly progressing, necrotic skin lesions, aggressive course, and poor prognosis.[96] Lesions show a markedly epidermotropic proliferation of CD8-positive T cells that usually are negative for CD30. This feature as well as the naïve, CD45RA-positive/CD45RO-negative phenotype of this aggressive lymphoma may be useful in distinguishing it from LyP.[72] Ultimately, however, the clinical features are paramount in this distinction.

The differential diagnosis of LyP type E, which shows large pleomorphic lymphocytes with angioinvasion, includes ENKTCL, nasal type; primary cutaneous gamma/delta T-cell lymphoma; and systemic PTCLs. LyP type E should be consistently negative for EBV, whereas EBV is positive in virtually all cases of ENKTCL.[13] CD30 expression is more variable in ENKTCL than LyP, but can be positive in the former. TCRβ is consistently expressed in LyP type E, and no cases with a γδ phenotype have been described.[13] As with other subtypes, distinction between LyP type E and an aggressive systemic lymphoma relies heavily on clinical information.

Pityriasis Lichenoides

Pityriasis lichenoides et varioliformis acuta (PLEVA) is an inflammatory condition, primarily of younger patients, that

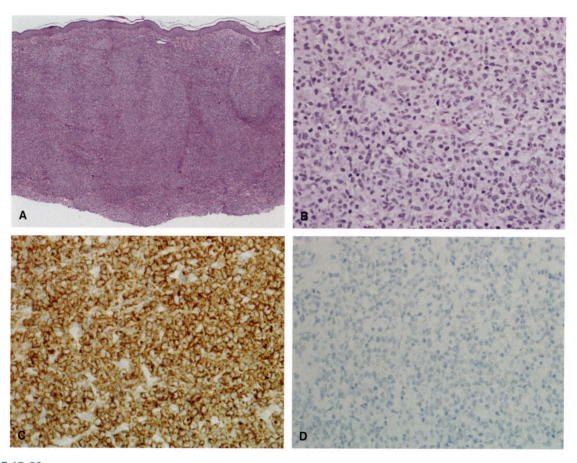

FIGURE 15-23. Secondary cutaneous involvement by systemic ALK-negative ALCL. There is a dermal infiltrate of large atypical lymphocytes (H&E: **A**, 4×; **B**, 40×) that is strongly and uniformly positive for CD30 by immunohistochemistry (**C**, 40×). ALK is negative (**D**, 40×). Distinction from primary cutaneous ALCL relies on the clinical history.

may present with lesions similar in clinical and histologic appearance to LyP type B and D.[97-100] Patients with PLEVA present with crops of erythematous macules and papules that may become pustular or necrotic and usually resolve permanently after a few weeks without scar formation.[100] On biopsy, lesions reveal a perivascular and diffuse lymphohistiocytic infiltrate, but typically lack the cytologic atypia seen in LyP.[97,98,100] The infiltrate typically is polymorphic, but neutrophils and eosinophils are uncommonly seen.[98] The presence of interface dermatitis with vacuolization in the junctional zone, necrotic keratinocytes, and extravasated red blood cells favor PLEVA over LyP.[98,99] Further complicating the distinction from LyP, T-cell clones often can be found in PLEVA.[101] Clinical features and thorough histopathologic evaluation allow distinction between PLEVA and LyP in most cases.

Other Reactive Conditions

Large CD30-positive cells can be seen amid a mixed inflammatory background in various reactive skin conditions, especially arthropod bites, viral infections, and drug reactions.[97] Cases of milker's nodule, herpes simplex virus, varicella zoster virus, molluscum, syphilis, tick bite, scabies, and leishmaniasis have all been reported to cause skin eruptions with proliferations of CD30-positive large cells. Various drug reactions also are well known for having dense cutaneous lymphoid infiltrates, often with large atypical cells. Drugs most often implicated include antiepileptics and chemotherapeutic agents.

CAPSULE SUMMARY

- Primary cutaneous CD30-positive T-cell lymphoproliferative disorders include primary cutaneous anaplastic large cell lymphoma (pcALCL) and lymphomatoid papulosis (LyP), which exist along a clinical and pathologic spectrum. While most cases can be classified as either pcALCL or LyP, borderline cases in which overlapping features preclude definitive classification exist.
- LyP is an indolent cutaneous lymphoproliferative disorder characterized clinically by a recurrent papulonodular eruption with a waxing and waning clinical course. There is an expanding number of recognized pathologic subtypes of LyP that show variable proportions of atypical CD30-positive T cells and reactive inflammatory cells. Despite marked variation in histologic appearance, the clinical behavior of these subtypes is similar.
- pcALCL resembles systemic ALCL but presents in the skin and is almost exclusively negative for the ALK protein and rearrangements involving the *ALK* gene. *DUSP22* rearrangements involving the locus are present in 28% of

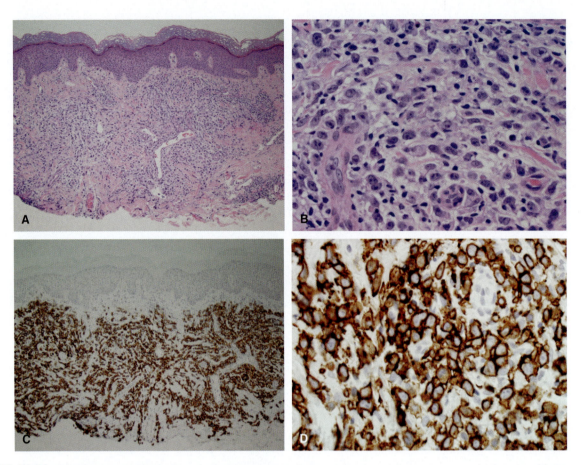

FIGURE 15-24. MF with large cell transformation and strong CD30 expression. This biopsy in a patient with confirmed MF shows a population of large atypical lymphocytes in the dermis without a significant epidermotropic component (H&E: **A**, 10×; **B**, 40×). The cells showed strong and uniform expression of CD30 by immunohistochemistry (**C**, 10×; **D**, 40×). The disease pursued an aggressive clinical course.

pcALCLs, making this the most common recurrent genetic abnormality in this disease. Cases of LyP with *DUSP22* rearrangements also have been described.
- The genomic landscape of primary cutaneous CD30-positive T-cell lymphoproliferative disorders has not been entirely elucidated, but early data suggest recurrent alterations in JAK-STAT pathway genes similar to those described in systemic ALCLs.
- Histopathologic overlap may occur between primary cutaneous CD30-positive T-cell lymphoproliferative disorders and large cell transformation of mycosis fungoides. Clinical history is essential and clonality studies may be useful in this setting.
- The myriad histopathologic patterns seen in LyP can mimic a variety of more aggressive lymphomas. Careful clinical history, physical examination, and staging are needed to avoid overtreatment in these cases.

References

1. Willemze R, Cerroni L, Kempf W, et al. The 2018 update of the WHO-EORTC classification for primary cutaneous lymphomas. *Blood*. 2019;133(16):1703-1714.
2. Willemze R, Paulli M, Kadin ME. Primary cutaneous CD30-positive T-cell lymphoproliferative disorders. In: Swerdlow S, Campo E, Harris N, et al, eds. *WHO Classification of Tumours of Haematopoietic and Lymphoid Tissues*. International Agency for Research on Cancer; 2017:392-396.
3. Kempf W, Kerl K, Mitteldorf C. Cutaneous CD30-positive T-cell lymphoproliferative disorders-clinical and histopathologic features, differential diagnosis, and treatment. *Semin Cutan Med Surg*. 2018;37(1):24-29.
4. Bekkenk MW, Geelen FA, van Voorst Vader PC, et al. Primary and secondary cutaneous CD30(+) lymphoproliferative disorders: a report from the Dutch Cutaneous Lymphoma Group on the long-term follow-up data of 219 patients and guidelines for diagnosis and treatment. *Blood*. 2000;95(12):3653-3661.
5. ten Berge RL, Oudejans JJ, Ossenkoppele GJ, et al. ALK expression in extranodal anaplastic large cell lymphoma favours systemic disease with (primary) nodal involvement and a good prognosis and occurs before dissemination. *J Clin Pathol*. 2000;53(6):445-450.
6. Kadin ME, Pinkus JL, Pinkus GS, et al. Primary cutaneous ALCL with phosphorylated/activated cytoplasmic ALK and novel phenotype: EMA/MUC1+, cutaneous lymphocyte antigen negative. *Am J Surg Pathol*. 2008;32(9):1421-1426.
7. Oschlies I, Lisfeld J, Lamant L, et al. ALK-positive anaplastic large cell lymphoma limited to the skin: clinical, histopathological and molecular analysis of 6 pediatric cases. A report from the ALCL99 study. *Haematologica*. 2013;98(1):50-56.
8. Melchers RC, Willemze R, van de Loo M, et al. Clinical, histologic, and molecular characteristics of anaplastic lymphoma kinase-positive primary cutaneous anaplastic large cell lymphoma. *Am J Surg Pathol*. 2020;44(6):776-781.

9. Gao C, McCormack CJ, van der Weyden C, et al. The importance of differentiating between mycosis fungoides with CD30-positive large cell transformation and mycosis fungoides with coexistent primary cutaneous anaplastic large cell lymphoma. *J Am Acad Dermatol.* 2021;84(1):185-187.
10. Cieza-Diaz DE, Prieto-Torres L, Rodriguez-Pinilla SM, et al. Mycosis fungoides associated with lesions in the spectrum of primary cutaneous CD30+ lymphoproliferative disorders: the same process or 3 coexisting lymphomas? *Am J Dermatopathol.* 2019;41(11):846-850.
11. El Shabrawi-Caelen L, Kerl H, Cerroni L. Lymphomatoid papulosis: reappraisal of clinicopathologic presentation and classification into subtypes A, B, and C. *Arch Dermatol.* 2004;140(4):441-447.
12. Macaulay WL. Lymphomatoid papulosis. A continuing self-healing eruption, clinically benign--histologically malignant. *Arch Dermatol.* 1968;97(1):23-30.
13. Kempf W, Kazakov DV, Schärer L, et al. Angioinvasive lymphomatoid papulosis: a new variant simulating aggressive lymphomas. *Am J Surg Pathol.* 2013;37(1):1-13. doi:10.1097/PAS.1090b1013e3182648596.
14. Saggini A, Gulia A, Argenyi Z, et al. A variant of lymphomatoid papulosis simulating primary cutaneous aggressive epidermotropic CD8+ cytotoxic T-cell lymphoma. Description of 9 cases. *Am J Surg Pathol.* 2010;34(8):1168-1175.
15. Bertolotti A, Pham-Ledard AL, Vergier B, Parrens M, Bedane C, Beylot-Barry M. Lymphomatoid papulosis type D: an aggressive histology for an indolent disease. *Br J Dermatol.* 2013;169(5):1157-1159.
16. Karai LJ, Kadin ME, Hsi ED, et al. Chromosomal rearrangements of 6p25.3 define a new subtype of lymphomatoid papulosis. *Am J Surg Pathol.* 2013;37(8):1173-1181.
17. Kempf W, Kazakov DV, Baumgartner H-P, Kutzner H. Follicular lymphomatoid papulosis revisited: a study of 11 cases, with new histopathological findings. *J Am Acad Dermatol.* 2013;68(5):809-816.
18. Liu HL, Hoppe RT, Kohler S, Harvell JD, Reddy S, Kim YH. CD30+ cutaneous lymphoproliferative disorders: the Stanford experience in lymphomatoid papulosis and primary cutaneous anaplastic large cell lymphoma. *J Am Acad Dermatol.* 2003;49(6):1049-1058.
19. Savage KJ, Harris NL, Vose JM, et al. ALK-anaplastic large-cell lymphoma is clinically and immunophenotypically different from both ALK+ ALCL and peripheral T-cell lymphoma, not otherwise specified: report from the International Peripheral T-Cell Lymphoma Project. *Blood.* 2008;111(12):5496-5504.
20. Booken N, Goerdt S, Klemke C-D. Clinical spectrum of primary cutaneous CD30-positive anaplastic large cell lymphoma: an analysis of the Mannheim Cutaneous Lymphoma Registry. *J Dtsch Dermatol Ges.* 2012;10(5):331-339.
21. Kumar S, Pittaluga S, Raffeld M, Guerrera M, Seibel NL, Jaffe ES. Primary cutaneous CD30-positive anaplastic large cell lymphoma in childhood: report of 4 cases and review of the literature. *Pediatr Dev Pathol.* 2005;8(1):52-60.
22. Feldman AL, Flowers CR. Ethnic disparity in primary cutaneous CD30(+) T-cell lymphoproliferative disorders: an analysis of 1496 cases from the US National Cancer database. *Br J Haematol.* 2018;181(6):721-722.
23. Wang SS, Flowers CR, Kadin ME, et al. Medical history, lifestyle, family history, and occupational risk factors for peripheral T-cell lymphomas: the InterLymph Non-Hodgkin Lymphoma Subtypes Project. *J Natl Cancer Inst Monogr.* 2014;2014(48):66-75.
24. Miquel J, Fraitag S, Hamel-Teillac D, et al. Lymphomatoid papulosis in children: a series of 25 cases. *Br J Dermatol.* 2014;171(5):1138-1146.
25. Georgesen C, Magro C. Lymphomatoid papulosis in children and adolescents: a clinical and histopathologic retrospective cohort. *Ann Diagn Pathol.* 2020;46:151486.
26. Fletcher CL, Orchard GE, Hubbard V, Whittaker SJ, Edelson RL, Russell-Jones R. CD30+ cutaneous lymphoma in association with atopic eczema. *Arch Dermatol.* 2004;140(4):449-454.
27. Kadin ME, Hamilton RG, Vonderheid EC. Evidence linking atopy and staphylococcal superantigens to the pathogenesis of lymphomatoid papulosis, a recurrent CD30+ cutaneous lymphoproliferative disorder. *PLoS One.* 2020;15(2):e0228751.
28. Wang HH, Myers T, Lach LJ, Hsieh C-C, Kadin ME. Increased risk of lymphoid and nonlymphoid malignancies in patients with lymphomatoid papulosis. *Cancer.* 1999;86(7):1240-1245.
29. Rongioletti F. Frequency, risk factors and prognosis of systemic haematologic malignancies, cutaneous and other neoplasms in lymphomatoid papulosis: where are we now? *J Eur Acad Dermatol Venereol.* 2020;34(2):216-217.
30. AbuHilal M, Walsh S, Shear N. Associated hematolymphoid malignancies in patients with lymphomatoid papulosis: a Canadian retrospective study. *J Cutan Med Surg.* 2017;21(6):507-512.
31. Davis TH, Morton CC, Miller-Cassman R, Balk SP, Kadin ME. Hodgkin's disease, lymphomatoid papulosis, and cutaneous T-cell lymphoma derived from a common T-cell clone. *N Engl J Med.* 1992;326(17):1115-1122.
32. Kaul S, Belzberg M, Hughes JM, et al. Comorbidities in mycosis fungoides and racial differences in co-existent lymphomatoid papulosis: a cross-sectional study of 580 patients in an Urban Tertiary Care Center. *Medicines (Basel).* 2019;7(1).
33. Lucioni M, Ippoliti G, Campana C, et al. EBV positive primary cutaneous CD30+ large T-cell lymphoma in a heart transplanted patient: case report. *Am J Transplant.* 2004;4(11):1915-1920.
34. Feldman AL, Dogan A, Smith DI, et al. Discovery of recurrent t(6;7)(p25.3;q32.3) translocations in ALK-negative anaplastic large cell lymphomas by massively-parallel genomic sequencing. *Blood.* 2011;117(3):915-919.
35. Sekine Y, Ikeda O, Hayakawa Y, et al. DUSP22/LMW-DSP2 regulates estrogen receptor-alpha-mediated signaling through dephosphorylation of Ser-118. *Oncogene.* 2007;26(41):6038-6049.
36. Li JP, Yang CY, Chuang HC, et al. The phosphatase JKAP/DUSP22 inhibits T-cell receptor signalling and autoimmunity by inactivating Lck. *Nat Commun.* 2014;5:3618.
37. Maurus K, Appenzeller S, Roth S, et al. Recurrent oncogenic JAK and STAT alterations in cutaneous CD30-positive lymphoproliferative disorders. *J Invest Dermatol.* 2020;140(10):2023-2031.e2021.
38. Hu G, Dasari S, Asmann YW, et al. Targetable fusions of the FRK tyrosine kinase in ALK-negative anaplastic large cell lymphoma. *Leukemia.* 2018;32(2):565-569.
39. Crescenzo R, Abate F, Lasorsa E, et al. Convergent mutations and kinase fusions lead to oncogenic STAT3 activation in anaplastic large cell lymphoma. *Cancer Cell.* 2015;27(4):516-532.

40. van Kester MS, Tensen CP, Vermeer MH, et al. Cutaneous anaplastic large cell lymphoma and peripheral T-cell lymphoma NOS show distinct chromosomal alterations and differential expression of chemokine receptors and apoptosis regulators. *J Invest Dermatol*. 2010;130(2):563-575.
41. Shono Y, Suga H, Kamijo H, et al. Expression of CCR3 and CCR4 suggests a poor prognosis in mycosis fungoides and sezary syndrome. *Acta Derm Venereol*. 2019;99(9):809-812.
42. Braun FK, Hirsch B, Al-Yacoub N, et al. Resistance of cutaneous anaplastic large-cell lymphoma cells to apoptosis by death ligands is enhanced by CD30-mediated overexpression of c-FLIP. *J Invest Dermatol*. 2009;130(3):826-840.
43. Boddicker RL, Kip NS, Xing X, et al. The oncogenic transcription factor IRF4 is regulated by a novel CD30/NF-kappaB positive feedback loop in peripheral T-cell lymphoma. *Blood*. 2015;125:3118-3127.
44. Lohoff M, Mittrucker HW, Brustle A, et al. Enhanced TCR-induced apoptosis in interferon regulatory factor 4-deficient CD4(+) Th cells. *J Exp Med*. 2004;200(2):247-253.
45. Durkop H, Hirsch B, Hahn C, Foss HD, Stein H. Differential expression and function of A20 and TRAF1 in Hodgkin lymphoma and anaplastic large cell lymphoma and their induction by CD30 stimulation. *J Pathol*. 2003;200(2):229-239.
46. Yi S, Sun J, Qiu L, et al. Dual role of EZH2 in cutaneous anaplastic large cell lymphoma: promoting tumor cell survival and regulating tumor microenvironment. *J Invest Dermatol*. 2018;138(5):1126-1136.
47. Hapgood G, Pickles T, Sehn LH, et al. Outcome of primary cutaneous anaplastic large cell lymphoma: a 20-year British Columbia Cancer Agency experience. *Br J Haematol*. 2016;176(2):234-240.
48. Shinohara MM, Shustov A. How I treat primary cutaneous CD30(+) lymphoproliferative disorders. *Blood*. 2019;134(6):515-524.
49. Heald P, Subtil A, Breneman D, Wilson LD. Persistent agmination of lymphomatoid papulosis: an equivalent of limited plaque mycosis fungoides type of cutaneous T-cell lymphoma. *J Am Acad Dermatol*. 2007;57(6):1005-1011.
50. Onaindia A, Montes-Moreno S, Rodríguez-Pinilla SM, et al. Primary cutaneous anaplastic large cell lymphomas with 6p25.3 rearrangement exhibit peculiar histological features. *Histopathology*. 2014;66(6):846-855.
51. Willemze R, Jaffe ES, Burg G, et al. WHO-EORTC classification for cutaneous lymphomas. *Blood*. 2005;105(10):3768-3785.
52. Massone C, El-Shabrawi-Caelen L, Kerl H, Cerroni L. The morphologic spectrum of primary cutaneous anaplastic large T-cell lymphoma: a histopathologic study on 66 biopsy specimens from 47 patients with report of rare variants. *J Cutan Pathol*. 2008;35(1):46-53.
53. Mann KP, Hall B, Kamino H, Borowitz MJ, Ratech H. Neutrophil-rich, Ki-1-positive anaplastic large-cell malignant lymphoma. *Am J Surg Pathol*. 1995;19(4):407-416.
54. Gru AA, Bhagat G, Subtil A, et al. Spindle-cell (sarcomatoid) variant of cutaneous anaplastic large-cell lymphoma (C-ALCL): an unusual mimicker of cutaneous malignant mesenchymal tumors-A series of 11 cases. *Am J Surg Pathol*. 2020;45(6):796-802.
55. Kempf W, Kazakov DV, Paredes BE, Laeng HR, Palmedo G, Kutzner H. Primary cutaneous anaplastic large cell lymphoma with angioinvasive features and cytotoxic phenotype: a rare lymphoma variant within the spectrum of CD30+ lymphoproliferative disorders. *Dermatology*. 2013;227(4):346-352.
56. Samols MA, Su A, Ra S, et al. Intralymphatic cutaneous anaplastic large cell lymphoma/lymphomatoid papulosis: expanding the spectrum of CD30-positive lymphoproliferative disorders. *Am J Surg Pathol*. 2014;38(9):1203-1211.
57. de Bruin PC, Beljaards RC, van Heerde P, et al. Differences in clinical behaviour and immunophenotype between primary cutaneous and primary nodal anaplastic large cell lymphoma of T-cell or null cell phenotype. *Histopathology*. 1993;23(2):127-135.
58. DeCoteau JF, Butmarc JR, Kinney MC, Kadin ME. The t(2;5) chromosomal translocation is not a common feature of primary cutaneous CD30+ lymphoproliferative disorders: comparison with anaplastic large-cell lymphoma of nodal origin. *Blood*. 1996;87(8):3437-3441.
59. Attygalle AD, Cabecadas J, Gaulard P, et al. Peripheral T-cell and NK-cell lymphomas and their mimics; taking a step forward - report on the lymphoma workshop of the XVIth meeting of the European Association for Haematopathology and the Society for Hematopathology. *Histopathology*. 2014;64(2):171-199.
60. Kummer JA, Vermeer MH, Dukers D, Meijer CJ, Willemze R. Most primary cutaneous CD30-positive lymphoproliferative disorders have a CD4-positive cytotoxic T-cell phenotype. *J Invest Dermatol*. 1997;109(5):636-640.
61. Boulland ML, Wechsler J, Bagot M, Pulford K, Kanavaros P, Gaulard P. Primary CD30-positive cutaneous T-cell lymphomas and lymphomatoid papulosis frequently express cytotoxic proteins. *Histopathology*. 2000;36(2):136-144.
62. Massone C, Cerroni L. Phenotypic variability in primary cutaneous anaplastic large T-cell lymphoma: a study on 35 patients. *Am J Dermatopathol*. 2014;36(2):153-157.
63. Hsi AC, Lee SJ, Rosman IS, et al. Expression of helper T cell master regulators in inflammatory dermatoses and primary cutaneous T-cell lymphomas: diagnostic implications. *J Am Acad Dermatol*. 2015;72(1):159-167.
64. Feldman AL, Law M, Remstein ED, et al. Recurrent translocations involving the IRF4 oncogene locus in peripheral T-cell lymphomas. *Leukemia*. 2009;23(3):574-580.
65. Savage KJ. Peripheral T-cell lymphomas. *Blood Rev*. 2007;21(4):201-216.
66. Asano N, Oshiro A, Matsuo K, et al. Prognostic significance of T-cell or cytotoxic molecules phenotype in classical Hodgkin's lymphoma: a clinicopathologic study. *J Clin Oncol*. 2006;24(28):4626-4633.
67. Feldman AL, Law ME, Inwards DJ, Dogan A, McClure RF, Macon WR. PAX5-positive T-cell anaplastic large cell lymphomas associated with extra copies of the PAX5 gene locus. *Mod Pathol*. 2010;23(4):593-602.
68. Venkataraman G, Song JY, Tzankov A, et al. Aberrant T-cell antigen expression in classical Hodgkin lymphoma is associated with decreased event-free survival and overall survival. *Blood*. 2013;121(10):1795-1804.
69. Gru AA, Williams E, Junkins-Hopkins JM. An immune suppression-associated EBV-positive anaplastic large cell lymphoma with a BRAF V600E mutation. *Am J Surg Pathol*. 2019;43(1):140-146. doi:10.1097/PAS.0000000000001174.
70. de Souza A, Camilleri MJ, Wada DA, Appert DL, Gibson LE, el-Azhary RA. Clinical, histopathologic, and immunophenotypic features of lymphomatoid papulosis with CD8 predominance in 14 pediatric patients. *J Am Acad Dermatol*. 2009;61(6):993-1000.

71. Flann S, Orchard GE, Wain EM, Russell-Jones R. Three cases of lymphomatoid papulosis with a CD56+ immunophenotype. *J Am Acad Dermatol.* 2006;55(5):903-906.
72. Plaza JA, Feldman AL, Magro C. Cutaneous CD30-positive lymphoproliferative disorders with CD8 expression: a clinicopathologic study of 21 cases. *J Cutan Pathol.* 2013;40(2):236-247.
73. Rodríguez-Pinilla SM, Ortiz-Romero PL, Monsalvez V, et al. TCR-γ expression in primary cutaneous T-cell lymphomas. *Am J Surg Pathol.* 2013;37(3):375-384. doi:10.1097/PAS.0b013e318275d1a2.
74. Greisser J, Palmedo G, Sander C, et al. Detection of clonal rearrangement of T-cell receptor genes in the diagnosis of primary cutaneous CD30+ lymphoproliferative disorders. *J Cutan Pathol.* 2006;33(11):711-715.
75. Wada DA, Law ME, Hsi ED, et al. Specificity of IRF4 translocations for primary cutaneous anaplastic large cell lymphoma: a multicenter study of 204 skin biopsies. *Mod Pathol.* 2011;24(4):596-605.
76. Pham-Ledard A, Prochazkova-Carlotti M, Laharanne E, et al. IRF4 gene rearrangements define a subgroup of CD30-positive cutaneous T-cell lymphoma: a study of 54 cases. *J Invest Dermatol.* 2010;130(3):816-825.
77. Kiran T, Demirkesen C, Eker C, Kumusoglu H, Tuzuner N. The significance of MUM1/IRF4 protein expression and IRF4 translocation of CD30(+) cutaneous T-cell lymphoproliferative disorders: a study of 53 cases. *Leuk Res.* 2013;37(4):396-400.
78. Sciallis AP, Law ME, Inwards DJ, et al. Mucosal CD30-positive T-cell lymphoproliferations of the head and neck show a clinicopathologic spectrum similar to cutaneous CD30-positive T-cell lymphoproliferative disorders. *Mod Pathol.* 2012;25(7):983-992.
79. Csikesz CR, Knudson RA, Greipp PT, Feldman AL, Kadin M. Primary cutaneous CD30-positive T-cell lymphoproliferative disorders with biallelic rearrangements of DUSP22. *J Invest Dermatol.* 2013;133(6):1680-1682.
80. Feldman AL, Dogan A, Smith DI, et al. Characterizing translocations involving the DUSP22-IRF4 gene region in ALK-negative anaplastic large cell lymphomas using next generation sequencing. *Mod Pathol.* 2011;24(suppl 1):296A. (abst 1258).
81. Somja J, Bisig B, Bonnet C, Herens C, Siebert R, de Leval L. Peripheral T-cell lymphoma with t(6;14)(p25;q11.2) translocation presenting with massive splenomegaly. *Virchows Arch.* 2014;464(6):735-741.
82. Parrilla Castellar ER, Jaffe ES, Said JW, et al. ALK-negative anaplastic large cell lymphoma is a genetically heterogeneous disease with widely disparate clinical outcomes. *Blood.* 2014;124(9):1473-1480.
83. Vasmatzis G, Johnson SH, Knudson RA, et al. Genome-wide analysis reveals recurrent structural abnormalities of TP63 and other p53-related genes in peripheral T-cell lymphomas. *Blood.* 2012;120:2280-2289.
84. Chavan RN, Bridges AG, Knudson RA, et al. Somatic rearrangement of the TP63 gene preceding development of mycosis fungoides with aggressive clinical course. *Blood Cancer J.* 2014;4:e253.
85. Peters K, Knoll JHM, Kadin ME. Cytogenetic findings in regressing skin lesions of lymphomatoid papulosis. *Cancer Genet Cytogenet.* 1995;80(1):13-16.
86. Velusamy T, Kiel MJ, Sahasrabuddhe AA, et al. A novel recurrent NPM1-TYK2 gene fusion in cutaneous CD30-positive lymphoproliferative disorders. *Blood.* 2014;124(25):3768-3771.
87. Jaffe ES, Krenacs L, Raffeld M. Classification of cytotoxic T-cell and natural killer cell lymphomas. *Semin Hematol.* 2003;40(3):175-184.
88. van der Weyden CA, Pileri SA, Feldman AL, Whisstock J, Prince HM. Understanding CD30 biology and therapeutic targeting: a historical perspective providing insight into future directions. *Blood Cancer J.* 2017;7(9):e603.
89. Beissert S, Schwarz A, Schwarz T. Regulatory T cells. *J Invest Dermatol.* 2006;126(1):15-24.
90. Sun J, Yi S, Qiu L, et al. SATB1 defines a subtype of cutaneous CD30(+) lymphoproliferative disorders associated with a T-helper 17 cytokine profile. *J Invest Dermatol.* 2018;138(8):1795-1804.
91. Falini B, Pileri S, Zinzani PL, et al. ALK+ lymphoma: clinicopathological findings and outcome. *Blood.* 1999;93(8):2697-2706.
92. Stein H, Delsol G, Pileri SA, Weiss LM, Poppema S, Jaffe ES. Classical Hodgkin lymphoma, introduction. In: Swerdlow S, Campo E, Harris N, et al, eds. *WHO Classification of Tumours of Haematopoietic and Lymphoid Tissues.* International Agency for Research on Cancer; 2008:326-329.
93. Noe MH, Drake A, Link BK, Liu V. Papular mycosis fungoides: report of two patients, literature review, and conceptual re-appraisal. *J Cutan Pathol.* 2013;40(8):714-719.
94. Zackheim HS, Jones C, Leboit PE, Kashani-Sabet M, McCalmont TH, Zehnder J. Lymphomatoid papulosis associated with mycosis fungoides: a study of 21 patients including analyses for clonality. *J Am Acad Dermatol.* 2003;49(4):620-623.
95. Basarab T, Fraser-Andrews EA, Orchard G, Whittaker S, Russell-Jones R. Lymphomatoid papulosis in association with mycosis fungoides: a study of 15 cases. *Br J Dermatol.* 1998;139(4):630-638.
96. Nofal A, Abdel-Mawla MY, Assaf M, Salah E, Abd-Elazim H. Primary cutaneous aggressive epidermotropic CD8+ T cell lymphoma: a diagnostic and therapeutic challenge. *Int J Dermatol.* 2014;53(1):76-81.
97. Werner B, Massone C, Kerl H, Cerroni L. Large CD30-positive cells in benign, atypical lymphoid infiltrates of the skin. *J Cutan Pathol.* 2008;35(12):1100-1107.
98. Fernandes NF, Rozdeba PJ, Schwartz RA, Kihiczak G, Lambert WC. Pityriasis lichenoides et varioliformis acuta: a disease spectrum. *Int J Dermatol.* 2010;49(3):257-261.
99. Sarantopoulos GP, Palla B, Said J, et al. Mimics of cutaneous lymphoma: report of the 2011 society for Hematopathology/European association for Haematopathology workshop. *Am J Clin Pathol.* 2013;139(4):536-551.
100. Bowers S, Warshaw EM. Pityriasis lichenoides and its subtypes. *J Am Acad Dermatol.* 2006;55(4):557-572.
101. Dereure O, Levi E, Kadin ME. T-cell clonality in pityriasis lichenoides et varioliformis acuta: a heteroduplex analysis of 20 cases. *Arch Dermatol.* 2000;136(12):1483-1486.

Subcutaneous panniculitis-like T-cell lymphoma

Alejandro A. Gru, Laura Beth Pincus, and Yann Charlie-Joseph

DEFINITION

Subcutaneous panniculitis-like T-cell lymphoma (SPTCL) is a mature T-cell lymphoma primary to the skin with T-cell receptor (TCR) αβ expression, subcutaneous involvement, and sparing of the epidermis. It most commonly involves the extremities, occurs at different age groups (including children), and has an indolent clinical behavior.[1] Panniculitic T-cell lymphomas with expression of γδ TCR have distinct clinicopathologic features and are currently classified as primary cutaneous γδ T-cell lymphoma (PCGDTCL).[2]

EPIDEMIOLOGY

SPTCL is more common in women and has a predilection for younger individuals. The median age at presentation is 26 to 46.5 years (range 1-80).[3-6] Approximately, 50% of European cases occurred in individuals 21 to 40 years of age, and 19% of cases were 20-year-old or younger.[3] Numerous cases have now been reported in children where it represents 3.4% of all skin lymphomas.[7]

ETIOLOGY

The etiology of SPTCL remains unknown. It has been reported that up to 19% of cases of SPTCL have associated autoimmune disorders. These included systemic lupus erythematosus, juvenile rheumatoid arthritis, Sjögren disease, type 1 diabetes mellitus, idiopathic thrombocytopenia, multiple sclerosis, Raynaud disease, and Kikuchi-Fujimoto disease.[3,8] A study by Yi et al[9] showed a series of 11 cases of SPTCL initially diagnosed as autoimmune disorders including erythema nodosum, pyoderma gangrenosum, lupus erythematosus profundus/panniculitis, vasculitis, and inflammatory myopathy-like lesions. The authors speculated that cases with inflammatory myositis and/or Behçet disease represented paraneoplastic manifestations of SPTCL. Some of these cases (2/11) had elevation of antinuclear antibodies in the serum, antidouble–stranded DNA antibodies, and one case had an elevated antineutrophil cytoplasmic antibody. A study from the Mayo Clinic on a series of 21 patients revealed preceding diagnoses of autoimmune disorders in ~57% of cases. These included lupus erythematosus profundus/panniculitis, erythema nodosum, Weber–Christian disease, cellulitis, and granulomatous panniculitis of unknown etiology.[10] The association between SPTCL and lupus erythematosus profundus/panniculitis has led to the hypothesis that perhaps the two entities represent two ends of the same spectrum.[11,12] A series of five cases of SPTCL by Pincus et al[12] showed serologic and/or end-organ dysfunction (in addition to cutaneous changes of lupus erythematosus profundus/panniculitis) in all the patients. Some of the cases met 4 of 11 diagnostic criteria from the American College of Rheumatology for a diagnosis of lupus erythematosus. One of the patients had pancytopenia, lymphadenopathy, and partial control of the disease with antimalarial medications. It should be noted that some cases of lobular panniculitis with a CD8+ phenotype can occur in children in association with clonal populations of T-cells in the setting of congenital immune deficiency syndromes.[13] Rare cases in association with HIV[14] and sarcoidosis have also been documented.[15] The association between certain medications and development of SPTCL has been described in patients receiving etanercept,[16] rituximab, and cyclophosphamide.[17] Unusual presentations have been reported in patients with Down syndrome,[18] cervical cancer,[19] during pregnancy,[20] sickle cell disease,[21] and neurofibromatosis type 1.[22] Familial cases and mutations in the *HAVCR2* gene have recently been described in SPLTCL patients (see genetic and molecular findings). The *HAVCR2* gene encodes T-cell immunoglobulin mucin 3 (TIM-3) protein, a negative immune checkpoint paramount in diverse areas of immune regulation. These findings, together with improved responses to immunosuppressive regimens (in comparison to chemotherapy), are shifting the understanding of SPTCL from a disease regarded as a classic malignant lymphoma to a genetic disease related to immune dysregulation.[23-25]

CLINICAL PRESENTATION/PROGNOSIS

SPTCL was originally described by Gonzalez et al.[26] The typical skin lesions consist of subcutaneous nodules/tumors or erythematous plaques, which can vary in diameter from 1 to 20 cm or more (Fig. 16-1). Lesions are frequently multifocal (78%) and rarely ulcerate (6%-18%). They mostly present on the extremities, particularly legs, and less frequently on the trunk and face.[3] Facial lesions might be associated with extraocular muscle palsy.[27] They can clinically simulate other causes of panniculitis, such as erythema nodosum[28] or lupus erythematosus profundus/panniculitis. Other rare clinical presentations might mimic dermatomyositis,[29,30] morphea,[31] cellulitis,[32] facial edema,[33] venous stasis-like ulceration,[34] lipomembranous panniculitis,[35] eschar-like crusting,[36] erythromelalgia,[37] and alopecia.[38] Rare cases in the breast have been reported.[39,40] Lipoatrophy might be seen after resolution.[41]

Systemic symptoms have been reported to occur in a broad range of patients (from 36% to 100% of cases) depending on the study. These include fever, chills, night sweats, and weight loss.[6,42,43] Cytopenias and alterations in liver enzymes often occur. Hemophagocytic lymphohistiocytosis (HLH) is seen in 14% to 44% of cases and is associated with high mortality (46% at 5 years).[3,23,44,45] HLH is more prevalent in PCGDTCL (45%).[46,47] Less common clinical manifestations include lymphadenopathy, hepatosplenomegaly, pleural effusions, and bone marrow involvement.[10,48] However, in most cases of SPTCL without HLH, the systemic workup is usually negative for extracutaneous disease.[49,50] Transmission of the disease has been documented after allogeneic bone marrow transplantation[51] and cardiac transplantation.[52] Some cases show spontaneous resolution.[53]

The prognosis of SPTCL is excellent with a 5-year overall survival (OS) of >80% vs as low as 11% for PCGDTCL.[3,54] Approximately 60% of patients achieve complete remission (CR), and approximately 14% die of the disease. Most of the mortality is due to HLH, which usually develops late in the course of disease.[3] In the largest European study on SPTCL the 5-year OS in patients without HLH was 91% vs 46% in those with HLH.[3] Pediatric cases appear to have higher recurrence rates (>50%), but overall low mortality.[55] A fatal case with overlap features of lupus and hemophagocytosis has been reported.[56]

TREATMENT

There is no standardized therapeutic approach for patients with SPTCL. In the past, most patients were treated with chemotherapy, while most authorities currently utilize immunomodulating medications as first-line treatment.[5,44,57] Common chemotherapeutic agents include chlorambucil, fludarabine, gemcitabine, and CHOP or CHOP-like regimens.

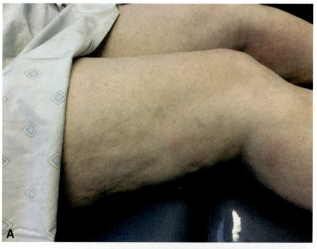
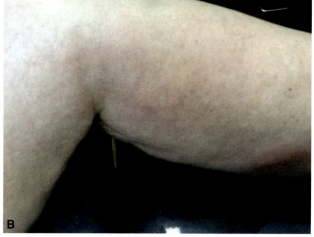
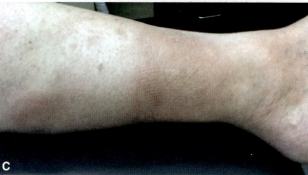

FIGURE 16-1. Subcutaneous panniculitis-like T-cell lymphoma. A and **B.** Erythematous nodules on the legs. **C.** Indurated and erythematous swelling simulating cellulitis. (Courtesy of H. Wong, MD, PhD and J. Hustings, MD.)

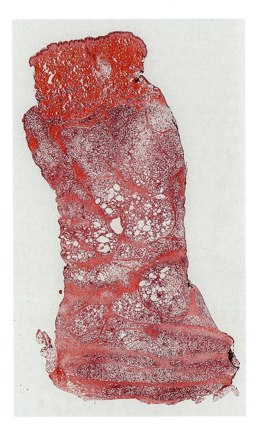

FIGURE 16-2. Subcutaneous panniculitis-like T-cell lymphoma. Predominantly lobular lymphoid infiltrates.

Immunomodulating medications include monotherapy or combinations of prednisone, cyclosporine A, methotrexate, cyclophosphamide, interferon-α, and hydroxychloroquine. Polychemotherapy has been reported to induce CR in 0% to 67% of cases.[3-5,58] By contrast, in a 2017 French cohort of 27 patients, CR after first-line treatment was reached in 81% of patients treated with immunosuppressive drugs alone, and only in 28% of patients with polychemotherapy, independently of the presence or absence of HLH.[44] Some authors, however, purport that chemotherapy may still be the preferred treatment for SPTCL cases, especially in the presence of HLH.[4] Bexarotene, a retinoid analog, and romidepsin, a histone deacetylase inhibitor, have also been used with good success in both adult and pediatric populations.[59-61] Pralatrexate, an antifolate, has additionally been reported to induce durable responses in a small group of patients.[62] There are also case reports of SPTCL successfully treated with ruxolitinib, a selective JAK1/JAK2 inhibitor, denileukin diftitox, a fusion protein of interleukin-2 and diphtheria toxin, and mycophenolate mofetil, a noncompetitive reversible inhibitor of inosine monophosphate dehydrogenase.[63-65] Most patients with relapses are treated with immunosuppressants and achieve >50% sustained clinical response.[66-78] Patients with solitary or few lesions might benefit from localized radiation therapy or surgical removal. Bone marrow transplantation in selected cases resulted in improved survival.[20,76,77] Rare cases with extensive cutaneous disease have been treated with a combination of chemotherapy and whole-body radiation therapy.[78] The use of graft-vs-tumor effect has been reported in a case of relapsed SPTCL following allotransplant and withdrawal of cyclosporine.[78,79] Pediatric series have highlighted the indolent course of SPTCL in some patients and have suggested a watchful waiting approach for their initial management, with treatment reserved for children who develop HLH.[80]

HISTOPATHOLOGY

SPTCL is characterized by a dense, adipotropic lymphoid infiltrate within subcutaneous lobules.[3,47,55,81-88] The infiltrate extends through the subcutaneous lobules and sometimes into the septae (Figs. 16-2–16-4). Extension of the infiltrate into the deep reticular dermis, surrounding and occasionally infiltrating sweat glands, hair follicles, and sebaceous glands can be seen.[70] Infiltration of the superficial epidermis and/or dermis is rare and, if present, should raise the diagnostic consideration of mycosis fungoides (MF) with a secondary panniculitic presentation or of PCGDTCL. Neoplastic lymphocytes are variable in size ranging from small to medium to large. In some cases, lymphocytes display irregular and hyperchromatic nuclei while in other cases lymphocytes are small and cytologically banal appearing. Mitotic figures can occasionally be found among the lymphocytes. Rimming of neoplastic cells around adipocytes is characteristic but not pathognomonic, since rimming can be seen in other conditions as well (see differential diagnosis section). Intravascular thrombi adjacent to tissue necrosis are not uncommon, whereas angiotropism and angiodestruction are exceedingly rare. Necrosis and karyorrhexis along with nonneoplastic inflammatory infiltrates (histiocytes, small lymphocytes, neutrophils) are often prominent, and may mask the underlying neoplastic process. In such scenarios, the presence of necrotic malignant lymphocytes (ghost cells) could be useful in identifying the atypical population, if they are present. Later stages might show epithelioid histiocytes, lipophages, granulomas, or lipomembranous changes.[35] Eosinophils and plasma cells are uncommon; however, the presence of plasma cells should raise the differential diagnosis of lupus erythematosus profundus/panniculitis or lupus erythematosus profundus/panniculitis/SPTCL overlap.[11,87-98] In the presence of intralobular histiocytes with phagocytosed red blood cells or apoptotic elements, workup for HLH should be considered.[97]

IMMUNOPHENOTYPE

Neoplastic cells express an αβ T-cytotoxic phenotype (βF1, CD3+, CD4−, CD8+, TIA-1+, perforin, granzyme B+).[3,47,55,81-86,98-100] Rare cases with a CD4−/CD8− phenotype have been described.[3,101] Recurrent lesions might lose βF1 expression; therefore, a negative TCRγ staining is necessary to confirm the diagnosis.[3] CD56 and CD30 are typically negative. Ki67 shows a high proliferation rate, in particular among lymphocytes rimming adipocytes (typically >50%).[102,103] Losses of CD2, CD5, and/or CD7 are seen in 10%, 50%, and 44% of cases, respectively.[3] CD45RO is usually positive and CD45RA is negative (Fig. 16-5). Epstein–Barr virus has been rarely documented in patients of Asian

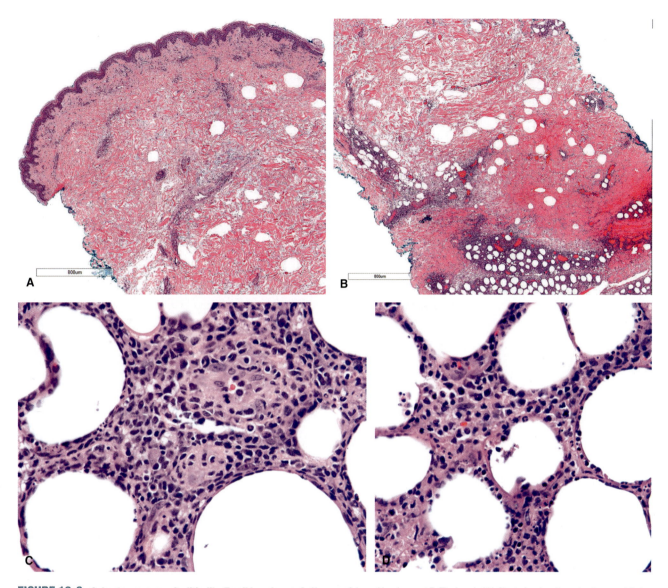

FIGURE 16-3. Subcutaneous panniculitis-like T-cell lymphoma. A. Absence of dermal involvement **B.** The lymphoid infiltrate involves the subcutaneous lobules and periadnexal dermal fat. **C** and **D.** Rimming of adipocytes by atypical cells. Note nuclear hyperchromasia and karyorrhectic debris.

descent.[43,66,100,104,105] Clusters of CD123-positive cells are present in a proportion of SPTCL cases (38.5% in one study), typically comprising a small percentage of the cellularity (mean of 2%).[103,106] c-Myc-positive cells were reported to be present in a percentage of 0.8% to 16% of the cellularity in a series of 23 cases of SPTCL.[107] P53 staining was found to be present in 18% of cases in a large French series.[44]

GENETIC AND MOLECULAR FINDINGS

Monoclonal TCR gene rearrangement is found in the majority of cases, ranging from 50% to 90%.[3,4,6,43,44,108,109] Improved detection of monoclonality can be achieved by microdissection techniques.[110] Chromosomal gains and losses as well as allelic *NAV3* aberrations have been described by comparative genome hybridization (CGH). The most common CGH findings are DNA copy number losses in chromosomes 1p (6/6 cases), 2p (5/6), 2q (4/6), 5p (5/6), 7p (4/6), 9q (5/6), 10q (5/6), 11q (5/6), 12q (5/6), 16 (5/6), 17q (4/6), 19 (4/6), 20 (6/6), and 22 (6/6) and gains in chromosomes 2q (5/6), 4q (5/6), 5q (4/6), 6q (4/6), and 13q (6/6).[109] Whole-exome sequencing of 10 cases of SPTCL revealed statistically significant enrichment of genes involved in the phosphoinositide 3-kinase/AKT/mechanistic/mammalian target of rapamycin and JAK-STAT signaling pathways. Furthermore, targeted sequencing in 18 cases in the same study showed mutations in epigenetic modifiers in 13 (72%) cases, involved in chromatin organization, DNA methylation, and histone modification.[111] High-throughput sequencing of SPTCL has additionally revealed potentially pathogenic variants in *ARID1B*, *KMT2D*, and *PLCG1* among other genes, further reinforcing the potential pathogenic role of epigenetic modifiers and TCR signaling

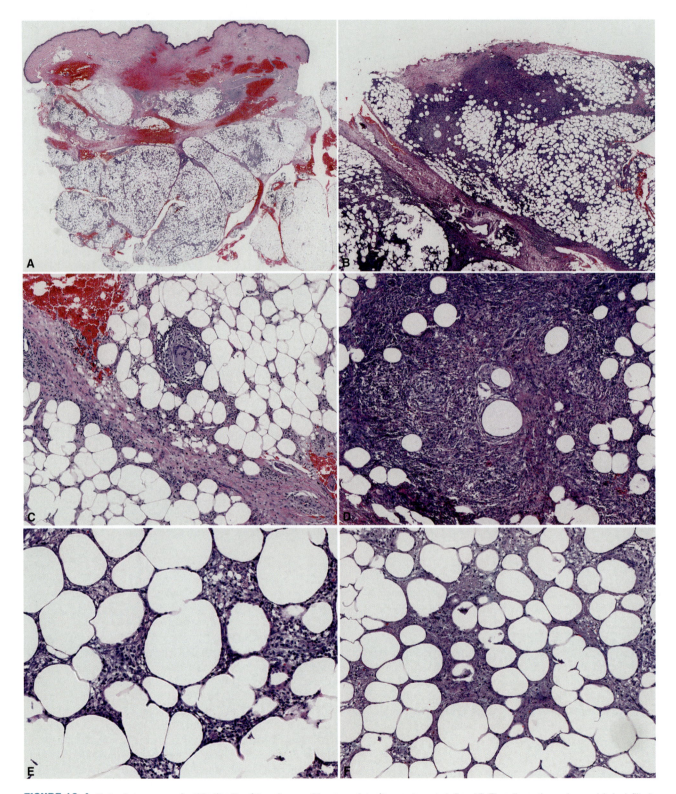

FIGURE 16-4. Subcutaneous panniculitis-like T-cell lymphoma with a granulomatous component. A and **B.** The adipose tissue shows a lobular infiltrate with nodularity. There is no dermal involvement. **C** and **D.** Nodular collections of epithelioid histiocytes and multinucleated giant cells. Adipocyte rimming by neoplastic cells **(E)** adjacent to necrosis **(F)**.

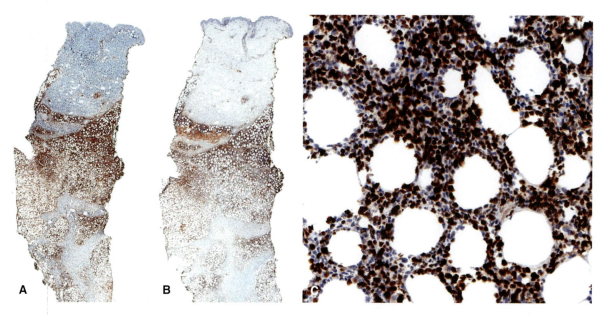

FIGURE 16-5. Subcutaneous panniculitis-like T-cell lymphoma. Lymphoma cells are CD8+ **(A)**, βF1+ **(B)**, and show a high Ki67 proliferation rate, particularly among rimming cells **(C)**.

proteins in SPTCL.[108] Mutations in *HAVCR2*, which encodes TIM-3, a negative checkpoint protein critical in the regulation of innate immunity and inflammatory responses, have recently been found in 59% of familial SPTCL, in 85% of sporadic Asian cases and in 25% of patients from a European study, with half of patients harboring mutations originating from East Asia or Polynesia. Furthermore, it appears that patients harboring the *HAVCR2* mutations have an increased frequency of HLH, and of significantly more severity than SPTCL patients without the mutation.[23-25]

POSTULATED CELL OF ORIGIN

Mature, Postthymic Cytotoxic T-Cells

DIFFERENTIAL DIAGNOSIS

The histologic differential diagnosis of SPTCL includes primarily the following: (A) Tumor-stage MF, (B) PCGDTCL, (C) Extranodal NK/T-cell lymphoma, nasal type (ENKTCL), (D) Blastic plasmacytoid dendritic cell neoplasm (BPDCN), and (E) Lupus erythematosus profundus/panniculitis.[112-133]

A. Tumor-stage MF might exhibit a panniculitic presentation, but typically has a CD4+ phenotype. By contrast CD8+ MF occurs mostly in children, where it lacks subcutaneous involvement.[114]
B. PCGDTCL is an aggressive disease with an average survival of 15 months.[113] Cases with more indolent clinical course have been recently described.[114] The lesions are typically widespread erythematous plaques or nodules, commonly ulcerated, and the patients often have elevated lactate dehydrogenase. As opposed to SPTCL, systemic presentations and bone marrow involvement (nearly a third of cases) are more frequent.[81,115,116] PCGDTCL characteristically exhibits a CD4−CD8−CD56+ phenotype, although CD8 expression might be observed in up to 50% of cases, and very rarely that of CD4. A sizable minority of cases are CD56-positive.[112,117,118] Immunohistochemical staining is positive for TCRγ, TIA-1, and negative for βF1. Subcutaneous involvement of fat lobules, epidermotropism, and pseudoepitheliomatous hyperplasia are frequent findings (Figs. 16-6–16-8). Pure panniculitic forms are rare.[117] EBER is present in up to 10% of cases.[43] Similar to SPTCL, some patients have comorbidities associated with immune suppression, including other lymphoproliferative conditions, immune dysregulation, other malignancies, and lupus erythematosus.[10,114,118] HLH is present in approximately 8% to 45% of cases.[3,116]
C. ENKTCL, nasal type might also show a panniculitic presentation.[116,119] EBER is invariably expressed. Similar to PCGDTCL, CD56 expression, angiocentricity, angiodestruction, and necrosis are frequently seen.[120] ENKTCL shows cytoplasmic staining for CD3 (CD3ε); both TCRαβ and TCRγδ are typically negative.
D. BPDCN, similar to ENKTCL, can also have significant involvement of the subcutis. Neoplastic cells are plasmacytoid dendritic cells of myeloid lineage which typically express CD4, CD56, CD123, TdT, TCL-1, and CD31, but lack expression of CD3 and CD8.[120-122,125]
E. There is a significant clinicopathologic overlap between SPTCL and lupus erythematosus profundus/panniculitis; it has been reported that around 20% of patients with SPTCL have a history of an autoimmune disorder and there is an increased prevalence of non-Hodgkin lymphoma in lupus erythematosus patients.[124,125] Lupus erythematosus profundus/panniculitis shows lymphoplasmacytic infiltrates within fat lobules (Figs. 16-9 and 16-10).[94,96] Interface changes and dermal mucin deposition

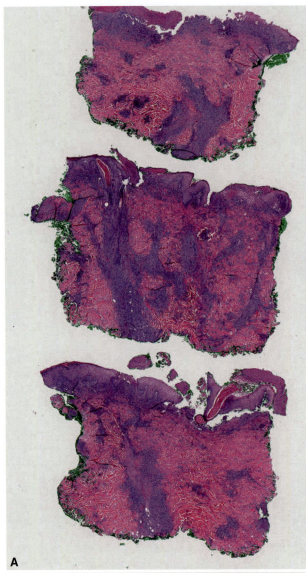

can be seen in half of the cases.[96] Criteria reported to be most useful in favor of lupus erythematosus profundus/panniculitis vs SPTCL include concurrent clinical and/or histopathologic features of lupus erythematosus, presence of reactive germinal centers, septal fibrosis, numerous plasma cells, and negative TCR clonality.[94] Other authors have included the lack of cytologic atypia, presence of subcutaneous hyaline necrosis, dermal mucin, and clusters of CD123+ plasmacytoid dendritic cells along with increased myxovirus resistance protein 1 expression, as attributes in favor of lupus erythematosus profundus/panniculitis (Fig. 16-11).[92,126] Nevertheless, a different study demonstrated the presence of clusters of CD123+ plasmacytoid dendritic cells, dermal mucin deposition, and plasma cell aggregations in a sizable proportion of SPTCL cases, thus casting doubt on their purported utility as discriminating attributes. By contrast, they found that a high Ki67 proliferation rate (greater than 25% in the lymphocytes rimming adipocytes) served as the most useful discriminating feature in favor of SPTCL.[103] Of note, TCR clonality should be interpreted with caution as clonal expansions of reactive T-cells are not uncommon in lupus erythematosus.[88]

Other hematologic malignancies that may less frequently involve the subcutis but should nonetheless be considered in the differential diagnosis of SPTCL include anaplastic large cell lymphoma, primary cutaneous CD4+ small/medium T-cell lymphoproliferative disorder, primary cutaneous aggressive epidermotropic CD8+ T-cell lymphoma, diffuse large B-cell lymphoma, lymphoplasmacytic lymphoma, myelogenous leukemia, and mantle cell lymphoma.[127-134]

CAPSULE SUMMARY

- SPTCL is a primary cutaneous T-cell lymphoma with αβ TCR expression, subcutaneous involvement, and epidermal sparing.
- Panniculitic T-cell lymphoma with γδ TCR phenotype has distinct clinicopathologic features and is classified as PCGDTCL.
- **Clinical features:** Nodules and plaques on extremities in different age groups (including children); indolent clinical behavior.
- Presence of hemophagocytosis is associated with worse prognosis and may require aggressive systemic therapy.
- Association with autoimmune disorders, including lupus, is common.
- **Histopathology:** Lobular panniculitis with atypia of lymphocytes, rimming of the adipocytes, and lack of epidermotropism.
- **Immunophenotype:** βF1+, CD8+, TIA-1+, granzyme B+, perforin+, Ki67high.
- **Differential diagnosis:** Lupus erythematosus profundus/panniculitis and cutaneous or systemic lymphomas with prominent panniculitic involvement.

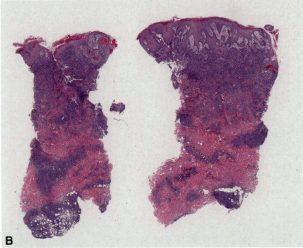

FIGURE 16-6. Primary cutaneous γδ T-cell lymphoma. A and B. Nodular and ulcerated lesions on the leg of a 56-year-old man. There is acanthosis, ulceration, and a diffuse dermal infiltrate extending superficially into the subcutaneous fat.

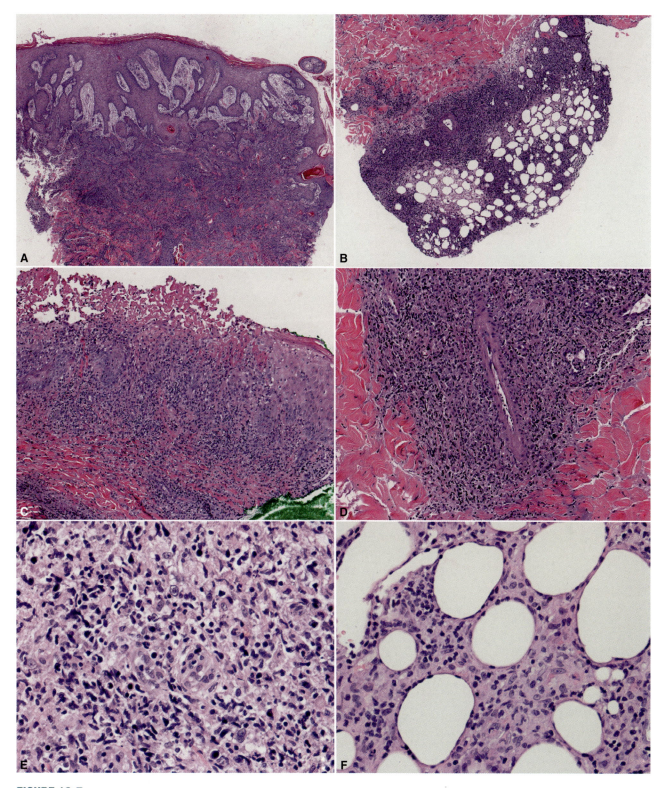

FIGURE 16-7. Primary cutaneous γδ T-cell lymphoma. A. There is prominent pseudoepitheliomatous hyperplasia. **B.** Lobular infiltration. **C.** Epidermal involvement adjacent to ulcer. **D.** Angiotropism. **E** and **F.** Medium-to-large lymphoma cells in a background of histiocytes. The malignant cells show nuclear irregularities and hyperchromasia.

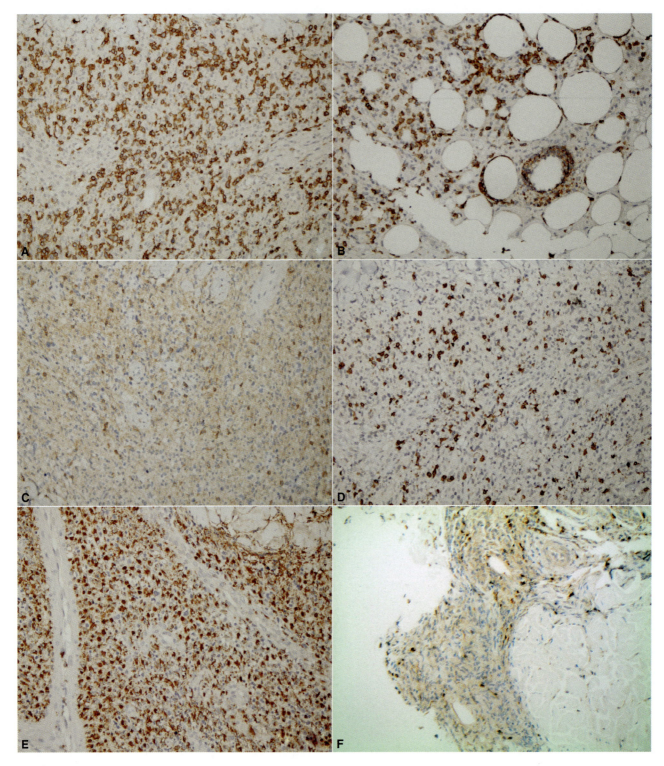

FIGURE 16-8. Primary cutaneous γδ T-cell lymphoma. Lymphoma cells are CD3+ **(A)**, CD56+ subset **(B)**, CD4− **(C)**, and CD8− **(D)**. CD68 **(E)** stains background histiocytes. βF1 **(F)** is negative, suggesting a γδ-phenotype.

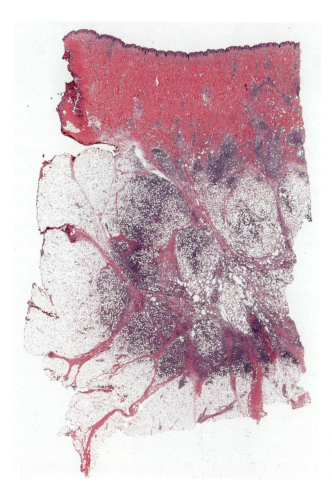

FIGURE 16-9. Lupus panniculitis (lupus profundus, subcutaneous lupus). There is lobular panniculitis with a superficial and deep perivascular infiltrates. No significant interface changes are present. The deep dermis shows nodular aggregates of lymphocytes with plasma cells. (Courtesy of Dr. Michael Arnold, Nationwide Children's Hospital, Columbus, OH.)

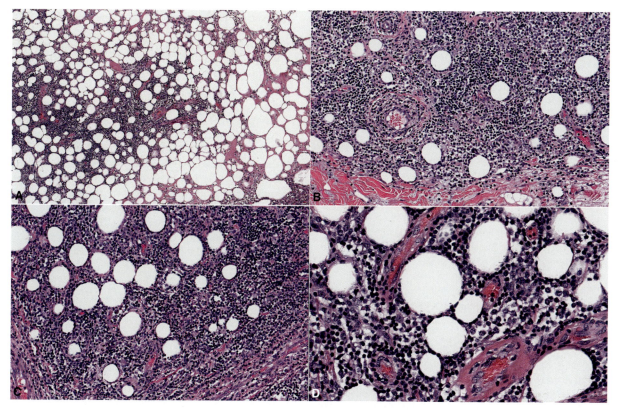

FIGURE 16-10. Lupus panniculitis. A. Hyaline necrosis. **B.** A relatively dense infiltrate involving the adipose tissue. **C** and **D.** Lymphoplasmacytic infiltrates with adipocyte rimming by small reactive lymphocytes. (Courtesy of Dr. Michael Arnold, Nationwide Children's Hospital, Columbus, OH.)

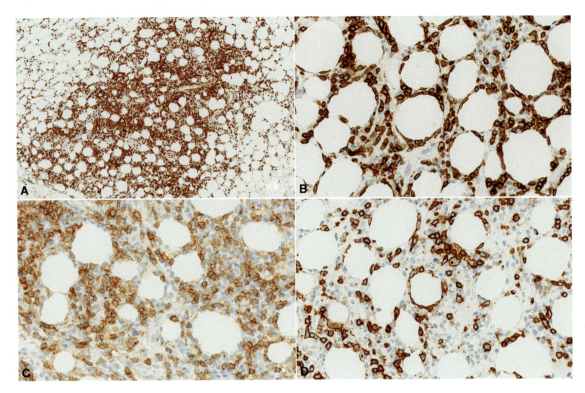

FIGURE 16-11. Lupus panniculitis. A and **B.** CD3 highlights T-cell infiltration of fat lobules with adipocyte rimming. CD4 **(C)** and CD8 **(D)** stains reveal a reactive T-cell population with preserved CD4:CD8 ratio. Rimming by cytotoxic T-cells is less pronounced. (Courtesy of Dr. Michael Arnold, Nationwide Children's Hospital, Columbus, OH.)

References

1. Jaffe ES, Gaulard P, Ralfiaer E. *Subcutaneous Panniculitis-like T-Cell Lymphoma*. International Agency for Research on Cancer; 2008.
2. Willemze R, Cerroni L, Kempf W, et al. The 2018 update of the WHO-EORTC classification for primary cutaneous lymphomas. *Blood.* 2019;133(16):1703-1714.
3. Willemze R, Jansen PM, Cerroni L, et al. Subcutaneous panniculitis-like T-cell lymphoma—definition, classification, and prognostic factors: an EORTC Cutaneous Lymphoma Group Study of 83 cases. *Blood.* 2008;111:838-845.
4. Ohtsuka M, Miura T, Yamamoto T. Clinical characteristics, differential diagnosis, and treatment outcome of subcutaneous panniculitis-like T-cell lymphoma: a literature review of published Japanese cases. *Eur J Dermatol.* 2017;27(1):34-41.
5. López-Lerma I, Peñate Y, Gallardo F, et al. Subcutaneous panniculitis-like T-cell lymphoma: clinical features, therapeutic approach, and outcome in a case series of 16 patients. *J Am Acad Dermatol.* 2018;79(5):892-898.
6. Rutnin S, Porntharukcharoen S, Boonsakan P. Clinicopathologic, immunophenotypic, and molecular analysis of subcutaneous panniculitis-like T-cell lymphoma: a retrospective study in a tertiary care center. *J Cutan Pathol.* 2019;46(1):44-51.
7. Moon HR, Lee WJ, Won CH, et al. Paediatric cutaneous lymphoma in Korea: a retrospective study at a single institution. *J Eur Acad Dermatol Venereol.* 2014;28(12):1798-1804.
8. Notaro E, Shustov A, Chen X, et al. Kikuchi-fujimoto disease associated with subcutaneous panniculitis-like T-cell lymphoma. *Am J Dermatopathol.* 2016;38(6):e77-80.
9. Yi L, Qun S, Wenjie Z, et al. The presenting manifestations of subcutaneous panniculitis-like T-cell lymphoma and T-cell lymphoma and cutaneous γδ T-cell lymphoma may mimic those of rheumatic diseases: a report of 11 cases. *Clin Rheumatol.* 2013;32:1169-1175.
10. Ghobrial IM, Weenig RH, Pittlekow MR, et al. Clinical outcome of patients with subcutaneous panniculitis-like T-cell lymphoma. *Leuk Lymphoma.* 2005;46(5):703-708.
11. Bosisio F, Boi S, Caputo V, et al. Lobular panniculitic infiltrates with overlapping histopathologic features of lupus panniculitis (Lupus Profundus) and subcutaneous T-cell lymphoma: a conceptual and practical dilemma. *Am J Surg Pathol.* 2015;39(2):206-211.
12. Pincus LB, LeBoit PE, McCalmont TH, et al. Subcutaneous panniculitis-like T-cell lymphoma with overlapping clinicopathologic features of lupus erythematosus: coexistence of 2 entities?. *Am J Dermatopathol.* 2009;31:520-526.
13. Bader-Meunier B, Rieux-Laucat F, Touzot F, et al. Inherited immunodeficiency: a new association with early-onset childhood panniculitis. *Pediatrics.* 2018;141(suppl 5):S496-S500.
14. Joseph LD, Panicker VK, Prathiba D, et al. Subcutaneous panniculitis-like T cell lymphoma in a HIV positive patient. *J Assoc Phys India.* 2005;53:314-316.
15. Iqbal K, Bott J, Greenblatt D, et al. Subcutaneous panniculitis-like T-cell lymphoma in association with sarcoidosis. *Clin Exp Dermatol.* 2011;36:677-679.
16. Michot C, Costes V, Gerard-Dran D, et al. Subcutaneous panniculitis-like T-cell lymphoma in a patient receiving etanercept for rheumatoid arthritis. *Br J Dermatol.* 2009;160:889-890.

17. Schmutz JL, Trechot P. Subcutaneous panniculitis-like T-cell lymphoma following treatment with rituximab and cyclophosphamide. *Ann Dermatol Venereol.* 2013;140:246-247.
18. Mixon B, Drach L, Monforte H, et al. Subcutaneous panniculitis-like T-cell lymphoma in a child with trisomy 21. *Fetal Pediatr Pathol.* 2010;29:380-384.
19. Swain M, Swarnalata G, Bhandari T. Subcutaneous panniculitis-like T-cell lymphoma in a case of carcinoma cervix. *Indian J Med Paediatr Oncol.* 2013;34:104-106.
20. Reimer P, Rudiger T, Muller J, et al. Subcutaneous panniculitis-like T-cell lymphoma during pregnancy with successful autologous stem cell transplantation. *Ann Hematol.* 2003;82:305-309.
21. Ma S, Zhao Y, Leudke C, et al. Subcutaneous panniculitis-like T-cell lymphoma in a 25-year-old male patient with sickle cell disease. *Pathol Res Pract.* 2019;215(8):152400.
22. Reich A, Butrym A, Mazur G, et al. Subcutaneous panniculitis-like T-cell lymphoma in type 1 neurofibromatosis: a case report. *Acta Dermatovenerol Croat.* 2014;22:145-149.
23. Gayden T, Sepulveda FE, Khuong-Quang DA, et al. Germline HAVCR2 mutations altering TIM-3 characterize subcutaneous panniculitis-like T cell lymphomas with hemophagocytic lymphohistiocytic syndrome. *Nat Genet.* 2018;50(12):1650-1657.
24. Polprasert C, Takeuchi Y, Kakiuchi N, et al. Frequent germline mutations of HAVCR2 in sporadic subcutaneous panniculitis-like T-cell lymphoma. *Blood Adv.* 2019;3(4):588-595.
25. Sonigo G, Battistella M, Beylot-Barry M, et al. HAVCR2 mutations are associated with severe hemophagocytic syndrome in subcutaneous panniculitis-like T-cell lymphoma. *Blood.* 2020;135(13):1058-1061.
26. Gonzalez CL, Medeiros LJ, Braziel RM, et al. T-cell lymphoma involving subcutaneous tissue. A clinicopathologic entity commonly associated with hemophagocytic syndrome. *Am J Surg Pathol.* 1991;15:17-27.
27. Leonard GD, Hegde U, Butman J, et al. Extraocular muscle palsies in subcutaneous panniculitis-like T-cell lymphoma. *J Clin Oncol.* 2003;21:2993-2995.
28. Risulo M, Rubegni P, Sbano P, et al. Subcutaneous panniculitis lymphoma: erythema nodosum-like. *Clin Lymphoma Myeloma.* 2006;7:239-241.
29. Chiu HY, He GY, Chen JS, et al. Subcutaneous panniculitis-like T-cell lymphoma presenting with clinicopathologic features of dermatomyositis. *J Am Acad Dermatol.* 2011;64:e121-e123.
30. Kaieda S, Idemoto A, Yoshida N, et al. A subcutaneous panniculitis-like T-cell lymphoma mimicking dermatomyositis. *Intern Med.* 2014;53:1455.
31. Troskot N, Lugovic L, Situm M, et al. From circumscribed scleroderma (morphea) to subcutaneous panniculitis-like T-cell lymphoma: case report. *Acta Dermatovenerol Croat.* 2004;12:289-293.
32. Tzeng HE, Teng CL, Yang Y, et al. Occult subcutaneous panniculitis-like T-cell lymphoma with initial presentations of cellulitis-like skin lesion and fulminant hemophagocytosis. *J Formos Med Assoc.* 2007;106:S55-S59.
33. Velez NF, Ishizawar RC, Dellaripa PF, et al. Full facial edema: a novel presentation of subcutaneous panniculitis-like T-cell lymphoma. *J Clin Oncol.* 2012;30:e233-e236.
34. Weenig RH, Daniel Su WP. Subcutaneous panniculitis-like T-cell lymphoma presenting as venous stasis ulceration. *Int J Dermatol.* 2006;45:1083-1085.
35. Weenig RH, Ng CS, Perniciaro C. Subcutaneous panniculitis-like T-cell lymphoma: an elusive case presenting as lipomembranous panniculitis and a review of 72 cases in the literature. *Am J Dermatopathol.* 2001;23:206-215.
36. Ghosh SK, Roy D, Mondal P, et al. Subcutaneous panniculitis-like T-cell lymphoma with unusual eschar-like crusting. *Dermatol Online J.* 2014;20(2):doj_21535.
37. Thomas J, Maramattom BV, Kuruvilla PM, et al. Subcutaneous panniculitis like T cell lymphoma associated with erythromelalgia. *J Postgrad Med.* 2014;60:335-337.
38. Torok L, Gurbity TP, Kirschner A, et al. Panniculitis-like T-cell lymphoma clinically manifested as alopecia. *Br J Dermatol.* 2002;147:785-788.
39. Gualco G, Chioato L, Harrington WJ Jr, et al. Primary and secondary T-cell lymphomas of the breast: clinico-pathologic features of 11 cases. *Appl Immunohistochem Mol Morphol.* 2009;17:301-306.
40. Jeong SI, Lim HS, Choi YR, et al. Subcutaneous panniculitis-like T-cell lymphoma of the breast. *Korean J Radiol.* 2013;14:391-394.
41. Santonja C, Gonzalo I, Feito M, et al. Lipoatrophic panniculitis of the ankles in childhood: differential diagnosis with subcutaneous panniculitis-like T-cell lymphoma. *Am J Dermatopathol.* 2012;34:295-300.
42. Kim Y, Coomarasamy C, Jarrett P. The epidemiology of subcutaneous panniculitis-like alpha-beta T-cell lymphoma in New Zealand. *Australas J Dermatol.* 2020;61(2):e196-e199.
43. Kong YY, Dai B, Kong JC, et al. Subcutaneous panniculitis-like T-cell lymphoma: a clinicopathologic, immunophenotypic, and molecular study of 22 Asian cases according to WHO-EORTC classification. *Am J Surg Pathol.* 2008;32:1495-1502.
44. Michonneau D, Petrella T, Ortonne N, et al. Subcutaneous panniculitis-like T-cell lymphoma: immunosuppressive drugs induce better response than polychemotherapy. *Acta Derm Venereol.* 2017;97(3):358-364.
45. Lee DW, Yang JH, Lee SM, et al. Subcutaneous panniculitis-like T-cell lymphoma: a clinical and pathologic study of 14 Korean patients. *Ann Dermatol.* 2011;23:329-337.
46. Koh MJ, Sadarangani SP, Chan YC, et al. Aggressive subcutaneous panniculitis-like T-cell lymphoma with hemophagocytosis in two children (subcutaneous panniculitis-like T-cell lymphoma). *J Am Acad Dermatol.* 2009;61:875-881.
47. Parveen Z, Thompson K. Subcutaneous panniculitis-like T-cell lymphoma: redefinition of diagnostic criteria in the recent World Health Organization-European Organization for Research and Treatment of Cancer classification for cutaneous lymphomas. *Arch Pathol Lab Med.* 2009;133:303-308.
48. Gao J, Gauerke SJ, Martinez-Escala ME, et al. Bone marrow involvement by subcutaneous panniculitis-like T-cell lymphoma: a report of three cases. *Mod Pathol.* 2014;27:800-807.
49. Babb A, Zerizer I, Naresh KN, et al. Subcutaneous panniculitis-like T-cell lymphoma with extracutaneous dissemination demonstrated on FDG PET/CT. *Am J Hematol.* 2011;86:375-376.
50. Huang CT, Yang WC, Lin SF. Positron-emission tomography findings indicating the involvement of the whole body skin in subcutaneous panniculitis-like T cell lymphoma. *Ann Hematol.* 2011;90:853-854.
51. Berg KD, Brinster NK, Huhn KM, et al. Transmission of a T-cell lymphoma by allogeneic bone marrow transplantation. *N Engl J Med.* 2001;345:1458-1463.
52. Bregman SG, Yeaney GA, Greig BW, Vnencak-Jones CL, Hamilton KS. Subcutaneous panniculitic T-cell lymphoma in a cardiac allograft recipient. *J Cutan Pathol.* 2005;32(5):366-370.

53. Kawachi Y, Furuta J, Fujisawa Y, et al. Indolent subcutaneous panniculitis-like T cell lymphoma in a 1-year-old child. *Pediatr Dermatol.* 2012;29:374-377.
54. Goyal A, Goyal K, Bohjanen K, et al. Epidemiology of primary cutaneous γδ T-cell lymphoma and subcutaneous panniculitis-like T-cell lymphoma in the U.S.A. from 2006 to 2015: a surveillance, epidemiology, and end results-18 analysis. *Br J Dermatol.* 2019;181(4):848-850.
55. Huppmann AR, Xi L, Raffeld M, et al. Subcutaneous panniculitis-like T-cell lymphoma in the pediatric age group: a lymphoma of low malignant potential. *Pediatr Blood Cancer.* 2013;60:1165-1170.
56. Ma L, Bandarchi B, Glusac EJ. Fatal subcutaneous panniculitis-like T-cell lymphoma with interface change and dermal mucin, a dead ringer for lupus erythematosus. *J Cutan Pathol.* 2005;32:360-365.
57. Kadin ME, Cualing HD. Subcutaneous pattern: subcutaneous lymphoproliferative disorders. In: Cualing HD, Kadin ME, Hoang MP, eds. *Cutaneous Hematopathology Approach to the Diagnosis of Atypical Lymphoid-Hematopoietic Infiltrates in Skin.* Springer; 2014.
58. West ES, Shinkai K, Ai WZ, et al. Remission of subcutaneous panniculitis-like T-cell lymphoma in a pregnant woman after treatment with oral corticosteroids as monotherapy. *JAAD Case Rep.* 2017;3(2):87-89.
59. Mehta N, Wayne AS, Kim YH, et al. Bexarotene is active against subcutaneous panniculitis-like T-cell lymphoma in adult and pediatric populations. *Clin Lymphoma Myeloma Leuk.* 2012;12:20-25.
60. Zhang X, Schlaak M, Fabri M, et al. Successful treatment of a panniculitis-like primary cutaneous T-cell lymphoma of the alpha/beta type with bexarotene. *Case Rep Dermatol.* 2012;4:56-60.
61. Bashey S, Krathen M, Abdulla F, et al. Romidepsin is effective in subcutaneous panniculitis-like T-cell lymphoma. *J Clin Oncol.* 2012;30:e221-e225.
62. Ong SY, Phipps C, Kaur H, et al. Pralatrexate induces long-term remission in relapsed subcutaneous panniculitis-like t-cell lymphoma. *Ann Acad Med Singap.* 2019;48(9):298-300.
63. Lévy R, Fusaro M, Guerin F, et al. Efficacy of ruxolitinib in subcutaneous panniculitis-like T-cell lymphoma and hemophagocytic lymphohistiocytosis. *Blood Adv.* 2020;4(7):1383-1387.
64. Hathaway T, Subtil A, Kuo P, Foss F. Efficacy of denileukin diftitox insubcutaneous panniculitis-like T-cell lymphoma. *Clin Lymphoma Myeloma.* 2007;7(8):541-545.
65. Heyman B, Beaven A. Mycophenolate mofetil for the treatment of subcutaneous panniculitis-like t-cell lymphoma: case report and review of the literature. *Clin Lymphoma Myeloma Leuk.* 2018;18(10):e437-e440.
66. Go SI, Lee WS, Kang MH, et al. Cyclosporine A treatment for relapsed subcutaneous panniculitis-like T-cell lymphoma: a case with long-term follow-up. *Korean J Hematol.* 2012;47:146-149.
67. Jung HR, Yun SY, Choi JH, et al. Cyclosporine in relapsed subcutaneous panniculitis-like T-cell lymphoma after autologous hematopoietic stem cell transplantation. *Cancer Res Treat.* 2011;43:255-259.
68. Mizutani S, Kuroda J, Shimura Y, et al. Cyclosporine A for chemotherapy-resistant subcutaneous panniculitis-like T cell lymphoma with hemophagocytic syndrome. *Acta Haematol.* 2011;126:8-12.
69. Rojnuckarin P, Nakorn TN, Assanasen T, et al. Cyclosporin in subcutaneous panniculitis-like T-cell lymphoma. *Leuk Lymphoma.* 2007;48:560-563.
70. Alaibac M, Berti E, Pigozzi B, et al. High-dose chemotherapy with autologous blood stem cell transplantation for aggressive subcutaneous panniculitis-like T-cell lymphoma. *J Am Acad Dermatol.* 2005;52:S121-S123.
71. Briki H, Bouaziz JD, Molinier-Frenkel V, et al. Subcutaneous panniculitis-like T-cell lymphoma αβ: complete sustained remission with corticosteroids and methotrexate. *Br J Dermatol.* 2010;163:1136-1138.
72. Chen R, Liu L, Liang YM. Treatment relapsed subcutaneous panniculitis-like T-cell lymphoma together HPS by Cyclosporin A. *Hematol Rep.* 2010;2:e9.
73. Go RS, Gazelka H, Hogan JD, et al. Subcutaneous panniculitis-like T-cell lymphoma: complete remission with fludarabine. *Ann Hematol.* 2003;82:247-250.
74. Jang MS, Baek JW, Kang DY, et al. Subcutaneous panniculitis-like T-cell lymphoma: successful treatment with systemic steroid alone. *J Dermatol.* 2012;39:96-99.
75. Nagai K, Nakano N, Iwai T, et al. Pediatric subcutaneous panniculitis-like T-cell lymphoma with favorable result by immunosuppressive therapy: a report of two cases. *Pediatr Hematol Oncol.* 2014;31:528-533.
76. Nakahashi H, Tsukamoto N, Yamane A, et al. Autologous peripheral blood stem cell transplantation to treat CHOP-refractory aggressive subcutaneous panniculitis-like T cell lymphoma. *Acta Haematol.* 2009;121:239-242.
77. Sakurai E, Satoh T, Akiko YA, et al. Subcutaneous panniculitis-like T-cell lymphoma (SPTCL) with hemophagocytosis (HPS): successful treatment using high-dose chemotherapy (BFM-NHL & ALL-90) and autologous peripheral blood stem cell transplantation. *J Clin Exp Hematopathol.* 2013;53:135-140.
78. Mukai HY, Okoshi Y, Shimizu S, et al. Successful treatment of a patient with subcutaneous panniculitis-like T-cell lymphoma with high-dose chemotherapy and total body irradiation. *Eur J Haematol.* 2003;70:413-416.
79. Yuan L, Sun L, Bo J, et al. Durable remission in a patient with refractory subcutaneous panniculitis-like T-cell lymphoma relapse after allogeneic hematopoietic stem cell transplantation through withdrawal of cyclosporine. *Ann Transplant.* 2011;16:135-138.
80. Johnston EE, LeBlanc RE, Kim J, et al. Subcutaneous panniculitis-like T-cell lymphoma: Pediatric case series demonstrating heterogeneous presentation and option for watchful waiting. *Pediatr Blood Cancer.* 2015;62(11):2025-2028.
81. Cerroni L, Gatter K, Kerl H, et al. *Skin Lymphoma: The Illustrated Guide.* Wiley-Blackwell; 2009.
82. Go RS, Wester SM. Immunophenotypic and molecular features, clinical outcomes, treatments, and prognostic factors associated with subcutaneous panniculitis-like T-cell lymphoma: a systematic analysis of 156 patients reported in the literature. *Cancer.* 2004;101:1404-1413.
83. Guitart J. Subcutaneous lymphoma and related conditions. *Dermatol Ther.* 2010;23:350-355.
84. Hahtola S, Burghart E, Jeskanen L, et al. Clinicopathological characterization and genomic aberrations in subcutaneous panniculitis-like T-cell lymphoma. *J Invest Dermatol.* 2008;128:2304-2309.

85. Jaffe ES, Nicolae A, Pittaluga S. Peripheral T-cell and NK-cell lymphomas in the WHO classification: pearls and pitfalls. *Mod Pathol.* 2013;26(suppl 1):S71-S87.
86. Quintanilla-Martinez L, Jansen PM, Kinney MC, et al. Non-mycosis fungoides cutaneous T-cell lymphomas: report of the 2011 Society for Hematopathology/European Association for Haematopathology workshop. *Am J Clin Pathol.* 2013;139:491-514.
87. Hoque SR, Child FJ, Whittaker SJ, et al. Subcutaneous panniculitis-like T-cell lymphoma: a clinicopathological, immunophenotypic and molecular analysis of six patients. *Br J Dermatol.* 2003;148:516-525.
88. Lozzi GP, Massone C, Citarella L, et al. Rimming of adipocytes by neoplastic lymphocytes: a histopathologic feature not restricted to subcutaneous T-cell lymphoma. *Am J Dermatopathol.* 2006;28:9-12.
89. Cassis TB, Fearneyhough PK, Callen JP. Subcutaneous panniculitis-like T-cell lymphoma with vacuolar interface dermatitis resembling lupus erythematosus panniculitis. *J Am Acad Dermatol.* 2004;50:465-469.
90. Fraga J, Garcia-Diez A. Lupus erythematosus panniculitis. *Dermatol Clin.* 2008;26:453-463, vi.
91. Gonzalez EG, Selvi E, Lorenzini S, et al. Subcutaneous panniculitis-like T-cell lymphoma misdiagnosed as lupus erythematosus panniculitis. *Clin Rheumatol.* 2007;26:244-246.
92. Li JY, Liu HJ, Wang L. Subcutaneous panniculitis-like T-cell lymphoma accompanied with discoid lupus erythematosus. *Chin Med J.* 2013;126:3590.
93. Liau JY, Chuang SS, Chu CY, et al. The presence of clusters of plasmacytoid dendritic cells is a helpful feature for differentiating lupus panniculitis from subcutaneous panniculitis-like T-cell lymphoma. *Histopathology.* 2013;62:1057-1066.
94. Massone C, Kodama K, Salmhofer W, et al. Lupus erythematosus panniculitis (lupus profundus): clinical, histopathological, and molecular analysis of nine cases. *J Cutan Pathol.* 2005;32:396-404.
95. Rose C, Leverkus M, Fleischer M, et al. Histopathology of panniculitis—aspects of biopsy techniques and difficulties in diagnosis. *J Dtsch Dermatol Ges.* 2012;10:421-425.
96. Weingartner JS, Zedek DC, Burkhart CN, et al. Lupus erythematosus panniculitis in children: report of three cases and review of previously reported cases. *Pediatr Dermatol.* 2012;29:169-176.
97. Ikeda E, Endo M, Uchigasaki S, et al. Phagocytized apoptotic cells in subcutaneous panniculitis-like T-cell lymphoma. *J Eur Acad Dermatol Venereol.* 2001;15:159-162.
98. Dargent JL, Roufosse C, Delville JP, et al. Subcutaneous panniculitis-like T-cell lymphoma: further evidence for a distinct neoplasm originating from large granular lymphocytes of T/NK phenotype. *J Cutan Pathol.* 1998;25:394-400.
99. Guizzardi M, Hendrickx IA, Mancini LL, et al. Cytotoxic gamma/delta subcutaneous panniculitis-like T-cell lymphoma: report of a case with pulmonary involvement unresponsive to therapy. *J Eur Acad Dermatol Venereol.* 2003;17:219-222.
100. Wang L, Yang Y, Liu W, et al. Subcutaneous panniculitis-like T-cell lymphoma: expression of cytotoxic-granule-associated protein TIA-1 and its relation with Epstein–Barr virus infection. *Chin J Pathol.* 2000;29:103-106.
101. Santucci M, Pimpinelli N, Massi D, et al. Cytotoxic/natural killer cell cutaneous lymphomas. Report of EORTC Cutaneous Lymphoma Task Force Workshop. *Cancer.* 2003;97:610-627.
102. Sen F, Rassidakis GZ, Jones D, et al. Apoptosis and proliferation in subcutaneous panniculitis-like T-cell lymphoma. *Mod Pathol.* 2002;15:625-631.
103. Sitthinamsuwan P, Pattanaprichakul P, Treetipsatit J, et al. Subcutaneous panniculitis-like t-cell lymphoma versus lupus erythematosus panniculitis: distinction by means of the peri-adipocytic cell proliferation index. *Am J Dermatopathol.* 2018;40(8):567-574.
104. Nemoto Y, Taniguchi A, Kamioka M, et al. Epstein–Barr virus-infected subcutaneous panniculitis-like T-cell lymphoma associated with methotrexate treatment. *Int J Hematol.* 2010;92:364-368.
105. Soylu S, Gul U, Kilic A, et al. A case with an indolent course of subcutaneous panniculitis-like T-cell lymphoma demonstrating Epstein–Barr virus positivity and simulating dermatitis artefacta. *Am J Clin Dermatol.* 2010;11:147-150.
106. Chen SJT, Tse JY, Harms PW, et al. Utility of CD123 immunohistochemistry in differentiating lupus erythematosus from cutaneous T cell lymphoma. *Histopathology.* 2019;74(6):908-916.
107. Fernandez-Pol S, De Stefano D, Kim J. Immunohistochemistry reveals an increased proportion of MYC-positive cells in subcutaneous panniculitis-like T-cell lymphoma compared with lupus panniculitis. *J Cutan Pathol.* 2017;44(11):925-930.
108. Salhany KE, Macon WR, Choi JK, et al. Subcutaneous panniculitis-like T-cell lymphoma: clinicopathologic, immunophenotypic, and genotypic analysis of alpha/beta and gamma/delta subtypes. *Am J Surg Pathol.* 1998;22:881-893.
109. Wan C, Xu C, Wang L, et al. Diagnostic significance of immunophenotyping and detection of gene rearrangement in subcutaneous panniculitis-like T-cell lymphoma. *Chin J Pathol.* 2008;37:390-394.
110. Hoffman D, Chaffins M, Cankovic M, et al. Manual microdissection technique in a case of subcutaneous panniculitis-like T-cell lymphoma: a case report and review. *J Cutan Pathol.* 2012;39:769-772.
111. Li Z, Lu L, Zhou Z, et al. Recurrent mutations in epigenetic modifiers and the PI3K/AKT/mTOR pathway in subcutaneous panniculitis-like T-cell lymphoma. *Br J Haematol.* 2018;181(3):406-410.
112. Castano E, Glick S, Wolgast L, et al. Hypopigmented mycosis fungoides in childhood and adolescence: a long-term retrospective study. *J Cutan Pathol.* 2013;40:924-934.
113. Tripodo C, Iannitto E, Florena AM, et al. Gamma-delta T-cell lymphomas. *Nat Rev Clin Oncol.* 2009;6:707-717.
114. Guitart J, Weisenburger DD, Subtil A, et al. Cutaneous γδ T-cell lymphomas: a spectrum of presentations with overlap with other cytotoxic lymphomas. *Am J Surg Pathol.* 2012;36:1656-1665.
115. Choi MY, Lechowicz MJ. Management of the cutaneous peripheral T-cell lymphomas: when subtypes matter. *Cancer J.* 2012;18:439-444.
116. Bekkenk MW, Jansen PM, Meijer CJ, et al. CD56+ hematological neoplasms presenting in the skin: a retrospective analysis of 23 new cases and 130 cases from the literature. *Ann Oncol.* 2004;15:1097-1108.
117. Willemze R, Meijer CJ. Classification of cutaneous T-cell lymphoma: from Alibert to WHO-EORTC. *J Cutan Pathol.* 2006;33(suppl 1):18-26.
118. Deonizio JM, Guitart J. Current understanding of cutaneous lymphoma: selected topics. *Dermatol Clin.* 2012;30:749-761, vii–viii.

119. Kim YC, Kim SC, Yang WI, et al. Extranodal NK/T-cell lymphoma with extensive subcutaneous involvement, mimicking subcutaneous panniculitis-like T cell lymphoma. *Int J Dermatol.* 2002;41:919-921.
120. Cota C, Vale E, Viana I, et al. Cutaneous manifestations of blastic plasmacytoid dendritic cell neoplasm-morphologic and phenotypic variability in a series of 33 patients. *Am J Surg Pathol.* 2010;34(1):75-87.
121. Salva KA, Haemel AK, Pincus LB, et al. Expression of CD31/PECAM-1 (platelet endothelial cell adhesion molecule 1) by blastic plasmacytoid dendritic cell neoplasms. *JAMA Dermatol.* 2014;150(1):73-76.
122. Sweet K. Blastic plasmacytoid dendritic cell neoplasm: diagnosis, manifestations, and treatment. *Curr Opin Hematol.* 2020;27(2):103-107.
123. Massone C, Chott A, Metze D, et al. Subcutaneous, blastic natural killer (NK), NK/T-cell, and other cytotoxic lymphomas of the skin: a morphologic, immunophenotypic, and molecular study of 50 patients. *Am J Surg Pathol.* 2004;28:719-735.
124. Bernatsky S, Boivin JF, Joseph L, et al. An international cohort study of cancer in systemic lupus erythematosus. *Arthritis Rheum.* 2005;52:1481-1490.
125. Bernatsky S, Ramsey-Goldman R, Rajan R, et al. Non-Hodgkin's lymphoma in systemic lupus erythematosus. *Ann Rheum Dis.* 2005;64:1507-1509.
126. Wang X, Magro CM. Human myxovirus resistance protein 1 (MxA) as a useful marker in the differential diagnosis of subcutaneous lymphoma vs. lupus erythematosus profundus. *Eur J Dermatol.* 2012;22(5):629-633.
127. Grogg KL, Jung S, Erickson LA, et al. Primary cutaneous CD4-positive small/medium-sized pleomorphic T-cell lymphoma: a clonal T-cell lymphoproliferative disorder with indolent behavior. *Mod Pathol.* 2008;21:708-715.
128. Kempf W, Kazakov DV, Kerl K. Cutaneous lymphomas – an update. Part 1: T-cell and natural killer/T-cell lymphomas and related conditions. *Am J Dermatopathol.* 2014;36:105-123.
129. Williams VL, Torres-Cabala CA, Duvic M. Primary cutaneous small- to medium-sized CD4+ pleomorphic T-cell lymphoma: a retrospective case series and review of the provisional cutaneous lymphoma category. *Am J Clin Dermatol.* 2011;12:389-401.
130. Nofal A, Abdel-Mawla MY, Assaf M, et al. Primary cutaneous aggressive epidermotropic CD8+ T-cell lymphoma: proposed diagnostic criteria and therapeutic evaluation. *J Am Acad Dermatol.* 2012;67:748-759.
131. Szepesi A, Csomor J, Rajnai H, et al. Primary cutaneous aggressive epidermotropic CD8+ T-cell lymphoma: report of two cases with no evidence of systemic disease. *Eur J Dermatol.* 2012;22:690-691.
132. Yoshizawa N, Yagi H, Horibe T, et al. Primary cutaneous aggressive epidermotropic CD8+ T-cell lymphoma with a CD15(+)CD30(−) phenotype. *Eur J Dermatol.* 2007;17:441-442.
133. Massone C, Lozzi GP, Egberts F, et al. The protean spectrum of non-Hodgkin lymphomas with prominent involvement of subcutaneous fat. *J Cutan Pathol.* 2006;33(6):418-425.
134. Laggis C, Miles R, Stephens DM, et al. Cutaneous mantle cell lymphoma histomorphologically mimicking subcutaneous panniculitis-like T-cell lymphoma: Case report. *J Cutan Pathol.* 2019;46(7):538-541.

Cutaneous CD4+ small to medium lymphoproliferative disorder and other proliferations with TFH phenotype

Sanam Loghavi, Farrah Bakr, Helmut Beltraminelli, Alistair M. Robson, and Michael T. Tetzlaff

DEFINITION

As implied by the name, primary cutaneous small/medium CD4-positive T-cell lymphoproliferative disorder (LPD) is a lesion confined to the skin and comprising predominantly small to intermediate-sized CD4+ T cells. The lesions are typically solitary (or only a few), and by definition, these patients do not have an antecedent history of patches and plaques typical of mycosis fungoides.[1,2] The postulated cell of origin is the skin homing follicular helper T cell.[3,4] Previously referred to as "Primary cutaneous small/medium CD4-positive T-cell lymphoma," this disease was considered a provisional entity in the 2008 edition of the World Health Organization (WHO)[5]; however, due to its indolent clinical course and similar clinicopathologic features to cutaneous pseudo-T-cell lymphoma or cutaneous lymphoid hyperplasia, it was since reclassified as a "lymphoproliferative disorder" in the latest iteration of the WHO classification.[1]

GENERAL FEATURES

Primary cutaneous CD4+ small/medium T-cell lymphoproliferative disorder accounts for ~2% of all primary cutaneous T-cell lymphomas[2] and does not show a gender predilection. Most patients are elderly, in their sixth and seventh decades of life, but it can occur at any age, including in children.[2,6-16]

CLINICAL FEATURES

Primary cutaneous CD4+ small/medium T-cell lymphoproliferative disorder is generally confined to the skin.[1,15,17,18] If widespread systemic disease is present, then diagnostic considerations should include previously undiagnosed mycosis fungoides (MF) or peripheral T-cell lymphoma (PTCL) not otherwise specified (NOS) (in particular, follicular helper T-cell lymphoma), with (secondary) cutaneous tumor formation and unrecognized systemic disease. Most patients present with an isolated erythematous, violaceous, pink or tan, cutaneous papule, plaque, or nodule, involving the head and neck region, trunk, or upper extremities (Fig. 17-1). Lesions can vary in size with papules of ~4 mm and plaques of up to 6 cm in the greatest dimension.[17] Suspected clinical diagnoses often list varied malignancies, notably including B-cell lymphoma.[4] Involvement of the lower extremities is uncommon.[3] The lesions are usually asymptomatic; however, pain and/or pruritus has been described in some cases.[3,10,12,14,15] Their clinical course is variable: lesions may be of sudden onset or may exhibit a more protracted course.[7,10,11,13-15,19] Occasional lesions may resolve spontaneously.[12,20] Sometimes they resolve, at least partially, after a skin biopsy. Rarely, patients have been reported to present with alopecia[14] or purpuric,[15] poikilodermic,[3] ulcerative,[3] or annular lesions.[21]

HISTOPATHOLOGIC FINDINGS

A recent large series suggested the presence of two principle histological patterns.[17] The most common pattern (pattern 1) is characterized by lesions that typically demonstrate involvement and effacement of the dermis with either nodular or diffuse distribution. Surface ulceration may be seen in larger lesions.[2,8,10,15,22] The tumor may involve adnexal[8] (Fig. 17-2) and vascular structures; angiodestruction was described in one series, although this predated the recognition of CD4+ lymphoproliferative disorder as an entity and included CD8+ and CD4− CD8− double-negative tumors[19]; if angiodestruction occurs, it is an exceptional event indeed. The lesions are typically "top heavy" in the dermis but may extend into the deep dermis and subcutaneous tissue (Figs. 17-3 and 17-4).[2,12] A less frequent pattern (pattern 2) is a subepidermal band-like infiltrate occupying the superficial dermis with a sharply demarcated lower border or with periadnexal distribution. Epidermotropism is rare and, if present, very focal (Fig. 17-3); the presence of focal epidermotropism is significantly higher in pattern 2. Adnexotropism is common[23]; folliculotropism is usually associated with follicular dystrophy or destruction; however, follicular mucinosis is not seen.

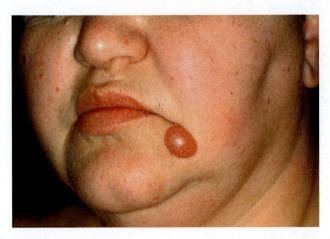

FIGURE 17-1. Clinical appearance of primary cutaneous CD4+ small/medium T-cell LPD. Solitary erythematous nodular lesion on the face of a 48-year-old woman.

Vascular changes including capillary hyperplasia, angiocentricity, and high endothelial venule formation is common and more often associated with pattern 1. Neurotropism is seen in up to 50% of cases.[17]

The majority of neoplastic cells are of small to medium size, with variable but appreciable atypia; however, a minor subset (<30%) may be large and exhibit more pronounced cytologic atypia (Fig. 17-6).[2,7] Pattern 1 lesions typically contain a larger proportion of large cells compared with pattern 2 lesions and show higher mitotic activity. The neoplastic CD4+ T cells are almost invariably accompanied by a variable admixture of CD8+ reactive T cells, histiocytes, eosinophils, polytypic plasma cells,[11,12] small B lymphocytes, and immunoblasts[3,4,6,8,9,11,12,15,22] as well as rare neutrophils.[12] An associated granulomatous reaction with multinucleated giant cells may be seen, mostly noted around follicular and adnexal structures. Tumor necrosis is not seen,[8,21,24] and formation of reactive secondary follicles is rare.[3,16,17]

It is important to appreciate that B cells are universally found in primary cutaneous small/medium CD4+ T-cell lymphoproliferative disorder (PCSM-LPD); moreover, they can account for up to 60% of the cell population[3,6,8,9,12,15,17,22,25-29]; these include small B cells and also immunoblasts, the latter scattered and typically surrounded by clusters of atypical CD4+ cells expressing PD-1 in a pseudorosette pattern.[3] The original defining criterion for PCSM-LPD states that these large cells must not make up more than 30% of the infiltrate[3,7,19]; however, tumors are reported with greater numbers, up to 40%,[17,25,30] which in some cases may reflect sampling bias of small partial biopsies (Fig. 17-7).

Of note, pattern 1 lesions more commonly involve the head and neck region and present as nodules and tumors, whereas pattern 2 lesions typically present as papules and plaques and more commonly involve the trunk.[17]

IMMUNOPHENOTYPE

The lesional cells express the pan T-cell marker CD3. By definition, the lesional cells are CD4+, CD8−, and CD30−.[1,6] They express T-cell receptor (TCR) αβ (β-F1) and are negative for TCR γδ.[31] Cytotoxic markers are not expressed.[19] Loss of pan T-cell antigens other than CD7 is unusual but may be seen.[4,7,8,10-13,15,32] The neoplastic cells express follicular helper T-cell markers including PD-1, CXCL13, ICOS, and BCL6 (variable and typically isolated to the medium/large cells); of these, PD-1 and Bcl-6 are the most widely expressed. PD1 is mostly expressed by atypical medium to large cells, frequently distributed in small clusters, whereas ICOS is also expressed by small lymphocytes. CXCL-13 is often positive in only a minor proportion of cells, and CD10 expression is typically negative (Fig. 17-5, 17-6, and 17-8).[3,4,9,17] Immunohistochemical studies for these markers may help highlight pseudorosette formation by neoplastic cells around CD20+ small B cells or CD30+ B immunoblasts.[3]

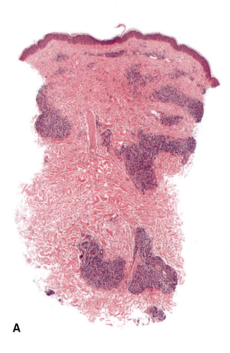
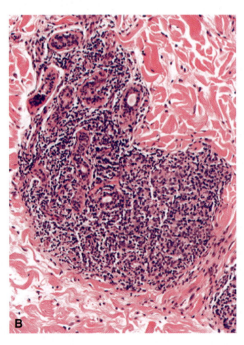

FIGURE 17-2. Primary cutaneous CD4+ small/medium T-cell LPD. A. Scanning magnification shows a variably dense dermal lymphoid infiltrate with periadnexal accentuation (hematoxylin and eosin [H&E]; 40×). **B.** Higher-power examination reveals a periadnexal infiltrate comprising predominantly medium-sized lymphocytes with hyperchromatic nuclei and no significant cytologic atypia (H&E; 200×).

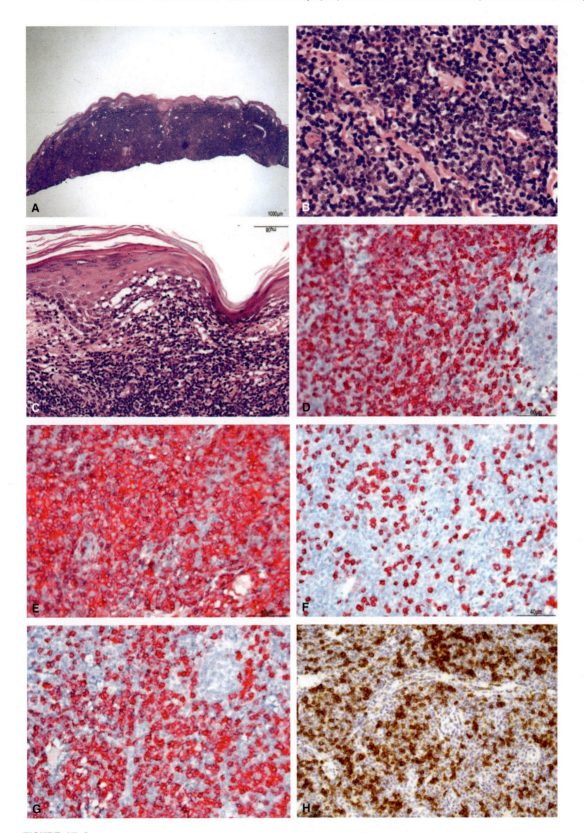

FIGURE 17-3. Primary cutaneous CD4+ small/medium T-cell LPD. A. Scanning magnification shows a dense pan-dermal lymphoid infiltrate (H&E; 20×); **B.** higher-power examination shows the infiltrate comprises a mixture of small and medium-sized lymphocytes, some with hyperchromatic nuclei and others with more vesicular appearing nuclear chromatin (H&E; 400×). **C.** Focal, minimal epidermotropism is present (H&E; 200×). Immunohistochemical studies demonstrate a predominance of CD3+ T cells (**D**, 400×). The CD3+ T cells are predominantly CD4+ (**E**, 400×). Few admixed CD8+ T cells (**F**, 400×) and numerous admixed CD20+ small B cells (**G**, 400×) are also present. Many of the lesional cells express PD-1 (**H**, 400×).

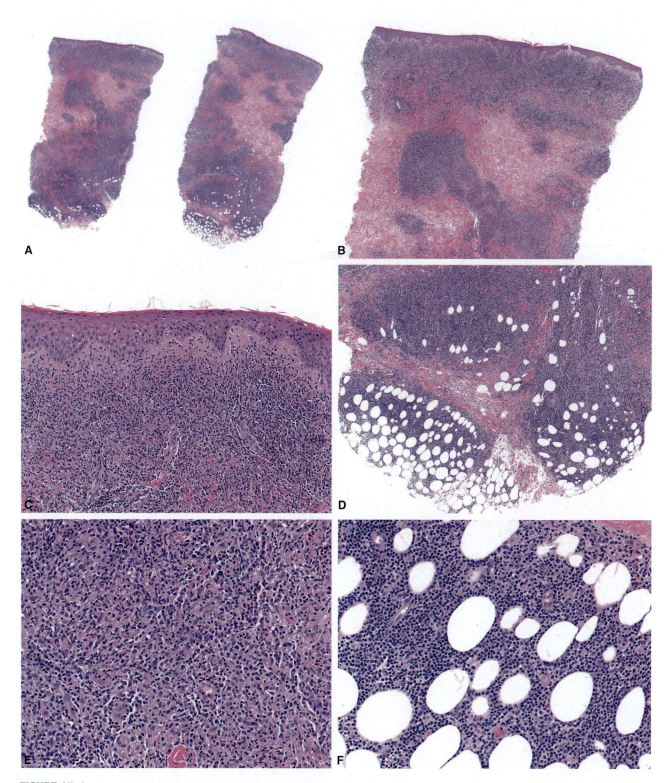

FIGURE 17-4. Primary cutaneous CD4+ small/medium T-cell LPD. A. Scanning magnification reveals a nodular, variably dense pan-dermal lymphoid infiltrate with extension into the subcutaneous adipose tissue (H&E; 40×). **B.** Higher-power examination reveals a superficial lymphoid infiltrate with a lichenoid and periadnexal/perivascular distribution (H&E; 100×). **C.** Epidermotropism is not prominent (H&E; 200×). **D.** The infiltrate extends to involve the subcutaneous adipose tissue (H&E; 100×). **E.** Higher-power examination of the superficial infiltrate reveals the infiltrate to comprise predominantly medium-sized lymphocytes with hyperchromatic nuclei, admixed with histiocytes, scattered eosinophils, and prominent endothelial cells (H&E; 400×). **F.** Higher-power examination reveals the subcutaneous infiltrate to comprise predominantly medium-sized lymphocytes with hyperchromatic nuclei, which entrap isolated adipocytes (H&E; 400×).

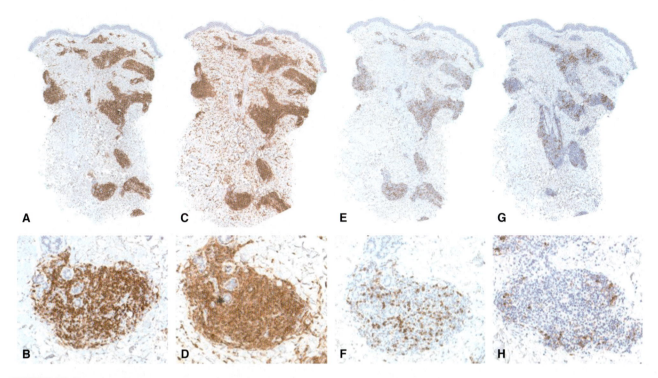

FIGURE 17-5. Immunophenotypic findings typical of primary cutaneous CD4+ small/medium T-cell LPD. Immunohistochemical studies demonstrate a predominance of CD3+ T cells (**A**, 40×; **B**, 200×) that are predominantly CD4+ (**C**, 40×; **D**, 200×) with scattered admixed reactive CD8+ T cells (**E**, 40×; **F**, 200×) and CD20+ B cells (**G**, 40×; **H**, 200×) throughout.

The frequent expression of follicular helper T-cell markers is believed to underlie the presence of numerous associated reactive B cells in the tumor.[16] There is no evidence of Epstein–Barr virus infection.[3,11,19,33] The Ki-67 proliferation index is typically low (usually ~5% and occasionally up to 20%).[4,8,11,32,34] Rare cases with relatively high proliferation index (~40%) have been described to still follow an indolent clinical course.[35] Larger studies are therefore required to determine the significance of the proliferative index in this lymphoproliferative disorder.

GENETIC AND MOLECULAR FINDINGS

Monoclonal T-cell receptor gene rearrangements are detected in 50% to 100% of cases.[3,6,8,10,13,31] In our experience, the diagnosis of primary cutaneous small/medium CD4-positive T-cell lymphoproliferative disorder would be unusual in the absence of a monoclonal T-cell receptor gene rearrangement, as the distinction from cutaneous lymphoid hyperplasia would be difficult in this setting. No recurrent chromosomal alterations have been identified.[36] Studies investigating the role of somatic gene mutations are sparse; a rare case with *DNMT3A* mutation has been described.[17]

DIFFERENTIAL DIAGNOSES

Primary cutaneous follicular helper T-cell lymphoma:[37] Occasionally, cutaneous T-cell lymphomas with a TFH phenotype, similar to CD4+ small/medium T-cell LPD, present with widespread skin lesions and large, rapidly growing tumors, contain more than 30% large tumor cells, and exhibit a high Ki-67 proliferation index. These lesions, which remain a poorly defined group of uncertain nosological status, should not be classified as CD4+ small/medium T-cell LPD due to their aggressive clinical course and are best classified as PTCL-NOS with a TFH phenotype.[19]

Cutaneous lymphoid hyperplasia with predominance of helper T cells: Similar to primary cutaneous small/medium T-cell LPD, these lesions also often present with an isolated cutaneous papule or nodule and are histologically composed of a heterogeneous population of lymphocytes, histiocytes, eosinophils, plasma cells, and occasional larger, atypical-appearing cells. Lack of spontaneous clinical resolution, demonstration of immunophenotypic aberrancy (in particular, loss of pan T-cell antigens), and/or monoclonal T-cell gene rearrangement support the diagnosis of primary cutaneous CD4+ small/medium T-cell LPD.[38,39] However, the distinction is not absolute, and since none of the aforementioned features are either entirely sensitive or specific, they should not be used in isolation to establish a diagnosis.[12,20]

Primary cutaneous marginal zone lymphoma (PCMZL): PCMZL is an important differential diagnosis, which may mimic PCSM-LPD owing to several overlapping clinicopathological features.[8,12,40-43] As noted above, B-cell lymphoma may be a suggested clinical differential diagnosis.[4] Each may present as a solitary lesion. In both PCSM-LPD and MZL, particularly the class-switched variant, there are often polymorphous dermal infiltrates comprising significant B- and T-cell populations; in PCSM-LPD B cells may account for up to 60% of the infiltrate.[3,8,9,12,17] Clonality assessment usually confirms these B cells as polyclonal,[3,15] but B-cell clones have been reported in 7 of 24 cases analyzed.[17,30] Importantly, all

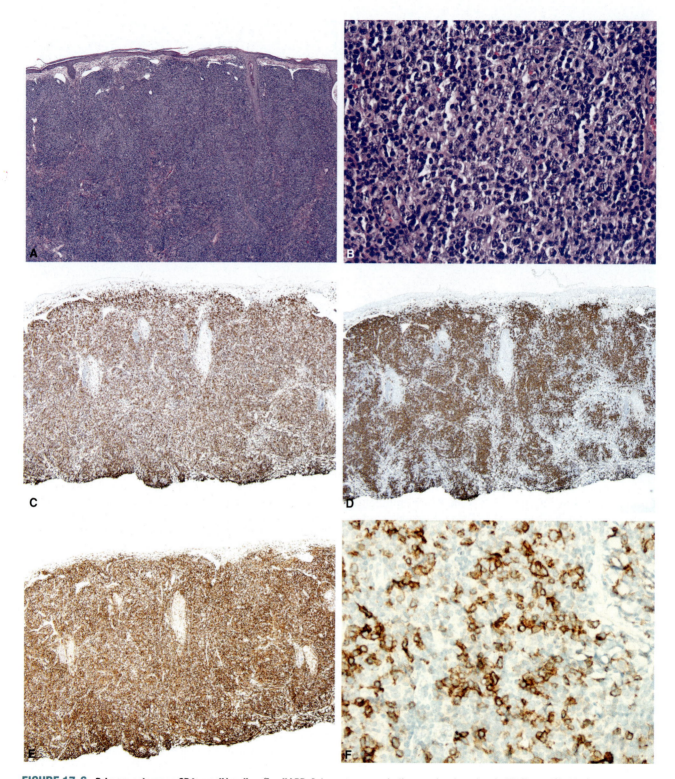

FIGURE 17-6. Primary cutaneous CD4+ small/medium T-cell LPD. A. Low-power examination reveals a dense lymphoid infiltrate diffusely effacing the dermis (H&E; 40×). **B.** Higher-power examination reveals a periadnexal infiltrate comprising predominantly medium-sized lymphocytes, some with hyperchromatic nuclei and others with more vesicular appearing nuclear chromatin (H&E; 400×). Immunohistochemical studies demonstrate a predominance of CD3+ T cells (100×) with numerous clusters of admixed CD20+ B cells (100×). The CD3+ T cells are predominantly CD4+ (100×) with a subset expressing PD-1 (100×).

cases of PCSM-LPD with B-cell clones reported to date had concomitant T-cell clones, an exceptional event in PCMZL. The neoplastic "centrocyte-like" cells of PCMZL can have an appearance similar to that of the small/medium lymphocytes in PCSM-LPD.[44] Plasma cells, seen in both conditions, are usually light chain restricted in PCMZL when present but polytypic in PCSM-LPD.[45] A further key distinguishing feature has been the TFH phenotype in a proportion of the T-cell population in PCSM-LPD, with the characteristic pattern of PD-1+ rosettes, which often surround B-cell blasts.[3] However,

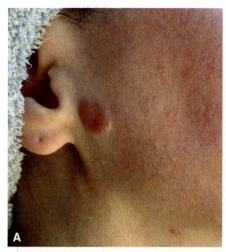
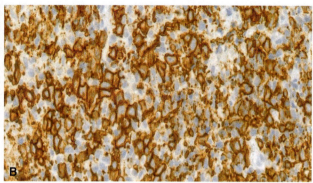

FIGURE 17-7. A. A primary cutaneous CD4+ small/medium T-cell LPD, which regressed over 2 months following partial biopsy. The pathology was of a diffuse population of CD4+ T cells expressing follicular T-helper markers including PD-1+ rosettes, but with expansive nodules of large cells and blasts **(B)** that had a CD20+ (inset) MUM-1+ phenotype. (Reprinted from Bakr F, Wain EM, Wong S, Palmer R, Robson A. Prominent blasts in primary cutaneous CD4+ small/medium T-cell lymphoproliferative disorder. A reconsideration of diagnostic criteria. *Am J Dermatopathol.* 2021;43(12):e190-e196, with permission.)

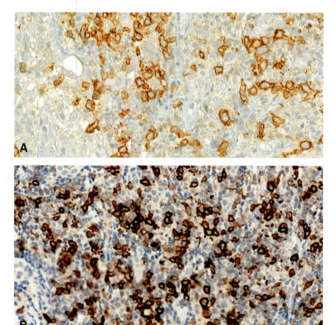

FIGURE 17-8. PD-1-positive cells in primary cutaneous CD4+ small/medium T-cell LPD adopt a characteristic rosette pattern **(A)**, which have been shown to surround B cells. This identical pattern is found in many cases of primary cutaneous marginal zone lymphoma **(B)**, which can be dominated by a T-cell infiltrate and so lead to diagnostic confusion. (A, Reprinted from Bakr F, Wain EM, Wong S, Palmer R, Robson A. Prominent blasts in primary cutaneous CD4+ small/medium T-cell lymphoproliferative disorder. A reconsideration of diagnostic criteria. *Am J Dermatopathol.* 2021;43(12):e190-e196, with permission. B, Reprinted from Robson A, Bakr F, Rashidghamat E, et al. Follicular T-helper cells in marginal zone lymphoma: Evidence of an organoid immune response. *Am J Dermatopathol.* 2021;43(12):e197-e203, with permission.)

these cells have been demonstrated in significant proportions in both PCMZL and nodal MZL.[41,42] Unsurprisingly, individual cases might pose a diagnostic challenge and indeed "overlap" tumors have been reported.[40] (see Chapter 32, Primary Cutaneous Marginal Zone Lymphoma).

<u>Mycosis fungoides</u>: Primary cutaneous CD4+ small/medium T-cell LPDs generally present clinically with isolated skin lesions on the head and neck and lack significant epidermotropism histopathologically. In contrast, patients with MF present with a history of multiple, erythematous, scaly patches and plaques typically affecting non-sun-exposed sites. Historically reported cases of MF Tumour d'Emblee, the rapid presentation of tumorous MF with dermal neoplastic cells, are commonly believed to have represented examples of a different then unrecognized aggressive lymphoma. Histopathologically, early lesions of MF are characterized by an epidermotropic infiltrate of small to medium-sized T cells. These distinctive clinical and histopathologic features most often facilitate the distinction of these two entities. Bosisio et al demonstrated that the tumor cells of MF can frequently (~55%) express T follicular helper antigens, including PD1, ICOS, CXCL13, and BCL6 and CD10.[46] This may present a challenge in distinguishing these two entities from one another purely on the basis of immunophenotypic features alone and reinforces that clinicopathologic correlation is critical for accurate diagnosis. Nevertheless, the neoplastic cells of MF showed diffuse expression of the TFH markers, and the characteristic mixed T- and B-cell populations, with a significant CD8+ "background" population, and rosetting or clusters of PD-1+ cells is not a feature of MF infiltrates.[46]

<u>Angioimmunoblastic T-cell lymphoma (AITL)</u>: Although there is some histopathologic and immunophenotypic overlap between AITL and primary cutaneous CD4+ small/medium T-cell LPD, their respective clinical presentations differ significantly. AITL may involve the skin but typically does so secondarily as these patients typically present with systemic disease, including prominent lymphadenopathy, anemia, hypergammaglobulinemia, elevated serum lactate dehydrogenase, and other systemic manifestations. In contrast to primary cutaneous CD4+ small/medium T-cell LPD, EBV-infected B cells are frequently seen in AITL.[47-49]

<u>Adult T-cell leukemia/lymphoma (ATLL)</u>: ATLL is endemic to several geographic regions including southwestern Japan, the Caribbean basin, and parts of Central Africa, whereas CD4+ small/medium T-cell lymphoma has no

specific regional distribution. The presence of marked cytologic atypia, especially with prominent epidermotropism and/or systemic involvement, should raise this differential diagnosis. PD-1 expression is a shared feature. Demonstration of human T-cell leukemia virus type-1 (HTLV1) infection, either by immunohistochemical or serologic studies would help establish the diagnosis of ATLL.[45]

Other

A case of cutaneous Richter transformation of chronic lymphocytic leukemia presenting in the skin misdiagnosed as primary cutaneous CD4+ small/medium T-cell LPD has been reported.[50] There was a significant background small lymphocyte population that expressed TFH markers, which partly obscured the diffuse large blasts of transformed CLL. The case reinforces the potential significance of blast populations in these tumors, and also the cautionary note that other lymphomas might include lymphoid populations that strongly express one or more TFH markers.

PROGNOSIS AND THERAPY

The clinical course of primary cutaneous CD4+ small/medium T-cell LPD is generally indolent. The reported overall 5-year survival is ~80% (with a reported range of 60%-100%)[17,51] but likely to be universally excellent. Cases with a reported adverse survival are believed by most authorities to represent inclusion of more aggressive systemic lymphomas (with secondary cutaneous involvement) that are best classified as PTCL NOS with TFH phenotype. Features that point toward PTCL-NOS include rapidly growing tumor nodules (≥5 cm), increased Ki-67 proliferation index (>22%-40%),[11,35] depletion of background CD8+ T cells, and increased number of CD30+ tumor cells.[11] Patients with limited disease can usually be treated successfully with local surgical excision, radiation therapy, and/or topical or intralesional steroids.[2,7,8,10,11,13,19,31,52,53] Spontaneous regression is seen in up to 32% of patients.[17]

References

1. Gaulard P, Berti E, Willemze R, Petrella T, Jaffe ES. Primary cutaneous CD4+ small/medium T-cell lymphoproliferative disorder. In: Swerdlow SH, Campo E, Harris NL, et al, eds. *WHO Classification of Tumours of Haematopoietic and Lymphoid Tissues*. IARC; 2017:401-402.
2. Willemze R, Jaffe ES, Burg G, et al. WHO-EORTC classification for cutaneous lymphomas. *Blood*. 2005;105(10):3768-3785.
3. Rodriguez Pinilla SM, Roncador G, Rodriguez-Peralto JL, et al. Primary cutaneous CD4+ small/medium-sized pleomorphic T-cell lymphoma expresses follicular T-cell markers. *Am J Surg Pathol*. 2009;33(1):81-90.
4. Ally MS, Prasad Hunasehally RY, Rodriguez-Justo M, et al. Evaluation of follicular T-helper cells in primary cutaneous CD4+ small/medium pleomorphic T-cell lymphoma and dermatitis. *J Cutan Pathol*. 2013;40(12):1006-1013.
5. Gaulard P, Berti E, Willemze R, Jaffe ES. Primary cutaneous peripheral T-cell lymphomas, rare subtypes. In: Swerdlow SH, Campo E, Harris NL, et al, eds. *WHO Classification of Tumours of Haematopoietic and Lymphoid Tissues*. IARC; 2008:304-305.
6. Baum CL, Link BK, Neppalli VT, Swick BL, Liu V. Reappraisal of the provisional entity primary cutaneous CD4+ small/medium pleomorphic T-cell lymphoma: a series of 10 adult and pediatric patients and review of the literature. *J Am Acad Dermatol*. 2011;65(4):739-748.
7. Beljaards RC, Meijer CJ, Van der Putte SC, et al. Primary cutaneous T-cell lymphoma: clinicopathological features and prognostic parameters of 35 cases other than mycosis fungoides and CD30-positive large cell lymphoma. *J Pathol*. 1994;172(1):53-60.
8. Beltraminelli H, Leinweber B, Kerl H, Cerroni L. Primary cutaneous CD4+ small-/medium-sized pleomorphic T-cell lymphoma: a cutaneous nodular proliferation of pleomorphic T lymphocytes of undetermined significance? A study of 136 cases. *Am J Dermatopathol*. 2009;31(4):317-322.
9. Cetinozman F, Jansen PM, Willemze R. Expression of programmed death-1 in primary cutaneous CD4-positive small/medium-sized pleomorphic T-cell lymphoma, cutaneous pseudo-T-cell lymphoma, and other types of cutaneous T-cell lymphoma. *Am J Surg Pathol*. 2012;36(1):109-116.
10. Friedmann D, Wechsler J, Delfau MH, et al. Primary cutaneous pleomorphic small T-cell lymphoma. A review of 11 cases. The French Study Group on Cutaneous Lymphomas. *Arch Dermatol*. 1995;131(9):1009-1015.
11. Garcia-Herrera A, Colomo L, Camos M, et al. Primary cutaneous small/medium CD4+ T-cell lymphomas: a heterogeneous group of tumors with different clinicopathologic features and outcome. *J Clin Oncol*. 2008;26(20):3364-3371.
12. Grogg KL, Jung S, Erickson LA, McClure RF, Dogan A. Primary cutaneous CD4-positive small/medium-sized pleomorphic T-cell lymphoma: a clonal T-cell lymphoproliferative disorder with indolent behavior. *Mod Pathol*. 2008;21(6):708-715.
13. Sterry W, Siebel A, Mielke V. HTLV-1-negative pleomorphic T-cell lymphoma of the skin: the clinicopathological correlations and natural history of 15 patients. *Br J Dermatol*. 1992;126(5):456-462.
14. Volks N, Oschlies I, Cario G, Weichenthal M, Folster-Holst R. Primary cutaneous CD4+ small to medium-size pleomorphic T-cell lymphoma in a 12-year-old girl. *Pediatr Dermatol*. 2013;30(5):595-599.
15. Williams VL, Torres-Cabala CA, Duvic M. Primary cutaneous small- to medium-sized CD4+ pleomorphic T-cell lymphoma: a retrospective case series and review of the provisional cutaneous lymphoma category. *Am J Clin Dermatol*. 2011;12(6):389-401.
16. Lan TT, Brown NA, Hristov AC. Controversies and considerations in the diagnosis of primary cutaneous CD4(+) small/medium T-cell lymphoma. *Arch Pathol Lab Med*. 2014;138(10):1307-1318.
17. Beltzung F, Ortonne N, Pelletier L, et al. Primary cutaneous CD4+ small/medium T-cell lymphoproliferative disorders: a clinical, pathologic, and molecular study of 60 cases presenting with a single lesion—a multicenter study of the French cutaneous lymphoma study group. *Am J Surg Pathol*. 2020;44(7):862-872.
18. Surmanowicz P, Doherty S, Sivanand A, et al. The clinical spectrum of primary cutaneous CD4+ small/medium-sized pleomorphic T-cell lymphoproliferative disorder: an updated systematic literature review and case series. *Dermatology (Basel, Switzerland)*. 2020;237:1-11.

19. Bekkenk MW, Vermeer MH, Jansen PM, et al. Peripheral T-cell lymphomas unspecified presenting in the skin: analysis of prognostic factors in a group of 82 patients. *Blood*. 2003;102(6):2213-2219.
20. Messeguer F, Gimeno E, Agusti-Mejias A, San Juan J. Primary cutaneous CD4+ small- to medium-sized pleomorphic T-cell lymphoma: report of a case with spontaneous resolution. Article in Spanish. *Actas Dermo-Sifiliográficas*. 2011;102(8):636-638.
21. Boussault P, Tucker ML, Weschler J, et al. Primary cutaneous CD4+ small/medium-sized pleomorphic T-cell lymphoma associated with an annular elastolytic giant cell granuloma. *Br J Dermatol*. 2009;160(5):1126-1128.
22. Leinweber B, Beltraminelli H, Kerl H, Cerroni L. Solitary small- to medium-sized pleomorphic T-cell nodules of undetermined significance: clinical, histopathological, immunohistochemical and molecular analysis of 26 cases. *Dermatology (Basel, Switzerland)*. 2009;219(1):42-47.
23. Pérez González YC, Llamas Velasco MDM, Díaz Recuero JL, et al. Adnexotropism as a histopathological clue for the diagnosis of primary cutaneous CD4+ small/medium-sized T-cell lymphoproliferative disorder. *Am J Dermatopathol*. 2020;42(5):383-384.
24. Scarabello A, Leinweber B, Ardigo M, et al. Cutaneous lymphomas with prominent granulomatous reaction: a potential pitfall in the histopathologic diagnosis of cutaneous T- and B-cell lymphomas. *Am J Surg Pathol*. 2002;26(10):1259-1268.
25. Magro CM, Olson LC, Fulmer CG. CD30+ T cell enriched primary cutaneous CD4+ small/medium sized pleomorphic T cell lymphoma: a distinct variant of indolent CD4+ T cell lymphoproliferative disease. *Ann Diagn Pathol*. 2017;30:52-58.
26. Topal IO, Goncu EK, Ozekinci S, Ayaz G, Aksaray F. Primary cutaneous CD4(+) small/medium-sized T-cell lymphoma of the face: successful treatment with radiation therapy. *J Dtsch Dermatol Ges*. 2016;14(5):522-524.
27. Keeling BH, Gavino ACP, Admirand J, Soldano AC. Primary cutaneous CD4-positive small/medium-sized pleomorphic T-cell lymphoproliferative disorder: report of a case and review of the literature. *J Cutan Pathol*. 2017;44(11):944-947.
28. Celebi Cherukuri N, Roth CG, Aggarwal N, Ho J, Gehris R, Akilov OE. Cutaneous small/medium CD4+ pleomorphic T-cell lymphoma-like nodule in a patient with erythema chronicum migrans. *Am J Dermatopathol*. 2016;38(6):448-452.
29. Sato-Sano M, Teixeira SP, Vargas JC, et al. Lenalidomide in the management of eosinophilic dermatosis of hematological malignancy. *J Dermatol*. 2019;46(7):618-621.
30. Bakr F, Wain EM, Wong S, Palmer R, Robson A. Prominent blasts in primary cutaneous CD4+ small/medium T-cell lymphoproliferative disorder. A reconsideration of diagnostic criteria. *Am J Dermatopathol*. 2021;43(12):e190-e196.
31. von den Driesch P, Coors EA. Localized cutaneous small to medium-sized pleomorphic T-cell lymphoma: a report of 3 cases stable for years. *J Am Acad Dermatol*. 2002;46(4):531-535.
32. James E, Sokhn JG, Gibson JF, et al. CD4+ primary cutaneous small/medium-sized pleomorphic T-cell lymphoma: a retrospective case series and review of literature. *Leuk Lymphoma*. 2015;56(4):951-957.
33. Choi M, Park SY, Park HS, Byun HJ, Cho KH. A case of primary cutaneous CD4 positive small/medium T cell lymphoma. *Ann Dermatol*. 2011;23(1):76-80.
34. Kempf W, Kazakov DV, Cozzio A, et al. Primary cutaneous CD8(+) small- to medium-sized lymphoproliferative disorder in extrafacial sites: clinicopathologic features and concept on their classification. *Am J Dermatopathol*. 2013;35(2):159-166.
35. Zhang L, Shao H. Primary cutaneous CD4 positive small/medium T-cell lymphoma with high proliferation index and CD30-positive large lymphoid cells. *J Cutan Pathol*. 2013;40(8):720-724.
36. Alberti-Violetti S, Torres-Cabala CA, Talpur R, et al. Clinicopathological and molecular study of primary cutaneous CD4+ small/medium-sized pleomorphic T-cell lymphoma. *J Cutan Pathol*. 2016;43(12):1121-1130.
37. Battistella M, Beylot-Barry M, Bachelez H, et al. Primary cutaneous follicular helper T-cell lymphoma. A new subtype of cutaneous T-cell lymphoma reported in a series of 5 cases. *Arch Dermatol*. 2012;148(7):832-839.
38. Bakels V, van Oostveen JW, van der Putte SC, Meijer CJ, Willemze R. Immunophenotyping and gene rearrangement analysis provide additional criteria to differentiate between cutaneous T-cell lymphomas and pseudo-T-cell lymphomas. *Am J Pathol*. 1997;150(6):1941-1949.
39. Bergman R. Pseudolymphoma and cutaneous lymphoma: facts and controversies. *Clin Dermatol*. 2010;28(5):568-574.
40. Bakr F, Wain EM, Barlow R, Robson A. Primary cutaneous CD4+ small/medium T-cell lymphoproliferative disorder or primary cutaneous marginal zone B-cell lymphoma? Two distinct entities with overlapping histopathological features. *Am J Dermatopathol*. 2021;43(12):e204-e212.
41. Robson A, Bakr F, Rashidghamat E, et al. Follicular T-Helper cells in marginal zone lymphoma: evidence of an organoid immune response. *Am J Dermatopathol*. 2021;43(12):e197-e203.
42. Egan C, Laurent C, Alejo JC, et al. Expansion of PD1-positive T Cells in nodal marginal zone lymphoma: a potential diagnostic pitfall. *Am J Surg Pathol*. 2020;44(5):657-664.
43. Goyal A, Moore JB, Gimbel D, et al. PD-1, S-100 and CD1a expression in pseudolymphomatous folliculitis, primary cutaneous marginal zone B-cell lymphoma (MALT lymphoma) and cutaneous lymphoid hyperplasia. *J Cutan Pathol*. 2015;42(1):6-15.
44. Cerroni L, Signoretti S, Höfler G, et al. Primary cutaneous marginal zone B-cell lymphoma: a recently described entity of low-grade malignant cutaneous B-cell lymphoma. *Am J Surg Pathol*. 1997;21(11):1307-1315.
45. Tokura Y, Sawada Y, Shimauchi T. Skin manifestations of adult T-cell leukemia/lymphoma: clinical, cytological and immunological features. *J Dermatol*. 2014;41(1):19-25.
46. Bosisio FM, Cerroni L. Expression of T-follicular helper markers in sequential biopsies of progressive mycosis fungoides and other primary cutaneous T-cell lymphomas. *Am J Dermatopathol*. 2015;37(2):115-121.
47. Mourad N, Mounier N, Briere J, et al. Clinical, biologic, and pathologic features in 157 patients with angioimmunoblastic T-cell lymphoma treated within the Groupe d'Etude des Lymphomes de l'Adulte (GELA) trials. *Blood*. 2008;111(9):4463-4470.
48. Weiss LM, Jaffe ES, Liu XF, Chen YY, Shibata D, Medeiros LJ. Detection and localization of Epstein-Barr viral genomes in angioimmunoblastic lymphadenopathy and angioimmunoblastic lymphadenopathy-like lymphoma. *Blood*. 1992;79(7):1789-1795.
49. Lin P, Hao S, Handy BC, Bueso-Ramos CE, Medeiros LJ. Lymphoid neoplasms associated with IgM paraprotein: a study of 382 patients. *Am J Clin Pathol*. 2005;123(2):200-205.

50. Rito M, Cabeçadas J, Costa Rosa J, Cravo M, Robson A. Cutaneous richter syndrome mimicking primary cutaneous CD4-positive small/medium T-cell lymphoma: case report and review of the literature. *Am J Dermatopathol.* 2018;40(4):286-290.
51. Willemze R, Cerroni L, Kempf W, et al. The 2018 update of the WHO-EORTC classification for primary cutaneous lymphomas. *Blood.* 2019;133(16):1703-1714.
52. Fink-Puches R, Zenahlik P, Back B, Smolle J, Kerl H, Cerroni L. Primary cutaneous lymphomas: applicability of current classification schemes (European Organization for Research and Treatment of Cancer, World Health Organization) based on clinicopathologic features observed in a large group of patients. *Blood.* 2002;99(3):800-805.
53. Grange F, Hedelin G, Joly P, et al. Prognostic factors in primary cutaneous lymphomas other than mycosis fungoides and the Sezary syndrome. The French Study Group on Cutaneous Lymphomas. *Blood.* 1999;93(11):3637-3642.

CHAPTER 18

Aggressive cytotoxic primary cutaneous T-cell lymphomas

Jacqueline M. Junkins-Hopkins and Ellen J. Kim

INTRODUCTION

Cytotoxic cutaneous T-cell lymphomas (CTCLs) are extremely rare non–mycosis fungoides (MF) cutaneous T-cell or natural killer (NK)-cell lymphomas that express cytotoxic markers (T-cell intracellular antigen-1 [TIA-1], granzyme B, and perforin). They have clinical and histologic features of cytotoxicity (ulceration, necrosis, angiodestruction) and typically exhibit an aggressive clinical course.[1] It is essential to note that cytotoxic markers can be expressed by other subtypes of CTCL, including indolent subtypes (such as CD8+ MF, subcutaneous panniculitis-like T-cell lymphoma [SPTCL], and primary cutaneous CD30+ lymphoproliferative disorders), and do not confer worse prognosis in those entities. Therefore, clinicopathologic correlation is essential to accurately identify true aggressive cytotoxic CTCLs. Furthermore, distinguishing subtypes of cytotoxic CTCLs from each other or advanced tumor MF is often very challenging due to extensive overlap of clinical and histologic features and often requires repeat evaluations and biopsies over time.[2] Historically, prior to the advent of a more extensive panel of immunohistochemical stains, some cases of previously described "tumor d'emblee" MF were likely actually aggressive cytotoxic CTCLs. This chapter will cover two subtypes of cytotoxic CTCLs: (1) primary cutaneous gamma-delta (γδ) T-cell lymphoma (PC GDTCL) and (2) primary cutaneous aggressive epidermotropic CD8+ cytotoxic TCL (PC AECTCL). Other aggressive CTCL subtypes such as peripheral T-cell lymphoma not otherwise specified, extranodal NK cell/T-cell lymphoma, and hydroa vacciniforme-like lymphoma are reviewed elsewhere in this book (see Chapters 19-21, respectively).

PRIMARY CUTANEOUS GAMMA-DELTA T-CELL LYMPHOMA

Definition

This is a rare subtype of cytotoxic CTCL that is characterized by cutaneous and/or subcutaneous infiltration by malignant lymphocytes expressing the γδ T-cell receptor (TCR) heterodimer.[3] It can present either as panniculitic plaques (early in its course with similar presentation as SPTCL) or as MF-like patches, plaques, or tumors, but with a tendency to develop necrosis and ulcerate more than classical MF. Until recently, identifying GDTCLs was limited by the lack of a reliable marker that could be used on routinely processed paraffin-embedded tissues.[4] Prior to the ability to demonstrate the γδ immunophenotype on paraffin sections with γM1, the diagnosis was inferred by documenting the lack of expression of the αβ TCR heterodimer by way of negative βF1 staining of the malignant population on paraffin-embedded sections. Documenting a positive γδ immunophenotype is preferred, but a diagnosis of PC GDTCL can accurately be made only in the appropriate clinical context of a cutaneous lymphoma that exhibits morphologic or systemic evidence of aggressive behavior or cytotoxicity, since γM1 can be expressed by other subtypes of CTCL (such as MF or type D lymphomatoid papulosis [LyP]).[5]

Epidemiology

The precise incidence of γδ CTCL is unknown, but this subtype accounts for <1% of all CTCLs and affects adults primarily, with most cases presenting between ages 50 and 60 years. A few pediatric cases have been reported,[6–8] including a 3-year-old.[6–8] Some series show a female predominance, but in others, males and females were equally affected.[8–10] While most patients in one large series were Caucasian, GDTCL is not restricted to this racial group.[8] In the largest US series of PC GDTCL patients reported to date, associated comorbidities included autoimmune diseases, such as lupus erythematosus (LE), other lymphoproliferative disorders, and other malignancies; and a small subset was associated with Epstein-Barr virus (EBV) expression (though the vast majority of PC GDTCL cases are EBV negative).

Etiology

PC GDTCL is sporadic and is not associated with specific genetic driver mutations. Precise etiology remains elusive, but immunosuppression and chronic antigenic stimulation may be risk factors for clonal expansion of γδ T-cells.[11]

Rarely, GDTCLs have been reported to arise in association with opportunistic infections in immunosuppressed patients,[12,13] or in the setting of immunosuppressive therapies.[14] EBV infection may play a role in a small subset of these patients.[15]

Clinical Presentation and Prognosis

The classical presentation of γδ CTCL is that of numerous or sometimes solitary or localized dermal and/or panniculitic pink or violaceous plaques that are frequently eroded, crusted, ulcerated, or necrotic. The median time of onset is approximately 2 months, with a range of 3 months to 20 years in one large series.[8] These are most common on the lower extremities, but can affect the trunk, arms, and face (panniculitic presentation)[9] (Figs. 18-1 and 18-2). Oral mucosal lesions have rarely been reported. Lesions may have epidermal change (scaling) and can mimic MF (Fig. 18-3) or psoriasis (Fig. 18-4), prior to becoming necrotic or ulcerated. Less commonly, it can mimic pyoderma or arthropod assault.[8] Constitutional symptoms may be present and include low-grade fevers, chills, fatigue, and night sweats. Disease progression can result in spread to extracutaneous sites, including the central nervous system. Gastrointestinal disease may be present at the time of skin diagnosis.[8] Nodal and hepatosplenic involvement by lymphoma is less common, although there is a subtype of γδ lymphoma that specifically homes to the liver and spleen (hepatosplenic T-cell lymphoma).

One distinct complication of the cytotoxic CTCLs is secondary hemophagocytic syndrome (HPS), more recently referred to as hemophagocytic lymphohistiocytosis (HLH).[16] HLH is a result of overactivation of T-cells and histiocytes in the reticuloendothelial system and presents with fever, hepatosplenomegaly, and lymphadenopathy. Lab tests will reveal pancytopenia, elevated lactate dehydrogenase, and liver function test elevations. Other abnormalities include elevated erythrocyte sedimentation rate, C-reactive protein, and ferritin. HLH is a poor prognostic sign, although the prognosis for PC GDTCL is poor even in the absence of HPS.[9]

The staging system used for γδ CTCL is different from that used for MF/Sézary syndrome. It is an anatomic staging system only (tumor-node-metastasis) without any associated numeric staging.[17]

Optimal therapies for γδ CTCL are unknown although numerous skin-directed and systemic therapies have been published, with mixed response. The most common regimen used is CHOP.[8,18–20] Systemic agents such as interferons and toll-like receptor agonists (imiquimod) should be avoided as they could stimulate further cytotoxicity of the tumor cells. Brentuximab vedotin (anti-CD30 therapy) has been reported to be successful in small case series and case reports.[21–24] Interestingly, some of the cases in the series of Talpur et al showed clinical responses with levels of CD30 expression below 10%. Based on the ECHELON-2 study,[25] patients with PC GDTCL are recommended to be treated with frontline BV-CHP if CD30 expression is present in more than 10% of the tumor cells. Allogeneic bone marrow transplant is useful in patients showing significant clinical responses.[26]

The prognosis of γδ CTCL is poor, with 5-year overall survival ranging from 0% to 34% in published studies.[3,8–10] A more recent retrospective series of 53 patients published by Guitart and colleagues demonstrated a 19.9% 5-year survival, with a median survival of 31 months. An MF-like clinical presentation followed a more indolent course when compared to the more aggressive panniculitic presentation.[8] PC GDTCL can occasionally have an initially indolent course, but then switch to a more aggressive course.[27–31]

Histology

Histologically, there is an infiltrate of atypical lymphocytes, with variable involvement of the dermis, epidermis, and subcutis. These histologic patterns may vary within the same patient and may be determined, in part, by the morphology of the lesion biopsied. The dermis is usually the epicenter, but a characteristic presentation of GDTCL is that of simultaneous epidermal, dermal, and subcutaneous involvement (Fig. 18-5). Perivascular, periadnexal, lichenoid, interstitial, nodular, and/or diffuse infiltrative patterns may be seen (Fig. 18-5).

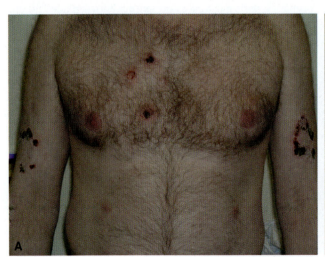 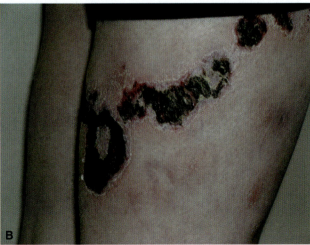

FIGURE 18-1. **A.** Primary cutaneous γδ T-cell lymphoma. **B.** Ulcerated plaques and nodules on the trunk and extremities with necrosis and hemorrhagic crusting.

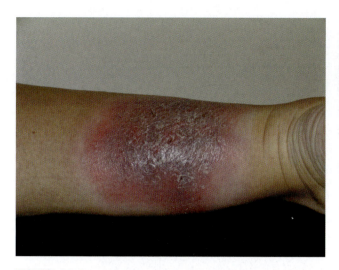

FIGURE 18-2. Primary cutaneous γδ T-cell lymphoma. Panniculitic plaques on the leg.

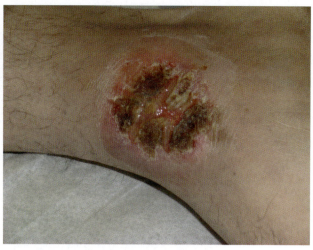

FIGURE 18-4. Primary cutaneous γδ T-cell lymphoma. Crusted and eroded psoriasiform plaque on the anterior ankle.

Extension into the subcutis is common. Karyorrhexis, necrosis, and emperipolesis can be observed. Similar to SPTCL, a lobular panniculitic infiltrate may demonstrate atypical T-cells encircling the adipocytes (rimming) (Fig. 18-6). Epidermal involvement takes on a variety of patterns. The lymphocytes are frequently noted at the base of the epidermis, and may be associated with dyskeratosis, extravasation and exocytosis of erythrocytes and lymphocytes, or a vacuolar interface dermatitis similar to LE (Fig. 18-7). The epidermal pattern may mimic MF (although Pautrier microabscesses are absent). Epidermotropism may be strikingly pagetoid throughout the entire thickness of the epidermis, simulating pagetoid reticulosis, or primary cutaneous AECTCL, and may involve adnexae. This latter presentation has been associated with gastrointestinal involvement.[8] Evidence of cytotoxicity may be manifest by dermal, epidermal, and/or subcutaneous necrosis, karyorrhexis, erythrocyte extravasation, and vascular invasion with fibrinoid necrosis. Necrosis is especially prominent when accompanied by angiodestruction. Other findings that may be encountered include neurotropism and prominent mucin deposition (Fig. 18-8). γδ CTCL cytomorphology can be variable. Many cases show a monotonous infiltrate of medium-sized lymphocytes, while in other cases, pleomorphism is present, with the infiltrate being composed of small, medium, and/or large lymphocytes. The nuclei are irregular or elongate with indented chromatin-dense or vesicular nuclei and scant slightly granular cytoplasm[8] (Fig. 18-9). Eosinophils and plasma cells are rarely seen, but may be present, especially if there is an adnexotropic component.[8] A histiocytic component may be present, and at times may be granulomatous, mimicking an infectious process. Or the histiocytes may simulate a benign process, such as traumatic panniculitis (Fig. 18-10).

Immunophenotype

Prior to 2009, there was no γδ antibody available for formalin-fixed paraffin-embedded (FFPE) tissue. Detection of γδ-expressing T-cells was possible only on frozen tissue or flow cytometry using TCR-δ1. Panniculitic cases of γδ CTCL were difficult to diagnose as it was difficult to obtain quality frozen sections from subcutaneous fat or to get sufficient number of tumor cells for flow cytometry. Lack of TCR αβ (βF1 loss) staining was often the only clue of potential PC GDTCL. Roullet and colleagues demonstrated in 2009 an immunohistochemical stain that worked on FFPE tissue (γM1),[4] allowing a more definitive diagnosis of GDTCL on routine biopsy specimens. Clone H-41 from Santa Cruz reliably labels TCR delta chain (Jungbluth et al[32]) and similarly allows a "positive" detection of γδ phenotype.

The immunophenotype of γδ CTCL is typically as follows: CD3+/CD2+/γM1+/H41+/TIA-1+/granzyme B+/perforin+/CD56+/CD4−/CD8−/CD5−/βF1−/CD45RA+/CD7−/+ (Figs. 18-11 and 18-12). Some cases can be CD8+. CD30 is typically negative. Evaluation for EBV is typically negative by

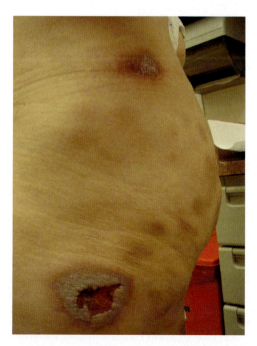

FIGURE 18-3. Primary cutaneous γδ T-cell lymphoma. MF-like presentation with plaques on buttocks and some plaques with prominent ulceration.

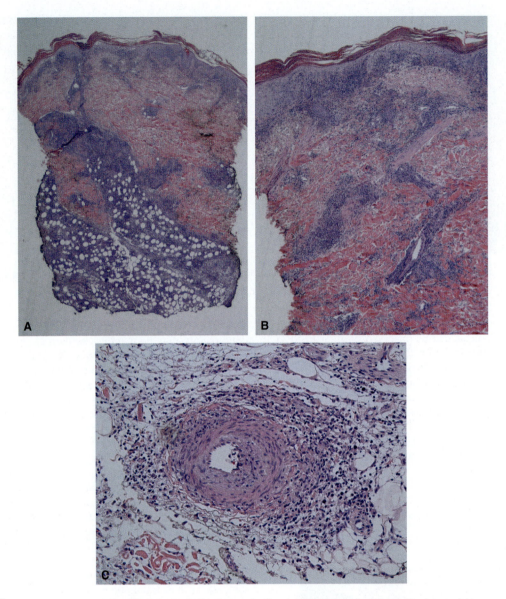

FIGURE 18-5. Primary cutaneous γδ T-cell lymphoma. A. Simultaneous involvement of epidermis, dermis, and subcutaneous fat is a common presentation (H and E, ×20). **B.** A lichenoid, perivascular, and interstitial pattern is seen in this biopsy (H and E, ×50). **C.** Angiocentrism may be seen, as demonstrated here (H and E, ×200).

immunohistochemistry (latent membrane protein [LMP]) and in situ hybridization (Epstein-Barr virus encoded RNA [EBER]), although rare cases felt to represent GDTCL have demonstrated EBER positivity.[8] Rarely, both heterodimers may be negative by tissue immunohistochemistry, but demonstrable by flow cytometry.[8] A recent study by Agbay et al reveals antigenic modulation in nine cases of PC GDTCL.[33] Gain of reactivity occurred in seven (31.8%) and loss in three (13.6%); increased reactivity in four (18.2%) and decreased in eight (36.4%). Molecular analysis of TCRγ showed identically sized monoclonal rearrangements between biopsy pairs in 4/4 (100%) patients. The most frequently affected markers included CD7, CD30, CD56, TIA-1, and CD8. Notoriously, gain of CD30 expression was seen in 44.4% of cases, an interesting marker from a therapeutic perspective.

Genetic and Molecular Findings

There is a paucity of data with regard to molecular genetics of PC GDTCL. In one patient studied via spectral karyotyping and genome-wide single nucleotide polymorphism arrays, multiple cytogenetic abnormalities were detected including (1) chromosomal translocations (at 9p21, 14q11.2, 14q32.1, 16q23.1) that corresponded to loci involved in T-cell lymphoma tumorigenesis such as *WWOX*, *TCL* gene cluster, and *BCL11B* and (2) various genome copy number gains and losses affecting gene expression along RAS, PI3K/AKT/mTOR, MYC, and TP53 signaling pathways.[34]

A novel study by Daniels et al evaluated the genetic landscape of PC GDTCL in a cohort of 29 cases.[35] Genome-wide DNA, RNA, and TCR sequencing was performed. Like αβ

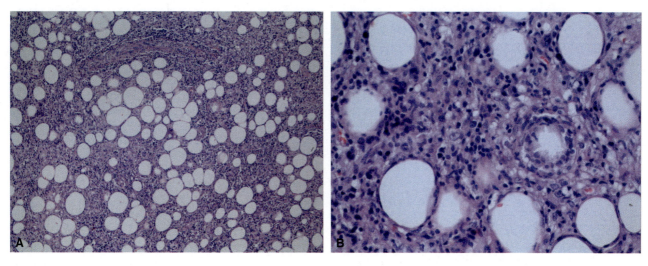

FIGURE 18-6. Primary cutaneous γδ T-cell lymphoma. A. Replacement of the fat lobule and disruption of the normal adipocyte architecture by malignant tumor cells (H and E, ×100). **B.** High-power view of subcutis, demonstrating a pleomorphic infiltrate of mostly intermediate-to-large hyperchromatic and atypical lymphocytes, admixed with larger cells and histiocytes. Some lymphocytes rim the adipocytes (H and E, ×400).

T-cells, γδ T-cells undergo VDJ recombination during development; however, unlike for αβ T-cells, the choice of Vγ and Vδ segments appears to predict tissue homing and effector function. The vast majority of γδ T-cells express either Vδ1 or Vδ2 TCRs. Vδ1 γδ T-cells predominate in mucosal interfaces such as the intestinal epithelia. Vδ2 cells represent the majority of circulating γδ T-cells in the blood. The initial presumption was one where all cases of PC GDTCL will have Vδ2 expression, but this did not happen. Indeed, they found that cases of PC GDTCL with an epidermotropic pattern had a Vδ1 phenotype, whereas more conventional cases with adipotropism had Vδ2 expression.

Vδ2 lymphomas have higher expression of Vδ2-specific genes (*IL12RB2, IL23R, CD26, RORC*). Vδ1 lymphomas have higher levels of *LEF1, TIGIT,* and *CCR8*. Their RNA-Seq analysis also showed enrichment in cytotoxic and inflammatory cytokines. Th1-associated genes (*IFNG* and *STAT4*) and Th17-associated genes (*IL26, IL23R, RORC*) were enriched in Vδ2 lymphomas. Hence, higher expression of pathways involving type I interferon or interferon-γ were noted in Vδ2 tumors. Vδ2 tumors displayed a more aggressive behavior with associated B symptoms, lymph node involvement, tumoral lesions, ulceration, and presence of HLH.

The mutational landscape also offered a new perspective in PC GDTCLs: mutations in the MAPK (*KRAS, NRAS, MAPK1*), MYC (*MYC, MYCN, FBXW7*), JAK/STAT—21% (*STAT3, STAT5B, JAK3, SOCS1*) and chromatin remodeling genes (*ARID1A, TRRAP, TET2, KMT2D*) were found in these tumors. Additional mutations in other genes frequently

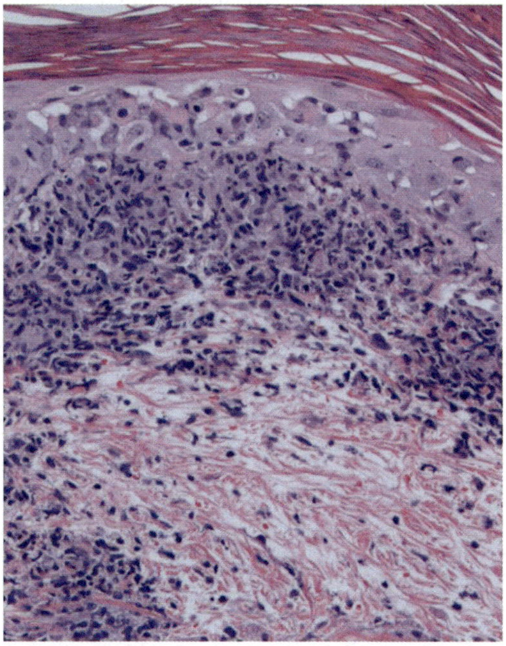

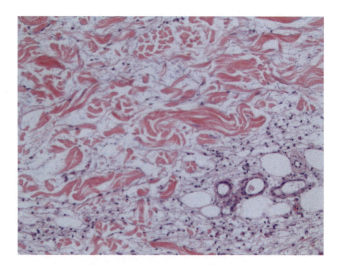

FIGURE 18-7. Primary cutaneous γδ lymphoma demonstrating a lichenoid tissue reaction with exocytosis, basal layer disruption, and dyskeratosis.

FIGURE 18-8. Primary cutaneous γδ lymphoma. Prominent hyaluronic acid (mucin) is splaying the dermal collagen bundles (H and E, ×200).

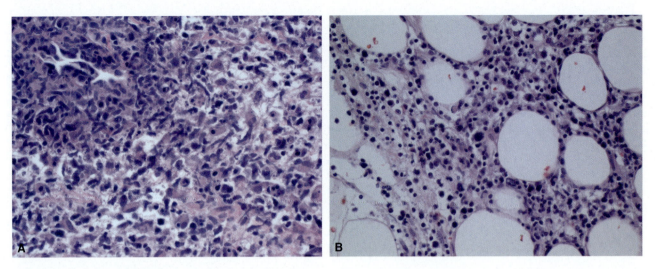

FIGURE 18-9. Primary cutaneous γδ lymphoma. A. High power demonstrating a pleomorphic infiltrate of atypical lymphocytes with intermediate-sized hyperchromatic nuclei, some of which have irregular indented or elongated nuclei and prominent cytoplasm (H and E, ×400). **B.** There is karyorrhexis. Rimming is not consistently present, in contrast to SPTCL (H and E, ×400).

seen in other T-cell lymphomas were also present (*CDKN2A, IDH2, TP53, TNFAIP3, FAS, PDCD1*). Copy number variations were also studied: recurrent arm level amplifications and deletions, including amplification of 1q (33%), 15q (33%), and 7q (39%) and deletions of 9p (22%) and 18q (22%) were identified. Deletions in *CDKN2A*, including biallelic deletions, were seen in 61% of cases. *ARID1A* was deleted in 28% of cases. Significantly recurrent amplifications included *TNFRSF1B* (amplified in 33%), which encodes the NF-kB pathway activating oncogene *TNFR2*, and *MAP4K4* (amplified in 17%), an activator of ERK signaling associated with poor outcomes in numerous cancers.

Postulated Cell of Origin

γδ T-cells comprise up to 5% of all T-cells in the body and are present in the skin and the gut primarily (where they can comprise up to 50% of mucosal site T-cells).[12] They are involved in innate and adaptive immunity for antimicrobial and antitumor surveillance. They are typically CD4-, CD8-, and express γδ TCR. In contrast to hepatosplenic GDTCLs, PC GDTCLs are composed of mature GD T-cells and express cytotoxic markers.

Differential Diagnosis

The clinical differential diagnosis for γδ CTCL that presents as dermal/subcutaneous plaques includes (1) inflammatory panniculitis (erythema nodosum, erythema induratum, lupus panniculitis, infectious panniculitis), (2) SPTCL—typically does not ulcerate, (3) cutaneous polyarteritis nodosa or other medium/large vessel vasculitis, (4) cutaneous metastases or lymphoma cutis or leukemia cutis, (5) other cytotoxic CTCLs (aggressive epidermotropic cytotoxic CD8+

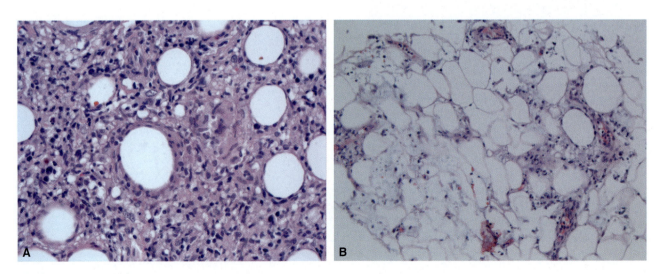

FIGURE 18-10. Primary cutaneous γδ lymphoma. A. Some areas may show prominent histiocytes, with multinucleated giant cells, simulating a granulomatous process (H and E, ×200). **B.** The histiocytes may predominate over the atypical lymphocytes, mimicking a benign panniculitis (H and E, ×200).

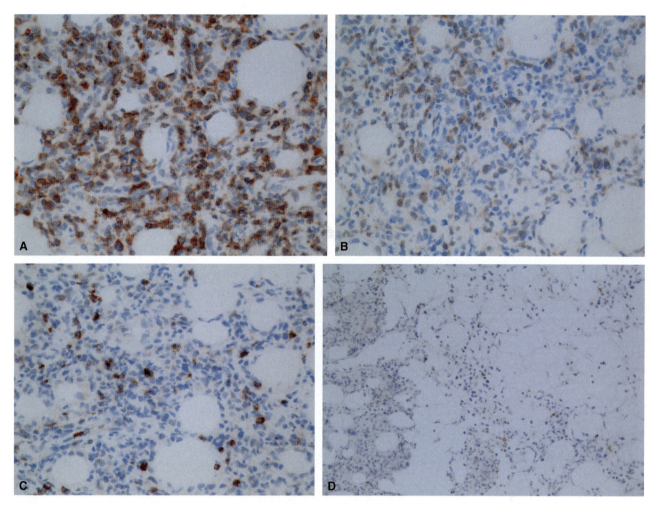

FIGURE 18-11. Primary cutaneous γδ lymphoma is frequently negative for CD4, CD8, and CD5. Immunohistochemical stains CD3 **(A)**; CD4 **(B)**; CD8 **(C)**; CD5 **(D)**.

CTCL, extranodal NK/T-cell lymphoma, MF), (6) aggressive advanced MF/CTCL, and (7) other aggressive lymphomas, such as diffuse large B-cell lymphoma, leg type.

The histologic differential includes other cytotoxic T-cell lymphomas, including SPTCL, extranodal NK/T-cell lymphoma, nasal type, and AECTCL (discussed below), as well as blastic plasmacytoid dendritic cell neoplasm, and nonmalignant conditions, such as lupus panniculitis and infection. However, a key distinction must be made between cases of conventional MF which have a γδ either at diagnosis or upon disease progression and conventional cases of PC GDTCL. Phenotypic switch of cases of MF to a γδ pattern has been documented in the literature.[36–38] Merrill et al[39] documented a large series of cases (27 biopsies from 13 patients) with epidermotropic PC GDCTL and compared them to cases of conventional PC-GDTCL. The results were indeed stunning: the epidermotropic variants have a much better prognosis, and median survival was not reached, compared to a median survival of 10 months for conventional PC-GDTCL. These results are supported by the molecular findings from Daniels et al described previously, based on the differences of Vδ1 and Vδ2 tumors. These findings bring up an important diagnostic dilemma: are epidermotropic tumors accurate examples of PC-GDTCL or should only conventional cases without significant epidermotropism be accurately classified as such?

Demonstrating a γδ immunophenotype directly (preferred) or indirectly with negative βF1 staining is the only definitive way to confirm a diagnosis of GDTCL, since there is much overlap with the other lymphoma subtypes, in addition to a careful review of the clinical, morphologic, and immunophenotypic findings. Flow cytometry may offer diagnostic information if tissue immunohistochemistry is not possible. However, there are rare examples of other CTCL subtypes, including LyP, PC-ALCL, and MF, that express a γδ immunophenotype,[40] and yet do not behave in an aggressive fashion typical of GDTCL. Additionally, infections may rarely present with clinical, histologic, and immunophenotypic features that mimic GDTCL. Such a case has been reported with *Stenotrophomonas maltophilia*, requiring tissue culture and response to antibiotics to confirm the diagnosis.[41]

SPTCL is a close mimicker of GDTCL, and in fact, prior to 2005, "SPTCL" was an umbrella term for both αβ and γδ cases of CTCL that affected the panniculus.[9] In 2005, the WHO-EORTC classification system for CTCL made a

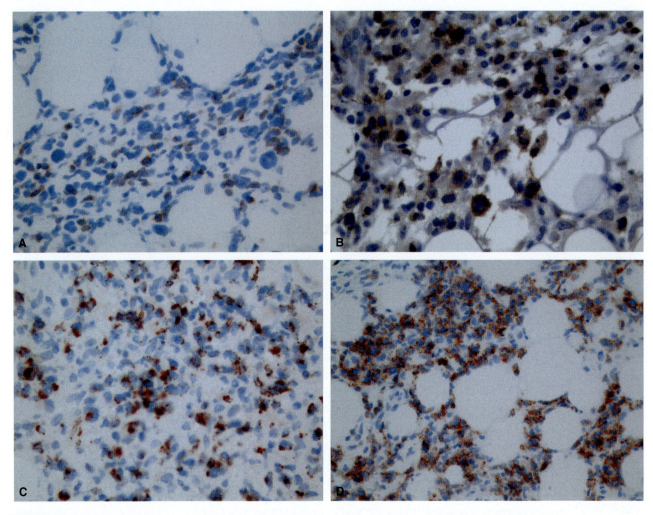

FIGURE 18-12. Primary cutaneous γδ lymphoma. Immunohistochemistry: The tumor cells are negative for βF1 **(A)** and positive for γδ **(B)**, TIA-1 **(C)**, and CD56 **(D)**.

distinction between the two, based on the different prognoses and clinical course, and defined by the immunophenotype of the tumor cell. Thus, the γδ TCR immunophenotype (γM1+/βF1−) defines the more aggressive primary cutaneous GD T-cell lymphoma, frequently associated with fatal HLH, and in contrast, βF1+/γM1− T-cells characterize the αβ T-cell of the more indolent SPTCL.[3] By light microscopy, extensive necrosis, angiodestruction, or involvement of epidermis and dermis by tumor cells favors GDTCL over SPTCL, which is typically confined to the subcutis or periadnexal fat. Identifying tumor cells that are CD4−/CD5−/CD8−/CD56+ also strongly supports GDTCL over the CD8+ SPTCL. Ultimately, because SPTCL and GDTCL have similar clinical and histologic features, these require differentiation with βF1 and γM1 immunohistochemistry, documenting αβ and γδ immunophenotypes, respectively.

NK/T-cell lymphoma, nasal type, shows overlap with GDTCL, including CD56 and cytotoxic immunophenotype, necrosis, and angiodestruction. Aside from a handful of cases demonstrating evidence of EBV, GDTCL is typically negative for EBV (EBER by in situ hybridization is preferred over LMP, due to frequent negative staining in the latter). In addition to CD56 and EBV positivity, NK/T-cell lymphoma, nasal type, is favored by the presence of CD3ε+/CD3 surface (−) immunophenotype and germline configuration of the *TCR* gene, in contrast to monoclonal *TCR* rearrangement seen in GDTCL. Nasal/nasopharyngeal/peri-nasal facial involvement also favors this diagnosis, but because NK/T-cell lymphoma, nasal type, may have extrafacial disease, location cannot always definitively discriminate these entities.

Hydroa vacciniforme-like lymphoproliferative disorder is a rare cytotoxic sometimes CD56+ lymphoma that has some overlap with GDTCL, but the clinical presentation helps to distinguish this, with photo-distributed occurrence in kids and young adults typically from Central and South America. Documenting EBV also will help to confirm this diagnosis. Some cases can also have γδ expression. There may be tight overlap with lupus panniculitis, especially in cases with prominent mucin and interface changes, causing considerable difficulty in diagnosis.[42] These cases of borderline atypical lymphocytic panniculitis should be followed closely, as some of these may evolve into bona fide GDTCL. On rare occasions, hepatosplenic T-cell lymphomas can show cutaneous dissemination.[43] Discriminating the latter from cases of PC GDTCL require a strong clinicopathologic correlate.

CAPSULE SUMMARY

- PC GDTCL is an aggressive cytotoxic CTCL that is heterogeneous in its clinical and histologic presentation.
- Clinical findings: panniculitic and/or dermal nodules, plaques, or tumors; MF-like patches, with a tendency toward ulceration and necrosis; or less commonly, pyoderma or bite-like reactions.
- Histology: combined panniculitic, epidermal, and dermal involvement is the most characteristic. Ulceration, necrosis, karyorrhexis, and angiocentricity/destruction can be seen. Hemophagocytic lymphohistiocytosis can be seen in up to half of PC GDTCL cases.
- Immunophenotype: the atypical T-cells express CD3, CD56, TIA-1, γM1, and various cytotoxic markers (TIA-1, perforin, granzyme B), but are negative for βF1 and frequently lack CD4, CD8, CD5, CD30, and EBV positivity.
- Optimal therapies for PC GDTCL are unknown, and thus, while some patients have an initial indolent course, most cases of PC GDTCL have an overall poor prognosis with a 0% to 34% 5-year survival.

AGGRESSIVE EPIDERMOTROPIC CD8+ CYTOTOXIC CUTANEOUS T-CELL LYMPHOMA

Definition

Primary cutaneous aggressive epidermotropic cytotoxic CD8+ T-cell lymphoma (PC AECTCL) is a rare, aggressive, and usually fatal cutaneous lymphoma that is currently a provisional entity in the WHO 2017 classification system.[1] Originally described in 1999, by Berti et al (thus, also referred to as Berti lymphoma), AECTCL is characterized by a short history of widespread ulcerated, crusted, or necrotic papules, nodules, plaques/tumors with a predilection for mucosal sites.[44] In a minority of cases, it can be preceded by MF-like lesions.[1,45] AECTCL is further defined by the biopsy findings, which include a markedly epidermotropic, typically pagetoid, atypical pleomorphic CD8+/CD4− T-cell infiltrate expressing at least one cytotoxic marker (TIA-1, granzyme B, or perforin), and often is CD45RA+/CD45RO−, and frequently CD7+. Historically, AECTCL cases were likely included in Ketron-Goodman disease, the generalized subtype of pagetoid reticulosis, described in 1931.

Epidemiology

There is no known ethnic or geographical predilection for this entity. The incidence is extremely low, representing less than 1% of CTCLs. There is a male predominance, and in the largest series reported to date, the mean age was 54.5 years (range, 27-87 years).[46] Very rarely pediatric cases of PC AECTCL have been reported.[47,48]

Etiology

This is a sporadic lymphoma and the etiology is unknown. There are a few case reports associated with HIV[49] or HTLV infection,[50] prior to treatment with immunosuppressive therapy (adalimumab)[51] and following TNF-alpha inhibitor therapy.[52]

A case is reported in a patient with homozygous mutations in the *SAMHD1* gene.[53]

Clinical Presentation and Prognosis

PC AECTCL classically presents with widespread plaques, papulonodules, and tumors, often with early ulceration, necrosis, and/or hemorrhagic crusting (see Fig. 18-1). Other morphologies include annular lesions, pustules, and a macular-papular eruption of the face, hands, and feet. There is usually a short duration of onset with no preceding patches or thin plaques, but in some cases can be preceded by MF-like lesions.[1] Initial presentations can mimic erythema multiforme[54] and be confused with Mucha-Habermann disease[55] leading some to speculate that previously fatal examples of Mucha-Habermann might include examples of undiagnosed PC AECTCL. An unusual case with widespread superficial pustules is reported.[56] Presentation with solitary or oligolesional tumors is also described, often on acral locations, sometimes clinically mimicking extranodal NK-type lymphoma or blastic plasmacytoid dendritic cell neoplasms (see Figs. 18-2 and 18-3); oligolesional tumors can mimic pyoderma gangrenosum (see Figs. 18-4–18-6). Early dissemination of these initially localized presentations is the almost invariable subsequent clinical course. Early ulceration (as opposed to the late pattern seen in tumors of MF) is a characteristic of the disease. One of the authors from this book has encountered a rare example of a process localized to the oral mucosa of the lips, with tongue and partial lymph node involvement, in the absence of widespread disseminated skin disease.

While there is no specific anatomic predilection, acral sites are frequently involved, and in contrast to most of the other CTCL subtypes, mucosal and genital involvement is common (Figs. 18-13–18-15).[57] The course is aggressive, in contrast to patients with MF, though a few reports of AECTCL with an initially indolent course have been published. In some series and case reports, there is a chronic (>6 month) history of ill-defined skin disease, either

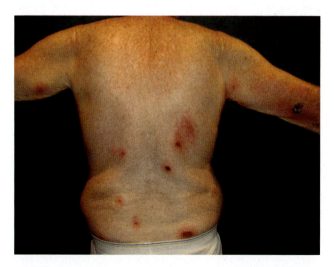

FIGURE 18-13. Primary cutaneous aggressive epidermotropic CD8+ T-cell lymphoma. Scattered ulcerated nodules on trunk and extremities.

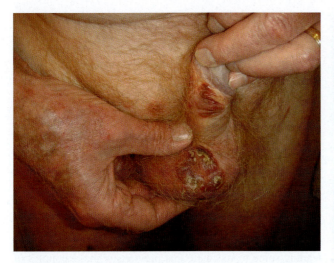

FIGURE 18-14. **Primary cutaneous aggressive epidermotropic CD8+ T-cell lymphoma.** Psoriasiform plaques on the genitals.

papulo-squamous, psoriasiform, or eczematous disease, prior to an acute aggressive presentation.[45,58–62] A more protracted prodromal[56] or a preexisting history of CD8+ MF 48 has been reported although it clearly raises the possibility that such cases were an aggressive end-stage of MF rather than PC AECTCL.

Optimal treatment remains unknown; because the course of disease is aggressive, systemic chemotherapy is often used, with some reported successes,[54,64,65] but in most cases, patients fail to respond or relapse. Stem cell transplantation is the best therapeutic approach when there is complete response after chemotherapy. There is rapid progression with early spread to the central nervous system and viscera, especially the lung. Bone marrow involvement is less common and spread to lymph nodes is rarely seen. Skin-directed and systemic therapies have been reported with variable success. Robson and colleagues reported a median survival of 12 months for their series of 18 patients. Others quote a 5-year survival of 18%. Success has been reported with allogenic hematopoietic stem cell transplantation[45,66,67] and one case with cord blood transplantation[68]; early intervention with these strategies is increasingly advised. Geller et al[69] reported low levels of C-C chemokine receptor 4 expression in PC AECTCL in comparison to CD8+ MF,[69] and it is therefore questionable whether mogamulizumab-targeted therapy has a role to play in combating this disease.

Histology

As indicated by the name, the hallmark of this entity is striking pagetoid epidermotropism of atypical CD8+ cytotoxic T-cells[3,44,70] (Fig. 18-16). In contrast to MF, Pautrier microabscesses are not common. The adnexae may be involved, although follicular mucinosis and destruction are not typical features. Syringotropism may be florid.[46,71] The epidermal changes are dictated by the lesion biopsied. Epidermal hyperkeratosis and acanthosis with ulceration or erosion are common, but atrophy may also be observed (Figs. 18-16–18-19). Numerous necrotic keratinocytes and spongiosis may result in blister formation. Marked ulceration accounts for some cases having a clinical presentation

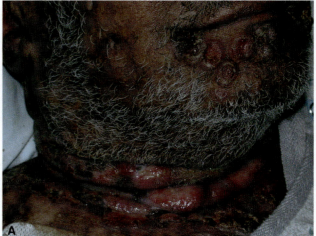

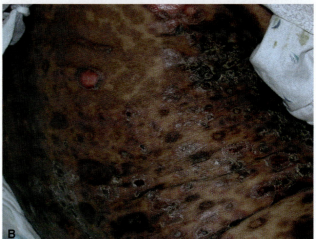

FIGURE 18-15. Primary cutaneous aggressive epidermotropic CD8+ T-cell lymphoma, generalized psoriasiform plaques, and ulcerated nodules on face **(A)** and trunk **(B)**.

mimicking pyoderma gangrenosum,[72,73] and biopsies should include the intact epidermis adjacent to the ulcer to facilitate diagnosis. The infiltrate, typically moderately pleomorphic with medium-sized to large atypical lymphocytes, may also involve the dermis with a nodular or diffuse pattern, extending to the subcutis (Figs. 18-17 and 18-18). Histologic signs of cytotoxicity, including epidermal necrosis/ulceration, dermal necrosis, karyorrhexis, and angiocentricity with or without destruction, may be present, but angiocentricity is less prominent in this entity as compared to γδ CTCL.[74] Exclusive panniculitic involvement is not common, in contrast to γδ CTCL or SPTCL, the latter of which is also characterized by a CD8 and cytotoxic immunophenotype. Rimming of subcutaneous fat spaces has been reported.[54]

Immunophenotype

The immunophenotypes of all cases are CD3+CD8+βF1+ γM1− H41− and CD4− EBV−[46,74] (see Fig. 18-19). Cases will express at least one cytotoxic marker such as TIA-1, granzyme B, or perforin. Ki-67 staining is often high (>75%). A significant subset of cases will express CD45RA and lack CD45RO, CD2, CD5, and γM1. CD7 and CD56 may or

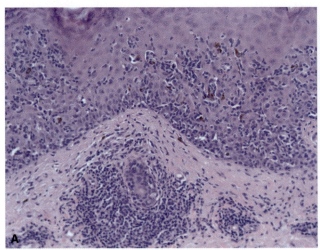
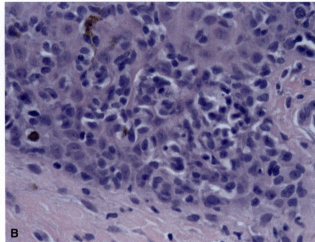

FIGURE 18-16. Aggressive epidermotropic cytotoxic CTCL. **A.** There is epidermal hyperplasia with a strikingly epidermotropic infiltrate of atypical lymphocytes. **B.** Higher-power view demonstrating atypical lymphocytes peppering all layers of the epidermis (H and E, ×400).

may not be expressed. CD30 is usually negative, but may rarely be positive, and has been associated with a response to brentuximab.[63,66] An important differential diagnosis of PC AECTCL is LyP type D.[75–77] Thus, it is important to recognize that CD30 expression may be seen in the former[63] and rare cases of LyP can lack CD30 expression.[78] Clinical correlation is an essential component of diagnosis.

Aberrant expression of CD15 has been reported.[79] While focal expression of Bcl-6 can be seen, other TFH markers are typically negative.[80] Cases with partial expression of CD8[81,82] reinforce the view that otherwise identical CD8(-) cases[45,83,84] could be aberrant phenotypes of the same disease and subsumed under a more generic "primary cutaneous aggressive epidermotropic cytotoxic lymphoma" diagnostic label.

These clinical and pathological features have been combined by some authors[46,54] to suggest a set of classical diagnostic criteria (Table 18-1).

Genetic and Molecular Findings

Comparative genomic hybridization has identified various chromosomal gains/deletions. These have included the short arm of chromosome 17 in the region of the p53 gene.[85] Generally, the copy number alterations affect regions found abnormal in other aggressive lymphomas, are unlikely to represent driver events, and simply reflect genomic instability.[86]

Very recently, Bastidas-Torres et al performed a comprehensive genomic study using WGS and RNA-seq in 12 patients with PC AECTCL.[87] Recurrent rearrangements were present in a large proportion of cases. The altered genes included cell cycle regulatory genes (*MYC, RB1*), chromatin remodeling (*BAZ1A*), and JAK-STAT pathway (*JAK2, PTPRC, SH2B3*). Fusion genes in *JAK2* were present in 3/12 patients. *SH2B3* deletions at 12q24.12 were mutually exclusive with the *JAK2* fusions. The *SH2B3* encodes a protein that antagonizes JAK2 signaling. Alterations in such pathway were seen in 7/12 patients. Two of the cases with *JAK2* fusions also carried *MYC* translocations. Chromosomal alterations were also present, and a large number and proportion of copy number changes. The most common altered cancer genes were *CDKN2A/B* at 9p21.3 (10/12 patients), *ARID1A* at 1p36.11 (5/12 patients), and *ELF1* at 13q14.11 (5/12 patients). Pathogenic mutations in *JAK3* or *STATB5* were seen in 4 additional patients. Overall, 9/12 patients had either structural or small-scar genetic alterations impacting the JAK2-SH2B3 signaling axis, whereas the remaining 3 patients carried pathogenic indels/SNVs in other JAK-STAT pathway genes.

Another recent molecular study by Lee et al[88] revealed further molecular insights in the alterations of the JAK-STAT pathway in PC AECTCL. Five of six patients carried *JAK2* fusions, and another patient carried a novel *ABL1* fusion. Monoclonal TCR gene rearrangements can be detected.

Postulated Cell of Origin

The immunophenotype of this tumor (CD8+CD45RA+ with downregulation of CD2, CD5) suggests a naïve T-cell phenotype. In addition, these cells express HLA-G, a nonclassical HLA type Ib molecule, which may act to downregulate host antitumor immunity.[89]

Differential Diagnosis

The clinicopathologic differential diagnosis includes other cytotoxic CTCLs such as PC GDTCL or extranodal NK/T-cell lymphoma and PTCL/CTCL NOS. Advanced plaque/tumor MF less often enters the differential, due to the short duration of disease onset of AECTCL, in contrast to the indolent lesions of MF. Histologically, the differential diagnosis includes indolent or nonaggressive disorders such as type D LyP or pagetoid reticulosis (Woringer-Kolopp) and γδ CTCL. LyP D, characterized by a similar CD8+ cytotoxic immunophenotype, can only be distinguished by documenting a self-resolving papulonodule, clinically. Pagetoid reticulosis has a distinctive clinical presentation of an indolent psoriasiform or verrucous plaque on acral skin. The epidermotropic lymphocytes are also CD8+ and express cytotoxic

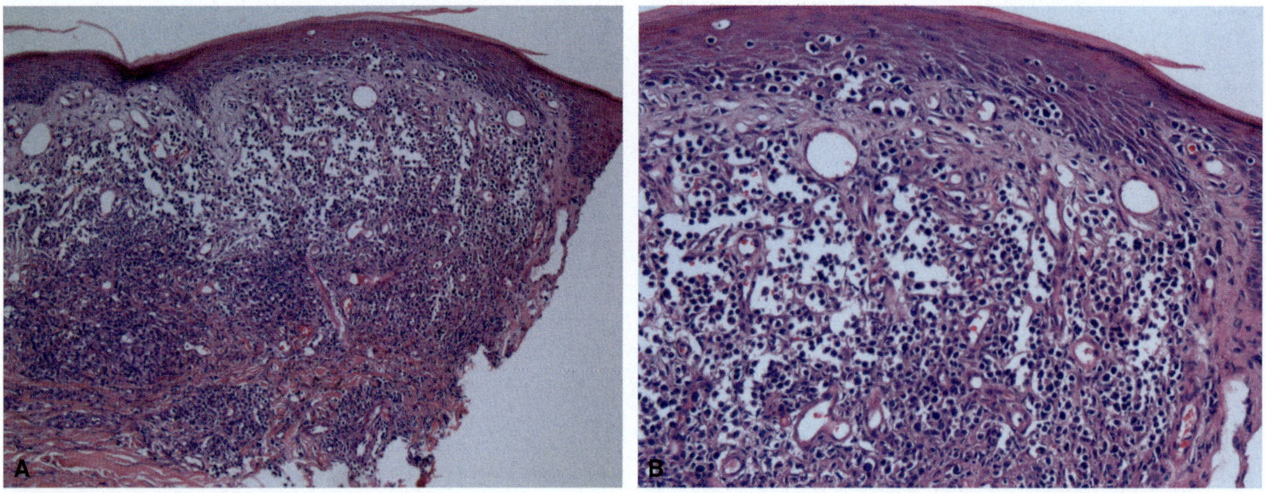

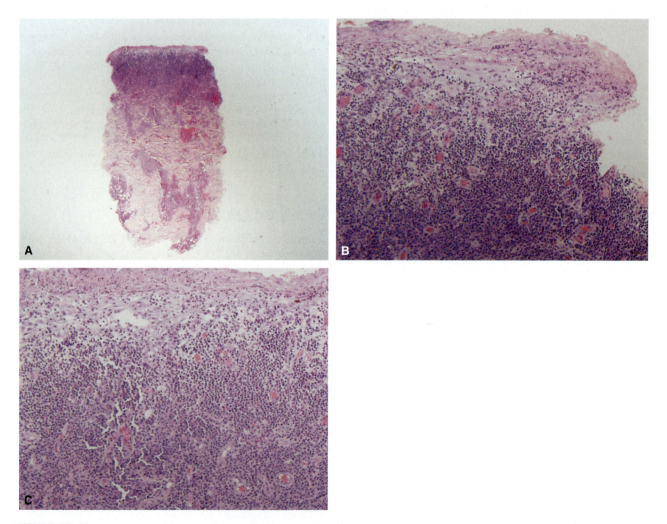

FIGURE 18-17. **Aggressive epidermotropic cytotoxic CTCL. A.** There is both an epidermotropic and dermal infiltrate of atypical lymphocytes (H and E, ×100). **B.** Medium-power view demonstrating hyperchromatic lymphocytes with perinuclear halos peppering the lower epidermis and dermis (H and E, ×200).

FIGURE 18-18. **Aggressive epidermotropic cytotoxic CTCL.** There may be epidermal atrophy with extension into the dermis. **A.** The infiltrate involves the epidermis, dermis, and superficial subcutaneous fat (H and E, ×20). **B.** The epidermis is atrophic and eroded (H and E, ×100). **C.** Higher power of epidermotropic and dermal atypical infiltrate (H and E, ×200).

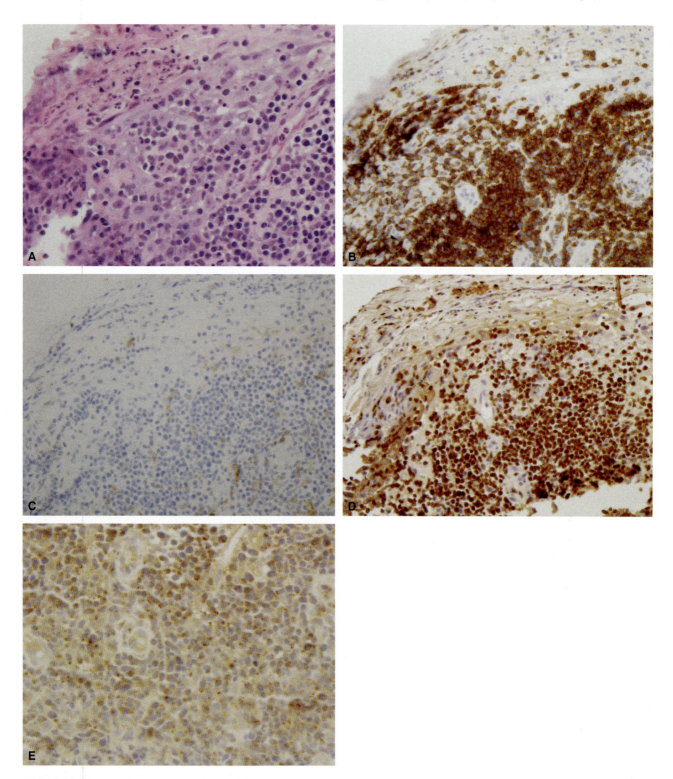

FIGURE 18-19. Aggressive epidermotropic cytotoxic CTCL. A. There is marked epidermotropism of atypical lymphocytes, with epidermal erosion and scale-crust (H and E, ×200). The malignant lymphocytes are positive for CD8 **(B)**, negative for CD4 **(C)**, and express βF1 **(D)** and TIA-1 positive cytotoxic granules in their cytoplasm **(E)** (**B–E** immunohistochemistry, ×200).

markers, and so one should rely on the clinical presentation to differentiate this from AECTCL. Some cases of γδ CTCL may show striking epidermotropism, or may have immunophenotypic overlap that includes positivity for CD8, CD7, and CD45RA, similar to AECTCL. These are differentiated by demonstrating γM1 on the T-cells. The presence of circulating physiological CD8⁺ γδ T-cells suggests, however, that CD8⁺ variants of γδ lymphoma may exist; classification of lymphomas arising from these as either AECTCL or γδ CTCL then likely becomes somewhat arbitrary and, in any event, does not alter the need for aggressive treatment since both have attendant poor prognoses.

CAPSULE SUMMARY

- AE CD8+ CTCL is a very rare, aggressive CTCL that presents with eroded or crusted plaques/tumors, with a short duration of onset, rapid clinical progression, and poor prognosis.
- Neoplastic cells have a striking epidermotropism that can histologically mimic type D LyP or pagetoid reticulosis.
- Epidermal hyperkeratosis and acanthosis with ulceration or erosion are common.
- The CD3+CD8+βF1+ T-cells express at least one cytotoxic marker and often express CD45RA and/or CD7 and lack CD45RO, CD30, or γM1.
- Accurate diagnosis of this condition requires careful assessment of clinical presentation and behavior. Due to its rarity, pathophysiology of this sporadic disorder remains unknown and optimal therapy remains unknown.
- The clinical, histological and immunophenotypic features are summarized in Table 18-1.

TABLE 18-1 Classical Features of Aggressive Epidermotropic CD8+ Cutaneous T-Cell Lymphoma

Clinical	Histological	Immunophenotype
Generalized ulcerated plaques and tumors	Epidermotropism mimicking LyP type D or pagetoid reticulosis	CD3+CD8+ Positivity for either TIA-1, Granzyme-B or perforin
+/− mucosal involvement	Acanthosis and hyperkeratosis Lack of Pautrier's microabscess Signs of cytotoxicity: Necrotic keratinocytes—ulceration Angiodestruction Dermal necrosis Karyoprrhexis	BetaF1+ or γδ−
Solitary tumorous lesions	Monomorphic atypia	One of either CD2−, CD5−, or CD45RA+
No immunosuppression	Diffuse or nodular dermal tumor No subcutaneous fat involvement No angiodestruction	EBV−

References

1. Berti E, Gaulard P, Willemze R, et al. Primary cutaneous peripheral T-cell lymphomas, rare subtypes. In: Swerdlow SH, Campo E, Harris NL, et al., eds. *WHO Classification of Tumours of Haematopoeitic and Lymphoid Tissues*. IARC Press; 2017:399-400.
2. Cerroni L. *Skin Lymphoma, the Illustrated Guide*. 4th ed. Wiley Blackwell; 2014.
3. Willemze R, Jaffe ES, Burg G, et al. WHO-EORTC classification for cutaneous lymphomas. *Blood*. 2005;105:3768-3785.
4. Roullet M, Gheith SM, Mauger J, et al. Percentage of T cells in panniculitis by paraffin immunohistochemical analysis. *Am J Clin Pathol*. 2009;131:820-826.
5. Rodriguez-Pinilla SM, Ortiz-Romero PL, Monsalvez V, et al. TCR-gamma expression in primary cutaneous T-cell lymphomas. *Am J Surg Pathol*. 2013;37:375-384.
6. Kerbout M, Mekouar F, Bahadi N, et al. A rare pediatric case of cutaneous gamma/delta T-cell lymphoma. *Ann Biol Clin (Paris)*. 2014;72:483-485.
7. Soon CW, Link M, Kim YH, et al. Primary cutaneous gamma-delta T-cell lymphoproliferative disorder in a 3-year-old boy. *Am J Dermatopathol*. 2015;37:567-569.
8. Guitart J, Weisenburger DD, Subtil A, et al. Cutaneous gamma-delta T-cell lymphomas: a spectrum of presentations with overlap with other cytotoxic lymphomas. *Am J Surg Pathol*. 2012;36:1656-1665.
9. Willemze R, Jansen PM, Cerroni L, et al. Subcutaneous panniculitis-like T-cell lymphoma: definition, classification, and prognostic factors – an EORTC Cutaneous Lymphoma Group Study of 83 cases. *Blood*. 2008;111:838-845.
10. Toro JR, Liewehr DJ, Pabby N, et al. Gamma-delta T-cell phenotype is associated with significantly decreased survival in cutaneous T-cell lymphoma. *Blood*. 2003;101:3407-3412.
11. Kelsen J, Dige A, Christensen M, et al. Frequency and clonality of peripheral gammadelta T cells in psoriasis patients receiving anti-tumour necrosis factor-alpha therapy. *Clin Exp Immunol*. 2014;177:142-148.
12. Tripodo C, Iannitto E, Florena AM, et al. Gamma-delta T-cell lymphomas. *Nat Rev Clin Oncol*. 2009;6:707-717.
13. Gardner RV, Velez MC, Ode DL, et al. Gamma/delta T-cell lymphoma as a recurrent complication after transplantation. *Leuk Lymphoma*. 2004;45:2355-2359.
14. Koens L, Senff NJ, Vermeer MH, et al. Cutaneous gamma/delta T-cell lymphoma during treatment with etanercept for rheumatoid arthritis. *Acta Derm Venereol*. 2009;89:653-654.
15. Garcia-Herrera A, Song JY, Chuang SS, et al. Nonhepatosplenic gammadelta T-cell lymphomas represent a spectrum of aggressive cytotoxic T-cell lymphomas with a mainly extranodal presentation. *Am J Surg Pathol*. 2011;35:1214-1225.
16. Avinoach I, Halevy S, Argov S, et al. Gamma/delta T-cell lymphoma involving the subcutaneous tissue and associated with a hemophagocytic syndrome. *Am J Dermatopathol*. 1994;16:426-433.
17. Kim YH, Willemze R, Pimpinelli N, et al. TNM classification system for primary cutaneous lymphomas other than mycosis fungoides and Sézary syndrome: a proposal of the International Society for Cutaneous Lymphomas (ISCL) and the cutaneous lymphoma Task Force of the European Organization of Research and Treatment of Cancer (EORTC). *Blood*. 2007;110:479-484.
18. Avarbock AB, Loren AW, Park JY, et al. Lethal vascular leak syndrome after denileukin diftitox administration to a patient with cutaneous gamma/delta T-cell lymphoma and occult cirrhosis. *Am J Hematol*. 2008;83:593-595.
19. Nakashima H, Sugaya M, Minatani Y, et al. Cutaneous gamma/delta T-cell lymphoma treated with retinoid and narrowband ultraviolet B. *Clin Exp Dermatol*. 2009;34:e345-e346.
20. Terras S, Moritz RK, Ditschkowski M, et al. Allogeneic haematopoietic stem cell transplantation in a patient with

cutaneous gamma/delta-T-cell lymphoma. *Acta Derm Venereol*. 2013;93:360-361.
21. Talpur R, Chockalingam R, Wang C, Tetzlaff MT, Duvic M. A Single-Center Experience With Brentuximab Vedotin in Gamma Delta T-Cell Lymphoma. *Clin Lymphoma Myeloma Leuk*. 2016;16:e15-9.
22. Rubio-Gonzalez Belen, Zain Jasmine, Garcia Lino, Rosen Steven T, Querfeld Christiane. Cutaneous Gamma-Delta T-Cell Lymphoma Successfully Treated With Brentuximab Vedotin. *JAMA Dermatol*. 2016;152:1388-1390.
23. Lastrucci I, Grandi V, Gozzini A, et al. Complete remission with brentuximab vedotin in a case of primary cutaneous gamma-delta T-cell lymphoma relapsed after allogeneic stem cell transplantation. *Int J Dermatol*. 2021;60:778-780.
24. Voruz Sophie, Leval Laurence de, Cairoli Anne. Successful salvage therapy for refractory primary cutaneous gamma-delta T-cell lymphoma with a combination of brentuximab vedotin and gemcitabine. *Exp Hematol Oncol*. 2021;10:32. doi: 10.1186/s40164-021-00225-2.
25. Horwitz Steven, O'Connor Owen A, Pro Barbara, et al. Brentuximab vedotin with chemotherapy for CD30-positive peripheral T-cell lymphoma (ECHELON-2): a global, double-blind, randomised, phase 3 trial. *Lancet*. 2019;393:229-240.
26. Isufi Iris, Seropian Stuart, Gowda Lohith, et al. Outcomes for allogeneic stem cell transplantation in refractory mycosis fungoides and primary cutaneous gamma Delta T cell lymphomas. *Leuk Lymphoma*. 2020;61:2955-2961. doi: 10.1080/10428194.2020.1790555.
27. Hosler GA, Liegeois N, Anhalt GJ, et al. Transformation of cutaneous gamma/delta T-cell lymphoma following 15 years of indolent behavior. *J Cutan Pathol*. 2008;35:1063-1067.
28. Harrington L, Sokol L, Holdener S, et al. Cutaneous gamma-delta T-cell lymphoma with central nervous system involvement: report of a rarity with review of literature. *J Cutan Pathol*. 2014;41:936-943.
29. Alexander RE, Webb AR, Abuel-Haija M, et al. Rapid progression of primary cutaneous gamma-delta T-cell lymphoma with an initial indolent clinical presentation. *Am J Dermatopathol*. 2014;36:839-842.
30. Kempf W, Kazakov DV, Scheidegger PE, et al. Two cases of primary cutaneous lymphoma with a gamma/delta+ phenotype and an indolent course: further evidence of heterogeneity of cutaneous gamma/delta+ T-cell lymphomas. *Am J Dermatopathol*. 2014;36:570-577.
31. Endly DC, Weenig RH, Peters MS, et al. Indolent course of cutaneous gamma-delta T-cell lymphoma. *J Cutan Pathol*. 2013;40:896-902.
32. Jungbluth AA, Frosina D, Fayad M, et al. Immunohistochemical detection of G/Dlymphocytes in formalin fixed paraffin embedded tissues. *Appl Immunohistochem Mol Morph*. 2019;27:581-583.
33. Agbay Rose Lou Marie C, Torres-Cabala Carlos A, Patel Keyur P, et al. Immunophenotypic Shifts in Primary Cutaneous γδ T-Cell Lymphoma Suggest Antigenic Modulation: A Study of Sequential Biopsy Specimens. *Am J Surg Pathol*. 2017;41:431-445. doi: 10.1097/PAS.0000000000000786.
34. Yamamoto-Sugitani M, Kuroda J, Shimura Y, et al. Comprehensive cytogenetic study of primary cutaneous gamma-delta T-cell lymphoma by means of spectral karyotyping and genome-wide single nucleotide polymorphism array. *Cancer Genet*. 2012;205:459-464.
35. Daniels Jay, Doukas Peter G, Escala Maria E Martinez, et al. Cellular origins and genetic landscape of cutaneous gamma delta T cell lymphomas. *Nat Commun*. 2020;11:1806. doi: 10.1038/s41467-020-15572-7.
36. Tomasini Dario, Croci Giorgio Alberto, Hotz Annamaria, et al. Gamma/delta T-cell lymphoma with mycosis fungoides-like clinical course transforming to "T-cell-receptor-silent" aggressive lymphoma: Description of one case. *J Cutan Pathol*. 2021;48:1197-1203.
37. Prillinger Knut Erich, Trautinger Franz, Kitzwögerer Melitta, Eder Johanna. Two faces of gamma-delta mycosis fungoides: before and after renal transplantation. *BMJ Case Rep*. 2017;2017:bcr2016216990.
38. Kash Natalie, Massone Cesare, Fink-Puches Regina, Cerroni Lorenzo. Phenotypic Variation in Different Lesions of Mycosis Fungoides Biopsied Within a Short Period of Time From the Same Patient. *Am J Dermatopathol*. 2016;38:541-5.
39. Merrill E Dean, Agbay Rose, Miranda Roberto N, et al. Primary Cutaneous T-Cell Lymphomas Showing Gamma-Delta (γδ) Phenotype and Predominantly Epidermotropic Pattern are Clinicopathologically Distinct From Classic Primary Cutaneous γδ T-Cell Lymphomas. *Am J Surg Pathol*. 2017;41:204-215.
40. Pulitzer Melissa, Geller Shamir, Kumar Erica et al. T-cell receptor-δ expression and γδ+ T-cell infiltrates in primary cutaneous γδ T-cell lymphoma and other cutaneous T-cell lymphoproliferative disorders. *Histopathology*. 2018;73:653-662. doi: 10.1111/his.13671. Epub 2018 Jul 27.
41. Kash N, Vin H, Danialan R, et al. Stenotrophomonas maltophilia with histologic features mimicking cutaneous gamma/delta T-cell lymphoma. *Int J Infect Dis*. 2015;30:7-9.
42. Aguilera P, Mascaro JM Jr, Martinez A, et al. Cutaneous gamma/delta T-cell lymphoma: a histopathologic mimicker of lupus erythematosus profundus (lupus panniculitis). *J Am Acad Dermatol*. 2007;56:643-647.
43. Santonja Carlos, Carrasco Loreto, de Los Ángeles Pérez-Sáenz María, Rodríguez-Pinilla Socorro-María. A Skin Plaque Preceding Systemic Relapse of Gamma-Delta Hepatosplenic T-Cell Lymphoma. *Am J Dermatopathol*. 2020;42:364-367.
44. Berti E, Tomasini D, Vermeer MH, et al. Primary cutaneous CD8-positive epidermotropic cytotoxic T cell lymphomas. A distinct clinicopathological entity with an aggressive clinical behavior. *Am J Pathol*. 1999;155:483-492.
45. Guitart J, Martinez-Escala E, Subtil A, et al. Primary cutaneous aggressive epidermotropic cytotoxic T-cell lymphomas: reappraisal of a provisional entity in the 2016 WHO classification of cutaneous lymphomas. *Mod Pathol*. 2017;30:761-772.
46. Robson A, Assaf C, Bagot M, et al. Aggressive epidermotropic cutaneous CD8+ lymphoma: a cutaneous lymphoma with distinct clinical and pathological features. Report of an EORTC Cutaneous Lymphoma Task Force Workshop. *Histopathology*. 2015;67:425-441.
47. Kikuchi Y, Kashii Y, Gunji Y, et al. Six-year-old girl with primary cutaneous aggressive epidermotropic CD8+ T-cell lymphoma. *Pediatr Int*. 2011;53:393-396.
48. Wang L, Gao T, Wang G. Primary cutaneous CD8+ cytotoxic T-cell lymphoma involving the epidermis and subcutis in a young child. *J Cutan Pathol*. 2015;42:271-275.
49. Karkouche R, Ingen-Housz-Oro S, Le Gouvello S, et al. Primary cutaneous aggressive epidermotropic CD8+ T-cell lymphoma with KIR3DL2 and NKp46 expression in a human immunodeficiency virus carrier. *J Cutan Pathol*. 2015;42:199-205.
50. Ohmatsu H, Sugaya M, Fujita H, et al. Primary cutaneous CD8+ aggressive epidermotropic cytotoxic T-cell lymphoma in a human T-cell leukaemia virus type-1 carrier. *Acta Derm Venereol*. 2010;90:324-325.

51. Jacks SM, Taylor BR, Rogers RPIII, et al. Rapid deterioration in a patient with primary aggressive cutaneous epidermotropic CD8+ cytotoxic T-cell ('Berti') lymphoma after administration of adalimumab. *J Am Acad Dermatol*. 2014;71:e86-e87.
52. Toussaint F, Erdmann M, Grosch E, et al. Transient response to nivolumab and relapse after infliximab in a patient with primary cutaneous CD8-positive aggressive epidermotropic cytotoxic T-cell lymphoma. *Brit J Dermatol*. 2021;184:345-347.
53. Merati M, Buethe DJ, Cooper KD, et al. Aggressive CD81 epidermotropic cutaneous T-cell lymphoma associated with homozygous mutation in SAMHD1. *JAAD Case Rep*. 2015;1:227-229.
54. Nofal A, Abdel-Mawla MY, Assaf M, et al. Primary cutaneous aggressive epidermotropic CD8+ T cell lymphoma: a diagnostic and therapeutic challenge. *Int J Dermatol*. 2014;53:76-81.
55. Sheng N, Li Z, Su W, et al. A case of primary cutaneous aggressive epidermotropic CD8+ cytotoxic T-cell lymphoma misdiagnosed as febrile ulceronecrotic Mucha-Habermann disease. *Acta Derm Venereol*. 2016;96:136-137.
56. Ito Y, Goto M, Hatano Y et al. Epidermotropic CD8+ cytotoxic T-cell lymphoma exhibiting a transition from the indolent to the aggressive phase, accompanied by emergence of CD7+ cells and formation of neutrophilic pustules. *Clin Exp Dermatol*. 2012;37:128-131.
57. Gormley RH, Hess SD, Anand D, et al. Primary cutaneous aggressive epidermotropic CD8+ T-cell lymphoma. *J Am Acad Dermatol*. 2010;62:300-307.
58. Moon J, Park JS, Cho KH. A case of primary cutaneous aggressive epidermotropic CD8+ cytotoxic T-cell lymphoma. *Ann Dermatol*. 2018;30:255-257.
59. Sanchez AR, Sambucety PS, Garcia CP, et al. Atypical presentation of primary cutaneous CD8 positive aggressive epidermotropic cytotoxic T-cell lymphoma. *Indian Dermatol Online*. 2019;10:298-299.
60. Geller S, Myskowski PL, Pulitzer M. NK/T-cell lymphoma, nasal type, γδ T-cell lymphoma, and CD8-positive epidermotropic T-cell lymphoma—clinical and histopathologic features, differential diagnosis, and treatment. *Semin Cutan Med Surg*. 2018;37:30-38.
61. Geller S, Myskowski PL, Pulitzer M, et al. Cutaneous T-cell lymphoma (CTCL), rare subtypes: five case presentations and review of the literature. *Chin Clin Oncol*. 2019;8:5.
62. Webber NK, Harwood C, Goldsmith P, et al. Aggressive epidermotropic cutaneous CD8+ (Berti's) lymphoma. *Clin Exp Dermatol*. 2010;35:e210-212.
63. Cyrenne BM, Subtil A, Girardi M, et al. Primary cutaneous aggressive epidermotropic cytotoxic CD8+ T-cell lymphoma: long-term remission after brentuximab vedotin. *Int J Dermatol*. 2017;56:1448-1450.
64. Rolland M, Dinulescu M, Saillard C et al. Nodules ulcérés du visage révélant un lymphome T cutané épidermotrope CD8+ cytotoxique agressif. *Ann Dermatol Vénéréol*. 2020;147:764-768.
65. Al Aoun SM, Iqbal S, AlHalouli TM, et al. Durable remission of a patient with primary cutaneous CD8+ aggressive epidermotropic cytotoxic T-cell lymphoma. *Hematol Oncol Stem Ther*. 2018;28:30096-30097.
66. Cyrenne BM, Gibson JF, Subtil A, et al. Transplantation in the treatment of primary cutaneous aggressive epidermotropic cytotoxic CD8-positive T-cell lymphoma. *Clin Lymphoma Myeloma Leuk*. 2018;18:e85-93.
67. Wehkamp U, Glaeser D, Oschlies I, et al. Successful stem cell transplantation in a patient with primary cutaneous aggressive cytotoxic epidermotropic CD8+ T-cell lymphoma. *Br J Dermatol*. 2015;173:869-871.
68. Ichikawa S, Fukuhara N, Hatta S, et al. Successful cord blood stem cell transplantation for primary cutaneous CD8-positive aggressive epidermotropic cytotoxic T-cell lymphoma complicated with Cerebral infiltration. *Intern Med*. 2018;57:2051-2055.
69. Geller S, Hollmann TJ, Horwitz SM, et al. C-C chemokine receptor 4 expression in CD8+ cutaneous T-cell lymphomas and lymphoproliferative disorders, and its implications for diagnosis and treatment. *Histopathology*. 2020;76:222-232.
70. Santucci M, Pimpinelli N, Massi D, et al. Cytotoxic/natural killer cell cutaneous lymphomas. Report of EORTC cutaneous lymphoma task force workshop. *Cancer*. 2003;97:610-627.
71. Saruta H, Ohata C, Muto I, et al. Hematopoietic stem cell transplantation in advanced cutaneous T-cell lymphoma. *J Dermatol*. 2017;44:1038-1042.
72. Deenen NJ, Koens L, Jaspars EH, et al. Pitfalls in diagnosing primary cutaneous aggressive epidermotropic CD8+ T-cell lymphoma. *Br J Dermatol*. 2019;180:411-412.
73. Wang Y, Li T, Wu LS, et al. Primary cutaneous aggressive epidermotropic CD8+ cytotoxic T-cell lymphoma clinically simulating pyoderma gangrenosum. *Clin Exp Dermatol*. 2009;34:e261-262.
74. Nofal A, Abdel-Mawla MY, Assaf M, et al. Primary cutaneous aggressive epidermotropic CD8+ T-cell lymphoma: proposed diagnostic criteria and therapeutic evaluation. *J Am Acad Dermatol*. 2012;67:748-759.
75. Saggini A, Gulia A, Argenyi Z, et al. A variant of lymphomatoid papulosis simulating primary cutaneous aggressive epidermotropic CD8+ cytotoxic T-cell lymphoma. Description of 9 cases. *Am J Surg Pathol*. 2010;34:1168-1175.
76. Andersen RM, Larsen MS, Svenstrup T, et al. Lymphomatoid papulosis type D or an aggressive epidermotropic CD8+ cytotoxic T-cell lymphoma? *Acta Derm Venereol*. 2014;94:474-475.
77. Tsujiwaki M, Abe R, Ohguchi Y et al. Recurrent course and CD30 expression of atypical T lymphocytes distinguish lymphomatoid papulosis from primary cutaneous aggressive epidermotropic CD8+ cytotoxic T-cell lymphoma. *Acta Derm Venereol*. 2014;94:613-614.
78. Simo OC, Warren SJ, Mark L, et al. CD8-positive lymphomatoid papulosis (type D): some lesions may lack CD30 expression and overlap histologically with mycosis fungoides. *Int J Dermatol*. 2019;58:800-805.
79. Yoshizawa N, Yagi H, Horibe T, et al. Primary cutaneous aggressive epidermotropic CD8+ T-cell lymphoma with a CD15+CD30– phenotype. *Eur J Dermatol*. 2007;17:441-442.
80. Bosisio FM, Cerroni L. Expression of T-follicular helper markers in sequential biopsies of progressive mycosis fungoides and other primary cutaneous T-cell lymphomas. *Am J Dermatopathol*. 2015;37:115-121.
81. Bruggen MC, Kerl K, Haralambieva E, et al. Aggressive rare T-cell lymphomas with manifestation in the skin: a monocentric cross-sectional case study. *Acta Derm Venereol*. 2018;98:835-841.
82. Plachouri KM, Weishaupt C, Metze D, et al. Complete durable remission of a fulminant primary cutaneous aggressive epidermotropic CD81 cytotoxic T-cell lymphoma after autologous and allogeneic hematopoietic stem cell transplantation. *JAAD*. 2017;3:196-199.
83. Yamamoto M, Nakada T, Iijima M. Primary cutaneous T-cell lymphoma, unspecified, exhibiting an aggressive clinical course and a cytotoxic phenotype. *Int J Dermatol*. 2008;47:720-722.

84. Miyauchi T, Abe R, Morita Y, et al. CD4/CD8 Double-negative T-cell lymphoma: a variant of primary cutaneous CD8+ aggressive epidermotropic cytotoxic T-cell lymphoma? *Acta Derm Venereol.* 2015;95:1024-1025.
85. Kato K, Oh Y, Takita J, et al. Molecular genetic and cytogenetic analysis of a primary cutaneous CD8-positive aggressive epidermotropic cytotoxic T-cell lymphoma. *Int J Hematol.* 2016;103:196-201.
86. Fanoni D, Corti L, Alberti-Violetti S, et al. Array-based CGH of primary cutaneous CD8+ aggressive epiderm-tropic cytotoxic T-cell lymphoma. *Genes Chromosomes Cancer.* 2018;57:622-629.
87. Torres Armando N Bastidas, Cats Davy, Out-Luiting Jacoba J. Deregulation of JAK2 signaling underlies primary cutaneous CD8+ aggressive epidermotropic cytotoxic T-cell lymphoma. *Haematologica.* 2022;107:702-714.
88. Lee Katie, Evans Mark G, Yang Lei, et al. Primary cytotoxic T-cell lymphomas harbor recurrent targetable alterations in the JAK-STAT pathway. *Blood.* 2021;138:2435-2440.
89. Urosevic M, Kamarashev J, Burg G, et al. Primary cutaneous CD8+ and CD56+ T-cell lymphomas express HLA-G and killer-cell inhibitory ligand, ILT2. *Blood.* 2004;103:1796-1798.

Primary cutaneous peripheral T-cell lymphoma, not otherwise specified

Alistair M. Robson, Andy C. Hsi, Amy C. Musiek, and András Schaffer

DEFINITION

Peripheral T-cell lymphoma, not otherwise specified (PTCL-NOS) denotes a heterogeneous group of non-Hodgkin lymphomas that, by definition, do not correspond to any T-cell lymphoma entities defined by the World Health Organization (WHO) criteria.[1] Cutaneous presentation of PTCL-NOS is usually secondary to lymphomatous spread of an extracutaneous disease. Primary cutaneous PTCL-NOS is designated when there is no evidence of extracutaneous involvement within 6 months of diagnosis.[2] Historical inclusion of some CD8+ cases, arising predominantly at acral sites,[3-6] would no longer be included in this category since the provisional inclusion of primary cutaneous acral CD8+ lymphoma in the updated version of the WHO classification.[7]

EPIDEMIOLOGY

PTCL-NOS is relatively common and represents ~30% of PTCLs in Western countries, but primary cutaneous PTCL-NOS is exceedingly rare, accounting for only 2% of all primary cutaneous T-cell lymphoma (CTCL) and B-cell lymphoma.[8,9] Similar to other primary CTCLs, primary cutaneous PTCL-NOS generally occurs in older adults and has a higher prevalence in males.[9,10] Treatment has usually consisted of multiagent chemotherapy, often with disappointing results.[9]

ETIOLOGY

Unknown.

CLINICAL PRESENTATION/PROGNOSIS/TREATMENT

Primary cutaneous PTCL-NOS presents as solitary or generalized papules, plaques, or nodules, with or without ulceration. Solitary lesions may have a predilection for the legs and arms (Fig. 19-1).[9,11-13] Historically, primary cutaneous PTCL-NOS is believed to have a poor prognosis, with a reported median overall survival of 2.4 years and a disease-specific 5-year survival of 16% in one study of 9 cases.[9,11] However, clinically indolent cases, including those with resolution after excision, have been reported.[9,12,14-16] Furthermore, two recent publications suggest that the prognosis may not be as dismal as has traditionally been thought. A European study of 30 patients with primary cutaneous PTCL-NOS reported 3-year and 5-year survivals of 61% and 54%, respectively.[13] A further European Organisation for Research and Treatment of Cancer study of primary cutaneous CD8+ proliferations included 11 patients with CD8+ PTCL-NOS, 55% of whom were alive without disease after a mean follow-up of 25 months with only one death from lymphoma recorded.[17] There is evidence that cases with considerable (>30%) large cell populations have a significantly worse prognosis in comparison to those with predominantly small- or medium-sized cells.[10,11,18-21] While this percentage of large cells within the infiltrate should not be considered a defining feature of this category, it has been assumed to be so in several series, likely accounting for the reported association of PTCL-NOS with a poor prognosis. However, the original study assessing peripheral PTCL-NOS with large cells had done so as a *prognostic* not diagnostic assessment; this study included cases of peripheral PTCL-NOS with majority small/medium cell populations,[18] not all of which can be accounted for by the then unrecognized CD4+ small–medium lymphoproliferative disorder, often with a less aggressive clinical course, a finding repeated in more recent series.[12,13,16,17]

HISTOLOGY

1. As the definition is one of exclusion, there are no unifying features to the histological appearance. Thus, there may be small, medium, and/or large cells with a nodular or diffuse pattern, sometimes extending significantly into the subcutaneous tissue. Focal epidermotropism may be

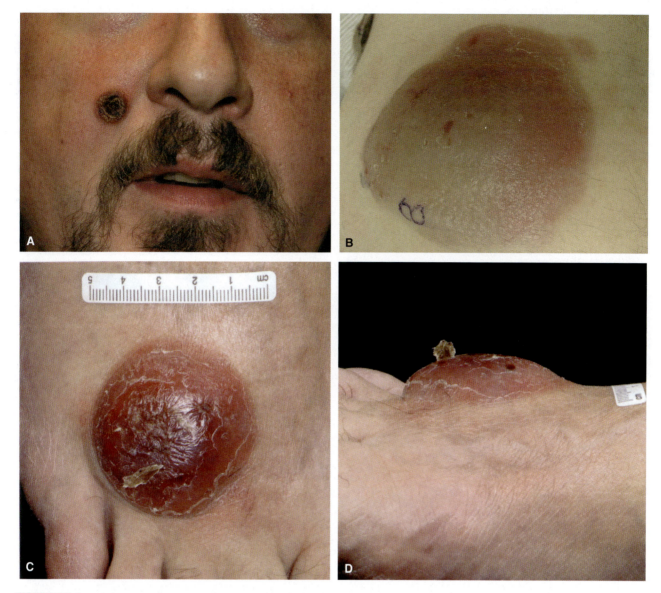

FIGURE 19-1. Clinical presentations of primary cutaneous PTCL-NOS. **A.** Solitary nodule on the face with central ulceration. **B.** Large, erythematous nodule on the abdomen. **C** and **D.** Infiltrated tumor on the dorsum of the foot. (C and D Reproduced from Martin et al courtesy of J Cutan Pathol.)[13]

evident.[9,11,12,16] Ulceration is common.[16] Angiocentricity and adnexal involvement, including folliculotropism, are occasionally seen (Fig. 19-2A–G).[22]

2. Given the association between a significant (>30%) large cell population and poor prognosis, it is probably prudent to record this feature when present.

IMMUNOPHENOTYPE

Neoplastic cells are mostly CD4+ T-cells with loss of one or more pan–T-cell markers (CD2, CD3, CD5, and CD7). One series reported that 78% of cases were CD4+CD8− and 22% were CD4−CD8− dual-negative.[11] Nevertheless, CD8+ and CD4/CD8+ (double-positive) cases are reported. CD30 expression is negative, or restricted to only scattered reactive cells.[9,11] Uniform CD30 expression denotes cutaneous anaplastic large-cell lymphoma.[23] Approximately, a third of PTCL-NOS express at least one cytotoxic marker (granzyme B and/or TIA-1).[11] CD52 and CD56 expressions are variable. Expression of follicular T-helper–associated antigens, including PD-1, CXCL13, BCL6, and CD10, is negative.[24] Proliferation index measured by Ki-67 expression is generally high (>50%). However, cases with clinically indolent behavior may have only <10% proliferation.[15] Interestingly, aberrant CD20 expression by CD79a− PAX5− neoplastic cells is not infrequently found, demonstrated in 18% in one recent series.[12,13]

GENETIC AND MOLECULAR FINDINGS

A monoclonal rearrangement of T-cell receptor, detected by PCR, is usually found.[11,15]

Category-specific genetic abnormalities have not been defined. Analysis with array-based comparative genomic hybridization showed large, complex chromosomal gains and losses in various regions including gains of 6p, 7q, 8p, 8q, 11p, 11q, 12q, 14q, 17q, 19p, and 19q. Losses of 8p and 9p were

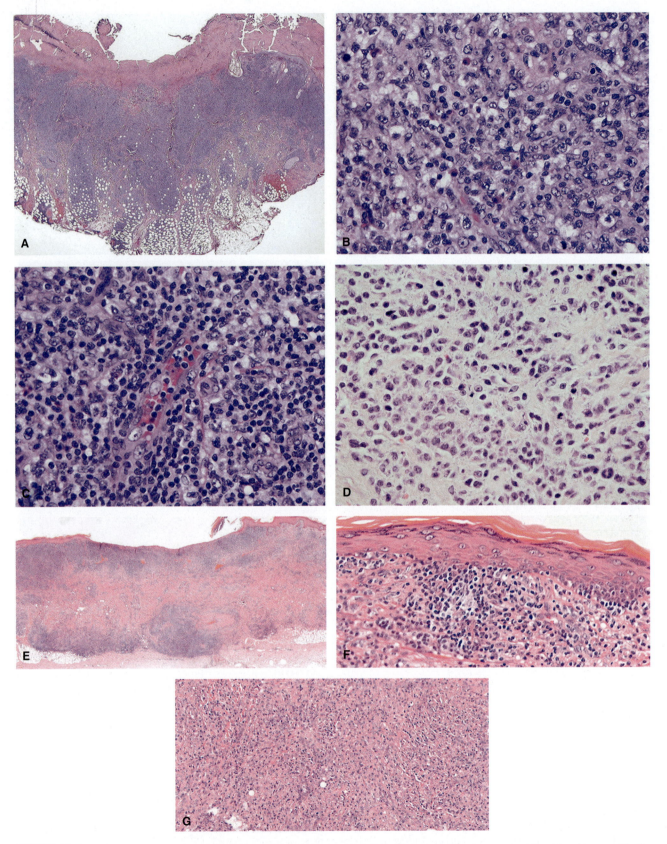

FIGURE 19-2. Histologic and immunophenotypic features of primary cutaneous PTCL-NOS. A. Hematoxylin and eosin (H&E) staining at low magnification (20×) shows ulceration of the epidermis with dense lymphocytic infiltrates involving the superficial and deep dermis as well as the subcutaneous adipose tissue. **B.** High magnification (630×) shows that the lesion is composed of medium-to-large pleomorphic immunoblasts with scattered small cells. **C.** Angiocentricity is evident in this field, with a more prominent population of small-to-medium–sized cells. **D.** A diffuse population of small-medium sized cells. **E.** Ulceration and a dense mononuclear cell infiltrate, within a fibrotic dermis. **F.** The solitary tumor is formed of moderately sized often histiocytoid mononuclear cells with admixed lymphocytes, lymphoplasmacytoid and plasma cells. **G.** Marked epidermotropism flanking the ulcer.) (E-G. Reproduced from Rolim et al 2021 courtesy of Am J Dermatopath.)[17]

less frequently observed.[25] Whether primary cutaneous tumors can be stratified into two prognostically significant groups determined by either high GATA-3 or T-bet expression, as demonstrated in nodal peripheral TCL NOS, remains to be established (Fig. 19-3).[26-28]

POSTULATED CELL OF ORIGIN

High expressions of either T-bet- or GATA-3-associated genes suggest that PTCL-NOS and therefore perhaps some primary cutaneous PTCL-NOS may derive from T_H1 and T_H2 cells.

DIFFERENTIAL DIAGNOSIS

Primary Cutaneous T-Cell Lymphomas

The diagnosis of CTCLs requires the interpretation of both clinical and pathological features; histology alone cannot be solely relied upon. Similarly, because PTCL-NOS lacks any unifying histological features, many other forms of CTCL may constitute legitimate differential diagnoses. These include plaque/tumor stages of mycosis fungoides, CD30+ anaplastic large cell lymphoma, aggressive cytotoxic lymphomas, and lymphomas composed of small or medium cell types. These are excluded by attention to the clinical setting, against which the histology and immunohistochemical prolife are interpreted. For the diagnostic features of these specific entities, or other diagnoses that may be considered in individual cases, please see the relevant entries elsewhere in this book. Once these are satisfactorily excluded, and the absence of systemic disease confirmed by appropriate staging investigations, a diagnosis of primary cutaneous peripheral TCL NOS is made by default.

CAPSULE SUMMARY

- Primary cutaneous PTCL-NOS is diagnosed when the clinicopathologic features do not fit into any of the defined subtypes of CTCL. Absence of extracutaneous disease for 6 months after the initial presentation is required for diagnosis.
- Presents as solitary or generalized nodules with or without ulceration. There is no particular site predilection.
- The prognosis is often poor, particularly if there is a significant large cell population, with a 5-year survival of <20%. Localized small/medium cell lymphomas may have a better outlook.
- Neoplastic cells vary from small, medium-to-large pleomorphic or immunoblastic with clonal TCR rearrangement, possibly originated from either T_H1 or T_H2 lymphocytes.
- The tumor cells are typically CD4+ with loss of one or more pan–T-cell markers. Focal CD30 positivity can be seen; PD-1, CXCR13, BCL-6, and CD10 expressions are absent.

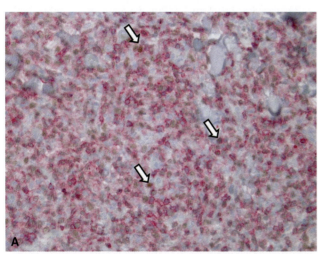
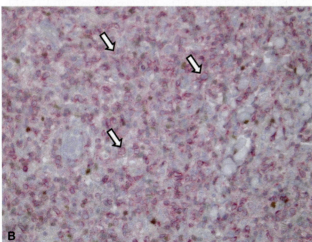

FIGURE 19-3. T-bet and GATA-3 expressions in primary cutaneous PTCL-NOS. CD3+ (*red*) T-cells are diffusely GATA-3+ with weak-to-moderate intensity (A) (*arrows*) and are T-bet− (B) (*arrows*). GATA-3 staining is significantly less prominent than that in tumor-stage MF (original magnification: 400×).

References

1. Swerdlow SH, Campo E, Pileri SA, et al. The 2016 revision of the World Health Organization classification of lymphoid neoplasms. *Blood*. 2016;127(20):2375-2390.
2. Pileri SA, Weisenburger DD, Sng I, et al. Peripheral T-cell lymphoma, NOS. In: Swerdlow S, Campo E, Harris NL, et al. eds. *WHO Classification of Tumours of the Haematopoietic and Lymphoid Tissue*. 4th ed. IARC; 2017:403-407.
3. Willemze R, Dreyling M; ESMO Guidelines Working Group. Primary cutaneous lymphoma: ESMO clinical recommendations for diagnosis, treatment and follow-up. *Ann Oncol*. 2009;20(suppl 4):115.
4. Beltraminelli H, Mullegger R, Cerroni L. Indolent CD8+ lymphoid proliferation of the ear: a phenotypic variant of the small-medium pleomorphic cutaneous T-cell lymphoma? *J Cutan Pathol*. 2010;37(1):81-84.
5. Petrella T, Maubec E, Cornillet-Lefebvre P, et al. Indolent CD8-positive lymphoid proliferation of the ear: a distinct primary cutaneous T-cell lymphoma? *Am J Surg Pathol*. 2007;31(12):1887-1892.
6. Ryan AJ, Robson A, Hayes BD, et al. Primary cutaneous peripheral T-cell lymphoma, unspecified with an indolent clinical course: a distinct peripheral T-cell lymphoma? *Clin Exp Dermatol*. 2010;35(8):892-896.

7. Petrella T, Gaulard P, Berti E et al. Primary cutaneous acral CD8+ T-cell lymphoma. In: Swerdlow S, Campo E, Harris NL et al. eds. *WHO Classification of Tumors of the Haematopoietic and Lymphoid Tissue*. 4th ed. IARC; 2017:400-401
8. Ally MS, Robson A. A review of the solitary cutaneous T-cell lymphomas. *J Cutan Pathol*. 2014;41(9):703-714.
9. Rizvi MA, Evens AM, Tallman MS, et al. T-cell non-Hodgkin lymphoma. *Blood*. 2006;107(4):1255-1264.
10. Willemze R, Jaffe ES, Burg G, et al. WHO-EORTC classification for cutaneous lymphomas. *Blood*. 2005;105(10):3768-3785.
11. Bekkenk MW, Vermeer MH, Jansen P, et al. Peripheral T-cell lymphomas unspecified presenting in the skin: analysis of prognostic factors in a group of 82 patients. *Blood*. 2003;102:2213-2219.
12. Weaver J, Mahindra AK, Pohlman B, et al. Non-mycosis fungoides cutaneous T-cell lymphoma: reclassification according to the WHO-EORTC classification. *J Cutan Pathol*. 2010;37(5):516-524.
13. Martin B, Stefanato CM, Whittaker S, et al. CD20+ primary cutaneous T-cell lymphoma. *J Cutan Pathol*. 2011;38(8):663-669.
14. Kempf W, Mitteldorf C, Battistella M, et al. Primary cutaneous peripheral T-cell lymphoma, not otherwise specified (NOS): results of a multicenter EORTC cutaneous lymphoma taskforce study on the clinico-pathological and prognostic features. *J Eur Acad Dermatol Venereol*. 2021;35(3):658-668.
15. Madan V, Cox NH. Primary cutaneous peripheral T-cell lymphoma, unspecified, that completely regressed after skin biopsy. *Br J Dermatol*. 2007;156(4):785-786.
16. Watabe H, Kawakami T, Murakami N, et al. Primary cutaneous peripheral T-cell lymphoma, unspecified, with CD8-positive phenotype. *Int J Dermatol*. 2006;45(11):1385-1387.
17. Rolim I, Bakshi A, West E, et al. Solitary CD8-positive primary cutaneous peripheral T-cell lymphoma: a question of classification. *Am J Dermatopathol*. 2021;43(9):e107-e110.
18. Kempf W, Petrella T, Willemze R, et al. Clinical, histopathological and prognostic features of primary cutaneous acral CD8+ T-cell lymphoma and other dermal CD8+ cutaneous lymphoproliferations—results of an EORTC Cutaneous Lymphoma Group Workshop. *Br J Dermatol*. 2022;186(5):887-897. doi:10.1111/bjd.20973
19. Beljaards R, Meijer CJLM, van Der Putte SCJ, et al. Primary cutaneous T-cell lymphoma: clinicopathological features and prognostic parameters of 35 cases other than mycosis fungoides and CD30-positive large cell lymphoma. *J Pathol*. 1994;172:53-60.
20. Willemze R, Kerl H, Sterry W, et al. EORTC classification for primary cutaneous lymphomas: a proposal from the cutaneous lymphoma study group of the European Organization for Research and Treatment of Cancer. *Blood*. 1997;90(1):354-371.
21. Grange F, Hedelin G, Joly P et al. Prognostic factors in primary cutaneous lymphomas other than mycosis fungoides and the Sezary syndrome. *Blood*. 1999;93(11):3637-3642.
22. Fink-Puches R, Zenahlik P, Back B, et al. Primary cutaneous lymphomas: applicability of current classification schemes (European Organization for Research and Treatment of Cancer, World Health Organization) based on clinicopathologic features observed in a large group of patients. *Blood*. 2002;99(3):800-805.
23. Paulli M, Berti E. Cutaneous T-cell lymphomas (including rare subtypes). Current concepts. II. *Haematologica*. 2004;89(11):1372-1388.
24. Went P, Agostinelli C, Gallamini A, et al. Marker expression in peripheral T-cell lymphoma: a proposed clinical-pathologic prognostic score. *J Clin Oncol*. 2006;24(16):2472-2479.
25. Cetinozman F, Jansen PM, Willemze R. Expression of programmed death-1 in primary cutaneous CD4-positive small/medium-sized pleomorphic T-cell lymphoma, cutaneous pseudo-T-cell lymphoma, and other types of cutaneous T-cell lymphoma. *Am J Surg Pathol*. 2012;36(1):109-116.
26. van Kester MS, Tensen CP, Vermeer MH, et al. Cutaneous anaplastic large cell lymphoma and peripheral T-cell lymphoma NOS show distinct chromosomal alterations and differential expression of chemokine receptors and apoptosis regulators. *J Invest Dermatol*. 2010;130(2):563-575.
27. Iqbal J, Wright G, Wang C, et al. Gene expression signatures delineate biological and prognostic subgroups in peripheral T-cell lymphoma. *Blood*. 2014;123(19):2915-2923.
28. Wang T, Feldman AL, Wada DA, et al. GATA-3 expression identifies a high-risk subset of PTCL, NOS with distinct molecular and clinical features. *Blood*. 2014;123(19):3007-3015.

CHAPTER 20

Primary cutaneous CD8+ acral lymphoproliferative disorder

Alistair M. Robson, Farrah Bakr, Melissa Pulitzer, and Werner Kempf

DEFINITION

Primary cutaneous acral CD8+ lymphoma was afforded provisional status for the first time in the World Health Organization revised lymphoma classification in 2016.[1] This designates a dermal tumor having nonactivated, cytotoxic T-cell immunophenotype, with a low proliferation index, frequent clonal gene rearrangements, and characteristic architectural and cytologic features. Petrella et al first drew attention to this distinct clinicopathological entity arising on the ears, which had malignant histological features but often a bland clinical presentation and indolent clinical course, therefore originally termed "indolent CD8+ lymphoid proliferation of the ear."[2] Subsequent case reports and small series confirmed the predilection for the ear but widened the reported anatomic locations, albeit almost always affecting acral sites, including nose, feet, and hands.[3-14] This period of increasing recognition of the tumor saw a proliferation of alternative labels, including indolent CD8+ lymphoid proliferation of the face,[15,16] indolent small/medium-sized CD8+ lymphoid proliferations with predilection for the ear and face,[17] and primary cutaneous CD8+ small/medium-sized pleomorphic T-cell lymphoma, ear-type.[18] The finding of such lesions at extrafacial sites stimulated new proposals, including extrafacial indolent CD8+ cutaneous lymphoid proliferation,[19] primary cutaneous CD8+ small medium lymphoproliferative disease of extrafacial sites.[20] Rare examples of multiple lesions affecting nonauricular sites nevertheless followed an innocuous clinical course. Initial claims that acral CD8+ lymphoma and small-medium CD4+ lymphoproliferative disease are immunophenotypic variants of the same disease[21] have rescinded with greater recognition of both entities and their distinct pathologies.

EPIDEMIOLOGY

Epidemiologic features are difficult to define, as the reported cases number fewer than 100.[17] Within this small group, there appears to be an approximately 2:1 male:female predominance with a wide age distribution among adults (29-87years).[19,22] No ethnic predilection has been described. Geographically, cases have been reported mostly from European and North American centers, with Israel and China reporting a single case each.[21,23]

ETIOLOGY

The almost invariant indolent clinical course has led authors to speculate if acral CD8+ lymphoma is a true lymphoma, a reactive or "intermediate" process,[16] but the cells are cytologically malignant and clonal and often have an abnormal immunophenotype. Furthermore, although as yet no systemic spread or fatalities have been reported, there are some reports of a less indolent clinical course, with recurrent disease or more widespread and locally destructive lesions.[3,4,24-27] The neoplastic cells have a CD3+, CD8+, TIA-1+ nonactivated cytotoxic T-lymphocyte signature. Physiologically, cytotoxic T lymphocytes are effectors in the primary host epithelial immune surveillance process, which involves both skin and mucosal barriers. Interestingly, there is a precedence for histologically malignant but clinically indolent cytotoxic T- or natural killer (NK)-cell proliferations at other epithelial sites, including various regions of the gastrointestinal tract.[28-31] Corresponding cytotoxic T-cell lymphomas frequently localize to the same regions of skin and mucosa, suggesting a reaction to a local chronic antigen stimulus, for example, enteropathy-associated T-cell lymphoma in response to gliadin as an antigenic stimulus. The preferential localization of this nonactivated cytotoxic T-cell subset to auricular and other acral skin sites, such as the nose and distal extremities, has led to the consideration of sources of antigen introduction such as arthropod bite, ear piercing, *Borrelia* infection, or other nonlocalized infectious agents such as HIV, which might cause an autoantigenic reaction via antigenic mimicry. However, most cases have no reported history of any of these possible sources and no candidate antigen has been identified.

CLINICAL PRESENTATION AND PROGNOSIS

Patients present typically with a solitary slow-growing papule, nodule, or plaque. Rarely lesions are multiple. At least five cases of bilateral and symmetric presentations have been reported.[2,4,32] Reports describe dome-shaped or poorly defined nonulcerated tumors ranging from 0.5 to 3cm in diameter, with a marked predilection for the ear, including both pinna and auricle (Fig. 20-1), and less commonly involving the face

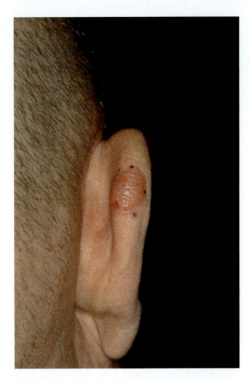

FIGURE 20-1. A "classic" dome-shaped, erythematous nodule on the posterior helix of the ear.

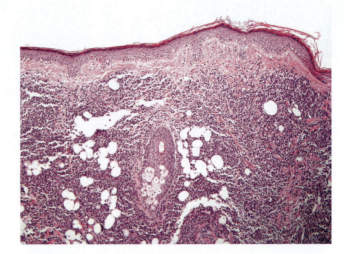

FIGURE 20-2. The small to medium-sized lymphocytes are arranged in a typically dense, diffuse pan-dermal infiltrate with a grenz zone (sparing of the epidermis).

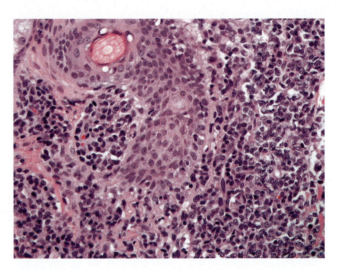

FIGURE 20-3. Hair follicles and other skin adnexal structures are characteristically surrounded by, but not invaded or destroyed by, the infiltrates, with rare exceptions.

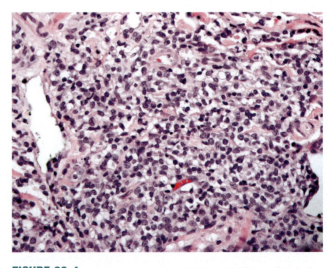

FIGURE 20-4. Lymphocytes are monomorphic and small to medium in size, with a paucity of other inflammatory cells.

(eyelid, nose),[3,15,16,33] hand,[3,4] shoulder, buttock, lower leg,[20] and foot.[4,19,21] Staging shows no evidence of extracutaneous disease. Typically, after radiation or surgical therapy, lesions do not recur, and the occasional recurrences respond well to subsequent treatment, with no distant spread or deaths due to disease reported. Maubec etal detailed a relapse after 7 years and reviewed the literature, concluding that recurrences were more frequent in younger patients.[34] One patient with ongoing repeated recurrences at multiple acral sites has been reported,[4] several patients have been described with unusually striking or multiple cutaneous tumors,[25-27] and there is a single case report documenting deep aggressive local growth and regional spread after 35years.[24] These observations suggest that sequelae may arise a lengthy interval after the initial presentation and that much longer follow-up might yet reveal a small subset of tumors to be more aggressive than originally believed.

HISTOLOGY

The most common histologic silhouette is of a nonulcerated dense pan-dermal infiltrate extending from a well-delineated grenz zone into the deep dermis (Fig. 20-2) or adipose tissues, with or without compression or destruction of hair follicles and eccrine glands, and without notable adnexal epitheliotropism (Figs. 20-3 and 20-5). However, focal infiltration and partial destruction of epithelial structures have been exceptionally described.[32] Occasional reports have identified epidermotropism and Pautrier-like microabscesses, although these are focal and the exception (Fig. 20-5).[3] Interface dermatitis, angiocentrism, or germinal centers are not identified. The lesional clearly atypical lymphocytes are usually monomorphic or mildly pleomorphic and are invariably small to

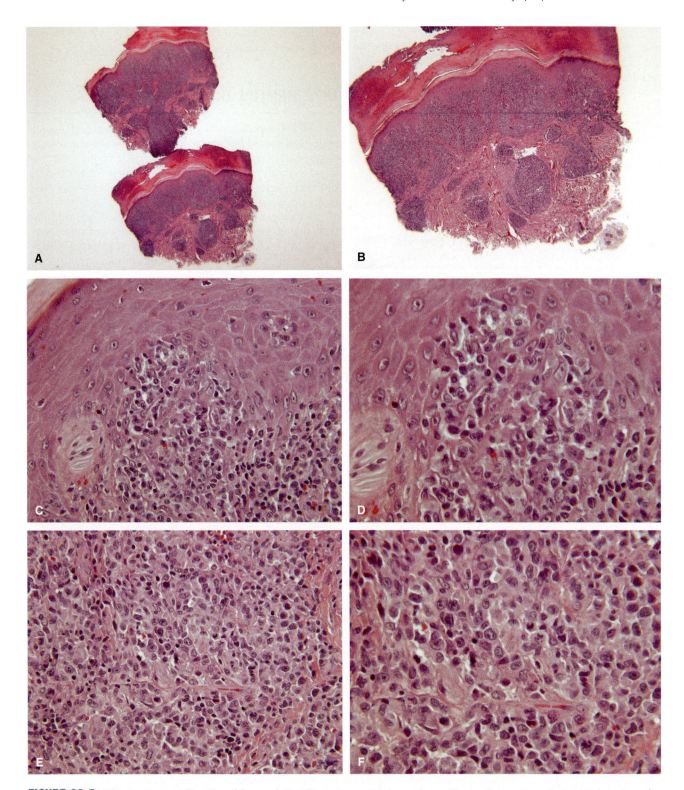

FIGURE 20-5. CD8⁺ lymphoid proliferation of the acral sites. This lesion presented on a 24-year-old man with a papule on the tip of his index finger. The lesion showed spontaneous resolution after 6weeks. **A** and **B** show prominent dermal infiltrate with epidermotropism. **C** and **D** highlight the epidermotropic population of cells with irregular nuclear borders. **E** and **F** illustrate the population of cells, predominantly medium in size, with nuclear contour irregularities and variable prominent nucleoli. Rare admixed mitotic figures are seen.

medium in size (Figs. 20-4 and 20-5). They may be blast-like or may show slightly irregular nuclear contours, but they do not exhibit cerebriform atypia. Signet ring/horseshoe cell variants have been reported, similar to the hallmark cells of anaplastic large-cell lymphoma (ALCL).[23,35] Other inflammatory cell populations rarely seen include plasma cells and histiocytes, occasionally in the form of granulomas.[16] Neutrophils and eosinophils are usually absent and are sparsely scattered when present.[16] Necrosis, ulceration, or angiodestructive features are absent.

IMMUNOPHENOTYPE

The atypical T lymphocytes express CD3, CD8, TIA-1, βF1, and CD45RO, characteristic of a clonal skin-homing nonactivated cytotoxic T cell (see Figs. 20-6A and 20-7). They do not express CD4, CD30, CD56, TDT, or PD-1,[16] ICOS, CXCL13, TCRγ-M1, or EBER-ISH.[3] Exceptionally they show CD45RA, perforin, or granzyme B expression (see Fig. 20-6B), usually only focally, indicative of an activated cytotoxic T-cell immunophenotype.[3] There is often loss of one or more of CD2, CD5, or CD7 (Figs. 20-6 and 20-7). CD99 is usually expressed. The MIB-1/Ki-67 proliferation index is typically less than 25% and often is less than 10%. Scarce reactive CD20+ B cells are commonly found.[2] Wobser et al reported a characteristic dot-like (Golgi) pattern of CD68 immunopositivity and suggested this was a very useful diagnostic feature of acral CD8+ lymphoma (Fig. 20-8).[36] An EORTC study of 31 cases of acral lymphoma included a comparison with examples of CD8+ peripheral T-cell lymphoma NOS and similarly concluded this pattern was highly sensitive and specific for the diagnosis.[37] Nevertheless, one PTCL NOS tumor in the study, and a further tumor reported separately,[38] documented similar dot-like CD68 expression indicating it can be rarely found in other diagnoses.

GENETIC AND MOLECULAR FINDINGS

Most cases described harbor monoclonal rearrangements of either T-cell receptor (TCR)-γ, or both TCRβ and TCRγ chains; however, monoclonality has not been used as a defining characteristic for inclusion within this group of diseases and polyclonality does not exclude the diagnosis. Identical T-cell clones are not present in peripheral blood.

DIFFERENTIAL DIAGNOSIS

Acral CD8+ lymphoma is a very distinct clinicopathological entity and should seldom be confused with alternative diagnoses. Differential diagnoses may include atypical reactive CD8+ infiltrates, such as those seen in various immune-compromised states (either congenital or acquired), and other lymphomas with a CD8+ phenotype.

Nonneoplastic but atypical CD8+ dermal infiltrates are well documented in various states of immunodeficiency. These include congenital disorders (Bruton X-linked agammaglobulinemia and common variable immunodeficiency)[20,37,39] and acquired (posttransplant and HIV)[37,40] states. Eruptions in these conditions vary but, in general, involve the development of multiple papules or plaques, often bilateral and on extremities and trunk, and respond well to adjustments in the patient's immunomodulating treatment and applied steroids. Cytological atypia is variable but usually mild, T-cell clones may be found, and some cases report an activated rather than constitutive cytotoxic phenotype. Significant numbers of admixed macrophages are often found, imparting a pale aspect to the infiltrate, in contrast to acral CD8+ lymphoma.

Acral CD8+ lymphoma can readily be distinguished from most other forms of CD8+ lymphoma. CD8+ variants of mycosis fungoides (MF) do not differ from the classical disease and present with the characteristic patches and plaques (see Chapter 13). Pagetoid reticulosis (Woringer-Kolopp), a subtype of MF, is a solitary often acral lesion, and with a CD8+ phenotype, but with conspicuous pagetoid epidermotropism and little dermal component, in direct reversal of the pattern found in acral CD8+ lymphoma. Nonpagetoid reticulosis solitary MF, an exceptional diagnosis indeed,[41] requires a typical clinical lesion and hallmark epidermotropic lymphoid cells, either as Pautrier microabscesses or tagging along the basal layer, neither found, or prominent, in the vast majority of acral CD8+ lymphomas. Although subcutaneous panniculitis-like T-cell lymphoma has a CD8+ phenotype, its markedly different clinical and pathological features (see Chapter 16)

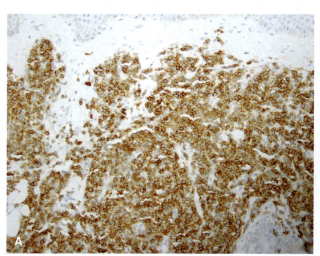
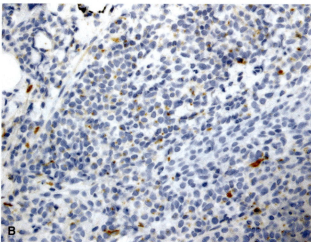

FIGURE 20-6. **A.** CD8 shows diffuse positivity. **B.** Granzyme B may occasionally label these tumors, despite the "quiescent" cytotoxic T-cell categorization.

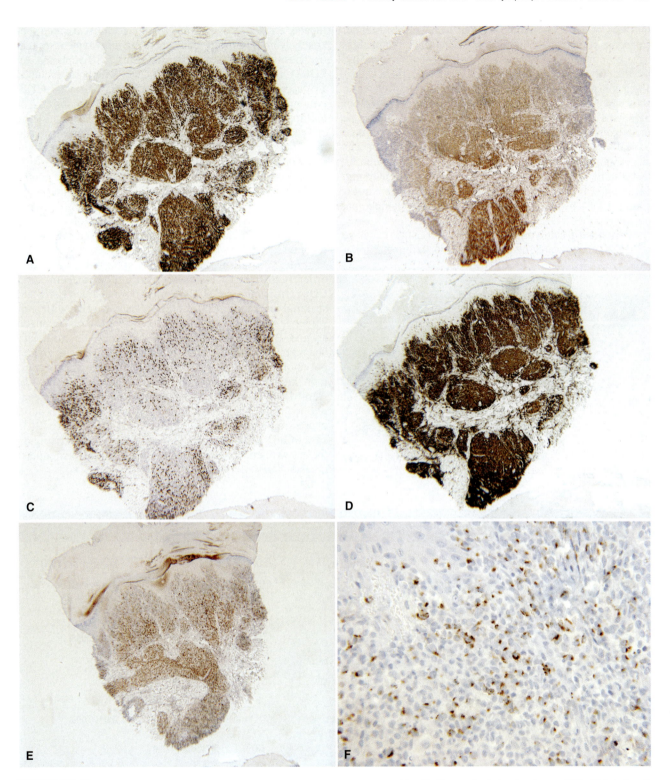

FIGURE 20-7. The lesional cells are positive for CD3 **(A)** and show focal aberrant loss of CD5 **(B)**. The neoplastic lymphocytes are CD4- **(C)** but strongly express CD8 **(D)**. MUM1 is diffusely positive **(E)**, and lesional cells, also stain for the cytotoxic marker TIA-1 **(F)**.

do not allow confusion. As some acral CD8+ lymphomas remit spontaneously, CD30+ lymphoproliferative disease may be a clinical consideration, but the absence of CD30 expression excludes this possibility.

Two lymphomas, however, can be more problematic. A solitary presentation of aggressive epidermotropic CD8+ ("Berti") lymphoma (AETCL) and a CD8+ variant of peripheral T-cell lymphoma NOS. The typical presentation of AETCL is of widespread ulcerated and often hemorrhagic plaques and tumors, markedly distinct from acral CD8+ lymphoma. However, rare cases do present with an initial solitary tumor, or oligolesional tumors. Histologically, most AETCL have a characteristically pagetoid epidermotropism, an often hemorrhagic dermal infiltrate with vasculocentricity, sometimes syringotropism; there is usually necrosis. These contrast significantly with the uniform diffuse dermal "clean" infiltrate of acral lymphoma without damage to bystander cutaneous components. Although rare acral CD8+ lymphomas have been noted to be epidermotropic, usually only focally[3] the majority are not, and in contrast to AETCL, there is usually a conspicuous grenz zone. Furthermore, the cells have an activated cytotoxic signature, with widespread expression of granzyme B and perforin (see Chapter 18). AETCL may be more likely to be CD45RA+, rather than CD45RO+, as is more typically seen in acral CD8+ lymphoma, and AETCL generally demonstrates a high proliferation index, while the indolent lesions usually have a Ki67 index below 25%, with rare exceptions.[3,42] If there should be doubt, the dot-like expression of CD68 by neoplastic cells in acral CD8+ lymphoma, not yet reported in AE CTCL,[36] may be useful.

Peripheral T-cell lymphoma NOS (PTCL NOS) can have a CD8+ phenotype and, by definition, lacks defining criteria. Indeed, acral CD8+ lymphoma is only recently classified separately from this group. Thus, there are individual cases that may be difficult to distinguish from acral CD8+ lymphoma. An EORTC report of 31 cases of acral CD8+ lymphoma included 11 cases of CD8+ PTCL NOS. In contrast to acral CD8+ lymphoma, PTCL NOS were rapidly evolving solitary or multiple (8 of 11) tumors, often consisting of medium-large cells having moderate-severe cytological pleomorphism, and more often with significant, albeit sometimes focal epidermotropism; granzyme B and/or perforin were expressed, and the proliferative fraction manifested by mitotic counts or Ki67 index, higher (>50%). Nevertheless, some range was observed and not all cases are clear-cut; furthermore, one case displayed the dot-like CD68 expression typical of acral CD8+ lymphoma, an exceptional finding previously reported.[37,38]

Finally, small-medium CD4+ lymphoproliferative disorder (CSMPTCL) is readily distinguished from acral CD8+ lymphoma. CSMPTCL presents a characteristic and strikingly mixed infiltrate of CD4+ T and B cells, with conspicuous expression of follicular T-helper cells arranged around B-cell immunoblasts. A constant but minority "background" CD8+ population is evident. There is greater polymorphism, with plasma cells and macrophages common, and a more inflammatory diathesis (see Chapter 17). Acral CD8+ lymphoma almost always is completely negative for follicular T-helper markers, with only focal bcl-6 expression reported in a single atypical case.[43] Recently, a case of otherwise classic CD8+ acral lymphoma arising on the ear with coexpression of CD4 and CD8 by the neoplastic cells was reported[44] (Table 20-1).

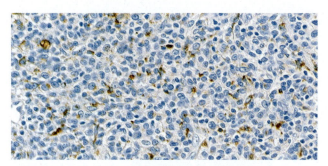

FIGURE 20-8. CD68 expression by some neoplastic cells, with the highly sensitive and specific dot-like pattern.

TABLE 20-1 Differential Diagnosis of Primary Cutaneous CD8+ Acral Lymphoma

	Clinical Features	Histopathology	Immunohistochemistry	Molecular (TCR)
CD8+ SMLPD	Solitary nodule/tumor, no patches or plaques	Not epidermotropic, +grenz zone, not cerebriform	CD3+, CD8+, CD45RO+/RA+, TIA-1+, CD30−, CD56−, γMI−	Monoclonal or polyclonal
CD8+ MF	Indolent, with patches and plaques, often, young age, hypopigmented or unilesional (PR)	Epidermotropic lichenoid, paucicellular, cerebriform small cells	CD3+, CD8+, CD45RO+, +/− cytotoxic markers, CD30+/−	Monoclonal
CD30+ ALCL	Single or few nodules	Large, hallmark cells, not epidermotropic	CD4+ mostly, CD30+ in >75% of cells, loss of CD2.CD3, CD45RO−, often cytotoxic marker+	Monoclonal
Primary cutaneous PTCL-NOS, aggressive variants	Typically widespread tumors unless CSMp TCL, which are CD4	May be nonepitheliotropic with a grenz zone, but have large cells, pleomorphic	CD4 or CD8+, +/− TFH markers (BCL-6, PD-1, CD10, CXCL13)+/−, CD30+/−	Monoclonal
CD8+ AETCL	Patch, plaque, tumor, ulcers	Epidermotropic, large cells, angiocentrism, necrosis, and ulceration	CD8+, CD45RO−, CD45RA+, TIA-1+, perforin+, GZB+	Monoclonal

References

1. Berti E, Gaulard P, Willemze R, et al. Primary cutaneous peripheral T-cell lymphomas, rare subtypes. In: Swerdlow SH, Campo E, Harris NL, et al, eds. *WHO Classification of Tumours of Haematopoeitic and Lymphoid Tissues.* IARC Press; 2017:400.
2. Petrella T, Maubec E, Cornillet-Lefebvre P, et al. Indolent CD8-positive lymphoid proliferation of the ear: a distinct primary cutaneous T-cell lymphoma? *Am J Surg Pathol.* 2007;31(12):1887-1892. doi:10.1097/PAS.0b013e318068b527
3. Greenblatt D, Ally M, Child F, et al. Indolent CD8(+) lymphoid proliferation of acral sites: a clinicopathologic study of six patients with some atypical features. *J Cutan Pathol.* 2013;40(2):248-258. doi:10.1111/cup.12045
4. Kluk J, Kai A, Koch D, et al. Indolent CD8-positive lymphoid proliferation of acral sites: three further cases of a rare entity and an update on a unique patient. *J Cutan Pathol.* 2016;43:125-136.
5. Swick BL, Baum CL, Venkat AP, et al. Indolent CD8+ lymphoid proliferation of the ear: report of two cases and review of the literature. *J Cutan Pathol.* 2011;38(2):209-215. doi:10.1111/j.1600-0560.2010.01647.x
6. Girisha BS, Srinivas T, Noronha TM, et al. A case of an indolent CD8-positive lymphoid proliferation of the ear. *Indian J Dermatol.* 2018;63(4):342-345.
7. Ormerod E, Murigu T, Pawade J, et al. Primary cutaneous acral CD8+ T-cell lymphoma of the ear: a case report. *J Cutan Pathol.* 2019;46:790-793.
8. Butsch F, Kind P, Bräuninger W. Bilateral indolent epidermotropic CD8-positive lymphoid proliferations of the ear. *J Dtsch Dermatol Ges.* 2012;10(3):195-196.
9. Tjahjono LA, Davis MDP, Witzig TE, et al. Primary cutaneous acral CD8+ T-cell lymphoma—a single center review of 3 cases and recent literature review. *Am J Dermatopathol.* 2019;41(9):644-648.
10. Virmani P, Jawed S, Myskowsk PL, et al. Long-term followup and management of small/medium-sized CD4+ T cell lymphoma and CD8+ lymphoid proliferation of acral sites: a multi-center experience. *Int J Dermatol.* 2016;55(11):1248-1254.
11. Fika Z, Karkos PD, Badran K, et al. Primary cutaneous aggressive epidermotropic CD8 positive cytotoxic T-cell lymphoma of the ear. *J Laryngol Otol.* 2007;121:503-505.
12. Nguyen CV, Miller DD, Hylwa SA. Changing nodule on the right helix. *Int J Dermatol.* 2017;56(5):483-485.
13. Valois A, Bastien C, Granel-Broca F, et al. Indolent lymphoma of the ear. *Ann Dermatol Venereol.* 2012;139(12):818-823.
14. Ryan AJA, Robson A, Hayes BD, et al. Primary cutaneous peripheral T-cell lymphoma, unspecified with an indolent clinical course: a distinct peripheral T-cell lymphoma? *Clin Exp Dermatol.* 2010;35(8):892-896.
15. Suchak R, O'Connor S, McNamara C, et al. Indolent CD8-positive lymphoid proliferation on the face: part of the spectrum of primary cutaneous small-/medium-sized pleomorphic T-cell lymphoma or a distinct entity? *J Cutan Pathol.* 2010;37(9):977-981. doi:10.1111/j.1600-0560.2009.01448.x
16. Hagen JW, Magro CM. Indolent CD8+ lymphoid proliferation of the face with eyelid involvement. *Am J Dermatopathol.* 2014;36(2):137-141. doi:10.1097/DAD.0b013e318297f7fd
17. Li JY, Guitart J, Pulitzer MP, et al. Multicenter case series of indolent small/medium-sized CD8+ lymphoid proliferations with predilection for the ear and face. *Am J Dermatopathol.* 2014;36(5):402-408. doi:10.1097/DAD.0b013e3182a74c7a
18. Geraud C, Goerdt S, Klemke CD. Primary cutaneous CD8+ small/medium-sized pleomorphic T-cell lymphoma, ear-type: a unique cutaneous T-cell lymphoma with a favourable prognosis. *Br J Dermatol.* 2011;164(2):456-458. doi:10.1111/j.1365-2133.2010.10105.x
19. Wobser M, Petrella T, Kneitz H, et al. Extrafacial indolent CD8-positive cutaneous lymphoid proliferation with unusual symmetrical presentation involving both feet. *J Cutan Pathol.* 2013;40(11):955-961. doi:10.1111/cup.12213
20. Kempf W, Kazakov DV, Cozzio A, et al. Primary cutaneous CD8(+) small- to medium-sized lymphoproliferative disorder in extrafacial sites: clinicopathologic features and concept on their classification. *Am J Dermatopathol.* 2013;35(2):159-166. doi:10.1097/DAD.0b013e31825c3a33
21. Khamaysi Z, Ben-Arieh Y, Epelbaum R, et al. Pleomorphic CD8+ small/medium size cutaneous T-cell lymphoma. *Am J Dermatopathol.* 2006;28(5):434-437. doi:10.1097/01.dad.0000210389.36724.dd
22. Petrella T. Indolent CD8+ lymphoid proliferation of the ear. *Ann Dermatol Venereol.* 2012;139(12):789-790. doi:10.1016/j.annder.2012.10.579
23. Li XQ, Zhou XY, Sheng WQ, et al. Indolent CD8+ lymphoid proliferation of the ear: a new entity and possible occurrence of signet ring cells. *Histopathology.* 2009;55(4):468-470. doi:10.1111/j.1365-2559.2009.03383.x
24. Alberti Violetti S, Fanoni D, Provasi M, et al. Primary cutaneous acral CD8 positive T-cell lymphoma with extra-cutaneous involvement: a long-standing case with an unexpected progression. *J Cutan Pathol.* 2017;44:964-968.
25. Eich D, Eich HT, Otte H, et al. Photodynamische therapie kutaner T-zell lymphoma in besonderer lokalisation Der. *Hautarzt.* 1999;50:109-114.
26. Le Loarer F, Barete S, Vallat L, et al. Primary cutaneous CD8+ T-cell lymphoma masquerading as acral vascular syndrome. *Acta Derm Venereol.* 2014;94:317-319.
27. Kutlubay Z, Engin B, Kote E, et al. A case of CD8+ small/medium-sized pleomorphic T-cell lymphoma: clinical and histopathological differential diagnosis. *Brit J Dermatol.* 2014;170:204-205.
28. Mansoor A, Pittaluga S, Beck PL, et al. NK-cell enteropathy: a benign NK-cell lymphoproliferative disease mimicking intestinal lymphoma: clinicopathologic features and follow-up in a unique case series. *Blood.* 2011;117:1447.
29. Takeuchi K, Yokoyama M, Ishizawa S, et al. Lymphomatoid gastropathy: a distinct clinicopathologic entity of self-limited pseudomalignant NK-cell proliferation. *Blood.* 2010;116:5631.
30. Ranheim EA, Jones C, Zehnder JL, et al. Warnke Spontaneously relapsing clonal, mucosal cytotoxic T-cell lymphoproliferative disorder: case report and review of the literature. *Am J Surg Pathol.* 2000;24:296.
31. Egawa N, Fukayama M, Kawaguchi K, et al. Relapsing oral and colonic ulcers with monoclonal T-cell infiltration. A low grade mucosal T-lymphoproliferative disease of the digestive tract. *Cancer.* 1995;75:1728.
32. Beltraminelli H, Mullegger R, Cerroni L. Indolent CD8+ lymphoid proliferation of the ear: a phenotypic variant of the small-medium pleomorphic cutaneous T-cell lymphoma? *J Cutan Pathol.* 2010;37(1):81-84. doi:10.1111/j.1600-0560.2009.01278.x
33. Milley S, Bories N, Balme B, et al. Indolent CD8+ lymphoid proliferation on the nose. *Ann Dermatol Venereol.* 2012;139(12):812-817. doi:10.1016/j.annder.2012.09.012

34. Maubec E, Marinho E, Laroche L, et al. Primary cutaneous acral CD8+ T-cell lymphomas relapse more frequently in younger patients. *Brit J Haematol*. 2019;185:598-601.
35. Vaillant L, Monegier du Sorbier C, Arbeille B, et al. Cutaneous T cell lymphoma of signet ring cell type: a specific clinico-pathologic entity. *Acta Derm Venereol*. 1993;73(4):255-258.
36. Wobser M, Roth S, Reinartz T, et al. CD68 expression is a discriminative feature of indolent cutaneous CD8-positive lymphoid proliferation and distinguishes this lymphoma subtype from other CD8-positive cutaneous lymphomas. *Brit J Dermatol*. 2015;172(6):1573-1580.
37. Kempf W, Petrella T, Willemze R, et al. Clinical, histopathological and prognostic features of primary cutaneous acral CD8+ T-cell lymphoma and other dermal CD8+ cutaneous lymphoproliferations—Results of an EORTC Cutaneous Lymphoma Taskforce Workshop. *Br J Dermatol*. 2022;186(5):887-897.
38. Rolim I, Bakshi A, West R, et al. Solitary CD8-positive primary cutaneous peripheral T-cell lymphoma; a question of classification. *Am J Dermatopathol*. 2021;43(9):e107-e110.
39. Gualdi G, Lorenzi L, Arisi M, et al. Acral lympho-histiocytic dermatitis in X-linked agammaglobulinemia: a case report showing clonal CD8+ T cells with indolent clinical behaviour. *J Eur Acad Dermatol Venereol*. 2016;30:446-556.
40. Baykal C, Buyukbabani N, Seckin D, et al. Cutaneous atypical papular CD8+ lymphoproliferative disorder at acral sites in a renal transplant patient. *Clin Exp Derm*. 2017;42:902-905.
41. Ally M, Pawade J, Tanaka M, et al. Solitary mycosis fungoides: a distinct clinicopathologic entity with a good prognosis. *J Am Acad Dermatol*. 2012;67(4):736-744.
42. Zeng W, Nava VE, Cohen P, et al. Indolent CD8-positive T-cell lymphoid proliferation of the ear: a report of two cases. *J Cutan Pathol*. 2012;39(7):696-700. doi:10.1111/j.1600-0560.2012.01917.x
43. Prieto-Torres L, Camacho-Garcia D, Piris MA, et al. Atypical BCL6/GATA3+ primary cutaneous acral CD8-positive T-cell lymphoma: a diagnostic challenge. *Am J Dermatopathol*. 2021;43(2):137-140.
44. Toberer F, Christopoulos P, Lasitschka F, et al. Double-positive CD8/CD4 primary cutaneous acral T-cell lymphoma. *J Cutan Pathol*. 2019;46:231-233.

CHAPTER 21

Granulomatous CD8-positive lymphoproliferative disorder associated with immunodeficiency

Werner Kempf and Christina Mitteldorf

INTRODUCTION AND DEFINITION

Patients with acquired immunodeficiency in the context of organ transplantation or human immunodeficiency virus (HIV) infection have an increased risk of developing malignant lymphomas. Similarly, patients with congenital forms of immunodeficiency such congenital variable immunodeficiency (CVID) syndrome also are prone to develop lymphoproliferations in various organs.[1] In addition to the lymphocytic proliferation, a granulomatous component may be present. Most commonly granulomatous infiltrates in congenital forms of immunodeficiency are found in the lungs, lymph nodes, and liver.[2] The skin is rarely involved.[3] Only very few reports on CD8-predominant cutaneous lymphoproliferations in patients with congenital forms of immunodeficiency exist.[3-8] In 2001, clonal CD8+ infiltrates in the skin in a patient with CVID were reported by Marzano and coworkers.[4] A small series on four patients with generalized papulonodular skin lesions and granulomatous and clonal CD8-positive T cells was described by Gammon et al who proposed the term CD8-positive granulomatous cutaneous T-cell lymphoma (CD8+ G-CTCL).[5]

The pathogenetic mechanisms underlying the formation of granulomatous CD8+ infiltrates are not yet elucidated. Mutations in various genes, however, were identified in patients with congenital forms of immunodeficiency; for example, mutations of the TACI (Transmembrane activator and calcium-modulating cyclophilin ligand interactor; TNF super receptor family 13B) genes were found in some patients with CVID and CD8-positive T-cell lymphoproliferations but have not been systematically investigated in patients with cutaneous CD8-positive lymphoproliferations. Aggressive forms of CD8-positive lymphomas involving the skin have been observed in a patient with a RAG (Recombination Activating Gene) mutation.[8,9] It is important for pathologists and dermatopathologists to be aware of and to identify CD8+ T-cell granulomatous lymphoproliferative disorder (CD8+ G-LPD) as the diagnosis may prompt further investigations for underlying immunodeficiency.

EPIDEMIOLOGY

Owing to the rarity of CD8+ G-LPD data on the exact prevalence in patients with congenital immunodeficiency are lacking.

CLINICAL PRESENTATION AND PROGNOSIS

Most patients present with asymptomatic red to brownish or violaceous papules or plaques[5] (Fig. 21-1). In most patients, the extremities are affected and represent the site of predilection. The lesions are slow growing and longstanding. There is no tendency for ulceration.

The therapeutic approach to CD8+ G-LPD has still to be determined. Response to systemic steroids and hydroxychloroquine has been reported but did not prevent recurrence or progression of the lesions.[6] Progression may require chemotherapy, but an effective therapy for CD8+ G-LPD has still to be identified.

Granulomatous CD8+ cutaneous lymphoproliferations are at least initially indolent, but longstanding and often therapy resistant.[5] In some patients, however, progression to overt CD8+ T-cell lymphoma may occur and lead to a fatal outcome.[5]

HISTOLOGY

CD8+ G-LPD is characterized by dermal multinodular and confluent infiltrates with a paler aspect on hematoxylin and eosin (H&E) stains compared with predominantly lymphocytic infiltrates due to their high number of histiocytes (Figs. 21-2 and 21-3). The infiltrates are composed of mostly small lymphocytes with dense chromatin and round to slightly elongated nuclei with subtle to moderate nuclear atypia (Fig. 21-4). Few medium-sized lymphocytes can be found. The histiocytes may form small granulomatous foci without necrosis. There is no epidermotropism or folliculotropism of the lymphocytes. Eosinophils are usually not admixed, whereas a few plasma cells can be found. Angiocentric growth is absent.

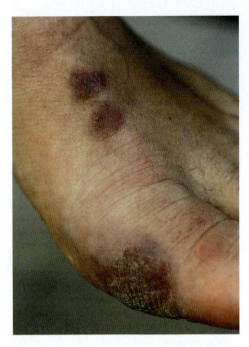

FIGURE 21-1. CD8-positive granulomatous lymphoproliferative disorder, clinical presentation: multiple papulonodular violaceous to brownish papules and small plaques on the legs.

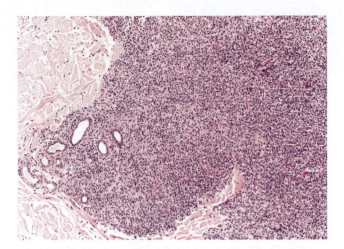

FIGURE 21-3. CD8-positive granulomatous lymphoproliferative disorder, histology: pale aspect of the infiltrates due to the prominent histiocytic component (H&E magnification, X200).

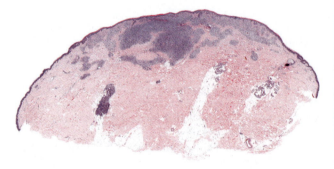

FIGURE 21-2. CD8-positive granulomatous lymphoproliferative disorder, histology: dermal nodular lymphocytic and histiocyte-rich infiltrate (H&E magnification, X2).

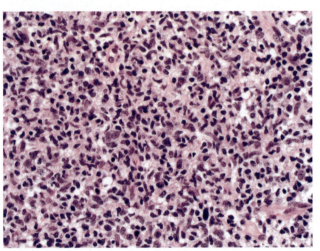

FIGURE 21-4. CD8-positive granulomatous lymphoproliferative disorder, histology: Atypical small to medium-sized lymphocytes with mild nuclear atypia admixed with numerous histiocytes (H&E magnification, X400).

IMMUNOPHENOTYPE

Immunophenotyping reveals that the majority of the lymphocytes expresses CD8, usually accounting for 70% to 80% of the lymphocytic component, embedded in a dense infiltrate of CD68-positive histiocytes (Fig. 21-5). The CD8-positive lymphocytes express TIA-1 but are negative for granzyme B or perforin (Fig. 21-6). Usually, the proliferative activity of the lymphocytes is low (ie, 5%-10%) (Fig. 21-7). In contrast to many lymphomas arising in primary or acquired immunodeficiency, no association of CD8+ G-LPD with Epstein-Barr virus can be demonstrated based on immunohistochemistry or in situ hybridization.

GENETIC AND MOLECULAR FINDINGS

Clonality assays may reveal monoclonal rearrangement of T-cell receptor beta or gamma genes by polymerase chain reaction.[4-6,8] It has to be emphasized that diagnosis and prognostic assessment of CD8+ G-LPD should not rely on the detection or absence of a T-cell clone.

Differential Diagnosis

The spectrum of differential diagnoses of CD8+ G-LPD spans indolent as well as highly malignant lymphomas, and also infectious diseases and inflammatory granulomatous skin disorders.

Primary cutaneous acral CD8-positive T-cell lymphoproliferative disorder (CD8+ acral LPD)

This lymphoproliferation is listed as a provisional entity in the WHO 2016/2017 and the updated WHO-EORTC classification 2018 and was originally referred to as primary cutaneous acral CD8-positive T-cell lymphoma.[10,11] It manifests usually with a solitary, rarely also with bilateral nonulcerated nodule(s) at acral sites, typically ears, hands, and feet.[12] Histologically, there are dense dermal monotonous infiltrates of small to mostly medium-sized lymphocytes with moderate nuclear

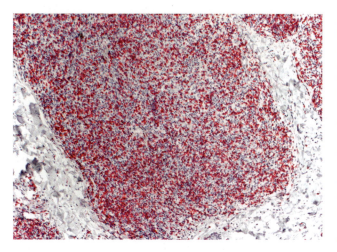

FIGURE 21-5. CD8-positive granulomatous lymphoproliferative disorder, immunohistochemistry: expression of CD8 by the majority of the lymphocytes.

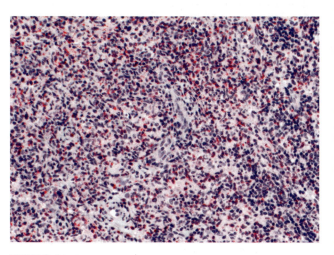

FIGURE 21-6. CD8-positive granulomatous lymphoproliferative disorder, immunohistochemistry: expression of TIA-1 by the atypical lymphocytes.

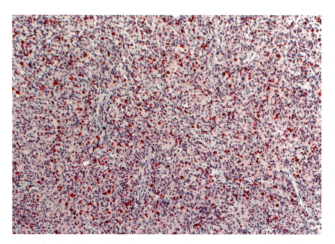

FIGURE 21-7. CD8-positive granulomatous lymphoproliferative disorder, immunohistochemistry: proliferative activity by approximately 10% of the lymphocytes.

atypia. Epidermotropism is absent or only focally present. The lymphocytes express CD8 and TIA-1 but are negative for granzyme B and perforin as in CD8-positive G-LPD. The proliferative activity is low, that is, less than 5% of the tumor cells. There is a diffuse admixture of histiocytes, which is less prominent than in CD8+ G-LPD. Immunohistochemistry reveals a unique staining pattern for CD68 and related antigens with a characteristic perinuclear dot-like pattern in tumor cells.[13] This feature has so far only been seen in **CD8+ acral LPD** but not in other CD8+ lymphoproliferations and therefore is of diagnostic value. The prognosis of **CD8+ acral LPD** is excellent.[12] Surgical excision and/or radiotherapy represent the first-line treatment if regression after incisional biopsy does not occur. The clinical presentation with a solitary nodule, the monotonous infiltrates and the characteristic dot-like pattern in the CD68 stain allow to distinguish **CD8+ acral LPD** from CD8+ G-LPD.

Granulomatous Mycosis Fungoides

Granulomatous mycosis fungoides (MF) may show similar histological features as CD8+ G-CTCL but differs clinically by the presence of hyperpigmented patches and plaques in contrast to the predominantly papular presentation in CD8+ G-LPD.[14] Histologically, either a sarcoid-like pattern with epithelioid cell granulomas or a granulomatous infiltrate mimicking granuloma annulare is found in granulomatous MF, whereas the granulomatous component in CD8+ G-LPD is diffuse.[14,15] Moreover, tumor cells in granulomatous MF most commonly shows a CD4-positive phenotype, although very rare cases of CD8-positive granulomatous MF exist. Of note, epidermotropism is found in only half of the cases of granulomatous MF and is therefore of limited diagnostic value for the distinction of granulomatous MF from CD8+ G-LPD.[14] In addition, nuclear atypia is not a characteristic finding in granulomatous MF, which contributes to the delay in diagnosing granulomatous MF. Clonality is helpful as an adjunctive diagnostic marker as clonal T cells are found in 90% of granulomatous MF but only very rarely in granuloma annulare or sarcoidosis.[14,16] The clinical presentation of granulomatous MF with patches and plaques is crucial in the differentiation from CD8+ G-LPD. The prognosis of granulomatous MF has still to be clarified as there are contradicting data in the literature regarding an impaired prognosis. In a multicenter study, a 5-year survival rate of only 66% was reported.[14] The treatment of granulomatous MF follows the recommendations for plaque-stage MF including systemic treatment with interferon, bexarotene, and psoralen-UVA light treatment.

CD8+ Aggressive Epidermotropic Cutaneous T-Cell Lymphoma

This very rare, but highly aggressive cytotoxic T-cell lymphoma differs from CD8+ G-LPD by the rapid evolution of necrotic and ulcerated plaques and nodules, a strongly epidermotropic infiltrate of medium-sized lymphocytes with nuclear atypia and rapid progression with fatal outcome.[17,18] The clinical presentation (ulceration, rapid onset) and the prominent epidermotropism allow differentiation from CD8+ G-LPD. (see Chapter 18).

CD8+ Cutaneous Pseudolymphoma

Various infections such as with herpes simplex virus, varicella zoster virus, HIV, treponema pallidum, and *Borrelia* sp. can result in infiltrates of CD8+ lymphocytes.[19] CD8+ infiltrates seem not to be exclusively limited to patients with infections, as similar findings were also described in a renal transplant recipient.[20] Histologically, diffuse dermal infiltrates of CD8+ small lymphocytes with admixture of small to medium cells with nuclear atypia are found. In addition, vacuolization in the junctional zone and exocytosis of CD8+ lymphocytes into the lower third of the epidermis is present, which mimics MF. The clinical presentations include localized or disseminated papules or small plaques.[21-23] In HIV-infected patients, the CD8+ skin infiltrates seem to be related to severe immunodeficiency as they occur in advanced HIV infection with low numbers of CD4+ cells. The predominance of CD8+ lymphocytes and detection of nuclear atypia of the lymphocytes may give rise to the suspicion of a T-cell lymphoma. The course of the cutaneous CD8+ pseudolymphoma is benign and lesions resolve after treatment of the underlying infection, but regression of the lesions may be protracted. In HIV-infected patients remission of the CD8+ papular eruption can be achieved when patients receive highly active antiretroviral therapy, and in moderately immunosuppressed patients methotrexate was shown to be effective.[24,25]

Sarcoidosis

The number of lymphocytes in sarcoidosis is lower than in CD8+ G-LPD. Moreover, a lower CD4+/CD8+ ratio was found in the cutaneous granulomatous infiltrates of patients with a primary immunodeficiency disorder as compared with the patients with cutaneous sarcoidosis.[26] Nuclear atypia of the lymphocytes in sarcoidosis is absent. Monoclonal rearrangement of T-cell receptor genes is not found in sarcoidosis.[16]

DIAGNOSIS

Diagnosis is based on the combination of histiocyte-rich or granulomatous infiltrates with a high number of CD8+ T cells, with or without nuclear atypia, in the context of primary immunodeficiency.[27] The term CD8+ G-LPD as proposed by Gammon et al can be used to refer to such constellations, but one has to be aware that this term is not included and not recommended in the current revised WHO classification or in the updated WHO-EORTC classification for primary cutaneous lymphomas.[10,11] The term CD8+ granulomatous CTCL as part of primary immunodeficiency-associated lymphoproliferative disorders better reflects the at least initially indolent biologic behaviour of this disease.

CONCLUSION

The presence of multiple papular and/or plaque-like skin lesions with granulomatous infiltrates and a predominance of CD8-positive T cells should prompt the search for congenital forms of immunodeficiency.

References

1. Riaz IB, Faridi W, Patnaik MM, Abraham RS. A systematic review on predisposition to lymphoid (B and T cell) Neoplasias in patients with primary Immunodeficiencies and Immune Dysregulatory disorders (Inborn Errors of Immunity). *Front Immunol*. 2019;10:777.
2. Ardeniz O, Cunningham-Rundles C. Granulomatous disease in common variable immunodeficiency. *Clin Immunol*. 2009;133(2):198-207.
3. Gregoriou S, Trimis G, Charissi C, Kalogeromitros D, Stefanaki K, Rigopoulos D. Cutaneous granulomas with predominantly CD8(+) lymphocytic infiltrate in a child with severe combined immunodeficiency. *J Cutan Med Surg*. 2008;12(5):246-248.
4. Marzano AV, Berti E, Alessi E, Caputo R. Clonal CD8 infiltration of the skin in common variable immunodeficiency: a prelymphomatous stage? *J Am Acad Dermatol*. 2001;44(4):710-713.
5. Gammon B, Robson A, Deonizio J, Arkin L, Guitart J. CD8(+) granulomatous cutaneous T-cell lymphoma: a potential association with immunodeficiency. *J Am Acad Dermatol*. 2014;71(3):555-560.
6. Amann VC, Dreier J, Ignatova D, et al. Disseminated primary cutaneous CD8+ small/medium-sized pleomorphic T-cell lymphoma responding to hydroxychloroquine. *Acta Derm Venereol*. 2015;95(5):602-603.
7. Gualdi G, Lorenzi L, Arisi M, et al. Acral lympho-histiocytic dermatitis in X-linked agammaglobulinemia: a case report showing clonal CD8(+) T cells with indolent clinical behaviour. *J Eur Acad Dermatol Venereol*. 2016;30(3):461-463.
8. Avitan-Hersh E, Stepensky P, Zaidman I, Nevet MJ, Hanna S, Bergman R. Primary cutaneous clonal CD8+ T-cell lymphoproliferative disorder associated with immunodeficiency due to RAG1 mutation. *Am J Dermatopathol*. 2020;42(1):e11-e5.
9. Schuetz C, Huck K, Gudowius S, et al. An immunodeficiency disease with RAG mutations and granulomas. *N Engl J Med*. 2008;358(19):2030-2038.
10. Swerdlow SH, Campo E, Harris NL, et al. *WHO Classification of Tumours of Haematopoietic and Lymphoid Tissues*. IARC; 2017:10-12.
11. Willemze R, Cerroni L, Kempf W, et al. The 2018 update of the WHO-EORTC classification for primary cutaneous lymphomas. *Blood*. 2019;133(16):1703-1714.
12. Petrella T, Maubec E, Cornillet-Lefebvre P, et al. Indolent CD8-positive lymphoid proliferation of the ear: a distinct primary cutaneous T-cell lymphoma? *Am J Surg Pathol*. 2007;31(12):1887-1892.
13. Wobser M, Roth S, Reinartz T, Rosenwald A, Goebeler M, Geissinger E. CD68 expression is a discriminative feature of indolent cutaneous CD8-positive lymphoid proliferation and distinguishes this lymphoma subtype from other CD8-positive cutaneous lymphomas. *Br J Dermatol*. 2015;172(6):1573-1580.
14. Kempf W, Ostheeren-Michaelis S, Paulli M, et al. Granulomatous mycosis fungoides and granulomatous slack skin: a multicenter study of the cutaneous lymphoma histopathology Task Force Group of the European Organization for Research and treatment of Cancer (EORTC). *Arch Dermatol*. 2008;144(12):1609-1617.
15. LeBoit PE, Zackheim HS, White CJ. Granulomatous variants of cutaneous T-cell lymphoma. The histopathology of granulomatous mycosis fungoides and granulomatous slack skin. *Am J Surg Pathol*. 1988;12(2):83-95.
16. Pfaltz K, Kerl K, Palmedo G, Kutzner H, Kempf W. Clonality in sarcoidosis, granuloma annulare, and granulomatous mycosis fungoides. *Am J Dermatopathol*. 2011;33(7):659-662.
17. Berti E, Tomasini D, Vermeer MH, Meijer CJ, Alessi E, Willemze R. Primary cutaneous CD8-positive epidermotropic cytotoxic T cell lymphomas. A distinct clinicopathological entity with an aggressive clinical behavior. *Am J Pathol*. 1999;155(2):483-492.

18. Robson A, Assaf C, Bagot M, et al. Aggressive epidermotropic cutaneous CD8+ lymphoma: a cutaneous lymphoma with distinct clinical and pathological features. Report of an EORTC Cutaneous Lymphoma Task Force Workshop. *Histopathology*. 2015;67(4):425-441.
19. Mitteldorf C, Kempf W. Cutaneous pseudolymphoma-A review on the spectrum and a proposal for a new classification. *J Cutan Pathol*. 2020;47(1):76-97.
20. Bayal C, Büyükbani N, Seckin D, Yilmaz Z, Kempf W. Cutaneous atypical papular CD8+ lymphoproliferative disorder at acral sites in a renal transplant patient. *Clin Exp Dermatol*. 2016;42(8):902-905.
21. Longacre TA, Foucar K, Koster F, Burgdorf W. Atypical cutaneous lymphoproliferative disorder resembling mycosis fungoides in AIDS. Report of a case with concurrent Kaposi's sarcoma. *Am J Dermatopathol*. 1989;11(5):451-456.
22. Egbers RG, Do TT, Su L, Helfrich YR, Gudjonsson JE. Rapid clinical change in lesions of atypical cutaneous lymphoproliferative disorder in an HIV patient: a case report and review of the literature. *Dermatol Online J*. 2011;17(9):4.
23. Mitteldorf C, Plumbaum H, Zutt M, Schon MP, Kaune KM. CD8-positive pseudolymphoma in lues maligna and human immunodeficiency virus with monoclonal T-cell receptor-beta rearrangement. *J Cutan Pathol*. 2019;46(3):204-210.
24. Sbidian E, Battistella M, Rivet J, et al. Remission of severe CD8(+) cytotoxic T cell skin infiltrative disease in human immunodeficiency virus–infected patients receiving highly active antiretroviral therapy. *Clin Infect Dis*. 2010;51(6):741-748.
25. Ingen-Housz-Oro S, Sbidian E, Ortonne N, et al. HIV-related CD8+ cutaneous pseudolymphoma: efficacy of methotrexate. *Dermatology*. 2013;226(1):15-18.
26. de Jager M, Blokx W, Warris A, et al. Immunohistochemical features of cutaneous granulomas in primary immunodeficiency disorders: a comparison with cutaneous sarcoidosis. *J Cutan Pathol*. 2008;35(5):467-472.
27. Kempf W, Petrella T, Willemze R, et al. Clinical, histopathological and prognostic features of primary cutaneous acral CD8+ T-cell lymphoma and other dermal CD8+ cutaneous lymphoproliferations - Results of an EORTC Cutaneous Lymphoma Group Workshop. *Br J Dermatol*. 2022;186(5):887-897.

CHAPTER 22

An approach to the treatment of mycosis fungoides/Sézary syndrome and CD30 positive lymphoproliferative disorders

Pietro Quaglino, Egle Ramelyte, Andrea Roggo, Crystal Gao, Rein Willemze, Stephen Lade, and H. Miles Prince

INTRODUCTION AND BASIC PRINCIPLES

Primary cutaneous T-cell lymphomas (CTCLs) are a group of T-cell lymphomas that present in the skin with no evidence of extracutaneous disease at the time of first diagnosis.[1-3] CTCL is a rare malignancy with an incidence of <10 per 100,000 of the population per year. The diagnostic workflow to assess patients with suspected CTCL includes exploration of patient's history, clinical examination, and pathological analysis of skin and blood samples.

The World Health Organization (WHO)–European Organisation for Research and Treatment of Cancer (EORTC) classification 2018 defines subtypes of CTCL according to clinicopathological characteristics and prognosis. Mycosis fungoides (MF) is the most common subgroup and comprises about 40% of all CTCL cases.[1-3] In MF, four variants can be distinguished named classical MF, folliculotropic MF, pagetoid reticulosis, and granulomatous slack skin.[1-3] MF typically occurs in sun-protected areas of the skin building patches, plaques, or, eventually, tumors.[1-4] Staging of patients is crucial for risk and prognosis assessment and for further planning of the treatment. The staging system of MF according to the TNM system denotes to tumor-node-metastasis and classifies according to skin, lymph node, and visceral involvement.[5] A clinical presentation with plaques and patches is classified as T1 (<10% body surface) or T2 (>10% body surface). With escalating severity, patients can suffer from tumor stage disease (T3) or erythroderma (T4). Involvement of lymph nodes (N 0/1) and visceral metastasis (M0/1) are central aspects to be assessed in clinical assessment or with imaging modalities.[6] About 71.5% of patients are diagnosed in the early stage of disease with 9.7% to 11.6% risk for progression. The majority suffer from a prolonged, indolent clinical course with initial skin involvement.[1-6] Sézary syndrome (SS) is rare and accounts for 2% of all CTCL cases. SS presents with the involvement of skin, lymph nodes, and blood by a malignant T-cell clone. The disease is associated with a poor prognosis, and overall survival (OS) rates vary from 7.5 to 22.4 months.[1-6]

The treatment of MF and SS is based on a multimodal approach through the involvement of different specialists, including hematologists, dermatologists, and radiotherapists. The objectives of the treatment are to control symptoms, maintain quality of life, and improve survival by maximally reducing the tumor burden. Treatment strategies vary from "wait-and-see" to skin-directed therapies (SDTs) (eg, topical steroids, nitrogen mustard, phototherapy, radiotherapy [RT]), systemic therapies (eg, immune modifiers, antimetabolites, retinoids, epigenetic regulators, monoclonal antibodies, chemotherapy), and allogeneic hematopoietic stem cell transplantation. Although there are several well-recognized therapies for the treatment of MF/SS, there are no curative remedies and a there is a paucity of effective regimens that provide long-term responses and disease outcome control.[1-3,7-9] (Table 22-1).

The choice of therapy to be carried out is mainly based on the stage of the disease and other prognostic factors, such as the presence of folliculotropic MF or transformation into large cells. Other variables to be evaluated for therapeutic choice are the severity of symptoms (itching, ulceration of tumor nodules), the degree of response to therapies, the time and duration of the response, any side effects arising during treatment, comorbidity, and accessibility to various treatments.[9,20] Early-stage disease is mainly treated by SDTs and advanced-stage disease with systemic regimens including chemotherapy. For early-stage MF European guidelines[21] recommend SDT as first line, which includes topical corticosteroids (TCSs), chlormethine gel, phototherapy, and RT. In patients with few symptoms, a wait-and-see strategy or use of topical treatments upon discretion is not uncommon. Patients refractory to SDT may be considered for systemic options. Immune modifiers (typically bexarotene or interferon alpha) are evaluated

TABLE 22-1 Summary of MF Treatment Results From the Main Studies

Stage	No of Pts	Regimen	Study	Response Rate	Follow-Up Data
IA-IB-IIA	251	Narrowband UVB	Review[10]	87.6%; CR 62.2%	29%-80% relapses
IA-IB-IIA	527	PUVA	Review[10]	90.9%; CR 73.8%	40%-50% relapses
IB-IIIA	33	Low-dose TSET	Pooled 3 phase-II trials[11]	88%; CR 27%	Median duration clinical benefit: 70.7w
IA-IIB	98	PUVA + IFN vs Acitretin + IFN	Randomized[12]	CR 70% in PUVA + IFN vs 38% in IFN + acitretin	Shorter time to CR in PUVA + IFN
IB-IIA	93	Bexarotene + PUVA	Phase III randomized vs PUVA alone[13]	77% Bexa-PUVA vs 71% PUVA; Trend toward fewer PUVA sessions to CR in Bexa-PUVA	mDOR 9.7 mo for Bexa-PUVA vs 5.8 mo for PUVA
CD30+ve MF/pcALCL	64	Brentuximab vedotin	III randomized vs Bexarotene or MTX (ALCANZA)[14]	56.3 vs 12.5% (ORR4);	mPFS: 16.7 vs 3.5 mo
IIB, IVA, IVB	49	Pegylated liposomal doxorubicine	Prospective multicenter phase II[15]	40.8%; CR 6.1%	mTTP: 7.43 mo, mDOR: 6 mo
IB-IV MF/SS, PTCLU	32	Gemcitabine	Phase II multicenter[42]	75%; CR 22%	Median CR duration 10 mo
SS/ Erythrodermic MF	407	ECP	Review[17]	Median RR 63% (range 31%-86%); Median CR 20% (0%-62%)	mDOR 22 mo (up to 11 y)
MF/SS Ib-IV (1 previous systemic)	372	Mogamulizumab	III randomized vs Vorinostat[18]	28 vs 5%; RR in SS 37%; 68% in the blood	mPFS 7.7 vs 3.1 mo; $P < .0001$
IA-IB-IIA	260	Mechlorethamine gel vs ointment	Randomized, observer-blinded[19]	Gel vs ointment 58.5 vs 47.7% (noninferiority)	90% responses at least 10 months

CR, complete response; ECP, extracorporeal photopheresis; IFN, interferon; mDOR, median duration of response; mPFS, median progression-free survival; mTTP, median time to progression; MTX, methotrexate; pcALCL, primary cutaneous anaplastic large-cell lymphoma; PTCLU, peripheral T-cell lymphoma unspecified; PUVA, psoralen plus UVA; TSET, total skin electron therapy.

before chemotherapy. There are few randomized controlled trials in early-stage MF, and guidelines list treatments in no particular order of preference. Stage IIB disease is most frequently treated by total-skin electron-beam RT, bexarotene, and gemcitabine; erythrodermic and SS patients by extracorporeal photochemotherapy; and stage IVA2 by polychemotherapy. Chemotherapy as first treatment is associated with a higher risk of death and/or change of therapy, and thus other options should be preferable as a first treatment approach. Maintenance treatments with skin directed or systemic therapy once remission has been achieved with the aim to maintain response and prevent relapse should be always considered particularly in advanced disease.[22]

SKIN-DIRECTED THERAPIES

Topical Corticosteroids

TCSs are often prescribed for patients with early-stage MF with thin patches or plaques. Despite the frequent use of TCS, evidence for TCS from literature data is limited.[23-25]

Zackheim et al published the largest prospective study of 79 patients affected by MF stage T1 or T2 with the majority using class 1 (very potent) TCS mostly twice daily. Complete remission was achieved in 63% and partial remission in 31%, with a total response rate (RR) of 94% in the T1 group. The responses for T2 patients were 25% complete response (CR) and 57% partial response (PR) for a total RR of 82%. The duration of response is rarely prolonged and, with discontinuation of TCS therapy, only 37% of T1 patients and 18% of T2 patients remained in complete remission during a median follow-up period of 9 months.[25]

Based on limited data, the recommendation is to use high-potency TCS over less potent topical steroids. Toxicity is negligible if precautions normally associated with the use of these topical agents in chronic skin conditions are followed.

PHOTOTHERAPY

In early- or advanced-stage MF with limited skin spreading, phototherapy using either UVA or UVB is a valuable treatment option.

Ultraviolet A (UVA) rays penetrate deeper into the dermis than ultraviolet B (UVB) rays. Overall, UVA rays are more effective in treating thicker plaques and can be successful in UVB-refractory MFs. The British Association of Dermatologists recommends psoralen-UVA (PUVA) as the first-line treatment of choice for the stage of plaque MF.[10] The National Comprehensive Cancer Network (NCCN) also recommends PUVA for early or advanced MF if the plaques are thicker.[26]

When used for MF, PUVA therapy often involves prescribing 8-methoxypsoralen (MOP) administered 2 to 3 times per week, as oral administration. The doses of UVA rays are initially low (0.5 J/cm^2) and subsequently increased during each treatment, until a CR is achieved or the maximum tolerated dose is reached. A common treatment schedule includes two to four sessions per week, until the skin clears up; sessions are then reduced to once every 2 to 4 weeks for no more than 1 year. Other treatment schemes can be applied according to the United States Cutaneous Lymphoma Consortium (USCLC) guidelines.[27] High cumulative dosages of PUVA are associated with an increased risk of nonmelanocytic skin cancers, particularly squamous cell carcinoma (SCC). An increased incidence of melanoma is controversially discussed.[28] A meta-analysis showed that patients with psoriasis who had been exposed to PUVA at high doses (more than 200 treatments or more than 2000 J/cm^2) had a 14-fold higher risk of developing SCC than low-dose patients (less than 100 treatments or less than 1000 J/cm^2).[29] Given this increased risk of skin cancer, the 2015 British Association of Dermatologists and British Photodermatology Group guidelines for the safe and effective use of PUVA therapy recommend limiting cumulative exposure to 1200 J/cm^2 and/or 250 sessions.[10] According to the same guidelines, maintenance therapy should be avoided, as it is rarely effective in preventing relapse. Maintenance PUVA may be considered to prevent MF from relapsing promptly and in rare cases of refractory MF for symptomatic benefit.

Broadband ultraviolet B (290-320 nm, bbUVB) is rarely in clinical use today, as it has been replaced by narrowband UVB lamps (TL-01: 311-312 nm, nbUVB). The RRs in patients with early-stage MF treated with bbUVB and nbUVB are high and comparable; however, nbUVB has fewer side effects such as erythema. Unlike UVA, the use of UVB does not require the ingestion of psoralens. Treatment with UVB also has a lower risk of carcinogenesis than UVA. There is consensus in the literature that UVB therapy is less effective and has shorter remission durations than PUVA, particularly for thicker plaques. Nevertheless, only limited data are available in few comparative studies.[27,30]

The current practice of using guidelines for psoriasis to treat patients with MF/SS is a challenge due to the objectives of prolonging survival and preventing disease progression specific to CTCL compared with a mainly symptom-oriented therapy in psoriasis.[30] In a recent consensus-based Delphi survey among Italian centers, phototherapy was confirmed to represent the mainstay of therapy for early stage MF with extended skin involvement or for cases poorly responsive to topical steroid therapy; nbUVB should be used as a monotherapy in most cases, but PUVA, and combinations with the so-called biologic response modifiers (retinoids, IFNs), can be taken in consideration if folliculotropism or a lack of response is observed. There is consensus about the use of the treatment schedules proposed by USCLC for nbUVB and PUVA induction and consolidation phases. The consolidation phase may allow improvement in the RRs and possibly reduce the rates of early relapse, but there is not enough evidence to recommend it as conventional standard. The decision should be made based on a patient's history.[27]

Total Skin Electron Beam Therapy

Total skin electron beam therapy (TSEBT) is based on the delivery to the skin of electrons generated in a linear accelerator and attenuated to penetrate the skin to a limited depth. In this way, toxicity of the internal organs, and in particular of the bone marrow, is avoided. TSEBT can be used for patients with MF with large patches and plaques at any stage. Several retrospective studies have shown that TSEBT has one of the highest overall RRs.[27-29] A retrospective cohort study demonstrated that stage IA patients treated with TSEBT achieved a 97% CR rate. TSEBT was also effective in generalized (T2) and nodular (T3) patchy or patchy MF, as demonstrated by a 75% T2 and 47% T3 CR. For more advanced MF (T4) or SS, TSEBT can be used and combined with systemic therapies. Typically, 30 to 36 Gy is given over 8 to 10 weeks. TSEBT tends to be applied only once, but repeated treatments are often possible at lower doses without severe toxicity. Acute adverse effects are dose dependent and include local skin reactions, pain, nail loss, and anhidrosis. Long-term effects including telangiectasias, alopecia, and secondary skin cancers have been reported in patients who received multiple TSEBTs.[11,31,32]

Radiation therapy represents a fundamental part of the treatment approach, either as the sole treatment or as part of a multimodality approach. The International Lymphoma Radiation Oncology Group developed specific guidelines based on the literature review of available evidence and consensus through multinational meetings.[33]

In particular, in recent years, based on the evidence that the standard-dose (36-Gy) TSEBT is highly effective but associated with relevant skin toxicity, a new low-dose regimen of TSEBT (12 Gy) has been developed. The original data from the Stanford trials reported the clinical activity of low-dose TSEBT from the pooled analysis of three clinical trials in which patients with stage IB to IIIA MF were treated with TSEBT (12 Gy, 1 Gy per fraction over 3 weeks).

The overall RR was 88% (29/33), with 9 patients with CR. Median time to response was 7.6 weeks, and median duration of clinical benefit was 70.7 weeks. The safety profile was favorable, the treatment was well tolerated, and toxicities were mild and reversible, allowing retreatment if clinically needed.[34]

Data from the Stanford group were also confirmed by the UK group in a series of 103 patients[35] with a CR rate of 18% and a PR rate of 69%. The median response duration was 11.8 months and median progression-free survival (PFS) 13.2 months for all patients. The clinical benefit duration was longer in patients with stage IB plaque disease with respect to tumor stage. Overall, the treatment was well tolerated with lower toxicity than the standard dosages.

SYSTEMIC THERAPIES

Retinoids (Including Bexarotene)

Retinoids are derivatives of vitamin A (retinoic acid): isotretinoin, etretinate, and recently also bexarotene and alitretinoin. Retinoids have been used in the treatment of CTCL alone or in combination since the early 1980s. The drug induces apoptosis by the downregulation of survivin, an inhibitor of apoptosis.[36] In a retrospective large study from a Greek series of 128 patients, 28 (21.9%) patients received acitretin monotherapy, while 100 (78.1%) concomitantly received phototherapy ($n = 65$; 50.8%). The overall RR was 77.3%, with 44.5% complete responses. A trend toward better response was observed in the combination arm compared with patients receiving acitretin alone.[13]

Bexarotene is the only retinoid that has been specifically developed and received approval for the treatment of CTCL.[12,15,16,37,38] Oral bexarotene can be considered as first-line treatment for patients with stage 1B and higher, as monotherapy or at a reduced dose in combination with PUVA. It has an overall RR of 45%. In clinical practice, bexarotene has been used as primary systemic therapy and has also shown efficacy in patients with extracutaneous involvement. It is usually given at a daily dose of 300 mg/m^2, and treatment is continued indefinitely in patients who have a good drug response. Among the main side effects are hypothyroidism and hypertriglyceridemia. It is essential to carefully monitor the serum and thyroid parameters. Although not approved and less studied, other retinoids such as acitretin and isotretinoin are also used in clinical practice.

The EORTC 21011 was a randomized phase III study comparing combined bexarotene and PUVA versus PUVA alone in patients with MF stage IB and IIA. The study was prematurely closed due to low accrual and lack of significant difference in RR or response duration. However, in the combination arm (PUVA and bexarotene), a trend toward fewer PUVA sessions and lower UVA dose required to achieve CCR was observed, even if this did not achieve statistical significance due to insufficient power.[38]

Interferon

Interferon alpha (IFN-α) is one of the most widely used first-line treatments and arguably the most effective single-agent therapy in the treatment of CTCL. Its use should be considered in all patients with MF/SS, but tolerability can be a concern. Among the most prominent side effects of IFN-α are hypothyroidism, weight loss, anorexia, and mood changes[39]

Type 1 interferons (alpha/beta) act partly through a cell surface receptor that activates JAK/STAT signaling, and also with direct cytotoxic effects. Recent studies have shown that IFN-α can also mediate its effects through the modulation of tumor-associated M2 macrophages. The use of IFN-α in CTCL was first reported in 1984. A long-term follow-up study of IFN-α showed an initial CR rate of 41%. However, relapse was observed in 57% of patients over a mean period of 7.5 months, regardless of clinical stage.[40] IFN-α can be used in combination with other agents such as bexarotene. It has also been shown to be moderately effective in combination with PUVA and nbUVB phototherapy, while the combination with retinoids does not appear to increase RRs.

In a randomized clinical trial, comparing the association of IFN plus PUVA versus IFN plus acitretin, the results support the superiority of IFN plus PUVA. This combination induced more complete remissions in patients with CTCL stages I and II.[41]

CHEMOTHERAPY

For the treatment of non-Hodgkin's lymphoma since the 1970s, conventional single-agent chemotherapy and combination chemotherapy with the CHOP regimen (Cyclophosphamide-Hydroxydaunorubicin-Oncovin-Prednisone or Prednisolone) have been used. At the same time, a number of other combinations and single agents have been tried in CTCL with varying but generally short-lived success. Pegylated liposomal doxorubicin (PLD) and gemcitabine can be highlighted as having promising results and acceptable toxicity.[1-3,7-9]

In 2012, the EORTC Cutaneous Lymphoma Group published the results of a prospective single-arm multicenter trial investigating the activity and safety of PLD in a clearly defined patient population with advanced MF. Eligible patients had stage IIB, IVA, or IVB MF, refractory or recurrent after at least two previous systemic therapies. The primary endpoint was RR. In total, 49 patients were enrolled. The RR was 40.8% with three patients (6.1%) who experienced CR and 17 patients (34.7%) with PR. A 50% or greater reduction of cutaneous manifestations was observed in 26 (60.5%) of 43 assessable patients. Two early deaths were reported, resulting from related cardiovascular toxicity and disease progression. Grade 3 or 4 nonhematologic/nonbiochemical toxicities included cardiac symptoms (2%), allergy/hypersensitivity (2%), constitutional symptoms (4%), hand and foot reaction (2%), other dermatologic toxicity (6%), other gastrointestinal toxicity (4%), infection (4%), pulmonary embolism (2%), and cardiac ischemia (2%). Median time to progression and median duration of response were 7.4 and 6 months, respectively.[17]

Gemcitabine is a widely used treatment option for MF. However, although its activity is well documented, literature data are difficult to compare with PLD. RR range between 62% and 75% according to different reports with varying inclusion criteria.[42-44] Concerning side effects, the original report by Marchi et al[42] identified a favorable toxicity profile, whereas the French group[44] reported severe hematologic toxicities in 30% of patients, serious infection complications in 26% of patients, and other serious adverse events in 26% of patients.

Data about the clinical activity of multiagent chemotherapy do not seem to be superior to monochemotherapy in terms of RR and remission duration even if weighted by more severe side effects. One single-institution study reported a 40% RR with a median remission duration of 5.7 months in patients with CTCL treated with COP (cyclophosphamide, vincristine, and prednisone) or CHOP (cyclophosphamide, doxorubicin, vincristine, and prednisone).[45]

Extracorporeal Photochemotherapy

Extracorporeal photochemotherapy (ECP), also called photopheresis, extracorporeal photopheresis, or extracorporeal photoimmunotherapy, is a form of phototherapy in which circulating mononuclear cells are separated by a method based on leukapheresis, mixed with 8-MOP, exposed to UVA light (1-2 J/cm^2), which activates 8-MOP causing DNA crosslinking, and reinfused to the patient.

ECP was approved in 1988 by the US Food and Drug Administration for the palliative treatment of patients with CTCL and plays a very important role in the treatment of SS.[46-48] European consensus guidelines recommend ECP as a first-line treatment for MF and SS. As monotherapy, RRs to ECP are around 63% (43%-100%), with CR rates of 20%. The addition of other immunomodulatory therapies such as bexarotene, IFN-α, localized RT and TSEB, chemotherapy, or the combination of bexarotene and IFN-alpha may increase RRs in specific patients. The first improvement is usually seen after several months.

In a retrospective cohort study enrolling 98 patients from an US referral center, treated with at least 3 months of extracorporeal photopheresis and 1 or more systemic immunostimulatory agents, 30% had CR and 45% had PR.[49]

ALLOGENEIC TRANSPLANTATION

Allogeneic hematopoietic stem cell transplantation (allo-HSCT) represents the only potentially curative treatment approach in advanced-stage MF/SS. Its clinical activity is mediated through the induction of a graft-versus-lymphoma reaction.[50-53]

The report from the European Society for Blood and Marrow Transplantation in an updated series of 113 patients demonstrated that allo-HSCT induced a sustained clinical benefit in a significant percentage of cases. The 5-year OS was 38%, even if the relapse rate (5-year PFS 26%) represented the major treatment failure. Patients with advanced stage disease or disease that was refractory or that relapsed/progressed after repeated therapeutic regimens and use of an unrelated donor were less likely to achieve a clinical benefit.[50]

Similar results were reported by the Center for the International Blood and Marrow Transplant[51] (5-year PFS of 17% and OS of 32% in 129 relapsed/refractory MF/SS) and the French Society of Bone Marrow Transplantation/Study Group of Cutaneous Lymphomas (31% PFS and 57% OS at 2 years in 37 pretreated patients).[45] SS was also suggested to experience a long-term outcome benefit.[52]

Allo-HSCT can therefore be considered a valid treatment option in young patients without comorbidities and aggressive advanced relapsed CTCL. Future studies will address the challenges to find the right timing of allo-HSCT in disease course, the early identification of best candidates, and the relevance of disease control before transplant.[53]

TREATMENT IN REAL LIFE PRACTICE: MYCOSIS FUNGOIDES

International guidelines (EORTC 2017, ESMO 2018, NCCN) report treatment options for the different stages without stipulating any particular order due to the paucity of evidence from clinical trials.[21,54,55]

The treatment strategy is driven by the distinct features of early and advanced MF.[1-3,7-9,20,56] In early MF,[14,18,57-59] the decision whether to treat or not depends on patient age, lesion site, symptoms, and disease kinetics. Therapy objective is not to induce the total eradication of skin lesions but a significant clinical and health-related quality of life (QoL) improvement.[57] Real-world data on early-stage treatment showed that first-line therapy was SDT in 81.6% (topical steroids and phototherapy) or expectant policy (7.3%). A group of patients (11.1%) received first-line systemic therapy (retinoids, IFN, or combination with phototherapy), mostly in plaque stage or folliculotropic MF. The RR to first-line SDT was superior to that of systemic treatments (73% vs 57%), meaning that it is conceivable to start with an SDT even in patients with worse prognostic factors.[58]

Patients with advanced MF have an unmet clinical need of effective treatments. Current medications have a low percentage and short duration of responses, lack effective maintenance, and induce side effects in elderly patients.[56,60] In a recent retrospective international study,[19] a wide heterogeneity of treatments was found, with more than 25 different first-line modalities and 38.9% of patients receiving four or more different approaches. MF stage IIB was most frequently treated by SDTs, bexarotene, and gemcitabine; patients with erythrodermic MF/SS were treated by ECP, and those with stage IVA2 were treated by polychemotherapy. A significant impact on disease course was found for first-line therapy: chemotherapy as first treatment was associated with higher death risk and/or change of therapy and thus other therapeutic options should be preferable as a first treatment approach, such as associations of immune modulators and SDT, or the new targeted agents.

In a retrospective chart review multicenter study conducted at 27 sites in Europe, the aim was to collect data in patients who received a first course of systemic therapy and relapsed or were refractory. In the first line (n = 147), patients were treated with different therapies, including single- and multiagent chemotherapy in 67 (46%), retinoids in 39 (27%), IFN in 31 (21%), ECP in 4 (3%), and new biological agents in 3 (2%). In the second line, the use of new biologics increased slightly. Third-line therapy was often based on chemotherapy.[61]

The majority of CTCL (in particular MF) follow an indolent disease course spanning over decades. It is important to carefully evaluate treatment options to preserve potential active agents for progressive cases. A possible treatment escalation in patch/plaque MF can be the change from phototherapy to interferons, retinoids, total skin electron therapy (TSET) up to monoclonal antibodies and chemotherapy for tumor stage. In situations of response, a downgrade of treatments is warranted (eg, phototherapy to treat residual patches). In CTCLs, there is the possibility of a rechallenge with an already used treating strategy or simply retreatment with the last performed agent leading to satisfactory results.[56]

TREATMENT IN REAL LIFE PRACTICE: SÉZARY SYNDROME

SS is characterized by an aggressive disease course, and concomitant impaired immune response status caused by altered T cells. The consequent high risk of relapsing infections and the severe QoL impairment due to itching are challenges in this chronic disease.[62] The first line of treatment according to international recommendations is ECP, which is particularly effective in patients with low blood tumor burden and very useful as maintenance after remissions obtained with more aggressive therapies.[21,46-48,54,55] ECP can be applied as a single therapy or in combination with other agents (retinoids/bexarotene, IFN, TSET). Multiagent chemotherapy treatments did not lead to a significant RR but resulted in side effects and systemic toxicity. Allo-HSCT, albeit in selected patients, currently represents the only treatment available with a truly curative intention.[50-53] In recent years, mogamulizumab, a monoclonal antibody targeting CCR4, was shown to have a significant effect in patients with high blood involvement leading to a rapid decrease of circulating atypical cells.[63]

NEW DRUGS: BRENTUXIMAB VEDOTIN, MOGAMULIZUMAB, TOPICAL MECHLORETHAMINE

The ALCANZA trial[64] was an international, open-label, randomized, phase III, multicenter trial enrolling adult patients with CD30-positive MF or primary cutaneous anaplastic large-cell lymphoma who had been previously treated. Patients were randomly assigned (1:1) to receive intravenous brentuximab vedotin (BV) or physician's choice (methotrexate [MTX] or bexarotene). BV is an antibody-drug conjugate linked to an antitubulin agent specifically targeting the CD30 surface marker. This study had a new primary endpoint defined as the proportion of patients in the intention-to-treat population achieving an objective global response lasting at least 4 months (ORR4). Among a total of 128 patients analyzed in the intention-to-treat population, ORR4 was significantly higher in the brentuximab group (56.3%) with respect to the physician choice (12.5%). The most common side effect was peripheral neuropathy seen in 67% of patients treated with brentuximab. According to the subtypes of patients, the drug showed a higher activity in patients with CD30+ anaplastic large-cell lymphoma and, among MF, in patients with tumor stage.[65]

The MAVORIC trial[63] was a phase III randomized trial comparing the anti-CCR4 antibody mogamulizumab with vorinostat. Enrolled Patients with MF/SS stage IB to IV had already been treated with at least one systemic therapy. In the MAVORIC trial, patients with SS were included while large-cell transformation was excluded. The number of patients was significantly higher in the MAVORIC trial than in the ALCANZA trial (372 vs 128). The study was able to demonstrate a significant longer PFS of the mogamulizumab arm with respect to vorinostat (median 7.7 vs 3.1; $P < .0001$). Moreover, the RR was significantly higher (28% vs 5%). The median duration of responses in the blood was 25.5 months and in the skin 20.6 months, with 20% of patients developing treatment-related adverse events. A specific post hoc analysis of the patients under mogamulizumab therapy demonstrated that patients with B1 or B2 score in the blood achieved a better response with respect to skin involvement compared with patients with B0, independently from the clinical cutaneous stage. In the same cohort, a higher benefit was confirmed in terms of disease outcome.[66]

The approval of topical mechlorethamine (CL) gel in the United States, European Union, and Israel was based on the results of a phase II, randomized 201 trial, which demonstrated that CL gel (equivalent to 0.02% CL) was noninferior to CL 0.02% ointment in patients with stages I to IIA MF.[67] The RR was 58.5% for the gel and 47.7% for the ointment based on the Composite Assessment of Index Lesion Severity and 46.9% versus 46.2% by the Modified Severity-Weighted Assessment Tool. Time-to-response was shorter for mechlorethamine gel ($P < 0.01$). Approximately 20.3% of patients in the gel treatment arm and 17.3% in the ointment treatment arm had to withdraw the treatment because of drug-related skin irritation. No systemic absorption of the study medication was detected. An open-label extension phase (study 202) evaluated the efficacy and safety of CL 0.04% in patients who did not achieve a CR after the completion of 12 months of treatment. The use of an increased CL dose and longer treatment period lead to increased clinical benefit without significant increased or unexpected toxicities.[68] The PROVe study was a prospective, observational study enrolling patients treated with chlormethine gel with the objective to analyze the effect of this topical drug in combination with other therapies. The primary endpoint was the proportion of patients with stage IA-IB disease receiving chlormethine + TCSs + other with ≥50% decrease in body surface area from baseline to 12 months. A total of 298 patients were included. At 12 months, 44.4% (chlormethine + TCSs + other) and 45.1% (patients receiving chlormethine + other treatment) of patients achieved a satisfying response. A significant correlation between responder status and lower post-baseline Skindex-29 scores was found.[69]

FUTURE PERSPECTIVES

The development of future strategies for the treatment in MF/SS will be based both on the availability of new drugs and on the results of ongoing clinical trials.[70-72]

Current drug development is focusing on finding new targetable driver mutations in CTCL. The most promising agents for new systemic therapies are monoclonal antibodies, histone deacetylase inhibitors (HDACis), proteasome inhibitors, immune-checkpoint inhibitors,[66] or chimeric antigen T-cell receptor strategies.

IPH4102 is a humanized monoclonal antibody that blocks the KIR3DL receptor and subsequently induces antibody-dependent cell cytotoxicity and phagocytosis. Recently, the results of an international, open-label, phase I, multicenter study evaluating IPH4102 in relapsed/refractory CTCL was reported with promising results[73] TELLOMAK, a multicohort phase II trial is currently ongoing to confirm the activity in other subtypes of T-cell lymphomas that express KIR3DL.

Immune-checkpoint inhibitors have been successfully used in melanoma treatment. Transformed cells of advanced CTCL show an altered PD-L1 expression and increased STAT3-activation in advanced stages of the disease.[74,75] So far, few patients have been included in early phase clinical trials.[76,77] Preliminary data from an ongoing phase II study with pembrolizumab in relapsed/refractory MF and SS show promising results and an overall response rate of 33%.[77]

HDAC is target epigenetic changes in CTCL. By inducing catalyzation of acetyl groups, active gene transcription is modified. Targeted genes are involved in carcinogenesis, the cell cycle, and regulation of apoptosis. Vorinostat (suberoylanilidehydroxamic acid) and romidepsin (depsipeptide) are currently evaluated HDACis with potential efficacy in CTCL and SS. In an earlier phase II trial, vorinostat was given at a dosage of 400 mg once a day and showed an RR of 30% in patients with advanced-stage disease. The drug was well tolerated, and patients profited from fewer clinical symptoms, such as pruritus relief or decreased lymphadenopathy.[78,79]

The development of new drugs requires detailed clinical examination and standardized documentation in clinical trials. Data collected in the PROCLIPI international registry of early-stage MF are very valuable to identify needs and associations in the clinics.[18] A consensus statement for clinical endpoints and response criteria in MF and SS[80] has been recently developed by International Society of Cutaneous Lymphomas (ISCL). EORTC proposed new flow cytometry–based criteria for responses in the blood, which still need prospective verification.[81] As a treatment end point, time to next treatment (TTNT) represents the interval from initiation of one treatment to initiation of the next line of therapy and can be used as surrogate marker for duration of clinical benefit.[82] Furthermore, evaluation of quality of life could be incorporated as an endpoint in clinical trials.

As a final consideration, a different therapeutic approach could also derive from the results of laboratory research, which are suggesting a different scenario in terms of disease spreading in patients with MF and SS. Recent data, using a whole-exome sequencing approach, indeed, clearly identified the presence of multiple neoplastic circulating clones in patients with early-stage MF, which continuously replenish the skin lesions increasing their heterogeneity with a tumor seeding mechanism. These findings could support the rational basis for the clinical use of systemic treatments even in the early stage of disease. Circulating neoplastic clones could represent a potential biomarker and a promising new target for therapy.[83]

TREATMENT OF CD30+ LYMPHOPROLIFERATIVE DISORDERS

Introduction

The CD30-positive lymphoproliferative disorders (CD30+ LPDs) comprise a spectrum of diseases ranging from the relatively benign lymphomatoid papulosis (LyP) to the potentially aggressive primary cutaneous anaplastic large-cell lymphoma (C-ALCL) and also "borderline" cases. Together, these account for approximately 30% of all cases of CTCL, being the second most common form of CTCL after MF.[84]

CD30 Antigen

The CD30 antigen is a transmembrane protein belonging to the tumor necrosis receptor superfamily and serves as a diagnostic marker in the majority of patients with LyP/C-ALCL. Its ligand (CD30L) is found on the surface of immune cells (neutrophils, lymphocytes, eosinophils, monocytes, and macrophages), and interaction between CD30/CD30L can lead to downstream effects ranging from uncontrolled proliferation to enhanced apoptosis of malignant cells.

A number of studies have suggested that CD30 overexpression confers a paradoxical antiproliferative effect in CD30+ LPDs, leading to either accelerated apoptosis or a CD30/CD30L inhibition of neoplastic proliferation (Fig. 22-1); this may account for the spontaneously regressing nature of lesions, as well as a benign clinical course.[86,87]

In healthy individuals, CD30 expression is generally restricted.[88-90] However, in CD30+ LPDs, rapid proliferation of tumor cells results in the marked upregulation and overexpression of CD30, which underscores it as an ideal target for immunotherapy.

TREATMENT APPROACH

There is a wide spectrum of management options for the relatively indolent CD30+ LPDs, with choice of therapy depending on factors such as extent of disease, staging, and treatment tolerability.

For example, many patients with LyP never require therapy, and when therapy is needed, low-dose MTX is the preferred first-line treatment. In patients with C-ALCL, surgical excision (SE) and RT are commonly used for solitary lesions, with systemic therapy being reserved for those with multifocal or advanced-stage disease.

Lymphomatoid Papulosis

Lymphomatoid papulosis is defined by its clinical presentation, typically as crops of recurrent, waxing and waning papules that spontaneously regress, in conjunction with paradoxical histopathological features of CD30-positive T-cell lymphoma.[91,92] Despite the presence of morphologically and immunophenotypically abnormal lesional cells, it generally behaves in a benign manner, with a 5-year disease-specific survival rate of almost 100%.[93,94]

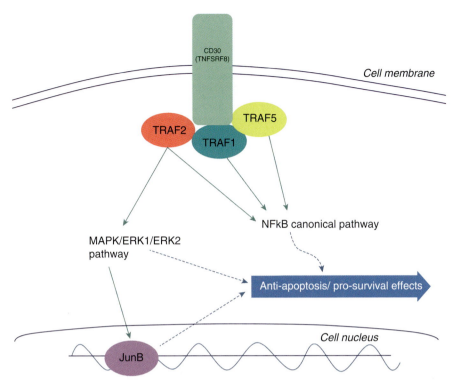

FIGURE 22-1. CD30 expression induces trimerization of tumor necrosis factor receptor–associated proteins (TRAFs), which mediate biological effects through activation of a number of downstream signaling pathways. (Reprinted by permission from Springer: from van der Weyden CA, Pileri SA, Feldman AL, Whisstock J, Prince HM. Understanding CD30 biology and therapeutic targeting: a historical perspective providing insight into future directions. *Blood Cancer J.* 2017;7:e603.)

TABLE 22-2 Malignancies Associated With LyP[96-98]

Common (>90% of Cases) https://pubmed.ncbi.nlm.nih.gov/21982062/	MF (38%-47.8%) C-ALCL (11.8%-37.2%) Hodgkin disease (8.7%-29.4%)
Uncommon (<10% of cases)	Chronic lymphocytic leukemia (5.9%) Systemic ALCL (<5%) B-cell lymphoma (<1%) Multiple myeloma (17.6%) Myelodysplastic syndrome (5.9%)

Multiple histological subtypes of LyP have been described, conventionally designated by an alphabetical lettering system. Different subtypes can occur concurrently in the same patient, either within the same crop of lesions or across different sites, in some cases likely reflecting varying histology during the usual resolution process. There are currently up to 10 recognized histological types, all characterized by strong CD30 positivity with the exception of type B, which demonstrates variable CD30 expression. *DUSP22* rearranged LyP also shows variable CD30 expression between large and small cell components, but it is not strictly considered a histological variant as it is defined by the chromosomal rearrangement. In most cases of LyP, the lesional cells are large and CD4 positive, but they may be small to medium sized and CD8 or gamma/delta positive, or CD4/CD8 double negative, and may vary markedly in number. Some cases demonstrate florid epidermotropism by atypical small to medium lymphocytes requiring distinction from either MF or aggressive cutaneous lymphoma. Other types are characterized variously by granulomatous inflammation, accumulation of intravascular tumor cells, folliculotropism, syringotropism, the presence of Reed-Sternberg-like tumor cells, or angiotropism with vascular damage. Although there is some association between histology and variations in clinical appearance, the different subtypes do not have prognostic significance. Understanding the protean nature of the pathology is therefore of interest primarily to aid recognition and to avoid misdiagnosis as an aggressive lymphoma.[95]

Up to 60% of patients with LyP develop a second neoplasm, either prior to diagnosis or during the course of the disease (Table 22-2),[99] the most common, also of T-cell lineage, MF and C-ALCL, accounting for >90% of secondary tumors in one series of 180 patients with LyP.[100] In a proportion of cases the two diseases are clonally related.[101,102]

Treatment Approach to LyP

Expectant Management—"Watch and Wait"

Given the relatively indolent nature of LyP and its naturally waxing and waning course, patients with limited lesions that are asymptomatic may not require any form of therapy.

Instead, an observant approach can be adopted, with regular monitoring until either spontaneous resolution of lesions or in the unlikely event of disease progression to more extensive disease or transformation to systemic lymphoma in 10% to 20% of patients.[94] In this setting, it is recommended that patients with LyP receive life-long follow-up given the risk of secondary malignancy, as well as the unpredictable timeline of its recurrence.[94]

Topical Agents

TCSs are often used as a first-line therapy in LyP and have been shown to offer improved disease control and hasten lesion regression.[94,103] However, recurrence is very frequent and complete remission (CR) has only been documented in up to 12% of patients.[103-106] It is often used in conjunction with other agents such as antibiotics or as an adjuvant to phototherapy.[104] The use of antibiotics has been reported, but their efficacy remains uncertain.[103,107]

Other topical therapies that have been reported for the treatment of LyP include topical nitrogen mustard,[104,108] bexarotene,[109] carmustine,[110,111] tacrolimus,[112,113] and imiquimod. However, at present there are limited data on the efficacy of these agents due to a lack of formal prospective trials.

Phototherapy

Another common treatment for LyP is phototherapy, in the form of PUVA or nbUVB. This is well tolerated, with an RR of up to 68% in patients treated with PUVA,[112,114-116] and PRs in 85.7% of patients treated with UVB.[104,117,118] Relapses are again common and occur shortly after cessation of treatment, with a time to relapse between 1 and 20 months.[119] Exposure to sunlight, with or without adjuvant agents such as topical steroids, was also demonstrated to be effective particularly in the pediatric population, with improvement in up to 57% in children.[94,118]

Chemotherapy

Monotherapy with low-dose MTX is the most widely utilized form of chemotherapy in patients with LyP.[94,120] The dosage varies depending on institutional protocols, ranging from 5 to 60 mg/wk, with oral administration of 20 to 30 mg/wk the most commonly used dosing regimen.[108,121] It is generally well tolerated, with mild side effects reported in up to 77% of patients. Hepatic fibrosis can occur, but generally only in a small proportion of patients who undergo long-term (>3 years) treatment.[94]

An early study by Vonderheid et al reported on 40 patients with LyP treated with 15 to 25 mg subcutaneous MTX weekly.[108] CR was achieved in 44% of patients, with a further 42% demonstrating minimal disease burden during treatment.[108] Following cessation of MTX, relapse occurred in 75% of patients over a follow-up period of 24 to 227 months.

A subsequent study by Newland et al demonstrated similar efficacy of low-dose MTX in a cohort of 53 patients with LyP, 25 of whom were treated with the regimen of 20 to 30 mg oral MTX weekly for a minimum of 6 months.[122] Of these, 44% of patients achieved CR, and a further 44% achieved a PR. Again, only a small proportion (24%) were successfully weaned from MTX, with 64% of patients remaining dependent on low-dose therapy (5-10 mg/wk). This demonstrates that, although MTX provides effective disease control, relapses are common and often occur shortly after cessation of treatment. Hence, the majority of patients require long-term maintenance therapy over months to years.[94,123,124]

MTX can be used repeatedly at subsequent relapse, and a relapse should not imply the need to switch to a second-line agent. Although a number of multiagent chemotherapy regimens have been trialed in LyP, none has been able to demonstrate prolonged disease control. In addition, multimodal chemotherapy often has extensive side effects. Hence, aggressive systemic therapy is not recommended in patients with LyP.

Other Treatment Options

Limited data are available on other treatment options such as immunomodulatory agents, antibiotics, and oral steroids. Varied responses have been seen with interferon alfa (IFN-α), retinoids, oral bexarotene, nicotinamide, and imiquimod, again with high rates of disease relapse within 3 to 4 weeks of treatment cessation.[94,125] Oral steroids were ineffective in all five reported cases.[103]

In a phase II trial by Duvic et al, the antibody drug conjugate BV demonstrated promising results in the treatment of LyP, with an overall RR of 100%. However, despite achieving rapid disease control upon commencement of BV, relapses were again common, with a median response duration of 26 weeks (range 6-44 weeks).[126] Thus, at present, BV would only be indicated for the very rare patient with extensive, refractory LyP requiring systemic therapy.

RT has been utilized, although there is no standardized technique or protocol available, and its efficacy is still widely debated.[127]

Although not commonly performed, SE can also be utilized for larger LyP lesions that more closely resemble nodular C-ALCL. This appears to be curative in the short term, although little data are available on the rate of recurrence.[128,129]

RECOMMENDATIONS IN THE TREATMENT OF LYP

1. Given its benign disease course and high rate of recurrence despite treatment, a "watch-and-wait" approach can be adopted for patients with asymptomatic disease.
2. Low-dose MTX monotherapy is a suitable first-line treatment option that is well tolerated; however, the majority of patients will require maintenance therapy as risk of relapse after cessation is high.
3. MTX can be used repeatedly at subsequent relapse, and a relapse should not imply the need to switch to a second-line agent.
4. Topical steroids can be given in conjunction with other treatments, for example, low-dose MTX, in order to hasten resolution of lesions and reduce disease burden.
5. In patients with larger/solitary lesions, RT or SE may be considered; in these cases, progression to C-ALCL should be investigated.
6. The histological subtype does not generally affect treatment strategy or outcome.
7. Up to as many as 60% of patients (more conservatively 4%-25%) may develop a second lymphoid neoplasm, even up to decades after the initial manifestation and resolution of LyP lesions. Therefore, the presence of

coexistent lymphomas (most commonly MF) should be investigated and treated accordingly.
8. It is recommended that patients with LyP receive lifelong follow-up due to the increased risk of further lymphoid neoplasms.

Primary Cutaneous Anaplastic Large-Cell Lymphoma

Primary cutaneous ALCL is defined as a skin-limited disease composed of large CD30-positive anaplastic cells. It accounts for ~9% of all CTCLs and tends to offer a better prognosis than its systemic counterpart.[2,130]

Clinically, C-ALCL tends to present with a solitary, fast-growing nodule usually on the trunk, face, or extremities (Fig. 22-2).[131] Multifocal C-ALCL is uncommon, occurring in approximately 20% of cases; although it is not thought to have a significant impact on disease prognosis, it has been found to be associated with a greater risk of progression to extracutaneous disease.[132,133]

Risk of Progression to Extranodal Disease

The risk of progression of C-ALCL to nodal or visceral disease has not been extensively studied to date. A cohort of 48 patients with C-ALCL at our Institution (Peter MacCallum Cancer Centre, Melbourne, Australia) were studied recently, a proportion of whom went on to develop nodal and visceral involvement.[134] The median age at diagnosis was 58 years, and 16% (7/48) of these patients progressed to nodal disease, representing an 8% risk of progression at 12 months (Fig. 22-3) and the median OS had not yet been reached. This is a very similar rate of progression observed in a Dutch series where they found a 12% progression to extracutaneous disease.[135] Importantly, we found that the risk of progression to nodal disease appeared to plateau after 8 years but once nodal involvement had occurred there was a very high risk of further progression to visceral disease within the next 24 months; three patients went on to develop organ involvement, representing a progression risk of 28.6% at 12 months ($P = .0031$).

The most common treatments for patients with C-ALCL with nodal disease in our cohort was localized RT and anthracycline-based chemotherapy. Of note, none of this patient group with extracutaneous ALCL received BV, due to lack of availability in Australia at that time. All three patients with subsequent visceral disease went on to receive allogeneic stem cell transplants, which appeared to be consistent with the treatment approach described in the Dutch series.[135]

Treatment Approach to C-ALCL

Treatment of C-ALCL is dependent upon extent of disease, that is, whether lesions

 i. are solitary (unifocal) vs multifocal;
 ii. have nodal involvement;
 iii. have visceral involvement;
 iv. are de novo or relapsed.

Surgical Excision

SE is a frequently utilized first-line therapy and is generally performed with curative intent.[94] There has been no standardized consensus with regards to margin of excision. So far, available studies have demonstrated a very favorable outcome. The relapse rate has been reported as 29% to 43% following SE alone, with time to relapse ranging from 2 to 76 months.[94,136]

Radiotherapy

RT is another key treatment strategy in C-ALCL.[137] Although there is no international consensus for radiation dosing for C-ALCL, doses ranging from 6 to 50 Gy have been reported.[137,138] Currently, the National Cancer Center Network recommends a minimal dose of 30 Gy; however, Million et al have reported that doses as low as 6 Gy can achieve CR, suggesting that a lower dose of radiation can be applied in some cases.[94,137,139] Some patients also undergo RT as an adjuvant to SE, and in these small studies high CR rates are reported.[94,136,140]

Chemotherapy

While localized therapies such as SE and RT are first line for patients with solitary or grouped lesions, those with more widespread disease may require more extensive treatment.

Low-dose MTX has become a treatment of choice for those with more extensive disease, although it demonstrates lesser efficacy than in LyP.[140] The modest efficacy of MTX was demonstrated in the ALCANZA study, a phase III trial comparing the efficacy of BV to physician's choice of either MTX or bexarotene; patients treated with physician's choice had an RR of only 12.5% with a short PFS of only 3.5 months.[64]

Other systemic agents that have been used in C-ALCL include imiquimod, etoposide, gemcitabine, and interferon-α and multiagent chemotherapy (see below).[94,141-143]

Previously, multiagent chemotherapy was recommended in those with multifocal disease. Various regimens were utilized, with CHOP (cyclophosphamide, doxorubicin, vincristine, and prednisolone) being the most common and yielding a CR rate of 85%. The overall CR rate of initial treatment with multiagent chemotherapy was 92%, although relapses

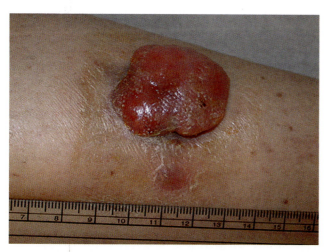

FIGURE 22-2. Primary cutaneous ALCL often presents as a solitary, fast-growing nodule. (Reprinted from Kempf W, Pfaltz K, Vermeer MH, et al. EORTC, ISCL, and USCLC consensus recommendations for the treatment of primary cutaneous CD30-positive lymphoproliferative disorders: lymphomatoid papulosis and primary cutaneous anaplastic large-cell lymphoma. *Blood.* 2011;118(15):4024-4035, with permission from Elsevier.)

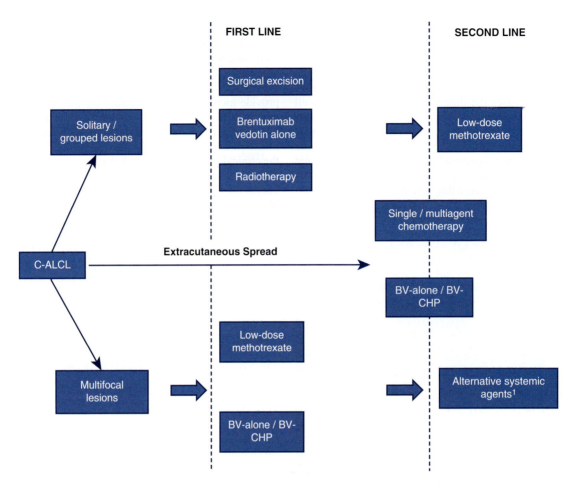

1. Other systemic agents include: isotretinoin; bexarotene; IFN-α; thalidomide; allogeneic stem cell transplant

FIGURE 22-6. The treatment algorithm for patients with C-ALCL is dependent upon disease burden and distribution of lesion.

RECOMMENDATIONS IN THE TREATMENT OF C-ALCL

1. Treatment for C-ALCL is guided by disease burden, that is, solitary/grouped lesions versus multifocal disease.
2. First-line treatment for localized C-ALCL is generally SE and/or RT.
3. In patients with multifocal disease, RT or low-dose MTX should be the initial approach.
4. Multiagent chemotherapy is no longer the treatment of choice for multifocal cutaneous-only disease and should only be used in cases of C-ALCL that is resistant to other treatment modalities or has extracutaneous spread.
5. BV has demonstrated significant efficacy in CD30+ LPDs and is generally well tolerated. It is the recommended single-agent therapy for patients with relapsed cutaneous-only C-ALCL.
6. Cutaneous-only C-ALCL progresses to nodal disease in about 12% to 16% of cases, but once nodal disease occurs, the risk of visceral progression is much higher, thus close monitoring for visceral and further nodal progression is required in patients who develop nodal C-ALCL.
7. For patients with nodal/visceral C-ALCL, treatment choices are BV alone or combined with multiagent therapy such as A-CHP.
8. Where cases of C-ALCL may be clinically atypical, careful clinicopathological correlation is required to distinguish from the much more aggressive CD30+ large-cell transformation of MF as patients with CD30+ LCT-MF demonstrate significantly poorer outcomes.

References

1. Willemze R, Kerl H, Sterry W, et al. EORTC classification for primary cutaneous lymphomas: a proposal from the cutaneous lymphoma study group of the European organization for research and treatment of cancer. *Blood*. 1997;90(1):354-371.
2. Willemze R, Jaffe ES, Burg G, et al. WHO-EORTC classification for cutaneous lymphomas. *Blood*. 2005;105(10):3768-3785.
3. Willemze R, Cerroni L, Kempf W, et al. The 2018 update of the WHO-EORTC classification for primary cutaneous lymphomas. *Blood*. 2019;133(16):1703.
4. Bobrowicz M, Fassnacht C, Ignatova D, Chang YT, Dimitriou F, Guenova E. Pathogenesis and therapy of primary cutaneous T-cell lymphoma: Collegium Internationale Allergologicum (CIA) update 2020. *Int Arch Allergy Immunol*. 2020;181(10):733-745.

5. Ahn CS, ALSayyah A, Sangüeza OP. Mycosis fungoides: an updated review of clinicopathologic variants. *Am J Dermatopathol.* 2014;36(12):933-951.
6. Wilcox RA. Cutaneous T-cell lymphoma: 2017 update on diagnosis, risk-stratification, and management. *Am J Hematol.* 2017;92:1085-1102.doi:10.1002/ajh.24876
7. Pulitzer M. Cutaneous T-cell lymphoma. *Clin Lab Med.* 2017;37(3):527-546. doi:10.1016/j.cll.2017.06.006
8. Larocca C, Kupper T. Mycosis fungoides and Sézary syndrome: an update. *Hematol Oncol Clin N Am.* 2019;33(1):103-120. doi:10.1016/j.hoc.2018.09.001
9. Horwitz SM, Olsen EA, Duvic M, Porcu P, Kim YH. Review of the treatment of mycosis fungoides and Sézary syndrome: a stage-based approach. *J Natl Compr Cancer Netw.* 2008;6(4):436-442.
10. Ling TC, Clayton TH, Crawley J, et al. British Association of Dermatologists and British Photodermatology Group guidelines for the safe and effective use of psoralen-ultraviolet A therapy 2015. *Br J Dermatol.* 2016;174(1):24-55. doi:10.1111/bjd.14317
11. Elsayad K, Susek KH, Eich HT. Total skin electron beam therapy as part of multimodal treatment strategies for primary cutaneous T-cell lymphoma. *Oncol Res Treat.* 2017;40(5):244-252. doi:10.1159/000475634
12. VäkEVä L, Annamari R, Hahtola S. Ten-year experience of bexarotene therapy for cutaneous T-cell lymphoma in Finland. *Acta Derm Venereol.* 2012;92(3):258-263.
13. Nikolaou V, Patsatsi A, Sidiropoulou P, et al. Monotherapy and combination therapy with acitretin for mycosis fungoides: results of a retrospective, multicentre study. *J Eur Acad Dermatol Venereol.* 2020;34(11):2534-2540.
14. Hodak E, Sherman S, Papadavid E, et al. Should we be imaging lymph nodes at initial diagnosis of early-stage mycosis fungoides? Results from the PROspective Cutaneous Lymphoma International Prognostic Index (PROCLIPI) international study. *Br J Dermatol.* 2021;184(3):524-553.
15. Abbott RA, Whittaker SJ, Morris SL, et al. Bexarotene therapy for mycosis fungoides and Sézary syndrome. *Br J Dermatol.* 2009;160(6):1299-1307.
16. Talpur R, Ward S, Apisarnthanarax R, et al. Optimizing bexarotene therapy for cutaneous T-cell lymphoma. *J Am Acad Dermatol.* 2002;47(5):672-684. doi:10.1067/mjd.2002.124607
17. Dummer R, Quaglino P, Becker JC, et al. Prospective international multicenter phase II trial of intravenous pegylated liposomal doxorubicin monochemotherapy in patients with stage IIB, IVA, or IVB advanced mycosis fungoides: final results from EORTC 21012. *J Clin Oncol.* 2012;30(33):4091-4097.
18. Scarisbrick JJ, Quaglino P, Prince HM, et al. The PROCLIPI international registry of early-stage mycosis fungoides identifies substantial diagnostic delay in most patients. *Br J Dermatol.* 2019;181(2):350-357.
19. Quaglino P, Maule M, Prince HM, et al. Global patterns of care in advanced stage mycosis fungoides/Sezary syndrome: a multicenter retrospective follow-up study from the Cutaneous Lymphoma International Consortium. *Ann Oncol.* 2017;28(10):2517-2525.
20. Scarisbrick JJ, Kim YH, Whittaker SJ, et al. Prognostic factors, prognostic indices and staging in mycosis fungoides and Sézary syndrome: where are we now? *Br J Dermatol.* 2014;170(6):1226-1236.
21. Trautinger F, Eder J, Assaf C, et al. European Organisation for Research and Treatment of Cancer consensus recommendations for the treatment of mycosis fungoides/Sézary syndrome - update 2017. *Eur J Cancer.* 2017;77:57-74. doi:10.1016/j.ejca.2017.02.027
22. Zinzani PL, Quaglino P, Violetti SA, et al. Critical concepts and management recommendations for cutaneous T-cell lymphoma: a consensus-based position paper from the Italian Group of Cutaneous Lymphoma. *Hematol Oncol.* 2021;39(3):275-283.
23. Lovgren ML, Scarisbrick JJ. Update on skin directed therapies in mycosis fungoides. *Chin Clin Oncol.* 2019;8(1):7. doi:10.21037/cco.2018.11.03
24. Nguyen CV, Bohjanen KA. Skin-directed therapies in cutaneous T-cell lymphoma. *Dermatol Clin.* 2015;33(4):683-696. doi:10.1016/j.det.2015.05
25. Zackheim HS, Kashani-Sabet M, Amin S. Topical corticosteroids for mycosis fungoides. Experience in 79 patients. *Arch Dermatol.* 1998;134(8):949-954.
26. Horwitz SM, Ansell SM, Ai WZ, et al. NCCN guidelines Insights: T-cell lymphomas, version 2.2018. *J Natl Compr Cancer Netw.* 2018;16(2):123-135. doi:10.6004/jnccn.2018.0007
27. Grandi V, Baldo A, Berti E, et al. Italian expert-based recommendations on the use of photo(chemo)therapy in the management of mycosis fungoides: results of an e-Delphi consensus. *Photodermatol Photoimmunol Photomed.* 2021;37(4):334-342.
28. Nijsten TEC, Stern RS. The increased risk of skin cancer is persistent after discontinuation of psoralen+ultraviolet A: a cohort study. *J Invest Dermatol.* 2003;121(2):252-258. doi:10.1046/j.1523-1747.2003.12350.x
29. Stern RS, Lunder EJ. Risk of squamous cell carcinoma and methoxsalen (psoralen) and UV-A radiation (PUVA). A meta-analysis. *Arch Dermatol.* 1998;134:121582-121585. doi:10.1001/archderm.134.12.1582
30. Olsen EA, Hodak E, Anderson T, et al. Guidelines for phototherapy of mycosis fungoides and Sézary syndrome: a consensus statement of the United States Cutaneous Lymphoma Consortium. *J Am Acad Dermatol.* 2016;74(1):27-58. doi:10.1016/j.jaad.2015.09.033
31. Chowdhary M., Chhabra A.M, Kharod S., Marwaha G. Total skin electron beam therapy in the treatment of mycosis fungoides: a review of conventional and low-dose regimens. *Clin Lymphoma Myeloma Leuk.* December 2016;16(12):662-671. doi:10.1016/j.clml.2016.08.019.
32. Lindahl LM, Kamstrup MR, Petersen PM, et al. Total skin electron beam therapy for cutaneous T-cell lymphoma: a nationwide cohort study from Denmark. *Acta Oncol.* November 2011;50(8):1199-1205.
33. Specht L, Dabaja B, Illidge T, Wilson LD, Hoppe RT, International Lymphoma Radiation Oncology Group. Modern radiation therapy for primary cutaneous lymphomas: field and dose guidelines from the International Lymphoma Radiation Oncology Group. *Int J Radiat Oncol Biol Phys.* May 1, 2015;92(1):32-39.
34. Hoppe RT, Harrison C, Tavallaee M, et al. Low-dose total skin electron beam therapy as an effective modality to reduce disease burden in patients with mycosis fungoides: results of a pooled analysis from 3 phase-II clinical trials. *J Am Acad Dermatol.* February 2015;72(2):286-292.

35. Morris S, Scarisbrick J, Frew J, et al. The results of low-dose total skin electron beam radiation therapy (TSEB) in patients with mycosis fungoides from the UK cutaneous lymphoma group. *Int J Radiat Oncol Biol Phys*. November 1, 2017;99(3):627-633.
36. Zhang C, Duvic M. Retinoids: therapeutic applications and mechanisms of action in cutaneous T-cell lymphoma. *Dermatol Ther*. 2003;16(4):322-330.
37. Duvic M, Hymes K, Heald P, et al. Bexarotene is effective and safe for treatment of refractory advanced-stage cutaneous T-cell lymphoma: multinational phase II-III trial results. *J Clin Oncol*. 2001;19(9):2456-2471.
38. Whittaker S, Ortiz P, Dummer R, et al. Efficacy and safety of bexarotene combined with psoralen-ultraviolet A (PUVA) compared with PUVA treatment alone in stage IB-IIA mycosis fungoides: final results from the EORTC Cutaneous Lymphoma Task Force phase III randomized clinical trial (NCT00056056). *Br J Dermatol*. September 2012;167(3):678-687.
39. Spaccarelli N, Rook AH. The Use of interferons in the treatment of cutaneous T-cell lymphoma. *Dermatol Clin*. October 2015;33(4):731-745. Epub 2015 Aug 20. doi:10.1016/j.det.2015.05.008.
40. Jumbou O, N'Guyen JM, Tessier MH, Legoux B, Dréno B. Long-term follow-up in 51 patients with mycosis fungoides and Sézary syndrome treated by interferon-alfa. *Br J Dermatol*. 1999;140(3):427-431. doi:10.1046/j.1365-2133.1999.02704.x.
41. Stadler R, Otte HG, Luger T, et al. Prospective randomized multicenter clinical trial on the use of interferon -2a plus acitretin versus interferon-2a plus PUVA in patients with cutaneous T-cell lymphoma stages I and II. *Blood*. November 15, 1998;92(10):3578-3581.
42. Marchi E, Alinari L, Tani M, et al. Gemcitabine as frontline treatment for cutaneous T-cell lymphoma: phase II study of 32 patients. *Cancer*. 2005;104:2437-2441.
43. Duvic M, Talpur R, Wen S, et al. Phase II evaluation of gemcitabine monotherapy for cutaneous T-cell lymphoma. *Clin Lymphoma Myeloma*. 2006;7:51-58.
44. Jidar K, Ingen-Housz-Oro S, Beylot-Barry M, et al. Gemcitabine treatment in cutaneous T-cell lymphoma: a multicentre study of 23 cases. *Br J Dermatol*. 2009;161:660-663.
45. Fierro MT, Quaglino P, Savoia P, et al. Systemic polychemotherapy in the treatment of primary cutaneous lymphomas: a clinical follow-up study of 81 patients treated with COP or CHOP. *Leuk Lymphoma*. 1998;31:583-588.
46. Knobler R, Arenberger P, Arun A, et al. European dermatology forum - updated guidelines on the use of extracorporeal photopheresis 2020 - part 1. *J Eur Acad Dermatol Venereol*. 2020;34(12):2693-2716.
47. Quaglino P, Knobler R, Fierro MT, et al. Extracorporeal photopheresis for the treatment of erythrodermic cutaneous T-cell lymphoma: a single center clinical experience with long-term follow-up data and a brief overview of the literature. *Int J Dermatol*. 2013;52(11):1308-1318. doi:10.1111/ijd.12121
48. Sanyal S, Child F, Alfred A, et al. National audit of extracorporeal photopheresis in cutaneous T-cell lymphoma. *Br J Dermatol*. 2018;178(2):569-570.
49. Raphael BA, Shin DB, Suchin KR, et al. High clinical response rate of Sezary syndrome to immunomodulatory therapies: prognostic markers of response. *Arch Dermatol*. 2011;147(12):1410-1415. doi:10.1001/archdermatol.2011.232
50. Domingo-Domenech E, Duarte RF, Boumedil A, et al. Allogeneic hematopoietic stem cell transplantation for advanced mycosis fungoides and Sezary syndrome. An updated experience of the Lymphoma Working Party of the European Society for Blood and Marrow Transplantation. *Bone Marrow Transplant*. 2021;56(6):1391-1401.
51. Lechowicz MJ, Lazarus HM, Carreras J, et al. Allogeneic hematopoietic cell transplantation for mycosis fungoides and Sezary syndrome. *Bone Marrow Transplant*. 2014;49(11):1360-1365.
52. de Masson A, Beylot-Barry M, Bouaziz JD, et al. Allogeneic stem cell transplantation for advanced cutaneous T-cell lymphomas: a study from the French Society of bone marrow transplantation and French study group on cutaneous lymphomas. *Haematologica*. 2014;99(3):527-534.
53. Dumont M, Peffault de Latour R, Ram-Wolff C, Bagot M, de Masson A. Allogeneic hematopoietic stem cell transplantation in cutaneous T-cell lymphomas. *Cancers*. 2020;12(10).
54. Mehta-Shah N, Horwitz SM, Ansell S, et al. NCCN guidelines Insights: primary cutaneous lymphomas, version 2.2020. *J Natl Compr Canc Netw*. 2020;18(5):522-536.
55. Willemze R, Hodak E, Zinzani PL, Specht L, Ladetto M, Committee EG. Primary cutaneous lymphomas: ESMO Clinical Practice Guidelines for diagnosis, treatment and follow-up. *Ann Oncol*. 2018;29(suppl 4):iv30-iv40.
56. Dummer R, Vermeer MH, Scarisbrick JJ, et al. Cutaneous T cell lymphoma. *Nat Rev Dis Primers*. 2021;7(1):61. doi:10.1038/s41572-021-00296-9
57. Molloy K, Jonak C, Woei AJF, et al. Characteristics associated with significantly worse quality of life in mycosis fungoides/Sezary syndrome from the Prospective Cutaneous Lymphoma International Prognostic Index (PROCLIPI) study. *Br J Dermatol*. 2020;182(3):770-779.
58. Quaglino P, Prince HM, Cowan R, et al. Treatment of early-stage mycosis fungoides: results from the PROspective Cutaneous Lymphoma International Study (PROCLIPI study). *Br J Dermatol*. 2021;184(4):722-730.
59. Scarisbrick JJ, Quaglino P, Prince HM, Kim YH, Willemze R, investigators P. Ethnicity in mycosis fungoides: white patients present at an older age and with more advanced disease. *Br J Dermatol*. 2019;180(5):1264-1265.
60. Stadler R, Scarisbrick JJ. Maintenance therapy in patients with mycosis fungoides or Sezary syndrome: a neglected topic. *Eur J Cancer*. 2021;142:38-47.
61. Assaf C, Waser N, Bagot M, et al. Contemporary treatment patterns and response in relapsed/refractory cutaneous T-cell lymphoma (CTCL) across five European Countries. *Cancers*. 2021;14(1):145.
62. Olsen EA, Rook AH, Zic J, et al. Sezary syndrome: immunopathogenesis, literature review of therapeutic options, and recommendations for therapy by the United States Cutaneous Lymphoma Consortium (USCLC). *J Am Acad Dermatol*. 2011;64(2):352-404.
63. Kim YH, Bagot M, Pinter-Brown L, et al. Mogamulizumab versus vorinostat in previously treated cutaneous T-cell lymphoma (MAVORIC): an international, open-label, randomised, controlled phase 3 trial. *Lancet Oncol*. 2018;19(9):1192-1204.
64. Prince HM, Kim YH, Horwitz SM, et al. Brentuximab vedotin or physician's choice in CD30-positive cutaneous T-cell lymphoma (ALCANZA): an international, open-label, randomised, phase 3, multicentre trial. *Lancet*. 2017;390(10094):555-566.

65. Kim YH, Prince HM, Whittaker S, et al. Dummer RResponse to brentuximab vedotin versus physician's choice by CD30 expression and large cell transformation status in patients with mycosis fungoides: an ALCANZA sub-analysis. *Eur J Cancer*. 2021;148:411-421.
66. Cowan RA, Scarisbrick JJ, Zinzani PL, et al. Efficacy and safety of mogamulizumab by patient baseline blood tumour burden: a post hoc analysis of the MAVORIC trial. *J Eur Acad Dermatol Venereol*. 2021;35(11):2225-2238.
67. Lessin SR, Duvic M, Guitart J, et al. Topical chemotherapy incutaneous T-cell lymphoma: positive results of a randomized, controlled, multicenter trial testing the efficacy and safety of anovel mechlorethamine, 0.02%, gel in mycosis fungoides. *JAMA Dermatol*. 2013;149(1):25-32.
68. Querfeld C, Kim YH, Guitart J, Scarisbrick J, Quaglino P. Use of chlormethine 0.04% gel for mycosis fungoides after treatment with topical chlormethine 0.02% gel: a phase 2 extension study. *J Am Acad Dermatol*. 2021;30. S0190-9622(21)02194-0
69. Kim EJ, Guitart J, Querfeld C, et al. The PROVe study: US real-world experience with chlormethine/mechlorethamine gel in combination with other therapies for patients with mycosis fungoides cutaneous T-cell lymphoma. *Am J Clin Dermatol*. 2021;22(3):407-414.
70. Cristofoletti C, Narducci MG, Russo G. Sezary syndrome, recent biomarkers and new drugs. *Chin Clin Oncol*. 2019;8(1):2.
71. Quaglino P, Fava P, Pileri A, et al. Phenotypical markers, molecular mutations, and immune microenvironment as targets for new treatments in patients with mycosis fungoides and/or Sezary syndrome. *J Invest Dermatol*. 2021;141(3):484-495.
72. Ramelyte E, Dummer R, Guenova E. Investigative drugs for the treatment of cutaneous T-cell lymphomas (CTCL): an update. *Expert Opin Investig Drugs*. 2019;28(9):799-809.
73. Bagot M, Porcu P, Marie-Cardine A, et al. IPH4102, a first-in-class anti-KIR3DL2 monoclonal antibody, in patients with relapsed or refractory cutaneous T-cell lymphoma: an international, first-in-human, open-label, phase 1 trial. *Lancet Oncol*. 2019;20(8):1160-1170. doi:10.1016/S1470-2045(19)30320-1
74. Munir S, Andersen G, Woetmann A, et al. Cutaneous T cell lymphoma cells are targets for immune checkpoint ligand PD-L1-specific, cytotoxic T cells. *Leukemia*. 2013;27:2251-2253. doi:10.1038/leu.2013.118
75. Klemke CD, Booken N, Weiss C, et al. Histopathological and immunophenotypical criteria for the diagnosis of Sezary syndrome in differentiation from other erythrodermic skin diseases: a European Organisation for research and treatment of cancer (EORTC) cutaneous lymphoma task force study of 97 cases. *Br J Dermatol*. 2015;173(1):93-105.
76. Roccuzzo G, Giordano S, Fava P, et al. Immune check point inhibitors in primary cutaneous T-cell lymphomas: biologic Rationale, clinical results and future perspectives. *Front Oncol*. 2021;11:733770. doi:10.3389/fonc.2021.733770
77. Khodadoust MS, Rook AH, Porcu P, et al. Pembrolizumab in relapsed and refractory mycosis fungoides and Sezary syndrome: a multicenter phase II study. *J Clin Oncol*. 2020;38(1):20-28.
78. Olsen EA, Kim YH, Kuzel TM, et al. Phase IIb multicenter trial of vorinostat in patients with persistent, progressive, or treatment refractory cutaneous T-cell lymphoma. *J Clin Oncol*. 2007;25(21):3109-3115.
79. Whittaker SJ, Demierre MF, Kim EJ, et al. Final results from a multicenter, international, pivotal study of romidepsin in refractory cutaneous T-cell lymphoma. *J Clin Oncol*. 2010;28(29):4485-4491.
80. Olsen EA, Whittaker S, Willemze R, et al. Primary cutaneous lymphoma: recommendations for clinical trial design and staging update from the ISCL, USCLC, and EORTC. *Blood*. 2021. blood.2021012057. doi:10.1182/blood.2021012057
81. Scarisbrick JJ, Hodak E, Bagot M, et al. Blood classification and blood response criteria in mycosis fungoides and Sezary syndrome using flow cytometry: recommendations from the EORTC cutaneous lymphoma task force. *Eur J Cancer*. 2018;93:47-56. doi:10.1016/j.ejca.2018.01.076
82. Campbell BA, Scarisbrick JJ, Kim YH, Wilcox RA, McCormack C, Prince HM. Time to next treatment as a meaningful endpoint for trials of primary cutaneous lymphoma. *Cancers*. 2020;12(8):2311. doi:10.3390/cancers12082311
83. Iyer A, Hennessey D, O'Keefe S, et al. Skin colonization by circulating neoplastic clones in cutaneous T-cell lymphoma. *Blood*. 2019;134(18):1517-1527. doi:10.1182/blood.2019002516
84. Swerdlow SH, Campo E, Pileri SA, et al. The 2016 revision of the World Health Organization classification of lymphoid neoplasms. *Blood*. 2016;127(20):2375-2390.
85. van der Weyden CA, Pileri SA, Feldman AL, Whisstock J, Prince HM. Understanding CD30 biology and therapeutic targeting: a historical perspective providing insight into future directions. *Blood Cancer J*. 2017;7:e603.
86. Gruss H, Boiani N, Williams D, Armitage R, Smith C, Goodwin R. Pleiotropic effects of the CD30 ligand on CD30-expressing cells and lymphoma cell lines. *Blood*. 1994;83(8):2045-2056.
87. Mori M, Manuelli C, Pimpinelli N, et al. CD30-CD30 ligand interaction in primary cutaneous CD30+ T-cell lymphomas: a clue to the pathophysiology of clinical regression. *Blood*. 1999;94(9):3077-3083.
88. Piris M, Brown DC, Gatter KC, Mason DY. CD30 expression in non-Hodgkin's lymphoma. *Histopathology*. 1990;17(3):211-218.
89. De Bruin PC. CD30 expression in normal and neoplastic lymphoid tissue: biological aspects and clinical implications. *Leukemia*. 1995;9:1620.
90. Del Prete G, De Carli M, D'Elios MM, et al. CD30-mediated signaling promotes the development of human T helper type 2-like T cells. *J Exp Med*. 1995;182(6):1655-1661.
91. Macaulay WL. Lymphomatoid papulosis: a continuing self-healing eruption, clinically benign—histologically malignant. *Arch Dermatol*. 1968;97(1):23-30.
92. Kunishige JH, McDonald H, Alvarez G, Johnson M, Prieto V, Duvic M. Lymphomatoid papulosis and associated lymphomas: a retrospective case series of 84 patients. *Clin Exp Dermatol*. 2009;34(5):576-581.
93. Campo E, Swerdlow SH, Harris NL, Pileri S, Stein H, Jaffe ES. The 2008 WHO classification of lymphoid neoplasms and beyond: evolving concepts and practical applications. *Blood*. 2011;117(19):5019-5032.
94. Kempf W, Pfaltz K, Vermeer MH, et al. EORTC, ISCL, and USCLC consensus recommendations for the treatment of primary cutaneous CD30-positive lymphoproliferative disorders: lymphomatoid papulosis and primary cutaneous anaplastic large-cell lymphoma. *Blood*. 2011;118(15):4024-4035.
95. Karai LJ, Kadin ME, Hsi ED, et al. Chromosomal rearrangements of 6p25.3 define a new subtype of lymphomatoid papulosis. *Am J Surg Pathol*. 2013;37(8):1173-1181.
96. de Souza A, el-Azhary RA, Camilleri MJ, Wada DA, Appert DL, Gibson LE. In search of prognostic indicators for lymphomatoid papulosis: a retrospective study of 123 patients. *J Am Acad Dermatol*. 2012;66(6):928-937.

97. Melchers RC, Willemze R, Bekkenk MW, et al. Frequency and prognosis of associated malignancies in 504 patients with lymphomatoid papulosis. *J Eur Acad Dermatol Venereol.* 2020;34(2):260-266.
98. Beljaards R, Willemze R. The prognosis of patients with lymphomatoid papulosis associated with malignant lymphomas. *Br J Dermatol.* 1992;126(6):596-602.
99. Cordel N, Tressières B, D'Incan M, et al. Frequency and risk factors for associated lymphomas in patients with lymphomatoid papulosis. *Oncologist.* 2016;21(1):76-83.
100. Wieser I, Tetzlaff MT, Torres Cabala CA, Duvic M. Primary cutaneous CD30(+) lymphoproliferative disorders. *J Dtsch Dermatol Ges.* 2016;14(8):767-782.
101. de la Garza Bravo MM, Patel KP, Loghavi S, et al. Shared clonality in distinctive lesions of lymphomatoid papulosis and mycosis fungoides occurring in the same patients suggests a common origin. *Hum Pathol.* 2015;46(4):558-569.
102. Chott A, Vonderheid EC, Olbricht S, Miao N-N, Balk SP, Kadin ME. The same dominant T cell clone is present in multiple regressing skin lesions and associated T cell lymphomas of patients with lymphomatoid papulosis. *J Invest Dermatol.* 1996;106(4):696-700.
103. Sanchez NP, Pittelkow MR, Muller SA, Banks PM, Winkelmann RK. The clinicopathologic spectrum of lymphomatoid papulosis: study of 31 cases. *J Am Acad Dermatol.* 1983;8(1):81-94.
104. Nijsten T, Curiel-Lewandrowski C, Kadin ME. Lymphomatoid papulosis in children: a retrospective cohort study of 35 cases. *Arch Dermatol.* 2004;140(3):306-312.
105. Kagaya M, Kondo S, Kamada A, Yamada Y, Matsusaka H, Jimbo K. Localized lymphomatoid papulosis. *Dermatology.* 2002;204(1):72-74.
106. Paul MA, Krowchuk DP, Hitchcock MG, Jorizzo JL. Lymphomatoid papulosis: successful weekly pulse superpotent topical corticosteroid therapy in three pediatric patients. *Pediatr Dermatol.* 1996;13(6):501-506.
107. el-Azhary RA, Gibson LE, Kurtin PJ, Pittelkow MR, Muller SA. Lymphomatoid papulosis: a clinical and histopathologic review of 53 cases with leukocyte immunophenotyping, DNA flow cytometry, and T-cell receptor gene rearrangement studies. *J Am Acad Dermatol.* 1994;30(2 part 1):210-218.
108. Vonderheid EC, Sajjadian A, Kadin ME. Methotrexate is effective therapy for lymphomatoid papulosis and other primary cutaneous CD30-positive lymphoproliferative disorders. *J Am Acad Dermatol.* 1996;34(3):470-481.
109. Krathen RA, Ward S, Duvic M. Bexarotene is a new treatment option for lymphomatoid papulosis. *Dermatology.* 2003;206(2):142-147.
110. Zackheim HS, Epstein EH, Jr, Crain WR. Topical carmustine therapy for lymphomatoid papulosis. *Arch Dermatol.* 1985;121(11):1410-1414.
111. Zackheim HS, Epstein EH, Jr, Crain WR. Topical carmustine (BCNU) for cutaneous T cell lymphoma: a 15-year experience in 143 patients. *J Am Acad Dermatol.* 1990;22(5):802-810.
112. Korpusik D, Ruzicka T. Clinical course and therapy of lymphomatoid papulosis. Experience with 17 cases and literature review. *Hautarzt.* 2007;58(10):870-881.
113. Miquel J, Fraitag S. HamelmelDermatologie, Venerologie, und verwsis in children: a series of 25 cases. *Br J Dermatol.* 2014;171(5):1138-1146.
114. Wantzin GL, Thomsen K. PUVA-treatment in lymphomatoid papulosis. *Br J Dermatol.* 1982;107(6):687-690.
115. Volkenandt M, Kerscher M, Sander C, Meurer M, Rocken M. PUVA-bath photochemotherapy resulting in rapid clearance of lymphomatoid papulosis in a child. *Arch Dermatol.* 1995;131(9):1094.
116. Fernández-de-Misa R, Hernández-Machín B, Servitje O, et al. First-line treatment in lymphomatoid papulosis: a retrospective multicentre study. *Clin Exp Dermatol.* 2018;43(2):137-143.
117. Van Neer FJ, Toonstra J, Van Voorst Vader PC, Willemze R, Van Vloten WA. Lymphomatoid papulosis in children: a study of 10 children registered by the Dutch Cutaneous Lymphoma Working Group. *Br J Dermatol.* 2001;144(2):351-354.
118. de Souza A, Camilleri MJ, Wada DA, Appert DL, Gibson LE, el-Azhary RA. Clinical, histopathologic, and immunophenotypic features of lymphomatoid papulosis with CD8 predominance in 14 pediatric patients. *J Am Acad Dermatol.* 2009;61(6):993-1000.
119. Calzavara-Pinton P, Venturini M, Sala R. Medium-dose UVA1 therapy of lymphomatoid papulosis. *J Am Acad Dermatol.* 2005;52(3 pt 1):530-532.
120. Bruijn MS, Horváth B, van Voorst Vader PC, Willemze R, Vermeer MH. Recommendations for treatment of lymphomatoid papulosis with methotrexate: a report from the Dutch Cutaneous Lymphoma Group. *Br J Dermatol.* 2015;173(5):1319-1322.
121. Everett MA. Treatment of lymphomatoid papulosis with methotrexate. *Br J Dermatol.* 1984;111(5):631.
122. Newland KM, McCormack CJ, Twigger R, et al. The efficacy of methotrexate for lymphomatoid papulosis. *J Am Acad Dermatol.* 2015;72(6):1088-1090.
123. Bekkenk MW, Geelen FA, van Voorst Vader PC, et al. Primary and secondary cutaneous CD30(+) lymphoproliferative disorders: a report from the Dutch Cutaneous Lymphoma Group on the long-term follow-up data of 219 patients and guidelines for diagnosis and treatment. *Blood.* 2000;95(12):3653-3661.
124. Kadin ME. Current management of primary cutaneous CD30+ T-cell lymphoproliferative disorders. *Oncology (Williston Park, NY).* 2009;23(13):1158-1164.
125. Rodrigues M, McCormack C, Yap LM, et al. Successful treatment of lymphomatoid papulosis with photodynamic therapy. *Australas J Dermatol.* 2009;50(2):129-132.
126. Duvic M, Tetzlaff MT, Gangar P, Clos AL, Sui D, Talpur R. Results of a phase II trial of brentuximab vedotin for CD30+ cutaneous T-cell lymphoma and lymphomatoid papulosis. *J Clin Oncol.* 2015;33(32):3759-3765.
127. Kaufmann T, Nisce LZ, Silver RT. Lymphomatoid papulosis: case report of a patient managed with radiation therapy and review of the literature. *Am J Clin Oncol.* 1992;15(5):412-416.
128. de Souza A, Gibson LE, Wada DA, et al. Resolution of CD8+ lymphomatoid papulosis after surgical excision of the type AB-thymoma. *Am J Dermatopathol.* 2009;31(5):475-479.
129. Martinez-Cabriales SA, Walsh S, Sade S, Shear NH. Lymphomatoid papulosis: an update and review. *J Eur Acad Dermatol Venereol.* 2020;34(1):59-73.
130. Querfeld C, Khan I, Mahon B, Nelson BP, Rosen ST, Evens AM. Primary cutaneous and systemic anaplastic large cell lymphoma: clinicopathologic aspects and therapeutic options. *Oncology (Williston Park, NY).* 2010;24(7):574-587.
131. Willemze R, Beljaards RC. Spectrum of primary cutaneous CD30 (Ki-1)-positive lymphoproliferative disorders: a proposal for classification and guidelines for management and treatment. *J Am Acad Dermatol.* 1993;28(6):973-980.

132. Shehan JM, Kalaaji AN, Markovic SN, Ahmed I. Management of multifocal primary cutaneous CD30 anaplastic large cell lymphoma. *J Am Acad Dermatol*. 2004;51(1):103-110.
133. Lakshmi P, Reddy I, Ala M. Multifocal primary cutaneous anaplastic lymphoma. *J Dr NTR Univ Health Sci*. 2016;5(3):230-233.
134. Gao C, McCormack CJ, van der Weyden C, et al. The importance of differentiating between mycosis fungoides with CD30-positive large cell transformation and mycosis fungoides with coexistent primary cutaneous anaplastic large cell lymphoma. *J Am Acad Dermatol*. 2021;84(1):185-187.
135. Scarisbrick JJ. Brentuximab vedotin therapy for CD30-positive cutaneous T-cell lymphoma: a targeted approach to management. *Future Oncol*. 2017;13(27):2405-2411.
136. Hapgood G, Pickles T, Sehn LH, et al. Outcome of primary cutaneous anaplastic large cell lymphoma: a 20-year British Columbia Cancer Agency experience. *Br J Haematol*. 2017;176(2):234-240.
137. Million L, Yi EJ, Wu F, et al. Radiation therapy for primary cutaneous anaplastic large cell lymphoma: an international lymphoma radiation oncology group multi-institutional experience. *Int J Radiat Oncol Biol Phys*. 2016;95(5):1454-1459.
138. Yu JB, McNiff JM, Lund MW, Wilson LD. Treatment of primary cutaneous CD30+ anaplastic large-cell lymphoma with radiation therapy. *Int J Radiat Oncol Biol Phys*. 2008;70(5):1542-1545.
139. Gentile MS, Martinez-Escala ME, Thomas TO, et al. Single-fraction radiotherapy for CD30+ lymphoproliferative disorders. *Biomed Res Int*. 2015;2015:629587.
140. Melchers RC, Willemze R, Bekkenk MW, et al. Evaluation of treatment results in multifocal primary cutaneous anaplastic large cell lymphoma: report of the Dutch Cutaneous Lymphoma Group. *Br J Dermatol*. 2018;179(3):724-731.
141. Calista D, Riccioni L, Bagli L, Valenzano F. Long-term remission of primary cutaneous neutrophil-rich CD30+ anaplastic large cell lymphoma treated with topical imiquimod. A case report. *J Eur Acad Dermatol Venereol*. 2016;30(5):899-901.
142. Ehst BD, Dréno B, Vonderheid EC. Primary cutaneous CD30+ anaplastic large cell lymphoma responds to imiquimod cream. *EJD European journal of dermatology*. 2008;18(4):467-468.
143. Didona B, Benucci R, Amerio P, Canzona F, Rienzo O, Cavalieri R. Primary cutaneous CD30+ T-cell lymphoma responsive to topical imiquimod (Aldara®). *Br J Dermatol*. 2004;150(6):1198-1201.
144. Desai A, Telang GH, Olszewski AJ. Remission of primary cutaneous anaplastic large cell lymphoma after a brief course of brentuximab vedotin. *Ann Hematol*. 2013:1-2.
145. Melchers RC, Willemze R, Vermaat JSP, et al. Outcomes of rare patients with a primary cutaneous CD30+ lymphoproliferative disorder developing extracutaneous disease. *Blood*. 2020;135(10):769-773.
146. Horwitz S, O'Connor OA, Pro B, et al. Brentuximab vedotin with chemotherapy for CD30-positive peripheral T-cell lymphoma (ECHELON-2): a global, double-blind, randomised, phase 3 trial. *Lancet*. 2019;393(10168):229-240.
147. Benner MF, Jansen PM, Vermeer MH, Willemze R. Prognostic factors in transformed mycosis fungoides: a retrospective analysis of 100 cases. *Blood*. 2012;119(7):1643-1649.
148. Kang SK, Chang SE, Choi JH, Sung KJ, Moon KC, Koh JK. Coexistence of CD30D30med mycosis fungoides: a retrospective analysis of 100 cases. *Clin Exp Dermatol*. 2002;27(3):212-215.
149. Kadin ME. CD30-rich transformed mycosis fungoides or anaplastic large cell lymphoma? How to get it right. *Br J Dermatol*. 2015;172(6):1478-1479.
150. Fauconneau A, Pham-Ledard A, Cappellen D, et al. Assessment of diagnostic criteria between primary cutaneous anaplastic large-cell lymphoma and CD30-rich transformed mycosis fungoides; a study of 66 cases. *Br J Dermatol*. 2015;172(6):1547-1554.
151. Elder D, Massi D, Scolyer R, Willemze R. *WHO Classification of Skin Tumours*. vol. 11, 4th ed. IARC Press: WHO; 2018.
152. Hsi AC, Lee SJ, Rosman IS, et al. Expression of helper T cell master regulators in inflammatory dermatoses and primary cutaneous T-cell lymphomas: diagnostic implications. *J Am Acad Dermatol*. 2015;72(1):159-167.
153. Collins K, Gu J, Aung PP, et al. Is immunohistochemical expression of GATA3 helpful in the differential diagnosis of transformed mycosis fungoides and primary cutaneous CD30-positive T cell lymphoproliferative disorders? *Virchows Arch*. 2021:479(2):377-383.
154. Mitteldorf C, Robson A, Tronnier M, Pfaltz MC, Kempf W. Galectin-3 expression in primary cutaneous CD30-positive lymphoproliferative disorders and transformed mycosis fungoides. *Dermatology*. 2015;231(2):164-170.

PART IV PRIMARY CUTANEOUS NK/T-CELL MALIGNANCIES

CHAPTER 23

Extranodal natural killer/T-cell lymphoma, nasal type

Carlos Barrionuevo-Cornejo and Leticia Quintanilla-Martinez

DEFINITION

Extranodal natural killer (NK)/T-cell lymphoma, nasal type (ENKTL) is an aggressive, extranodal necrotizing tumor associated with Epstein-Barr virus (EBV) infection. It has predilection for extranodal involvement, including the nasopharyngeal region, skin, gastrointestinal tract, testis, and central nervous system.[1-4] Morphologically, ENKTL is characterized by an infiltrate of small to large lymphoid cells usually arranged in an angiocentric and angiodestructive pattern with prominent coagulative necrosis and karyorrhexis. ENKTL can have either an NK-cell or a cytotoxic T-cell phenotype. A strict definition of primary cutaneous NKTL (CNKTL) requires absence of nasopharyngeal involvement as the primary source of the tumor.

EPIDEMIOLOGY

This neoplasm is rare in Western countries but prevalent in Asia (China, Japan, Korea, and Southeast Asia),[5-8] South America (México, Peru, Brazil),[9-11] and Central America, suggesting that ethnic background (ie, genetic risk factors) may have a role in the pathogenesis of these lymphomas.[12,13] Occasional case series have also been reported from Europe and North America.[14,15] It is more common in males, with a male-to-female ratio of 2:1, and usually affects middle-aged adults, with a median age of 49 to 53 years.[3]

ETIOLOGY

There is very strong evidence of a pathogenic association between EBV infection and ENKTL. The pattern of viral latency is of type II. The type II latency pattern includes the expression of the EBV nuclear antigen 1 (EBNA-1) and latent membrane protein 1 (LMP-1), while the EBNA-2 is negative. EBV-associated messenger RNA (EBER) is invariably positive in all latency patterns.[13,16-19] The EBV is present in a clonal episomal form.[12,13,20,21] Gene expression profiling has shown patterns different from normal NK cells, and several oncogenic pathways are activated including Notch-1, Wnt, JAK/STAT, AKT, and nuclear factor-κB (NF-κB).[22] Most studies have also shown different subtypes of EBV associated with the ENKTL in Asia (subtype A) when compared with Western countries, including South and Central America (subtype B).[10,13,23,24]

CLINICAL PRESENTATION AND PROGNOSIS

Bearing in mind that many ENKTLs spread to the skin, nasopharyngeal involvement as the primary source of the tumor must be excluded. Often, it is necessary to undertake comprehensive reviews of the nasal and nasopharyngeal regions using positron emission tomography/computed tomography.[25-27]

CNKTL usually presents as erythematous plaques, nodules, or as multiple tumors, often with hemorrhage and ulceration, preferentially on the face, trunk, and extremities[2,28-30] (Fig. 23-1). Some cutaneous lesions can mimic cellulitis or granulomatous panniculitis.[31] Approximately, 40% of the cases have evidence of extracutaneous dissemination at diagnosis, 60% have widespread lesions, and 20% have locoregional involvement.[29,30] Systemic symptoms such as fever, malaise, and weight loss may be present, and some cases are accompanied by a hemophagocytic syndrome.[2,32]

The median survival for CNKTL is about 15 months. Patients with extracutaneous disease at presentation have a shorter survival as compared with those without extracutaneous involvement. Usually, CNKTL has a less aggressive clinical course and better outcomes when compared with the ENKTL with cutaneous dissemination.[30] Age, gender, extent of cutaneous involvement, and initial response to therapy do not seem to influence survival. Moreover, patients with

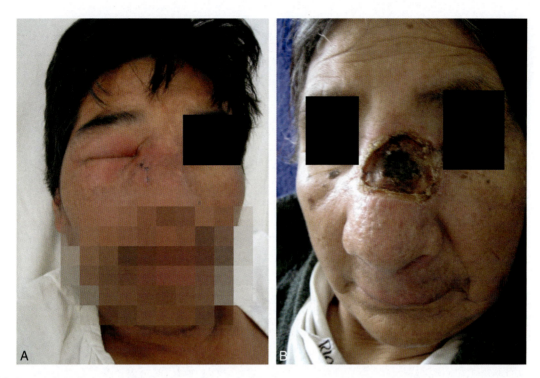

FIGURE 23-1. **Clinical presentation of ENKTL. A.** Erythematous plaques on the right eye and expansion of the nasal bridge. **B.** Ulcerated lesion on the nose.

coexpression of CD30 tend to have a less favorable outcome.[33] CD38 expression in ENKTL correlates with a poor outcome and indicates the potential role of this epitope as a therapeutic target.[34] Another prognostic marker for ENKTL is circulating plasma EBV-DNA, which is derived from apoptotic and necrotic cells, thus serving as a marker of tumor load.[35] Other routine histopathologic parameters have no prognostic impact.[4,10]

HISTOLOGY

The neoplastic cells infiltrate the epidermis, dermis, appendages, and subcutis (Fig. 23-2A, B). Pautrier microabscess formation has been described.[36] The epidermis can be ulcerated or intact or show pseudoepitheliomatous hyperplasia.[37] Malignant lymphocytes exhibit variable size, with mild to moderate nuclear pleomorphism, and nuclear hyperchromasia[1,2] (Fig. 23-2C, D). There is angiocentricity and fibrinoid angiodestruction with necrosis of the surrounding tissue[4,30,38,39] (Fig. 23-3).

IMMUNOPHENOTYPE

The immunophenotypes of CNKTL and ENKTL are identical. Most cases show an NK phenotype, with expression of CD3ε, CD2, CD56, and cytotoxic molecules such as TIA-1, perforin, and granzyme B (Fig. 23-4A–C). Tumor cells are negative for surface CD3, CD4, CD8, CD5, CD16, CD57, TCRγδ, and BF1 (TCRαβ). Usually, neoplastic cells also express CD43, CD25, CD45-RO, FAS, and HLA-DR, and sometimes CD30 and CD7. Some cases may show positivity for LMP-1, but all cases show the presence of EBV by in situ hybridization for EBV-encoded RNA (EBER) (Fig. 23-4D). About 10% of cases have a cytotoxic CD8+ and CD56- T-cell phenotype along with EBER positivity.[1-3,40]

GENETIC AND MOLECULAR FINDINGS

Several cytogenetic aberrations have been described in ENKTL. The most common recurrent cytogenetic alteration is the loss of 6q21-25 (20%-43%) resulting in the loss of tumor suppression genes such as *PRDM1*, *HACE1*, and *FOXO3*.[41-43] Other recurrent chromosomal alterations include losses of 11q24-q25 (20%-40%), 13q14 (15%-60%), 17p13 (20%-40%), and i(6) (p10), and gains in 1q21-q44 (20%-50%), 2q13-q32 (25%-42%), 6p25-p11 (25%-40%), 7q11-q36 (20%-60%), 17q21 (20%-50%), and 20q11 (30%-50%). The most recurrently mutated genes include members of the JAK-STAT signaling pathway (*STAT3*, *JAK3*, *STAT5B*),[44] followed by epigenetic modifiers (*KMT2D*, *ARID1A*, *EP300*), tumor suppressor genes (*TP53*, *BCOR*, *MGA*), and the RNA helicase gene *DDX3X*.[45-49] Epigenetic alterations such as methylation in cell cycle regulators, histone modifications, and deregulated miRNA are also described.[50-56] Gene expression profiling has also demonstrated upregulation of *BIRC5* encoding for survivin, *MYC*, *PD-L1*, *RUNX3*, *AURKA*, and *PDGFRA*.[57,58]

Based on molecular integrated analysis, a new molecular classification has been proposed. This classification

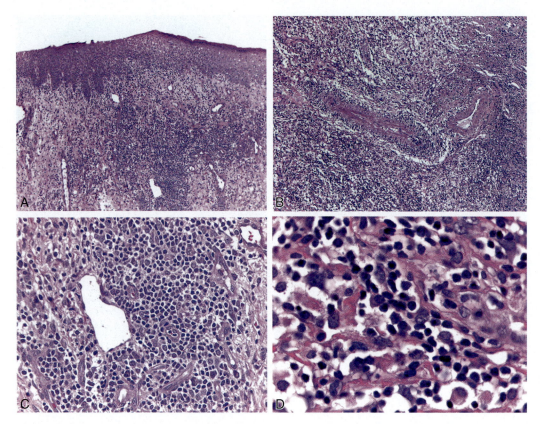

FIGURE 23-2. Epidermotropic and dermal lymphocytic infiltrates **(A)** with subcutaneous extension **(B)**. Medium-sized neoplastic lymphocytes **(C)** with nuclear hyperchromasia and irregular nuclear contours **(D)**.

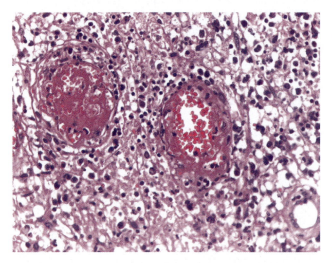

FIGURE 23-3. Angiocentric growth and angiodestruction with tissue necrosis.

stratifies cases in three molecular subgroups. The first group, TSIM subtype (alterations in Tumor Suppressors and Immune Modulators) is characterized by activation-through mutations of the JAK-STAT signaling pathway, *TP53* mutations, del6q21, NK-cell mediated cytotoxicity, immune surveillance, PD-L1 overexpression, and genomic instability. Interestingly, this group has the higher NK cell gene expression. The second group, MB subtype (*MGA* mutations and LOH of the *BRDT* locus), consists of cases with *MGA* mutations, a tumor suppressor gene related to MYC overexpression, and *BRDT* enhances oncogenic functions of cancer drivers including *MYC*. This suggests that the overexpression of *MYC* is critically in this subtype. The third group, HEA subtype (mutations in *HDAC1*, *EP300* and *ARID1A*), is linked to epigenetic changes leading to NF-κB and T-cell receptor (TCR) signaling pathways. In this group the T-cell gene expression signature predominates. The molecular subtypes correlate well with the cell of origin (NK vs T cell).[59]

POSTULATED CELL OF ORIGIN

They are activated NK cells and, less commonly, cytotoxic T lymphocytes. Although there are some phenotypic dissimilarities between ENKTLs of the T-cell and NK-cell types, there are no major clinicopathologic differences to distinguish these two groups for clinical purposes.[60]

DIFFERENTIAL DIAGNOSIS

The main differential diagnosis of CNKTL is hydroa vacciniforme lymphoproliferative disorder (HV-LPD) as the entities share some morphologic and phenotypic characteristics,

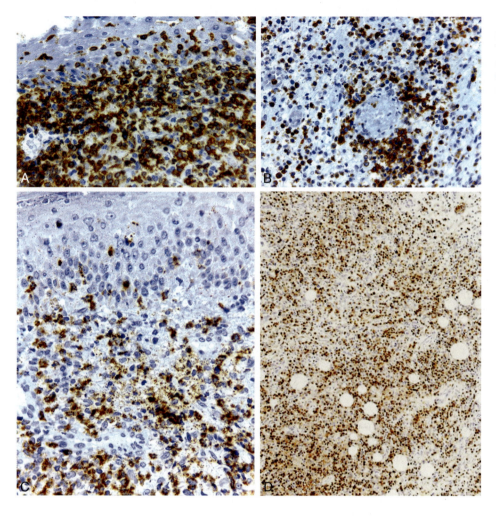

FIGURE 23-4. Neoplastic cells are highlighted by CD3 **(A)**, CD56 **(B)**, and TIA-1 **(C)**. Note the angiocentric arrangement of CD56+ cells **(B)**. EBV infection is detected by positive EBER in situ hybridization **(D)**.

besides their association with EBV. In contrast to CNKTL, HV-LPD tends to affect the pediatric population and has a less aggressive clinical course. Some cases of HVLL can progress to NKTL.[61-63]

Subcutaneous panniculitis-like T-cell lymphoma (SPTCL) is another differential diagnosis to consider. Although clinical features may be similar because of the nodular appearance of the lesions, SPTCL shows almost exclusive involvement of the subcutaneous tissue, without dermal and epidermal dissemination. SPTCL has a cytotoxic CD8+ phenotype and lacks EBV and CD56 expression. Cases previously described as "SPTCL" with CD56 and TCRγδ expression are now classified as primary cutaneous γδ T-cell lymphomas (GDTCLs). GDTCL can also show angiotropism and angiodestruction and occasionally be linked to EBV. However, GDTCL characteristically expresses TCRγδ and lacks BF1, whereas NKTL is typically negative for both markers.

Primary cutaneous aggressive epidermotropic CD8+ cytotoxic T-cell lymphoma is rare and clinically characterized by sudden eruptions of localized or disseminated papules, nodules, and tumors with central ulceration and necrosis. Histologically, this entity shows marked, pagetoid epidermotropism. Tumor cells exhibit a CD8+TIA-1+CD3+CD7+BF1+ cytotoxic T-cell phenotype and lack EBV.[1,3,32,36]

CAPSULE SUMMARY

- CNKTL is an aggressive lymphoma usually of NK or, less frequently, CD8+ cytotoxic T-cell phenotype.
- CNKTL presents as ulcerated tumors, plaques, or nodules on the face, arms, and trunk and has a poor prognosis.
- Neoplastic cells are small to medium in size with pleomorphic, irregularly shaped nuclei. Angiocentric and angiodestructive growth pattern is characteristic.
- Neoplastic cells express CD56, CD3ε, CD2, CD5, TIA-1, perforin, granzyme B, and sometimes LMP-1, CD30, and CD7. They are negative for CD4, CD8, CD5, CD57, CD16, and TCRγ and TCRBF1. A subset of cases may have a cytotoxic CD8+ profile. All cases are positive for EBER.
- No specific chromosomal translocation but complex cytogenetic aberrations have been described.
- Mutations affecting the JAK/STAT pathways and other genetic alterations may be useful for targeted therapies.

ACKNOWLEDGMENTS

I wish to thank Dr. Daniela Duenas for her contribution to the photomicrographs and also Dr. Francisco Bravo for his contribution to clinical pictures.

References

1. Chan JKC, Quintanilla-Martinez L, Ferry JA, et al. Extranodal NK/T-cell lymphoma, nasal type. In: Swerdlow SH, Campo E, Harris NL, et al., eds. *WHO Classification of Tumours of Haematopoietic and Lymphoid Tissues*. 4th ed. IARC; 2008:285-288.
2. Kohler S, Iwatsuki K, Jaffe ES, et al. Extranodal NK/T-cell lymphoma, nasal type. In: LeBoit PE, Burg G, Weedon D, et al., eds. *WHO Classification of Tumours. Pathology & Genetics of Skin Tumours*. IARC; 2005:191-192.
3. Jaffe ES, Harris NE, Vardiman JW, et al., eds. *Hematopathology*. Elsevier; 2011.
4. Mraz-Gernhard S, Nantkunan Y, Hoppe RT, et al. Natural killer/natural killer-like T cell lymphoma, CD56+, presenting in the skin: an increasingly recognized entity with an aggressive course. *J Clin Oncol*. 2001;19:2179-2188.
5. Au WY, Ma SY, Chim CS, et al. Clinicopathologic features and treatment outcome of mature T-cell and natural Killer-cell lymphomas diagnosed according to the World Health Organization according to the World Health Organization classification scheme: a single center experience of 10 years. *Ann Oncol*. 2005;16(2):206-214.
6. Lymphoma Study Group of Japanese Pathologists. The World Health Organization Classification of malignant lymphomas in Japan: incidence of recently recognized entities. *Pathol Int*. 2000;50:696-702.
7. Takata K, Hong ME, Sitthinamsuwan P, et al. Primary cutaneous NK/T-cell lymphoma, nasal type and CD56-positive peripheral T-cell lymphoma: a cellular lineage and clinicopathologic study of 60 patients from Asia. *Am J Surg Pathol*. 2015;39(1):1-12.
8. Jae HH, Young-Hyeh K, Yun KK, et al. Characteristics of cutaneous lymphomas in Korea according to the new WHO-EORTC Classification: report of a nationwide study. *Korean J Pathol*. 2014;48:126-132.
9. Aviles A, Dıaz NR, Neri N, et al. Angiocentric nasal T/natural killer cell lymphoma: a single centre study of prognostic factors in 108 patients. *Clin Lab Haematol*. 2000;22(4):215-220.
10. Barrionuevo C, Zaharia M, Martinez MT, et al. Extranodal NK/T-cell lymphoma, nasal type: study of clinicopathologic and prognosis factors in a series of 78 cases from Peru. *Appl Immunohistochem Mol Morphol*. 2007;15(1):38-44.
11. Gualco G, Domeny-Duarte P, Chioato L, et al. Clinicopathologic and molecular features of 122 Brazilian cases of nodal and extranodal NK/T-cell lymphoma, nasal type, with EBV subtyping analysis. *Am J Surg Pathol*. 2011;35(8):1195-1203.
12. Arber DA, Weiss LM, Albujar PF, et al. Nasal lymphomas in Peru. High incidence of T-cell immunophenotype and Epstein–Barr virus infection. *Am J Surg Pathol*. 1993;17:392-399.
13. Elenitoba-Johnson KS, Zarate-Osorno A, Meneses A, et al. Cytotoxic granular protein expression, Epstein–Barr virus strain type, and latent membrane protein-1 oncogene deletions in nasal T-lymphocyte/natural killer cell lymphomas from Mexico. *Mod Pathol*. 1998;11:754-761.
14. Jaccard A, Gachard N, Marin B, et al. GELA and GOELAMS Intergroup. Efficacy of L-asparaginase with methotrexate and dexamethasone (AspaMetDex regimen) in patients with refractory or relapsing extranodal NK/T-cell lymphoma, a phase 2 study. *Blood*. 2011;117(6):1834-1839.
15. Li S, Feng X, Li T, et al. Extranodal NK/T-cell lymphoma, nasal type: a report of 73 cases at MD Anderson Cancer Center. *Am J Surg Pathol*. 2013;37(1):14-23.
16. Chiang AK, Wong KY, Liang AC, et al. Comparative analysis of Epstein–Barr virus gene polymorphisms in nasal T/NK-cell lymphomas and normal nasal tissues: implications on virus strain selection in malignancy. *Int J Cancer*. 1999;80:356-364.
17. Dirnhofer S, Angeles-Angeles A, Ortiz-Hidalgo C, et al. High prevalence of a 30-base pair deletion in the Epstein–Barr virus (EBV) latent membrane protein 1 gene and of strain type B EBV in Mexican classical Hodgkin's disease and reactive lymphoid tissue. *Hum Pathol*. 1999;30:781-787.
18. Kuo TT, Shih LY, Tsang NM. Nasal NK/T cell lymphoma in Taiwan: a clinicopathologic study of 22 cases, with analysis of histologic subtypes, Epstein–Barr virus LMP-1gene association, and treatment modalities. *Int J Surg Pathol*. 2004;12:375-387.
19. Tai YC, Kim LH, Peh SC. High frequency of EBV association and 30-bp deletion in the LMP-1 gene in CD56 lymphomas of the upper aerodigestive tract. *Pathol Int*. 2004;54:158-166.
20. Quintanilla-Martinez L, Franklin JL, Guerrero I, et al. Histological and immunophenotypic profile of nasal NK/T cell lymphomas from Peru: high prevalence of p53 overexpression. *Hum Pathol*. 1999;30:849-855.
21. van Gorp J, Weiping L, Jacobse K, et al. Epstein–Barr virus in nasal T-cell lymphomas (polymorphic reticulosis/midline malignant reticulosis) in western China. *J Pathol*. 1994;173:81-87.
22. Tse E, Kwong YL. How I treat NK/T-cell lymphomas. *Blood*. 2013;121(25):4997-5005.
23. Peh SC, Kim LH, Poppema S. Frequent presence of subtype A virus in Epstein–Barr virus-associated malignancies. *Pathology*. 2002;34:446-450.
24. Suzumiya J, Ohshima K, Takeshita M, et al. Nasal lymphomas in Japan: a high prevalence of Epstein–Barr virus type A and deletion within the latent membrane protein gene. *Leuk Lymphoma*. 1999;35:567-578.
25. Au WY, Weisenburger DD, Intragumtornchai T, et al. International Peripheral T-Cell Lymphoma Project. Clinical differences between nasal and extranasal natural killer/T-cell lymphoma: a study of 136 cases from the International Peripheral T-Cell Lymphoma Project. *Blood*. 2009;113(17):3931-3937.
26. Khong PL, Pang CB, Liang R, et al. Fluorine-18 fluorodeoxyglucose positron emission tomography in mature T-cell and natural killer cell malignancies. *Ann Hematol*. 2008;87(8):613-621.
27. Kwong YL, Anderson BO, Advani R, et al; Asian Oncology Summit. Management of T-cell and natural-killer-cell neoplasms in Asia: consensus statement from the Asian Oncology Summit 2009. *Lancet Oncol*. 2009;10(11):1093-1101.
28. Bekkenk MW, Jansen PM, Meijer CJLM, et al. CD56 hematological neoplasms presenting in the skin: a retrospective analysis of 23 new cases and 130 cases from the literature. *Ann Oncol*. 2004;15:1097-1108.
29. Gniadecki R, Rossen K, Ralfkier E, et al. CD56+ Lymphoma with skin involvement clinicopathologic features and classification. *Arch Dermatol*. 2004;140(4):427-436.
30. Choi YL, Park JH, Namkung JH, et al. Extranodal NK/T-cell lymphoma with cutaneous involvement: "nasal" vs. "nasal-type" subgroups—a retrospective study of 18 patients. *Br J Dermatol*. 2009;160(2):333-337.

31. Sitthinamsuwan P, Pongpruttipan T, Chularojmontri L, et al. Extranodal NK/T cell lymphoma, nasal type, presenting with primary cutaneous lesion mimicking granulomatous panniculitis: a case report and review of literature. *J Med Assoc Thai*. 2010;93(8):1001-1007.
32. Jaffe ES, Nicolae A, Pittaluga S. Peripheral T-cell and NK-cell lymphomas in the WHO classification: pearls and pitfalls. *Mod Pathol*. 2013;26:S71-S87.
33. Li P, Jiang L, Zhang X, et al. CD30 expression is a novel prognostic indicator in extranodal natural killer/T-cell lymphoma, nasal type. *BMC Cancer*. 2014;28(14):890.
34. Wang L, Wang H, Li PF, et al. CD38 expression predicts poor prognosis and might be a potential therapy target in extranodal NK/T cell lymphoma, nasal type. *Ann Hematol*. 2015;94(8):1381-1388.
35. Au WY, Pang A, Choy C, et al. Quantification of circulating Epstein–Barr virus (EBV) DNA in the diagnosis and monitoring of natural killer cell and EBV-positive lymphomas in immunocompetent patients. *Blood*. 2004;104(1):243-249.
36. Quintanilla-Martinez L, Jansen PM, Kinney MC, et al. Non–mycosis fungoides cutaneous T-Cell lymphomas: report of the 2011 Society for Hematopathology/European Association for Haematopathology workshop. *Am J Clin Pathol*. 2013;139:491-514.
37. Ling YH, Zhu CM, Wen SH, et al. Pseudoepitheliomatous hyperplasia mimicking invasive squamous cell carcinoma in extranodal natural killer/T-cell lymphoma: a report of 34 cases. *Histopathology*. 2015;67(3):404-409.
38. Chan JK, Sin VC, Wong KF, et al. Nonnasal lymphoma expressing the natural killer cell marker CD56: a clinicopathologic study of 49 cases of an uncommon aggressive neoplasm. *Blood*. 1997;89:4501-4513.
39. Natkunam Y, Smoller BR, Zehnder JL, et al. Aggressive cutaneous NK and NK-like T-cell lymphomas: clinicopathologic, immunohistochemical, and molecular analyses of 12 cases. *Am J Surg Pathol*. 1999;23:571-581.
40. Hsi ED. *Hematopathology*. 2nd ed. Elsevier; 2012.
41. Nakashima Y, Tagawa H, Suzuki R, et al. Genome-wide array-based comparative genomic hybridization of natural killer cell lymphoma/leukemia: different genomic alteration patterns of aggressive NK-cell leukemia and extranodal Nk/T-cell lymphoma, nasal type. *Genes Chromosomes Cancer*. 2005;44(3):247-255.
42. Huang Y, de Reyniès A, de Leval L, et al. Gene expression profiling identifies emerging oncogenic pathways operating in extranodal NK/T-cell lymphoma, nasal type. *Blood*. 2010;115(6):1226-1237.
43. Ng SB, Chung TH, Kato S, et al. Epstein-Barr virus-associated primary nodal T/NK-cell lymphoma shows a distinct molecular signature and copy number changes. *Haematologica*. 2018;103(2):278-287.
44. Küçük C, Jiang B, Hu X, et al. Activating mutations of STAT5B and STAT3 in lymphomas derived from γδ-T or NK cells. *Nat Commun*. 2015;6:6025.
45. Quintanilla-Martinez L, Kremer M, Keller G, et al. p53 Mutations in nasal natural killer/T-cell lymphoma from Mexico: association with large cell morphology and advanced disease. *Am J Pathol*. 2001;159(6):2095-2105.
46. Lee S, Park HY, Kang SY, et al. Genetic alterations of JAK/STAT cascade and histone modification in extranodal NK/T-cell lymphoma nasal type. *Oncotarget*. 2015;6(19):17764-17776.
47. Montes-Mojarro IA, Chen BJ, Ramirez-Ibarguen AF, et al. Mutational profile and EBV strains of extranodal NK/T-cell lymphoma, nasal type in Latin America. *Mod Pathol*. 2020;33(5):781-791.
48. Jiang L, Gu ZH, Yan ZX, et al. Exome sequencing identifies somatic mutations of DDX3X in natural killer/T-cell lymphoma. *Nat Genet*. 2015;47(9):1061-1066.
49. Dobashi A, Tsuyama N, Asaka R, et al. Frequent BCOR aberrations in extranodal NK/T-Cell lymphoma, nasal type. *Genes Chromosomes Cancer*. 2016;55(5):460-471.
50. Iqbal J, Weisenburger DD, Chowdhury A, et al; International Peripheral T-cell Lymphoma Project. Natural killer cell lymphoma shares strikingly similar molecular features with a group of non-hepatosplenic γδ T-cell lymphoma and is highly sensitive to a novel aurora kinase A inhibitor in vitro. *Leukemia*. 2011;25(2):348-358.
51. Ng SB, Selvarajan V, Huang G, et al. Activated oncogenic pathways and therapeutic targets in extranodal nasal-type NK/T cell lymphoma revealed by gene expression profiling. *J Pathol*. 2011;223(4):496-510.
52. Paik JH, Jang JY, Jeon YK, et al. MicroRNA-146a downregulates NFκB activity via targeting TRAF6 and functions as a tumor suppressor having strong prognostic implications in NK/T cell lymphoma. *Clin Cancer Res*. 2011;17(14):4761-4771.
53. Ng SB, Yan J, Huang G, et al. Dysregulated microRNAs affect pathways and targets of biologic relevance in nasal-type natural killer/T-cell lymphoma. *Blood*. 2011;118(18):4919-4929.
54. Yan J, Ng SB, Tay JL, et al. EZH2 overexpression in natural killer/T-cell lymphoma confers growth advantage independently of histone methyltransferase activity. *Blood*. 2013;121(22):4512-4520.
55. Nagato T, Ohkuri T, Ohara K, et al. Programmed death-ligand 1 and its soluble form are highly expressed in nasal natural killer/T-cell lymphoma: a potential rationale for immunotherapy. *Cancer Immunol Immunother*. 2017;66(7):877-890.
56. Chang Y, Cui M, Fu X, et al. MiRNA-155 regulates lymphangiogenesis in natural killer/T-cell lymphoma by targeting BRG1. *Cancer Biol Ther*. 2019;20(1):31-41.
57. Drieux F, Ruminy P, Abdel-Sater A, et al. Defining signatures of peripheral T-cell lymphoma with a targeted 20-marker gene expression profiling assay. *Haematologica*. 2020;105(6):1582-1592.
58. Montes-Mojarro IA, Fend F, Quintanilla-Martinez L. EBV and the pathogenesis of NK/T cell lymphoma. *Cancers (Basel)*. 2021;13(6):1414.
59. Xiong J, Cui BW, Wang N, et al. Genomic and transcriptomic characterization of natural killer T cell lymphoma. *Cancer Cell*. 2020;37(3):403-419.e6.
60. Pongpruttipan T, Sukpanichnant S, Assanasen T. Extranodal NK/T-cell lymphoma, nasal type, includes cases of natural killer cell and αβ, γδ, and αβ/γδ T-cell origin: a comprehensive clinicopathologic and phenotypic study. *Am J Surg Pathol*. 2012;36(4):481-499.
61. Barrionuevo C, Anderson VM, Zevallos-Giampietri E, et al. Hydroa-like cutaneous T-cell lymphoma: a clinicopathologic and molecular genetic study of 16 pediatric cases from Peru. *Appl Immunohistochem Mol Morphol*. 2002;10(1):7-14.
62. Rodríguez-Pinilla SM, Barrionuevo C, Garcia J, et al. EBV-associated cutaneous NK/T-cell lymphoma: review of a series of 14 cases from Peru in children and young adults. *Am J Surg Pathol*. 2010;34(12):1773-1782.
63. Quintanilla-Martinez L, Ridaura C, Nagl F, et al. Hydroa vacciniforme-like lymphoma: a chronic EBV+ lymphoproliferative disorder with risk to develop a systemic lymphoma. *Blood*. 2013;122(18):3101-3110.

CHAPTER 24

Hydroa vacciniforme lymphoproliferative disorder

Jose A. Plaza and J. Martin Sangueza

DEFINITION

Historically, hydroa vacciniforme (HV) has been defined as a rare photodermatosis characterized by recurrent vesicles on sun-exposed skin that resolve with varioliform scarring.[1,2] HV is usually seen in children, and there is an association with latent Epstein-Barr virus (EBV) infection.[2-6] Systemic symptoms are not observed, and the disease often resolves spontaneously in adolescence.[2,6] A similar but more aggressive form of the disease characterized by systemic symptoms (including fever, lymphadenopathy, and hepatosplenomegaly) was described in Latin America and Asia and associated with EBV infection. In such cases, the term "HV-like lymphoma" was suggested and incorporated for the first time in the 2008 WHO classification.[7-9] However, given the broad clinical spectrum of the disease and the lack of reliable histomorphology or molecular criteria to predict its behavior, the term "HV-like lymphoproliferative disorder (HV-LPD)" was proposed and included in the 2017 WHO classification.[10-13] HV-LPD is a chronic EBV-positive disorder that mainly affects children and young adults with a risk of developing a systemic lymphoma. The clinical presentation of HV-LPD ranges from a self-limited photodermatosis ("classic" HV-LPD) to a more aggressive systemic disorder ("systemic" HV-LPD).[8,14] Cutaneous symptoms include edema, blisters, ulcers, and scars on the face, trunk, and extremities. In severe cases, the skin lesions may involve the subcutaneous fat, leaving scars and areas of necrosis. In the past, the disease has also been referred to as edematous scarring vasculitis panniculitis, angiocentric cutaneous T-cell lymphoma of childhood, and severe hydroa vacciniforme.

EPIDEMIOLOGY

HV-LPD has a limited geographical distribution and has been mainly described in Central and South America, Mexico, and Asia, with recent cases reported in India. It is rare in Caucasians. The mean age is 10 to 15 years, and there is a slight male predilection with a ratio of 2:1.

ETIOLOGY

EBV infections are usually acquired during childhood or adolescence, and the virus establishes a permanent latent state in B lymphocytes of immunocompetent hosts.[15] While EBV usually infects B cells (Western countries), it rarely infects T cells and/or natural killer (NK) cells.[8,16] EBV is closely associated to classic Hodgkin lymphoma, extranodal NK/T-cell lymphoma, Burkitt lymphoma, and posttransplant lymphoproliferative disorder.[16,17] The exact mechanism by which EBV infects T or NK cells is not entirely understood; however, it is likely to take place during primary infection. The proliferation of EBV-infected T and NK cells has been related to the development of EBV-associated T and NK cell lymphoproliferative disorders, which are highly prevalent in Asian and indigenous populations of Latin America and affect all age groups.[9] EBV-associated T/NK-cell lymphoproliferative disorders are rare and usually occur in patients without apparent immunodeficiency and are closely linked to chronic active EBV (CAEBV) infection.[18] CAEBV infection comprised heterogeneous disorders, including HV, hypersensitivity to mosquito bites, EBV-associated hemophagocytic syndrome, NK/T-cell lymphoma, and NK-cell leukemia. It is unclear whether HV-LPD arises de novo or belongs to a part of the spectrum of classic HV. The fact that both entities are associated with EBV and that T-cell clonality is the main criterion for distinguishing HV-LPD from HV favors the latter hypothesis. It has been postulated that CAEBV infection in patients with HV with particular genetic predispositions followed by subsequent environmental triggers can lead to malignant transformation of lymphocytes characterized by persistent clonal populations with a cytotoxic T-cell or NK-cell phenotype. In HV-LPD, well-described triggers include inflammatory stimuli secondary to mosquito bites or sunlight exposure. Initially, affected individuals may develop a self-limiting disease with local recurrence, but certain patients undergo a more aggressive behavior.

CLINICAL FEATURES

Classic HV-LPD is characterized by a photo distributed vesicular eruption (including the head, neck, and extremities) that evolves to blisters and ulcers leaving characteristic varioliform scars (Fig. 24-1). Skin lesions show a seasonal variation, with recurrences seen more often in the spring and summer (reflecting their photosensitivity character).[8,19-22] Some cases resolve in adolescence, and few cases have a more protracted course. The clinical course is variable, and patients may have recurrent skin lesions for as long as 10 to 15 years before developing systemic involvement. In the systemic form of HV-LPD, the lesions are not clearly exacerbated by sun exposure and as the disease progresses there are severe and extensive skin lesions associated with fever, weight loss, asthenia, hepatosplenomegaly, and lymphadenopathy.[8,9,12,14] Skin lesions show deep ulcerations, necrosis, and facial edema (periocular) (Figs. 24-2–24-4). Marked facial edema is a typical sign of the disease, often with persistent eyelid compromise, which may be unilateral or bilateral.[23] The periorbital swelling can be prominent and may represent the first clinical manifestation (Fig. 24-3B). Both

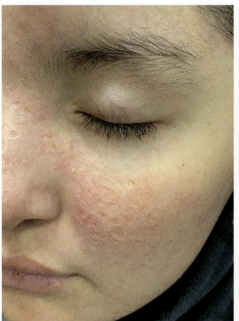
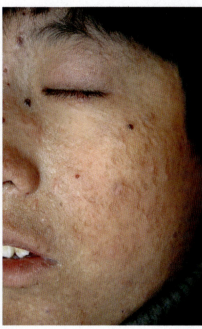

FIGURE 24-1. Two photos of hydroa vacciniforme showing classic vesicles on sun-exposed skin resolving with varioliform scarring.

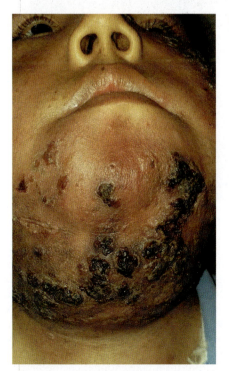

FIGURE 24-2. One image of HV-like lymphoproliferative disorder showing facial necrotic papulovesicular lesions with crusting and facial edema.

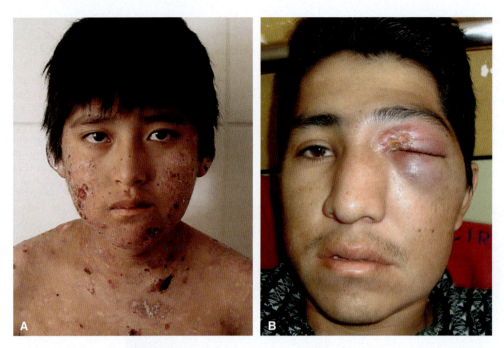

FIGURE 24-3. **HV-like lymphoproliferative disorder. A.** A young patient with classic photo distributed necrotic papulovesicular lesions with crusting. **B.** Marked periorbital edema ulceration and with progressive edema in the nose and the upper cheek.

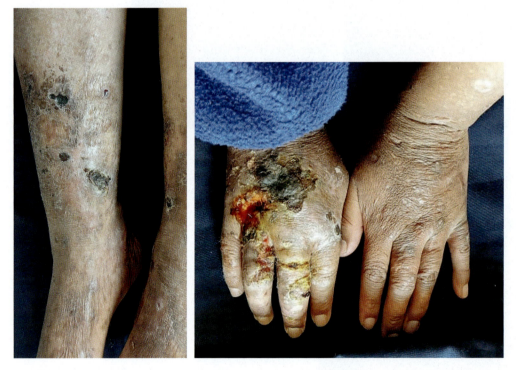

FIGURE 24-4. HV-like lymphoproliferative disorder showing extensive ulcerated lesions on extremities.

sun-exposed and nonexposed body sites can be involved, typically with lesions on the face as well as on the upper and lower extremities (Fig. 24-4). Although it is not entirely clear whether the lesions in HV-LPD are exacerbated by sun exposure, symptoms appear to be highly associated with hypersensitivity to mosquito bites.[24] Clinical progression is heralded by a lack of improvement with photo protection, severe facial and lip swelling, systemic complications, and increase in the number of EBV+ cells. Patients with systemic involvement exhibit a variable clinical course but often have fatal outcomes.[24] There are cases with a peculiar clinical presentation including prominent lip or periorbital edema associated with systemic symptoms. HV-LPD was initially considered a disease with poor prognosis; however, the poor clinical outcome is thought to be largely due to infections and liver failure from conventional chemotherapy that was partially effective.[20,25] Recent clinical studies suggest that systemic HV-LPD can be successfully treated with immunomodulators (eg, thalidomide) and in severe cases with hematopoietic stem cell transplantation.[26,27] In indolent cases, a conservative approach is recommended; however, the challenge for the clinicians following such cases is when to draw the line between an inflammatory condition and a lymphomatous process requiring aggressive therapy. T-cell clonality, number of EBV-positive cells, and/or the density of the infiltrate do not correlate with the clinical course.

HISTOPATHOLOGY

Histologically, cases show epidermal spongiosis with vesiculation and variable necrosis. Within the dermis, there is a mixture of acute and chronic inflammatory cells composed of a dense and diffuse lymphohistiocytic infiltrate admixed with neutrophils, small lymphocytes, plasma cells, and, in some cases, rare eosinophils[8,21,22] (Fig. 24-5). The small to intermediate size atypical lymphocytes have enlarged and pleomorphic nuclei with inconspicuous nucleoli, but large cells can be noted in some cases (Fig. 24-6). In some cases, the lymphocytic infiltrate shows a superficial and deep perivascular pattern. In advanced cases, the epidermis is ulcerated and epidermotropism can be present. Other epidermal findings include dyskeratosis, spongiosis, blisters, intracorneal neutrophilic microabscesses, and ulcerations with serum crusts. The dense atypical dermal population of lymphocytes can extend into the subcutaneous adipose tissue, mimicking subcutaneous panniculitis-like T-cell lymphoma (SCPTCL); such cases tend to have an NK/T-cell phenotype[8,21] (Fig. 24-7). Subcutaneous involvement could be a sign of more risk of severe disease, and it helps to differentiate HV-LPD from lymphomatoid papulosis (LyP).[23] Cases with adnexal involvement and infiltration of small nerve bundles can be

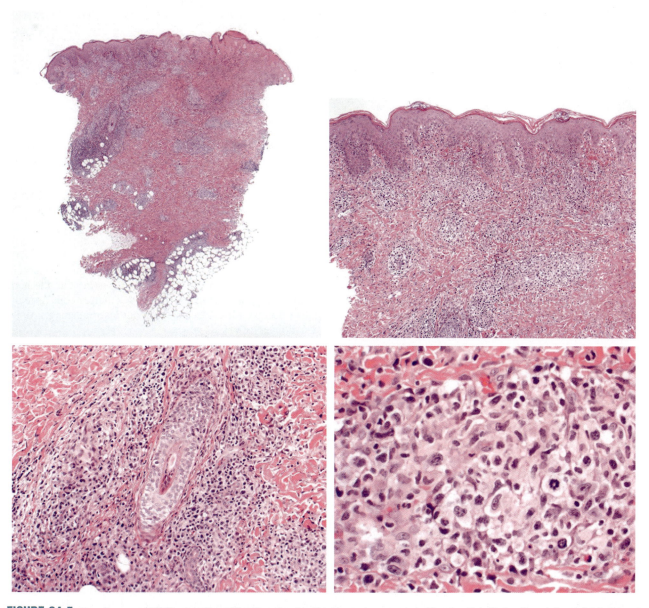

FIGURE 24-5. Four images of HV-like lymphoproliferative disorder. This biopsy shows an atypical lymphocytic infiltrate with periadnexal distribution and subcutaneous involvement. The atypical infiltrate is composed of medium-sized lymphocytes with enlarged, oval, and pleomorphic nuclei. Rare mitoses are noted.

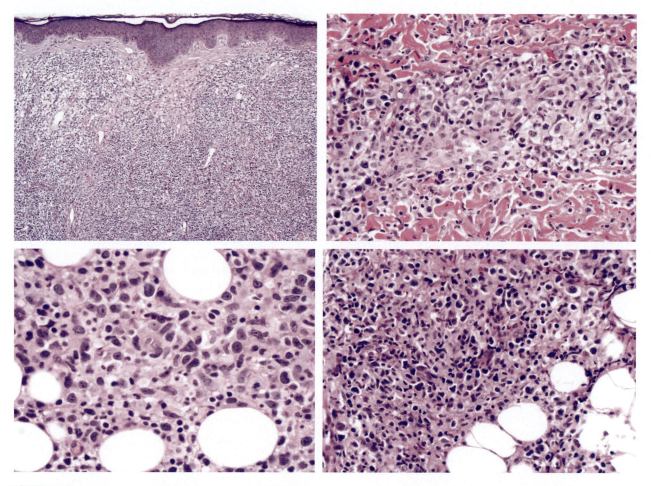

FIGURE 24-6. Four images of HV-like lymphoproliferative disorder. This biopsy shows a diffuse atypical lymphocytic infiltrate occupying the entire dermis. The atypical infiltrate is composed of medium to large-sized lymphocytes. There are inflammatory cells (reactive lymphocytes, histiocytes, and plasma cells) admixed with the atypical lymphocytes.

present. In most cases, there is angiotropism with angiodestruction.[28] It is important to note that, in some of these cases, the histopathologic findings can be mild and subtle, making a diagnosis of HV-LPD more difficult.

IMMUNOPHENOTYPE

Neoplastic lymphocytes in HV-LPD have a classic cytotoxic prolife showing CD8, TIA-1, granzyme B, or perforin expression[12,16,22] (Fig. 24-8). In some rare occasions, the lymphocytes will have a CD4+ T-helper or CD4−CD8− dual-negative phenotype or an NK phenotype (CD56+).[8,29,30] In cases with an NK/T-cell phenotype, the lymphocytic infiltrate often involves the subcutis, mimicking SCPTCL. In situ hybridization EBV-encoded small nonpolyadenylated RNA (EBER) is positive, with variable numbers of cells expressing EBER[8,29] (Fig. 24-8C and D). Proliferation index measured by Ki-67 can vary from low to as high as 50%. It has been suggested that a high number of EBER+ cells is directly proportional to the Ki-67 index and implies a more aggressive behavior, highlighted by increased cellular atypia and epidermal necrosis. CD5, CD7, CD43, and activation markers CD25 and CD30 display variable expression. CD57, ALK, TdT, EMA, and p53 are negative. Other negative markers include PD1, BCL-6, and FOXP3, suggesting that the neoplastic lymphocytes are not follicular T-helper cells or regulatory T cells. Most cases have clonal rearrangements of the T-cell receptor (TCR) genes.

GENETIC AND MOLECULAR FINDINGS

Polymerase chain reaction (PCR) analyses have demonstrated clonal rearrangements of the β, γ, and δ loci of the TCRs in the EBV+ neoplastic cells in HV-LPD. Both the $\alpha\beta$ and $\gamma\delta$ phenotypes have been observed. EBER is positive, with variable numbers of positive cells.[14,31] Although LMP1 is often negative by immunohistochemistry, it can be detected in most cases by PCR in peripheral blood, indicating type II EBV latency.[32]

POSTULATED CELL OF ORIGIN

The presumed cell of origin is CD8+ cytotoxic T cells in HV-LPD. Derivation from CD4+ T-helper cells has been reported.[12,33]

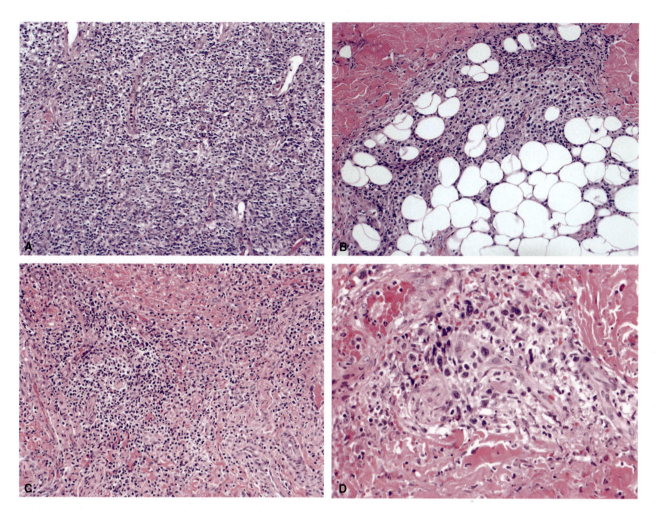

FIGURE 24-7. HV-like lymphoproliferative disorder. A. Dense polymorphous atypical lymphocytic infiltrate. **B.** The atypical lymphocytic infiltrate invades in the subcutis. **C.** Interstitial lymphocytic infiltrate. **D.** Angiocentric infiltration.

DIFFERENTIAL DIAGNOSIS

Histologically, the diagnosis of HV-LPD needs to be always correlated clinically as by morphology and immunophenotype alone it can mimic other T-cell lymphomas.[8,16]

Extranodal NK/T-cell lymphoma, nasal type: Aggressive, EBV-associated lymphoma that may be morphologically indistinguishable from HV-LPD. EBER positivity is seen in all cases. The immunohistochemical profile shows an NK phenotype with expression of CD2, CD56, Cd7, CD3ε, and cytotoxic markers (such as TIA-1, granzyme B, and perforin) but lacks T-cell surface markers such as CD3, CD4, CD8, CD5, BF1 (TCRαβ), and TCRγδ. The EBV infection of the tumor cells leads to overexpression of PD-L1 in the vast majority of cases.[30]

Subcutaneous panniculitis-like T-cell lymphoma (SCPTCL): May have overlapping histopathologic features with HV-LPD, especially when the latter infiltrates the subcutaneous tissue. However, SCPTCL does not involve the epidermis, and the classic rimming of adipocytes by neoplastic lymphocytes is not a feature of HV-LPD. SCPTCL is not EBV related and is mostly seen in adults with subcutaneous nodules in the extremities. Immunohistochemically, most cases of SCPTCL are positive for TCR-α/β, CD3, CD8, and cytotoxic proteins, while CD4 is negative. Cases with CD30 and CD56 expression have been reported.

Primary cutaneous γδ T-cell lymphoma (PCGD-TCL): Aggressive lymphoma that occurs in older individuals. It presents with rapidly progressing plaques and necrotic nodules most frequently located on the extremities. Epidermotropism as well as angiocentricity with angiodestruction can be present, along with rare EBV positivity by EBER. Immunohistochemistry in PCGD-TCL reveals TCR gamma/delta+, CD3+, CD4−, CD8−, CD56+, and betaF1- immunophenotype. Malignant cells also characteristically express cytotoxic proteins such Granzyme B, TIA-1, and perforin.

CAPSULE SUMMARY

- Hydroa vacciniforme lymphoproliferative disorder (HV-LPD) is a chronic EBV-positive skin disease that is mainly seen in South and Central America, Mexico, and Asia.
- It mainly affects children and young adults with a risk of developing a systemic lymphoma.
- The clinical presentation ranges from an indolent, self-limited photodermatosis (classic HV-LPD) to a more

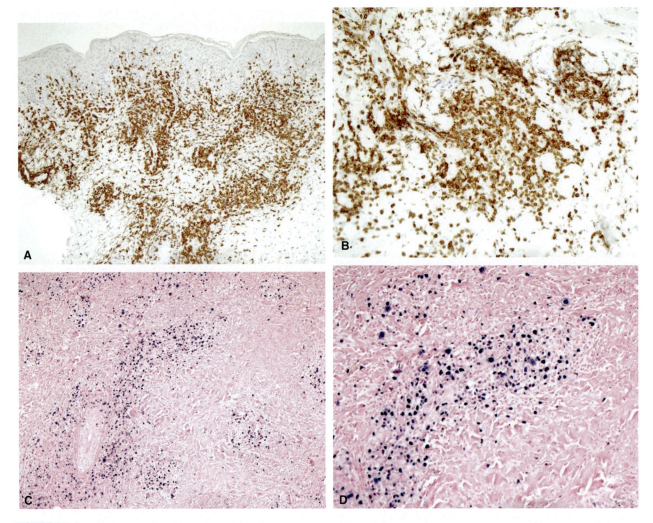

FIGURE 24-8. HV-like lymphoproliferative disorder. A. CD3 shows an atypical T-cell lymphocytic infiltrate in dermis with focal epidermotropism. **B.** CD8 highlights the atypical T cells. **C** and **D.** EBER shows a strong positivity in the atypical T cells.

aggressive systemic disorder with lymphadenopathy and hepatosplenomegaly in (systemic HV-LPD).
- The neoplastic lymphocytes are small to medium in size with a perivascular, periadnexal, and interstitial distribution, occasionally extending into the subcutis. Epidermotropism and angiotropism are common.
- Most cases are CD8$^+$ cytotoxic T cell expressing TIA-1, granzyme B, or perforin. In some rare occasions, the lymphocytes will have a CD4$^+$ T-helper or CD4$^-$CD8$^-$ dual-negative phenotype or an NK phenotype (CD56$^+$).
- Histologically, HV-LPD can mimic other aggressive CTCLs; thus, clinical correlation is essential for appropriate classification.

References

1. Sonnex TS, Hawk JL. Hydroa vacciniforme: a review of ten cases. *Br J Dermatol*. 1988;118(1):101-108.
2. Gupta G, Man I, Kemmett D. Hydroa vacciniforme: a clinical and follow-up study of 17 cases. *J Am Acad Dermatol*. 2000;42(2 pt 1):208-213.
3. Quintanilla-Martinez L, Fend F. Deciphering hydroa vacciniforme. *Blood*. 2019;133(26):2735-2737.
4. Iwatsuki K, Ohtsuka M, Akiba H, Kaneko F. Atypical hydroa vacciniforme in childhood: from a smoldering stage to Epstein-Barr virus-associated lymphoid malignancy. *J Am Acad Dermatol*. 1999;40(2 pt 1):283-284.
5. Oh SJ, Lee J, Park JH, et al. Hydroa vacciniforme-like lymphoproliferative disorder in Korea: prognostic implication of clinical signs and whole blood Epstein-Barr virus DNA. *Ann Dermatol*. 2021;33(3):222-227.
6. Iwatsuki K, Miyake T, Hirai Y, Yamamoto T. Hydroa vacciniforme: a distinctive form of Epstein-Barr virus-associated T-cell lymphoproliferative disorders. *Eur J Dermatol*. 2019;29(1):21-28.
7. Quintanilla-Martinez LKH, Jaffe ES, *EBV positive T-cell lymphoproliferative disorders of childhood*. In: *WHO Classification of Tumours of Haematopoietic and Lymphoid Tissues 2008*. IARC press; 2008:278-260.
8. Sangueza M, Plaza JA. Hydroa vacciniforme-like cutaneous T-cell lymphoma: clinicopathologic and immunohistochemical study of 12 cases. *J Am Acad Dermatol*. 2013;69(1):112-119.
9. Barrionuevo C, Anderson VM, Zevallos-Giampietri E, et al. Hydroa-like cutaneous T-cell lymphoma: a clinicopathologic and molecular genetic study of 16 pediatric cases from Peru. *Appl Immunohistochem Mol Morphol*. 2002;10(1):7-14.

10. Wang X, Liang Y, Yang Y, et al. Hydroa vacciniforme-like lymphoproliferative disorder: a clinicopathological, immunohistochemical, and prognostic study of 24 cases in China. *J Dermatol.* 2021;48:1315-1326.
11. Ordonez-Parra J, Cortes MM, Tamayo-Buendía MM, GómezAMI. Hydroa vacciniforme-like lymphoproliferative disorder (HV-LPD) is an Epstein-Barr virus (EBV) associated disease. *An Bras Dermatol.* 2021;96(3):388-390.
12. Guo N, Chen Y, Wang Y, et al. Clinicopathological categorization of hydroa vacciniforme-like lymphoproliferative disorder: an analysis of prognostic implications and treatment based on 19 cases. *Diagn Pathol.* 2019;14(1):82.
13. Sundram U. Cutaneous lymphoproliferative disorders: what's new in the revised 4th Edition of the World Health Organization (WHO) classification of lymphoid neoplasms. *Adv Anat Pathol.* 2019;26(2):93-113.
14. Quintanilla-Martinez L, Ridaura C, Nagl F, et al. Hydroa vacciniforme-like lymphoma: a chronic EBV+ lymphoproliferative disorder with risk to develop a systemic lymphoma. *Blood.* 2013;122(18):3101-3110.
15. Mendoza N, Diamantis M, Arora A, et al. Mucocutaneous manifestations of Epstein-Barr virus infection. *Am J Clin Dermatol.* 2008;9(5):295-305.
16. Montes-Mojarro IA, Kim WY, Fend F, Quintanilla-Martinez L. Epstein-Barr virus positive T and NK-cell lymphoproliferations: morphological features and differential diagnosis. *Semin Diagn Pathol.* 2020;37(1):32-46.
17. Gru AA, Jaffe ES. Cutaneous EBV-related lymphoproliferative disorders. *Semin Diagn Pathol.* 2017;34(1):60-75.
18. Suzuki K, Ohshima K, Karube K, et al. Clinicopathological states of Epstein-Barr virus-associated T/NK-cell lymphoproliferative disorders (severe chronic active EBV infection) of children and young adults. *Int J Oncol.* 2004;24(5):1165-1174.
19. Xie Y, Wang T, Wang L. Hydroa vacciniforme-like lymphoproliferative disorder: a study of clinicopathology and whole-exome sequencing in Chinese patients. *J Dermatol Sci.* 2020;99(2):128-134.
20. Xue R, Elbendary A, Liu H, Chen Y, Cleaver N, Elston DM. Hydroa vacciniforme-like lymphoma: clinicopathologic description, treatment, and outcome. *J Am Acad Dermatol.* 2021;85(3):752-755.
21. Liu Y, Ma C, Wang G, Wang L, et al. Hydroa vacciniforme-like lymphoproliferative disorder: clinicopathologic study of 41 cases. *J Am Acad Dermatol.* 2019;81(2):534-540.
22. Magaña M, Massone C, Magaña P, Cerroni L. Clinicopathologic features of hydroa vacciniforme-like lymphoma: a series of 9 patients. *Am J Dermatopathol.* 2016;38(1):20-25.
23. Plaza JA, Sangueza M. Hydroa vacciniforme-like lymphoma with primarily periorbital swelling: 7 cases of an atypical clinical manifestation of this rare cutaneous T-cell lymphoma. *Am J Dermatopathol.* 2015;37(1):20-25.
24. Miyake T, Yamamoto T, Hirai Y, et al. Survival rates and prognostic factors of Epstein-Barr virus-associated hydroa vacciniforme and hypersensitivity to mosquito bites. *Br J Dermatol.* 2015;172(1):56-63.
25. Wang X, Wang P, Wang A, Xu Y, Wang L, Chen Z. Hydroa vacciniforme-like lymphoproliferative disorder in an adult invades the liver and bone marrow with clear pathological evidence: a case report and literature review. *BMC Infect Dis.* 2021;21(1):17.
26. Beltran BE, Maza I, Moisés-Alfaro CB, et al. Thalidomide for the treatment of hydroa vacciniforme-like lymphoma: report of four pediatric cases from Peru. *Am J Hematol.* 2014;89(12):1160-1161.
27. Ruan Y, Shen XY, Shi R, Zhao XQ, Zheng J. Hydroa vacciniforme-like lymphoproliferative disorder treated with intravenous immunoglobulin: long-term remission without haematopoietic stem cell transplantation or chemotherapy. *Acta Derm Venereol.* 2020;100(13):adv00192.
28. Magana M, SangüezaP, Gil-BeristainJ, et al. Angiocentric cutaneous T-cell lymphoma of childhood (hydroa-like lymphoma): a distinctive type of cutaneous T-cell lymphoma. *J Am Acad Dermatol.* 1998;38(4):574-579.
29. Doeden K, Molina-Kirsch H, Perez E, Warnke R, Sundaram U. Hydroa-like lymphoma with CD56 expression. *J Cutan Pathol.* 2008;35(5):488-494.
30. Wang GN, Cui Y, Zhao WG, et al. Clinicopathological analysis of the hydroa vacciniforme-like lymphoproliferative disorder with natural killer cell phenotype compared with cutaneous natural killer T-cell lymphoma. *Exp Ther Med.* 2018;16(6):4772-4778.
31. Tanaka C, Hasegawa M, Fujimoto M, et al. Phenotypic analysis in a case of hydroa vacciniforme-like eruptions associated with chronic active Epstein-Barr virus disease of gammadelta T cells. *Br J Dermatol.* 2012;166(1):216-218.
32. Demachi A, Nagata H, Morio T, et al. Characterization of Epstein-Barr virus (EBV)-positive NK cells isolated from hydroa vacciniforme-like eruptions. *Microbiol Immunol.* 2003;47(7):543-552.
33. Kim YJ, Choi ME, Lee WJ, Chang SE, Choi JH, Lee MW. The face of CD4(+) hydroa vacciniforme-like lymphoproliferative diseases: the shadow of systemic T-cell lymphoma. *Ann Dermatol.* 2019;31(Suppl):S17-S19.

CHAPTER 25

Natural killer–cell leukemias/lymphomas

Aharon G. Freud and Madelie Sellers

INTRODUCTION

Natural killer (NK) cells comprise a third major lineage of lymphocytes that are distinct from B cells and T cells but share many phenotypic and functional features with cytotoxic CD8+ T cells (see Chapter 3). Among their characteristic features are large granular lymphocyte morphology, a CD3−CD2+CD7+CD56+CD16+/− surface immunophenotype, and germline configuration of T-cell receptor (TCR) genes. In healthy peripheral blood specimens, NK cells may be subdivided into two major subsets: a CD56^{bright}CD16$^{dim/neg}$ subset that are circulating NK cells and a more predominant CD56^{dim}CD16+ subset. The CD56^{bright} NK-cell subset preferentially localizes to extramedullary sites such as secondary lymphoid tissues and the uterus where it likely plays roles in immunomodulation through the robust secretion of cytokines. The CD56^{dim} NK-cell subset shows more capacity for natural perforin-mediated cytotoxicity and likely functions as direct killers of tumor- or pathogen-infected cells.[1]

Neoplasms derived from NK cells are generally rare diseases, representing less than 1% of non-Hodgkin lymphoma (NHL), except in Asia and Central and South America, where they represent 3% to 6%. In the latest World Health Organization (WHO) classification of tumors of hematopoietic and lymphoid tissues (2017), three systemic neoplasms of mature NK-cell origin are included[2,3]: (1) chronic lymphoproliferative disorders of NK cells (CLPD-NK); (2) aggressive NK-cell leukemia (ANKL); and (3) extranodal NK/T-cell lymphoma, nasal type (ENKL), which is mainly a neoplasm of mature NK cells and also includes some T cell–derived lymphomas.[4,5] CLPD-NK is an indolent neoplasm rarely associated with transformation to an aggressive clinical course. In contrast, ANKL and ENKL are aggressive diseases with generally poor outcomes. Both ANKL and ENKL are associated with infection of the neoplastic cells by the Epstein-Barr virus (EBV).

In the older literature, a so-called blastic NK-cell lymphoma or CD4+CD56+ hematodermic neoplasm that characteristically involved not only the skin but also other sites was thought to be NK cell derived. However, it is now established that this neoplasm also expresses CD68 and CD123 (the interleukin [IL]-3 receptor) and originates from a plasmacytoid dendritic cell; it is no longer considered a type of NK-cell neoplasm and is referred to as blastic plasmacytoid dendritic cell neoplasm (see Chapter 56).

EXTRANODAL NK/T-CELL LYMPHOMA, NASAL TYPE

Definition

ENKL is a unique form of mature NK/T-cell lymphoma that is characterized by extranodal (frequently upper aerodigestive) infiltration by EBV-infected cytotoxic lymphocytes associated with vascular destruction and prominent necrosis. As the name of this disease implies (NK/T instead of NK), some cases originate from EBV-infected cytotoxic T cells.

Epidemiology

ENKL is rare in the United States and Europe and among those of European descent (<1% of NHL) but tends to be more prevalent in East Asian countries as well as among Native American populations in Mexico and South and Central America (up to 20% of NHL). It occurs most often in adults with a male predominance.[6,7]

Etiology

EBV plays an etiological role in the development of ENKL irrespective of the patient's origin.[3,8] A clonal episomal form of EBV is present with type II latency pattern (EBV nuclear antigen [EBNA]-1+, EBNA-2−, latent membrane protein [LMP]-1+), and it commonly shows a 30-bp deletion in the gene encoding LMP-1.[3,9] Most studies show that EBV is typically subtype A in Asia and subtype B in Western countries.[3,10,11] Extranodal NK/T-cell lymphomas can occur in the setting of immunosuppression, including following hematopoietic stem cell transplantation.[3] A low frequency of HLA-A*0201 allele has been reported in patients with ENKL,[12] suggesting that immune surveillance, likely associated with EBV infection, is important in the pathogenesis of the disease.

Clinical Presentation and Prognosis

ENKL characteristically has an extranodal presentation mostly in the upper aerodigestive tract including the nasal cavity, nasopharynx, paranasal sinuses, and palate. However, some cases show an extranasal presentation. Lymph nodes can also be involved. Patients present with symptoms associated with local tumor infiltration. Typical nasal-type ENKL may show localized disease early on but eventually may disseminate rapidly to various extranasal sites including the skin, gastrointestinal tract, testis, or cervical lymph nodes. Involvement of these sites may be associated with ulceration, perforation, and symptoms associated with a mass lesion. Systemic symptoms (fever, weight loss, malaise, and night sweats) can be present. ENKL may also be associated with the hemophagocytic syndrome.[3,13]

Historically, the prognosis is generally poor, although initial response to therapy is variable. Some patients respond to therapy and can achieve complete remission, whereas others die of disseminated disease despite aggressive therapy (WHO). The survival rate is 30% to 40%,[14,15] but in recent years it has improved with more intensive therapy including upfront radiotherapy and SMILE (dexamethaSone, Methotrexate, Ifosfamide, L-asparaginase, and Etoposide) regimen.[16] Unfavorable prognostic factors include advanced stage (III or IV), bone marrow (BM) or skin involvement, and high levels of EBV DNA in the serum.[3,14,17] Although the neoplastic cells of ENKL can range from small mature-appearing lymphocytes to large transformed cells, the prognostic importance of cytologic grade is unclear.

Histology

Histologic features of ENKL are similar irrespective of the site of involvement and characteristically include an angiocentric and angiodestructive growth pattern with coagulative necrosis, admixed apoptotic bodies, and fibrinoid change in blood vessels even in the absence of angioinvasion (Fig. 25-1).[3] Mucosal sites may show florid pseudoepitheliomatous hyperplasia of the overlying epithelium and/or ulceration with mucosal glands commonly widely spaced or absent.[3] The neoplastic infiltrate is composed of atypical lymphoid cells that may be small or medium sized to large or anaplastic, but in most cases the lymphoma is composed of medium-sized cells or a mixture of small and large cells. The chromatin is typically granular, although it may have a vesicular appearance in very large cells. Nucleoli are typically small and inconspicuous. Mitotic figures may be frequent, and the cells often have azurophilic cytoplasmic granules that appear ultrastructurally as electron-dense membrane-bound granules. Admixed small lymphocytes, histiocytes, and some granulocytes are often present in the background.[4,18]

Immunophenotype

ENKL is thought most commonly to derive from NK cells and less commonly from cytotoxic T cells (Figs. 25-2–25-5). Consistent with this is the fact that most cases show expression of NK-associated antigens including CD2, CD56, and cytolytic granules (granzyme B, TIA1, and perforin). Except for the minority of cases derived from T cells, ENKL will be negative for surface CD3 expression yet positive for cytoplasmic CD3 subunits including CD3ε and CD3ζ. As such, ENKL will be positive for CD3 when using polyclonal anti-CD3 antibodies for immunohistochemistry (IHC). ENKL is also typically positive for CD43, CD45RO, HLA-DR, CD25, and FAS (CD95) and negative for CD4, CD5, CD8, TCRδ, βF1, CD16, and CD57.[9,19] In situ hybridization studies for EBV-encoded RNA (EBER) are routinely used in clinical practice to confirm EBV infection.

Genetic and Molecular Findings

The TCR and immunoglobulin heavy chain (IGH) genes are in germline configurations in ENKL derived from NK cells. No specific genetic mutations have been identified, although del(6)(q21q25) and i(6)(p10) are common chromosomal abnormalities. Aberrant methylation of promoter CpG regions of multiple genes, in particular p73, has been reported.[20]

Skin Involvement

ENKL in the skin can represent either primary cutaneous disease (20% of primary cutaneous lymphoma in South Korea[10]; see Chapter 19) or cutaneous involvement by systemic ENKL. There appear to be no major clinical, epidemiologic, or histologic differences between primary and secondary cutaneous disease, although patients with ENKL that is restricted to the skin appear to have a better prognosis and response to therapy.[21,22] In patients with nasal-type ENKL and secondary cutaneous involvement, poor survival is associated with a high international prognostic index score.[14,21-23] Cutaneous involvement by systemic ENKL occurs in ~10% of patients and may present as multiple erythematous maculopapular lesions, cellulitis, abscess-like swelling, subcutaneous nodules, or ulceration.[13,21,24] Lesions are most commonly distributed throughout the extremities and trunk (especially the lower extremities).[21] The diagnosis relies on recognizing the typical histologic and immunophenotypic features described above for nasal-type ENKL including detection of EBER by in situ hybridization analysis (see Fig. 25-1).

Differential Diagnosis

The differential diagnosis, particularly for cutaneous involvement by ENKL, includes other EBV-associated T-cell or NK-cell lymphoproliferative disorders such as EBV+ peripheral T-cell lymphoma, not otherwise specified (PTCL-NOS), chronic active EBV infection, systemic EBV+ T-cell and NK-cell lymphoproliferative disease of childhood, and hydroa vacciniforme–like lymphoproliferative disorder, which also occurs predominantly in children. ANKL (described in the next section) is also in the

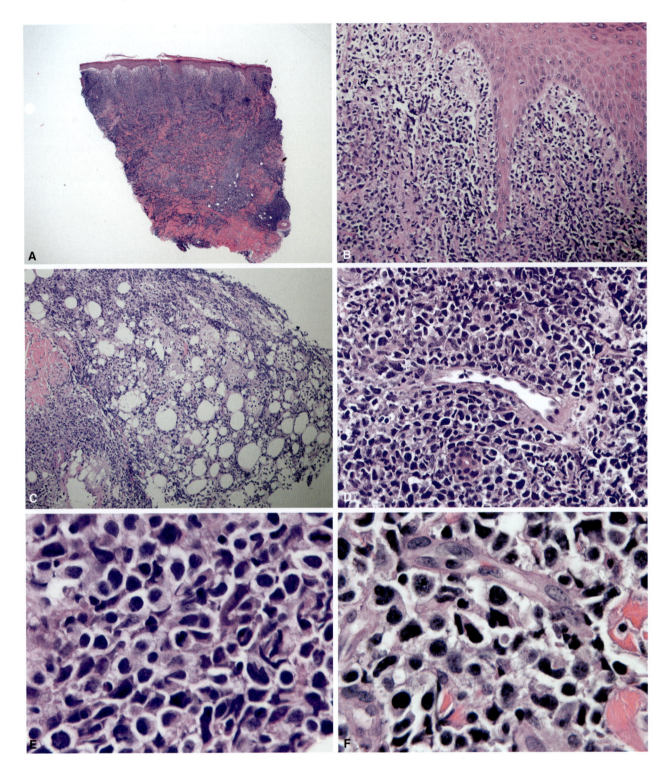

FIGURE 25-1. Extranodal NK/T-cell lymphoma involving the skin. A and **B** (low and intermediate magnifications—20× and 200×). There is a diffuse dermal infiltrate with an overall relative sparing of the surface epidermis. Occasional atypical cells show tagging along the entrance of an eccrine duct. **C** (intermediate magnification—100×). The infiltrate shows extension into the adipose tissue. **D** (high magnification—400×). Extensive angiotropism is present. **E** and **F** (high magnifications—600× and 1000×). The malignant cells are medium to large and show marked nuclear hyperchromasia and a moderate amount of cytoplasm with fine granules.

differential diagnosis, but ANKL rarely involves the skin, and so the clinical features and sites of involvement usually aid in distinguishing between ENKL and ANKL. The distinction of PTCL-NOS from ENKL is typically based on the EBV status, following the recommendations of the WHO classification. ENKLs are invariably EBV+, whereas PTCL-NOS in the setting of CD56 expression is EBV−. A recent study has shown no significant differences in survival when comparing primary cutaneous ENKL versus CD56+ PC PTCL. In addition, a differential diagnosis of

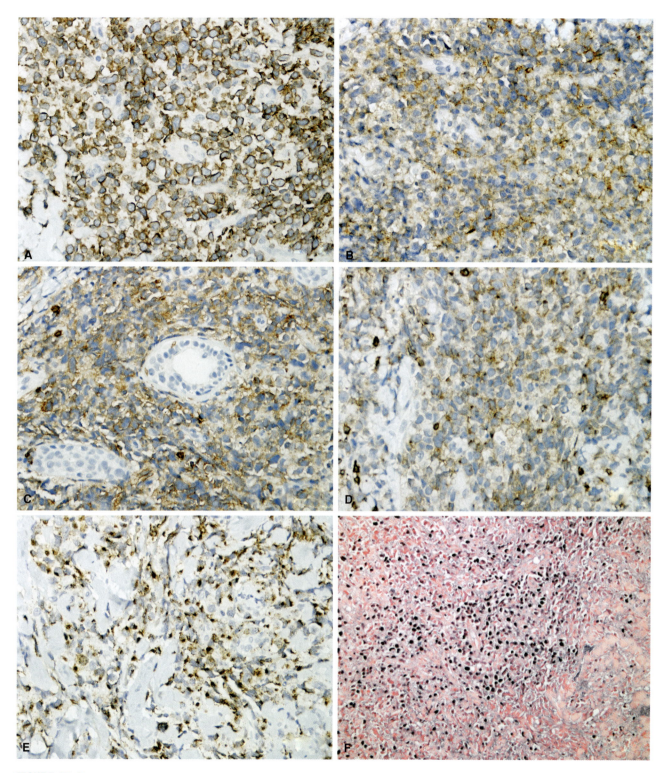

FIGURE 25-2. Extranodal NK/T-cell lymphoma involving the skin—IHC. The malignant lymphocytes are positive for CD3 **(A)**, CD56 **(B)**, CD8 **(C)**, and partially for CD7 **(D)**. **E.** Granzyme B is also diffusely positive in the tumor cells. **F.** Strong and diffuse expression of EBER is present.

primary cutaneous γδ T-cell lymphoma (PCGDL) should be considered, as those can also be CD56⁺. An additional difficulty arises from the fact that rarely PCGDL can be EBV+, making the distinction from ENKL completely arbitrary. Helping in the differential between PCGDL and ENKL is the fact that PCGDL shows γδ TCR expression and TCR gene rearrangement, whereas ENKL shows germline status of the TCR.

AGGRESSIVE NK-CELL LEUKEMIA

Definition

ANKL is a rare disease characterized by the proliferation of neoplastic NK cells almost always associated with EBV infection and associated with an aggressive clinical course and multiorgan involvement.

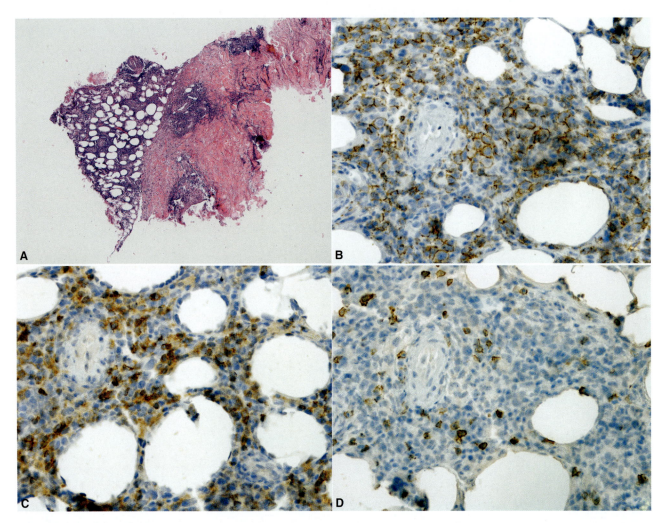

FIGURE 25-3. **Extranodal NK/T-cell lymphoma involving the skin. A** (low magnification—40×). There is a diffuse infiltrate particularly prominent in the adipose tissue. In this case, there is a more classic immunophenotype with CD56 coexpression **(B)**, but negative for CD4 **(C)** and CD8 **(D)**. EBER was also positive (not shown).

Epidemiology

There is a higher prevalence among individuals of Asian descent. There may be a slight male predominance, and the disease usually manifests in the third or fourth decade.[25]

Etiology

As with ENKL, there is a strong association with EBV infection and ANKL suggesting a pathogenic role of the virus. Likewise, the virus is in clonal episomal form and in a pattern suggestive of latency type II.[26]

Clinical Presentation and Prognosis

Patients with ANKL usually present with fever, constitutional symptoms, hepatosplenomegaly, and lymphadenopathy. The disease may be complicated by coagulopathy, hemophagocytic syndrome, and/or multiorgan failure. Sites of involvement are most commonly peripheral blood, bone marrow, liver, and spleen, but any organ may be involved. However, in contrast to ENKL, skin lesions in ANKL are uncommon. Laboratory studies often show anemia, neutropenia, thrombocytopenia, and elevated lactate dehydrogenase. High levels of Fas ligand may be detected in the serum.[18,27] The number of circulating leukemia cells is variable. Anthracycline-containing chemotherapy regimens are commonly offered as the initial therapy, and some patients may receive a stem cell transplant. Nonetheless, most cases have a fulminant clinical course; the median survival is less than 2 months, and the relapse rate is very high even after transplantation.[25,28-30]

Histology

The cytologic features of ANKL vary; the leukemia cells may range from normal-appearing large granular lymphocytes to markedly atypical cells with large irregular nuclei, open chromatin, and prominent nucleoli. Cytoplasmic granules are often present. In BM tissue sections, the neoplastic cells are often interstitially distributed and intermixed with reactive histiocytes. Hemophagocytosis may be prominent. Involved tissue sections typically show diffuse or patchy destructive infiltrates composed of a monotonous population of atypical lymphoid cells variably associated with admixed apoptotic bodies, necrosis, and angioinvasion.[4]

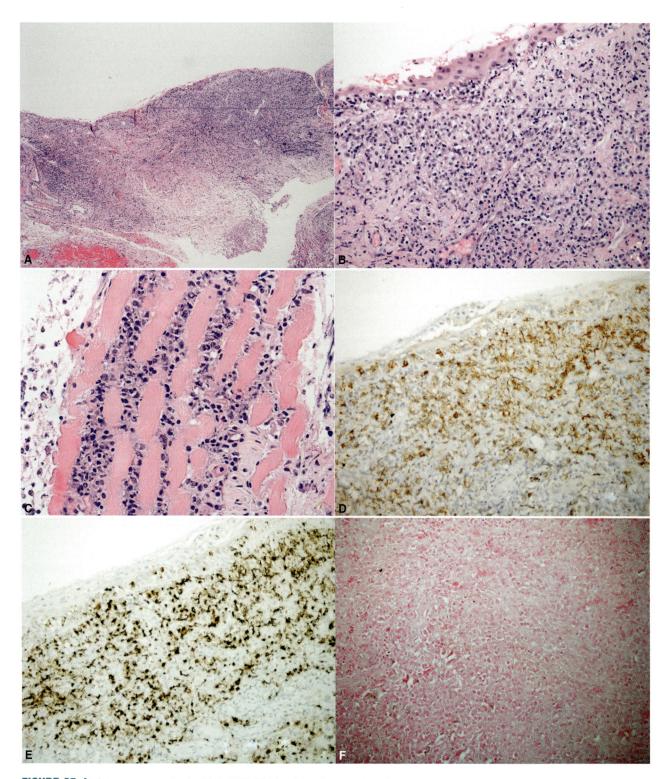

FIGURE 25-4. Cutaneous extension by CD56+ PTCL-NOS involving the orbit. **A** and **B** (low and intermediate magnifications—40× and 200×). There is a submucosal infiltrate with areas of epidermotropism. **C** (high magnification—400×). Diffuse infiltrate into the muscle fibers is noted. Marker karyorrhexis is present. The infiltrate is positive for CD56 **(D)** and granzyme B **(E)**, whereas it is negative for EBER **(F)**, a feature that puts this lymphoma under the category of PTCL-NOS.

Immunophenotype

The neoplastic cells in ANKL are usually CD2+, surface CD3−, cytoplasmic CD3+, and CD56+. They are also characteristically positive for cytotoxic molecules, and CD16 is reportedly expressed in ~75% of cases.[25] Most cases of ANKL are CD57−.[18]

Genetic and Molecular Findings

TCR and IGH genes are in the germline configurations. Therefore, if clinically applicable, clonality may be established by the demonstration of a clonal cytogenetic abnormality that occurs in 77% of cases.[7,31,32] Chromosomal abnormalities include del(6) (q21q25), 11q−, 7p−, 17p−, and 1q+; 6q− is more frequent in ENKL, whereas the other abnormalities listed above are more frequent in ANKL.[33]

Skin Involvement

As mentioned above, ANKL rarely involves the skin. Reported clinical and morphologic features of skin lesions in ANKL overlap with those associated with secondary cutaneous involvement by ENKL. ANKL shows similar immunophenotypic features to those of ENKL except that ENKL is typically CD16−, whereas CD16 is 75% positive in ANKL.[25]

Differential Diagnosis

The differential diagnosis of skin involvement by ANKL includes primary or secondary ENKL as well as PTCL-NOS, chronic active EBV infection, systemic EBV+ T-cell and NK-cell lymphoproliferative disease of childhood, and hydroa vacciniforme–like lymphoproliferative disorder. Other neoplastic infiltrates may be excluded by the detection of EBER by in situ hybridization.

CHRONIC LYMPHOPROLIFERATIVE DISORDERS OF NK CELLS

Definition

CLPD-NK is a provisional diagnosis in the 2017 WHO and defined as a chronic proliferation of NK cells in peripheral blood without any identified cause.[3,4,34] Typically, NK cells are present at a concentration of greater than 2×10^9/L for more than 6 months. Bone marrow and peripheral blood are primarily involved. The neoplastic cells are not infected by EBV.

Epidemiology

The disease occurs predominantly in adults (median age of 60 years) with no gender or ethnic predilection.[35]

Etiology

The etiology is unknown in CLPD-NK. Chronic viral or other antigenic stimulation has been postulated as an inciting factor leading to the outgrowth of a clonal NK-cell population.[2,36] Indeed as in the case of T-cell large granular lymphocytic leukemia (T-LGLL), there is a relatively high association with autoimmune disease.[37] There is as yet no evidence of direct NK-cell infection by EBV as there is for ENKL and ANKL.

Clinical Presentation and Prognosis

Most patients are asymptomatic, and the increase in NK-cell large granular lymphocytes is detected incidentally. However, some patients present with signs and symptoms associated with cytopenias (mainly neutropenia and anemia). Lymphadenopathy, hepatosplenomegaly, and other organ system involvement are rare or unreported. Sometimes, other medical conditions (solid tumors, hematologic neoplasms, vasculitis, splenectomy, neuropathy, and autoimmune disorders) may occur in association with CLPD-NK.[35] Most patients follow an indolent clinical course and may not require therapeutic intervention. Patients with cytopenias, recurrent infections, and (rarely) cytogenetic abnormalities do worse and may be treated with immunosuppressive agents.[38] Rare cases of transformation into an acute and aggressive disease similar to ENKL have been reported.[39]

Morphology

The NK cells in CLPD-NK show typical large granular lymphocyte morphology characterized by small-to-intermediate-size cells with round-to-mildly irregular nuclear contours, condensed chromation, moderate amounts of slightly basophilic cytoplasm, and coarse azurophilic cytoplasmic granules. Bone marrow involvement may be very subtle, and an increase or atypical infiltration of NK cells within sinusoids and/or in the interstitium may only be identifiable upon immunohistochemical analysis.[40] For T-LGLL, which shows many overlapping features with CLPD-NK, the detection of atypical clusters of granzyme B+ lymphocytes is helpful in making the diagnosis.[41,42]

Immunophenotype

The typical immunophenotype detected in CLPD-NK is that of a mature CD16+ NK cell showing expression of CD2, cytoplasmic CD3, and cytolytic granules. CD56 expression may be weak or absent as can the expression of other pan–NK-cell markers such as CD335 (NKp46).[43] Other NK- and T-cell–associated antigens, including CD2, CD7, and CD57, are variably expressed. The expression of the major histocompatibility complex–binding receptors, CD94/NKG2A and killer immunoglobulin-like receptors (KIRs), shows altered and restricted patterns of expression.[42]

Genetic and Molecular Findings

Most reported cases of CLPD-NK show a normal karyotype. TCR and IGH genes are in the germline configurations. Mutations in signal transducer and activator of transcription (STAT3) molecules have been reported in approximately one-third of cases.[44,45]

Skin Involvement

Skin involvement either rarely occurs or has been underreported in CLPD-NK.[2] CLPD-NK shares many morphologic, immunophenotypic, and clinical features with T-LGLL, which is associated with skin lesions in ~20% of cases.[46-48] Skin lesions associated with T-LGLL vary and can manifest as petechiae, edema, erythroderma, purpura, and/or nodules.[49-52] A case of T-LGLL presenting with generalized pruritus has also been reported.[53]

Differential Diagnosis

Clonal CLPD-NK should be distinguished from reactive LGL expansions that can occur in the settings of splenectomy, viral infections, stem cell or BM transplantation, autoimmune disease, and certain drugs (eg, imatinib), among others. Detection of a restricted CD94/NKG2A and/or KIR pattern of expression helps to distinguish CLPD-NK from these reactive expansions.[41] The clinical features and absence of EBV infection exclude ANKL and ENKL.

NK-CELL ENTEROPATHY LYMPHOPROLIFERATIVE DISORDER

In 2011, Mansoor et al reported a series of eight patients with NK-cell enteropathy (NKE).[54] Such patients complained of vague abdominal distress and had biopsy findings confirming the presence of an abnormal population of lymphocytes filling the lamina propia of the mucosa and in some stages destruction of the glands. In general, there was absence of significant epitheliotropism, a feature that was useful to separate apart this process from the enteropathy associated T-cell lymphoma, a process in intimate association with celiac sprue. This population of cells had an NK-cell phenotype (CD3, CD56, CD2, CD7), lacked evidence of EBV infection, had germline rearrangement of the T-cell receptor, and had a very indolent clinical course. Indeed, many of such patients were originally diagnosed as having a NK/T-cell lymphoma and subsequently received chemotherapy. The study reported no instances of mortality or disease progression in five patients over a median follow-up of 30 months. Takeuchi et al reported a similar cohort of patients with a so-called lymphomatoid gastropathy in 2010.[55] In their series the infiltrates were limited to the mucosa of the stomach and in some cases had areas of necrosis. T-cell clonality also showed no rearrangement of the TCR. More recently, Gru et al reported a case of enteropathy-like NK-cell lymphoproliferative disorder presenting in the vaginal mucosa (Figs. 25-5 and 25-6).

The molecular nature of NKE is poorly understood; however, a recent study by Xiao et al revealed the presence of *JAK3 K563_C565del* mutations in 3/10 patients with NKE (30%).[56] The authors speculated that such mutations can lead to activations downstream of STAT3 and STAT5 signaling pathways. These results suggest a clonal and "neoplastic" origin of this process, at least in a subset of cases. Interestingly, *JAK3* mutations are not specific for this process and have been reported in a variety of T- and NK-cell lymphomas.

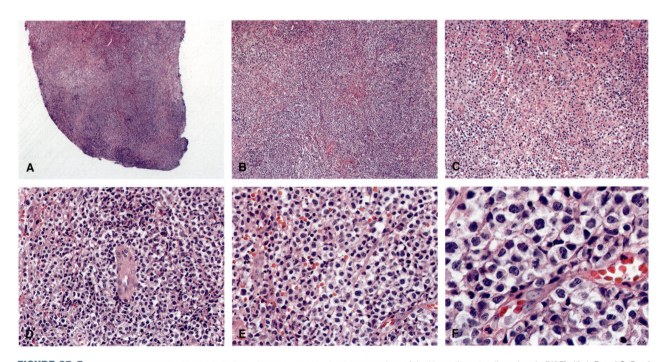

FIGURE 25-5. NK-cell enteropathy-like LPD. **A.** The infiltrate extends to the deeper portions of the biopsy (hematoxylin and eosin [H&E], 40×). **B** and **C.** Focal areas of necrosis are seen in the infiltrate (H&E, 100× and 200×). **D.** The atypical lymphocytic infiltrate exhibits angiotropism in the absence of angionecrosis (H&E, 400×). **E** and **F.** The cytologic features of this infiltrate are characterized by the presence of medium and large cells, with ample cytoplasm, fine granularity, and some nuclear contour irregularities. Mitotic figures are present (H&E, 600× and 1000×). Obtained with permission.

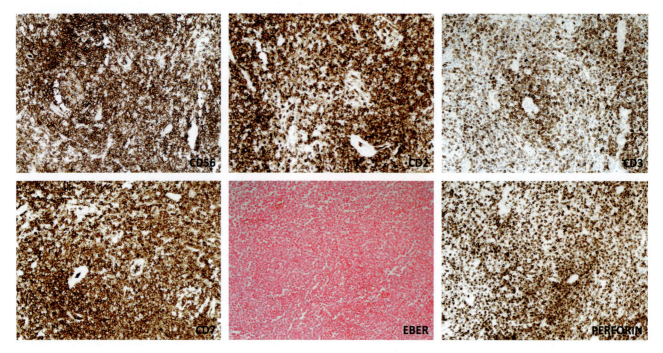

FIGURE 25-6. NK-cell enteropathy-like LPD—immunophenotype. Immunophenotypic features of the infiltrate. The atypical lymphoid cells are positive for CD56, CD2, CD3 (partial and with a cytoplasmic character), and CD7. EBER is negative in the lesional cells. Most of the cells show expression of the cytotoxic marker perforin. Obtained with permission.

References

1. Caligiuri MA. Human natural killer cells. *Blood.* 2008;112(3):461-469.
2. Semenzato G, Marino F, Zambello R. State of the art in natural killer cell malignancies. *Int J Lab Hematol.* 2012;34(2):117-128.
3. Swerdlow S, Campo E, Harris NL, et al. (eds.). *WHO Classification of Tumors of Haematopoietic and Lymphoid Tissue.* revised 4th ed. International Agency for Research on Cancer; 2017.
4. Liang X, Graham DK. Natural killer cell neoplasms. *Cancer.* 2008;112(7):1425-1436.
5. Kinney MC, Jones D. Cutaneous T-cell and NK-cell lymphomas: the WHO-EORTC classification and the increasing recognition of specialized tumor types. *Am J Clin Pathol.* 2007;127(5):670-686.
6. Greer JP, Mosse CA. Natural killer-cell neoplasms. *Curr Hematol Malig Rep.* 2009;4(4):245-252.
7. Lima M. Aggressive mature natural killer cell neoplasms: from epidemiology to diagnosis. *Orphanet J Rare Dis.* 2013;8:95.
8. Harabuchi Y, Takahara M, Kishibe K, et al. Extranodal natural killer/T-cell lymphoma, nasal type: basic science and clinical progress. *Front Pediatr.* 2019;7:141.
9. Kuo TT, Shih LY, Tsang NM. Nasal NK/T cell lymphoma in Taiwan: a clinicopathologic study of 22 cases, with analysis of histologic subtypes, Epstein–Barr virus LMP-1 gene association, and treatment modalities. *Int J Surg Pathol.* 2004;12(4):375-387.
10. Jang MS, Kang DY, Park JB, et al. Cutaneous T-cell lymphoma in Asians. *ISRN Dermatol.* 2012;2012:575120.
11. Chen XY, Pepper SD, Arrand JR. Prevalence of the A and B types of Epstein–Barr virus DNA in nasopharyngeal carcinoma biopsies from southern China. *J Gen Virol.* 1992;73(pt. 2):463-466.
12. Kanno H, Kojya S, Li T, et al. Low frequency of HLA-A*0201 allele in patients with Epstein–Barr virus-positive nasal lymphomas with polymorphic reticulosis morphology. *Int J Cancer.* 2000;87(2):195-199.
13. Chan JK, Sin VC, Wong KF, et al. Nonnasal lymphoma expressing the natural killer cell marker CD56: a clinicopathologic study of 49 cases of an uncommon aggressive neoplasm. *Blood.* 1997;89(12):4501-4513.
14. Chim CS, Ma SY, Au WY, et al. Primary nasal natural killer cell lymphoma: long-term treatment outcome and relationship with the International Prognostic Index. *Blood.* 2004;103(1):216-221.
15. Barrionuevo C, Zaharia M, Martinez MT, et al. Extranodal NK/T-cell lymphoma, nasal type: study of clinicopathologic and prognosis factors in a series of 78 cases from Peru. *Appl Immunohistochem Mol Morphol.* 2007;15(1):38-44.
16. Yamaguchi M, Suzuki R, Kwong YL, et al. Phase I study of dexamethasone, methotrexate, ifosfamide, l-asparaginase, and etoposide (SMILE) chemotherapy for advanced-stage, relapsed or refractory extranodal natural killer (NK)/T-cell lymphoma and leukemia. *Cancer Sci.* 2008;99(5):1016-1020.
17. Huang WT, Chang KC, Huang GC, et al. Bone marrow that is positive for Epstein–Barr virus encoded RNA-1 by in situ hybridization is related with a poor prognosis in patients with extranodal natural killer/T-cell lymphoma, nasal type. *Haematologica.* 2005;90(8):1063-1069.
18. Chan JK. Natural killer cell neoplasms. *Anat Pathol (Chic IL).* 1998;3:77-145.
19. Hasserjian RP, Harris NL. NK-cell lymphomas and leukemias: a spectrum of tumors with variable manifestations and immunophenotype. *Am J Clin Pathol.* 2007;127(6):860-868.
20. Siu LL, Chan JK, Wong KF, et al. Specific patterns of gene methylation in natural killer cell lymphomas: p73 is consistently involved. *Am J Pathol.* 2002;160(1):59-66.

21. Lee WJ, Jung JM, Won CH, et al. Cutaneous extranodal natural killer/T-cell lymphoma: a comparative clinicohistopathologic and survival outcome analysis of 45 cases according to the primary tumor site. *J Am Acad Dermatol.* 2014;70(6):1002-1009.
22. Suzuki R. NK/T-cell lymphomas: pathobiology, prognosis and treatment paradigm. *Curr Oncol Rep.* 2012;14(5):395-402.
23. Kim TM, Park YH, Lee SY, et al. Local tumor invasiveness is more predictive of survival than International Prognostic Index in stage I(E)/II(E) extranodal NK/T-cell lymphoma, nasal type. *Blood.* 2005;106(12):3785-3790.
24. Radonich MA, Lazova R, Bolognia J. Cutaneous natural killer/T-cell lymphoma. *J Am Acad Dermatol.* 2002;46(3):451-456.
25. Suzuki R, Suzumiya J, Nakamura S, et al. Aggressive natural killer-cell leukemia revisited: large granular lymphocyte leukemia of cytotoxic NK cells. *Leukemia.* 2004;18(4):763-770.
26. Kawa-Ha K, Ishihara S, Ninomiya T, et al. CD3-negative lymphoproliferative disease of granular lymphocytes containing Epstein–Barr viral DNA. *J Clin Invest.* 1989;84(1):51-55.
27. Kato K, Ohshima K, Ishihara S, et al. Elevated serum soluble Fas ligand in natural killer cell proliferative disorders. *Br J Haematol.* 1998;103(4):1164-1166.
28. Ito T, Makishima H, Nakazawa H, et al. Promising approach for aggressive NK cell leukaemia with allogeneic haematopoietic cell transplantation. *Eur J Haematol.* 2008;81(2):107-111.
29. Kwong YL. The diagnosis and management of extranodal NK/T-cell lymphoma, nasal-type and aggressive NK-cell leukemia. *J Clin Exp Hematop.* 2011;51(1):21-28.
30. Suzuki R. Treatment of advanced extranodal NK/T cell lymphoma, nasal-type and aggressive NK-cell leukemia. *Int J Hematol.* 2010;92(5):697-701.
31. Ryder J, Wang X, Bao L, et al. Aggressive natural killer cell leukemia: report of a Chinese series and review of the literature. *Int J Hematol.* 2007;85(1):18-25.
32. Wong KF, Zhang YM, Chan JK. Cytogenetic abnormalities in natural killer cell lymphoma/leukaemia—is there a consistent pattern? *Leuk Lymphoma.* 1999;34(3/4):241-250.
33. Nakashima Y, Tagawa H, Suzuki R, et al. Genome-wide array-based comparative genomic hybridization of natural killer cell lymphoma/leukemia: different genomic alteration patterns of aggressive NK-cell leukemia and extranodal NK/T-cell lymphoma, nasal type. *Genes Chromosomes Cancer.* 2005;44(3):247-255.
34. Oshimi K. Leukemia and lymphoma of natural killer lineage cells. *Int J Hematol.* 2003;78(1):18-23.
35. Lima M, Almeida J, Montero AG, et al. Clinicobiological, immunophenotypic, and molecular characteristics of monoclonal CD56−/+dim chronic natural killer cell large granular lymphocytosis. *Am J Pathol.* 2004;165(4):1117-1127.
36. Loughran TP Jr, Hadlock KG, Yang Q, et al. Seroreactivity to an envelope protein of human T-cell leukemia/lymphoma virus in patients with CD3− (natural killer) lymphoproliferative disease of granular lymphocytes. *Blood.* 1997;90(5):1977-1981.
37. Rabbani GR, Phyliky RL, Tefferi A. A long-term study of patients with chronic natural killer cell lymphocytosis. *Br J Haematol.* 1999;106(4):960-966.
38. Oshimi K, Yamada O, Kaneko T, et al. Laboratory findings and clinical courses of 33 patients with granular lymphocyte-proliferative disorders. *Leukemia.* 1993;7(6):782-788.
39. Huang Q, Chang KL, Gaal KK, et al. An aggressive extranodal NK-cell lymphoma arising from indolent NK-cell lymphoproliferative disorder. *Am J Surg Pathol.* 2005;29(11):1540-1543.
40. Tefferi A. Chronic natural killer cell lymphocytosis. *Leuk Lymphoma.* 1996;20(3/4):245-248.
41. Morice WG. The immunophenotypic attributes of NK cells and NK-cell lineage lymphoproliferative disorders. *Am J Clin Pathol.* 2007;127(6):881-886.
42. Morice WG, Kurtin PJ, Leibson PJ, et al. Demonstration of aberrant T-cell and natural killer-cell antigen expression in all cases of granular lymphocytic leukaemia. *Br J Haematol.* 2003;120(6):1026-1036.
43. Freud AG, Zhao S, Wei S, et al. Expression of the activating receptor, NKp46 (CD335), in human natural killer and T-cell neoplasia. *Am J Clin Pathol.* 2013;140(6):853-866.
44. Ishida F, Matsuda K, Sekiguchi N, et al. STAT3 gene mutations and their association with pure red cell aplasia in large granular lymphocyte leukemia. *Cancer Sci.* 2014;105(3):342-346.
45. Jerez A, Clemente MJ, Makishima H, et al. STAT3 mutations unify the pathogenesis of chronic lymphoproliferative disorders of NK cells and T-cell large granular lymphocyte leukemia. *Blood.* 2012;120(15):3048-3057.
46. Pandolfi F, Loughran TP Jr, Starkebaum G, et al. Clinical course and prognosis of the lymphoproliferative disease of granular lymphocytes. a multicenter study. *Cancer.* 1990;65(2):341-348.
47. Semenzato G, Zambello R, Starkebaum G, et al. The lymphoproliferative disease of granular lymphocytes: updated criteria for diagnosis. *Blood.* 1997;89(1):256-260.
48. Zambello R, Teramo A, Gattazzo C, et al. Are T-LGL leukemia and NK-chronic lymphoproliferative disorder really two distinct diseases? *Transl Med UniSa.* 2014;8:4-11.
49. van Steensel MA, van Gelder M, van Marion AM, et al. T-cell large granular lymphocytic leukaemia with an uncommon clinical and immunological phenotype. *Acta Derm Venereol.* 2009;89(2):172-174.
50. Kim J, Park CJ, Jang S, et al. A case of CD4(+)T-cell large granular lymphocytic leukemia. *Ann Lab Med.* 2013;33(3):196-199.
51. Herling M, Khoury JD, Washington LT, et al. A systematic approach to diagnosis of mature T-cell leukemias reveals heterogeneity among WHO categories. *Blood.* 2004;104(2):328-335.
52. Magro CM, Morrison CD, Heerema N, et al. T-cell prolymphocytic leukemia: an aggressive T cell malignancy with frequent cutaneous tropism. *J Am Acad Dermatol.* 2006;55(3):467-477.
53. Mallo S, Coto P, Caminal L, et al. Generalized pruritus as presentation of T-cell large granular lymphocyte leukaemia. *Clin Exp Dermatol.* 2008;33(3):348-349.
54. Mansoor A, Pittaluga S, Beck PL, Wilson WH, Ferry JA, Jaffe ES. NK-cell enteropathy—a benign NK-cell lymphoproliferative disease mimicking intestinal lymphoma: clinicopathologic features and follow-up in a unique case series. *Blood.* 2011;117(5):1447-1452.
55. Takeuchi K, Yokoyama M, Ishizawa S. Lymphomatoid gastropathy: a distinct clinicopathologic entity of self-limited pseudomalignant NK-cell proliferation. *Blood.* 2010;116(25):5631-5637.
56. Xiao W, Gupta GK, Yao J, et al. Recurrent somatic JAK3 mutations in NK-cell enteropathy. *Blood.* 2019;134(12):986-991.

PART V — SYSTEMIC T- AND NK-CELL LYMPHOMAS WITH CUTANEOUS DISSEMINATION

CHAPTER 26

Systemic anaplastic large cell lymphoma

Alejandro A. Gru and Werner Kempf

DEFINITION

Anaplastic lymphoma kinase positive (ALK⁺) anaplastic large cell lymphoma (ALCL) is a mature T-cell lymphoma with expression of CD30 and ALK1 and translocation of the *ALK1* gene.[1] ALCL with similar morphologic and phenotypic features but lacking ALK1 expression and translocation of the *ALK1* gene is a separate and provisional category in the current World Health Organization (WHO) classification (ALK⁻ ALCL).[2]

EPIDEMIOLOGY

ALK⁺ ALCL is the second most common (25%) subtype of peripheral T-cell lymphoma (PTCL) and accounts for 5% of non-Hodgkin lymphomas (NHLs). It is the most common subtype of PTCL in children and accounts for 10% to 30% of all pediatric lymphomas.[3-5] ALK⁻ ALCL represents 40% to 50% of all ALCLs and occurs in the older population, predominantly in the sixth decade of life.[2] ALK⁻ ALCL is rare in infants, children, and young individuals (<10%).[6-8] The median age at diagnosis in pediatric patients is approximately 10.2 to 11.0 years. ALK⁻ ALCL shows a slight male predominance.

CLINICAL PRESENTATION AND PROGNOSIS

Most cases of ALK⁺ ALCL present with lymphadenopathy. The most common extranodal site is the skin (26%).[9-12] Other affected sites include bone, lung, liver, and soft tissues.[1] A leukemic presentation is rare and more frequent in the small cell variant.[13] The bone marrow is affected in a small percentage (10% to 30%) of cases.[14] Affected individuals with ALK⁻ ALCL also present with lymphadenopathy and extranodal involvement.[8,15] Approximately 17% of ALK⁻ ALCL cases have cutaneous involvement.[8] Most patients have advanced disease (stage III or IV) and B-symptoms.

The cutaneous manifestation of ALK⁺ ALCL can be precipitated by insect bites.[16,17] Lesions resemble typical arthropod bite reactions without clinical resolution. Most patients with ALK⁺ ALCL or ALK⁻ have pink papulonodular lesions.[18-20] The lesions are more frequently solitary and rarely multiple (Figs. 26-1A,B and 26-2). Rare cases of isolated cutaneous ALCL (C-ALCL), ALK⁺ have been reported.[21] Some uncommon clinical appearances include generalized erythroderma,[22] orbital lesions,[23] and ichthyosis.[24]

The prognoses of ALK⁺ ALCL, ALK⁻ ALCL, and PTCLs not otherwise specified (PTCL-NOS) are significantly different. ALK⁺ ALCL has a good prognosis with a 5-year survival rate of 70% to 80% in contrast to 49% and 32% 5-year survival rates for ALK⁻ ALCL and PTCL-NOS, respectively.[8,25]

A recently described form of ALCL occurring in association with breast implants has a more indolent behavior. Some of these patients can present with skin ulceration.[26-30] Removal of the implants appears to be curative.[29]

HISTOLOGY

ALCL is typified by "hallmark" cells: large neoplastic cells with a pleomorphic, horseshoe-shaped nuclei, prominent central Golgi zone, and abundant pale cytoplasm.[31] A wreath-like appearance of the nuclei can also be seen. Mitoses are common. Lymphoma cells are frequently located in perivascular spaces. Several histologic variants are recognized by the WHO classification: (a) lymphohistiocytic (10% to 20%), (b) small cell (5% to 10%),[32] (c) Hodgkin-like (3%),[33] and (d) nodular sclerosing variants (<5%). More uncommon variants include multinucleated giant cells and sarcomatoid and myxoid forms.[1,3-5] In ALK⁻ ALCL, the cytology of the tumor cells is identical to that of ALK⁺ ALCL, but the tumor cells tend to

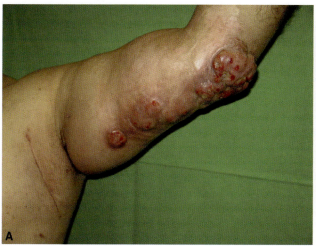
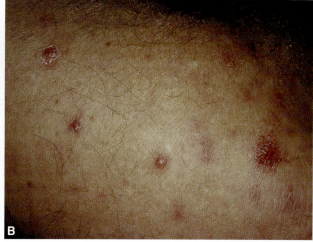

FIGURE 26-1. **Anaplastic large cell lymphoma, systemic.** Large ulcerated nodules in the arm **(A)** and trunk **(B)**.

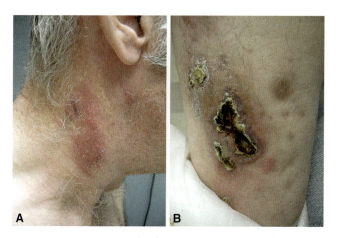

FIGURE 26-2. **A case of ALK⁻ ALCL with an intravascular distribution and cutaneous dissemination. A.** Erythematous, indurated, plaque with "pustules" on the right lateral neck. **B.** Erythematous, crusted, multinodular plaque on the right leg. (From Deetz CO, Gilbertson KG II, Anadkat MJ, et al. A rare case of intravascular large T-cell lymphoma with an unusual T helper phenotype. *Am J Dermatopathol*. 2011;33(8):e99–e102, with permission.)

be larger and more pleomorphic. Small cell–predominant ALK⁻ ALCL is uncommon and should be classified as PTCL-NOS.[6]

Cutaneous involvement by ALCL is usually manifested by a superficial and deep mostly nodular dermal infiltration with extension into the adipose tissue (Figs. 26-3–26-6). The features are similar to primary C-ALCL. Ulceration and acanthosis can occur, whereas epidermotropism is infrequent. Uncommon systemic variants with skin involvement include myxoid[34] and small cell forms.[13,32] The small cell variant is frequently associated with widespread disseminated disease, and initial biopsies may be from sites such as skin, liver, or body cavities.[6] The pyogenic variant (Fig. 26-7) contains numerous neutrophils and histiocytes, which can potentially mask the tumor cells, which may be present as scattered element with a dense background of inflammatory cells. Some of these cases follow an indolent clinical course similar to lymphomatoid papulosis or C-ALCL.[35-37] Some cases can also show a predominantly intravascular dissemination pattern, which can potentially mimic an intravascular B-cell lymphoma (Fig. 26-8). Rare examples of breast-implant associated ALCL with skin dissemination have been reported.[38]

IMMUNOPHENOTYPE

The immunophenotype of ALK⁺ ALCL is characterized by the presence of CD30 and ALK expression. Strong membranous and Golgi staining pattern for CD30 in virtually every cell is characteristic. Treatment with the anti-CD30 agent brentuximab vedotin can cause a drastic reduction in the degree of CD30 expression.[39] In the majority of the cases, there is a loss of multiple T-cell antigens, including CD3, CD5, and CD7.[40] CD2 and CD4 are frequently preserved. Some cases can be positive for T-cell receptors (TCRs). Cytotoxic markers (perforin, TIA-1, and granzyme B) are usually expressed (see Fig. 26-4).[41] The majority of systemic ALCLs are positive for epithelial membrane antigen (EMA), and rare cases can be CD15⁺.[42] Cytokeratins, PAX5, CD13, and CD33 can be aberrantly expressed. The cellular localization of the ALK expression correlates with the pattern of translocation: the *NPM/ALK* fusion leads to both nuclear and cytoplasmic ALK staining. The ALK staining patterns in less-common translocation variants include diffuse cytoplasmic (eg, *TPM3, ATIC, TFG, TPM4, MYH9, ALO17*), granular cytoplasmic (*CLTC*), or membranous (*MSN*). ALK⁻ ALCL shows strong and diffuse expression of CD30 (see Figs. 26-3–26-6). The pattern can be membranous, Golgi, and/or cytoplasmic. The strong and diffuse character is often a helpful clue to distinguish ALK⁻ ALCL from PTCL-NOS. Lack of multiple pan–T-cell antigens and the expression of cytotoxic markers are characteristic. EMA and clusterin can be positive, but less frequent than in ALK⁺ ALCL.[8]

Rare ALCLs have a CD8⁺ phenotype (see Fig. 26-4). Approximately 85% to 90% of ALCLs have a detectable clonal T-cell gene rearrangement, and the remainder of cases are considered "null cell type" (see Fig. 26-6).[4,7,40,41] Approximately 10% of cases show clonal *IGH* gene rearrangement. The majority of ALK⁺ ALCL cases express CD25 and CD99.[43] Rare cases express cytokeratins[44] and human

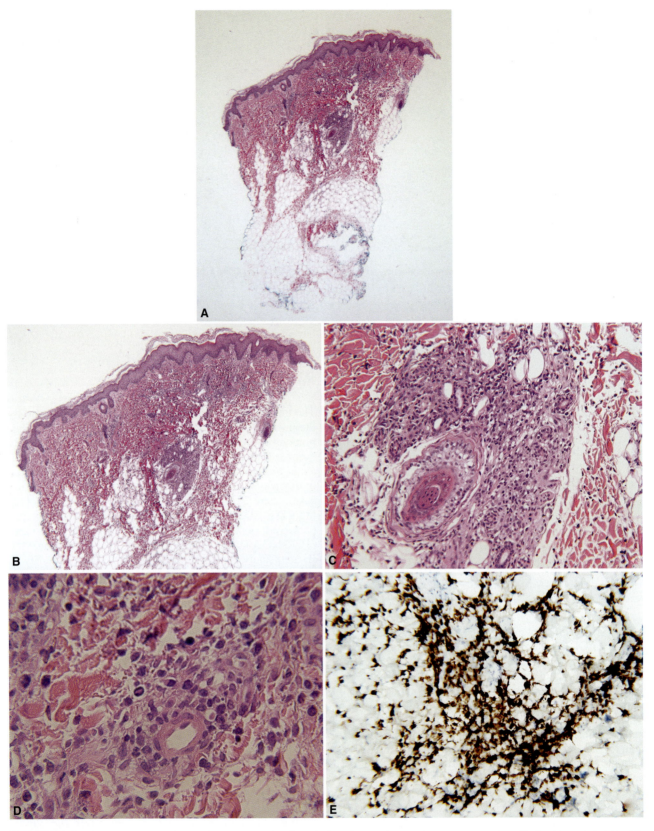

FIGURE 26-3. **ALK+ ALCL, "small cell variant," with cutaneous dissemination. A** and **B.** Perifollicular infiltrate resembling folliculitis (20× and 40×). **C** and **D.** The infiltrate is composed of small mononuclear cells with marked hyperchromasia and variably prominent nucleoli (200× and 400×). **E.** The tumor cells are strongly positive for ALK1.

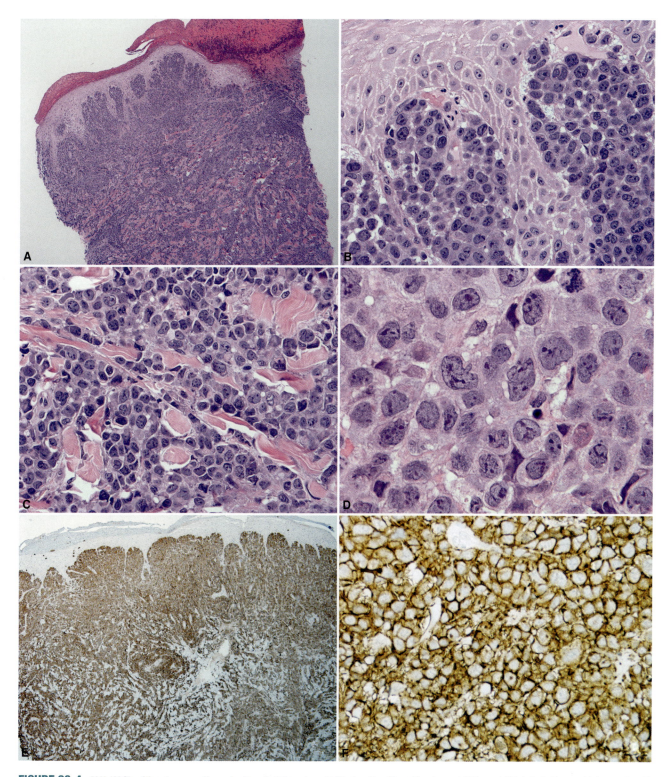

FIGURE 26-4. ALK⁻ ALCL with cutaneous dissemination. A. Diffuse dermal infiltrate with epidermal involvement (200× and 400×). **B–D.** Pleomorphic large cells with irregular nuclear membranes and prominent nucleoli. **E** and **F.** Malignant cells are diffusely positive for CD3 and CD30.

chorionic gonadotropin (HCG).[45] Cases with *DUSP22* translocations are typically positive for LEF-1.[46]

POSTULATED CELL OF ORIGIN

Mature postthymic T cell.

GENETIC AND MOLECULAR FINDINGS

ALK⁺ ALCL have rearrangements of the *ALK* gene at 2p23 with various partner genes, most typically the nucleophosmin (*NPM*) at 5q35.[47,48] Some translocations can be cryptic by conventional cytogenetic methods. Other translocation partners include non-muscle tropomyosin (*TPM3*, 1q25 and *TPM4*, 19p13.1); amino

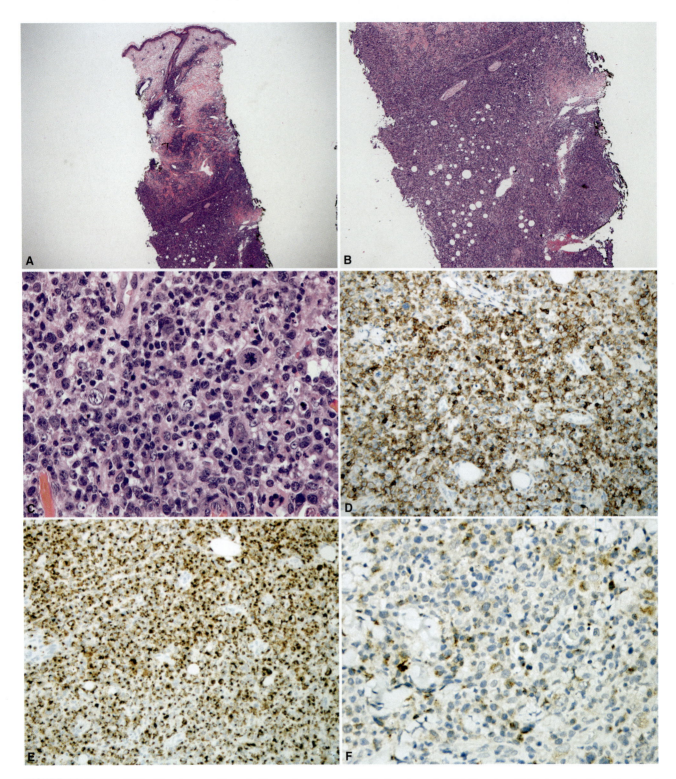

FIGURE 26-5. ALK⁻ ALCL with cutaneous dissemination and uncommon (CD8⁺) phenotype. **A** and **B.** Deep dermal infiltrate sparing the epidermis and extending into the adipose tissue (20× and 40×). **C.** The infiltrate is composed of large and pleomorphic cells with numerous mitoses, including atypical forms (400×). Malignant cells are positive for CD8 **(D)**, granzyme B **(E)**, and EMA **(F)**.

terminus of 5-aminoimidazole-4-carboxamide ribonucleotide formyltransferase/IMP cyclohydrolase gene (*ATIC*, 2q35); TRK-fused gene (*TFG*, 3q21); clathrin heavy polypeptide gene (*CLTC*, 17q23); moesin gene (*MSN*, Xq11-12); myosin heavy chain 9 gene (*MYH9*, 22q11.2); and ALK lymphoma oligomerization partner on chromosome 17 (*ALO17*, 17q25).[1,6]

Rearrangements of the *DUSP22-IRF4* locus have been described in ALK⁻ ALCL and in approximately one-third of C_ALCL.[49-51] The most common partner is *FRA7H* at 7q32. 6p25.3 rearrangements are mutually exclusive of ALK translocations. They are classically seen in C-ALCL but can be seen in ALK⁻ ALCL in 18% of cases. We have also reported the unusual occurrence of

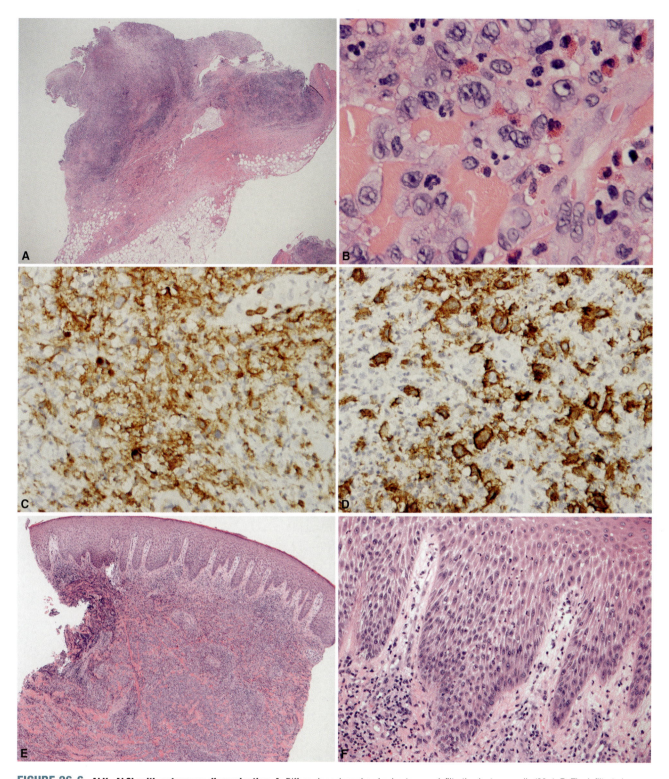

FIGURE 26-6. ALK⁻ ALCL with cutaneous dissemination. A. Diffuse deep dermal and subcutaneous infiltration by tumor cells (20×). **B.** The infiltrate is composed of frequent eosinophils and the classic "hallmark" cells (600×). The malignant cells are positive for CD4 **(C)** and CD30 **(D)**, a more typical phenotype of ALCL. **E.** Prominent psoriasiform hyperplasia (40×) and **(F)** epidermotropism by smaller cells (200×).

a case of anaplastic large cell lymphoma with cutaneous lesions that occurred in association with the use of a JAK-inhibitor (tofacitinib), who developed widespread disseminated disease including lung metastases. The tumor showed the presence of a driving *BRAF V600* mutation, and cytogenetic aberrations were similar between the skin and lung tumors.[52]

DIFFERENTIAL DIAGNOSIS

Distinction of ALK⁻ ALCL from Hodgkin lymphoma (HL) can be challenging in lymph nodes and skin. Cutaneous presentation by HL typically occurs in the setting of preexistent nodal disease. In contrast to ALCL, HL is mostly PAX5⁺, but

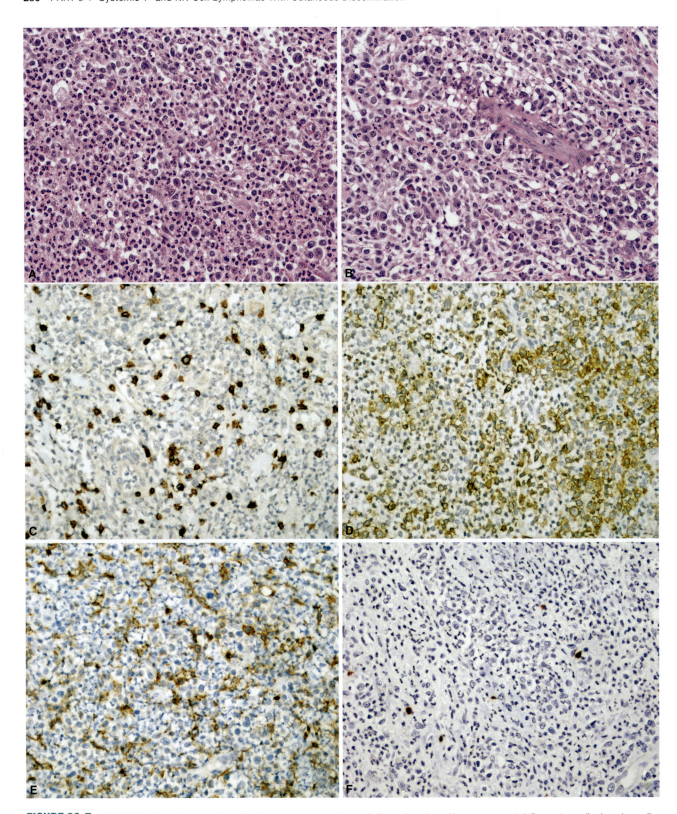

FIGURE 26-7. **ALK⁻ ALCL with cutaneous dissemination, uncommon patterns. A.** Pyogenic variant with numerous acute inflammatory cells obscuring malignant cells (200×). **B.** Angiotropic pattern (40×). This case shows a "null" phenotype: tumor cells are negative for CD3 **(C)**, CD4 **(E)**, and CD8 **(F)** but positive for CD30 **(D)**.

ALCL may aberrantly express PAX5. In addition, *TCR* gene rearrangement is more typical of ALCL and only rarely seen in HL. HL can show aberrant expression of T-cell markers. BCL-6 is expressed in most cases of HL, and approximately 50% of ALCL, and is of little significance to distinguish between the two entities. Similarly, fascin and clusterin can be expressed in both entities. Cytotoxic markers are more typical of ALCL, but TIA-1 can be seen in 15% of HL.[6]

Cutaneous involvement by angioimmunoblastic T-cell lymphoma (AITL) is relatively common and presents in up to 50% of patients. AITL is a PTCL of T follicular helper phenotype, with expression of markers (PD-1, BCL-6, CD10, CXCL13)

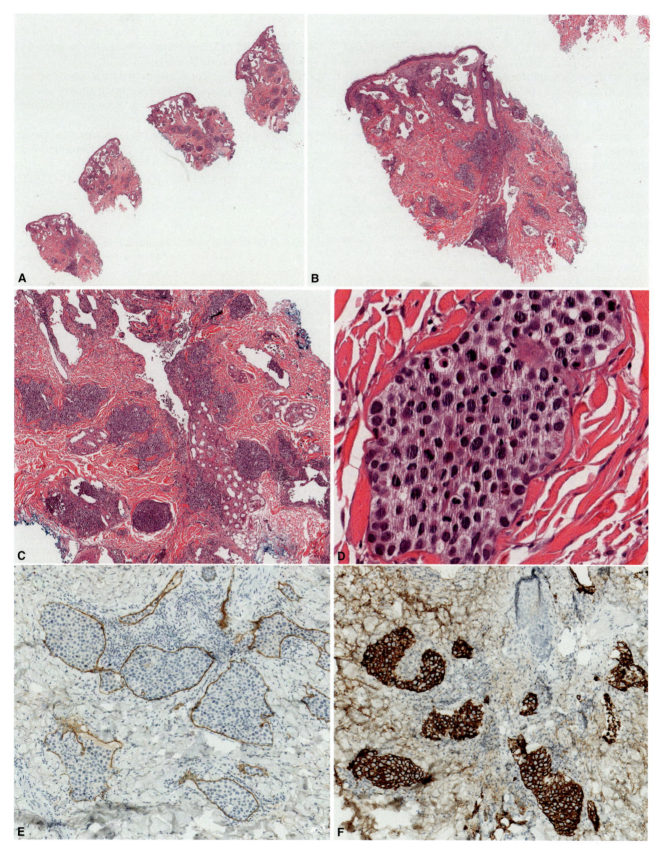

FIGURE 26-8. **ALK⁻ ALCL with cutaneous dissemination and an intravascular distribution. A–D.** Dilated lymphatic channels filled with neoplastic cells (10× and 20×, 200× and 400×, respectively). **E.** D2-40 immunostain highlighting lymphatic channels. **F.** CD30 diffusely staining lymphoma cells.

of germinal center origin, and those are typically negative in ALCL.[6] AITL can express CD30, but in fewer numbers than in ALCL. In addition, AITL is Epstein-Barr virus (EBV)-related, and most ALCLs are EBV–. Gene-expression profiling might improve the classification of AITL and ALCL.[53]

C-ALCL needs to be distinguished as it differs from systemic ALCL by an indolent clinical course. Most patients are adults, usually 50 to 60 years of age.[54,55] The histology of the lesion is similar or identical to systemic ALCLs. In 20% of cases, a morphologic variant is seen (eg, pyogenic variant, small cell variant). The infiltrate extends from the dermis into the subcutis.[6,56-58] Admixed acute inflammatory cells can be prominent giving rise to neutrophil-rich (so called pyogenic) and eosinophilic-rich variants. Pseudoepitheliomatous hyperplasia and epidermotropism can be present, features that are not typical in systemic ALCL. Some cases exhibit an intravascular distribution.[35,37,59] Similar to its systemic counterpart, C-ALCL shows diffuse and strong CD30 expression, variable loss of pan–T-cell antigens, and some expression of cytotoxic markers. C-ALCLs express cutaneous lymphocyte antigen (CLA), which is absent in systemic ALCL. Contrary to systemic ALCL, EMA expression in C-ALCL is usually focal and seen only in 20% to 30% of cases. Survivin expression is often present in systemic ALCL, but not in C-ALCL.[60] Expression of ALK in C-ALCL is very rare. ALK+ ALCL seems to carry a favorable prognosis, although some cases showed progression with involvement of lymph nodes.[61,62] A study evaluating common markers in C-ALCL, BI-ALCL, and s-ALCL was done looking at common biomarkers: P53, P63, MUM1, MYC, GATA3, p-STAT3, PD1, and PDL1 protein expression and *DUP22, TP53, TP63, MYC, and PDL1* chromosomal aberrations. Compared with C-ALCL, MUM1 expression was higher in S-ALCL, but no other differences were seen between the remaining markers.[63] In addition, C-ALCL can develop locoregional nodal involvement, which is associated with a less favorable outcome. A study looking at clonal similarities in patients who had lesions of LyP or C-ALCL who later develop lymph node involvement typically show clonal relationship between the tumors.[64]

The morphologic and immunophenotypic distinction of ALCL from PTCL is a challenging one. However, it is of extraordinary importance, though, owing to survival differences and possibly treatment options as ALCL shows a better prognosis and is amenable to more treatment options when compared with PTCL-NOS. Expression of CD30 in PTCL-NOS is typically focal and by less than 30% of the tumor cells as opposed to the diffuse strong expression in systemic and cutaneous ALCL. Compared with ALK– ALCL, PTCL-NOS is more frequently CD2+, CD3+, CD4+, and CD43+ and less often expresses EMA or cytotoxic proteins.[8] In difficult cases, gene-expression profiling might facilitate the differential diagnosis.[65,66]

On rare occasions, ALCL can be indistinguishable from melanoma,[58] carcinomas,[44] or atypical fibrous histiocytoma.[67] Rare cases with intravascular distribution (see Fig. 26-7) can mimic intravascular B-cell lymphoma.[68]

CAPSULE SUMMARY

- Systemic ALCL is a mature CD30+ T-cell lymphoma.
- The presence or absence of *ALK1* gene rearrangement and ALK1 protein expression defines two subgroups with distinct clinical and prognostic features.
- ALK+ ALCL typically occurs in children, whereas ALK– ALCL affects adults in their sixth decade of life. The prognosis of ALK+ ALCL is better, whereas the prognosis of ALK– ALCL is worse.
- Cutaneous involvement is manifested by a superficial and deep cutaneous infiltration with extension into the adipose tissue. These features are similar to those seen in primary C-ALCL.
- Hallmark cells ("horseshoe cells") are pathognomonic: large cells with U- or C-shaped nuclei surrounding an eosinophilic Golgi area.
- Immunophenotype: CD30+, EMA+, granzyme+, TIA-1+, ALK1+/–.

References

1. Delsol G, Falini B, Muller-Hermelink HK, et al. *Anaplastic Large Cell Lymphoma (ALCL), ALK-Positive*. International Agency for Research on Cancer; 2008.
2. Mason DY, Harris NL, Delsol G, et al. *Anaplastic Large Cell Lymphoma, ALK-Negative*. International Agency for Research on Cancer; 2008.
3. Benharroch D, Meguerian-Bedoyan Z, Lamant L, et al. ALK-positive lymphoma: a single disease with a broad spectrum of morphology. *Blood*. 1998;91(6):2076-2084.
4. Falini B, Pileri S, Zinzani PL, et al. ALK+ lymphoma: clinico-pathological findings and outcome. *Blood*. 1999;93(8):2697-2706.
5. Ferreri AJ, Govi S, Pileri SA, et al. Anaplastic large cell lymphoma, ALK-positive. *Crit Rev Oncol Hematol*. 2012;83(2):293-302.
6. Kinney MC, Higgins RA, Medina EA. Anaplastic large cell lymphoma: twenty-five years of discovery. *Arch Pathol Lab Med*. 2011;135(1):19-43.
7. Medeiros LJ, Elenitoba-Johnson KS. Anaplastic large cell lymphoma. *Am J Clin Pathol*. 2007;127(5):707-722.
8. Savage KJ, Harris NL, Vose JM, et al. ALK—anaplastic large-cell lymphoma is clinically and immunophenotypically different from both ALK+ ALCL and peripheral T-cell lymphoma, not otherwise specified: report from the International Peripheral T-Cell Lymphoma Project. *Blood*. 2008;111(12):5496-5504.
9. Ando K, Tamada Y, Shimizu K, et al. ALK-positive primary systemic anaplastic large cell lymphoma with extensive cutaneous manifestation. *Acta Derm Venereol*. 2010;90(2):198-200.
10. Chan DV, Summers P, Tuttle M, et al. Anaplastic lymphoma kinase expression in a recurrent primary cutaneous anaplastic large cell lymphoma with eventual systemic involvement. *J Am Acad Dermatol*. 2011;65(3):671-673.
11. Hosoi M, Ichikawa M, Imai Y, et al. A case of anaplastic large cell lymphoma, ALK positive, primary presented in the skin and relapsed with systemic involvement and leukocytosis after years of follow-up period. *Int J Hematol*. 2010;92(4):667-668.
12. Pulitzer M, Ogunrinade O, Lin O, et al. ALK-positive (2p23 rearranged) anaplastic large cell lymphoma with localization to the skin in a pediatric patient. *J Cutan Pathol*. 2015;42(3):182-187.
13. Bayle C, Charpentier A, Duchayne E, et al. Leukaemic presentation of small cell variant anaplastic large cell lymphoma: report of four cases. *Br J Haematol*. 1999;104(4):680-688.
14. Fraga M, Brousset P, Schlaifer D, et al. Bone marrow involvement in anaplastic large cell lymphoma. Immunohistochemical detection of minimal disease and its prognostic significance. *Am J Clin Pathol*. 1995;103(1):82-89.

15. Ferreri AJ, Govi S, Pileri SA, et al. Anaplastic large cell lymphoma, ALK-negative. *Crit Rev Oncol Hematol.* 2013;85(2):206-215.
16. Lamant L, Pileri S, Sabattini E, et al. Cutaneous presentation of ALK-positive anaplastic large cell lymphoma following insect bites: evidence for an association in five cases. *Haematologica.* 2010;95(3):449-455.
17. Piccaluga PP, Ascani S, Orcioni FG, et al. Anaplastic lymphoma kinase expression as a marker of malignancy. Application to a case of anaplastic large cell lymphoma with huge granulomatous reaction. *Haematologica.* 2000;85(9):978-981.
18. Hoshina D, Arita K, Mizuno O, et al. Skin involvement in ALK-negative systemic anaplastic large-cell lymphoma. *J Am Acad Dermatol.* 2012;67(4):e159-e160.
19. Marschalko M, Eros N, Hollo P, et al. Secondary ALK negative anaplastic large cell lymphoma in a patient with lymphomatoid papulosis of 40 years duration. *Am J Dermatopathol.* 2010;32(7):708-712.
20. Querfeld C, Khan I, Mahon B, et al. Primary cutaneous and systemic anaplastic large cell lymphoma: clinicopathologic aspects and therapeutic options. *Oncology.* 2010;24(7):574-587.
21. Oschlies I, Lisfeld J, Lamant L, et al. ALK-positive anaplastic large cell lymphoma limited to the skin: clinical, histopathological and molecular analysis of 6 pediatric cases. A report from the ALCL99 study. *Haematologica.* 2013;98(1):50-56.
22. Hanafusa T, Igawa K, Takagawa S, et al. Erythroderma as a paraneoplastic cutaneous disorder in systemic anaplastic large cell lymphoma. *J Eur Acad Dermatol Venereol.* 2012;26(6):710-713.
23. Mencia-Gutierrez E, Gutierrez-Diaz E, Salamanca J, et al. Cutaneous presentation on the eyelid of primary, systemic, CD30+, anaplastic lymphoma kinase (ALK)-negative, anaplastic large-cell lymphoma (ALCL). *Int J Dermatol.* 2006;45:766-769.
24. Rodis DG, Liatsos GD, Moulakakis A, et al. Paraneoplastic cerebellar degeneration: initial presentation in a patient with anaplastic T-cell lymphoma, associated with ichthyosiform cutaneous lesions. *Leuk Lymphoma.* 2009;50(8):1369-1371.
25. Bajor-Dattilo EB, Pittaluga S, Jaffe ES. Pathobiology of T-cell and NK-cell lymphomas. *Best Pract Res Clin Haematol.* 2013;26(1):75-87.
26. Aladily TN, Medeiros LJ, Alayed K, et al. Breast implant-associated anaplastic large cell lymphoma: a newly recognized entity that needs further refinement of its definition. *Leuk Lymphoma.* 2012;53(4):749-750.
27. Aladily TN, Medeiros LJ, Amin MB, et al. Anaplastic large cell lymphoma associated with breast implants: a report of 13 cases. *Am J Surg Pathol.* 2012;36(7):1000-1008.
28. Brody GS, Deapen D, Taylor CR, et al. Anaplastic large cell lymphoma (ALCL) occurring in women with breast implants: analysis of 173 cases. *Plast Reconstr Surg.* 2015;135(3):695-705.
29. Taylor CR, Siddiqi IN, Brody GS. Anaplastic large cell lymphoma occurring in association with breast implants: review of pathologic and immunohistochemical features in 103 cases. *Immunohistochem Mol.* 2013;21(1):13-20.
30. Thompson PA, Prince HM. Breast implant-associated anaplastic large cell lymphoma: a systematic review of the literature and mini-meta analysis. *Curr Hematol Malig Rep.* 2013;8(3):196-210.
31. Feldman AL, Dogan A. *Peripheral T-Cell Lymphomas*; 2014.
32. Kinney MC, Collins RD, Greer JP, et al. A small-cell-predominant variant of primary Ki-1 (CD30)+ T-cell lymphoma. *Am J Surg Pathol.* 1993;17(9):859-868.
33. Vassallo J, Lamant L, Brugieres L, et al. ALK-positive anaplastic large cell lymphoma mimicking nodular sclerosis Hodgkin's lymphoma: report of 10 cases. *Am J Surg Pathol.* 2006;30(2):223-229.
34. Gable AD, Clark SH, Magro CM. Myxoid variant of anaplastic large cell lymphoma involving the skin: a case report. *J Cutan Pathol.* 2012;39(8):787-790.
35. Samols MA, Su A, Ra S, et al. Intralymphatic cutaneous anaplastic large cell lymphoma/lymphomatoid papulosis: expanding the spectrum of CD30-positive lymphoproliferative disorders. *Am J Surg Pathol.* 2014;38(9):1203-1211.
36. Kempf W, Keller K, John H, et al. Benign atypical intravascular CD30+ T-cell proliferation: a recently described reactive lymphoproliferative process and simulator of intravascular lymphoma—report of a case associated with lichen sclerosus and review of the literature. *Am J Clin Pathol.* 2014;142(5):694-699.
37. Metcalf RA, Bashey S, Wysong A, et al. Intravascular ALK-negative anaplastic large cell lymphoma with localized cutaneous involvement and an indolent clinical course: toward recognition of a distinct clinicopathologic entity. *Am J Surg Pathol.* 2013;37(4):617-623.
38. Ducastel N, Cimpean IM, Theate I, Vanhooteghem O. Breast erythema and nodular skin metastasis as the first manifestation of breast implant-associated anaplastic large cell lymphoma. *Rare Tumors.* 2021;13:20363613211028498.
39. Goyal A, Patel S, Goyal K, Morgan EA, Foreman RK. Variable loss of CD30 expression by immunohistochemistry in recurrent cutaneous CD30+ lymphoid neoplasms treated with brentuximab vedotin. *J Cutan Pathol.* 2019;46(11):823-829. doi:10.1111/cup.13545. Epub 2019 Aug 2.
40. Foss HD, Anagnostopoulos I, Araujo I, et al. Anaplastic large-cell lymphomas of T-cell and null-cell phenotype express cytotoxic molecules. *Blood.* 1996;88(10):4005-4011.
41. Foss HD, Demel G, Anagnostopoulos I, et al. Uniform expression of cytotoxic molecules in anaplastic large cell lymphoma of null/T cell phenotype and in cell lines derived from anaplastic large cell lymphoma. *Pathobiology.* 1997;65(2):83-90.
42. Rosso R, Paulli M, Magrini U, et al. Anaplastic large cell lymphoma, CD30/Ki-1 positive, expressing the CD15/Leu-M1 antigen. Immunohistochemical and morphological relationships to Hodgkin's disease. *Virchows Arch A Pathol Anat Histopathol.* 1990;416(3):229-235.
43. Buxton D, Bacchi CE, Gualco G, et al. Frequent expression of CD99 in anaplastic large cell lymphoma: a clinicopathologic and immunohistochemical study of 160 cases. *Am J Clin Pathol.* 2009;131(4):574-579.
44. Nguyen TT, Kreisel FH, Frater JL, et al. Anaplastic large-cell lymphoma with aberrant expression of multiple cytokeratins masquerading as metastatic carcinoma of unknown primary. *J Clin Oncol.* 2013;31(33):e443-e445.
45. Leong MY, English M, McMullan D, et al. Aberrant expression of beta-HCG in anaplastic large cell lymphoma. *Pediatr Dev Pathol.* 2008;11(3):230-234.
46. Ravindran A, Feldman AL, Ketterling RP, et al. Striking association of lymphoid enhancing factor (LEF1) overexpression and DUSP22 rearrangements in anaplastic large cell lymphoma. *Am J Surg Pathol.* 2021;45(4):550-557. doi:10.1097/PAS.0000000000001614. PMID: 33165091.
47. de Leval L. Molecular classification of ganglionic T cell lymphomas: pathological and diagnostic implications. *Bull Mem Acad R Med Belg.* 2010;165:99.

48. de Leval L, Bisig B, Thielen C, et al. Molecular classification of T-cell lymphomas. *Crit Rev Oncol Hematol.* 2009;72(2):125-143.
49. Feldman AL, Dogan A, Smith DI, et al. Discovery of recurrent t(6;7)(p25.3;q32.3) translocations in ALK-negative anaplastic large cell lymphomas by massively parallel genomic sequencing. *Blood.* 2011;117(3):915-919.
50. Feldman AL, Law M, Remstein ED, et al. Recurrent translocations involving the IRF4 oncogene locus in peripheral T-cell lymphomas. *Leukemia.* 2009;23(3):574-580.
51. Wada DA, Law ME, Hsi ED, et al. Specificity of IRF4 translocations for primary cutaneous anaplastic large cell lymphoma: a multicenter study of 204 skin biopsies. *Mod Pathol.* 2011;24(4):596-605.
52. Gru AA, Williams E, Junkins-Hopkins JM. An immune suppression-associated EBV-positive anaplastic large cell lymphoma with a BRAF V600E mutation. *Am J Surg Pathol.* 2019;43(1):140-146. doi:10.1097/PAS.0000000000001174.
53. Piccaluga PP, Tabanelli V, Pileri SA. Molecular genetics of peripheral T-cell lymphomas. *Int J Hematol.* 2014;99:219-226.
54. Benner MF, Willemze R. Applicability and prognostic value of the new TNM classification system in 135 patients with primary cutaneous anaplastic large cell lymphoma. *Arch Dermatol.* 2009;145(12):1399-1404.
55. Booken N, Goerdt S, Klemke CD. Clinical spectrum of primary cutaneous CD30-positive anaplastic large cell lymphoma: an analysis of the Mannheim Cutaneous Lymphoma Registry. *J Dtsch Dermatol Ges.* 2012;10(5):331-339.
56. Kunishige JH, McDonald H, Alvarez G, et al. Lymphomatoid papulosis and associated lymphomas: a retrospective case series of 84 patients. *Clin Exp Dermatol.* 2009;34(5):576-581.
57. Plaza JA, Feldman AL, Magro C. Cutaneous CD30-positive lymphoproliferative disorders with CD8 expression: a clinicopathologic study of 21 cases. *J Cutan Pathol.* 2013;40:236-247.
58. Pulitzer M, Brady MS, Blochin E, et al. Anaplastic large cell lymphoma: a potential pitfall in the differential diagnosis of melanoma. *Arch Pathol Lab Med.* 2013;137(2):280-283.
59. Foss HD, Marafioti T, Stein H. The many faces of anaplastic large cell lymphoma. *Pathologe.* 2000;21(2):124-136.
60. Goteri G, Simonetti O, Rupoli S, et al. Differences in survivin location and Bcl-2 expression in CD30+ lymphoproliferative disorders of the skin compared with systemic anaplastic large cell lymphomas: an immunohistochemical study. *Br J Dermatol.* 2007;157(1):41-48.
61. Geller S, Canavan TN, Pulitzer M, et al. ALK-positive primary cutaneous anaplastic large cell lymphoma: a case report and review of the literature. *Int J Dermatol* 2018;57(5):515-520. PMID: 29057463.
62. Melchers RC, Willemze R, van de Loo M, et al. Clinical, histologic, and molecular characteristics of anaplastic lymphoma kinase-positive primary cutaneous anaplastic large cell lymphoma. *Am J Surg Pathol.* 2020;44(6):776-781.
63. Anna G, Alame M, Olivier D, et al. Systemic, primary cutaneous, and breast implant-associated ALK-negative anaplastic large-cell lymphomas present similar biologic features despite distinct clinical behavior. *Virchows Arch.* 2019;475(2):163-174. doi:10.1007/s00428-019-02570-4. Epub 2019 Apr 6.
64. Xerri L, Adélaïde J, Morgan A, et al. Common origin of sequential cutaneous CD30+ lymphoproliferations with nodal involvement evidenced by genome-wide clonal evolution. *Histopathology.* 2019;74(4):654-662. doi:10.1111/his.13783. Epub 2019 Jan 31.
65. Iqbal J, Wright G, Wang C, et al. Gene expression signatures delineate biological and prognostic subgroups in peripheral T-cell lymphoma. *Blood.* 2014;123(19):2915-2923.
66. Bird JE, Leitenberger JJ, Solomon A, et al. Fatal ALK-negative systemic anaplastic large cell lymphoma presenting with disseminated cutaneous dome-shaped papules and nodules. *Dermatol Online J.* 2012;18(5):5.
67. Szablewski V, Laurent-Roussel S, Rethers L, et al. Atypical fibrous histiocytoma of the skin with CD30 and p80/ALK1 positivity and ALK gene rearrangement. *J Cutan Pathol.* 2014;41:715-719.
68. Deetz CO, Gilbertson KGII, Anadkat MJ, et al. A rare case of intravascular large T-cell lymphoma with an unusual T helper phenotype. *Am J Dermatopathol.* 2011;33(8):e99-e102.

T-cell prolymphocytic leukemia

Alejandro A. Gru

DEFINITION

T-cell prolymphocytic leukemia (T-PLL) is a mature neoplasm of T cells with peripheral blood involvement. It is the most common subtype of mature T-cell leukemia in the Western Hemisphere.[1-4]

EPIDEMIOLOGY

T-PLL is a rare aggressive disorder, accounting for 2% of the mature lymphoid leukemias. The median age at presentation is 65 years. It was originally classified in the 1970s as a variant of chronic lymphocytic leukemia but later reclassified as a distinct entity.[2,3]

ETIOLOGY

The etiologic factors are unclear. The rare association with the human T-cell lymphotropic virus (HTLV) infection has been reported[5]; however, these cases likely represent adult T-cell leukemia/lymphoma (ATLL) in the current World Health Organization classification.

CLINICAL PRESENTATION AND PROGNOSIS

Almost half of the patients present with hepatosplenomegaly and lymphadenopathy.[6] Peripheral blood has a characteristic high lymphocytosis (>100 × 10^9/L) with more than 90% of cells being prolymphocytes.[2,3,6-8] Cases with moderate lymphocytosis have also been described.[4] A minority of patients (~15%) may be asymptomatic at diagnosis, and this "indolent" phase can persist for a variable length of time, which may extend to several years. Skin involvement is identified in 20% to 50% of cases. It typically occurs in the setting of high white blood cell (WBC) counts and does not appear to impact on survival.[9-13] The average 5-year survival without skin involvement is 13.2 months and ~10 months with skin disease.[11] A slight male predominance is present in patients with skin disease.[9] Concurrent involvement of the skin at the time of T-PLL diagnosis is frequent,[14] and, in rare occasions, cutaneous involvement may herald the diagnosis of T-PLL.[15] Facial erythema, periorbital edema, and conjunctival injection are common. Erythrodermic presentations have been reported.[12,14,16-19] Cutaneous nodules tend to be linear and symmetrical in distribution and have a petechial/purpuric quality[20] (Fig. 27-1).[21] Some cases also present with leonine facies (also seen in chronic lymphocytic leukemia). Recent atypical presentations mimicking a vasculitis and perniosis have been described[22,23] (Figs. 27-2 and 27-3). The clinical presentation may mimic dermatomyositis or lymphomatoid contact dermatitis[24,25] in some cases. Anemia and thrombocytopenia are seen in half of patients. Pleuroperitoneal effusions and central nervous system involvement may also occur. Some cases can also resemble dermatomyositis.[26]

HISTOLOGY

T-PLL has a broad morphologic spectrum (Figs. 27-4 and 27-5). Most cases show a predominance of large prolymphocytes with round nuclei, condensed chromatin, prominent nucleoli, and basophilic, agranular cytoplasm. In some cases, cytoplasmic blebs can be present. In 20% of cases, neoplastic cells are small with inconspicuous nucleoli ("small cell variant"). In 5% of cases, lymphoma cells show cerebriform nuclei similar to those seen in Sézary syndrome (SS) ("cerebriform variant").[1-3,6,8] In the bone marrow, there are diffuse and interstitial infiltrates, which are usually accompanied by reticulin fibrosis. In the lymph nodes, there is an abnormal paracortical expansion of neoplastic T cells.

Histopathology of the skin shows prominent superficial perivascular and interstitial infiltrates of prolymphocytes

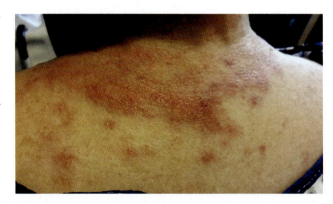

FIGURE 27-1. T-PLL purpuric and erythematous papules and plaques on the neck.

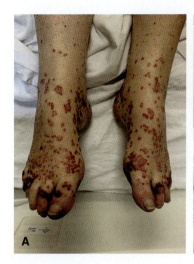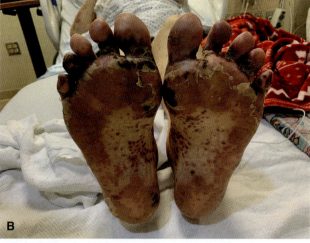

FIGURE 27-2. T-PLL, vasculitic presentation. Annular and solitary scaly red-purple papules with darker violaceous papules distally on the dorsal feet with blanching toe erythema **(A)**. Violaceous erythema on the soles, and lateral and inferior plantar feet with red-purple pinpoint macules and papules in addition to desquamation and scattered darker violaceous papules on the toes **(B)**. Targetoid dark violaceous papules can be appreciated on the bilateral fifth toes.

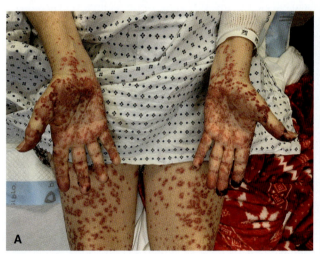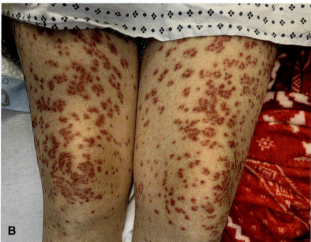

FIGURE 27-3. T-PLL, vasculitic presentation. Numerous red-purple scaly papules, some with annular configuration and collarette of scale, on the thighs and palmar hands with areas of desquamation and purple patches on the palmar hand **(A)**. There are darker violaceous papules on the distal fingertips. **B.** Close-up view of anterior thighs and knees.

with a grenz zone.[27] Epidermotropism can be seen in some cases (Fig. 27-6). Petechial lesions show extravasated red blood cells without vasculitis.[9,11,12,14,28,29] Prolymphocytes in cutaneous lesions tend to exhibit prominent nuclear clefts and cerebriform morphology.[9] Skin involvement by the small cell variant has also been described.[30]

IMMUNOPHENOTYPE

Immunophenotypically, T-PLL is a mature T-cell leukemia with a CD2+CD3+CD7+ phenotype (Fig. 22-7). As opposed to SS, CD7 and CD26 show retained expression. TdT is always negative. Nearly 80% of cases express CD4: 65% are CD4+CD8−, 21% CD4+CD8+, 17% CD8+CD4−,[6] and 3.4% CD4−CD8−. Rare cases show a phenotypic switch from CD4 to CD8.[1,31] Most cases have high levels of CD52 expression, providing a rational for treatment with alemtuzumab.[4,7,32-34] CD25, CD38, and HLA-DR are variably expressed.[35] Nearly all cases will have rearrangements of the TCR-β or TCR-γ genes. TCL-1 overexpression can be seen in cases with inv.[14,36] An interesting finding is the expression of S100 in cases of T-PLL.[37] BCL-2 is also strongly expressed.

POSTULATED CELL OF ORIGIN

Coexpression of CD4 and CD8, weak membrane CD3, and strong CD7 suggests that T-PLL represents an intermediate differentiation stage between a cortical thymocyte and a circulating mature T cell.

GENETIC AND MOLECULAR FINDINGS

Inversion (14)(q11;q32) and tandem t(14;14) translocations are present in more than two-thirds of the cases,[3,7,38] and 20% of patients have a t(X;14) translocation.[9] The rearrangements

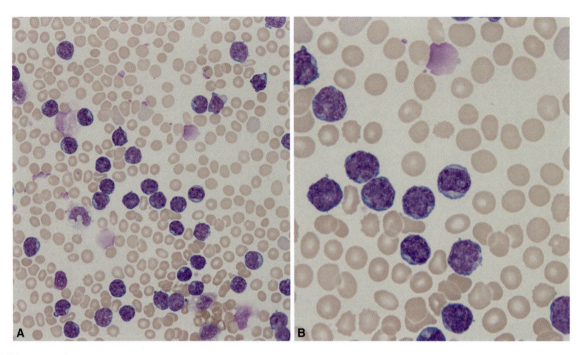

FIGURE 27-4. A and **B.** T-PLL peripheral blood smear shows medium-sized prolymphocytes with irregular nuclear borders, moderate cytoplasm, and prominent nucleoli.

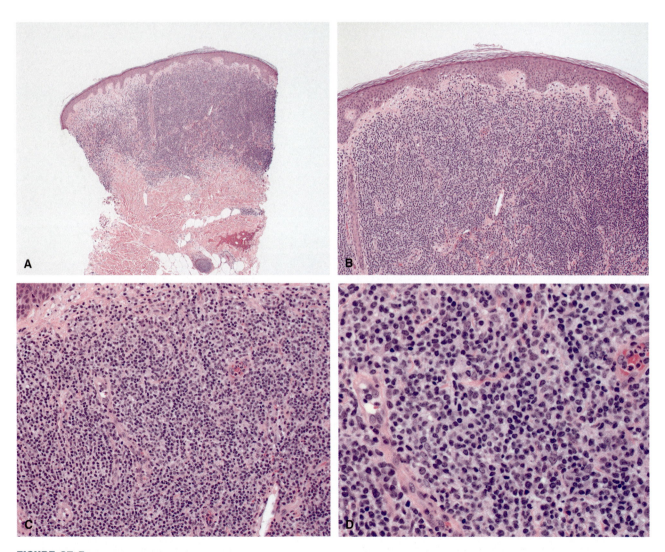

FIGURE 27-5. Cutaneous involvement by T-PLL. A and **B.** Dermal perivascular infiltrates sparing the epidermis (40× and 100×, respectively). **C** and **D.** Monotonous infiltrate in the dermis (200× and 400×, respectively).

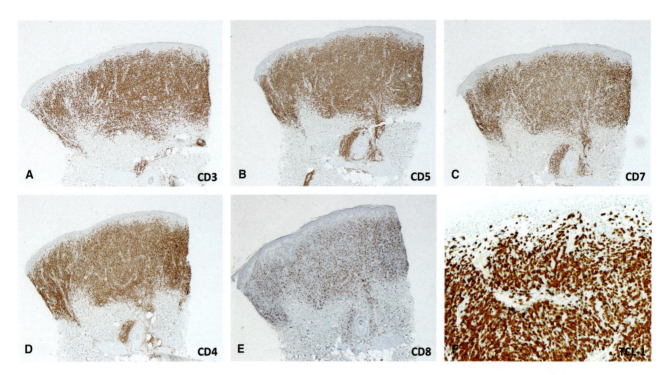

FIGURE 27-6. Cutaneous involvement by T-PLL, immunohistochemistry. The malignant lymphocytes show expression of CD3 **(A)**, CD5 **(B)**, and CD7 **(C)**. No aberrant loss of CD7 is noted. The lymphocytes are positive for CD4 **(D)** and negative for CD8 **(E)**. Strong expression of TCL-1 is present **(F)**.

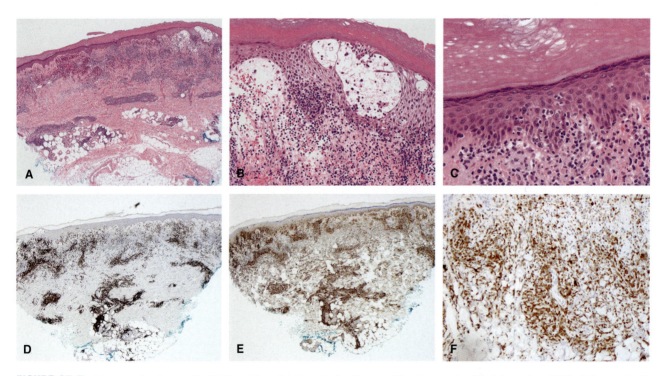

FIGURE 27-7. Cutaneous involvement by T-PLL, epidermotropic variant with vasculitic changes. A and **B.** A dense dermal infiltrate is present with prominent dermal edema and hemorrhage (40x and 200x). **B** and **C.** Prominent epidermotropism is present (200× and 400×). The infiltrate is positive for TCR-beta **(D)**, CD99 **(E)**, and S100 **(F)**.

involve the *TCR-α* and protooncogene *TCL-1*. TCL1A has been shown to promote cell proliferation and survival by acting as a coactivator of protein kinase B (Akt).[9] Abnormalities involving both arms of chromosome 8 (iso8q) with overexpression of the c-myc oncoprotein or copy number gains of the *MYC* gene are frequent. 14q abnormality and trisomy 8q are common in Western countries, but they are rarely seen in Japan.[39] 11q23 abnormalities are frequently detected (64%) by conventional cytogenetics.

Mutations of the *ATM*, *JAK1*, and *JAK3* genes are found in up to 34% of cases, respectively.[9,40-42] Activating mutations of *IL2RG*, *JAK1/3*, and *STAT5B* genes leading to constitutive STAT5 signaling are recurrent with a total frequency of up to 75% in T-PLL.[41,43-45] Mutations in *EZH2*, *FBXW10*, and

CHEK2 may further contribute to the pathogenesis of T-PLL putatively through their functions in epigenetic regulation, proteasome degradation, and DNA repair, pathways, respectively.[45,46] Complex karyotypes are observed in 70% to 80% of cases. Abnormalities of chromosome 8 including 8idic(8)(p11), t(8;8)(p11-12;q12), and trisomy 8q are seen in 70% to 80% of cases. Deletions in 12p13 and 22q, gains in 8q24 (*MYC*), and abnormalities of chromosomes 5p, 6, and 17 have also been described.[3,47,48]

DIFFERENTIAL DIAGNOSIS

Mimics of T-PLL include cutaneous lymphomas with peripheral blood involvement such as SS, erythrodermic mycosis fungoides (MF), and ATLL.

The diagnosis of SS is more typically favored in the presence of generalized erythroderma. The infiltrate in SS could also be sparse and tends to be more superficial than in T-PLL. As opposed to T-PLL, in SS there is very frequently loss of CD7. In addition, coexpression of CD4+/CD8+ or CD4-/CD8+ is never present in cases of SS. The classic cytogenetic aberrations of T-PLL are not typical of SS.[49]

Erythrodermic MF is regarded as the leukemic form of MF. Patients have long-standing cutaneous patches on sun-protected skin that progress to plaques and tumors. The immunophenotype is similar to that of SS.

Most cases of ATLL occur in endemic areas in association with HTLV-1 infection. ATLL has an aggressive clinical course, striking leukocytosis, and hypercalcemia. Circulating neoplastic cells have classic nuclear lobation ("flower-like" cells). ATLL has a CD3+CD4+CD8-CD25+CD52- phenotype. Coexpression of CD4 and CD8 is rare. Cutaneous lesions with epidermotropism are present in nearly 50% of cases and are indistinguishable from MF.

Rare cases of cutaneous involvement in the course of T-cell large-granular lymphocytic leukemia (T-LGL) have been reported.[50-52] As opposed to T-PLL, T-LGL is a very indolent disease, sometimes in association with autoimmune disorders and frequently with low WBC counts. The morphology of the cells reveals the presence of large granular lymphocytes in the peripheral blood. The immunophenotype is one of a CD8+, CD57+ cytotoxic leukemia. Expression of cytotoxic markers granzyme, TIA-1, and perforin is frequently seen. Rare examples showing the coexistence of both CLL and T-PLL have been reported.[22,53]

Treatment is usually based on protocols containing alemtuzumab (anti-CD52 therapy), pentostatin, venetoclax (anti-BCL2), and, in some cases, brentuximab vedotin.[54-58]

CAPSULE SUMMARY

- T-PLL is a rare aggressive disorder, accounting for 2% of mature lymphoid leukemias in adults and frequently associated with lymphadenopathy and splenomegaly.
- Skin involvement is identified in 20% to 50% of cases.
- Facial involvement with or without periorbital edema and petechiae are characteristic.
- Skin biopsies show perivascular and interstitial infiltrates in the superficial dermis. The epidermis is spared.
- Prolymphocytes are medium-sized cells with fine chromatin, moderate to abundant cytoplasm, and prominent nucleoli.
- The most common immunophenotype is CD4+/CD8-CD7+CD52+.
- The classic cytogenetic aberrations in T-PLL include inv(14) and t(14;14) rearrangement.

References

1. Catovsky D, Muller-Hermelink HK, Ralfkiaer E. *T-cell Prolymphocytic Leukaemia*. 4th ed. International Agency for Research on Cancer; 2008.
2. Dearden CE. T-cell prolymphocytic leukemia. *Med Oncol.* 2006;23(1):17-22.
3. Dearden CE. T-cell prolymphocytic leukemia. *Clin Lymphoma Myeloma.* 2009;9(suppl 3):S239-S243.
4. Dearden C. How I treat prolymphocytic leukemia. *Blood.* 2012;120(3):538-551.
5. Kojima K, Hara M, Sawada T, et al. Human T-lymphotropic virus type I provirus and T-cell prolymphocytic leukemia. *Leuk Lymphoma.* 2000;38(3/4):381-386.
6. Chen X, Cherian S. Immunophenotypic characterization of T-cell prolymphocytic leukemia. *Am J Clin Pathol.* 2013;140(5):727-735.
7. Dungarwalla M, Matutes E, Dearden CE. Prolymphocytic leukaemia of B- and T-cell subtype: a state-of-the-art paper. *Eur J Haematol.* 2008;80(6):469-476.
8. Khot A, Dearden C. T-cell prolymphocytic leukemia. *Exp Rev Anticancer Ther.* 2009;9(3):365-371.
9. Hsi AC, Robirds DH, Luo J, et al. T-cell prolymphocytic leukemia frequently shows cutaneous involvement and is associated with gains of MYC, loss of ATM, and TCL1A rearrangement. *Am J Surg Pathol.* 2014;38(11):1468-1483.
10. Herling M, Valbuena JR, Jones D, et al. Skin involvement in T-cell prolymphocytic leukemia. *J Am Acad Dermatol.* 2007;57(3):533-534.
11. Magro CM, Morrison CD, Heerema N, et al. T-cell prolymphocytic leukemia: an aggressive T cell malignancy with frequent cutaneous tropism. *J Am Acad Dermatol.* 2006;55(3):467-477.
12. Matutes E, Brito-Babapulle V, Swansbury J, et al. Clinical and laboratory features of 78 cases of T-prolymphocytic leukemia. *Blood.* 1991;78(12):3269-3274.
13. Valbuena JR, Herling M, Admirand JH, et al. T-cell prolymphocytic leukemia involving extramedullary sites. *Am J Clin Pathol.* 2005;123(3):456-464.
14. Mallett RB, Matutes E, Catovsky D, et al. Cutaneous infiltration in T-cell prolymphocytic leukaemia. *Br J Dermatol.* 1995;132(2):263-266.
15. Serra A, Estrach MT, Marti R, et al. Cutaneous involvement as the first manifestation in a case of T-cell prolymphocytic leukaemia. *Acta Derm Venereol.* 1998;78(3):198-200.
16. De Belilovsky C, Guillaume JC, Gilles E, et al. Cutaneous manifestations of T-cell prolymphocytic leukemia. *Ann Dermatol Venereol.* 1989;116(11):889-891.
17. Dessart P, Lemaire P, Le Du K, et al. T-cell prolymphocytic leukemia: potential diagnostic pitfalls. *Ann Dermatol Venereol.* 2014;141(12):777-781.
18. Zanelli M, Panico L, Manfra I, Zizzo M, Sanguedolce F, Ascani S. T-cell prolymphocytic leukemia: Insidious onset followed by aggressive course with cutaneous involvement. *Int J Lab Hematol.* 2021;43(5):892-894.

19. Hasan F, Parashar Y, Rao RN, Kashyap R. Leonine facies: a unique presentation of T-prolymphocytic leukemia. *Indian J Pathol Microbiol*. 2021;64(4):817-819.
20. Dybjer A, Hellquist L, Johansson B, et al. Seropositive polyarthritis and skin manifestations in T-prolymphocytic leukemia/Sézary cell leukemia variant. *Leuk Lymphoma*. 2000;37(3/4):437-440.
21. Kaminska EC, Yu Z, Kress J, et al. Erythematous eruption with marked conjunctival injection—quiz case. Diagnosis: leukemia cutis with conjunctival involvement in the setting of T-cell prolymphocytic leukemia (T-PLL). *Arch Dermatol*. 2012;148(10):1199.
22. Edmonds N, Guerra R, Noland MMB, Schenck O, Krasner B, Gru AA. An unusual case of T-cell prolymphocytic leukemia mimicking a cutaneous vasculitis. *J Cutan Pathol*. 2021;48(10):1311-1316. doi:10.1111/cup.14079
23. Leckey BD, Jr, Kheterpal MK, Selim MA, Al-Rohil RN. Cutaneous involvement by T-cell prolymphocytic leukemia presenting as livedoid vasculopathy. *J Cutan Pathol*. 2021;48(7):975-979.
24. Nousari HC, Kimyai-Asadi A, Huang CH, et al. T-cell chronic lymphocytic leukemia mimicking dermatomyositis. *Int J Dermatol*. 2000;39(2):144-146.
25. Abraham S, Braun RP, Matthes T, et al. A follow-up: previously reported apparent lymphomatoid contact dermatitis, now followed by T-cell prolymphocytic leukaemia. *Br J Dermatol*. 2006;155(3):633-634.
26. Ingrasci G, Diaz-Perez J, Verne S, Romanelli P, Yosipovitch G. Cutaneous presentation of T-cell prolymphocytic leukemia mimicking dermatomyositis. *Am J Dermatopathol*. 2021;43(7):521-524.
27. Jevremovic D, Morice WG. Leukaemias of mature T-cells and natural killer cells. In: Orazi A, Weiss L, Foucar K, et al. eds. *Knowles' Neoplasic Hematopathology*. 3rd ed. Wolters Kluwer/Lippincott Williams & Wilkins; 2014.
28. Thomas A, Dompmartin A, Troussard X, et al. Cutaneous localization of T-cell prolymphocytic leukemia. *Ann Dermatol Venereol*. 1995;122(8):526-529.
29. Ventre MO, Bacelieri RE, Lazarchick J, et al. Cutaneous presentation of T-cell prolymphocytic leukemia. *Cutis*. 2013;91(2):87-91.
30. Jeong KH, Lew BL, Sim WY. Generalized leukaemia cutis from a small cell variant of T-cell prolymphocytic leukaemia presenting with exfoliative dermatitis. *Acta Derm Venereol*. 2009;89(5):509-512.
31. Tse E, So CC, Cheung WW, et al. T-cell prolymphocytic leukaemia: spontaneous immunophenotypical switch from CD4 to CD8 expression. *Ann Hematol*. 2011;90(4):479-481.
32. Dearden C. The role of alemtuzumab in the management of T-cell malignancies. *Semin Oncol*. 2006;33(2 suppl 5):S44-S52.
33. Wiktor-Jedrzejczak W, Dearden C, de Wreede L, et al. Hematopoietic stem cell transplantation in T-prolymphocytic leukemia: a retrospective study from the European Group for Blood and Marrow Transplantation and the Royal Marsden Consortium. *Leukemia*. 2012;26(5):972-976.
34. Lu L, Peters J, Roome C, et al. Cost-effectiveness of alemtuzumab for T-cell prolymphocytic leukemia. *Int J Technol Assess Health Care*. 2012;28(3):241-248.
35. Osuji N, Matutes E, Catovsky D, et al. Histopathology of the spleen in T-cell large granular lymphocyte leukemia and T-cell prolymphocytic leukemia: a comparative review. *Am J Surg Pathol*. 2005;29(7):935-941.
36. Foucar K. Mature T-cell leukemias including T-prolymphocytic leukemia, adult T-cell leukemia/lymphoma, and Sézary syndrome. *Am J Clin Pathol*. 2007;127(4):496-510.
37. Aggarwal N, Pongpruttipan T, Patel S, et al. Expression of S100 protein in CD4-positive T-cell lymphomas is often associated with T-cell prolymphocytic leukemia. *Am J Surg Pathol*. 2015;39(12):1679-1687.
38. Feldman AL, Law M, Grogg KL, et al. Incidence of TCR and TCL1 gene translocations and isochromosome 7q in peripheral T-cell lymphomas using fluorescence in situ hybridization. *Am J Clin Pathol*. 2008;130(2):178-185.
39. Kameoka J, Takahashi N, Noji H, et al. T-cell prolymphocytic leukemia in Japan: is it a variant? *Int J Hematol*. 2012;95(6):660-667.
40. Boultwood J. Ataxia telangiectasia gene mutations in leukaemia and lymphoma. *J Clin Pathol*. 2001;54(7):512-516.
41. Bellanger D, Jacquemin V, Chopin M, et al. Recurrent JAK1 and JAK3 somatic mutations in T-cell prolymphocytic leukemia. *Leukemia*. 2014;28(2):417-419.
42. Bergmann AK, Schneppenheim S, Seifert M, et al. Recurrent mutation of JAK3 in T-cell prolymphocytic leukemia. *Genes Chromosomes Cancer*. 2014;53(4):309-316.
43. Wahnschaffe L, Braun T, Timonen S, et al. JAK/STAT-activating genomic Alterations are a hallmark of T-PLL. *Cancers (Basel)*. 2019;11(12):1833. doi:10.3390/cancers11121833
44. López C, Bergmann AK, Paul U, et al. Genes encoding members of the JAK-STAT pathway or epigenetic regulators are recurrently mutated in T-cell prolymphocytic leukemia. *Br J Haematol*. 2016;173(2):265-273. doi:10.1111/bjh.13952
45. Kiel MJ, Velusamy T, Rolland D, et al. Integrated genomic sequencing reveals mutational landscape of T-cell prolymphocytic leukemia. *Blood*. 2014;124(9):1460-1472. doi:10.1182/blood-2014-03-559542
46. Schrader A, Crispatzu G, Oberbeck S, et al. Actionable perturbations of damage responses by TCL1/ATM and epigenetic lesions form the basis of T-PLL. *Nat Commun*. 2018;9(1):697. doi:10.1038/s41467-017-02688-6
47. Urbankova H, Holzerova M, Balcarkova J, et al. Array comparative genomic hybridization in the detection of chromosomal abnormalities in T-cell prolymphocytic leukemia. *Cancer Genet Cytogenet*. 2010;202(1):58-62.
48. Delgado P, Starshak P, Rao N, et al. A comprehensive update on molecular and cytogenetic abnormalities in T-cell prolymphocytic leukemia (T-pll). *J Assoc Genet Technol*. 2012;38(4):193-198.
49. Diwan AH, Prieto VG, Herling M, et al. Primary Sézary syndrome commonly shows low-grade cytologic atypia and an absence of epidermotropism. *Am J Clin Pathol*. 2005;123(4):510-515.
50. Duarte AF, Nogueira A, Mota A, et al. Leg ulcer and thigh telangiectasia associated with natural killer cell CD56(−) large granular lymphocyte leukemia in a patient with pseudo-Felty syndrome. *J Am Acad Dermatol*. 2010;62(3):496-501.
51. Sia PI, Figueira E, Kuss B, et al. T-cell large granular lymphocyte leukemia in the lower eyelid. *Ophthal Plast Reconstr Surg*. Published online 2014. doi:10.1097/IOP.0000000000000297
52. van Steensel MA, van Gelder M, van Marion AM, et al. T-cell large granular lymphocytic leukaemia with an uncommon clinical and immunological phenotype. *Acta Derm Venereol*. 2009;89(2):172-174.
53. Sakhdari A, Tang G, Ginsberg LE, et al. Composite chronic lymphocytic leukemia/small lymphocytic lymphoma and T-prolymphocytic leukemia presenting with lymphocytosis, skin lesions, and generalized lymphadenopathy. *Case Rep Pathol*. 2019;2019:4915086.

54. Senchak J, Pickens P. Brentuximab vedotin therapy for cutaneous lesions in T-prolymphocytic leukemia: a case report. *Hematol Rep.* 2016;8(3):6593.
55. Bose P, Konopleva MY. T-PLL: another check on the venetoclax list? *Blood.* 2017;130(23):2447-2448.
56. Herbaux C., Kornauth C., Poulain S., et al. BH3 profiling identifies ruxolitinib as a promising partner for venetoclax to treat T-cell prolymphocytic leukemia. *Blood.* 2021;137(25):3495-3506. doi:10.1182/blood.2020007303.
57. Colon Ramos A, Tarekegn K, Aujla A, Garcia de de Jesus K, Gupta S. T-cell prolymphocytic leukemia: an overview of current and future approaches. *Cureus.* 2021;13(2):e13237.
58. Sud A, Dearden C. T-Cell prolymphocytic leukemia. *Hematol Oncol Clin North Am.* 2017;31(2):273-283.

CHAPTER 28

Skin manifestations of angioimmunoblastic T-cell lymphoma

Nicolas Ortonne

DEFINITION

Angioimmunoblastic T-cell lymphoma (AITL) was first recognized as a "new" specific entity during the 1970s, characterized by a peculiar clinical picture that could suggest a drug hypersensitivity reaction and a distinct histopathology of affected lymph nodes. Then the disease was referred to as "immunoblastic lymphadenopathy" or "angioimmunoblastic lymphadenopathy with dysproteinemia" because its neoplastic nature was not recognized.[1,2] Soon after, AITL was mentioned as a specific subtype among peripheral T-cell lymphoma (PTCL) in the successive lymphoma classifications.[3,4]

AITL is the most frequent PTCL in Western countries, clinically characterized by systemic involvement with constitutional symptoms (fever, night sweats, and weight loss) and polyadenopathy. Spleen, liver, bone marrow, and skin are the most frequent sites of secondary involvement.

POSTULATED CELL OF ORIGIN

Gene expression profiling studies have demonstrated the derivation of AITL from the follicular helper T-cell (TFH) subset. Thus, it is now widely accepted that the neoplastic cells in AITL can be regarded as the malignant counterpart of normal TFH lymphocytes.[5,6]

CLINICAL PRESENTATION/PROGNOSIS

AITL is one of the most common peripheral T-cell lymphomas (PTCLs) found in Western countries and accounts for approximately 15% to 20% of PTCLs.

AITL has a characteristic clinical presentation that contributes to its recognition as a specific clinicopathological entity. The most distinctive clinical and biological features of AITL are summarized in Table 28-1.[7-9] This lymphoma typically presents with systemic symptoms (fever, night sweats, and weight loss) and generalized lymphadenopathy. In addition to having lymph node (LN) swelling, patients with AITL commonly have splenomegaly, as well as bone marrow involvement. They may present with polyarthritis. Most patients have abnormal laboratory tests, including eosinophilia and hypergammaglobulinemia. AITL is usually associated with autoimmune biological manifestations in contrast to most other PTCL subtypes. Production of various autoantibodies (eg, rheumatoid factor, antinuclear antibodies) and autoimmune cytopenias are not unusual, with hemolytic anemia (positive direct antiglobulin) being the most common event. These autoimmune manifestations evolve in parallel with the lymphoma and often respond to the lymphoma-directed treatments.

Altogether, the prevalence of hypergammaglobulinemia, autoimmune manifestations, and proliferation of EBV+ B cells suggest that AITL drives B-cell dysfunctions. This may be related to the fact that the tumor cells of AITL have T follicular helper functions, in agreement with their phenotypic characteristics. Neoplastic T cells may actually interact with B cells and promote the development of EBV-infected cells and autoimmune clones, which normally would be under control. The development of monoclonal gammapathies, B-cell lymphoproliferations, or even diffuse large B-cell lymphomas in patients with AITL represents the most severe consequences of such abnormal B-T-cell interaction.

Up to 50% of patients with AITL have skin manifestations (Table 28-1). Skin manifestations may reveal the disease explaining why patients with AITL are sometimes first referred to dermatologists. It is therefore important to accurately diagnose AITL in skin biopsies. Several studies have described the morphological and phenotypic characteristics of cutaneous AITL.[10-15] They mostly present as a nonspecific rash (Fig. 28-1A and B), mimicking a viral exanthem or a drug reaction. The skin rashes, which may fluctuate in intensity, were initially considered to be reactive by nature but have later been shown to represent infiltration of the skin by the lymphoma. Patients

TABLE 28-1 Clinical Features of AITL According to Published Series

	Mourad et al	Lachenal et al	Tokunaga et al
Number of patients	157	77	207
Mean age (y-o)	62	64	67
Skin rash	44%	45%	7%
B symptoms	72%	77%	60%
Ann Arbor stages III-IV	81%	92%	90%
BM involvement	47%	60%	29%
IPI score >2	89%	87%	89%
Anemia (Hb < 12 g/dL):	65%	51%	61%
DAT +	33%	58%	46%
Hypergamma (>12 g/L)	50%	51%	54%
LDH >1N	66%	71%	75%
Overall survival	5 yr: 33%	3 yr: 49%	5 yr: 41%

BM, bone marrow; DAT, direct antiglobulin test; IPI, international prognostic index; LDH, lactate dehydrogenase.

with such rashes often have pruritus.[16] Papular and nodular or even tumoral lesions (Fig. 28-1C), erythroderma (Fig. 28-1D), as well as urticarial and petechial or purpuric patches can also be seen in a significant number of cases.[15,16] Autoimmune skin manifestations may also develop in patients with AITL. Cases associated with IgA-mediated bullous disease, IgA-mediated paraneoplastic pemphigus, or IgA-mediated leukocytoclastic vasculitis have been reported.[17,18] Although frequent, the presence of skin manifestations bears no prognostic value in patients with AITL, unless EBV+ B cells are present.[15]

The majority of patients with AITL have a poor prognosis,[3,10,19] with a 5-year survival rate of 30% and a median survival of less than 36 months.

HISTOLOGY

In the LNs, the prototypical aspects of AITL have been extensively described[4] and variably include the following features: (1) an effacement of the normal lymph node architecture, usually with disappearance of B-cell follicles; (2) a frequent spreading of lymphoma throughout the lymph node capsule, without effacement of the cortical sinuses; (3) a meshwork of high endothelial venules; (4) a polymorphic infiltrate comprising small lymphocytes, eosinophils, plasma cells, histiocytes or epithelioid cells, and scattered large B-cells, which most often show an immunoblast-like cytology but may in some instances resemble Reed–Sternberg cells; (5) a hyperplastic meshwork of follicular dendritic cells; and (6) a variable number of atypical small to medium-sized T cells, which typically have abundant clear cytoplasm. Various patterns are actually described, which are regarded as different stages of lymphoma development.[20] Patients with pattern 1 show limited nodal involvement and hyperplastic follicles, while those with patterns 2 and 3 show the typical histopathological aspects of AITL with or without regressed follicles.

The first clinical-pathological descriptions of skin manifestations of AITL were published in the 1980s.[21] On histopathological grounds, skin manifestations of AITL are highly variable from one case to another and often strongly differ from those observed in the LNs. Of note, a minimal lymphocytic infiltration may be seen in many instances, so that the histopathological picture may first appear as nonspecific, as previously highlighted by several authors.[16,21] To date, five case series have reported the histopathological spectrum and phenotypic characteristics of cutaneous AITL (Table 28-2).[11-15] According to these studies, the majority of cutaneous infiltrates of AITL can be classified into four groups, as illustrated in Fig. 28-2: (1) light perivascular infiltrates, with no identifiable atypical lymphocytes (pattern 1), making the differential diagnosis from an inflammatory dermatitis challenging on hematoxylin and eosin (H&E)-stained slides; (2) atypical perivascular infiltrates morphologically suggestive of a cutaneous T-cell lymphoma (pattern 2); (3) a dense dermal infiltrate reminiscent of the neoplastic infiltrate seen in nodal AITL (pattern 3); and (4) dermal lymphocytic vasculitis with extravasated red blood cells.

Epidermotropism is not a common feature but may be seen in individual cases. Occasionally, a dense monomorphic infiltrate consisting of large lymphoid T cells with a TFH phenotype, which may represent a "cytological transformation" as reported in nodal AITL, may be observed.[20] Regarding inflammatory cells, plasma cells are more common than eosinophils.[13,14] A proliferation of high endothelial venules can be seen, especially in samples with patterns 2 and 3. Although the presence of a CD21+/CD23+ meshwork of follicular dendritic cells is said to be of diagnostic value,[22] this feature has not been studied in large series of samples. A prominent granulomatous reaction,[14,23] sometimes with necrosis,[24] is another rare and misleading feature.

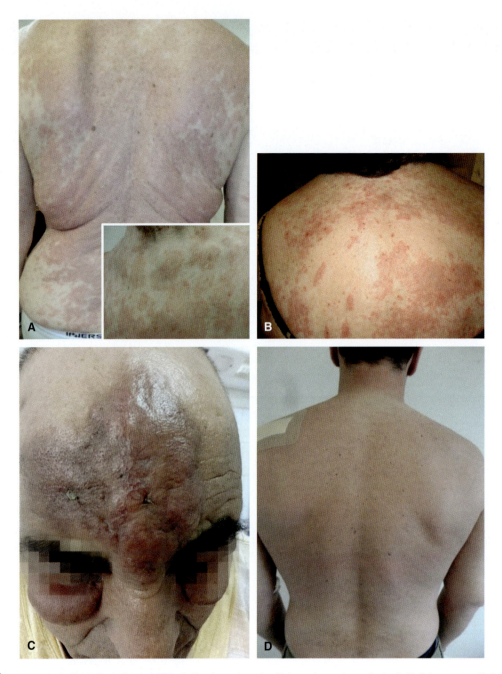

FIGURE 28-1. Dermatological manifestations of AITL. A. Maculopapular rash with purpuric papules on the back. **B.** Cutaneous manifestations of AITL, presenting as a widespread urticarial maculopapular rash, closely resembling a drug reaction. **C.** Large infiltrated plaque on the forehead of a patient with an EBV+ AITL. **D.** Slightly infiltrated erythroderma.

Immunophenotype

The neoplastic T-cells of AITL usually display a TCRαβ, CD4+ T-cell phenotype with expression of at least two TFH markers. These include TCR costimulatory receptors (CD278/PD1, CD279/ICOS),[25,26] chemokines and chemokine receptors (CXCL13, CXCR5),[12,27] germinal center markers (CD10, SAP, and BCL6),[28] and the transcription factor c-Maf.[29] All phenotypic studies performed to date have shown that the neoplastic TFH cells in the skin maintain a TFH phenotype. TFH markers can thus be reliably used for the diagnosis of lymphoid infiltrates in the skin, including cases with subtle infiltrates that may be confused with an inflammatory condition (pattern 1 or 2). As described for LNs,[25,26] PD1 and ICOS appeared to be the most sensitive markers, followed by CXCL13 and CD10, as shown in Table 28-2. The low frequency of CD10 antigen expression in extranodal infiltrates of AITL, including the skin, was highlighted in a study.[30] The variable expression of CD10 reported in published series may reflect the difficulty to assess CD10+ T cells in skin infiltrates, in which numerous CD10+ dendritic cells are usually present. As in most PTCLs, pan-T-cell antigen losses can be observed in cutaneous AITL. CD7 is the most frequently lost antigen, but CD3,[13] CD2, and CD5[14] can also be lost.

As in LNs, scattered EBV-positive B cells can also be identified (Table 28-2) and are helpful for the diagnosis in difficult cases. Interestingly, Lee et al have shown that the frequency of EBV positivity in tumor tissue was

TABLE 28-2 Histopathological and Phenotypic Features of Cutaneous AITL According to Published Series

	Number of Skin Samples	Morphological pattern[a]	Eo/PC (%)	Prevalence of TFH Markers				EBV (%)	B-Cell LPD (No. of Patients)	Molecular Findings in the Skin	
				CD10	CXCL13	PD1	ICOS			T-Cell Clone (%)	Mutations (%)
Martel et al	14	1:14% 2:43% 3:28.5% 4:14%	NE	ND	ND	ND	ND	ND	0	64%	ND
Ortonne et al	15	1:33% 2:33% 3:33% 4:0%	0%/27%	13.5%	80%	ND	ND	40%	1 (EBV+)	87.5%	ND
Leclaire Alirkilicarslan et al	41	1:27% 2:31.5% 3:10% 4:7%	15%/32%	84%	94%	97.5%	26%	4 (2 EBV+ & 2 MP)	100%	RHOA:p.G17V: 78% IDH2 p.R172: 19%
Oishi et al	19	1:26% 2:47% 3:26% 4:0%	26%/47%	37%	ND	100%	ND	17%	1 (EBV+)	82%	ND
Lee et al	42	1:47%; 6% 2:28.6% 3:11.9% 4:11.9%	NE	71.4%	ND	83.3%	ND	45%	NE	66.6%	ND

[a]According to Martel et al: 1: perivascular infiltrate without atypical lymphocytes, 2: perivascular infiltrate with atypical cells, 3: dense lymphomatous infiltrate, and 4: lymphocytic vasculitis.
All data are expressed in percent of positive samples, except for associated B-cell LPD.
LPD, lymphoproliferative disorder; MP, monotypic plasmacytoid LPD; ND, not done, NE, not evaluated.

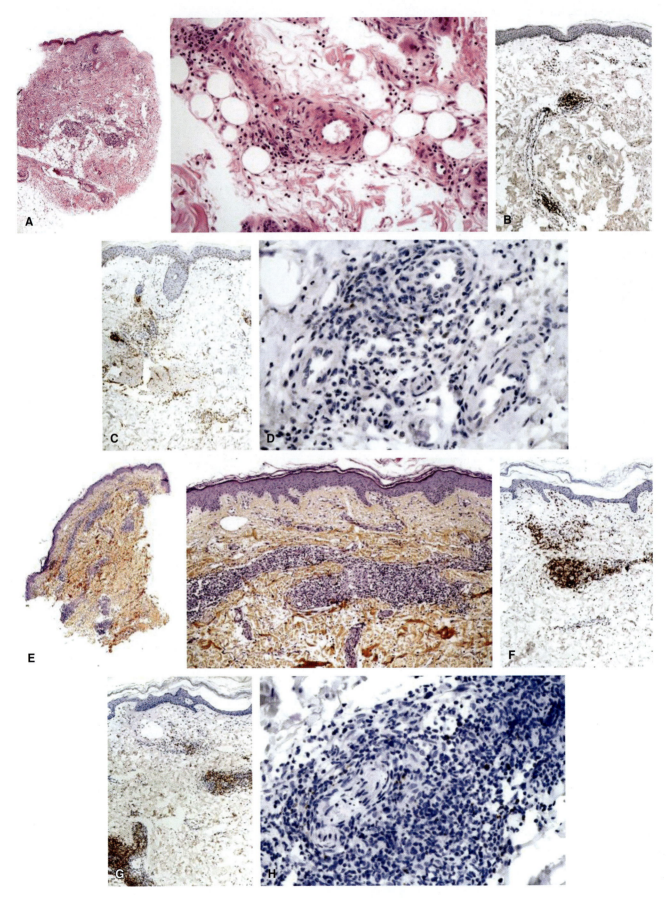

FIGURE 28-2. Cont'd

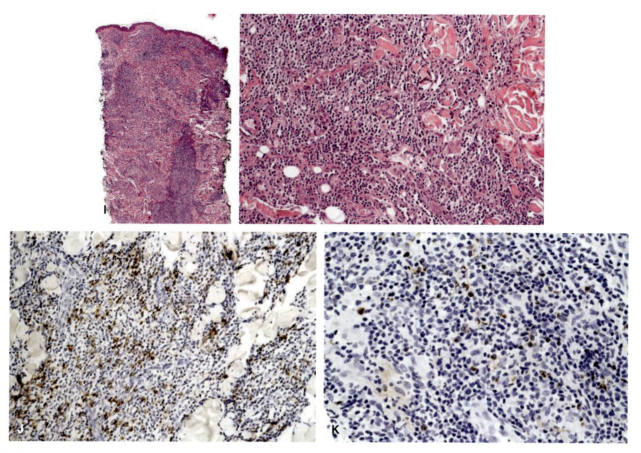

FIGURE 28-2. **Morphological spectrum of cutaneous AITL. A. Pattern 1.** Light perivascular lymphocytic infiltrate involving the superficial and deep dermis with no obvious lymphocytic atypia. H&E (5 × and 400 ×). **B.** CD5 staining showing a light perivascular T-cell infiltrate. Immunohistochemistry (100 ×). **C.** A proportion of T cells express CD10. Immunohistochemistry (100 ×). **D.** Scattered CXCL13+ lymphocytes are admixed with neutrophils. Immunohistochemistry (400 ×). **E. Pattern 2.** Moderately dense lymphocytic infiltrate in which atypical elongated clear lymphocytes are identified. H&E (5 × and 100 ×). **F.** Moderately dense lymphocytic infiltrate identified with CD3 staining. Immunohistochemistry (100 ×). **G.** Strong expression of PD1 by the T-cell infiltrate. Immunohistochemistry (100 ×). **H.** Numerous CXCL13+ T cells are seen. Immunohistochemistry (200 ×). **I. Pattern 3.** Dense lymphocytic infiltrate involving the entire dermis, consisting of clear lymphocytes admixed with eosinophils, normal-appearing lymphocytes, and vessels with high endothelial cells, reminiscent of nodal AITL. H&E (5 × and 10 ×). **J.** Scattered atypical lymphocytes with clear cytoplasm showing PD1 expression. Immunohistochemistry (100 ×). **K.** Numerous CXCL13+ lymphocytes are seen. Immunohistochemistry (200 ×).

significantly higher in patients with skin involvement than in patients without skin involvement and that patients with EBV+ B cells in the skin were older. In addition, they reported that skin manifestations with EBV+ B cells were more frequently papular or nodular in appearance.[15] In this series, the overall survival of patients with EBV+ cutaneous AITL was significantly worse than for patients without cutaneous involvement.

The occurrence of B-cell lineage lymphoproliferative disorders within AITL infiltrates is a well-described phenomenon in the literature,[31,32] including in cutaneous infiltrates.[12,13] EBV+ lymphoproliferative disorders, sometimes with features of diffuse large B-cell lymphoma, can be associated with the malignant T-cell infiltrates of AITL (Fig. 28-3). In patients with an associated EBV+ lymphoproliferative disorder, the neoplastic B-cell component is hypothesized to be derived from the scattered EBV+ B blasts of the tumor microenvironment, which have been shown to have a restricted Ig repertoire.[31,33]

The possible presence of an EBV- monotypic plasma cell component mimicking a plasma cell neoplasm and obscuring the AITL component has been reported in LNs of patients with AITL, as shown in Figure 28-4.[32,34,35] Monoclonal plasmocytoid cells were identified in the skin biopsies in two patients from one series.[13]

Genetics and Molecular Findings

Beside oncogene alterations, the identification of a T-cell clone can help to differentiate AITL skin lesions from inflammatory conditions.[11,12] Although several different T-cell clones may be identified in a single patient with AITL, a dominant T-cell clone was actually reported in skin infiltrates of AITL in 64% to 100% of cases, among published series (Table 28-2). The use of next-generation sequencing studies may increase the ability to detect clonal rearrangements of the TCR in skin infiltrates of AITL. To the best of our knowledge, this new approach has not been studied yet in large cohorts of samples, neither in LNs nor in skin infiltrates.

The mutational profile of AITL neoplastic cells has been recently deciphered, based on whole exome sequencing and more targeted studies performed on case series. In contrast to

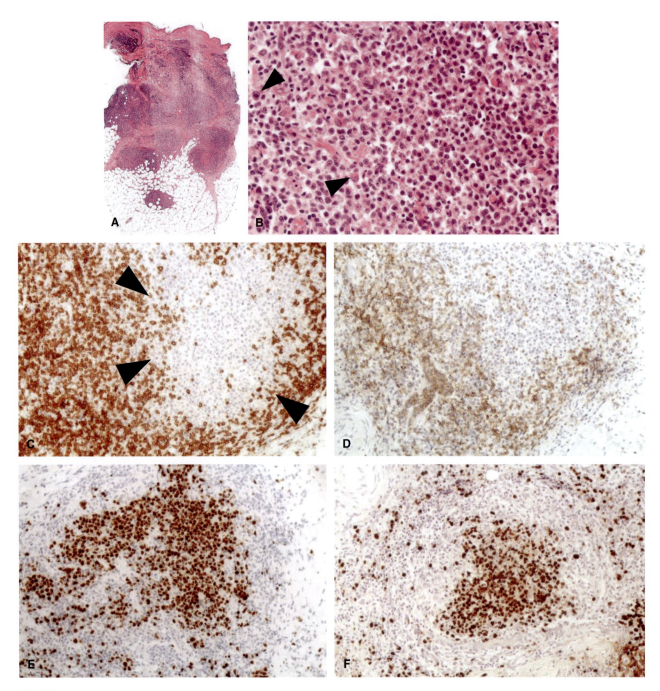

FIGURE 28-3. **EBV+ large B-cell lymphoproliferation associated with cutaneous AITL. A.** Dense lymphocytic infiltrate involving the entire dermis and expanding into the hypodermis. H&E (5 ×). **B.** Atypical dermal infiltrate of small lymphocytes with slightly irregular borders and large atypical lymphocytes with blastoid appearance (arrowheads). H&E (200 ×). **C.** Numerous small, but slightly atypical, CD3+ T cells surrounding aggregates of B cells (arrowheads). Immunohistochemistry (100 ×). **D.** Most of the T cells express PD1. Immunohistochemistry (100 ×). **E.** Aggregates of B cells highlighted by PAX5 staining. Immunohistochemistry (100 ×). **F.** The aggregates of atypical immunoblast-like B cells strongly express EBER. In situ hybridization (200 ×).

many other PTCL subtypes, AITL is associated with recurrent molecular alterations, including hot-spot mutations, targeting mostly *TET2*, *DNMT3A*, *IDH2*, and *RHOA* genes. *TET2*, *DNMT3A*, and *IDH2* genes encode epigenetic regulators.[36-39] Among the mutations involving the *IDH2 gene*, p.R172K is the most prevalent and may be identified in situ using monoclonal antibodies specific for the mutated protein (Fig. 28-5).[13] The *RHOA* gene encodes a GTPase that normally interacts with the actin cytoskeleton downstream of TCR signaling. The mutation almost constantly results in an amino acid substitution at p.G17V,[40-42] reported in up to 70% of cases. Functional studies have shown that the *RHOA* p.G17V mutation may play a role in the pathogenesis of AITL[43] but has no prognostic impact.[42,44] The mutated *RHOA* gene encodes an abnormal protein that can interact with Vav1. The RHOA p.G17V mutation is actually mutually exclusive with *VAV1* gene alterations (activating mutations or rearrangements), which also lead to Vav1 activation.[45] The hierarchy of those mutational events has been studied in *AITL*. *RHOA* and *IDH2* mutations appear to be confined to tumor cells. By contrast,

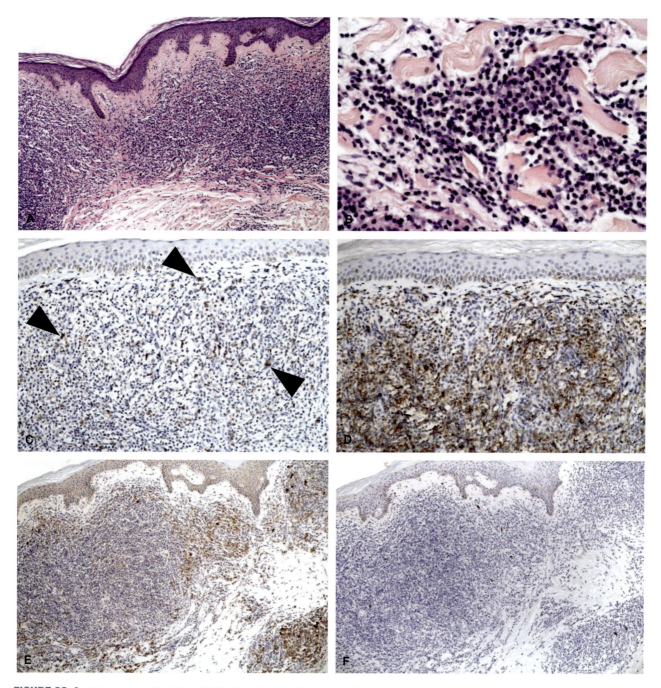

FIGURE 28-4. Cutaneous manifestation of AITL with a plasmocytic lymphoproliferative component with monotypic Kappa light chain expression. **A.** Dense lymphocytic infiltrate mainly organized around dermal vessels and adnexae. H&E (5 ×). **B.** Sheets of plasmocytoid lymphocytes are present at the periphery of the infiltrate. H&E (400 ×). **C-D.** Many lymphocytes are CXCL13+ (**C**, arrowheads) and express PD1 (**D**). Immunohistochemistry (100 ×). **E-F.** In situ hybridization studies showing that the plasmocytoid cells surrounding the neoplastic T cells have kappa light chain restriction. In situ hybridization for Kappa (**E**) and Lambda (**F**) (200 × & 100 ×).

TET2 and *DNMT3A* mutations may be found in normal cells of the tumor microenvironment, including CD8+ T cells or B cells, and in CD34+ precursors.[36,46] *RHOA* and *IDH2* mutations may thus be secondary to other critical molecular events that first occur in "premalignant" lymphocyte precursors or stem cells, reflecting clonal hematopoiesis, and follow a multistep process.[47] In keeping with this, different T-cell clones harboring the same inactivating *TET2* mutation have been identified in AITL infiltrates.[48]

The hot-spot mutations of *RHOA* and *IDH2* genes make them good candidates for a diagnostic assay in AITL.[40] Actually, their presence was demonstrated in skin infiltrates of AITL, including cases presenting with pattern 1 or 2, using allele-specific polymerase chain reaction, highlighting the high sensitivity of this molecular technique.[13] In this study, the frequency of *RHOA* p.G17V mutation in the skin was close to that previously described in LN samples. Although there are no commercially available panels dedicated to the diagnosis of PTCL to date, many laboratories have designed their own panels covering *TET2*, *DNMT3A*, *RHOA*, and *IDH2* genes,[49] which are nowadays used in routine practice.

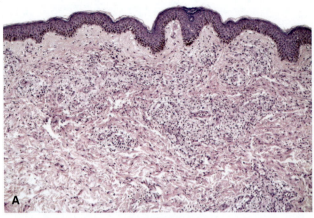
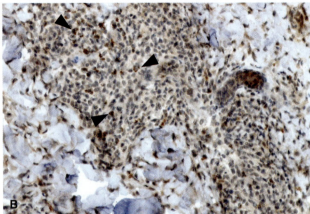

FIGURE 28-5. Cutaneous AITL with *IDH2* R172K mutation. **A.** Dermal infiltrate of small elongated atypical lymphocytes associated with hyperplastic small vessels (pattern 2). **B.** Detection of the R172K IDH2 mutant protein in scattered lymphocytes (arrowheads) within the skin infiltrate. Immunohistochemistry (400 ×).

Differential Diagnosis

The histopathological diagnosis of AITL in the skin may be highly challenging, especially in cases with minimal lymphocytic infiltration mimicking an inflammatory condition, and because other lymphomas may share similar clinicopathological features.

Cutaneous AITL presenting as a maculopapular rash can be difficult to distinguish from a drug reaction, in particular a drug rash with eosinophilia and systemic symptoms (DRESS). Indeed, DRESS syndrome often presents with an erythroderma or a maculopapular rash, is often associated with lymphadenopathy and EBV reactivation, and may show atypical cells in the dermal infiltrates.[50] In addition, inflamed LNs from patients with DRESS syndrome may mimic AITL at the histological level.[51] In case of erythroderma, cutaneous AITL has to be distinguished from other erythrodermic conditions, including T-cell lymphomas such as erythrodermic mycosis fungoides and Sézary syndrome (SS). Clues for the diagnoses are summarized in Table 28-3. In most instances, SS is characterized by lymphocytic infiltrates involving the superficial dermis containing small to medium-sized atypical lymphocytes with hyperchromatic nuclei, and with rare eosinophils and plasma cells. To note, TFH markers may be expressed in SS infiltrates. Both PD1[52,53] and ICOS[54] are actually expressed in most cases, while CXCL13 was shown to be so in a subset of samples.[55]

In patients with papular or nodular lesions, it is important to accurately distinguish cutaneous AITL from other lymphomas or lymphoproliferative disorders of the TFH lineage presenting in the skin. They include primary cutaneous CD4+ small/medium T-cell lymphoproliferative disorder (PCSMLPD) and cutaneous PTCL, NOS. PCSMLPD was recognized as a new specific entity in the World Health Organization classification.[10] PCSMLPD and cutaneous AITL share pathological and immunophenotypic features, including the expression of TFH markers (CXCL13, PD1, and ICOS). They, however, strongly differ clinically, the former presenting as a solitary tumor with indolent behavior. Patients with pure cutaneous TFH lymphomas presenting with multiple skin lesions should be diagnosed as "peripheral T-cell lymphomas, not otherwise specified (PTCL, NOS)." Few authors have reported such cases, and the term "cutaneous T-cell lymphomas showing a TFH phenotype (CTFHL)" was proposed to designate this group of cutaneous lymphomas.[56-58] Le Tourneau et al, Battistella et al, and Buder et al have jointly reported eight cases of patients presenting with multiple rapidly growing papules, plaques, and nodules who showed relative resistance to many treatment modalities including polychemotherapy (PCT). The lesions followed a different course compared with PCSMLPD, with chronic evolution and resistance to treatments including chemotherapies. Therefore, differentiation between cutaneous AITL, CTFHL, and PCSMLPD is necessary because they appear to be different diseases, and this requires clinical information and staging.

Patients with associated B-cell lymphoproliferative disorder may be misdiagnosed as having a B-cell lymphoma,[59] including a marginal zone B-cell lymphoma in case of monotypic plasma cell infiltrates, or a diffuse large B-cell lymphoma in case of EBV+ lymphoproliferations.

Treatment

As for most PTCLs, the management of patients with AITL is highly challenging and there is no specific approach.

Regarding skin manifestations, although the benefit of skin-targeted therapies has been reported in isolated case reports,[60] there is no specific treatment.

Until recently, conventional PCT with cyclophosphamide, doxorubicine hydrochloride (Hydroxydaunorubicin), vincristine (Oncovin) and Prednisone (CHOP) or CHOP-like regimens was the sole treatment option. A complete or partial remission may actually be obtained with PCT in a subset of patients but sustained remission is rare. Overall, it is considered that one-third of patients will be cured, one-third will transiently respond to treatment but ultimately relapse, and one-third will be refractory to treatment.[61] Various other PCT regimens have been studied, and among them, the association of Gemcitabine, Cisplatin, and Methylprednisolone has given encouraging results in relapsed and refractory patients.[62] Until now, CHOP thus remains the standard treatment.

As compared with conventional PCT, the benefits of autologous stem-cell transplantation as first-line treatment for younger patients and allogenic stem-cell transplantation in case of relapse remain controversial.[63] Other treatment modalities are under evaluation in phase 2 trials, such as 5-Azacytidine,[64] and may help to treat patients in the future.

TABLE 28-3 Differential Diagnosis of AITL Presenting With Erythroderma or a Maculopapular Rash

Diagnosis	Erythroderma	Systemic Symptoms	ADP	Atypical Lymphocytes in Blood	Hypereo	Inflammatory Features	Epidermo-tropism	Vasculitis	Atypical Lymphocytes	T-Cell Ag Loss	Phenotype of Atypical Cells	EBV+ B Cells	Skin T-Cell Clone	Blood T-Cell Clone
AITL	+	+	+	Rare	+	Rare	Rare	Possible	Frequent	Possible	$CD4^+$, $CXCL13^+$, $PD1^+$	Possible	+	−
Sézary	+	+	+	+(Sézary cells)	Rare	Rare	Frequent	−	Frequent	Possible (CD7>CD2)	$CD4^+$, $PD1^+$ $KIR3DL2^+$	−	+	+
PCSMLPD	−	−	−	−	−	Rare	Possible	−	+	Rare	$CD4^+$, $PD1^+$	−	+	−
DRESS	Frequent	+	+	Frequent (hyperbaso-philic)	+	Frequent	Frequent	−	Possible	-	$CD8>CD4$ $perf/GrB^+$	Rare	Rare	Rare

PCSMLPD, primary cutaneous $CD4^+$ small/medium T-cell lymphoproliferative disorder.

CAPSULE SUMMARY

- AITL is the most frequent PTCL in Western countries and follows an aggressive course.
- Nearly 50% of patients have skin lesions that can be the first clinical manifestation of the disease, mostly presenting as a pruritic and nonspecific rash resembling a drug reaction.
- Skin infiltrates can either present as slight perivascular lymphocytic infiltrates (pattern 1), perivascular infiltrates with atypical cells (pattern 2), dense lymphomatous infiltrates (pattern 3), or lymphocytic vasculitis (pattern 4).
- Neoplastic T cells maintain a TFH phenotype in the skin and the expression of several markers of this lineage (CXCL13, BCL6, PD1, ICOS) in addition to CD10 is an aid for the diagnosis in skin biopsies.
- A dominant T-cell clone as well as mutations commonly associated with AITL such as *RHOA* p.G17V and *IDH2* p.R172K are usually present in skin infiltrates of AITL, in agreement with their neoplastic nature.
- EBV+ B cells are commonly seen in skin infiltrates of AITL, and their presence is associated with a papular or nodular presentation and with a worse prognosis.
- The main differential diagnoses include viral exanthem and drug reactions, Sézary syndrome, and primary cutaneous CD4+ small/medium T-cell lymphoproliferative disorder.

ACKNOWLEDGMENTS

Acknowledgments to Dr Justin Deschamps for reviewing the English throughout the manuscript.

References

1. Lukes RJ, Tindle BH. Immunoblastic lymphadenopathy. A hyperimmune entity resembling Hodgkin's disease. *N Engl J Med*. 1975;292:1-8.
2. Frizzera G, Moran EM, Rappaport H. Angio-immunoblastic lymphadenopathy. Diagnosis and clinical course. *Am J Med*. 1975;59:803-818.
3. Weltgesundheitsorganisation; Swerdlow SH; International Agency for Research on Cancer, eds. WHO Classification of Tumours of Haematopoietic and Lymphoid Tissues: [... Reflects the Views of a Working Group that Convened for an Editorial and Consensus Conference at the International Agency for Research on Cancer (IARC), Lyon, October 25-27, 2007]. 4th ed. Lyon: Internat. Agency for Research on Cancer; 2008.
4. Swerdlow S, Campo E, Jaffe ES, et al. *WHO Classification of Tumours of Haematopoietic and Lymphoid Tissues*. 4th rev ed. International Agency for Research on Cancer; 2017.
5. de Leval L, Rickman DS, Thielen C, et al. The gene expression profile of nodal peripheral T-cell lymphoma demonstrates a molecular link between angioimmunoblastic T-cell lymphoma (AITL) and follicular helper T (TFH) cells. *Blood*. 2007;109:4952-4963.
6. Piccaluga PP, Agostinelli C, Califano A, et al. Gene expression analysis of angioimmunoblastic lymphoma indicates derivation from T follicular helper cells and vascular endothelial growth factor deregulation. *Cancer Res*. 2007;67:10703-10710.
7. Mourad N, Mounier N, Brière J, et al. Clinical, biologic, and pathologic features in 157 patients with angioimmunoblastic T-cell lymphoma treated within the Groupe d'Etude des Lymphomes de l'Adulte (GELA) trials. *Blood*. 2008;111:4463-4470.
8. Lachenal F, Berger F, Ghesquières H, et al. Angioimmunoblastic T-cell lymphoma: clinical and laboratory features at diagnosis in 77 patients. *Medicine (Baltim)*. 2007;86:282-292.
9. Tokunaga T, Shimada K, Yamamoto K, et al. Retrospective analysis of prognostic factors for angioimmunoblastic T-cell lymphoma: a multicenter cooperative study in Japan. *Blood*. 2012;119:2837-2843.
10. Swerdlow SH, Campo E, Pileri SA, et al. The 2016 revision of the World Health Organization classification of lymphoid neoplasms. *Blood*. 2016;127:2375-2390.
11. Martel P, Laroche L, Courville P, et al. Cutaneous involvement in patients with angioimmunoblastic lymphadenopathy with dysproteinemia: a clinical, immunohistological, and molecular analysis. *Arch Dermatol*. 2000;136:881-886.
12. Ortonne N, Dupuis J, Plonquet A, et al. Characterization of CXCL13+ neoplastic t cells in cutaneous lesions of angioimmunoblastic T-cell lymphoma (AITL). *Am J Surg Pathol*. 2007;31:1068-1076.
13. Leclaire Alirkilicarslan A, Dupuy A, Pujals A, et al. Expression of TFH markers and detection of RHOA p.G17V and IDH2 p.R172K/S mutations in cutaneous localizations of angioimmunoblastic T-cell lymphomas. *Am J Surg Pathol*. 2017;41:1581-1592.
14. Oishi N, Sartori-Valinotti JC, Bennani NN, et al. Cutaneous lesions of angioimmunoblastic T-cell lymphoma: clinical, pathological, and immunophenotypic features. *J Cutan Pathol*. 2019;46:637-644.
15. Lee WJ, Won KH, Choi JW, et al. Cutaneous angioimmunoblastic T-cell lymphoma: epstein-Barr virus positivity and its effects on clinicopathologic features. *J Am Acad Dermatol*. 2019;81:989-997.
16. Balaraman B, Conley JA, Sheinbein DM. Evaluation of cutaneous angioimmunoblastic T-cell lymphoma. *J Am Acad Dermatol*. 2011;65:855-862.
17. Colmant C, Camboni A, Dekeuleneer V, et al. Linear IgA dermatosis in association with angioimmunoblastic T-cell lymphoma infiltrating the skin: a case report with literature review. *J Cutan Pathol*. 2020;47:251-256.
18. Sugaya M, Nakamura K, Asahina A, et al. Leukocytoclastic vasculitis with IgA deposits in angioimmunoblastic T cell lymphoma. *J Dermatol*. 2001;28:32-37.
19. de Leval L, Parrens M, Le Bras F, et al. Angioimmunoblastic T-cell lymphoma is the most common T-cell lymphoma in two distinct French information data sets. *Haematologica*. 2015;100:e361-364.
20. Attygalle AD, Kyriakou C, Dupuis J, et al. Histologic evolution of angioimmunoblastic T-cell lymphoma in consecutive biopsies: clinical correlation and insights into natural history and disease progression. *Am J Surg Pathol*. 2007;31:1077-1088.
21. Seehafer JR, Goldberg NC, Dicken CH, et al. Cutaneous manifestations of angioimmunoblastic lymphadenopathy. *Arch Dermatol*. 1980;116:41-45.
22. Patterson. *Weedon's Skin Pathology*. Elsevier Health Sciences; 2020.
23. Suarez-Vilela D, Izquierdo-Garcia FM. Angioimmunoblastic lymphadenopathy-like T-cell lymphoma: cutaneous clinical onset with prominent granulomatous reaction. *Am J Surg Pathol*. 2003;27:699-700.
24. Jayaraman AG, Cassarino D, Advani R, et al. Cutaneous involvement by angioimmunoblastic T-cell lymphoma: a unique histologic presentation, mimicking an infectious etiology. *J Cutan Pathol*. 2006;33(suppl 2):6-11.

25. Roncador G, García Verdes-Montenegro J-F, Tedoldi S, et al. Expression of two markers of germinal center T cells (SAP and PD-1) in angioimmunoblastic T-cell lymphoma. *Haematologica*. 2007;92:1059-1066.
26. Marafioti T, Paterson JC, Ballabio E, et al. The inducible T-cell co-stimulator molecule is expressed on subsets of T cells and is a new marker of lymphomas of T follicular helper cell-derivation. *Haematologica*. 2010;95:432-439.
27. Dupuis J, Boye K, Martin N, et al. Expression of CXCL13 by neoplastic cells in angioimmunoblastic T-cell lymphoma (AITL): a new diagnostic marker providing evidence that AITL derives from follicular helper T cells. *Am J Surg Pathol*. 2006;30:490-494.
28. Attygalle A, Al-Jehani R, Diss TC, et al. Neoplastic T cells in angioimmunoblastic T-cell lymphoma express CD10. *Blood*. 2002;99:627-633.
29. Murakami YI, Yatabe Y, Sakaguchi T, et al. c-Maf expression in angioimmunoblastic T-cell lymphoma. *Am J Surg Pathol*. 2007;31:1695-1702.
30. Attygalle AD, Diss TC, Munson P, et al. CD10 expression in extranodal dissemination of angioimmunoblastic T-cell lymphoma. *Am J Surg Pathol*. 2004;28:54-61.
31. Willenbrock K, Bräuninger A, Hansmann M-L. Frequent occurrence of B-cell lymphomas in angioimmunoblastic T-cell lymphoma and proliferation of Epstein-Barr virus-infected cells in early cases. *Br J Haematol*. 2007;138:733-739.
32. Attygalle AD, Cabeçadas J, Gaulard P, et al. Peripheral T-cell and NK-cell lymphomas and their mimics; taking a step forward—report on the lymphoma workshop of the XVIth meeting of the European Association for Haematopathology and the Society for Hematopathology. *Histopathology*. 2014;64:171-199.
33. Bräuninger A, Spieker T, Willenbrock K, et al. Survival and clonal expansion of mutating "forbidden" (immunoglobulin receptor-deficient) Epstein-Barr virus-infected b cells in angioimmunoblastic t cell lymphoma. *J Exp Med*. 2001;194:927-940.
34. Huppmann AR, Roullet MR, Raffeld M, et al. Angioimmunoblastic T-cell lymphoma partially obscured by an Epstein-Barr virus-negative clonal plasma cell proliferation. *J Clin Oncol*. 2013;31:e28-e30.
35. Balagué O, Martínez A, Colomo L, et al. Epstein-Barr virus negative clonal plasma cell proliferations and lymphomas in peripheral T-cell lymphomas: a phenomenon with distinctive clinicopathologic features. *Am J Surg Pathol*. 2007;31:1310-1322.
36. Quivoron C, Couronné L, Della Valle V, et al. TET2 inactivation results in pleiotropic hematopoietic abnormalities in mouse and is a recurrent event during human lymphomagenesis. *Cancer Cell*. 2011;20:25-38.
37. Odejide O, Weigert O, Lane AA, et al. A targeted mutational landscape of angioimmunoblastic T-cell lymphoma. *Blood*. 2014;123:1293-1296.
38. Couronné L, Bastard C, Bernard OA. TET2 and DNMT3A mutations in human T-cell lymphoma. *N Engl J Med*. 2012;366:95-96. doi:10.1056/NEJMc1111708
39. Cairns RA, Iqbal J, Lemonnier F, et al. IDH2 mutations are frequent in angioimmunoblastic T-cell lymphoma. *Blood*. 2012;119:1901-1903.
40. Sakata-Yanagimoto M, Enami T, Yoshida K, et al. Somatic RHOA mutation in angioimmunoblastic T cell lymphoma. *Nat Genet*. 2014;46:171-175.
41. Palomero T, Couronné L, Khiabanian H, et al. Recurrent mutations in epigenetic regulators, RHOA and FYN kinase in peripheral T cell lymphomas. *Nat Genet*. 2014;46:166-170.
42. Vallois D, Dobay MPD, Morin RD, et al. Activating mutations in genes related to TCR signaling in angioimmunoblastic and other follicular helper T-cell-derived lymphomas. *Blood*. 2016;128:1490-1502.
43. Yoo HY, Sung MK, Lee SH, et al. A recurrent inactivating mutation in RHOA GTPase in angioimmunoblastic T cell lymphoma. *Nat Genet*. 2014;46:371-375.
44. Ondrejka SL, Grzywacz B, Bodo J, et al. Angioimmunoblastic T-cell lymphomas with the RHOA p.Gly17Val mutation have classic clinical and pathologic features. *Am J Surg Pathol*. 2016;40:335-341.
45. Fujisawa M, Sakata-Yanagimoto M, Nishizawa S, et al. Activation of RHOA-VAV1 signaling in angioimmunoblastic T-cell lymphoma. *Leukemia*. 2017;32(3):694-702.
46. Nguyen TB, Sakata-Yanagimoto M, Asabe Y, et al. Identification of cell-type-specific mutations in nodal T-cell lymphomas. *Blood Cancer J*. 2017;7:e516.
47. Sakata-Yanagimoto M. Multistep tumorigenesis in peripheral T cell lymphoma. *Int J Hematol*. 2015;102:523-527.
48. Yao W-Q, Wu F, Zhang W, et al. Angioimmunoblastic T-cell lymphoma contains multiple clonal T-cell populations derived from a common TET2 mutant progenitor cell. *J Pathol*. 2020;250:346-357.
49. Dupuy A. Multiple ways to detect IDH2 mutations in angioimmunoblastic T cell lymphoma: from immunohistochemistry to Next Generation Sequencing. *J Mol Diagn*. 2018;20(5):677-685.
50. Ortonne N, Valeyrie-Allanore L, Bastuji-Garin S, et al. Histopathology of drug rash with eosinophilia and systemic symptoms syndrome: a morphological and phenotypical study. *Br J Dermatol*. 2015;173:50-58.
51. Rim MY, Hong J, Yo I, et al. Cervical lymphadenopathy mimicking angioimmunoblastic T-cell lymphoma after dapsone-induced hypersensitivity syndrome. *Korean J Pathol*. 2012;46:606-610.
52. Cetinözman F, Jansen PM, Vermeer MH, et al. Differential expression of programmed death-1 (PD-1) in Sézary syndrome and mycosis fungoides. *Arch Dermatol*. 2012;148:1379-1385.
53. Samimi S, Benoit B, Evans K, et al. Increased programmed death-1 expression on CD4+ T cells in cutaneous T-cell lymphoma: implications for immune suppression. *Arch Dermatol*. 2010;146:1382-1388.
54. Amatore F, Ortonne N, Lopez M, et al. ICOS is widely expressed in cutaneous T-cell lymphoma and its targeting promotes potent killing of malignant cells. *Blood Adv*. 2020;4(20):5203-5214.
55. Picchio MC, Scala E, Pomponi D, et al. CXCL13 is highly produced by Sézary cells and enhances their migratory ability via a synergistic mechanism involving CCL19 and CCL21 chemokines. *Cancer Res*. 2008;68:7137-7146.
56. Battistella M, Beylot-Barry M, Bachelez H, et al. Primary cutaneous follicular helper T-cell lymphoma: a new subtype of cutaneous T-cell lymphoma reported in a series of 5 cases. *Arch Dermatol*. 2012;148:832-839.
57. Le Tourneau A, Audouin J, Molina T, et al. Primary cutaneous follicular variant of peripheral T-cell lymphoma NOS. A report of two cases. *Histopathology*. 2010;56:548-551.
58. Buder K, Poppe LM, Bröcker EB, et al. Primary cutaneous follicular helper T-cell lymphoma: diagnostic pitfalls of this new lymphoma subtype. *J Cutan Pathol*. 2013;40:903-908.

59. Szablewski V, Dereure O, René C, et al. Cutaneous localization of angioimmunoblastic T-cell lymphoma may masquerade as B-cell lymphoma or classical Hodgkin lymphoma: a histologic diagnostic pitfall. *J Cutan Pathol.* 2019;46:102-110.
60. Tartar D, Konia T, Fung M, et al. Treatment of cutaneous angioimmunoblastic T-cell lymphoma with Fractionated Carbon Dioxide Laser. *Dermatol Surg.* 2016;42:560-562.
61. Abouyabis AN, Shenoy PJ, Sinha R, et al. A systematic review and meta-analysis of front-line anthracycline-based chemotherapy regimens for peripheral T-cell lymphoma. *ISRN Hematol.* 2011;2011:623924.
62. Gleeson M, Peckitt C, To YM, et al. CHOP versus GEM-P in previously untreated patients with peripheral T-cell lymphoma (CHEMO-T): a phase 2, multicentre, randomised, open-label trial. *Lancet Haematol.* 2018;5:e190-e200.
63. Fossard G, Broussais F, Coelho I, et al. Role of up-front autologous stem-cell transplantation in peripheral T-cell lymphoma for patients in response after induction: an analysis of patients from LYSA centers. *Ann Oncol.* 2018;29:715-723.
64. Lemonnier F, Dupuis J, Sujobert P, et al. Treatment with 5-azacytidine induces a sustained response in patients with angioimmunoblastic T-cell lymphoma. *Blood.* 2018;132(21):2305-2309.

CHAPTER 29

Adult T-cell leukemia/lymphoma

Melissa Pulitzer

DEFINITION

Adult T-cell leukemia/lymphoma (ATLL) is an aggressive peripheral T-cell malignancy of a mature helper-T/regulatory-phenotype, which develops after chronic infection with human T-lymphotropic virus-1 (HTLV-1). The cells usually express CD4 and the IL-2 receptor CD25. Malignant T-cells in ATLL may present primarily in the skin or systemically with secondary skin involvement. Classification of ATLL as leukemia or lymphoma depends on the presentation as either infiltration of the blood by neoplastic cells or as infiltrative disease of the lymphoid organs, respectively.[1]

EPIDEMIOLOGY

ATLL most often occurs in patients from areas endemic for HTLV-1, with onset at approximately age 60 in patients of Japanese origin,[2] versus age 40 in South and Central American and Caribbean patients.[3,4] In Japan, there is a three times increased incidence of HTLV-1 infection in women; however, there is a marked predilection for the development of ATLL in men with a 3- to 5-fold higher risk versus females and a 6% to 7% lifetime risk for men vs 2% to 3% in women.[5] HTLV-1 prevalence in many parts of the world is difficult to ascertain, with estimates of 5 to 20 million carriers worldwide, mostly in pockets of endemic areas with ranges from 1% to 40% including southwest Japan, the Caribbean basin,[3] regions of South America including Peru,[6] Colombia, French Guyana and Brazil (mostly within populations of African > Japanese ancestry but also small tribes of South Amerindian and ancient Andean ancestry), equatorial Africa such as South Gabon, Australo-Melanesia, and small groups in the Middle East such as the Mashhad region of Iran. Romania and Southern Italy are rare European countries with endemic HTLV-1,[7] and within the United States, areas of higher prevalence include particular regions of NY (primarily within an African American population,[8] with a distinctively lower male:female ratio), LA, and Miami. Transmission of HTLV-1 is most often vertical (mother to child via breast milk). Other means of transmission include sexual intercourse and blood transfusion of packed red blood cells. Antibodies to HTLV-1 are found in 6% to 37% of healthy adults aged over 40 in endemic areas in Japan and are increasing in nonendemic areas in Japan and the United States, suggesting spread by move of carriers.[9] The seroprevalence of HTLV-1 in the United States is reportedly 0.01% to 0.03%.[10]

Up to 5% of HTLV-1 carriers will develop ATLL, usually after a latency of 2 to 4 decades following infection early in life. Earlier exposure to virus is associated with a higher risk of malignancy. Additional risk factors include high viral load, age, family history of ATLL or HTLV-1 associated myelopathy/tropical spastic paraparesis, and immunocompromise.[11] Overall lifetime risk of progression to ATLL is 2.1% in women and 6.6% in men.[12] Worldwide, in 2012,[13,14] the GLOBOCAN database of the IARC estimated 3000 new cases of ATLL, from 2100 in 2008[14] and 3340 in 2002.[15] In the United States, the incidence of ATLL is approximately one per million individuals per year (300 per year, with an age-adjusted incidence of 0.05 in males, and 0.03 in females per 100,000 per year).[8] In endemic areas of Japan, ATLL is estimated to represent as many as 16.8% of all non-Hodgkin lymphoma, representing the most common T-cell NHL in the country.[16]

ETIOLOGY

ATLL was described as a clinical entity in Japan in 1977 by Uchiyama, Takatsuki, and others.[17,18] Shortly thereafter, retrovirus particles that were later identified as HTLV-1 were isolated from a patient with cutaneous T-cell lymphoma in the United States,[19] resulting in the confirmation of the Japanese syndrome as a virally associated lymphoproliferative disease.

HTLV-1 is a single-stranded RNA virus with a diploid genome, which infects human CD4+ helper T-cells, undergoes reverse transcription to proviral DNA, and randomly integrates into the host genome. Early in infection, HTLV-1 is thought to spread via cell-to-cell conjugation, viral budding, and the formation of an extracellular viral assembly, which can easily transmit to adjacent immune cells.[20] Over time, viral burden increases as the virus induces clonal proliferations of infected cells in most HTLV-1 carriers. Clones each exhibit a different integration site of provirus and can persist for decades. Insertion of provirus into cellular genomic DNA near transcriptional start sites of cellular genes,[21] or near activating epigenetic markers, may confer a survival advantage for those clones, influencing the number of clones expressed.[22,23] Over time, the high relative abundance of a clone of cells with a single viral integration site constitutes "monoclonality," correlating with neoplasia. Although no

TABLE 29-1 Genes Harboring Provirus[14]		
CD46	CASP8	BCL2
ITGA4	CDKN2A	IL6ST
DPYSL2	GTF21	HGF
RAP2A	TACR1	

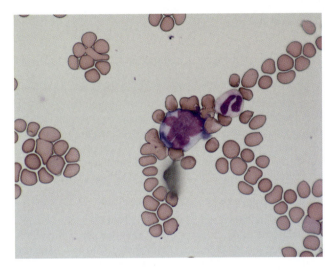

FIGURE 29-1. A classic "flower cell" of adult T-cell leukemia, showing multilobated nuclei, in a background of atypical monolobated lymphocytes and erythrocytes from a peripheral smear. (Photo courtesy of Mikhail Roshal, MD.)

specific viral integration hot spots have been identified, some genes are more frequently affected than others (Table 29-1).[23]

The provirus itself encodes products, which promote cellular transformation, including the retroviral long terminal repeats gag, pol, env, and a unique pX region. The latter encodes a 40-kDa cell-transforming oncoprotein Tax and human basic zipper factor HBZ, which are implicated in proliferation. The resultant HTLV-1 proteins are often silenced in both HTLV-1 carriers and ATLL patients, allowing infected cells to evade the host response[24] by interactions with the host microenvironment[25] or by other epigenetic mechanisms.[26] Phylogenetic analyses have suggested that ATL-associated HLA alleles HLA-A*26 and HLA-A*36 confer a natural host status to carriers via a low immune responsiveness to the virus, which explains subpopulations of ATL patients in disparate geographic locales who exhibit similar disease course.[27]

CLINICAL PRESENTATION AND PROGNOSIS

Although as many as 31% of patients may present with disease limited to the skin,[4] more commonly there is systemic involvement at presentation. This includes widespread lymph node and marrow or other extranodal (lung, liver, GI) involvement, elevated lactate dehydrogenase (LDH), and/or hypercalcemia, with or without skin lesions. Eventually, skin involvement develops in ~50% of all patients. Peripheral blood may show anemia, thrombocytopenia, leukocytosis, neutrophilia, and/or eosinophilia. Flower cells (Fig. 29-1) or occasional blast-like lymphoma cells may be present. Some of these findings may vary according to the geographic region, for example, less hypercalcemia and concomitantly less osteolysis have been identified in Caribbean patients.[4]

The spectrum of ATLL presentations was originally delineated by the Shimoyama classification, which divides ATLL presentations into acute, chronic, lymphomatous, and smoldering types[28,29] (Table 29-2). Over time, the acute and lymphomatous forms have come to be known as the most aggressive forms of the disease with median survival of 8.3 and 10.6 months, respectively.[30] The chronic and smoldering forms are less aggressive (31.5 and 55 months MS, respectively). Chronic ATLL with a high LDH may be categorized as "unfavorable chronic." Hypercalcemia is considered an adverse prognostic marker.[31] Serum soluble interleukin-2 receptor appears to be an independent prognostic factor for chronic and smoldering subtypes, which can sometimes progress to a more aggressive type of ATLL. Not only do the chronic and smoldering subtypes have a more protracted course, but they also show more frequent skin involvement (43%-72%).[32] When the skin is the *only* organ involved (all types considered), the prognosis is better—with a caveat below.[33] There is controversy as to whether skin involvement in patients with extracutaneous disease is a poor prognostic factor, with some authors finding an adverse impact of skin involvement,[34] and others finding no survival difference.

Among patients with skin involvement, smoldering ATLL with a deep versus superficial infiltrate may have a worse overall survival.[34] Moreover, the type of clinical skin eruption in smoldering ATLL was shown to be an independent prognostic factor although smoldering disease was the variant most commonly marked by patch lesions[35] (Table 29-3). Patch and plaque disease were linked to better outcomes; erythrodermic presentations correlated with shorter survival (present in typically acute ATLL).[36] Extranodal primary cutaneous ATLL with no leukemic component had previously been subdivided into erythematous-papular and tumoral types.[37,38] Worse outcomes were identified for primary cutaneous ATLL compared to smoldering ATLL overall and a worse outcome for the tumoral versus erythemopapular type was specifically identified. Thus, recently, cases of primary cutaneous tumoral ATL without leukemic, lymph node, or other lesions, which had been recognized to have worse outcomes than smoldering ATLL without skin lesions,[36] are recommended to be recognized with the designation "lymphoma type of ATL, extranodal primary cutaneous variant" within the revised ATLL International Consensus meeting report,[39] a fifth clinical type in the Shimoyama classification.[38] These tumors grow rapidly, and as with erythrodermic types, have been shown to have a 5-year survival rate of 0%; thus, this categorization allows for more appropriately aggressive ATL protocols.

Beyond the common nodules, tumors, papules, plaques, and macules[35] of ATLL (Fig. 29-2), clinical presentations also include subcutaneous tumors, erythroderma, purpura, alopecia, and folliculitis (Fig. 29-3). Although all types can mimic other cutaneous lymphomas, the clinical differential diagnoses also include a wide range of nonlymphomatous entities.[4]

TABLE 29-2 Shimoyama Classification of Adult T-Cell Leukemia/Lymphoma[18,19]

Type	% cases	Blood	LYMPH nodes	SKIN	Systemic	Median/2-Y/4-Y Survival
Acute	60%	Leukocytosis, atypical lymphocytes, polylobated flower cells, eosinophilia	LAD	50% of cases tumor, patch, plaque, erythroderma	HSMG, LDH, hypercalcemia w/wo osteolysis, renal, fever, cough, neuropsychiatric	6 mo/16.7%/5%
Chronic	15%	Leukocytosis, >10% lymphocytes, fewer atypical cells	Mild LAD	Common	Mild HSMG, normal to elevated calcium	24 mo/52.4%/26.9%
Lymphoma	20%	Aleukemic, no lymphocytosis, rare circulating leukemia cells	Marked LAD	Rare cases	+/− elevated calcium	10 mo/21.3%/5.7%
Smoldering	5%	Normal WBC, <5% atypical lymphocytes	No or minimal LAD	Most cases	Lung, no or minimal HMSG, normal calcium/LDH	24 mo/77.7%/62.8%

HSMG, hepatosplenomegaly; LAD, lymphadenopathy; LDH, lactate dehydrogenase; WBC, white blood count.

TABLE 29-3 Clinical Lesion Stratification for Adult T-Cell Leukemia/Lymphoma[23]

Type of Lesion	Prognosis[a]
Nodulotumoral	Most severe
Erythroderma	Most severe
Multipapular	Intermediate
Plaque	Least severe
Patch	Least severe
Purpuric	Unknown

[a]Prognostic significance of skin lesion type in otherwise extracutaneous disease. It has been suggested that the most "severe type" of skin lesions should be noted, when multiple types of skin eruption exist in a given patient.

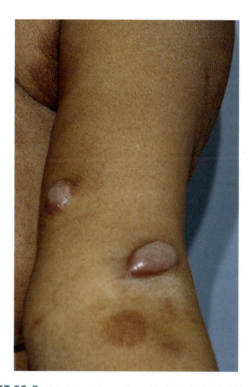

FIGURE 29-2. Plaques and tumors in a patient with ATLL, mimicking MF.

Patients with all subtypes of ATLL are susceptible to superimposed infection owing to impaired cellular immunity. Such infections range from tuberculosis to crusted scabies,[17] *Pneumocystis carinii*, fungi, viruses, and parasites. Fungal infections of the skin including tinea and candida are seen in 50% of ATLL patients, are often intractable with treatment, and exhibit little inflammation, consistent with defective innate immunity to these organisms.[40] *Strongyloides stercoralis* is often seen in HTLV-1 patients (16.3% in HTLV-1+ vs 7.6% in HTLV-1−)[41] and may have bearing on susceptibility to development of clonal disease.

Initial diagnosis of ATLL is made by clinical presentation and confirmation of HTLV-1 seropositivity. Enzyme-linked immunosorbent assay (ELISA) screening is the test most commonly used for diagnosis of HTLV-1.[38] If positive, often

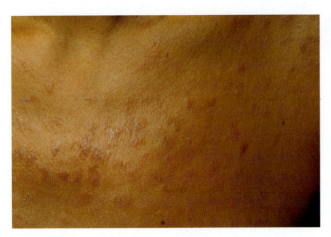

FIGURE 29-3. Follicular papules in a patient with folliculitis-like ATLL.

after duplicate testing, serum is tested by either immunoblot assay (typically Western blot) or enzyme immunoassay INNO-LIA for confirmation.[5] If cases are indeterminate by ELISA/blot/EI sequence, then polymerase chain reaction (PCR) is used to look for proviral DNA in peripheral blood mononuclear cells (PBMCs). When blood is not available, other biologic fluids which can be used for HTLV-1 testing include breast milk, urine, and saliva. Predictors of the evolution of clinical disease include rising or high proviral load (PVL) (typically rising over decades from <0.001% to >100%), which is assessed by quantitative of digital droplet PCR of PBMCs or leukocyte concentrates, lymph nodes, or skin.[5] The risk of disease is increased with PVL >4% in Japan or >10% in the United Kingdom.[42] Another major determinant of risk may be the absolute number of clones,[15] which is determined by the efficiency of host cytotoxic T-lymphocyte response to virus.[43,44]

Regarding therapies, clinically aggressive subtypes (acute, lymphoma, and unfavorable chronic) are managed as subtypes of aggressive non-Hodgkin lymphoma, often with allogeneic stem cell transplant and/or multiagent chemotherapy, although the use of investigational agents has grown (alemtuzumab ± AI (8), belinostat ± AZT (3), bortezomib (1), brentuximab vedotin (6), denileukin diftitox (2), mogamulizumab (2), valproic acid/AZT (1), vorinostat-AZT (1) zidovudine/interferon), whereas indolent types (favorable chronic and smoldering) are treated similar to CLL,[45-47] often with watchful waiting. Skin lesions of indolent ATLL can sometimes be treated by topical steroids, UV light, radiation, systemic steroids, oral retinoids, interferon, or single-agent chemotherapy.[48] While mogamulizumab has been approved in Japan for the treatment of ATLL, the studies conducted in the United States showed less significant responses.[49]

HISTOLOGY

Histopathologic features of ATLL are well defined for nodal disease per WHO classification schema from 2008 (Table 29-4). In the skin, architectural patterns are described as perivascular, nodular, or diffuse[20] (Fig. 29-4A–C). Lichenoid and interstitial patterns are not uncommon (Fig. 29-5). The findings are most often those of an epidermotropic, pleomorphic, large-cell lymphoma with high-grade features including cells with multilobation, angiocentrism (Fig. 29-6), perineural invasion, and marked adnexotropism, including follicular mucinosis[4,50,51] (Fig. 29-7). Pautrier-like microabscesses are common and tend to be larger and more pleomorphic (than cases of typical mycosis fungoides)[4] (Fig. 29-8). The chronic type of ATLL may be less florid in its presentation. Of note, patients whose biopsies show one type of morphology in skin lesions can show different findings in subsequent biopsies.[52]

TABLE 29-4 WHO Morphologic Classification for Adult T-Cell Leukemia/Lymphoma

Type a	Pleomorphic small-cell type[a]
Type b	Pleomorphic medium-cell type[b]
Type c	Pleomorphic large-cell type
Type d	Anaplastic large-cell lymphoma-like type[c]
	Angioimmunoblastic lymphoma (AITL) type[d]

[a]Small cells approximate the size of normal blood lymphocytes.
[b]Medium and large cells may be cerebriform and may contain Reed–Sternberg-like or bizarre large cells.
[c]ALCL-type tumors may contain multinucleated or cerebriform mononuclear cells, often with prominent nucleoli (as in "flower cells") and abundant cytoplasm.
[d]The least common AITL type is characterized by high endothelial venules, plasma cells, and eosinophils with medium-sized lymphocytes.[20]

IMMUNOPHENOTYPE CHECK CURRENT WHO

Neoplastic lymphocytes are typically positive for CD2, CD3, CD4, CD5, CD45RO, and CD25 (IL-2 receptor) with a CD4:CD8 ratio greater than 20:1[4,53] (Fig. 29-9). CD7 and CD8 are usually negative.[53] CD3 may be decreased. CD30 may be present in over half of ATLL lesions, particularly in the Caribbean population (54% vs Japanese 19%).[4] Rare CD8+ variants show no survival difference[54] and CD56 positivity is rare, possibly correlating with advanced cases and poor outcomes.[55] CD99 was reported in four out of six tumors tested and may yet be useful as an ancillary test.[56] Both PD-1 and PD-1-L may be positive in neoplastic and nonneoplastic CD4+ T-cells in ATLL patients, possibly contributing to tumor-related immunosuppression.[25,57] ATLL shows a high frequency of CCR4 expression in the blood and skin, which may facilitate lymph node invasion by binding nodal and epidermal CCL17 and CCL22.[58] FOXp3 transcription factor, an indicator of the T_{reg} phenotype, may serve to suppress the activation or proliferation of other CD4+ and CD8+ T-cells and is frequently positive in subsets of ATLL. As with CD30, FOXp3 has been noted in the Caribbean population in which 62% of cases were FOXp3+. This was found to correlate with CD25 expression.[52] Moreover, FOXp3 is also reported to label inversely to CD30+.[59] FOXp3 is expressed less often in most Japanese studies, ranging from 30% to 68%[59-61] and may correlate with the presence of more Epstein-Barr virus positive cells.[59]

Tumor-associated macrophages of the alternatively activated phenotype M2 (CD163+, IL10+, and chemokine ligand+)[62] may induce angiogenesis, immunosuppression,

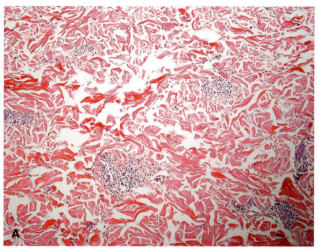
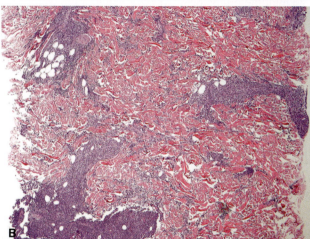
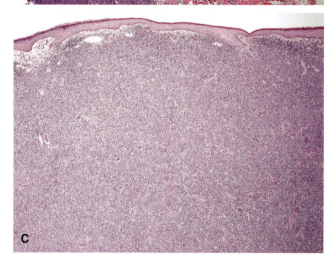

FIGURE 29-4. The most common histopathologic patterns seen in cutaneous involvement by ATLL are perivascular **(A)**, nodular **(B)**, and diffuse **(C)**.

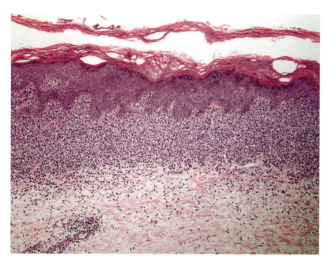

FIGURE 29-5. Lichenoid patterns of infiltration are common in plaque-type disease.

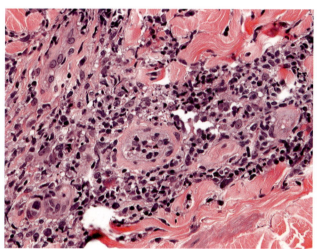

FIGURE 29-6. Malignant T-cells are pleomorphic and tend to localize to the blood vessels (angiocentrism).

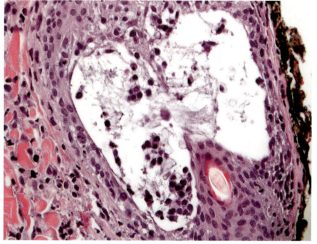

FIGURE 29-7. Follicular mucin is seen in up to 10% of cases and is associated with folliculotropic large atypical lymphocytes.

and invasion and may be associated with progression of ATLL. The percentage of CD163+ cells in infiltrates was an independent prognostic factor on multivariate analysis,[63] and a higher ratio of CD163-to-CD68+ macrophages in ATLL may correlate with worse survival.[63] The use of HBZ and tax RNA scope in situ hybridization (ISH) probes have been shown to be useful in confirming the diagnosis in the absence of viral integration studies.[64]

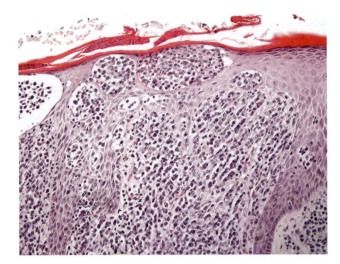

FIGURE 29-8. Unlike in MF, Pautrier-like microabscesses in ATLL tend to be large and composed of hyperchromatic large lymphocytes without cerebriform atypia.

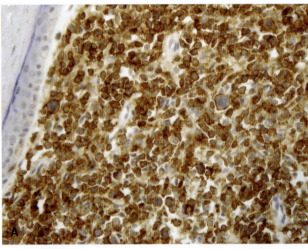
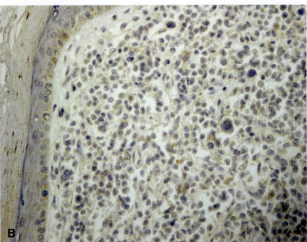

FIGURE 29-9. CD4 is typically diffuse and strong in labeling pattern **(A)**, whereas CD8 tends to be absent, with few to no positive intervening reactive cells **(B)**.

GENETIC AND MOLECULAR FINDINGS

The molecular mechanisms of transformation in ATLL are thought to include a multistep process in which the virus induces a chronic T-lymphoproliferative state, with accumulation of genetic defects that allow for the development of monoclonal neoplasia over time. Although PCR usually shows monoclonal T-cell receptor gene rearrangements in ATLL, supporting a diagnosis of lymphoma, such findings are not specific for ATLL. Demonstration of proviral integration within host genomes is more specific, but it is not usually performed outside a research setting in the United States. Patterns of viral integration, as assessed by Southern blot, have been shown to correlate with survival and include the following variants: defective "D-type" integration, complete/monoclonal "C-type" integration, and multiple/oligoclonal "M-type" integration, which correlate with median survivals of 6.8, 24.4, and 33.3 months, respectively.[65]

Viral genetics have been well studied. Tax is a transactivator and oncoprotein which enhances and represses transcription of viral and cellular gene products, interfering with DNA repair and affecting proliferation.[66] Tax is involved in deregulation of cell growth, apoptosis, repression of β polymerase, DNA repair, and inactivation of mitotic arrest defective protein, which predispose cells to chromosomal instability.[1,67] By immunohistochemistry and ISH, Tax is present only in 40% of ATLL,[68] and to a lesser extent in acute ATLL. The HBZ factor interacts with Tax and NF-κB/p65 in leukemogenesis, appears to deregulate function of cellular factors,[69] and blocks apoptosis.[70] Unlike Tax, HBZ appears to be present in all ATLL cases.[71] HBZ RNA further induces TIGIT and CCR4 on ATLL cells which may contribute to malignant cell infiltration.[72]

The ATLL cell karyotype is complex, suggesting that the disease is a single entity which acquires a variety of different molecular abnormalities, with clonal selection occurring as a consequence of clonal evolution.[73,74] Gene expression profiling has shown that the major functional categories of genes that are altered in ATLL include those involving T-cell homeostasis and activation and cell cycle/proliferation (Table 29-5). Such studies showed differential patterns for ATLL compared to mycosis fungoides (MF)[75] and peripheral T-cell lymphoma, not otherwise specified (PTCL-NOS),[76] allowing for reclassification of four PTCL-NOS cases[76] as ATLL in one study. Overall numbers of alterations were noted to be greater in acute versus chronic ATLL, and acute ATLL showed more losses of CDKN2A/p16 INK4a and CDKN2B/ARF p14, as well as loss of CD58, implicating an immune escape mechanism of neoplasia.[77] Gain of RXRA was the most frequent alteration found in chronic ATLL, whereby gain of RXRA and loss of ITGB1, CCDC7, or CD68 were significantly associated with early progression to acute type. Several somatic mutations have been identified in ATLL patient samples, including gain-of-function alterations in T-cell receptor/NF-kappa B signaling, alterations in immune evasion–related molecules, and alterations in transcription factors, transcriptional coregulators, chemokine receptors, epigenetic regulators, and tumor suppressors[78-84]

TABLE 29-5 Histopathologic Differential Diagnosis of Adult T-Cell Leukemia/Lymphoma

	Clinical Features	Histopathology	Immunohistochemistry	Molecular
MF/SS	Patches/plaques/tumors	Epidermotropic cerebriform cell, interfollicular sparing in FMF	CD4:CD8 3:1–10:1, CCR10+, CD25−, or faint	TCR monoclonal No viral integration
ALCL	Single or few nodules	Large, hallmark cells, nucleoli, nonepidermotropic	Loss of CD2, CD3, CD45RO−, often cytotoxic marker+	TCR monoclonal No viral integration
PTCL-NOS	Typically widespread tumors	Nonepidermotropic/ nonfolliculotropic, noncerebriform	CD4 or CD8+	TCR monoclonal No viral integration
CD8+ AETCL	Patches, plaques, tumors, ulcers	Epidermotropic, intermediate-sized cells	CD8+, CD45RO−, CD45RA+, cytotoxic marker+	TCR monoclonal No viral integration

AETCL, aggressive epidermotropic; ALCL, anaplastic large-cell lymphoma; FMF, follicular mycosis fungoides; LPD, lymphoproliferative disorder; MF/SS, mycosis fungoides/Sézary syndrome; PTCL-NOS, peripheral T-cell lymphoma not otherwise specified; SMPTCL, small–medium pleomorphic T-cell lymphoma; T-cell lymphoma TCR, T-cell receptor.

(Table 29-5). Point mutations in p53 were found in 25% of acute ATLL patients, correlating with a significantly shorter overall survival.[81] *CCR4* mutations have been identified and are hypothesized to alter the migration of ATLL cells as well as enhance AKT activation with ligand engagement.[78] Epigenetic alterations including H3K27 trimethylation and CpG island DNA hypermethylation, which may impact NF-kappa B and MHC class I signaling, are commonly identified in ATLL cases.[82,85]

Microsatellite alterations and loss of heterozygosity have been found in aggressive and indolent ATLL and are not necessarily correlative or prognostic.[79,86,87] Downregulation of miR-145 may be associated with worsened survival (per multivariate analysis in patients with aggressive-type ATLL).[88]

DIFFERENTIAL DIAGNOSIS

The differential diagnosis includes both benign and malignant lymphoid proliferations. Recognition that the patient is from an endemic area may facilitate the earlier diagnosis of ATLL. However, certain inflammatory skin conditions may occur in patients who are infected with HTLV-1, including HTLV-related infective dermatitis. These patients typically present as children, with a seborrheic dermatitis-like or lichenoid rash, chronic nasal discharge/crusting of the nares with *Staphylococcus aureus* or β hemolytic streptococci infection, lymphadenopathy, anemia, and pruritus. Histopathologic changes show a spongiotic and/or lichenoid partially intraepidermal lymphoid infiltrate without cytologic atypia, which is typically CD8+ with minimal to absent labeling for CD4, CD25, CD30, and FOXp3.[89] Other benign skin diseases which affect patients with ATLL are diverse and include xerosis, acquired ichthyosis, seborrheic dermatitis, dermatophytosis, scabies, bacterial skin infections, and verruca vulgaris.[28,90,91] The clinical and histologic distinction of these entities is straightforward, when classic. If nonclassic, the identification of an epidermotropic, destructive, and high-grade infiltrate with cytologic atypia and the characteristic immunophenotype should favor a diagnosis of ATLL.

Distinguishing ATLL from other cutaneous lymphomas including MF/Sézary syndrome (SS), anaplastic large-cell lymphoma, and peripheral T-cell lymphoma, unspecified may be more challenging (Table 29-6). In contrast to MF, the initial lesions of ATLL are more often of acute onset with rapid progression and are nodular, papular, or even tumoral. Smoldering presentations of ATLL are more difficult to differentiate from MF and may require additional biopsies and serology for diagnosis. As with other cutaneous lymphoma, ATLL may show either small or large cells; however, larger cells are very common, suggestive of a high-grade lymphoma. Marked epitheliotropic, angiodestructive, and perineural infiltrates are seen, with frequently identified multilobated lymphocytes. CD4:CD8 ratios are high, and strong CD25 and/or strong CD30 expression may favor the possibility of ATLL, particularly in a patch-/plaque-stage lesion. Epidermotropism is more often maintained in tumor-stage ATLL versus tumor-stage MF. In folliculotropic lesions, interfollicular involvement of the epidermis and Pautrier-like microabscesses are more commonly seen in ATLL versus follicular MF. Flow cytometry can be helpful, as it demonstrates that the CD3+ T-cells are uniformly CD4+ and CD8− (Fig. 29-10). Gene expression profiling shows promise in the distinction of MF versus ATLL, in the demonstration of a differential gene expression pattern,[65] but is not currently in use as a clinical assay.

TABLE 29-6 Molecular Genetic Alterations Described in Adult T-Cell Leukemia/Lymphoma

Alteration	Acute	Chronic	Either
Copy number gains	1q, 4q	RXRA	Trisomy 3, 7, 21, 14q,[60,61] 7q, 3p, 14q32[58] MYC, REL1, NOTCH1[63]
Copy number losses	CDKN2A/B, CD58[65]	ITGB1, CCDC7, or CD68	13q, 6q, chromosome Y,[77-80] 6q15-21[81]
Somatic mutations	TP53, p15/INK4b, and P16/Ink4a[69]		Notch1, Jak3, FAS, and p53[62,63]

Also see reference 62.

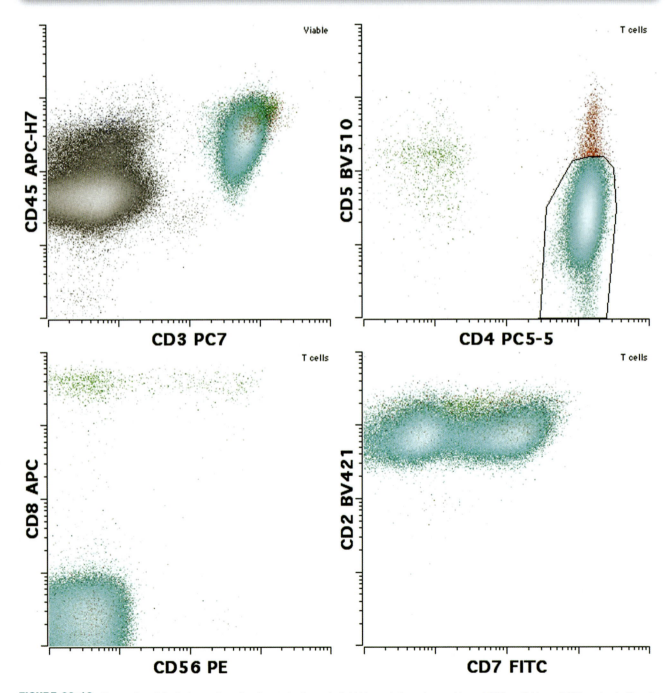

FIGURE 29-10. Flow cytometric features. Here, the abnormal cells are in *light blue* and show abnormal loss of CD5, partial loss of CD7, and reduction of expression of CD3 and CD45 compared to the residual normal T-cells (*red* and *green*). They are positive for CD4 and negative for CD8 and CD56. (Photo courtesy of Mikhail Roshal, MD.)

References

1. Nicot C. Current views in HTLV-I-associated adult T-cell leukemia/lymphoma. *Am J Hematol*. 2005;78(3):232-239.
2. Shimoyama M, Abe T, Miyamoto K, et al. Chromosome aberrations and clinical features of adult T cell leukemia-lymphoma not associated with human T cell leukemia virus type I. *Blood*. 1987;69(4):984-989.
3. Hanchard B. Adult T-cell leukemia/lymphoma in Jamaica: 1986-1995. *J Acquir Immune Defic Syndr Hum Retrovirol*. 1996;13(suppl 1):S20-S25.
4. Marchetti MA, Pulitzer MP, Myskowski PL, et al. Cutaneous manifestations of human T-cell lymphotrophic virus type-1-associated adult T-cell leukemia/lymphoma: a single-center, retrospective study. *J Am Acad Dermatol*. 2015;72(2):293-301.e2.
5. Cassar O, Gessain A. Serological and molecular methods to study epidemiological aspects of human T-cell lymphotropic virus type 1 infection. In: *Human T-Lymphotropic Viruses: Methods and Protocols*, Casoli C, Editor. 2017, Springer New York. pp. 3-24.
6. Chabay P, Lens D, Hassan R, et al. Lymphotropic viruses EBV, KSHV and HTLV in Latin America: epidemiology and associated malignancies. A literature-based study by the RIAL-CYTED. *Cancers*. 2020;12(8):2166.
7. Manzari V, Gradilone A, Barillari G, et al. HTLV-I is endemic in southern Italy: detection of the first infectious cluster in a white population. *Int J Cancer*. 1985;36(5):557-559.
8. Yamamoto JF, Goodman MT. Patterns of leukemia incidence in the United States by subtype and demographic characteristics, 1997-2002. *Cancer Causes Control*. 2008;19(4):379-390.
9. Chihara D, Ito H, Katanoda K, et al. Increase in incidence of adult T-cell leukemia/lymphoma in non-endemic areas of Japan and the United States. *Cancer Sci*. 2012;103(10):1857-1860.
10. Proietti FA, Carneiro-Proietti ABF, Catalan-Soares BC, Murphy EL. Global epidemiology of HTLV-I infection and associated diseases. *Oncogene*. 2005;24(39):6058-6068.
11. Iwanaga M. Epidemiology of HTLV-1 infection and ATL in Japan: an update. *Front Microbiol*. 2020;11:1124.
12. Matutes E. Adult T-cell leukaemia/lymphoma. *J Clin Pathol*. 2007;60(12):1373-1377.
13. Plummer M, de Martel C, Vignat J, Ferlay J, Bray F, Franceschi S. Global burden of cancers attributable to infections in 2012: a synthetic analysis. *Lancet Glob Health*. 2016;4(9):e609-616.
14. de Martel C, Ferlay J, Franceschi S, et al. Global burden of cancers attributable to infections in 2008: a review and synthetic analysis. *Lancet Oncol*. 2012;13(6):607-615.
15. Parkin DM. The global health burden of infection-associated cancers in the year 2002. *Int J Cancer*. 2006;118(12):3030-3044.
16. Miyoshi H, Ohshima K. Epidemiology of malignant lymphoma and recent progress in research on adult T-cell leukemia/lymphoma in Japan. *Int J Hematol*. 2018;107(4):420-427.
17. Hlela C, Bittencourt A. Infective dermatitis associated with HTLV-1 mimics common eczemas in children and may Be a prelude to severe systemic diseases. *Dermatol Clin*. 2014;32(2):237-248.
18. Uchiyama T, Yodoi J, Sagawa K, Takatsuki K, Uchino H. Adult T-cell leukemia: clinical and hematologic features of 16 cases. *Blood*. 1977;50(3):481-492.
19. Poiesz BJ, Ruscetti FW, Gazdar AF, Bunn PA, Minna JD, Gallo RC. Detection and isolation of type C retrovirus particles from fresh and cultured lymphocytes of a patient with cutaneous T-cell lymphoma. *Proc Natl Acad Sci U S A*. 1980;77(12):7415-7419.
20. Pais-Correia AM, Sachse M, Guadagnini S, et al. Biofilm-like extracellular viral assemblies mediate HTLV-1 cell-to-cell transmission at virological synapses. *Nat Med*. 2009;16(1):83-89.
21. Doi K, Wu X, Taniguchi Y, et al. Preferential selection of human T-cell leukemia virus type I provirus integration sites in leukemic versus carrier states. *Blood*. 2005;106(3):1048-1053.
22. Gillet NA, Malani N, Melamed A, et al. The host genomic environment of the provirus determines the abundance of HTLV-1-infected T-cell clones. *Blood*. 2011;117(11):3113-3122.
23. Cook LB, Melamed A, Niederer H, et al. The role of HTLV-1 clonality, proviral structure, and genomic integration site in adult T-cell leukemia/lymphoma. *Blood*. 2014;123(25):3925-3931.
24. Miyatake Y, Oliveira ALA, Jarboui MA, et al. Protective roles of epithelial cells in the survival of adult T-cell leukemia/lymphoma cells. *Am J Pathol*. 2013;182(5):1832-1842.
25. Kinpara S, Hasegawa A, Utsunomiya A, et al. Stromal cell-mediated suppression of human T-cell leukemia virus type 1 expression in vitro and in vivo by type I interferon. *J Virol*. 2009;83(10):5101-5108.
26. Taniguchi Y, Nosaka K, Yasunaga JI, et al. Silencing of human T-cell leukemia virus type I gene transcription by epigenetic mechanisms. *Retrovirology*. 2005;2:64.
27. Sonoda S, Li HC, Tajima K. Ethnoepidemiology of HTLV-1 related diseases: ethnic determinants of HTLV-1 susceptibility and its worldwide dispersal. *Cancer Sci*. 2011;102(2):295-301.
28. Jabbour M, Tuncer H, Castillo J. Hematopoietic SCT for adult T-cell leukemia/lymphoma: a review. *Bone Marrow Transpl*. 2011;46(8):1039-1044.
29. Qayyum S, Choi JK, Adult T-cell leukemia/lymphoma. *Arch Pathol Lab Med*. 2014;138(2):282-286.
30. Katsuya H, Ishitsuka K, Utsunomiya A, et al. Treatment and survival among 1594 patients with ATL. *Blood*. 2015;126(24):2570-2577.
31. Bazarbachi A, Plumelle Y, Carlos Ramos J, et al. Meta-analysis on the use of zidovudine and interferon-alfa in adult T-cell leukemia/lymphoma showing improved survival in the leukemic subtypes. *J Clin Oncol*. 2010;28(27):4177-4183.
32. Ohshima K. Pathological features of diseases associated with human T-cell leukemia virus type I. *Cancer Sci*. 2007;98(6):772-778.
33. Amano M, Setoyama M, Grant A, Kerdel FA. Human T-lymphotropic Virus 1 (HTLV-1) infection—dermatological implications. *Int J Dermatol*. 2011;50(8):915-920.
34. Setoyama M, Katahira Y, Kanzaki T. Clinicopathologic analysis of 124 cases of adult T-cell leukemia/lymphoma with cutaneous manifestations: the smouldering type with skin manifestations has a poorer prognosis than previously thought. *J Dermatol*. 1999;26(12):785-790.
35. Tokura Y, Sawada Y, Shimauchi T. Skin manifestations of adult T-cell leukemia/lymphoma: clinical, cytological and immunological features. *J Dermatol*. 2014;41(1):19-25.
36. Sawada Y, Hino R, Hama K, et al. Type of skin eruption is an independent prognostic indicator for adult T-cell leukemia/lymphoma. *Blood*. 2011;117(15):3961-3967.
37. Amano M, Kurokawa M, Ogata K, et al. New entity, definition and diagnostic criteria of cutaneous adult T-cell leukemia/lymphoma: human T-lymphotropic virus type 1 proviral DNA load can distinguish between cutaneous and smoldering types. *J Dermatol*. 2008;35(5):270-275.
38. Bittencourt AL, Oliveira Mde F. Cutaneous manifestations associated with HTLV-1 infection. *Int J Dermatol*. 2010;49(10):1099-1110.

39. Cook LB, Fuji S, Hermine O, et al. Revised adult T-cell leukemia-lymphoma International Consensus meeting report. *J Clin Oncol*. 2019;37(8):677-687.
40. Bunn PA, Schechter GP, Jaffe E, et al. Clinical course of retrovirus-associated adult T-cell lymphoma in the United States. *N Engl J Med*. 1983;309(5):257-264.
41. Hirata T, Kinjo N, Kishimoto K, et al. Impairment of host immune response against strongyloides stercoralis by human T cell lymphotropic virus type 1 infection. *Am J Trop Med Hyg*. 2006;74(2):246-249.
42. Demontis MA, Hilburn S, Taylor GP. Human T cell lymphotropic virus type 1 viral load variability and long-term trends in asymptomatic carriers and in patients with human T cell lymphotropic virus type 1-related diseases. *AIDS Res Hum Retrovir*. 2013;29(2):359-364.
43. Macnamara A, Rowan A, Hilburn S, et al. HLA class I binding of HBZ determines outcome in HTLV-1 infection. *PLoS Pathog*, 2010;6(9):e1001117.
44. Bangham CRM. CTL quality and the control of human retroviral infections. *Eur J Immunol*. 2009;39(7):1700-1712.
45. Tobinai K, Hotta T. Clinical trials for malignant lymphoma in Japan. *Jpn J Clin Oncol*. 2004;34(7):369-378.
46. Watanabe T. The strategy of treatment for malignant lymphoma: conventional-dose chemotherapy versus high-dose therapy followed by hematopoietic stem cell transplantation. [Article in Japanese]. *Rinsho Ketsueki*. 2004;45(1):39-47.
47. Ishida M, Iwai M, Yoshida K, Kagotani A, Okabe H. Adult T-cell leukemia/lymphoma accompanying follicular mucinosis: a case report with review of the literature. *Int J Clin Exp Pathol*. 2013;6(12):3014-3018.
48. Ishitsuka K, Tamura K. Human T-cell leukaemia virus type I and adult T-cell leukaemia-lymphoma. *Lancet Oncol*. 2014;15(11):e517-e526.
49. Phillips AA, Fields PA, Hermine O, et al. Mogamulizumab versus investigator's choice of chemotherapy regimen in relapsed/refractory adult T-cell leukemia/lymphoma. *Haematologica*. 2019;104(5):993-1003.
50. Wada T, Yoshinaga E, Oiso N, Kawara S, Kawada A, Kozuka T. Adult T-cell leukemia–lymphoma associated with follicular mucinosis. *J Dermatol*. 2009;36(12):638-642.
51. Camp BJ, Busam KJ, Brownell I, Koehne G, Hedvat C, Pulitzer MP. Donor-derived lymphomatoid papulosis in a stem-cell transplantation recipient. *J Clin Oncol*. 2011;29(35):e855-e858.
52. Yao J, Gottesman SRS, Ayalew G, Braverman AS, Axiotis CA. Loss of Foxp3 is associated with CD30 expression in the anaplastic large cell subtype of adult T-cell leukemia/lymphoma (ATLL) in US/caribbean patients. *Am J Surg Pathol*. 2013;37(9):1407-1412.
53. Juncà J, Botín T, Vila J, Navarro JT, Millá F. Adult T-cell leukemia/lymphoma with an unusual CD1a positive phenotype. *Cytometry B Clin Cytometry*. 2013;86(4):292-296.
54. Bittencourt AL, Barbosa HS, Vieira MDG, Farré L. Adult T-cell leukemia/lymphoma (ATL) presenting in the skin: clinical, histological and immunohistochemical features of 52 cases. *Acta Oncol*. 2009;48(4):598-604.
55. Sugimoto KJ, Shimada A, Wakabayashi M, et al. CD56-positive adult T-cell leukemia/lymphoma: a case report and a review of the literature. *Med Mol Morphol*. 2014;48(1):54-59.
56. Lin TH, Wu HC, Hsieh YC, Tseng CE, Ichinohasama R, Chuang SS. CD4 and CD8 double-negative adult T-cell leukemia/lymphoma with monomorphic cells expressing CD99: a diagnostic challenge in a country non-endemic for human T-cell leukemia virus. *Pathol Int*. 2013;63(2):132-137.
57. Shimauchi T, Kabashima K, Nakashima D, et al. Augmented expression of programmed death-1 in both neoplastic and non-neoplastic CD4+ T-cells in adult T-cell leukemia/lymphoma. *Int J Cancer*. 2007;121(12):2585-2590.
58. Shimauchi T, Imai S, Hino R, Tokura Y. Production of thymus and activation-regulated chemokine and macrophage-derived chemokine by CCR4+ adult T-cell leukemia cells. *Clin Cancer Res*. 2005;11(6):2427-2435.
59. Ohshima K, Niino D, Karube K. Microenvironment of adult T-cell leukemia/lymphoma-associated nodal lesions. *Int J Hematol*. 2014;99(3):240-248.
60. Karube K, Aoki R, Sugita Y, et al. The relationship of FOXP3 expression and clinicopathological characteristics in adult T-cell leukemia/lymphoma. *Mod Pathol*. 2008;21(5):617-625.
61. Roncador G, Garcia JF, Garcia JF, et al. FOXP3, a selective marker for a subset of adult T-cell leukaemia/lymphoma. *Leukemia*. 2005;19(12):2247-2253.
62. Cacciatore M, Guarnotta C, Calvaruso M, et al. Microenvironment-centred dynamics in aggressive B-cell lymphomas. *Adv Hematol*. 2012;2012:138079.
63. Komohara Y, Niino D, Saito Y, et al. Clinical significance of CD163+tumor-associated macrophages in patients with adult T-cell leukemia/lymphoma. *Cancer Sci*. 2013;104(7):945-951.
64. Yamada K, Miyoshi H, Yoshida N, et al. Human T-cell lymphotropic virus HBZ and tax mRNA expression are associated with specific clinicopathological features in adult T-cell leukemia/lymphoma. *Mod Pathol*. 2021;34(2):314-326. doi:10.1038/s41379-020-00654-0
65. Tsukasaki K, Tsushima H, Yamamura M, et al. Integration patterns of HTLV-I provirus in relation to the clinical course of ATL: frequent clonal change at crisis from indolent disease. *Blood*. 1997;89(3):948-956.
66. Ko NL, Taylor JM, Bellon M, et al. PA28γ is a novel corepressor of HTLV-1 replication and controls viral latency. *Blood*. 2013;121(5):791-800.
67. Wang W, Zhou J, Shi J, et al. Human T-cell leukemia virus type 1 Tax-deregulated autophagy pathway and c-FLIP expression contribute to resistance against death receptor-mediated apoptosis. *J Virol*. 2014;88(5):2786-2798.
68. Takeda S, Maeda M, Morikawa S, et al. Genetic and epigenetic inactivation of tax gene in adult T-cell leukemia cells. *Int J Cancer*. 2004;109(4):559-567.
69. Mukai R, Ohshima T. HTLV-1 HBZ positively regulates the mTOR signaling pathway via inhibition of GADD34 activity in the cytoplasm. *Oncogene*. 2013;33(18):2317-2328.
70. Tanaka-Nakanishi A, Yasunaga J, Takai K, Matsuoka M. HTLV-1 bZIP factor suppresses apoptosis by attenuating the function of FoxO3a and altering its localization. *Cancer Res*. 2013;74(1):188-200.
71. Shimizu-Kohno K, Satou Y, Arakawa F, et al. Detection of HTLV-1 by means of HBZ gene in situ hybridization in formalin-fixed and paraffin-embedded tissues. *Cancer Sci*. 2011;102(7):1432-1436.
72. Bangham CRM, Matsuoka M. Human T-cell leukaemia virus type 1: parasitism and pathogenesis. *Philos Trans R Soc Lond B Biol Sci*. 2017;372(1732):20160272. doi:10.1098/rstb.2016.0272
73. Tsukasaki K, Utsunomiya A, Fukuda H, et al. VCAP-AMP-VECP compared with biweekly CHOP for adult T-cell leukemia-lymphoma: Japan clinical oncology group study JCOG9801. *J Clin Oncol*. 2007;25(34):5458-5464.

74. Tsukasaki K. Genetic instability of adult T-cell leukemia/lymphoma by comparative genomic hybridization analysis. *J Clin Immunol*. 2002;22(2):57-63.
75. Hashikawa K, Yasumoto S, Nakashima K, et al. Microarray analysis of gene expression by microdissected epidermis and dermis in mycosis fungoides and adult T-cell leukemia/lymphoma. *Int J Oncol*. 2014;45(3):1200-1208.
76. Iqbal J, Wright G, Wang C, et al. Gene expression signatures delineate biological and prognostic subgroups in peripheral T-cell lymphoma. *Blood*. 2014;123(19):2915-2923.
77. Yoshida N, Karube K, Utsunomiya A, et al. Molecular characterization of chronic-type Adult T-cell leukemia/lymphoma. *Cancer Res*. 2014;74(21):6129-6138.
78. Nakagawa M, Schmitz R, Xiao W, et al. Gain-of-function CCR4 mutations in adult T cell leukemia/lymphoma. *J Exp Med*. 2014;211(13):2497-2505.
79. Magalhães M, Oliveira PD, Bittencourt AL, Farre L. Microsatellite alterations are also present in the less aggressive types of adult T-cell leukemia-lymphoma. *PLoS Neglected Trop Dis*, 2015;9(1):e0003403.
80. Elliott NE, Cleveland SM, Grann V, Janik J, Waldmann TA, Davé UP. FERM domain mutations induce gain of function in JAK3 in adult T-cell leukemia/lymphoma. *Blood*. 2011;118(14):3911-3921.
81. Magalhaes M, Oliveira PD, Bittencourt AL, Farre L. Point mutations inTP53but not inp15Ink4bandp16Ink4agenes represent poor prognosis factors in acute adult T cell leukemia/lymphoma. *Leuk Lymphoma*. 2015;56(12):3434-3436.
82. Kataoka K, Nagata Y, Kitanaka A, et al. Integrated molecular analysis of adult T cell leukemia/lymphoma. *Nat Genet*. 2015;47(11):1304-1315. doi:10.1038/ng.3415
83. Kogure Y, Kataoka K. Genetic alterations in adult T-cell leukemia/lymphoma. *Cancer Sci*. 2017;108(9):1719-1725.
84. Licata MJ, Janakiram M, Tan S, et al. Diagnostic challenges of adult T-cell leukemia/lymphoma in North America - a clinical, histological, and immunophenotypic correlation with a workflow proposal. *Leuk Lymphoma*. 2018;59(5): 1188-1194.
85. Yamagishi M, Watanabe T. Molecular hallmarks of adult T cell leukemia. *Front Microbiol*. 2012;3:334. doi:10.3389/fmicb.2012.00334
86. Hayami Y. Microsatellite instability as a potential marker for poor prognosis in adult T cell leukemia/lymphoma. *Leuk Lymphoma*, 1999;32(3-4):345-349.
87. Hatta Y, Yamada Y, Tomonaga M, Miyoshi I, Said JW, Koeffler HP. Microsatellite instability in adult T-cell leukaemia. *Br J Haematol*. 1998;101(2):341-344.
88. Xia H, Yamada S, Aoyama M, et al. Prognostic impact of microRNA-145 down-regulation in adult T-cell leukemia/lymphoma. *Hum Pathol*. 2014;45(6):1192-1198.
89. Torres-Cabala CA, Curry JL, Li Ning Tapia EM, et al. HTLV-1-associated infective dermatitis demonstrates low frequency of FOXP3-positive T-regulatory lymphocytes. *J Dermatol Sci*. 2015;77(3):150-155.
90. GonÇAlves DU, Lambertucci JR, De Freitas Carneiro Proietti AB, Martins ML, Proietti FA, Guedes ACM. Dermatologic lesions in asymptomatic blood donors seropositive for human T cell lymphotropic virus TYPE-1. *Am J Trop Med Hyg*. 2003;68(5):562-565.
91. Brites C, Weyll M, Pedroso C, Badaró R. Severe and Norwegian scabies are strongly associated with retroviral (HIV-1/HTLV-1) infection in Bahia, Brazil. *AIDS*. 2002;16(9):1292-1293.

PART VI PRIMARY CUTANEOUS B-CELL LYMPHOPROLIFERATIVE DISORDERS

CHAPTER 30

Approach to the diagnosis of cutaneous B-cell lymphomas

Alejandro A. Gru and Elaine S. Jaffe

INTRODUCTION

The diagnosis of cutaneous B-cell lymphomas (CBCLs) requires a careful evaluation of the clinical features, as well as a comprehensive histologic and immunophenotypic analysis. It is important that oncologists, dermatologists, and pathologists speak a common language. While many cutaneous lymphomas have distinctive features, there is also overlap with other nodal and extranodal lymphomas, so that cutaneous lymphomas must be viewed in a broader context.[1-3]

Several factors can affect the way one approaches a diagnosis of CBCL: (1) the same disease can have different names in different sites; (2) "organ-specific diagnoses" may impede understanding of diseases common to diverse anatomic sites (e.g., extranodal marginal zone lymphoma [MZL] vs cutaneous immunocytoma); (3) some primary "cutaneous lymphomas" may be systemic, and the skin may be the first clinical presentation of the disease (e.g., intravascular large B-cell lymphoma, EBV+ diffuse large B-cell lymphoma [DLBCL]); (4) a diagnosis of large B-cell lymphoma on the skin might not reflect the true clinical behavior of the disease (e.g., many cutaneous follicle center lymphomas show a significant component of large cells, and that does not correlate with the clinical behavior or need for systemic therapy); (5) common algorithms to use in the distinction of DLBCL subtypes might not apply adequately to large B-cell lymphomas on the skin (e.g., Hans algorithm). Nevertheless, the site of presentation of a lymphoproliferative disorder is a signpost for some of the underlying biologic features of the disease.

APPROACH TO THE DIAGNOSIS OF CUTANEOUS B-CELL LYMPHOMAS — HISTOLOGIC CLUES

Table 30-1 summarizes the more common primary and secondary CBCLs. The diagnosis of B-cell lymphomas in the skin should always start with the question of: is the infiltrate in question a reactive condition or neoplastic? We now understand that some instances of cutaneous lymphoid hyperplasia represent examples of primary cutaneous follicle center lymphoma (PCFCL) and primary cutaneous marginal zone lymphoma (PCMZL)[4,5] and vice versa. Molecular studies can be useful ancillary techniques for the detection of a clonal B-cell expansion, but should not be used to define an infiltrate as neoplastic.[6] Cutaneous findings in Lyme disease can be typically confused with PCMZL. In fact, many of the cases of PCMZL in Europe have been linked to the infection by *Borrelia burgdorferi*,[7-9] a feature that has not been seen in the United States. In Lyme disease, there is typically a superficial and deep perivascular and interstitial lymphoplasmacytic infiltrate with the formation of germinal centers.[10] Other causes of B-pseudolymphomatous reactions occur in the setting of contact dermatitis, arthropod bite reactions, cutaneous adverse manifestations to specific medications, tattoos, vaccinations, and infections, among other causes.[11] The histology in those pseudolymphomas revealed dermal lymphoid, follicle-like structures with predominantly CD20+ cells, and variable number of germinal centers[12-14] (Fig. 30-1). The presence of follicular aggregates of B-cells, under these circumstances, is referred to as cutaneous lymphoid hyperplasias or "lymphocytoma cutis" and many of them are idiopathic in nature.

The presence of normal-appearing germinal centers should not be used as an excuse to define something as reactive. MZL frequently has reactive or atrophic germinal centers admixed with the neoplastic infiltrate.[15-17] The germinal centers tend to show a more atrophic pattern in well-established lesions of PCMZL.[18] Furthermore, the abundance of B-cells in a mixed infiltrate might not necessarily imply a diagnosis of a B-cell lymphoma.[19,20] For example, subsets of T-cell lymphomas with a follicular T-helper (T_{FH}) phenotype can be accompanied by a large number of B-cells and plasma cells and potentially mimic B-cell lymphomas. T cell lymphomas with prominent B-cell infiltrates include primary cutaneous CD4+ small to

TABLE 30-1 Primary Cutaneous B-Cell Lymphomas and Systemic B-Cell Lymphomas With Cutaneous Dissemination

Primary Cutaneous B-Cell Lymphomas and Lymphoproliferative Conditions	Systemic B-Cell Lymphomas With Cutaneous Dissemination
Primary cutaneous follicle center lymphoma	Chronic lymphocytic leukemia
Primary cutaneous diffuse large B-cell lymphoma, leg type	Mantle cell lymphoma
Cutaneous marginal zone lymphoma	Follicular lymphoma
EBV+ diffuse large B-cell lymphoma	Plasmablastic lymphoma
Plasmablastic lymphoma	Multiple myeloma
EBV+ mucocutaneous ulcer	Primary effusion lymphoma
Intravascular B-cell lymphoma	Diffuse large B-cell lymphoma
	Lymphomatoid granulomatosis
	Burkitt lymphoma
	ALK-positive large B-cell lymphoma
	Classic Hodgkin lymphoma
	High-grade B-cell lymphomas

medium T-cell lymphoproliferative disorder, mycosis fungoides with a T_{FH} phenotype, and nodal T-cell lymphomas T-follicular helper phenotype (which include angioimmunoblastic T-cell lymphoma) (Fig. 30-2).[21]

Tables 30-2 and 30-3 summarize a concise clinical, histologic, and molecular approach to common primary cutaneous and secondary CBCLs, respectively.

ANATOMIC LOCATION OF THE INFILTRATE

The location and clinical appearance of the lesion are of capital importance in the arrival to a specific diagnosis. Most of the cases of PCFCL typically present as a solitary nodule or plaque in the head and neck region or the trunk. In contrast, PCMZL typically presents in the trunk and extremities, as multiple papules, nodules, or plaques, and tends to spare the head and neck.[7,15,22] The more aggressive and uncommon variant of CBCL, primary cutaneous diffuse large B-cell lymphoma, leg type (DLBCL-LT), usually presents as solitary or multiple nodules in the legs. One should also remember that 10% to 20% of DLBCL-LT present outside the extremities.[2,3-31] The anatomic location sometimes can have more important prognostic significance than the size of the cells. One should be aware that a lesion that occurs in the head and neck should be favored to be a low-grade lymphoma (even in the context of aggressive cytologic features) and high-grade lymphoma if present in the legs (even if it is of low-grade cytology). In PCFCL, there is frequently a prominent stromal reaction with fibrosis, a feature that is commonly missing in cases of DLBCL-LT.[23,24,32,33]

GROWTH PATTERNS OF B-CELL INFILTRATES

The different histologic subtypes of CBCL typically have some different growth patterns that allow for a possible diagnostic distinction: PCFCL shows a predominantly follicular, diffuse, or combined pattern of growth in the dermis. PCMZL is usually nodular or diffuse in growth, but can also show small-appearing follicles with germinal centers, and is more typically bottom-heavy. PCMZL frequently has adnexotropic extension (Fig. 30-3). DLBCL-LT shows a diffuse growth pattern in the dermis. All of them share the presence of a grenz zone that separates the infiltrate from the surface epidermis. However, the epidermotropic character of lymphocytes, perhaps a diagnostic paradigm of most of the cutaneous T-cell lymphomas, can also be very rarely encountered in certain B-cell lymphomas, particularly PCMZL, EBV-DLBCL, and DLBCL-LT (Fig. 30-4).[34-38]

The morphology and cellular types are also different across CBCLs: PCFCL shows a mixture of centrocytes and centroblasts, with more frequent centroblasts in the diffuse variants. Some cases can show spindle cell morphology and may lead to a diagnostic consideration of a nonhematopoietic neoplasm (Fig. 30-5). The spindle cell variant was originally named as Crosti disease or reticulohistiocytoma.[39] PCZMLs are composed of an admixture of monocytoid B-cells, centrocyte-like cells, lymphoplasmacytic cells, plasma cells, and occasional large immunoblasts.[18] In contrast, DLBCL-LT shows sheets of large immunoblasts in the dermis.[24] Intravascular large B-cell lymphomas also have a predominance of immunoblasts within

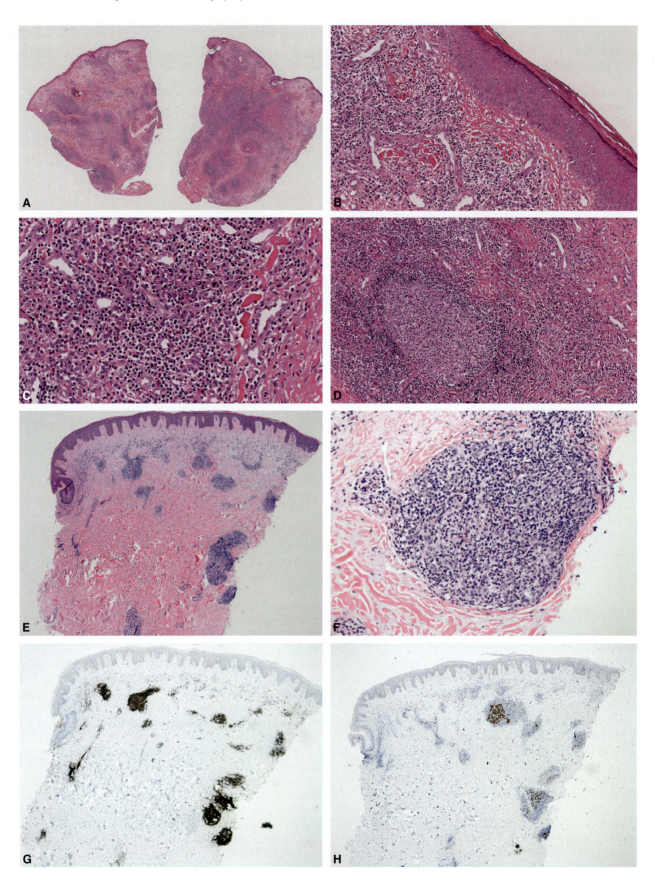

FIGURE 30-1. **A–D.** Angiolymphoid hyperplasia with eosinophilia (ALHE). Nodular aggregates of lymphocytes with the presence of germinal center formation (more common in Kimura disease). Increased vascularity and endothelial swelling is typical (20×, 100×, and 200×). **E** and **F.** Cutaneous idiopathic lymphoid hyperplasia with focal germinal center formation (40× and 200×). **G.** CD20 is positive in follicles of B-cells. **H.** Ki67 is very high in the germinal centers.

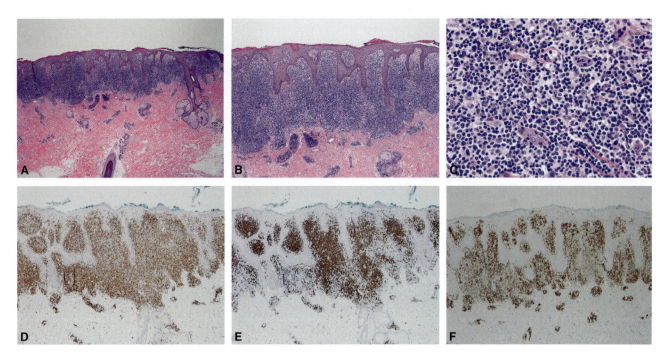

FIGURE 30-2. Primary cutaneous CD4⁺ small to medium T-cell lymphoproliferative disorder. **A** and **B.** Diffuse and vaguely nodular infiltrate that spares the epidermis (40× and 100×). **C.** The infiltrate contains scattered medium and large cells with irregular nuclear borders (400×). The infiltrate shows a mixture of CD3⁺ T-cells **(D)** and numerous background CD20⁺ B-cells **(E)** which can raise the diagnostic possibility of a B-cell lymphoma. CD4 is diffusely positive in most of the cells (not shown), which also stain for the follicular T-helper marker PD-1 **(F)**.

TABLE 30-2 Common Primary Cutaneous B-Cell Lymphomas

Subtype	Location/Clinical	Age	Morphology	Immunophenotype	Molecular Features
Primary cutaneous follicle center lymphoma (PCFCL)	Head and neck, trunk (plaques, papules, nodules, and tumors)	55 median	Nodular, diffuse, nodular, and diffuse Centrocytes, centroblasts, and spindle cells	CD20⁺, HGAL⁺, LMO2⁺, BCL6⁺, CD10⁻/⁺ (+ in nodular pattern more frequently), BCL2⁻/⁺ MUM1⁻, CD21⁺ in follicles IgM⁻, IgD⁻	1p36del *TNFRSF14* mutations (28%) Rare t(14; 18) *IGH::BCL2* (~8%)
Primary cutaneous diffuse large B-cell lymphoma, leg type (DLBCL-LT)	Legs (10%-20%) outside this location; nodules and tumors +/− ulceration	76 median	Diffuse immunoblasts	CD20⁺, BCL-6⁺, MUM1⁺, BCL-2⁺,, FOXP1⁺, CD10⁻ IgM⁺, IgD⁺	*MYD88*, *CD79b*, *TNFAIP3/A20*, and *CARD11* mutations *MYC* translocations; *BCL2* amplifications 9p21.3 deletion (loss of *CDKN2A* and *CDKN2B*)
Primary cutaneous marginal zone lymphoma (PCZML)	Trunk and extremities (papulonodular rash)	55 median	Nodular or diffuse. Presence of GCs, monocytoid cells, plasma cells, centrocyte-like cells	CD20⁺, CD10⁻, BCL-6⁻, CD43⁻, IgG or IgM, CD5⁻, intact or disrupted FDC, CD138 (if PCs), IgG4+	Rare cases with t(14; 18) *IGH::MALT1*

TABLE 30-2 Common Primary Cutaneous B-Cell Lymphomas *continued*

Subtype	Location/Clinical	Age	Morphology	Immunophenotype	Molecular Features
Intravascular large B-cell lymphoma (IVLBCL)	Trunk and extremities (macules, nodules, and plaques)	67 median	Intravascular immunoblasts. Western variant (++ skin) vs Asian variant (++ hemophagocytosis)	CD20+, MUM1+, BCL6+/−, CD5+/−, BCL-2+	*MYD88, RAC2, CD79B, SETD1B* mutations *PD-L1/L2* rearrangements (38%)
Plasmablastic lymphoma (PBL)	Oral cavity (tumor) and skin	30-40 (in HIV), second peak 70-80 (no HIV)	Plasmablasts	CD20 and CD19−, CD138+, CD79a+, EMA+, CD30+, EBER+, CD10−/+, CD56−/+	*MYC* rearrangements (50%) *NRAS, KRAS, BRAF, STAT3, TP53* mutations
EBV-mucocutaneous ulcer (EBV-MCU)	Oropharyngeal mucosa, perianal skin (ulcers)	77 median	Diffuse Immunoblasts, RS cells, RS variants, necrosis.	PAX5+, OCT2+, MUM1+, CD45+/−, CD30+, CD15+/−, CD20+/−	EBER+

TABLE 30-3 Systemic B-Cell Lymphomas With Frequent Cutaneous Dissemination

Subtype	Location/Clinical	Age	Morphology	Immunophenotype	Molecular Features
Chronic lymphocytic leukemia (CLL)	Head and neck (papules, plaques, nodules, and tumors)	60 median	Perivascular and periadnexal nodular and diffuse infiltrate of small lymphocytes. Rare Richter transformation	CD19+, CD20+, CD5+, CD23+, BCL-1−, CD43+	Trisomy 12 (30%), deletion 13q14 (25%-50%), deletion 11q23 (10%-20%)
Mantle cell lymphoma	Trunk, head, and neck, extremities (nodules and tumors)	60	Nodular or nodular and diffuse. Small- to medium-sized lymphocytes. Blastoid and pleomorphic variants more frequent	CD19+, CD20+, CD5+, CD43+, BCL1+, SOX11+, CD23−, MUM1+	t(11; 14) *IGH::CCND1*
Diffuse large B-cell lymphoma	Variable, trunk and extremities more common (nodules and tumors, +/− ulceration)	Variable, typically 50-70 EBV-DLBCL 80-90	Diffuse infiltrate of large cells. Geographic necrosis (EBV-associated) Immunoblasts; Hodgkin-like cells (EBV); plasmablasts	CD19+, CD20+, CD5+/− (association with extranodal disease); CD30+/− Different groups ABC (MUM1+) vs GCT (CD10+ or BCL6+/MUM1−)	Variable *MYC, BCL2,* and *BCL6* translocations EBER: plasmablastic and EBV-DLBCL HHV8: primary effusion lymphoma *ALK* rearrangements

(Continued)

TABLE 30-3 Systemic B-Cell Lymphomas With Frequent Cutaneous Dissemination *continued*

Subtype	Location/Clinical	Age	Morphology	Immunophenotype	Molecular Features
Lymphomatoid granulomatosis	Variable, trunk and extremities (nodules and tumors, −/+ ulceration)	40-60	Angiocentric +/− angiodestruction, lymphohistiocytic panniculitis Immunoblasts, Hodgkin-like cells	CD19+, CD20+, CD30+, EBER used for grading, CD15−	EBER
Plasma cell myeloma	Trunk and extremities (nodules, tumors, and plaques)—very advanced stage	59 median	Diffuse; +/− amyloid Malignant plasma cells and plasmablasts more frequent	CD20, CD138+, CD38+, EMA+/−, CD56+, BCL1+/−	Deletion of 13q, 17p−/p53 deletion or translocations t(4; 14) and t(14; 16)

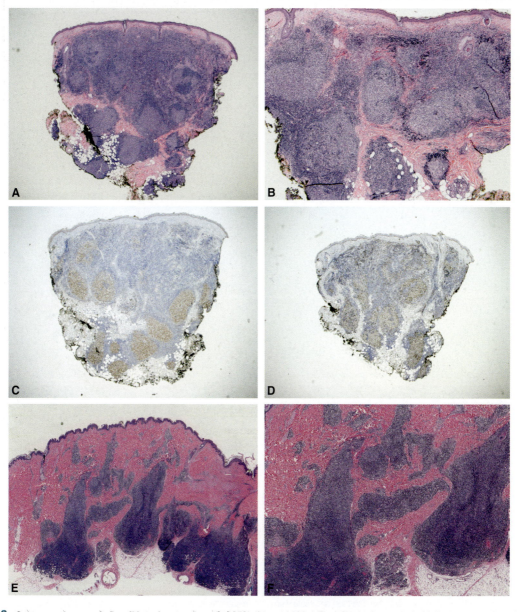

FIGURE 30-3. **Cutaneous low-grade B-cell lymphomas.** **A** and **B.** PCFCL (20× and 100×). The infiltrate shows a typical follicular pattern throughout the dermis. The follicles are positive for BCL-6 **(C)**, while negative for BCL-2 **(D)**. **E** and **F.** Cutaneous marginal zone lymphoma (10× and 100×). As opposed to PCFCL, in MZL the infiltrate is heavier in the bottom part of the biopsy, frequently shows adnexotropism, and sometimes has associated entrapped germinal centers.

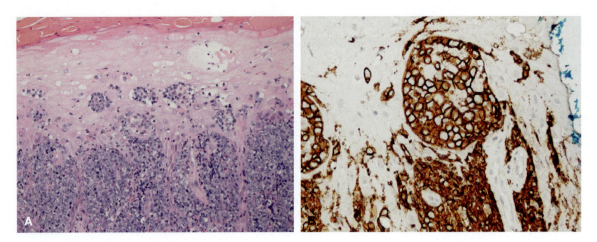

FIGURE 30-4. **Epidermotropic B-cell lymphomas. A.** Presence of epidermotropism in a case of diffuse large B-cell lymphoma, leg type (200×). **B.** CD20 is positive in the large cells.

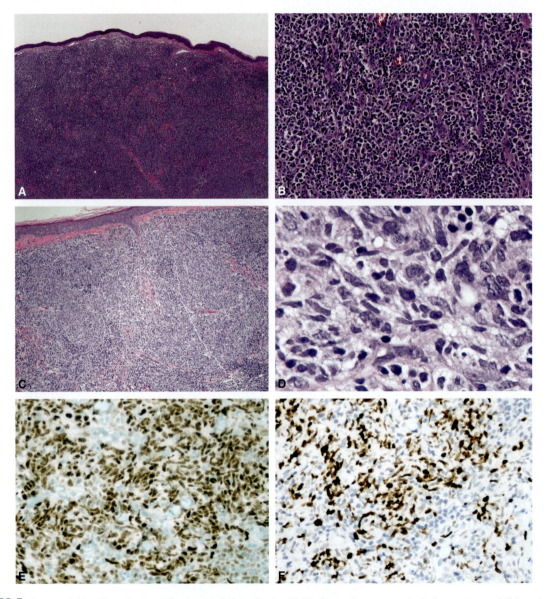

FIGURE 30-5. **Low-grade B-cell lymphomas with numerous large cells. A** and **B.** The figures show an example of primary cutaneous follicle center lymphoma with numerous large cells in the scalp (40× and 200×). The location should warrant a "reconsideration and avoidance" for the use of large cell lymphoma. **C** and **D.** The figures show an example of PCFCL with spindle cell appearance (so-called Crosti lymphoma) (40× and 600×). Spindle cells have a high proliferation index by Ki67 **(E)** and are positive for BCL-6 **(F)**.

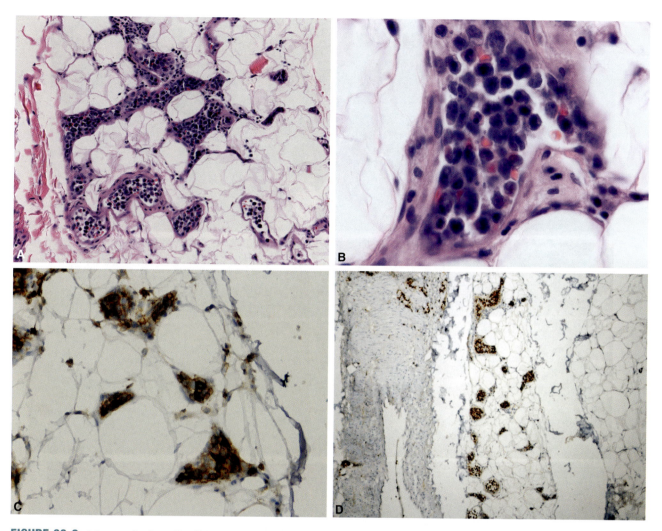

FIGURE 30-6. Intravascular large B-cell lymphoma. **A** and **B**. Aggregates of large cells confined to the vascular spaces with immunoblastic appearance (40× and 600×). The malignant cells are positive for CD20 **(C)** and have a high Ki67 proliferation index **(D)**.

the vessels[40] (Fig. 30-6). Plasmablastic lymphomas show the presence of plasmablasts: immature-appearing large cells, with large vesicular nuclei, very prominent nucleoli, and moderate-to-abundant cytoplasm[41] (Fig. 30-7). Other types of cells that can be seen in large B-cell lymphomas of the skin include Reed–Sternberg cells and variants among cases of EBV+ large B-cell lymphomas[42] and the so-called EBV–mucocutaneous ulcer[43,44] (Fig. 30-8). Rare Hodgkin-like cells can also occur in cases of PCFCL[45] and MZL (particularly cases with EBV+ cells).[46-49,77,78] Systemic B-cell lymphomas that are CD5+, such as DLBCL, high-grade histologic variants of mantle cell lymphoma, and Richter transformation, can also occur in the skin (Fig. 30-9).

A MOLECULAR APPROACH IN THE DIAGNOSIS OF B-CELL LYMPHOMAS OF THE SKIN

A standard testing for proving clonality of a lymphoid infiltrate always starts with the use of in situ hybridization (ISH) for κ and λ cytoplasmic light chains. Such testing is particularly useful in lymphomas with plasma cell differentiation, and PCZML in particular. More recent methodologies, particularly ultrasensitive RNA scope ISH, allow for better identification of light chains restriction within B-cells and plasma cells.[50,51] Nonetheless, cytoplasmic light chains restriction can also be proven in other forms of cutaneous lymphoproliferative disorders. Flow cytometry is often times of limited value, particularly because an adequate cell extraction of the lesional cells from the skin is oftentimes difficult.[52]

While immunoglobulin heavy chain gene rearrangements by polymerase chain reaction are a very helpful tool to confirm a diagnosis of clonality of B-cell lymphomas, not all cases will be clonal by this confirmatory testing. Indeed, PCMZL has been shown to be clonal in 70% to 75% of cases.[53,54] The use of novel platforms, such as next-generation sequencing assays for the confirmation of clonality, might prove to be more valuable in the future.

The t(14; 18) *IGH::BCL2* translocation is one of the most common molecular signatures characteristic of follicular lymphomas. However, the translocation can also be present in a smaller proportion of PCFCL[55-59] (approximately 8%). Such translocation carries no prognostic significance and should not be interpreted as a marker of cutaneous dissemination of a systemic FL. More recently, 1p36 deletions were identified

34. Lee BA, Jacobson M, Seidel G. Epidermotropic marginal zone lymphoma simulating mycosis fungoides (dagger). *J Cutan Pathol*. 2013;40:569-572.
35. Magro CM, Momtahen S, Lee BA, et al. Epidermotropic B-cell lymphoma: a unique subset of CXCR3-positive marginal zone lymphoma. *Am J Dermatopathol*. 2016;38:105-112.
36. Wu S, Subtil A, Gru AA. Epidermotropic Epstein-Barr virus-positive diffuse large B-cell lymphoma: a series of 3 cases of a very unusual high-grade lymphoma. *Am J Dermatopathol*. 2021;43(1):51-56.
37. Boudreaux BW, Patel MH, Brumfiel CM, et al. Primary cutaneous epidermotropic marginal zone B-cell lymphoma treated with total skin electron beam therapy. *JAAD Case Rep*. 2021;15:15-18.
38. Magro CM, Momtahen S, Coleman M, Grossman ME. Epidermotropic CXCR3 positive marginal zone lymphoma: a distinctive clinical histopathological entity potentially originating in the skin; it does not always indicate splenic marginal zone lymphoma. *Dermatol Online J*. 2019;25(7):13030/qt4207n83g.
39. Cerroni L, El-Shabrawi-Caelen L, Fink-Puches R, et al. Cutaneous spindle-cell B-cell lymphoma: a morphologic variant of cutaneous large B-cell lymphoma. *Am J Dermatopathol*. 2000;22:299-304.
40. Orwat DE, Batalis NI. Intravascular large B-cell lymphoma. *Arch Pathol Lab Med*. 2012;136:333-338.
41. Morscio J, Dierickx D, Nijs J, et al. Clinicopathologic comparison of plasmablastic lymphoma in HIV-positive, immunocompetent, and posttransplant patients: single-center series of 25 cases and meta-analysis of 277 reported cases. *Am J Surg Pathol*. 2014;38:875-886.
42. Kempf W, Kazakov DV, Mitteldorf C. Cutaneous lymphomas—an update. Part 2: B-cell lymphomas and related conditions. *Am J Dermatopathol*. 2014;36:197-208; quiz 209-110.
43. Dojcinov SD, Venkataraman G, Raffeld M, et al. EBV positive mucocutaneous ulcer—a study of 26 cases associated with various sources of immunosuppression. *Am J Surg Pathol*. 2010;34:405-417.
44. Hart M, Thakral B, Yohe S, et al. EBV-positive mucocutaneous ulcer in organ transplant recipients: a localized indolent posttransplant lymphoproliferative disorder. *Am J Surg Pathol*. 2014;38:1522-1529.
45. Aldarweesh FA, Treaba DO. Primary cutaneous follicle centre lymphoma with Hodgkin and Reed-Sternberg like cells: a case report and review of the literature. *Case Rep Hematol*. 2017;2017:9549428.
46. Leus HJ, Robin V, Molina TJ, Forsyth R, Dehou MF. Marginal zone lymphoma associated with Reed-Sternberg cells: a challenge for the pathologist. *Ann Pathol*. 2021;41(2):212-215.
47. Prieto-Torres L, Manso R, Cieza-Díaz DE, et al. Large cells with CD30 expression and hodgkin-like features in primary cutaneous marginal zone B-cell lymphoma: a study of 13 cases. *Am J Surg Pathol*. 2019;43(9):1191-1202.
48. Gibson SE, Swerdlow SH, Craig FE, et al. "EBV-positive extranodal marginal zone lymphoma of mucosa-associated lymphoid tissue in the posttransplant setting: a distinct type of posttransplant lymphoproliferative disorder?" *Am J Surg Pathol*. 2011;35(6):807-815.
49. Gong S, Crane GM, McCall CM, et al. "Expanding the Spectrum of EBV-positive marginal zone lymphomas: a lesion associated with diverse immunodeficiency settings." *Am J Surg Pathol*. 2018;42(10):1306-1316.
50. Craddock AP, Kane WJ, Raghavan SS, Williams ES, Gru AA, Gradecki SE. Use of ultrasensitive RNA in situ hybridization for determining clonality in cutaneous B-cell lymphomas and lymphoid hyperplasia decreases Subsequent use of molecular testing and is cost-effective. *Am J Surg Pathol*. 2022;46(7):956-962.
51. Guo L, Wang Z, Anderson CM, et al. Ultrasensitive automated RNA in situ hybridization for kappa and lambda light chain mRNA detects B-cell clonality in tissue biopsies with performance comparable or superior to flow cytometry. *Mod Pathol*. 2018;31(3):385-394.
52. Schafernak KT, Variakojis D, Goolsby CL, et al. Clonality assessment of cutaneous B-cell lymphoid proliferations: a comparison of flow cytometry immunophenotyping, molecular studies, and immunohistochemistry/in situ hybridization and review of the literature. *Am J Dermatopathol*. 2014;36:781-795.
53. Cho-Vega JH, Vega F, Rassidakis G, et al. Primary cutaneous marginal zone B-cell lymphoma. *Am J Clin Pathol*. 2006;125(suppl):S38-S49.
54. Servitje O, Gallardo F, Estrach T, et al. Primary cutaneous marginal zone B-cell lymphoma: a clinical, histopathological, immunophenotypic and molecular genetic study of 22 cases. *Br J Dermatol*. 2002;147:1147-1158.
55. Abdul-Wahab A, Tang SY, Robson A, et al. Chromosomal anomalies in primary cutaneous follicle center cell lymphoma do not portend a poor prognosis. *J Am Acad Dermatol*. 2014;70:1010-1020.
56. Bergman R, Kurtin PJ, Gibson LE, et al. Clinicopathologic, immunophenotypic, and molecular characterization of primary cutaneous follicular B-cell lymphoma. *Arch Dermatol*. 2001;137:432-439.
57. Kim BK, Surti U, Pandya A, et al. Clinicopathologic, immunophenotypic, and molecular cytogenetic fluorescence in situ hybridization analysis of primary and secondary cutaneous follicular lymphomas. *Am J Surg Pathol*. 2005;29:69-82.
58. Mirza I, Macpherson N, Paproski S, et al. Primary cutaneous follicular lymphoma: an assessment of clinical, histopathologic, immunophenotypic, and molecular features. *J Clin Oncol*. 2002;20:647-655.
59. Pham-Ledard A, Cowppli-Bony A, Doussau A, et al. Diagnostic and prognostic value of BCL2 rearrangement in 53 patients with follicular lymphoma presenting as primary skin lesions. *Am J Clin Pathol*. 2015;143:362-373.
60. Dijkman R, Tensen CP, Jordanova ES, et al. Array-based comparative genomic hybridization analysis reveals recurrent chromosomal alterations and prognostic parameters in primary cutaneous large B-cell lymphoma. *J Clin Oncol*. 2006;24:296-305.
61. Zhou XA, Yang J, Ringbloom KG, et al. Genomic landscape of cutaneous follicular lymphomas reveals 2 subgroups with clinically predictive molecular features. *Blood Adv*. 2021;5(3):649-661.
62. Barasch NJK, Liu YC, Ho J, et al. The molecular landscape and other distinctive features of primary cutaneous follicle center lymphoma. *Hum Pathol*. 2020;106:93-105.
63. Gángó A, Bátai B, Varga M, et al. Concomitant 1p36 deletion and TNFRSF14 mutations in primary cutaneous follicle center lymphoma frequently expressing high levels of EZH2 protein. *Virchows Arch*. 2018;473(4):453-462.
64. Szablewski V, Ingen-Housz-Oro S, Baia M, Delfau-Larue MH, Copie-Bergman C, Ortonne N. Primary cutaneous follicle center lymphomas expressing BCL2 protein frequently

harbor BCL2 gene Break and may present 1p36 deletion: a study of 20 cases. *Am J Surg Pathol.* 2016;40(1):127-136.
65. Schreuder MI, Hoefnagel JJ, Jansen PM, et al. FISH analysis of MALT lymphoma-specific translocations and aneuploidy in primary cutaneous marginal zone lymphoma. *J Pathol.* 2005;205:302-310.
66. Hallermann C, Kaune KM, Gesk S, et al. Molecular cytogenetic analysis of chromosomal breakpoints in the IGH, MYC, BCL6, and MALT1 gene loci in primary cutaneous B-cell lymphomas. *J Invest Dermatol.* 2004;123:213-219.
67. Carlsen ED, Swerdlow SH, Cook JR, Gibson SE. "Class-switched primary cutaneous marginal zone lymphomas are frequently IgG4-positive and have features distinct from IgM-positive cases." *Am J Surg Pathol.* 2019;43(10):1403-1412.
68. Gibson SE, Swerdlow SH. How I diagnose primary cutaneous marginal zone lymphoma. *Am J Clin Pathol.* 2020;154(4):428-449.
69. Menguy S, Laharanne E, Prochazkova-Carlotti M, et al. "Challenges in assessing MYC rearrangement in primary cutaneous diffuse large B-cell lymphoma, leg-type." *Am J Surg Pathol.* 2020;44(3):424-427. (MYC is controversial.)
70. Schrader AMR, de Groen RAL, Willemze R, et al. Cell-of-origin classification using the Hans and Lymph2Cx algorithms in primary cutaneous large B-cell lymphomas. *Virchows Arch.* 2022;480(3):667-675.
71. Gros A, Menguy S, Bobée V, et al. Integrative diagnosis of primary cutaneous large B-cell lymphomas supports the relevance of cell of origin profiling. *PLoS One.* 2022;17(4):e0266978.
72. Pham-Ledard A, Beylot-Barry M, Barbe C, et al. High frequency and clinical prognostic value of MYD88 L265P mutation in primary cutaneous diffuse large B-cell lymphoma, leg-type. *JAMA Dermatol.* 2014;150:1173-1179.
73. Lucioni M, Pescia C, Bonometti A, et al. Double expressor and double/triple hit status among primary cutaneous diffuse large B-cell lymphoma: a comparison between leg type and not otherwise specified subtypes. *Hum Pathol.* 2021;111:1-9.
74. Menguy S, Beylot-Barry M, Parrens M, et al. Primary cutaneous large B-cell lymphomas—relevance of the 2017 World Health Organization classification: clinicopathological and molecular analyses of 64 cases. *Histopathology.* 2019;74(7):1067-1080.
75. Schrader AMR, Jansen PM, Vermeer MH, Kleiverda JK, Vermaat JSP, Willemze R. High incidence and clinical significance of MYC rearrangements in primary cutaneous diffuse large B-cell lymphoma, leg type. *Am J Surg Pathol.* 2018;42(11):1488-1494.
76. Jaffe ES. "Navigating the cutaneous B-cell lymphomas: avoiding the rocky shoals." *Mod Pathol.* 2020;33(suppl 1):96-106.
77. Pham-Ledard A, Prochazkova-Carlotti M, Andrique L, et al. Multiple genetic alterations in primary cutaneous large B-cell lymphoma, leg type support a common lymphomagenesis with activated B-cell-like diffuse large B-cell lymphoma. *Mod Pathol.* 2014;27:402-411.
78. Senff NJ, Zoutman WH, Vermeer MH, et al. Fine-mapping chromosomal loss at 9p21: correlation with prognosis in primary cutaneous diffuse large B-cell lymphoma, leg type. *J Invest Dermatol.* 2009;129:1149-1155.

CHAPTER 31

Primary cutaneous follicle center B-cell lymphoma

Antonio Subtil and Michi M. Shinohara

DEFINITION

Primary cutaneous follicle center lymphoma (PCFCL) is a neoplastic proliferation of germinal center B cells in the skin. PCFCL is one of the three main subtypes of primary cutaneous B-cell lymphomas (CBCLs) recognized by the 2005 World Health Organization (WHO)/European Organization for the Research and Treatment of Cancer (EORTC) cutaneous lymphoma task force[1,2] and the 2008 WHO classification (Table 31-1).[3] The current WHO classification defines PCFCL as a tumor of neoplastic follicle center cells, including centrocytes and variable numbers of centroblasts, with a follicular, follicular and diffuse, or diffuse growth pattern.[4] PCFCL is the most frequently encountered of the CBCLs and falls in a low-grade, indolent category along with primary cutaneous marginal zone B-cell lymphoma (PCMZL). By definition, PCFCL is limited to the skin at the time of diagnosis, without evidence of systemic or nodal involvement, and as such represents a distinct entity from systemic or nodal follicular lymphoma (FL). As with other types of CBCL, initial staging includes a complete history and physical examination, laboratory studies (complete blood cell count with differential, comprehensive metabolic panel, and lactate dehydrogenase), and radiologic evaluation (computerized tomography [CT] scan of chest, abdomen, and pelvis with contrast or a positron emission tomography with CT [PET/CT]).[5]

EPIDEMIOLOGY

PCFCL is the most common subtype of CBCL, accounting for 1/3 to 1/2 of all CBCLs.[1,2,6,7] PCFCL occurs primarily in adults, with an age range of 17 to 89 years (median 51-58 years) and a slight male predominance.[2,6] Since the adoption of the 2005 WHO/EORTC classification for CBCLs, many cases previously thought to be primary cutaneous diffuse large B-cell lymphoma (PCDLBCL) would now be reclassified as PCFCL,[2] a distinction that is critical because of prognostic implications and therapeutic approach.

ETIOLOGY

The etiology of PCFCL is unknown. *Borrelia burgdorferi* DNA can be identified within tissue from a minority of PCFCL cases in endemic areas in Europe[8]; however, this finding has not been confirmed in nonendemic areas including the United States.[9] Screening for *B. burgdorferi* is not currently recommended as part of the evaluation of patients with suspected PCFCL.[5] Causal connection to oncogenic bacterial or viral infections has also not been established. Hepatitis C viral DNA can be demonstrated in as many as 30% of cases of PCFCL, although the clinical relevance is unknown[10]; a similar situation exists for human herpes virus 8.[11] Epstein-Barr virus DNA has not been demonstrated in PCFCL.[12]

Clinical Presentation and Prognosis

The clinical presentation of PCFCL is of solitary or clustered smooth, erythematous to violaceous infiltrated papules, plaques, nodules, or tumors, usually on the head and neck or trunk[2,13] (Fig. 31-1). Widespread or multifocal involvement can occur but is uncommon (15% of cases).[2] Ulceration is rare but may occur in longstanding cases.[14] PCFCL occurring on the scalp is a particularly common presentation (Fig. 31-2) and can demonstrate relatively subtle erythema (Fig. 31-3), hypochromasia,[15] or isolated telangiectasias.[16] A few distinct clinical variants of PCFCL have been described; "Crosti lymphoma" or "reticulohistiocytoma of the dorsum" presents with figurate, annular erythematous plaques surrounding infiltrated central plaques on the trunk.[17] A miliary or agminated presentation on the face and trunk can mimic benign entities such as rosacea, insect bites, or folliculitis[18,19] (Fig. 31-4). Regardless of the clinical variant or extent of involvement, PCFCL has an excellent prognosis, with a 5-year survival of ≥95%.[2,20] Recurrences are relatively common, occurring in 20% to 50% of patients,[1,6] but do not negatively impact the long-term outcome. Subsequent extracutaneous involvement is uncommon, observed in about 10% of cases in the largest case series.[2,6] An exception to the generally excellent prognosis is PCFCL occurring on the leg, which has been associated with a less favorable 5-year survival of 41%.[2]

TABLE 31-1 Comparison of Primary Cutaneous B-Cell Lymphomas

	Follicle Center Lymphoma	Marginal Zone Lymphoma	Diffuse Large B-Cell Lymphoma, Leg Type
Growth pattern	Follicular Follicular and diffuse Diffuse	Periadnexal, diffuse and nodular	Diffuse
Plasmacytic differentiation	−	+	−
Kappa/lambda IHC/ISH	Not helpful	Light chain restriction in vast majority of cases	Usually not helpful
CD21 IHC	Positive in follicular and in follicular/diffuse cases	Positive if lymphoid follicles are present	Negative (absent follicular dendritic cell meshworks)
BCL2 IHC	Usually negative in neoplastic cells (may be positive in up to 20% of cases)	Positive	Usually positive (may be negative in 10% of cases)
MUM1 IHC	−	Positive in plasma cells	Usually positive (may be negative in 10% of cases)
Ki-67 proliferative index	Variable (usually <50%)	Low (if present, reactive lymphoid follicles exhibit high Ki-67)	High (>50%)

IHC, immunohistochemistry; ISH, in situ hybridization.

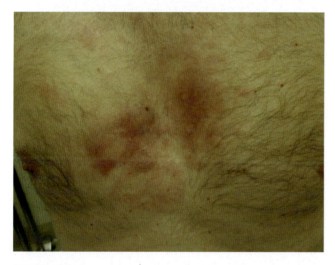

FIGURE 31-1. Clustered erythematous to violaceous papules, plaques, and nodules of PCFCL occurring on the trunk.

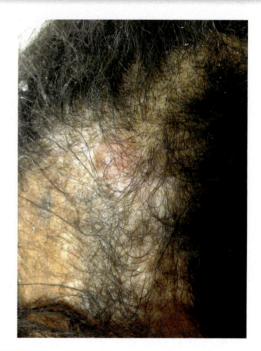

FIGURE 31-2. Erythematous nodule of PCFCL on the scalp.

HISTOLOGY

PCFCLs are composed of a mixture of centrocytes, with smaller, cleaved (elongated) nuclei, and centroblasts, with larger, noncleaved (round) nuclei and visible peripheral nucleoli (Fig. 31-5). Follicular, diffuse and follicular, or diffuse growth patterns are seen, with variable mixtures sometimes present within the same lesion. Evaluation of growth pattern may be affected by limited sampling. The epidermis is spared, and a Grenz zone is nearly always present[21,22] (Fig. 31-6A). Lymphoid infiltrates are perivascular and periadnexal and can extend into the fat[21] in what has been described as a "bottom heavy" appearance.[23] As opposed to systemic FL, grading of PCFCL according to the WHO classification is not reflective of the clinical behavior of the disease and is no longer routinely reported.

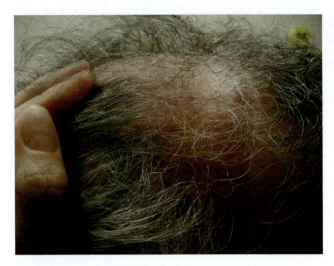

FIGURE 31-3. PCFCL presenting as diffuse erythema with subtle induration of the scalp.

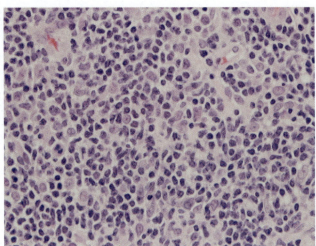

FIGURE 31-5. Centrocytes (small, cleaved) and centroblasts (larger, round) in PCFCL.

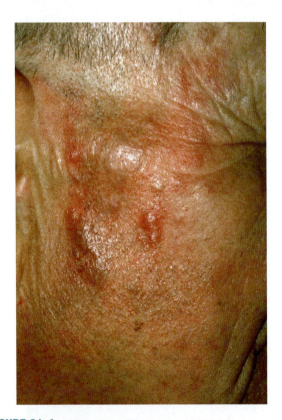

FIGURE 31-4. PCFCL with acneiform papules, mimicking acne or rosacea.

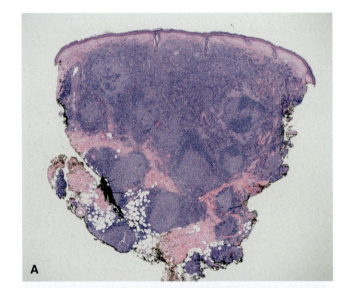

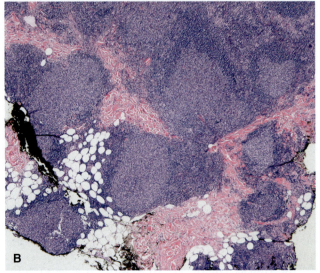

FIGURE 31-6. Low power of follicular type PCFCL, with a "bottom heavy" dense lymphocytic infiltrate **(A)** demonstrating distorted lymphoid follicles **(B)**. (Hematoxylin and eosin [H&E]).

The follicular pattern of PCFCL demonstrates distorted, variably sized follicles throughout the dermis and sometimes into the subcutaneous fat (Fig. 31-6). The most reliable feature of neoplastic follicles in PCFCL is a lack of tingible body macrophages, found in the majority of cases.[23,24] Other features of neoplastic follicles are crowding, variable size, reduced or absent mantle zones, and a lack of polarization, without distinct dark and light zones[24] (Fig. 31-7). The nodularity of this growth pattern is due to the follicular architecture produced by prominent follicular dendritic cell meshworks. Reactive

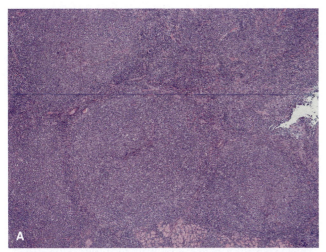

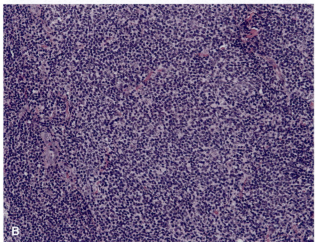

FIGURE 31-7. Follicular-type PCFCL showing crowded and distorted follicles with no discernible mantle zones **(A)**. Higher power **(B)** highlights a lack of polarization and absence of tingible body macrophages. (H&E).

lymphoid follicles at the periphery[22] and T-cell infiltrates can be prominent, particularly in the interfollicular zone and stroma of early lesions.[20] Other inflammatory cells, such as eosinophils and plasma cells, are less frequently seen.[23,24]

The diffuse pattern was the first type of PCFCL recognized and is more frequently encountered than the follicular type.[2,20,23,25] The diffuse pattern is usually present in larger nodules and tumors of PCFCL but can be seen in smaller, early lesions and, in contrast to nodal FL, is a distinct histologic type that does not represent progression from a follicular pattern.[26] Morphologically, diffuse PCFCL shows a proliferation of centrocytes with a smaller subset of centroblasts in a nodular or sheet-like pattern, extending throughout the dermis and often into the subcutaneous fat. Well-formed follicular structures and follicular dendritic cell meshworks are absent[26] (Figs. 31-8 and 31-9). The diffuse pattern of PCFCL can be difficult to distinguish from PCDLBCL, particularly when there is an abundance of centroblasts (see Differential, below, and Fig. 31-5).

A spindle-cell or sarcomatoid variant of CBCL has also been described, with many of these cases demonstrating follicle center origin.[27-31] Spindle-cell follicle center lymphoma shows nodules or fascicles of spindled cells (ie, composed primarily of centrocytes), often with focal areas of more typical-appearing centroblasts admixed with centrocytes. The spindled cells can be monomorphic or take on pleomorphic shapes, including "boomerang" or "spermatozoa" morphology[27,28] (Fig. 31-10). Spindled and mucinous morphology has also been reported.[32] Thickened collagen bundles can be present, and differentiation from other spindle-cell neoplasms can be challenging and requires immunohistochemical stains.[28]

Other rare morphologic findings described in PCFCL include follicular mucinosis,[33] clear cell,[34] multilobated, and Reed-Sternberg or Hodgkin-like cells.[35]

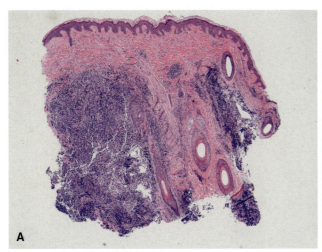 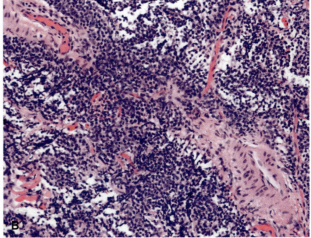

FIGURE 31-8. Diffuse-type PCFCL with a perivascular and periadnexal infiltrate without discernible follicles in the superficial dermis **(A)** and sheet-like growth in the deeper dermis **(B)**. (H&E).

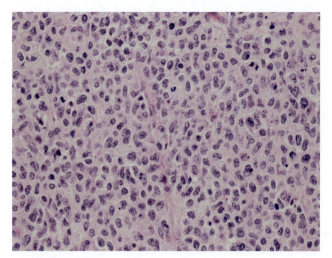

FIGURE 31-9. Diffuse-type PCFCL comprising mostly medium-sized, cleaved centrocytes. (H&E).

IMMUNOPHENOTYPE

The immunophenotype of PCFCL can be assessed by immunohistochemical (IHC) staining, or less commonly by flow cytometry,[36] and reflects a germinal center B-cell origin, with neoplastic B cells universally expressing CD20, CD79a,[20] PAX5 (paired box gene 5),[37] PU.1,[38] and the germinal center marker Bcl-6[39,40] (Fig. 31-11). The germinal center marker CD10 is variably positive depending on the growth pattern, with relatively consistent staining seen within neoplastic follicles in the follicular growth pattern and less frequent (about 1/3 of cases) staining in the diffuse pattern[2,23,24,26] (Fig. 31-12). Newer germinal center markers stathmin 1 (STMN1), LIM-only transcription factor 2 (LMO2), human germinal center–associated lymphoma (HGAL), and activation-induced cytidine deaminase (AID) are also frequently expressed in PCFCL.[41] CD21 highlights irregular follicular contours or disrupted follicular dendritic cell (FDC) networks in follicular pattern PCFCL[24] but may be sparse or even absent in diffuse pattern PCFCL.[26,40] Neoplastic follicles have a reduced (<50%) proliferative rate as assessed by Ki-67/MIB-1 staining when compared with reactive germinal centers, which typically show >90% Ki-67 staining[24] (Fig. 31-11D).

Staining for the antiapoptotic protein Bcl-2 is seen in only a minority (10%-20%) of cases of PCFCL[2,12,23,42,43] and can be helpful in distinguishing from nodal FL, where Bcl-2 staining is usually present[13,42,44] (Fig. 31-13). Positive Bcl-2 staining (defined as >50%), when present, has been associated with a worse prognosis in diffuse large B-cell lymphoma, including PCFCL.[45] Of note, Bcl-2 is normally present in reactive lymphocytes of primary follicles as well as in T follicular helper cells and mantle zone B cells of secondary follicles; therefore, immunostaining must be interpreted with this in mind.

Immunoglobulin (Ig) light chain restriction with κ or λ can be demonstrated in the majority of cases of PCFCL when staining is performed on frozen sections[13] or by flow cytometry,[36] but a low yield from paraffin-fixed sections is typical.[23,46] Immunoglobulin heavy chain (IgM or IgD) expression is rarely positive, except in cases of PCFCL occurring on the leg.[46]

MUM-1 (Multiple myeloma-1) is a member of the interferon regulatory factor family of transcription factors and plays a role in B-cell lymphomagenesis.[47] Expression of MUM-1 (as defined by nuclear staining in ≥30% of cells) is seen in <10% of PCFCL.[2,12] FOX-P1 (Forkhead box-P1)

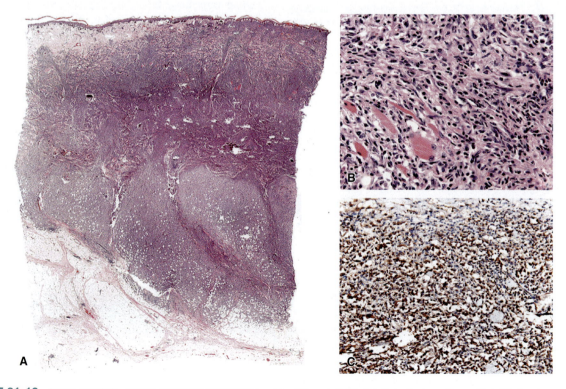

FIGURE 31-10. Spindle cell PCFCL, showing distorted lymphoid follicles and sheet like growth **(A)**. Spindled cells show pleomorphism **(B)**; the presence of Bcl-6 immunostaining supports a germinal center origin **(C)**.

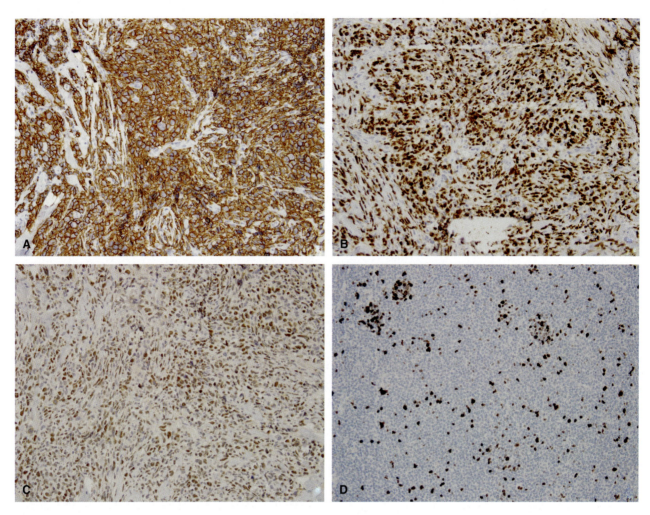

FIGURE 31-11. Immunostaining pattern of PCFCL, showing strong staining for CD20 **(A)**, PAX5 **(B)**, and Bcl-6 **(C)**, with a low Ki-67 proliferative rate within neoplastic lymphoid follicles (<50%) **(D)**.

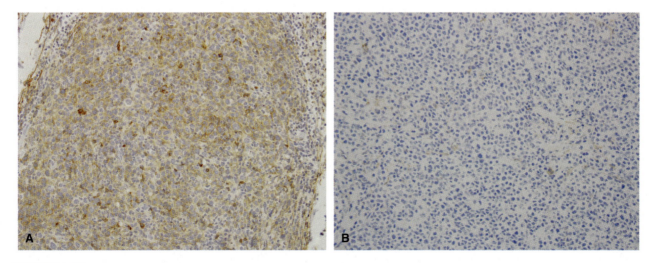

FIGURE 31-12. CD10 staining is variable in PCFCL depending on the growth pattern; strong positive staining in follicular type **(A)** and negative in diffuse type **(B)**.

transcription factor is also uncommonly found in PCFCL, with positivity (>90% strong nuclear staining) seen in <10% of cases[2]; there is some evidence that FOX-P1 may predict a worse prognosis when it is present.[12]

CD30 is expressed in activated lymphocytes and is found in a proportion of nodal FL as well as the CD30+ lymphoproliferative disorders. Diffuse and strong CD30 expression has been reported in otherwise typical cases of PCFCL.[48]

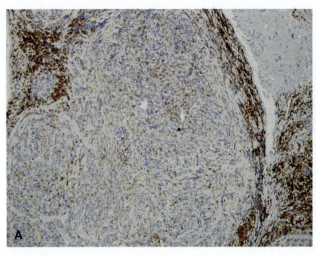 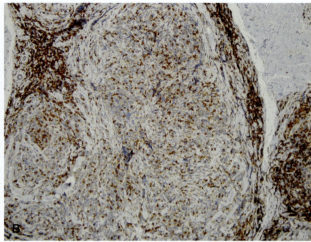

FIGURE 31-13. Bcl-2 is usually negative (<50% staining) in PCFCL **(A)** but should be interpreted along-side a T-cell marker **(B)**.

PD-1 (Programmed death-1) is highly expressed in the follicular helper-type T cells that play a role in the formation and cell maturation of germinal centers. PD-1 does not appear to be expressed in the neoplastic B cells of PCFCL but can be seen in infiltrating reactive T cells.[49]

Genetic and Molecular Findings

A B-cell clone with monoclonal gene rearrangement at J_H (*IGH*) can be demonstrated in over half of cases of PCFCL when assessed by polymerase chain reaction (PCR),[23,24] with the same B-cell clone in different neoplastic follicles in the same specimen.[23] False-negative PCR may occur due to somatic hypermutation. A higher sensitivity and specificity are found when *IGH* and *IGK* genes are both assessed.[50] Flow cytometry is also a sensitive method for demonstrating clonality in PCFCL.[36]

Numerous chromosomal aberrations can be seen in PCFCL. Comparative genomic hybridization shows both chromosomal gains and deletions, including amplifications at 2p and 12q and deletion of 14q.[51,52]

The interchromosomal translocation between *BCL2* on chromosome 18 and the immunoglobulin heavy locus (*IGH*) on chromosome 14 [t(14:18) (q32;q21)] is seen in the majority of nodal FL,[44] usually resulting in aberrant Bcl-2 expression demonstrable by IHC.[53] The t(14;18) translocation can be assayed by PCR or fluorescence in situ hybridization (FISH), with the translocation found in PCFCL only rarely by PCR.[13,22,42,50,51] FISH shows a higher detection rate, with 8% to 41% (most series in the 8%-10% range) of PCFCL showing t(14;18).[54-58] The presence of the t(14;18) translocation in PCFCL does not appear to affect the overall or disease-specific survival,[54] although there may be an association with secondary extracutaneous spread.[57] While it may occur in a small subset of PCFCLs, the presence of the t(14;18) translocation would raise the possibility of cutaneous dissemination by systemic FL.

Translocations between *BCL6* and *IGH* [t(3;14) (q27;q32)][55] and *BCL2* and *MALT1*[54] have also been rarely demonstrated in PCFCL. 1p36 deletions (with accompanying mutations in the tumor suppressor *TNFRSF14*) have also been reported.[56] Translocations affecting the *MYC* loci have not been found, in contrast to systemic FL, double-hit lymphoma, Burkitt lymphoma, and PCDLBCL-leg type.[59] Therefore, the identification of a MYC rearrangement would raise the possibility of a different lymphoma than PCFCL.

Gene expression profiling of PCFCL shows upregulation of genes (*SPINK2*, *LCK*, and *SLAM*) in a germinal center B cell–like pattern.[60] Next-generation sequencing of PCFCL shows a distinct mutational profile compared with nodal FL, with mutations in *TNFAIP3* detected more frequently in PCFCL, and *CREBBP*, *KMT2D*, and *BCL2* mutations found more in FL.[61]

MicroRNAs (miRs) are small sequences of noncoding RNA that can, in some circumstances, act as oncogenes. The miR cluster designated miR-17-92 is overexpressed in systemic B-cell lymphomas and is thought to play a role in lymphoma progression and treatment resistance.[62,63] Battistella et al[64] confirmed overexpression of the oncogenic miR-17-92 cluster in CBCL and linked high expression of miR-20a and miR-20b to worse prognosis. The tumor suppressor PTEN is a possible target for miRs in PCFCL, with decreased expression in one-third of cases.[64] Several studies have confirmed differential expression profiles of miRs in PCFCL compared with PCDLBCL-leg type, suggesting that this may be a helpful tool for differentiating between these entities in difficult cases and also identifying those cases with poor prognostic features.[64,65]

POSTULATED CELL OF ORIGIN

Mature germinal center B cells.

DIFFERENTIAL DIAGNOSIS

The main differential diagnosis for PCFCL includes cutaneous lymphoid hyperplasia (CLH), PCMZL, PCDLBCL-leg type, and secondary nodal FL. The spindle cell variant of PCFCL can also prompt a differential diagnosis of other spindle cell neoplasms in the skin (spindle cell melanoma, fibrohistiocytic lesions, etc.).

Differentiating PCFCL from CLH is a frequently encountered clinical scenario, particularly for small, solitary, or early lesions. Features that are in favor of the diagnosis of PCFCL include distorted, crowded follicles with diminished to absent mantle zones, reduced tingible body macrophages, and a low (<50%) proliferative rate.[24] Features that favor CLH are a "top heavy" appearance, with the majority of the infiltrate in the superficial and mid dermis, well-spaced lymphoid follicles with preserved mantle zones, a regular follicular dendritic network outlined by CD21, and the presence of reactive, polytypic plasma cells.[66] A Ki-67 immunostain is a helpful tool in these circumstances, as it will highlight a low proliferative rate in PCFCL and high proliferative rate in reactive germinal centers.[24] Although the presence of a monoclonal B-cell clone favors PCFCL, B-cell clonality studies are neither 100% sensitive nor specific and should not be solely relied upon to establish or exclude the diagnosis of PCFCL.[50]

The follicular type of PCFCL must also be differentiated from PCMZL variants with abundant reactive germinal centers or prominent immunoblasts. Reactive germinal centers in PCMZL can be distinguished from the neoplastic germinal centers of PCFCL by the features mentioned in the above discussion of CLH. PCMZL often shows plasmacytic differentiation, with lymphoplasmacytoid and plasma cells frequently present[1] (Table 31-1). Neoplastic marginal zone B cells express Bcl-2, without expression of the germinal center markers Bcl-6 and CD10.[1,24] These cells may occasionally colonize reactive lymphoid follicles, thus mimicking Bcl-2-positive follicular lymphoma. The absence of Bcl-6 expression and the lack of centrocytes are helpful in the differential with this variant of MZBCL. As reactive T cells in PCFCL also express Bcl-2, utilization of a pan-T-cell marker (such as CD2 or CD3) is recommended to aid in interpretation. Table 31-1 summarizes some of the main morphologic and immunohistochemical differences between PCFCL and PCMZL.

Of considerable importance is differentiating PCFCL with a diffuse growth pattern from PCDLBCL-leg type (see Table 31-1 and Fig. 31-5), as the latter has a significantly worse prognosis.[1] PCDLBCL-leg type is characterized by diffuse sheets of centroblasts and immunoblasts,[1] without the remnants of follicular dendritic cell networks (ie, negative CD21) and robust reactive T-cell infiltrates that can be seen in PCFCL.[2] Immunophenotyping is mandatory; Bcl-2, MUM-1, and FOX-P1 expression favors PCDLBCL-leg type, as most cases of PCDLBCL-leg type demonstrate this pattern by immunostaining.[2,38] Cytoplasmic IgM and IgD staining are also seen in most cases of PCDLBCL-leg type and infrequently in PCFCL.[67] Bcl-6 is not helpful in differentiating PCDLBCL-leg type from PCFCL, as it is often present in both entities[2,38,68]; Ki-67 proliferative rates may be similar in both entities.[68] Positive p63 staining is seen more frequently in PCDLBCL-leg type[69] but can also be present in PCFCL, with frequency rates depending on the clone of antibody used.[68,69] Utilization of a panel of immunostains is recommended, rather than relying on one stain in isolation. Cases remain in which definitive distinction on the basis of morphology and immunohistochemistry between PCFCL with a diffuse growth pattern and PCDLBCL-leg type is extremely challenging (Fig. 31-14).

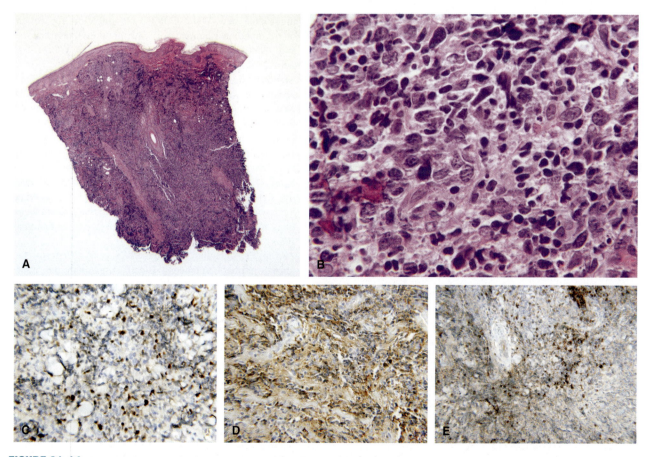

FIGURE 31-14. A challenging case of diffuse-type PCFCL, mimicking PCDLBCL-leg type. There is sheet-like growth of large, pleomorphic, centroblast-like cells **(A** and **B)**. IgM **(C)** and IgD **(D)** show patchy cytoplasmic staining. MUM-1 **(E)** stains a subset of cells but does not demonstrate the diffuse, strong staining typically seen in PCDLBCL-leg type.

TABLE 31-2 Comparison of Primary Cutaneous Follicle Center Lymphoma and Secondary Cutaneous Involvement by Systemic/nodal follicular Lymphoma

	Primary Cutaneous Follicle Center Lymphoma	Systemic/Nodal Follicular Lymphoma
BCL2 IHC	Usually negative in neoplastic cells (may be positive in up to 20% of cases)	Usually positive (may be negative in up to 30% of cases, particularly grade 3)
CD10 IHC	Variable (expression is more frequent in follicular growth pattern than in diffuse)	Usually positive (may be negative in a subset of grade 3 cases)
BCL6 IHC	Positive	Positive
Grading	Not done	1-2 (low-grade), 3A, 3B (based on the number of centroblasts per high-power microscopic field)
Initial staging workup (gold standard)	Skin-only disease	Evidence of systemic disease

IHC, immunohistochemistry.

Bcl-2 expression is seen in most cases of nodal FL,[53] and the presence of Bcl-2 staining in a cutaneous follicular B-cell lymphoma should strongly raise suspicion for skin involvement by nodal FL (Table 31-2). Bcl-2 expression is not diagnostic of nodal FL; however, as 10% to 20% of cases of PCFCL show Bcl-2 positivity,[2,12,23,42,43] although cases of nodal FL may show more intense Bcl-2 staining.[58] Likewise, the absence of Bcl-2 does not exclude nodal FL; as many as 30% of nodal FLs are negative for Bcl-2 by IHC.[70,71] Most cases of Bcl-2 negative systemic follicular lymphoma represent higher-grade tumors.[70] Nevertheless, complete staging, including radiologic evaluation with a CT or PET/CT scan of chest, abdomen, and pelvis is recommended in all cases of suspected PCFCL regardless of Bcl-2 expression status.[5]

CAPSULE SUMMARY

Clinical: Violaceous papules, nodules, or plaques; predilection for the scalp and upper trunk. Five-year survival ≥95%, except when involving the leg.

Histology: Nodular infiltrates of centrocytes and centroblasts in a follicular, follicular and diffuse, or diffuse pattern. Reactive T-cell infiltrates common.

Immunophenotype: CD20+, Pax5+, Bcl6+, CD10+/-, Bcl2-, MUM-1-

Genetic and Molecular Findings: Monoclonal J_H gene rearrangements; usually negative for t(14;18).

Postulated Cell of Origin: Mature germinal center B-cells.

Differential diagnosis: CLH, PCMZL, PCDLBCL-leg type, and nodal FL.

ACKNOWLEDGMENTS

Dr. Alejandro Gru and Dr. Oliver Chang for providing histologic images.

References

1. Willemze R, Jaffe ES, Burg G, et al. WHO-EORTC classification for cutaneous lymphomas. *Blood*. 2005;105(10):3768-3785.
2. Senff NJ, Hoefnagel JJ, Jansen PM, et al. Reclassification of 300 primary cutaneous B-Cell lymphomas according to the new WHO-EORTC classification for cutaneous lymphomas: comparison with previous classifications and identification of prognostic markers. *J Clin Oncol*. 2007;25(12):1581-1587.
3. Swerdlow SH, Campo E, Harris NL, et al. *WHO Classification of Tumours of Haematopoietic and Lymphoid Tissues*. IARC; 2008.
4. NCCN Clinical Practice Guidelines in Oncology (NCCN Guidelines), Primary Cutaneous Lymphomas. National Comprehensive Cancer Network. Published 2022. Updated June 8, 2022. Accessed July 10, 2022. https://www.nccn.org/professionals/physician_gls/pdf/primary_cutaneous.pdf
5. Senff NJ, Noordijk EM, Kim YH, et al. European Organization for Research and treatment of Cancer and International Society for cutaneous lymphoma consensus recommendations for the management of cutaneous B-cell lymphomas. *Blood*. 2008;112(5):1600-1609.
6. Zinzani PL, Quaglino P, Pimpinelli N, et al. Prognostic factors in primary cutaneous B-cell lymphoma: the Italian study Group for cutaneous lymphomas. *J Clin Oncol*. 2006;24(9):1376-1382.
7. Bradford PT, Devesa SS, Anderson WF, Toro JR. Cutaneous lymphoma incidence patterns in the United States: a population-based study of 3884 cases. *Blood*. 2009;113(21):5064-5073.
8. Cerroni L, Zochling N, Putz B, Kerl H. Infection by Borrelia burgdorferi and cutaneous B-cell lymphoma. *J Cutan Pathol*. 1997;24(8):457-461.
9. Ponzoni M, Ferreri AJ, Mappa S, et al. Prevalence of Borrelia burgdorferi infection in a series of 98 primary cutaneous lymphomas. *Oncol*. 2011;16(11):1582-1588.
10. Michaelis S, Kazakov DV, Schmid M, Dummer R, Burg G, Kempf W. Hepatitis C and G viruses in B-cell lymphomas of the skin. *J Cutan Pathol*. 2003;30(6):369-372.

11. Zochling N, Putz B, Wolf P, Kerl H, Cerroni L. Human herpesvirus 8-specific DNA sequences in primary cutaneous B-cell lymphomas. *Arch Dermatol*. 1998;134(2):246-247.
12. Kodama K, Massone C, Chott A, Metze D, Kerl H, Cerroni L. Primary cutaneous large B-cell lymphomas: clinicopathologic features, classification, and prognostic factors in a large series of patients. *Blood*. 2005;106(7):2491-2497.
13. Bergman R, Kurtin PJ, Gibson LE, Hull PR, Kimlinger TK, Schroeter AL. Clinicopathologic, immunophenotypic, and molecular characterization of primary cutaneous follicular B-cell lymphoma. *Arch Dermatol*. 2001;137(4):432-439.
14. Fierro MT, Marenco F, Novelli M, Fava P, Quaglino P, Bernengo MG. Long-term evolution of an untreated primary cutaneous follicle center lymphoma of the scalp. *Am J Dermatopathol*. 2010;32(1):91-94.
15. Massone C, Fink-Puches R, Cerroni L. Atypical clinical presentation of primary and secondary cutaneous follicle center lymphoma (FCL) on the head characterized by macular lesions. *J Am Acad Dermatol*. 2016;75(5):1000-1006.
16. Ingen-Housz-Oro S, Jones M, Ortonne N, Haioun C, Chosidow O. Extensive telangiectases of the scalp: atypical presentation of primary cutaneous follicle centre lymphoma. *Br J Haematol*. 2012;158(3):297.
17. Berti E, Alessi E, Caputo R, Gianotti R, Delia D, Vezzoni P. Reticulohistiocytoma of the dorsum. *J Am Acad Dermatol*. 1988;19(2 Pt 1):259-272.
18. Massone C, Fink-Puches R, Laimer M, Rutten A, Vale E, Cerroni L. Miliary and agminated-type primary cutaneous follicle center lymphoma: report of 18 cases. *J Am Acad Dermatol*. 2011;65(4):749-755.
19. Barzilai A, Feuerman H, Quaglino P, et al. Cutaneous B-cell neoplasms mimicking granulomatous rosacea or rhinophyma. *Arch Dermatol*. 2012;148(7):824-831.
20. Willemze R, Kerl H, Sterry W, et al. EORTC classification for primary cutaneous lymphomas: a proposal from the cutaneous lymphoma study Group of the European Organization for Research and treatment of Cancer. *Blood*. 1997;90(1):354-371.
21. Garcia CF, Weiss LM, Warnke RA, Wood GS. Cutaneous follicular lymphoma. *Am J Surg Pathol*. 1986;10(7):454-463.
22. Franco R, Fernandez-Vazquez A, Rodriguez-Peralto JL, et al. Cutaneous follicular B-cell lymphoma: description of a series of 18 cases. *Am J Surg Pathol*. 2001;25(7):875-883.
23. Cerroni L, Arzberger E, Putz B, et al. Primary cutaneous follicle center cell lymphoma with follicular growth pattern. *Blood*. 2000;95(12):3922-3928.
24. Leinweber B, Colli C, Chott A, Kerl H, Cerroni L. Differential diagnosis of cutaneous infiltrates of B lymphocytes with follicular growth pattern. *Am J Dermatopathol*. 2004;26(1):4-13.
25. Cerroni L, Kerl H. Primary cutaneous follicle center cell lymphoma. *Leuk Lymphoma*. 2001;42(5):891-900.
26. Gulia A, Saggini A, Wiesner T, et al. Clinicopathologic features of early lesions of primary cutaneous follicle center lymphoma, diffuse type: implications for early diagnosis and treatment. *J Am Acad Dermatol*. 2011;65(5):991-1000.
27. Jghaimi F, Hocar O, Akhdari N, Amal S, Belaabidia B. Primary cutaneous spindle-cell B-cell lymphoma of follicle center cell origin. *Am J Dermatopathol*. 2013;35(8):871-873.
28. Cerroni L, El-Shabrawi-Caelen L, Fink-Puches R, LeBoit PE, Kerl H. Cutaneous spindle-cell B-cell lymphoma: a morphologic variant of cutaneous large B-cell lymphoma. *Am J Dermatopathol*. 2000;22(4):299-304.
29. Rozati S, Kerl K, Kempf W, et al. Spindle-cell variant of primary cutaneous follicle center lymphoma spreading to the hepatobiliary tree, mimicking Klatskin tumor. *J Cutan Pathol*. 2013;40(1):56-60.
30. Garrido MC, Rios JJ, Riveiro-Falkenbach E, Escamez PJ, Ronco MA, Rodriguez-Peralto JL. Primary cutaneous spindle cell B-cell lymphoma of follicle origin mimicking acne rosacea. *Am J Dermatopathol*. 2014;37(6):e64-e67.
31. Charli-Joseph Y, Cerroni L, LeBoit PE. Cutaneous spindle-cell B-cell lymphomas: most are neoplasms of follicular center cell origin. *Am J Surg Pathol*. 2015;39(6):737-743.
32. Li L, Majerowski J, Sokumbi O. Cutaneous spindled follicle center cell lymphoma with abundant mucin: a diagnostic pitfall. *J Cutan Pathol*. 2020;47(4):394-397.
33. Garrido MC, Riveiro-Falkenbach E, Rodriguez-Peralto JL. Primary cutaneous follicle center lymphoma with follicular mucinosis. *JAMA Dermatol*. 2014;150(8):906-907.
34. Cassisa A, Colpani F, Rinaldi R, Cima L. Primary cutaneous follicle center lymphoma clear cell variant: expanding the spectrum of cutaneous clear cell neoplasms. *Am J Dermatopathol*. 2018;40(11):849-853.
35. Dilly M, Ben-Rejeb H, Vergier B, et al. Primary cutaneous follicle center lymphoma with Hodgkin and Reed-Sternberg-like cells: a new histopathologic variant. *J Cutan Pathol*. 2014;41(10):797-801.
36. Schafernak KT, Variakojis D, Goolsby CL, et al. Clonality assessment of cutaneous B-cell lymphoid proliferations: a comparison of flow cytometry immunophenotyping, molecular studies, and immunohistochemistry/in situ hybridization and review of the literature. *Am J Dermatopathol*. 2014;36(10):781-795.
37. Kempf W, Kazakov DV, Mitteldorf C. Cutaneous lymphomas an update. Part 2: B-cell lymphomas and related conditions. *Am J Dermatopathol*. 2014;36(3):197-208; quiz 209-110.
38. Hoefnagel JJ, Mulder MM, Dreef E, et al. Expression of B-cell transcription factors in primary cutaneous B-cell lymphoma. *Mod Pathol*. 2006;19(9):1270-1276.
39. Hoefnagel JJ, Vermeer MH, Jansen PM, Fleuren GJ, Meijer CJ, Willemze R. Bcl-2, Bcl-6 and CD10 expression in cutaneous B-cell lymphoma: further support for a follicle centre cell origin and differential diagnostic significance. *Br J Dermatol*. 2003;149(6):1183-1191.
40. de Leval L, Harris NL, Longtine J, Ferry JA, Duncan LM. Cutaneous b-cell lymphomas of follicular and marginal zone types: use of Bcl-6, CD10, Bcl-2, and CD21 in differential diagnosis and classification. *Am J Surg Pathol*. 2001;25(6):732-741.
41. Verdanet E, Dereure O, René C, et al. Diagnostic value of STMN1, LMO2, HGAL, AID expression and 1p36 chromosomal abnormalities in primary cutaneous B cell lymphomas. *Histopathology*. 2017;71(4):648-660.
42. Child FJ, Russell-Jones R, Woolford AJ, et al. Absence of the t(14;18) chromosomal translocation in primary cutaneous B-cell lymphoma. *Br J Dermatol*. 2001;144(4):735-744.
43. Cerroni L, Volkenandt M, Rieger E, Soyer HP, Kerl H. bcl-2 protein expression and correlation with the interchromosomal 14;18 translocation in cutaneous lymphomas and pseudolymphomas. *J Invest Dermatol*. 1994;102(2):231-235.
44. Weiss LM, Warnke RA, Sklar J, Cleary ML. Molecular analysis of the t(14;18) chromosomal translocation in malignant lymphomas. *N Engl J Med*. 1987;317(19):1185-1189.

45. Grange F, Petrella T, Beylot-Barry M, et al. Bcl-2 protein expression is the strongest independent prognostic factor of survival in primary cutaneous large B-cell lymphomas. *Blood.* 2004;103(10):3662-3668.
46. Koens L, Vermeer MH, Willemze R, Jansen PM. IgM expression on paraffin sections distinguishes primary cutaneous large B-cell lymphoma, leg type from primary cutaneous follicle center lymphoma. *Am J Surg Pathol.* 2010;34(7):1043-1048.
47. Gaidano G, Carbone A. MUM1: a step ahead toward the understanding of lymphoma histogenesis. *Leukemia.* 2000;14(4):563-566.
48. Kempf W, Kazakov DV, Rutten A, et al. Primary cutaneous follicle center lymphoma with diffuse CD30 expression: a report of 4 cases of a rare variant. *J Am Acad Dermatol.* 2014;71(3):548-554.
49. Cetinozman F, Koens L, Jansen PM, Willemze R. Programmed death-1 expression in cutaneous B-cell lymphoma. *J Cutan Pathol.* 2014;41(1):14-21.
50. Morales AV, Arber DA, Seo K, Kohler S, Kim YH, Sundram UN. Evaluation of B-cell clonality using the BIOMED-2 PCR method effectively distinguishes cutaneous B-cell lymphoma from benign lymphoid infiltrates. *Am J Dermatopathol.* 2008;30(5):425-430.
51. Hallermann C, Kaune KM, Siebert R, et al. Chromosomal aberration patterns differ in subtypes of primary cutaneous B cell lymphomas. *J Invest Dermatol.* 2004;122(6):1495-1502.
52. Dijkman R, Tensen CP, Jordanova ES, et al. Array-based comparative genomic hybridization analysis reveals recurrent chromosomal alterations and prognostic parameters in primary cutaneous large B-cell lymphoma. *J Clin Oncol.* 2006;24(2):296-305.
53. Tsujimoto Y, Finger LR, Yunis J, Nowell PC, Croce CM. Cloning of the chromosome breakpoint of neoplastic B cells with the t(14;18) chromosome translocation. *Science.* 1984;226(4678):1097-1099.
54. Abdul-Wahab A, Tang SY, Robson A, et al. Chromosomal anomalies in primary cutaneous follicle center cell lymphoma do not portend a poor prognosis. *J Am Acad Dermatol.* 2014;70(6):1010-1020.
55. Streubel B, Scheucher B, Valencak J, et al. Molecular cytogenetic evidence of t(14;18)(IGH;BCL2) in a substantial proportion of primary cutaneous follicle center lymphomas. *Am J Surg Pathol.* 2006;30(4):529-536.
56. Gángó A, Bátai B, Varga M, et al. Concomitant 1p36 deletion and TNFRSF14 mutations in primary cutaneous follicle center lymphoma frequently expressing high levels of EZH2 protein. *Virchows Arch.* 2018;473(4):453-462.
57. Pham-Ledard A, Cowppli-Bony A, Doussau A, et al. Diagnostic and prognostic value of BCL2 rearrangement in 53 patients with follicular lymphoma presenting as primary skin lesions. *Am J Clin Pathol.* 2015;143(3):362-373.
58. Servitje O, Climent F, Colomo L, et al. Primary cutaneous vs secondary cutaneous follicular lymphomas: a comparative study focused on BCL2, CD10, and t(14;18) expression. *J Cutan Pathol.* 2019;46(3):182-189.
59. Hallermann C, Kaune KM, Gesk S, et al. Molecular cytogenetic analysis of chromosomal breakpoints in the IGH, MYC, BCL6, and MALT1 gene loci in primary cutaneous B-cell lymphomas. *J Invest Dermatol.* 2004;123(1):213-219.
60. Hoefnagel JJ, Dijkman R, Basso K, et al. Distinct types of primary cutaneous large B-cell lymphoma identified by gene expression profiling. *Blood.* 2005;105(9):3671-3678.
61. Barasch NJK, Liu YC, Ho J, et al. The molecular landscape and other distinctive features of primary cutaneous follicle center lymphoma. *Hum Pathol.* 2020;106:93-105.
62. Fassina A, Marino F, Siri M, et al. The miR-17-92 microRNA cluster: a novel diagnostic tool in large B-cell malignancies. *Lab Invest.* 2012;92(11):1574-1582.
63. Rao E, Jiang C, Ji M, et al. The miRNA-17 approximately 92 cluster mediates chemoresistance and enhances tumor growth in mantle cell lymphoma via PI3K/AKT pathway activation. *Leukemia.* 2012;26(5):1064-1072.
64. Battistella M, Romero M, Castro-Vega LJ, et al. The high expression of the microRNA 17-92 cluster and its paralogs, and the downregulation of the target gene PTEN, is associated with primary cutaneous B-cell lymphoma progression. *J Invest Dermatol.* 2015;135(6):1659-1667.
65. Koens L, Qin Y, Leung WY, et al. MicroRNA profiling of primary cutaneous large B-cell lymphomas. *PLoS One.* 2013;8(12):e82471.
66. Bergman R, Khamaysi K, Khamaysi Z, Ben Arie Y. A study of histologic and immunophenotypical staining patterns in cutaneous lymphoid hyperplasia. *J Am Acad Dermatol.* 2011;65(1):112-124.
67. Demirkesen C, Tuzuner N, Esen T, Lebe B, Ozkal S. The expression of IgM is helpful in the differentiation of primary cutaneous diffuse large B cell lymphoma and follicle center lymphoma. *Leuk Res.* 2011;35(9):1269-1272.
68. Menguy S, Beylot-Barry M, Parrens M, et al. Primary cutaneous large B-cell lymphomas relevance of the 2017 World Health Organization classification: clinicopathological and molecular analyses of 64 cases. *Histopathology.* 2019;74(7):1067-1080.
69. Robson A, Shukur Z, Ally M, et al. Immunocytochemical p63 expression discriminates between primary cutaneous follicle centre cell and diffuse large B cell lymphoma-leg type, and is of the TAp63 isoform. *Histopathology.* 2016;69(1):11-19.
70. Marafioti T, Copie-Bergman C, Calaminici M, et al. Another look at follicular lymphoma: immunophenotypic and molecular analyses identify distinct follicular lymphoma subgroups. *Histopathology.* 2013;62(6):860-875.
71. Schraders M, de Jong D, Kluin P, Groenen P, van Krieken H. Lack of Bcl-2 expression in follicular lymphoma may be caused by mutations in the BCL2 gene or by absence of the t(14;18) translocation. *J Pathol.* 2005;205(3):329-335.

CHAPTER 32

Primary cutaneous marginal zone B-cell lymphoma

Katalin Ferenczi, Farrah Bakr, and Alistair M. Robson

DEFINITION

Primary cutaneous marginal zone B-cell lymphomas (PCMZLs) are indolent low-grade B-cell lymphomas of the skin. PCMZLs have been regarded as the cutaneous counterpart of marginal zone lymphomas (MZLs) occurring at extranodal sites, in particular the mucosa-associated lymphoid tissue, so-called MALT lymphomas, in light of overlapping morphologic features and indolent clinical behavior. Recent data, however, indicate that primary cutaneous MZL and noncutaneous MZL (so-called MALT lymphoma) have distinct characteristics with respect to eliciting factors, immunoglobulin and chemokine receptor expression pattern, frequency of translocations, and systemic dissemination. In the 2005 World Health Organization–European Organization for Research and Treatment of Cancer (WHO-EORTC) classification of primary cutaneous lymphomas, cutaneous marginal zone B-cell lymphomas represent a separate entity.[1] However, the distinct features that separate cutaneous MZL from other extranodal marginal zone B-cell lymphomas are not well reflected in the WHO 2016 classification, as PCMZLs are not categorized separately but included in the broad group of extranodal marginal zone B-cell lymphomas of MALT type.[2] The term SALT (skin-associated lymphoid tissue) has also formerly been used for these tumors. They incorporate cases previously regarded as primary cutaneous immunocytoma and primary cutaneous plasmacytoma (PCP); these entities are now considered plasma cell–rich variants of PCMZL.[3] Cutaneous marginal zone B-cell lymphomas also include cases previously designated as cutaneous follicular lymphoid hyperplasia with monotypic plasma cells.[4] It remains to be elucidated whether some cases reported as PCMZL characterized by γ light chain restriction, indolent course, and spontaneous remission in children and young individuals represent marginal zone hyperplasia of the skin, a cutaneous counterpart of atypical marginal zone hyperplasia of MALT as found in the appendix and tonsils.[5]

EPIDEMIOLOGY

Primary cutaneous MZLs account for ~7% of all primary cutaneous lymphomas and represent between 20% and 40% of all primary cutaneous B-cell lymphomas.[1,6,7] The disease affects middle-aged individuals, with the median age at diagnosis of 55 years. Primary cutaneous MZLs with marked plasmacytic differentiation, previously regarded as immunocytomas, tend to be more common in the elderly. PCMZL is rare in children and young adults.[8,9] Men are almost twice as frequently affected as women. The incidence rate of cutaneous marginal zone B-cell lymphoma is higher among non-Hispanic whites than in other races.[6]

ETIOLOGY

The etiology and pathogenesis of PCMZLs are not entirely understood. It has long been thought that the inflammatory microenvironment and host immune response may play a role in the development of extranodal MZLs. MZLs, irrespective of the primary site, originate from B-cells in the marginal zone, the portion of the follicle with the highest rate of chronic antigenic exposure that typically function as a first line of defense against microbial pathogens. Chronic antigenic stimulation leading to persistent lymphoid hyperplasia and subsequent development of MZL has been suggested to play a role in the pathogenesis of MALT lymphomas. The pathogenic role of chronic antigenic stimulation, infection, or autoimmunity has been well documented in MALT lymphomas, such as the association between gastric MALT lymphoma and *Helicobacter pylori* infection, and MALT lymphomas of the salivary gland and thyroid and Sjögren syndrome and Hashimoto thyroiditis, respectively. Extranodal MZLs in general are thought to arise on a background of chronic inflammation characterized by a T_H1 cytokine profile, expression of CXCR3, and predominant expression of IgM. In contrast, the vast majority of primary cutaneous MZLs are characterized by a T_H2 cytokine profile, absence of CXCR3, and expression of the class-switched immunoglobulins IgG, IgA, and IgE.[10] These findings suggest that primary cutaneous MZL may develop in an inflammatory environment that is different from noncutaneous extranodal MZL. However, a small subset of cutaneous MZLs, so-called "nonclass-switched" PCMZLs, express CXCR3 and IgM similar to extranodal MZLs.[10] Whereas class-switched cases of PCMZLs do not appear to be associated with infectious agents, the small, nonclass-switched subset has been linked to *Borrelia burgdorferi* infection.[11]

Long-term antigenic stimulation caused by *B. burgdorferi* infection has been hypothesized to play a role in the development of a subset of cutaneous MZL in Europe. Earlier reports from certain endemic areas in Europe documented the development of PCMZL from infiltrates associated with *B. burgdorferi* infection, and antibiotic treatment in some cases resulted in regression of the tumors.[1,12-14] Detection of *Borrelia*-specific DNA sequences has been reported in 10%–42% of cutaneous MZL with higher detection rates in certain endemic areas in Europe.[12,15,16] These findings, however, were never confirmed in Asian or North American PCMZL patients.[17,18] Recent large studies from East Asia, the United States, Germany, and Italy similarly failed to show any evidence of *Borrelia*-specific sequences in patients with cutaneous MZL using polymerase chain reaction (PCR).[19-21]

A common antigen, however, may be involved in the antigenic stimulation and development of some cases of cutaneous MZL in the United States as suggested by findings showing the use of similar V_H gene segments and conserved complementarity determining region 3 sequences in PCMZL skin lesions.[22]

Other antigenic, infectious, or inflammatory factors that have been reported in association with the development of PCMZL include tattoos, tick bites, leishmania,[23] herpes simplex virus type 1 infection, and vaccinations, such as influenza and hepatitis C.[24] Chronic inflammation arising in the setting of autoimmune diseases, such as Sjögren syndrome or Hashimoto thyroiditis, and certain medications, such as antidepressants and antihistamines, have also been implicated.[25]

The clonally restricted response to antigenic triggers in neoplastic transformation and lymphomagenesis is also suggested by reports showing a bias in the immunoglobulin variable (IgV) repertoire with preferential usage of certain IgVH genes and the pattern of somatic hypermutations.[26] Aberrant somatic hypermutation, a mechanism associated with the induction of genetic instability, has been described in cutaneous MZL.[27] This genetic instability might account for stepwise DNA mutations culminating in the development of MZL.

CLINICAL PRESENTATION AND PROGNOSIS

PCMZLs clinically present as solitary or multiple red to violaceous papules, nodules (<3 cm), or plaques most often localized on the trunk (Fig. 32-1) and upper extremities or, less frequently, the head and neck. Rare, unusual clinical variants, such as anetodermic[28] or agminated form resembling rosacea, have been described.[29] The anetodermic form of PCMZL may be associated with antiphospholipid antibodies.[30]

Primary cutaneous MZL is an indolent but persistent disease and ~50% of PCMZL cases will show cutaneous relapses.[31] Patients with multifocal disease have shorter disease-free survival than those with single or localized lesions.[31] The disease typically remains confined to the skin; rarely, extracutaneous disease with systemic involvement by marginal zone B-cell lymphoma can occur. Extracutaneous spread is seen in less than 10% of the patients, and it is more commonly seen in the nonclass-switched subtype of

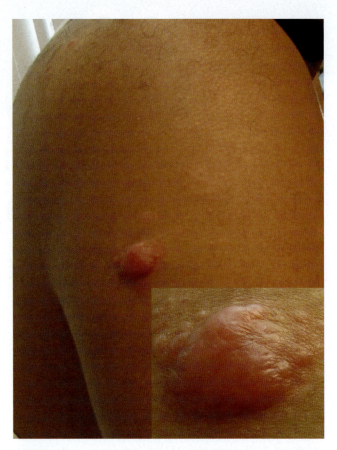

FIGURE 32-1. Primary cutaneous marginal zone lymphoma. Red nodule on the arm.

the disease. Significant association with gastrointestinal tract disorders, certain autoimmune conditions, and systemic malignancies has been reported.[32] Although relapses are common, prognosis is excellent with a 5-year disease-specific survival rate of over 98%.[1,33-35]

HISTOLOGY

Histology shows a nodular or diffuse mononuclear cell infiltrate centered in the dermis, which may extend into the subcutaneous fat (Figs. 32-2 and 32-3). The epidermis is spared, and a zone of uninvolved dermis (grenz zone) is often present (Fig. 32-4). Periadnexal tracking by neoplastic cells surrounding eccrine glands and hair follicles is frequently seen[36] (Fig. 32-5). It has been suggested that the presence of infiltration of the follicular epithelium or eccrine ducts could provide a helpful clue for MZL.[25] Substantial subcutaneous extension and involvement in MZL is more commonly seen in secondary cutaneous MZL.[37] Reactive germinal centers with distinct surrounding mantle zones are frequently present (Fig. 32-2), but as the disease progresses, the follicles can become colonized by neoplastic B-cells and the distinct germinal center–mantle zone demarcation will be absent, and the germinal centers become atrophic. In one of the author's experience, some cases can show Castleman-like features with atrophic follicles, onion-skinning of the mantle zone, and a permeative and fibrotic vessel. Some cases of MZL may show epidermotropism,[38,39] usually more limited in

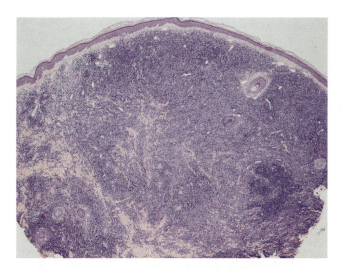

FIGURE 32-2. Primary cutaneous marginal zone lymphoma. Dense nodular lymphoid infiltrate involving the dermis and extending into subcutaneous tissue. Note the presence of a reactive germinal center in the reticular dermis (H&E, 4×).

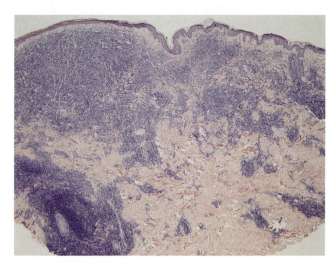

FIGURE 32-3. Primary cutaneous marginal zone lymphoma. Diffuse dermal mononuclear infiltrate showing perifollicular accentuation (H&E, 4×).

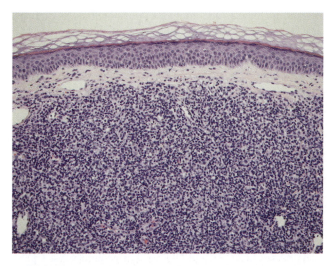

FIGURE 32-4. Primary cutaneous marginal zone lymphoma. The dermal infiltrate is separated from the epidermis by a grenz zone in the superficial dermis (H&E, 20×).

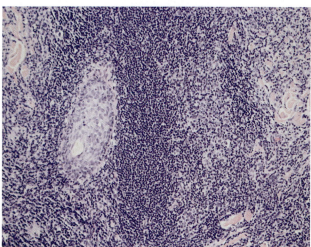

FIGURE 32-5. Primary cutaneous marginal zone lymphoma. Periadnexal distribution of the neoplastic cells is often seen (H&E, 20×).

extent than mycosis fungoides, and always lacking Pautrier microabscesses. The presence of epidermotropism should prompt careful review to exclude the possibility of a systemic MZL with secondary skin dissemination.[40,41]

The infiltrate is polymorphous, composed of small- to medium-sized lymphocytes, plasma cells, lymphoplasmacytoid cells, and often considerable numbers of reactive T-cells (Fig. 32-6). Marginal zone B-cells or centrocyte-like cells are small- to medium-sized lymphocytes with indented nuclei, inconspicuous nucleoli, and abundant pale cytoplasm (Fig. 32-7). The number of neoplastic B-cells within the infiltrate can be variable, but at times is very low.[2] Admixed T-cells are numerous, often comprising 50%–70% of the infiltrate. A predominance of B-cells is seen in the rare, nonclass-switched IgM+ subtype of PCMZL. Prominent plasmacytic differentiation is not uncommon, particularly immediately beneath the epidermis or at the tumor periphery. Plasma cells and lymphoplasmacytoid cells are often found in the superficial dermis and at the periphery of the infiltrates (Fig. 32-8A,B). Plasma cells may demonstrate atypia or binucleation (Fig. 32-9A). Periodic acid–Schiff-positive immunoglobulin-containing intranuclear inclusions

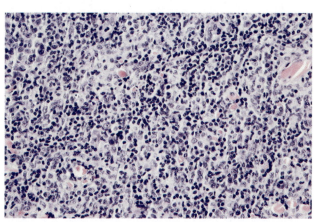

FIGURE 32-6. Primary cutaneous marginal zone lymphoma. The infiltrate is mixed composed of small- to medium-sized lymphocytes, reactive T-cells, and plasma cells (H&E, 40×).

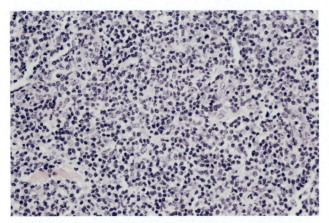

FIGURE 32-7. Primary cutaneous marginal zone lymphoma. Marginal zone B-cells (centrocyte-like cells) with abundant pale cytoplasm (H&E, 40×).

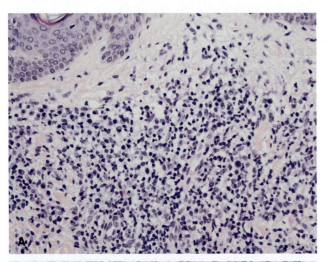

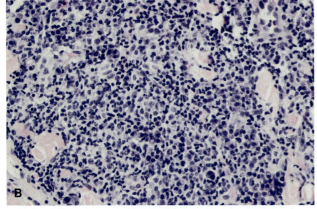

FIGURE 32-8. Primary cutaneous marginal zone lymphoma. Plasma cells in the papillary dermis **(A)** and reticular dermis **(B)**.

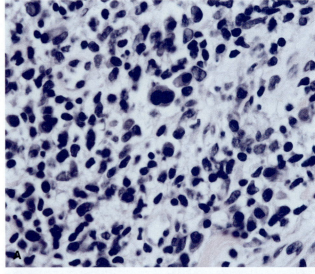

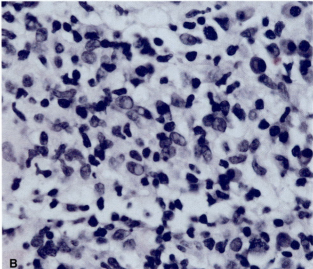

FIGURE 32-9. Primary cutaneous marginal zone lymphoma. Atypical binucleated plasma cells **(A)** and Dutcher bodies **(B)** (H&E, 100×).

the presence of eosinophils is not unusual, a moderate-to-marked increase in the number of eosinophils was reported as a feature of Asian but not European or US cutaneous MZL cases.[19] Prieto-Torres et al reported a series of 13 cases of MZL in the skin with increased number of CD30+ cells with Hodgkin-like appearance. Such cases showed a higher incidence of advanced disease and locoregional recurrence in approximately 69% of cases.[43]

IMMUNOPHENOTYPE

The immunophenotype of the neoplastic cells in MZL is that of normal marginal zone B-cells. Neoplastic cells express B-cell associated antigens CD19, CD20, CD22, CD79a (Fig. 32-11), and BCL-2 (Fig. 32-12) and are negative for CD5, CD23, cyclin D1, CD10, and BCL-6 (Table 32-1). Plasma cells express CD138 and CD79a, but generally not CD20. The proportion of admixed reactive CD3+ T-cells within the infiltrate can represent anywhere from 29%–80% of

(Dutcher bodies) may be present in cases with predominance of lymphoplasmacytoid cells (Fig. 32-9B). Eosinophilic, immunoglobulin-containing intracytoplasmic inclusions (Russell bodies) may occasionally be seen in cases with abundant plasma cells. Occasionally, a predominance of monocytoid B-cells instead of lymphoplasmacytic cells or plasma cells is present.[42] Within the infiltrate, occasional centroblasts and a few eosinophils can be seen (Fig. 32-10A,B). Whereas

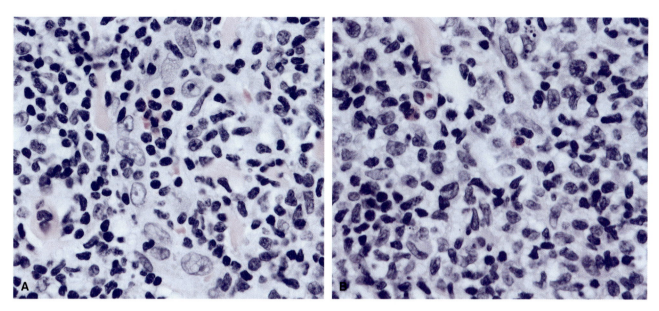

FIGURE 32-10. Primary cutaneous marginal zone lymphoma. A. Occasional centroblasts can be seen admixed with marginal zone B-cells and small lymphocytes. **B.** Marginal zone B-cells admixed with eosinophils (H&E, 100×).

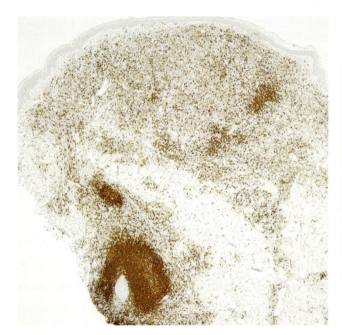

FIGURE 32-11. Primary cutaneous marginal zone B-cell lymphoma. CD20 highlights tumor cells within the dermis (H&E, 4×).

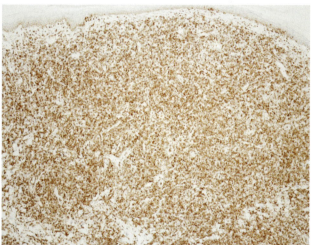

FIGURE 32-12. Primary cutaneous marginal zone B-cell lymphoma. Note diffuse BCL-2 expression by the dermal infiltrate.

the infiltrate (mean 67%) and outnumber B-cells (Fig. 32-13A,B).[45] Occasionally, the prominent T-cell component may obscure the neoplastic B-cells within the infiltrate. Although classically a hallmark of primary cutaneous CD4+ small/medium T-cell lymphoproliferative disorder (PCSM-LPD), there is evidence that a significant proportion of the T-cells seen in MZL, including PCMZL, display a follicular T helper (TFH) phenotype.[45-47] The most widely expressed TFH markers in PCMZL, as seen in PCSM-LPD, are PD-1 and Bcl-6, and may be present in substantial numbers (20%–40%). The distribution of TFH cells in MZL includes germinal centers of lymphoid follicles and the interstitial (interfollicular) compartment.[46]

Reactive or atrophic germinal centers are BCL-2−, BCL-6+, and CD10+ (Fig. 32-14A,B). Staining with Ki-67 helps highlight proliferating cells at the margin of the nodules. CD21 immunostaining shows regular and irregular networks of follicular dendritic cells in reactive follicles. Increased numbers of plasmacytoid dendritic cells (CD123+) have been reported in PCMZL when compared with very few to absent plasmacytoid dendritic cells in primary cutaneous follicle center lymphoma (PCFCL) and primary cutaneous large B-cell lymphoma (PCLBCL), respectively, and the use of CD123 has been suggested as an adjunctive marker in the diagnosis of PCMZL.[48] Aberrant nuclear BCL-10 has been reported in 36%–46% of PCMZL, and it has been observed particularly in locally aggressive tumors.[49-51] An aberrant phenotype demonstrating CD23 and/or CD5 expression associated with the development of large-cell foci, in the setting

TABLE 32-1 Marginal Zone B-Cell Lymphoma

Clinical
- Solitary or multiple red papules, nodules, or plaques
- Rare clinical presentations: anetodermic and agminated form (resembling rosacea)
- Trunk and upper extremities; less often on head and neck

Histology
- Nodular or diffuse infiltrate in dermis, may involve subcutaneous fat
- Epidermis spared, grenz zone often present
- Heterogeneous infiltrate: marginal zone B-cells, plasma cells, lymphoplasmacytoid cells, often numerous reactive T-cells
- Plasma cells often found at the periphery of the infiltrates
- Intranuclear inclusions (Dutcher bodies) may be seen
- Neoplastic cells often involve the adnexal epithelium
- Reactive germinal centers often seen

Immunophenotype
- B-cell–associated antigens: $CD19^+$, $CD20^+$, $CD22^+$, $CD79a^+$
- CD20 is lost after rituximab therapy
- $BCL-2^+$ $CD5^-$, $CD23^-$, $CD10^-$, BCL-6, and cyclin D1
- Very rare $CD23^+$ and/or $CD5^+$ phenotype may be seen in blastic transformation[44]
- Plasma cells: $CD138^+$, $CD79a^+$, and CD20
- Demonstrate monotypic intracytoplasmic expression of Ig light chain (κ or λ)
- Reactive germinal centers: BCL-2
- Other
- Class-switched PCMZL (majority): IgG, IgA, or IgE, CXCR3
- Nonclass-switched (small subset): IgM^+, $CXCR3^+$

Cell of Origin
- Postgerminal center B-cells

Molecular Features
- Clonal IgH gene rearrangement

Genetics
- t(14;18)(q32;q21) IGH and MALT-1
- t(3;14)(p14;q32) IGH and FOXP1
- t(11;18)(q21;q21) AP12/MALT

of cutaneous MZL, could indicate large-cell transformation. This type of blastic transformation in PCMZL is exceedingly rare and portends worse prognosis.[44]

Recent studies indicate that on the basis of immunoglobulin expression, two types of PCMZL can be distinguished, the more common class-switched (90%) and the nonclass-switched (10%) forms.[10] The more frequent class-switched form of the disease demonstrates expression of IgG and to a lesser extent IgA or IgE and lacks CXCR3.[10,11,52] In particular, high frequency (39%) of IgG4 expression has been described in PCMZL with plasmacytic differentiation.[53] In contrast, the nonclass-switched PCMZL is characterized by CXCR3 and IgM expression.

Immunoglobulin light chain restriction is considered an important diagnostic criterion in the diagnosis of PCMZL. Plasma cells in PCMZL show monotypic cytoplasmic immunoglobulin kappa (κ) or lambda (λ) light chain expression on paraffin sections (Fig. 32-15), and a ratio of 5:1–10:1 is considered monoclonal by most experts. Immunohistochemical staining in PCMZL lesions reveals a monotypic intracytoplasmic light chain expression of Ig in ~75% of the cases.[32,54] In situ hybridization is another sensitive method used for the detection of monotypic light chain expression in PCMZL. Immunohistochemistry and in situ hybridization are considered superior to both flow cytometry and PCR for determining clonality in PCMZL,[32,55] but it is important to note that these methods indicate monotypia of light chain as a surrogate for monoclonality, an accepted diagnostic feature, rather than proving a clonal population per se. Interestingly, the monotypic light chain may differ between lesions removed from distinct anatomic sites from the same patient. The monotypic production of light chain is the basis for rare cases of PCMZL with amyloid deposition. Such "amyloidomas" (Fig. 32-16) may be associated with the neoplastic B-cell population or arise as naked extracellular cutaneous deposits.[56] Such cases do not imply systemic amyloidosis which seldom if ever arises from cutaneous MZL. More recently, ultrasensitive bright-field RNA in situ hybridization (BRISH) has been introduced for the evaluation of light chains restriction, not only in the plasma cells but also in the B-cells. BRISH appears to be more sensitive than conventional FISH (fluorescence in situ hybridization) and reduces the rates of additional molecular testing by PCR methodologies.[57] Rare examples of MZL with EBV expression can be seen in association with immunodeficiencies.[58]

GENETIC AND MOLECULAR FINDINGS

Demonstration of rearrangement of the immunoglobulin heavy chain (IgH) genes using the internationally accepted BIOMED-2 PCR-based protocol is considered a useful adjunctive test in the diagnosis of PCMZL.[59] Molecular analysis reveals clonal IgH gene rearrangements in about 80% of the patients.[2,60] As some cutaneous MZL cases harbor only a few neoplastic B-cells within large numbers of reactive lymphocytes, PCR studies can be falsely negative.[11] False-negative PCR rate could also be due to somatic hypermutation of the IgH variable region genes.[61] Deep sequencing

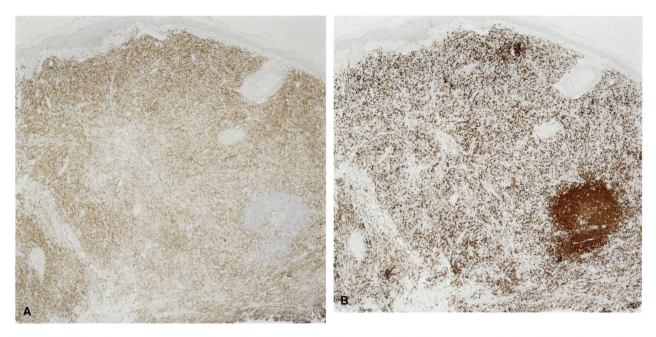

FIGURE 32-13. Primary cutaneous marginal zone B-cell lymphoma. A. CD3 immunostain highlights numerous reactive T-cells. **B.** Occasionally, T-cells can outnumber CD20+ B-cells within the infiltrate.

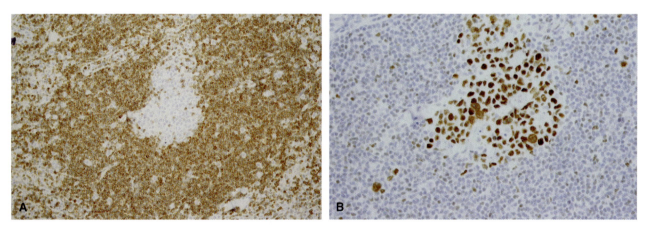

FIGURE 32-14. Primary cutaneous marginal zone B-cell lymphoma. Reactive germinal centers are BCL-2− **(A)** and BCL-6+ **(B)**.

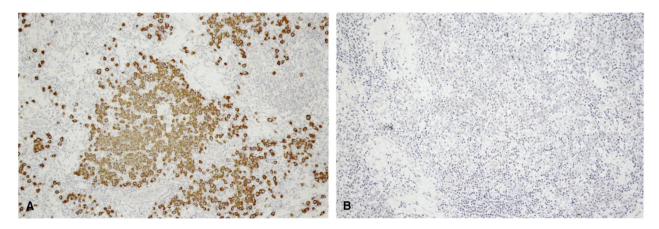

FIGURE 32-15. Primary cutaneous marginal zone B-cell lymphoma. A. Monotypic cytoplasmic expression of κ light chain. **B.** λ light chain expression is absent.

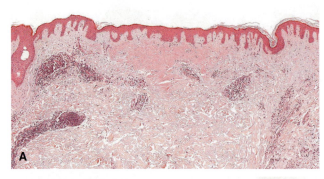
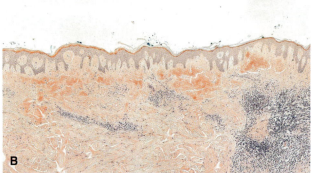

FIGURE 32-16. A. Perivascular infiltrate of lymphocytes and plasma cells, which were light chain restricted, with a band of amorphous eosinophilic material in the superficial dermis. **B.** Congo red confirms the presence of amyloid.

shows a very low percentage of clonal B-cells in cases with CD30+ Hodgkin-like cells.[62]

Cytogenetic and molecular analyses have shown that 25% or fewer cases of PCMZLs harbor the t(14;18)(q32;q21) translocation involving IGH and MALT-1 gene.[63,64] Other translocations reported in a subset of PCMZL include t(3;14)(p14;q32) involving the IGH and FOXP1 genes and t(11;18)(q21;q21) AP12/MALT (Table 32-1).[64,65] The FOXP1 gene has an important role in B-cell development, and the oncogenic activity of the IgH/MALT-1 and AP12/MALT may play a role in the induction of NF-κB activation.[66]

The t(14;18) IGH/BCL-2 translocation, originally described as mainly restricted to follicular lymphoma and diffuse large B-cell lymphoma,[64] has also been detected in a subset of PCMZL.[63] Trisomy 3 has also been reported in a small subset of PCMZL cases.[67] Overexpression of microRNAs 155 and 150 is a feature characteristic of PCMZL and may predict longer progression-free survival.[68] Recent studies have shown a high proportion of *FAS* mutations in cases of MZL (63%–68%).[69,70] Such damaging mutations result in impaired apoptosis. Other mutations that have been reported included *SLAMF1, SPEN,* and *NCOR2.*

POSTULATED CELL OF ORIGIN

Tumor cells in cutaneous MZL have a post-germinal center phenotype. This is supported by detection of IgV gene mutations produced by somatic hypermutations, a hallmark of germinal center B-cells in cutaneous B-cell lymphomas.[71] Most extranodal MZLs are nonclass-switched and express IgM, whereas the vast majority of cutaneous MZLs express class-switched immunoglobulins IgG, IgA, or IgE and only a small subset express IgM. On the basis of these findings, a dual origin for cutaneous MZL has been recently proposed: germinal center for the more common class-switched cases and the marginal zone for the rare nonclass-switched subset.[66,72]

DIFFERENTIAL DIAGNOSIS

Distinction between cutaneous lymphoid hyperplasia (CLH) and cutaneous marginal zone B-cell lymphoma is a common histologic challenge owing to significant overlap in clinical, histologic, and immunophenotypic features. CLH usually has a less dense, more polymorphous, "top-heavy," and polyclonal infiltrate predominantly involving the upper dermis.[73] However, these features cannot be relied upon to differentiate a reactive lymphoid hyperplasia from cutaneous B-cell lymphoma, as the histologic features may be strikingly similar. PCMZL often has a background of reactive lymphocytes, and CLH can present with a dense and florid inflammatory infiltrate.[73] Features that would favor PCMZL over a reactive process include the presence of multifocal and relapsing disease and monoclonality.[74] Clonality in itself is insufficient for rendering a diagnosis of lymphoma as benign lymphoid infiltrates can harbor clonal gene rearrangements.[75] Some authors feel that clonal CLH may represent a spectrum in the lymphoid dyscrasias, representing a link between inflammation and neoplasia and the two processes may represent evolutionary steps.[76]

PCSM-LPD and PCMZL share a number of clinicopathological features which can represent a diagnostic challenge.[45-47,77] Clinically, they both follow an indolent course and present with solitary or multiple papules or nodules. Histologically, they are characterized by polymorphous dermal infiltrates that include variable proportions of atypical lymphoid cells, plasma cells, macrophages, and eosinophils. The neoplastic "centrocyte-like" cells of PCMZL can have a similar appearance to the small/medium lymphocytes of PCSM-LPD.[78] Plasma cells are seen in both conditions but are light chain restricted in PCMZL while polytypic in PCSM-LPD.[42,79] A striking similarity is the mixed populations of B- and T-cells, often in similar proportions. In PCSM-LPD, the infiltrate comprises predominantly of T-cells, but B-cells can make up a considerable fraction, from 10% to 60%, thus dominating the phenotype.[80-83] Clonality assessment usually confirms these B-cells as polyclonal,[81] but B-cell clones have been reported in 6 of 23 cases tested within a large series.[83] Similarly, in PCMZL, B-cells comprise the majority of the infiltrate, but T-cells can account for a significant proportion, from 50% to 75%.[82] The T-cell population is most often polyclonal, but T-cell oligoclones may be detected. The presence of TFH as a significant proportion of the T-cell population is a defining feature of PCSM-LPD, in which PD-1+ T-cells characteristically surround a B-cell immunoblast forming rosette-like clusters,[81] but the demonstration of appreciable numbers of these cells and PD-1+ rosettes in PCMZL, and nodal MZL,[46,47] both of which may have a dominant CD4+ T-cell population (Fig. 32-17), underlines the diagnostic challenge in some tumors, such that misdiagnoses can be made. Bakr et al described two tumors with markedly dominant CD4+

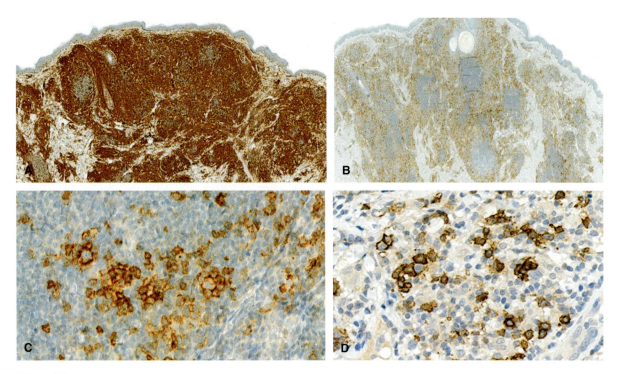

FIGURE 32-17. A. Immunohistochemistry demonstrates diffuse CD4 expression by a heavy T-cell infiltrate in this marginal zone lymphoma, with **(B)** appreciable PD-1 expression. **C** and **D**. Rosettes of PD-1+ T-cells are readily identified, some surrounding negative likely B-cells, as characteristically seen in cases of small medium CD4+ lymphoproliferative disorder.

T-cell populations, one with appreciable atypia, in which the monotypic plasma cell population—a minority of one of the tumors—indicated the correct diagnosis of PCMZL.[77] In this respect, the finding of B-cell clones in PCSM-LPD by Beltzung may present further diagnostic challenges, but, importantly, all cases that had a B-cell clone were accompanied by the finding of a T-cell clonal population.[83]

Nevertheless, helpful diagnostic tests in these cases are molecular studies of IgH gene and TCR gene rearrangement studies as detection of clonal TCR gene rearrangements would be more consistent with a cutaneous T-cell lymphoma.

Primary cutaneous MZL with marked plasmacytic differentiation has to be distinguished from *plasmacytoma* associated with myeloma. The latter is composed almost entirely of mature plasma cells with rare scattered lymphocytes. Nuclear atypia, mitotic figures are often seen, and sometimes amyloid deposits are noted.[84] Plasmacytomas in patients with multiple myeloma are CD19−, CD20−, and CD38+ and often express the NK-cell marker CD56. Features that would favor MZL over a plasmacytoma are the presence of lymphoid follicles, B-cells, and/or follicular dendritic cells.[79] PCP, in the absence of multiple myeloma, has been subsumed into the PCMZL diagnostic category since the 2005 WHO-EORTC consensus classification,[3] although the only rationale proffered for this nosological sleight of hand was diagnostic difficulty in some cases. As plasmacytoma exists as an entity at all other anatomic sites, this position has been challenged, with reports of cutaneous tumors having features of plasmacytoma without evidence of PCMZL.[85]

Distinction of PCMZL from cutaneous involvement by B-cell chronic lymphocytic leukemia (B-cell CLL) can be difficult. In B-cell CLL, the skin can be the first site of presentation in the elderly, and both entities may show similar architectural patterns. Plasma cells and light chain restriction may be seen in B-cell CLL. However, the phenotype of malignant cells in B-cell CLL is CD5+, CD23+, and CD43+, in contrast to PCMZL in which tumor cells are CD5− and CD43−.[86,87]

The histologic and immunophenotypic features in primary cutaneous MZL and systemic MZL secondarily involving the skin may be indistinguishable. However, PCMZL is more commonly seen in younger patients and has a predilection for the trunk and extremities, whereas extranodal MZL lymphoma with secondary cutaneous involvement favors the head and neck regions and affects older patients.[36] Subtle histologic differences may include the more frequent presence of germinal centers in primary cutaneous MZL.[36]

Cutaneous involvement by lymphoplasmacytoid B-cell lymphomas, including Waldenstrom's macroglobulinemia, may be particularly challenging. Clinical history and staging investigations clearly play an important role. Furthermore, analysis of *MYD88* for somatic mutation, present in 90% of cases but in smaller fractions of nodal MZL or extranodal MALT lymphomas, is useful. Mutations have only rarely been identified in PCMZL, and these appear restricted to IgM, ie, nonclass switched tumors.[88]

The differential diagnosis includes other primary cutaneous B-cell lymphomas, such as PCFCL. In cutaneous marginal zone B-cell lymphoma, the composition of the infiltrate is heterogeneous with marginal zone B-cells, monotypic plasma cells, and reactive T-cells versus an infiltrate composed of centrocytes and few centroblasts in cutaneous follicle center cell lymphoma. Occasionally it may be difficult to distinguish PCFCL, which is typically CD10(-), from primary cutaneous MZL. Furthermore, widespread BCL-6 expression, albeit often weak/variable, is commonly found in PCMZL as a consequence of the admixed TFH population (Fig. 32-18).[46]

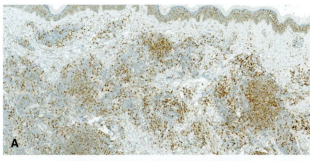
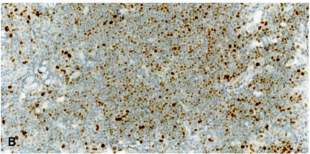

FIGURE 32-18. The presence of sometimes numerous follicular T-helper cells, which express Bcl-6, in MZL can cause diagnostic difficulty. **A.** Diffuse expression within a typical MZL. **B.** Bcl-6 positivity is typically variable in intensity throughout the population.

CAPSULE SUMMARY

PCMZL is an indolent lymphoma characterized by an infiltrate composed of marginal zone B-cells (small-to-medium–sized lymphocytes), plasma cells, lymphoplasmacytoid cells, and numerous reactive T-cells. The postulated normal counterpart to PCMZL is a postgerminal center B-cell. The neoplastic cells express CD20, CD22, CD79a, and BCL-2 and are typically negative for CD3, CD5, CD10, and BCL-6. Some cases of PCMZL may overlap considerably with PCSM-LPD owing to polymorphous, mixed B- and T-cell populations; the latter also displaying a TFH phenotype in the minority of the infiltrate. There is cytoplasmic expression of immunoglobulin with light chain restriction as well as monoclonal IgH gene rearrangements.

Two distinctive subsets of PCMZL have been described: the more common class-switched (expressing IgG, IgA, IgE) and the rare nonclass-switched subtype (IgM$^+$). The latter demonstrates features overlapping with extranodal marginal zone (MALT) lymphomas and shows more common extracutaneous involvement.

PCMZL is an indolent lymphoma with excellent prognosis, but recurrences are common.

References

1. Willemze R, Jaffe ES, Burg G, et al. WHO-EORTC classification for cutaneous lymphomas. *Blood*. 2005;105(10):3768-3785.
2. Swerdlow SH, Campo E, Pileri SA, et al. The 2016 revision of the World Health Organization classification of lymphoid neoplasms. *Blood*. 2016;127(20):2375-2390.
3. Slater DN. The new World Health Organization-European Organization for Research and Treatment of Cancer classification for cutaneous lymphomas: a practical marriage of two giants. *Br J Dermatol*. 2005;153(5):874-880.
4. Schmid U, Eckert F, Griesser H, et al. Cutaneous follicular lymphoid hyperplasia with monotypic plasma cells. A clinicopathologic study of 18 patients. *Am J Surg Pathol*. 1995;19(1):12-20.
5. Guitart J, Gerami P. Is there a cutaneous variant of marginal zone hyperplasia?. *Am J Dermatopathol*. 2008;30(5):494-496.
6. Bradford PT, Devesa SS, Anderson WF, et al. Cutaneous lymphoma incidence patterns in the United States: a population-based study of 3884 cases. *Blood*. 2009;113(21):5064-5073.
7. Senff NJ, Hoefnagel JJ, Jansen PM, et al. Reclassification of 300 primary cutaneous B-cell lymphomas according to the new WHO-EORTC classification for cutaneous lymphomas: comparison with previous classifications and identification of prognostic markers. *J Clin Oncol*. 2007;25(12):1581-1587.
8. Fink-Puches R, Chott A, Ardigo M, et al. The spectrum of cutaneous lymphomas in patients less than 20 years of age. *Pediatr Dermatol*. 2004;21(5):525-533.
9. Kempf W, Kazakov DV, Buechner SA, et al. Primary cutaneous marginal zone lymphoma in children: a report of 3 cases and review of the literature. *Am J Dermatopathol*. 2014;36(8):661-666.
10. van Maldegem F, van Dijk R, Wormhoudt TA, et al. The majority of cutaneous marginal zone B-cell lymphomas expresses class-switched immunoglobulins and develops in a T-helper type 2 inflammatory environment. *Blood*. 2008;112(8):3355-3361.
11. Edinger JT, Kant JA, Swerdlow SH. Cutaneous marginal zone lymphomas have distinctive features and include 2 subsets. *Am J Surg Pathol*. 2010;34(12):1830-1841.
12. Goodlad JR, Davidson MM, Hollowood K, et al. Primary cutaneous B-cell lymphoma and Borrelia burgdorferi infection in patients from the Highlands of Scotland. *Am J Surg Pathol*. 2000;24(9):1279-1285.
13. Garbe C, Stein H, Dienemann D, et al. Borrelia burgdorferi-associated cutaneous B cell lymphoma: clinical and immunohistologic characterization of four cases. *J Am Acad Dermatol*. 1991;24(4):584-590.
14. Roggero E, Zucca E, Mainetti C, et al. Eradication of Borrelia burgdorferi infection in primary marginal zone B-cell lymphoma of the skin. *Hum Pathol*. 2000;31(2):263-268.
15. de la Fouchardiere A, Vandenesch F, Berger F. Borrelia-associated primary cutaneous MALT lymphoma in a nonendemic region. *Am J Surg Pathol*. 2003;27(5):702-703.
16. Cerroni L, Zochling N, Putz B, et al. Infection by Borrelia burgdorferi and cutaneous B-cell lymphoma. *J Cutan Pathol*. 1997;24(8):457-461.
17. Li TJ, Yu SF. Clinicopathologic spectrum of the so-called calcifying odontogenic cysts: a study of 21 intraosseous cases with reconsideration of the terminology and classification. *Am J Surg Pathol*. 2003;27(3):372-384.
18. Nihal M, Mikkola D, Qian Z, et al. The clonality of tumor-infiltrating lymphocytes in African Kaposi's sarcoma. *J Cutan Pathol*. 2001;28(4):200-205.
19. Takino H, Li C, Hu S, et al. Primary cutaneous marginal zone B-cell lymphoma: a molecular and clinicopathological study of cases from Asia, Germany, and the United States. *Mod Pathol*. 2008;21(12):1517-1526.
20. Goteri G, Ranaldi R, Simonetti O, et al. Clinicopathological features of primary cutaneous B-cell lymphomas from an academic regional hospital in central Italy: no evidence of Borrelia burgdorferi association. *Leuk Lymphoma*. 2007;48(11):2184-2188.

21. Ponzoni M, Ferreri AJ, Mappa S, et al. Prevalence of Borrelia burgdorferi infection in a series of 98 primary cutaneous lymphomas. *Oncologist*. 2011;16(11):1582-1588.
22. Bahler DW, Kim BK, Gao A, et al. Analysis of immunoglobulin V genes suggests cutaneous marginal zone B-cell lymphomas recognise similar antigens. *Br J Haematol*. 2006;132(5):571-575.
23. Tomasini C, Moneghini L, Barbui AM. Chronic amastigote-negative cutaneous leishmaniasis: a clinical, histopathologic and molecular study of 27 cases with emphasis on atypical and pseudolymphomatous presentations. *J Cutan Pathol*. 2017;44:530-537.
24. Willemze R. Primary cutaneous B-cell lymphoma: classification and treatment. *Curr Opin Oncol*. 2006;18(5):425-431.
25. Magro CM, Crowson AN, Mihm MC Jr. *The Cutaneous Lymphoid Proliferations: A Comprehensive Textbook of Lymphocytic Infiltartes of the Skin*. Vol. 1. 1st ed.: Wiley; 2007.
26. Perez M, Pacchiarotti A, Frontani M, et al. Primary cutaneous B-cell lymphoma is associated with somatically hypermutated immunoglobulin variable genes and frequent use of VH1-69 and VH4-59 segments. *Br J Dermatol*. 2010;162(3):611-618.
27. Deutsch AJ, Fruhwirth M, Aigelsreiter A, et al. Primary cutaneous marginal zone B-cell lymphomas are targeted by aberrant somatic hypermutation. *J Invest Dermatol*. 2009;129(2):476-479.
28. Kasper RC, Wood GS, Nihal M, et al. Anetoderma arising in cutaneous B-cell lymphoproliferative disease. *Am J Dermatopathol*. 2001;23(2):124-132.
29. Barzilai A, Feuerman H, Quaglino P, et al. Cutaneous B-cell neoplasms mimicking granulomatous rosacea or rhinophyma. *Arch Dermatol*. 2012;148(7):824-831.
30. Hodak E, Feuerman H, Barzilai A, et al. Anetodermic primary cutaneous B-cell lymphoma: a unique clinicopathological presentation of lymphoma possibly associated with antiphospholipid antibodies. *Arch Dermatol*. 2010;146(2):175-182.
31. Servitje O, Muniesa C, Benavente Y, et al. Primary cutaneous marginal zone B-cell lymphoma: response to treatment and disease-free survival in a series of 137 patients. *J Am Acad Dermatol*. 2013;69(3):357-365.
32. Guitart J, Deonizio J, Bloom T, et al. High incidence of gastrointestinal tract disorders and autoimmunity in primary cutaneous marginal zone B-cell lymphomas. *JAMA Dermatol*. 2014;150(4):412-418.
33. Senff NJ, Willemze R. The applicability and prognostic value of the new TNM classification system for primary cutaneous lymphomas other than mycosis fungoides and Sézary syndrome: results on a large cohort of primary cutaneous B-cell lymphomas and comparison with the system used by the Dutch Cutaneous Lymphoma Group. *Br J Dermatol*. 2007;157(6):1205-1211.
34. Hoefnagel JJ, Dijkman R, Basso K, et al. Distinct types of primary cutaneous large B-cell lymphoma identified by gene expression profiling. *Blood*. 2005;105(9):3671-3678.
35. Bessell EM, Humber CE, O'Connor S, et al. Primary cutaneous B-cell lymphoma in Nottinghamshire U.K.: prognosis of subtypes defined in the WHO-EORTC classification. *Br J Dermatol*. 2012;167(5):1118-1123.
36. Gerami P, Wickless SC, Querfeld C, et al. Cutaneous involvement with marginal zone lymphoma. *J Am Acad Dermatol*. 2010;63(1):142-145.
37. Bailey EM, Ferry JA, Harris NL, et al. Marginal zone lymphoma (low-grade B-cell lymphoma of mucosa-associated lymphoid tissue type) of skin and subcutaneous tissue: a study of 15 patients. *Am J Surg Pathol*. 1996;20(8):1011-1023.
38. Boudreaux BW, Patel MH, Brumfiel CM, et al. Primary cutaneous epidermotropic marginal zone B-cell lymphoma treated with total skin electron beam therapy. *JAAD Case Rep*. 2021;15:15-18.
39. Magro CM, Momtahen S, Coleman M, Grossman ME. Epidermotropic CXCR3 positive marginal zone lymphoma: a distinctive clinical histopathological entity potentially originating in the skin – it does not always indicate splenic marginal zone lymphoma. *Dermatol Online J*. 2019;25(7).
40. Magro CM, Momtahen S, Lee BA, Swanson DL, Pavlovic MD. Epidermotropic B-cell lymphoma: a unique subset of CXCR3-positive marginal zone lymphoma. *Am J Dermatopathol*. 2016;38(2):105-112.
41. Baykal C, Erdem S, Kılıç S, Nalçacı M, Büyükbabani N. Epidermotropic skin involvement of splenic marginal zone B-cell lymphoma: a diagnostic challenge. *J Cutan Pathol*. 2017;44(3):312-314.
42. Burg G, Kempf W, Cozzio A, et al. WHO/EORTC classification of cutaneous lymphomas 2005: histological and molecular aspects. *J Cutan Pathol*. 2005;32(10):647-674.
43. Prieto-Torres L, Manso R, Elisabeth Cieza-Díaz D, et al. Large cells with CD30 expression and Hodgkin-like features in primary cutaneous marginal zone B-cell lymphoma: a study of 13 cases. *Am J Surg Pathol*. 2019;43(9):1191-1202. doi:10.1097/PAS.0000000000001287
44. Magro CM, Yang A, Fraga G. Blastic marginal zone lymphoma: a clinical and pathological study of 8 cases and review of the literature. *Am J Dermatopathol*. 2013;35(3):319-326.
45. Goyal A, Moore JB, Gimbel D, et al. PD-1, S-100, and CD1a expression in pseudolymphomatous folliculitis, primary cutaneous marginal zone B-cell lymphoma (MALT lymphoma), and cutaneous lymphoid hyperplasia. *J Cutan Pathol*. 2015;42(1):6-15.
46. Robson A, Bakr F, Rashid E, et al. Follicular T-helper cells in marginal zone lymphoma: evidence of an organoid immune response. *Am J Dermpathol*. 2021. 43, e197.
47. Egan C, Laurent C, Alejo JC, et al. Expansion of PD1-positive T cells in nodal marginal zone lymphoma. *Am J Surg Pathol*. 2020;44:657-664.
48. Kutzner H, Kerl H, Pfaltz MC, et al. CD123-positive plasmacytoid dendritic cells in primary cutaneous marginal zone B-cell lymphoma: diagnostic and pathogenetic implications. *Am J Surg Pathol*. 2009;33(9):1307-1313.
49. Li C, Inagaki H, Kuo TT, et al. Primary cutaneous marginal zone B-cell lymphoma: a molecular and clinicopathologic study of 24 Asian cases. *Am J Surg Pathol*. 2003;27(8):1061-1069.
50. Gronbaek K, Ralfkiaer E, Kalla J, et al. Infrequent somatic Fas mutations but no evidence of Bcl10 mutations or t(11;18) in primary cutaneous MALT-type lymphoma. *J Pathol*. 2003;201(1):134-140.
51. Gallardo F, Bellosillo B, Espinet B, et al. Aberrant nuclear BCL10 expression and lack of t(11;18)(q21;q21) in primary cutaneous marginal zone B-cell lymphoma. *Hum Pathol*. 2006;37(7):867-873.
52. Vermeer MH, Willemze R. Recent advances in primary cutaneous B-cell lymphomas. *Curr Opin Oncol*. 2014;26(2):230-236.
53. Brenner I, Roth S, Puppe B, et al. Primary cutaneous marginal zone lymphomas with plasmacytic differentiation show frequent IgG4 expression. *Mod Pathol*. 2013;26(12):1568-1576.

54. Servitje O, Gallardo F, Estrach T, et al. Primary cutaneous marginal zone B-cell lymphoma: a clinical, histopathological, immunophenotypic and molecular genetic study of 22 cases. *Br J Dermatol*. 2002;147(6):1147-1158.
55. Schafernak KT, Variakojis D, Goolsby CL, et al. Clonality assessment of cutaneous B-cell lymphoid proliferations: a comparison of flow cytometry immunophenotyping, molecular studies, and immunohistochemistry/in situ hybridization and review of the literature. *Am J Dermatopathol*. 2014;36(10):781-795.
56. Ueberdiek S, Kempf W, Kretschmer L, et al. AL-amyloidoma of the skin – a rare manifestation of primary cutaneous marginal zone lymphoma. *Am J Dermatopathol*. 2019;41:518-521.
57. Craddock AP, Kane WJ, Raghavan SS, Williams ES, Gru AA, Gradecki SE. Use of ultrasensitive RNA in situ hybridization for determining clonality in cutaneous B-cell lymphomas and lymphoid hyperplasia decreases subsequent use of molecular testing and is cost-effective. *Am J Surg Pathol*. 2022. 10.1097/PAS.0000000000001868.
58. Gong S, Crane GM, McCall CM, et al. Expanding the spectrum of EBV-positive marginal zone lymphomas: a lesion associated with diverse immunodeficiency settings. *Am J Surg Pathol*. 2018;42(10):1306-1316.
59. Senff NJ, Noordijk EM, Kim YH, et al. European Organization for Research and Treatment of Cancer and International Society for Cutaneous Lymphoma consensus recommendations for the management of cutaneous B-cell lymphomas. *Blood*. 2008;112(5):1600-1609.
60. Child FJ, Woolford AJ, Calonje E, et al. Molecular analysis of the immunoglobulin heavy chain gene in the diagnosis of primary cutaneous B cell lymphoma. *J Invest Dermatol*. 2001;117(4):984-989.
61. Cho-Vega JH, Vega F, Rassidakis G, et al. Primary cutaneous marginal zone B-cell lymphoma. *Am J Clin Pathol*. 2006;125(suppl):S38-S49.
62. Di Napoli A, Rogges E, Noccioli N, et al. Deep sequencing of immunoglobulin genes identifies a very low percentage of monoclonal B cells in primary cutaneous marginal zone lymphomas with CD30-positive Hodgkin/Reed-Sternberg-like cells. *Diagnostics*. 2022;12(2):290. 10.3390/diagnostics12020290
63. Palmedo G, Hantschke M, Rutten A, et al. Primary cutaneous marginal zone B-cell lymphoma may exhibit both the t(14;18)(q32;q21) IGH/BCL2 and the t(14;18)(q32;q21) IGH/MALT1 translocation: an indicator for clonal transformation towards higher-grade B-cell lymphoma?. *Am J Dermatopathol*. 2007;29(3):231-236.
64. Streubel B, Lamprecht A, Dierlamm J, et al. T(14;18)(q32;q21) involving IGH and MALT1 is a frequent chromosomal aberration in MALT lymphoma. *Blood*. 2003;101(6):2335-2339.
65. Streubel B, Vinatzer U, Lamprecht A, et al. T(3;14)(p14.1;q32) involving IGH and FOXP1 is a novel recurrent chromosomal aberration in MALT lymphoma. *Leukemia*. 2005;19(4):652-658.
66. Fernandez-Flores A. Current concepts on cutaneous MALT lymphomas. *Am J Dermatopathol*. 2013;35(4):477-484.
67. de la Fouchardiere A, Gazzo S, Balme B, et al. Cytogenetic and molecular analysis of 12 cases of primary cutaneous marginal zone lymphomas. *Am J Dermatopathol*. 2006;28(4):287-292.
68. Monsalvez V, Montes-Moreno S, Artiga MG, et al. MicroRNAs as prognostic markers in indolent primary cutaneous B-cell lymphoma. *Mod Pathol*. 2013;26(2):171-181.
69. Vela V, Juskevicius D, Dirnhofer S, Menter T, Tzankov A. Mutational landscape of marginal zone B-cell lymphomas of various origin: organotypic alterations and diagnostic potential for assignment of organ origin. *Virchows Arch*. 2022, 480, 403. doi:10.1007/s00428-021-03186-3
70. Maurus K, Appenzeller S, Roth S, et al. Panel sequencing shows recurrent genetic FAS alterations in primary cutaneous marginal zone lymphoma. *J Invest Dermatol*. 2018;138(7):1573-1581. 10.1016/j.jid.2018.02.015. Epub 2018 Feb 23.
71. Walsh SH, Rosenquist R. Immunoglobulin gene analysis of mature B-cell malignancies: reconsideration of cellular origin and potential antigen involvement in pathogenesis. *Med Oncol*. 2005;22(4):327-341.
72. Fernandez-Flores A. Is there a narrow connection between the two subsets of cutaneous MALT lymphomas and the dynamics of the follicle?. *Am J Dermatopathol*. 2013;35(2):283-284.
73. Gilliam AC, Wood GS. Cutaneous lymphoid hyperplasias. *Semin Cutan Med Surg*. 2000;19(2):133-141.
74. Kempf W, Kazakov DV, Mitteldorf C. Cutaneous lymphomas: an update. Part 2 – B-cell lymphomas and related conditions. *Am J Dermatopathol*. 2014;36(3):197-208; quiz 209-210.
75. Böer A, Tirumalae R, Bresch M, et al. Pseudoclonality in cutaneous pseudolymphomas: a pitfall in interpretation of rearrangement studies. *Br J Dermatol*. 2008;159(2):394-402.
76. Pimpinelli N. New aspects in the biology of cutaneous B-cell lymphomas. *J Cutan Pathol*. 2006;33(suppl 1):6-9.
77. Bakr F, Wain M, Barlow R, et al. Primary cutaneous CD4+ small/medium T-cell lymphoproliferative disorder or primary cutaneous marginal zone B-cell lymphoma? Two distinct entities with overlapping histopathological features. *Am J Dermatopathol*. 2021. 43, e204.
78. Cerroni L, Signoretti S, Hofler G, et al. Primary cutaneous marginal zone BN-cell lymphoma: a recently described entity of low-grade malignant cutaneous B-cell lymphoma. *Am J Surg Pathol*. 1997;21(11):1307-1315.
79. Geyer JT, Ferry JA, Longtine JA, et al. Characteristics of cutaneous marginal zone lymphomas with marked plasmacytic differentiation and a T cell-rich background. *Am J Clin Pathol*. 2010. 133(1):59-69.
80. Beltraminelli H, Leinweber B, Cerroni L. Primary cutaneous CD4+ small-/medium-sized pleomorphic T-cell lymphoma: a cutaneous nodular proliferation of pleomorphic T lymphocytes of undetermined significance? A Study of 136 Cases. *Am J Dermatopathol*. 2009;31:317-322.
81. Pinilla S, Roncador G, Peralto JLR, et al. Primary cutaneous CD4+ small/medium-sized pleomorphic T-cell lymphoma expresses follicular T-cell markers. *Am J Surg Pathol*. 2009;33:81-90.
82. Cetinozman F, Jansen P, Willemze R. Expression of programmed death-1 in primary cutaneous CD4-positive small/medium-sized pleomorphic T-cell lymphoma, cutaneous pseudo-T-cell lymphoma, and other types of cutaneous T-cell lymphoma. *Am J Surg Pathol*. 2012;36:109-116.
83. Beltzung F, Ortonne N, Pelletier L, et al. Primary cutaneous CD4+ small/medium T-cell lymphoproliferative disorders: a clinical, pathologic, and molecular study of 60 cases presenting with a single lesion – a multicenter study of the French Cutaneous Lymphoma Study Group. *Am J Surg Pathol*. 2020;44:862-872.
84. Deonizio JM, Guitart J. Current understanding of cutaneous lymphoma: selected topics. *Dermatol Clin*. 2012;30(4):749-761, vii–viii.

85. Robson A, Kempf W, Kolm I, et al. A problem of classification: 2 cases of EBV+ primary cutaneous plasmacytomas arising in immunocompetent elderly patients. *Am J Dermatopathol.* 2021. 43, e237.
86. Kash N, Fink-Puches R, Cerroni L. Cutaneous manifestations of B-cell chronic lymphocytic leukemia associated with Borrelia burgdorferi infection showing a marginal zone B-cell lymphoma-like infiltrate. *Am J Dermatopathol.* 2011;33(7):712-715.
87. Levin C, Mirzamani N, Zwerner J, et al. A comparative analysis of cutaneous marginal zone lymphoma and cutaneous chronic lymphocytic leukemia. *Am J Dermatopathol.* 2012;34(1):18-23.
88. Wobser M, Maurus K, Roth S, et al. Myeloid differentiation primary response 88 mutations in a distinct type of cutaneous marginal-zone lymphoma with a non-class switched immunoglobulin M immunophenotype. *Brit J Dermatol.* 2017; 177: 564-566.

Primary cutaneous diffuse large B-cell lymphoma

Christina MItteldorf, Alejandro A. Gru, and José Cabeçadas

DEFINITION

According to the current World Health Organization (WHO) classification only two entities are listed as primary cutaneous large B-cell lymphomas: primary cutaneous diffuse large B-cell lymphoma, leg type (PCDLBCL-LT) and EBV-positive mucocutaneous ulcer (EBVMCU) (REF WHO).[1-5] PCDLBCL-LT is a primary cutaneous large B-cell lymphoma composed exclusively of centroblasts and immunoblasts, most commonly occurring in the legs of elderly individuals (WHO).[6] EBVMCU is a newly recognized clinicopathological entity, occurring in patients with age-related or iatrogenic immunosuppression, often with Hodgkin-like features, found in the cutaneous mucosal transitions.[1-6]

As rare forms of DLBCL the WHO classification of skin tumors mentioned also diffuse large B-cell lymphoma—not otherwise specified (NOS), intravascular large B-cell lymphoma, ALK+ diffuse large B-cell lymphoma, and T-cell rich large B-cell lymphoma. It is noteworthy that most primary cutaneous DLBCL (PCDLBCL) and secondary forms of systemic lymphomas with cutaneous dissemination share similar clinicopathologic and immunophenotypic features.

EPIDEMIOLOGY

PCDLBCL-LT typically affects the legs of elderly individuals with a mean age of 77 years. PCDLBCL-LT is more common in females with a ratio of 1.6:1.[2] PCDLBCL-LT accounts for approximately 10% to 15% of cases of primary cutaneous B-cell lymphomas. Rare cases can occur in younger individuals.[3,4] EBVMCU is a recently described B-cell lymphoproliferative disease of unestablished incidence that manifests with isolated sharply demarcated ulceration most commonly in the oropharynx, skin, and gastrointestinal tract. A third of the affected patients have drug-related immunosuppression, but age-related immune impairment is also a common feature. It has a slight male dominance and usually occurs in patients older than 70 years.[5,6]

ETIOLOGY

The mechanisms that drive the lymphomagenesis of PCDLBCL-LT are not well understood. Recent genetic and molecular analysis performed in these groups has revealed a common genetic origin with its nodal counterpart.[7] Rare cases with infection of HHV-6 and HHV-8 have been reported.[8] More recently, cases of diffuse large B-cell lymphoma (DLBCL) presenting in and outside the skin have been found in association with the use of methotrexate (MTX).[5,9-13] It appears that some or most of these are associated with Epstein-Barr virus (EBV) infection. Interestingly, the fact that many of these large proliferations of cells regress upon discontinuation of MTX has led to the hypothesis that some of these should be separated as MTX-related B-cell lymphoproliferative disorders. These subjects also present at a mean age of 76 years, and the time interval between the use of MTX and the development of the lesions is ~4 years.

CLINICAL PRESENTATION/PROGNOSIS

The series from Grange et al[2] showed that the most common clinical features of PCDLSCL-LT include cutaneous nodules or tumors, deeply infiltrated plaques, large subcutaneous tumors, and more infrequently leg ulcers[14] (Fig. 33-1). However, in 10% to 20% of cases, other parts of the body are affected.[2,15-22] About 13.3% have lesions on the trunk, 15.0% on the arm, 18.3% on the head, and 71.7% on the leg. The lesions can be unifocal in one-third of cases, but more than one lesion is seen in the majority of cases, and approximately another third of cases have more than five lesions clinically. Large ulcerations with infiltrative borders have led to the misdiagnosis of chronic venous ulcers and stasis.[23] Upon recurrence or in the evolution of the disease, the clinical lesions usually retain the tropism for the legs. A case of isolated relapse in the lungs has been reported.[24] During the early phases, the lesions can have an annular configuration and might resemble erythema chronicum migrans or gyrate erythemas.[25,26] Other uncommon

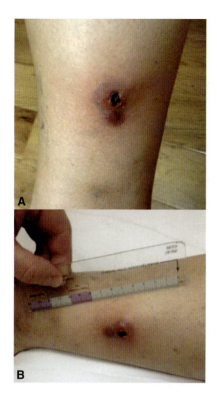

FIGURE 33-1. Primary cutaneous diffuse large B-cell lymphoma, leg type. **A** and **B.** Clinically, the lesions consist of solitary nodules in the legs with a purple color and more frequently do not reveal ulceration.

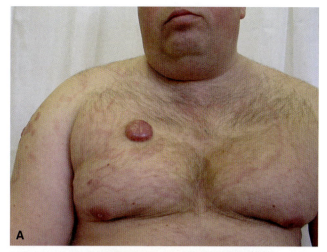
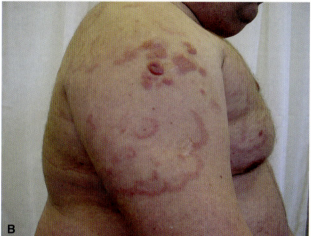
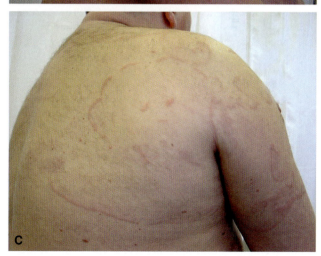

FIGURE 33-2. Primary cutaneous diffuse large B-cell lymphoma, leg type. **A–C.** Unusual clinicopathologic presentation of PCDLBCL-LT, with multiple nodules and widespread garland-like lesions. (From Belousova IE, Vanecek T, Skreg SV, et al. Unusual clinicopathological presentation of primary cutaneous diffuse large B-cell lymphoma, leg type, with multiple nodules and widespread garland-like lesions. *Am J Dermatopathol.* 31(4):370-374, with permission.)

clinical presentations have included garland-like lesions on the chest[27] (Fig. 33-2); telangiectatic lesions[28] (Fig. 33-3); postexcision from Jessner-like infiltrate on the shoulder[9]; postradiation,[29] postburn,[30] dermatomyositis-like,[31] multiple nodules in the leg with a lymphangitic pattern (mimicking infection from sporotrichosis)[32]; chronic lymphedema-like,[33] mononeuritis multiplex,[34] bluish-reddish multicolored rainbow pattern[35]; and a solitary nodule in the breast.[36] Rarely, cases might not be palpable clinically and can present as fever of unknown origin.[37] The presence of B symptoms is seen in 10% of cases, and nearly 12% have elevated lactate dehydrogenase (LDH) levels in the blood. Rare cases have been reported to show spontaneous resolution without treatment[38] and POEMS-like syndrome,[39] and in association with hemophagocytic syndrome.[40] PCDLBCL-LT can also occur in association with HIV infection[41] and in renal transplant recipients[42,43] and can be associated with intravascular cryoglobulin deposits.[44] A case revealing dissemination to the paranasal sinuses has also been reported.[45]

Although, by definition, these lymphomas are limited to the skin at presentation, they often spread to extracutaneous sites, most commonly to the lymph nodes, the bone marrow, bone,[46] the central nervous system,[2,16,47-50] and other organs (for example, eye,[50] ureters[51]). A single case of isolated relapse in the lungs has been reported.[27]

In contrast to other cutaneous B-cell lymphomas (CBCLs), the prognosis of PCDLBCL-LT is poor with a 5-year survival rate of 55% (20%-60%).[52-54] Zinzani et al[16] have reported a survival of 73% in 51 patients from Italy. A more recent study from Grange et al[47] in France (n = 115) has shown an increased survival from 55% to 74% and 46% to 66% at 3 and 5 years, respectively. The appearance of multiple lesions, location on the leg (in contrast to non-leg location), the location on both legs (involvement of one leg vs. both legs: 5-year survival rate 45% vs. 36%), the loss of expression of p16 (p16 negative vs positive: 5-year

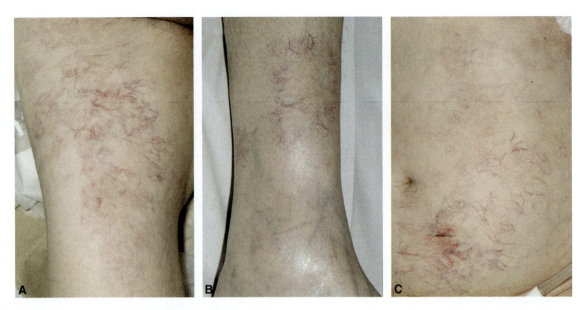

FIGURE 33-3. PCDLBCL-LT: Unusual clinical presentation with telangiectasia. A and **B** show lesions in the extremities, whereas **C** shows lesions in the abdomen. (From Shim TN, El-Daly H, Carr RA, et al. Cutaneous telangiectasia and cauda equina syndrome: a presentation of diffuse large B-cell lymphoma. *Am J Dermatopathol.* 2013;35(4):507-510, with permission.)

survival rate 43% vs 70%), activated apoptosis cascade, and MYC expression (>40%) are prognostically unfavorable prognostic markers.[55-57] Sex, B symptoms, BCL-2 expression, MUM1/IRF4 expression, performance status, serum LDH level, duration of lesions before diagnosis, and variables related to therapy have no effect on survival.[2] The data about prognostic impact of *MYC* rearrangement are controversial. An inactivation of the *CDKN2A* gene have been also described to be associated with an unfavorable diagnosis (*n* = 64, loss of *CDKN2A* in 67%). A reduced progression-free survival and specific survival and therapy resistance was associated with mutation that targets one of the B-cell receptor signaling genes, *CARD11* or *CD79 A/B*.[56,58,59]

HISTOLOGY

The typical histologic features of DLBCL-LT show a diffuse infiltrate in the entire dermis, often extending into the subcutaneous tissue (Fig. 33-4). Plaza et al[60] published a large series of 79 cases of DLBCL: in their series they found 11.4% of cases with a sclerosing pattern with thickened interconnective bands of connective tissue in the dermis, surrounded by groups of large lymphoid cells, admixed with smaller cells. A similar proportion of cases show large areas of geographic necrosis. More uncommon patterns represented in their series included anaplastic morphology (Figs. 33-5 and 33-6) (7.6%), angioinvasion (7.6%), a starry-sky pattern (mimicking Burkitt or Burkitt-like lymphomas, 6.3%), admixed inflammation (6.3%), spindle cells (6.3%), a histiocytoid appearance (5.1%), pseudosarcomatous areas (3.8%), multilobated cells (3.8%), and epidermotropism (2.5%). The presence of epidermotropic cells can sometimes simulate the presence of Darier nests (Pautrier microabscesses). Rare cases can also show a band-like infiltrate that could potentially mimic mycosis fungoides. Cytologically, the neoplastic cells consist predominantly of large cells with round nuclei and variable prominent nucleoli. The so-called spindle cell pattern[61-65] has been favored by some authors to represent variants of primary cutaneous follicle center lymphoma (PCFCL) with diffuse areas. Some cases can also relapse with an intravascular component, mimicking intravascular large B-cell lymphoma.[65] The presence of starry-sky areas should also raise the consideration of cutaneous involvement by Burkitt lymphoma, or involvement by B-cell lymphoma, unclassifiable, with intermediate features between DLBCL and Burkitt lymphoma.[67] Both of these lymphomas usually show an extraordinarily high proliferation index. In cases of PCDLBCL-LT exhibiting a significant reactive T-cell infiltrate, occasional epithelioid granulomas (histiocytic cells) can be found, reflecting a local paraneoplastic granulomatous diathesis.[60] In the latter series, cutaneous perineural invasion was a relatively infrequent phenomenon, but in our experience, this appears to be more common than what has been reported.

IMMUNOPHENOTYPE

In addition to traditional B-cell markers (CD19, CD20, CD22, CD79a, PAX-5), PCDLBCL-LT classically expresses BCL-2, MUM1/IRF4, and FOXP1[68] (Fig. 33-7). However, this immunophenotype is not specific to PCDLBCL-LT and may also be seen in other DLBCLs that secondarily involve the skin. Follicular dendritic networks are typically lacking on PCDLBCL-LT; however, Plaza et al[69] have shown that in nearly 12.5% of cases focal dendritic networks can be seen using CD21 or CD35 immunostains. The importance of using MUM1/IRF4 and BCL-2 in the diagnosis of this disease has entered into debate, as the WHO describes that in nearly 10% of cases those markers can be absent.[1] The study from Plaza et al[69] has shown that MUM1/IRF4 was present in only 60% of PCDLBCL-LT. In the current WHO classification of skin tumors, primary cutaneous cases which have morphological features of DLBCL, but didn't meet the criteria of primary

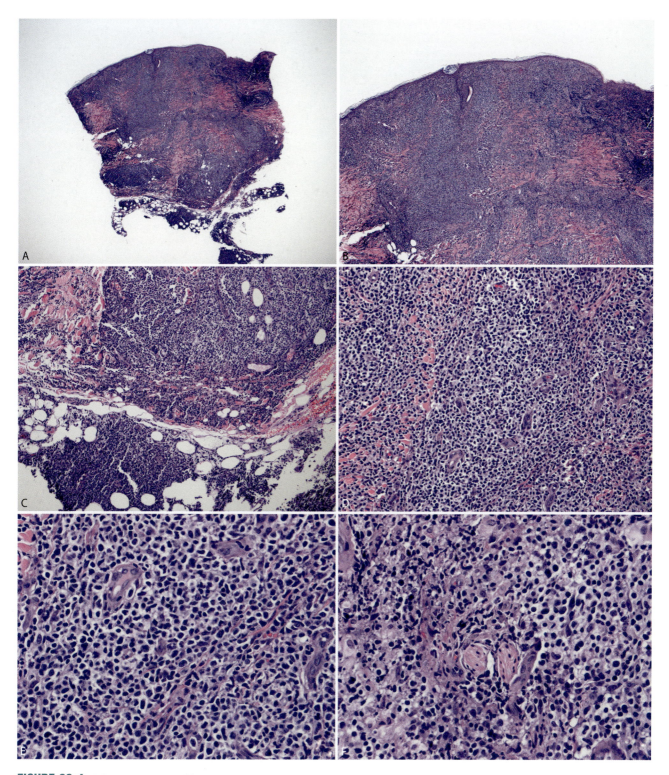

FIGURE 33-4. Primary cutaneous diffuse large B-cell lymphoma, leg type. There is a diffuse infiltrate in the dermis, relatively sparing the epidermis and extending to the adipose tissue (**A** and **B**, 20× and 100×). The infiltrate extends to the adipose tissue in a diffuse manner (**C**, 200×). The infiltrate is composed of medium to large cells with hyperchromasia and areas with perineural arrangement (**D–F**, 400×).

cutaneous follicle center cell lymphoma or PCDLBCL-LT should be diagnosed as primary cutaneous DLBCL-NOS.[1] Others have shown a lack of prognostic significance upon the expression of those markers[2,15,70] when the clinical and histologic diagnosis otherwise fits the criteria for PCDLBCL-LT. Most cases show weak expression of BCL-6 but lack of CD10. IgM strong expression with or without IgD coexpression (only 50%) is present in PCDBCL-LT, and the staining could have a potential role to distinguish it from PCFCL.[71] Expression of CD30 can also occur in some cases.[72,73] Similar nodal counterparts are classified as "anaplastic variants."[74] A better prognosis of cases expressing CD30 has been reported in nodal cases,

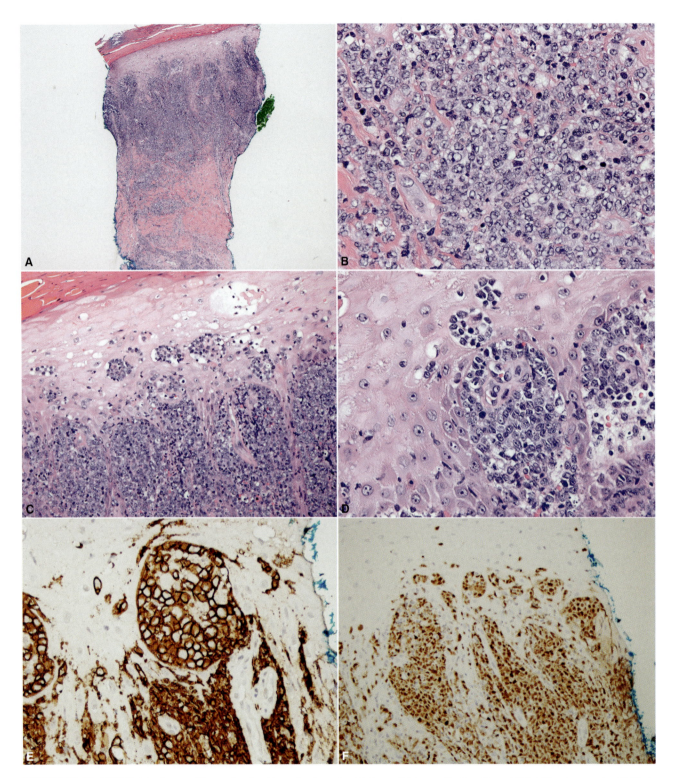

FIGURE 33-5. PCDLBCL-LT—A case with prominent epidermotropism. A and **B** (low and high magnification, 20× and 400×). There is a prominent infiltrate composed of large cells with vesicular nuclei and prominent nucleoli. **C** and **D** (medium and high magnifications, 200× and 400×). Prominent epidermotropism and "Pautrier microabscesses" are present. The tumor cells are positive for CD20 **(E)** and MUM1/IRF4 **(F)** highlighting the epidermotropic component.

but there is an absence of data regarding PCDLBCL-LT.[75,76] Expression of MYC is seen in more than 55% of cases.[7] This is not related to MYC rearrangements. PD-1 expression is very rarely seen in LT lymphoma.[77] However, PD-1 can be seen with certain frequency in T cells in the background of PCFCL. Therefore, PD-1 might be another marker that can help discriminating between the two entities.[78] PD-L1 was found in the tumor microenvironment of PCDLBCL-LT, which seem to be relevant for treatment with immune checkpoint inhibitors.[79,80] EBV positivity has been rarely described[81] and should raise the possibility of an EBV-related DLBCL. Overexpression of FOXP1 can be related to numerical gains

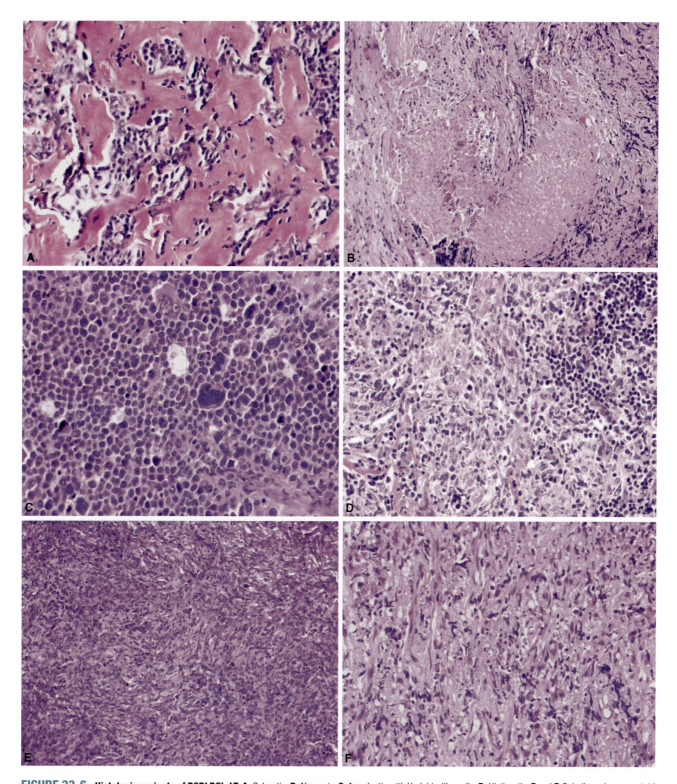

FIGURE 33-6. Histologic variants of PCDLBCL-LT. A. Sclerotic. **B.** Necrosis. **C.** Anaplastic with Hodgkin-like cells. **D.** Histiocytic. **E** and **F.** Spindle and sarcomatoid forms. (From Plaza JA, Kacerovska D, Stockman DL, et al. The histomorphologic spectrum of primary cutaneous diffuse large B-cell lymphoma: a study of 79 cases. *Am J Dermatopathol.* 2011;33(7):649-655; quiz 656-658, with permission.)

of the gene but not to translocations.[82] The presence of FOXP3 expression and abundance of T-cell regulatory cells have been linked to a better prognosis.[83] MUM1/IRF4 expression is not linked to an *IRF4* rearrangement.[84] OCT-2 expression (more frequently seen in PCDLBCL-LT) can help distinguish this from PCFCL. Novel markers such as TCL-1 and BLIMP1 have been reported in PCDLBCL-LT.[85]

GENETIC AND MOLECULAR FINDINGS

The most interesting observations in the group of primary cutaneous large B-cell lymphoma (PCLBCL), leg type, are high-level DNA amplifications of chromosome 18q21 and deletions of chromosome 9p21.3, findings demonstrated using array comparative genome hybridization. High-level

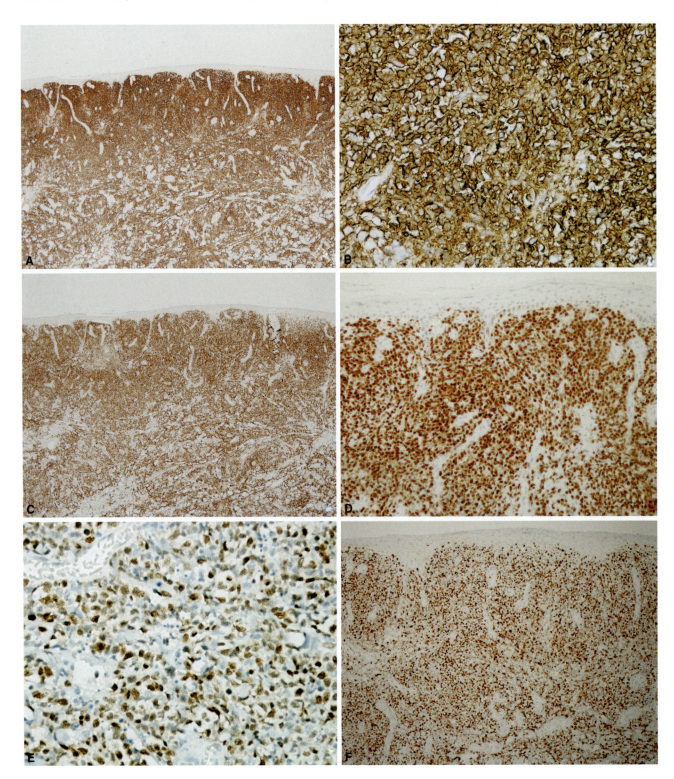

FIGURE 33-7. Primary cutaneous diffuse large B-cell lymphoma, leg type—immunohistochemistry. The atypical large cells are positive for CD20 (**A** and **B**), BCL-2 (**C**), PAX5 (**D**), and MUM1/IRF4 (**E**) and show a very high (70%-80%) proliferation index, as measured by Ki67 (**F**).

DNA amplifications of chromosome 18q21.31-q21.33 encompassing the *BCL-2* and *MALT1* genes were detected in 8 (67%) of 12 PCLBCL, leg type, but in only 2 (11%) of 19 PCFCLs.[86,87] High-level DNA amplification of a small region of chromosome 2p16.1 containing both the *BCL11A* and *c-REL* genes was seen in only 3 of 12 PCLBCL, leg type, cases, and it is particularly more common in PCFCL. Although in PCFCL transcription repressor *BCL11A* is always coamplified with *c-REL*, two of three PCLBCL, leg type, cases showed amplification of only the *BCL11A* but not of the *c-REL* gene. Activation and amplification of the *MALT1* gene are particularly more common in DLBCL of nongerminal center origin. Deletion of a small region on chromosome 9p21.3 containing the *CDKN2A* and *CDKN2B* gene loci was detected in 8 of 12 patients with PCLBCL, leg type, but not in any of the patients with PCFCL. Most interestingly, all seven patients with PCLBCL, leg type, who died as a result of their lymphoma had a homozygous deletion of 9p21.3 (five cases), promoter hypermethylation of the *CDKN2A* gene (one case), or hemizygous deletion combined with *CDKN2A* hypermethylation (one case). In contrast, none of the cases of PCFCL show alterations in the *c-REL* gene. Loss of p16, therefore, can be considered as a useful marker in determination of the prognosis. In the large study by Senff et al,[58] inactivation of the CDKN2a pathway was also linked to a worse outcome. Amplification of *c-REL* is frequently found in nodal and extranodal DLBCL, transformed follicular lymphomas (FLs), and Hodgkin lymphoma.[88-90] Kaune et al[91] have also shown that alterations of the RB and p53 pathways, in addition to CDKN2A, are frequently seen in PCDLBCL-LT. A translocation of the t(8;14) has also been reported in two of six cases of PCDLBCL-LT.[92] Some of the cytogenetic aberrations could be potentially missed by fluorescent in situ hybridization studies.[93,94]

The most recent study by Pham-Ledard et al[7] observed an abnormal genetic profile for at least one gene studied among *BCL-2, BCL-6, MYC, CDKN2A, BLIMP1*, or *MYD88* in 22 of 23 patients (96%). There were no cases of double-hit or triple-hit lymphomas. The most frequent genetic alterations included the p.L265P *MYD88* mutation (c.794 T4C) occurring in 11 of 18 informative cases (61%) and the 6q deletions involving *BLIMP1* in 11 of 18 informative cases (61%; interstitial deletion in five cases, 6q deletion including BLIMP in six cases). The *MYD88* mutation[95,96] was also associated with a worse prognosis. In their study, alterations of CDKN2A were only seen in 25% of cases. *BCL-6* and *MYC* rearrangements occurred in 22% and 13% of cases, respectively. There were no de novo cutaneous cases with double-hit or triple-hit rearrangements. Altogether, the cytogenetic alterations observed in their series demonstrate PCLBCL, leg type, to be similar to its activated B-cell (ABC) nodal counterpart as no double-hit lymphoma was observed. The hallmark of ABC-type nodal DLBCL is the constitutive activation of the NF-κβ signaling pathway that promotes cell survival, proliferation, and inhibition of apoptosis. Activating mutations in the Toll/IL-1 receptor domain of *MYD88* were shown to drive prosurvival NF-κB signaling effects transactivating *IRF4* and *CARD11* in an oncogenic loop.[97] A recent small cohort from Koens et al[97] showed alterations of the NF-κB signaling pathways in most (70%) of PCDLBCL-LT.

Mareschal et al. found that *MYD88L265P* variant was associated with copy neutral loss of herozygosity or variants in the copy number in 60%. Other frequent losses were HIST1H1E (41%), TBL1XR1 (33%), MYC (26%), CREBBP (26%) and IRF4 (21%).[98] Durchame et al. found that that a mutation that targets BCR signaling genes (*CARD11* or *CD79A/B*) was associated with a reduced progression-free and disease specific survival. Moreover, they found that *CD79B* and *MYD88* were the earliest and among the most mutated genes.[59] Genetic analysis on systemic DLBCL showed, that they can subdivided in five clusters (C1–C5) and a group of unclassifiable DLBCL (C0). The described mutations in PCDLBCL-LT share genetic similarities to the C1 subgroup and with central nervous system and testicular DLBCL.[99,100]

POSTULATED CELL OF ORIGIN

Postgerminal center B cells.[101-104]

DIFFERENTIAL DIAGNOSIS

The differential diagnosis of PCDLBCL-LT is broad, and multiple cutaneous and systemic B-cell lymphomas with secondary cutaneous dissemination are included. To exclude secondary cutaneous involvement, staging procedures are essential. Perhaps, the most important differential diagnosis from both clinical and therapeutic standpoints represents PCFCL (Figs. 33-8 and 33-9). PCFCL is an indolent CBCL of germinal center origin that most typically presents in the head and neck or trunk. Rare presentations in the leg have been described, and debate persists whether these lesions are more aggressive and should be managed differently from typical PCFCL.[2,15,47] In addition, those rare cases with leg presentation tend to more frequently have IgM and MUM1/IRF4 coexpression. PCFCL can have a nodular, nodular/diffuse, or diffuse growth pattern, the latter more likely to be confused with PCDLBCL-LT. Admixture of T cells is often seen, and these features can be useful to distinguish it from PCDLBCL-LT.[78] The number of PD-1 positive T-cells is also higher in PCFCL than in PCDLBCL-LT. In addition to pan–B-cell markers (CD19, CD20, CD22, CD79a, PAX-5), PCFCLs express BCL-6 and less commonly CD10. BCL-2 is more typically negative but can be positive in a subset of cases. MUM1/IRF4 expression, when present, usually stains a relatively small subset of cells. This is in contrast to PCDLBCL-LT, which classically has strong diffuse BCL-2 and MUM1/IRF4 expression. Strong expression of CD10 and BCL-2 usually supports a diagnosis of systemic FL with secondary cutaneous dissemination.[13,48,55,105-107] If present on a large-cell lymphoma, it is most likely a reflection of cutaneous dissemination of a systemic DLBCL of germinal center origin, as PCDLBCL-LT is a disease with a nongerminal center immunophenotype.[104] Residual follicular dendritic networks (CD21, CD23, or CD35) can be seen in PCFCL but not usually in PCDLBCL-LT. As previously noted, IgM with or without coexpression of IgD is a useful marker to distinguish from PCFCL (the only caveat is, be aware that low percentages of both markers can still be seen in the setting of PCFCL and should not be interpreted as transformation or PCDLBCL-LT).[71,108] Another important differential pattern in between the two is the frequent lack of surface immunoglobulins and RNA cytoplasmic expression in PCFCL, but their presence in PCDLBCL-LT. At a molecular level, there is a high percentage (80%-100%) of cases of PCDLBCL-LT with chromosomal aberrations, and high-level DNA amplification of 18q21.31-q21.31, including the *BCL2* and *MALT1* genes. In contrast, PCFCL shows alteration of the *BCL11A* and *c-REL* genes. The translocation t(14;18) characteristic of systemic FL, and 10% to 41% of PCFCL, is never found in cases of PCDLBCL-LT.[109]

A recent study using microRNA (miRNA) profiling has also established differences between PCFCL and PCDLBCL-LT.[110] Cluster analysis of the complete microRNome could not distinguish between the two subtypes, but 16 single microRNAs were found to be differentially expressed. Higher expression of miR-9-5p, miR-31-5p,

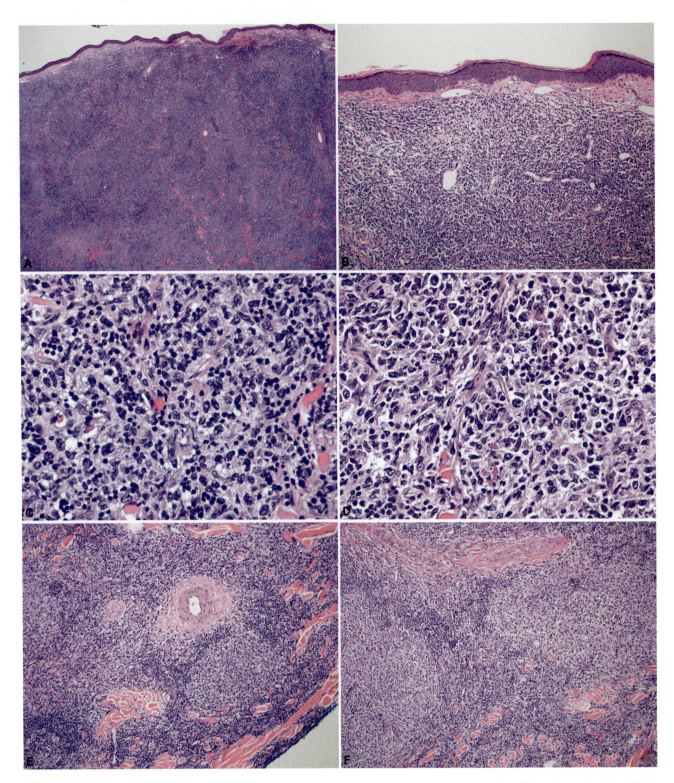

FIGURE 33-8. **Patient with history of PCFCL and early large-cell transformation. A** and **B** (20× and 100×). There is a diffuse and vaguely nodular infiltrate that spares the epidermis. **C** and **D** (400×). The infiltrate is composed of areas with sheets of larger cells with vesicular nuclei and prominent nucleoli. Frequent mitoses are also seen. **E** and **F** (200×). Areas with a more nodular pattern are present, without definitive germinal centers.

miR-129-2-3p, and miR-214-3p was seen in PCFCL as compared with PCLBCL-LT. MicroRNAs previously described to have higher expression in ABC-type as compared with germinal center B-cell–type nodal DLBCL were not differentially expressed between PCFCL and PCLBCL-LT.[110] Another study has shown that PCFCLs are characterized by a relatively intense cellular cytotoxic immune response and that PCLBCL leg types are characterized by constitutive activation of the intrinsic-mediated apoptosis pathway, with concomitant downstream inhibition of this apoptosis pathway.[111]

Intravascular B-cell lymphoma (IBL) is a rare extranodal B-cell lymphoma characterized by the intravascular growth

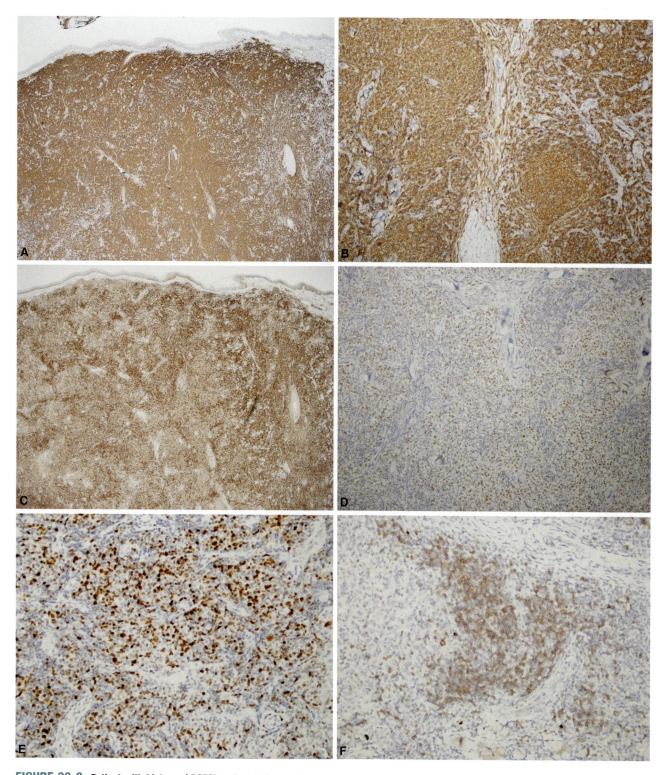

FIGURE 33-9. **Patient with history of PCFCL and early large-cell transformation, Immunohistochemistry.** The diffuse infiltrate is positive for CD20 (**A** and **B**) and also has aberrant expression of BCL-2 (**C**), an unusual pattern for cases of PCFCL. Germinal center differentiation is supported by BCL-6 expression (**D**). The areas of large cells show expression of MUM1/IRF4/IRF4 (**E**) and IgM (**F**), features in support of early changes of transformation.

of large cells especially in small capillaries and venules. Skin involvement manifests with livedo-like reticular erythema, panniculitis, or painful telangiectasias simulating inflammatory diseases or with nodules.[106,112-114] In addition to the B-cell markers CD20 and PAX5, the tumor cells express BCL-2 and can be positive for CD5 and CD10. The pure intravascular localization helps to distinguish this from PCDLBCL-LT. However, it should be noted that extranodal involvement by systemic DLBCL and PCDLBCL-LT could also be accompanied by the presence of prominent collections of intravascular cells.[60]

Similarly, cases of primary effusion B-cell lymphoma (PEL) can occur in the skin and have a predominantly

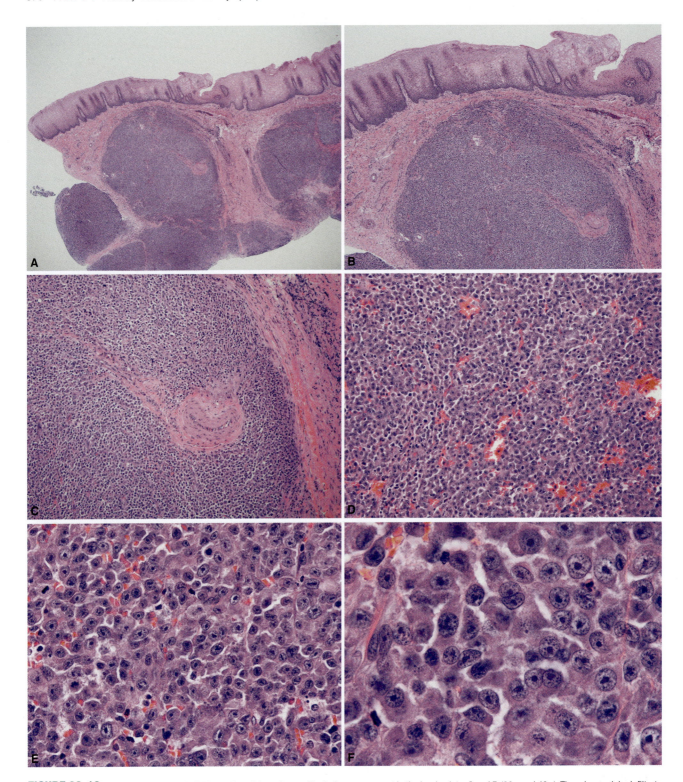

FIGURE 33-10. **Primary mucosal ALK1 large B-cell lymphoma.** The lesion was present in the hard palate. **A** and **B** (20× and 40×). There is a nodular infiltrate in the submucosa. **C** (200×). A perivascular localization is present in some areas. **D–F** (200×, 400×, and 1000×). The malignant cells show features of immature plasma cells or plasmablasts, with eccentric nuclei, abundant cytoplasm, and prominent nucleoli. Frequent mitoses are seen.

intravascular distribution mimicking IBL.[115-117] PEL can present initially in the skin and is a disease related to HHV-8 infection. PEL has a plasmablastic morphology and lacks pan–B-cell markers expression (CD19, CD20, and CD79a). These cells rarely express surface or cytoplasmic immunoglobulins. Expression of plasma cell markers CD38 and CD138 is typical. EBV can be seen in ~78% of cases,[118] and the proliferation index, as measured by Ki67, is extraordinarily high. To this day only one case of ALK+ DLBCL have been described in a cutaneous site, and the authors have come in contact with an isolated case presenting in a mucosal surface.[118] In addition to the hallmark ALK-1 positivity, the

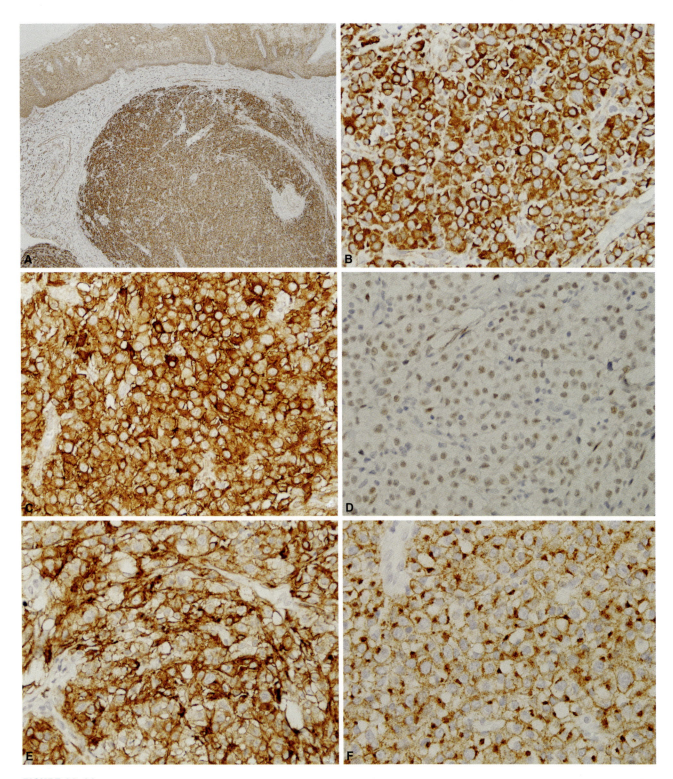

FIGURE 33-11. Primary mucosal ALK1 large B-cell lymphoma—immunohistochemistry. The malignant cells are positive for CD38 (a plasma cell marker; **A** and **B**), EMA **(C)**, weakly for PAX5 **(D)** and CD10 **(E)**, and strongly for ALK1 **(F)**. The pattern seen for ALK expression is suggestive of a variant translocation (nucleolar and cytoplasmic).

tumors also show typical IgA expression and a lack of B-cell markers[120] (Figs. 33-10 and 33-11).

The previously named EBV+ DBLCL of the elderly is nowadays called EBV-positive diffuse large B-cell lymphoma, NOS. Although the disease typically presents in patients older than 50 years of age, also younger people can be affected. The disease presents without any documented predisposing immunodeficiency and it is believed to be related with immunosenescence.[16,51,121] It represents the highest proportion of DLBCLs in people older than 90 years. Extranodal presentations are seen in 70% of cases, and the skin might be the only site of involvement in 20% of cases. Morphologically, it is characterized by the presence of geographic necrosis, as well as a mixture of malignant cells with features of centroblasts, immunoblasts, and Hodgkin-like cells, in addition to a rich inflammatory background. Like PCDLBCL-LT, it expresses MUM1/IRF4. Unlike PCDLBCL-LT, EBV+ DLBCL-NOS is, by definition, EBV positive.

PBL usually presents in the setting of HIV infection and immunosuppression (eg, transplant) and in elderly individuals. The main presentation is usually in the oral cavity. To date, less than 30 cases of PBL have been documented in the skin.[106,122-124] Occasional large tumor nodules in the legs have been reported mimicking PCDLBCL-LT.

Another diagnostic category, which also encompasses DLBCL, includes posttransplant lymphoproliferative disorders (PTLDs). PTLD represents a spectrum of lymphoid diseases, ranging from early lesions, such as plasmacytic hyperplasia, to monomorphic neoplasms (DLBCL). Fifty cases of primary cutaneous B-cell PTLD were recently reviewed[125-128]: like PCDLBCL-LT, they typically present in the legs of older male individuals. However, they present several years after transplant and most of them are associated with EBV. Some cases can have a plasmacytoma-like appearance.

Lymphomatoid granulomatosis (LyG) is another EBV-driven B-cell proliferation. Patients with HIV, iatrogenic immunomodulation, and congenital immune deficiencies (eg, Wiskott-Aldrich syndrome) are at particular risk for the development of LyG.[48,106,129-131] Most patients also have pulmonary involvement (>90%) and central nervous system dissemination. Cutaneous involvement is present in 25% to 50% of cases of LyG. Patients typically present with nodules, papules, and plaques, which frequently ulcerate (as opposed to PCDLBCL-LT). Most patients have a poor prognosis, the disease having a median survival of 2 years; however, a waxing-and-waning course or even spontaneous remissions may be seen. Morphologically, LyG is characterized by an angiocentric and angiodestructive, large, EBV+ B-cell infiltrate, often with a mixed background of small lymphocytes, plasma cells, and histiocytes. Necrosis and periadnexal involvement are common. A lymphohistiocytic panniculitis with fat necrosis is frequently present. The angiocentricity and the number of EBER+ cells are the main distinguishing feature from PCDLBCL-LT. Grading of these lesions is based on the number of EBER+ cells. Grade 3 lesions (>50 EBER+/high-power field) can be hard to distinguish from DLBCL. However, sheets of large cells are not usually a feature of LyG. A case of EBV-negative LyG was reported in the skin.[121] Because of overlapping clinical and histomorphologic features, a differentiation of secondary cutaneous infiltrates of Mantle cell lymphoma (MCL) from PCDLBCL-LT can be challenging. Although ML is typically composed of monomorphic small to medium-sized lymphocytes, a blastoid variant can also occur. As in DLBCL-LT the tumor cells express BCL-2, most commonly also MUM-1/IRF4 (83%), and IgM (82%), and lack CD10 (25%) and BCL6 (0%). The expression of Cyclin D1 (100%) and the presence of t(11;14) (100%) allows a distinction. In Cyclin D1 negative cases, expression of SOX-11 in MCL is also helpful.[132,133]

TREATMENT

A study from Grange et al in France has shown an improvement in survival rates in mainly two groups of patients: (1) treated from 1988 to 2003 and (2) treated from 2004 to 2010.

The main differences in the groups evoke a change from a pure treatment with radiation (earlier on the first group)[2,134,135] to a rituximab-based regimen containing polychemotherapy.[136-145] During 2002 to 2005, it was demonstrated that addition of rituximab to CHOP regimen improved response rates, short-term survival, and long-term outcome without increasing toxic effects in patients aged 60 to 80 years with DLBCL. Many difficulties often encountered with these patients are related to the presence of other diseases, diminished organ function, and altered drug metabolism. In day-to-day practice, this resulted in frequent replacement of the standard rituximab-CHOP regimen with rituximab regimens including lower doses (rituximab–mini-CHOP) or no anthracycline. Recent alternatives to mini-CHOP regimens include rituximab plus pegylated doxorubicin, with preliminary good results in individuals who are less likely to benefit from a more aggressive chemotherapeutic regimen.[146] Single-agent rituximab and local radiotherapy has also been used for palliative care.[147] A study from Hamilton et al[148] showed (on a CHOP-based regimen) that nearly 50% or more of the patients in their series (n = 25) received adjuvant radiation treatment. Limb perfusion using Melphalan has been used in an isolated case report with good clinical response.[149] Yttrium-90 ibritumomab tiuxetan radioimmunotherapy has been used post rituximab in a series of 10 patients, most of whom had relapsed DLBCL-LT.[150] Lenalidomide monotherapy has also been used with some success in relapsed cases.[151] In a study with single agent lenalidomide, 26% of the patients (n = 19) responded. A higher overall-response was associated with the absence of a MYD88L265P mutation.[152] A recent phase II clinical trial of interferon-γ gene transfer with TG1042 showed local responses in the two cases of CBCL examined (one disseminated primary cutaneous marginal zone lymphoma and one PCDLBCL-LT), lending support for further developing this novel interferon-γ gene transfer in CBCL.[153] Some PCDLBCL-LT patients have been already successful treated with the Bruton's tyrosine kinase inhibitor Ibrutinib. One patient developed progressive nodal disease and novel genomic changes occurred during the therapy were found.[154,155]

CAPSULE SUMMARY

- PCDLBCL-LT typically affects the legs of elderly individuals with a mean age of 77 years.
- However, in 10% to 20% of cases, other parts of the body are affected.
- The most common treatment modality is a rituximab-based regimen comprising polychemotherapy and mini-CHOP.
- Molecular studies show striking differences between this entity and PCFCL, and PCDLBCL-LT is considered a disease of postgerminal origin analogous to nodal nongerminal center DLBCL.
- The typical histologic features of DLBCL-LT show a diffuse infiltrate in the entire dermis, often extending into the subcutaneous tissue.
- In addition to traditional B-cell markers (CD19, CD20, CD22, CD79a, PAX-5), PCDLBCL-LT classically expresses BCL-2, MUM1/IRF4, and FOXP1.
- The differential diagnosis includes systemic large B-cell lymphomas, and more recently subtypes of DLBCL that can present or occur only in the skin (PBL, IBL, PTLD,

PEL, LyG, B-cell lymphomas with intermediate features between DLBCL and BL).
- EBV+ mucocutaneous ulcer and MTX-related lymphoproliferative disorders are recently described entities occurring more frequently in the setting of immunosuppression and are characterized by the presence of Hodgkin-like cells, a Hodgkin-like phenotype, and a very indolent behavior that often does not require chemotherapy.

References

1. Willemze R, Vergier B, Duncan LM, et al. *Primary Cutaneous Diffuse Large B-Cell Lymphoma, Leg Type.* 5th ed. International Agency for Research on Cancer; 2017:303-304.
2. Mondal SK, Mandal PK, Roy S, et al. Primary cutaneous large B-cell lymphoma, leg type: report of two cases and review of literature. *Indian J Med Paediatr Oncol.* 2012;33(1):54-57.
3. Ferenczi K. Cutaneous B-cell lymphoma: important diagnostic tools. *G Ital Dermatol Venereol.* 2010;145(3):361-373.
4. Rausch T, Cairoli A, Benhattar J, et al. EBV+ cutaneous B-cell lymphoproliferation of the leg in an elderly patient with mycosis fungoides and methotrexate treatment. *APMIS.* 2013;121(1):79-84.
5. Gaulard P, Swerdlow SH, Harris NL et al. *EBV+ Mucocutaneous Ulcer.* 5th ed. International Agency for Research on Cancer; 2017:307-308.
6. Grange F, Beylot-Barry M, Courville P, et al. Primary cutaneous diffuse large B-cell lymphoma, leg type: clinicopathologic features and prognostic analysis in 60 cases. *Arch Dermatol.* 2007;143(9):1144-1150.
7. Pham-Ledard A, Prochazkova-Carlotti M, Andrique L, et al. Multiple genetic alterations in primary cutaneous large B-cell lymphoma, leg type support a common lymphomagenesis with activated B-cell-like diffuse large B-cell lymphoma. *Mod Pathol.* 2014;27(3):402-411.
8. Nakayama-Ichiyama S, Yokote T, Iwaki K, et al. Co-infection of human herpesvirus-6 and human herpesvirus-8 in primary cutaneous diffuse large B-cell lymphoma, leg type. *Br J Haematol.* 2011;155(4):514-516.
9. Brouillard C, Granel-Brocard F, Montagne K, et al. An atypical presentation of primary cutaneous diffuse B-cell lymphoma, leg type. *Ann Dermatol Venereol.* 2011;138(8/9):601-604.
10. Koens L, Senff NJ, Vermeer MH, et al. Methotrexate-associated B-cell lymphoproliferative disorders presenting in the skin: a clinicopathologic and immunophenotypical study of 10 cases. *Am J Surg Pathol.* 2014;38(7):999-1006.
11. Matsumoto Y, Horiike S, Maekawa S, et al. Rheumatoid arthritis/methotrexate-associated primary cutaneous diffuse large B-cell lymphoma, leg type. *Intern Med.* 2014;53(11):1177-1181.
12. Slater DN. The new World Health Organization-European Organization for Research and Treatment of Cancer classification for cutaneous lymphomas: a practical marriage of two giants. *Br J Dermatol.* 2005;153(5):874-880.
13. Swerdlow SH, Quintanilla-Martinez L, Willemze R, et al. Cutaneous B-cell lymphoproliferative disorders: report of the 2011 Society for Hematopathology/European Association for Haematopathology workshop. *Am J Clin Pathol.* 2013;139(4):515-535.
14. Khan JA, Usman F, Abbasi S, et al. Diffuse large B-cell lymphoma presenting as a chronic leg ulcer: the importance of repeat tissue biopsy. *Ann R Coll Surg Engl.* 2011;93(4):e9-e10.
15. Kodama K, Massone C, Chott A, et al. Primary cutaneous large B-cell lymphomas: clinicopathologic features, classification, and prognostic factors in a large series of patients. *Blood.* 2005;106(7):2491-2497.
16. Zinzani PL, Quaglino P, Pimpinelli N, et al. Prognostic factors in primary cutaneous B-cell lymphoma: the Italian study group for cutaneous lymphomas. *J Clin Oncol.* 2006;24(9):1376-1382.
17. Dongre A, Kar S, Gondse S, et al. Primary cutaneous diffuse large B cell lymphoma, leg type. *Indian J Dermatol Venereol Leprol.* 2011;77(2):212-214.
18. Patrizi A, Raone B, Sabattini E, et al. Primary cutaneous large B-cell lymphoma, leg type, localized on the dorsum. *Case Rep Dermatol.* 2009;1(1):87-92.
19. Gopal MM, Malik A. Primary cutaneous diffuse large B-cell lymphoma of the upper limb: a fascinating entity. *Indian J Dermatol.* 2013;58(5):366-368.
20. Hallermann C, Niermann C, Fischer RJ, et al. New prognostic relevant factors in primary cutaneous diffuse large B-cell lymphomas. *J Am Acad Dermatol.* 2007;56(4):588-597.
21. Pandolfino TL, Siegel RS, Kuzel TM, et al. Primary cutaneous B-cell lymphoma: review and current concepts. *J Clin Oncol.* 2000;18(10):2152-2168.
22. Vermeer MH, Willemze R. Recent advances in primary cutaneous B-cell lymphomas. *Curr Opin Oncol.* 2014;26(2):230-236.
23. Suss A, Simon JC, Sticherling M. Primary cutaneous diffuse large B-cell lymphoma, leg type, with the clinical picture of chronic venous ulceration. *Acta Derm Venereol.* 2007;87(2):169-170.
24. Chen YF, Li YC, Chen LM, et al. Primary cutaneous diffuse large B cell lymphoma relapsed solely as a huge lung tumor mimicking a primary pulmonary lymphoma. *Int J Hematol.* 2010;91(1):112-116.
25. Ekmekci TR, Koslu A, Sakiz D, et al. Primary cutaneous large B-cell lymphoma, leg type, presented with a migratory lesion. *J Eur Acad Dermatol Venereol.* 2007;21(7):1000-1001.
26. Marchesi A, Leone F, Menicanti C, et al. A 'migrant' mass of the forehead: diagnosis and treatment. *J Plast Reconstr Aesthet Surg.* 2013;66(11):e310-e312.
27. Belousova IE, Vanecek T, Skreg SV, et al. Unusual clinicopathological presentation of primary cutaneous diffuse large B-cell lymphoma, leg type, with multiple nodules and widespread garland-like lesions. *Am J Dermatopathol.* 2009;31(4):370-374.
28. Shim TN, El-Daly H, Carr RA, et al. Cutaneous telangiectasia and cauda equina syndrome: a presentation of diffuse large B-cell lymphoma. *Am J Dermatopathol.* 2013;35(4):507-510.
29. Chaudhuri AA, Xavier MF. Primary cutaneous diffuse large B cell lymphoma, leg type (PCDLBCL-LT) in the setting of prior radiation therapy. *J Gen Intern Med.* 2015;30(3):371-372.
30. Meziane M, Hesse S, Chetaille B, et al. Cutaneous large B-cell leg-type lymphoma occurring on a leg burn. *Ann Dermatol Venereol.* 2009;136(11):791-794.
31. Levy A, Randall MB, Henson T. Primary cutaneous B-cell lymphoma, leg type restricted to the subcutaneous fat arising in a patient with dermatomyositis. *Am J Dermatopathol.* 2008;30(6):578-581.
32. Evans KG, Abraham RM, Mihova D, et al. Acute onset of leg nodules in a sporotrichoid pattern—quiz case. Diagnosis: primary cutaneous diffuse large B-cell lymphoma, leg type (PCLBCL-LT). *Arch Dermatol.* 2012;148(10):1199-1200.
33. Gonzalez-Vela MC, Gonzalez-Lopez MA, Val-Bernal JF, et al. Cutaneous diffuse large B-cell lymphoma of the leg associated with chronic lymphedema. *Int J Dermatol.* 2008;47(2):174-177.

34. Ho SL, Tang BY, Chai J, et al. Cutaneous large B-cell lymphoma of the leg: presenting initially as mononeuritis multiplex. *Singapore Med J.* 2009;50(5):e158-e160.
35. Huang CT, Yang WC, Liu YC, et al. Primary cutaneous diffuse large B-cell lymphoma, leg type, with unusual clinical presentation of bluish-reddish multicolored rainbow pattern. *J Clin Oncol.* 2011;29(17):e497-e498.
36. Bertaud S, Dindyal S, Kaur C, et al. Diffuse primary large B cell lymphoma of leg type presenting on the breast: a rare case of surgical excision. *BMJ Case Rep.* 2011;2011:bcr0520114286. doi:10.1136/bcr.05.2011.4286
37. Antic D, Petrovic N, Pelemis M, et al. "Invisible" primary cutaneous diffuse large B-cell lymphoma, leg type, as a cause of fever of unknown origin. *J Clin Oncol.* 2013;31(17):e276-e279.
38. Alcantara-Gonzalez J, Gonzalez-Garcia C, Fernandez-Guarino M, et al. Spontaneous regression of primary diffuse large B-cell lymphoma, leg type. *Actas Dermosifiliogr.* 2014;105(1):78-83.
39. Nakayama S, Yokote T, Kobayashi K, et al. Primary cutaneous diffuse large B-cell lymphoma, leg type, with features simulating POEMS syndrome. *Eur J Haematol.* 2010;84(1):79-83.
40. Jamil A, Nadzri N, Harun N, et al. Primary cutaneous diffuse large B-cell lymphoma leg type presenting with hemophagocytic syndrome. *J Am Acad Dermatol.* 2012;67(5):e222-e223.
41. Kawakami T, Mizoguchi M, Soma Y. Primary cutaneous diffuse large B-cell lymphoma, leg type in an elderly man with human immunodeficiency virus encephalopathy. *Acta Derm Venereol.* 2009;89(5):534-535.
42. Zhao J, Han B, Shen T, et al. Primary cutaneous diffuse large B-cell lymphoma (leg type) after renal allograft. *Eur J Haematol.* 2008;81(2):163.
43. Zhao J, Han B, Shen T, et al. Primary cutaneous diffuse large B-cell lymphoma (leg type) after renal allograft: case report and review of the literature. *Int J Hematol.* 2009;89(1):113-117.
44. Lacoste C, Duong TA, Dupuis J, et al. Leg ulcer associated with type I cryoglobulinaemia due to incipient B-cell lymphoma. *Ann Dermatol Venereol.* 2013;140(5):367-372.
45. Shaikh AJ, Masood N, Ahsan A, et al. Primary cutaneous B cell lymphoma—leg type (NEW EORTC—WHO classification), with nasal sinuses involvement. *J Pakistan Med Assoc.* 2008;58(5):274-276.
46. Lipowicz S, Beylot-Barry M, Choquet S, et al. Bone involvement in two cases of thoracic primary cutaneous diffuse large B-cell lymphoma, leg type. *Eur J Dermatol.* 2011;21(5):744-749.
47. Grange F, Joly P, Barbe C, et al. Improvement of survival in patients with primary cutaneous diffuse large B-cell lymphoma, leg type, in France. *JAMA Dermatol.* 2014;150(5):535-541.
48. Hristov AC. Primary cutaneous diffuse large B-cell lymphoma, leg type: diagnostic considerations. *Arch Pathol Lab Med.* 2012;136(8):876-881.
49. Aoki K, Arima H, Tabata S, et al. Central nervous system involvement of primary cutaneous diffuse large B cell lymphoma-leg type diagnosed according to the WHO 2008 classification. *Ann Hematol.* 2012;91(12):1975-1976.
50. Rozati S, Kempf W, Ostheeren-Michaelis S, et al. Cutaneous diffuse large B-cell lymphoma, leg type, with bilateral intraocular involvement and infiltration to the CNS. *J Clin Oncol.* Published online 2014. doi:10.1200/JCO.2013.51.6559
51. Salem AB, Nfoussi H, Kchir N. Ureteral spread of a primary cutaneous diffuse large B-cell lymphoma, leg type. *Indian J Urol.* 2014;30(2):222-224.
52. Bessell EM, Humber CE, O'Connor S, et al. Primary cutaneous B-cell lymphoma in Nottinghamshire U.K.: prognosis of subtypes defined in the WHO-EORTC classification. *Br J Dermatol.* 2012;167(5):1118-1123.
53. Hallermann C, Niermann C, Fischer RJ, et al. Survival data for 299 patients with primary cutaneous lymphomas: a monocentre study. *Acta Derm Venereol.* 2011;91(5):521-525. doi:10.2340/00015555-1112
54. Senff NJ, Willemze R. The applicability and prognostic value of the new TNM classification system for primary cutaneous lymphomas other than mycosis fungoides and Sézary syndrome: results on a large cohort of primary cutaneous B-cell lymphomas and comparison with the system used by the Dutch Cutaneous Lymphoma Group. *Br J Dermatol.* 2007;157(6):1205-1211.
55. Kempf W, Denisjuk N, Kerl K, et al. Primary cutaneous B-cell lymphomas. *J German Soc Dermatol.* 2012;10(1):12-22; quiz 23.
56. Schrader AMR, Jansen PM, Vermeer MH, Kleiverda JK, Vermaat JSP, Willemze R. High incidence and clinical significance of MYC rearrangements in primary cutaneous diffuse large B-cell lymphoma, leg type. *Am J Surg Pathol.* 2018;42(11):1488-1494. doi:10.1097/PAS.0000000000001132
57. Kim YJ, Won CH, Chang SE, Choi JH, Lee MW, Lee WJ. MYC protein expression is associated with poor prognosis in cutaneous diffuse large B-cell lymphoma. *Australas J Dermatol.* 2018;59(3):e240-e242. doi:10.1111/ajd.12705
58. Senff NJ, Zoutman WH, Vermeer MH, et al. Fine-mapping chromosomal loss at 9p21: correlation with prognosis in primary cutaneous diffuse large B-cell lymphoma, leg type. *J Invest Dermatol.* 2009;129(5):1149-1155.
59. Ducharme O, Beylot-Barry M, Pham-Ledard A, et al. Mutations of the B-cell receptor pathway confer chemoresistance in primary cutaneous diffuse large B-cell lymphoma leg type. *J Invest Dermatol.* 2019;139(11):2334-2342.e8. doi:10.1016/j.jid.2019.05.008
60. Plaza JA, Kacerovska D, Stockman DL, et al. The histomorphologic spectrum of primary cutaneous diffuse large B-cell lymphoma: a study of 79 cases. *Am J Dermatopathol.* 2011;33(7):649-655; quiz 656-658.
61. Cerroni L, El-Shabrawi-Caelen L, Fink-Puches R, et al. Cutaneous spindle-cell B-cell lymphoma: a morphologic variant of cutaneous large B-cell lymphoma. *Am J Dermatopathol.* 2000;22(4):299-304.
62. Ferrara G, Bevilacqua M, Argenziano G. Cutaneous spindle B-cell lymphoma: a reappraisal. *Am J Dermatopathol.* 2002;24(6):526-527; author reply 527-528.
63. Goodlad JR. Spindle-cell B-cell lymphoma presenting in the skin. *Br J Dermatol.* 2001;145(2):313-317.
64. Nagatani T, Miyazawa M, Matsuzaki T, et al. A case of cutaneous B-cell lymphoma with a storiform stromal reaction. *J Dermatol.* 1993;20(5):298-303.
65. Ries S, Barr R, LeBoit P, et al. Cutaneous sarcomatoid B-cell lymphoma. *Am J Dermatopathol.* 2007;29(1):96-98.
66. Kamath NV, Gilliam AC, Nihal M, et al. Primary cutaneous large B-cell lymphoma of the leg relapsing as cutaneous intravascular large B-cell lymphoma. *Arch Dermatol.* 2001;137(12):1657-1658.
67. Magro CM, Wang X, Subramaniyam S, et al. Cutaneous double-hit B-cell lymphoma: an aggressive form of B-cell lymphoma with a propensity for cutaneous dissemination. *Am J Dermatopathol.* 2014;36(4):303-310.

68. Hoefnagel JJ, Mulder MM, Dreef E, et al. Expression of B-cell transcription factors in primary cutaneous B-cell lymphoma. *Mod Pathol.* 2006;19(9):1270-1276.
69. Plaza JA, Kacerovska D, Sangueza M, et al. Can cutaneous low-grade B-cell lymphoma transform into primary cutaneous diffuse large B-cell lymphoma? An immunohistochemical study of 82 cases. *Am J Dermatopathol.* 2014;36(6):478-482.
70. Senff NJ, Hoefnagel JJ, Jansen PM, et al. Reclassification of 300 primary cutaneous B-cell lymphomas according to the new WHO-EORTC classification for cutaneous lymphomas: comparison with previous classifications and identification of prognostic markers. *J Clin Oncol.* 2007;25(12):1581-1587.
71. Koens L, Vermeer MH, Willemze R, et al. IgM expression on paraffin sections distinguishes primary cutaneous large B-cell lymphoma, leg type from primary cutaneous follicle center lymphoma. *Am J Surg Pathol.* 2010;34(7):1043-1048.
72. Herrera E, Gallardo M, Bosch R, et al. Primary cutaneous CD30 (Ki-1)-positive non-anaplastic B-cell lymphoma. *J Cutan Pathol.* 2002;29(3):181-184.
73. Magro CM, Nash JW, Werling RW, et al. Primary cutaneous CD30+ large cell B-cell lymphoma: a series of 10 cases. *Appl Immunohistochem Mol Morphol.* 2006;14(1):7-11.
74. Stein H, Chan JKC, Warnke RA. *Diffuse Large B-Cell Lymphoma, Not Otherwise Specified.* International Agency for Research on Cancer; 2008.
75. Hu S, Xu-Monette ZY, Balasubramanyam A, et al. CD30 expression defines a novel subgroup of diffuse large B-cell lymphoma with favorable prognosis and distinct gene expression signature: a report from the International DLBCL Rituximab-CHOP Consortium Program Study. *Blood.* 2013;121(14):2715-2724.
76. Slack GW, Steidl C, Sehn LH, et al. CD30 expression in de novo diffuse large B-cell lymphoma: a population-based study from British Columbia. *Br J Haematol.* 2014;167(5):608-617.
77. Mitteldorf C, Bieri M, Wey N, et al. Expression of programmed death-1 (CD279) in primary cutaneous B-cell lymphomas with correlation to lymphoma entities and biological behaviour. *Br J Dermatol.* 2013;169(6):1212-1218. doi:10.1111/bjd.12579
78. Cetinozman F, Koens L, Jansen PM, et al. Programmed death-1 expression in cutaneous B-cell lymphoma. *J Cutan Pathol.* 2014;41(1):14-21.
79. Mitteldorf C, Berisha A, Pfaltz MC, et al. Tumor microenvironment and checkpoint molecules in primary cutaneous diffuse large B-cell lymphoma-new therapeutic targets. *Am J Surg Pathol.* 2017;41(7):998-1004. doi:10.1097/PAS.0000000000000851
80. Menguy S, Prochazkova-Carlotti M, Beylot-Barry M, et al. PD-L1 and PD-L2 are differentially expressed by macrophages or tumor cells in primary cutaneous diffuse large B-cell lymphoma, leg type. *Am J Surg Pathol.* 2018;42(3):326-334. doi:10.1097/PAS.0000000000000983
81. Gaitonde S, Kavuri S, Alagiozian-Angelova V, et al. EBV positivity in primary cutaneous large B-cell lymphoma with immunophenotypic features of leg type: an isolated incident or something more significant? *Acta Oncol.* 2008;47(3):461-464.
82. Espinet B, Garcia-Herrera A, Gallardo F, et al. FOXP1 molecular cytogenetics and protein expression analyses in primary cutaneous large B cell lymphoma, leg-type. *Histol Histopathol.* 2011;26(2):213-221.
83. Felcht M, Heck M, Weiss C, et al. Expression of the T-cell regulatory marker FOXP3 in primary cutaneous large B-cell lymphoma tumour cells. *Br J Dermatol.* 2012;167(2):348-358.
84. Pham-Ledard A, Prochazkova-Carlotti M, Vergier B, et al. IRF4 expression without IRF4 rearrangement is a general feature of primary cutaneous diffuse large B-cell lymphoma, leg type. *J Invest Dermatol.* 2010;130(5):1470-1472.
85. Laurenti L, De Padua L, D'Arena G, et al. New and old monoclonal antibodies for the treatment of chronic lymphocytic leukemia. *Mini Rev Med Chem.* 2011;11(6):508-518.
86. Dijkman R, Tensen CP, Jordanova ES, et al. Array-based comparative genomic hybridization analysis reveals recurrent chromosomal alterations and prognostic parameters in primary cutaneous large B-cell lymphoma. *J Clin Oncol.* 2006;24(2):296-305.
87. Gimenez S, Costa C, Espinet B, et al. Comparative genomic hybridization analysis of cutaneous large B-cell lymphomas. *Exp Dermatol.* 2005;14(12):883-890.
88. Houldsworth J, Olshen AB, Cattoretti G, et al. Relationship between REL amplification, REL function, and clinical and biologic features in diffuse large B-cell lymphomas. *Blood.* 2004;103(5):1862-1868.
89. Martin-Subero JI, Gesk S, Harder L, et al. Recurrent involvement of the REL and BCL11A loci in classical Hodgkin lymphoma. *Blood.* 2002;99(4):1474-1477.
90. Martinez-Climent JA, Alizadeh AA, Segraves R, et al. Transformation of follicular lymphoma to diffuse large cell lymphoma is associated with a heterogeneous set of DNA copy number and gene expression alterations. *Blood.* 2003;101(8):3109-3117.
91. Kaune KM, Neumann C, Hallermann C, et al. Simultaneous aberrations of single CDKN2A network components and a high Rb phosphorylation status can differentiate subgroups of primary cutaneous B-cell lymphomas. *Exp Dermatol.* 2011;20(4):331-335.
92. Belaud-Rotureau MA, Marietta V, Vergier B, et al. Inactivation of p16INK4a/CDKN2A gene may be a diagnostic feature of large B cell lymphoma leg type among cutaneous B cell lymphomas. *Virchows Arch.* 2008;452(6):607-620.
93. Wiesner T, Obenauf AC, Geigl JB, et al. 9p21 deletion in primary cutaneous large B-cell lymphoma, leg type, may escape detection by standard FISH assays. *J Invest Dermatol.* 2009;129(1):238-240.
94. Wiesner T, Streubel B, Huber D, et al. Genetic aberrations in primary cutaneous large B-cell lymphoma: a fluorescence in situ hybridization study of 25 cases. *Am J Surg Pathol.* 2005;29(5):666-673.
95. Pham-Ledard A, Beylot-Barry M, Barbe C, et al. High frequency and clinical prognostic value of MYD88 L265P mutation in primary cutaneous diffuse large B-cell lymphoma, leg-type. *JAMA Dermatol.* 2014;150(11):1173-1179.
96. Pham-Ledard A, Cappellen D, Martinez F, et al. MYD88 somatic mutation is a genetic feature of primary cutaneous diffuse large B-cell lymphoma, leg type. *J Invest Dermatol.* 2012;132(8):2118-2120.
97. Koens L, Zoutman WH, Ngarmlertsirichai P, et al. Nuclear factor-κB pathway-activating gene aberrancies in primary cutaneous large B-cell lymphoma, leg type. *J Invest Dermatol.* 2014;134(1):290-292.
98. Mareschal S, Pham-Ledard A, Viailly PJ, et al. Identification of somatic mutations in primary cutaneous diffuse large B-cell lymphoma, leg type by massive parallel sequencing. *J Invest Dermatol.* 2017;137(9):1984-1994. doi:10.1016/j.jid.2017.04.010
99. Chapuy B, Stewart C, Dunford AJ, et al. Molecular subtypes of diffuse large B cell lymphoma are associated with

distinct pathogenic mechanisms and outcomes. *Nat Med.* 2018;24(5):679-690. doi:10.1038/s41591-018-0016-8.
100. Chapuy B, Roemer MG, Stewart C, et al. Targetable genetic features of primary testicular and primary central nervous system lymphomas. *Blood.* 2016;127(7):869-881. doi:10.1182/blood-2015-10-673236.
101. Aarts WM, Willemze R, Bende RJ, et al. VH gene analysis of primary cutaneous B-cell lymphomas: evidence for ongoing somatic hypermutation and isotype switching. *Blood.* 1998;92(10):3857-3864.
102. Dijkman R, Tensen CP, Buettner M, et al. Primary cutaneous follicle center lymphoma and primary cutaneous large B-cell lymphoma, leg type, are both targeted by aberrant somatic hypermutation but demonstrate differential expression of AID. *Blood.* 2006;107(12):4926-4929.
103. Perez M, Pacchiarotti A, Frontani M, et al. Primary cutaneous B-cell lymphoma is associated with somatically hypermutated immunoglobulin variable genes and frequent use of VH1-69 and VH4-59 segments. *Br J Dermatol.* 2010;162(3):611-618.
104. Gellrich S, Rutz S, Golembowski S, et al. Primary cutaneous follicle center cell lymphomas and large B cell lymphomas of the leg descend from germinal center cells. A single cell polymerase chain reaction analysis. *J Invest Dermatol.* 2001;117(6):1512-1520.
105. Khamaysi Z, Ben-Arieh Y, Izhak OB, et al. The applicability of the new WHO-EORTC classification of primary cutaneous lymphomas to a single referral center. *Am J Dermatopathol.* 2008;30(1):37-44.
106. Kempf W, Kazakov DV, Mitteldorf C. Cutaneous lymphomas: an update, part 2—B-cell lymphomas and related conditions. *Am J Dermatopathol.* 2014;36(3):197-208; quiz 209-210.
107. Sokol L, Naghashpour M, Glass LF. Primary cutaneous B-cell lymphomas: recent advances in diagnosis and management. *Cancer Control.* 2012;19(3):236-244.
108. Demirkesen C, Tuzuner N, Esen T, et al. The expression of IgM is helpful in the differentiation of primary cutaneous diffuse large B cell lymphoma and follicle center lymphoma. *Leuk Res.* 2011;35(9):1269-1272.
109. Suarez AL, Pulitzer M, Horwitz S, et al. Primary cutaneous B-cell lymphomas, part I: clinical features, diagnosis, and classification. *J Am Acad Dermatol.* 2013;69(3):329.e1–329.e13; quiz 341-342.
110. Koens L, Qin Y, Leung WY, et al. MicroRNA profiling of primary cutaneous large B-cell lymphomas. *PLoS One.* 2013;8(12):e82471.
111. van Galen JC, Hoefnagel JJ, Vermeer MH, et al. Profiling of apoptosis genes identifies distinct types of primary cutaneous large B cell lymphoma. *J Pathol.* 2008;215(3):340-346.
112. Feldmann R, Schierl M, Sittenthaler M, et al. Intravascular large B-cell lymphoma of the skin: typical clinical manifestations and a favourable response to rituximab-containing therapy. *Dermatology.* 2009;219(4):344-346.
113. Orwat DE, Batalis NI. Intravascular large B-cell lymphoma. *Arch Pathol Lab Med.* 2012;136(3):333-338.
114. Wahie S, Dayala S, Husain A, et al. Cutaneous features of intravascular lymphoma. *Clin Exp Dermatol.* 2011;36(3):288-291.
115. Crane GM, Ambinder RF, Shirley CM, et al. HHV-8-positive and EBV-positive intravascular lymphoma: an unusual presentation of extracavitary primary effusion lymphoma. *Am J Surg Pathol.* 2014;38(3):426-432.
116. Crane GM, Xian RR, Burns KH, et al. Primary effusion lymphoma presenting as a cutaneous intravascular lymphoma. *J Cutan Pathol.* 2014;41(12):928-935.
117. Pielasinski U, Santonja C, Rodriguez-Pinilla SM, et al. Extracavitary primary effusion lymphoma presenting as a cutaneous tumor: a case report and literature review. *J Cutan Pathol.* 2014;41(9):745-753.
118. Kim Y, Leventaki V, Bhaijee F, et al. Extracavitary/solid variant of primary effusion lymphoma. *Ann Diagn Pathol.* 2012;16(6):441-446.
119. Kempf W, Torricelli R, Zettl A, Zimmermann AK, Berisha A, Ghielmini M. Primary cutaneous anaplastic lymphoma kinase-positive large B-cell lymphoma. *Am J Dermatopathol.* 2019;41(8):602-605.
120. Valera A, Colomo L, Martinez A, et al. ALK-positive large B-cell lymphomas express a terminal B-cell differentiation program and activated STAT3 but lack MYC rearrangements. *Mod Pathol.* 2013;26(10):1329-1337.
121. Messana K, Marburger T, Bergfeld W. EBV-negative cutaneous lymphomatoid granulomatosis with concomitant EBV-positive pulmonary involvement: a potential diagnostic and prognostic pitfall. *Am J Dermatopathol.* 2015;37(9):707-711.
122. Corti M, Villafane MF, Bistmans A, et al. Oral cavity and extra-oral plasmablastic lymphomas in AIDS patients: report of five cases and review of the literature. *Int J STD AIDS.* 2011;22(12):759-763.
123. Horna P, Hamill JR Jr, Sokol L, et al. Primary cutaneous plasmablastic lymphoma in an immunocompetent patient. *J Am Acad Dermatol.* 2013;69(5):e274-e276.
124. Morscio J, Dierickx D, Nijs J, et al. Clinicopathologic comparison of plasmablastic lymphoma in HIV-positive, immunocompetent, and posttransplant patients: single-center series of 25 cases and meta-analysis of 277 reported cases. *Am J Surg Pathol.* 2014;38(7):875-886.
125. Wang E, Stoecker M. Primary cutaneous giant cell plasmacytoma in an organ transplant recipient: a rare presentation of a posttransplant lymphoproliferative disorder. *Am J Dermatopathol.* 2010;32(5):479-485.
126. Molina-Ruiz AM, Pulpillo A, Lasanta B, et al. A rare case of primary cutaneous plasmacytoma-like lymphoproliferative disorder following renal transplantation. *J Cutan Pathol.* 2012;39(7):685-689.
127. Salama S, Todd S, Cina DP, et al. Cutaneous presentation of post-renal transplant lymphoproliferative disorder: a series of four cases. *J Cutan Pathol.* 2010;37(6):641-653.
128. Seckin D. Cutaneous lymphoproliferative disorders in organ transplant recipients: update 2014. *G Ital Dermatol Venereol.* 2014;149(4):401-408.
129. Beaty MW, Toro J, Sorbara L, et al. Cutaneous lymphomatoid granulomatosis: correlation of clinical and biologic features. *Am J Surg Pathol.* 2001;25(9):1111-1120.
130. Katzenstein AL, Doxtader E, Narendra S. Lymphomatoid granulomatosis: insights gained over 4 decades. *Am J Surg Pathol.* 2010;34(12):e35-e48.
131. McNiff JM, Cooper D, Howe G, et al. Lymphomatoid granulomatosis of the skin and lung. An angiocentric T-cell-rich B-cell lymphoproliferative disorder. *Arch Dermatol.* 1996;132(12):1464-1470.
132. Wehkamp U, Pott C, Unterhalt M, et al. Skin involvement of mantle cell lymphoma may mimic primary cutaneous diffuse large B-cell lymphoma, leg type. *Am J Surg Pathol.* 2015;39(8):1093-1101.

133. Hsi AC, Hurley MY, Lee SJ, et al. Diagnostic utility of SOX11 immunohistochemistry in differentiating cutaneous spread of mantle cell lymphoma from primary cutaneous B-cell lymphomas. *J Cutan Pathol*. 2016;43(4):354-361.
134. Senff NJ, Hoefnagel JJ, Neelis KJ, et al. Results of radiotherapy in 153 primary cutaneous B-Cell lymphomas classified according to the WHO-EORTC classification. *Arch Dermatol*. 2007;143(12):1520-1526.
135. Sumida H, Sugaya M, Miyagaki T, et al. Frequent relapse and irradiation strategy in primary cutaneous diffuse large B-cell lymphoma, leg-type. *Acta Derm Venereol*. 2013;93(1):97-98.
136. Coiffier B, Lepage E, Briere J, et al. CHOP chemotherapy plus rituximab compared with CHOP alone in elderly patients with diffuse large-B-cell lymphoma. *N Engl J Med*. 2002;346(4):235-242.
137. Feugier P, Van Hoof A, Sebban C, et al. Long-term results of the R-CHOP study in the treatment of elderly patients with diffuse large B-cell lymphoma: a study by the Groupe d'Etude des Lymphomes de l'Adulte. *J Clin Oncol*. 2005;23(18):4117-4126.
138. Mounier N, Briere J, Gisselbrecht C, et al. Rituximab plus CHOP (R-CHOP) overcomes bcl-2—associated resistance to chemotherapy in elderly patients with diffuse large B-cell lymphoma (DLBCL). *Blood*. 2003;101(11):4279-4284.
139. Thieblemont C, Coiffier B. Lymphoma in older patients. *J Clin Oncol*. 2007;25(14):1916-1923.
140. Brandenburg A, Humme D, Terhorst D, et al. Long-term outcome of intravenous therapy with rituximab in patients with primary cutaneous B-cell lymphomas. *Br J Dermatol*. 2013;169(5):1126-1132.
141. Fernandez-Guarino M, Ortiz-Romero PL, Fernandez-Misa R, et al. Rituximab in the treatment of primary cutaneous B-cell lymphoma: a review. *Actas Dermosifiliogr*. 2014;105(5):438-445.
142. Grange F, Maubec E, Bagot M, et al. Treatment of cutaneous B-cell lymphoma, leg type, with age-adapted combinations of chemotherapies and rituximab. *Arch Dermatol*. 2009;145(3):329-330.
143. Guyot A, Ortonne N, Valeyrie-Allanore L, et al. Combined treatment with rituximab and anthracycline-containing chemotherapy for primary cutaneous large B-cell lymphomas, leg type, in elderly patients. *Arch Dermatol*. 2010;146(1):89-91.
144. Paulli M, Lucioni M, Maffi A, et al. Primary cutaneous diffuse large B-cell lymphoma (PCDLBCL), leg-type and other: an update on morphology and treatment. *G Ital Dermatol Venereol*. 2012;147(6):589-602.
145. Posada Garcia C, Florez A, Pardavila R, et al. Primary cutaneous large B-cell lymphoma, leg type, successfully treated with rituximab plus chemotherapy. *Eur J Dermatol*. 2009;19(4):394-395.
146. Fabbri A, Cencini E, Alterini R, et al. Rituximab plus liposomal pegylated doxorubicin in the treatment of primary cutaneous B-cell lymphomas. *Eur J Haematol*. 2014;93(2):129-136.
147. Fenot M, Quereux G, Brocard A, et al. Rituximab for primary cutaneous diffuse large B-cell lymphoma-leg type. *Eur J Dermatol*. 2010;20(6):753-757.
148. Hamilton SN, Wai ES, Tan K, et al. Treatment and outcomes in patients with primary cutaneous B-cell lymphoma: the BC Cancer Agency experience. *Int J Radiat Oncol Biol Phys*. 2013;87(4):719-725.
149. Kobold S, Killic N, Lutkens T, et al. Isolated limb perfusion with melphalan for the treatment of intractable primary cutaneous diffuse large B-cell lymphoma leg type. *Acta Haematol*. 2010;123(3):179-181.
150. Maza S, Gellrich S, Assaf C, et al. Yttrium-90 ibritumomab tiuxetan radioimmunotherapy in primary cutaneous B-cell lymphomas: first results of a prospective, monocentre study. *Leuk Lymphoma*. 2008;49(9):1702-1709.
151. Savini P, Lanzi A, Foschi FG, et al. Lenalidomide monotherapy in relapsed primary cutaneous diffuse large B cell lymphoma-leg type. *Ann Hematol*. 2014;93(2):333-334.
152. Beylot-Barry M, Mermin D, Maillard A, et al. A single-arm phase II trial of lenalidomide in relapsing or refractory primary cutaneous large b-cell lymphoma, leg type. *J Invest Dermatol*. 2018;138(9):1982-1989.
153. Dummer R, Eichmuller S, Gellrich S, et al. Phase II clinical trial of intratumoral application of TG1042 (adenovirus-interferon-gamma) in patients with advanced cutaneous T-cell lymphomas and multilesional cutaneous B-cell lymphomas. *Mol Ther*. 2010;18(6):1244-1247.
154. Fox LC, Yannakou CK, Ryland G, et al. Molecular mechanisms of disease progression in primary cutaneous diffuse large B-cell lymphoma, leg type during ibrutinib therapy. *Int J Mol Sci*. 2018;19(6):1758.
155. Pang A, Au-Yeung R, Leung RYY, Kwong YL. Addictive response of primary cutaneous diffuse large B cell lymphoma leg type to low-dose ibrutinib. *Ann Hematol*. 2019;98(10):2433-2436.

CHAPTER 34

Lymphomatoid granulomatosis

Yasmin Hambaroush and Alejandro A. Gru

DEFINITION

Lymphomatoid granulomatosis (LyG) is a rare angiocentric and angiodestructive Epstein–Barr virus (EBV)–associated B-cell lymphoproliferative disorder (LPD) with a predilection for the lung, central nervous system (CNS), and, less frequently, the skin.[1-5]

EPIDEMIOLOGY

Originally described by Liebow[6] in 1972 in the lungs, it primarily affects adults in the fourth to sixth decades of life and has a male predominance of 2:1. Unlike other LPDs, many patients with LyG have no clearly defined underlying immunodeficiency. In a large multicenter case series of cutaneous posttransplant LPD (PTLD), only one case of LyG was found.[7]

ETIOLOGY

LyG is linked to EBV infection. LyG patients have serologic evidence of past EBV exposure and low viral loads by polymerase chain reaction (PCR) analysis (~18 copies/10^6 genome equivalents). On the contrary, patients with PTLD usually show high EBV viremia. The typical latency pattern of EBV infection in LyG is type III.[8,9] EBV-infected B-cells may avoid immune surveillance due to dysfunctional T-cell or NK-cell responses.[2] Patients with an underlying acquired or inherited immunodeficiency syndrome may be diagnosed with LyG (eg, Wiskott–Aldrich syndrome, cartilage hair hypoplasia,[10] X-linked lymphoproliferative syndrome, HIV/AIDS, solid organ transplant) under the current WHO classification. Electron microscopy reveals features of endothelial necrosis and regeneration.[11] The angiocentric and angiodestructive infiltrate is characterized by numerous T-helper memory cells.[12] EBV-induced chemokines, such as inducible protein 10 (IP-10) and Mig, have been implicated in mediating the vascular damage in pulmonary LyG and most likely the skin.[13,14]

CLINICAL PRESENTATION AND PROGNOSIS

Most patients present with respiratory symptoms, and usually show multiple, bilateral lung infiltrates or nodules.[15] The lungs are virtually always involved.[1] Skin involvement is present in approximately 34% of cases.[15-19] Rare cases of only skin involvement have been reported.[20] Other organs such as the kidneys (19%), CNS (40%), liver (17%), and spleen (10%) are also commonly affected. The lymph nodes[21] and bone marrow are usually spared. Cutaneous lesions of LyG have been seen in association with Wiskott–Aldrich syndrome, myeloproliferative disorders, and in posttransplant settings.[22-25] A history of lymphoma, leukemia, biliary cirrhosis, chronic hepatitis, and others can be seen in some patients.[1,26] Constitutional symptoms, including fever, weight loss, fatigue, and/or night sweats, are common complaints (80% of cases).[14,27] The clinical lesions can precede, coincide, or follow the pulmonary disease with the latter two scenarios being the most typical.

The cutaneous lesions of LyG are typically dermal or subcutaneous nodules. The lesions occur in the extremities, trunk, and head and neck regions. A third of these cases show ulceration.[28] Plaques (Fig. 34-1) or lichen sclerosus–like presentations had been reported in 15% and 10% of the cases, respectively.[14] More uncommon clinical presentations include alopecia,[14] necrobiosis lipoidica-like,[29] facial edema, papules, folliculitis-like lesions,[30] annular lesions,[31] angioedema,[32] and eschar-like violaceous nodules.[33] Rarely, the disease can present in children.[24,34] Cases secondary to azathioprine, imatinib, and methotrexate therapy have been described.[35-38] A rare isolated cutaneous form with indolent clinical course had been also reported following heart–lung transplantation.[25] An unusual EBV-cutaneous LyG in a patient with coexistent EBV+ lung LyG had been also seen.[39] We have also reported the occurrence of LyG with midline septal necrosis and punched out ulcers mimicking extranodal NK/T-cell lymphoma (ENKL)[40] (Fig. 34-2).

Treatment of LyG is usually based on the grading of the lesions, with grade 1 lesions usually treated by rituximab, corticosteroids, interferon (IFN)-alpha; high-grade lesions are usually treated with a combination of chemo-immunotherapy. Dose-adjusted EPOCH-R has been used with an overall response rate of 77% and 41% of patients going into complete remission (CR).[41] Approximately, one-third of patients experienced a durable remission with a 5-year progression free survival (PFS) and overall survival (OS) of 28% and 66%, respectively, with most of the remaining patients relapsing with low-grade disease. Similar findings were noted in another small retrospective study at Moffitt Cancer Center that evaluated 11 LyG patients (45% grade 3) treated with other rituximab-based therapies, mainly

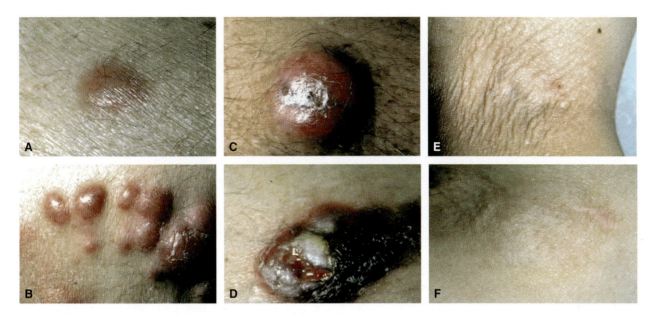

FIGURE 34-1. Clinical spectrum in cutaneous LyG. **A.** Erythematous papule. **B.** Multiple dermal nodules. **C.** Plum-colored dermal/subcutaneous tumor. **D.** Indurated subcutaneous nodule with necrosis and central ulceration. **E.** Atrophic plaque with prominent skin folds. **F.** A lichen sclerosus–like lesion showing hypopigmentation and a shiny texture. (Reprinted from Beaty MW, Toro J, Sorbara L et al. Cutaneous lymphomatoid granulomatosis: correlation of clinical and biologic features. *Am J Surg Pathol.* 2001;25(9):1111-1120, with permission.)

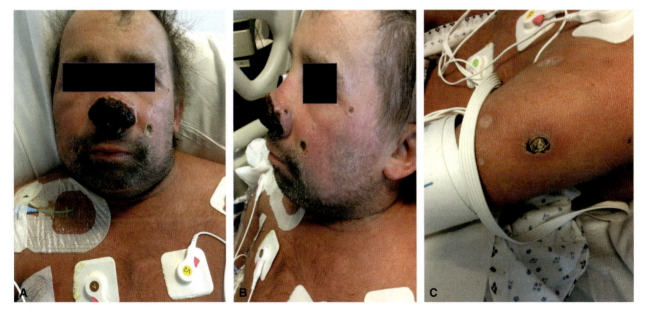

FIGURE 34-2. Cutaneous LyG mimicking extranodal NK/T-cell lymphoma. **A.** Extensive necrosis of the nose and midline septum is noted. **B.** Numerous punched-out ulcers on the face are also present. **C.** Similar ulcerated lesions are seen on the extremities.

cyclophosphamide, doxorubicin, vincristine, and prednisone (R-CHOP). Response to therapy was achieved in approximately two-thirds of patients, with one-third attaining a CR; median PFS and OS were ~1 and ~2 years, respectively.[42]

The clinical course of LyG is variable, ranging from spontaneous regression[43,44] to progression to EBV+ diffuse large B-cell lymphoma (DLBCL). Overall, the survival rate for LyG is poor with an average of 2 years of survival following the initial diagnosis.[1,2,16] Death typically results from progressive pulmonary insufficiency.[14]

HISTOLOGY

Cutaneous LyG is histologically characterized by a lymphocytic or polymorphous lymphohistiocytic infiltrate, without multinucleated giant cells. The infiltrates have a periadnexal and/or perivascular–angiocentric distribution with angionecrosis. The subcutaneous tissue shows a lymphohistiocytic panniculitis, often with poorly formed granulomas (Figs. 34-3 and 34-4). Sarcoidal or necrotizing granulomas are not present.[14] Occasional mild reactive lymphocyte exocytosis can be

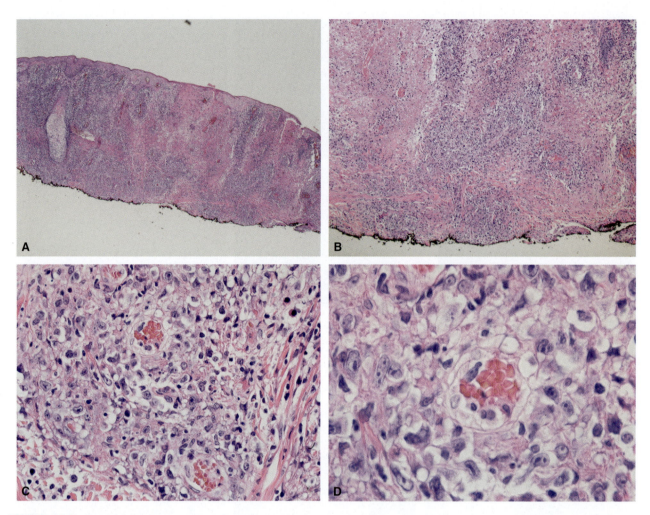

FIGURE 34-3. Cutaneous LyG, histopathologic findings. A. A notable angiocentric infiltrate in the dermis is present (40×). **B.** The angioncentric infiltrate is also accompanied by coagulative necrosis (100×). **C** and **D.** A malignant angiotropic infiltrate is seen composed of numerous large immunoblastic cells with prominent nucleoli (400× and 600×).

seen in the epidermis, but without the histologic atypia associated with mycosis fungoides. The dermal infiltrate often has a superficial and deep distribution. Angiodestruction, necrosis, and atypical lymphoid cells surrounding the vessels are seen (Fig. 34.5). The large cells have an immunoblastic appearance with nuclear hyperchromasia, pleomorphism, and prominent nucleoli. Some cases have Hodgkin-like cells, although classic Reed-Sternberg cells are not present. The histologic grading is based on the number of large atypical cells. In low-grade lesions, they are few and scattered, while in the high-grade lesions they form aggregates or sheets. Angiodestruction is not typical in papular lesions, but is often seen in nodules.[14] Admixed plasma cells, histiocytes, and occasional eosinophils can be seen. LyG in extracutaneous sites shows similar angiocentric, atypical lymphohistiocytic infiltrates. Infarcts in the lungs and CNS are common[1,26] (Figs. 34.6 and 34.7).

IMMUNOPHENOTYPE

The large atypical cells are CD20+ B-cells, which are outnumbered by background CD3+ T-cells. Some of the T-cells show a cytotoxic profile (TIA-1, CD8+, granzyme B). However, the background T-cells are predominantly CD4+ (over CD8+).[2,14,16] CD30 is positive in ~50% of cases. CD15 is invariably negative. A subset of these cells may express EBV LMP1. EBNA2 is also frequently positive, consistent with EBV latency type III. Staining for kappa and lambda light chains is of limited value, although rare cases may show light chain restriction in plasma cells.

GRADING

The original grading scheme (grades 1-3) was proposed by Lipford et al[45] Grading is based on the number of neoplastic large B-cells. The new WHO classification[1,3] has incorporated the use of in situ hybridization (ISH) for EBV (EBER) for grading: grade 1 is composed of a polymorphous infiltrate with "absent or rare" large lymphoid cells and less than five EBV-positive cells per high-power field by ISH. EBV-positive cells may be absent in some cases. Grade 2 contains "occasional large lymphoid cells" that may form "small clusters" in a polymorphous background with 5 to 20, and "occasionally" up to 50 EBV-positive cells per high-power field. In grade 3, large atypical B-cells are "readily identified" and "can form larger aggregates," and EBV-positive cells are "extremely numerous" comprising greater than 50 per

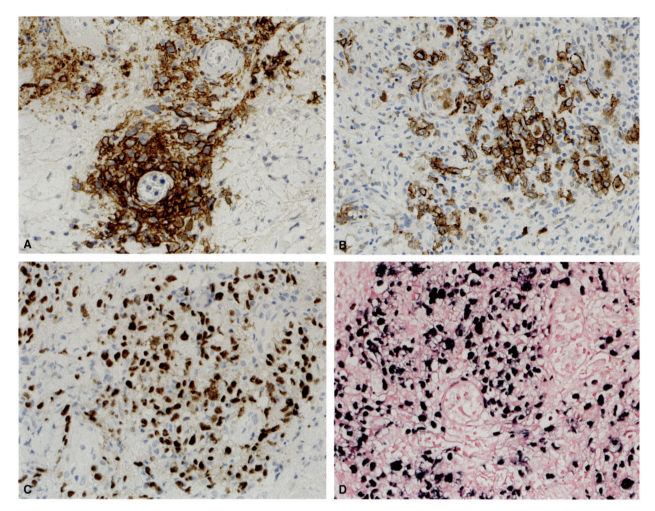

FIGURE 34-4. Cutaneous LyG, immunophenotypic findings. The infiltrate is positive for CD20 **(A)**, CD30 **(B)**, and PAX-5 **(C)**. Numerous EBV+ cells are seen, establishing the diagnosis of a high-grade LyG **(grade 3, D)**.

high-power field and can form "confluent sheets." Necrosis is more common in grade 2 and 3 lesions. CD20+ "ghost cells" are often present in grade 2 and 3 lesions.

Lesions in the skin are less often positive for EBER than those in the lungs (23% vs >90%).[2,14,46] In the series from Beaty et al,[14] only 37% of cases were EBV+; none of the plaque lesions were positive for EBV. Multiple cutaneous lesions in the same patient might show different EBV expression. Since plaque lesions and necrotic areas are typically negative for EBER ISH, skin biopsies should include nonulcerated nodules or papules, rather than ulcerated lesions or plaques. Discordant grading between pulmonary and cutaneous LYG lesion has have been observed and might be a potential diagnostic and prognostic pitfall.[47]

Due to inconsistent EBV expression in cutaneous LyG, grading of lesions in the skin is often not encouraged.[1,2,14,26,46,48]

GENETIC AND MOLECULAR FINDINGS

The lack of consistent EBV expression in the cutaneous manifestations of LyG suggests that at least in part cutaneous LyG is an epiphenomenon of the systemic disease and has a different pathobiology.[1,2,14,26,46] Therefore, grading of skin lesions might not be appropriate. Grading of LyG is further complicated by the fact that using PCR-based methods, no significant difference in the percent of EBV was seen when comparing the three grades.[48] Additionally, EBER can be positive in small and large cells, and this factor has not been taken into consideration in the WHO grading. Interestingly, the presence of cutaneous lesions did not coincide directly with the presence of active disease in the lung.

Whether LyG is a type of lymphoma or an inflammatory process still remains somewhat unanswered. Although most grade 2 and all grade 3 cases could be categorized morphologically as "lymphoma," the nosology of grade 1 LyG remains elusive, because atypical cells are scant, necrosis can be absent, and ISH is often negative for EBV. Despite these facts, it is known that cases of grade 1 LyG can further progress with time to grade 2 or 3[26,49,50] and grade 1 lesions can coexist with higher-grade ones. Progression to a higher grade along with variability from site to site suggests that differences in grades may be more a reflection of sampling inequities or variation in stage at presentation rather than an indication of differences in the nature of the disease.[1,51]

Clonality studies by PCR reveal clonal populations of B-cells in ~25% of cases. The clonality rates correlate with increase in relationship to the histologic grade of LyG (8% grade 1 vs 69% grade 3).[2] Rarely, clonal populations of

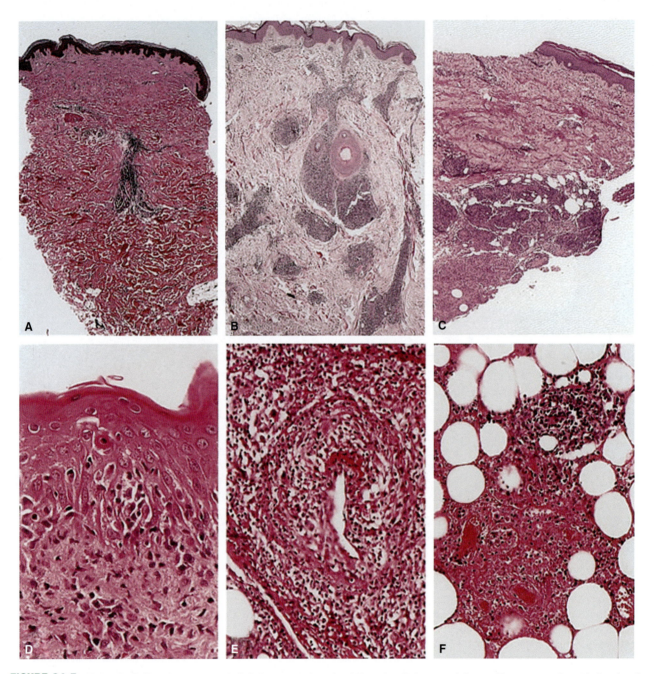

FIGURE 34-5. Histologic findings in cutaneous LyG. A. Low-power view of an indurated, well-demarcated plaque with a sparse angiocentric, lymphocytic infiltrate involving the upper dermis and sparing the deeper dermis and adipose tissue. **B.** An erythematous papule containing a moderate angiocentric and periadnexal lymphocytic infiltrate involving the superficial and deep dermis but sparing the subcutis. **C.** A nodular lesion exhibiting lobular panniculitis. **D.** A papular lesion containing a superficial dermal infiltrate with exocytosis of lymphocytes into the epidermis. This case also manifested a marked deep dermal and subcutaneous lymphohistiocytic infiltrate. EBV was identified in scattered cells. A nodular lesion with lymphohistiocytic panniculitis, vasculitis **(E)**, and focal necrosis **(F)**. (Reprinted from Beaty MW, Toro J, Sorbara L et al. Cutaneous lymphomatoid granulomatosis: correlation of clinical and biologic features. *Am J Surg Pathol.* 2001;25(9):1111-1120, with permission.)

T cells can be identified. These rates are similar in the skin.[14] In LyG patients with EBV-positive biopsies that show clonal B-cell proliferation, therapeutic options including antiviral therapy may be beneficial.[27,52]

The pathogenesis of tissue necrosis and vascular damage in LYG and other EBV+ B-LPDs is hypothesized to be both chemokine-mediated and directly related to invasion of inflammatory cells responding to EBV infection. Prior studies have implicated induction of the CXC chemokines CXCL9 and CXCL10 (formerly known as the monokine induced by IFN-γ [Mig] and IFN-γ IP-10). CXCL9 and CXCL10 localize to the reactive cells in the viable tissue surrounding areas of necrosis, suggesting that cells in the tumor microenvironment and not the malignant cells themselves are the principal source of chemokines, resulting in vascular damage and necrosis. Thus, the host immune response to EBV is a principal cause of the vasculitic changes that are such a typical feature of the disease.[13,53]

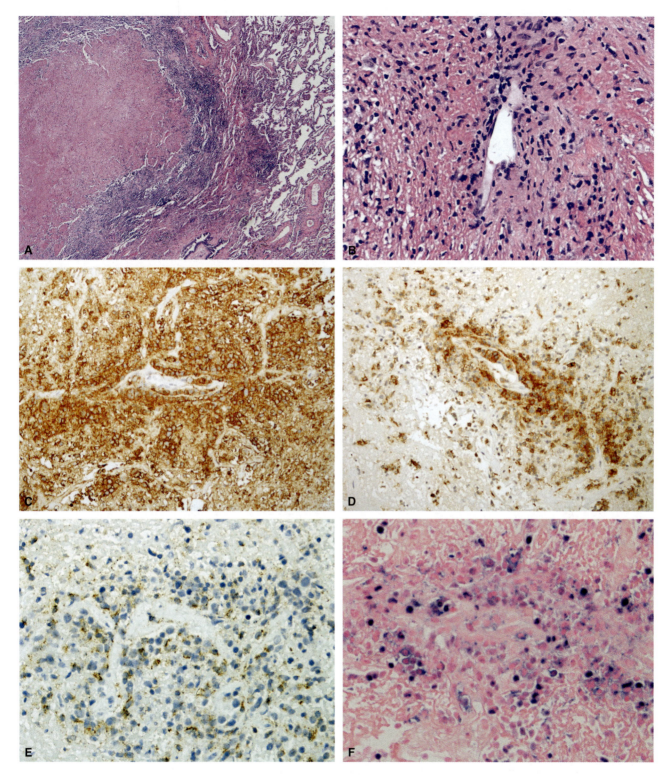

FIGURE 34-6. Lung involvement in LyG. A. Pulmonary infarct (20×). **B.** Angiocentric infiltrates with scattered atypical large cells and fibrinoid necrosis of the vessel (400×). Atypical large cells are positive for CD30 **(C)**, CD20 **(D)**, and the EBV-associated protein LMP1 **(E)** and EBER **(F)**. EBER **(F)** is positive in approximately 20 to 30 cells per high-power field (grade 2).

DIFFERENTIAL DIAGNOSIS

The differential diagnosis for LyG includes inflammatory disorders such as granulomatosis with polyangiitis, EBV-associated B-cell LPDs such as PTLD, senile or age-related B-cell LPD, Hodgkin lymphoma, EBV-positive DLBCL, and T-cell or NK-cell lymphomas (ie, ENKL, nasal type; peripheral T-cell lymphoma, not otherwise specified). Clinicopathologic correlation is imperative. Some important factors that pathologists should consider when diagnosing LyG are as follows: (1) is there a transplant history? (2) is there morphology of DLBCL? and (3) when the histologic

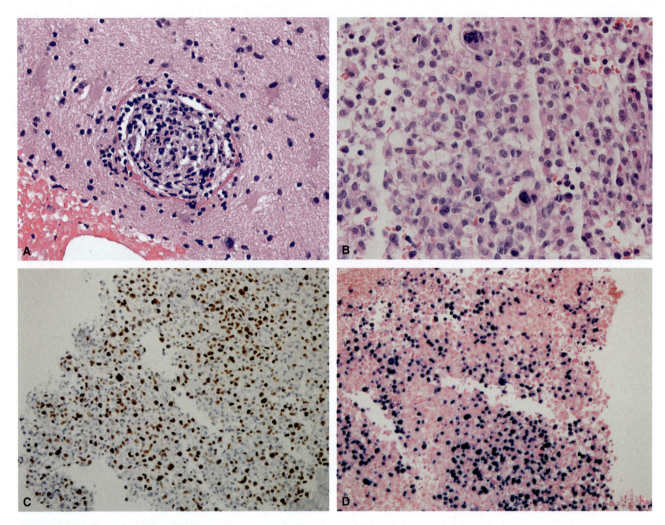

FIGURE 34-7. CNS involvement in LyG. **A.** Grade 1 lesion. **B.** Grade 3 lesion. Higher-grade forms are composed of sheets of large cells frequently showing Hodgkin-like cells. Note elevated Ki67 **(C)** proliferation index in high-grade lesions. EBER **(D)** shows >50+ cells per high-power field.

features of cutaneous LyG are seen, is there coexistent lung disease? If the answer to (1) is yes, then a diagnosis of PTLD is preferred; if the answer to (2) is yes, then one should establish such morphology, as there is significant subjectivity between grade 3 and DLBCL; if the answer to (3) is no, then a diagnosis of LyG should be put into question very strongly! Only rare cases[54,55] of isolated cutaneous LyG have been reported in the absence of lung lesions, acknowledging the fact that cutaneous LyG can precede in time the diagnosis in other organs.

Granulomatosis with polyangiitis (Wegener granulomatosis, WG) shares similar clinical and histologic findings with LyG. Like LyG, WG typically involves the lungs and the skin.[56] The clinical patterns include purpura, papules, vesicles, nodules, and ulcers. While both entities can produce necrosis and granulomatous inflammation, vasculitis in WG is accompanied by a mixed infiltrate of neutrophils, eosinophils, and plasma cells. Intramural neutrophils in LyG vasculitis are not typical. WG lacks atypical B-cells and EBV stains are negative. Additionally, the most typical histologic pattern seen in active WG is leukocytoclastic vasculitis without granulomatosis.[57] Similar to WG, Churg–Strauss disease, and rarely sarcoidosis, can manifest with necrotizing angiitis and lung disease.[58,59]

EBV+ mucocutaneous ulcer (EBV MCU) is characterized by shallow ulcers in the skin and mucosal sites, including the gastrointestinal tract of immunocompromised individuals. There is a polymorphous infiltrate with plasmacytoid-appearing apoptotic cells and large atypical B-cells with a Hodgkin-like appearance. Similar to LyG, angioinvasion and necrosis can also be present. In contrast to EBV MCU, LyG does not involve mucosal sites.[60-62]

EBV+ DLBCL can also present as nodules and plaques. Polymorphous lesions show a mixture of centroblasts, immunoblasts, and Hodgkin-like cells in a background of mixed inflammatory cells. There is frequent necrosis and angiocentricity. Monomorphous lesions exhibit sheets of large cells, more typical of classical DLBCL. There is strong and diffuse expression of EBV. Large cells can be CD30+.[63-66] As opposed to LyG, most cases of EBV-DLBCL show nodal involvement.

Lesions of EBV+ polymorphic PTLD are relatively T-cell "poor," lack angioinvasion/angiodestruction, and show prominent plasmacytoid differentiation. As opposed to LyG, high EBV viremia is typical.[5] Cases with overlap have been reported.[22]

Angiocentricity and angiodestruction can also be seen in ENKL, primary cutaneous γδ T-cell lymphoma (PCGDL), and other T-cell LPDs (eg, transformed mycosis fungoides). Similar to LyG, ENKL is also associated with EBV expression but is more frequent in the upper aerodigestive tract and orbit and rarely involves the lungs. Nodular and ulcerated lesions are typical, but the immunophenotype reveals strong CD56 and cytoplasmic CD3ε expression. Cytotoxic markers (TIA-1, perforin, granzyme B) are also positive. Some of the preliminary studies on cutaneous LyG did note an increased number of NK cells, findings that have not been observed since.[67]

PCGDL shows γδ TCR expression and typically lacks EBV.

CAPSULE SUMMARY

- LyG is a very rare angiocentric and angiodestructive EBV-associated B-cell LPD with a predilection for the lungs, CNS, and, less frequently, the skin.
- **Clinical findings in the skin:** Dermal or subcutaneous nodules, papules, and plaques. Ulceration is seen in about a third of the cases.
- **Skin histology:** Periadnexal and/or angiocentric lymphocytic or lymphohistiocytic infiltrates, with varying number of large atypical cells, angiodestruction, and necrosis. Multinucleate giant cells might be seen.
- **Immunophenotype:** Large atypical CD20+ EBER+ B-cells and background CD3+ T-cells.
- Histologic grading is based on the number of large atypical EBER+ cells.

References

1. Katzenstein AL, Doxtader E, Narendra S. Lymphomatoid granulomatosis: insights gained over 4 decades. *Am J Surg Pathol*. 2010;34(12):e35-e48.
2. Song JY, Pittaluga S, Dunleavy K, et al. Lymphomatoid granulomatosis—a single institute experience: pathologic findings and clinical correlations. *Am J Surg Pathol*. 2015;39(2):141-156.
3. Pittaluga S, Wilson WH, Jaffe ES. *Lymphomatoid Granulomatosis*. 4th ed. International Agency for Research on Cancer; 2008.
4. Gru AA, Jaffe ES. Cutaneous EBV-related lymphoproliferative disorders. *Semin Diagn Pathol*. 2017;34(1):60-75. doi:10.1053/j.semdp.2016.11.003
5. Srivali N, Thongprayoon C, Cheungpasitporn W, Ungprasert P. Lymphomatoid granulomatosis mimicking vasculitis. *Ann Hematol*. 2016;95(2):345-346. doi:10.1007/s00277-015-2507-8
6. Liebow AA, Carrington CR, Friedman PJ. Lymphomatoid granulomatosis. *Hum Pathol*. 1972;3(4):457-558.
7. Seckin D. Cutaneous lymphoproliferative disorders in organ transplant recipients: update 2014. *G Ital Dermatol Venereol*. 2014;149(4):401-408.
8. Taniere P, Thivolet-Bejui F, Vitrey D, et al. Lymphomatoid granulomatosis—a report on four cases: evidence for B phenotype of the tumoral cells. *Eur Respir J*. 1998;12(1):102-106.
9. Hall LD, Eminger LA, Hesterman KS, et al. Epstein–Barr virus—dermatologic associations and implications, Part I: mucocutaneous manifestations of Epstein–Barr virus and nonmalignant disorders. *J Am Acad Dermatol*. 2015;72(1):1-19.
10. Sathishkumar D, Gach JE, Ogboli M, et al. Cartilage hair hypoplasia with cutaneous lymphomatoid granulomatosis. *Clin Exp Dermatol*. 2018;43(6):713-717. doi:10.1111/ced.13543
11. Murphy GF, Harrist TJ, Sato S, et al. Microvascular injury in lymphomatoid granulomatosis involving the skin. An ultrastructural study. *Arch Dermatol*. 1981;117(12):804-808.
12. Savoia P, Novelli M, Bertero M, et al. Adhesion molecules in lymphomatoid granulomatosis. *Dermatology*. 1994;189(1):9-15.
13. Teruya-Feldstein J, Jaffe ES, Burd PR, et al. The role of Mig, the monokine induced by interferon-gamma, and IP-10, the interferon-gamma-inducible protein-10, in tissue necrosis and vascular damage associated with Epstein–Barr virus-positive lymphoproliferative disease. *Blood*. 1997;90(10):4099-4105.
14. Beaty MW, Toro J, Sorbara L, et al. Cutaneous lymphomatoid granulomatosis: correlation of clinical and biologic features. *Am J Surg Pathol*. 2001;25(9):1111-1120.
15. Eminger LA, Hall LD, Hesterman KS, et al. Epstein–Barr virus—dermatologic associations and implications: part II. Associated lymphoproliferative disorders and solid tumors. *J Am Acad Dermatol*. 2015;72(1):21-34.
16. Rysgaard CD, Stone MS. Lymphomatoid granulomatosis presenting with cutaneous involvement: a case report and review of the literature. *J Cutan Pathol*. 2015;42(3):188-193.
17. Kempf W, Kazakov DV, Mitteldorf C. Cutaneous lymphomas—an update, Part 2: B-cell lymphomas and related conditions. *Am J Dermatopathol*. 2014;36(3):197-208.
18. Magro CM, Tawfik NH, Crowson AN. Lymphomatoid granulomatosis. *Int J Dermatol*. 1994;33(3):157-160.
19. Minars N, Kay S, Escobar MR. Lymphomatoid granulomatosis of the skin. A new clinocopathologic entity. *Arch Dermatol*. 1975;111(4):493-496.
20. Kuriyama S, Majima Y, Egawa Y, Suzuki Y, Moriki T, Tokura Y. Cutaneous lymphomatoid granulomatosis with long-term absence of lung involvement. *J Dermatol*. 2019;46(2):e69-e70. doi:10.1111/1346-8138.14548
21. Takeshita M, Akamatsu M, Ohshima K, et al. Angiocentric immunoproliferative lesions of the lymph node. *Am J Clin Pathol*. 1996;106(1):69-77.
22. Kwon EJ, Katz KA, Draft KS, et al. Posttransplantation lymphoproliferative disease with features of lymphomatoid granulomatosis in a lung transplant patient. *J Am Acad Dermatol*. 2006;54(4):657-663.
23. Park JH, Lee DY, Ko YH. Cutaneous lesion of lymphomatoid granulomatosis in a Korean woman with secondary myelofibrosis. *J Dermatol*. 2011;38(10):1012-1014.
24. Sebire NJ, Haselden S, Malone M, et al. Isolated EBV lymphoproliferative disease in a child with Wiskott–Aldrich syndrome manifesting as cutaneous lymphomatoid granulomatosis and responsive to anti-CD20 immunotherapy. *J Clin Pathol*. 2003;56(7):555-557.
25. Tas S, Simonart T, Dargent J, et al. Primary and isolated cutaneous lymphomatoid granulomatosis following heart-lung transplantation. *Ann Dermatol Venereol*. 2000;127(5):488-491.
26. Katzenstein AL, Carrington CB, Liebow AA. Lymphomatoid granulomatosis: a clinicopathologic study of 152 cases. *Cancer*. 1979;43(1):360-373.
27. McNiff JM, Cooper D, Howe G, et al. Lymphomatoid granulomatosis of the skin and lung. An angiocentric T-cell-rich B-cell lymphoproliferative disorder. *Arch Dermatol*. 1996;132(12):1464-1470.

28. Wood ML, Harrington CI, Slater DN, et al. Cutaneous lymphomatoid granulomatosis: a rare cause of recurrent skin ulceration. *Br J Dermatol*. 1984;110(5):619-625.
29. Akagi M, Taniguchi S, Ozaki M, et al. Necrobiosis-lipoidica-like skin manifestation in lymphomatoid granulomatosis (Liebow). *Dermatol*. 1987;174(2):84-92.
30. Carlson KC, Gibson LE. Cutaneous signs of lymphomatoid granulomatosis. *Arch Dermatol*. 1991;127(11):1693-1698.
31. Brodell RT, Miller CW, Eisen AZ. Cutaneous lesions of lymphomatoid granulomatosis. *Arch Dermatol*. 1986;122(3):303-306.
32. Torrelo A, Martin M, Rocamora A, et al. Lymphomatoid granulomatosis presenting as angioedema. *Postgrad Med J*. 1992;68(799):366-368.
33. Fischer R, Shaath T, Meade C, et al. An eschar and violaceous nodules as the presenting signs of lymphomatoid granulomatosis. *Dermatol Online J*. 2014;20(11).
34. Tacke ZC, Eikelenboom MJ, Vermeulen RJ, et al. Childhood lymphomatoid granulomatosis: a report of 2 cases and review of the literature. *J Pediatr Hematol Oncol*. 2014;36(7):e416-e422.
35. Connors W, Griffiths C, Patel J, et al. Lymphomatoid granulomatosis associated with azathioprine therapy in Crohn disease. *BMC Gastroenterol*. 2014;14:127.
36. Ochi N, Yamane H, Yamagishi T, et al. Methotrexate-induced lymphoproliferative disease: Epstein–Barr virus-associated lymphomatoid granulomatosis. *J Clin Oncol*. 2013;31(20):e348-e350.
37. Yamakawa T, Kurosawa M, Yonezumi M, et al. Methotrexate-related lymphomatoid granulomatosis successfully treated with discontinuation of methotrexate and radiotherapy to brain. *[Rinsho ketsueki] Jpn J Clin Hematol*. 2014;55(3):321-326.
38. Yazdi AS, Metzler G, Weyrauch S, et al. Lymphomatoid granulomatosis induced by imatinib-treatment. *Arch Dermatol*. 2007;143(9):1222-1223.
39. Messana K, Marburger T, Bergfeld W. EBV-negative cutaneous lymphomatoid granulomatosis with concomitant EBV-positive pulmonary involvement: a potential diagnostic and prognostic pitfall. *Am J Dermatopathol*. Published online ahead of print August 21, 2014. doi:10.1097/DAD.0000000000000198
40. Pollack K, Guffey D, & Gru AA. Necrotic plaque on the distal nose with diffuse crateriform nodules. *JAMA Dermatol*. 2019;155(1):113-114. doi:10.1001/jamadermatol.2018.2552
41. Melani C, Roschewski M, Pittaluga S, et al. Phase II study of interferon-alpha and DA-EPOCH+/−R in lymphomatoid granulomatosis [abstract]. *Blood*. 2018;132(suppl 1). Abstract 785.
42. Chavez JC, Sandoval-Sus J, Horna P, et al. Lymphomatoid granulomatosis: a single institution experience and review of the literature. *Clin Lymphoma Myeloma Leuk*. 2016;16(suppl):S170-S174.
43. Aoki T, Harada Y, Matsubara E, et al. Long-term remission after multiple relapses in an elderly patient with lymphomatoid granulomatosis after rituximab and high-dose cytarabine chemotherapy without stem-cell transplantation. *J Clin Oncol*. 2013;31(22):e390-e393.
44. James WD, Odom RB, Katzenstein AL. Cutaneous manifestations of lymphomatoid granulomatosis. Report of 44 cases and a review of the literature. *Arch Dermatol*. 1981;117(4):196-202.
45. Lipford EH Jr, Margolick JB, Longo DL, et al. Angiocentric immunoproliferative lesions: a clinicopathologic spectrum of post-thymic T-cell proliferations. *Blood*. 1988;72(5):1674-1681.
46. Angel CA, Slater DN, Royds JA, et al. Epstein–Barr virus in cutaneous lymphomatoid granulomatosis. *Histopathology*. 1994;25(6):545-548.
47. Yang M, Rosenthal AC, Ashman JB, Yang M. "The role and pitfall of F18-FDG PET/CT in surveillance of high grade pulmonary lymphomatoid granulomatosis." *Curr Probl Diagn Radiol*. 2021;50(3):443-449. doi:10.1067/j.cpradiol.2019.02.002
48. Katzenstein AL, Peiper SC. Detection of Epstein–Barr virus genomes in lymphomatoid granulomatosis: analysis of 29 cases by the polymerase chain reaction technique. *Mod Pathol*. 1990;3(4):435-441.
49. Koss MN, Hochholzer L, Langloss JM, et al. Lymphomatoid granulomatosis: a clinicopathologic study of 42 patients. *Pathology*. 1986;18(3):283-288.
50. Guinee DG Jr, Perkins SL, Travis WD, et al. Proliferation and cellular phenotype in lymphomatoid granulomatosis: implications of a higher proliferation index in B cells. *Am J Surg Pathol*. 1998;22(9):1093-1100.
51. Nair BD, Joseph MG, Catton GE, et al. Radiation therapy in lymphomatoid granulomatosis. *Cancer*. 1989;64(4):821-824.
52. Gangar P, Venkatarajan S. Granulomatous lymphoproliferative disorders: granulomatous slack skin and lymphomatoid granulomatosis. *Dermatol Clin*. 2015;33(3):489-496. doi:10.1016/j.det.2015.03.013
53. Melani C, Jaffe ES, Wilson WH. Pathobiology and treatment of lymphomatoid granulomatosis, a rare EBV-driven disorder. *Blood*. 2020;135(16):1344-1352. doi:10.1182/blood.2019000933
54. Tawfik NH, Magro CM, Crowson AN, et al. Lymphomatoid granulomatosis presenting as a solitary cutaneous lesion. *Int J Dermatol*. 1994;33(3):188-189.
55. Tong MM, Cooke B, Barnetson RS. Lymphomatoid granulomatosis. *J Am Acad Dermatol*. 1992;27(5 pt 2):872-876.
56. Gibson LE. Granulomatous vasculitides and the skin. *Dermatol Clin*. 1990;8(2):335-345.
57. Frances C, Du LT, Piette JC, et al. Wegener's granulomatosis. Dermatological manifestations in 75 cases with clinicopathologic correlation. *Arch Dermatol*. 1994;130(7):861-867.
58. Poonawalla T, Colome-Grimmer MI, Kelly B. Ulcerative sarcoidosis in the legs with granulomatous vasculitis. *Clin Exp Dermatol*. 2008;33(3):282-286.
59. Wei CH, Huang YH, Shih YC, et al. Sarcoidosis with cutaneous granulomatous vasculitis. *Australas J Dermatol*. 2010;51(3):198-201.
60. Dojcinov SD, Venkataraman G, Raffeld M, et al. EBV positive mucocutaneous ulcer—a study of 26 cases associated with various sources of immunosuppression. *Am J Surg Pathol*. 2010;34(3):405-417.
61. Hart M, Thakral B, Yohe S, et al. EBV-positive mucocutaneous ulcer in organ transplant recipients: a localized indolent posttransplant lymphoproliferative disorder. *Am J Surg Pathol*. 2014;38(11):1522-1529.
62. McGinness JL, Spicknall KE, Mutasim DF. Azathioprine-induced EBV-positive mucocutaneous ulcer. *J Cutan Pathol*. 2012;39(3):377-381.
63. Rausch T, Cairoli A, Benhattar J, et al. EBV+ cutaneous B-cell lymphoproliferation of the leg in an elderly patient

with mycosis fungoides and methotrexate treatment. *APMIS*. 2013;121(1):79-84.
64. Suarez AL, Pulitzer M, Horwitz S, et al. Primary cutaneous B-cell lymphomas, Part I: clinical features, diagnosis, and classification. *J Am Acad Dermatol*. 2013;69(3):329.e1–329.e13; quiz 341-342.
65. Swerdlow SH, Quintanilla-Martinez L, Willemze R, et al. Cutaneous B-cell lymphoproliferative disorders: report of the 2011 society for hematopathology/European association for haematopathology workshop. *Am J Clin Pathol*. 2013;139(4):515-535.
66. Hristov AC. Primary cutaneous diffuse large B-cell lymphoma, leg type: diagnostic considerations. *Arch Pathol Lab Med*. 2012;136(8):876-881.
67. Rooney N, Slater D, Clark A, et al. Natural killer cells in lymphomatoid granulomatosis. *Br J Dermatol*. 1984;110(2):248-249.

CHAPTER 35

Mucocutaneous EBV- and HHV-8 associated lymphoproliferative disorders in acquired immunodeficiency

Alejandro A. Gru, Melissa Pulitzer, and András Schaffer

INTRODUCTION

This chapter reviews mucocutaneous lymphoproliferative disorders (LPDs) in the setting of various types of acquired immunosuppression, including iatrogenic immunosuppression, human immunodeficiency virus (HIV) infection, and immunosenescence in elderly. These entities are commonly linked to Epstein-Barr virus (EBV) and less frequently to human herpes virus 8 (HHV-8), although there are cases without known viral etiology. The clinicopathological spectrum of these entities ranges from reactive lymphoid hyperplasia to indolent or even aggressive lymphomas. The EBV-driven plasmablastic lymphoma, is discussed under systemic B-cell lymphomas (Chapter 39).

CUTANEOUS POSTTRANSPLANT LYMPHOPROLIFERATIVE DISORDERS

Definition

EBV-associated cutaneous posttransplant lymphoproliferative disorders (PTLDs) occur in solid organ and less frequently in hematopoietic stem cell transplant patients. Their clinical course varies from lymphoid hyperplasia to aggressive lymphomas that are typically more aggressive than their counterparts in immune-competent individuals. Association with EBV viremia is common. In the skin, they frequently present as tumors or plaques and histological features reminiscent of primary cutaneous B- and T-cell lymphomas.

Epidemiology

PTLDs occur in 1% to 16% of solid organ transplantation (SOT) recipients and the majority (70%) of them are EBV related. The risk of PTLD correlates with the level and duration of immunosuppression required for the transplanted organ, as well as the age and EBV serostatus of the recipient.[1-4] EBV-naive patients who acquire a primary EBV infection after transplantation are at the highest risk for developing PTLD.[5,6] Furthermore, the use of T-cell depleting agents such as OKT3 and polyclonal antithymocyte globulins are associated with PTLD after SOT.[7] In contrast, alemtuzumab, a monoclonal antibody directed against the CD52 surface marker found on B and T cells and other leukocytes has not been clearly associated with an increased risk of PTLD. Thus, additional depletion of B cells may reduce the risk of B-cell proliferative disease.[8]

In a single center study, the incidence of PTLD was 0.8% for bone marrow transplants, 1.4% for renal transplants, 1.8% for cardiac transplants, 4.5% for lung transplants, and up to 10% in combined heart and lung transplant recipients.[9] Since the rates of PTLD are higher in cardiac and lung transplant recipients, many of whom are pediatric patients, cutaneous PTLD has been described with some frequency in childhood.[10-12]

Primary cutaneous PTLD is extraordinarily rare. Data from two transplant centers in France reported 7.5 primary cutaneous PTLD/1000 total primary cutaneous lymphomas/year, and 0.7 cutaneous PTLD/1000 SOT (excluding intestinal-transplant patients)/year.[13] A subgroup of cases shows banal plasmacytoid morphology, immunoglobulin light-chain expression, and presence or absence of detectable EBV. This primary cutaneous plasmacytoma-like PTLD is a subtype of monomorphic B-cell PTLD.[14-20]

Clinical Presentation

While PTLD may occur any time after SOT, the risk of developing PTLD is the highest in the first year after transplantation. Extranodal dissemination of PTLD is frequent and typically involves the central nervous system, lung, and liver.

Skin involvement is less common and often presents in analogy to primary cutaneous lymphomas. B-cell cutaneous PTLD presents as single or multiple macules/patches

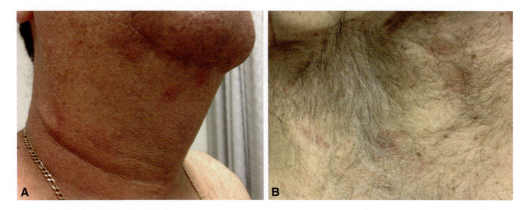

FIGURE 35-1. Cutaneous monomorphic PTLD—Primary cutaneous plasmacytoma-like PTLD. Red to violaceous macules and plaques on the neck and chest in a patient on cyclosporine immunosuppression and 15 years following kidney transplantation (**A** and **B**). (Photo courtesy of Dr. Ellen Kim, Hospital of University of Pennsylvania, Philadelphia, PA.)

(Fig. 35-1A and B) or nodules, with or without ulceration, and sometimes as tumors. The lesions are typically located on the legs, face, oral mucosa, and scalp.[13] A single case with intertriginous erythematous plaques had been also described.[15] T-cell PTLD cases diagnosed as mycosis fungoides-like PTLD usually present as infiltrated plaques in the trunk and upper and lower extremities, followed by the buttocks and the face. Some cases presented as papules, alopecia, and comedo-like lesion. Cases diagnosed as anaplastic large cell lymphoma PTLD presented as tumors or plaques with frequent ulceration. The lesions were typically located in the extremities, face, buttocks, and trunk. Rare cases of Sezary syndrome usually present as generalized erythroderma.

Histology

Most of noncutaneous PTLD are of B cell origin, and 12.5% to 14% of cases exhibit a T-cell phenotype.[9,21] Seckin et al showed that EBV was present in 16.6% of T-cell PTLDs and 90.9% of B-cell PTLDs in cutaneous sites.[13] A large meta-analysis from Herreman et al showed that only a third of T-cell PTLD are related to EBV.[22]

PTLD has been grouped by the 2017 World Health Organization (WHO) Classification into six major morphological categories: plasmacytic hyperplasia, infectious mononucleosis-like PTLD, florid follicular hyperplasia, polymorphic PTLD, monomorphic PTLD and classic Hodgkin lymphoma-like PTLD.[23]

Approximately 22% of PTLD cases show cutaneous involvement, mostly in the setting of renal transplantation.[1] A significant portion of cutaneous cases (30%-60%) are of T-cell phenotype.[24-30] Among cutaneous B-cell PTLDs, most cases were designated as diffuse large B-cell lymphoma (Fig. 35-2) or plasmacytoma[1,31] (Figs. 35-1 and 35-3), some cases were classified as plasmablastic lymphoma,[10,12] and less frequently lymphomatoid granulomatosis (LyG).[13] Cutaneous T-cell PTLDs were typically classified as mycosis fungoides, cutaneous anaplastic large cell lymphoma (C-ALCL), and rarely adult T-cell leukemia / lymphoma, lymphomatoid papulosis (Fig. 35-4), and cutaneous peripheral T-cell lymphoma.[13] Rare cases in the skin have shown an ambiguous B- and T-cell phenotype mimicking mycosis fungoides.[11] A case with atypical Hodgkin cells and Reed-Sternberg-like cells had been also described.[32]

Immunophenotype

The immunophenotype varies according to the PTLD subtype. Primary cutaneous plasmacytoma-like PTLD shows strong CD79 expression, plasma cell marker expression (CD138, CD38), light chain restriction, d EBER positivity, and lack of CD20 and HHV-8 expression (Fig. 35-3). Diffuse large B-cell lymphoma (DLBCL)-PTLD is positive for B-cell markers (CD20, CD19, CD79a, PAX5) and shows a nongerminal center phenotype (MUM1+, variable BCL-6, CD10−) (Fig. 35-2). Plasmablastic lymphomas are negative for B-cell surface antigens (CD20, CD19) and positive for plasma cell markers (CD138, CD38, CD79a, MUM1) and have a very high Ki67 labeling index (>90%).[1,4,22,28] EBV/EBER expression is seen in almost all B cell–type PTLDs corresponding to DLBCL, plasmacytoma, plasmablastic lymphoma, and LyG.[13,31]

Mycosis fungoides–like PTLD characteristically shows a CD4+ phenotype, with expression of CD2, CD3, and CD5 but variable loss of CD7. C-ALCL-like PTLD is often CD4+ as well, with variable expression of CD3, CD5, and CD7. Most cases are positive for CD2 and CD30. Some cases can be EMA positive. C-ALCL-like PTLD characteristically shows expression of the cytotoxic markers TIA-1 and Granzyme-B. Rare cases show EBV/EBER expression.[13]

Genetics

Early PTLD lesions are polyclonal, while monomorphic PTLDs exhibit clonal B-cell or T-cell gene rearrangement. Polymorphic PTLDs are usually monoclonal and rarely oligoclonal. Several nonrandom chromosomal alterations involving lymphoma-associated oncogenes such as BCL-1, BCL-2, MYC, RAS, and TP53 had been described in polymorphic and monomorphic PTLD but not in early PTLD lesions.[33,34] The presence of somatic hypermutation within the BCL-6 gene had been associated with shortened disease survival and refractoriness to reduced immunosuppression or surgical excision.[35]

Therapy

Early lesions are most often seen in children or young adults and respond well to immunosuppression reduction.[36] In contrast, monomorphic PTLD might not respond to decrease

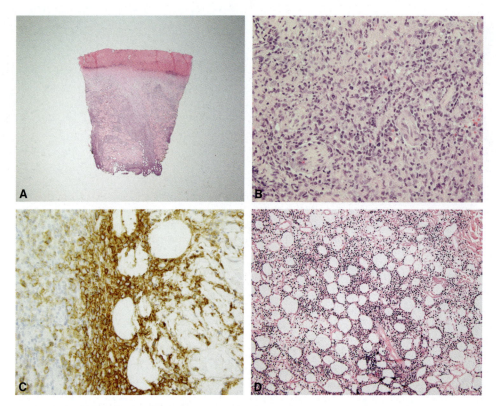

FIGURE 35-2. Cutaneous monomorphic PTLD—Diffuse large B-cell lymphoma. The biopsy shows a deep dermal-based infiltrate with sparing of the epidermis (**A**, 20×). The infiltrate is composed of sheets of large cells with vesicular nuclei and prominent nucleoli (**B**, 200×). The large cells are diffusely positive for CD20 **(C)** and EBER **(D)**.

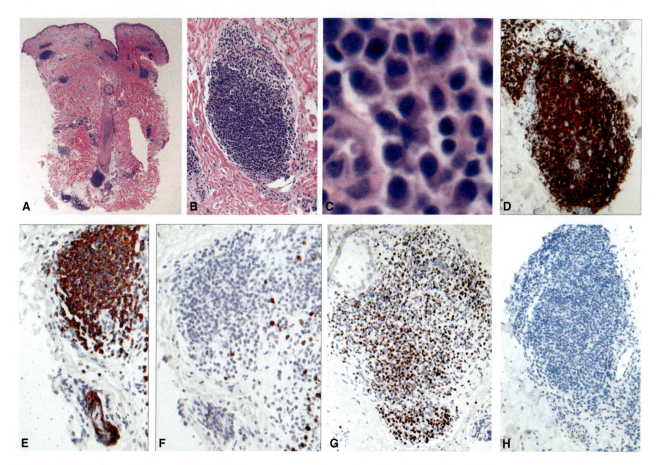

FIGURE 35-3. Cutaneous Monomorphic PTLD—Primary cutaneous plasmacytoma-like PTLD. A–C. Superficial and deep dermal perivascular infiltrates without epidermotropism. The infiltrates are composed of monotonous, benign-appearing plasma cells. Plasma cells express CD79a **(D)** and show a markedly elevated lambda **(E)** to kappa **(F)** ratio. EBER stains the majority of plasma cells **(G)**. HHV-8 stain is negative **(H)**.

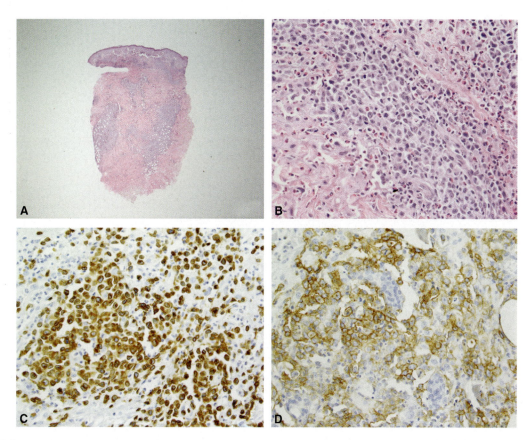

FIGURE 35-4. Lymphomatoid papulosis (LyP) arising from donor-derived lymphocytes. There is an epidermal and dermal-based infiltrate with areas of epidermotropism (**A**, 20×). Large cells are present in the dermis with a background rich in acute inflammatory cells and eosinophils (**B**, 200×). The infiltrate is composed of T cells, which are positive for CD3 **(C)** and CD30 **(D)**.

in immune suppression and require cytotoxic therapies. In localized disease, radiation or surgical excision may lead to remission. Other treatment strategies include antiviral therapy, systemic chemotherapy, and rituximab. In general, PTLDs presenting in the skin usually respond well to reduction of immunosuppression with topical Imiquimod (5% cream)[15] and show a favorable prognosis. However, aggressive neoplasms warrant additional therapy like chemotherapy and antiviral therapy.[9,14,37]

EBV+ CHRONIC MUCOCUTANEOUS ULCER

Definition

EBV-positive chronic mucocutaneous ulcer (EBVMCU) is defined as solitary, sharply defined ulcerative lesions in the skin, oral cavity, or gastrointestinal tract in patients with iatrogenic or age-related immunosuppression, although cases in solid organ transplant recipients had been described. EBVMCU is characterized by indolent B-cell proliferation, Hodgkin-like phenotype, lack of EBV-DNA in peripheral blood, and self-limited, indolent clinical course.

Epidemiology

EBVMCU had been described in patients with immunosuppression secondary to azathioprine, cyclosporine, or methotrexate or in patients with age-related immunosenescence.[38-42] Recently, cases have also been reported in patients after solid and allogeneic bone marrow transplantation.[43,44] EBVMCU is slightly more frequent in women with a mean age of 80 years.

Clinical

Patients typically present with solitary, sharply demarcated ulcers in the oropharyngeal mucosa (buccal mucosa, tongue, tonsils) and less frequently in the large bowel, rectum, or skin lesions in the lips, arms, and chest (Fig. 35-5). Isolated regional lymphadenopathy can occur, but systemic adenopathy is never present. Spontaneous resolution of the lesions occurs in approximately 25% of cases. Disease-associated mortality had not yet been reported.[41]

Histology

Microscopic examination shows shallow, sharply circumscribed mucosal or cutaneous ulcers with adjacent mucosal or epidermal acanthosis including pseudoepitheliomatous changes. The underlying polymorphous infiltrate includes a mixture of lymphocytes, atypical large B-cell immunoblasts with Hodgkin-like morphology, plasma cells, histiocytes, and eosinophils (Fig. 35-6). The presence of Hodgkin-like cells, plasmacytoid apoptotic cells, and tissue necrosis is pathognomonic. The lesion is usually delineated by a rim

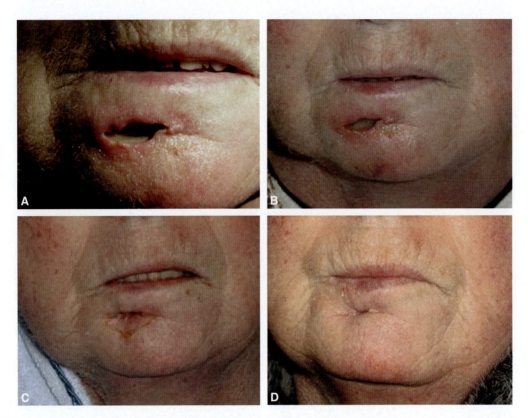

FIGURE 35-5. EBV-positive mucocutaneous ulcer—clinical presentations. EBV-positive mucocutaneous ulcer in a patient treated with methotrexate (MTX) for rheumatoid arthritis. Spontaneous resolution after withdrawal of MTX. **A.** At presentation the ulcer had perforated from the buccal sulcus onto the skin surface of the lower lip. Ulcer healing **(B)** 2 weeks, **(C)** 4 weeks, and **(D)** 8 weeks after withdrawal of MTX. (Obtained with permission. Dojcinov SD, Venkataraman G, Raffeld M, Pittaluga S, Jaffe ES. EBV positive mucocutaneous ulcer--a study of 26 cases associated with various sources of immunosuppression. Am J Surg Pathol. 2010;34(3):405-417.)

of small lymphocytes.[41,42,45,46] Cases with small lymphocytic infiltration without atypical lymphocytes mimicking reactive ulceration had been described (Fig. 35-8).[47]

Immunohistochemistry

Large cells are EBER+, PAX-5+, OCT-2+, MUM-1+, BOB-1+/−, CD45+/− (Fig. 35-7). Reduced or absent expression of CD20 can be seen in a third of cases. The Hodgkin-like cells are CD30+ with CD15 coexpression in 43% of cases. Rimming reactive lymphocytes are CD3+ T cells. The small lymphocyte variant of EBVMCU shows EBER positivity in small B cells (Fig. 35-8).

Genetics

B- and T-cell clonality are present in 39% and 38% of cases, respectively.

Differential Diagnosis

Ulcerating cutaneous and mucosal lesions might be encountered in advanced stages of classical Hodgkin lymphoma (cHL), DLBCL, and LyG. In contrast to cHL, EBVMCU shows plasmacytoid apoptotic cells, tissue necrosis, and CD30+CD15- large cells that are more frequently positive for CD45 and B-cell markers. Perilesional expansion of CD8+ T cells is more characteristic of EBVMCU than cHL.[41,44,48-50] LyG is an angiocentric and angiodestructive lymphoproliferative disease of B-cell origin. The infiltrate has a significant histiocytic and T-cell component along with scattered atypical EBER+ B cells.

METHOTREXATE-ASSOCIATED B-CELL LYMPHOPROLIFERATIVE DISORDERS

Definition

The WHO Classification of Hematological Malignancies recognizes a subset of LPDs that develop in patients on chronic methotrexate (MTX) therapy. Majority of the nodal MTX-LPDs are B-cell lymphomas,[51] both EBV related and unrelated, present as DLBCL,[52] and less frequently Hodgkin lymphoma, LyG,[53] and other entities. MTX-associated T-cell LPDs are rare and include angioimmunoblastic T-cell lymphoma (AITL),[54] extranodal NK/T-cell lymphoma,[55] and peripheral T-cell lymphoma not otherwise specified.[56]

Cutaneous MTX-LPDs are rare and mostly manifests as multiple plaques or tumors with ulceration on the lower legs, DLBCL, and rarely as subcutaneous panniculitis-like T-cell lymphoma (SPTCL).[57] Differentiation of MTX-LPD from primary cutaneous B-cell lymphomas, particularly DLBCL leg type, primary cutaneous follicle center cell lymphoma (PCFCL), EBV+ DLBCL of elderly, and nodal DLBCL is extremely important as MTX-LPD may show spontaneous regression after the withdrawal of MTX therapy.[58,59]

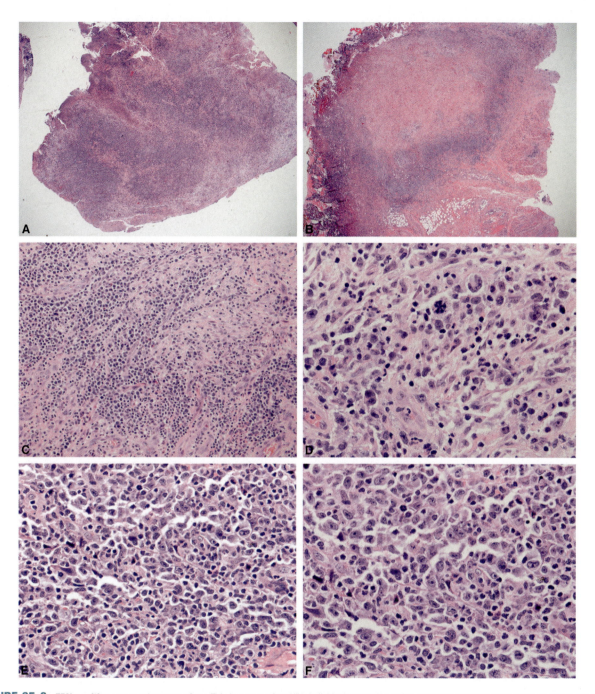

FIGURE 35-6. EBV-positive mucocutaneous ulcer. This is a case of an HIV+ individual presenting with a nonhealing ulcer in the rectum (**A** and **B**, 20×). The surface mucosa is ulcerated with no residual mucosal surface. Areas of necrosis with a rim of lymphoid cells at the periphery of the sharply demarcated ulcer are notable (**C**, 200×). Ulcer bed with mixed inflammatory cells including histiocytes and eosinophils (**D**, 400×). Numerous immunoblasts, histiocytes, and Hodgkin-like cells are seen. Mitotic figures are also appreciated (**E** and **F**, 400×). Numerous immunoblasts and large cells with vesicular nuclei and prominent nucleoli are present. Admixed neutrophils are also present. (Obtained with permission. Dojcinov SD, Venkataraman G, Raffeld M, Pittaluga S, Jaffe ES. EBV positive mucocutaneous ulcer--a study of 26 cases associated with various sources of immunosuppression. *Am J Surg Pathol.* 2010;34(3):405-417.)

Epidemiology

The association of the immunosuppressive drug methotrexate with B-cell lymphoproliferative disorders (MTX-LPDs) was originally described in 1985, more than 30 years after MTX had been reported to successfully treat rheumatoid arthritis and psoriasis.[58,60-64] Cutaneous MTX-LPD usually develops in elderly (mean 76 years old), slightly more commonly in women, and approximately 4 years after the initiation of MTX treatment.[58] Most patients are treated for rheumatoid arthritis and less commonly for lupus, dermatomyositis, psoriatic arthritis, or juvenile rheumatoid arthritis.[58]

Clinical

Approximately 50% of the patients with cutaneous MTX-LPD have multiple skin lesions. The lesions typically present as plaques, tumors, and nodules in the head and neck, trunk, or extremities (Fig. 35-9).[41,58,62]

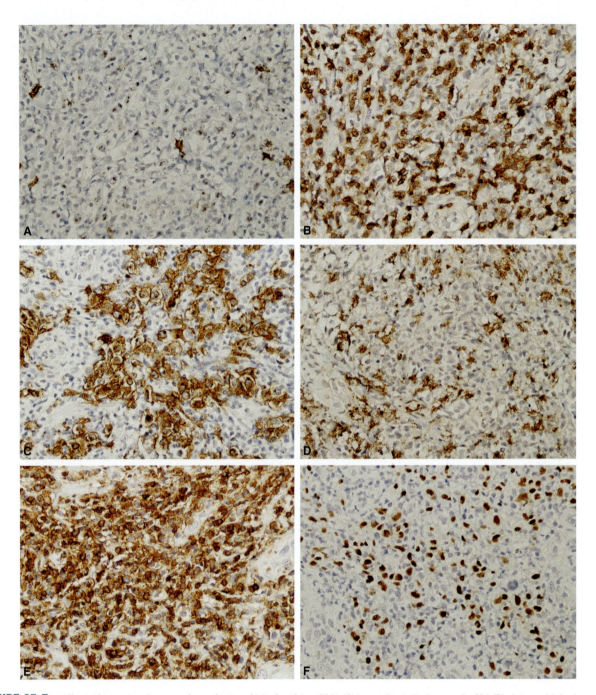

FIGURE 35-7. EBV-positive mucocutaneous ulcer—immunohistochemistry. CD20 **(A)** is negative in the larger cells. CD3 **(B)** shows a rich background of small T cells. CD30 **(C)** is diffusely positive in the larger cells. CD15 **(D)** is negative. The majority of the lymphocytes are positive for CD45 **(E)**, including the larger cells. PAX5 **(F)** shows a strong pattern of staining among the larger cells. This phenotype differs from cHL in the expression of CD45, the absence of CD15, and the focal strong PAX-5 expression. Similar to cHL large cells in EBVMCU are negative for CD20 and positive for CD30. (Obtained with permission. Dojcinov SD, Venkataraman G, Raffeld M, Pittaluga S, Jaffe ES. EBV positive mucocutaneous ulcer--a study of 26 cases associated with various sources of immunosuppression. *Am J Surg Pathol.* 2010;34(3):405-417.)

Histology

The histological spectrum is broad. The most common presentation (~50% of cases) is that of diffuse large B-cell lymphoma with large immunoblasts-like cells in a sheet-like or, less frequently, perivascular and/or perifollicular distribution (Fig. 35-10). Hodgkin-like cells can be seen in EBV-infected cases.[41,58,62] The histological features of MTX-induced Hodgkin lymphoma, LyG, AITL, and SPTCL are indistinguishable to those seen in immune-competent individuals.

Immunohistochemistry

EBV+ and EBV− cases show significant immunohistochemical staining differences. Lesional cells in EBV-positive diffuse large B-cell lymphoma are CD30+ and MUM1+, with variable loss of B-cell markers CD20 and CD79a. EBV-negative cases lack CD30 but show strong nuclear MYC and FOXP1 expression[65] (Fig. 35-10). BCL-2 and BCL-6 are positive in the majority of the cases, independent of the EBV status. Only a minority of cases showed retained

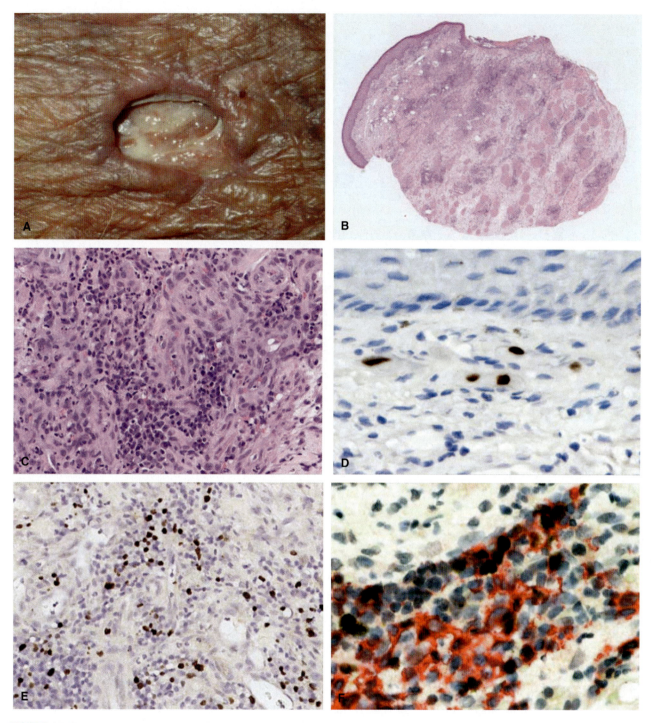

FIGURE 35-8. Small-lymphocyte variant EBV-positive mucocutaneous ulcer. A. Scrotal ulcer in a 77-year-old man treated with prednisone for refractory dermatitis herpetiformis. **B.** Punch biopsy shows superficial and deep perivascular inflammation in the periphery of the ulcer. **C.** Small lymphocyte infiltration, mixed with plasma cells and neutrophils. **D.** Rare CMV-positive cells in the superficial dermis next to ulcer. **E.** Small perivascular lymphocytes are positive for EBER. **F.** Double staining of EBER (brown) and CD20 (red). Nuclear EBER positivity is observed in part of small B cells with cytoplasmic CD20 expression. (Reprinted from Fujimoto M, Kaku Y, Hirata M, Usui S, Yamada Y, Haga H. EBV-positive mucocutaneous ulcer with small lymphocytic infiltration mimicking nonspecific ulceration. *Am J Surg Pathol*. 2021;45(5):694-700.)

follicular dendritic cell meshwork by CD35 or CD23/CD21 stains. Hodgkin-like cells and Reed Sternberg cells in MTX-induced Hodgkin lymphoma express CD30, CD15, and the B-cell marker PAX-5. EBER is usually positive. Immunoblasts in MTX-induced LyG also show CD30 and PAX-5 expression along with EBER positivity. According to a single report, malignant T cells in MTX-induced SPTCL show a CD3+CD8+CD8− EBER+ phenotype.[57]

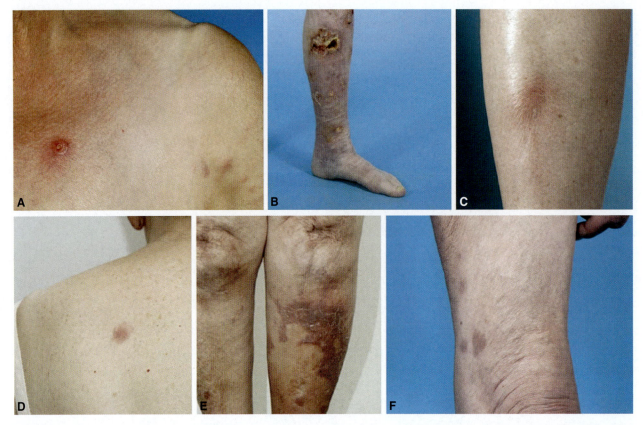

FIGURE 35-9. Cutaneous methotrexate-associated B-cell lymphoproliferative disorder. Clinical findings. **A.** generalized plaques and small tumors, with focal ulceration. **B.** extensive lesions on the lower left leg with marked ulceration. **C.** deep nodules on the right leg clinically resemble erythema nodosum. **D.** small nonulcerating nodules on the trunk and extensive plaques on the left lower leg **(E)**. **F.** multiple small plaques on arms and legs. (Obtained with permission. Koens L, Senff NJ, Vermeer MH, Willemze R, Jansen PM. Methotrexate-associated B-cell lymphoproliferative disorders presenting in the skin: A clinicopathologic and immunophenotypical study of 10 cases. Am J Surg Pathol. 2014;38(7):999-1006.)

Genetics

Nearly all B-cell lymphoma cases, irrespective of EBV status, show a monoclonal rearrangement of the IGH gene.

Differential Diagnosis

Differentiation of EBV⁺ cutaneous MTX-LPD from PCFCL is straightforward. MTX-LPD typically presents as multiple lesions on the leg, often with ulceration. Lesional cells are composed of MUM-1⁺, FOXP-1⁺, BCL-2⁺, EBER⁺ centroblasts with minimal preservation of the FDC meshwork. In contrast, PCFCL manifests on the head and neck (mostly on the scalp) and comprises centrocytes that are negative for BCL-2, MUM-1, and FOXP-1.

Distinction of EBV- cutaneous MTX-LPD from primary cutaneous diffuse large B-cell lymphoma leg type (PCDLBCL-LT) is more challenging. While both cases mostly present in elderly women, most cases of PCDLBCL-LT are unifocal on the lower leg and lack ulceration. Neoplastic cells in PCDLBCL-LT strongly express B-cell markers CD79a or CD20 and are devoid of Hodgkin-like cells or EBV. Despite these differences, a biological overlap between these two entities might exist as PCDLBCL-LT in association with MTX has been previously reported.[61]

Some of the clinicopathological features of cutaneous EBV⁺ MTX-LPD and EBV⁺ MCU overlap, such as reversible clinical course and decreased CD20 expression. Nonetheless, these entities appear to be distinct as EBV⁺ MCU shows solitary sharply circumscribed ulcers as opposed to the multifocality of cutaneous lesions in EBV⁺ MTX-LPD.

Distinction from EBV⁺ DLBCL can be challenging as both entities present on the leg of elderly patients.

Treatment

Discontinuation of MTX, with or without additional radiotherapy, is sufficient to achieve complete resolution in some cases.[51]

CASTLEMAN DISEASE

Definition

Castleman disease (CD) (angiolymphoid follicular hyperplasia, giant lymph node hyperplasia) is a rare B-cell lymphoproliferative disease characterized by lymph node enlargement and vascular hyperplasia.[66] Lymph nodes in the mediastinum or pulmonary hilus are commonly involved.

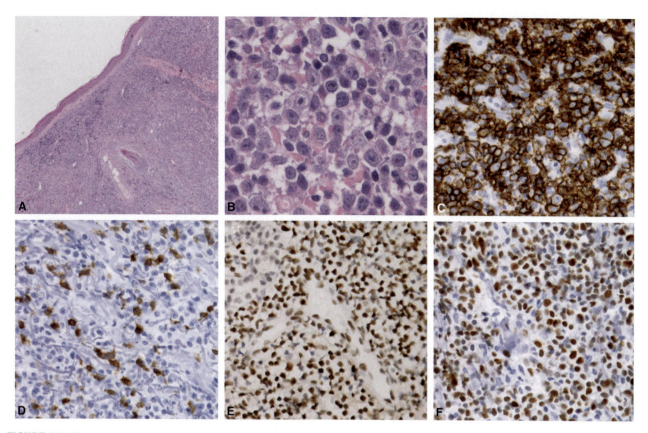

FIGURE 35-10. Cutaneous methotrexate-associated B-cell lymphoproliferative disorder. Histological findings. **A.** Diffuse growth of tumor cells in the dermis. **B.** The tumor cells exhibit an immunoblastic morphology with a large central nucleolus and round nuclear contour. **C.** The tumor cells are CD20 positive. **D.** Only few CD3+ T lymphocytes are present. FOXP1 **(E)** and MYC **(F)** showed diffuse and strong nuclear staining. (Obtained with permission. Koens L, Senff NJ, Vermeer MH, Willemze R, Jansen PM. Methotrexate-associated B-cell lymphoproliferative disorders presenting in the skin: A clinicopathologic and immunophenotypical study of 10 cases. Am J Surg Pathol. 2014;38(7):999-1006.)

There are three clinical subtypes: unicentric, HHV-8 positive multicentric, and HHV-8 negative multicentric CD. Three histological subtypes are recognized: hyaline vascular (HV-CD), plasma cell (PC-CD), and mixed types.[67] CD has been associated with cutaneous lesions including paraneoplastic pemphigus, POEMS syndrome, and amyloidosis. Only few cases of cutaneous CD had been reported. While the clinical course of CD is indolent, patients are at increased risk of developing large B-cell lymphoma, Kaposi sarcoma, and follicular dendritic cell tumors.

Epidemiology

Most cases of CD are reported in HIV-negative patients, only 5% to 10% of patients with CD are HIV infected. Most CD in HIV-infected patients present as HHV-8-positive multicentric CD (MCD).[68,69] HHV-8 positive MCD can be rarely detected in HIV-negative patients as well. HHV-8 is typically negative in localized CD.[70]

Few cases of HHV-8-positive MCD had been described in solid organ transplant patients.[71,72]

Cutaneous involvement had been reported in 11 cases of MCD with a slight female predominance.[73-84] The average age of presentation is 58 years (range: 36 ~ 72 years).[85]

Clinical

Patients with multicentric CD manifest with lymphadenopathies, hyperproteinemia, and hypergammaglobulinemia, and systemic symptoms (fever, weight loss, and anemia) occur. Both the unicentric and multicentric forms of plasma cell CD can be associated with POEMS syndrome (Crow-Fukase syndrome), a rare medical condition characterized by polyneuropathy, organomegaly, endocrinopathy, M-spike, and skin changes.[86] Between 11% to 30% of patients with POEMS have documented CD or Castleman-like changes.[87-89] It is presumed that these numbers can be conservative, as most patients with POEMS do not undergo a lymph node biopsy. A study of 30 patients with POEMS showed that 19 of 32 biopsied lymph nodes showed typical changes of CD.[90]

Patients with CD, especially the multicentric variant, have an increased risk of developing nodal lymphomas.[91] Mantle cell lymphoma, diffuse large B-cell lymphoma, and Hodgkin disease are the most common malignant complications. Cases of CD with associated follicular dendritic cell sarcoma had been also described.[92]

Cutaneous involvement by CD is very rare with less than 15 cases reported in the literature.[73-84] The cutaneous presentation includes multiple erythematous to brownish nodules and plaques predominantly on the back, but involvement of the face, trunk, and extremities had been described (Fig. 35-11). Patients may also present with slowly growing mass, often asymptomatic, or with symptoms that are related to the local mass effect of the lesion.[93]

Besides POEM syndrome, other rare cutaneous manifestations in CD include paraneoplastic pemphigus,[94] Kaposi sarcoma,[95] follicular dendritic cell sarcoma,[96] and HHV-8-positive plasmablastic lymphoma.[95]

Histology

Histologically, CD is subdivided into three forms: hyaline vascular type (90%), plasma cell type (10%), and mixed forms.[67,87-89] The hyaline vascular CD represents 80% to 90% of solitary CD (Fig. 35-11). The plasma cell and mixed CD are less frequent and more commonly seen in the setting of HIV infection and MCD.

The involved skin shows similar features to those present in lymph nodes (Figs. 35-11 and 35-12). The hyaline vascular subtype shows atrophic and hyalinized germinal centers, devoid of centrocytes and centroblasts, and contain prominent follicular dendritic cells, which can show dysplastic or atypical features. Multiple germinal centers can be seen within a follicle with an expanded mantle zone composed of concentric small lymphocytes (onion-skinning). There is increased interfollicular vascularity with hyalinized vessels that often penetrate the germinal centers ("lollipop" lesions). The number of CD123+ plasmacytoid dendritic cells is increased.[79,97]

The plasma cell variant of CD (PC-CD) shows variably hyperplastic germinal centers along with prominent interfollicular vascularity and sheets of usually polyclonal but sometimes monoclonal plasma cells.[79,98] Most cutaneous cases showed plasma cell–rich infiltrates, and only one case presented with hyaline vascular histology.[99]

Immunophenotype

The immunophenotype of CD is similar to that of reactive lymphoid follicles. CD21, CD23, CD35, and CAN.42 highlight expanded follicular dendritic cell meshwork. CD90 or CD105 or α-smooth muscle actin (α-SMA) detects the hyperplasia of fibroblastic reticular cells. Plasma cells in PC-CD are polyclonal, although cases with monoclonal plasma cells may be observed.

Pathogenesis

The pathogenesis of CD is not well understood. It has been suggested that MCD arises in the setting of immune dysregulation, which has been supported by the strong association with HHV-8 and HIV infections.[100] The role of HHV-8 and interleukin (IL)-6 in the pathogenesis of PC-CD has been long recognized. In patients with PC-CD, high levels of IL-6 have been demonstrated, which likely contributes to the systemic symptoms. Furthermore, HHV-8 encodes a viral IL-6, which can induce endogenous secretion of human IL-6 contributing to the plasmacytosis, and vascular endothelial growth factor (VEGF) promoting angiogenesis.[79]

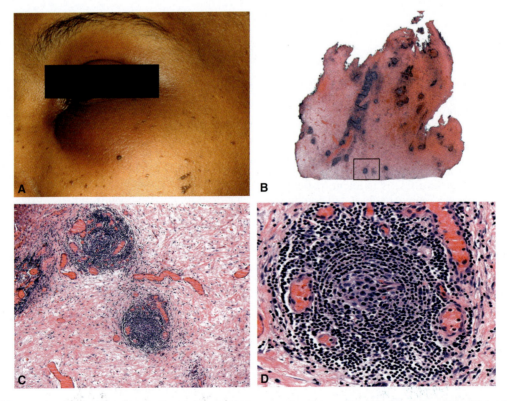

FIGURE 35-11. Cutaneous Castleman disease. Clinical findings. **A.** Nodular and erythematous swelling in the left cheek and infraorbital region. **B.** Small lymphoid follicles throughout the dermis. **C.** Atrophic germinal centers are noted with vessels inserting into the abnormal follicles. **D.** Proliferation of small hyalinized vessels and "onion-rimming" of lymphocytes surrounding the atrophic follicles. (Courtesy of Dr. Jason Lee, Thomas Jefferson University Hospital, Philadelphia, PA.)

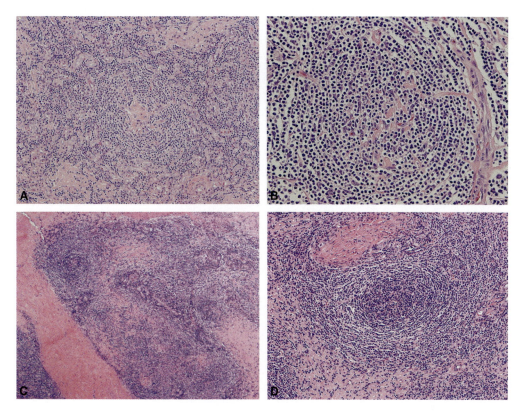

FIGURE 35-12. Nodal Castleman disease, hyaline vascular type. A and **B.** atrophic germinal centers and a classic "lollipop" lesion. Hyalinized vessels penetrate into an atrophic follicle with increased number of FDCs. **C** (40×) showing a background of fibrosis. **D** (200×) showing a concentric mantle zone of lymphocytes rimming around an atrophic follicle.

The pathogenesis of HV-CD is unrelated to HHV-8 and IL-6 and appears to be directly linked to FDC dysplasia/dysregulation. It is presumed that the dysplastic changes seen in FCD are the initiating factor in CD development and can potentially transform into follicular dendritic cell sarcoma (Fig. 35-13).

Differential Diagnosis

The differential diagnosis of CD includes lymphoproliferative lesions that are associated with either vascular pathology or prominent plasmacytic infiltrates. The former group includes angiolymphoid hyperplasia with eosinophilia (ALHE), Kimura disease (KD), AITL, and sinus histiocytosis with massive lymphadenopathy. Plasma cell–rich entities include cutaneous and systemic plasmacytosis (CSP), primary or secondary syphilis, osteosclerotic myeloma (POEMS syndrome), and primary cutaneous marginal zone lymphoma (PCMZBL). Differentiating CD from these diseases can be achieved by clinical correlation, immunohistochemistry, and in situ hybridization for kappa and lambda immunoglobulin (Ig) light chains.

Positive immunohistochemistry for HHV-8 is a definitive finding of CD.[101,102]

ALHE is a benign vascular neoplasm composed of proliferation of histiocytoid endothelial cells and a prominent mixed inflammatory infiltrate of reactive T and B lymphocytes, plasma cells, and eosinophils. Lymphadenopathy and peripheral eosinophilia are absent. Cases that lack the lymphohistiocytic infiltrate and eosinophils had been recognized.[103]

KD is distinct from ALHE. Clinically, KD shows lymphadenopathy and peripheral eosinophilia. Histologically, KD has prominent lymphoid follicles and lack protuberant endothelial cells.

The presence of clonally expanded T cells with follicular T helper cell phenotype (positivity for CD10, BCL-6, CXCL-13, and ICOS), EBV/EBER expression, and arborizing thickened capillaries is diagnostic of AITL.

Osteosclerotic myeloma, a plasma cell neoplasm, exhibits bone marrow fibrosis and lymph node changes similar to the plasma cell variant of CD. This entity presents in association with polyneuropathy, organomegaly, endocrinopathy, monoclonal gammopathy, and skin changes such as glomeruloid hemangiomas (POEMS).

B cell predominance with nongerminal center phenotype, BCL-2 expression, and monoclonal lambda or kappa Ig light chain expression excludes the diagnosis of CD and favors PCMZBL.

Differentiating CD from CSP can be difficult. CSP is a rare disease described mainly in individuals of Japanese descent.[73,104] Watanabe et al described a series of patients with a skin rash, lymphadenopathy, and polyclonal hypergammaglobulinemia and bone marrow plasmacytosis.[102] CSP is more common in men and can rarely present in patients of European origin. The skin manifestations of CSP are fairly uniform and usually consist of multiple, persistent, asymptomatic, or mildly pruritic, smooth, or slightly scaly patches, infiltrated plaques, or nodules, with

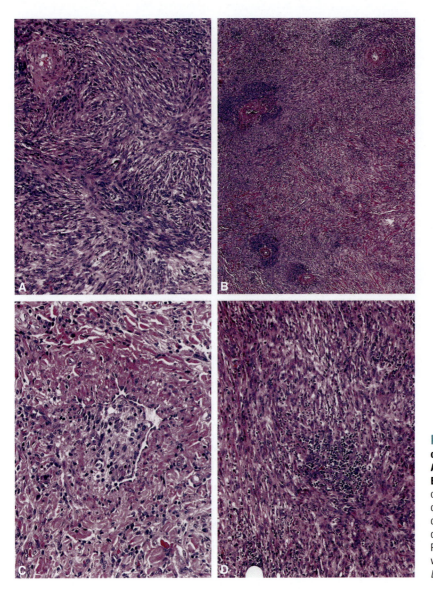

FIGURE 35-13. Follicular dendritic cell sarcoma developing in the setting of cutaneous CD. **A.** Spindle cells are arranged in a short fascicular pattern. **B.** Perivascular accentuation and concentric arrangement of the neoplastic cells around a blood vessel (upper right corner). **C.** Subendothelial extension of the neoplastic cells. **D.** Lymphoid cells intermingled among the spindle cells. (Obtained with permission. Kazakov DV, Morrisson C, Plaza JA, Michal M, Suster S. Sarcoma arising in hyaline-vascular Castleman disease of skin and subcutis. *Am J Dermatopathol.* 2005;27(4):327-332.)

violaceous-to-brownish color symmetrically distributed on the trunk, face, and proximal extremities.[104] The distribution of lesions in some cases can be reminiscent of the "Christmas tree" pattern described for pityriasis rosea and small patch parapsoriasis. Facial involvement can also lead to a diagnostic consideration of lupus erythematosus or rosacea. Lymphadenopathy (54%) and liver (9%) or splenomegaly (12%) can be seen. The histopathologic findings characteristically show a dermal infiltrate composed of mature PCs without atypia and variable numbers of admixed lymphocytes and histiocytes. The epidermis is minimally affected, with only mild acanthosis and basal hyperpigmentation. The pattern of the infiltrate is usually perivascular and/or periadnexal in the upper to mid dermis, but diffuse involvement is seen in 22% of cases.[104] Nearly 40% of cases show the presence of follicles and germinal centers. In most cases the plasma cells are polyclonal.[105] Increased IL-6 levels, similar to CD, are seen in CSP.[104,105] Many cases of CSP have marked elevations of IgG4, and therefore CSP has been proposed as part of the spectrum of cutaneous IgG4+ disorders.[83]

CAPSULE SUMMARY

Cutaneous PTLD

- Clinical: The duration and degree of immune suppression are the major determinants in the development of PTLD. Most PTLD is seen in kidney transplant patients. About a fifth of PTLD cases show cutaneous involvement. Most cutaneous B-PTLD cases clinically present as tumors or nodules, whereas T-PTLD cases manifest either as MF or C-ALCL.
- Histology: PTLD can present in six histologic patterns: plasmacytic hyperplasia, infectious mononucleosis-like, florid follicular hyperplasia, polymorphous and monomorphous PTLD, and Hodgkin lymphoma–like PTLD. Cutaneous B-cell PTLD (90.9%) is EBV related and shows histological features of DLBCL. About 30% to 60% of cutaneous PTLD has a T-cell phenotype, the majority of which lacks EBV (83.4%) and pathologically present as MF or C-ALCL. Primary cutaneous plasmacytoma-like PTLD is a rare variant that can present decades after solid organ transplantation.

EBV-Positive Mucocutaneous Ulcer
- Clinical: Solitary, sharply defined ulcers in the skin and oral mucosa in immunosuppressed patients.
- Histology: ulcer, tissue necrosis, and a polymorphous infiltrate with a mixture of lymphocytes, atypical large B-cell immunoblasts with Hodgkin-like morphology, plasma cells, plasmacytoid apoptotic cells, histiocytes, and eosinophils. Cases with small lymphocytic infiltration lack cytological atypia and pose diagnostic challenge.
- Immunohistochemistry: lesional cells are $CD30^+$, EBV^+ $CD20^{low}$ without CD15 expression.
- The clinical course is generally indolent and self-limited, responding well to cessation of immunosuppression.

MTX-Related Lymphoproliferative Disorders
- Clinical: cutaneous findings include generalized or multifocal plaques, nodules with or without ulceration.
- Histology: about 50% of cases present as diffuse large B-cell lymphoma with large immunoblasts-like cells in a sheet like distribution.
- Immunohistochemistry:
  - EBV^+ MTX-LPD: $CD30^+$ and $MUM1^+$, with variable loss of B-cell markers CD20 and CD79a.
  - EBV–MTX-LPD: CD30- with strong nuclear MYC and FOXP1 expression.[67]
- BCL-2 and BCL-6 are positive in the majority of the cases, independent of the EBV status.

Castleman Disease
- Clinical: CD has three clinical forms: unicentric, $HHV-8^+$ multicentric, and $HHV-8^-$ multicentric. Cutaneous presentation of CD is extraordinarily rare with less than 15 cases reported in the literature.
- Histology: *Hyalin-vascular type* cases show atrophic and hyalinized germinal centers. Centrocytes and centroblasts are absent; the follicular dendritic cell meshwork is prominent and shows dysplastic features. Expanded mantle zone with concentric small lymphocytes (onion-skinning). Increased interfollicular vascularity with hyalinized vessels penetrating germinal centers (lollipop). The *plasma cell variant* of CD shows hyperplastic germinal centers, prominent interfollicular vascularity, and sheets of usually polyclonal but sometimes monoclonal plasma cells.
- Cutaneous associations of CD include POEMS syndrome, paraneoplastic pemphigus, Kaposi sarcoma, and follicular dendritic cell sarcoma.

References

1. Salama S, Todd S, Cina DP, Margetts P. Cutaneous presentation of post-renal transplant lymphoproliferative disorder: a series of four cases. *J Cutan Pathol*. 2010;37(6):641-653.
2. Opelz G, Henderson R. Incidence of non-Hodgkin lymphoma in kidney and heart transplant recipients. *Lancet*. 1993;342(8886-8887):1514-1516.
3. Penn I. Cancers complicating organ transplantation. *N Engl J Med*. 1990;323(25):1767-1769.
4. Swerdlow SH, Webber SA, Chadburn A, Ferry JA. *Post-Transplant Lymphoproliferative Disorders*. 4th ed. International Agency for Research on Cancer; 2008.
5. Knight JS, Tsodikov A, Cibrik DM, Ross CW, Kaminski MS, Blayney DW. Lymphoma after solid organ transplantation: risk, response to therapy, and survival at a transplantation centre. *J Clin Oncol*. 2009;27:3354-3362.
6. Dharnidharka VR, Lamb KE, Gregg JA, Meier-Kriesche HU. Associations between EBV serostatus and organ transplant type in PTLD risk: an analysis of the SRTR national registry data in the United States. *Am J Transplant*. 2012;12:976-983.
7. Caillard S, Dharnidharka V, Agodoa L, Bohen E, Abbott K. Posttransplant lymphoproliferative disorders after renal transplantation in the United States in era of modern immunosuppression. *Transplantation*. 2005;80(9):1233-1243.
8. Kirk AD, Cherikh WS, Ring M, et al. Dissociation of depletional induction and post-transplant lymphoproliferative disease in kidney recipients treated with alemtuzumab. *Am J Transplant*. 2007;7:2619-2625.
9. Leblond V, Sutton L, Dorent R, et al. Lymphoproliferative disorders after organ transplantation: a report of 24 cases observed in a single center. *J Clin Oncol*. 1995;13(4):961-968.
10. Apichai S, Rogalska A, Tzvetanov I, Asma Z, Benedetti E, Gaitonde S. Multifocal cutaneous and systemic plasmablastic lymphoma in an infant with combined living donor small bowel and liver transplant. *Pediatr Transplant*. 2009;13(5):628-631.
11. Mills KC, Sangueza OP, Beaty MW, Raffeld M, Pang CS. Composite B-cell and T-cell lineage post-transplant lymphoproliferative disorder of the lung with unusual cutaneous manifestations of mycosis fungoides. *Am J Dermatopathol*. 2012;34(2):220-225.
12. Hernandez C, Cetner AS, Wiley EL. Cutaneous presentation of plasmablastic post-transplant lymphoproliferative disorder in a 14-month-old. *Pediatr Dermatol*. 2009;26(6):713-716.
13. Seckin D, Barete S, Euvrard S, et al. Primary cutaneous post-transplant lymphoproliferative disorders in solid organ transplant recipients: a multicenter European case series. *Am J Transplant*. 2013;13(8):2146-2153.
14. Molina-Ruiz AM, Pulpillo A, Lasanta B, Zulueta T, Andrades R, Requena L. A rare case of primary cutaneous plasmacytoma-like lymphoproliferative disorder following renal transplantation. *J Cutan Pathol*. 2012;39(7):685-689.
15. Traboulsi D, Wink J, Wong R, et al. Cutaneous plasmacytoma-like posttransplant lymphoproliferative disorder after renal transplantation with response to imiquimod 5% cream and reduced immunosuppression. *JAAD Case Rep*. 2019;5(12):1071-1074.
16. Richendollar BG, Hsi ED, Cook JR. Extramedullary plasmacytoma-like posttransplantation lymphoproliferative disorders: clinical and pathologic features. *Am J Clin Pathol*. 2009;132(4):581-588.
17. McFarlane R, Hurst S, Sabath D, George E, Argenyi Z. A rare case of plasmacytoma-like post-transplant lymphoproliferative disorder presenting in the skin of a lung transplant patient. *J Cutan Pathol*. 2008;35(6):599-602.
18. Willoughby V, Werlang-Perurena A, Kelly A, Francois J, Donner LR. Primary cutaneous plasmacytoma (posttransplant lymphoproliferative disorder, plasmacytoma-like) in a heart transplant patient. *Am J Dermatopathol*. 2006;28(5):442-445.
19. Tessari G, Fabbian F, Colato C. Primary cutaneous plasmacytoma after rejection of a transplanted kidney: case report and review of the literature. *Int J Hematol*. 2004;80(4):361-364.
20. Pacheco TR, Hinther L, Fitzpatrick J. Extramedullary plasmacytoma in cardiac transplant recipients. *J Am Acad Dermatol*. 2003;49(5):255-258.
21. Penn I. The changing pattern of posttransplant malignancies. *Transplant Proc*. 1991;23(1 pt 2):1101-1103.

22. Herreman A, Dierickx D, Morscio J, et al. Clinicopathological characteristics of posttransplant lymphoproliferative disorders of T-cell origin: single-center series of nine cases and meta-analysis of 147 reported cases. *Leuk Lymphoma*. 2013;54(10):2190-2199.
23. Swerdlow SH, Campo E, Harris NL, et al. (eds). *WHO Classification of Tumours of Haematopoietic and Lymphoid Tissues*. Revised 4th ed. IARC; 2017.
24. Albrecht H, Woodroof JM, Reyes R, Powers BC, Fraga GR. CD30 expression in cutaneous B-cell and post-transplant peripheral T-cell lymphoma: report of 2 cases. *Dermatol Online J*. 2014;20(7):13030/qt24t0s15d.
25. Belloni-Fortina A, Montesco MC, Piaserico S, et al. Primary cutaneous CD30+ anaplastic large cell lymphoma in a heart transplant patient: case report and literature review. *Acta Derm Venereol*. 2009;89(1):74-77.
26. Chiu LS, Choi PC, Luk NM, Chang M, Tang WY. Spontaneous regression of primary cutaneous Epstein-Barr virus-positive, CD30-positive anaplastic large T-cell lymphoma in a heart-transplant recipient. *Clin Exp Dermatol*. 2009;34(5):e21-24.
27. Coyne JD, Banerjee SS, Bromley M, Mills S, Diss TC, Harris M. Post-transplant T-cell lymphoproliferative disorder/T-cell lymphoma: a report of three cases of T-anaplastic large-cell lymphoma with cutaneous presentation and a review of the literature. *Histopathology*. 2004;44(4):387-393.
28. Lok C, Viseux V, Denoeux JP, Bagot M. Post-transplant cutaneous T-cell lymphomas. *Crit Rev Oncol-Hematol*. 2005;56(1):137-145.
29. Lucioni M, Ippoliti G, Campana C, et al. EBV positive primary cutaneous CD30+ large T-cell lymphoma in a heart transplanted patient: case report. *Am J Transplant*. 2004;4(11):1915-1920.
30. Santos-Briz A, Romo A, Antunez P, et al. Primary cutaneous T-cell lymphoproliferative disorder of donor origin after allogeneic haematopoietic stem-cell transplantation. *Clin Exp Dermatol*. 2009;34(8):e778-781.
31. Crombie JL, LaCasce AS. Epstein Barr virus associated B-cell lymphomas and Iatrogenic lymphoproliferative disorders. *Front Oncol*. 2019;9:109.
32. Robinson C, Burroughs S, Addis B, Mason J. Cutaneous post-transplant lymphoproliferative disorder with atypical Hodgkin and Reed-Sternberg-like cells. *Histopathology*. 2007;50(3):403-404.
33. http://www.ncbi.nlm.nih.gov/pubmed/16041261
34. http://www.ncbi.nlm.nih.gov/pubmed/16216037
35. http://www.ncbi.nlm.nih.gov/pubmed/9746767
36. Starzl TE, Nalesnik M A, Porter KA, et al. Reversibility of lymphomas and lymphoproliferative lesions developing under cyclosporin-steroid therapy. *Lancet*. 1984;1(8377):583-587.
37. Seckin D. Cutaneous lymphoproliferative disorders in organ transplant recipients: update 2014. *G Ital Dermatol venereol Organo Uff Soc Ital Dermatol Sifilogr*. 2014;149(4):401-408.
38. Bunn B, van Heerden W. EBV-positive mucocutaneous ulcer of the oral cavity associated with HIV/AIDS. *Oral Surg Oral Med Oral Pathol Oral Radiol*. 2015;120(6):725-732.
39. Moran NR, Webster B, Lee KM, et al. Epstein Barr virus-positive mucocutaneous ulcer of the colon associated Hodgkin lymphoma in Crohn's disease. *World J Gastroenterol*. 2015;21(19):6072-6076.
40. Magalhaes M, Ghorab Z, Morneault J, Akinfolarin J, Bradley G. Age-related Epstein-Barr virus-positive mucocutaneous ulcer: a case report. *Clin Case Rep*. 2015;3(7):531-534.
41. Dojcinov SD, Venkataraman G, Raffeld M, Pittaluga S, Jaffe ES. EBV positive mucocutaneous ulcer—a study of 26 cases associated with various sources of immunosuppression. *Am J Surg Pathol*. 2010;34(3):405-417.
42. Stojanov IJ, Woo SB. Human papillomavirus and Epstein-Barr virus associated conditions of the oral mucosa. *Semin Diagn Pathol*. 2015;32(1):3-11.
43. Nelson AA, Harrington AM, Kroft S, Dahar MA, Hamadani M, Dhakal B. Presentation and management of post-allogeneic transplantation EBV-positive mucocutaneous ulcer. *Bone Marrow Transplant*. 2016;51(2):300-302.
44. Hart M, Thakral B, Yohe S, et al. EBV-positive mucocutaneous ulcer in organ transplant recipients: a localized indolent posttransplant lymphoproliferative disorder. *Am J Surg Pathol*. 2014;38(11):1522-1529.
45. Asano N, Yamamoto K, Tamaru J, et al. Age-related Epstein-Barr virus (EBV)-associated B-cell lymphoproliferative disorders: comparison with EBV-positive classic Hodgkin lymphoma in elderly patients. *Blood*. 2009;113(12):2629-2636.
46. Shimoyama Y, Asano N, Kojima M, et al. Age-related EBV-associated B-cell lymphoproliferative disorders: diagnostic approach to a newly recognized clinicopathological entity. *Pathol Int*. 2009;59(12):835-843.
47. Fujimoto M, Kaku Y, Hirata M, Usui S, Yamada Y, Haga H. EBV-Positive mucocutaneous ulcer with small lymphocytic infiltration mimicking nonspecific ulceration. *Am J Surg Pathol*. 2021;45(5):694-700.
48. Kempf W, Kazakov DV, Mitteldorf C. Cutaneous lymphomas: an update. Part 2—B-cell lymphomas and related conditions. *Am J Dermatopathol*. 2014;36(3):197-208; quiz 209-110.
49. McGinness JL, Spicknall KE, Mutasim DF. Azathioprine-induced EBV-positive mucocutaneous ulcer. *J Cutan Pathol*. 2012;39(3):377-381.
50. Swerdlow SH, Quintanilla-Martinez L, Willemze R, Kinney MC. Cutaneous B-cell lymphoproliferative disorders: report of the 2011 Society for hematopathology/European association for haematopathology workshop. *Am J Clin Pathol*. 2013;139(4):515-535.
51. http://www.bloodjournal.org/content/99/11/3909?sso-checked=true
52. http://www.ncbi.nlm.nih.gov/pubmed/20210795
53. http://www.ncbi.nlm.nih.gov/pubmed/23733760
54. http://www.sciencedirect.com/science/article/pii/S0344033809000910
55. http://www.ncbi.nlm.nih.gov/pubmed/26459854
56. https://jrheum.com/subscribers/07/02/322.html
57. Nemoto Y, Taniguchi A, Kamioka M, et al. Epstein-Barr virus-infected subcutaneous panniculitis-like T-cell lymphoma associated with methotrexate treatment. *Int J Hematol*. 2010;92:364-368.
58. Koens L, Senff NJ, Vermeer MH, Willemze R, Jansen PM. Methotrexate-associated B-cell lymphoproliferative disorders presenting in the skin: a clinicopathologic and immunophenotypical study of 10 cases. *Am J Surg Pathol*. 2014;38(7):999-1006.
59. EBV+ DLBCL of elderly. http://www.ncbi.nlm.nih.gov/pmc/articles/PMC3779382/
60. Hashimoto K, Nagao T, Saito T, Kinoshita H. Methotrexate-associated lymphoproliferative disorders of the tongue developing in patients with rheumatoid arthritis: a report of 2 cases and a review. *Oral Surg Oral Med Oral Pathol Oral Radiol*. 2015;119(1):e1-5.

61. Matsumoto Y, Horiike S, Maekawa S, et al. Rheumatoid arthritis/methotrexate-associated primary cutaneous diffuse large B-cell lymphoma, leg type. *Intern Med.* 2014;53(11):1177-1181.
62. Pastor-Nieto MA, Kilmurray LG, Lopez-Chumillas A, et al. Methotrexate-associated lymphoproliferative disorder presenting as oral ulcers in a patient with rheumatoid arthritis. [Article in Spanish]. *Actas Dermosifiliogr.* 2009;100(2):142-146.
63. Yamada K, Oshiro Y, Okamura S, et al. Clinicopathological characteristics and rituximab-plus cytotoxic therapies in patients with rheumatoid arthritis and methotrexate-associated large B-lymphoproliferative disorders. *Histopathology.* 2014.
64. Weinstein A, Marlowe S, Korn J, Farouhar F. Low-dose methotrexate treatment of rheumatoid arthritis. Long-term observations. *Am J Med.* 1985;79(3):331-337.
65. http://www.ncbi.nlm.nih.gov/pubmed/24805861
66. Castleman B, Iverson L, Menendez VP. Localized mediastinal lymphnode hyperplasia resembling thymoma. *Cancer.* 1956;9(4):822-830.
67. Knowles DM, Cesarman E, Chadburn A, et al. Correlative morphologic and molecular genetic analysis demonstrates three distinct categories of posttransplantation lymphoproliferative disorders. *Blood.* 1995;85(2):552-565.
68. Talat N, Schulte KM. Castleman's disease: systematic analysis of 416 patients from the literature. *Oncologist.* 2011;16(9):1316-1324.
69. Soumerai JD, Sohani AR, Abramson JS. Diagnosis and management of Castleman disease. *Cancer Control.* 2014;21(4):266-278.
70. Fajgenbaum DC, van Rhee F, Nabel CS. HHV-8-negative, idiopathic multicentric Castleman disease: novel insights into biology, pathogenesis, and therapy. *Blood.* 2014;123(19):2924-2933.
71. Ariza-Heredia EJ, Razonable RR. Human herpes virus 8 in solid organ transplantation. *Transplantation.* 2011;92(8):837-844.
72. Bonatti HJ, Axt J, Hunter EB, et al. Castleman disease in a pediatric liver transplant recipient: a case report and literature review. *Pediatr Transplant.* 2012;16(6):E229-E234.
73. Chen H, Xue Y, Jiang Y, Zeng X, Sun JF. Cutaneous and systemic plasmacytosis showing histopathologic features as mixed-type Castleman disease: a case report. *Am J Dermatopathol.* 2012;34(5):553-556.
74. Kayasut K, Le Tourneau A, Rio B, et al. Are multicentric Castleman's disease with cutaneous plasmacytosis and systemic plasmacytosis the same entity? *Histopathology.* 2006;49(5):557-558.
75. Grossin M, Crickx B, Aitken G, Belaich S, Bocquet L. Subcutaneous localizations of Castleman's pseudolymphoma. Review of the literature apropos of a case. [Article in French]. *Annales de dermatologie et de venereologie.* 1985;112(6-7):497-506.
76. Kubota Y, Noto S, Takakuwa T, Tadokoro M, Mizoguchi M. Skin involvement in giant lymph node hyperplasia (Castleman's disease). *J Am Acad Dermatol.* 1993;29(5 pt 1):778-780.
77. Lattes R, Pachter MR. Benign lymphoid masses of probable hamartomatous nature. Analysis of 12 cases. *Cancer.* 1962;15:197-214.
78. Munoz J, Naing A, Qi M, Kurzrock R. Cutaneous castleman disease. *Br J Haematol.* 2012;157(6):652.
79. Naghashpour M, Cualing HD, Szabunio M, Bui MM. Hyaline-vascular castleman disease: a rare cause of solitary subcutaneous soft tissue mass. *Am J Dermatopathol.* 2010;32(3):293-297.
80. Park HY, Lee JJ, Lee JB, et al. Castleman's disease with cutaneous involvement manifesting as multiple violaceous plaques on entire body. *Ann Dermatol.* 2011;23(suppl 2):S169-S174.
81. Skelton HG, Smith KJ. Extranodal multicentric Castleman's disease with cutaneous involvement. *Mod Pathol.* 1998;11(1):93-98.
82. Sleater J, Mullins D. Subcutaneous Castleman's disease of the wrist. *Am J Dermatopathol.* 1995;17(2):174-178.
83. Takeuchi M, Sato Y, Takata K, et al. Cutaneous multicentric Castleman's disease mimicking IgG4-related disease. *Pathol Res Pract.* 2012;208(12):746-749.
84. Cardenas V, Vitiello M, Miteva M, Amano M, Romanelli P, Kerdel FA. An unusual case of cutaneous hyaline-vascular Castleman's disease with multicentric involvement and systemic symptoms. *Int J Dermatol.* 2011;50(8):1030-1032.
85. http://www.ncbi.nlm.nih.gov/pmc/articles/PMC3229057/pdf/ad-23-S169.pdf
86. Shi X, Hu S, Yu X, et al. Clinicopathologic analysis of POEMS syndrome and related diseases. *Clin Lymphoma Myeloma Leuk.* 2015;15(1):e15-21.
87. Dispenzieri A. POEMS syndrome. *Blood Rev.* 2007;21(6):285-299.
88. Dispenzieri A. How I treat POEMS syndrome. *Blood.* 2012;119(24):5650-5658.
89. Dispenzieri A. POEMS syndrome: update on diagnosis, risk-stratification, and management. *Am J Hematol.* 2012;87(8):804-814.
90. Nakanishi T, Sobue I, Toyokura Y, et al. The Crow-Fukase syndrome: a study of 102 cases in Japan. *Neurology.* 1984;34(6):712-720.
91. http://onlinelibrary.wiley.com/store/10.1002/ajh.10022/asset/10022_ftp.pdf?v=1&t=ij5v60wh&s=b80e2f786037763a14f737b69fd2577d678c8536
92. http://onlinelibrary.wiley.com/doi/10.1002/(SICI)1096-8652(199810)59:2%3C161::AID-AJH10%3E3.0.CO;2-C/epdf
93. Komatsuda A, Wakui H, Togashi M, Sawada K. IgA nephropathy associated with Castleman disease with cutaneous involvement. *Am J Med Sci.* 2010;339(5):486-490.
94. http://www.ncbi.nlm.nih.gov/pubmed/14674890
95. Liu W, Lacouture ME, Jiang J, et al. KSHV/HHV8-associated primary cutaneous plasmablastic lymphoma in a patient with Castleman's disease and Kaposi's sarcoma. *J Cutan Pathol.* 2006;33(suppl 2):46-51.
96. Kazakov DV, Morrisson C, Plaza JA, Michal M, Suster S. Sarcoma arising in hyaline-vascular castleman disease of skin and subcutis. *Am J Dermatopathol.* 2005;27(4):327-332.
97. Tomasini D, Zampatti C, Serio G. Castleman's disease with numerous mantle zone lymphocytes with clear cytoplasm involving the skin: case report. *J Cutan Pathol.* 2009;36(8):887-891.
98. Okuyama R, Harigae H, Moriya T, et al. Indurated nodules and plaques showing a dense plasma cell infiltrate as a cutaneous manifestation of Castleman's disease. *Br J Dermatol.* 2007;156(1):174-176.
99. http://www.ncbi.nlm.nih.gov/pubmed/19586499
100. Stebbing J, Adams C, Sanitt A, et al. Plasma HHV8 DNA predicts relapse in individuals with HIV-associated multicentric Castleman disease. *Blood.* 2011;118(2):271-275.
101. Higashi Y, Kanekura T, Sakamoto R, Mochitomi Y, Kanzaki T. Multicentric Castleman disease with cutaneous

manifestations: report of 2 cases and comparison with systemic plasmacytosis. *Dermatology*. 2007;214(2):170-173.
102. Shadel BN, Frater JL, Gapp JD, Hurley MY. Cutaneous and systemic plasmacytosis in an Asian male born in the North American continent: a controversial entity potentially related to multicentric Castleman disease. *J Cutan Pathol*. 2010;37(6):697-702.
103. http://www.ncbi.nlm.nih.gov/pubmed/7065665
104. Haque M, Hou JS, Hisamichi K, et al. Cutaneous and systemic plasmacytosis vs. cutaneous plasmacytic castleman disease: review and speculations about pathogenesis. *Clin Lymphoma Myeloma Leuk*. 2011;11(6):453-461.
105. Honda R, Cerroni L, Tanikawa A, Ebihara T, Amagai M, Ishiko A. Cutaneous plasmacytosis: report of 6 cases with or without systemic involvement. *J Am Acad Dermatol*. 2013;68(6):978-985.

CHAPTER 36

An approach to the treatment of primary cutaneous B-Cell lymphomas

Pablo L. Ortiz-Romero and Mariana Cravo

INTRODUCTION

Primary cutaneous B-cell lymphomas (CBCLs) are a heterogeneous group of diseases characterized by B-cell proliferations that clinically present on the skin without extracutaneous involvement at diagnosis. CBCLs account for 20% to 25% of all primary cutaneous lymphomas. According to Surveillance, Epidemiology and End Results Program (SEER), the yearly incidence is around three cases per million of inhabitants.[1]

CBCL classification includes five main entities: primary cutaneous marginal zone lymphoma (PCMZL), primary cutaneous follicle center lymphoma (PCFCL), primary cutaneous large B-cell lymphoma, leg type (PCDLBCL, LT), and intravascular large B-cell lymphoma, and recently EBV+ mucocutaneous ulcer has been included as a new provisional entity. PCMZL is not considered an independent entity by the World Health Organization (WHO) but is included in the group of extranodal marginal zone lymphomas of mucosa-associated lymphoid tissue (MALT lymphomas). Table 36-1 shows the relative frequency and the 5-year disease-specific survival of CBCL.[2,3]

Staging of CBCL is performed using the International Society for Cutaneous Lymphomas (ISCL)–European Organization of Research and Treatment of Cancer(EORTC) TNM classification system for primary cutaneous lymphomas other than mycosis fungoides and Sézary syndrome.[4]

A summary of this staging system is shown in Table 36-2.

For diagnosis of CBCL clinic-pathologic and immunohistochemical correlation are mandatory. Molecular studies may help in securing a diagnosis. This topic will be reviewed in a different chapter.

PRIMARY CUTANEOUS MARGINAL ZONE LYMPHOMA

PCMZL represents around 7% to 9% of all cutaneous lymphomas and 26% to 50% of all CBCL. The mean age at presentation is 55 years and is twice more frequent in males than in females.[2,5-9]

Clinical Features

PCMZL usually presents as multiple or occasionally solitary papules, nodules, or plaques appearing mostly on the trunk

TABLE 36-1 Relative Frequency and 5-Year Disease-Specific Survival of CBCL[2]

CBCL	% (from Total Primary Cutaneous Lymphomas)	5-y DSS (%)
PCMZL	9	99
PCFCCL	12	95
PCDLBCL, LT	5	56
EBV+ mucocutaneous ulcer (provisional)	<1	100
Intravascular large B-cell lymphoma	<1	72

CBCL, primary cutaneous B-cell lymphoma; DSS, disease-specific survival; EVB, Epstein-Barr virus; PCDLBCL, LT, primary cutaneous large B-cell lymphoma, leg type; PCFCCL, primary cutaneous follicle center cell lymphoma; PCMZL, primary cutaneous marginal zone lymphoma.

TABLE 36-2 ISCL/EORTC Proposal on TNM Classification of Cutaneous Lymphoma Other Than Mycosis Fungoides/Sézary Syndrome

Classification
T
T1: Solitary skin involvement
T1a: a solitary lesion <5 cm diameter
T1 b: a solitary >5 cm diameter
T2: Regional skin involvement: multiple lesions limited to 1 body region or 2 contiguous body regions
T2a: all-disease-encompassing in a <15-cm-diameter circular area
T2b: all-disease-encompassing in a >15- and <30-cm-diameter circular area
T2c: all-disease-encompassing in a >30-cm-diameter circular area
T3: Generalized skin involvement
T3a: multiple lesions involving 2 noncontiguous body regions
T3b: multiple lesions involving ≥3 body regions
N
N0: No clinical or pathologic lymph node involvement
N1: Involvement of 1 peripheral lymph node region that drains an area of current or prior skin involvement
N2: Involvement of 2 or more peripheral lymph node regions or involvement of any lymph node region that does not drain an area of current or prior skin involvement
N3: Involvement of central lymph nodes
M
M0: No evidence of extracutaneous non–lymph node disease
M1: Extracutaneous non–lymph node disease present

and upper extremities. Lesions are often violaceous in color and rarely ulcerate. Extracutaneous dissemination is exceptional; however, cutaneous relapses are frequent, especially in patients with multiple skin lesions. Behavior is usually indolent with disease-specific survival >99%. The cause is unknown, but chronic antigenic stimulation may play a role as some cases have been related to *Borrelia burgdorferi* infection (mostly cases from central Europe); development of PCMZL on tattoos, tick bites, or vaccines has also been reported.

Diagnostic Workup

After diagnosis, a complete review of symptoms, particularly the evaluation for B symptoms and organ-specific symptoms, should be pursued. However, the authors have yet to encounter a case of PCMZL with systemic symptoms. Laboratory studies should include a complete blood cell count with differential. Biochemistry investigations in serum should include lactate dehydrogenase (LDH) and electrophoresis (serum protein electrophoresis, urine protein electrophoresis) to exclude monoclonal gammopathy. In cases with leukocytosis, flow cytometry is recommended. In endemic areas for *B. burgdorferi*, infection should be studied by serology and/or polymerase chain reaction. For those patients to be treated with rituximab, serologies for hepatitis B and C (HBV, HCV), HIV, and purified protein derivative (PPD) are mandatory.[10,11]

Bone marrow biopsy is considered optional and of very limited value.[10] However, in a paper published by Senff et al, 2 of 82 patients with PCMZL had bone marrow infiltration. In one of them, bone marrow was the only extracutaneous involvement.[12] Bone marrow biopsy is necessary to study any unexplained cytopenias but should not be performed as routine workup after the diagnosis is made.

Image studies (positron emission tomography [PET]–computed tomography [CT] or CT scan) should be considered in cases with multiple lesions, systemic symptoms, or frequent relapses. The choice between PET-CT and CT scan should be based on the knowledge of the amount of irradiation delivered by the specific machine of the center studying the patient. In some centers, irradiation of PET-CT is double than that of a CT scan, but almost the opposite can occur in other hospitals.

Prognosis

The prognosis of PCMZL is excellent, with a 5-year disease-specific survival close to 100%. As relapses are frequent, a prognostic index has been developed by the IESLG11 group. This index gives 1 point each to a high LDH, more than two skin lesions, and the presence of nodular lesions (rather than only plaques, macules, or papules). Three groups with different relapse risk were defined: low (0 point), intermediate (1 point), and high (2-3 points). Progression-free survival (PFS) and disease-free survival (DFS) were statistically different among the three groups. No significant differences were found in overall survival (OS).[13] With respect to this prognostic index, a high LDH is extremely rare in PCMZL and of questionable utility, as the authors of this chapter have never found a case with this abnormality.

Treatment

Although a "wait and see" approach is totally acceptable for PCMZL, most patients prefer to be treated. Very importantly, wait and see requires a close and watchful follow-up of the patient. For solitary or low numbers of lesions, surgical excision is the treatment of choice. Radiotherapy for larger lesions that would leave big scars is also an excellent option but should be used cautiously in young patients. Complete responses (CRs) are achieved in almost every treated case, but relapses are frequent (46%). Radiation doses are usually between 30 and 45 Gy, but doses as low as 10 Gy may be sufficient.[10,14,15] Surgical or radiation margins are not well defined. Surgically, in the authors' experience, less than 1 cm is sufficient. Reported margins for external radiation are between 1 and 5 cm. Intralesional injection of corticosteroids in depot formulation is frequently used for small lesions (maximum 1-1.5 cm in diameter). CRs are frequent and can last more than 4 years.[16]

In cases with associated *B. burgdorferi* infection, systemic antibiotics should be recommended as CRs have been reported (especially with systemic cephalosporins).[10,17,18] The use of intralesional interferon (IFN) alpha has also been reported to achieve success in a very limited number of cases. Nearly all patients responded with 25% of relapses.[19] Unfortunately, IFN alpha is no longer available in most countries. No reports of the use of intralesional or systemic pegylated IFN are available in the literature.

Intralesional rituximab[20] is used with a dosage of three injections per week, 1 week a month. Around 10 mg per lesion is injected every time, but it is variable depending on the lesion size. Almost all patients respond with around 60% to 70% of CRs. Intralesional injections are very painful, so prior local anesthetic is recommended. Transient inflammation (wheal-like) occurs frequently after injection and can occur as a distant reaction of noninjected lesions before disappearance. Other adverse events are usually mild and include urticaria, fever, transient rash, nausea, and malaise. Severe reduction of B cells within weeks of the first injection is frequent, even with low cumulative dosage. Assessment and prevention of hepatitis B and C or tuberculosis reactivation is strongly recommended. Responses are prolonged with a median duration around 6 months.[20]

Systemic rituximab is useful, especially in cases with multiple disseminated lesions. The usual dose is 375 mg/m^2 weekly, four to eight intravenous infusions. The largest series included 25 cases.[21] Overall response rate (ORR) was seen in 98% of the patients with 64% CRs. Median PFS reached 58 months and median time to next treatment 60 months.

Adverse events occurred in 32% of the cases, mostly grade 1 or 2, with pruritus, erythema, urticaria, nausea, vomiting, chest discomfort, diarrhea, angioedema, grade 3 dyspnea, dysarthria, weakness, and confusion.

Chlorambucil as a single-agent chemotherapeutic treatment has been used (particularly in Europe) for patients with multiple disseminated lesions. The recommendation is to use it for a limited time (maximum 3 months). All reported patients respond with >60% having CRs.[10,22] Multiagent chemotherapy is rarely indicated in PCMZL, being too aggressive therapy for an indolent condition. Reported cases achieve CR in 85% of the cases, but relapses occur as frequently as in other treatments.[10]

PRIMARY CUTANEOUS FOLLICLE CENTER LYMPHOMA

PCFCL represents around 9% to 11% of all cutaneous lymphomas and 32% to 57% of all CBCLs. It usually affects middle-aged adults, and the sex distribution has a male/female ratio of 1.5:1.[2,5-9]

Clinical Features

PCFCL presents lesions clinically undistinguishable from PCMZL but is more often localized on the head and neck, rather than the trunk. Between 15% and 25% of the cases present with multiple lesions. As PCMZL, lesions are usually violaceous in color and rarely ulcerate. Very importantly, lesions on the back are frequently surrounded by smaller lesions, even tiny papules that may be misdiagnosed as folliculitis or other conditions. Untreated, those lesions develop large tumors months or years later. This is the origin of the classical entity known as "Crosti reticulohistiocytoma of the dorsum." Extracutaneous disseminations are uncommon. Behavior is indolent with 5-year specific survival >95%.[2,3,7]

Diagnostic Workup

A complete review of symptoms, specifically looking for B symptoms and organ-specific symptoms, should be pursued. Laboratory studies should include a complete blood cell count with differential. Biochemistry investigations should include serum LDH and electrophoresis to exclude monoclonal gammopathy. In cases with leukocytosis, flow cytometry is recommended. For those patients to be treated with rituximab, serologies for HBV, HCV, HIV, and PPD are mandatory. Imaging (CT scan or PET-CT trying to irradiate the patient as less as possible) is recommended. In cases with lesions on the head, the study should include evaluation of the neck region. Bone marrow has been considered optional but in one study, 22/192 cases (11%) presented bone marrow involvement. In nine of those 22, bone marrow was the only extracutaneous involvement.[11,12] An argument can be made for the staging evaluation of the bone marrow in patients who have systemic symptoms, multiple lesions clinically (specifically outside the head and neck region), and particularly when lesions are BCL-2 positive.

Prognosis

The prognosis is excellent with 95% disease-specific survival (DSS) at 10 years; however, OS drops to around 40% in those cases with lesions present on the legs. The presence of multiple lesions does not worsen the outcome. Cutaneous relapses are seen in around 30% of the cases (less frequent than PCMZL); nevertheless, relapses do not mean progression. About 10% of the patients have extracutaneous dissemination.[8,23,24]

Treatment

Similarly to PCMZL, for patients with solitary or a limited number of lesions, the treatments of choice are surgery and/or radiotherapy, depending on the size of the lesions clinically. Radiotherapy is highly effective with 99% of CRs. Reported doses are around 30 Gy with variable margins (0.5-5 cm).[14,15,25] The relapse rate is around 47% but can be as high as 76%.[10,26] Intralesional IFN alpha has been reported in a limited number of cases. All reported patients achieved CR with a relapse rate of approximately 30%.[10] As mentioned above, unfortunately, IFN alpha is no longer available in most countries.

Intralesional rituximab[10,20] is used according to the same protocol for PCMZL. Adverse events and recommendations for the prevention of infection reactivations are also the same. An 80% response rate is reported albeit with relapses between 22% and 40%.

Systemic rituximab is useful, especially in cases with multiple disseminated lesions. The reported protocol is the same as in PCMZL. The largest series described 29 cases.[21] ORR was 96% with 72% of CRs. Median PFS reached 78 months and median time to next treatment, 85 months. Adverse events occurred in 38% of the cases, mostly grade 1 or 2, with similar conditions appearing in the treatment of PCMZL with systemic rituximab.

Multiagent chemotherapy should be recommended only for those cases with very extensive cutaneous disease or rare cases with extracutaneous dissemination. Senff et al systematically reviewed the literature and found 85% of CRs with 44% of relapses. The most frequently used regimen was CHOP. Cyclophosphamide, vincristine sulfate, prednisone seems less effective.[10] Combination radiotherapy of the involved fields with CHOP has also been reported. CRs were documented in all treated patients with 14% relapses. The combination of Rituximab + CHOP (doxorubicin, vincristine, cyclophosphamide, prednisone) (R-CHOP) has also been reported, but experience is very limited. Given the worse prognosis for patients with PCFCL having lesions arising on the legs, the current recommendation is to use the same treatment as for PCDLBCL, LT.[10]

PRIMARY CUTANEOUS DIFFUSE LARGE B-CELL LYMPHOMA, LEG TYPE

PCDLBCL, LT represents about 2.6% to 6% of all cutaneous lymphoma (CL)[2,5,27-29] and 10% to 20% of CBCL.[5,27,30-33] In contrast to indolent cutaneous lymphomas, PCDLBCL, LT normally affects elderly female patients[2,32,34] (men/women ratio 1:2 to 1:4),[5,27,33] although this finding is not consistently reported.[30,35] The median age at presentation is 70 to 82 years.[5,27,30,36]

Clinical Features

It is clinically characterized by rapidly progressive solitary or multiple tumors and also nodules or infiltrated plaques, usually erythematous to violaceous, that can ulcerate, involving one or both lower legs.[32,34,37] Other sites are involved in 10% to 20% of cases.[5,27,31-35,37] Rare clinical variants have been reported, including presentations mimicking cellulitis and sporotrichosis,[38] and arising in association with chronic lymphoedema.[39] Spontaneous remission is extremely rare, having been reported only in a few cases.[40] Involvement of multiple sites, on one or both legs, is associated with a significantly inferior disease-specific survival.[23,34] In cases of systemic disease, patients may have B symptoms such as fever, night sweats, and weight loss.[31]

Extracutaneous dissemination is frequent,[27,32-34] and while some studies showed that patients with leg involvement had higher rates of extracutaneous spread and worse prognosis than those with lesions at other sites (33% vs 18%),[5,31,36] other studies did not duplicate this finding.[8,24,41]

Classification and Diagnostic Workup

PCDLBCL, LT follows the EORTC/ISCL consensus classification,[4] and the diagnostic workup should include laboratory tests (complete blood count with differential, comprehensive metabolic panel); PET-CT/CT of the chest, abdomen, and pelvis; bone marrow biopsy; and peripheral blood flow cytometry.[5,10,37]

Prognosis

This subtype of CBCL is considered aggressive, and its natural history more closely resembles that of systemic diffuse large B-cell lymphoma (DLBCL).[34] It is associated with a 5-year disease-specific survival of approximately 50%.[27,31-34] The presence of multiple lesions, location on the leg, and age over 75 years correlate with a worse prognosis.[5] Also, dual BCL-2 and MYC expression is associated with inferior survival, as well as the presence of a somatic $MYD88_{L265P}$ mutation.[34,37] Some authors have also found high expression of MUM1 and FOXP1 and the deletion of the $CDKN2A$ locus on chromosome 9p21 to be negative prognostic factors.[33]

Treatment

Owing to its aggressive behavior, this subtype of CBCL is better approached in similar fashion to its systemic counterpart, with the recommended first-line treatment being polychemotherapy (CHOP) in combination with intravenous rituximab (R)[5,10,30-33,37,41,42] followed by localized radiotherapy.[42,43] The R-CHOP combination has shown to have a 60% to 90% response rate and a 3-year disease-specific survival rate of 80% to 90%[5] and is, in terms of OS rates, significantly superior to all other possible combinations[37,44] (Fig. 36-1). This combination of radiotherapy and chemotherapy may yield a better outcome than cases treated only with chemotherapy[5] but relapse occurs in about 56% of cases.[42]

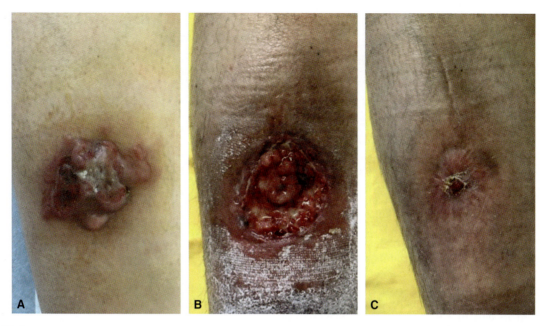

FIGURE 36-1. Female patient with PCDLBCL, LT **(A)** at presentation, **(B)** immediately after R-CHOP × 6 + RT, **(C)** 3 months after the end of treatment.

Nevertheless, one of the biggest challenges in the treatment of PCDLCBL, LT is the fact that it mainly affects elderly people who frequently have comorbidities that render CHOP-like regimens intolerable due to cardiac and hematological side effects (R-mini-CHOP). There is the frequent need to use modified age-adapted R-CHOP regimens in this population. If polychemotherapy is contraindicated, disease control can be achieved with rituximab monotherapy in combination with local radiotherapy.[10,29,42] A further option is the use of pegylated liposomal doxorubicin (PLD) with or without rituximab, having good results and safety profile.[28,30,32,33] In palliative settings, in cases with solitary or confined lesions, treatments such as radiotherapy as monotherapy[30,37,42] and surgery can also be used.[30,37] The former has showed CR rates of 88% but a relapse rate of 58% with extracutaneous progression occurring in approximately 30% of cases.[10]

Unfortunately, there are no universally accepted recommendations for the treatment of recalcitrant or recurrent disease.[37] In this situation, several different treatment options have been described, in the setting of clinical trials and case reports, such as isolated PLD,[45] PLD or gemcitabine in combination with rituximab,[46] isolated limb perfusion with melphalan,[47] lenalidomide,[48,49] bendamustine + rituximab,[50-52] ibrutinib,[53] immune check point inhibitors like nivolumab[54] and pembrolizumab associated with rituximab and lenalidomide,[55] and also stem cell transplantation.[56]

PLD in monotherapy or combined with rituximab seems to be an effective, well-tolerated treatment.[30,45,46] Lenalidomide inhibits cell signaling engaging NF-kB and IFN-κB pathways exhibiting both antiproliferative and antiangiogenic effects[57] and its efficacy has been shown in relapsing and refractory DLBCL, with a good safety profile even in the elderly.[49] A case report of its effectiveness in association with dexamethasone in a case of relapsed PCDLBCL, LT has been published,[40] and a multicenter, single-arm, phase II clinical trial was conducted to assess the benefits and safety of this drug in relapsed or refractory disease.[49] Nineteen patients were included in this study, and the 6-month ORR was 26.3%, with 1 CR and 4 partial responses (PRs) and median PFS of 4 months. The study also showed that reduced doses tended to be associated with higher 6-month ORR and PFS. A higher overall response under treatment was seen in the absence of the $MYD88_{L265P}$ mutation. The authors concluded that the use of reduced doses of this drug may allow prolonged responses in some patients and is a therapeutic option in relapsed/refractory disease.[49]

The Bruton tyrosine kinase (BTK) is an important signaling molecule of the B-cell receptor signaling pathway,[32] and therefore, the use of BTK inhibitors such as ibrutinib may have a role in the treatment of this disease, in the absence of associated *CARD11* or *PIM1* mutations that have been correlated with resistance to this drug.[58,59] Two case reports have been published where this drug was used in refractory previously heavily treated disease, with both patients achieving CR, although one of them progressed to nodal disease after 2 months.[53,60]

Further new treatment options for this disease are needed, and there is in fact a growing number of new monoclonal antibodies, checkpoint inhibitors, BKT inhibitors, and other small molecules being studied and used in DLBCL that could potentially play a role in the treatment of PCBLBCL, LT. Therefore, randomized clinical trials should be performed to evaluate their efficacy in this subtype of CBCL.

INTRAVASCULAR LARGE B-CELL LYMPHOMA

This rare subtype of CBCL represents <1% of all CLs,[2] being diagnosed in less than 1 per million adults.[30] It also typically affects older patients (median age 67 years)[5,27,30,35] with no gender prevalence.[30,35] It is defined by collections of large lymphoma cells within the small to medium-sized blood vessels lumina[2,30] and has a propensity to involve the brain, lungs, and skin, creating intraluminal microthrombi.[2,27,31,33,41]

Clinical Features

Two clinical variants of intravascular large B-cell lymphoma have been described: the Asian and the Western. The former is characterized by hemophagocytic lymphohistiocytosis, whereas the latter presents with involvement of the skin and the central nervous system (CNS).[5,61,62] The majority of patients often show disseminated disease,[33] but in 25% of the Western subtype cases patients present with skin-limited involvement at the time of diagnosis. This variation is more common in women, and its prognosis is substantially better when compared with patients with systemic disease.[2,35,63]

This lymphoma subtype normally presents in the skin but one-third to half of patients may not develop skin lesions.[5,31,63] Cutaneous manifestations present as maculopapular eruptions, nodules, violaceous plaques, ulcerated tumors, painful telangiectasias, purpura, livedo reticularis, and cellulitis-like infiltration[5,27,30,31,33] located on the upper arms, thighs, and legs, and also on the lower abdomen and breasts.[31,63]

Most patients present with constitutional symptoms,[5] and neurological complaints are described in about 34% of patients.[63]

Classification and Diagnostic Workup

Conventional staging with PET/CT frequently fails to disclose extracutaneous disease, and this subtype of lymphoma usually does not involve lymph nodes.[27] Diagnostic workup should follow those recommended for PCDLBCL, LT, and also MRI of the CNS, due to the frequency of its involvement. Nevertheless, imaging is often directed by the patient's symptoms and signs.[31]

Prognosis

The prognosis of both Asian and Western variants is poor with a mean 3-year survival of 30% and median survival of 5 months.[5,63] The cutaneous-limited presentation has a better prognosis, with a 3-year survival of 56%.[63] The following factors have been found to be negative prognostic indicators: poor performance status (PS), advanced disease, elevated serum LDH, and B symptoms.[5,61]

Treatment

The standard treatment is multiagent chemotherapy combined with rituximab (R-CHOP), although this recommendation is based on retrospective reviews and case reports as clinical trials are not available.[5,30,33] CNS treatment with methotrexate should also be performed in cases with CNS involvement.[31,33] Stem cell transplantation ought to be considered in young patients with good PS.[5,64]

EBV-POSITIVE MUCOCUTANEOUS ULCER (PROVISIONAL)

This EBV-driven lymphoproliferative disorder accounts for less than 1% of all CL and is still a provisional entity in the latest WHO-EORTC classification of CL.[2] It is associated with immunodeficiency in the setting of iatrogenic immunosuppression or age-related immune senescence.[2,27,33]

Clinical Features

It characteristically presents as a solitary, sharply demarcated ulcer in the skin, oropharyngeal mucosa, or gastrointestinal tract of immunosuppressed individuals.[2,27,33]

Prognosis

It has an excellent prognosis with a 5-year disease-specific survival of 100%.[2]

Treatment

It has an indolent behavior, with a self-limited course,[2,27,33] showing spontaneous regression in 45% of cases.[65] Therefore, reduction of the immunosuppression is the first-line treatment, whenever feasible.[2,33] Other treatment options include rituximab or other specific treatment against EBV.[66]

References

1. Smith BD, Smith GL, Cooper DL, Wilson LD. The cutaneous B-cell lymphoma prognostic index: a novel prognostic index derived from a population-based registry. *J Clin Oncol*. 2005;23(15):3390-3395. doi:10.1200/JCO.2005.08.137
2. Willemze R, Cerroni L, Kempf W, et al. The 2018 update of the WHO-EORTC classification for primary cutaneous lymphomas. *Blood*. 2019;133(16):1703-1714. doi:10.1182/blood-2018-11-881268
3. Swerdlow S, Campo E, Harris N, Jaffe E, Pileri S, Stein H. *Weltgesundheitsorganisation. WHO Classification of Tumours of Haematopoietic and Lymphoid Tissues*. 4th revised Edition. International Agency for Research of Cancer; 2017.
4. Kim YH, Willemze R, Pimpinelli N, et al. TNM classification system for primary cutaneous lymphomas other than mycosis fungoides and Sézary syndrome: a proposal of the International Society for cutaneous lymphomas (ISCL) and the cutaneous lymphoma Task Force of the European Organization of research and treatment of Cancer (EORTC). *Blood*. 2007;110(2):479-484. doi:10.1182/blood-2006-10-054601
5. Goyal A, LeBlanc RE, Carter JB. Cutaneous B-cell lymphoma. *Hematol Oncol Clin N Am*. 2019;33(1):149-161. doi:10.1016/j.hoc.2018.08.006
6. Peñate Y, Servitje O, Machan S, et al. Registro de linfomas cutáneos primarios de la AEDV: primer año de funcionamiento. *Actas Dermosifiliogr*. 2018;109(7):610-616. doi:10.1016/j.ad.2018.03.006
7. Willemze R. WHO-EORTC classification for cutaneous lymphomas. *Blood*. 2005;105(10):3768-3785. doi:10.1182/blood-2004-09-3502

8. Zinzani PL, Quaglino P, Pimpinelli N, et al. Prognostic factors in primary cutaneous B-cell lymphoma: the Italian study group for cutaneous lymphomas. *J Clin Oncol.* 2006;24(9):1376-1382. doi:10.1200/JCO.2005.03.6285
9. Bradford PT, Devesa SS, Anderson WF, Toro JR. Cutaneous lymphoma incidence patterns in the United States: a population-based study of 3884 cases. *Blood.* 2009;113(21):5064-5073. doi:10.1182/blood-2008-10-184168
10. Senff NJ, Noordijk EM, Kim YH, et al. European Organization for research and treatment of Cancer and International Society for cutaneous lymphoma consensus recommendations for the management of cutaneous B-cell lymphomas. *Blood.* 2008;112(5):1600-1609. doi:10.1182/blood-2008-04-152850
11. *NCCN Guidelines, Primary Cutaneous Lymphomas V2.* 2021. https://www.nccn.org/professionals/physician_gls/pdf/primary_cutaneous.pdf
12. Senff NJ, Kluin-Nelemans HC, Willemze R. Results of bone marrow examination in 275 patients with histological features that suggest an indolent type of cutaneous B-cell lymphoma. *Br J Haematol.* 2008;142(1):52-56. doi:10.1111/j.1365-2141.2008.07159.x
13. Mian M, Marcheselli L, Luminari S, et al. CLIPI: a new prognostic index for indolent cutaneous B cell lymphoma proposed by the International Extranodal Lymphoma Study Group (IELSG 11). *Ann Hematol.* 2011;90(4):401-408. doi:10.1007/s00277-010-1083-1
14. Senff NJ. Results of radiotherapy in 153 primary cutaneous B-cell lymphomas classified according to the WHO-EORTC classification. *Arch Dermatol.* 2007;143(12):1520-1526. doi:10.1001/archderm.143.12.1520
15. Eich HT, Eich D, Micke O, et al. Long-term efficacy, curative potential, and prognostic factors of radiotherapy in primary cutaneous B-cell lymphoma. *Int J Radiat Oncol Biol Phys.* 2003;55(4):899-906. doi:10.1016/S0360-3016(02)04199-8
16. Perry A, Vincent BJ, Parker SRS. Intralesional corticosteroid therapy for primary cutaneous B-cell lymphoma. *Br J Dermatol.* 2010;163(1):223-225. doi:10.1111/j.1365-2133.2010.09798.x
17. Roggero E, Zucca E, Mainetti C, et al. Eradication of Borrelia burgdorferi infection in primary marginal zone B-cell lymphoma of the skin. *Hum Pathol.* 2000;31(2):263-268. doi:10.1016/S0046-8177(00)80233-6
18. Kütting B, Bonsmann G, Metze D, Luger TA, Cerroni L. Borrelia burgdorferi—associated primary cutaneous B cell lymphoma: complete clearing of skin lesions after antibiotic pulse therapy or intralesional injection of interferon alfa-2a. *J Am Acad Dermatol.* 1997;36(2):311-314. doi:10.1016/S0190-9622(97)80405-7.
19. Cozzio A, Kempf W, Schmid-Meyer R, et al. Intra-lesional low-dose interferon α2a therapy for primary cutaneous marginal zone B-cell lymphoma. *Leuk Lymphoma.* 2006;47(5):865-869. doi:10.1080/10428190500399698
20. Peñate Y, Hernández-Machín B, Pérez-Méndez LI, et al. Intralesional rituximab in the treatment of indolent primary cutaneous B-cell lymphomas: an epidemiological observational multicentre study. The Spanish Working Group on Cutaneous Lymphoma. *Br J Dermatol.* 2012;167(1):174-179. doi:10.1111/j.1365-2133.2012.10902.x
21. Muniesa C, Domingo-Domenech E, Fornons-Servent R, et al. Systemic rituximab for the treatment of the indolent forms of primary cutaneous B-cell lymphomas: data from the spanish primary cutaneous lymphoma registry. *J Am Acad Dermatol.* 2020;83(5):1535-1538. doi:10.1016/j.jaad.2020.07.028
22. Stanway A, Rademaker M, Kennedy I, Newman P. Cutaneous B-cell lymphoma of nails, pinna and nose treated with chlorambucil. *Australas J Dermatol.* 2004;45(2):110-113. doi:10.1111/j.1440-0960.2004.00057.x
23. Grange F, Bekkenk MW, Wechsler J, et al. Prognostic factors in primary cutaneous large B-cell lymphomas: a European multicenter study. *J Clin Oncol.* 2001;19(16):3602-3610. doi:10.1200/JCO.2001.19.16.3602
24. Senff NJ, Hoefnagel JJ, Jansen PM, et al. Reclassification of 300 primary cutaneous B-cell lymphomas according to the new WHO–EORTC classification for cutaneous lymphomas: comparison with previous classifications and Identification of prognostic markers. *J Clin Oncol.* 2007;25(12):1581-1587. doi:10.1200/JCO.2006.09.6396
25. Smith BD, Glusac EJ, McNiff JM, et al. Primary cutaneous B-cell lymphoma treated with radiotherapy: a comparison of the European Organization for research and treatment of cancer and the WHO classification systems. *J Clin Oncol.* 2004;22(4):634-639. doi:10.1200/JCO.2004.08.044
26. Piccinno R, Caccialanza M, Berti E. Dermatologic radiotherapy of primary cutaneous follicle center cell lymphoma. *Eur J Dermatol.* 2003;13(1):49-52.
27. Pinter-Brown LC. Diagnosis and management of cutaneous B-cell lymphoma. *Dermatol Clin.* 2015;33(4):835-840. doi:10.1016/j.det.2015.05.003
28. Lima M. Cutaneous primary B-cell lymphomas: from diagnosis to treatment. *An Bras Dermatol.* 2015;90(5):687-706. doi:10.1590/abd1806-4841.20153638
29. Fernández-Guarino M, Ortiz-Romero PL, Fernández-Misa R, Montalbán C. Rituximab in the treatment of primary cutaneous B-cell lymphoma: a review. *Actas Dermo-Sifiliográficas.* 2014;105(5):438-445. doi:10.1016/j.ad.2012.10.021
30. Malachowski SJ, Sun J, Chen PL, Seminario-Vidal L. Diagnosis and management of cutaneous B-cell lymphomas. *Dermatol Clin.* 2019;37(4):443-454. doi:10.1016/j.det.2019.05.004
31. Chen ST, Barnes J, Duncan L. Primary cutaneous B-cell lymphomas- clinical and histopathologic features, differential diagnosis, and treatment. *Semin Cutan Med Surg.* 2018;37(1):49-55. doi:10.12788/j.sder.2018.014
32. Dumont M, Battistella M, Ram-Wolff C, Bagot M, de Masson A. Diagnosis and treatment of primary cutaneous b-cell lymphomas: State of the art and perspectives. *Cancers.* 2020;12(6):1-21. doi:10.3390/cancers12061497
33. Vitiello P, Sica A, Ronchi A, Caccavale S, Franco R, Argenziano G. Primary cutaneous B-cell lymphomas: an update. *Front Oncol.* 2020;10. doi:10.3389/fonc.2020.00651
34. Wilcox RA. Cutaneous B-cell lymphomas: 2019 update on diagnosis, risk stratification, and management. *Am J Hematol.* 2018;93(11):1427-1430. doi:10.1002/ajh.25224
35. Hope CB, Pincus LB. Primary cutaneous B-cell lymphomas with large cell predominance–primary cutaneous follicle center lymphoma, diffuse large B-cell lymphoma, leg type and intravascular large B-cell lymphoma. *Semin Diagn Pathol.* 2017;34(1):85-98. doi:10.1053/j.semdp.2016.11.006
36. Grange F, Beylot-Barry M, Courville P, et al. Primary cutaneous diffuse large B-cell lymphoma, leg type clinicopathologic features and prognostic analysis in 60 cases. *Arch Dermatol.* 2007;143:1144-1150. https://jamanetwork.com/

37. Nicolay JP, Wobser M. B-Zell-Lymphome der Haut – pathogenese, Diagnostik und Therapie. *J Dtsch Dermatol Ges.* 2016;14(12):1207-1225. doi:10.1111/ddg.13164
38. Long V, Liang MW, Lee JSS, Lim JHL. Two instructive cases of primary cutaneous diffuse large B-cell lymphoma (leg type) mimicking cellulitis and sporotrichosis. *JAAD Case Rep.* 2020;6(9):815-818. doi:10.1016/j.jdcr.2020.06.043
39. Marasca C, Fabbrocini G, Cinelli E, Fontanella G, Marasca D, Zagaria O. A case of a primary cutaneous diffuse large B-cell lymphoma, leg type. *Int Wound J.* 2020;17(2):514-515. doi:10.1111/iwj.13298
40. Al Dhafiri M, Sicre de Fontbrune F, Marinho E, et al. Effectiveness of lenalidomide in relapsed primary cutaneous diffuse large B-cell lymphoma, leg type. *Clin Case Rep.* 2019;7(5):964-967. doi:10.1002/ccr3.2137
41. Hope CB, Pincus LB. Primary cutaneous B-cell lymphomas. *Clin Lab Med.* 2017;37(3):547-574. doi:10.1016/j.cll.2017.05.009
42. Lang CCV, Ramelyte E, Dummer R. Innovative therapeutic approaches in primary cutaneous B cell lymphoma. *Front Oncol.* 2020;10:1163. doi:10.3389/fonc.2020.01163
43. Specht L, Dabaja B, Illidge T, Wilson LD, Hoppe RT. Modern radiation therapy for primary cutaneous lymphomas: field and dose guidelines from the International lymphoma radiation Oncology group. *Int J Radiat Oncol Biol Phys.* 2015;92(1):32-39. doi:10.1016/j.ijrobp.2015.01.008
44. Grange F, Joly P, Barbe C, et al. Improvement of survival in patients with primary cutaneous diffuse large B-cell lymphoma, leg type, in France. *JAMA Dermatol.* 2014;150(5):535-541. doi:10.1001/jamadermatol.2013.7452
45. Pulini S, Rupoli S, Goteri G, et al. Efficacy and safety of pegylated liposomal doxorubicin in primary cutaneous B-cell lymphomas and comparison with the commonly used therapies. *Eur J Haematol.* 2009;82(3):184-193. doi:10.1111/j.1600-0609.2008.01197.x
46. Fabbri A, Cencini E, Alterini R, et al. Rituximab plus liposomal pegylated doxorubicin in the treatment of primary cutaneous B-cell lymphomas. *Eur J Haematol.* 2014;93(2):129-136. doi:10.1111/ejh.12315
47. Kobold S, Killic N, Lütkens T, Bokemeyer C, Fiedler W. Isolated limb perfusion with melphalan for the treatment of Intractable primary cutaneous diffuse large B-cell lymphoma leg type. *Acta Haematol.* 2010;123(3):179-181. doi:10.1159/000294963
48. Savini P, Lanzi A, Foschi FG, Marano G, Stefanini GF. Lenalidomide monotherapy in relapsed primary cutaneous diffuse large B cell lymphoma-leg type. *Ann Hematol.* 2014;93(2):333-334. doi:10.1007/s00277-013-1787-0
49. Beylot-Barry M, Mermin D, Maillard A, et al. A single-arm phase II trial of lenalidomide in relapsing or refractory primary cutaneous large B-cell lymphoma, leg type. *J Invest Dermatol.* 2018;138(9):1982-1989. doi:10.1016/j.jid.2018.03.1516
50. Ohmachi K, Niitsu N, Uchida T, et al. Multicenter phase II study of bendamustine plus rituximab in patients with relapsed or refractory diffuse large B-cell lymphoma. *J Clin Oncol.* 2013;31(17):2103-2109. doi:10.1200/JCO.2012.46.5203
51. Zeremski V, Jentsch-Ullrich K, Kahl C, et al. Is bendamustine-rituximab a reasonable treatment in selected older patients with diffuse large B cell lymphoma? Results from a multicentre, retrospective study. *Ann Hematol.* 2019;98(12):2729-2737. doi:10.1007/s00277-019-03819-3
52. Hong JY, Yoon DH, Suh C, et al. Bendamustine plus rituximab for relapsed or refractory diffuse large B cell lymphoma: a multicenter retrospective analysis. *Ann Hematol.* 2018;97(8):1437-1443. doi:10.1007/s00277-018-3317-6
53. Gupta E, Accurso J, Sluzevich J, Menke DM, Tun HW. Excellent outcome of Immunomodulation or Bruton's tyrosine kinase inhibition in highly refractory primary cutaneous diffuse large B-cell lymphoma, leg type. *Rare Tumors.* 2015;7(4):6067. doi:10.4081/rt.2015.6067
54. Lesokhin AM, Ansell SM, Armand P, et al. Nivolumab in patients with relapsed or refractory hematologic malignancy: preliminary results of a phase Ib study. *J Clin Oncol.* 2016;34(23):2698-2704. doi:10.1200/JCO.2015.65.9789
55. di Raimondo C, Abdulla FR, Zain J, Querfeld C, Rosen ST. Rituximab, lenalidomide and pembrolizumab in refractory primary cutaneous diffuse large B-cell lymphoma, leg type. *Br J Haematol.* 2019;187(3):e79-e82. doi:10.1111/bjh.16211
56. Massone C, Fink-Puches R, Wolf I, Zalaudek I, Cerroni L. Atypical clinicopathologic presentation of primary cutaneous diffuse large B-cell lymphoma, leg type. *J Am Acad Dermatol.* 2015;72(6):1016-1020. doi:10.1016/j.jaad.2015.02.1134
57. Chanan-Khan AA, Cheson BD. Lenalidomide for the treatment of B-cell malignancies. *J Clin Oncol.* 2008;26(9):1544-1552. doi:10.1200/JCO.2007.14.5367
58. Kuo HP, Ezell SA, Hsieh S, et al. The role of PIM1 in the ibrutinib-resistant ABC subtype of diffuse large B-cell lymphoma. *Am J Cancer Res.* 2016;6:2489-2501. Accessed June 3, 2021. www.ajcr.us/
59. Wilson WH, Young RM, Schmitz R, et al. Targeting B cell receptor signaling with ibrutinib in diffuse large B cell lymphoma. *Nat Med.* 2015;21(8):922-926. doi:10.1038/nm.3884
60. Fox L, Yannakou C, Ryland G, et al. Molecular mechanisms of disease progression in primary cutaneous diffuse large B-cell lymphoma, leg type during ibrutinib therapy. *Int J Mol Sci.* 2018;19(6):1758. doi:10.3390/ijms19061758
61. Murase T, Yamaguchi M, Suzuki R, et al. Intravascular large B-cell lymphoma (IVLBCL): a clinicopathologic study of 96 cases with special reference to the immunophenotypic heterogeneity of CD5. *Blood.* 2007;109(2):478-485. doi:10.1182/blood-2006-01-021253
62. Shimada K, Kinoshita T, Naoe T, Nakamura S. Presentation and management of intravascular large B-cell lymphoma. *Lancet Oncol.* 2009;10(9):895-902. doi:10.1016/S1470-2045(09)70140-8
63. Ferreri AJM, Campo E, Seymour JF, et al. Intravascular lymphoma: clinical presentation, natural history, management and prognostic factors in a series of 38 cases, with special emphasis on the "cutaneous variant." *Br J Haematol.* 2004;127(2):173-182. doi:10.1111/j.1365-2141.2004.05177.x
64. Orwat DE, Batalis NI. Intravascular large B-cell lymphoma. *Arch Pathol Lab Med.* 2012;136(3):333-338. doi:10.5858/arpa.2010-0747-RS
65. Dojcinov SD, Venkataraman G, Raffeld M, Pittaluga S, Jaffe ES. EBV positive mucocutaneous ulcer—a study of 26 cases associated with various Sources of immunosuppression. *Am J Surg Pathol.* 2010;34(3):405-417. doi:10.1097/PAS.0b013e3181cf8622
66. Grimm KE, O'Malley DP. Aggressive B cell lymphomas in the 2017 revised WHO classification of tumors of hematopoietic and lymphoid tissues. *Ann Diagn Pathol.* 2019;38:6-10. doi:10.1016/j.anndiagpath.2018.09.014

PART VII SYSTEMIC B-CELL LYMPHOMAS WITH CUTANEOUS DISSEMINATION

CHAPTER 37

Systemic follicular lymphoma, marginal zone lymphomas, and lymphoplasmacytic lymphoma

Alejandro A. Gru and Antonio Subtil

FOLLICULAR LYMPHOMA

Definition

Systemic follicular lymphoma (sFL) is defined by the WHO as a neoplasm composed of follicle center (germinal center) B-cells (typically both centrocytes and centroblasts), which usually has at least a partially follicular growth pattern.[1] sFL is the most common subtype of non-Hodgkin lymphomas (NHLs), accounting for approximately 45% of cases.[2] While most patients present with disseminated disease, sFL has an overall good prognosis with a 5-year survival of 75%.

Cutaneous Involvement by Systemic Follicular Center Cell Lymphoma

Almost 4% of sFL cases involve the skin.[3-6] Cutaneous dissemination invariably occurs after the diagnosis of nodal disease. The typical interval between the original diagnosis of lymphoma and skin involvement is 3–7 years. Most of the cutaneous lesions in sFL present on the head and neck.[4] Rare cases with rosacea-like clinical presentation had been described.[7] Cases of sFL with cutaneous recurrences had been reported.[8] Bone marrow infiltration is usually present at the time of skin involvement. Unlike primary cutaneous follicle center lymphoma (PCFCL), the prognosis of sFL depends on the histologic grade: the 5-year survival is 60% in high-grade (grade 3) and 100% in low-grade disease (grade 1–2).[3] Skin involvement does not appear to influence clinical outcome. sFL needs to be distinguished from PCFCL, as the latter carries an excellent prognosis and only rarely requires systemic treatment (Table 37-1).

Histopathology

sFL with cutaneous involvement is characterized by a dermal-based infiltrate with sparing of the epidermis (Fig. 37-1). The infiltrate shows a follicular and/or diffuse pattern (50%). Grading of lesions is mandatory for sFL, as this can determine the prognosis of the tumors. Grading of sFL is based on the number of centroblasts per 40X high-power field (counting 10 HPF, 0.159 mm^2). Grade 3 lesions reveal more than 15 centroblasts/HPF. Grade 3A contains both centrocytes and centroblasts, while grade 3B lacks centrocytes. Fewer than 15 centroblasts/HPF are found in grade 1–2 (low grade). Grading of PCFCL is of no value and should not be performed in any case. The morphologic pattern of PCFCL is similar to that of sFL. The so-called spindle cell variant is unique to PCFCL and not associated with sFL.

Immunophenotype

The immunophenotype of sFL is characterized by B-cell antigenic expression (CD20, CD19) and markers of germinal center differentiation (CD10, BCL6, LMO-2) (Fig. 37-2). BCL2 expression by centrocytes and centroblasts is considered the hallmark of the disease. However, BCL2 and CD10 are often negative in high-grade cases.[9] Cases with a follicular growth pattern show retained follicular dendritic networks, demonstrated by CD21, CD23, or CD35. MUM1 is typically positive in high-grade lesions and only stains background plasma cells in low-grade follicular lymphoma (FL). CD30 can be seen in approximately 30% of cases.[10]

Nearly all cases of low-grade FL and higher grade FL show the t(14;18) translocation affecting the *IGH* and *BCL2* genes. This translocation is only seen in a small fraction of cases of PCFCL (10%–20%).[2]

TABLE 37-1 Comparison of Primary Cutaneous Follicle Center Lymphoma and Secondary Cutaneous Involvement by Systemic/Nodal Follicular Lymphoma

	Primary Cutaneous Follicle Center Lymphoma	Systemic/Nodal Follicular Lymphoma
BCL2 IHC	Usually negative in neoplastic cells (may be positive in up to 20% of cases)	Usually positive (may be negative in up to 30% of cases, particularly grade 3)
CD10 IHC	Variable (expression is more frequent in follicular growth pattern than in diffuse)	Usually positive (may be negative in a subset of grade 3 cases)
BCL6 IHC	Positive	Positive
Grading	Not done	1–2 (low grade), 3A, 3B (based on the number of centroblasts per high-power microscopic field)
Initial staging workup (gold standard)	Skin-only disease	Evidence of systemic disease

IHC, immunohistochemistry.

As opposed to sFL, most cases of PCFCL are negative for BCL2.[11] Additionally, CD10 can be negative in cases with a diffuse growth pattern. MUM1 is invariably negative in PCFCL. Follicular dendritic cell networks are retained in cases with a nodular growth, but lost in diffuse patterns. Ki67 can be markedly elevated in PCFCL, particularly those with a large number of centroblasts. Increased proliferation has no prognostic significance in PCFCL, as opposed to sFL.

Genetics

The t(14;18)(q32;q21), *IGH::BCL2* translocation is present in 90% of low-grade FL, but is less frequent in high-grade FL. Other common cytogenetic aberrations include loss of 1p, 6q, 10q, and 17p and gains of chromosomes 1, 6p, 7, 8, 12q, 18, and X. Fluorescent in situ hybridization (FISH) detects ~85% of the *IGH::BCL2* translocation. This translocation is only seen in a small fraction of cases of PCFCL (10%–20%).[2] Rare cases of sFL may develop transformation into a double-hit lymphoma (high-grade B-cell lymphoma with *MYC* and *BCL2* and/or *BCL6* rearrangements).[1] A recent study by Zhu et al[12] revealed novel insights into the molecular profiling that can separate apart PCFCL from sFL with secondary skin dissemination: a total of 30 cases of PCFCL and 10 of sFL and performed whole-exome sequencing on 18 specimens of PCFCL and 6 of SCFL. Although the sFLs universally expressed BCL2 and had *BCL2* rearrangements, 73% of the PCFCLs lacked BCL2 expression, and only 8% of skin-restricted PCFCLs had *BCL2* rearrangements. sFLs showed low proliferation fractions, whereas 75% of PCFCLs had proliferation fractions >30%. Of the sFLs, 67% had characteristic loss-of-function *CREBBP* or *KMT2D* mutations vs none in skin-restricted PCFCL. Both sFL and skin-restricted PCFCL showed frequent *TNFRSF14* loss-of-function mutations and copy number loss at chromosome 1p36.

CAPSULE SUMMARY

- sFL is the most common subtype of systemic NHL, accounting for approximately 45% of cases.
- The t(14;18)(q32;q21), *IGH::BCL2* translocation is present in 90% of low-grade FL, but is less frequent in high-grade FL.
- Almost 4% of sFL cases involve the skin. Skin dissemination invariably occurs after the diagnosis of nodal disease is made.
- As opposed to PCFCL, grading of sFL is important in prognostic stratification.
- As opposed to PCFCL, sFL is strongly BCL2+ and CD10+ in most cases. Ki67 also shows prognostic information in sFL, but not in PCFCL.
- Staging is the gold standard for final differentiation between sFL and PCFCL.

SYSTEMIC MARGINAL ZONE LYMPHOMAS

Definition

Marginal zone lymphoma (MZL) is defined as a low-grade lymphoma composed of small lymphocytes, lymphocytes with plasmacytic differentiation, monocytoid cells, and plasma cells.[13] Diffuse sheets of large transformed cells are absent. It represents approximately 25% of cutaneous B-cell lymphomas. Systemic MZL is divided into nodal, splenic, and extranodal (MALT lymphoma) subtypes.[14]

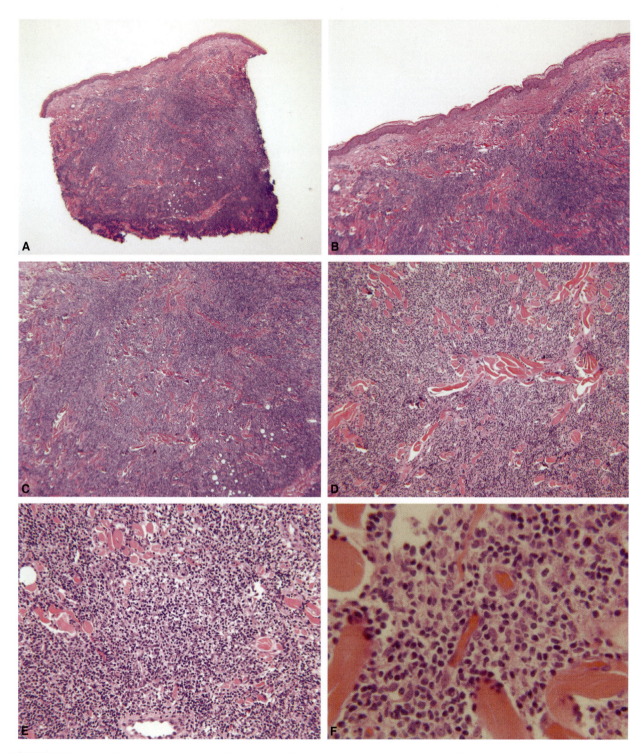

FIGURE 37-1. Systemic follicular lymphoma with cutaneous dissemination. There is a predominantly diffuse and vaguely nodular dermal infiltrate that shows sparing of the epidermis (**A** and **B**, 20× and 100×). The infiltrate dissects through the collagen fibers (**C** and **D**, 100× and 200×). The infiltrate is composed of predominantly centrocytes with no significant number of centroblasts. A histiocyte-rich infiltrate is also present in the background (**E** and **F**, intermediate-to-high magnifications—200× and 400×).

Cutaneous Involvement in MZL

Cutaneous involvement is present in approximately 12% of patients with systemic MZL.[15] Cutaneous lesions typically occur as multiple red nodules on the head and neck (Fig. 37-3). In contrast, primary cutaneous MZL (PCMZL) has a predilection for the trunk and extremities. Nearly 20% of PCMZL can show generalized skin lesions.[16] MZL can occur more frequently in the setting of hepatitis C virus (HCV) infection, and rarely may present as lipoatrophy.[17]

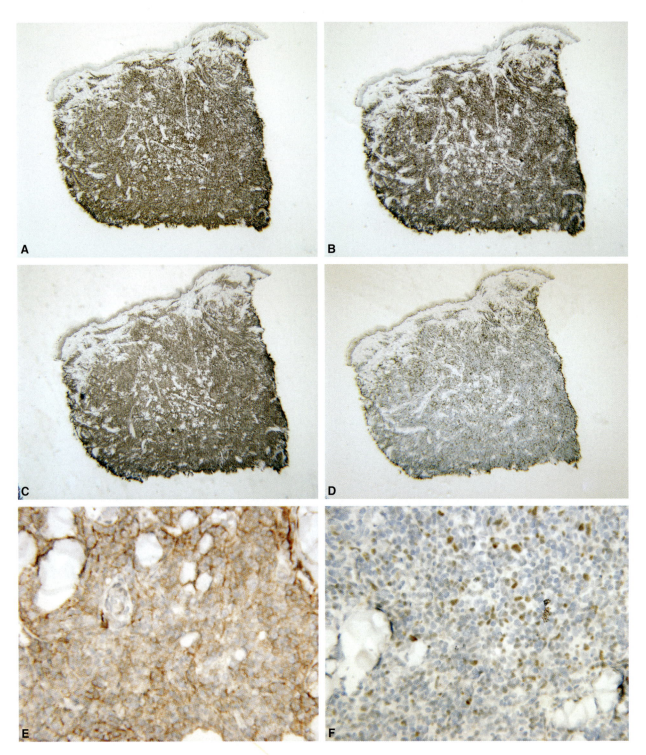

FIGURE 37-2. Systemic follicular lymphoma with cutaneous dissemination—Immunohistochemistry. The infiltrate is positive for PAX5 **(A)** and shows aberrant coexpression of BCL-2 **(C)**. CD3 **(B)** is positive in smaller T-cells in the background. Ki67 **(D)** shows a relatively low (<20%) proliferation index. The atypical cells are positive for CD10 **(E)** and BCL-6 **(F)**, indicating a germinal center phenotype.

Histopathology

The histopathologic features and immunophenotype are nearly identical in PCMZL and secondary cutaneous MZL (SCMZL). The infiltrates are typically patchy and/or vertically oriented and follow adnexal structures. In some cases, the infiltrate can involve the piloerector muscles. The infiltrate shows a mixture of monocytoid lymphocytes and plasmacytoid cells with focal aggregates of mature-appearing plasma cells. As opposed to PCMZL, SCMZL lacks germinal centers. Additionally, SCMZL shows a higher number of B-cells as compared to PCMZL. Very rarely, cases of MZL can be associated with epidermotropism, potentially mimicking mycosis fungoides.[18]

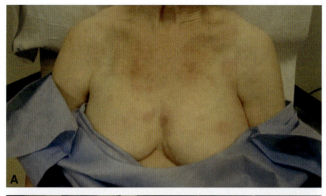
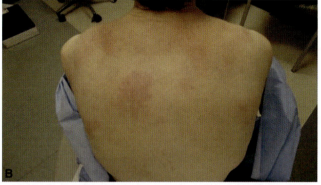

FIGURE 37-3. Splenic marginal zone lymphoma with cutaneous dissemination. Numerous pink patches and indurated smooth plaques that were 2–5 cm in size with overlying telangiectasias on the chest (**A**) and back (**B**). (Reprinted from Cohen JM, Nazarian RM, Ferry JA, et al. Rare presentation of secondary cutaneous involvement by splenic marginal zone lymphoma: report of a case and review of the literature. *Am J Dermatopathol.* 2015;37:e1–e4, with permission.)

Immunophenotype

The immunophenotype of PCMZL and SCMZL is similar. Lymphoma cells are CD5−, CD19+, CD20+, PAX5+, and BCL2+ and negative for germinal center markers CD10, BCL6, LMO-2, and GCET. Expression of CD43 and CD23 has been described,[15] a feature that can also be present in a small subset of PCMZL. IgG4 has recently been proposed as a good marker of PCMZL with plasmacytic differentiation.[19]

Because PCMZL and SCMZL share many histologic, immunophenotypic, and clinical findings, adequate staging procedures should be performed. Blastic transformation (≥30% of large cells in the infiltrate) in PCMZL can mimic systemic disease as it is often associated with extracutaneous dissemination and sometimes nodal involvement.[20,21] Furthermore, Wenzel et al[22] suggested that aberrant CD5 expression in extranodal MZL of the head and neck may be a prognostic marker for recurrent disease, early dissemination, leukemia progression, and aggressive clinical behavior.

In splenic marginal zone lymphoma (SMZL), there is splenomegaly with or without associated lymphadenopathy,[23] and frequent peripheral blood and bone marrow involvement.[24] Very rarely, SMZL can disseminate into the skin[25,26] (Figs. 37-4–37-6). At times, autoimmune disorders can be seen in association with SMZL. The immunophenotype (BCL2+, CD5−, CD10−, CD43−, CD23−, cyclin D1−, IgD−) is similar to other cases of MZL. Some cases of SMZL can show epidermotropism and mimic a cutaneous T-cell lymphoma.[26] Mutations in Kruppel-like factor 2 have been found in nearly half of the cases of SMZL, but are not present in other indolent low-grade B-cell lymphomas.[27-29] As opposed to hairy cell leukemia, which can share histopathologic and

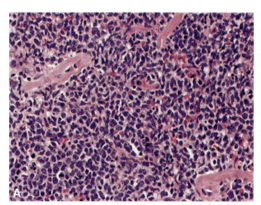
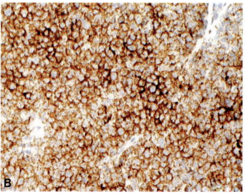

FIGURE 37-4. Splenic marginal zone lymphoma with cutaneous dissemination. Left chest skin punch biopsy specimen showing a dense atypical dermal lymphoid infiltrate (**A**, 200×) composed of numerous small- and medium-sized B-cells with scant-to-moderate cytoplasm, irregular nuclear contours, and coarse chromatin (**B**, CD20 immunostain, 200×). (Reprinted from Cohen JM, Nazarian RM, Ferry JA, et al. Rare presentation of secondary cutaneous involvement by splenic marginal zone lymphoma: report of a case and review of the literature. *Am J Dermatopathol.* 2015;37:e1–e4, with permission.)

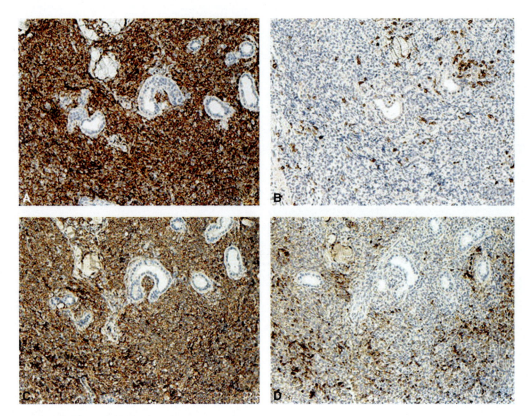

FIGURE 37-5. **Splenic marginal zone lymphoma with cutaneous dissemination.** Left chest skin punch biopsy specimen showing that the neoplastic cells are CD79a+ B-cells (**A**, CD79a stain, 400×) that lack CD5 expression; scattered CD5+ T-cells are present (**B**, CD5 stain, 400×). The neoplastic B-cells demonstrate positive immunohistochemical staining for immunoglobulin M (**C**, IgM, 400×) but are negative for immunoglobulin G (**D**, IgG, 400×). (Reprinted from Cohen JM, Nazarian RM, Ferry JA, et al. Rare presentation of secondary cutaneous involvement by splenic marginal zone lymphoma: report of a case and review of the literature. *Am J Dermatopathol.* 2015;37:e1–e4, with permission.)

immunophenotypic findings, SMZL does not reveal the *BRAF V600E* mutation.

Genetics

FISH studies for translocations t(11;18) and t(1;14) have proven to be helpful in some cases of systemic MZL but not in PCMZL.

CAPSULE SUMMARY

- MZL is defined as a low-grade B-cell lymphoma composed of small lymphocytes, lymphoplasmacytic cells, and plasma cells.
- Cutaneous involvement is present in approximately 12% of patients with systemic MZL and usually as multiple red nodules in the head and neck. MZL may occur in association with HCV.
- Because systemic MZL and PCMZL share clinical, histopathologic, and immunophenotypic findings, adequate staging procedures should be done to exclude nodal or extranodal and extracutaneous disease.
- SMZL is characteristically associated with marked splenomegaly, with or without lymphadenopathy, and on rare occasions, cutaneous dissemination.

LYMPHOPLASMACYTIC LYMPHOMA (WITH OR WITHOUT WALDENSTRÖM MACROGLOBULINEMIA)

Definition

Lymphoplasmacytic lymphoma (LPL) is defined by the WHO as a neoplasm of small B lymphocytes, plasmacytoid lymphocytes, and plasma cells, usually involving bone marrow and sometimes lymph nodes and spleen, which does not fulfill the criteria for any of the other small B-cell lymphomas that can also have plasmacytic differentiation.[1] While IgM paraproteinemia and *MYD88* mutation are both present in the majority of cases, neither is specific for LPL nor required for the diagnosis. A large subset of LPL patients meets criteria for Waldenström macroglobulinemia, which is currently defined as LPL with bone marrow involvement and an IgM monoclonal gammopathy of any concentration.[1] IgM paraprotein is uncommon in plasma cell myeloma, which usually has an IgG, IgA, or light chain paraprotein.[1,30]

Epidemiology and Clinical Findings

LPL represents approximately 2% of the hematologic malignancies in the United States, and the majority of patients are men in the seventh decade of life.[31] LPL patients exhibit bone

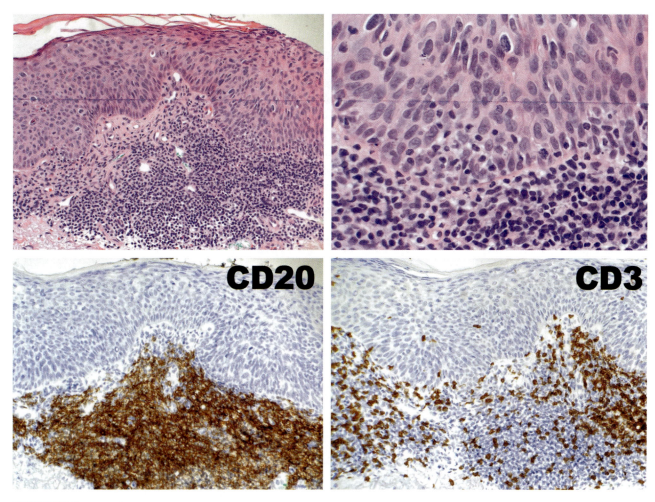

FIGURE 37-6. Splenic marginal zone lymphoma with cutaneous dissemination. Forearm skin biopsy from a patient with splenomegaly and prior diagnosis of splenic marginal zone lymphoma showing incidental skin involvement in association with squamous cell carcinoma in situ (200×). While the infiltrate is predominantly dermal, there is focal exocytosis of lymphocytes in the epidermis (400×). The atypical lymphoid infiltrate consists of CD20+ B-cells, while CD3+ T-cells are rare (200×).

marrow involvement and anemia, which can be associated with fatigue and weakness. Lymphadenopathy, splenomegaly, and/or hyperviscosity may occur in up to one third of LPL patients.[1] In some cases, IgM paraproteinemia can lead to the development of type I (monoclonal) cryoglobulinemia, which manifests histologically as a thrombotic vasculopathy with frequent cutaneous involvement.

Cutaneous Findings and Histopathology

Cutaneous manifestations in LPL are rare and can be seen either as direct extension of LPL into the skin or as cutaneous macroglobulinosis (CM) with dermal deposits of IgM paraprotein in the dermis.[31-34] Cutaneous spread of LPL manifests as nodules, plaques, or ulcerated lesions on the trunk, face, neck, and scalp.[34] The typical histopathologic findings reveal a lymphoplasmacytic infiltrate in the dermis, with a perivascular, periadnexal, and interstitial distribution. Dutcher bodies (PAS+ intranuclear pseudoinclusions) are common (Fig. 37-7).

CM is a less common cutaneous manifestation of LPL and is more frequent in men. Cutaneous lesions often appear prior to the diagnosis of LPL. Most patients present with

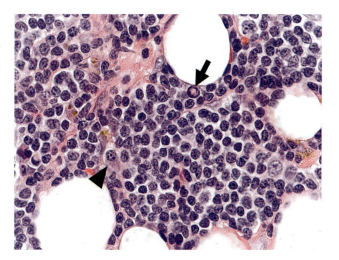

FIGURE 37-7. Lymphoplasmacytic lymphoma with cutaneous dissemination (400×). Abdominal skin biopsy from a patient with anemia and IgM paraproteinemia showing a dense infiltrate with an admixture of small noncleaved lymphocytes and plasma cells (arrowhead). Dutcher body formation is present (arrow). *MYD88* mutation was identified via PCR. Bone marrow biopsy demonstrated a similar lymphoplasmacytic infiltrate.

TABLE 37-2 Comparison of Systemic Follicular Lymphoma, Systemic Marginal Zone Lymphomas, and Lymphoplasmacytic Lymphoma

	Systemic Follicular Lymphoma	Systemic Marginal Zone Lymphomas	Lymphoplasmacytic Lymphoma
Subtypes	Nodal, duodenal-type, pediatric-type, testicular	Splenic, nodal, extranodal (MALT)	With or without Waldenström macroglobulinemia
Cytomorphology of neoplastic cells	Centrocytes and centroblasts (variable admixture)	Small noncleaved lymphocytes, lymphoplasmacytoid cells, plasma cells	Small noncleaved lymphocytes, lymphoplasmacytoid cells, plasma cells
Plasmacytic differentiation	Very rare	Common	Common
Dutcher bodies	Very rare	Occasional	Common
Lymphoid follicles	Neoplastic	Generally absent. If present, reactive or colonized follicles	Generally absent. If present, reactive or colonized follicles
BCL6 IHC	+++	Negative (may be focally positive if reactive follicles are present)	Negative (may be focally positive if reactive follicles are present)
Kappa/lambda IHC/ISH	Not helpful	Light chain restriction in majority of cases	Light chain restriction in majority of cases
MYD88 (L265P) mutation PCR	–	Rarely present	Present in vast majority (>90%)

IHC, immunohistochemistry; ISH, in situ hybridization; MALT, mucosa-associated lymphoid tissue; PCR, polymerase chain reaction.

skin-colored papules on the knees, buttocks, and extensor surfaces of the upper and lower extremities. In CM, there are dense, eosinophilic, amorphous PAS-positive deposits that fill the dermis. This material stains positive for IgM and is typically negative for amyloid stains such as Congo Red or thioflavin T.[31] Increased dermal vascularity with a glomeruloid pattern can be seen.[33]

Laboratory Findings

The early disease stage is manifested by low levels of IgM paraproteinemia (<3 g/L and <10% bone marrow infiltration by lymphoplasmacytic cells), referred to as monoclonal gammopathy of undetermined significance (MGUS). Indolent cases of LPL are characterized by the absence of signs and symptoms of end-organ damage. As the disease progresses, the bone marrow infiltration becomes more prominent; there are higher levels of IgM in the serum, which may ultimately lead to the development of organ failure and symptoms of hyperviscosity.

Immunophenotype

LPL has a relative nonspecific pattern: the B-cells demonstrate pan B-cell marker expression (CD19, CD20, CD22, CD79a, PAX-5). Most cases lack CD5, CD10, and CD23. However, rare cases can be positive for CD5 and CD23. Rare cases can also be positive for CD10. The plasma cell component of the infiltrate can be demonstrated with the use of CD138 and MUM1. In situ hybridization (ISH) or immunohistochemistry (IHC) for kappa and lambda reveals clonal populations of plasma cells and plasmacytoid lymphocytes. This immunophenotype does not help to distinguish LPL from MZL. Indeed, an IgM paraprotein can also be present in the setting of MZL. *MYD88* (L265P) mutations have been found to be relatively specific in the group of patients with LPL and IgM MGUS.[35-39] None of the patients with MZL and IgM expression have that particular mutation (Table 37-2). Rare cases of SMZL and a small subset of DLBCL can also share that mutation.[1]

CAPSULE SUMMARY

- LPL is a B-cell lymphoma with plasmacytic differentiation that secretes IgM.
- Cutaneous manifestations of LPL include direct cutaneous extension and dermal deposition of IgM paraprotein (CM).
- Cutaneous dissemination of LPL shows papules and nodules involving the face and trunk. In CM, there are skin-colored papules on the knees, buttocks, and extensor surfaces of the upper and lower extremities.
- Infiltrates show a variable admixture of small B lymphocytes, plasmacytoid lymphocytes, and plasma cells. Dutcher bodies are frequent.

- The immunophenotype of LPL includes expression of CD20, CD79a, and PAX5. While most cases lack CD5, CD10, and CD23, aberrant phenotypes are not rare. Light chain restriction can often be demonstrated with kappa and lambda IHC or ISH.
- *MYD88* mutations have been found in the vast majority of LPL cases (>90%).

References

1. Swerdlow SH, et al. (Eds.). *WHO Classification of Tumors of Hematopoietic and Lymphoid Tissues* (Revised 4th ed.). IARC; 2017.
2. Harris NL, Swerdlow SH, Jaffe ES, et al. *Follicular Lymphoma.* International Agency for Research on Cancer; 2008.
3. Dabski K, Banks PM, Winkelmann RK. Clinicopathologic spectrum of cutaneous manifestations in systemic follicular lymphoma. A study of 11 patients. *Cancer.* 1989;64:1480-1485.
4. Franco R, Fernandez-Vazquez A, Mollejo M, et al. Cutaneous presentation of follicular lymphomas. *Mod Pathol.* 2001;14:913-919.
5. Garcia CF, Weiss LM, Warnke RA, et al. Cutaneous follicular lymphoma. *Am J Surg Pathol.* 1986;10:454-463.
6. Moreira E, Lisboa C, Alves S, et al. Cutaneous lesions as the first manifestation of systemic follicular lymphoma in an HIV patient. *Dermatol Online J.* 2008;14:17.
7. Sahil M, Prins C, Kaya G, et al. Case report: unusual clinical presentation of a follicular lymphoma [in French]. *Rev Med Suisse.* 2014;10:744, 746-748.
8. Palacios Abufon A, Acebo Marinas E, Gardeazabal Garcia J, et al. Systemic follicular lymphoma with cutaneous manifestations and exclusively cutaneous recurrence [in Spanish]. *Actas Dermosifiliogr.* 2012;103:253-255.
9. Hoeller S, Bihl MP, Zihler D, et al. Molecular and immunohistochemical characterization of B-cell lymphoma-2-negative follicular lymphomas. *Hum Pathol.* 2012;43:405-412.
10. Gardner LJ, Polski JM, Evans HL, et al. CD30 expression in follicular lymphoma. *Arch Pathol Lab Med.* 2001;125:1036-1041.
11. Servitje O, Climent F, Colomo L, et al. Primary cutaneous vs secondary cutaneous follicular lymphomas: a comparative study focused on BCL2, CD10, and t(14;18) expression. *J Cutan Pathol.* 2019;46(3):182-189.
12. Zhou XA, Yang J, Ringbloom KG, et al. *Blood Adv.* 2021;5(3):649-661.
13. Isaacson PG, Piris MA, Berger F, et al. *Splenic B-Cell Marginal Zone Lymphoma.* International Agency for Research on Cancer; 2008.
14. Bathelier E, Thomas L, Balme B, et al. Marginal zone B-cell lymphoma affecting the skin: histological and phenotypic study of 49 cases [in French]. *Ann Dermatol Venereol.* 2008;135:748-752.
15. Gerami P, Wickless SC, Querfeld C, et al. Cutaneous involvement with marginal zone lymphoma. *J Am Acad Dermatol.* 2010;63:142-145.
16. Servitje O, Muniesa C, Benavente Y, et al. Primary cutaneous marginal zone B-cell lymphoma: response to treatment and disease-free survival in a series of 137 patients. *J Am Acad Dermatol.* 2013;69:357-365.
17. Beck K, Paul J, Sawardekar S, et al. Secondary cutaneous marginal zone B-cell lymphoma presenting as lipoatrophy in a patient with hepatitis C. *J Dermatol Case Rep.* 2014;8:46-49.
18. Lee BA, Jacobson M, Seidel G. Epidermotropic marginal zone lymphoma simulating mycosis fungoides. *J Cutan Pathol.* 2013;40:569-572.
19. Brenner I, Roth S, Puppe B, et al. Primary cutaneous marginal zone lymphomas with plasmacytic differentiation show frequent IgG4 expression. *Mod Pathol.* 2013;26:1568-1576.
20. Magro CM, Yang A, Fraga G. Blastic marginal zone lymphoma: a clinical and pathological study of 8 cases and review of the literature. *Am J Dermatopathol.* 2013;35:319-326.
21. Ferry JA, Yang WI, Zukerberg LR, et al. CD5+ extranodal marginal zone B-cell (MALT) lymphoma. A low grade neoplasm with a propensity for bone marrow involvement and relapse. *Am J Clin Pathol.* 1996;105:31-37.
22. Wenzel C, Dieckmann K, Fiebiger W, et al. CD5 expression in a lymphoma of the mucosa-associated lymphoid tissue (MALT)-type as a marker for early dissemination and aggressive clinical behaviour. *Leuk Lymphoma.* 2001;42:823-829.
23. Kurtin PJ. Indolent lymphomas of mature B lymphocytes. *Hematol Oncol Clin North Am.* 2009;23:769-790.
24. Mollejo M, Algara P, Mateo MS, et al. Splenic small B-cell lymphoma with predominant red pulp involvement: a diffuse variant of splenic marginal zone lymphoma?. *Histopathology.* 2002;40:22-30.
25. Cohen JM, Nazarian RM, Ferry JA, et al. Rare presentation of secondary cutaneous involvement by splenic marginal zone lymphoma: report of a case and review of the literature. *Am J Dermatopathol.* 2015;37:e1-e4.
26. Gomez-de la Fuente E, Villalon LB, Calzado-Villarreal L, et al. Splenic marginal zone B-cell lymphoma with epidermotropic skin involvement [in Spanish]. *Actas Dermosifiliogr.* 2012;103:427-431.
27. Clipson A, Wang M, de Leval L, et al. KLF2 mutation is the most frequent somatic change in splenic marginal zone lymphoma and identifies a subset with distinct genotype. *Leukemia.* 2015;29(5):1177-1185.
28. Martinez N, Almaraz C, Vaque JP, et al. Whole-exome sequencing in splenic marginal zone lymphoma reveals mutations in genes involved in marginal zone differentiation. *Leukemia.* 2014;28:1334-1340.
29. Piva R, Deaglio S, Fama R, et al. The Kruppel-like factor 2 transcription factor gene is recurrently mutated in splenic marginal zone lymphoma. *Leukemia.* 2015;29(2):503-507.
30. Swerdlow SH, Berger F, Pileri SA, et al. *Lymphoplasmacytic Lymphoma.* International Agency for Research on Cancer; 2008.
31. Camp BJ, Magro CM. Cutaneous macroglobulinosis: a case series. *J Cutan Pathol.* 2012;39:962-970.
32. Spicknall KE, Dubas LE, Mutasim DF. Cutaneous macroglobulinosis with monotypic plasma cells: a specific manifestation of Waldenström macroglobulinemia. *J Cutan Pathol.* 2013;40:440-444.
33. del Olmo J, Espana A, Idoate MA, et al. Waldenström macroglobulinemia associated with cutaneous lesions and type I cryoglobulinemia [in Spanish]. *Actas Dermosifiliogr.* 2008;99:138-144.
34. Libow LF, Mawhinney JP, Bessinger GT. Cutaneous Waldenström's macroglobulinemia: report of a case and overview of the spectrum of cutaneous disease. *J Am Acad Dermatol.* 2001;45:S202-S206.
35. Gachard N, Parrens M, Soubeyran I, et al. IGHV gene features and MYD88 L265P mutation separate the three

marginal zone lymphoma entities and Waldenström macroglobulinemia/lymphoplasmacytic lymphomas. *Leukemia*. 2013;27:183-189.

36. Jimenez C, Sebastian E, Chillon MC, et al. MYD88 L265P is a marker highly characteristic of, but not restricted to, Waldenström's macroglobulinemia. *Leukemia*. 2013;27:1722-1728.

37. Treon SP, Xu L, Yang G, et al. MYD88 L265P somatic mutation in Waldenström's macroglobulinemia. *N Engl J Med*. 2012;367:826-833.

38. Xu L, Hunter ZR, Yang G, et al. MYD88 L265P in Waldenström macroglobulinemia, immunoglobulin M monoclonal gammopathy, and other B-cell lymphoproliferative disorders using conventional and quantitative allele-specific polymerase chain reaction. *Blood*. 2013;121:2051-2058.

39. Shekhar R, Naseem S, Binota J, et al. Frequency of MYD88 L256P mutation and its correlation with clinico-hematological profile in mature B-cell neoplasm. *Hematol Oncol Stem Cell Ther*. 2021;14:231.

CHAPTER 38

Intravascular large B-cell lymphoma

Alejandro A. Gru and Maxime Battistella

DEFINITION

Intravascular large B-cell lymphoma (IVLBCL) is a rare subtype of extranodal large B-cell lymphoma characterized by the confinement of lymphoma cells within the lumina of small vessels, particularly capillaries.[1,2] Although IVLBCL typically presents as disseminated disease with multiorgan involvement and poor prognosis, a unique isolated cutaneous variant with better prognosis is recognized. Rare cases of intravascular T- and natural killer (NK)-cell lymphomas have been reported, but they are considered a different entity.

VARIANTS

The Western variant shows a higher prevalence of cutaneous disease, a younger age, and a more indolent clinical course. Approximately 26% of these cases include cases with skin-limited disease.[3] The Asian variant is more frequently linked to hemophagocytosis (HPC) and less commonly has cutaneous involvement.[3-5]

EPIDEMIOLOGY

IVLBCL is very rare, with an estimated frequency of ~1 person per million. IVLBCL occurs slightly more frequently in men (male-to-female ratio of 1.1:1) and most often in the setting of advanced age (median age 67 years; range, 41-85 years).[6] Ferreri et al[3] showed that the cutaneous variant, which comprises 10 (26%) of 38 IVLBCL patients in Europe, is characterized by the exclusive limitation of tumors to the skin at presentation and has an invariably female predominance.

Diagnostic delay can be quite pronounced. In fact, in some of the original case series, the diagnosis was made only on autopsy specimens.[7] Most cases, nowadays, are diagnosed on routine biopsies.

ETIOLOGY

The etiology of IVLBCL is unclear. The most distinctive property of intravascular lymphoma (IVL) cells is their tendency to grow within blood vessel lumina without substantial extravasation. Neoplastic B cells in IVL may be able to adhere to endothelial cells, but they seem to lack critical adhesion molecules, such as CD29 (β1 integrin subunit), for extravasation. Besides adhesion, other molecular defects in diapedesis have also been implicated.[8] The relationship of IVL and infectious organisms is not clear. It has been suggested that the "Asian variant," which is typically linked to HPC, could be related to the endemic presence of helminthic infections, as suggested by the detection of serum antibodies to *Fasciola* and *Anisakis* in some patients.[9] Association with HHV-8 infection or blastomycosis has also been reported.[10,11]

Approximately 15% of cases of IVLBCL have an association with preceding or concomitant neoplastic disorders. IVLBCL is most frequently associated with non-Hodgkin lymphomas, particularly diffuse large B-cell lymphoma (DLBCL).[12,13] Less frequent associations include chronic lymphocytic leukemia and follicular and mucosa-associated lymphoid tissue lymphomas. Association with nonhematopoietic neoplasms such as renal cell carcinoma, meningioma, angioleiomyomas, and cutaneous hemangiomas has also been described.[14,15] Interestingly, in those cases associated with other malignancies, IVL cells are present also, if not preferentially, within tumor-associated vessels, thus suggesting the expression of particular molecules by this cancer-associated endothelium. IVL colonizing cutaneous hemangiomas has been reported in a number of reports.[16-21]

CLINICAL PRESENTATION/PROGNOSIS

IVL can involve virtually any organ and, because of this, protean clinical manifestations have been described. An isolated cutaneous variant comprising 26% of patients with IVL has been recently identified.[3,22] This variant is associated with a 3-year survival rate of 56%, compared with the survival rate of 22% seen in disseminated cases.[22] Patients with the cutaneous variant are younger and lack peripheral blood cytopenias.

Systemic symptoms such as fever, weight loss, and night sweats are seen in ~55% of cases.[8] The patients usually present nonspecific symptoms and show a marked deterioration in their performance status. In some cases, a persistent fever of unknown origin leads to a bone marrow biopsy with the subsequent diagnosis of IVL.[7,23]

Cutaneous lesions are present in 40% of cases and are more common in the Western variant. The lesions are typically nodules and/or plaques (49%) or macules (22.5%) of red (31%) or blue to livid (19%) color on the leg (35%), the thigh (41%), and the trunk (31%). Telangiectasis is present in only 20% of the patients. Edema (27.5%) of the legs and pain (24%) may be accompanying features.[24] Other unusual clinical presentations described in the skin include purpuric lesions with leukocytoclastic vasculitis,[25] erythema nodosum–like forms,[26,27] retiform purpura,[28] generalized telangiectasias,[29,30] and inflammatory lymphedema.[31]

Bone marrow involvement is very frequently seen in the Asian subtype and often accompanied by HPC (61%), symptomatic anemia (66%), thrombocytopenia (58%), and sometimes leukopenia (27%), neurologic manifestations, or cutaneous lesions.[3-6,32-35] Approximately 14% of cases (most commonly in the Asian variant) show a monoclonal paraprotein.[6]

In the Western variant, ~32% of cases have bone marrow involvement, hepatosplenic infiltration, and thrombocytopenia. Central nervous system (CNS) involvement is seen in ~34% of cases. Symptoms attributable to CNS involvement vary, with sensory and motor deficits, meningoradiculitis, paresthesias, aphasia, dysarthria, hemiparesis, seizures, myoclonus, transient visual loss, vertigo, sensory neuropathy, and altered conscious states.[36,37] Rare cases can present as mononeuritis multiplex.[38,39] Prostatic acid phosphatase as a diagnostic and potential prognostic marker of IVL has been proposed[40,41] recently.

Other clinical abnormalities include respiratory symptoms, with frequent dyspnea and associated pleural effusions.[33] Involvement of endocrine organs, particularly adrenal[33,42-44] and pituitary[45] glands, is common. Other commonly involved organs include thyroid,[46] prostate,[47,48] vulva,[49] gallbladder,[50] lung,[51] breast,[52] eye (choroides),[53] and uterus.[54]

HPC is linked to disseminated disease, higher soluble levels of IL-2, and lower albumin concentration, and also less peripheral blood involvement and lower creatinin levels.[6] Although HPC does not appear to have prognostic value, its presence increases the likelihood of stage IV disease (100% vs 76%), fever (92% vs 42%), jaundice (17% vs 0%), hepatic involvement (58% vs 26%), splenic involvement (58% vs 26%), marrow involvement (75% vs 30%), thrombocytopenia (83% vs 32%), elevated alanine aminotransferase levels (42% vs 6%), and high bilirubin levels (42% vs 2%).[3]

Tumors with an *MYD88* mutation and alterations and rearrangement of immune evasion–related genes have displayed poorer outcomes.[55]

TREATMENT

The most common treatment modality for IVLBCL is combination chemotherapy. Cyclophosphamide, Adriamycin, Oncovin, and prednisone (CHOP) and CHOP-like chemotherapy have achieved positive objective responses; however, anthracycline-based chemotherapy has been associated with superior remission and overall survival rates.[1,4,32,33,56-58] The prognosis still remains dismal, and on the cohort of patients treated with anthracycline regimens, the mean survival was 12 to 13 months.[3] The addition of rituximab to other chemotherapeutic agents has been shown to improve survival significantly.[59-63] One analysis found complete remission in 11 of 12 patients with no relapses at a median follow-up of 15 months.[3] Autologous bone marrow transplantation can potentially improve survival in some cases.[4,6,33,64-66] Although radiotherapy has been used with some success,[58,67] systemic therapy is still the recommended choice in patients with localized skin disease.[22] Detection of PD-L1 expression in a subset of IVLBCL lymphoma cases may identify patients who might benefit from targeted anti-PD-1 or anti-PD-L1 antibodies.[68]

HISTOLOGY

Numerous skin biopsies may be required to obtain a diagnostic sample. Sets of random skin biopsies from clinically unaffected skin were found to be sensitive (sensitivity of 83% vs 92% for trephine bone marrow biopsy) in achieving a definitive diagnosis.[42,69-72] Sampling normal skin in at least three sites, skin lesions, and angiomas, when present, is a reasonable approach. Sampling should be done to a depth of at least 4 mm and include adequate subcutaneous tissue.[73]

Lymphoma cells are confined within the lumina of small to medium-sized vessels. Large arteries and veins are spared (Fig. 38-1A,B). Associated fibrin thrombi and ischemic necrosis are frequent histologic findings.[6] Lymphoma cells are usually large, but small-cell variants have been described (Fig. 38-2).[1] They have scant cytoplasm, prominent nucleoli, and frequent mitotic figures. Cohesion of lymphoma cells might simulate lymphovascular invasion from a carcinoma. Limited extravasation into the surrounding parenchyma and lymphangiectasia in the superficial dermis owing to vascular obstruction have been reported.[24,35]

Sinusoidal involvement in the liver and bone marrow[74] and the red pulp of the spleen is common.[6,35] Lymphoma cells in the peripheral blood can be rarely detected.

IMMUNOPHENOTYPE

IVLBCL cells may have germinal center (20%) or non–germinal center (80%) phenotypes.[57] They express the following markers (Fig. 38-3): CD79a (100%), CD20 (96%), MUM1/IRF4 (95%), BCL-2 (91%), CD19 (85%), immunoglobulin κ light chain (71%), CD5 (38%), BCL-6 (26%), immunoglobulin λ light chain (18%), CD10 (12%), and CD23 (4%).[1,6,35,75] CD22, CD43, CD45, and HLA-DR are also frequently expressed.[1] The frequency of CD5 expression varies from 22% to 75%.[75-77] A subset of IVLBCL expresses PD-L1, in both the classic form as well as the HPS variant.[78] PD-L1 is expressed irrespective of CD5 expression.[68]

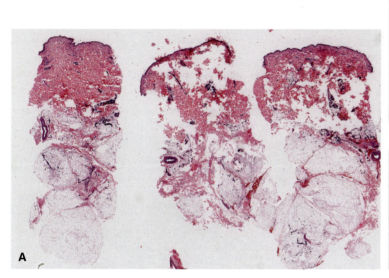
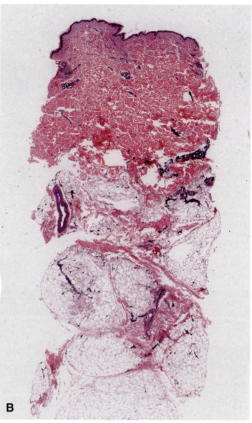

FIGURE 38-1. IVLBCL. A and **B.** Subtle intravascular infiltrates in the deep dermis and subcutis.

GENETIC AND MOLECULAR FINDINGS

Somatic hypermutations occur in approximately 74% to 99.4% of cases.[79] There is no known specific chromosomal alteration. Genetic changes reported in both IVLBCL and other B-cell lymphomas include −6 or 6q- and +18 or dup(18q), with a minimally deleted region located at 6q21–q23 and a commonly amplified region located at 18q13–q23.[80] Cytogenetic changes in isolated case reports include t(3;14)(q27; q32),[81] triplication of the *MLL* and *BCL-2* genes,[82,83] t(14;19)(q32;q13),[84] and gains of 11q and trisomy 18 in a CD5+ case.[85]

The pathogenesis of IVLBCL includes defective transendothelial migration by lymphoma cells owing to the lack of adhesion receptors such as CD29 (β1 integrin) and CD54 (ICAM-1 or CD11a ligand) or aberrant expression of CD11a and CXCR3.[8,75,86]

Recent studies identified significantly enriched driver mutations in the B-cell receptor/NF-κB signaling pathways, including *CD79B* (67%), *MYD88* (57%), *IRF4* (38%), *ITPKB* (14%), *NFKBIE* (14%), and *TNFAIP3* (24%); *PIM1* (95%) and *IGLL5* (90%); *PRDM1* (43%) and *TOX* (33%). Other common mutational targets included histone/chromatin modification factors, such as *SETD1B* (57%), *KMT2D* (24%), and *EP300* (14%). IVLBCL harbor *PD-L1/PD-L2* rearrangements at a high frequency, and SVs in *PD-L1/PD-L2* likely correlate with overexpression of PD-L1/PD-L2 protein.

POSTULATED CELL OF ORIGIN

The high frequency of somatically hypermutated immunoglobulin *genes* suggests a post–germinal center B-cell origin. In a case report, using microarray molecular classification, IVLBCL showed molecular similarity to non-GCB DLBCL.[87] A case report of IVL with a T-cell phenotype in association with HTLV-1 infection has been reported.[88] This case likely represents an intravascular variant of adult T-cell leukemia/lymphoma according to the current World Health Organization (WHO) classification. Rare cases with T- or NK-cell phenotypes and Epstein-Barr virus positivity have also been described.[8]

DIFFERENTIAL DIAGNOSIS

The following entities might have morphologic overlap with IVLBCL: lymphomatoid granulomatosis (LG), intralymphatic histiocytosis, Melkerson-Rosenthal syndrome, other lymphomas with intravascular dissemination, and CD30+ intravascular lymphoid proliferations.

LG often has cutaneous involvement and angioinvasion mimicking IVL. In contrast to IVLBCL, LG characteristically exhibits extravascular spread, frequent Hodgkin-like morphology, EBER expression, and angiodestruction.

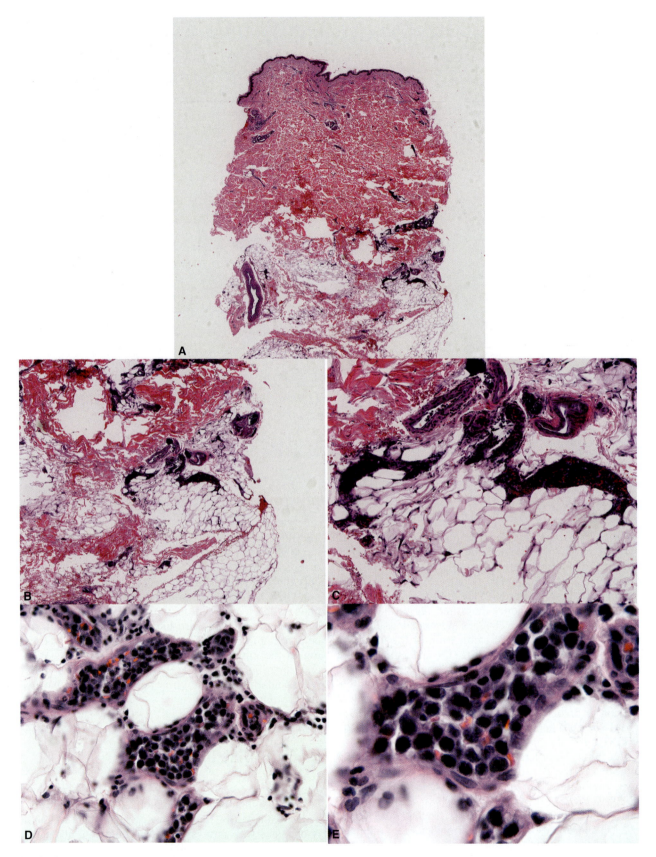

FIGURE 38-2. IVLBCL—histologic findings. A–C (40×, 100×, and 200×). There is a predominantly intravascular infiltrate without significant extravasation into the surrounding tissue. **D** and **E** (400× and 600×). The intravascular lymphoid population is composed of medium to large cells with hyperchromasia and variable nucleoli.

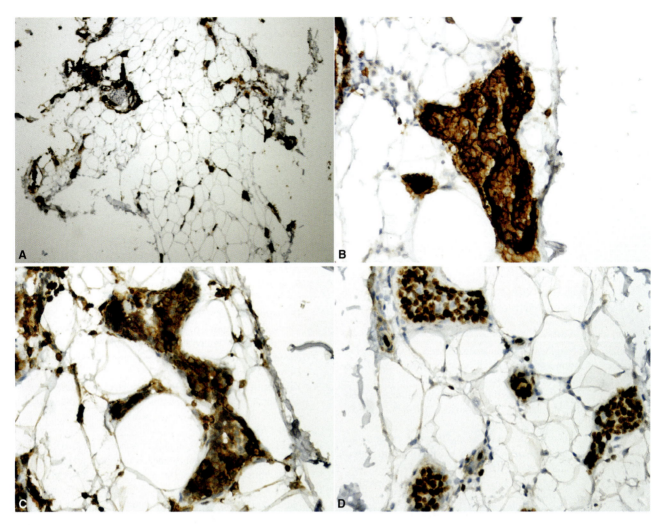

FIGURE 38-3. IVLBCL. The malignant cells are positive for CD20 (**A** and **B**) and CD45 (**C**) and show a high proliferation index by Ki67 (**D**) (>80%).

Intravascular neoplastic lymphocytes of B-cell chronic lymphocytic leukemia, mantle cell lymphoma, and splenic marginal zone lymphoma are small-sized and have a distinct immunophenotype allowing straightforward distinction from IVLBCL.[35]

In intralymphatic histiocytosis, there is a vascular and intralymphatic expansion of histiocytic cells, which are positive for CD68, CD163, and CD31 but negative for B-cell markers.[89] In Melkersson-Rosenthal syndrome, multiple granulomata are present, with occasional intralymphatic distribution. The patients typically have lesions in the face and genital areas.[90]

CD5+ DLBCL represents a broad category of large-cell lymphomas and can show an intravascular growth in ~19% of cases that do not meet the criteria for IVLBCL.[76] Most of these cases express BCL-2 and MUM1 and show a non–germinal center phenotype (activated B-cell type).

Indolent intravascular CD30+ lymphoproliferative disorder is believed to be a variant of cutaneous anaplastic large-cell lymphoma and expresses pan–T-cell antigens along with CD30.[68,91,92] Similar intravascular findings can be observed in CD30+ pseudolymphoma in the setting of phenytoin hypersensitivity (personal observation).

Finally, the differential diagnosis should also include nonhematopoietic tumors with prominent dermal intravascular component such as intravascular breast carcinoma and melanoma.

CAPSULE SUMMARY

- IVLBCL is a type of extranodal large B-cell lymphoma with tumor cells confined within the lumina of capillaries.
- Lymphoma cells have a post-germinal center B-cell phenotype. Coexpression of CD5 can be seen in a third of cases.
- The Western variant typically shows cutaneous involvement, occurs in younger individuals, and has a better prognosis. A third of cases exhibit isolated cutaneous involvement only.
- The Asian variant is more frequently associated with HPC. Cutaneous involvement is less common.
- The prognosis is overall poor, with a mean survival of 13 months.
- Skin findings include plaques and nodules. Most cases need numerous skin biopsies to demonstrate lymphoma.
- About 20% of diagnoses are made postmortem.

References

1. Orwat DE, Batalis NI. Intravascular large B-cell lymphoma. *Arch Pathol Lab Med*. 2012;136(3):333-338.
2. Nakamura N, Ponzoni M, Campo E. *Intravascular Large B-Cell Lymphoma*. International Agency for Research on Cancer; 2008.
3. Ferreri AJ, Dognini GP, Campo E, et al. Variations in clinical presentation, frequency of hemophagocytosis and clinical behavior of intravascular lymphoma diagnosed in different geographical regions. *Haematologica*. 2007;92(4):486-492.
4. Chihara T, Wada N, Ikeda J, et al. Frequency of intravascular large B-cell lymphoma in Japan: study of the Osaka lymphoma study group. *J Hematol Oncol*. 2011;4:14.
5. Fung KM, Chakrabarty JH, Kern WF, et al. Intravascular large B-cell lymphoma with hemophagocytic syndrome (Asian variant) in a Caucasian patient. *Int J Clin Exp Pathol*. 2012;5(5):448-454.
6. Murase T, Yamaguchi M, Suzuki R, et al. Intravascular large B-cell lymphoma (IVLBCL): a clinicopathologic study of 96 cases with special reference to the immunophenotypic heterogeneity of CD5. *Blood*. 2007;109(2):478-485.
7. Wick MR, Mills SE, Scheithauer BW, et al. Reassessment of malignant "angioendotheliomatosis." Evidence in favor of its reclassification as "intravascular lymphomatosis." *Am J Surg Pathol*. 1986;10(2):112-123.
8. Ponzoni M, Ferreri AJ. Intravascular lymphoma: a neoplasm of "homeless" lymphocytes? *Hematol Oncol*. 2006;24(3):105-112.
9. Murase T, Tashiro K, Suzuki T, et al. Detection of antibodies to Fasciola and Anisakis in Japanese patients with intravascular lymphomatosis. *Blood*. 1998;92(6):2182-2183.
10. Ferry JA, Sohani AR, Longtine JA, et al. HHV8-positive, EBV-positive Hodgkin lymphoma-like large B-cell lymphoma and HHV8-positive intravascular large B-cell lymphoma. *Mod Pathol*. 2009;22(5):618-626.
11. Harket A, Oukabli M, Al Bouzidi A, et al. Cutaneous blastomycosis revealing intravascular B-cell lymphoma: a case in Morocco. *Med Trop*. 2007;67(3):278-280.
12. Kamath NV, Gilliam AC, Nihal M, et al. Primary cutaneous large B-cell lymphoma of the leg relapsing as cutaneous intravascular large B-cell lymphoma. *Arch Dermatol*. 2001;137:1657-1658.
13. Ponzoni M, Campo E, Ferreri AJ. Intravascular lymphoma occurring in patients with other non-Hodgkin lymphomas. *Clin Adv Hematol Oncol*. 2010;8(9):641-642.
14. Ho CW, Mantoo S, Lim CH, et al. Synchronous invasive ductal carcinoma and intravascular large B-cell lymphoma of the breast: a case report and review of the literature. *World J Surg Oncol*. 2014;12:88.
15. Muftah S, Xu Z, El Gaddafi W, et al. Synchronous intravascular large B-cell lymphoma within meningioma. *Neuropathology*. 2012;32(1):77-81.
16. Cerroni L, Zalaudek I, Kerl H. Intravascular large B-cell lymphoma colonizing cutaneous hemangiomas. *Dermatology*. 2004;209(2):132-134.
17. Nixon BK, Kussick SJ, Carlon MJ, et al. Intravascular large B-cell lymphoma involving hemangiomas: an unusual presentation of a rare neoplasm. *Mod Pathol*. 2005;18(8):1121-1126.
18. Wahie S, Dayala S, Husain A, et al. Cutaneous features of intravascular lymphoma. *Clin Exp Dermatol*. 2011;36(3):288-291.
19. Ishida M, Hotta M, Hodohara K, et al. A case of intravascular large B-cell lymphoma colonizing in senile hemangioma. *J Cutan Pathol*. 2011;38(2):251-253.
20. Wang J, Wang CH, Xu JY, et al. Intravascular lymphomatosis arising in angioleiomyoma: a case report. *Zhonghua Bing Li Xue Za Zhi*. 2006;35(6):377-378.
21. Smith ME, Stamatakos MD, Neuhauser TS. Intravascular lymphomatosis presenting within angiolipomas. *Ann Diagn Pathol*. 2001;5(2):103-106.
22. Ferreri AJ, Campo E, Seymour JF, et al. Intravascular lymphoma: clinical presentation, natural history, management and prognostic factors in a series of 38 cases, with special emphasis on the "cutaneous variant." *Br J Haematol*. 2004;127(2):173-183.
23. Gual-Tarrada N, Selva-O'Callaghan A, Ruiz-Marcellan C. Intravascular large B-cell lymphoma, a cause of fever of unknown origin in the elderly. *J Am Geriatr Soc*. 2012;60(2):375-376.
24. Roglin J, Boer A. Skin manifestations of intravascular lymphoma mimic inflammatory diseases of the skin. *Br J Dermatol*. 2007;157(1):16-25.
25. Cardinali C, Santini S, di Leo A, et al. Generalized B-cell non Hodgkin's lymphoma in association with leukocytoclastic vasculitis and disseminated intravascular coagulation. *Dermatol Online J*. 2006;12(3):15.
26. Kiyohara T, Kumakiri M, Kobayashi H, et al. A case of intravascular large B-cell lymphoma mimicking erythema nodosum: the importance of multiple skin biopsies. *J Cutan Pathol*. 2000;27(8):413-418.
27. Lu PH, Kuo TT, Yu KH, et al. Intravascular large B-cell lymphoma presenting in subcutaneous fat tissue and simulating panniculitis clinically. *Int J Dermatol*. 2009;48(12):1349-1352.
28. Kruse L, Buescher L, Nietert E. Intravascular B-cell lymphoma presenting as retiform purpura. *J Am Acad Dermatol*. 2012;67(5):e238-e240.
29. Niiyama S, Amoh Y, Katsuoka K. Generalized telangiectasia as the manifestation of intravascular large B-cell lymphoma complicated with breast cancer. *Eur J Dermatol*. 2012;22(4):566-567.
30. Saleh Z, Kurban M, Ghosn S, et al. Generalized telangiectasia: a manifestation of intravascular B-cell lymphoma. *Dermatology*. 2008;217(4):318-320.
31. Pallure V, Dandurand M, Stoebner PE, et al. Intravascular B-cell lymphoma with febrile inflammatory lymphoedema of the lower limbs and lower back. *Ann Dermatol venereol*. 2008;135(4):299-303.
32. Koyano S, Hashiguchi S, Tanaka F. Literature review of intravascular lymphomatosis [in Japanese]. *Brain Nerve*. 2014;66(8):927-946.
33. Matsue K, Asada N, Takeuchi M, et al. A clinicopathological study of 13 cases of intravascular lymphoma: experience in a single institution over a 9-yr period. *Eur J Haematol*. 2008;80(3):236-244.
34. Hong JY, Kim HJ, Ko YH, et al. Clinical features and treatment outcomes of intravascular large B-cell lymphoma: a single-center experience in Korea. *Acta Haematol*. 2014;131(1):18-27.
35. Ponzoni M, Ferreri AJ, Campo E, et al. Definition, diagnosis, and management of intravascular large B-cell lymphoma: proposals and perspectives from an international consensus meeting. *J Clin Oncol*. 2007;25(21):3168-3173.

36. Aznar AO, Montero MA, Rovira R, et al. Intravascular large B-cell lymphoma presenting with neurological syndromes: clinicopathologic study. *Clin Neuropathol.* 2007;26(4):180-186.
37. Brunet V, Marouan S, Routy JP, et al. Retrospective study of intravascular large B-cell lymphoma cases diagnosed in Quebec: a retrospective study of 29 case reports [published correction appears in Medicine (Baltimore). 2017 May;96(20):e7018]. *Medicine (Baltim).* 2017;96(5):e5985. doi:10.1097/MD.0000000000005985
38. Lynch KM, Katz JD, Weinberg DH, et al. Isolated mononeuropathy multiplex—a rare manifestation of intravascular large B-cell lymphoma. *J Clin Neuromuscul Dis.* 2012;14(1):17-20.
39. Shimada K, Murase T, Matsue K, et al. Central nervous system involvement in intravascular large B-cell lymphoma: a retrospective analysis of 109 patients. *Cancer Sci.* 2010;101(6):1480-1486.
40. Kishi Y, Kami M, Kusumi E, et al. Prostatic acid phosphatase: a possible diagnostic marker of intravascular large B-cell lymphoma. *Haematologica.* 2004;89(5):ECR13.
41. Seki K, Miyakoshi S, Lee GH, et al. Prostatic acid phosphatase is a possible tumor marker for intravascular large B-cell lymphoma. *Am J Surg Pathol.* 2004;28(10):1384-1388.
42. Raza M, Qayyum S, Raza S, et al. Intravascular B-cell lymphoma: an elusive diagnosis. *J Clin Oncol.* 2012;30(15):e144-e145.
43. Srivatsa S, Sharma J, Logani S. Intravascular lymphoma: an unusual diagnostic outcome of an incidentally detected adrenal mass. *Endocr Pract.* 2008;14(7):884-888.
44. Venizelos I, Tamiolakis D, Petrakis G. High grade primary adrenal intravascular large B-cell lymphoma manifesting as Addison disease. *Rev Esp Enferm Dig.* 2007;99(8):471-474.
45. Anila KR, Nair RA, Koshy SM, et al. Primary intravascular large B-cell lymphoma of pituitary. *Indian J Pathol Microbiol.* 2012;55(4):549-551.
46. Stonecypher M, Yan Z, Wasik MA, et al. Intravascular large B cell lymphoma presenting as a thyroid mass. *Endocr Pathol.* 2014;25(3):359-360.
47. Ozsan N, Sarsik B, Yilmaz AF, et al. Intravascular large B-cell lymphoma diagnosed on prostate biopsy: a case report. *Turk J Haematol.* 2014;31(4):403-407.
48. Wakim JJ, Levenson BM, Mathews D, et al. Management of an unusual case of intravascular large B-cell lymphoma of the penis, prostate, and bones with CNS relapse. *J Clin Oncol.* 2013;31(17):e288-e290.
49. Zizi-Sermpetzoglou A, Petrakopoulou N, Tepelenis N, et al. Intravascular T-cell lymphoma of the vulva, CD30 positive: a case report. *Eur J Gynaecol Oncol.* 2009;30(5):586-588.
50. Tajima S, Waki M, Yamazaki H, et al. Intravascular large B-cell lymphoma manifesting as cholecystitis: report of an Asian variant showing gain of chromosome 18 with concurrent deletion of chromosome 6q. *Int J Clin Exp Pathol.* 2014;7(11):8181-8189.
51. Liu C, Lai N, Zhou Y, et al. Intravascular large B-cell lymphoma confirmed by lung biopsy. *Int J Clin Exp Pathol.* 2014;7(9):6301-6306.
52. Monteiro M, Duarte I, Cabecadas J, et al. Intravascular large B-cell lymphoma of the breast. *Breast.* 2005;14(1):75-78.
53. Lee HB, Pulido JS, Buettner H, et al. Intravascular B-cell lymphoma (angiotropic lymphoma) with choroidal involvement. *Arch Ophthalmol.* 2006;124(9):1357-1359.
54. Xia Y, Wang Y, Jiang Y, et al. Primary intravascular large B cell lymphoma of the endometrium. *Acta Histochem.* 2014;116(5):993-996.
55. Shimada K, Yoshida K, Suzuki Y, et al. Frequent genetic alterations in immune checkpoint-related genes in intravascular large B-cell lymphoma. *Blood.* 2021;137(11):1491-1502. doi:10.1182/blood.2020007245
56. Bessell EM, Humber CE, O'Connor S, et al. Primary cutaneous B-cell lymphoma in Nottinghamshire U.K.: prognosis of subtypes defined in the WHO-EORTC classification. *Br J Dermatol.* 2012;167(5):1118-1123.
57. Masaki Y, Dong L, Nakajima A, et al. Intravascular large B cell lymphoma: proposed of the strategy for early diagnosis and treatment of patients with rapid deteriorating condition. *Int J Hematol.* 2009;89(5):600-610.
58. Suarez AL, Querfeld C, Horwitz S, et al. Primary cutaneous B-cell lymphomas, part II: therapy and future directions. *J Am Acad Dermatol.* 2013;69(3):343.e1-343.e11; quiz 355-356.
59. Ferreri AJ, Dognini GP, Bairey O, et al. The addition of rituximab to anthracycline-based chemotherapy significantly improves outcome in "Western" patients with intravascular large B-cell lymphoma. *Br J Haematol.* 2008;143(2):253-257.
60. Ferreri AJ, Dognini GP, Govi S, et al. Can rituximab change the usually dismal prognosis of patients with intravascular large B-cell lymphoma? *J Clin Oncol.* 2008;26(31):5134-5136; author reply 5136-5137.
61. Horvath B, Demeter J, Eros N, et al. Intravascular large B-cell lymphoma: remission after rituximab-cyclophosphamide, doxorubicin, vincristine, and prednisolone chemotherapy. *J Am Acad Dermatol.* 2009;61(5):885-888.
62. Shimada K, Matsue K, Yamamoto K, et al. Retrospective analysis of intravascular large B-cell lymphoma treated with rituximab-containing chemotherapy as reported by the IVL study group in Japan. *J Clin Oncol.* 2008;26(19):3189-3195.
63. Feldmann R, Schierl M, Sittenthaler M, et al. Intravascular large B-cell lymphoma of the skin: typical clinical manifestations and a favourable response to rituximab-containing therapy. *Dermatology.* 2009;219(4):344-346.
64. Kato K, Ohno Y, Kamimura T, et al. Long-term remission after high-dose chemotherapy followed by auto-SCT as consolidation for intravascular large B-cell lymphoma. *Bone Marrow Transplant.* 2014;49(12):1543-1544.
65. Sawamoto A, Narimatsu H, Suzuki T, et al. Long-term remission after autologous peripheral blood stem cell transplantation for relapsed intravascular lymphoma. *Bone Marrow Transplant.* 2006;37(2):233-234.
66. Shimada K, Kinoshita T, Naoe T, et al. Presentation and management of intravascular large B-cell lymphoma. *Lancet Oncol.* 2009;10(9):895-902.
67. Sips GJ, Amory CF, Delman BN, et al. Intravascular lymphomatosis of the brain in a patient with myelodysplastic syndrome. *Nat Rev Neurol.* 2009;5(5):288-292.
68. Metcalf RA, Bashey S, Wysong A, et al. Intravascular ALK-negative anaplastic large cell lymphoma with localized cutaneous involvement and an indolent clinical course: toward recognition of a distinct clinicopathologic entity. *Am J Surg Pathol.* 2013;37(4):617-623.
69. Barnett CR, Seo S, Husain S, et al. Intravascular B-cell lymphoma: the role of skin biopsy. *Am J Dermatopathol.* 2008;30(3):295-299.

70. Kong YY, Dai B, Sheng WQ, et al. Intravascular large B-cell lymphoma with cutaneous manifestations: a clinicopathologic, immunophenotypic and molecular study of three cases. *J Cutan Pathol*. 2009;36(8):865-870.
71. Matsue K, Asada N, Odawara J, et al. Random skin biopsy and bone marrow biopsy for diagnosis of intravascular large B cell lymphoma. *Ann Hematol*. 2011;90(4):417-421.
72. Namekawa M, Nakano I. Diagnosis of intravascular lymphoma: usefulness of random skin biopsies. *Brain Nerve*. 2011;63(5):451-458.
73. Tung JK, Rozenbaum D, Rrapi R, et al. Skin biopsy in the diagnosis of intravascular lymphoma: a retrospective diagnostic accuracy study. *J Am Acad Dermatol*. published online July 24, 2021;S0190-9622(21)02168-X. doi:10.1016/j.jaad.2021.07.024
74. Sajid RM, Qureshi A. Involvement of bone marrow with intravascular large B-cell lymphoma. *Hematol/Oncol Stem Cell Ther*. 2010;3(1):39-41.
75. Kanda M, Suzumiya J, Ohshima K, et al. Intravascular large cell lymphoma: clinicopathological, immuno-histochemical and molecular genetic studies. *Leuk Lymphoma*. 1999;34(5-6):569-580.
76. Yamaguchi M, Seto M, Okamoto M, et al. De novo CD5+ diffuse large B-cell lymphoma: a clinicopathologic study of 109 patients. *Blood*. 2002;99(3):815-821.
77. Yegappan S, Coupland R, Arber DA, et al. Angiotropic lymphoma: an immunophenotypically and clinically heterogeneous lymphoma. *Mod Pathol*. 2001;14(11):1147-1156.
78. Gupta GK, Jaffe ES, Pittaluga S. A study of PD-L1 expression in intravascular large B cell lymphoma: correlation with clinical and pathological features. *Histopathology*. 2019;75(2):282-286. doi:10.1111/his.13870
79. Kanda M, Suzumiya J, Ohshima K, et al. Analysis of the immunoglobulin heavy chain gene variable region of intravascular large B-cell lymphoma. *Virchows Arch*. 2001;439(4):540-546.
80. Khoury H, Lestou VS, Gascoyne RD, et al. Multicolor karyotyping and clinicopathological analysis of three intravascular lymphoma cases. *Mod Pathol*. 2003;16(7):716-724.
81. Cui J, Liu Q, Cheng Y, et al. An intravascular large B-cell lymphoma with a t(3;14)(q27;q32) translocation. *J Clin Pathol*. 2014;67(3):279-281.
82. Deisch J, Fuda FB, Chen W, et al. Segmental tandem triplication of the MLL gene in an intravascular large B-cell lymphoma with multisystem involvement: a comprehensive morphologic, immunophenotypic, cytogenetic, and molecular cytogenetic antemortem study. *Arch Pathol Lab Med*. 2009;133(9):1477-1482.
83. Yamamoto K, Okamura A, Yakushijin K, et al. Tandem triplication of the BCL2 gene in CD5-positive intravascular large B cell lymphoma with bone marrow involvement. *Ann Hematol*. 2014;93(10):1791-1793.
84. Kobayashi T, Ohno H. Intravascular large B-cell lymphoma associated with t(14;19)(q32;q13) translocation. *Intern Med*. 2011;50(18):2007-2010.
85. Yamamoto K, Yakushijin K, Okamura A, et al. Gain of 11q by an additional ring chromosome 11 and trisomy 18 in CD5-positive intravascular large B-cell lymphoma. *J Clin Exp Hematop*. 2013;53(2):161-165.
86. Kato M, Ohshima K, Mizuno M, et al. Analysis of CXCL9 and CXCR3 expression in a case of intravascular large B-cell lymphoma. *J Am Acad Dermatol*. 2009;61(5):888-891.
87. Bauer WM, Aichelburg MC, Griss J, et al. Molecular classification of tumour cells in a patient with intravascular large B-cell lymphoma. *Br J Dermatol*. 2018;178(1):215-221. doi:10.1111/bjd.15841
88. Shimokawa I, Higami Y, Sakai H, et al. Intravascular malignant lymphomatosis: a case of T-cell lymphoma probably associated with human T-cell lymphotropic virus. *Hum Pathol*. 1991;22(2):200-202.
89. Bakr F, Webber N, Fassihi H, et al. Primary and secondary intralymphatic histiocytosis. *J Am Acad Dermatol*. 2014;70(5):927-933.
90. Elias MK, Mateen FJ, Weiler CR. The Melkersson–Rosenthal syndrome: a retrospective study of biopsied cases. *J Neurol*. 2013;260(1):138-143.
91. Kempf W, Keller K, John H, et al. Benign atypical intravascular CD30+ T-cell proliferation: a recently described reactive lymphoproliferative process and simulator of intravascular lymphoma—report of a case associated with lichen sclerosus and review of the literature. *Am J Clin Pathol*. 2014;142(5):694-699.
92. Samols MA, Su A, Ra S, et al. Intralymphatic cutaneous anaplastic large cell lymphoma/lymphomatoid papulosis: expanding the spectrum of CD30-positive lymphoproliferative disorders. *Am J Surg Pathol*. 2014;38(9):1203-1211.

CHAPTER 39

Cutaneous involvement in systemic diffuse large B-cell lymphomas

Alejandro A. Gru and Yvonne Perner

DIFFUSE LARGE B-CELL LYMPHOMA

The overall landscape of systemic B-cell lymphomas with a large-cell component has undergone major changes in the most recent World Health Organization (WHO) classification.[1,2] At this stage, it is much speculated that subsequent modifications will occur in the next few years, mostly based on the molecular findings of each diagnostic category. The paradigm of diffuse large-cell lymphoma as a distinct entity is altered by the numerous subcategories that can be potentially included under this term. It is important to emphasize that certain prognostic biomarkers have played a significant role in the distinction between germinal center types (GCTs) and nongerminal center (activated B-cell type, ABC) using gene expression profiles. Diffuse large B-cell lymphomas (DLBCLs) with GCT have a better prognosis than those of ABC.[3,4] It is now widely recommended that a panel of several markers must be performed upon the diagnosis of systemic DLBCL, even when there is cutaneous dissemination by the disease. Several algorithms have been employed and, among them, the Hans algorithm is one of the most widely used for the cell of origin (COO) classification.[5] Under the Hans algorithm, cases with CD10 expression, or CD10−, MUM1−, BCL-6+ are classified as GCT. Cases that are CD10− and MUM1+ are categorized as ABC (Fig. 39-1). The use of such algorithm is, however, subject to potential misclassifications in approximately 15% to 20% of cases, when comparing with gene expression profiling.[5] Other algorithms such as the ones developed by Muris et al[6] and Choi et al[7] have been used with success. In addition to such markers, fluorescent in situ hybridization (FISH) also plays an important role, as cases with an *MYC*[8,9] or *BCL-6*[10] rearrangements tend to have a more aggressive behavior and worse prognosis. The cell of origin using immunohistochemistry and/or gene expression profiling (GEP) has an importance in defining both prognostic and therapeutic subgroups. COO using GEP is more reliable than immunohistochemistry (IHC)-based algorithms.

DLBCL, not otherwise specified (DLBCL, NOS) encompasses all cases of nodal and extranodal large B-cell lymphoma that do not belong to a specific diagnostic category. It is not a single disease but a collection of morphologically, genetically, and clinically different malignant lymphoproliferative disorders. The very recent article from the international consensus classification of malignant lymphomas and the WHO classification has suggested to de-emphasize the role of certain subsets of DLBCL (CD5+ DLBCL, double expressors BCL-2+/MYC⁰) for the diagnosis of DLBCL. These variants have (weak) adverse prognostic impact and do not reflect true biological subgroups but rather represent the end results of different biological pathways.[1,2,11-17]

Recently, molecular/cytogenetic profiling studies have independently identified five to seven new functional genetic subgroups of DLBCL, strongly emphasizing the validity of this concept, but failing to classify all cases.[18-20] The C1 cluster exhibited *BCL6*SVs in combination with mutations in the *NOTCH2* and NF-κB pathways. Most of them are classified as ABC by Hans. Notably, **C1 (cluster 1) DLBCLs** exhibited multiple genetic bases of immune escape, including inactivating mutations in *B2M, CD70, FAS*, and SVs of *PD-L1 and PD-L2*. The **C5 cluster** also corresponds to the ABC category by COO and is associated with the typical *MYD88*^{L265} mutation, not seen in C1. C5 also showed mutations of *CD79B* and *TBL1XR1*. The **C3 (cluster 3) DLBCLs** harbored *BCL2* mutations and *IGH::BCL2* translocations. C3 DLBCLs also exhibited frequent mutations in chromatin modifiers, *KMT2D, CREBBP*, and *EZH2*. C3 genetic alterations have been described in follicular lymphoma (FL) and de novo GCB-type B-cell lymphoma, and 95% of cases fell under the GCB category. It also includes the double hit cases (*BCL2-R and MYC-R*). **C4 (cluster 4) DLBCLs** were characterized by mutations in four linker and four core histone genes, multiple immune evasion molecules (*CD83, CD58, and CD70*), BCR/Pi3K signaling intermediates (*RHOA, GNA13*, and *SGK1*), NF-κB modifiers (*CARD11, NFKBIE*, and *NFKBIA*), and RAS/JAK/STAT pathway members (*BRAF* and *STAT3*). C4 DLBCLs were primarily of the GCB subtype. C4 differed from C3 in the lack of *BCL-2* translocations and higher

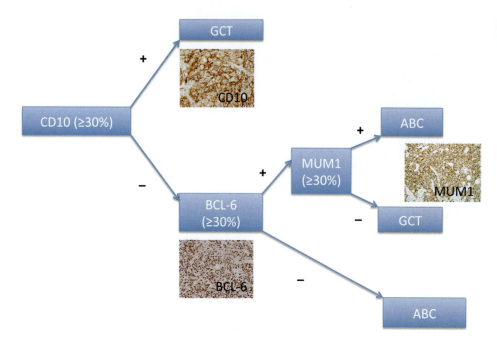

FIGURE 39-1. Hans algorithm for subclassification of GCT versus ABC in DLBCL.

prevalence of *PTEN* and *RHOA* mutations. They also lacked the mutations in chromatin modifiers but exhibited mutations in H1 linker histones (sometimes present in FL). **C2 (cluster 2) DLBCLs** harbored frequent biallelic inactivation of *TP53* by mutations and 17p copy loss. Loss of *CDKN2A* and *RB1* are also common to this cluster. This cluster typically included both GCB and ABC types by COO. More frequent CNVs are also common.

Schmitz et al performed an independent clustering analysis of cases of DLBCL into seven major subtypes.[21] The **MCD** subtype corresponded to the C5 cluster. This group included most cases of primary central nervous system lymphoma and primary testicular lymphomas. An **N1** subtype was also described, characterized by *NOTCH1* mutations and a poor prognosis. A **BN2** subtype corresponded to the C1 cases, shared the mutational landscape of marginal zone lymphomas, but was not enriched in transformed MZLs. The **ST2** grouped together with the C4 cluster.

De novo CD5-positive diffuse large B-cell lymphoma (CD5+ DLBCL) appears to represent an immunophenotypic variant of DLBCL associated with worse prognosis.[11,22,23] It is estimated that between 5% and 10% of DLBCL will express CD5. CD5+DLBCL is associated with advanced-stage (III or IV) and frequent nodal and extranodal disease. Approximately 75% of cases have extranodal involvement, and the skin is a frequent site of manifestation.[24-26] Histologically, the cases have a centroblastic or immunoblastic appearance, and some can also have intravascular dissemination (Fig. 39-2). This should be distinguished with intravascular large B-cell lymphoma (IVL) that in 30% to 40% of cases can have associated CD5 expression. The immunophenotype of the cells is more typical of a postgerminal center pattern, with BCL-6 and MUM1 expression. However, 10% to 20% of cases have a germinal center phenotype.[11] The prognosis of this disease is poor and worse than cases of CD5− DLBCL.[11,23,26]

CD5+ DLBCL must be distinguished from Richter transformation of chronic lymphocytic leukemia (CLL) and from the pleomorphic variant of mantle cell lymphoma (MCL). In Richter, there is typically a preceding history of CLL/small lymphocytic lymphoma with the classic cytogenetic aberrations of the disease (trisomy 12, del13q, etc.). In MCL, there is typically a rearrangement of the BCL-1 gene with high expression of BCL-1 by IHC. In addition, most cases of MCL are SOX11 positive, features that help to distinguish them from CLL and DLBCL. Vela-Chavez et al[27] previously reported a series of cases of DLBCL with low-level expression of BCL-1 in the tumor cells but that typically lack a rearrangement of the gene.

In the former WHO classification from 2016, a provisional entity by the name of Burkitt-like lymphoma with 11q aberration was introduced, as a lesion with pathologic findings of Burkitt lymphoma (BL) but lacking the *MYC* translocation.[28] Such cases are more common in children and young adults and have a good prognosis. Subsequently, other pathologic studies revealed morphologic variability with cases having a predominance of large cells. Importantly, genetic studies also suggest these cases are distinct from BL and closer to conventional DLBCL with germinal center B-cell derivation harboring more complex karyotypes and absence of typical BL mutations. Hence, in the International Consensus Classification (ICC) consensus, and **high-grade B-cell lymphoma with 11q aberrations** for the WHO classification, is the preferred nomenclature. FISH, cytogenetic, of SNP arrays studies are mandatory for such diagnostic confirmation.

Another provisional diagnostic category in the current ICC and WHO classification is the **HHV-8- and EBV-negative primary effusion-based lymphoma**.[29-31] The characteristic findings include presentation in elderly, HIV-negative patients with medical conditions that lead to fluid overload, suggesting chronic serosal stimulation in pathogenesis. Most cases have been reported from Japan (60%) and often have a history of hepatitis C infection. These patients usually have good prognosis with reported spontaneous regression or cure with drainage alone. Most cases

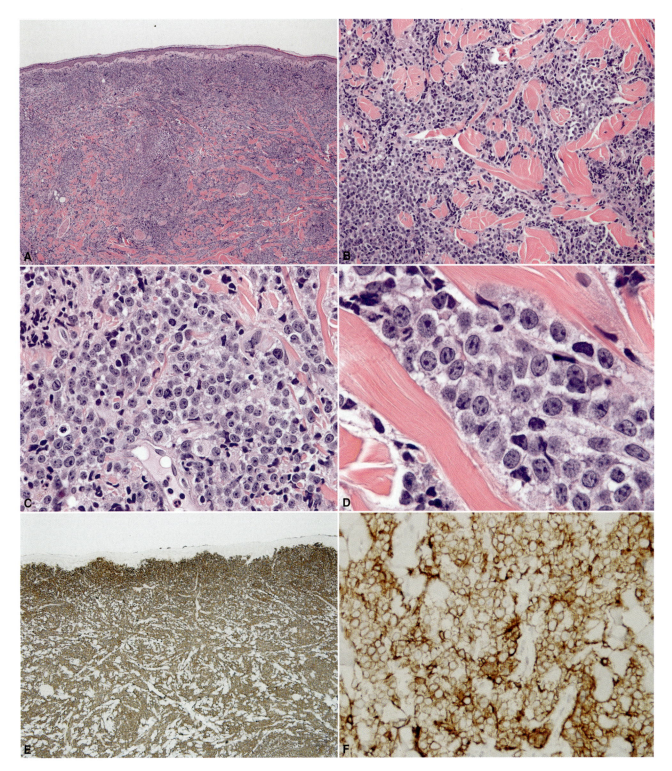

FIGURE 39-2. CD5⁺ DLBCL with cutaneous dissemination. A. 40× magnification reveals a diffuse dermal-based infiltrate with sparing of the epidermis. **B.** 200× magnification shows that the infiltrate dissects through the collagen fibers. **C** and **D.** (400× and 600×). The malignant cells are large with vesicular nuclei and prominent nucleoli. Some of them show an immunoblastic appearance. The tumor cells are positive for CD20 **(E)** and CD5 **(F)**.

show centroblastic morphology, express at least one B-cell marker, and show a GCB gene expression profile. Such lesions typically do not involve the skin.[29]

Large B-cell lymphoma with *IRF4* rearrangement has now been upgraded to a definite diagnostic category[32]; it is most common in children and young adults and usually has at least a partially follicular growth pattern. However, the same disease can be seen uncommonly in adults. FISH for *IRF4-R* must be performed for diagnosis. Cases lacking demonstrable rearrangements should have evidence of either IGH or IGK/IGL breaks. Detection of *IRF4* mutation may support the diagnosis. *IRF4-R* can occur in other aggressive

B-cell lymphomas associated with *BCL2-R* or *MYC-R*, mainly in adults, and in this context is not specific for the entity. DLBCL-LT do not have IRF translocations.[33]

HIGH-GRADE B-CELL LYMPHOMAS AND GRAY ZONE LYMPHOMAS

The 2016 WHO classification included two categories of high-grade B-cell lymphoma (HGBCL): HGBCL, NOS and HGBCL with *MYC and BCL2* and/or *BCL6* rearrangements ("double-hit" or "triple-hit", HGBCL-DH/TH).[28,34-37] Histopathologically they share an intermediate to large cell morphology, often a Burkitt-like pattern, and the aforementioned translocations (Figs. 39-3 and 39-4). HGBCL-DH now comprises two groups: HGBCL with *MYC and BCL2* rearrangements (with or without *BCL6* rearrangement) (HGBCL-DH-BCL2) and a new provisional entity, HBGBL with *MYC and BCL6* rearrangements (HGBCL-DH-BCL6). HGBCL-DH-BCL2 and HGBCL-DH-BCL6 entities continue to exclude FL and the morphology (large cell or high-grade cytology) should be reported.[38-48] Studies performed since the 2016 WHO classification support HGBCL-DH-BCL2 as an aggressive lymphoma of GCB origin with distinct biology from other GCB-DLBCL, NOS and HGBCL-DH-BCL6. It can occur in patients with or without prior FL. Data to support distinct biology in the HGBCL-DH-BCL6 cases are less compelling; however, it has been retained as a provisional entity to allow for continued study based on poor outcomes seen in some studies. Another less common category included in this subgroup is HGBCL, NOS. It remains in this classification as a diagnosis of exclusion for tumors that are not HGBCL-DH but that have intermediate-sized cells, often with blastoid or Burkitt-like cytology, but cannot be classified as DLBCL or BL. These cases are rare, and the diagnosis should only be made on well-fixed and preserved specimens as large cell cytology must be excluded.[49] DLBCL with starry-sky morphology and/or high proliferation index do not merit recategorization as HGBCL, NOS. Some cases of HGBCL can show expression of the immature marker TdT. Those were in the past classified as B lymphoblastic lymphomas (B-ALL).[50] In the more recent classification schemes, TdT+ mature HGBCL are allowed and must be separated from B-ALLs. Their mutational landscape supports their classification as mature lymphomas.[51]

The former diagnostic category of B-cell lymphoma, unclassifiable, with features intermediate between DLBCL and classic Hodgkin lymphoma (CHL) (former gray zone lymphomas), has now been changed to the preferred term mediastinal gray zone lymphomas (MGZLs). Such changes may share histologic and immunophenotypic overlap with cases of primary mediastinal large B-cell lymphoma.[52-55] A diagnosis of MGZL requires both morphological (high tumor cell density) and immunophenotypic criteria (at least two B-cell markers with strong expression) (Figs. 39-5 and 39-6). Cases of otherwise typical nodular sclerosis CHL, with variable expression of CD20, are still designated as CHL, although a close biological relationship to primary mediastinal large B-cell lymphoma remains. Clinical and genomic data indicate that most nonmediastinal GZLs are distinct from MGZLs and as such these cases should be diagnosed as DLBCL, NOS. Finally, nearly all EBV-positive DLBCL, while they may contain admixed Hodgkin/Reed-Sternberg-like cells, differ at the genomic level from MGZL and should be retained within the category of EBV-positive DLBCL.

EBV+ DIFFUSE LARGE B-CELL LYMPHOMA, NOS

EBV+ diffuse large B-cell lymphoma (EBV-DLBCL) has been renamed from the prior WHO classification (formerly known as EBV+ diffuse large B-cell lymphoma of the elderly) as a distinct entity that occurs in patients with a wide range of age, but typically in individuals who are older than 50 years and without any known immunodeficiency or previous lymphoma diagnosis.[56-58] Patients who are younger than 45 years appear to have a better prognosis. It appears likely that changes in the immune status related to the aging process are linked to this lymphoma subtype. EBV-DLBCL appears to be more common in certain areas of Asia and Mexico and more infrequent in Western countries.[59] The disease has a striking predilection for extranodal sites (70%), and particularly the skin, lung, tonsils, and stomach.[59-62] In individuals 90 years or older, it represents 20% to 30% of all B-cell lymphomas.[59] An important factor affecting the definition of such lymphoproliferative disorder is linked to the fact that the definition of this entity has struggled with different cutoff points for the number of EBV+ cells but currently requires expression of EBV in >80% of the tumor cells.[59] Clinically, patients can present with lymphadenopathy and cutaneous plaques and tumors.[56,63] Lesions are usually nonulcerated. Because sometimes lesions can present in the legs, a diagnosis of DLBCL leg type (LT) is often entertained. Some cases of EBV-DLBCL can occur as a complication or during the progression of cases of angioimmunoblastic T-cell lymphoma.[64] A rare case of this entity was associated with the use of mogamulizumab in the treatment of adult T-cell leukemia/lymphoma.[65]

Histologically, EBV-DLBCL presents with two distinctive patterns: polymorphous and monomorphous types (Figs. 39-7 and 39-8), but often a combination of the two can be present.[56] A more recent series showed the monomorphic pattern to be slightly more prevalent (55%).[66] A granulomatous reaction can be seen in a small subset of cases (45%). Such patterns do not have any prognostic significance. We have recently reported the presence of epidermotropism in a series of three cases of EBV-DLBCL (Figs. 39-9 and 39-10).[67] The polymorphous variant is classically associated with a mixture of immunoblasts, plasmablasts, and centroblasts and the presence of cells with Hodgkin or Hodgkin-like appearance. The background cells include small lymphocytes, histiocytes, and plasma cells. The monomorphic variant is characterized by the presence of sheets of immunoblastic-appearing cells. Classically, lymph nodes show areas of necrosis with a geographic pattern, but such phenomenon is less common in the skin.[62] The tumor cells express B-cell antigens (CD20, CD19, CD79a, PAX5), but some cases can have loss of CD20, as opposed to the majority of the other systemic DLBCLs. EBV-DLBCL has a nongerminal center phenotype (activated B-cell type) with expression of MUM1, and lack of expression of CD10 and BCL-6. CD30 shows

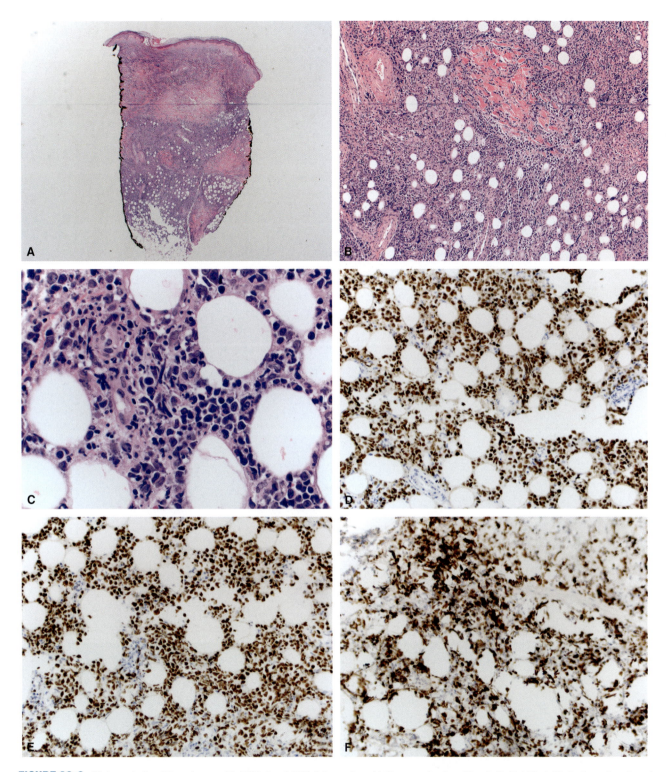

FIGURE 39-3. High-grade B-cell lymphoma with *BCL2-R* and *MYC-R*. Dense dermal infiltrate sparing the epidermis (**A**, 40×). The infiltrate shows deep dermal and subcutaneous extension (**B**, 100×). It is composed of intermediate-sized cells with a very high number of mitotic figures (**C**, 600×). The malignant cells are positive for PAX-5 (**D**) and MYC (**E**) and have a high proliferation by Ki67 (**F**).

variable expression in the cells but more frequently is seen in a high proportion of cases. The detection of EBV is a prerequisite for the diagnosis, typically in >80% of the tumor cells (Fig. 39-11). Some cases can show expression of LMP-1 and EBNA2, which suggest a latency III type of infection, similar to posttransplant lymphoproliferative disorders.[62] EBV-DLBCL shows activation of the NF-κB pathway and has a monoclonal immunoglobulin light chains restriction. PD-L1 is upregulated and diffusely positive in these tumors, a feature that can be associated with PD-L1 amplification.

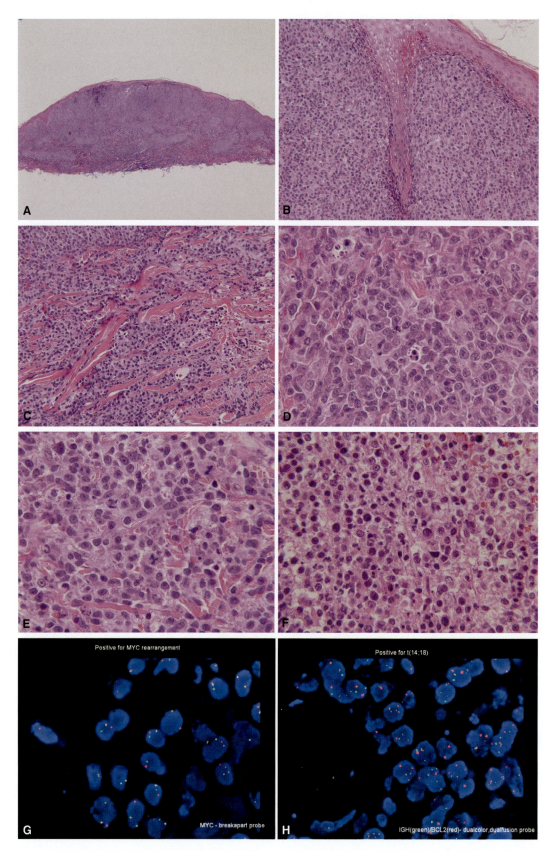

FIGURE 39-4. Cutaneous involvement by double-hit lymphoma. A. Low-power magnification (40×). A shave biopsy of the nodule shows a malignant lymphoid infiltrate throughout the dermis without epidermal involvement. **B.** The grenz zone is much attenuated and in areas difficult to see. **C** and **D.** (200× and 400×, respectively). The malignant lymphoid infiltrate has a substantial large-cell component and shows an interstitial distribution. The malignant cells have vesicular nuclei and prominent nucleoli. Mitosis and apoptosis are very frequently observed. **E.** The large-cell component contrasts the "starry-sky" pattern seen in other areas **(F)** of the biopsy, more typical of a classic BL. FISH studies show a "double-hit" lymphoma with both an MYC **(G)** and IGH-BCL2 **(H)** rearrangements.

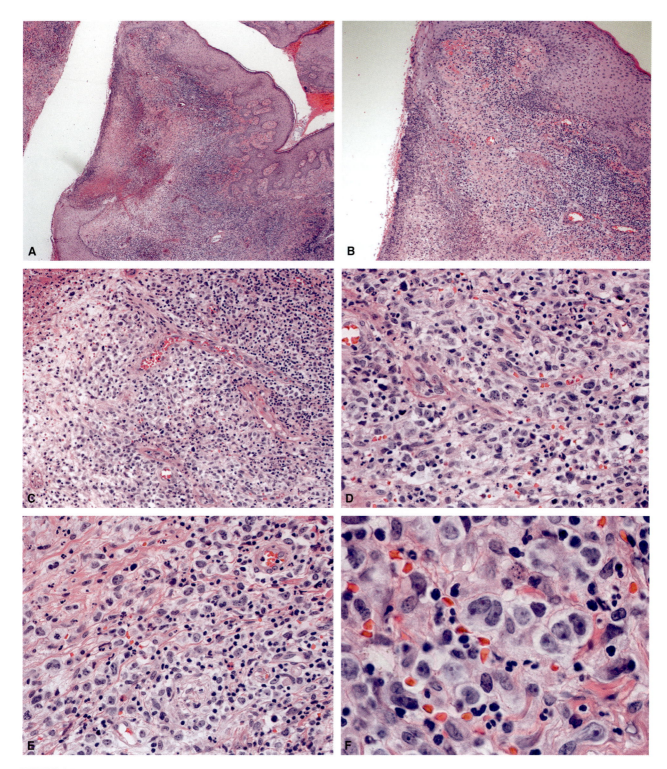

FIGURE 39-5. Skin involved by gray zone lymphoma by direct extension. (**A** and **B**) The skin shows an ulcerated surface appearance with an atypical lymphoid infiltrate underneath the ulceration (hematoxylin and eosin [H&E] stain, original magnification ×20 and ×40); (**C**) the infiltrate is composed of sheets of large mononuclear cells (H&E stain, original magnification ×200); (**D** and **E**) the neoplastic cells are immersed in a rich background of inflammatory cells that include neutrophils and eosinophils (H&E stain, original magnification ×400); (**F**) the same Hodgkin RS cells and variants are also present in the skin (H&E stain, original magnification x600). (From Subtil A, Gru AA. Secondary cutaneous involvement by direct extension in high-grade B-cell lymphomas. *J Cutan Pathol*. 2021;48(4):541-546.)

The latter findings suggest a possible role for the use of PD-1 blockade in the management of these tumors. Most cases lack rearrangements of the *BCL-2, BCL-6, and MYC* genes.

The differential diagnosis includes DLBCL, NOS, CHL, and DLBCL-LT, which typically do not show high levels of EBV expression. Cutaneous dissemination by BL can also be linked to high levels of EBV expression in the malignant cells. But, as opposed to EBV-DLBCL, the cells are smaller, are typically more homogeneous, have a germinal center phenotype (BCL-2$^-$, BCL-6$^+$, and CD10$^+$), are CD30$^-$, and

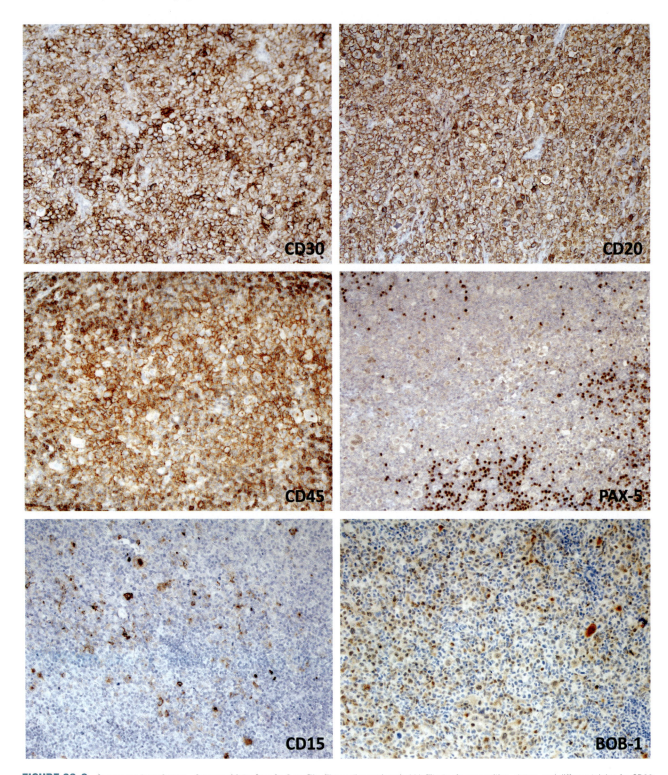

FIGURE 39-6. Gray zone lymphoma—immunohistochemical profile. The malignant lymphoid infiltrate shows positive, strong, and diffuse staining for CD30, CD20, and CD45. PAX-5 shows a dim staining pattern in the large lymphoma cells. CD15 and BOB-1 are positive in a subset of the large malignant cells. (From Subtil A, Gru AA. Secondary cutaneous involvement by direct extension in high-grade B-cell lymphomas. *J Cutan Pathol.* 2021;48(4):541-546.)

have a much higher Ki67 (~100%). CHLs can also be EBV⁺. The expression of B-cell markers in >50% of the tumor cells, extranodal presentation, and/or EBV latency III favors the diagnosis of EBV-positive DLBCL, NOS. Extended B-cell antibody panels are critical in this setting.

Plasmablastic lymphoma (PBL) can also have significant overlap with EBV-DLBCL. In fact, some cases with a monomorphic plasmablastic morphology might be impossible to distinguish on the basis of the histologic or immunophenotypic profile.[68] However, PBL has also diffuse EBV⁺

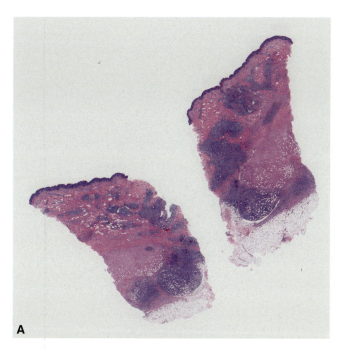
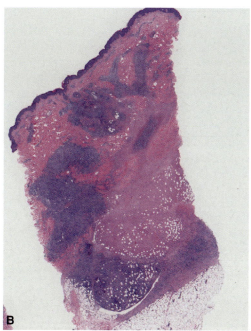

FIGURE 39-7. **EBV⁺ diffuse large B-cell lymphoma. A** and **B** (H&E, 10× and 20×). There is a vaguely nodular and diffuse infiltrate extending into the subcutaneous tissue with an area of deep dermal necrosis. The infiltrate shows sparing of the surface epidermis.

but is more frequently negative for B-cell markers such as CD20, CD19, and PAX5. It has been shown that such distinction might be an important one, as cases of EBV-DLBCL have a worse prognosis compared with PBL.[64] Other lymphomas with a plasmablastic appearance such as primary serous effusion lymphoma and diffuse large B-cell lymphoma associated with Castleman disease can be distinguished on the basis of their association with human herpes virus-8 (HHV-8). ALK⁺ DLBCL also has a plasmablastic appearance but invariably shows expression of ALK1 and a rearrangement of the gene. EBV⁺ mucocutaneous ulcers are also seen in association with immune suppression, and in mucosal sites (oral cavity and anal region). Although they can share similarities with the polymorphous variant of EBV-DLBCL, they differ in the clinical context where the tumors occur.

Another variant of EBV⁺-associated large B-cell lymphoma represents the so-called fibrin-associated DLBCL or diffuse large B-cell lymphoma associated with chronic inflammation (DLBCL-CI). Some examples of DLBCL associated with breast implant seromas have been described with an indolent behavior. Patients with DLBCL-CI typically have a longstanding history of pyothorax with associated respiratory symptoms and can present with a tumor in the chest wall. The interval between the onset of pyothorax and this lymphoma is ~37 years. This subtype shares the immunophenotype with EBV-DLBCL and commonly has *MYC* amplification.

The prognosis of EBV-DLBCL is very poor with a median survival of ~2 years.[56,59-62] A recent study showed a median overall survival of 88 months, worse than that of cases of DLBCL-LT.[66] The treatment of the disease is complicated further by the advanced age of this population and the limited tolerability of aggressive chemotherapeutic regimens. Most of the treatment modalities include anti-CD20 (rituximab), and some have used anti-CD30 with some success (brentuximab). Experimental protocols targeting the NF-κB pathway with bortezomib are underway.

PLASMABLASTIC LYMPHOMA

PBL is an aggressive non-Hodgkin lymphoma showing terminal B-cell (plasmablastic) differentiation and a propensity to arise in the oral cavity of immunocompromised individuals.[69,70] The revised 2016 WHO edition describes PBL as a diffuse proliferation of large neoplastic cells most of which resemble B-cell immunoblasts, but in which all tumor cells have a plasma cell immunophenotype, and places PBL in a category of its own, separate from conventional diffuse large B-cell lymphoma.[71,72]

An accurate incidence of this tumor is difficult to reference. It shows a predilection for immunocompromised individuals and is far more common in HIV-positive individuals where it is believed to account for between 2% and 2.6% of all HIV-related lymphomas.[73] PBL is also described in immunocompetent individuals, albeit less commonly. The tumor occurs with greater frequency in males, in both oral and extraoral locations, where tumor prevalence among males and females is reported between 5.7:1 and 4:1 in these respective locations.[69] It is predominantly a tumor of adulthood, the mean age at presentation being around 50 years. HIV-positive individuals present approximately a decade earlier and in immunocompetent individuals, the presentation is not infrequently beyond the age of 60 years, raising the possible role of immune senescence.[73-77] PBL is uncommon in children, with approximately 20 cases reported in

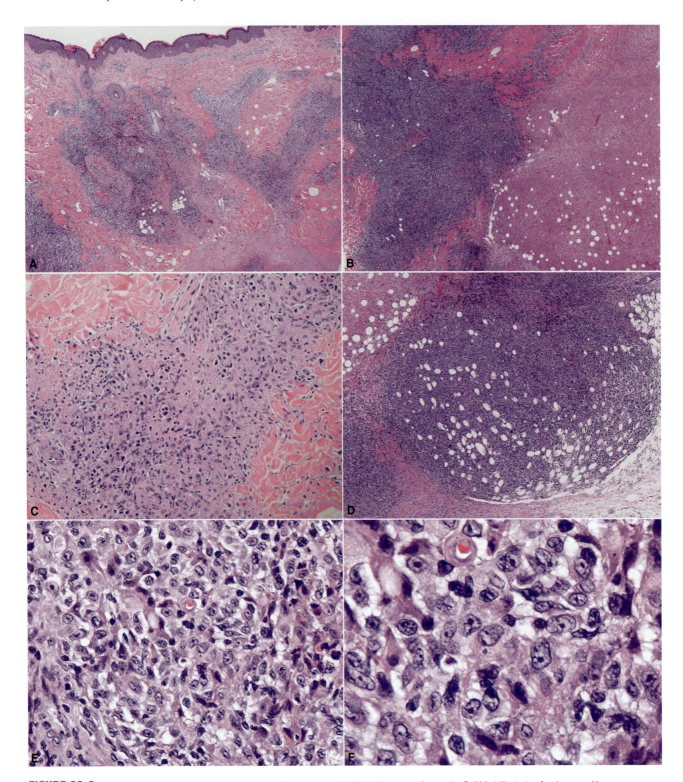

FIGURE 39-8. **EBV⁺ diffuse large B-cell lymphoma. A** and **B** (100× each) highlight the areas of necrosis. **C** (200×) illustrates focal areas with a vague granulomatous pattern. **D** (100×) shows the infiltrate in the adipose tissue. **E** and **F** (400× and 600×) show diffuse sheets of large cells with an immunoblastic appearance and prominent nucleoli.

the literature.[78,79] The disease occurs primarily within the oral cavity and is well described, although less frequently in lymph nodes and a variety of extranodal locations.

Cutaneous presentation is rarely reported.

PBL occurs most frequently in the context of immune suppression where it has a strong association with Epstein-Barr virus (EBV) infection, in up to 75% of cases.[79] It is also well documented to occur in immunocompetent individuals, although much less frequently.[80] HIV infection remains the most common state of immunodeficiency in which it arises. Of the variety of other immunodeficient states, it is well described in iatrogenically induced immune

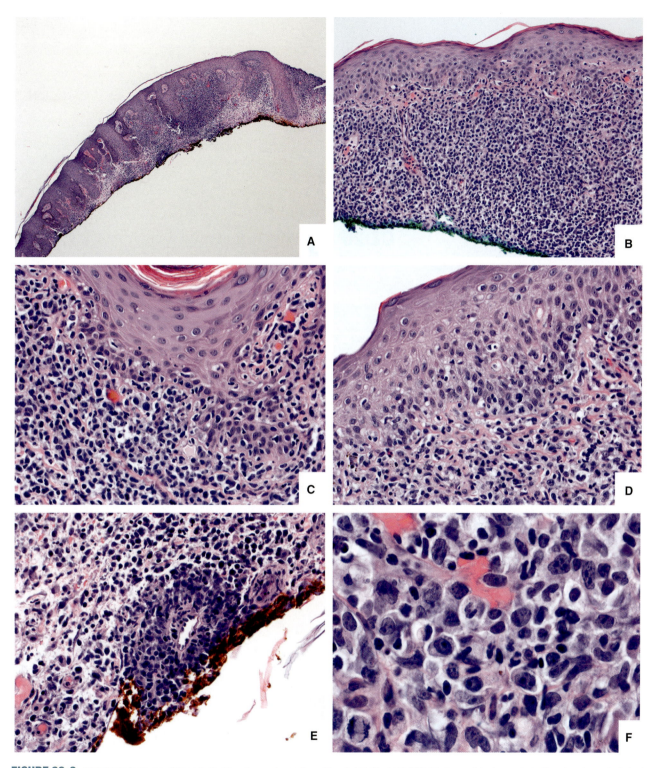

FIGURE 39-9. Histologic features of Case 1. Sections show a dense, dermal lymphoid infiltrate (**A**, H&E, 20×) comprising large, atypical lymphocytes and admixed inflammatory cells (**B**, H&E, 100×). At higher magnification, significant pleomorphism is observed and atypical lymphocytes are present within the epidermis and vessel walls (**C–E**, H&E, 200×). Cytomorphologically, the infiltrate comprises a mixture of immunoblastic and centroblastic cells, constituting the polymorphous variant (**F**, H&E, 400×). (From Wu S, Subtil A, Gru AA. Epidermotropic Epstein-Barr virus-positive diffuse large b-cell lymphoma: a series of 3 cases of a very unusual high-grade lymphoma. *Am J Dermatopathol.* 2021;43(1):51-56.)

dysregulation following bone marrow and solid organ transplantation.[80-83] Long-term use of corticosteroids, cyclosporine, azathioprine, mycophenolate mofetil, and TNFα antagonists has been implicated in this context.[84] PBL has also been reported in patients receiving immunomodulatory therapy for autoimmune diseases such as rheumatoid arthritis, psoriasis, dermatomyositis, and inflammatory bowel disease,[75,80,85] and in the setting of immune senescence in the elderly.[80] Rarely, it has been documented following transformation from a small B-cell non-Hodgkin lymphoma,

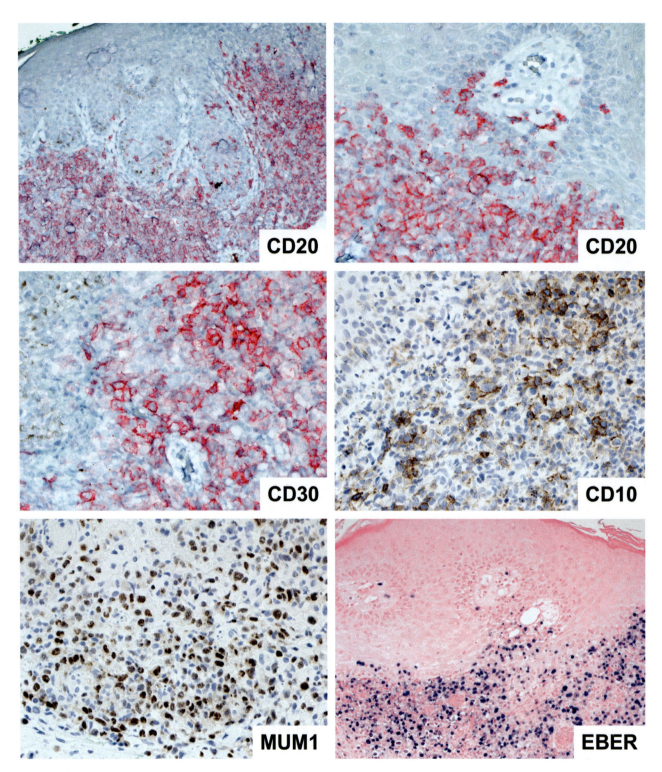

FIGURE 39-10. Immunohistochemical features of Case 1. CD20 is diffusely positive in the large, atypical cells (100×). At higher magnification, CD20-positive cells are seen within the epidermis (400×). CD30 is strongly and diffusely positive within the infiltrate (400×). CD10 is positive in small subset of cells (200×), and MUM1 is diffusely positive (200×), consistent with a nongerminal center DLBCL by Hans algorithm. EBER is diffusely positive, including within the epidermotropic malignant lymphocytes (100×). (From Wu S, Subtil A, Gru AA. Epidermotropic Epstein-Barr virus-positive diffuse large b-cell lymphoma: a series of 3 cases of a very unusual high-grade lymphoma. *Am J Dermatopathol.* 2021;43(1):51-56.)

such as FL and small lymphocytic lymphoma/chronic lymphocytic leukemia.[80,86-88]

EBV DNA expression, as determined by in situ hybridization for EBV-encoded small RNA (EBER) is commonly expressed in tumor cells in 50% to 75% of PBL, with a higher frequency in HIV-positive cases.[74,89] The EBV latency pattern is not fully elucidated and appears to be heterogeneous. EBV latent membrane protein 1 (LMP1) is mostly negative, indicating a type I latency pattern, apart from posttransplant cases where a type II latency pattern is more common.[73,74]

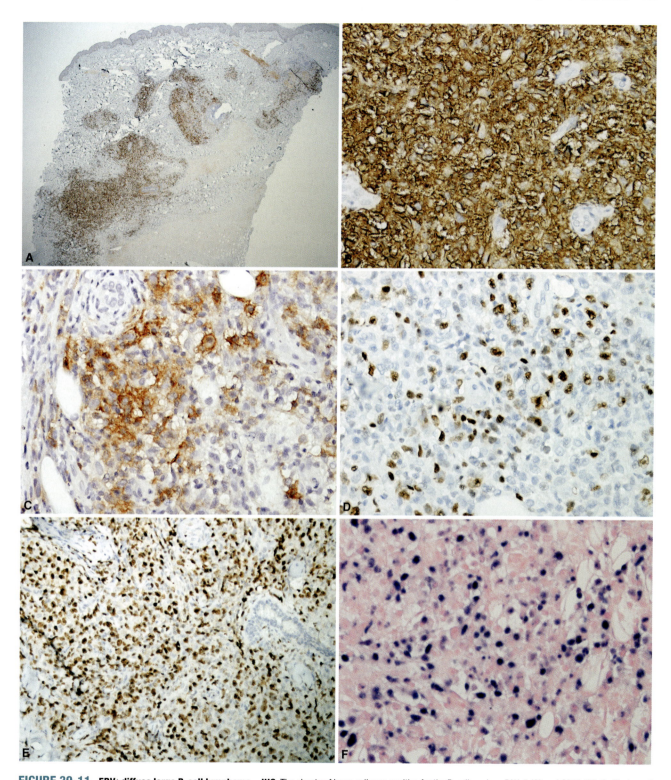

FIGURE 39-11. EBV+ diffuse large B-cell lymphoma—IHC. The sheets of large cells are positive for the B-cell markers PAX-5 **(A)** and CD20 **(B)**. **C.** Clusters of large cells are positive for CD30. **D.** MUM1 is positive in a subset of the large cells. **E.** Ki67 is markedly elevated within the larger cells (70%-80%). **F.** EBER is diffusely positive in the malignant infiltrate.

A noncanonical pattern of type II latency expression has been recently described.[16] Coexpression of HHV-8-associated protein latency-associated nuclear antigen-1 (LANA-1) is not seen in PBL and, when present, should prompt consideration of primary effusion lymphoma (PEL) (and its extracavitary variant), to which it bears close morphological and immunophenotypic resemblance. A less likely diagnostic consideration by virtue of quite different histological appearances is HHV-8/EBER-associated germinotropic lymphoproliferative disorder, and PBL arising in the context of multicentric plasma-cell variant Castleman disease. These are the only other lymphoid proliferations currently known to coexpresses EBER and HHV-8.[90]

Originally described to occur in the oral cavity of adults (gingiva, followed by palate and floor of mouth) with acquired immunodeficiency syndrome, PBL may also arise in a variety of extraoral locations, notably the nasal and paranasal sinuses, anogenital region, gastrointestinal tract, lymph nodes, skin, and soft tissues.[69,91-93] Primary nodal disease is uncommon, being reported with a variable frequency of 11% to 15%, this dependent on the clinical setting in which PBL arises.[73] Oral presentation is more frequent in HIV-positive patients,[94] whereas cutaneous and nodal involvement is more readily seen in the posttransplant setting.[81] Primary nasal presentation is reported to occur more commonly in immunocompetent individuals.[73,95-97] When occurring in children, it is mostly seen in lymph nodes, in the setting of retroviral disease.[74,78,79] Rarely, it occurs as a primary cutaneous neoplasm, where it has been described as ulcerative and infiltrative purple nodular lesions or erythematous infiltrated plaques, mostly on the lower legs.[74,87,98,99]

PBL that arises in the context of immunodeficiency secondary to HIV infection or organ transplantation usually presents with stage 3 or 4 disease.[73] Primary bone marrow disease is exceptionally rare.[100] It has a dismal prognosis, and the median survival in untreated cases is 3 months.[101] Intensive chemotherapy is associated with a median survival of 14 months.[102] Poor prognostic features include age over 60 years, advanced stage at clinical presentation, and no treatment.[102] MYC/IgH gene rearrangement is associated with poor median overall survival of 3 months.[103]

There are single case reports in the literature of spontaneous regression of PBL with the commencement of **highly active antiretroviral therapy (HAART) in HIV-positive cases.**[104] Regression of PBL has been reported following diminished methotrexate dosage in a patient with rheumatoid arthritis.[105] Chemotherapy is currently the main treatment modality for PBL, particularly in the context of systemic disease, although overall treatment response is poor. A combination of radiation therapy and chemotherapy for palliation of locally advanced disease is reported in the literature, with numbers being too low to make inferences regarding efficacy.[106] Given the overall poor prognosis of patients with PBL, an established standard of care for this disease is required. Cyclophosphamide, doxorubicin, vincristine, and prednisone (CHOP) is considered inadequate therapy, and current guidelines recommend more intensive regimens, such as infusional EPOCH (etoposide, prednisone, vincristine, cyclophosphamide, and doxorubicin).

HyperCVAD (cyclophosphamide, vincristine, doxorubicin, and dexamethasone) alternating with high-dose methotrexate and cytarabine is also suggested, as is high-dose therapy with autologous stem cell rescue in first complete remission in selected patients.[107] Improved survival rates have been reported with the use of bortezomib in combination with infusion adjusted EPOCH, but case numbers are small and, here too, predictions regarding efficacy are uncertain.[108]

Pathologically, irrespective of site, the tumor is composed of a diffuse proliferation of large lymphoma cells that display plasmablastic cytological characteristics with a conspicuous acidophilic nucleolus, vesicular chromatin, and in some instances a paranuclear hof. The cytoplasm is amphophilic to eosinophilic, mitotic activity is brisk, and interspersed tingible body macrophages may be numerous (Fig. 39-12). While a plasmablastic morphology is considered typical, some tumors have a closer resemblance to centroblasts. There may be admixed plasma cells that are interpreted as plasmacytic differentiation. Cutaneous involvement shows extensive dermal and subcuticular infiltration, and surface ulceration is a frequent finding.

PBL is by definition negative or, at most, weakly positive for CD45, CD20, and PAX5 in small numbers of tumor cells (<5%).[109,110] It has a plasmacytic immunophenotype and expresses CD38, CD138 (syndecan1), IRF4 (interferon regulatory factor-4)/MUM1 in 60% to 100% of tumor cells and is usually positive for XBP1 (X-box binding protein).[76,111] There is CD56 expression in up to 25% of cases, CD79a expression in 40%, and CD10 expression in 20%, and there is a uniformly high Ki67 expression in excess of 90%.[110,112] EMA and CD30 are frequently positive and MYC protein is overexpressed in up to 73% of cases.[89] Light chain restriction has been documented in up to 43% of cases.[73,111] BCL6 expression is usually negative as a consequence of BCL6 downregulation, which is required to complete the process of terminal differentiation to plasma cell maturity.[113,114] BCL2 is infrequently positive.[74] Lineage infidelity with aberrant expression of T-cell markers CD2, CD3, CD4, or CD7 is infrequent but well documented in both PBL and plasmablastic plasma cell myeloma, probably the most important consideration in the differential diagnosis of PBL.[74,115] Tumor suppressor gene protein expression is similar to that of plasmablastic plasma cell myeloma, with loss of p16 and p27 expression. There is positive staining for p53 suggesting a p53 mutation, as wildtype p53 is usually undetectable by immunohistochemistry.[74]

PBL is a karyotypically complex tumor: a *MYC* rearrangement is documented in 50% of PBL and is associated with MYC protein over expression in up to 73% of cases.[89,116,117] The immunoglobulin (Ig) gene region is the most frequent partner, reportedly involved in up to 85% of cases.[103] The t(8;14) translocation that typifies BL is the most frequently encountered translocation in PBL.[88,110] The majority of lymphomas with *MYC* rearrangements have a germinal center phenotype. In contrast, PBL has an activation status phenotype.

MYC amplification is reported in 11%, with fewer numbers showing *MYC* deletion.[109]

While PBL shows no arrangements with *BCL2, BCL6, MALT1,* and *PAX5,* in 31% to 41% of cases there are frequent gains of these loci.[89,103] In up to 30%, these gains involve three or more loci.

Concurrent copy number gains, most frequently of chromosome 3 (specifically 3q [BCL6 is located at 3q27] and 18q [BCL2 is located at 18q21]), were previously reported by Valera et al in 2010, in approximately 30% of PBL. This contrasts with DLBCL where gains of chromosomes 3q and 18q are generally mutually exclusive, 3q gains occurring in DLBCL of GCB phenotype and gains in 18q occurring in DLBCL of ABC phenotype. This difference supports the belief that PBL is genetically distinct from DLBCL. More recently, copy number gains have been recorded in chromosome 1q (43%) and the whole of chromosome 7 (28%).[80]

As with other lymphomas in the differential diagnosis of PBL, notably ALK-positive large B-cell lymphoma, PEL, HHV-8-positive diffuse large B-cell lymphoma, NOS and EBV-positive mucocutaneous ulcer, gene expression

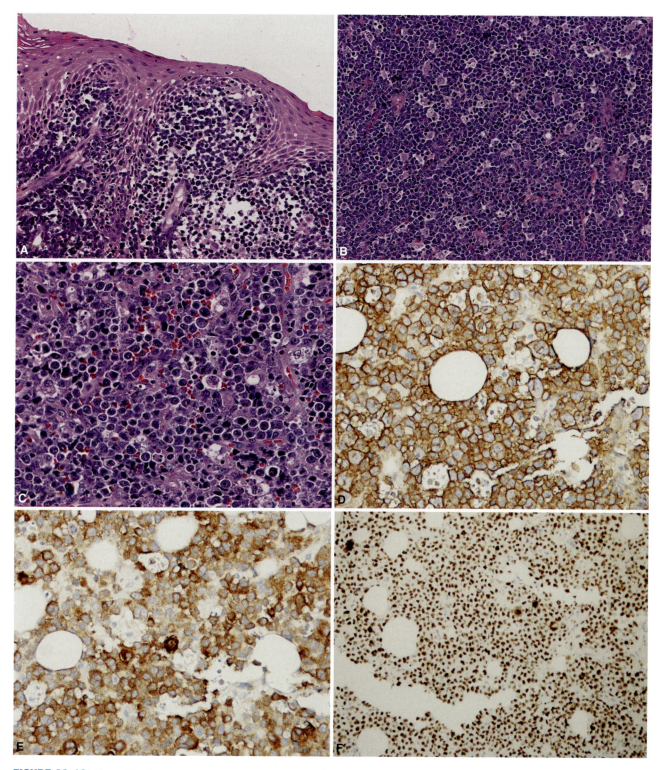

FIGURE 39-12. Plasmablastic lymphoma. A. 200× magnification shows that the malignant infiltrate focally extends to the surface mucosa in a case of PBL presenting in a patient with HIV. **B** and **C.** (200× and 400×). A "starry-sky" pattern is present, with numerous medium to large cells with a plasmablastic appearance, numerous mitoses, apoptotic bodies, and admixed macrophages. The tumor cells are positive for CD138 **(D)** and EMA **(E)** and show a high (>90%) proliferation index by Ki67 **(F)**.

profiling studies of PBL show upregulation of genes associated with plasmacytic differentiation, namely, X-box binding protein-1 (XBP1), PR domain zinc finger protein-1 (*PRDM1*), also known as BLIMP1 and interleukin-21 receptor (IL21R). In contrast, PBL shows low expression of genes for the B-cell receptor signaling pathway, such as *CD79a, CD79b, BCL6, BLK, LYN, SYK, RTPRC, PAX5, SPI-B, CSK, PIK3CD, SWAP70,* and *REL*.[118]

More recent literature on mutational analysis of PBL by whole exome sequencing indicates that PBL is overall more closely aligned to multiple myeloma than to other mature B-cell malignancies. It appears to be quite distinct from diffuse large B-cell lymphoma of both germinal center and activation status phenotype. Recurrent mutations in genes of the JAK-STAT3, MAPK-ERG, and Notch signaling pathways are reported.[80] The most frequent of these involves the JAK-STAT3 pathway, with 62% of cases showing mutations in at least 1 of 5 genes involved in this pathway.[80] Gain-of-function mutations in the RAS-MAPK pathway are seen in 28% of cases, with mutations in the *RAS* gene family being most common.

MicroRNA profiling for PBL, BL, and EMPC by Ambrosio et al in 2017 identified cellular miRNAs that were differentially expressed, showing partial alignment to either extramedullary plasma cell neoplasms or BL.[88] Furthermore, miRNAs discriminating HIV-positive cases from HIV-negative cases were found. A percentage of PBL escape the antitumor host immune response by manipulating immune checkpoint pathways. This results in diminished T-cell proliferation, decreased cytotoxicity and cytokine production, as well as an increased susceptibility to apoptosis.[119]

Immune checkpoint protein programmed cell death-1 (PD-1) and programmed cell death-ligand 1 (PDL-1) have been shown to be expressed in the histiocytic cells of the microenvironment of PBL in 60% to 72% of cases, and in the tumor cells in PBL in 22.5% and 5% of cases, respectively. This has been documented in both EBV-positive and -negative cases, indicating that there are probably several potential pathways of PBL immune escape.[89,119]

Synergy with EBV may be operative in this instance, in that EBV is able to take control of the PD1 pathway, allowing for persistent viral infection in host cells. As PBL is often positive for EBV infection, this may provide a target for immune checkpoint therapy in PBL.

PBL arises from a B lymphocyte that has undergone preterminal differentiation to a plasmablast, having exited the germinal center and undergone somatic hypermutation, with transition of the transcriptional program to that of a plasma cell.[120,121] While this particular cell is rare in normal lymphoid tissue, it is readily recognized in clonally expanded virally stimulated reactive lymph nodes caused principally by EBV and HIV. In this context, plasmablasts are evident in disorders such as HHV-8-positive multicentric Castleman disease (MCD) and Kaposi sarcoma–associated herpesvirus (KSHV)- and EBV-associated germinotropic lymphoproliferative disorder.[109]

A host of lymphoid neoplasms showing plasmacytic and plasmablastic differentiation may involve the skin, the majority of which represent secondary cutaneous involvement by primary disease elsewhere, either nodal or extranodal. Aggressive lymphoid neoplasms included here are EBV+ diffuse large B-cell lymphoma, plasmablastic extramedullary plasmacytoma and plasmablastic multiple myeloma, ALK+ large B-cell lymphoma, HHV-8/EBV+ PEL (and the extracavitary variant of PEL), and KSHV-associated diffuse large B-cell lymphoma arising in the context of multicentric plasma cell variant of Castleman disease.

EBV+ diffuse large B-cell lymphoma is a rare tumor, occurring most frequently in immunocompetent Asian individuals over the age of 50 years, with a mean age of onset of 71 years. Extranodal presentation is frequent, and the tumor is highly aggressive, showing a poor response to conventional treatment.[122] These tumors are positive for CD45, CD20, and often CD30, and they are defined by EBER expression. Cutaneous plasmacytoma is usually a late manifestation of multiple myeloma and is associated with a heavy tumor burden, plasma cell leukemia, and a poor prognosis.[123,124] Primary cutaneous plasmacytoma is very rare. It appears to be more aggressive than noncutaneous extramedullary plasmacytoma, with a 40% disease-related mortality.[125]

ALK+ large B-cell lymphoma is also a rare tumor occurring primarily as generalized nodal or mediastinal disease. It is composed of immunoblast-type lymphoid cells, often showing a sinusoidal growth pattern, and most cases are CD20 and CD30 negative.[126] PEL is a rare EBV and HHV-8-driven tumor that occurs primarily in the context of HIV infection. Rarely, it presents with soft tissue disease, or as a soft tissue primary, the extracavitary variant of PEL. There is considerable morphological and immunophenotypic overlap with PBL, with both tumors being negative for CD20 and ALK-1 and both expressing MUM1, CD138, EMA, EBER, and MYC in excess of 50% of cases. In distinction to PBL, CD45 is almost always expressed in PEL, as is CD30 and most usefully, HHV-8.[127]

HHV-8-associated diffuse large B-cell lymphoma, not otherwise specified (NOS) arising in the context of multicentric plasma cell variant Castleman disease usually occurs in HIV-positive individuals and presents with nodal and rarely splenic disease. The hallmarks of plasma cell variant Castleman disease are usually evident within lymph node biopsies. While having a plasmablastic morphology, these tumors express CD45 and CD20, are positive for HHV-8, but lack EBER expression.[128]

Lymphoplasmacytic lymphoma, FL, and marginal zone lymphoma displaying plasmacytic differentiation are low-grade neoplasms that, although showing plasmacytic features, should not be readily mistaken for PBL. Isolated cases of small lymphocytic lymphoma and FL showing Richter transformation to PBL have been described.[86,129] EBV+ mucocutaneous ulcer usually presents in mucocutaneous sites of individuals with immune dysregulation, with less frequent cutaneous presentation in the form of ulcerated nodules. Although the infiltrate includes cells with a plasmablastic or Reed-Sternberg-like morphology, the inflammatory background of plasma cells, mature lymphocytes, and eosinophils in the early stages of this condition bears greater resemblance to Hodgkin lymphoma than PBL. The large atypical cells in this condition express CD20, CD30 and, in approximately 50% of cases, CD15. They are EBER positive.[121] Rarely, EBER and HHV-8-positive primary cutaneous PBL has been described to occur in the setting of posttransplantation.

PRIMARY EFFUSION LYMPHOMA

PEL is an unusual form of non-Hodgkin lymphoma etiologically related to HHV-8 that usually presents as a lymphomatous effusion in the body cavities but without associated tumor masses (classic PEL). EBV-positive and HHV-8-positive lymphomas are often clinically aggressive in immunocompromised individuals and include PEL presenting as an effusion or mass lesion, germinotrophic lymphoproliferative disorder, and rare cases of multicentric Castleman-associated PBL or microlymphomas. PEL represents ~4% of the lymphomas in patients with HIV, but only 0.3% of all lymphomas in immunodeficient individuals.[130-132] PEL is more frequent in homosexuals and in advanced stages of immunosuppression (median CD4 count is approximately 100/L). The more typical clinical presentations are represented by the presence of B symptoms (fever, weight loss, night sweats) and effusion involving the body cavities (pleural, pericardial, or peritoneal). However, the solid variant forms tumor masses in different sites,[133] the skin being one of them.[134]

Histologically, these tumors have a plasmablastic appearance and can be accompanied by an intravascular pattern of dissemination, like IVL (Figs. 39-13 and 39-14). The immunophenotype of the malignant cells is characterized by the absence of pan-B-cell antigens (CD19, CD20, PAX5, CD79a), expression of plasma cell markers (CD138, CD38, vCD38), and also MUM1 expression. OCT2 and BOB-1 are expressed in a small subset of cases.[135] Aberrant expression of T-cell markers is seen in 50% of cases, CD3 being the most common one. Some have shown expression of CD79a in 23% of cases of PEL[136] as well as CD30.[137] PELs are linked to HHV-8 infection, and serologic titers of HHV-8 can be followed to monitor disease recurrence and progression. Aberrant expression of T-cell markers can also occur.[138-140] It is often difficult to determine clonality, as many of these cases lack surface of cytoplasmic light chain expression and rearrangements of the IGH gene. The proliferation rate is very high and averages 70% to 90% of the cells. EBV is reportedly positive in ~78% of cases. More recent cases of EBV$^-$ HHV-8-negative cases of PEL have been introduced in the more recent classifications schemes. A recent series of 19 cases of PEL revealed the following mutations: *B2M* ($n = 2$), *CD58* ($n = 1$), *EP300* ($n = 1$), *TNFAIP3* ($n = 1$), *AID1A* ($n = 1$), and *TP53* ($n = 1$).[135] Survival is similar between EBV$^+$ and EBV$^-$ cases (~60% at 2 years).

The presence of PEL in the skin is exceptional but well documented.[141-143] A recent case report has been documented on a patient presenting with a panniculitic appearance.[144] Other studies have shown that the extent of extracavitary involvement in PEL might be underestimated. In one series, 9 of 29 patients with PEL who presented with a classic cavitary lesion also had lymphoma in solid tissues including the pericardium, lymph nodes, gastrointestinal tract, and skin.[145] In half of the cases, the solid lesions preceded the development of positive effusions by a period of weeks to months.[133] The prognosis of PEL is poor in most cases, with more than 90% of the patients succumbing after a median survival of 3 months.[131] Of the total of seven cases documented on the skin, only one of the cases was EBV$^-$.

CUTANEOUS INVOLVEMENT IN BURKITT LYMPHOMA

BL has three specific forms: (1) an endemic variant occurring in certain regions of Africa, with a strong relationship to EBV and frequent extranodal presentations (face, gastrointestinal and gynecologic tracts); (2) a sporadic form presenting in children and young adults of the Western hemisphere, and with a much lower relationship to EBV (15%-30% of cases); and (3) a form associated to immunodeficiencies, particularly in the setting of HIV (and associated to EBV in up to 40% of cases).[146]

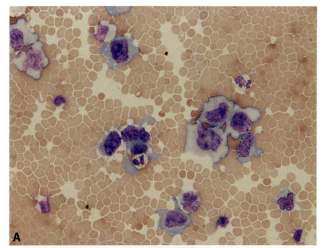
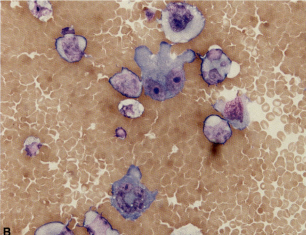
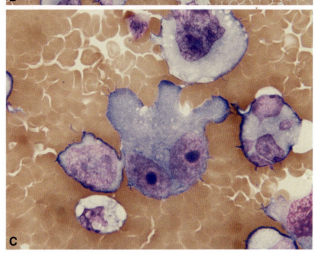

FIGURE 39-13. Primary effusion lymphoma. This is a serous effusion fluid illustrating highly pleomorphic tumor cells, predominantly large in size, with coarse chromatin and very prominent nucleoli. Some of them also show a plasmablastic appearance. Some of the cells are multinucleated (**A–C**, 4003, 6003, and 10,003, respectively).

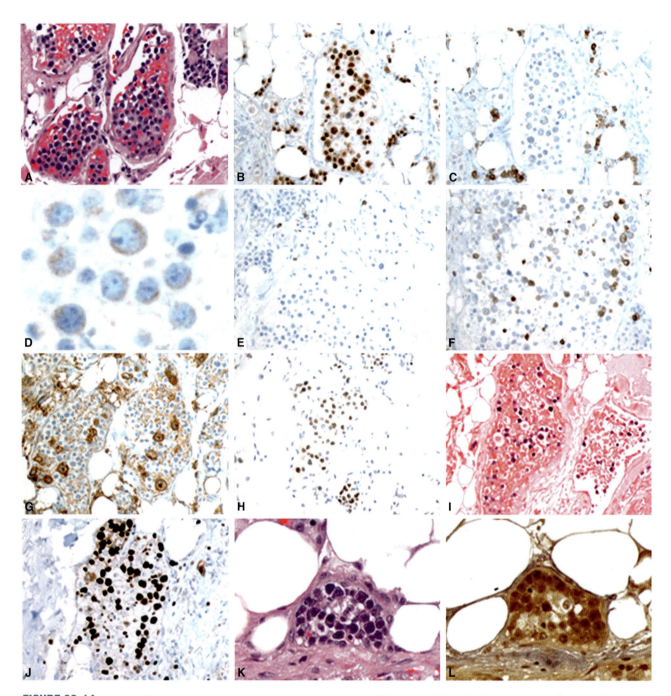

FIGURE 39-14. Primary effusion lymphoma. Immunostains and in situ hybridization (ISH) reveal an HHV-8+, EBV+ B-cell lymphoma with aberrant T-cell marker expression. The atypical cells (**A**, H&E) are positive for MUM-1 (**B**) and have dim expression of CD79a (**C** and **D**), but are negative for CD20 (**E**), CD19, Pax-5, and CD138 (not shown). The tumor cells also express dim cytoplasmic CD3 (**F**), dim CD4 (**G**), and CD45-RO (not shown), but are negative for CD5, CD7, CD8, CD56, and TIA-1 (not shown). An immunostain for HHV-8 (LANA-1) (**H**) and an ISH for EBV (EBER) (**I**) are positive in the neoplastic cells, which are restricted to the intravascular compartment. **J.** The tumor cells have a high Ki67 proliferation index. The neoplastic cells (**K**, H&E) also show expression of viral IL-6 (**L**). (From Crane GM, Ambinder RF, Shirley CMet al. HHV-8-positive and EBV-positive intravascular lymphoma: an unusual presentation of extracavitary primary effusion lymphoma. *Am J Surg Pathol.* 2014;38:426-432, with permission.)

Cutaneous involvement by BL has been documented previously[147-151] and occurs invariably as a secondary dissemination of the systemic disease. From the Surveillance, Epidemiology, and End Results (SEER) data, approximately 0.23% of cases of BL have skin disease.[152,153] While there are isolated reports of skin and soft tissue involvement, these cases were in the setting of an immunodeficiency state and were felt to be the result of either iatrogenic tumor seeding after nodal biopsies, for which there is limited prospective evidence of such a mechanism, or local spread from intrathoracic lymph nodes in the setting of recurrent disease. BL arising in the soft tissue of the lower extremity and chest wall has been reported during relapse in a child.[149] The suggestion is that hematogenous or lymphatic dissemination of malignant cells may be the mechanism underlying the development of skin and soft tissue involvement.[147,149]

Histologically, BL presents as diffuse sheets of medium-sized cells with blastoid appearance, numerous mitosis, and apoptotic cells. Background histiocytes engulfing some of the apoptotic cells provide the classic description of the so-called starry-sky pattern. The tumor cells show pan-B-cell antigens (CD20, CD19) and have a germinal center phenotype (CD10, BCL-6) but characteristically lack BCL-2 expression. The Ki67 is extraordinarily high and approaches 99% of the cells. BL is characterized by a rearrangement of the *MYC* gene, usually with the *IGH* gene with a t(8;14)(q24;q32). Variant translocations include a t(2;8)(p12;q24) (*IGK/MYC*) and t(8;22)(q24q11) (*MYC/IGL*).

T-CELL HISTIOCYTE-RICH LARGE B-CELL LYMPHOMA

The WHO has introduced this category of large B-cell lymphoma that is accompanied by a background rich in small T cells and histiocytes. The B-cell infiltrate must not exceed 10% of the total cells.[154] Cutaneous involvement is exceedingly rare in such entity but occasionally reported. We agree with Cerroni that we have not encountered in our series such cases, and most of the so-called THRBCLs (T-cell histiocyte-rich large B-cell lymphomas) represent examples of primary cutaneous follicle-center lymphoma (PCFCL) with a rich background of T cells and a more diffuse architecture.[155] Invariably, all the "cutaneous" cases of THRBCL have an excellent prognosis.

The reported cases of THRBCL present as nodules, plaques, and papules in the trunk and head and neck; this is one of extraordinarily high coincidence with the locations of where PCFCL arises.[156-160] Histologically, there is an admixture of small lymphocytes and rare occasional larger cells. The immunophenotype of the cells is linked to BCL-6 expression and background CD3+ T cells and CD68+ or CD163+ macrophages.[163] The nodal variants of THRBCL are aggressive forms that require intensive chemotherapy, usually in the form of R-CHOP, whereas most of these cutaneous cases are treated with surgical excision, radiation, or rituximab therapy.[159]

References

1. Campo E, Jaffe ES, Cook JR, et al. The international consensus classification of mature lymphoid neoplasms: a report from the clinical advisory committee. *Blood*. Published online 2022. blood.2022015851.
2. Alaggio R, Amador C, Anagnostopoulos I, et al. The 5th edition of the World Health Organization classification of Haematolymphoid tumours: lymphoid neoplasms. *Leukemia*. 2022;22:1-29.
3. Alizadeh AA, Eisen MB, Davis RE, et al. Distinct types of diffuse large B-cell lymphoma identified by gene expression profiling. *Nature*. 2000;403:503-511.
4. Rosenwald A, Wright G, Chan WC, et al. The use of molecular profiling to predict survival after chemotherapy for diffuse large-B-cell lymphoma. *N Engl J Med*. 2002;346:1937-1947.
5. Hans CP, Weisenburger DD, Greiner TC, et al. Confirmation of the molecular classification of diffuse large B-cell lymphoma by immunohistochemistry using a tissue microarray. *Blood*. 2004;103:275-282.
6. Muris JJ, Meijer CJ, Vos W, et al. Immunohistochemical profiling based on Bcl-2, CD10 and MUM1 expression improves risk stratification in patients with primary nodal diffuse large B cell lymphoma. *J Pathol*. 2006;208:714-723.
7. Choi WW, Weisenburger DD, Greiner TC, et al. A new immunostain algorithm classifies diffuse large B-cell lymphoma into molecular subtypes with high accuracy. *Clin Cancer Res*. 2009;15:5494-5502.
8. Tzankov A, Xu-Monette ZY, Gerhard M, et al. Rearrangements of MYC gene facilitate risk stratification in diffuse large B-cell lymphoma patients treated with rituximab-CHOP. *Mod Pathol*. 2014;27:958-971.
9. Zhou K, Xu D, Cao Y, et al. C-MYC aberrations as prognostic factors in diffuse large B-cell lymphoma: a meta-analysis of epidemiological studies. *PLoS One*. 2014;9:e95020.
10. Akyurek N, Uner A, Benekli M, et al. Prognostic significance of MYC, BCL2, and BCL6 rearrangements in patients with diffuse large B-cell lymphoma treated with cyclophosphamide, doxorubicin, vincristine, and prednisone plus rituximab. *Cancer*. 2012;118:4173-4183.
11. Xu-Monette ZY, Tu M, Jabbar KJ, et al. Clinical and biological significance of de novo CD5+ diffuse large B-cell lymphoma in western countries. *Oncotarget*. 2015;6(8):5615-5633. .
12. Durani U, Ansell SM. CD5+ diffuse large B-cell lymphoma: a narrative review. *Leuk Lymphoma*. 2021;62:3078-3086.
13. Hu B, Nastoupil LJ, Loghavi S, et al. De novo CD5+ diffuse large B-cell lymphoma, NOS: clinical characteristics and outcomes in rituximab era. *Leuk Lymphoma*. 2020;61:328-336.
14. Tzankov A, Leu N, Muenst S, et al. Multiparameter analysis of homogeneously R-CHOP-treated diffuse large B cell lymphomas identifies CD5 and FOXP1 as relevant prognostic biomarkers: report of the prospective SAKK 38/07 study. *J Hematol Oncol*. 2015;8:70.
15. Meriranta L, Pasanen A, Alkodsi A, Haukka J, Karjalainen-Lindsberg ML, Leppa S. Molecular background delineates outcome of double protein expressor diffuse large B-cell lymphoma. *Blood Adv*. 2020;4:3742-3753.
16. Staiger AM, Ziepert M, Horn H, et al. Clinical impact of the cell-of-origin classification and the MYC/BCL2 dual expresser status in diffuse large B-cell lymphoma treated within prospective clinical trials of the German high-grade non-Hodgkin's lymphoma study group. *J Clin Oncol*. 2017;35:2515-2526.
17. Bartlett NL, Wilson WH, Jung SH, et al. Dose-adjusted EPOCH-R compared with R-CHOP as frontline therapy for diffuse large B-cell lymphoma: clinical outcomes of the Phase III Intergroup trial Alliance/CALGB 50303. *J Clin Oncol*. 2019;37:1790-1799.
18. Chapuy B, Stewart C, Dunford AJ, et al. Molecular subtypes of diffuse large B cell lymphoma are associated with distinct pathogenic mechanisms and outcomes. *Nat Med*. 2018;24:679-690.
19. Wright GW, Huang DW, Phelan JD, et al. A probabilistic classification tool for genetic subtypes of diffuse large B cell lymphoma with therapeutic Implications. *Cancer Cell*. 2020;37:551-568 e14.
20. Lacy SE, Barrans SL, Beer PA, et al. Targeted sequencing in DLBCL, molecular subtypes, and outcomes: a Haematological Malignancy Research Network report. *Blood*. 2020;135:1759-1771.
21. Schmitz R, Wright GW, Huang DW, et al. Genetics and pathogenesis of diffuse large B-cell lymphoma. *N Engl J Med*. 2018;378:1396-1407.

22. Westin J, McLaughlin P. De novo CD5+ diffuse large B-cell lymphoma: a distinct subset with adverse features, poor failure-free survival and outcome with conventional therapy. *Leuk Lymphoma*. 2010;51:161-163.
23. Yamaguchi M, Nakamura N, Suzuki R, et al. De novo CD5+ diffuse large B-cell lymphoma: results of a detailed clinicopathological review in 120 patients. *Haematologica*. 2008;93:1195-1202.
24. Dargent JL, Lespagnard L, Feoli F, et al. De novo CD5-positive diffuse large B-cell lymphoma of the skin arising in chronic limb lymphedema. *Leuk Lymphoma*. 2005;46:775-780.
25. Igawa T, Sato Y, Takata K, et al. De novo CD5-positive diffuse large B-cell lymphomas show high specificity for cyclin D2 expression. *Diagn Pathol*. 2013;8:81.
26. Jain P, Fayad LE, Rosenwald A, et al. Recent advances in de novo CD5+ diffuse large B cell lymphoma. *Am J Hematol*. 2013;88:798-802.
27. Vela-Chavez T, Adam P, Kremer M, et al. Cyclin D1 positive diffuse large B-cell lymphoma is a post-germinal center-type lymphoma without alterations in the CCND1 gene locus. *Leuk Lymphoma*. 2011;52:458-466.
28. Swerdlow SH, Campo E, Pileri SA, et al. The 2016 revision of the World Health Organization classification of lymphoid neoplasms. *Blood*. 2016;127(20):2375-2390.
29. Kaji D, Ota Y, Sato Y, et al. Primary human herpesvirus 8-negative effusion-based lymphoma: a large B-cell lymphoma with favorable prognosis. *Blood Adv*. 2020;4:4442-4450.
30. Kubota T, Sasaki Y, Shiozawa E, Takimoto M, Hishima T, Chong JM. Age and CD20 expression are significant prognostic factors in human herpes virus-8-negative effusion-based lymphoma. *Am J Surg Pathol*. 2018;42:1607-1616.
31. Alexanian S, Said J, Lones M, Pullarkat ST. KSHV/HHV8-negative effusion-based lymphoma, a distinct entity associated with fluid overload states. *Am J Surg Pathol*. 2013;37:241-249.
32. Ramis-Zaldivar JE, Gonzalez-Farre B, Balague O, et al. Distinct molecular profile of IRF4- rearranged large B-cell lymphoma. *Blood*. 2020;135:274-286.
33. Pham-Ledard A, Prochazkova-Carlotti M, Vergier B, et al. IRF4 expression without IRF4 rearrangement is a general feature of primary cutaneous diffuse large B-cell lymphoma, leg type. *J Invest Dermatol*. 2010;130(5):1470-1472.
34. Li S, Lin P, Fayad LE, et al. B-cell lymphomas with MYC/8q24 rearrangements and IGH@BCL2/t(14;18)(q32;q21): an aggressive disease with heterogeneous histology, germinal center B-cell immunophenotype and poor outcome. *Mod Pathol*. 2012;25:145-156.
35. Lin P, Dickason TJ, Fayad LE, et al. Prognostic value of MYC rearrangement in cases of B-cell lymphoma, unclassifiable, with features intermediate between diffuse large B-cell lymphoma and Burkitt lymphoma. *Cancer*. 2012;118:1566-1573.
36. Zhao XF, Hassan A, Perry A, et al. C-MYC rearrangements are frequent in aggressive mature B-cell lymphoma with atypical morphology. *Int J Clin Exp Pathol*. 2008;1:65-74.
37. Magro CM, Wang X, Subramaniyam S, et al. Cutaneous double-hit B-cell lymphoma: an aggressive form of B-cell lymphoma with a propensity for cutaneous dissemination. *Am J Dermatopathol*. 2014;36(4):303-310.
38. Cucco F, Barrans S, Sha C, et al. Distinct genetic changes reveal evolutionary history and heterogeneous molecular grade of DLBCL with MYC/BCL2 double-hit. *Leukemia*. 2020;34:1329-1341.
39. Evrard SM, Pericart S, Grand D, et al. Targeted next generation sequencing reveals high mutation frequency of CREBBP, BCL2 and KMT2D in high-grade B-cell lymphoma with MYC and BCL2 and/or BCL6 rearrangements. *Haematologica*. 2019;104:e154-e157.
40. Kunstner A, Witte HM, Riedl J, et al. Mutational landscape of high-grade B-cell lymphoma with MYC-, BCL2 and/or BCL6 rearrangements characterized by whole-exome sequencing. *Haematologica*. Published online 2021.
41. Ennishi D, Jiang A, Boyle M, et al. Double-hit gene expression signature defines a distinct subgroup of germinal center B-cell-like diffuse large B-cell lymphoma. *J Clin Oncol*. 2019;37:190-201.
42. Sha C, Barrans S, Cucco F, et al. Molecular high-grade B-cell lymphoma: defining a poor-risk group that requires different approaches to therapy. *J Clin Oncol*. 2019;37:202-212.
43. Hilton LK, Tang J, Ben-Neriah S, et al. The double-hit signature identifies double-hit diffuse large B-cell lymphoma with genetic events cryptic to FISH. *Blood*. 2019;134:1528-1532.
44. Li S, Desai P, Lin P, et al. MYC/BCL6 double-hit lymphoma (DHL): a tumour associated with an aggressive clinical course and poor prognosis. *Histopathology*. 2016;68:1090-1098.
45. Pillai RK, Sathanoori M, van Oss SB, Swerdlow SH. Double-hit B-cell lymphomas with BCL6 and MYC translocations are aggressive, frequently extranodal lymphomas distinct from BCL2 double-hit Bcell lymphomas. *Am J Surg Pathol*. 2013;37:323-332.
46. Rosenwald A, Bens S, Advani R, et al. Prognostic significance of MYC rearrangement and translocation partner in diffuse large B-cell lymphoma: a study by the Lunenburg lymphoma biomarker consortium. *J Clin Oncol*. 2019;37:3359-3368.
47. Ye Q, Xu-Monette ZY, Tzankov A, et al. Prognostic impact of concurrent MYC and BCL6 rearrangements and expression in de novo diffuse large B-cell lymphoma. *Oncotarget*. 2016;7:2401-2416.
48. Johnson SM, Umakanthan JM, Yuan J, et al. Lymphomas with pseudo-double-hit BCL6-MYC translocations due to t(3;8)(q27;q24) are associated with a germinal center immunophenotype, extranodal involvement, and frequent BCL2 translocations. *Hum Pathol*. 2018;80:192-200.
49. Huttl KS, Staiger AM, Richter J, et al. The "Burkitt-like" immunophenotype and genotype is rarely encountered in diffuse large B cell lymphoma and high-grade B cell lymphoma, NOS. *Virchows Arch*. 2021;479:575-583.
50. Nanua S, Bartlett NL, Hassan A, et al. Composite diffuse large B-cell lymphoma and precursor B lymphoblastic lymphoma presenting as a double-hit lymphoma with MYC and BCL2 translocation. *J Clin Pathol*. 2011;64:1032-1034.
51. Bhavsar S, Liu Y, Gibson SE, Moore EM, Swerdlow SH. Mutational landscape of TdT+ large B-cell lymphomas supports their distinction from B-lymphoblastic neoplasms. A multiparameter study of a rare and aggressive entity. *Am J Surg Pathol*. 2022;46:71-82.
52. Wilson WH, Pittaluga S, Nicolae A, et al. A prospective study of mediastinal gray-zone lymphoma. *Blood*. 2014;124:1563-1569.
53. Pittaluga S, Nicolae A, Wright GW, et al. Gene expression profiling of mediastinal gray zone lymphoma and its relationship to primary mediastinal B-cell lymphoma and classical Hodgkin lymphoma. *Blood Cancer Discov*. 2020;1:155-161.
54. Chapuy B, Stewart C, Dunford AJ, et al. Genomic analyses of PMBL reveal new drivers and mechanisms of sensitivity to PD-1 blockade. *Blood*. 2019;134:2369-2382.

55. Sarkozy C, Hung SS, Chavez EA, et al. Mutational landscape of gray zone lymphoma. *Blood*. 2021;137:1765-1776.
56. Nakamura S, Jaffe ES, Swerdlow SH. *EBV Positive Diffuse Large B-Cell Lymphoma of the Elderly*. International Agency for Research on Cancer; 2008.
57. Mo XL, Zhou MY, Ye QR. Primary cutaneous Epstein-Barr virus-positive diffuse large B-cell lymphoma, not otherwise specified, in a non immuno compromised young man: a case report. *J Cutan Pathol*. 2020;47(4):387-389.
58. Malpica L, Marques-Piubelli ML, Beltran BE, Chavez JC, Miranda RN, Castillo JJ. EBV-positive diffuse large B-cell lymphoma, not otherwise specified: 2022 update on diagnosis, risk-stratification, and management. *Am J Hematol*. 2022;97(7):951-965.
59. Shimoyama Y, Yamamoto K, Asano N, et al. Age-related Epstein–Barr virus-associated B-cell lymphoproliferative disorders: special references to lymphomas surrounding this newly recognized clinicopathologic disease. *Cancer Sci*. 2008;99:1085-1091.
60. Shimoyama Y, Asano N, Kojima M, et al. Age-related EBV-associated B-cell lymphoproliferative disorders: diagnostic approach to a newly recognized clinicopathological entity. *Pathol Int*. 2009;59:835-843.
61. Shimoyama Y, Oyama T, Asano N, et al. Senile Epstein–Barr virus-associated B-cell lymphoproliferative disorders: a mini review. *J Clin Exp Hematopathol*. 2006;46:1-4.
62. Asano N, Yamamoto K, Tamaru J, et al. Age-related Epstein–Barr virus (EBV)-associated B-cell lymphoproliferative disorders: comparison with EBV-positive classic Hodgkin lymphoma in elderly patients. *Blood*. 2009;113:2629-2636.
63. De Unamuno Bustos B, Zaragoza Ninet V, Ballester Sanchez R, et al. Epstein–Barr virus-positive diffuse large B-cell lymphoma in an elderly patient. *Clin Exp Dermatol*. 2014;39:484-487.
64. Poon F, Ieremia E, Collins G, Matin RN. Epstein-Barr virus-induced cutaneous diffuse large B-cell lymphoma in a patient with angioimmunoblastic T-cell lymphoma. *Am J Dermatopathol*. 2019;41(12):927-930.
65. Kamachi K, Shindo T, Miyahara M, et al. Epstein-Barr virus-related diffuse large B-cell lymphoma in mogamulizumab-treated adult T-cell leukemia with incomplete T-cell reconstitution. *Int J Hematol*. 2019;109(2):221-227.
66. Jung JM, Na HM, Won CH, et al. Cutaneous Epstein-Barr virus-positive diffuse large B-cell lymphoma, not otherwise specified: a systematic review and comparative analysis with Epstein-Barr virus-negative, leg type. *J Am Acad Dermatol*. 2022;86(1):221-225.
67. Wu S, Subtil A, Gru AA. Epidermotropic epstein-barr virus-positive diffuse large B-cell lymphoma: a series of 3 cases of a very unusual high-grade lymphoma. *Am J Dermatopathol*. 2021;43(1):51-56. doi:10.1097/DAD.0000000000001718
68. Liu F, Asano N, Tatematsu A, et al. Plasmablastic lymphoma of the elderly: a clinicopathological comparison with age-related Epstein–Barr virus-associated B cell lymphoproliferative disorder. *Histopathology*. 2012;61:1183-1197.
69. Delecluse HJ, Anagnostopoulos I, Dallenbach F, et al. Plasmablastic lymphomas of the oral cavity: a new entity associated with the human immunodeficiency virus infection. *Blood*. 1997;89(4):1413-1420. doi:10.1182/blood.v89.4.1413
70. Jaffe ES, Pittaluga S. Aggressive B-cell lymphomas: a review of new and old entities in the WHO classification. *Hematology Am Soc Hematol Educ Prog*. 2011;2011:506-514.
71. Campo E, Stein HN. Plasmablastic lymphoma. In: Swerdlow S, Campo E, Harris NL, et al. eds. *WHO Classification of Tumours of the Haematopoietic and Lymphoid Tissue*. 4th ed. IARC; 2017:321-322.
72. Stein H, Harris NL, Campo E. *Plasmablastic Lymphoma*. International Agency for Research on Cancer; 2008.
73. Morscio J, Dierickx D, Nijs J, et al. Clinicopathologic comparison of plasmablastic lymphoma in HIV-positive, immunocompetent, and posttransplant patients: single-center series of 25 cases and meta-analysis of 277 reported cases. *Am J Surg Pathol*. 2014;38:875-886.
74. Castillo JJ, Bibas M, Miranda RN. The biology and treatment of plasmablastic lymphoma. *Blood*. 2015;125(15):2323-2330. doi:10.1182/blood-2014-10-567479
75. Tchernonog E, Faurie P, Coppo P, et al. Clinical characteristics and prognostic factors of plasmablastic lymphoma patients: analysis of 135 patients from the LYSA group. *Ann Oncol*. 2017;28(4):843-848. doi:10.1093/annonc/mdw684
76. Harmon CM, Smith LB. Plasmablastic lymphoma a review of clinicopathologic features and differential diagnosis. *Arch Pathol Lab Med*. 2016;140(10):1074-1078. doi:10.5858/arpa.2016-0232-RA
77. Shayanfar N, Babaheidarian P, Rahmani H, et al. Epidermodysplasia verruciformis associated with plasmablastic lymphoma and hepatitis B virus infection. *Acta Dermatovenerol Croat*. 2012;20:267-271.
78. Pather S, MacKinnon D, Padayachee RS. Plasmablastic lymphoma in pediatric patients: clinicopathologic study of three cases. *Ann Diagn Pathol*. 2013;17(1):80-84. doi:10.1016/j.anndiagpath.2012.08.005
79. Goedhals J, Stones DK, Botha MC. Plasmablastic lymphoma in childhood: a report of two cases. *SAJCH South African J Child Heal*. 2014;8(1):39-40. doi:10.7196/SAJCH.613
80. Liu Z, Filip I, Gomez K, et al. Genomic characterization of HIV-associated plasmablastic lymphoma identifies pervasive mutations in the JAK–STAT pathway. *Blood Cancer Discov*. 2020;1(1):112-125. doi:10.1158/2643-3230.bcd-20-0051
81. Black CL, Foster-Smith E, Lewis ID, et al. Post-transplant plasmablastic lymphoma of the skin. *Australas J Dermatol*. 2013;54:277-282.
82. Jordan LB, Lessells AM, Goodlad JR. Plasmablastic lymphoma arising at a cutaneous site. *Histopathology*. 2005;46:113-115.
83. Apichai S, Rogalska A, Tzvetanov I, et al. Multifocal cutaneous and systemic plasmablastic lymphoma in an infant with combined living donor small bowel and liver transplant. *Pediatr Transplant*. 2009;13:628-631.
84. Chen DB, Song QJ, Chen YX, Chen YH, Shen DH. Clinicopathologic spectrum and EBV status of post-transplant lymphoproliferative disorders after allogeneic hematopoietic stem cell transplantation. *Int J Hematol*. 2013;97(1):117-124. doi:10.1007/s12185-012-1244-1
85. Teruya-Feldstein J, Chiao E, Filippa DA, et al. CD20-negative large-cell lymphoma with plasmablastic features: a clinically heterogenous spectrum in both HIV-positive and -negative patients. *Ann Oncol*. 2004;15(11):1673-1679. doi:10.1093/annonc/mdh399
86. Martinez D, Valera A, Perez NS, et al. Plasmablastic transformation of low-grade b-cell lymphomas: report on 6 cases. *Am J Surg Pathol*. 2013;37(2):272-281. doi:10.1097/PAS.0b013e31826cb1d1

87. Marques SA, Abbade LPF, Guiotoku MM, et al. Primary cutaneous plasmablastic lymphoma revealing clinically unsuspected HIV infection. *An Bras Dermatol*. 2016;91(4):507-509. doi:10.1590/abd1806-4841.20164764
88. Ambrosio MR, Mundo L, Gazaneo S, et al. MicroRNAs sequencing unveils distinct molecular subgroups of plasmablastic lymphoma. *Oncotarget*. 2017;8(64):107356-107373. doi:10.18632/oncotarget.22219
89. Laurent C, Fabiani B, Do C, et al. Immune-checkpoint expression in epstein-barr virus positive and negative plasmablastic lymphoma: a clinical and pathological study in 82 patients. *Haematologica*. 2016;101(8):976-983. doi:10.3324/haematol.2016.141978
90. Bhavsar T, Lee JC, Perner Y, et al. KSHV-associated and EBV-associated germinotropic lymphoproliferative disorder: new findings and review of the literature. *Am J Surg Pathol*. 2017;41(6):795-800. doi:10.1097/PAS.0000000000000823
91. Corti M, Villafane MF, Bistmans A, et al. Oral cavity and extra-oral plasmablastic lymphomas in AIDS patients: report of five cases and review of the literature. *Int J STD AIDS*. 2011;22(12):759-763. doi:10.1258/ijsa.2011.011235
92. Sarode SC, Sarode GS, Patil A. Plasmablastic lymphoma of the oral cavity: a review. *Oral Oncol*. 2010;46(3):146-153. doi:10.1016/j.oraloncology.2009.12.009
93. Verma S, Nuovo GJ, Porcu P, Baiocchi RA, Crowson AN, Magro CM. Epstein-Barr virus- and human herpesvirus 8-associated primary cutaneous plasmablastic lymphoma in the setting of renal transplantation. *J Cutan Pathol*. 2005;32(1):35-39. doi:10.1111/j.0303-6987.2005.00258.x
94. Liu W, Lacouture ME, Jiang J, et al. KSHV/HHV8-associated primary cutaneous plasmablastic lymphoma in a patient with Castleman's disease and Kaposi's sarcoma. *J Cutan Pathol*. 2006;33(suppl 2):46-51.
95. Dales JP, Harket A, Bagneres D, et al. Plasmablastic lymphoma in a patient with HIV infection: an unusual case located in the skin. *Ann Pathol*. 2005;25:45-49.
96. Horna P, Hamill JR, Jr, Sokol L, et al. Primary cutaneous plasmablastic lymphoma in an immunocompetent patient. *J Am Acad Dermatol*. 2013;69:e274-e276.
97. Jambusaria A, Shafer D, Wu H, et al. Cutaneous plasmablastic lymphoma. *J Am Acad Dermatol*. 2008;58:676-678.
98. Tavares MDL, Magalhães TC, de Moraes FMB, Piñeiro-Maceira J, Ramos-e-Silva M. Plasmablastic lymphoma: a rare and exuberant cutaneous emergence in an immunocompetent patient. *Int J Dermatol*. 2015;54(5):e175-e178. doi:10.1111/ijd.12705
99. Mani SSR, Kodiatte T, Jagannati M. A rare presentation of plasmablastic lymphoma as cutaneous nodules in an immunocompromised patient. *Int J STD AIDS*. 2017;28(6):623-625. doi:10.1177/0956462416675037
100. Al Shaarani M, Shackelford RE, Master SR, et al. Plasmablastic lymphoma, a rare entity in bone marrow with unusual immunophenotype and challenging differential diagnosis. *Case Rep Hematol*. 2019;2019:1-9. doi:10.1155/2019/1586328
101. Castillo JJ, Winer ES, Stachurski D, et al. Prognostic factors in chemotherapy-treated patients with HIV-associated plasmablastic lymphoma. *Oncol*. 2010;15(3):293-299. doi:10.1634/theoncologist.2009-0304
102. Castillo JJ, Winer ES, Stachurski D, et al. Clinical and pathological differences between human immunodeficiency virus-positive and human immunodeficiency virus-negative patients with plasmablastic lymphoma. *Leuk Lymphoma*. 2010;51(11):2047-2053. doi:doi:10.3109/10428194.2010.516040.
103. Valera A, Balagué O, Colomo L, et al. IG/MYC rearrangements are the main cytogenetic alteration in plasmablastic lymphomas. *Am J Surg Pathol*. 2010;34(11):1686-1694. doi:10.1097/PAS.0b013e3181f3e29f
104. Armstrong R, Bradrick J, Liu YC. Spontaneous regression of an HIV-associated plasmablastic lymphoma in the oral cavity: a case report. *J Oral Maxillofac Surg*. 2007;65(7):1361-1364. doi:10.1016/j.joms.2005.12.039
105. García-Noblejas A, Velasco A, Cannata-Ortiz J, Arranz R. Remisión espontánea de un linfoma no Hodgkin plasmablástico asociado a metotrexato tras disminución de la dosis del fármaco. *Med Clin*. 2013;140(12):569-570. doi:10.1016/j.medcli.2012.10.001
106. Phipps C, Yeoh KW, Lee YS, et al. Durable remission is achievable with localized treatment and reduction of immunosuppression in limited stage EBV-related plasmablastic lymphoma. *Ann Hematol*. 2017;96(11):1959-1960. doi:10.1007/s00277-017-3109-4
107. National Comprehensive Cancer Network. *NCCN Clinical Practice Guidelines in Oncology: B-Cell Lymphomas*. 2021.
108. Castillo JJ, Reagan JL, Sikov WM, Winer ES. Bortezomib in combination with infusional dose-adjusted EPOCH for the treatment of plasmablastic lymphoma. *Br J Haematol*. 2015;169(3):352-355. doi:10.1111/bjh.13300
109. Montes-Moreno S, Martinez-Magunacelaya N, Zecchini-Barrese T, et al. Plasmablastic lymphoma phenotype is determined by genetic alterations in MYC and PRDM1. *Mod Pathol*. 2017;30(1):85-94. doi:10.1038/modpathol.2016.162
110. Chen BJ, Chuang SS. Lymphoid neoplasms with plasmablastic differentiation: a comprehensive review and diagnostic approaches. *Adv Anat Pathol*. 2020;27(2):61-74. doi:10.1097/PAP.0000000000000253
111. Vega F, Chang CC, Medeiros LJ, et al. Plasmablastic lymphomas and plasmablastic plasma cell myelomas have nearly identical immunophenotypic profiles. *Mod Pathol*. 2005;18(6):806-815. doi:10.1038/modpathol.3800355
112. Chao C, Silverberg MJ, Xu L, et al. A comparative study of molecular characteristics of diffuse large B-cell lymphoma from patients with and without human immunodeficiency virus infection. *Clin Cancer Res*. 2015:21(6):1429-1437. doi:10.1158/1078-0432.CCR-14-2083
113. Boy S, van Heerden M, Pool R, Willem P, Slavik T. Plasmablastic lymphoma versus diffuse large B cell lymphoma with plasmablastic differentiation: proposal for a novel diagnostic scoring system. *J Hematop*. 2015;8(1):3-11. doi:10.1007/s12308-014-0227-y
114. Diehl SA, Schmidlin H, Nagasawa M, et al. STAT3-Mediated up-regulation of BLIMP1 is coordinated with BCL6 down-regulation to control human plasma cell differentiation. *J Immunol*. 2008;180(7):4805-4815. doi:10.4049/jimmunol.180.7.4805
115. Suzuki Y, Yoshida T, Nakamura N, et al. CD3- and CD4-Positive plasmablastic lymphoma: a literature review of Japanese plasmablastic lymphoma cases. *Intern Med*. 2010;49(16):1801-1805. doi:10.2169/internalmedicine.49.3164
116. Chisholm KM, Bangs CD, Bacchi CE, et al. Expression profiles of MYC protein and MYC gene rearrangement in lymphomas. *Am J Surg Pathol*. 2015;39:294-303.

117. Taddesse-Heath L, Meloni-Ehrig A, Scheerle J, et al. Plasmablastic lymphoma with MYC translocation: evidence for a common pathway in the generation of plasmablastic features. *Mod Pathol.* 2010;23:991-999.
118. Chapman J, Gentles AJ, Sujoy V, et al. Gene expression analysis of plasmablastic lymphoma identifies downregulation of B-cell receptor signaling and additional unique transcriptional programs. *Leukemia.* 2015;29(11):2270-2273. doi:10.1038/leu.2015.109
119. Gravelle P, Péricart S, Tosolini M, et al. EBV infection determines the immune hallmarks of plasmablastic lymphoma. *OncoImmunology.* 2018;7(10):1-11. doi:10.1080/2162402X.2018.1486950
120. Hsi ED, Lorsbach RB, Fend F, Dogan A. Plasmablastic lymphoma and related disorders. *Am J Clin Pathol.* 2011;136(2):183-194. doi:10.1309/AJCPV1I2QWKZKNJH
121. Gaulard P, Swerdlow SH, Harris NL, et al. EBV-positive mucocuntaeous ulcer. In: Swerdlow S, Campo E, Harris NL, et al, eds. *WHO Classification of Tumours of the Hematopoietic and Lymphoid Tissue.* 4th ed. IARC; 2017:307-308.
122. Zhou Y, Xu Z, Lin W, et al. Comprehensive genomic profiling of EBV-positive diffuse large B-cell lymphoma and the expression and clinicopathological correlations of some related genes. *Front Oncol.* 2019;9. doi:10.3389/fonc.2019.00683
123. Usmani SZ, Heuck C, Mitchell A, et al. Extramedullary disease portends poor prognosis in multiple myeloma and is over-represented in high-risk disease even in the era of novel agents. *Haematologica.* 2012;97(11):1761-1767. doi:10.3324/haematol.2012.065698
124. Chung A, Liedtke M. Cutaneous plasmablastic plasmacytoma. *Blood.* 2019;134(23):2116. doi:10.1182/blood.2019002821
125. Wong KF, Chan JKC, Li LPK, Yau TK. Primary cutaneous plasmacytoma - report of two cases and review of the literature. *Am J Dermatopathol.* 1994;16(4):392-397. doi:10.1097/00000372-199408000-00006
126. Campo E. In: Swerdlow S, Campo E, et al, eds. *WHO Classification of Tumours of the Haematopoietic and Lymphoid Tissue.* 4th ed. IARC; 2017.
127. Hu Z, Pan Z, Chen W, et al. Primary effusion lymphoma: a clinicopathological study of 70 cases. *Cancers (Basel).* 2021;13(4):1-14. doi:10.3390/cancers13040878
128. Chadburn A, Said J, Gratzinger D, et al. HHV8/KSHV-positive lymphoproliferative disorders and the spectrum of plasmablastic and plasma cell neoplasms. *Am J Clin Pathol.* 2017;147(2):171-187. doi:10.1093/ajcp/aqw218
129. Ouansafi I, He B, Fraser C, et al. Transformation of follicular lymphoma to plasmablastic lymphoma with c-myc gene rearrangement. *Am J Clin Pathol.* 2010;134(6):972-981. doi:10.1309/AJCPWY1SGJ9IEAOR
130. Patel S, Xiao P. Primary effusion lymphoma. *Arch Pathol Lab Med.* 2013;137:1152-1154.
131. Wu W, Youm W, Rezk SA, et al. Human herpesvirus 8-unrelated primary effusion lymphoma-like lymphoma: report of a rare case and review of 54 cases in the literature. *Am J Clin Pathol.* 2013;140:258-273.
132. Aguilar C, Laberiano C, Beltran B, Diaz C, Taype-Rondan A, Castillo JJ. Clinicopathologic characteristics and survival of patients with primary effusion lymphoma. 2020;61(9):2093-2102. doi:10.1080/10428194.2020.1762881
133. Kim Y, Leventaki V, Bhaijee F, et al. Extracavitary/solid variant of primary effusion lymphoma. *Ann Diagn Pathol.* 2012;16:441-446.
134. Inoue S, Miyamoto T, Yoshino T, et al. Primary effusion lymphoma with skin involvement. *J Clin Pathol.* 2006;59:1221-1222.
135. Calvani J, Gérard L, Fadlallah J, et al. A comprehensive clinicopathologic and molecular study of 19 primary effusion lymphomas in HIV-infected patients. *Am J Surg Pathol.* 2022;46(3):353-362. doi:10.1097/PAS.0000000000001813
136. Pan ZG, Zhang QY, Lu ZB, et al. Extracavitary KSHV-associated large B-cell lymphoma: a distinct entity or a subtype of primary effusion lymphoma? Study of 9 cases and review of an additional 43 cases. *Am J Surg Pathol.* 2012;36:1129-1140.
137. Bhatt S, Ashlock BM, Natkunam Y, et al. CD30 targeting with brentuximab vedotin: a novel therapeutic approach to primary effusion lymphoma. *Blood.* 2013;122:1233-1242.
138. Boulanger E, Hermine O, Fermand JP, et al. Human herpesvirus 8 (HHV-8)-associated peritoneal primary effusion lymphoma (PEL) in two HIV-negative elderly patients. *Am J Hematol.* 2004;76:88-91.
139. Carbone A, Gloghini A, Vaccher E, et al. Kaposi's sarcoma-associated herpesvirus/human herpesvirus type 8-positive solid lymphomas: a tissue-based variant of primary effusion lymphoma. *J Mol Diagn.* 2005;7:17-27.
140. Dong HY, Wang W, Uldrick TS, et al. Human herpesvirus 8- and Epstein–Barr virus-associated solitary B cell lymphoma with a T cell immunophenotype. *Leuk Lymphoma.* 2013;54:1560-1563.
141. Crane GM, Ambinder RF, Shirley CM, et al. HHV-8-positive and EBV-positive intravascular lymphoma: an unusual presentation of extracavitary primary effusion lymphoma. *Am J Surg Pathol.* 2014;38:426-432.
142. Crane GM, Xian RR, Burns KH, et al. Primary effusion lymphoma presenting as a cutaneous intravascular lymphoma. *J Cutan Pathol.* 2014;41(12):928-935.
143. Pielasinski U, Santonja C, Rodriguez-Pinilla SM, et al. Extracavitary primary effusion lymphoma presenting as a cutaneous tumor: a case report and literature review. *J Cutan Pathol.* 2014;41:745-753.
144. Saggini A, Di Prete M, Facchetti S, Rapisarda VM, Anemona L. Panniculitis-like presentation of extracavitary primary effusion lymphoma. *Am J Dermatopathol.* 2020;42(6):446-451. doi:10.1097/DAD.0000000000001539
145. Chadburn A, Hyjek E, Mathew S, et al. KSHV-positive solid lymphomas represent an extra-cavitary variant of primary effusion lymphoma. *Am J Surg Pathol.* 2004;28:1401-1416.
146. Leoncini L, Raphael M, Stein H, et al. *Burkitt Lymphoma.* International Agency for Research on Cancer; 2008.
147. Berk DR, Cheng A, Lind AC, et al. Burkitt lymphoma with cutaneous involvement. *Dermatol Online J.* 2008;14:14.
148. Fuhrmann TL, Ignatovich YV, Pentland A. Cutaneous metastatic disease: burkitt lymphoma. *J Am Acad Dermatol.* 2011;64:1196-1197.
149. Lu R. Primary burkitt lymphoma of the chest wall. *Case Rep Hematol.* 2012;2012:746098.
150. Pettey AA, Walsh JS. Cutaneous involvement with Burkitt-like lymphoma. *Am J Dermatopathol.* 2007;29:184-186.
151. Rogers A, Graves M, Toscano M, et al. A unique cutaneous presentation of Burkitt lymphoma. *Am J Dermatopathol.* 2014;36:997-1001.
152. Goyal N, Rubin N, Goyal A. Differential survival of systemic B-cell lymphomas initially diagnosed in the skin: a population-based study of 883 patients. *Arch Dermatol Res.* Published online November 15, 2021. doi:10.1007/s00403-021-02293-0

153. Thakkar D, Lipi L, Misra R, Yadav SP. Skin involvement in Burkitt's lymphoma. *Hematol Oncol Stem Cell Ther*. 2018;11(4):251-252.
154. De Wolf-Peters C, Delabie J, Campo E, et al. *T-Cell/Histiocyte-rich Large B-Cell Lymphoma*. International Agency for Research on Cancer; 2008.
155. Cerroni L, Gatter K, Kerl H, et al. *Skin Lymphoma: The Illustrated Guide*. Wiley-Blackwell; 2009.
156. Arai E, Sakurai M, Nakayama H, et al. Primary cutaneous T-cell-rich B-cell lymphoma. *Br J Dermatol*. 1993;129:196-200.
157. Dommann SN, Dommann-Scherrer CC, Zimmerman D, et al. Primary cutaneous T-cell-rich B-cell lymphoma. A case report with a 13-year follow-up. *Am J Dermatopathol*. 1995;17:618-624.
158. Dunphy CH, Nahass GT. Primary cutaneous T-cell-rich B-cell lymphomas with flow cytometric immunophenotypic findings. Report of 3 cases and review of the literature. *Arch Pathol Lab Med*. 1999;123:1236-1240.
159. Li S, Griffin CA, Mann RB, et al. Primary cutaneous T-cell-rich B-cell lymphoma: clinically distinct from its nodal counterpart? *Mod Pathol*. 2001;14:10-13.
160. Sander CA, Kaudewitz P, Kutzner H, et al. T-cell-rich B-cell lymphoma presenting in skin. A clinicopathologic analysis of six cases. *J Cutan Pathol*. 1996;23:101-108.
161. Kambayashi Y, Fujimura T, Tsukada A, et al. Extranodal T-cell/histiocyte-rich large B-cell lymphoma presenting primarily on the skin. *Acta Derm Venereol*. 2012;92:637-639.

CHAPTER 40

Cutaneous mantle cell lymphoma

José Cabeçadas and Alejandro A. Gru

DEFINITION

Mantle cell lymphoma (MCL) is a mature B-cell non-Hodgkin lymphoma (NHL) comprising approximately 3% to 10% of the systemic B-cell NHL.[1-4] It has a distinctive pathologic, immunophenotypic, and molecular genetic profile and is often accompanied by an aggressive clinical course.[5] First described by K. Lennert in 1973 as "diffuse germinocytoma,"[6] this was later included in the 1974 Kiel classification as centrocytic lymphoma; MCL is defined in the current World Health Organization (WHO) classification as a "B-cell neoplasm generally composed of monomorphic small-to-medium–sized lymphoid cells with irregular nuclear contours and a *CCND1* translocation."[3,7]

Although traditionally considered a very aggressive lymphoma, two indolent variants, in situ mantle cell neoplasia and leukemic nonnodal mantle cell lymphoma are now recognized.[3]

MICROSCOPY, IMMUNOPHENOTYPE, AND GENETIC PROFILE

Classically mantle cell lymphoma is a monomorphic proliferation of small to medium-sized transformed cells resembling centrocytes, with dispersed chromatin and inconspicuous nucleoli. Four variants are recognized: two of them, pleomorphic and blastoid, are associated with an aggressive clinical course. The other two, small cell and marginal zone–like, may have a better prognosis. Nevertheless, only a moderate agreement was shown among laboratories in cytology assessment.[8] Hyalinized small-caliber vessels are common as well as scattered epithelioid histiocytes.[9] True plasmacytic differentiation is very rare and mainly occurs in the SOX11-negative subtype.[10]

The growth pattern is usually vaguely nodular, but mantle zone, diffuse, and follicular patterns may be present, sometimes in the same sample.

IMMUNOPHENOTYPE

The immunophenotype of MCL includes the expression of pan-B-cell antigens such as CD19, CD20, CD79, and PAX5, together with surface IgM/IgD. Like chronic lymphocytic leukemia (CLL), CD5 is positive but CD23 is usually negative (few cases may be positive for CD23). Absence of CD5 has been reported in 5% to 17% of cases of MCL[11,12] (Figs. 40-1 and 40-2). Aberrant expression of BCL-6 can be seen in about 10% of cases, but CD10 coexpression is rarely seen. Nonetheless, the presence of CD10 is more common in blastoid cases variants and also reported on those involving the skin.[13,14] MUM1 expression is infrequently expressed.[15] The majority of cases of MCL (>95%) are positive for cyclin D1 (BCL-1), but negative cases have been described.[16] In this particular scenario, SOX11 has emerged as a useful marker to help in the diagnosis of the disease, being positive in 93% to 95% of cases.[17,18] Staining for SOX11 in CCND1-negative cases, together with CD5 expression in the tumor cells, could help clarify the diagnosis. However, SOX11 expression is not unique to MCL as can also be seen in lymphoblastic lymphomas, Burkitt lymphoma, hairy cell leukemia, and T-cell prolymphocytic leukemia.[19,20] SOX-11 cases usually are associated with a classic morphology, higher proportion of CD23, and CD200 expression.[21]

IG genes are clonally rearranged and IGV genes are hypermutated in 15% to 40% of cases. A biased usage of the IGHV genes supports the possibility of an antigenic drive.[22-24]

MCL has a distinctive cytogenetic translocation with the presence of the t(11;14) (q13;q32) rearrangement, which juxtaposes the *CCND1* gene on chromosome 11 with the immunoglobulin heavy chain gene (*IGH*) on chromosome 14, resulting in the characteristic overexpression of the BCL-1 protein.[25,26] Rarely *CCND1* is translocated with the IG-light chains genes.[24]

Other cyclins are rarely involved in an immunoglobulin translocation, and this needs to be investigated by fluorescence in situ hybridization.[23,24]

Loss of TP53 is an independent prognostic factor and may be detected by IHC.[8] Ki67 and TP53 stains should be performed as their results are incorporated in the clinical decision for mantle cell lymphoma international prognostic index (MIPI).[8,29]

Other genetic and epigenetic alterations are emerging with an impact in our understanding of the disease.[30]

CUTANEOUS DISEASE

Extranodal involvement is frequent in MCL, particularly in the bone marrow, gastrointestinal tract, and Waldeyer ring. Cutaneous involvement by MCL typically occurs in the

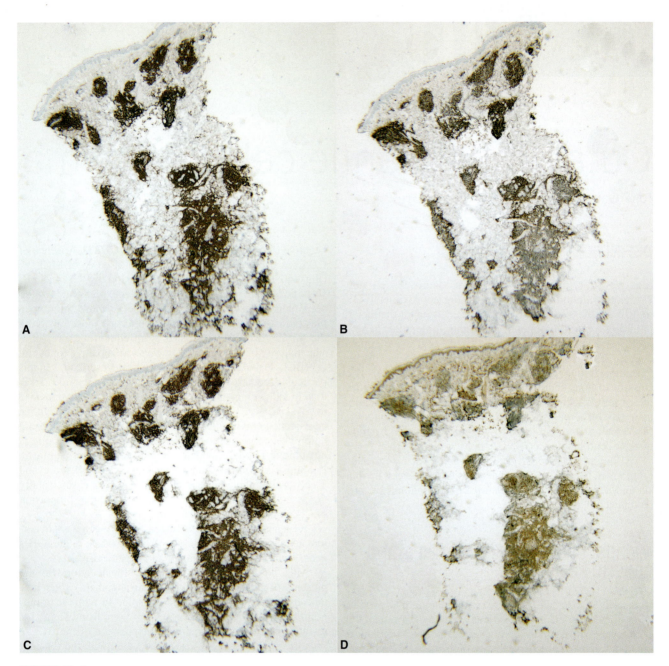

FIGURE 40-1. Cutaneous MCL—immunohistochemistry. The infiltrate is positive for CD20 **(A)**, CD5 **(C)**, and cyclin D1 **(D)**. CD3 **(B)** is expressed by reactive bystander T cells.

setting of systemic disease with less than 100 cases that have been previously described in the literature. It is said that cutaneous dissemination can be present in up to 17% of patients with stage IV disease.[31] Primary cutaneous involvement by MCL has been the subject of isolated case reports.[1,31-37] A primary cutaneous lymphoma, according to the WHO–EORTC definition,[38,39] is one that presents in the skin with no evidence of extracutaneous disease at the time of presentation. A total of five cases of primary cutaneous MCL are described, and of those, three were classified as blastoid variants, one of the reported more aggressive forms of the disease. None of these cases developed systemic involvement after more than 20 months of clinical follow-up. Motegi et al[40] reviewed the documented cases of cutaneous involvement by MCL. Of the 17 cases described, 14 patients exhibited skin lesions at the time of the initial diagnosis. The most common skin locations included the trunk (most common site), followed by the face, arms, thighs, legs, and scalp. The lesions were frequently described as nodular, but other cutaneous presentations included macular, maculopapular, tumoral, plaques, and subcutaneous nodules (Fig. 40-3A–C).[40] We have also found similar locations being most common in the extremities and the face (data not published) where most of the cases presented as nodules or tumors. In addition to the neoplastic dissemination to the skin, occasional paraneoplastic syndromes with cutaneous manifestations have been associated to MCL. Crops of pruritic papules throughout the body have been described in this setting. The biopsies of these lesions show a mixed inflammatory infiltrate with foci of folliculitis and the presence of eosinophils.[41-43]

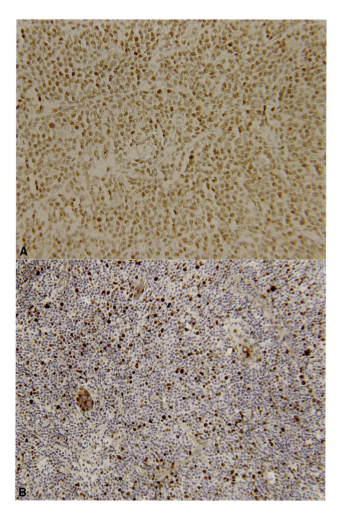

FIGURE 40-2. Cutaneous MCL—immunohistochemistry. A. Strong nuclear positivity for Cyclin D1 is appreciated in the neoplastic cells. **B.** The Ki67 is relatively low (<30%) in this classic variant of MCL with cutaneous dissemination.

HISTOPATHOLOGIC CHANGES

In all the cases of cutaneous involvement by MCL, the lymphoid infiltrate is typically centered in the dermis with sparing of the epidermis, and a grenz zone between the dermal infiltrate and the epidermis. In addition, a perivascular and periadnexal distribution is present (Fig. 40-4). A nodular or nodular and diffuse character is the predominant pattern seen. In the classic histologic variant, a population of small to medium-sized lymphocytes with irregular nuclear borders, coarse chromatin, and inconspicuous nucleoli is present. Mitotic figures can be present but are sparse. Nearly half of cases show pleomorphic morphology. Cases diagnosed as such have a variable-sized population of lymphocytes, but with a predominantly medium-to-large cell population. The abnormal cells also have irregular nuclear borders, with vesicular nuclei and prominent nucleoli. Mitotic figures are abundant. Some cases have a blastoid morphology. Blastoid MCL is characterized by small to medium-sized cells with finely dispersed chromatin and variable prominent nucleoli. Mitotic figures are also frequent[44] (Fig. 40-5).

A previous study by Sen et al. reported that the blastoid morphology was overrepresented[26] among cases of cutaneous MCL (Fig. 40-6). It has been described that cases of blastoid MCL show expression of cutaneous lymphocyte-associated antigen (CLA), a cell-surface glycoprotein that binds to E-selectin on endothelial cells and mediates lymphocyte entry into the dermis[45] and is expressed normally by a subset of circulating memory T cells, normal T cells in inflammatory skin disorders, and most cutaneous T-cell lymphomas.[46] However, subsequent studies failed to reveal expression of CLA in cutaneous MCL. The blastoid variant and TP53 alterations in MCL are associated with higher proliferation rates and worse overall survival of the disease.[47] In a study of 59 patients with MCL, the median survival was 50 months for patients with conventional MCL and 18 months for those with blastoid morphology. We have also found (data not published) a higher rate of pleomorphic and classic variants among cutaneous MCL ($n = 7$) and did not see a significant difference in prognosis when comparing with the more conventional variants. A single case with composite features of MCL and anaplastic large T-cell lymphoma has been recently described.[48]

A more recent study by Kim et al[49] evaluated the clinical and pathologic features of 37 cases of MCL involving the skin. The authors found that most patients have multiple skin nodules clinically (81%) and that skin disease preceded the diagnosis of systemic MCL in one-third of cases. Seventy-three percent of cases have pleomorphic blastoid variants. EZH2 overexpression occurred more frequently in cases with higher Ki67 proliferation index (which corresponded to those blastoid or pleomorphic variants).

DIFFERENTIAL DIAGNOSIS

The differential diagnosis of MCL in the skin includes other cutaneous B-cell lymphoid proliferations such as reactive lymphoid hyperplasias, primary cutaneous B-cell lymphomas, and other systemic B-cell lymphomas/leukemias with secondary skin dissemination. The reactive lymphoid proliferations of B cells typically have a more superficial dermal distribution (top heavy), are not associated with aberrant antigenic expression, and do not show the presence of clonal B-cell proliferations. In contrast, B-cell lymphomas show a more prominent infiltrate in the mid to deeper portions of the dermis (bottom heavy). Cutaneous lymphoid hyperplasia (CLH) in this form may be idiopathic or may arise in response to a wide variety of foreign antigens, including arthropod bites, stings and infestations, tattoos, vaccinations, trauma, injection of foreign substances, pierced ear jewelry, and drugs. Some cases of CLH might be attributed to the infection by *Borrelia burgdorferi*, particularly within endemic regions. Nonetheless, most cases of CLH are idiopathic in nature.

A recent study of MCL[50] expanded an old observation[51] and identified an unusual series of cases, mimicking extranodal marginal zone lymphomas. According to these authors, "EMCL" (extranodal mantle cell lymphomas) may be a subset with preferential involvement of Waldeyer ring and gastrointestinal tract, mimicking the clinicopathologic features of EMZL. These cases share the morphologic and phenotypic features of the nodal form of MCL and the indolent course of the indolent variant of MCL.[50,51] No such cases are

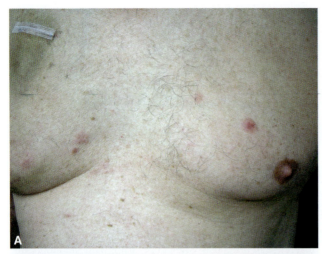
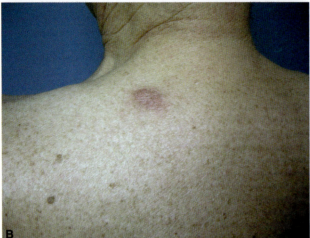
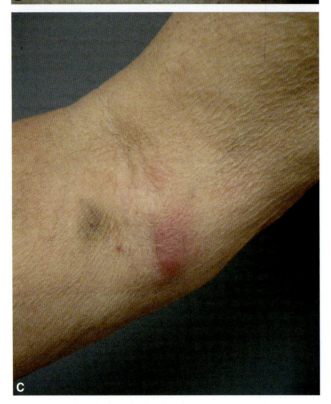

FIGURE 40-3. Cutaneous MCL—clinical features. A–C. Cutaneous nodules are present in the chest, back, and arms. Lesions are invariably multiple and have an erythematous surface.

reported in the skin, but confusion with cutaneous MZL is of importance.

Cutaneous marginal zone lymphoma (see Chapter 37) is a relatively indolent B-cell lymphoproliferative disorder of monotonous population of monocytoid B cells, or B cells with a plasmacytoid differentiation. In some cases, the plasma cell differentiation can be so extreme that cases can be confused with plasma cell neoplasms involving the skin. Primary cutaneous follicle center lymphoma usually has at least some areas with a nodular/follicular growth pattern, in addition to having a germinal center phenotype (CD10 and/or BCL-6 expression). In contrast, MCL does not have a germinal center profile (with the exception of cases with partial BCL-6 expression) and is CD5- and CCND1-positive. Cutaneous diffuse large B-cell lymphoma (DLBCL), leg type, or secondarily disseminated large B-cell lymphomas can create diagnostic problems with the pleomorphic variants of MCL. It is important to highlight that the expression of CD5 can be seen in up to 10% to 15% of cases of DLBCL.[52] CD5 coexpression can also be seen in intravascular B-cell lymphomas, which frequently are associated with cutaneous dissemination. However, intravascular lymphomas have a very peculiar intravascular compartmentalization, a phenomenon not seen in MCL. In addition, rare cases of DLBCL can be associated with cyclin D1 expression.[53] In this respect, none of those cases show the *CCND1* rearrangement seen in MCL, a feature that helps to distinguish between them. Some novel provisional categories of lymphomas report double-hit cytogenetic aberrations with *CCND1* and *MYC* rearrangements. Few of these cases show aberrant coexpression of BCL-6 and CD10 in addition to CCND1. These rare cases are typically leukemic at presentation with an average survival of only 8 months. None of these systemic disorders have been documented so far in cutaneous sites. The blastoid variant of MCL can also be confused with B-lymphoblastic leukemia/lymphoma, although the cutaneous dissemination of this immature B-cell process is very uncommon and shows a phenotype with expression of immature markers CD34 and/or TdT, none of which should be seen in MCL. Cutaneous involvement by chronic lymphocytic leukemia/small lymphocytic lymphoma is common in the setting of more advanced disease. In addition, CLL/SLL also has CD5 coexpression. However, CLL/SLL is typically CD23 positive and FMC7 negative and lacks CyclinD1 expression.[54]

PROGNOSIS AND TREATMENT

The prognosis of MCL is the poorest among patients with B-cell lymphoma, but some subgroups of patients can survive for years with little or no treatment (eg, indolent leukemia).

The mean survival time as measured from the time of the diagnosis to death or last clinical follow-up is 63.5 months (range, 26-182 months). The mean time to recurrence as measured from the diagnosis to first clinical recurrence is 43.6 months (range, 11-132 months). The mean time of the diagnosis to the diagnosis of cutaneous involvement by MCL is 34.83 months (range, 1-132 months). The skin is the most common first site of recurrence of the disease in the majority of patients. All patients are typically treated with systemic chemotherapy (typically R-CHOP (rituximab, cyclophosphamide, doxorubicin hydrochloride (hydroxydaunorubicin), vincristine sulfate (Oncovin), and prednisone) regimens). Some cases have shown clinical responses to radiotherapy and the novel tyrosine-kinase inhibitor ibrutinib[55] and lenalidomide.[56]

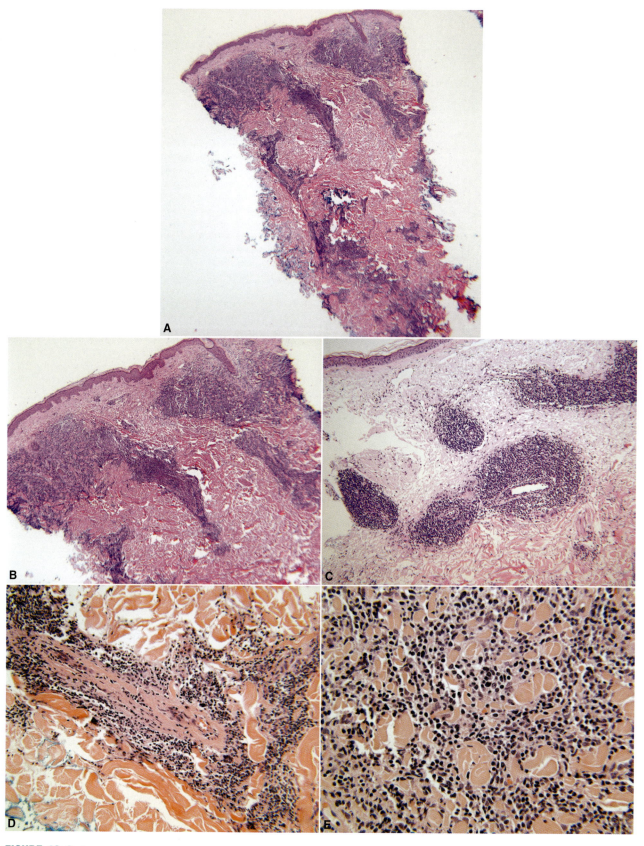

FIGURE 40-4. Cutaneous MCL—histologic features. A and **B** (40× and 100×) show a nodular, superficial and deep, perivascular infiltrate that spares the epidermis. **C** (200×) shows a prominent perivascular character of the infiltrate. **D** and **E** (400×) show periadnexal extension and interstitial infiltration of the malignant cells dissecting through the collagen fibers. The atypical lymphoid cells are predominantly small to medium in size and show features of the classic variant of MCL.

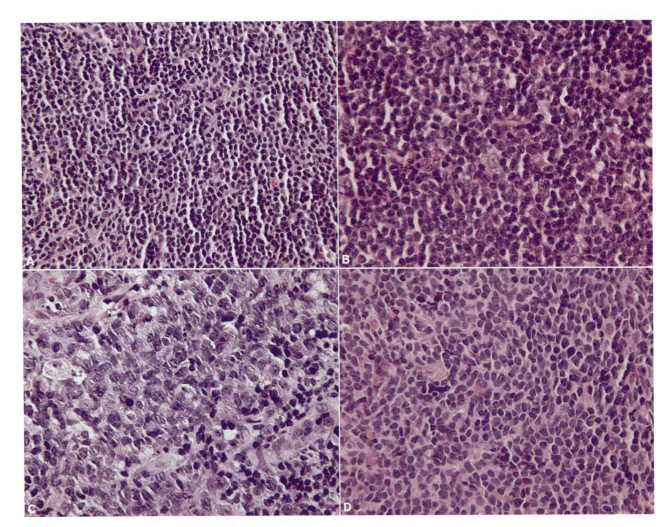

FIGURE 40-5. Cutaneous MCL—histologic variants. A. Classic variant, composed of intermediate-sized cells with irregular nuclear borders and admixed histiocytes. **B** and **C.** Pleomorphic variants. In these, cells are typically larger and show higher number of mitotic figures and nuclear pleomorphism. **D.** Blastoid variant. In this form, the cells are typically small or intermediate in size and have fine and "blastic" chromatin with nucleoli. The cells resemble lymphoblastic processes.

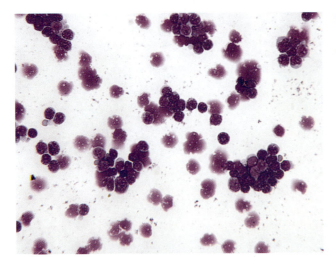

FIGURE 40-6. Cutaneous MCL, blastoid variant—touch imprint. The cytologic smear shows intermediate-sized cells with irregular nuclear borders and fine chromatin.

CAPSULE SUMMARY

- MCL is a B-cell NHL that comprises approximately 3% to 10% of the systemic B-cell NHL. It has a distinctive cytogenetic translocation with the presence of the t(11;14)(q13;q32) rearrangement, which juxtaposes the *CCND1* gene on chromosome 11 with the immunoglobulin heavy chain gene (*IGH*) on chromosome 14, resulting in the characteristic overexpression of Cyclin D1.
- Cutaneous involvement by MCL typically occurs in the setting of systemic disease with only 18 cases that have been previously described in the literature, and in ~17% of cases with stage IV disease.
- In all the cases of cutaneous involvement by MCL, the lymphoid infiltrate is typically centered in the dermis with sparing of the epidermis, and a grenz zone between the dermal infiltrate and the epidermis.
- The tissue immunophenotype of MCL includes the expression of CyclinD1, CD5, and FMC7 with absence of CD23. In CCND1-negative cases, SOX11 is a useful marker to help in the diagnosis of the disease being positive in 93% to 95% of cases.

References

1. Estrozi B, Sanches JA Jr, Varela PC, et al. Primary cutaneous blastoid mantle cell lymphoma-case report. *Am J Dermatopathol*. 2009;31(4):398-400.
2. A clinical evaluation of the international lymphoma study group classification of non-Hodgkin's lymphoma. The non-Hodgkin's lymphoma classification project. *Blood*. 1997;89:3909-3918.
3. Swerdlow SH, Campo E, Harris NL, et al. *WHO Classification of Tumours of the Hematopoietic and Lymphoid Tissues*. International Agency for Research on Cancer; 2017:285-290.
4. Swerdlow SH, Williams ME. From centrocytic to mantle cell lymphoma: a clinicopathologic and molecular review of 3 decades. *Hum Pathol*. 2002;33(1):7-20.
5. Ghielmini M, Zucca E. How I treat mantle cell lymphoma. *Blood*. 2009;114(8):1469-1476.
6. Gerard-Marchant R. Current nosologic concepts in malignant non-Hodgkin lymphomas. *Anna Anat Pathol*. 1974;19(2):149-162.
7. Fernandez V, Salamero O, Espinet B, et al. Genomic and gene expression profiling defines indolent forms of mantle cell lymphoma. *Cancer Res*. 2010;70(4):1408-1418.
8. Croci GA, Hoster E, BeàS, et al. Reproducibility of histologic prognostic parameters for mantle cell lymphoma: cytology, Ki67, p53 and SOX11. *Virchows Arch*. 2020;477(2):259-267. doi:10.1007/s00428-020-02750-7
9. Argatoff LH, Connors JM, Klasa RJ, Horsman DE, Gascoyne RD. Mantle cell lymphoma: A clinicopathologic study of 80 cases. *Blood*. 1997;89(6):2067-2078.
10. Ribera-Cortada I, Martinez D, Amador V, et al. Plasma cell and terminal B-cell differentiation in mantle cell lymphoma mainly occur in the SOX11-negative subtype. *Mod Pathol*. 2015;28(11):1435-1447. doi:10.1038/modpathol.2015.99
11. Liu Z, Dong HY, Gorczyca W, et al. CD5− mantle cell lymphoma. *Am J Clin Pathol*. 2002;118(2):216-224.
12. Gao J, Peterson L, Nelson B, et al. Immunophenotypic variations in mantle cell lymphoma. *Am J Clin Pathol*. 2009;132(5):699-706.
13. Phelps A, Gorgan M, Elaba Z, et al. CD10-positive blastoid mantle cell lymphoma with secondary cutaneous involvement. *J Cutan Pathol*. 2013;40(8):765-767.
14. Phelps A, Elaba Z, Murphy MJ. Blastoid mantle cell lymphoma with cutaneous involvement and aberrant immunophenotype. *Am J Dermatopathol*. 2014;36(6):526-527.
15. Gualco G, Weiss LM, Harrington WJ, Bacchi CE. BCL6, MUM1, and CD10 expression in mantle cell lymphoma. *Appl Immunohistochem Mol Morphol*. 2010;18(2):103-108. doi:10.1097/PAI.0b013e3181bb9edf
16. Fu K, Weisenburger DD, Greiner TC, et al. Cyclin D1-negative mantle cell lymphoma: a clinicopathologic study based on gene expression profiling. *Blood*. 2005;106(13):4315-4321.
17. Gru AA, Hurley MY, Salavaggione AL, et al. Cutaneous mantle cell lymphoma: a clinicopathologic review of 10 cases. *J Cutan Pathol*. 2016;43(12):1112-1120. doi:10.1111/cup.12802
18. Hsi AC, Hurley MY, Lee SJ, et al. Diagnostic utility of SOX11 immunohistochemistry in differentiating cutaneous spread of mantle cell lymphoma from primary cutaneous B-cell lymphomas. *J Cutan Pathol*. 2016;43(4):354-361.
19. Zeng W, Fu K, Quintanilla-Fend L, et al. Cyclin D1-negative blastoid mantle cell lymphoma identified by SOX11 expression. *Am J Surg Pathol*. 2012;36(2):214-219.
20. Mozos A, Royo C, Hartmann E, et al. SOX11 expression is highly specific for mantle cell lymphoma and identifies the cyclin D1-negative subtype. *Haematologica*. 2009;94(11):1555-1562.
21. Xu J, Wang L, Li J, et al. SOX11-negative mantle cell lymphoma: clinicopathologic and prognostic features of 75 patients. *Am J Surg Pathol*. 2019;43(5):710-716. doi:10.1097/PAS.0000000000001233
22. de Boer CJ, Schuuring E, Dreef E, et al. Cyclin D1 protein analysis in the diagnosis of mantle cell lymphoma. *Blood*. 1995;86(7):2715-2723.
23. Thorsélius M, Walsh S, Eriksson I, et al. Somatic hypermutation and Vh gene usage in mantle cell lymphoma. *Eur J Haematol*. 2002;68(4):217-224.
24. Orchard J, Garand R, Davis Z, et al. A subset of t(11;14) lymphoma with mantle cell features displays mutated IgVH genes and includes patients with good prognosis, nonnodal disease. *Blood*. 2003;101(12):4975-4981.
25. Thelander EF, Rosenquist R. Molecular genetic characterization reveals new subsets of mantle cell lymphoma. *Leuk Lymphoma*. 2008;49(6):1042-1049.
26. Sen F, Medeiros LJ, Lu D, et al. Mantle cell lymphoma involving skin: cutaneous lesions may be the first manifestation of disease and tumors often have blastoid cytologic features. *Am J Surg Pathol*. 2002;26(10):1312-1318.
27. Martín-Garcia D, Navarro A, Valdés-Mas R, et al. CCND2 and CCND3 hijack immunoglobulin light-chain enhancers in cyclin D1− mantle cell lymphoma. *Blood*. 2019;133(9):940-951. doi:10.1182/blood-2018-07-862151
28. Salaverria I, Royo C, Carvajal-Cuenca A, et al. CCND2 rearrangements are the most frequent genetic events in cyclin D1 - mantle cell lymphoma. *Blood*. 2013;121(8):1394-1402.
29. Navarro A, Beà S, Jares P, Campo E. Molecular pathogenesis of mantle cell lymphoma. *Hematol Oncol Clin N Am*. 2020;34(5):795-807. doi:10.1016/j.hoc.2020.05.002
30. Lynch DW, Verma R, Larson E, et al. Primary cutaneous mantle cell lymphoma with blastic features: report of a rare case with special reference to staging and effectiveness of chemotherapy. *J Cutan Pathol*. 2012;39(4):449-453.
31. Zattra E, Zambello R, Marino F, et al. Primary cutaneous mantle cell lymphoma. *Acta Derm Venereol*. 2011;91(4):474-475.
32. Mazzuoccolo LD, Castro Perez GA, Sorin I, et al. Primary cutaneous mantle cell lymphoma: a case report. *Case Rep Dermatol Med*. 2013;2013:394596.
33. Hoster E, Rosenwald A, Berger F, et al. Prognostic value of Ki-67 index, cytology, and growth pattern in mantle-cell lymphoma: Results from randomized trials of the european mantle cell lymphoma network. *J Clin Oncol*. 2016;34(12):1386-1394.
34. Cesinaro AM, Bettelli S, Maccio L, et al. Primary cutaneous mantle cell lymphoma of the leg with blastoid morphology and aberrant immunophenotype: a diagnostic challenge. *Am J Dermatopathol*. 2014;36(2):e16-e18.
35. Canpolat F, Tas E, Albayrak Sonmez A, et al. Cutaneous presentation of mantle cell lymphoma. *Acta Derm Venereol*. 2010;90(5):548-550.
36. Bertero M, Novelli M, Fierro MT, et al. Mantle zone lymphoma: an immunohistologic study of skin lesions. *J Am Acad Dermatol*. 1994;30(1):23-30.
37. Hamad N, Armytage T, McIlroy K, et al. Primary cutaneous mantle-cell lymphoma: a case report and literature review. *J Clin Oncol*. Published online April 14, 2014. doi:10.1200/JCO.2012.47.2829

38. Willemze R, Jaffe ES, Burg G, et al. WHO-EORTC classification for cutaneous lymphomas. *Blood*. 2005;105(10):3768-3785.
39. Burg G, Kempf W, Cozzio A, et al. WHO/EORTC classification of cutaneous lymphomas 2005: histological and molecular aspects. *J Cutan Pathol*. 2005;32(10):647-674.
40. Motegi S, Okada E, Nagai Y, et al. Skin manifestation of mantle cell lymphoma. *Eur J Dermatol*. 2006;16(4):435-438.
41. Murphy PT, Gilmore R, Mitra S. Another case of paraneoplastic cutaneous syndrome preceding indolent mantle cell lymphoma. *Acta Haematol*. 2006;116(3):228.
42. Nemets A, Ronen M, Lugassy G. Chronic paraneoplastic cutaneous syndrome preceding an indolent variant of mantle cell lymphoma: favorable response to rituximab. *Acta Haematol*. 2006;115(1-2):113-116.
43. Farber MJ, La Forgia S, Sahu J, et al. Eosinophilic dermatosis of hematologic malignancy. *J Cutan Pathol*. 2012;39(7):690-695.
44. Wehkamp U, Pott C, Unterhalt M, et al. Skin involvement of mantle cell lymphoma may mimic primary cutaneous diffuse large B-cell lymphoma, leg type. *Am J Surg Pathol*. 2015;39(8):1093-1101. doi:10.1097/PAS.0000000000000445
45. Marti RM, Campo E, Bosch F, et al. Cutaneous lymphocyte-associated antigen (CLA) expression in a lymphoblastoid mantle cell lymphoma presenting with skin lesions. Comparison with other clinicopathologic presentations of mantle cell lymphoma. *J Cutan Pathol*. 2001;28(5):256-264.
46. Lu D, Duvic M, Medeiros LJ, et al. The T-cell chemokine receptor CXCR3 is expressed highly in low-grade mycosis fungoides. *Am J Clin Pathol*. 2001;115(3):413-421.
47. Slotta-Huspenina J, Koch I, de Leval L, et al. The impact of cyclin D1 mRNA isoforms, morphology and p53 in mantle cell lymphoma: p53 alterations and blastoid morphology are strong predictors of a high proliferation index. *Haematologica*. 2012;97(9):1422-1430.
48. Leduc CP, Blandino II, Alhejaily A, et al. Composite mantle cell and primary cutaneous anaplastic large cell lymphoma: case report and review of the literature. *Am J Dermatopathol*. 2015;37(3):232-236.
49. Kim DH, Medeiros LJ, Aung PP, Young KH, Miranda RN, Ok CY. Mantle cell lymphoma involving skin: a clinicopathologic study of 37 cases. *Am J Surg Pathol*. 2019;43(10):1421-1428. doi:10.1097/PAS.0000000000001312
50. Rattotti S, Croci G, Ferretti VV, et al. Mantle cell lymphoma mimicking mucosa-associated lymphoid tissue (MALT) lymphomas: a pathological characterization (on behalf of the Fondazione Italiana Linfomi (FIL)—postgraduate Master course). *Blood*. 2017;130(suppl 1):4049.
51. Shibata K, Shimamoto Y, Nakano S, Miyahara M, Nakano H, Yamaguchi M. Mantle cell lymphoma with the features of mucosa-associated lymphoid tissue (MALT) lymphoma in an HTLV-I-seropositive patient. *Ann Hematol*. 1995;70(1):47-51. doi:10.1007/BF01715382
52. Jain P, Fayad LE, Rosenwald A, et al. Recent advances in de novo CD5+ diffuse large B cell lymphoma. *Am J Hematol*. 2013;88(9):798-802.
53. Vela-Chavez T, Adam P, Kremer M, et al. Cyclin D1 positive diffuse large B-cell lymphoma is a post-germinal center-type lymphoma without alterations in the CCND1 gene locus. *Leuk Lymphoma*. 2011;52(3):458-466.
54. Yoshino T, Tanaka T, Sato Y. Differential diagnosis of chronic lymphocytic leukemia/small lymphocytic lymphoma and other indolent lymphomas, including mantle cell lymphoma. *J Clin Exp Hematop*. 2020;60(4):124-129.
55. Mancebo SE, Smith JR, Intlekofer AM, et al. Treatment response of cutaneous mantle cell lymphoma to brutinib and radiotherapy. *Clin Lymphoma Myeloma Leuk*. 2015;15(6):e113-e115.
56. Mishchenko E, Attias D, Tadmor T. Response of cutaneous lesion of mantle cell lymphoma to lenalidomide. *Int J Hematol*. 2014;100(1):1-2.

CHAPTER 41

Cutaneous manifestations of chronic lymphocytic leukemia/small lymphocytic lymphoma

Alejandro A. Gru and Maxime Battistella

DEFINITION

Chronic lymphocytic leukemia/small lymphocytic lymphoma (CLL/SLL) is the most common adult leukemia in Europe and North America, with a reported incidence of 3 to 5 cases per 100,000[1,2] and is more commonly seen in elderly individuals. Most patients are asymptomatic, while others can present with fatigue, fever, easy bruising, and generalized lymphadenopathy. The incidence of CLL has increased during the past decade.[3] Patients with CLL are at increased risk of other malignancies, including squamous cell carcinoma, basal cell carcinoma, malignant melanoma, and Merkel cell carcinoma. They are also prone to cutaneous infections, especially viral infections, and have exaggerated reactions to insect bites.[4]

CUTANEOUS MANIFESTATIONS

Cutaneous lesions in patients with CLL are less common in comparison with T-cell leukemias or lymphomas. However, skin manifestations can occur in up to 25% of patients with CLL.[2] The cutaneous manifestations of the disease can be secondary to seeding by leukemic cells (leukemia/lymphoma cutis, LC) and other malignant diseases or nonmalignant disorders. Leukemia cutis generally arises months after the onset of leukemia. However, it may occasionally precede the hematologic manifestations by several months. In a study by Cerroni et al,[5] describing 42 CLL patients, the mean duration of CLL before skin manifestation was 39 months. A more recent study from different French centers reported a lapse of 5.4 years before the development of skin lesions.[6] However, 16.7% of the patients developed skin lesions as the first sign of disease. When skin involvement does occur, it is most commonly found on the face (Fig. 41-1).[1,5,7,8] Earlobe lesions are present in 26% of cases. LC usually manifests as a solitary grouped or generalized papules, plaques, nodules, or large tumors. Some cases can also present as a papulovesicular (Fig. 41-2A,B) or granuloma annulare–like eruptions.[9,10]

The lesions can arise at sites of scars from herpes zoster or herpes simplex virus (HSV) eruptions.[11] Rare cases have occurred in association with granuloma annulare,[12] actinic granulomas,[13] or dermatofibromas.[14] The skin lesions occur in patients before starting systemic therapy in 2/3 of cases and present after treatment in 1/3. Systemic therapy usually led to resolution of the skin lesions in most cases. It is not uncommon to see leukemic infiltrates of CLL/SLL on excisional specimens performed for biopsy-proven carcinomas (Fig. 41-3),[15,16] melanoma,[17] and Merkel cell carcinomas.[18-20] It is also relatively common to see the coexistence of CLL/SLL in association with metastasis on sentinel or excisional biopsies of patients with melanoma (Fig. 41-4).[17] Patients with coexistent CLL and Merkel cell carcinoma or melanoma have a worse prognosis, when compared to patients without CLL.[21] Such association has not been reported in cases associated with cutaneous squamous cell carcinoma.[22,23] On rare occasions, the coexistence of a nonmelanoma skin cancer and a diagnosis of CLL can lead to the diagnosis of the disease by the first time.[24] An association between Merkel cell polyomavirus infection in T-cells of CLL has also been detected.[25,26] The prognosis of LC in the course of CLL is controversial. Isolated case reports showing the coexistence of CLL and Sézary syndrome are available.[27] While most authors agree that LC is associated with a worse prognosis,[28,29] others have claimed the opposite.[5]

HISTOPATHOLOGY AND IMMUNOPHENOTYPE

Histologically, LC presents as a patchy perivascular and periadnexal, nodular and diffuse, and band-like types of infiltration in the skin (Figs. 41-5 and 41-6). Overlap of these histologic patterns can be seen. Cytologically, the leukemic cells are typically small, uniform lymphocytes, with scant cytoplasm and coarsely clumped chromatin. Prolymphocytes, cells with finely dispersed chromatin, more abundant cytoplasm, and distinctive nucleoli can also be present. Additional inflammatory

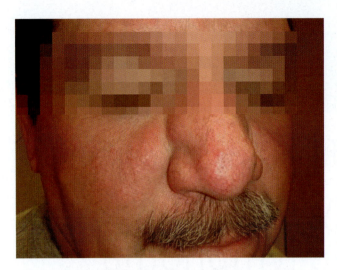

FIGURE 41-1. Nodules and plaques on the forehead (so-called facies leontina). (Courtesy of Ellen Kim, MD, University of Pennsylvania.)

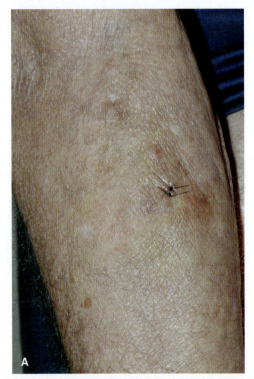

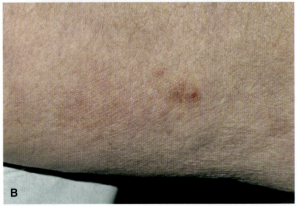

FIGURE 41-2. A and **B.** Small papules in the arms and thigh of a patient with cutaneous involvement by CLL.

cells such as eosinophils, plasma cells, and histiocytes can also be seen.[2,5,30] Walther et al[15] have also shown the peculiar association of CLL in the skin in association with scars. On some occasions, scattered atrophic germinal centers can be seen, and such pattern can mimic primary cutaneous marginal zone lymphoma[31] (Figs. 41-7 and 41-8).

Neoplastic B-cells are CD20+, CD19+, PAX-5+, LEF-1+, and CD200+ and show aberrant coexpression of CD5, CD43, and CD23. CLL cells lack CD79b, CD10, BCL-6, BCL-1 (cyclin D1), and FMC7 expression (Figs. 41-6 and 41-8). A word of caution should be used with PAX5, as Merkel cell carcinoma and other neuroendocrine carcinomas can also express this marker. This is particularly important when PAX5 is the sole B-cell lineage specific marker such as in patients treated with rituximab (anti-CD20 mAb) whose leukemic cells lack CD20 expression.[32] Flow cytometry shows dim surface light chains expression and dim-to-moderate expression of CD20. Cutaneous involvement by CLL can rarely show biclonality.[33] *IGHV* mutations are seen in a large proportion of cases (57%). A very interesting finding reported from a French study is the presence of a t(14;18) translocation in 18.5% of cases.[6] Other molecular alterations identified in CLL cases with skin involvement include trisomy 12(31%), 13q deletion (30%), 11q deletion (13%), and 17p deletions (9%). The most frequently mutated genes include *NOTCH1* (22.5%), *TP53* (20%), *SF3B1* (12.5%), and *BIRC3* (12.5%). Mutations in the NOTCH pathway occurred in 33% of cases. Rare cases (1%-3%) of CLL can have *BRAF V600E* mutations.[34]

DIFFERENTIAL DIAGNOSIS

The differential diagnosis includes *primary cutaneous B-cell lymphomas*, such as primary cutaneous follicle center lymphoma (PCFCL), and marginal zone B-cell lymphoma (PCMZL) and other systemic lymphomas with secondary cutaneous manifestations (follicular and mantle cell lymphoma [MCL] among others). PCFCL has a germinal center phenotype with BCL-6 and/or CD10 expression, markers not typically seen in CLL. A rare case of PCFCL has been reported in a patient with preexistent history of CLL.[35] PCMZL can show substantial overlap with CLL; however, PCMZL is typically negative for CD5 and CD23. In addition, PCMZL often shows cytoplasmic light chains restriction within the plasma cell population, a feature that can be analyzed with the use of in situ hybridization studies.[1] Among the systemic lymphomas, MCLs are also CD5+. However, as opposed to CLL, they are typically cyclin D1 (BCL-1) and SOX-11 positive and carry the t(11;14) translocation.[36-40] They are also LEF-1 and CD200-. It is also important to highlight that second skin lymphomas in patients with CLL can also occur. A recent series of 12 cases of patients with CLL showed the secondary occurrence of mycosis fungoides/Sézary syndrome and cutaneous marginal zone lymphomas, among the most common subtypes.[41] Composite lymphomas with coexistence of both CLL and primary cutaneous B-cell lymphomas have been reported (eg, PCFCL).[42,43]

Richter Transformation

The presence of large cells in the setting of CLL always brings the diagnostic consideration of Richter (large-cell)

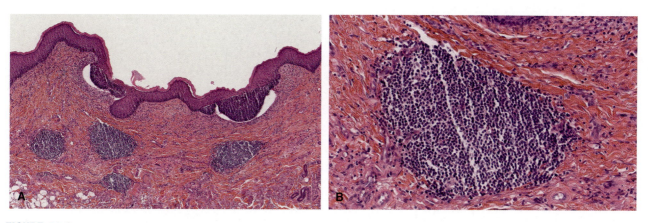

FIGURE 41-3. Coexistence of CLL and BCC. A. This excisional biopsy shows the classic changes of a superficial variant of basal cell carcinoma with an atypical nodular lymphocytic infiltrate (100×). **B.** The infiltrate is composed of a monotonous population of small lymphocytes.

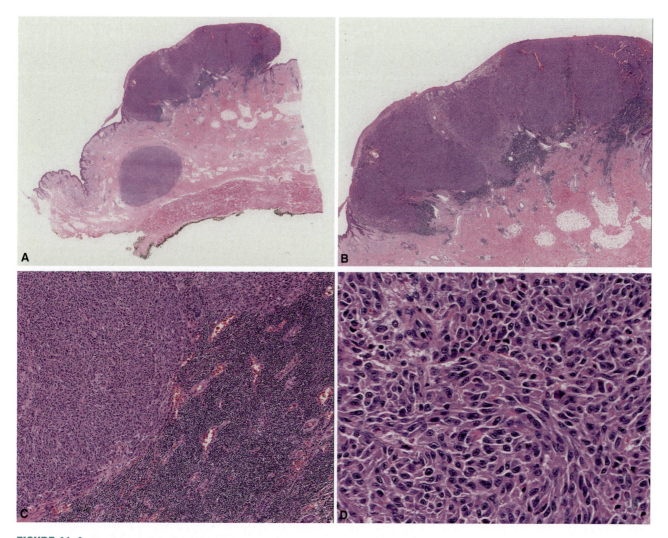

FIGURE 41-4. Coexistence of melanoma and CLL. There is a malignant nodular epithelioid and spindle proliferation with an associated separate satellite nodule from the main mass (**A** and **B**, 20× and 40×). A lymphoid infiltrate in the dermis is composed of monotonous small cells (**C**, 100×). The areas of malignant melanoma show variable degrees of nuclear pleomorphism (**D**, 200×).

transformation (RS), which has unequivocally an ominous prognosis.[2] RS is clinically characterized by an abrupt onset of fever, weight loss, night sweats, progressive lymphadenopathy, and elevated LDH levels. Skin involvement by RS is extraordinarily rare, with only a handful of cases reported.[2,28,29]

Cutaneous RS presents after a mean duration of 37 months in CLL with multiple cutaneous nodules. It may or may not be associated with a peripheral blood lymphocytosis and 75% of cases had a fatal outcome (24-129 months) after the diagnosis.[28] A rare case appears to have been precipitated

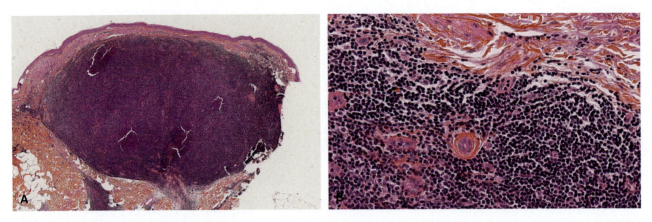

FIGURE 41-5. Cutaneous involvement by CLL. A. Leukemic cells are present as a dense nodular lymphocytic infiltrate sparing the epidermis (40×). **B.** Small, hyperchromatic, monomorphic neoplastic cells are seen with coarsely clumped chromatin (400×).

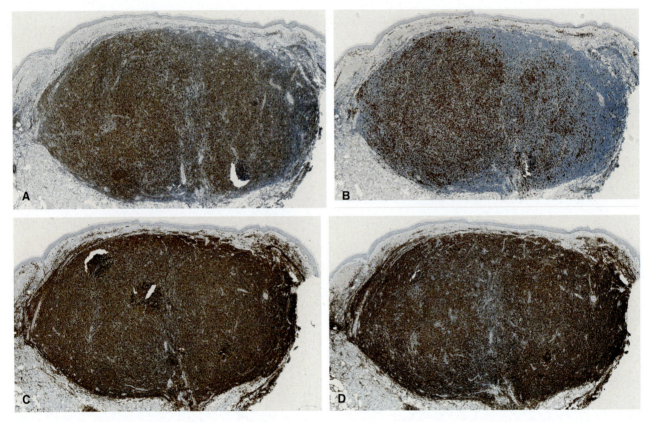

FIGURE 41-6. Cutaneous involvement by CLL—Immunophenotypic findings. The atypical infiltrate is positive for CD20 **(A)**. CD3 is positive in background T-cells **(B)**. The lymphoma cells show coexpression of CD5 **(C)** and CD23 **(D)**.

by the cutaneous infection of HSV.[44] The histologic features consist of a dense dermal infiltrate, with a perivascular and periadnexal distribution, composed predominantly of large cells (Fig. 41-9). Numerous mitoses are typically present in the large-cell infiltrate. The immunophenotype of the large cell is typically CD20, CD79a positive with variable CD30 expression. About 50% of cases can be EBV positive.[28] RS is frequently associated with CD38 expression and IGHV4-39 rearrangements.[45] The most common chromosomal numerical aberrations in RS include trisomy 12 and 11q23 deletions.[28] The response to treatment with CHOP chemotherapy or combination with other regimens is only 40% and the mean survival is 2 to 5 months.[46] However, Yu et al[29] reported a relatively better prognosis when compared to systemic RS, with an average survival of 6.7 years. The differential diagnosis includes other large B-cell lymphomas, but an emphasis should be placed to separate it from diffuse large B-cell lymphoma (DLBCL), leg type and CD5+ DLBCLs.[47] Maeshima et al[48] reported nine cases of secondary CD5+ DLBCL of non-Richter's syndrome, two of which presented in cutaneous sites. Five of these cases gained CD5 during the clinical course of the disease (originally CD5− tumors). We have also previously reported the strange association between CLL and lymphomatoid papulosis and CLL and EDV, a histologic caveat that can potentially lead to a presumptive diagnosis of RS.[49]

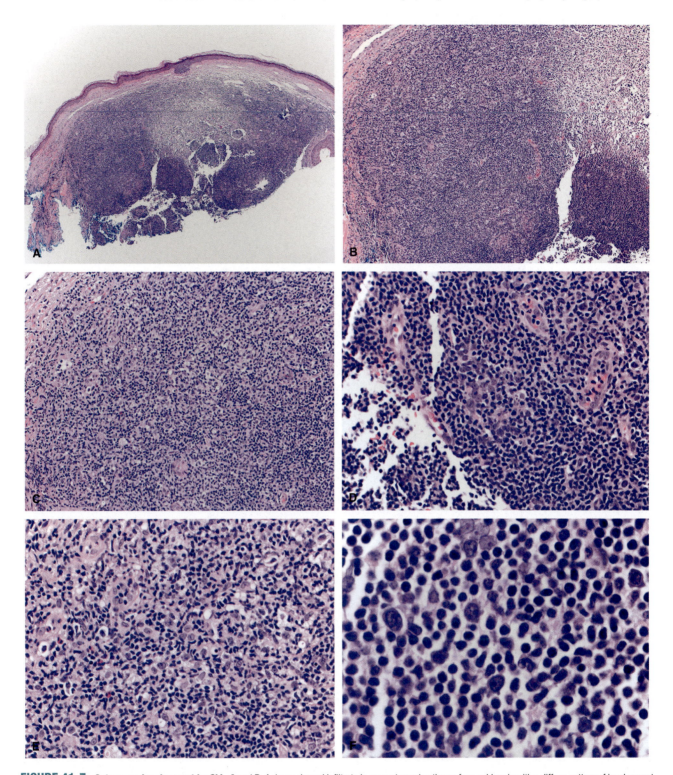

FIGURE 41-7. Cutaneous involvement by CLL. A and **B.** A dense dermal infiltrate is present, sparing the surface epidermis with a diffuse pattern of involvement (40× and 100×). **C.** An increased number of larger cells is also present (200×). **D.** There is an atrophic germinal center (400×). **E.** Closer magnification shows an increased number of paraimmunoblasts (400×). **F.** The conventional cytomorphologic changes of classic CLL cells are seen with lymphocytes with "soccer ball" chromatin of very small size and few larger prolymphocytes (600×).

Another potential diagnostic consideration is cutaneous infiltrates in the setting of acute myeloid or lymphoblastic leukemias. The original large study by Longacre and Smoller[50] showed that nearly 40% to 50% of the cases of leukemia cutis were related to CLL. As opposed to myeloid disorders, CLL is negative for CD34 and other markers of myeloid differentiation, such as lysozyme or myeloperoxidase. As opposed to lymphoblastic infiltrates, CLL is typically negative for TdT and CD34, and the proliferation rate is very low (typically less than 5%), whereas most cases of B- or T-lymphoblastic leukemia have immature markers (CD34, TdT, CD1a) and have a high proliferation index. Rare cases of coexisting myeloid and lymphoid infiltrates of CLL have been described.[51]

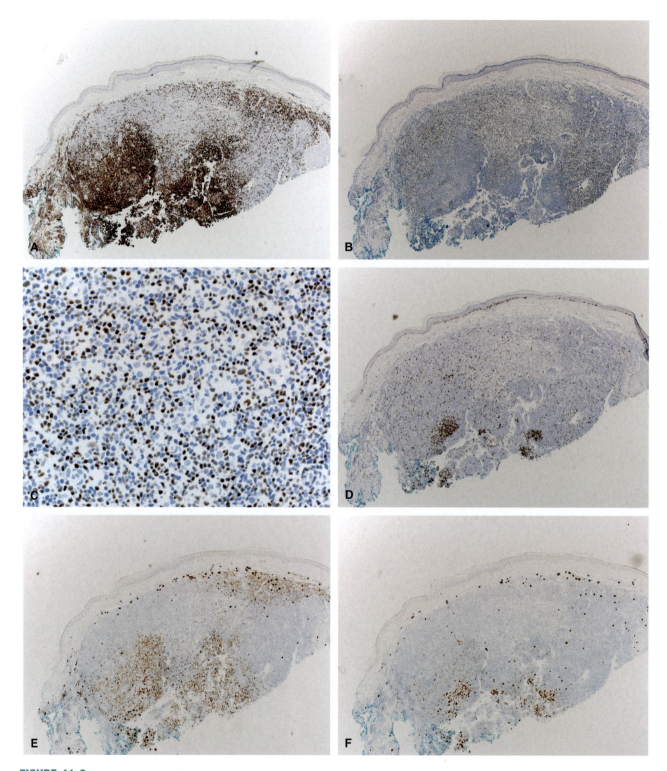

FIGURE 41-8. **Cutaneous involvement by CLL—Immunophenotypic findings.** Some of the atypical cells are positive for CD23 **(A)**. LEF-1 is also positive in the neoplastic infiltrate **(B** and **C)**. Ki67 shows a high proliferative rate in the atrophic germinal centers **(D)**. RNA scope ultrasensitive in situ hybridization for kappa **(E)** and lambda **(F)** shows kappa-restricted B-cells.

CUTANEOUS NONNEOPLASTIC IMMUNE INFILTRATES IN CLL

Immune dysregulation in CLL can be associated with nonleukemic cutaneous manifestations. These include pseudolymphomatous infiltrates that are likely exaggerated immune reaction to insect bites,[4] vasculitis,[50] paraneoplastic pemphigus,[52] exfoliative erythroderma, vesicullobulous eruptions, urticaria, Sweet syndrome, vasculitis, erythema nodosum, bullous pemphigoid, pyoderma gangrenosum, interstitial granulomatous dermatitis, and others.[53] The risk of skin cancers is also markedly increased in patients with CLL/SLL.[2,54] The more recently described eosinophilic

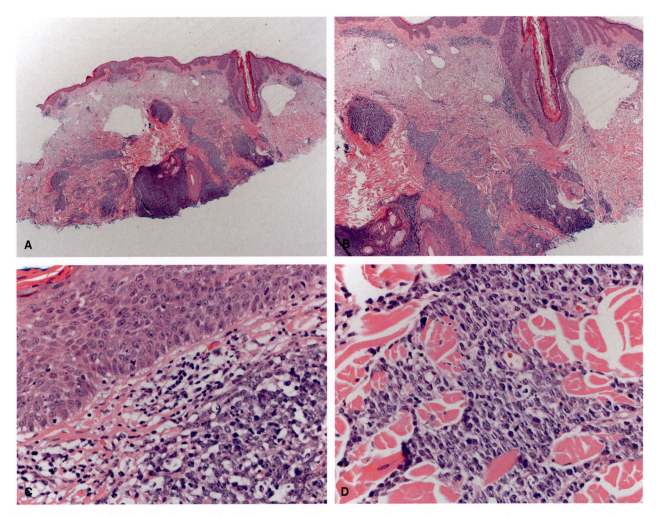

FIGURE 41-9. Richter's transformation of CLL with skin involvement. A. A malignant infiltrate in the dermis is present with a nodular arrangement (40×). **B.** The abnormal nodules extend to the deep reticular dermis (100×). **C.** Closer inspection shows sheets of malignant large lymphoma cells underneath the epidermis with changes of squamous cell carcinoma in situ (400×). **D.** The large lymphoma cells show vesicular nuclei and prominent nucleoli with numerous mitoses and apoptotic cells (400×).

dermatosis of hematologic malignancy has also been seen in CLL/SLL.[55] Patients with CLL/SLL also can present in association with mycosis fungoides–[56-58] Sézary syndrome,[27,57] cutaneous NK-cell lymphoma,[57] and peripheral T-cell lymphoma, NOS.[57] It is believed that nonneoplastic autoimmune disorders, arising in conjunction with CLL, represent a phenomenon of malignant lymphocytic reaction to antigenic stimulation. In some cases, neoplastic B-cells within the skin may not be secondary to proliferation and expansion of the malignant clone but more closely related to cutaneous recruitment of circulating cells in the course of immunologic reactions such as elicited by cutaneous trauma, fungal infection, or drug hypersensitivity.[30] Cutaneous manifestations in association with current biologic therapies for CLL are also relatively common. The most frequent manifestations seen with the use of the BTK inhibitor ibrutinib include bruising, ecchymoses, and petechiae.[59] Nail and hair changes are also common, as skin infections (opportunistic infections including herpes simplex and herpes zoster virus reactivations, and *Staphylococcus aureus* superinfection), folliculitis, and other types of rashes. An unusual subtype of mixed septal and lobular panniculitis, presenting in association with the Bruton tyrosine kinase inhibitor ibrutinib has been reported (Fig. 41-10).[60] Aphthous-like ulcerations with stomatitis, neutrophilic dermatosis, peripheral edema, and skin cracking can also occur. The incidence of those side effects appears to be similar with newer generations of BTK inhibitors like acalabrutinib and zanubrutinib. Some of these cases had the coexistence of leukemic subcutaneous deposits of CLL and the hypersensitivity to the medication.

The mechanisms of cutaneous involvement by CLL are poorly understood. However, leukemic infiltrates in patients with high tumor burden (very marked lymphocytosis in the peripheral blood) could be attracted by the local release of cytokines. This is one of the mechanisms proposed for the localization of those infiltrates in and around scars: epidermal trauma is believed to induce the release of IL-1 from injured keratinocytes, which activates a cytokine cascade that recruits leukocyte chemotactic factors such as IL-3, IL-6, and granulocyte colony-stimulating factor. IL-1 also functions to increase vascular permeability, enabling leukemic cells to involve the dermis.

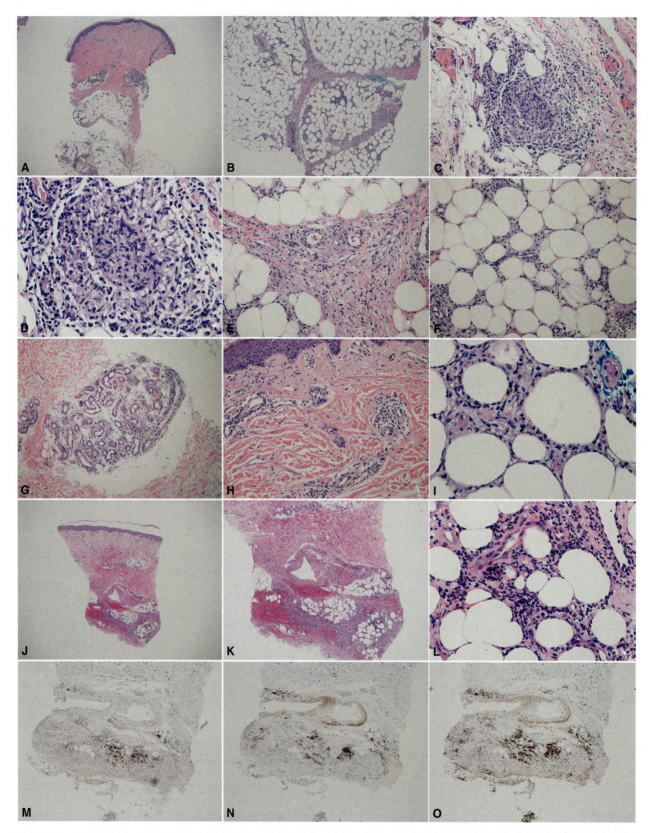

FIGURE 41-10. Cutaneous manifestations of ibrutinib therapy in the setting of CLL. **A** and **B**. Lobular and septal panniculitis (20× and 40×, respectively). **C** and **D**. Loosely formed epithelioid granulomas are seen, which have some resemblance to the Miescher's radial granulomas seen in cases of erythema nodosum (20× and 40×). **E** and **F**. Septal and lobular inflammation containing predominantly lymphocytes along with fewer histiocytes and eosinophils (200×). **G** and **H**. Periadnexal and perivascular infiltrates (100×). **I**. Focal areas with leukocytoclasis (400×). **J** and **K**. Lobular and septal inflammatory infiltrates—(20× and 40×). **L**. The infiltrate involves the subcutaneous lobule and includes neutrophils and numerous lymphocytes (400×). Immunohistochemistry (400×) (40×, each figure) for CD3 **(M)**, PAX5 **(N)**, and CD5 **(O)** reveals that there is low-level involvement by a population of B-cells with coexpression of CD5. This immunophenotype is compatible with CLL/SLL.

CUTANEOUS INFECTIONS IN CLL

Another subtype of complications that can be seen in CLL patients are infections, which represent one of the leading causes of mortality in this patient population.[2] The pathogenesis of infections in CLL is multifactorial and involves disease- and therapy-related factors, such as immunoglobulin deficiency, abnormal T-cell function, and neutropenia. This immune dysregulation can be further compounded by current CLL medications, such as ibrutinib. We have observed (data not published) cases of EBV reactivation in this cohort, with large-cell infiltrates, suspicious for RS. However, contrary to RS, they responded to therapy against the EBV viremia. This brings the important point of performing EBER in situ hybridization studies in all cases of CLL where patients are undergoing treatment with tyrosine kinase inhibitors.

A correlation between very low CD4 counts after therapy with fludarabine (FA) and reactivation of herpes zoster has been observed. Herpetic infections in this cohort are quite severe and occur typically while the patients undergo immunosuppressive therapy.[2] Byrd et al[61,62] performed a prospective study of infections in 21 patients with indolent lymphoid malignancies receiving FA. 12 (57%) of these patients developed herpes infections including herpes zoster in 9 and HSV infection in 3 at a median of 8 months following initiation of FA. Patients undergoing therapy with the anti-CD52 antibody alemtuzumab (Campath) are usually under prophylaxis with antiviral agents.

Other uncommon cutaneous infections that can present in CLL patients include disseminated molluscum contagiosum,[63] bacillary angiomatosis,[64] leishmaniasis, and mycobacterial infections of the MAC (mycobacterium avium complex) group.[65]

PROGNOSIS

The prognosis of LC in the course of CLL is controversial. While most authors agree that LC is associated with a worse prognosis,[28,29] others have claimed the opposite.[5] Cerroni et al[5] found a 66.6% 5-year survival in patients with LC and CLL. They also supported the hypothesis that local antigenic stimulation with recruitment of the leukemic cells to the affected skin areas was probably the cause of the leukemic infiltrate. In counterpart, Su et al[66] found that 12 of their 16 patients died within a mean interval of ~16 months of developing leukemia cutis involving CLL. They concluded that this represents a dissemination of systemic leukemia to the skin and is associated with a very poor prognosis, although the patients with CLL had a longer survival period than those with granulocytic or myeloid leukemias. It is clear, though, that the development of RS[29] is associated with high mortality and poor outcome, regardless of the site where RS presents.

CAPSULE SUMMARY

- CLL/SLL is the most common adult leukemia in Europe and North America, but cutaneous infiltrates are less frequent, when comparing to leukemic deposits of myeloid or T-cell malignancies. However, skin manifestations can occur in up to 25% of patients with CLL.
- 16.7% of the patients developed skin lesions as the first sign of disease. When skin involvement does occur, it is most commonly found on the face. LC usually manifests as a solitary grouped or generalized papules, plaques, nodules, or large tumors.
- Histologically, LC presents as a patchy perivascular and periadnexal, nodular and diffuse, and band-like types of infiltration in the skin. The immunophenotype includes expression of CD20, CD19, CD5, LEF-1+, and CD43, but absence of BCL-1 expression.
- RS is an ominous manifestation of CLL, which can also present in cutaneous sites, and is associated with a very poor outcome.
- Differential diagnosis includes primary and secondary cutaneous B-cell lymphomas and myeloid and lymphoblastic leukemias.
- The prognosis of CLL with LC is controversial, as frequently the infiltrate presents as a "bystander" outflow in the setting of cytokine stimulation and attraction of the leukemic cells to a localized lesion.

References

1. Levin C, Mirzamani N, Zwerner J, et al. A comparative analysis of cutaneous marginal zone lymphoma and cutaneous chronic lymphocytic leukemia. *Am J Dermatopathol*. 2012;34:18-23.
2. Robak E, Robak T. Skin lesions in chronic lymphocytic leukemia. *Leuk Lymphoma*. 2007;48:855-865.
3. Levi F, Randimbison L, Te VC, et al. Non-Hodgkin's lymphomas, chronic lymphocytic leukaemias and skin cancers. *Br J Cancer*. 1996;74:1847-1850.
4. Bairey O, Goldschmidt N, Ruchlemer R, et al. Insect-bite-like reaction in patients with chronic lymphocytic leukemia: a study from the Israeli Chronic Lymphocytic Leukemia Study Group. *Eur J Haematol*. 2012;89:491-496.
5. Cerroni L, Zenahlik P, Hofler G, et al. Specific cutaneous infiltrates of B-cell chronic lymphocytic leukemia: a clinicopathologic and prognostic study of 42 patients. *Am J Surg Pathol*. 1996;20:1000-1010.
6. Lazarian G, Munger M, Quinquenel A, et al. Clinical and biological characteristics of leukemia cutis in chronic lymphocytic leukemia: a study of the French innovative leukemia organization (FILO). *Am J Hematol*. 2021;96(9):E353-E356.
7. Kaddu S, Smolle J, Cerroni L, et al. Prognostic evaluation of specific cutaneous infiltrates in B-chronic lymphocytic leukemia. *J Cutan Pathol*. 1996;23:487-494.
8. Jasim ZF, Cooke N, Somerville JE, et al. Chronic lymphocytic leukaemia skin infiltrates affecting prominent parts of the face and the scalp. *Br J Dermatol*. 2006;154:981-982.
9. Rosman IS, Nunley KS, Lu D. Leukemia cutis in B-cell chronic lymphocytic leukemia presenting as an episodic papulovesicular eruption. *Dermatol Online J*. 2011;17:7.
10. Sokumbi O, Gibson LE, Comfere NI, et al. Granuloma annulare-like eruption associated with B-cell chronic lymphocytic leukemia. *J Cutan Pathol*. 2012;39:996-1003.
11. Hapgood G, Mooney E, Dinh HV, et al. Leukaemia cutis in chronic lymphocytic leukaemia following varicella zoster virus reactivation. *Intern Med J*. 2012;42:1355-1358.
12. Hadian Y, Beroukhim K, Fung MA, Schulman JM. Granuloma annulare-like eruption in chronic lymphocytic leukemia. *Dermatol Online J*. 2020;26(9):13030/qt6cz076w4.

13. Kauffman JA, Ivan D, Cutlan JE, et al. Actinic granuloma occurring in an unusual association with cutaneous B-cell chronic lymphocytic leukemia. *J Cutan Pathol.* 2012;39:294-297.
14. Maughan C, Kolker S, Markus B, et al. Leukemia cutis coexisting with dermatofibroma as the initial presentation of B-cell chronic lymphocytic leukemia/small lymphocytic lymphoma. *Am J Dermatopathol.* 2014;36(1):e14-e15.
15. Walther BS, Gibbons G, Chan EF, et al. Leukemia cutis (involving chronic lymphocytic leukemia) within excisional specimens: a series of 6 cases. *Am J Dermatopathol.* 2009;31:162-165.
16. Catteau X, Dehou MF, Dargent JL, et al. Chronic lymphocytic leukemia mimicking recurrent carcinoma of the breast: case report and review of the literature. *Pathol Res Pract.* 2011;207:514-517.
17. Farma JM, Zager JS, Barnica-Elvir V, et al. A collision of diseases: chronic lymphocytic leukemia discovered during lymph node biopsy for melanoma. *Ann Surg Oncol.* 2013;20:1360-1364.
18. Barroeta JE, Farkas T. Merkel cell carcinoma and chronic lymphocytic leukemia (collision tumor) of the arm: a diagnosis by fine-needle aspiration biopsy. *Diagn Cytopathol.* 2007;35:293-295.
19. Craig PJ, Calonje JE, Harries M, et al. Incidental chronic lymphocytic leukaemia in a biopsy of Merkel cell carcinoma. *J Cutan Pathol.* 2009;36:706-710.
20. Zhang H, Gupta G, Yang XY, et al. A unique case of merkel cell carcinoma and chronic lymphocytic leukaemia presenting in a single cutaneous lesion (collision tumour). *BMJ Case Rep.* 2009;2009:bcr09.2008.1016. doi:10.1136/bcr.09.2008.1016
21. Brewer JD, Shanafelt TD, Otley CC, et al. Chronic lymphocytic leukemia is associated with decreased survival of patients with malignant melanoma and Merkel cell carcinoma in a SEER population-based study. *J Clin Oncol.* 2012;30:843-849.
22. Lai M, Pampena R, Cornacchia L, et al. Cutaneous squamous cell carcinoma in patients with chronic lymphocytic leukemia: a systematic review of the literature. *Int J Dermatol.* 2022;61(5):548-557.
23. Maxfield L, Gaston Ii DA, Sanghvi A. Chronic lymphocytic leukemia and infiltrates seen during excision of nonmelanoma skin cancer. *Cutis.* 2019;103(2):E23-E26.
24. Valdes-Rodriguez R, Bryer B, Gru AA. A story of a pimple: newly diagnosed chronic lymphocytic leukemia in a basal cell carcinoma biopsy. *J Cutan Pathol.* 2021;48(1):192-194.
25. Cimino PJ Jr, Bahler DW, Duncavage EJ. Detection of Merkel cell polyomavirus in chronic lymphocytic leukemia T-cells. *Exp Mol Pathol.* 2013;94:40-44.
26. Teman CJ, Tripp SR, Perkins SL, et al. Merkel cell polyomavirus (MCPyV) in chronic lymphocytic leukemia/small lymphocytic lymphoma. *Leuk Res.* 2011;35:689-692.
27. Karsai S, Hou JS, Telang G, et al. Sézary syndrome coexisting with B-cell chronic lymphocytic leukemia: case report and review of the literature. *Dermatology.* 2008;216:68-75.
28. Duong T, Grange F, Auffret N, et al. Cutaneous Richter's syndrome, prognosis, and clinical, histological and immunohistological patterns: report of four cases and review of the literature. *Dermatology.* 2010;220:226-233.
29. Yu L, Bandhlish A, Fullen DR, et al. Cutaneous Richter syndrome: report of 3 cases from one institution. *J Am Acad Dermatol.* 2012;67:e187-e193.
30. Plaza JA, Comfere NI, Gibson LE, et al. Unusual cutaneous manifestations of B-cell chronic lymphocytic leukemia. *J Am Acad Dermatol.* 2009;60:772-780.
31. LeBlanc RE, Carter JB, Kaur P, Lansigan F. Small lymphocytic lymphoma mimicking primary cutaneous marginal zone lymphoma with colonization of germinal center follicles. *J Cutan Pathol.* 2021;48(1):72-76.
32. Papalas JA, McKinney MS, Kulbacki E, et al. Merkel cell carcinoma with partial B-cell blastic immunophenotype: a potential mimic of cutaneous richter transformation in a patient with chronic lymphocytic lymphoma. *Am J Dermatopathol.* 2014;36:148-152.
33. Singh A, Graziano S, Vajpayee N. Biclonal chronic lymphocytic leukemia presenting as skin lesion. *Am J Dermatopathol.* 2014;36:260-262.
34. Johnstone KJ, Strutton GM. A rare pitfall in the molecular interpretation of BRAF V600E status in melanoma in the setting of BRAF V600E-mutated chronic lymphocytic leukemia/small lymphocytic lymphoma. *J Cutan Pathol.* 2019;46(6):455-456. doi:10.1111/cup.13440
35. Konda S, Beckford A, Demierre MF, et al. Primary cutaneous follicle center lymphoma in the setting of chronic lymphocytic leukemia. *Indian J Dermatol Venereol Leprol.* 2011;77:314-317.
36. Sen F, Medeiros LJ, Lu D, et al. Mantle cell lymphoma involving skin: cutaneous lesions may be the first manifestation of disease and tumors often have blastoid cytologic features. *Am J Surg Pathol.* 2002;26:1312-1318.
37. Cesinaro AM, Bettelli S, Maccio L, et al. Primary cutaneous mantle cell lymphoma of the leg with blastoid morphology and aberrant immunophenotype: a diagnostic challenge. *Am J Dermatopathol.* 2014;36(2):e16-e18.
38. Fernandez V, Salamero O, Espinet B, et al. Genomic and gene expression profiling defines indolent forms of mantle cell lymphoma. *Cancer Res.* 2010;70:1408-1418.
39. Mozos A, Royo C, Hartmann E, et al. SOX11 expression is highly specific for mantle cell lymphoma and identifies the cyclin D1-negative subtype. *Haematologica.* 2009;94:1555-1562.
40. Zeng W, Fu K, Quintanilla-Fend L, et al. Cyclin D1-negative blastoid mantle cell lymphoma identified by SOX11 expression. *Am J Surg Pathol.* 2012;36:214-219.
41. Liu YA, Finn AJ, Subtil A. Primary cutaneous lymphomas in patients with chronic lymphocytic leukemia/small lymphocytic lymphoma (CLL/SLL): a series of 12 cases. *J Cutan Pathol.* 2021;48(5):617-624.
42. Wang HY, Hinds BR. Cutaneous composite small lymphocytic lymphoma and primary cutaneous follicle center lymphoma. *Blood.* 2019;134(8):717.
43. Khan AM, Munir A, Raval M, Mehdi S. Blastic plasmacytoid dendritic cell neoplasm in the background of myeloproliferative disorder and chronic lymphocytic leukaemia. *BMJ Case Rep.* 2019;12(7):e230332.
44. Izquierdo FM, Suárez-Vilela D, de la Hera-Magallanes A, Honrado E. Chronic lymphocytic leukemia and Richter transformation skin involvement recruited by herpesvirus infection. *J Cutan Pathol.* 2021;48(5):713-716.
45. Rossi D, Cerri M, Capello D, et al. Biological and clinical risk factors of chronic lymphocytic leukaemia transformation to Richter syndrome. *Br J Haematol.* 2008;142:202-215.
46. Zarco C, Lahuerta-Palacios JJ, Borrego L, et al. Centroblastic transformation of chronic lymphocytic leukaemia with

primary skin involvement—cutaneous presentation of Richter's syndrome. *Clin Exp Dermatol.* 1993;18:263-267.
47. Miyazaki K, Yamaguchi M, Suzuki R, et al. CD5-positive diffuse large B-cell lymphoma: a retrospective study in 337 patients treated by chemotherapy with or without rituximab. *Ann Oncol.* 2011;22:1601-1607.
48. Maeshima AM, Taniguchi H, Nomoto J, et al. Secondary CD5+ diffuse large B-cell lymphoma not associated with transformation of chronic lymphocytic leukemia/small lymphocytic lymphoma (Richter syndrome). *Am J Clin Pathol.* 2009;131:339-346.
49. Hibler J, Salavaggione AL, Martin A, et al. A unique case of concurrent chronic lymphocytic leukemia/small lymphocytic lymphoma and lymphomatoid papulosis in the same biopsy. *J Cutan Pathol.* 2015;42(4):276-284.
50. Longacre TA, Smoller BR. Leukemia cutis. Analysis of 50 biopsy-proven cases with an emphasis on occurrence in myelodysplastic syndromes. *Am J Clin Pathol.* 1993;100:276-284.
51. Miller MK, Strauchen JA, Nichols KT, et al. Concurrent chronic lymphocytic leukemia cutis and acute myelogenous leukemia cutis in a patient with untreated CLL. *Am J Dermatopathol.* 2001;23:334-340.
52. van Mook WNK, Fickers MM, Theunissen PH, et al. Paraneoplastic pemphigus as the initial presentation of chronic lymphocytic leukemia. *Ann Oncol.* 2001;12:115-118.
53. Fried LJ, Criscito MC, Stevenson ML, Pomeranz MK. Chronic lymphocytic leukemia and the skin: implications for the dermatologist. *Int J Dermatol.* 2022;61(5):519-531.
54. Onajin O, Brewer JD. Skin cancer in patients with chronic lymphocytic leukemia and non-Hodgkin lymphoma. *Clin Adv Hematol Oncol.* 2012;10:571-576.
55. Farber MJ, La Forgia S, Sahu J, et al. Eosinophilic dermatosis of hematologic malignancy. *J Cutan Pathol.* 2012;39:690-695.
56. Barzilai A, Trau H, David M, et al. Mycosis fungoides associated with B-cell malignancies. *Br J Dermatol.* 2006;155:379-386.
57. Chang MB, Weaver AL, Brewer JD. Cutaneous T-cell lymphoma in patients with chronic lymphocytic leukemia: clinical characteristics, temporal relationships, and survival data in a series of 14 patients at Mayo Clinic. *Int J Dermatol.* 2014;53(8):966-970.
58. Metzman MS, Stevens SR, Griffiths CE, et al. A clinical and histologic mycosis fungoides simulant occurring as a T-cell infiltrate coexisting with B-cell leukemia cutis. *J Am Acad Dermatol.* 1995;33:341-345.
59. Sibaud V, Beylot-Barry M, Protin C, Vigarios E, Recher C, Ysebaert L. Dermatological toxicities of Bruton's tyrosine kinase inhibitors. *Am J Clin Dermatol.* 2020;21(6):799-812. doi:10.1007/s40257-020-00535-x
60. Fabbro SK, Smith SM, Duvobsky JA, et al. Panniculitis in patients undergoing treatment with the Bruton tyrosine kinase inhibitor ibrutinib for lymphoid leukemias. *JAMA Oncol.* 2015;1(5):684-686.
61. Flynn JM, Andritsos L, Lucas D, et al. Second malignancies in B-cell chronic lymphocytic leukaemia: possible association with human papilloma virus. *Br J Haematol.* 2010;149:388-390.
62. Perkins JG, Flynn JM, Howard RS, et al. Frequency and type of serious infections in fludarabine-refractory B-cell chronic lymphocytic leukemia and small lymphocytic lymphoma: implications for clinical trials in this patient population. *Cancer.* 2002;94:2033-2039.
63. Pitini V, Arrigo C, Barresi G. Disseminated molluscum contagiosum in a patient with chronic lymphocytic leukaemia after alemtuzumab. *Br J Haematol.* 2003;123:565.
64. Milde P, Brunner M, Borchard F, et al. Cutaneous bacillary angiomatosis in a patient with chronic lymphocytic leukemia. *Arch Dermatol.* 1995;131:933-936.
65. Nannini EC, Keating M, Binstock P, et al. Successful treatment of refractory disseminated *Mycobacterium avium* complex infection with the addition of linezolid and mefloquine. *J Infect.* 2002;44:201-203.
66. Su WP, Buechner SA, Li CY. Clinicopathologic correlations in leukemia cutis. *J Am Acad Dermatol.* 1984;11:121-128.

CHAPTER 42

Cutaneous plasma-cell neoplasms

Liaqat Ali, Jozef Malysz, and José Cabeçadas

DEFINITION

Plasma-cell neoplasms (PCNs) include a spectrum of diseases that range from clinically indolent entities, such as monoclonal gammopathy of unknown significance, to locally invasive neoplasms, including solitary plasmacytoma of bone and extraosseous plasmacytoma, such as primary cutaneous plasmacytoma, and finally to systemic neoplasms with aggressive clinical course such as multiple myeloma (MM) and plasma cell leukemia.

EPIDEMIOLOGY

Skin involvement by PCN is rare, occurring in less than 4% of patients with MM, and has been described only as single case reports and small case series.[1,2] IgA- and IgD-expressing tumors appear to have more frequent cutaneous involvement than other types of myeloma.[3] African American males are more commonly affected.[4] Cutaneous lesions may represent direct extension from underlying bone lesions or present as metastatic MM lesion. Primary cutaneous plasmacytomas that do not arise from underlying bone lesions are exceedingly rare.[5]

CLINICAL FEATURES

Most patients with primary cutaneous plasmacytomas are elderly or middle-aged with mean age 59.5 years.[6] The clinical manifestations include solitary or clustered erythematous papules, nodules, or subcutaneous plaques[7] (Figs. 42-1A,B–42-3). Some of them are not related to direct cutaneous infiltration by neoplastic plasma cells, but rather due to deposition of paraproteins they produce, as in the case of amyloidosis and cryoglobulinemia. Patients with PCN seem to have an increased risk of developing a second primary malignancy, likely secondary to chronic immunosuppression.[8]

In myeloma, skin lesions rarely develop early in the course of the disease or even during its first manifestation[7,9,10]; most commonly cutaneous involvement appears late in the course. It is believed that cutaneous dissemination by MM occurs in the advanced stages, when the overall tumoral mass approximates 2 to 3 kg.[11] The prognosis at this stage is dismal with average overall survival of less than 1 year.[12] Other cutaneous manifestations described in association with MM are listed in Table 42-1.[13]

HISTOLOGY

Microscopic examination of skin lesions of MM usually demonstrates dermal-based nodular (Fig. 42-4A,B) and/or diffuse interstitial infiltrates of neoplastic plasma cells with sparing of the epidermis.[7] The diffuse interstitial pattern is characterized by sheets and cords of neoplastic plasma cells infiltrating the dermis and subcutis. In some cases, the neoplastic cells can be easily identified as plasma cells showing intermediate-sized coarse, clumped chromatin, abundant cytoplasm, perinuclear hof, and variable nucleoli. The neoplastic tumor cells show variable maturation with occasional morphologic atypia including binucleation and multinucleation (Fig. 42-4C).[1] In some cases, given the degree of atypia, the recognition of a plasma cell neolasm can be very challenging (Fig. 42-4D). In such cases, the tumor cells are large with pleomorphic vesicular nuclei, prominent nucleoli, and granular eosinophilic cytoplasm, best characterized as plasmablasts. In those cases, mitotic activity is usually increased. A distinct grenz zone is commonly seen.[1] Intracytoplasmic inclusions (Russell bodies) and intranuclear inclusions (Dutcher bodies), although not usually prominent, may sometimes be present (Fig. 42-5A–D).[14,15]

IMMUNOPHENOTYPE

Neoplastic plasma cells stain positive for CD138 (Fig. 42-6A), CD38, CD79a, and frequently for CD56 (Fig. 42-6B). They are usually negative for B-lymphocytic markers such as CD19 and CD20; however, plasma cells can be CD20 positive in 10% of myelomas. Monotypic light chain restriction can be documented by κ and λ immunohistochemistry or in situ hybridization studies (Fig. 42-6C,D).

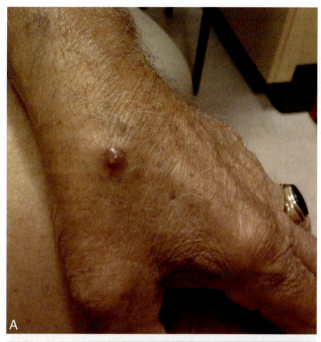
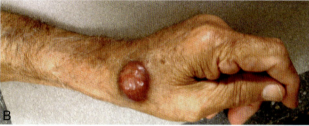

FIGURE 42-1. **A.** Clinical photograph of a patient with cutaneous tumor nodule on the wrist; skin involvement in MM. **B. Progression of the same tumor nodule 6 weeks later.**

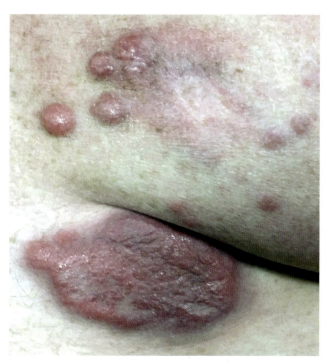

FIGURE 42-2. Papules, nodules, and a large plaque on the chest wall.

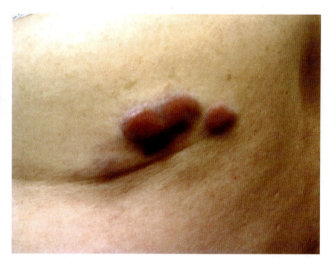

FIGURE 42-3. Indurated plaque on the left side of abdomen; skin involvement from systemic multiple myeloma.

TABLE 42-1 Cutaneous Manifestations of Multiple Myeloma

Extramedullary cutaneous plasmacytomas
Cutaneous amyloidosis
Pyoderma gangrenosum
Leukocytoclastic vasculitis
Necrobiotic xanthogranuloma
Scleromyxedema
Sweet syndrome
Subcorneal pustular dermatosis
POEMS syndrome
Scleredema
Angioedema with C1 inhibitor deficiency
Plane xanthomas
Follicular hyperkeratosis

The tumor cells may additionally exhibit aberrant immunohistochemical markers such as EMA and CD43, but these stains are not reliable in the workup of plasma cell infiltrates. A study comparing immunophenotypic profiles between extramedullary plasmacytomas and MMs revealed that extramedullary plasmacytomas revealed infrequent expression of CD56 and CyclinD1, showed weaker staining for BCL-2, and did not have overexpression of p53, while most systemic myeloma cases showed CD56 expression and stronger staining for BCL-2 and may show CyclinD1 coexpression and p53 overexpression.[16]

CYTOGENETIC STUDIES

Cytogenetic features play a very important role in predicting biologic behavior and prognosis in MM. Complex karyotype, deletion of 13q, 17p-/p53 deletion, or translocations t(4;14)

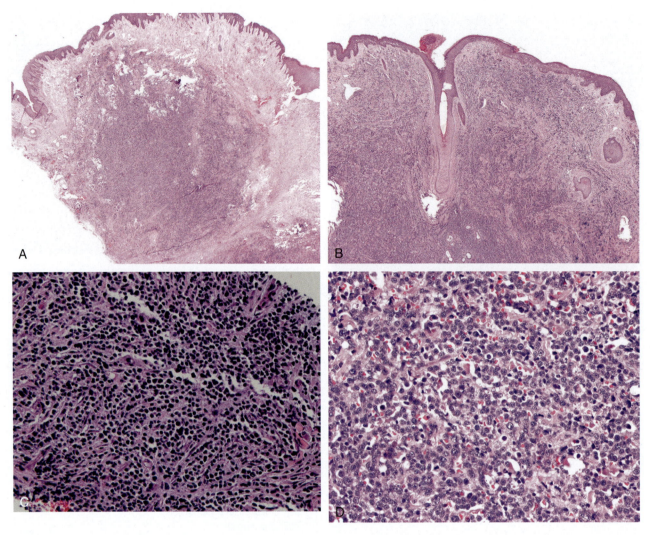

FIGURE 42-4. A. Low-power magnification showing nodular dermal plasma cell lesion. **B.** Diffuse dermal involvement of the entire dermis by neoplastic plasma cells. **C.** Intermediate magnification depicting only mild morphologic atypia with relatively easy recognition of plasma cells. **D.** Highly atypical plasma cell lesion, where recognition of plasma cells by morphology alone is very difficult.

and t(14;16) by fluorescent in situ hybridization (FISH) are unfavorable findings.[17-20] These patients have a poor response to induction chemotherapy and, overall, a more aggressive clinical course. Owing to their importance in prognosis, the cytogenetic and FISH results have been integrated in defining the revised International Staging System (ISS) for MM. Patients harboring 17p deletion, t(4;14), or t(14;16) are currently classified as having stage III disease, regardless of other clinical information.[21]

DIFFERENTIAL DIAGNOSIS OF PLASMA CELL–RICH INFILTRATES IN THE SKIN

The differential diagnosis includes other hematolymphoid and nonhematolymphoid neoplasms as well as some plasma cell–rich reactive infiltrates. Any hematolymphoid neoplasm with plasmacytoid cytomorphologic features could lead to an erroneous histologic impression. The list of differential diagnoses could be exhaustingly long; however, most pertinent entities with plasmacytoid cytologic features are discussed here[6] and these include the following:

1. Primary cutaneous marginal zone lymphoma (PCMZL), plasmacytic variant
2. Plasmablastic lymphoma (PBL), involving skin or mucous membranes
3. Pretibial lymphoplasmacytic plaque (PLP)
4. Castleman disease (CD), plasma cell variant
5. Cutaneous and systemic plasmacytosis (C/SP)

Clinical presentation and history along with morphology and an array of appropriate immunohistochemical markers will resolve most differential dilemmas.

PCMZL (see Chapter 32) is considered an extranodal lymphoma of mucosa-associated lymphoid tissue (MALT-type), composed of small B cells, lymphoplasmacytoid cells, and plasma cells. Tumors with plasmacytic differentiation may display an unusually prominent nodular or

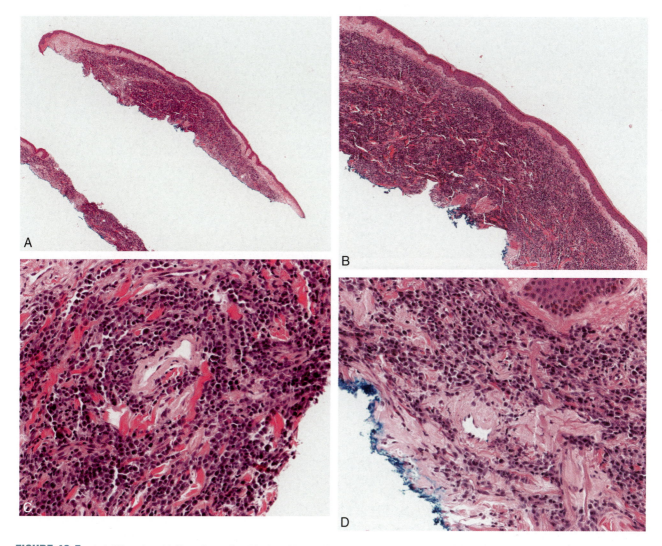

FIGURE 42-5. **A.** A diffuse dermal infiltrate is noted on this shave biopsy with cutaneous involvement by multiple myeloma. **B.** The infiltrate spares the epidermis with a grenz zone. **C.** The neoplastic plasma cells are small, and some of them show a characteristic perivascular pattern. The vessel shows dense amorphous eosinophilic material in the wall, compatible with amyloid. **D.** Other small vessels in the dermis also reveal amyloid deposition, which were positive for Congo red (not shown).

sheet-like proliferation of monotypic plasma cells, resembling primary extramedullary plasmacytoma (PEMP). In PCMZL, the predominant cell type is a centrocyte-like or monocytoid small B cell. Other cells include lymphoplasmacytoid cells and scattered plasma cells; the plasma cell component may be prominent in some cases. Since the neoplastic cells are B lymphocytes, they will be CD19+, CD20+, CD45+, BCL-2+. Plasma cells with strong CD138 expression will be scattered among neoplastic B cells and may or not show light chain restriction. Up to one-third of patients with PCMZL will have M-protein. Most cases of previously reported cutaneous PEMP, in fact, are likely examples of PCMZL with marked plasmacytic differentiation, based on retrospective evaluation of a benign course and favorable prognosis.[22]

PBL (see Chapter 39) is an uncommon B-cell lymphoma with the highest incidence in HIV-positive individuals, as well as patients with other immunodeficiency states. The most frequent sites of involvement are oral mucosa and other mucosal sites (sinonasal, ocular, gastrointestinal). Less commonly skin, soft tissue, and bone may be involved. Lesions are histologically characterized by sheets of cells with plasmablastic and/or immunoblastic morphology. Neoplastic cells in majority of cases are CD20−, CD138+, EBER+, and CD56−. However, positivity of EBV alone along with plasmablastic morphology is not sufficient for a diagnosis of PBL as myeloma progressing to EBV-positive plasmacytoma does occur.[22]

PLP is a recently described clinicopathologic entity that presents as a solitary lesion on the pretibial area of young children. The histology is characterized by a prominent plasma cell infiltrate, and the lesion exhibits a chronic, benign course. Histologic features may closely resemble those seen in C/SP or cutaneous lesions of plasmacytic CD, with mixed populations of CD20+ B cells and CD138+ plasma cells with polytypic κ and λ light chains. The clinical presentation and absence of systemic manifestations are essential in differentiating it from neoplastic conditions.[23,24]

CD is an uncommon hematologic disorder characterized by lymphadenopathy. It is felt to be a reactive process induced by an immunologic reaction to an infectious

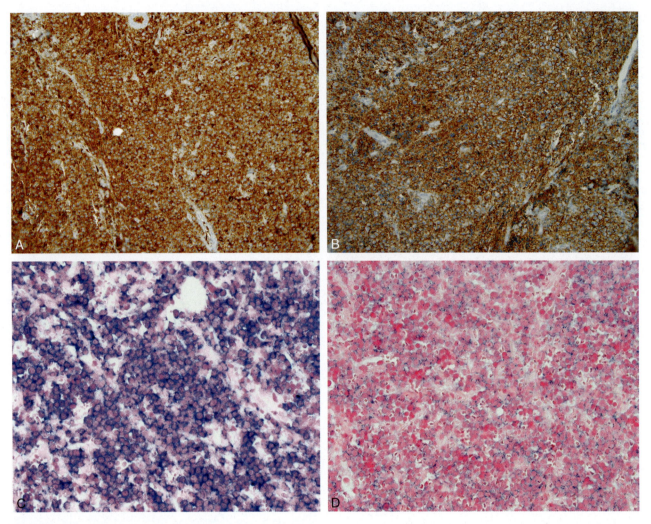

FIGURE 42-6. **A.** Neoplastic plasma cells highlighted by CD138. **B.** Diffuse positive staining for CD56. **C.** In situ hybridization κ stain clearly shows κ light chain restriction. **D.** In situ hybridization λ stain is virtually negative.

organism, particularly HHV-8, or a drug.[25] The reactive lymphoid cells in CD produce an excess of interleukin (IL)-6, leading to hypergammaglobulinemia and vascular proliferation.[26] Cutaneous lesions of CD typically present with multiple scattered nodules and indurated plaques involving the trunk and extremities.[27] Although cutaneous involvement by CD is rare, this entity should be considered in any patient with cutaneous lesions containing a prominent plasma cell infiltrate. The presence of lymphadenopathy, elevated serum levels of IL-6, and polyclonal hypergammaglobulinemia and absence of M-protein or marrow involvement support the CD diagnosis.[28]

C/SP is an exceedingly rare reactive lymphoproliferative disorder that primarily affects Japanese individuals (see Chapter 35). Like multicentric plasmacytic CD, this condition is characterized by a polyclonal plasma cell infiltrate involving the skin and frequently multiple lymph nodes with accompanying hypergammaglobulinemia. Like CD, elevated serum IL-6 likely plays a central role in pathogenesis. Unlike CD, C/SP is not associated with HHV-8 and presents primarily in the skin with numerous lesions.[29,30] Nonetheless, some authors consider C/SP and HHV-8–negative multicentric plasmacytic CD to be part of the same spectrum of plasma cell–rich reactive lymphoproliferative disorders.[29]

CAPSULE SUMMARY

- Cutaneous PCNs are rare and include extraosseous plasmacytomas and cutaneous involvement by MM.
- In patients with myeloma, cutaneous involvement occurs in late stages of the disease because of extramedullary dissemination or as a direct extension from underlying bone lesions.
- Morphology and immunohistochemical staining pattern are essential in recognition of cutaneous plasmacytic infiltrates; light chain restriction and abnormal phenotype (aberrant coexpression of CD56, CD117, and CyclinD1) allow confirmation of the neoplastic nature of the plasma cells involving the skin.
- FISH techniques allow demonstration of 17p-/p53 deletion, t(4;14) and t(14;16) abnormalities, providing useful information that defines high-risk patients.

References

1. Patterson JW, Parsons JM, White RM, et al. Cutaneous involvement of multiple myeloma and extramedullary plasmacytoma. *J Am Acad Dermatol*. 1988;19:879-890.
2. Panse G, Subtil A, McNiff JM, et al. Cutaneous involvement in plasma cell myeloma: clinicopathologic findings in a series of ten cases. *Am J Clin Pathol*. 2021;155(1):106-116. doi:10.1093/ajcp/aqaa122
3. Kato N, Kimura K, Yasukawa K, et al. Metastatic cutaneous plasmacytoma: a case report associated with IgA lambda multiple myeloma and a review of the literature of metastatic cutaneous plasmacytomas associated with multiple myeloma and primary cutaneous plasmacytoma. *J Dermatol*. 1999;26:587-594.
4. Alberts DS, Lynch P. Cutaneous plasmacytomas in multiple myeloma. *Arch Dermatol*. 1978;114:1784-1787.
5. Alexiou C, Kau RJ, Dietzfelbinger H, et al. Extramedullary plasmacytoma: tumor occurrence and therapeutic concepts. *Cancer*. 1999;85(11):2305-2314.
6. Wong KF, Chan JK, Li LP, et al. Primary cutaneous plasmacytoma—report of two cases and review of the literature. *Am J Dermatopathol*. 1994;16(4):392.
7. Malysz J, Talamo G, Zhu J, et al. Cutaneous involvement in multiple myeloma (MM): a case series with clinicopathologic correlation. *J Am Acad Dermatol*. 2016;74:878-884. doi:10.1016/j.jaad.2015.12.028
8. Costa LJ, Godby KN, Chhabra S, et al. Second primary malignancy after multiple myeloma-population trends and cause-especific mortality. *Br J Haematol*. 2018;182:513-520.
9. Cholongitas E, Pipili C, Katsogridakis K, et al. Plasmacytic infiltrates of the skin as the first clinical manifestation of multiple myeloma. *Int J Dermatol*. 2007;46:1323-1324.
10. Torne R, Su WPD, Winkelmann RK, et al. Clinicopathologic study of cutaneous plasmacytoma. *Int J Dermatol*. 1990;29:562-566.
11. Requena L. Specific cutaneous involvement in patients with multiple myeloma. A clinicopathological, immunohistochemical and cytogenetic study of 40 cases [in Spanish]. *Actas Dermosifiliogr*. 2005;96(7):424-440.
12. Jurczyszyn A, Olszewska-Szopa M, Hungria V, et al. Cutaneous involvement in multiple myeloma: a multi-institutional retrospective study of 53 patients. *Leuk Lymphoma*. Published online January 4, 2016.
13. Kois JM, Sexton FM, Lookingbill DP. Cutaneous manifestations of multiple myeloma. *Arch Dermatol*. 1991;127:69-74.
14. Requena L, Kutzner H, Palmedo G, et al. Cutaneous involvement in multiple myeloma: a clinicopathologic, immunohistochemical, and cytogenetic study of 8 cases. *Arch Dermatol*. 2003;139:475-486.
15. Muscardin LM, Pulsoni A, Cerroni L. Primary cutaneous plasmacytoma: report of a case and review of the literature. *J Am Acad Dermatol*. 2000;43:962-965.
16. Kremer M, Ott G, Nathrath M, et al. Primary extramedullary plasmacytoma and multiple myeloma: phenotypic differences revealed by immunohistochemical analysis. *J Pathol*. 2005;205(1):92-101.
17. Tricot G, Barlogie B, Jagannath S, et al. Poor prognosis in multiple myeloma is associated only with partial or complete deletions of chromosome 13 or abnormalities involving 11q and not with other karyotype abnormalities. *Blood*. 1995;86:4250-4256.
18. Tricot G, Sawyer JR, Jagannath S, et al. Unique role of cytogenetics in the prognosis of patients with myeloma receiving high-dose therapy and autotransplants. *J Clin Oncol*. 1997;15:2659-2666.
19. Konigsberg R, Zojer N, Ackermann J, et al. Predictive role of interphase cytogenetics for survival of patients with multiple myeloma. *J Clin Oncol*. 2000;18:804-812.
20. Swerdlow SH, Campo E, Harris NL, et al. *WHO Classification of Tumors of Hematopoietic and Lymphoid Tissues*. IARC Press; 2008:256-260.
21. Palumbo A, Avet-Loiseau H, Oliva S, et al. Revised international staging system for multiple myeloma: a report from International Myeloma Working Group. *J Clin Oncol*. 2015;33(26):2863-2869.
22. Walsh NM, Kutzner H, Requena L, et al. Plasmacytic cutaneous pathology: a review. *J Cutan Pathol*. 2019;46:698-708.
23. Fried I, Wiesner T, Cerroni L. Pretibial lymphoplasmacytic plaque in children. *Arch Dermatol*. 2010;146:95-96.
24. Gilliam AC, Mullen RH, Oviedo G, et al. Isolated benign primary cutaneous plasmacytosis in children: two illustrative cases. *Arch Dermatol*. 2009;145:299-302.
25. Soulier J, Grollet L, Oksenhendler E, et al. Kaposi's sarcoma-associated herpesvirus-like DNA sequences in multicentric Castleman's disease. *Blood*. 1995;86:1276-1280.
26. Casper C. The aetiology and management of Castleman disease at 50 years: translating pathophysiology to patient care. *Br J Haematol*. 2005;129:3-17.
27. Kubota Y, Noto S, Takakuwa T, et al. Skin involvement in giant lymph node hyperplasia (Castleman's disease). *J Am Acad Dermatol*. 1993;29:778-780.
28. Okuyama R, Harigae H, Moriya T, et al. Indurated nodules and plaques showing a dense plasma cell infiltrate as a cutaneous manifestation of Castleman's disease. *Br J Dermatol*. 2007;156:174-176.
29. Haque M, Hou JS, Hisamichi K, et al. Cutaneous and systemic plasmacytosis vs. cutaneous plasmacytic Castleman disease: review and speculations about pathogenesis. *Clin Lymphoma Myeloma Leuk*. 2011;11:453-461.
30. Leonard AL, Meehan SA, Ramsey D, et al. Cutaneous and systemic plasmacytosis. *J Am Acad Dermatol*. 2007;56:S38-S40.

Cutaneous involvement by Hodgkin's lymphoma

Alejandro A. Gru, András Schaffer, and Maxime Battistella

DEFINITION

Hodgkin lymphoma (HL) is a clonal lymphoproliferative disease of germinal center B-cell origin. Lymph nodes of the cervical (75% of cases), mediastinal, axillary, and paraaortic regions are the commonest sites of involvement. HL lesions contain a small number of large mononuclear or multinuclear neoplastic cells, which are admixed with nonneoplastic inflammatory and accessory cells. HL is composed of two separate disease entities: classic HL (CHL) and nodular lymphocyte predominant HL (NLPHL). These groups differ in their clinical presentation and histologic, immunophenotypic, and genetic features. Cutaneous dissemination is exceedingly rare and had been described in classic CHL and rarely in NLPHL. Isolated case reports of "primary HL" are anecdotal. Diagnosing cutaneous HL is problematic as it shows morphologic and immunophenotypic overlap with primary cutaneous CD30+ lymphoproliferative diseases, such as lymphomatoid papulosis (LyP) or cutaneous anaplastic large-cell lymphoma (cALCL). Furthermore, nodal extension of CD30+ lymphoproliferations should be differentiated from CHL.

EPIDEMIOLOGY

HL accounts for about 15% to 30% of all lymphomas.[1-3] The age-adjusted incidence rate in the United States is approximately 3 to 4 per 100,000 population.[4] In the United States, there are approximately 9000 cases of CHL diagnosed each year. CHL accounts for about 90% to 95% of HLs in Western countries and displays a characteristic bimodal age distribution curve with peaks at 15 to 35 years of age and in the elderly.[1-3] NLPHL comprises about 3% to 8% of HLs and occurs in all age groups with a peak in the third decade.[2,3]

The incidence of CHL is higher in patients with history of infectious mononucleosis (4-fold) or HIV (6- to 20-fold).[5-7] Furthermore, a paradoxical increase in HL incidence had been observed in HIV patients receiving combination antiretroviral therapy, or in patients receiving allogeneic bone marrow transplantation, suggesting that immune reconstitution may underpin the pathogenesis in some cases.[7,8]

ETIOLOGY

Epstein–Barr virus (EBV) is detected in 25% to 75% of CHLs, while NLPHL is generally considered EBV negative.[9,10] The EBV genome is detected in the neoplastic cells in the EBV+ cases. Rare cases of NLPHL may be EBV positive in both children and adults.[11] Evidence of EBV infection is more prevalent in the mixed cellularity and lymphocyte-depleted variants, in HIV-associated cases and in patients from tropical countries.[1,12-14] Critical advances in the treatment of HL have occurred over the last 2 decades (including combination of chemotherapy and radiotherapy, monoclonal antibodies, and immunotherapy), which have led to cure rates exceeding 80%.[15-17]

CUTANEOUS DISSEMINATION

First described by the German physician Grosz in 1906, cutaneous HL is an exceedingly rare manifestation of the nodal disease (0.5%-7.5% of cases).[18] It occurs when the neoplastic cells from the systemic lymphoma invade the skin. Nonetheless, cutaneous symptoms such as pruritus can be seen in up to 40% of patients with HL.[19] The most recent studies showed an incidence of <0.5% of skin infiltration.[20] The incidence of cutaneous HL decreased over the last decades in part owing to improved therapy, including autologous stem cell transplantation for systemic disease.[18,21-26] Cutaneous dissemination is associated with an aggressive clinical course.[20]

The pathomechanism of cutaneous dissemination is unclear. While hematogenous spread and direct extension from involved lymph nodes had been proposed, the likeliest route of spread is retrograde lymphatogenous. This is supported by the predilection of skin lesions for anatomical sites such as axilla and chest, which overlie affected draining lymph nodes that lack histologic evidence of extranodal extension.[20] Cutaneous dissemination had been described only for CHL, most commonly for the nodular sclerosis variant.[27] The exceedingly rare case of NLPHL with cutaneous extension has been reported on one occasion.[28] We recently reported the largest case series of CHL with cutaneous dissemination (n = 25 cases).[29]

The isolated case reports of "primary HL" are anecdotal and most likely represent examples of LyP or ALCL, rather than de novo cutaneous disease.[30-33]

CLINICAL PRESENTATION

Cutaneous dissemination of CHL typically affects the skin of the chest and axilla, which are the draining areas of the most commonly affected lymph nodes. The clinical presentation includes single or agminated papules,[20,34] plaques,[35] sinus tracts,[36,37] nodules,[38] or tumors (with or without ulceration).[39] Cases with generalized erythroderma had been described.[40-42] In our experience, a single lesion, usually a tumor, nodule, or infiltrative plaque was observed in 56% of cases and multiple lesions were present in 28% of cases. Regarding the clinical location, 28% presented in the head and neck region (7/25), 28% on the trunk (7/25), 20% in the inguinal or axillary folds (5/25), and 16% on the extremities (4/25). The interval between the clinical (first) diagnosis of HL and development of skin lesions ranged between 6 and 108 months (average 33.75 months). Cutaneous lesions were present in 28% of cases upon the diagnosis of CHL (5/18), as a manifestation of relapse in 67% of cases (12/18), and during the disease progression in 5% (1/18). Most patients (86%-12/14) had a diagnosis of stage IV disease at first diagnosis.[29] Four patients had received allogeneic bone marrow transplant as a form of therapy (18%). Disease overall survival was estimated as an average of 62.14 months after the diagnosis of cutaneous disease (n = 8): five patients died of disease, two were alive without disease (complete response), and one showed disease progression but was lost to follow-up.

Paraneoplastic dermatoses are found in 3% and 50% of patients and include hyperpigmentation,[43] pruritus,[19] acquired ichthyosis,[44] herpes zoster,[45] alopecia,[46] and disseminated granuloma annular.[47,48]

ASSOCIATION WITH OTHER MALIGNANCIES

A significant subset of patients with CD30+ lymphoproliferative disorders (LPDs), such as LyP, has a higher risk for the development of CHL.[49-53] Conversely, patients with CHL might develop other malignancies including melanoma,[54] granulomatous slack skin, and follicular mucinosis.[55-57] In our cohort, other comorbidities were present in 16% of cases and included the history of chronic lymphocytic leukemia, ALK-negative anaplastic large-cell lymphoma, marginal zone lymphoma, and malignant melanoma. The rare association of CHL and coexistence of mycosis fungoides has been documented in the past.[58,59]

HISTOPATHOLOGY

The hallmark cell of CHL is the Reed–Sternberg (RS) cell. The classic RS cell is large with hyperlobulated nucleus that might appear multinucleated. Mono- or binucleated forms also exist. The mononuclear variant is called the Hodgkin cell. The nuclei of these variants show pale chromatin, thickened nuclear membrane, and large, eosinophilic, viral inclusion–like nucleolus (owl's eye appearance) (Fig. 43-1). Additionally, mummified cells with collapsed basophilic nucleus and lack of nucleolus are invariably found (Fig. 43-1). They are thought to represent degenerate RS and Hodgkin cells. RS cells and their variants are sparsely dispersed among numerous bystander inflammatory cells, most commonly small lymphocytes, plasma cells, neutrophils, histiocytes, and eosinophils (Fig. 43-1).[1,60] RS-like cells and variants can be seen in a range of different disorders, particularly in LyP and cALCL (see Differential Diagnosis), and therefore they are not diagnostic of HL.

In the skin, CHL manifests as a dermal-based infiltrate that commonly extends into the adipose tissue. The epidermis is spared in most cases.[19,20,60] The lesion shows nodular or interstitial growth with frequent adnexal involvement. The inflammatory infiltrate can be potentially mistaken for ruptured cyst or hair follicle.

In our large cohort of cases of CHL with skin dissemination, a diagnosis of CHL not otherwise specified in 60% of cases (15/25), nodular sclerosis type in 24% (6/25) (Fig. 43.2), mixed cellularity in 12% (3/25) (Fig. 43-3), and lymphocyte depleted in 4% (1/25) was done. Cutaneous involvement was manifested by a neoplastic infiltrate of cells involving the dermis in all cases and with subcutaneous extension in 50% of cases (Fig. 43-4). Necrosis was present in 24% of cases (6/25), surface ulceration in 25% of cases (5/25) (Fig. 43-4), and fibrosis in 24% of cases (6/25).[29]

IMMUNOHISTOCHEMISTRY

CHL: CD30+ and PAX-5+ in nearly all cases. CD15+ in 75% to 85% of cases (Fig. 43-5). OCT-2 expression is variable.[61] Only 20% to 30% of CHLs are positive for CD20, which is a marker of better prognosis and response to rituximab. B-cell–specific transcriptional coactivators BOB1, CD45, CD79a, ALK, and EMA are negative. CD68 highlights background histiocytes, which appears to correlate with clinical outcome.[62] EBER in situ hybridization can be positive.[1,20,35,60] In our cohort of cutaneous CHL, immunophenotypic evaluation showed expression of CD30 in all cases (100%), while CD15 expression was noted in 74% of cases (17/23) and PAX-5 in 88% (15/17). The latter showed the characteristic dim pattern of expression seen in CHL. Expression of CD20 was seen in 27% of cases (6/22), and typically in a focal or weak pattern. CD3 was negative in all cases. LMP-1 expression was seen in 38% of cases (5/13) and EBER in 17% (2/12). MUM-1 was also positive in all cases tested (9/9).

NLPHL: PAX-5+, CD20+, OCT-2+, PU.1+, BOB-1+, BCL-6+, CD30−, CD15−, and EBER−.

GENETICS AND MOLECULAR FINDINGS

There is no significant role for routine molecular studies (Southern blot, polymerase chain reaction [PCR]) in the diagnosis of CHL. Due to the paucity of neoplastic cells (<1%), these techniques often yield either false-negative results or weak clonal bands. With appropriate single-cell enrichment,

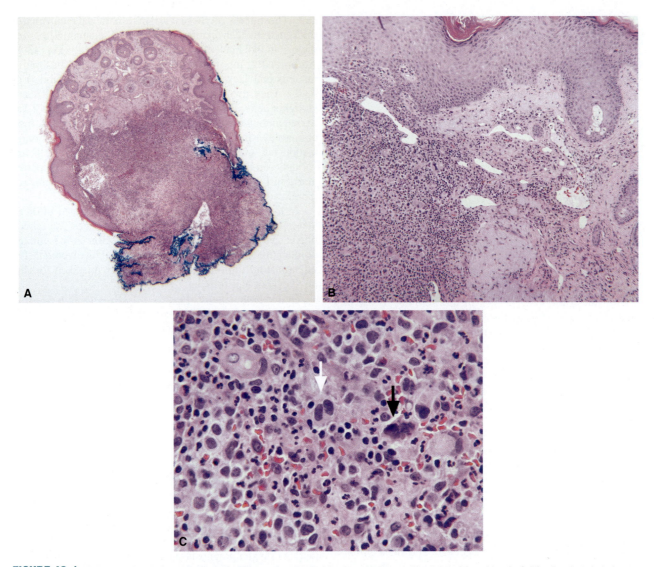

FIGURE 43-1. Cutaneous involvement by Hodgkin disease. A and **B.** Nodular dermal infiltrate with sparing of the epidermis. **C.** RS cell variants include mononuclear Hodgkin cells, binucleated RS cells with owl's eye appearance (*white arrow*), and multinucleated mummified cells (*black arrow*). Hodgkin cells contain a single, centrally placed eosinophilic nucleolus. Background inflammatory cells include small lymphocytes, neutrophils, histiocytes, and eosinophils.

or newer methods such as the BIOMED-2-based PCR assay, clonal immunoglobulin (Ig) rearrangement is seen in the majority of lesions.[63-65] Only rare cases show monoclonal T-cell receptor rearrangement, suggesting their T-cell derivation.[66]

Classic cytogenetic studies failed to demonstrate recurrent translocations in CHL.[67,68] Comparative genomic hybridization identified amplification of the 2p13 chromosomal region harboring the REL oncogene in 46% of cases.[69-71] REL encodes a lymphoid-specific transcription factor, which is a component of the nuclear factor (NF)-κB.[72] In addition, deletion of the *IκBα* gene and inactivating mutations in the *TNFAIP3* tumor suppressor gene lead to constitutive activation of NK-κB, a hallmark of CHL.[73-75] Constitutive activation of the JAK/STAT pathway by amplification of *JAK-2* gene and mutations in the JAK inhibitor SOCS-1 had been also described (50%).[69,76,77] This consecutively leads to the accumulation of various nuclear STATs in HL. Bona fide activating mutations of the nuclear shuttle protein XPO1 also contribute to the nuclear accumulation of STATs and have been found in 18% to 26% of the studied CHL cases.[78-80]

Interestingly, amplification of the 9p24 locus with increased PD-1 ligand expression has been noted in CHL, a mechanism shared by the primary mediastinal large B-cell lymphomas.[81] Such amplification occurs in 50% to 55% of cases of CHL and is associated with a poor response to conventional therapies, but they are an indicator for response and superior progression-free survival—to PD1/PDL1 immune checkpoint inhibition–based immunotherapy.[82]

Inactivating mutations of the beta 2 microglobulin gene (*B2M*) also play an instrumental role in immune evasion, influencing the assembly of MHC class I and thus altering tumor cell "visibility" for effector cells. *B2M* is the most commonly mutated or deleted gene in up to 70% of studied cHL cases.[78,83,84] Other mutations in the JAK-STAT pathway of relevance include *STAT6* (40%-50%)[80] and *CSF2RB* (20%).[78]

The PI3K/AKT/mTOR pathway is one of the key cell cycle regulators in cancer. Perturbations of this signaling cascade have been found in approximately 45% of CHLs. *GNA13*, which encodes the G13 protein alpha subunit, a tumor suppressor that inhibits AKT, is a recurrent target (25%) of

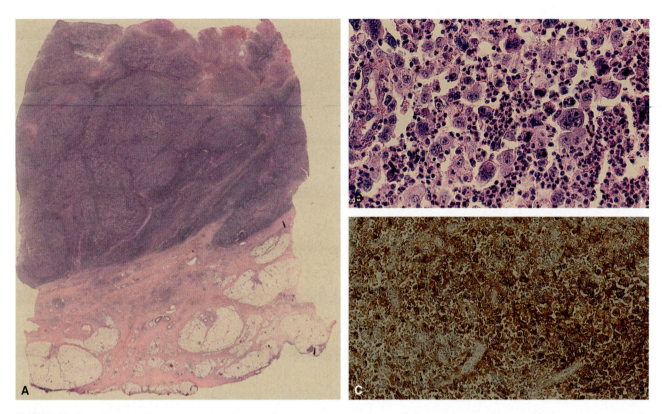

FIGURE 43-2. Cutaneous involvement by CHL, nodular sclerosis subtype. A. Numerous nodular aggregates of atypical lymphocytes are present in the deep reticular dermis (40×). **B.** Frequent Reed–Sternberg cells are identified (400×). The large lymphoma cells are strongly CD30+ **(C)**.

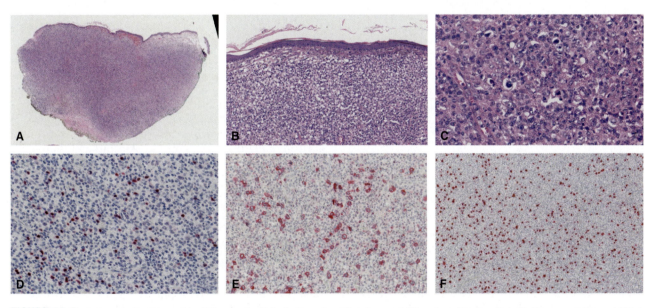

FIGURE 43-3. Cutaneous involvement by CHL, mixed cellularity type. A and **B.** A dense and diffuse dermal lymphocytic infiltrate is present (40× and 100×). **C.** Numerous mummified cells are present (400×). The large lymphoma cells are weakly positive for PAX-5 **(D)** and strongly positive for CD30 **(E)** and EBV **(F)**.

mutations in CHL. *ITPKB* mutations are found in slightly over 25% of CHL.[85] Other mutations of interest involving other pathways include *TP53* (10%),[80] *RBM38* (15%),[86] *ETV6* (15%),[78] *SPEN* (12.5%), *NOTCH1/2* (5%), and *FBXW7* (7.5%).[85] Promoter hypermethylation of seven cancer-related genes has been found in CHL: *CDKN2A* (77%), *RASSF1A* (59%), *CDH1* (51%), *DAPK* (45%), *GSTP1* (43%), *SHP1* (also called *PTPN6*) (38%), and *MGMT* (24%).[87]

Downregulation of B-cell–specific gene expression in Hodgkin and RS cells is a hallmark of CHL. The precise mechanism of this transcriptional deregulation is not entirely known. Amplification of ID2, an inhibitor of B-cell–specific transcription factor E2A, aberrant somatic hypermutation of the *PAX-5* gene, and silencing epigenetic alterations are a few possible molecular events underpinning this phenotype.[88-90]

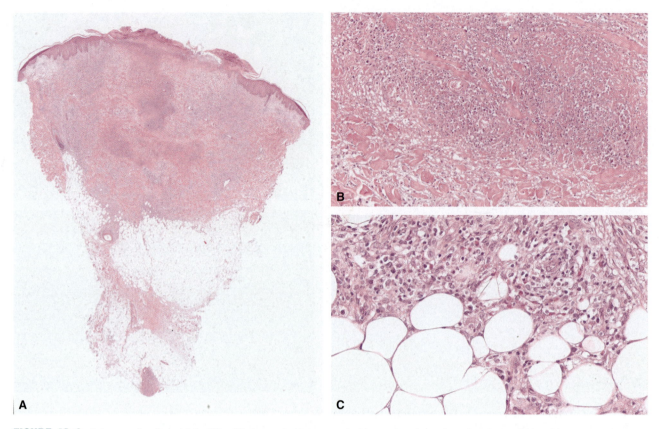

FIGURE 43-4. Cutaneous involvement by CHL with deep subcutaneous extension and surface ulceration. **A.** A malignant infiltrate is present in the dermis and subcutaneous tissue with surface ulceration (40×). **B.** Prominent areas of necrosis are seen (200×). **C.** Large atypical cells are seen in the subcutaneous tissue (400×).

POSTULATED CELL OF ORIGIN

The presence of clonal, somatically mutated Ig genes suggests that neoplastic RS cells are the progeny of germinal center B cells defective in Ig transcription.[63,91] In rare cases, RS cells originate from mature, postthymic peripheral T cells.[73,76]

DIFFERENTIAL DIAGNOSIS

CHL exhibits a significant morphologic and immunophenotypic overlap with primary cutaneous CD30+ T-cell lymphomas (TCLs). These lymphomas include CD30+ T-cell LPDs (CD30-T-LPDs), such as *LyP* and primary *cALCL* as well as *CD30+ tumor-stage mycosis fungoides*. The differentiation of these entities is further complicated by findings of de novo CHL in patients with CD30-T-PLD and mycosis fungoides.[49-53] Similar to CHL, RS-like or Hodgkin-like cells with a CD30+CD15+CD3− immunophenotype can be encountered in CD30+ TCL Fig. 43-6A–D).[60] Additionally, these primary cutaneous lymphomas could spread to draining lymph nodes and exhibit histologic features, such as capsular thickening and bands of fibrosis, and CD30+CD15+CD3− phenotype, that mimic nodal CHL (Figs. 43-6 and 43-7).[60] The lack of the B-cell marker PAX-5 and the presence of TCR clonality and sinusoidal involvement are the most reliable features to differentiate nodal CD30-T-LPD from CHL.[60]

Transformed mycosis fungoides with regional lymph node involvement can also share a similar immunophenotypic profile, posing a diagnostic challenge, as CHL can appear similar with aberrant expression of T-cell (1%-8%) and cytotoxic markers (3%-32%).[92-95]

EBV+ mucocutaneous ulcer (*EBVMCU*) is a novel form of LPD that occurs in the skin (around the mouth and other mucosal surfaces) and presents in patients with underlying immunosuppression (related to medications or advanced age). Such patients present with shallow ulcers that can resolve upon reduction of the immunosuppression. Histopathologically, EBVMCU shows an infiltrate that includes numerous Hodgkin-like cells, plasmacytoid apoptotic cells, and is accompanied by the background inflammatory cells seen in CHL (histiocytes, granulomas, neutrophils, and eosinophils). The immunophenotype of this disorder includes CHL-like marker expression, as the cells are CD30+, EBV+, and show CD15 expression in 42% of cases. There is variable expression of CD45 and PAX-5. As opposed to the cases of cutaneous HL, none of the EBVMCU patients have underlying HL.[96-101] Like the EBVMCU, cases of cutaneous PTLD containing Hodgkin-like elements have been reported in the literature.[102,103]

EBV-positive diffuse large B-cell lymphoma is an aggressive B-cell malignancy that usually presents in older individuals and is frequently associated with extranodal involvement. Extranodal disease with or without concurrent nodal disease is common, occurring in 50% to 70% of cases and most frequently involves the skin, lungs, tonsils, and stomach. The

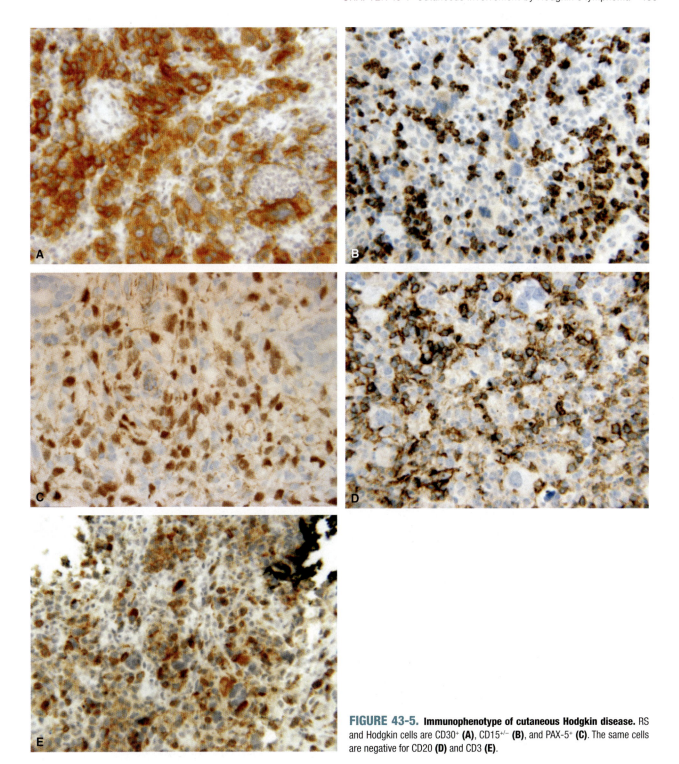

FIGURE 43-5. Immunophenotype of cutaneous Hodgkin disease. RS and Hodgkin cells are CD30+ **(A)**, CD15+/− **(B)**, and PAX-5+ **(C)**. The same cells are negative for CD20 **(D)** and CD3 **(E)**.

polymorphous variant of EBV+ DLBCL is comprised of a mixture of centroblasts, immunoblasts, RS-like cells, or pleomorphic cells and variable numbers of small lymphocytes and histiocytes. Geographic necrosis can also be present. As opposed to the cases of cutaneous HL, solid sheets of large EBV+ cells are seen. The malignant cells show strong (not weak) PAX-5 and CD30 expression, and are also positive for CD20 and CD79a, as opposed to CHL.[104-107]

Lastly, grey zone lymphoma (GZL) has been recently included as a distinct diagnostic category in the WHO classification. GZL displays overlapping features with CHL and primary mediastinal (thymic) large B-cell lymphomas. Sheets of large centroblasts or immunoblasts are seen, in addition to cells with features of RS or RS-variants. Expression of PAX-5, BOB-1, and OCT-2 is variable in GZL, but there is strong expression of at least one B-cell marker (CD20, CD79a, and

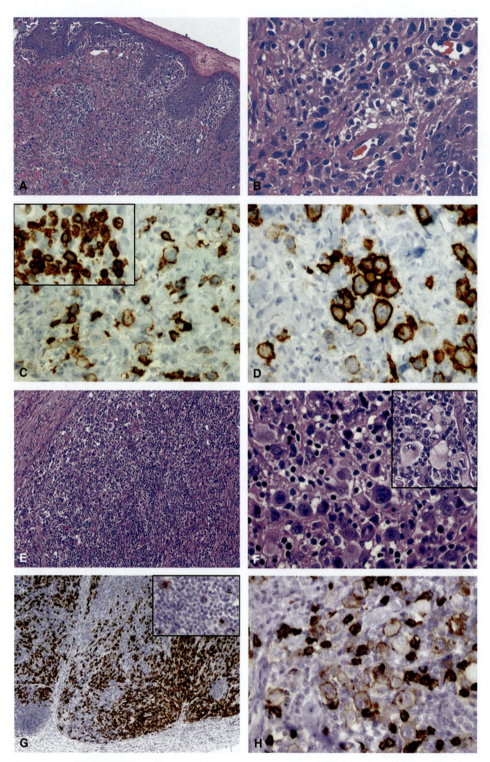

FIGURE 43-6. Cutaneous LyP with Hodgkin-like cells and nodal extension. A. Skin biopsy shows features of LyP with a dense dermal infiltrate composed of **(B)** atypical medium-to-large cells that are positive for CD8 **(C)** and CD3 (*inset*), as well as CD30 **(D)**. **E.** The same patient had an inguinal node containing a pleomorphic infiltrate with sinusoidal infiltration by **(F)** large Hodgkin-like cells that were positive for CD30 **(G)**, CD15 (*inset*), and CD8 **(H)**. (From Eberle FC, Mani H, Jaffe ES. Histopathology of Hodgkin's lymphoma. *Cancer J.* 2009;15:129-137, with permission.)

PAX-5). CD30 is positive, and there is variable expression of CD45 and CD15.[108,110] We have recently reported the occurrence of this entity in the skin via direct extension from a locally affected lymph node.[111]

Patients with CHL might develop granulomatous slack skin[55,56] or alopecia mucinosa/follicular mucinosis.[57] Granulomatous slack skin is a rare variant of mycosis fungoides with characteristic clinical findings of pendulous masses

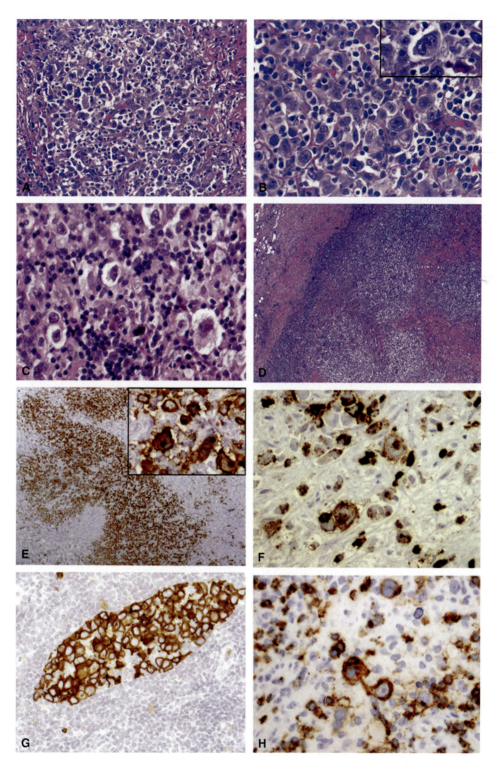

FIGURE 43-7. CD30-positive LPD with Hodgkin-like cells mimicking CHL in a lymph node. A and **B.** Tumor cells infiltrate in sheets and show variability in size, irregular nuclear contours, vesicular chromatin, and prominent nucleoli (*inset*) reminiscent of RS cells. **C.** Lacunar-like cells can be seen in some cases. **D.** Thickened capsule and broad bands of fibrosis can be seen, mimicking CHL, nodular sclerosis subtype. **E.** CD30 highlights the tumor cells forming nodular aggregates divided by dense fibrosis and (*inset*) the variability in cell size of the tumor cells. **F.** Hodgkin-like cells are positive for CD15 but negative for PAX-5 (not shown). **G.** Sinusoidal infiltration. **H.** Tumor cells are positive for T-cell–associated markers such as CD2. (From Eberle FC, Mani H, Jaffe ES. Histopathology of Hodgkin's lymphoma. *Cancer J.* 2009;15:129-137, with permission.)

in the axilla and groin (see Chapter 12). Histologically, it shows a dense, diffuse lymphohistiocytic infiltrate in the dermis with giant cells that enact elastophagocytosis. Follicular mucinosis shows mucinous degeneration of the follicular outer-root sheath. Perifollicular or intrafollicular lymphocytes with eosinophils can be seen. The presence of atypical folliculotropic T lymphocytes raises the differential diagnosis of folliculotropic mycosis fungoides (see Chapter 42).

Hodgkin-like cells had been also described in rare cases of cutaneous, nodal, and extranodal B-cell lymphoproliferations. Cases of primary cutaneous and nodal follicle center lymphomas, T-cell/histiocyte-rich large B-cell lymphoma, B-cell chronic lymphocytic leukemia, and transformed marginal zone lymphoma in the larynx had been shown to harbor CD30+ RS-like cells with variable CD15 staining.[112-115] These lymphomas, however, are rich in B-cells, strongly express CD20, and lack the mixed inflammatory background of eosinophils, neutrophils, and plasma cells typical of CHL.

Finally, reactive inflammatory conditions with enriched CD30+ immunoblasts might also enter the differential diagnosis and include pseudolymphomatous drug reactions, nodular scabies, atopic dermatitis, and infections.[20]

CAPSULE SUMMARY

- HL accounts for about 15% to 30% of all lymphomas. There are two clinicopathologic variants: CHL (90%-95% of cases) and NLPHL (3%-8% of cases).
- The commonest site of involvement is cervical lymph nodes.
- EBV is detected in 25% to 75% of CHL; NLPHL is generally considered EBV negative.
- Cutaneous dissemination is rare and only associated with CHL, not with NLPHL.
- Nodular sclerosis variant is the commonest subtype of CHL presenting in the skin.
- **Clinical:** Single or agminated papules and plaques on the chest, axilla corresponding to drainage areas of affected lymph nodes. Reactive dermatoses in up to 50% of patients.
- **Histopathology:** Nodular and diffuse dermal infiltrates frequently involving the subcutis. Rare, scattered RS cells and variants in the background of reactive lymphocytes, histiocytes, neutrophils, and eosinophils.
- **Immunophenotype:** RS cells—CD30+CD15+PAX-5+. Less frequent and weak expression of other B-cell markers include CD20, OCT-2, and BOB-1. CD45, CD79a, ALK, and EMA are usually negative.
- **Genetics and molecular findings:** Clonal Ig rearrangement in most cases. Lack of recurrent chromosomal translocations. Amplification of the *REL* gene on chromosome 2p13 in 46% of cases. Constitutive NF-κB activation, with frequent inactivating mutations in *IκBα* and *TNFAIP3* genes.
- **Cell of origin:** Germinal center B-cell with crippled Ig transcription. Mature, postthymic peripheral T-cell in very rare instances.
- **Differential diagnosis:** CD30+ lymphoproliferative disease, CD30+ transformed mycosis fungoides, rare B-cell lymphomas, and CD30+ pseudolymphomas.

References

1. Stein H, Delsol G, Pileri S, et al. *Classical Hodgkin Lymphoma*. International Agency for Research on Cancer; 2008.
2. Morton LM, Wang SS, Devesa SS, et al. Lymphoma incidence patterns by WHO subtype in the United States, 1992-2001. *Blood*. 2006;107:265-276.
3. Sant M, Allemani C, Tereanu C, et al. Incidence of hematologic malignancies in Europe by morphologic subtype: results of the HAEMACARE project. *Blood*. 2010;116:3724-3734.
4. Shenoy P, Maggioncalda A, Malik N, et al. Incidence patterns and outcomes for hodgkin lymphoma patients in the United States. *Adv Hematol*. 2011;2011:725219.
5. Hjalgrim H, Askling J, Sorensen P, et al. Risk of Hodgkin's disease and other cancers after infectious mononucleosis. *J Natl Cancer Inst*. 2000;92:1522-1528.
6. Jacobson CA, Abramson JS. HIV-associated Hodgkin's Lymphoma: prognosis and therapy in the era of cART. *Adv Hematol*. 2012;2012:507257.
7. Lanoy E, Rosenberg PS, Fily F, et al. HIV-associated Hodgkin lymphoma during the first months on combination antiretroviral therapy. *Blood*. 2011;118:44-49.
8. Rowlings PA, Curtis RE, Passweg JR, et al. Increased incidence of Hodgkin's disease after allogeneic bone marrow transplantation. *J Clin Oncol*. 1999;17:3122-3127.
9. Flavell KJ, Linford JA, Flavell JR, et al. Detection of Epstein–Barr virus in archival Hodgkin's disease specimens. *Mol Pathol*. 2000;53:162.
10. Flavell KJ, Murray PG. Hodgkin's disease and the Epstein–Barr virus. *Mol Pathol*. 2000;53:262-269.
11. Huppmann AR, Nicolae A, Slack GW, et al. EBV may be expressed in the LP cells of nodular lymphocyte-predominant Hodgkin lymphoma (NLPHL) in both children and adults. *Am J Surg Pathol*. 2014;38:316-324.
12. Carbone A, Spina M, Gloghini A, et al. Classical Hodgkin's lymphoma arising in different host's conditions: pathobiology parameters, therapeutic options, and outcome. *Am J Hematol*. 2011;86:170-179.
13. Weinreb M, Day PJ, Niggli F, et al. The consistent association between Epstein–Barr virus and Hodgkin's disease in children in Kenya. *Blood*. 1996;87:3828-3836.
14. Weinreb M, Day PJ, Niggli F, et al. The role of Epstein–Barr virus in Hodgkin's disease from different geographical areas. *Arch Dis Child*. 1996;74:27-31.
15. Aldinucci D, Borghese C, Casagrande N. Formation of the immunosuppressive microenvironment of classic hodgkin lymphoma and therapeutic approaches to counter it. *Int J Mol Sci*. 2019;20(10):2416. doi:10.3390/ijms20102416.
16. Shanbhag S, Ambinder RF. Hodgkin lymphoma: a review and update on recent progress. *CA Cancer J Clin*. 2018;68(2):116-132. doi:10.3322/caac.21438
17. Connors JM, Cozen W, Steidl C, et al. Hodgkin lymphoma. *Nat Rev Dis Primers*. 2020;6(1):61. doi:10.1038/s41572-020-0189-6
18. Smith JL Jr, Butler JJ. Skin involvement in Hodgkin's disease. *Cancer*. 1980;45:354-361.
19. Rubenstein M, Duvic M. Cutaneous manifestations of Hodgkin's disease. *Int J Dermatol*. 2006;45(3):251-256. doi:10.1111/j.1365-4632.2006.02675.x
20. Introcaso CE, Kantor J, Porter DL, et al. Cutaneous Hodgkin's disease. *J Am Acad Dermatol*. 2008;58:(2):295-298. doi:10.1016/j.jaad.2005.11.1055
21. Benninghoff DL, Medina A, Alexander LL, et al. The mode of spread of Hodgkin's disease to the skin. *Cancer*. 1970;26:1135-1140.
22. Gordon RA, Lookingbill DP, Abt AB. Skin infiltration in Hodgkin's disease. *Arch Dermatol*. 1980;116:1038-1040.
23. Silverman CL, Strayer DS, Wasserman TH. Cutaneous Hodgkin's disease. *Arch Dermatol*. 1982;118:918-921.
24. Tassies D, Sierra J, Montserrat E, et al. Specific cutaneous involvement in Hodgkin's disease. *Hematol Oncol*. 1992;10:75-79.
25. White RM, Patterson JW. Cutaneous involvement in Hodgkin's disease. *Cancer*. 1985;55:1136-1145.

26. Fernandez-Flores A. The early reports on cutaneous involvement by Hodgkin lymphoma. *Am J Dermatopathol.* 2009;31:853-854.
27. Cerroni L, Beham-Schmid C, Kerl H. Cutaneous Hodgkin's disease: an immunohistochemical analysis. *J Cutan Pathol.* 1995;22:229-235.
28. Chang KL, Kamel OW, Arber DA, Horyd ID, Weiss LM. Pathologic features of nodular lymphocyte predominance Hodgkin's disease in extranodal sites. *Am J Surg Pathol.* 1995;19(11):1313-1324. doi:10.1097/00000478-199511000-00012
29. Gru AA, Bacchi CE, Pulitzer M, et al. Secondary skin involvement in classic Hodgkin lymphoma: results of an international collaborative cutaneous lymphoma working group study of 25 patients. *J Cutan Pathol.* 2021;48(11):1367-1378. doi:10.1111/cup.14077
30. Guitart J, Fretzin D. Skin as the primary site of Hodgkin's disease: a case report of primary cutaneous Hodgkin's disease and review of its relationship with non-Hodgkin's lymphoma. *Am J Dermatopathol.* 1998;20:218-222.
31. Kumar S, Kingma DW, Weiss WB, et al. Primary cutaneous Hodgkin's disease with evolution to systemic disease. Association with the Epstein–Barr virus. *Am J Surg Pathol.* 1996;20:754-759.
32. Mukesh M, Shuttleworth D, Murray P. Primary cutaneous Hodgkin's lymphoma. *Clin Exp Dermatol.* 2009;34:e673-e675.
33. Sioutos N, Kerl H, Murphy SB, et al. Primary cutaneous Hodgkin's disease. Unique clinical, morphologic, and immunophenotypic findings. *Am J Dermatopathol.* 1994;16:2-8.
34. Llamas-Velasco M, Fraga J, Perez-Gala S, et al. Specific skin infiltration as first sign of localized stage Hodgkin's lymphoma involving an epitrochlear node. *Am J Dermatopathol.* 2015;37:499-502.
35. Khalifeh I, Hughey LC, Huang CC, et al. Solitary plaque on the scalp as a primary manifestation of Hodgkin lymphoma: a case report and review of the literature. *J Cutan Pathol.* 2009;36(suppl 1):80-85.
36. De Grip A, Schofield JB, Shotton JC. An unusual cutaneous presentation of Hodgkin's disease. *J Laryngol Otol.* 1999;113:765-768.
37. Erkilic S, Erbagci Z, Kocer NE, et al. Cutaneous involvement in Hodgkin's lymphoma: report of two cases. *J Dermatol.* 2004;31:330-334.
38. Jain S, Nigam S, Kumar N, et al. Cutaneous relapse in Hodgkin's disease: a case report. *Acta Cytol.* 2005;49:191-194.
39. Dhull AK, Soni A, Kaushal V. Hodgkin's lymphoma with cutaneous involvement. *BMJ Case Rep.* 2012;2012:bcr2012007599.
40. Marque M, Girard C, Bessis D, et al. Acute onset Hodgkin's disease following Lyell's syndrome. [Article in French]. *Ann Dermatol Venereol.* 2007;134:767-770.
41. Bartus CL, Parker SR. Hodgkin lymphoma presenting as generalized pruritus in an adolescent. *Cutis.* 2011;87:169-172.
42. Schoeffler A, Levy E, Weinborn M, et al. Stevens-Johnson syndrome and Hodgkin's disease: a fortuitous association or paraneoplastic syndrome? [Article in French]. *Ann Dermatol Venereol.* 2014;141:134-140.
43. Ackerman AB, Lantis LR. Acanthosis nigricans associated with Hodgkin's disease. Concurrent remission and exacerbation. *Arch Dermatol.* 1967;95:202-205.
44. Ghislain PD, Roussel S, Marot L, et al. Acquired ichthyosis disclosing Hodgkin's disease. Simultaneous recurrence. [Article in French]. *Presse Med.* 2002;31:1126-1128.
45. Sanli HE, Kocyigit P, Arica E, et al. Granuloma annulare on herpes zoster scars in a Hodgkin's disease patient following autologous peripheral stem cell transplantation. *J Eur Acad Dermatol Venereol.* 2006;20:314-317.
46. Garg S, Mishra S, Tondon R, et al. Hodgkin's lymphoma presenting as alopecia. *Int J Trichology.* 2012;4:169-171.
47. Dadban A, Slama B, Azzedine A, et al. Widespread granuloma annulare and Hodgkin's disease. *Clin Exp Dermatol.* 2008;33:465-468.
48. Macaya A, Servitje O, Moreno A, et al. Cutaneous granulomas as the first manifestation of Hodgkin's disease. *Eur J Dermatol.* 2003;13:299-301.
49. Kaudewitz P, Stein H, Plewig G, et al. Hodgkin's disease followed by lymphomatoid papulosis. Immunophenotypic evidence for a close relationship between lymphomatoid papulosis and Hodgkin's disease. *J Am Acad Dermatol.* 1990;22:999-1006.
50. Caya JG, Choi H, Tieu TM, et al. Hodgkin's disease followed by mycosis fungoides in the same patient. Case report and literature review. *Cancer.* 1984;53:463-467.
51. Clement M, Bhakri H, Monk B, et al. Mycosis fungoides and Hodgkin's disease. *J R Soc Med.* 1984;77:1037-1039.
52. Davis TH, Morton CC, Miller-Cassman R, et al. Hodgkin's disease, lymphomatoid papulosis, and cutaneous T-cell lymphoma derived from a common T-cell clone. *N Engl J Med.* 1992;326:1115-1122.
53. Simrell CR, Boccia RV, Longo DL, et al. Coexisting Hodgkin's disease and mycosis fungoides. Immunohistochemical proof of its existence. *Arch Pathol Lab Med.* 1986;110:1029-1034.
54. Gru AA, Lu D. Concurrent malignant melanoma and cutaneous involvement by classical Hodgkin lymphoma (CHL) in a 63 year-old man. *Diagn Pathol.* 2013;8:135.
55. DeGregorio R, Fenske NA, Glass LF. Granulomatous slack skin: a possible precursor of Hodgkin's disease. *J Am Acad Dermatol.* 1995;33:1044-1047.
56. Noto G, Pravata G, Miceli S, et al. Granulomatous slack skin: report of a case associated with Hodgkin's disease and a review of the literature. *Br J Dermatol.* 1994;131:275-279.
57. Stewart M, Smoller BR. Follicular mucinosis in Hodgkin's disease: a poor prognostic sign?. *J Am Acad Dermatol.* 1991;24:784-785.
58. Zanelli M, Ricci S, Sanguedolce F, et al. Cutaneous localization of classic Hodgkin lymphoma associated with mycosis fungoides: report of a rare event and review of the literature. *Life.* 2021;11(10):1069.
59. Chen Y, Nong L, Li X, Wang Y. Cutaneous composite lymphoma of mycosis fungoides and Hodgkin lymphoma: response to sequential therapy. *J Cutan Pathol.* 2020;47(9):829-833.
60. Eberle FC, Mani H, Jaffe ES. Histopathology of Hodgkin's lymphoma. *Cancer J.* 2009;15:129-137.
61. Cho RJ, McCalmont TH, Ai WZ, et al. Use of an expanded immunohistochemical panel to distinguish cutaneous Hodgkin lymphoma from histopathologic imitators. *J Cutan Pathol.* 2012;39:651-658.
62. Steidl C, Lee T, Shah SP, et al. Tumor-associated macrophages and survival in classic Hodgkin's lymphoma. *N Engl J Med.* 2010;362:875-885.
63. Kuppers R, Rajewsky K, Zhao M, et al. Hodgkin disease: hodgkin and Reed–Sternberg cells picked from histological sections show clonal immunoglobulin gene rearrangements and appear to be derived from B cells at various stages of development. *Proc Natl Acad Sci U S A.* 1994;91:10962-10966.

64. Marafioti T, Hummel M, Foss HD, et al. Hodgkin and Reed–Sternberg cells represent an expansion of a single clone originating from a germinal center B-cell with functional immunoglobulin gene rearrangements but defective immunoglobulin transcription. *Blood.* 2000;95:1443-1450.
65. Tapia G, Sanz C, Mate JL, et al. Improved clonality detection in Hodgkin lymphoma using the BIOMED-2-based heavy and kappa chain assay: a paraffin-embedded tissue study. *Histopathology.* 2012;60:768-773.
66. Muschen M, Rajewsky K, Brauninger A, et al. Rare occurrence of classical Hodgkin's disease as a T cell lymphoma. *J Exp Med.* 2000;191:387-394.
67. Atkin NB. Cytogenetics of Hodgkin's disease. *Cytogenet Cell Genet.* 1998;80:23-27.
68. Rowley JD. Chromosomes in Hodgkin's disease. *Cancer Treat Rep.* 1982;66:639-643.
69. Joos S, Kupper M, Ohl S, et al. Genomic imbalances including amplification of the tyrosine kinase gene JAK2 in CD30+ Hodgkin cells. *Cancer Res.* 2000;60:549-552.
70. Joos S, Menz CK, Wrobel G, et al. Classical Hodgkin lymphoma is characterized by recurrent copy number gains of the short arm of chromosome 2. *Blood.* 2002;99:1381-1387.
71. Martin-Subero JI, Gesk S, Harder L, et al. Recurrent involvement of the REL and BCL11A loci in classical Hodgkin lymphoma. *Blood.* 2002;99:1474-1477.
72. Gilmore TD, Gerondakis S. The c-Rel transcription factor in development and disease. *Genes Cancer.* 2011;2:695-711.
73. Kuppers R. Molecular biology of Hodgkin lymphoma. *Hematology Am Soc Hematol Educ Program.* 2009;2009:491-496.
74. Cabannes E, Khan G, Aillet F, et al. Mutations in the IkBa gene in Hodgkin's disease suggest a tumour suppressor role for IkappaBalpha. *Oncogene.* 1999;18:3063-3070.
75. Izban KF, Ergin M, Huang Q, et al. Characterization of NF-kappaB expression in Hodgkin's disease: inhibition of constitutively expressed NF-kappaB results in spontaneous caspase-independent apoptosis in Hodgkin and Reed-Sternberg cells. *Mod Pathol.* 2001;14:297-310.
76. Kuppers R, Engert A, Hansmann ML. Hodgkin lymphoma. *J Clin Invest.* 2012;122:3439-3447.
77. Weniger MA, Melzner I, Menz CK, et al. Mutations of the tumor suppressor gene SOCS-1 in classical Hodgkin lymphoma are frequent and associated with nuclear phospho-STAT5 accumulation. *Oncogene.* 2006;25:2679-2684.
78. Wienand K, Chapuy B, Stewart C, et al. Genomic analyses of flow-sorted Hodgkin Reed-Sternberg cells reveal complementary mechanisms of immune evasion. *Blood Adv.* 2019;3:4065-4080.
79. Camus V, Stamatoullas A, Mareschal S, et al. Detection and prognostic value of recurrent exportin 1 mutations in tumor and cell-free circulating DNA of patients with classical Hodgkin lymphoma. *Haematologica.* 2016;101:1094-1101. doi:10.3324/haematol.2016.145102
80. Tiacci E, Ladewig EM, Schiavoni G, et al. Pervasive mutations of JAK-STAT pathway genes in classical Hodgkin lymphoma. *Blood.* 2018;131:2454-2465. doi:10.1182/blood-2017-11-814913
81. Green MR, Monti S, Rodig SJ, et al. Integrative analysis reveals selective 9p24.1 amplification, increased PD-1 ligand expression, and further induction via JAK2 in nodular sclerosing Hodgkin lymphoma and primary mediastinal large B-cell lymphoma. *Blood.* 2010;116:3268-3277.
82. Roemer MGM, Redd RA, Cader FZ, et al. Major histocompatibility complex class II and programmed death ligand 1 expression predict outcome after programmed death 1 blockade in classic hodgkin lymphoma. *J Clin Oncol.* 2018;36:942-950.
83. Reichel J, Chadburn A, Rubinstein PG, et al. Flow sorting and exome sequencing reveal the oncogenome of primary Hodgkin and Reed-Sternberg cells. *Blood.* 2015;125:1061-1072. doi:10.1182/blood-2014-11-610436
84. Juskevicius D, Lorber T, Gsponer J, et al. Distinct genetic evolution patterns of relapsing diffuse large B-cell lymphoma revealed by genome-wide copy number aberration and targeted sequencing analysis. *Leukemia.* 2016;30:2385-2395. doi:10.1038/leu.2016.135
85. Spina V, Bruscaggin A, Cuccaro A, et al. Circulating tumor DNA reveals genetics, clonal evolution, and residual disease in classical Hodgkin lymphoma. *Blood.* 2018;131:2413-2425. doi:10.1182/blood-2017-11-812073
86. Zhang J, Xu E, Ren C, et al. Genetic ablation of Rbm38 promotes lymphomagenesis in the context of mutant p53 by downregulating PTEN. *Cancer Res.* 2018;78:1511-1521. doi:10.1158/0008-5472.CAN-17-2457
87. Dhiab MB, Ziadi S, Mestiri S, Gacem RB, Ksiaa F, Trimeche M. DNA methylation patterns in EBV-positive and EBV-negative Hodgkin lymphomas. *Cell Oncol.* 2015;38:453-462. doi:10.1007/s13402-015-0242-8
88. Liso A, Capello D, Marafioti T, et al. Aberrant somatic hypermutation in tumor cells of nodular-lymphocyte-predominant and classic Hodgkin lymphoma. *Blood.* 2006;108:1013-1020.
89. Renne C, Martin-Subero JI, Eickernjager M, et al. Aberrant expression of ID2, a suppressor of B-cell-specific gene expression, in Hodgkin's lymphoma. *Am J Pathol.* 2006;169:655-664.
90. Ushmorov A, Leithauser F, Sakk O, et al. Epigenetic processes play a major role in B-cell-specific gene silencing in classical Hodgkin lymphoma. *Blood.* 2006;107:2493-2500.
91. Kanzler H, Kuppers R, Hansmann ML, et al. Hodgkin and Reed–Sternberg cells in Hodgkin's disease represent the outgrowth of a dominant tumor clone derived from (crippled) germinal center B cells. *J Exp Med.* 1996;184:1495-1505.
92. Reddi DM, Sebastian S, Wang E. Acquisition of CD30 and CD15 accompanied with simultaneous loss of all pan-T-cell antigens in a case of histological transformation of mycosis fungoides with involvement of regional lymph node: an immunophenotypic alteration resembling classical Hodgkin lymphoma. *Am J Dermatopathol.* 2015;37(3):249-253. doi:10.1097/DAD.0b013e31828cf3d3
93. Eberle FC, Song JY, Xi L, et al. Nodal involvement by cutaneous CD30-positive T-cell lymphoma mimicking classical Hodgkin lymphoma. *Am J Surg Pathol.* 2012;36(5):716-725. doi:10.1097/PAS.0b013e3182487158
94. Subhawong AP, Subhawong TK, Ali SZ. Large cell transformation of mycosis fungoides on fine needle aspiration: an unusual case mimicking classical Hodgkin lymphoma. *Acta Cytol.* 2012;56(3):321-324. doi:10.1159/000335570
95. O'Malley DP, Dogan A, Fedoriw Y, Medeiros LJ, Ok CY, Salama ME. American registry of pathology expert opinions: immunohistochemical evaluation of classic Hodgkin lymphoma. *Ann Diagn Pathol.* 2019;39:105-110. doi:10.1016/j.anndiagpath.2019.02.001
96. Dojcinov SD, Venkataraman G, Raffeld M, Pittaluga S, Jaffe ES. EBV positive mucocutaneous ulcer—a study of 26 cases associated with various sources of immunosuppression. *Am J Surg Pathol.* 2010;34(3):405-417. doi:10.1097/PAS.0b013e3181cf8622

97. Ikeda T, Gion Y, Yoshino T, Sato Y. A review of EBV-positive mucocutaneous ulcers focusing on clinical and pathological aspects. *J Clin Exp Hematop*. 2019;59(2):64-71. doi:10.3960/jslrt.18039
98. Prieto-Torres L, Erana I, Gil-Redondo R, et al. The spectrum of EBV-positive mucocutaneous ulcer: a study of 9 cases. *Am J Surg Pathol*. 2019;43(2):201-210. doi:10.1097/PAS.0000000000001186
99. Willemze R, Cerroni L, Kempf W, et al. The 2018 update of the WHO-EORTC classification for primary cutaneous lymphomas. *Blood*. 2019;133(16):1703-1714. doi:10.1182/blood-2018-11-881268
100. Gru AA, Jaffe ES. Cutaneous EBV-related lymphoproliferative disorders. *Semin Diagn Pathol*. 2017;34(1):60-75. doi:10.1053/j.semdp.2016.11.003
101. Ikeda T, Gion Y, Sakamoto M, et al. Clinicopathological analysis of 34 Japanese patients with EBV-positive mucocutaneous ulcer. *Mod Pathol*. 2020;33(12):2437-2448. doi:10.1038/s41379-020-0599-8
102. Dunn C, Nguyen HP, Patel V, et al. Primary cutaneous Hodgkin-like polymorphic post-transplant lymphoproliferative disorder. *J Cutan Pathol*. 2019;46(5):358-362. doi:10.1111/cup.13427
103. Robinson C, Burroughs S, Addis B, Mason J. Cutaneous post-transplant lymphoproliferative disorder with atypical Hodgkin and Reed-Sternberg-like cells. *Histopathology*. 2007;50(3):403-404. doi:10.1111/j.1365-2559.2007.02597.x
104. Castillo JJ, Beltran BE, Miranda RN, Young KH, Chavez JC, Sotomayor EM. EBV-positive diffuse large B-cell lymphoma of the elderly: 2016 update on diagnosis, risk-stratification, and management. *Am J Hematol*. 2016;91(5):529-537. doi:10.1002/ajh.24370
105. Ok CY, Papathomas TG, Medeiros LJ, Young KH. EBV-positive diffuse large B-cell lymphoma of the elderly. *Blood*. 2013;122(3):328-340. doi:10.1182/blood-2013-03-489708
106. Castillo JJ, Beltran BE, Miranda RN, Paydas S, Winer ES, Butera JN. Epstein-barr virus-positive diffuse large B-cell lymphoma of the elderly: what we know so far. *Oncologist*. 2011;16(1):87-96. doi:10.1634/theoncologist.2010-0213
107. Park S, Lee J, Ko YH, et al. The impact of Epstein-Barr virus status on clinical outcome in diffuse large B-cell lymphoma. *Blood*. 2007;110(3):972-978. doi:10.1182/blood-2007-01-067769
108. Swerdlow SH; World Health Organization, International Agency for Research on Cancer. *WHO classification of tumours of haematopoietic and lymphoid tissues*. Revised 4th ed. *World Health Organization Classification of Tumours*. International Agency for Research on Cancer; 2017:585 pages.
109. Parker K, Venkataraman G. Challenges in the diagnosis of gray zone lymphomas. *Surg Pathol Clin*. 2019;12(3):709-718. doi:10.1016/j.path.2019.03.014
110. O'Malley DP, Fedoriw Y, Weiss LM. Distinguishing classical hodgkin lymphoma, gray zone lymphoma, and large B-cell lymphoma: a proposed Scoring System. *Appl Immunohistochem Mol Morphol*. 2016;24(8):535-540. doi:10.1097/PAI.0000000000000236
111. Subtil A, Gru AA. Secondary cutaneous involvement by direct extension in high-grade B-cell lymphomas. *J Cutan Pathol*. 2021;48(4):541-546. doi:10.1111/cup.13798
112. Bayerl MG, Bentley G, Bellan C, et al. Lacunar and Reed-Sternberg-like cells in follicular lymphomas are clonally related to the centrocytic and centroblastic cells as demonstrated by laser capture microdissection. *Am J Clin Pathol*. 2004;122:858-864.
113. Fung EK, Neuhauser TS, Thompson LD. Hodgkin-like transformation of a marginal zone B-cell lymphoma of the larynx. *Ann Diagn Pathol*. 2002;6:61-66.
114. Kanzler H, Kuppers R, Helmes S, et al. Hodgkin and Reed-Sternberg-like cells in B-cell chronic lymphocytic leukemia represent the outgrowth of single germinal-center B-cell-derived clones: potential precursors of Hodgkin and Reed-Sternberg cells in Hodgkin's disease. *Blood*. 2000;95:1023-1031.
115. Marie D, Houda BR, Beatrice V, et al. Primary cutaneous follicle center lymphoma with Hodgkin and Reed-Sternberg-like cells: a new histopathologic variant. *J Cutan Pathol*. 2014;41:797-801.

PART VIII CUTANEOUS REACTIVE INFILTRATES

CHAPTER 44

Pityriasis lichenoides chronica

Emily Y. Chu and Werner Kempf

DEFINITION, CLINICAL PRESENTATION, AND PROGNOSIS

Pityriasis lichenoides chronica (PLC) is a benign, self-limited, diffuse skin eruption composed of discrete red-brown scaly papules (Fig. 44-1). In darker-skinned patients, PLC may present instead with hypopigmented nonscaly macules and patches (Fig. 44-2).[1] Individual lesions typically last from weeks to several months, whereas the eruption persists from months to years in a given patient. PLC is thought to be closely related to a more severe condition, pityriasis lichenoides et varioliformis acuta (PLEVA), also known as Mucha-Habermann disease, and in fact may evolve from this more acute form. It may also arise independently of a preceding PLEVA eruption. Similar to PLEVA/Mucha-Habermann disease, an individual patient affected with PLC often has lesions in all stages of development, from those that are newly erupted to those that are in the resolution phase.

The lesions of PLC are most often diffusely distributed on the trunk and proximal extremities; however, segmental and acral presentations of this condition have been described.[2] The lesions are usually asymptomatic, although rarely patients complain of pruritus. PLC affects both children and adults. The incidence in women and men appears to be equal, without a predilection for one gender.[2]

PLC is felt to be an indolent condition. Progression from PLC to cutaneous lymphoma has been documented in the literature, but this occurs very rarely.[3,4] Resolution of the lesions, which may be spontaneous or aided by the use of topical or systemic medications, typically results in dyspigmentation, either hypo- or hyperpigmentation[5]; scarring is not commonly seen. Interestingly, it has been suggested in the literature that children with PLC tend to have a more difficult course as compared with adults, with higher lesion counts and a greater degree of dyspigmentation.[6] In addition, children may not be as responsive to therapy.

Occasionally, PLC has been reported to arise following use of systemic medications, including the TNF-α inhibitors adalimumab and infliximab.[7-9] PLC has also been associated with viral infections, including HIV and HHV-8.[10,11]

Several therapeutic options exist for the treatment of PLC. Patients may be successfully treated with mid- to high-potency topical steroids. The topical calcineurin inhibitor tacrolimus has also been reported to be effective for cases of PLC, at concentrations of 0.03% and 0.1%, and is particularly useful when a steroid-sparing agent is desired.[10,11]

Ultraviolet light therapy is generally efficacious in the treatment of PLC. A small study of narrow-band ultraviolet B (nbUVB) and psoralen plus ultraviolet A (PUVA) light therapy in patients with pityriasis lichenoides found that, of eight patients treated with nbUVB, seven had a complete response to therapy and one had a partial response (the mean number of treatment sessions was 37), whereas of seven PUVA-treated patients five had a complete response and two had a partial response (the mean number of treatment sessions was 40).[12]

Oral medications commonly used for the treatment of PLC include systemic antibiotics and methotrexate. Macrolide antibiotics including erythromycin and azithromycin as well as tetracycline are commonly utilized in this setting for their anti-inflammatory rather than antimicrobial properties. For children, erythromycin is the preferred treatment over tetracycline, as tetracycline dosing is contraindicated in children younger than 8 years out of concern for its adverse effects on secondary tooth development. Hapa et al[13] recently suggested that treatment duration for erythromycin should be at least 3 months, on the basis of their finding that treatment response rates improved to 83% in month 3 of therapy, compared with 64% and 73% in months 1 and 2, respectively.

Methotrexate has been employed successfully in some persistent cases of PLC. Of note, several cases of TNF inhibitor–induced PLC were reported to respond well to methotrexate.[7,9] Additional therapies to consider for more severe cases of PLC include systemic steroids, intravenous immunoglobulin (IVIG), and cyclosporine.[14,15]

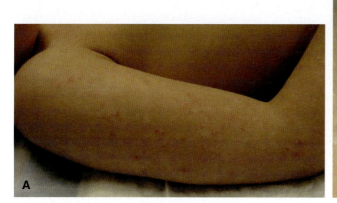
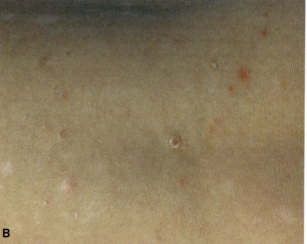

FIGURE 44-1. **A** and **B.** Discrete scaly pink-brown papules on the skin. Lesions in different stages of development can be seen, and hypopigmented macules are observed. (Courtesy of Dr. Leslie Castelo-Soccio.)

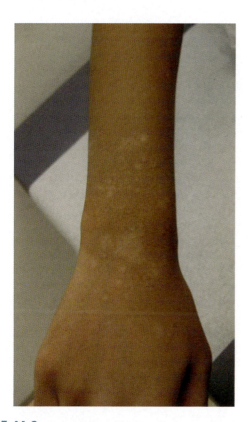

FIGURE 44-2. Hypopigmented nonscaly macules and small patches in a patient with a darker skin type. (Courtesy of Dr. Leslie Castelo-Soccio.)

HISTOPATHOLOGY

Under the microscope, PLC displays both interface lichenoid changes as well as mild spongiosis in the epidermis (Fig. 44-3). Lymphocytes approximate the dermal-epidermal junction, accompanied by basovacuolar change and scattered dyskeratotic keratinocytes in the epidermis. Small intraepidermal lymphocytes with regular nuclear contours are seen. There is variable ortho- and parakeratosis. The dermis typically shows a superficial perivascular lymphocytic infiltrate. Eosinophils are rarely present.[16] Fibrin deposition may be observed within vessel walls, but frank vasculitis is not seen. Other common histologic findings include the presence of extravasated red blood cells and/or melanophages in the upper dermis.

IMMUNOPHENOTYPE

Although PLEVA and PLC are thought to be closely related conditions, or even different manifestations of a single disorder by some,[17] they may manifest different immunophenotypes. The infiltrate of PLEVA has been found to more often display an elevated CD8:CD4 ratio, whereas the T lymphocytes in PLC show a predominance of CD4+ cells rather than CD8+ cells.[17,18] Moreover, T-cell intracellular antigen 1 (TIA-1) is more likely to be expressed in the T lymphocytes of PLEVA, compared with PLC, which shows increased expression of FOXP3, a marker of T regulatory cells.[18] Interestingly, one recent study found that four of 23 cases diagnosed as PLC with a benign clinical course showed a predominantly γδ T-cell phenotype, even though γδ T cells have more traditionally been associated with aggressive lymphomas[19] (Fig. 44-4).

A recent study by Borra et al[20] perhaps offers some meaningful insights into the classification of PL and related conditions. The authors included 66 patients diagnosed as PLEVA, atypical pityriasis lichenoides, lymphomatoid papulosis, and PL-like mycosis fungoides. The classic group of PLEVA did not progress to mycosis fungoides, lacked immunophenotypic aberrations, and showed monoclonal T cells in 46.2% of cases. The cases of atypical pityriasis lichenoides were composed of cases with abnormal phenotype (loss of CD2 and CD4, coexpression of CD4/CD8, expression of CD56, etc.) and had a higher rate of clonal TCR studies (52.6%). Of the 25 patients in this cohort, four showed progression to mycosis fungoides (Fig. 44-5).

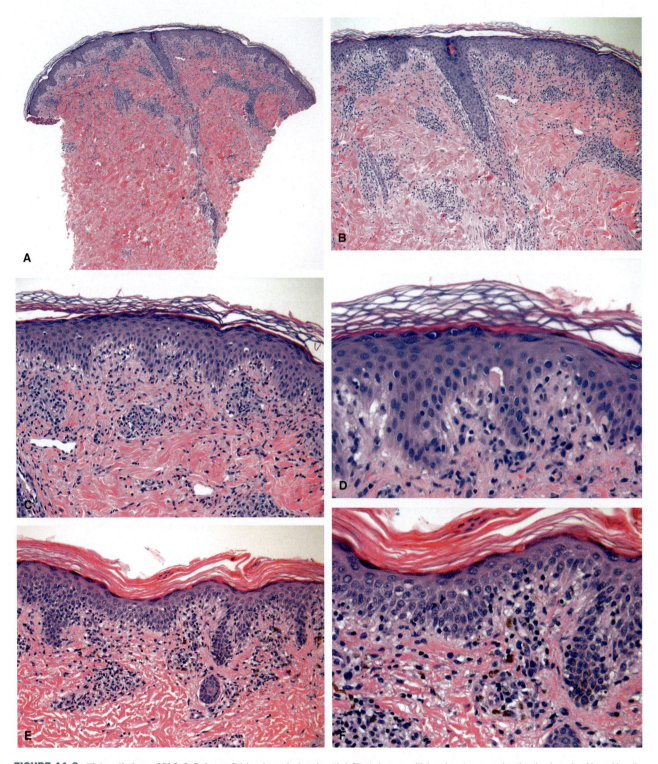

FIGURE 44-3. Histopathology of PLC. A–D. A superficial perivascular lymphocytic infiltrate is seen, with lymphocytes approximating the dermal-epidermal junction accompanied by basovacuolar change and scattered dyskeratotic keratinocytes. The lesional lymphocytes are small in size. Perivascular lymphocytic inflammation is also seen in the upper dermis. **E** and **F.** Parakeratosis and mild spongiosis are common features of PLC, in addition to the interface dermatitis.

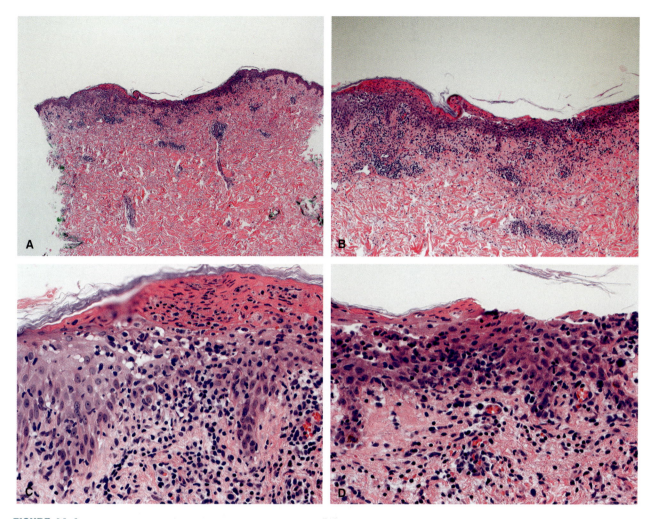

FIGURE 44-4. Histopathology of PL, unusual case. A–D. A band-like infiltrate is present in the superficial papillary and reticular dermis. Focal superficial epidermal necrosis is present. There are vacuolar interface changes and atypical intraepidermal lymphocytes. Superficial red blood cell extravasation is present.

GENETIC AND MOLECULAR FINDINGS

Clonal rearrangement of the T-cell receptor gene may be observed in PLC; on the basis of this finding, PLC has been classified as a T-cell dyscrasia.[21] A study by Magro et al.[17] found evidence of T-cell clonality in 33 of 35 patients with pityriasis lichenoides. The patients studied were interpreted to have either PLEVA or PLC considering both clinical and histopathologic findings, with the majority of the patients classified as having PLC. Other studies have found occasional clonal TCRγ gene rearrangement in their patients with PLC, in 1 of 13 and 3 of 6 patients, respectively.[22,23] By contrast, Kim et al[18] did not detect clonal TCRγ gene rearrangement in any of 13 patients with PLC. The differences in these studies may reflect some of the difficulties in differentiating PLC from early lesions of mycosis fungoides. A recent molecular analysis of TCR rearrangement has been done using next-generation sequencing. Raghavan et al[24] reported 7 of 12 patients (58%) and 9 of 17 biopsy specimens (53%) showed evidence of T-cell clonality. Two patients showed matching TRB clones from different anatomic sites.

DIFFERENTIAL DIAGNOSIS

The histopathologic changes of PLC closely resemble those of PLEVA, as both show lymphocyte exocytosis, interface dermatitis with basovacuolar alteration, mild spongiosis, a superficial lymphocytic infiltrate, and papillary dermal hemorrhage. However, the microscopic findings in PLC are typically more subtle than in PLEVA; the lymphocytic infiltrate of the latter is more intense in both the epidermal and dermal compartments, with a wedge-shaped perivascular lymphocytic inflammation extending into the reticular dermis. In addition, ulceration is not a characteristic observation in PLC but is seen with some frequency in more severe cases of PLEVA, often in conjunction with a serum crust containing neutrophils.

Some variants of mycosis fungoides may be difficult to distinguish from PLC, both clinically and histologically. A recent study detailed four patients with eventual diagnoses of papular mycosis fungoides, all of whom had small reddish-brown papules present between 5 and 25 years.[25] Based on initial clinicopathologic correlation, three of the four patients were initially felt to have pityriasis lichenoides, but additional biopsies in each case demonstrated characteristic findings

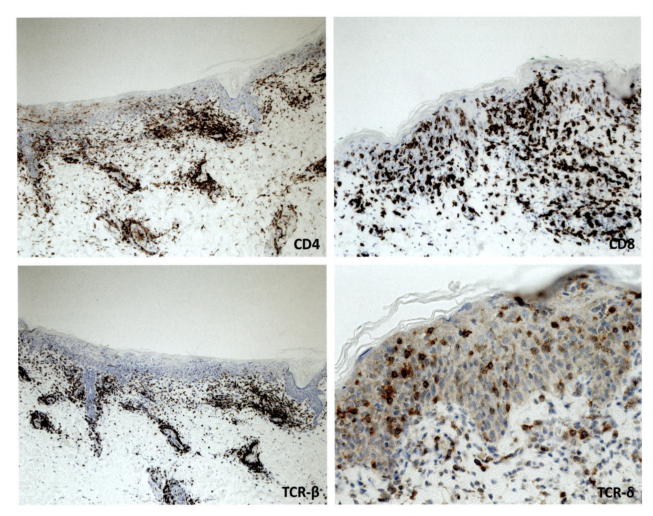

FIGURE 44-5. Histopathology of PL, unusual case. The infiltrate shows a predominance of CD8+ intraepidermal cells. Many of the atypical cells show a TCR-delta phenotype.

of mycosis fungoides on histology, including epidermotropism with lymphocyte atypia and elevated CD4:CD8 ratios. Hypopigmented mycosis fungoides often demonstrates overlapping histologic findings with PLC, and in these cases clinicopathologic correlation is essential.

References

1. Lane TN, Parker SS. Pityriasis lichenoides chronica in black patients. *Cutis*. 2010;85(3):125-129.
2. Bowers S, Warshaw EM. Pityriasis lichenoides and its subtypes. *J Am Acad Dermatol*. 2006;55(4):557-572; quiz 573-576.
3. Thomson KF, Whittaker SJ, Russell-Jones R, et al. Childhood cutaneous T-cell lymphoma in association with pityriasis lichenoides chronica. *Br J Dermatol*. 1999;141(6):1146-1148.
4. Tomasini D, Zampatti C, Palmedo G, et al. Cytotoxic mycosis fungoides evolving from pityriasis lichenoides chronica in a seventeen-year-old girl. Report of a case. *Dermatology*. 2002;205(2):176-179.
5. Koh WL, Koh MJ, Tay YK. Pityriasis lichenoides in an asian population. *Int J Dermatol*. 2013;52(12):1495-1499.
6. Wahie S, Hiscutt E, Natarajan S, et al. Pityriasis lichenoides: the differences between children and adults. *Br J Dermatol*. 2007;157(5):941-945.
7. Lopez-Ferrer A, Puig L, Moreno G, et al. Pityriasis lichenoides chronica induced by infliximab, with response to methotrexate. *Eur J Dermatol*. 2010;20(4):511-512.
8. Newell EL, Jain S, Stephens C, et al. Infliximab-induced pityriasis lichenoides chronica in a patient with psoriasis. *J Eur Acad Dermatol Venereol*. 2009;23(2):230-231.
9. Said BB, Kanitakis J, Graber I, et al. Pityriasis lichenoides chronica induced by adalimumab therapy for Crohn's disease: report of 2 cases successfully treated with methotrexate. *Inflamm Bowel Dis*. 2010;16(6):912-913.
10. Mallipeddi R, Evans AV. Refractory pityriasis lichenoides chronica successfully treated with topical tacrolimus. *Clin Exp Dermatol*. 2003;28(4):456-458.
11. Simon D, Boudny C, Nievergelt H, et al. Successful treatment of pityriasis lichenoides with topical tacrolimus. *Br J Dermatol*. 2004;150(5):1033-1035.
12. Farnaghi F, Seirafi H, Ehsani AH, et al. Comparison of the therapeutic effects of narrow band UVB vs. PUVA in patients with pityriasis lichenoides. *J Eur Acad Dermatol Venereol*. 2011;25(8):913-916.
13. Hapa A, Ersoy-Evans S, Karaduman A. Childhood pityriasis lichenoides and oral erythromycin. *Pediatr Dermatol*. 2012;29(6):719-724.

14. Garcia B, Connelly EA, Newbury R, et al. Pityriasis lichenoides and idiopathic thrombocytopenic purpura in a young girl. *Pediatr Dermatol*. 2006;23(1):21-23.
15. Griffiths JK. Successful long-term use of cyclosporin A in HIV-induced pityriasis lichenoides chronica. *J Acquir Immune Defic Syndr Hum Retrovirol*. 1998;18(4):396-397.
16. Sharon VR, Konia TH, Barr KL, et al. Assessment of the "no eosinophils" rule: are eosinophils truly absent in pityriasis lichenoides, connective tissue disease, and graft-vs.-host disease? *J Cutan Pathol*. 2012;39(4):413-418.
17. Magro C, Crowson AN, Kovatich A, et al. Pityriasis lichenoides: a clonal T-cell lymphoproliferative disorder. *Hum Pathol*. 2002;33(8):788-795.
18. Kim JE, Yun WJ, Mun SK, et al. Pityriasis lichenoides et varioliformis acuta and pityriasis lichenoides chronica: comparison of lesional T-cell subsets and investigation of viral associations. *J Cutan Pathol*. 2011;38(8):649-656.
19. Martinez-Escala ME, Sidiropoulos M, Deonizio J, et al. γδ T-cell-rich variants of pityriasis lichenoides and lymphomatoid papulosis: benign cutaneous disorders to be distinguished from aggressive cutaneous γδ T-cell lymphomas. *Br J Dermatol*. 2015;172(2):372-379.
20. Borra T, Custrin A, Saggini A, et al. Pityriasis lichenoides, atypical pityriasis lichenoides, and related conditions: A study of 66 cases. *Am J Surg Pathol*. 2018;42(8):1101-1112.
21. Guitart J, Magro C. Cutaneous T-cell lymphoid dyscrasia: a unifying term for idiopathic chronic dermatoses with persistent T-cell clones. *Arch Dermatol*. 2007;143(7):921-932.
22. Shieh S, Mikkola DL, Wood GS. Differentiation and clonality of lesional lymphocytes in pityriasis lichenoides chronica. *Arch Dermatol*. 2001;137(3):305-308.
23. Weinberg JM, Kristal L, Chooback L, et al. The clonal nature of pityriasis lichenoides. *Arch Dermatol*. 2002;138(8):1063-1067.
24. Raghavan SS, Wang JY, Gru AA, et al. Next-generation sequencing confirms T-cell clonality in a subset of pediatric pityriasis lichenoides. *J Cutan Pathol*. 2022;49(3):252-260.
25. de Unamuno Bustos B, Ferriols AP, Sanchez RB, et al. Adult pityriasis lichenoides-like mycosis fungoides: a clinical variant of mycosis fungoides. *Int J Dermatol*. 2014;53(11):1331-1338.

CHAPTER 45

Jessner lymphocytic infiltrate and tumid lupus erythematosus

Juanita Duran and Jose A. Plaza

DEFINITION

Lymphocytic infiltrate of the skin (LIS) (also known as Jessner lymphocytic infiltrate of the skin) and tumid lupus erythematosus (TLE) are uncommon and benign entities with overlapping clinical and histopathological features.[1,2] Owing to their shared traits, their characterization as separate entities has been controversial for decades. Some authors hypothesize they may represent the same disease covering a continued spectrum of changes.[1,3-5] LIS is a term that has been used to define papular lesions that involve sun-exposed areas such as the head and neck. It was initially described under the term cutaneous lymphoid hyperplasia along with lymphocytoma cutis and lymphomas; there is still debate as to whether this entity is a unique disease or part of a spectrum of cutaneous diseases, including lupus erythematosus (LE), polymorphous light eruption (PMLE), reticular erythematous mucinosis (REM), and possibly lymphoma.[1,2,6,7]

TLE has been classically recognized by most, under the Gilliam nomenclature and classification system, as one of the forms of chronic cutaneous lupus erythematosus.[8,9] Owing to its specific clinical and histological properties, characteristic course, and favorable prognosis it was proposed, in the Duesseldorf classification (2004), to subcategorize it under its own group as intermittent cutaneous lupus erythematosus.[9-11] In contrast to acute and subacute lupus-specific cutaneous lesions, TLE is infrequently associated with systemic lupus erythematosus (SLE).[12,13] The latter is also true for LIS.[14] Owing to this weak association with systemic involvement and a relative lack of serologic abnormalities in patients with TLE, some consider TLE to be a separate entity from lupus. TLE and LIS are mostly limited to the dermis, rarely associated with serologic titers, demonstrate photosensitivity (and respond to antimalarials), and leave no scarring or atrophy.[1,3,5] Owing to their many similarities, we will approach these entities together.

EPIDEMIOLOGY

LIS and TLE are uncommon skin disorders for which the literature lacks precise and up-to-date epidemiologic data. Onset of disease is usually seen in middle-aged adults (30-50 years of age), without gender bias (or slight female predominance according to some authors).[3,12,15,16] Both disorders have been rarely reported in children.[17,18]

ETIOLOGY

One of the proposed initiating stimuli in the pathophysiologic mechanism of these entities involves the presence of modified skin antigens due to the exposure to ultraviolet radiation (UVR). These antigens elicit an immune reaction by production of interleukins and interferons.[19]

Type I interferons (IFNs) are thought to play a vital role in the pathogenesis of many inflammatory skin diseases, including TLE and LIS.[20,21] These IFNs are known to be produced by plasmacytoid dendritic cells (PDCs). They aid in the amplification of the inflammatory process by induction of IFN-inducible chemokines and recruitment of activated leukocytes into the skin lesions. Two common IFN-inducible ligands described in TLE and LIS are CXCL9 and CXCL10. Interaction with their related receptor CXCR3 has been reported as at least one of the driving activating and maintenance pathways of the inflammatory process.[20,21] The expression of these proteins has been described to reflect the typical inflammatory pattern of TLE and LIS (perivascular and periadnexal).[5,20,21] A specific cascade of adhesion molecules is simultaneously enhanced helping with cell migration to the sites of injury. Some adhesion molecules reported by different authors include (1) intercellular adhesion molecule-1 (ICAM-1) and vascular adhesion molecule-1 (VCAM-1), upregulated by endothelial cell activation; (2) E-selectin, increases its levels secondary to cytokine stimulation, such as tumor necrosis factor α; (3) P-selectin, becomes exposed on endothelial cells by proinflammatory mediators, histamine being one of these known intermediaries.[22-24]

The skin-infiltrating/recruited cells, as a result of the proinflammatory cascade, are dominated by T lymphocytes, with the typical distribution of TLE and LIS mentioned above, perivascular and periadnexal.[20-22,25] Skin biopsy specimens from patients with TLE have shown a percentage of T lymphocytes, usually greater than 75%, with variable predominance of CD4$^+$ T cells (CD4:CD8, 1:1-5:1, mean 3:1).[12]

The lymphocytes have mainly a helper/inducer phenotype (CD45RO+), and most aberrantly express the major histocompatibility class II molecule (HLA-DR). Conversely, lymphocytes are predominantly CD8+ T cells in LIS and appear negative to HLA-DR.[12,19,22-24]

Although many details of the etiopathogenesis of TLE and LIS remain elusive, there is no doubt of the pathogenic role of CD4+ CD45RO+ T cells.

CLINICAL FEATURES

Patients with TLE and LIS usually present with asymptomatic erythematous and/or violaceous papules, plaques, or nodules distributed on sun-exposed areas (TLE, predominantly on the face and trunk; LIS, on face and back). The lesions are photo induced, but often the rash does not appear immediately and there may be a delay of a couple of weeks between UVR exposure and onset of the cutaneous symptoms. Both entities demonstrate a chronic or an intermittent/cyclical course, show no epidermal changes, resolve without scarring or atrophy, and lack extracutaneous involvement.[12] Half of patients with TLE and LIS have positive antinuclear antibody titers.[1,12,14] In patients with TLE, the low prevalence of SLE, the relative lack of serologic testing, and the very low prevalence of immunoglobulin deposition within the lesions have made it difficult to know whether TLE represents a variant of LE or a distinct entity. However, the presence of TLE cutaneous lesions in patients with other specific types of cutaneous LE is in favor of it being classified as a form of cutaneous LE. There have been some cases of long-standing TLE and LIS that have been reported to progress into DLE and SCLE.[15,26] TLE has been associated with the use of highly active antiretroviral therapy (HAART) for HIV infection.[27] Also, cases of LIS have been associated with medications, infection, tattoos, or arthropod bites.[28]

HISTOPATHOLOGY

The histopathological characteristics of TLE and LIS are indistinct. They show moderate to dense lymphocytic infiltrates confined to the dermis in a perivascular and periadnexal pattern (Figs. 45-1 and 45-2). The epidermis is generally not compromised, but cases of TLE and LIS with focal epidermal or interface change at the dermal epidermal junction have been reported (Fig. 45-3).[1,12,15] Dermal interstitial mucin has also been identified in both disorders.[1] In cases in which mucin deposition is focal and minimal, it can be highlighted with special stains (eg, alcian blue) (Fig. 45-4). Dermal edema is a finding mostly described in TLE.

IMMUNOPHENOTYPE

Immunohistochemical criteria include a predominance of T cells with a majority of CD4+ cells in TLE (in some cases there is a mixture of both CD4 and CD8+ T cells) and CD8+ in LIS.[12] The presence of PDCs, identified by CD123 and

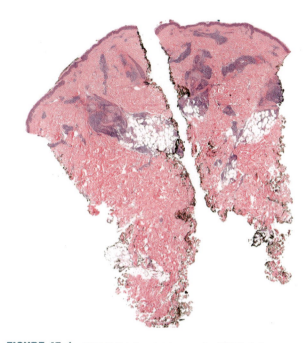

FIGURE 45-1. TLE/LIS: This is a classic example of TLE that shows a superficial and deep perivascular and periadnexal lymphocytic dermatitis.

CD2AP expression, is a useful adjunctive tool to distinguish TLE from several inflammatory skin diseases (including PMLE and lichen planopilaris) and low-grade cutaneous lymphomas. Large clusters of PDC are normally seen in cases of TLE and LIS.[29,30] Direct immunofluorescence (DIF) evaluation is usually negative or nonspecific.[3,12]

DIFFERENTIAL DIAGNOSIS

The main differential diagnoses to consider are PMLE, REM, and pseudolymphoma (Table 45-1).[31,32] PMLE is a common photodermatosis that is usually seen in young females as recurrent, erythematous papules and/or plaques following UVR light exposure. Lesions develop after a latent period of hours to days and commonly resolve within days healing without sequelae. The clinical distinction between PMLE and TLE can be difficult; however, TLE tends to show a delayed reaction after sun exposure and healing takes longer than in PMLE. Histologically, it shows a superficial and deep perivascular lymphohistiocytic infiltrate with characteristic papillary dermal edema, which is often marked (in rare cases can be absent). Owing to the marked papillary dermal edema, it can be associated with subepidermal vesicle formation. The histologic features of TLE are sometimes difficult to distinguish from PMLE. The presence of dermal mucin deposition should favor TLE/LIS, while the presence of subepidermal edema favors PMLE. CD123 may be helpful in distinguishing these two entities, as the clusters of PDC are more frequent and larger in cases of TLE than in PMLE. Most cases of PMLE are negative with DIF, and when immunoreactants are present only weak staining is noted (C3, IgG, IgM may be seen along the basement membrane zone). Careful clinicopathological correlation and serological

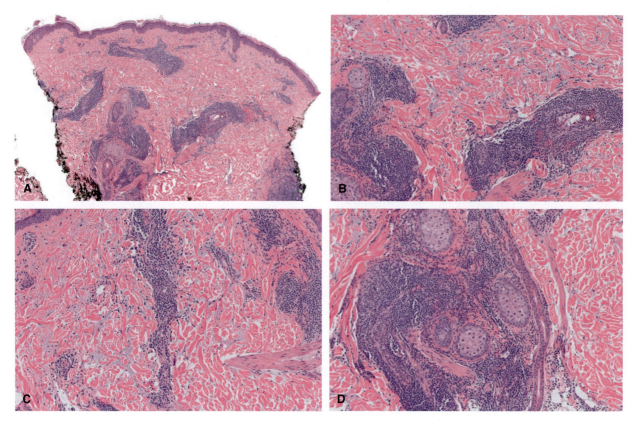

FIGURE 45-2. TLE/LIS: **A.** The biopsy shows a perivascular and perifollicular lymphocytic infiltrate without interface changes. **B.** Higher magnification of the perifollicular lymphocytic infiltrate. Note the chronic nature of the infiltrate without any eosinophils. **C.** The dermis shows brisk mucin deposits. **D.** Higher magnification of the periadnexal lymphocytic infiltrate.

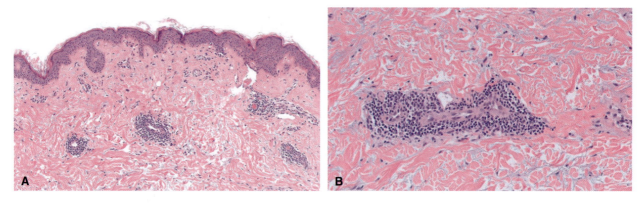

FIGURE 45-3. TLE/LIS: **A.** This example shows patchy vacuolar damage of the dermal-epidermal junction along with a perivascular lymphocytic infiltrate and mucin deposition in the dermis. **B.** Higher magnification showing a perivascular lymphocytic infiltrate with mucin deposition.

evaluation helps to distinguish these conditions. REM is also considered a variant of discoid lupus erythematosus or TLE by some authors, particularly because it can be induced by sun exposure, and antimalarials have been reported as its most effective therapy.[3,33] In contrast to TLE, young to middle-aged women are mostly affected, and there is a spectrum of skin lesions that range from erythematous, indurated papules to reticulated, macular erythema. Cutaneous lesions are mainly localized on the central chest or upper back. Histologically, REM shows a marked perivascular and often perifollicular infiltrate composed mainly of T-helper (CD4+) lymphocytes. Dermal mucin deposition is seen in the dermis; however, resolving lesions show only minimal to no dermal mucin deposits. Distinguishing between TLE and REM can be very difficult. Histologically, RME shows no epidermal changes and the DIF is usually negative. Some rare examples of REM can show granular IgM immunoglobulin deposition at the dermal epidermal junction. Cutaneous pseudolymphoma is described as a reactive lymphoid proliferation that histopathologically and/or clinically

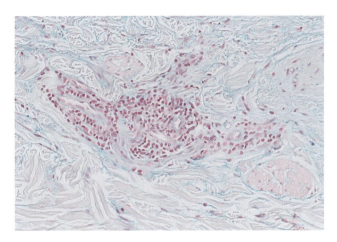

FIGURE 45-4. TLE/LIS: This is an example of alcian blue highlighting mucin deposition in dermis (alcian blue, 20×).

simulates cutaneous lymphomas.[32,34] This condition has been associated with a wide range of causes such as infections (*Borrelia*), drugs, and foreign agents. Pseudolymphoma of the skin has variable clinical presentation. It may be seen as a single or multiple erythematous dermal nodules, typically involving the face, chest, or upper extremities. It is not photosensitive, and the cutaneous lesions tend to persist without treatment. Histologically, it shows a dense perivascular and interstitial lymphoid proliferation without mucin deposits. In some cases and depending on the etiology, eosinophils can be noted and occasionally are seen in high numbers. Rarely, pseudolymphomas can be primarily perivascular and periadnexal and be confused with TLE/LIS; however, pseudolymphoma lacks mucin deposition in the dermis. Usually, CD123 will demonstrate small clusters of plasmacytoid dendritic cells in close relation to T cells and plasma cells, which contrasts with TLE/LIS in which the clusters tend to be larger in size and denser.

TABLE 45-1 Differential Diagnoses: PMLE, REM, and Pseudolymphoma

Disease	Localization	Clinical Features	Histopathological Characteristics
TLE and LIS	Sun-exposed areas	Erythematous and/or violaceous papules, plaques, or nodules Chronic/cyclical course	Dense lymphocytic infiltrate with perivascular/periadnexal pattern Interstitial mucin
PMLE	Sun-exposed areas	Papular, papulovesicular, or plaque-like lesions—monomorphous by patient Cyclical seasonal (summer, or sudden exposure to sun) pattern	Dense lymphocytic infiltrate with perivascular/periadnexal pattern Subepidermal edema No interstitial mucin
REM	Central chest and back	Reticulated macular erythema, indurated erythematous plaques	Dense lymphocytic infiltrate with perivascular/periadnexal pattern Marked interstitial mucin
Pseudolymphoma	Varies, nonspecific	Highly variable (nodules or plaques)	Simulate cutaneous lymphomas Do not fit any other diagnosis after clinical correlation

CAPSULE SUMMARY

- TLE and LIS lack standardized diagnostic criteria.
- Owing to their many similarities, including a favorable prognosis, TLE and LIS may be approached as a spectrum of changes rather than separate entities.
- Clinically, both entities can present with papules or plaques that have minimal to absent surface changes.
- Lesions in both conditions can appear on sun-exposed anatomic sites and can be induced or aggravated by light exposure.
- Both disorders are mostly confined to the dermis, with a perivascular and periadnexal pattern; show mucin deposition, photosensitivity; resolve without sequelae; and lack extracutaneous involvement.
- DIF is mostly negative in patients with TLE/LIS.
- Combined clinical and histopathological information are necessary for their accurate diagnosis.

References

1. Remy-Leroux V, Leonard F, Lambert D, et al. Comparison of histopathologic-clinical characteristics of Jessner's lymphocytic infiltration of the skin and lupus erythematosus tumidus: multicenter study of 46 cases. *J Am Acad Dermatol*. 2008;58(2):217-223.
2. Pereira A, Ferrara G, Calamaro P, et al. The histopathological spectrum of Pseudolymphomatous infiltrates in cutaneous lupus erythematosus. *Am J Dermatopathol*. 2018;40(4):247-253.
3. Kuhn A, Richter-Hintz D, Oslislo C, Ruzicka T, Megahed M, Lehmann P. Lupus erythematosus tumidus—a neglected subset of cutaneous Lupus erythematosus: report of 40 cases. *Arch Dermatol*. 2000;136(8):1033-1041.
4. Kuhn A, Sonntag M, Ruzicka T, Lehmann P, Megahed M. Histopathologic findings in lupus erythematosus tumidus: review of 80 patients. *J Am Acad Dermatol*. 2003;48(6):901-908.

5. Weber F, Schmuth M, Fritsch P, Sepp N. Lymphocytic infiltration of the skin is a photosensitive variant of lupus erythematosus: evidence by phototesting. *Br J Dermatol.* 2001;144(2):292-296.
6. Konttinen YT, Reitamo S, Ranki A, Segerberg-Konttinen M. T lymphocytes and mononuclear phagocytes in the skin infiltrate of systemic and discoid lupus erythematosus and Jessner's lymphocytic infiltrate. *Br J Dermatol.* 1981;104(2):141-145.
7. Williams CT, Harrington DW. *Jessner Lymphocytic Infiltration of the Skin.* StatPearls; 2021.
8. Kuhn A, Landmann A. The classification and diagnosis of cutaneous lupus erythematosus. *J Autoimmun.* 2014;48-49:14-19.
9. Rodriguez-Caruncho C, Bielsa I. Lupus erythematosus tumidus: a clinical entity still being defined. *Actas Dermosifiliogr.* 2011;102(9):668-674.
10. Schmitt V, Meuth AM, Amler S, et al. Lupus erythematosus tumidus is a separate subtype of cutaneous lupus erythematosus. *Br J Dermatol.* 2010;162(1):64-73.
11. Kuhn A, Bein D, Bonsmann G. The 100th anniversary of lupus erythematosus tumidus. *Autoimmun Rev.* 2009;8(6):441-448.
12. Alexiades-Armenakas MR, Baldassano M, Bince B, et al. Tumid lupus erythematosus: criteria for classification with immunohistochemical analysis. *Arthritis Rheum.* 2003;49(4):494-500.
13. Lenormand C, Lipsker D. Lupus erythematosus: significance of dermatologic findings. *Ann Dermatol Venereol.* 2021;148(1):6-15.
14. Lipsker D, Mitschler A, Grosshans E, Cribier B. Could Jessner's lymphocytic infiltrate of the skin be a dermal variant of lupus erythematosus? An analysis of 210 cases. *Dermatology.* 2006;213(1):15-22.
15. Vieira V, Del Pozo J, Yebra-Pimentel MT, Martinez W, Fonseca E. Lupus erythematosus tumidus: a series of 26 cases. *Int J Dermatol.* 2006;45(5):512-517.
16. Biazar C, Sigges J, Patsinakidis N, et al. Cutaneous lupus erythematosus: first multicenter database analysis of 1002 patients from the European Society of Cutaneous Lupus Erythematosus (EUSCLE). *Autoimmun Rev.* 2013;12(3):444-454.
17. Petersen MP, Vestergaard V, Bygum A. Jessner lymphocytic infiltration—rare in childhood. *Dermatol Online J.* 2017;23(10):13030.
18. Sonntag M, Lehmann P, Megahed M, Ruzicka T, Kuhn A. Lupus erythematosus tumidus in childhood. Report of 3 patients. *Dermatology.* 2003;207(2):188-192.
19. Kuhn A, Lehmann PM, Ruzicka T. *Cutaneous Lupus Erythematosus.* 1st ed. Springer; 2005.
20. Wenzel J, Zahn S, Mikus S, Wiechert A, Bieber T, Tuting T. The expression pattern of interferon-inducible proteins reflects the characteristic histological distribution of infiltrating immune cells in different cutaneous lupus erythematosus subsets. *Br J Dermatol.* 2007;157(4):752-757.
21. Flier J, Boorsma DM, van Beek PJ, et al. Differential expression of CXCR3 targeting chemokines CXCL10, CXCL9, and CXCL11 in different types of skin inflammation. *J Pathol.* 2001;194(4):398-405.
22. Kuhn A, Sonntag M, Lehmann P, Megahed M, Vestweber D, Ruzicka T. Characterization of the inflammatory infiltrate and expression of endothelial cell adhesion molecules in lupus erythematosus tumidus. *Arch Dermatol Res.* 2002;294(1-2):6-13.
23. Norris DA. Pathomechanisms of photosensitive lupus erythematosus. *J Invest Dermatol.* 1993;100(1):58S-68S.
24. Springer TA. Adhesion receptors of the immune system. *Nature.* 1990;346(6283):425-434.
25. Meller S, Winterberg F, Gilliet M, et al. Ultraviolet radiation-induced injury, chemokines, and leukocyte recruitment: an amplification cycle triggering cutaneous lupus erythematosus. *Arthritis Rheum.* 2005;52(5):1504-1516.
26. Stead J, Headley C, Ioffreda M, Kovarik C, Werth V. Coexistence of tumid lupus erythematosus with systemic lupus erythematosus and discoid lupus erythematosus: a report of two cases of tumid lupus. *J Clin Rheumatol.* 2008;14(6):338-341.
27. Chamberlain AJ, Hollowood K, Turner RJ, Byren I. Tumid lupus erythematosus occurring following highly active antiretroviral therapy for HIV infection: a manifestation of immune restoration. *J Am Acad Dermatol.* 2004;51(5 suppl):S161-S165.
28. Abbad N, Lanal T, Brenuchon C, Morel G, Deprez X. Etanercept-induced lymphocytic infiltration of Jessner-Kanof. *Arthritis Rheumatol.* 2018;70(3):449.
29. Tomasini D, Mentzel T, Hantschke M, et al. Plasmacytoid dendritic cells: an overview of their presence and distribution in different inflammatory skin diseases, with special emphasis on Jessner's lymphocytic infiltrate of the skin and cutaneous lupus erythematosus. *J Cutan Pathol.* 2010;37(11):1132-1139.
30. Vermi W, Lonardi S, Morassi M, et al. Cutaneous distribution of plasmacytoid dendritic cells in lupus erythematosus. Selective tropism at the site of epithelial apoptotic damage. *Immunobiology.* 2009;214(9-10):877-886.
31. Kuhn A, Bijl M. Pathogenesis of cutaneous lupus erythematosus. *Lupus.* 2008;17(5):389-393.
32. Mitteldorf C, Kempf W. Cutaneous pseudolymphoma-A review on the spectrum and a proposal for a new classification. *J Cutan Pathol.* 2020;47(1):76-97.
33. Cohen PR, Rabinowitz AD, Ruszkowski AM, DeLeo VA. Reticular erythematous mucinosis syndrome: review of the world literature and report of the syndrome in a prepubertal child. *Pediatr Dermatol.* 1990;7(1):1-10.
34. Rijlaarsdam JU, Willemze R. Cutaneous pseudolymphomas: classification and differential diagnosis. *Semin Dermatol.* 1994;13(3):187-196.

CHAPTER 46

Pigmented purpuric dermatoses

Casey A. Carlos

DEFINITION

The pigmented purpuric dermatoses (PPDs) are benign inflammatory conditions predominantly occurring in adults on the lower extremities. There are several variants, including Schamberg disease, purpura annularis telangiectoides of Majocchi, lichenoid purpura of Gougerot and Blum, lichen aureus, linear PPD, granulomatous PPD, and the eczematous variant of Doucas and Kapetenakis. These variants are separated by their clinical and histologic features and are unified by the histologic features of a perivascular lymphocytic infiltrate, absence of fibrinoid necrosis, and extravasated erythrocytes. Most are self-limited conditions, but more persistent variants are also reported. This subgroup is given the term persistent pigmented purpuric dermatoses (PPPDs).

EPIDEMIOLOGY AND CLINICAL PRESENTATION

The lichen aureus and lichenoid purpura variants are generally the variants that are challenging at times to differentiate from mycosis fungoides (MF). The lichenoid variant of PPD is uncommon. It typically occurs in middle-aged to older men on the lower extremities. It tends to be a chronic and occasionally pruritic dermatosis. Lesions are lichenoid purple to violaceous papules that fuse into plaques with a predominance for the hips, thighs, and legs (Fig. 46-1). Lichen aureus is also uncommon. It tends to occur as a solitary lesion or multiple lesions in a localized area and is asymptomatic. The lower extremity is the most commonly reported site of involvement, with some cases noting occurrence of lesions overlying perforating veins.

HISTOPATHOLOGY

The typical biopsy specimen will demonstrate a moderate-to-dense lichenoid lymphocytic infiltrate with extravasated erythrocytes (Fig. 46-2A,B). There is controversy about whether to categorize PPD into the lymphocytic vasculitis category. Historically, the lack of fibrinoid change in the vessels has been included as criteria for PPD; however, many authors consider this a vasculitis despite the lack of fibrinoid change.[1,2] Although true vasculitis may be lacking, the endothelial cells are often swollen. Some vessels may appear occluded from the swelling. In typical cases of PPD, the majority of the T cells are CD4+, small in size, and lack cytologic atypia. Lymphocytes and erythrocytes may be seen in the epidermis. Focal areas of spongiosis can be seen, especially in the eczematous variant. Hemosiderin laden macrophages may be seen within or surrounding the areas of inflammation (Fig. 46-2B).

DIFFERENTIAL DIAGNOSIS

There are several scenarios in which PPD and MF can overlap. First, patients with MF may present with PPD-like clinical lesions.[3-5] Second, there have been cases reported of patients with a long-standing diagnosis of PPD who later develop MF.[6] In fact, the first reported case of lichen aureus in the United States was later reported to have developed cutaneous T-cell lymphoma (CTCL).[7,8] Some of these cases are controversial as the diagnosis of early MF, especially on histology, can be quite challenging. Some experts consider these cases to be MF all along but lacking in definitive histology at the time of presentation. Third, there have been patients described to have clinical and histologic lesions of classical MF concomitant with PPD-like lesions that lack the histologic features of MF.[4,9,10]

Given the significant overlap in some of these cases, it can be challenging to differentiate between CTCL and PPD in some scenarios. A case of PPD with some overlapping features with MF is shown in Figure 46-3. Martínez et al[4] report clinical features that favor CTCL over PPD, which include a widespread distribution of the eruption, presence of features of parapsoriasis, and an age range between the second and fourth decades. Histologically, Toro et al[11] reviewed 56 patients (60 specimens) with persistent pigmented purpuric dermatitis. In this study, 29 of 56 patients demonstrated histologic patterns typically seen in MF. Features that were more commonly seen in patch stage MF included large collections of lymphocytes in the epidermis, many lymphocytes in the upper epidermis, and marked lymphocytic atypia. Features that favored PPPD included papillary dermal edema, extravasation of many erythrocytes in the papillary dermis, and the presence of erythrocytes in the epidermis. Some authors have reported that the presence of superficial dermal fibrosis favored MF; however, Toro et al found a significant number of cases of PPPD with papillary

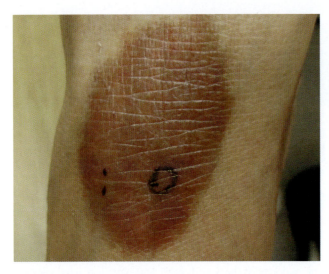

FIGURE 46-1. PPD, lichenoid variant. A purple-red plaque on the dorsal ankle.

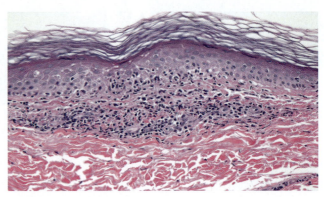

FIGURE 46-3. Histologic overlap between lichenoid PPD and MF. There is epidermotropism with lymphocytes tagging the dermal-epidermal junction. These lymphocytes are medium sized with subtle atypia. In the underlying dermis, there are rare extravasated erythrocytes and hemosiderin deposition.

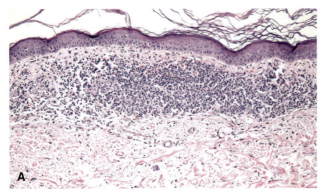
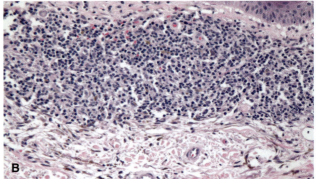

FIGURE 46-2. PPD, lichenoid variant. A. A dense lichenoid inflammatory infiltrate is seen in the superficial dermis with minimal epidermotropism. **B.** The infiltrate consists of small to medium-sized lymphocytes with admixed extravasated erythrocytes. There is prominent hemosiderin deposition within and surrounding the inflammatory infiltrate.

dermal fibrosis. Crowson et al have put forth the term "atypical pigmentary purpura" for these cases of PPD with some histologic features but no clear diagnosis of CTCL.

T-cell receptor gene rearrangement studies may not be diagnostic, although they can be helpful in cases that are polyclonal. Cases of CTCL with PPD-like presentation with identifiable clones have been reported.[12] However, several groups have identified cases of PPD, which also show monoclonality.[13] A decrease in T_{reg} cells has been reported in PPD, although not to the degree seen in true T-cell neoplasms.[14]

In addition to MF, PPD or PPPD must be differentiated from cutaneous small vessel vasculitis, medication-induced PPD, lichenoid allergic contact reaction, purpura from platelet dysfunction, venous stasis dermatitis, and hypergammaglobulinemic purpura of Waldenström.

References

1. Ratnam KV, Su WP, Peters MS. Purpura simplex (inflammatory purpura without vasculitis): a clinicopathologic study of 174 cases. *J Am Acad Dermatol*. 1991;25(4):642-647.
2. Weedon D. *Weedon's Skin Pathology*. Vol 1. 3rd ed. Churchill Livingstone; 2010:041.
3. Cather JC, Farmer A, Jackow C, et al. Unusual presentation of mycosis fungoides as pigmented purpura with malignant thymoma. *J Am Acad Dermatol*. 1998;39(5 Pt 2):858-863.
4. Martínez W, del Pozo J, Vázquez J, et al. Cutaneous T-cell lymphoma presenting as disseminated, pigmented, purpura-like eruption. *Int J Dermatol*. 2001;40(2):140-144.
5. Puddu P, Ferranti G, Frezzolini A, et al. Pigmented purpura-like eruption as cutaneous sign of mycosis fungoides with autoimmune purpura. *J Am Acad Dermatol*. 1999;40(2 Pt 2):298-299.
6. Georgala S, Katoulis AC, Symeonidou S, et al. Persistent pigmented purpuric eruption associated with mycosis fungoides: a case report and review of the literature. *J Eur Acad Dermatol Venereol*. 2001;15(1):62-64.
7. Waisman M, Waisman M. Lichen aureus. *Arch Dermatol*. 1976;112(5):696-697.
8. Farrington J. Lichen aureus. *Cutis*. 1970;6:1251-1253.
9. Barnhill RL, Braverman IM. Progression of pigmented purpura-like eruptions to mycosis fungoides: report of three cases. *J Am Acad Dermatol*. 1988;19(1 Pt 1):25-31.
10. Lipsker D, Cribier B, Heid E, et al. Cutaneous lymphoma manifesting as pigmented, purpuric capillaries [in French]. *Ann Dermatol Venereol*. 1999;126(4):321-326.

11. Toro JR, Sander CA, LeBoit PE. Persistent pigmented purpuric dermatitis and mycosis fungoides: simulant, precursor, or both? A study by light microscopy and molecular methods. *Am J Dermatopathol*. 1997;19(2):108-118.
12. Foo CC, Tang MB, Chong TK, et al. T-cell receptor-gamma gene analysis in evolving to advancing cutaneous T-cell lymphoma. *Australas J Dermatol*. 2007;48(3):156-160.
13. Plaza JA, Morrison C, Magro CM. Assessment of TCR-beta clonality in a diverse group of cutaneous T-cell infiltrates. *J Cutan Pathol*. 2008;35(4):358-365.
14. Solomon GJ, Magro CM. Foxp3 expression in cutaneous T-cell lymphocytic infiltrates. *J Cutan Pathol*. 2008;35(11):1032-1039.

CHAPTER 47

Chronic actinic dermatitis—actinic reticuloid

Sena J. Lee and András Schaffer

DEFINITION

Chronic actinic dermatitis (CAD) is a unifying term for chronic eczematous photodermatoses lasting for more than 3 months with abnormal sensitivity to a broad spectrum of wavelengths, including ultraviolet (UV) and often visible light. It encompasses persistent light reaction, photosensitive eczema, and photosensitivity dermatitis and presents as pruritic eczematous or lichenified patches or plaques in sun-exposed areas. Its most severe form is termed actinic reticuloid (AR), which can resemble cutaneous T-cell lymphoma (CTCL).

EPIDEMIOLOGY

CAD has been reported in Europe, Asia, and North America, with largest numbers observed in Northwestern Europe. Although AR, the most severe type, almost exclusively affects elderly men with history of chronic sun exposure through work or hobby, CAD as a whole showed a moderate preference of men over women at the ratio of 2.6:1 in a study conducted in the United States and Japan.[1,2] CAD has been reported in HIV+ patients and can present as the first sign of advanced asymptomatic HIV infection.[3-5] These HIV+ patients are younger than the general CAD population. There also have been sporadic reports of CAD in young patients with a history of atopic dermatitis.[6-8] Susceptibility for CAD has been found in all Fitzpatrick skin types. In the United States, predominantly affected types are V and VI.[1,2,9]

ETIOLOGY

The etiology of CAD remains unknown despite conjecture and debate over the last several decades. The most important diagnostic feature in CAD is decreased minimal erythema dose to broad spectrum of light, which is easily observed but difficult to explain. In many European patients, but not in those in the United States or Asia, a history of photoallergic contact dermatitis predates development of CAD. Sesquiterpene lactone mix from Compositae plant oleoresin was found to be an allergen in 25% to 36% of patients with CAD.[10,11] Patch testing with oleoresin extracts from daisy, dandelion, and thistle also produced similar results.[12] Photoallergy to sunscreens and fragrance was another common finding.[9]

It has been suggested that CAD is a delayed hypersensitivity reaction to a known or yet unidentified photoallergen. Predominance of CD8+ T cells and increased Langerhans cells in the inflammatory infiltrate of the CAD skin[13,14] are histologic features that are similar to allergic contact dermatitis. The presence of eosinophils, plasma cells, and fibrosis in skin biopsies suggests a possible role for type-2 helper T cell–derived cytokines (IL-4, IL-5, IL-6, IL-13) in the pathogenesis. Expression of adhesion molecules, such as E-selectin, VCAM-1, and ICAM-1, on dermal blood vessels for recruitment of inflammatory cells in CAD also supports this notion.[15] It has been postulated that allergic photocontact dermatitis became persistent light reaction, when an endogenous protein was modified into an autoantigen in the presence of the initial photoallergen. In support of this theory, photooxidation of the histidine moiety of human serum albumin was observed in the presence of tetrachlorosalicylanilide, an antimicrobial agent and preservative.[16] In another study, persistent light reaction was induced in guinea pigs after intradermal injection with Freund adjuvant and UVA radiation, suggesting concurrent dermatitis and UV radiation may be sufficient to create an endogenous photoallergen.[17] Elevated levels of kynurenic acid, which is involved in the tryptophan metabolic pathway, was suggested as a possible pathogenic mechanism,[18] but this hypothesis was later disputed by a tryptophan metabolism study.[19] Defective ability to respond to UV-induced oxidative stress in fibroblasts in CAD has also been suggested as the cause.[20] In summary, although causality is difficult to establish with these associated findings, AR may be best considered a delayed hypersensitivity reaction to an exogenous or endogenous photoallergen.

CLINICAL PRESENTATION AND PROGNOSIS

CAD affects sun-exposed areas, such as face, helices of ears, neck, forearms, and hands, with sparing of upper eyelids, postauricular creases, nasolabial folds, and finger

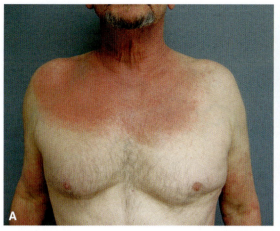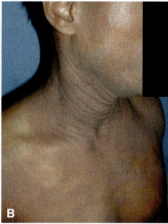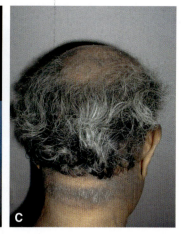

FIGURE 47-1. Clinical presentation of chronic actinic dermatitis and actinic reticuloid. Confluent erythematous rash involving sun-exposed areas in a patient with CAD **(A)**. Lichenified papules and plaques on sun-exposed skin in a patient with AR **(B and C)**. (Photo courtesy of Dr. Milan Anadkat **(A)**. Images **B** and **C** are reprinted from[13] with permission.)

webs. Initially, erythema, edema, pruritus, and burning sensation are observed. Over time, lichenified patches and plaques develop and may extend to nonexposed areas (Fig. 47-1).

In AR, infiltrated thickening of the skin with papules, plaques, and nodules or even erythroderma can occur and may give a similar appearance to Sezary syndrome. Generalized lymphadenopathy may also be observed, and Sezary cells can be found in the peripheral blood of patients with AR.

Despite similarities, predominance of CD8 T cells in affected skin and peripheral blood and absence of monoclonal T-cell receptor gene rearrangement can help distinguish CAD from erythrodermic mycosis fungoides or Sezary syndrome. Decreased minimal erythema dose to a broad spectrum of light is also an important distinguishing feature and diagnostic criterion for CAD.

Patients with CAD are treated with sun avoidance and photoprotection using protective clothing or sunscreens without offending allergens. Topical and systemic corticosteroids are often helpful. There have been reports of successful treatment with azathioprine, psoralen with UVA (PUVA), and UVB therapy. The course can be unpredictable, but the condition improves over time for the majority of patients with CAD.[21] A retrospective study conducted in New York of 40 patients with CAD via patient questionnaire and chart review in a 3- to 19-year follow-up period reported complete resolution in 35%, partial improvement in 55%, and either no change or worsening in 10% of the patients.[22] A Scottish cohort study of 178 patients reported resolution or significant improvement in 79% in a 15-year follow-up after initial diagnosis with phototesting.[21] Recently, dupilumab, a monoclonal antibody against IL-4/IL-14 emerged as a potential therapeutical alternative in a small cohort of patients.[23]

The risk of developing lymphoma in patients with AR became concerning after a few patients with AR developed lymphoma,[24-26] but a retrospective study of 231 patients with chronic actinic dermatitis, including AR, between 1971 and 1991, showed no increased incidence of lymphoma or other types of malignancies.[27] However, a study showed patients with nonmalignant erythroderma, including those with erythrodermic AR, have a decreased lifespan.[28]

HISTOLOGY

Skin biopsies demonstrate eczematous features including parakeratosis, acanthosis, spongiosis, solar elastosis, and prominent dermal fibroplasia. Dermal histiocytes are usually prominent with frequent angulated and oligonucleated forms (Montgomery cells). Most cases display a brisk lymphocytic infiltrate with subtle exocytosis, atypical lymphocytes, and increased numbers of Langerhans cells, eosinophils, and plasma cells (Fig. 47-2A–C).

IMMUNOPHENOTYPE

The majority of cases show a predominance of CD8+ T cells within the epidermis with a decreased CD4:CD8 ratio and preserved CD7 expression (Fig. 47-2D–G).[29,30] Dermal histiocytes, including Montgomery cells, are positive for factor XIIIa and S100 (Fig. 47-2 H,I).[13]

GENETICS

Polyclonal T-cell receptor gene rearrangement.[31]

CAPSULE SUMMARY

- CAD/AR is an uncommon chronic photodermatosis of unknown etiology.
- It commonly affects elderly men with all skin types.
- Sensitivity to UVA, UVB, and visible light by patch testing is diagnostic.

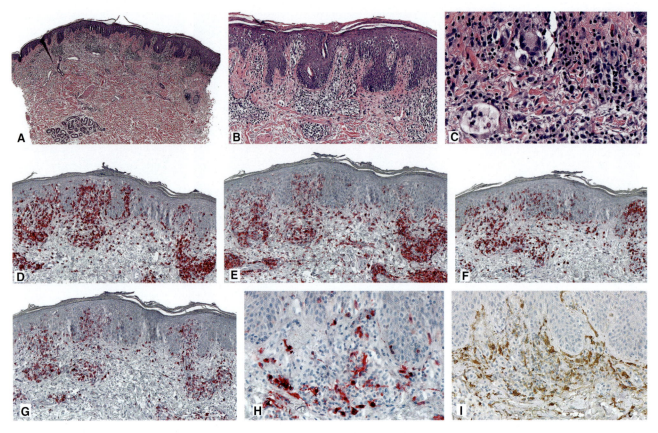

FIGURE 47-2. Histological findings in actinic reticuloid. Acanthosis, spongiosis, parakeratosis with superficial lymphocytic infiltrates, exocytosis, and prominent dermal histiocytes (**A–C**). Intraepidermal lymphocytes are predominantly CD8+ with slightly diminished CD7 expression (**D–F**). Dermal dendrocytes are positive for factor XIIIa and S100 (**G–I**).

- Clinical differential diagnosis includes drug-induced photosensitivity, atopic dermatitis, airborne contact dermatitis, allergic photocontact dermatitis, and eczematous variant of CTCL.
- Association with HIV infection has been described.
- Presence of dermal histiocytes with oligo- and multinucleated forms (Montgomery cells), eosinophils, plasma cells, and a low CD4:CD8 ratio favors CAD/AR over lymphoma.

References

1. Lim HW, Morison WL, Kamide R, Buchness MR, Harris R, Soter NA. Chronic actinic dermatitis. An analysis of 51 patients evaluated in the United States and Japan. *Arch Dermatol*. 1994;130(10):1284-1289.
2. Que SK, Brauer JA, Soter NA, Cohen DE. Chronic actinic dermatitis: an analysis at a single institution over 25 years. *Dermatitis*. 2011;22(3):147-154.
3. Wong SN, Khoo LS. Chronic actinic dermatitis as the presenting feature of HIV infection in three Chinese males. *Clin Exp Dermatol*. 2003;28(3):265-268.
4. Pappert A, Grossman M, DeLeo V. Photosensitivity as the presenting illness in four patients with human immunodeficiency viral infection. *Arch Dermatol*. 1994;130(5):618-623.
5. Meola T, Sanchez M, Lim HW, Buchness MR, Soter NA. Chronic actinic dermatitis associated with human immunodeficiency virus infection. *Br J Dermatol*. 1997;137(3):431-436.
6. Russell SC, Dawe RS, Collins P, Man I, Ferguson J. The photosensitivity dermatitis and actinic reticuloid syndrome (chronic actinic dermatitis) occurring in seven young atopic dermatitis patients. *Br J Dermatol*. 1998;138(3):496-501.
7. Creamer D, McGregor JM, Hawk JL. Chronic actinic dermatitis occurring in young patients with atopic dermatitis. *Br J Dermatol*. 1998;139(6):1112-1113.
8. Ogboli MI, Rhodes LE. Chronic actinic dermatitis in young atopic dermatitis sufferers. *Br J Dermatol*. 2000;142(4):845.
9. Beach RA, Pratt MD. Chronic actinic dermatitis: clinical cases, diagnostic workup, and therapeutic management. *J Cutan Med Surg*. 2009;13(3):121-128.
10. Menage H, Ross JS, Norris PG, Hawk JL, White IR. Contact and photocontact sensitization in chronic actinic dermatitis: sesquiterpene lactone mix is an important allergen. *Br J Dermatol*. 1995;132(4):543-547.
11. du PMH, Hawk JL, White IR. Sesquiterpene lactone mix contact sensitivity and its relationship to chronic actinic dermatitis: a follow-up study. *Contact Dermatitis*. 1998;39(3):119-122.
12. Dawe RS, Green CM, MacLeod TM, Ferguson J. Daisy, dandelion and thistle contact allergy in the photosensitivity dermatitis and actinic reticuloid syndrome. *Contact Dermatitis*. 1996;35(2):109-110.
13. Sidiropoulos M, Deonizio J, Martinez-Escala ME, Gerami P, Guitart J. Chronic actinic dermatitis/actinic reticuloid: a clinicopathologic and immunohistochemical analysis of 37 cases. *Am J Dermatopathol*. 2014;36(11):875-881.

14. Fujita M, Miyachi Y, Horio T, Imamura S. Immunohistochemical comparison of actinic reticuloid with allergic contact dermatitis. *J Dermatol Sci*. 1990;1(4):289-296.
15. Menage Hdu P, Sattar NK, Haskard DO, Hawk JL, Breathnach SM. A study of the kinetics and pattern of E-selectin, VCAM-1 and ICAM-1 expression in chronic actinic dermatitis. *Br J Dermatol*. 1996;134(2):262-268.
16. Kochevar IE, Harber LC. Photoreactions of 3,3',4',5-tetrachlorosalicylanilide with proteins. *J Invest Dermatol*. 1977;68(3):151-156.
17. Katsumura Y, Tanaka J, Ichikawa H, Kato S, Kobayashi T, Horio T. Persistent light reaction: induction in the guinea pig. *J Invest Dermatol*. 1986;87(3):330-333.
18. Swanbeck G, Wennersten G. Evidence for kynurenic acid as a possible photosensitizer in actinic reticuloid. *Acta Derm Venereol*. 1973;53(2):109-113.
19. Vonderheid EC, Sobel EL, Hoeldtke RD, Faerber GJ, Sardi VS. Kynurenic acid and xanthurenic acid excretion after tryptophan loading in actinic reticuloid. *Int J Dermatol*. 1987;26(1):33-41.
20. Giannelli F, Botcherby PK, Marimo B, Magnus IA. Cellular hypersensitivity to UV-A: a clue to the aetiology of actinic reticuloid? *Lancet*. 1983;1(8316):88-91.
21. Dawe RS, Crombie IK, Ferguson J. The natural history of chronic actinic dermatitis. *Arch Dermatol*. 2000;136(10):1215-1220.
22. Wolverton JE, Soter NA, Cohen DE. The natural history of chronic actinic dermatitis: an analysis at a single institution in the United States. *Dermatitis*. 2014;25(1):27-31.
23. Patel N, Konda S, Henry W. Dupilumab for the treatment of chronic actinic dermatitis. *Photodermatol Photoimmunol Photomed*. 2020;36:398-400.
24. Jensen NE, Sneddon IB. Actinic reticuloid with lymphoma. *Br J Dermatol*. 1970;82(3):287-291.
25. Thomsen K. The development of Hodgkin's disease in a patient with actinic reticuloid. *Clin Exp Dermatol*. 1977;2(2):109-113.
26. Ashinoff R, Buchness MR, Lim HW. Lymphoma in a black patient with actinic reticuloid treated with PUVA: possible etiologic considerations. *J Am Acad Dermatol*. 1989;21(5 pt 2):1134-1137.
27. Bilsland D, Crombie IK, Ferguson J. The photosensitivity dermatitis and actinic reticuloid syndrome: no association with lymphoreticular malignancy. *Br J Dermatol*. 1994;131(2):209-214.
28. Sigurdsson V, Toonstra J, Hezemans-Boer M, van Vloten WA. Erythroderma. A clinical and follow-up study of 102 patients, with special emphasis on survival. *J Am Acad Dermatol*. 1996;35(1):53-57.
29. Toonstra J, Henquet CJ, van Weelden H, van der Putte SC, van Vloten WA. Actinic reticuloid. A clinical photobiologic, histopathologic, and follow-u study of 16 patients. *J Am Acad Dermatol*. 1989;21(2 pt 1):205-214.
30. Toonstra J, Van der Putte SC, van Wichen DF, van Weelden H, Henquet CJ, van Vloten W. Actinic reticuloid: immunohistochemical analysis of the cutaneous infiltrate in 13 patients. *Br J Dermatol*. 1989;120(6):779-786.
31. Bakels V, van Oostveen JW, van der Putte SC, Meijer CJ, Willemze R. Immunophenotyping and gene rearrangement analysis provide additional criteria to differentiate between cutaneous T-cell lymphomas and pseudo-T-cell lymphomas. *Am J Pathol*. 1997;150(6):1941-1949.

CHAPTER 48

CD30 pseudolymphomas

Jacqueline M. Junkins-Hopkins and Werner Kempf

DEFINITION

Cutaneous pseudolymphomas (CPLs) are benign lymphocytic infiltrates of the skin, which microscopically and immunophenotypically simulate cutaneous lymphoma, and yet do not have clinical corroboration to confirm a malignant designation. CPLs may mimic many of the B- or T-cell lymphomas recognized by the World Health Organization–European Organization for Research and Treatment of Cancer classification scheme,[1] especially those falling under the subtype of CD30+ lymphoproliferative disorder (LPD). These include lymphomatoid papulosis (LyP) and anaplastic large cell lymphoma (ALCL). Other LPDs may express CD30,[1] such as mycosis fungoides (MF) that has undergone large cell transformation or the folliculotropic subtype, pagetoid reticulosis, NK-/T-cell lymphoma, nasal type, subcutaneous panniculitis-like T-cell lymphoma, intravascular (IV) T-cell lymphoma,[2] some B-cell lymphomas,[3] (see Fig. 48-1) and hematologic malignancies that may affect the skin secondarily, such as Hodgkin lymphoma, hydroa vacciniforme–like lymphoma,[4] adult T-cell leukemia/lymphoma, and angioimmunoblastic-like T-cell lymphoma.[5] Of these, CD30 CPL most frequently mimics either LyP or ALCL. CD30+ expression is seen on activated CD45RO+ memory T cells,[6] and as would be expected, scattered atypical CD30+ cells are found in a variety of benign inflammatory infiltrates, but do not usually present with critical mass to specifically mimic malignancy. Nevertheless, these may be met with anxiety and concern for a neoplastic lymphoproliferative process such as LyP; thus, this will also be discussed in this chapter.

EPIDEMIOLOGY

The epidemiology of CD30 CPL has not been formally evaluated. It is reported more frequently in adults of all ages; however, it may occur in children, including infants.[7] Several patients with herpesvirus-induced CPL have had a prior hematologic malignancy,[8] but this may be related to a tendency for this population to develop herpes infections. Additionally, HIV-infected individuals have been reported to have CD30 CPL,[9] and CD30 can be induced by stimulation with viruses, such as Epstein-Barr virus (EBV) and human T-cell lymphotropic virus types 1 and 2, suggesting susceptibility for CD30 expression by reactive infiltrates in virally infected individuals.[6] In fact, CD30+ cells were frequently noted in skin biopsies from individuals with HIV, especially in later-stage disease.[10] A remarkably high number of enlarged atypical, but reactive CD30 cells can be observed in molluscum contagiosum (MC) or parapoxvirus infections which represent another viral-induced CD30 PSL.[7,11,12] A number of patients reported to have CD30 CPL have had autoimmune disorders, but it is not clear whether this is related to immune dysregulation from their disease or their medications.

ETIOLOGY

CD30 CPLs may be caused by or associated with a variety of benign inflammatory conditions.[7-53] A list of these conditions is provided in Table 48-1. CD30 expression has also been documented in benign and malignant nonhematopoietic neoplasms.[3,54] The specific details of the immune dysregulation leading to the lymphoid dyscrasia in CD30 CPL have not been elucidated. Furthermore, the pathogenesis may differ among the entities. CD30 antigen, a cytokine receptor and transmembrane glycoprotein of the tumor necrosis factor superfamily, may be expressed in normal lymphoid tissue (germinal center B cells and some T and B peri/interfollicular blasts)[3] and by activated CD45+ RO memory T and B lymphocytes, in response to induction by various mitogens and virus stimulation.[6] CD30 is especially expressed by T lymphocytes producing T helper-2 (TH2)–type cytokines,[10,55] and investigators have shown a relationship between some TH2 diseases and CD30 expression.[55,56] Overexpression of CD30 and its ligand (CD153 or CD30L) has been documented in the dermal infiltrate of atopic dermatitis (AD), a TH2-mediated disease (in contrast to infiltrates of allergic dermatitis),[55] and soluble CD30 has been shown to be increased in the serum of atopic patients with active dermatitis.[56] Mast cells are also increased in AD biopsies, as well as other chronic inflammatory conditions, and in Hodgkin disease, a malignancy characterized by increased numbers of CD30 cells, cells expressing CD30L, and CD30+ Reed-Sternberg cells. In fact, mast cells represent a significant portion of these CD30L-expressing cells and are felt to play a role in tumor progression, through CD30-CD30L interactions. CD30L transduces signaling downstream that leads to cytokine production.[55] Mast cells

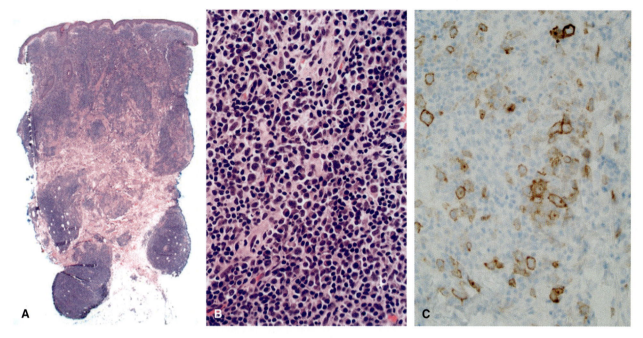

FIGURE 48-1. CD30 CPL. There are scattered large atypical lymphocytes amidst a mixed infiltrate of nonatypical lymphocytes and eosinophils. CD30 staining in marginal zone lymphoma. **A.** There is a dense diffuse and nodular lymphocytic infiltrate sparing the epidermis with a Grenz zone, which is unusual for lymphomatoid papulosis and anaplastic large cell lymphoma. **B.** There are sheets and clusters of plasma cells, which were monotypic for lambda (not shown), and clonal by IgH PCR. **C.** Numerous large lymphocytes stain positive for CD30 with a membranous and Golgi staining pattern. These are mostly solitary, but rare aggregates are present.

have been shown to release chemokines through a pathway distinct from the IgE-mediated degranulation pathway,[55] thus possibly playing a role in AD via interactions with CD30. The release of chemokines by mast cells may also play a role in defense against a variety of pathogens,[55] possibly explaining the presence of CD30 cells in other inflammatory and infectious conditions. HIV infection may also play a role in promoting the proliferation of activated T lymphocytes, due to induction of a TH2 cytokine profile by the virus.[10] A series of bone marrow transplant patients with eruption of lymphocyte recovery (ELR) had infiltrates with atypical CD30+ CD25+ activated T-cells, felt to be drug or viral induced (HHV6), further supporting this theory.[53] CD30 CPL has been associated with drugs that share a common structural feature of two noncoplanar rings that includes a heterocyclic amine ring and carbonyl group, which bridges or is external to the rings.[45] This suggests that certain molecular structures may contribute to the etiology of CD30 CPL.

CLINICAL PRESENTATION, COURSE, AND PROGNOSIS

The clinical presentation of CD30 CPL is determined by the cause. Papules, nodules, plaques, patches, hemangioma-like lesions, and rarely tumors have been reported. These may be crusted or ulcerated, and in the cases of drug, an exanthema may be present. A critical clinical feature is the lack of systemic "B" symptoms, negative laboratory/radiologic workup, and absence of other clinical features that are otherwise seen in lymphoma. The clinical course of the cutaneous lesions is also key, as these lesions tend to regress when the instigating agent is removed, or do not recur after surgical removal/medical therapy. This is in contrast to LyP, which waxes and wanes, before and after therapy is discontinued, despite complete regression. In general, the prognosis for CD30 CPL is excellent, provided there is no ongoing or significant immunosuppression that was responsible for the CPL.

TABLE 48-1 Inflammatory Conditions Associated With Expression of CD30

Infection
Viral
Herpes simplex virus/herpes zoster virus
Molluscum contagiosum
HIV
Epstein-Barr virus
Milker nodule
Verruca vulgaris
HTLV-1
Hepatitis B, C
Mycotic
Dermatophytosis (superficial and follicular)
Bacterial/atypical mycobacterial/spirochetal/parasitic
Rickettsia tsutsugamushi
Leishmania
Syphilis
Mycobacterial tuberculosis

TABLE 48-1 Inflammatory Conditions Associated With Expression of CD30 (Continued)
Inflammatory
Arthropod assault
Scabies and postscabietic nodules
Insect bite reactions
Spider bite reaction
Pityriasis lichenoides et varioliformis acuta
Atopic dermatitis
Tattoo
Pernio
Hidradenitis suppurativa
Gold acupuncture
Cyst rupture
Perirectal abscess
Scar post BCC excision
Hyper IgE syndrome
Chronic ulceration TUGSE[a]/Eosinophilic ulcer of the oral mucosa
Lichen sclerosis
Trauma
Eruption of lymphocyte recovery
Drugs
Carbamazepine
Lamotrigine
Gabapentin
Cefuroxime
Cefepime[b]
Terbinafine
Metronidazole
Piperacillin/tazobactam
Levofloxacin[b]
Atenolol
Metoprolol[b]
Amlodipine
Lisinopril/Valsartan
Losartan
Atorvastatin
Simvastatin
Sertraline
Gemcitabine
Decitabine
Cyclophosphamide
Sirolimus
Mycophenolic acid
Leuprolide/Lupron
Tocilizumab
Ipilimumab
Hepatobiliary iminodiacetic acid scintigraphy

[a]Traumatic ulcerative granuloma with stromal eosinophilia.
[b]drugs suspected.

HISTOLOGY

The histologic features are determined by the cause of the CD30 CPL. Selected presentations are discussed separately in this chapter. In general, scattered large atypical cells reside in a background of a variably dense dermal lymphocytic infiltrate (T more often than B) (Fig. 48-1). These have large vesicular nuclei, variably prominent nucleoli, and ample cytoplasm. Reed-Sternberg cytomorphology may be seen (see Chapter 14). Exocytosis into a variably acanthotic epidermis, or involvement of adnexae, especially in the cases of herpes virus infections, may be seen (Fig. 48-2). Angiocentricity frequently occurs in some CD30 CPL, especially in cases induced by drugs. Significant angiodestruction is rare, but mild vasculitis can be seen in some CD30 CPL, including those due to scabies mite infestation (Fig. 48-2A). There is a subtype that simulates IV lymphoma[32-35,57] (Fig. 48-3).

IMMUNOPHENOTYPE

The cells are decorated in a pattern similar to that of CD30 LPDs, characterized by a membranous and Golgi dot pattern of staining (Fig. 48-4). Plasma cells may be highlighted with CD30 antibody, but in a cytoplasmic pattern. Ki-67 is variable, but may reach at least 80%.[15] The CD30 staining in CPL is usually less intense than that of LyP and ALCL, and the cells tend to be scattered and are not apposed, nor in large clusters and sheets, in contrast to LyP and ALCL (Fig. 48-4). Nonetheless, exceptions exist, especially in cases of inflammatory MC[7,12] in which large aggregates may be seen (Fig. 48-5). CD30+ atypical cells may arise in the background of a dense infiltrate rich in neutrophils and eosinophils. This has been reported in insect bite reactions, spider bites, hidradenitis suppurativa, genital herpes virus infection, perirectal abscess, ruptured cyst, and rhinophyma.[9] The CD30+ cells tend to associate with small T and B lymphocytes (as opposed to the neutrophils and eosinophils) where these cells may represent up to approximately 25% of the lymphoid population. CD30+ cells have not been reported in infections, such as cellulitis and necrotizing fasciitis, and in Sweet syndrome.[9]

MOLECULAR FINDINGS

Gene rearrangement testing with polymerase chain reaction (PCR) analysis for the T-cell receptor (TCR) is nearly always polyclonal,[11] but monoclonality has rarely been reported in herpes virus infection[8] and in drug reactions.[41,46] One should use caution if attempting to use PCR to differentiate CD30 CPL from LyP, since a monoclonal T-cell population in LyP using standard PCR is only detected between 20% and 80% of cases studied.[58]

CELL OF ORIGIN

Activated CD45RO+ memory T cells.[6]

INFECTION-ASSOCIATED CD30 PSEUDOLYMPHOMA

Several infections, especially virally induced, have been reported to have CD30+ cells in their infiltrates. These are listed in Table 48-1. Selected subtypes are discussed below.

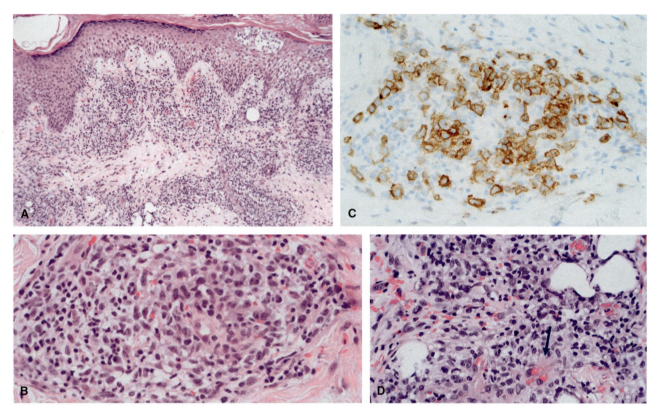

FIGURE 48-2. A. CD30 CPL due to nodular scabies. **A.** There is a dense angiocentric and band-like lymphocytic infiltrate with spongiosis and subcorneal fragments of a mite in the upper left of the image. **B.** There is a dense perivascular lymphocytic infiltrate, composed of cohesive aggregates of large atypical lymphocytes. **C.** CD30 immunohistochemical stain highlighting numerous the atypical lymphocytes in cohesive aggregates. **D.** Evidence of vasculitis, with erythrocyte extravasation, vascular disruption with early fibrinoid necrosis (arrow).

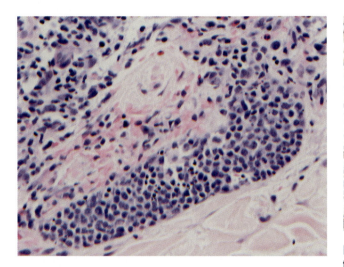

FIGURE 48-3. Intravascular CD30 CPL. Area adjacent to chronic folliculitis with a perifollicular lymphocytic and eosinophilic infiltrate and large atypical intravascular lymphocytes that stained positive for CD30.

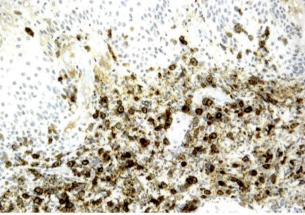

FIGURE 48-4. CD30 immunohistochemical stain demonstrating scattered, nonclustered CD30+ atypical lymphocytes in a pseudolymphomatous infiltrate. These have a membranous and cytoplasmic dot-staining pattern.

Herpes Virus Infection

Classical herpes virus infections present as clustered, dermatomal, or occasionally disseminated papules that are in various stages of vesiculation or crusting, with a limited, self-healing course of approximately 2 to 3 weeks. In cases of herpes simplex virus (HSV)-associated CD30 CPL, the lesions are often present for a longer period of time, and are not vesicular. Submitted diagnoses for these lesions may include mycotic infection, basal cell carcinoma, lymphoma, or pseudolymphoma.[8] Histopathologic features of classical herpes simplex virus/herpes zoster virus (HSV/VZV) infections include acantholytic vesicle or ulcer formation, epidermal and/or pilosebaceous necrosis, epithelial cell alteration that includes balloon-cell degeneration, eosinophilic intranuclear inclusions, ground glass nuclei, and/or multinucleated giant cell formation with molded nuclei, and lymphocytic inflammation that is usually superficial

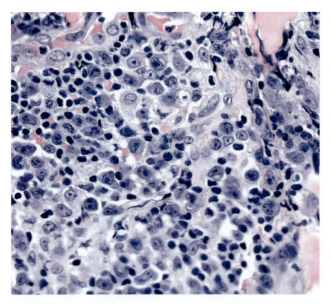

FIGURE 48-5. CD30 CPL due to ruptured molluscum contagiosum. There are large clusters of atypical cells with large vesicular nuclei, conspicuous nucleoli, and ample cytoplasm, simulating LyP-C or ALCL.

and deep, perifollicular, perineural, and rarely syringotropic. Lichenoid dermatitis and/or leukocytoclastic vasculitis may be seen. Both HSV and VZV may present in a clinically and histologically clandestine fashion, mimicking a variety of hematologic malignancies. These usually simulate LyP, but herpes may mimic other subtypes of T-cell lymphoma, including ALCL, NK-/T-cell lymphoma and other angiocentric presentations, and B-cell lymphoma. Patients with immunocompromised states, especially HIV disease, may be more at risk of such atypical presentations. Some patients have a prior history of hematologic malignancy or eczema herpeticum.[8] Pseudolymphomatous reactions are common in both HSV and VZV infections. In nearly half of cases, a dense lymphocytic infiltrate may be seen, and approximately 67% of these will have atypical lymphocytes.[8] Atypical lymphocytes can also be identified in less dense perivascular infiltrates of herpes virus infections (Fig. 48-6). These reactions have also occurred at sites of prior VZV vaccination.[14] Differentiating the specific viral cause is usually not possible, although the presence of herpes folliculitis may be more indicative of VZV than HSV.[8] The lymphocytes may exhibit angiotropism with vessel disruption and erythrocyte extravasation (Fig. 48-6) in

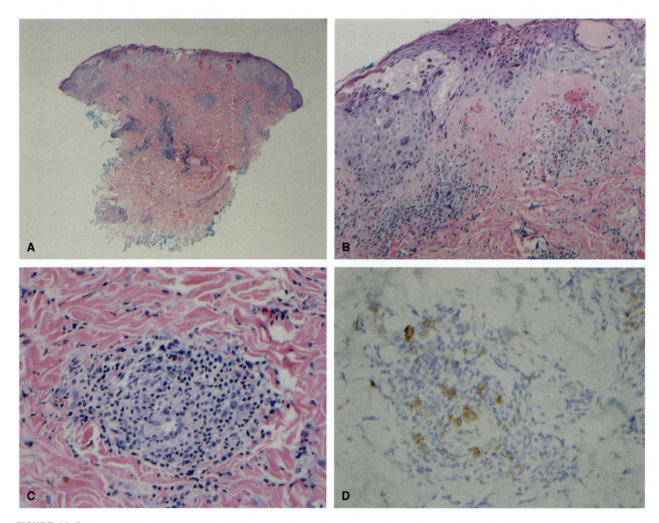

FIGURE 48-6. Herpes-induced CD30 CPL. **A.** Scanning view showing a wedge-shaped perivascular lymphocytic infiltrate with an overlying epidermal vesicle. **B.** Intraepidermal acantholytic vesicle with viral cytopathic changes and vessel disruption with erythrocyte extravasation. **C.** Perivascular lymphocytic infiltrate with atypical cells and rare eosinophils. **D.** CD30 stain highlights scattered large CD30+ lymphocytes.

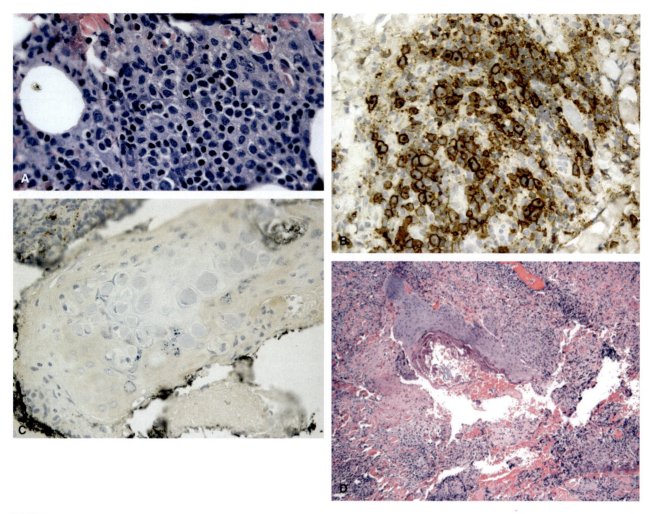

FIGURE 48-7. CD30 CPL due to ruptured molluscum contagiosum. A. There is a dense lymphocytic infiltrate with numerous large atypical cells, some of which are in clusters. **B.** These are positive for CD30. **C.** CD20 stain is negative, but shows hints of molluscum bodies in detached crusted epithelium. **D.** Deeper sections showing ruptured cystic epithelium with numerous molluscum bodies in the keratin horny layer.

at least a third of cases, but significant angiodestruction is rare. Granulomatous infiltrates are also rare, in contrast to postzoster lesions, which are known to be associated with granulomatous and lymphoid reactions. Numerous eosinophils, while typically not a feature of herpes virus infection, may rarely be numerous. The immunophenotype is usually that of a T-cell–rich infiltrate with CD30 decorating the large atypical cells, but rare cases of CD20-cell–rich lymphocytic infiltrates simulating B-cell lymphoma have been reported.[13] The presence of scattered CD30+ cells in this context may be a clue to the viral nature of the process. Within the dense infiltrates, CD30+ atypical lymphocytes are usually <5% and scattered (Fig. 48-6), differentiating this from LyP and ALCL, but these may range from 15% to 25% of the infiltrate, and present as clusters.[8] CD56/TIA1 positivity may also be seen. PCR is typically yields a polyclonal TCR rearrangement in CD30 CPL; however, rarely, a monoclonal TCR band associated with lymphocytic infiltrates containing clusters of CD30 positivity may be documented,[8] truly simulating LyP. Detection of HSV by PCR analysis or correlating with an appropriate clinical presentation, and/or presence of typical herpetic viral changes, is required to confirm pseudolymphoma in such instances (Fig. 48-6).

Molluscum Contagiosum

MC, an infection due to poxvirus infection, classically presents as discrete translucent to flesh-colored or pink umbilicated dome-shaped papules. MC occurs at all ages, but is common in children, in sexually active adults on the genitalia, or as disseminated papules in immunocompromised patients.[49] Less common presentations include cystic or polypoid lesions, eczematized plaques, or giant molluscum (often seen in HIV patients). Classical histopathologic features are those of exo- and endophytic acanthosis and the presence of eosinophilic to basophilic cytoplasmic viral inclusions that compress the nucleus, eventually becoming molluscum bodies. These accumulate in the horny layer, creating a centrally located plug that is eventually extruded. A protective ultrastructural membrane around the virions may contribute to a lack of significant host immune response to MC.[17] However, if irritated or traumatized, the lesions may clinically and histologically become inflamed, resulting in a brisk host response, characterized by a dense mixed inflammatory infiltrate, granulation tissue, and spongiosis. The epidermal invagination containing the molluscum bodies may be cystic,[16] absent, or inconspicuous in chronic or heavily inflamed cases, and additionally, there may be a brisk delayed hypersensitivity response, resulting in a dense infiltrate of pleomorphic and atypical lymphocytes, simulating lymphoma[7,11,15-17] (Fig. 48-7). The infiltrate is typically rich in T lymphocytes, which may be CD4+[11,17] or CD8+.[15] There is a variable component of CD30+ cells that are scattered amidst the infiltrate,[16,17] or may be numerous and in cohesive sheets, representing 30%[15] to 75%[11] of the infiltrate, presenting as sheets of anaplastic cells simulating LyP or ALCL (Fig. 48-7). The Ki67 rate may reach 90%, and expression of CD56 and cytotoxic markers may be seen, further mimicking an aggressive lymphoma. Usually, molluscum bodies can be found; thus, it is worth getting deeper levels or closely inspecting any detached crust or horn to exclude the possibility of MC pseudolymphoma (Fig. 48-7). If there is any doubt, PCR should yield a polyclonal TCR rearrangement.

Epstein-Barr Virus

Evidence of EBV can be seen in aggressive lymphoma, but also may be seen in immunodeficiency-related LPDs. Both malignant and benign infiltrates may demonstrate EBV and CD30 expression. A more extensive discussion of EBV-related disorders can be found in Chapter 46. It is important to note that, similar to other CD30 CPLs, immunodeficiency-related infiltrates of EBV/CD30+ LPDs may be histologically identical to lymphoma, yet may resolve without aggressive therapy or may undergo a benign course.[18] A variety of immunodeficiency states may be seen, including posttransplant and associated with medications, such as methotrexate (Fig. 48-8).The histologic features may include dermal and subcutaneous atypical lymphocytic infiltrates with vascular occlusion and tissue necrosis, and a predominance of either B, T, or both B and T expression in the atypical lymphocytes. Atypical CD30/EBV-positive lymphocytic infiltrates in patients who are posttransplant or on immunosuppressive agents such as methotrexate should be signed out descriptively and reassessed after discontinuation of the implicated medication. Because immune-deficient and posttransplant LPDs have an unpredictable course that includes progression to a fatal lymphoma, these should be handled more cautiously than conventional CD30 CPL.

Milker Nodule and Verruca Vulgaris

Milker nodules are caused by parapoxvirus and have a clinicopathologic presentation that varies with stage of the lesion. CD30+ infiltrates may be seen in these lesions. The lesions are usually solitary,[7] but may be multiple.[19] The incidence of CD30 CPL is hard to document, given that the patient may not always present for surgical evaluation. In an interesting "familial" case, three members of one household were infected by their family cow, resulting in erythematous dorsal hand plaques showing dense superficial and deep CD3- and CD4-positive infiltrates with a Ki-67 proliferative index of 70% and numerous scattered and clustered CD30+ infiltrates in each of their lesions. This was accompanied by acanthosis, papillary dermal edema with fibrin deposition, vascular proliferation, and an admixture of eosinophils and plasma cells. PCR was polyclonal in all three. The virus was documented by electron microscopy.[19]

Verruca vulgaris rarely has been reported to be associated with CD30 CPL[20] in an HIV negative patient. The infiltrate was CD3 and CD4 positive with 10% CD30+ cells. The viral-induced epidermal changes were still recognizable.

Mycotic Infections

Fungal infections, including superficial[21,22] and follicular[21] dermatophytosis, may less frequently be associated with pseudolymphomatous CD30+ infiltrates.[21,22] These have clinically presented with annular plaques simulating granuloma annulare or other nonfungal inflammatory diagnoses. In the cases reported, the lesions were present from 4 to 6 months. Histopathologically, these are characterized by a dense nodular CD4+ T lymphocytic infiltrate in the dermis and superficial subcutis, admixed with eosinophils, histiocytes, and atypical large or smaller pleomorphic lymphocytes. CD30 staining highlights scattered, nonclustered large lymphocytes. The lymphocytes may infiltrate the adnexal epithelium, especially if there is follicular involvement. PAS staining will identify the organism in most dermatophytic CD30 CPLs, but this finding may be focal, requiring sectioning to document the hyphae in some cases, especially if the hyphae are only intrafollicular.

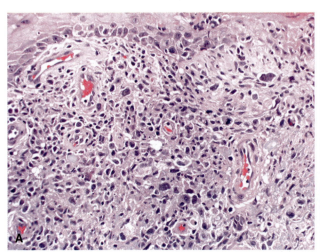
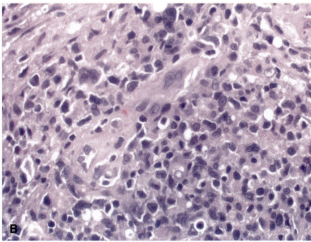

FIGURE 48-8. **Methotrexate induced CD30 ⁺EBV⁺lymphocytic infiltrate.** There are atypical hyperchromatic lymphocytes in the dermis. **A.** Medium power. **B.** High power.

Mycobacteria

In general, mycobacterial infections are not typically associated with CD30 CPL; however, a case was reported in which a patient with cutaneous and lymph node tuberculosis presented with facial papules, a biopsy of which showed a dense lymphocytic infiltrate, nearly 30% of which were CD30+, including many large atypical cells. Granulomas were not present. Neither bacilli nor DNA evidence of tuberculosis were detected, but the lesions cleared after antituberculous treatment.[24]

INFLAMMATORY DERMATOSES ASSOCIATED WITH CD30+ INFILTRATES

A variety of inflammatory dermatoses have been reported to contain atypical CD30+ lymphocytes in their infiltrates. These are listed in Table 48-1. Selected dermatoses are discussed below.

Arthropod Assault and Postscabetic Nodules

Host responses to infestation by *Sarcoptes scabiei* are variable in the acute stage, but in chronic nodular scabies, there is frequently a dense lymphocytic infiltrate that usually contains atypical CD30+ lymphocytes.[25] CD30+ cells may be seen in 33%[11] to 72%.[25] Comorbidities in these cases have included hepatitis C virus with interferon treatment and Hodgkin disease.[25] A history of antiscabietic therapy does not preclude a diagnosis of postscabetic CD30 CPL. Lesions that present under 3 months do not tend to contain these cells, but they are a consistent finding in older lesions. The histologic features include a dense perivascular and interstitial lymphocytic infiltrate with numerous eosinophils in the papillary and upper reticular dermis, which may extend deeper, imparting a wedge-shaped configuration (Fig. 48-9). A Sarcoptes mite is found less often with the chronic (>3 months) lesions. The infiltrate is CD3+/CD4+, although in HIV disease, CD8 lymphocytes may predominate in scabies infiltrates. The CD30 cells are scattered or in small noncohesive aggregates in the interstitium and around vessels. Occasionally, cohesive clusters of large atypical CD30+ lymphocytes can be found (Fig. 48-2A). Furthermore, evidence of vasculitis can be seen in lesions of nodular scabies, simulating the angiodestructive presentation of LyP (Fig. 48-2A). S100-positive dermal dendritic cells are present in the chronic lesions. PCR may rarely yield a monoclonal TCR gene rearrangement.[11]

Insect bite reactions are less likely to have CD30 positivity.[9] Other causes of arthropod assault, such as chronic tick-bite reaction and spider bite, may show CD30 expression. The latter may present with a prominent neutrophilic response with numerous and clustered CD30+ cells,[9] potentially simulating the neutrophil-rich variant of ALCL.

Pityriasis Lichenoides et Varioliformis Acuta

Pityriasis lichenoides et varioliformis acuta (PLEVA) presents with numerous to generalized erythematous papules that evolve through a crusting and variably vesicular, hemorrhagic, and/or necrotic stage. It is more common in kids than adults. Histologically, there is a wedge-shaped perivascular and band-like lymphocytic infiltrate that blurs the dermal-epidermal junction due to exocytosis. Depending on the lesion biopsied, the epidermis may show mild to moderate acanthosis, spongiosis that may form vesicles, parakeratosis, crust, vacuolar changes, and dyskeratosis. Microscopic hemorrhage into the papillary dermis, epidermis, and scale crust is a common feature. There may be angiocentricity. On the extreme end of the spectrum, epidermal necrosis, robust superficial and very deep infiltrates, and vasculitis are seen. This overlaps with LyP, but the absence of significant lymphocyte atypia and essentially no CD30 positivity are said to differentiate PLEVA from LyP. However, recent reports of CD30+ cells in PLEVA[26,50] have challenged this. These patients have typical unremitting clinical presentations consistent with PLEVA (vs the waxing and waning of LyP), without the presence of atypical large lymphocytes that characterize LyP. The CD30+ lymphocytes are present in the epidermal and dermal components, often with a CD8/TIA-1 immunophenotype, typical of PLEVA. The CD30+ cells are strictly small- to medium sized and range from 60% to 80% of the infiltrate in some cases. Even biopsies with only 15% to 20% CD30+ cells mimic LyP by forming clusters. Other features that overlap with LyP included lymphocytic vasculitis, prominent epidermotropism, and clonality (nearly 50% of those studied). Distinguishing PLEVA with CD30 positivity from LyP may be impossible, especially since rare variants of PLEVA (febrile ulceronecrotic Mucha-Haberman) may also have fever, systemic symptoms, and potential fatality. It is critical to follow patients with possible CD30+ PLEVA, since both pityriasis lichenoides and LyP may be associated with MF. Parvovirus B19 may rarely be positive, but it is not clear if this has clinical or pathogenic significance.

Atopic Dermatitis

As mentioned, cells expressing CD30 have been documented in biopsies of AD.[56] This upregulation may be related to the relationship between mast cells expressing CD30L.[55] These CD30+ mononuclear cells are located in the superficial dermis, coexpress CD4, and are few in number, without significant enlargement or atypia; thus, this does not constitute a true pseudolymphoma, but it is helpful to know that these cells may be present, potentially mimicking a CD30 LPD, such as LyP or MF with large cell transformation. Moreover, there is a potential relationship with AD and true CD30 LPD, as cases of with ALCL or LyP have been reported in patients with AD.[51] Many of these patients have had treatment with cyclosporine, and some experienced an unusually aggressive course.

Tattoo

Pseudolymphomatous reactions in tattoos may take the form of T- or B-cell infiltrates, and typically occur in red-inked portions of the tattoo[27]; however, pseudolymphoma localized to green, blue,[28] and black-ink tattoo has been reported.[29] CD30 CPL is rare and should be recognizable by the presence of pigment and fewer CD30+ cells (Fig. 48-10). On occasion, it may be difficult to distinguish this from regional LyP arising in a tattoo.[27] The lesions of pseudolymphoma tend to persist, while LyP spontaneously clears. It is important to follow the

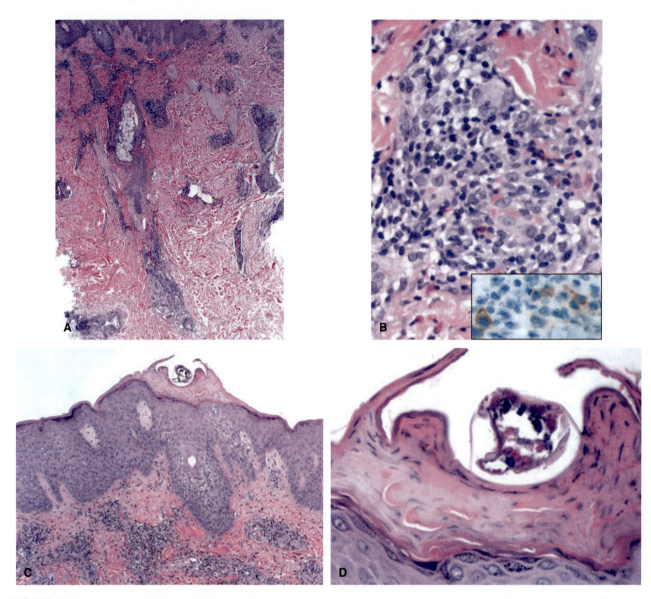

FIGURE 48-9. **Scabies with atypical CD30 [1] lymphocytes. A.** Scanning view showing a perivascular wedge-shaped lymphocytic infiltrate, without exocytosis. **B.** High power, demonstrating atypical large lymphocytes admixed with nonatypical lymphocytes, histiocytes, and numerous eosinophils. B inset. CD30 stains scattered atypical cells. **C.** There is a mite in the stratum corneum. Note: there is no significant exocytosis. **D.** High-power view of Sarcoptes mite.

patient closely, since rare cases of pseudolymphoma (B cell) have progressed to lymphoma.[59]

Pernio

Pernio (chilblains) clinically presents with painful dusky to violaceous papulonodular lesions on distal sites, especially fingers and toes, but also ears and nose, as a response to cold temperatures in susceptible individuals. This may be idiopathic, or associated with lupus erythematosus and other forms of autoimmune disease.[52] There is a superficial and deep perivascular and variably perieccrine lymphocytic infiltrate with papillary dermal edema, basal cell vacuolization, occasional necrotic keratinocytes, and variable mild lymphocytic vasculitis. Rarely, scattered atypical CD30+ lymphocytes have been reported in classic lesions of pernio.[7,31] The classic clinical presentation and other typical histologic features confirm a pernio diagnosis.

Eruption of Lymphocyte Recovery

ELR occurs in patients status post chemotherapy and bone marrow transplant who develop a self-resolving eruption 3 weeks after chemotherapy, after a time of aplasia, when the circulation becomes repopulated by lymphocytes. The maculopapular eruption involves the trunk and extremities and is often accompanied by a transient fever. Histopathologic features include a mild perivascular infiltrate of CD4+ lymphocytes with mild spongiosis and basal cell vacuolization. In a series of 12 patients (11 with acute myeloid leukemia) with ELR and atypical cells in perivascular or band-like infiltrates, 10 of 12 had CD30+ cells, with 6 mimicking a cutaneous T-cell lymphoma or Sézary syndrome.[53] The patients otherwise showed clinical features typical of ELR. Most of the atypical lymphocytes were positive for CD30, CD25, ICOS, and CD4 or CD8, without expression of cytotoxic proteins or PD1. In 75%, the atypical cells comprised 10%

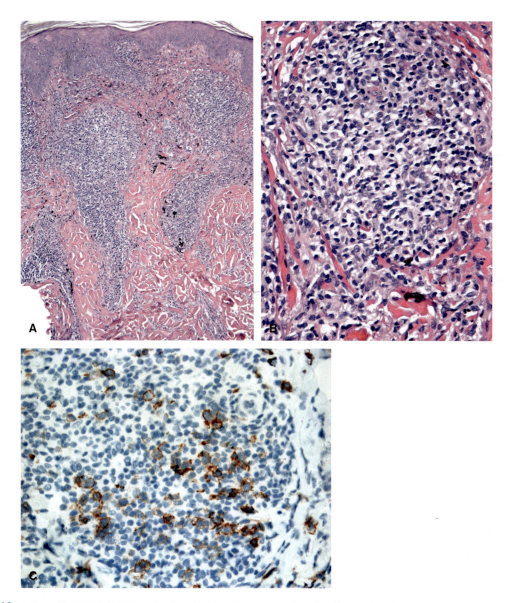

FIGURE 48-10. Tattoo with CD30 CPL. A. Scanning view showing a dense perivascular and nodular to diffuse dermal infiltrate, with scattered areas of red and black tattoo pigment. **B.** Higher power demonstrating large atypical lymphocytes amidst small lymphocytes, histiocytes, and macrophages with red tattoo pigment. **C.** CD30 marks scattered atypical large cells.

to 50% of the infiltrate. The atypia was prominent enough to prompt a potential diagnosis of cutaneous T-cell lymphoma, but mild spongiosis and dermal edema were common, epidermotropism was not a feature, and the studied cases were polyclonal. Furthermore, the clinical rash and circumstances easily differentiate CD30 CPL from LyP or other cutaneous T-cell lymphomas. All eruptions cleared spontaneously or with topical steroids within 3 days to 4 weeks.

Chronic Ulceration

Benign Atypical Intravascular CD30+ T-Cell Proliferation

Benign atypical IV CD30+ T-cell proliferation is the accumulation of benign but atypical large lymphocytes within lymphatic channels, simulating aggressive IV lymphoma (Fig. 48-3). This may occur in lesions with surface erosion or ulceration and/or with a history of trauma. This has been reported in association with pyogenic granuloma,[32] trauma-induced ulcer,[33,34] ulcerated lichen sclerosis,[35] and regressing keratoacanthoma.[57] The cells reside in lymphatics, based on D2-40+, CD31+ staining of the endothelial cells but can also be found in the perivascular areas. A case in which the intralymphatic atypical cells demonstrated the immunophenotype of an effector/memory-like regulatory T lymphocyte (CD4+/CD25+, with FoxP3 and CCR7+ cells) and some CD30+ cells led some to propose the IV lymphocytes to reflect an immune response, either locally or migrating to local lymph nodes.[32] A high proliferative index, up to 100%, contributes to a concern for malignant aggressive IV lymphoma. Polyclonal TCR PCR should confirm a benign process. There is often surrounding inflammatory changes of an otherwise benign process, further supporting a reactive process.

Traumatic Ulcerative Granuloma With Stromal Eosinophilia

Traumatic ulcerative granuloma with stromal eosinophilia (TUGSE), also reported under the term eosinophilic ulcer of the oral mucosa and a variety of other names, is a benign, self-limiting condition, which presents as a rapidly developing ulceration with indurated borders, ranging from a few millimeters to several centimeters. It typically occurs on the tongue, but buccal and other oral mucosal sites may be involved. It is seen most often in adults, but has a bimodal presentation; in infants, it is referred to as Riga-Fede disease.[36] The lesions are usually solitary, and heal without recurrence; however, synchronous and metachronous lesions have rarely been reported.[37] The duration of the lesion prior to presentation is usually several months to a year, but may rarely be only several days to weeks. The cause is unknown. Although most attribute the lesion to trauma, frequently, a history of trauma cannot be elicited. Furthermore, the histologic changes are more exuberant than that of a traumatic ulcer. There is a dense, diffuse polymorphous T- and B-lymphocytic infiltrate rich in eosinophils and mononuclear cells, extending through the tissue, throughout the skeletal muscle bundles (Fig. 48-11). The mononuclear cells are usually histiocytes; however, in a subset of these cases, there are scattered and clustered large CD30+ lymphocytes with atypical irregular nuclei, conspicuous nucleoli, and ample cytoplasm (Fig. 48-11). The stroma also shows a proliferation of endothelial cells and small vessels. Some have proposed a role for mast cells to explain the intense eosinophilic infiltrate that may be seen. Based on observations noted above, this may also explain the occasional occurrence of CD30 expression that may be quite prominent, simulating ALCL. There is frequently TIA1 positivity, with an admixture of CD4 and CD8 lymphocytes. Angiodestruction is rare. Ki-67 proliferation index ranges from 10% to 50% in the small and large lymphocytes. Most cases of TUGSE have had polyclonal T-cell gene rearrangements by PCR; however, monoclonal rearrangements have been reported.[36] The lesions are nonaggressive, usually resolving spontaneous or a few weeks after biopsy, without recurrence. Nonetheless, because the findings may be identical to ALCL or LyP, follow-up for recurrence is recommended after the initial diagnosis is rendered to exclude a CD30 LPD.

Drug-Induced CD30 Pseudolymphoma

A subset of drugs and other forms of therapy have been associated with CD30+ CPL (Table 48-1). Some of these drug-induced lymphoid dyscrasias may present with features

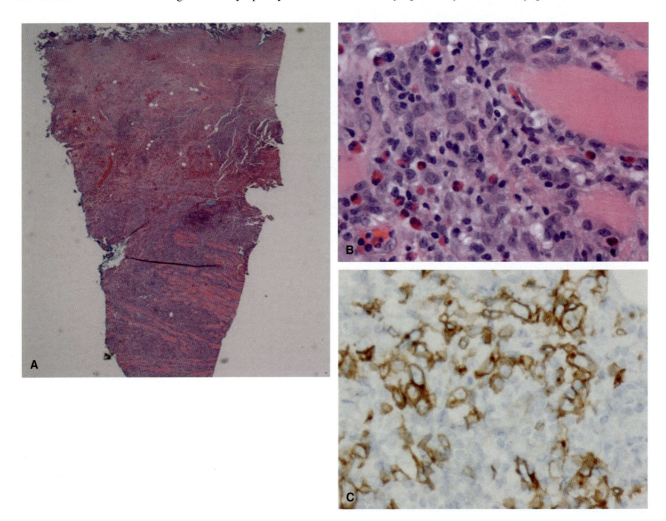

FIGURE 48-11. Traumatic ulcerative granuloma with stromal eosinophilia. A. This biopsy from the tongue shows surface ulceration with a dense diffuse infiltrate, extending into the deep tissue, where skeletal muscle is infiltrated. **B.** High power showing a mixed cell infiltrate dissecting skeletal muscle. There are numerous eosinophils admixed with large atypical lymphocytes, small lymphocytes, endothelial cells, and histiocytes. **C.** CD30 documents numerous atypical lymphocytes.

nearly identical to LyP, while others show an angiocentric lymphoid infiltrate with variably dense CD30+ atypical lymphocytes. CD30+ infiltrates have been reported in patients taking antiepileptics,[38,39,60] statins,[46] cephalosporin antibiotics,[39,40] fluoroquinolones,[39,46] terbinafine,[7] metronidazole,[46] piperacillin/tazobactam,[46] antihypertensives, including β-blockers,[41,46] calcium channel blockers,[39,42] angiotensin II receptor antagonists,[44,46] and antihypertensive/diuretic combinations,[46] selective serotonin reuptake inhibitors,[39,46] chemotherapeutic agents,[41,43,46] immunosuppressive agents,[46] hormonal therapy (leuprolide/Lupron),[41] biologics,[46,47] and checkpoint inhibitors,[48] after undergoing hepatobiliary iminodiacetic acid (HIDA) scintigraphy[45] or in situations in which a combination of potential offending agents have been implicated.[39,41,46] Drugs implicated in more than one instance include statins, ACE inhibitors (especially amlodipine), sertraline, and levofloxacin.

Several reported patients with CD30 CPL have had an underlying hematopoietic disorder,[39,46] possibly predisposing them to developing atypical lymphoid infiltrates. Some patients have a history of allergy or immune dysregulation. For instance, in a patient with prior positive patch test to gold and nickel, acupuncture with gold needles resulted in puncture site papules with a pseudolymphomatous T-cell infiltrate and scattered CD30+ large cells (vs the typical B-cell–rich gold-induced pseudolymphoma).[30] Immune modulatory agents, including biologic agents such as tumor necrosis alpha inhibitors[46] and tocilizumab,[47] have been reported to cause other types of pseudolymphomatous eruptions in addition to CD30 CPL.[47] A patient with a suspected CD30 CPL, manifested as a papular facial and truncal eruption associated with tocilizumab 7 days after the fifth administration, was reported. Histopathologically, there was a dense perivascular infiltrate of mostly CD4+ lymphocytes intermingled with eosinophils and scattered large CD30-positive lymphocytes. A lymphocyte stimulation test with tocilizumab in conjunction with resolution with drug discontinuation confirmed a pseudolymphoma.[47] The target inhibitor, ipilimumab, has also recently been reported to have caused a CD30 CPL.[48] A papular eruption occurred 5 weeks after starting the medication and progressed to coalescing plaques, with histological features of a psoriasiform epidermis, dermal edema, and a dense band-like and perivascular CD4-rich lymphocytic infiltrate with scattered large CD30+ cells. This nearly cleared in a month after stopping the drug. An antecedent viral infection may also contribute to a more robust dysregulated immune response,[46] resulting in a CD30 CPL and indeed human herpesvirus 6 was documented in blood samples of a patient with drug reaction with eosinophilia and systemic symptom (DRESS)–associated CD30 CPL due to lamotrigine[60]

These papular or papulonodular presentations are the most common, but the clinical lesions are heterogeneous and polymorphous and include discrete scattered papules, erythematous or purpuric macular/papular eruptions, urticarial lesions with desquamation, and erythema. Solitary annular plaques simulating carcinoma have also been described. A rare case of CD30 CPL presenting as DRESS syndrome was reportedly due to lamotrigine, started 40 days prior for somatization disorder.[60] In this instance, the syndrome-associated lymphadenopathy further simulated a cutaneous and systemic hematopoietic disorder, due to the presence of CD30+ nodal lymphocytes.[60] In some cases, the pseudolymphomatous eruption may arise after having a previous conventional drug hypersensitivity reaction.[44]

The offending agent is usually present for several weeks to several months prior to the onset of the CD30 CPL, but shorter times of onset are seen. After only 3 days (five doses), intravenous cefuroxime caused a papular rash with LyP type C histology.[40] Days following scintigraphy and exposure to the 99Tc-iminodiacetic acid HIDA scan complex, a patient developed 2mm painful and pruritic erythematous papules with atypical CD30+ cells representing <25% of the infiltrate on biopsy.[45] In a series of 20 cases of CD30 CPL, the onset of the eruption was a month or less from the initiation of the medication in nearly half of the cases. These cases suggest that CD30 CPLs may have a shorter duration of onset than T-cell drug–induced lymphoid dyscrasias not associated with CD30 immunophenotype.[46] Most drug-induced CD30 LPDs clear days, weeks, or months after removing the offending agent, and there is usually complete response to therapy. In contrast, LyP recurs despite initially responding to treatment.

The histologic findings are heterogeneous. Most cases present with lymphocytes distributed along the vascular plexus in a "wedge-shaped" pattern in the superficial or superficial and mid to deep dermis. Involvement of the deeper dermis, adipose tissue, nerves, and eccrine glands is not typical, in contrast to cases of LyP.[46] Small lymphocytes are admixed with large atypical immunoblastic lymphocytes and often eosinophils.[43,44,46] Erythrocyte extravasation may be seen. Extension into the interstitium, dense diffuse infiltrates,[43] or frank lichenoid patterns may be encountered. Some cases may show exocytosis or disruption of the epidermal interface, with frequent spongiosis, papillary dermal edema, and mild vacuolar interface dermatitis, but frank lichenoid tissue reactions and vesiculobullous lesions are not typically seen. There may be a combination of spongiosis and dense dermal inflammation (Fig. 48-12). Rarely, prominent epidermotropism[39] or Pautrier microabscesses[38] have been reported. A rare case of a granulomatous CD30+ CPL occurring 2 weeks after starting amlodipine was characterized by papulonodules, annular plaques, and peripheral eosinophilia. The biopsy showed a granulomatous infiltrate and a subpopulation of scattered nonatypical CD30+ lymphocytes.[61]

The percentage of large CD30+ cells in the lymphocyte population is also variable, ranging from scattered (<3% to 5%) to 30%, but up to nearly 100% of the large atypical cells stain for CD30+.[40] CD30+ cells are usually distributed around the vessels and surrounding intersitium, but may be identified in the epidermis.[56] There is frequent loss of CD7 expression, with either a CD4 or CD8 immunophenotype,[43] or the helper:suppressor ratio may be normal. Cytotoxic proteins, TIA-1 and granzyme, are not typically expressed, while this cytotoxic immunophenotype can be seen in LyP. In contrast, PD-1+ lymphocytes are reported to be present in CD30 CPL but not in LyP.[46] B cells are rare to absent, but coexpression of CD3, CD20, and CD30 may occur.[39] PCR may show polyclonal or monoclonal rearrangements; however, in a series of 20 cases of CD30 CPLs, none were monoclonal.[46] If the patient is felt to have a CD30 CPL and is on methotrexate, an immunodeficiency-related LPD should be considered instead, and the patient followed closely, as these patients may progress to true lymphoma. EBV+ staining will help identify these individuals. In general, evaluating for clonality is not necessary, since monoclonality will not confirm a

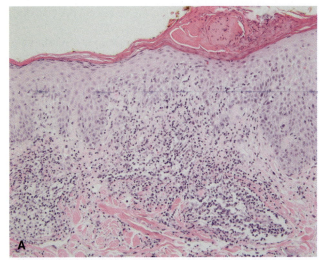

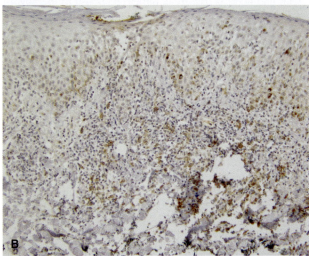

FIGURE 48-12. Drug-induced CD30⁺ lymphoid dyscrasia. A. The epidermis is acanthotic and spongiotic, with scale crust and mild exocytosis. There is a dense perivascular and lichenoid lymphocytic infiltrate with scattered atypical cells. **B.** CD30 highlights scattered CD30⁺ lymphocytes in the dermis and epidermis. (Slides A and B courtesy of Dr. Melissa Pulitzer.)

CD30 LPD. Additionally, the clinical presentation of a nonwaxing and waning and usually more widespread eruption in concert with histology showing concomitant inflammatory changes, such as papillary dermal edema, spongiosis without neutrophilic spongiosis or epidermotropism, and vacuolization, will point to CD30 CPL, allowing medication discontinuation to confirm the diagnosis.

CD30 EXPRESSION IN NEOPLASMS

CD30 expression via Ber-H2 antibody has been demonstrated in several benign and malignant neoplasms, and on normal exocrine pancreas tissue.[3] These include numerous mesenchymal neoplasms (leiomyoma, leiomyosarcoma, malignant fibrous histiocytoma [storiform/pleomorphic type], aggressive fibromatosis, synovial sarcoma, giant cell tumor of tendon sheath, rhabdomyosarcoma, Ewing sarcoma, atypical fibroxanthoma, osteosarcoma), selected carcinomas (embryonal carcinoma, rarely others), adnexal tumors (cutaneous lymphadenoma), and rarely melanoma. In some of these neoplasms, all or nearly all of the tumor cells are positive, with staining patterns that are surface, dot-like intracytoplasmic, or cytoplasmic. Assessment of morphology and application of other immunohistochemical markers allow differentiation from sarcomatous ALCL.

DIFFERENTIAL DIAGNOSIS

Differentiating the various causes of CD30 CPL from true lymphoma may be challenging, requiring correlation with the clinical presentation and course. Unfortunately, the lesion may be a solitary plaque or nodule with overlapping features of both true CD30 LPD and CD30 CPL. In fact, the submitted clinical diagnosis of herpes may occur less than 50% of the time.[8] In most cases, CD30⁺ cells in pseudolymphoma are scattered and separate from one another, without larger clustering. In *HSV/VZV CD30 CPL*, concentration of the infiltrate around and within a hair follicle, especially with necrotic folliculitis, should prompt pursuit of herpes viral cytopathic changes in the epidermis or follicle with deeper levels or immunohistochemical stains for HSV/VZV. PCR analysis for HSV/VZV may be required to confirm infection, and should be pursued if herpes is in the clinical differential diagnosis, yet immunohistochemical stains cannot confirm. One should be sure to distinguish herpes CD30 CPL from infiltration of herpetic scars by chronic lymphocytic leukemia.[62] Histologically, it may be difficult to distinguish *drug-induced* CD30 CPL from LyP. Concentration of the process along the vascular plexus, especially if neutrophils are absent, without significant exocytosis, is more typical of drug CD30 CPL than LyP. *Neutrophilic-rich CPL* may closely mimic pyodermic ALCL. The clinical presentation or culture should allow differentiation of benign abscesses from malignancy. Ultimately, since there may also be clinical overlap with LyP and CD30 CPL, and both may have a monoclonal TCR gene rearrangement, the diagnosis will rely on the clinical course. The lesions should clear with removal of the offending agent, and should not recur after initial response to therapeutic intervention. In contrast, the waxing and waning course of LyP will not be permanently altered by initial response to treatment.

CAPSULE SUMMARY

- CD30 CPLs are benign infiltrations of the skin, with cytomorphologic and immunophenotypic atypia that overlaps with cutaneous lymphoma, usually of the CD30 lymphoproliferative subtype (LyP or ALCL).
- CD30 CPLs occur at any age in association with infections, especially viral, chronic antigenic stimulation due to arthropod assault or exogenous agents, inflammatory and traumatic causes of chronic ulceration, and drugs.
- The clinical lesions and histological features are heterogenous, reflecting the variety of conditions associated with the pseudolymphoma.
- The CD30⁺ cells are large, with atypical nuclei, conspicuous nucleoli, and ample cytoplasm, identical to those seen in CD30 LPD, including a membranous and

dot-like staining pattern. Large cells are scattered separately throughout the infiltrate, but may be clustered, or may represent a third or more of the infiltrate, similar to LyP or ALCL.
- The T-cell infiltrate may have a normal immunophenotype or may show CD4 or CD8 predominance, ± loss of CD7, and may have monoclonal TCR gene rearrangements.
- Some nonhematopoietic malignant neoplasms may show diffuse expression of CD30, but the pattern of CD30 staining may be different. These entities have identifiable microscopic and immunophenotypic features to confirm the diagnosis.
- Correlation with the clinical presentation and medication history is critical to arriving at the appropriate diagnosis.

References

1. Willemze R, Jaffe ES, Burg G, et al. WHO-EORTC classification for cutaneous lymphomas. *Blood*. 2005;105:3768-3785.
2. Iacobelli J, Spagnolo DV, Tesfai Y, et al. Cutaneous intravascular anaplastic large T-cell lymphoma: a case report and review of the literature. *Am J Dermatopathol*. 2012;34:e133-e138.
3. Schwarting R, Gerdes J, Durkop H, et al. BER-H2: a new anti-Ki-1 (CD30) monoclonal antibody directed at a formol-resistant epitope. *Blood*. 1989;74(5):1678-1689.
4. Quintanilla-Martinez L, Ridaura C, Nagl F, et al. Hydroa vacciniforme-like lymphoma: a chronic EBV+ lymphoproliferative disorder with risk to develop a systemic lymphoma. *Blood*. 2013;122(18):3101-3110.
5. Sabattini E, Pizzi M, Tabanelli V, et al. CD30 expression in peripheral T-cell lymphomas. *Haematologica*. 2013;98(8):e81-e82.
6. Falini B, Pileri S, Pizzolo G, et al. CD30 (Ki-1) molecule: a new cytokine receptor of the tumor necrosis factor receptor superfamily as a tool for diagnosis and immunotherapy [Review]. *Blood*. 1995;85(1):1-14.
7. Werner B, Massone C, Kerl H, et al. Large CD30-positive cells in benign, atypical lymphoid infiltrates of the skin. *J Cutan Pathol*. 2008;35(12):1100-1107.
8. Leinweber B, Kerl H, Cerroni L. Histopathologic features of cutaneous herpes virus infections (herpes simplex, herpes varicella/zoster): a broad spectrum of presentations with common pseudolymphomatous aspects. *Am J Surg Pathol*. 2006;30(1):50-58.
9. Cepeda LT, Pieretti M, Chapman SF, et al. CD30-positive atypical lymphoid cells in common non-neoplastic cutaneous infiltrates rich in neutrophils and eosinophils. *Am J Surg Pathol*. 2003;27(7):912-918.
10. Smith KJ, Barrett TL, Neafie R, et al. Is CD30 immunostaining in cutaneous eruptions useful as a marker of Th1 to Th2 cytokine switching and/or as a marker of advanced HIV disease? *Br J Dermatol*. 1998;138:774.
11. Kempf W. CD30+ lymphoproliferative disorders: histopathology, differential diagnosis, new variants, and simulators. *J Cutan Pathol*. 2006;33(suppl 1):58-70.
12. Shalabi D, Ringe J, Lee JB, Nikbakht N. Molluscum contagiosum infection with features of primary cutaneous anaplastic large cell lymphoma. *Dermatol Online J*. 2019;25(11):13030/qt7vp863hz.
13. Fukamachi S, Kimura T, Kobayashi M, et al. Palmar pseudolymphoma associated with herpes simplex infection. *J Cutan Pathol*. 2010;37(7):808-811.
14. Porto DA, Comfere NI, Myers LM, et al. Pseudolymphomatous reaction to varicella zoster virus vaccination: role of viral in situ hybridization. *J Cutan Pathol*. 2010;37(10):1098-1102.
15. Guitart J, Hurt MA. Pleomorphic T-cell infiltrate associated with molluscum contagiosum. *Am J Dermatopathol*. 1999;21(2):178-180.
16. De Diego J, Berridi D, Saracibar N, et al. Cutaneous pseudolymphoma in association with molluscum contagiosum. *Am J Dermatopathol*. 1998;20:518-521.
17. Moreno-Ramírez D, García-Escudero A, Ríos-Martín JJ, et al. Cutaneous pseudolymphoma in association with molluscum contagiosum in an elderly patient. *J Cutan Pathol*. 2003;30:473-475.
18. Chai C, White WL, Shea CR, et al. Epstein–Barr virus-associated lymphoproliferative-disorders primarily involving the skin. *J Cutan Pathol*. 1999;26(5):242-247.
19. Rose C, Starostik P, Bröcker EB. Infection with parapoxvirus induces CD30-positive cutaneous infiltrates in humans. *J Cutan Pathol*. 1999;26(10):520-522.
20. Cesinaro AM, Maiorana A. Verruca vulgaris with CD30-positive lymphoid infiltrate: a case report. *Am J Dermatopathol*. 2002;24:60-62.
21. Kash N, Ginter-Hanselmayer G, Cerroni L. Cutaneous mycotic infections with pseudolymphomatous infiltrates. *Am J Dermatopathol*. 2010;32(5):514-517.
22. Murphy M. Intradermal CD30–positive mononuclear cells in superficial fungal infections of the skin. *Mycoses*. 2009;52:182-186.
23. Lee JS, Park MY, Kim YJ, et al. Histopathological features in both the eschar and erythematous lesions of Tsutsugamushi disease: identification of CD30+ cell infiltration in Tsutsugamushi disease. *Am J Dermatopathol*. 2009;31(6):551-556.
24. Massi D, Trotta M, Franchi A, et al. Atypical CD30+ cutaneous lymphoid proliferation in a patient with tuberculosis infection. *Am J Dermatopathol*. 2004;26(3):234-236.
25. Gallardo F, Barranco C, Toll A, et al. CD30 antigen expression in cutaneous inflammatory infiltrates of scabies: a dynamic immunophenotypic pattern that should be distinguished from lymphomatoid papulosis. *J Cutan Pathol*. 2002;29(6):368-373.
26. Kempf W, Kazakov DV, Palmedo G, et al. Pityriasis lichenoides et varioliformis acuta with numerous CD30(+) cells: a variant mimicking lymphomatoid papulosis and other cutaneous lymphomas. A clinicopathologic, immunohistochemical, and molecular biological study of 13 cases. *Am J Surg Pathol*. 2012;36(7):1021-1029.
27. Haus G, Utikal J, Geraud C, et al. CD30-positive lymphoproliferative disorder in a red tattoo: regional lymphomatoid papulosis type C or pseudolymphoma? *Br J Dermatol*. 2014;171(3):668-670.
28. Ploysangam T, Breneman DL, Mutasim DF. Cutaneous pseudolymphomas. *J Am Acad Dermatol*. 1998;38(6 pt 1):877-895.
29. Campolmi P, Bassi A, Bonan P, et al. Cutaneous pseudolymphoma localized to black tattoo. *J Am Acad Dermatol*. 2011;65(5):e155-e157.
30. Kim KJ, Lee MW, Choi JH, et al. CD30-positive T-cell-rich pseudolymphoma induced by gold acupuncture. *Br J Dermatol*. 2002;146(5):882-884.
31. Massey PR, Wanat KA, Stewart CL, et al. CD30 positive atypical lymphocytes in perniosis: a potential histopathologic

pitfall in a benign condition. *Am J Dermatopathol.* 2014;36(9):730-733.
32. Ardighieri L, Lonardi S, Vermi W, et al. Intralymphatic atypical T-cell proliferation in a cutaneous hemangioma. *J Cutan Pathol.* 2010;37:497-503.
33. Baum CL, Stone MS, Liu V. Atypical intravascular CD30+ T-cell proliferation following trauma in a healthy 17-year-old male: first reported case of a potential diagnostic pitfall and literature review. *J Cutan Pathol.* 2009;36:350-354.
34. Riveiro-Falkenbach E, Fernandez-Figueras MT, Rodriguez-Peralto JL. Benign atypical intravascular CD30(+) T-cell proliferation: a reactive condition mimicking intravascular lymphoma. *Am J Dermatopathol.* 2013;35:143-150.
35. Kempf W, Keller K, John H, et al. Benign atypical intravascular CD30+ T-cell proliferation: a recently described reactive lymphoproliferative process and simulator of intravascular lymphoma – report of a case associated with lichen sclerosus and review of the literature. *Am J Clin Pathol.* 2014;142(5):694-699.
36. Hirshberg A, Amariglio N, Akrish S, et al. Traumatic ulcerative granuloma with stromal eosinophilia: a reactive lesion of the oral mucosa. *Am J Clin Pathol.* 2006;126(4):522-529.
37. Damevska K, Gocev G, Nikolovska S. Eosinophilic ulcer of the oral mucosa: report of a case with multiple synchronous lesions. *Am J Dermatopathol.* 2014;36(7):594-596.
38. Nathan DL, Belsito DV. Carbamazepine-induced pseudolymphoma with CD-30 positive cells. *J Am Acad Dermatol.* 1998;38:806-809.
39. Pulitzer MP, Nolan KA, Oshman RG, et al. CD30+ lymphomatoid drug reactions. *Am J Dermatopathol.* 2013;35(3):343-350.
40. Saeed SA, Bazza M, Zaman M, et al. Cefuroxime induced lymphomatoid hypersensitivity reaction. *Postgrad Med.* 2000;76(899):577-579.
41. Magro CM, Crowson AN, Kovatich AJ, et al. Drug-induced reversible lymphoid dyscrasia: a clonal lymphomatoid dermatitis of memory and activated T cells. *Hum Pathol.* 2003;34(2):119-129.
42. Kabashima R, Orimo H, Hino R, et al. CD30-positive T-cell pseudolymphoma induced by amlodipine. *J Eur Acad Dermatol Venereol.* 2008;22(12):1522-1524.
43. Marucci G, Sgarbanti E, Maestri A, et al. Gemcitabine-associated CD8+CD30+ pseudolymphoma. *Br J Dermatol.* 2001;145(4):650-652.
44. Sawada Y, Yoshiki R, Kawakami C, et al. Valsartan-induced drug eruption followed by CD30+ pseudolymphomatous eruption. *Acta Derm Venereol.* 2010;90(5):521-522.
45. Rader RK, Stoecker WV, Hinton KA, et al. CD30+ reversible lymphoid dyscrasia (pseudolymphoma) following HIDA scintigraphy and the [Ring1]-[Ring2]-[C=O] generalized structure hypothesis. *J Am Acad Dermatol.* 2013;68(3):e99-e101.
46. Magro CM, Olson LC, Nguyen GH, de Feraudy SM. CD30 positive lymphomatoid angiocentric drug reactions: characterization of a series of 20 cases. *Am J Dermatopathol.* 2017;39(7):508-517.
47. Inoue A, Sawada Y, Ohmori S, et al. CD30-positive cutaneous pseudolymphoma caused by tocilizumab in a patient with rheumatoid arthritis: case report and literature review. *Acta Derm Venereol.* 2016;96(4):570-571.
48. Bush AE, Garcia A, Li J, Curry J, Chon SY. CD30(+) lymphomatoid skin toxicity secondary to ipilimumab. *JAAD Case Rep.* 2020;6(4):251-253.
49. Cribier B, Scrivener Y, Grosshans E. Molluscum contagiosum: histologic patterns and associated lesions. A study of 578 cases. *Am J Dermatopathol.* 2001;23(2):99-103.
50. Borra T, Custrin A, Saggini A, et al. Pityriasis lichenoides, atypical pityriasis lichenoides, and related conditions: a study of 66 cases. *Am J Surg Pathol.* 2018;42(8):1101-1112.
51. Nakamura S, Takeda K, Hashimoto Y, et al. Primary cutaneous CD30+ lymphoproliferative disorder in an atopic dermatitis patient on cyclosporine therapy. *Indian J Dermatol Venereol and Leprol.* 2011;77(2):253.
52. Boada A, Bielsa I, Fernández-Figueras MT, et al. Perniosis: clinical and histopathological analysis. *Am J Dermatopathol.* 2010;32(1):19-23.
53. Hurabielle C, Sbidian E, Beltraminelli H, et al. Eruption of lymphocyte recovery with atypical lymphocytes mimicking a primary cutaneous T-cell lymphoma: a series of 12 patients. *Hum Pathol.* 2018;71:100-108.
54. Mechtersheimer G, Moller P. Expression of Ki-1 antigen (CD30) in mesenchymal tumors. *Cancer.* 1990;66(8):1732-1737.
55. Fischer M, Harvima IT, Carvalho RF, et al. Mast cell CD30 ligand is upregulated in cutaneous inflammation and mediates degranulation-independent chemokine secretion. *J Clin Invest.* 2006;116(10):2748-2756.
56. Dummer W, Rose C, Bröcker EB. Expression of CD30 on T helper cells in the inflammatory infiltrate of acute atopic dermatitis but not of allergic contact dermatitis. *Arch Dermatol Res.* 1998;290(11):598-602.
57. Kailas A, Elston DM, Crater SE, Cerruto CA. Cutaneous intravascular CD30+ T-cell pseudolymphoma occurring in a regressing keratoacanthoma. *J Cutan Pathol.* 2018;45(4):296-298. Epub 2018 Feb 18.
58. Greisser J, Palmedo G, Sander C, et al. Detection of clonal rearrangement of T-cell receptor genes in the diagnosis of primary cutaneous CD30 lymphoproliferative disorders. *J Cutan Pathol.* 2006;33(11):711-755.
59. Sangueza OP, Yadav S, White CR Jr, et al. Evolution of B-cell lymphoma from pseudolymphoma. A multidisciplinary approach using histology, immunohistochemistry, and Southern blot analysis. *Am J Dermatopathol.* 1992;14(5):408-413.
60. Stephan F, Haber R, Kechichian E, Kamar F. Lamotrigine-induced hypersensitivity syndrome with histologic features of CD30+ lymphoma. *Ind J Dermatol.* 2016;61(2):235.
61. Cheong KW, Lim GZ, Tan KB, Lim JH. An instructive case of amlodipine-induced reversible granulomatous CD30(+) T-cell pseudolymphoma. *Australas J Dermatol.* 2020;61(3):e346-e350.
62. Cerroni L, Zenahlik P, Kerl H. Specific cutaneous infiltrates of B-cell chronic lymphocytic leukemia arising at the site of herpes zoster and herpes simplex scars. *Cancer.* 1995;76(1):26-31.

CHAPTER 49

Pseudolymphomatous reactions with associated cutaneous neoplastic proliferations

Sara C. Shalin and Bruce R. Smoller

INTRODUCTION

On occasion, neoplasms may be so infiltrated by inflammatory cells that a lymphomatous process is considered within the differential diagnosis. Such tumors range from epithelial to mesenchymal, benign to malignant, but the lymphoid infiltrate may be dense enough to obscure their true derivation. In such cases, the pathologist is tasked with remembering entities such as those discussed in this chapter to help arrive at the correct diagnosis. Importantly, it should be remembered that, while immunohistochemical stains often reveal and support the correct diagnosis, so too immunohistochemical stains may often complicate the situation. For example, large numbers of CD30-positive reactive lymphocytes may erroneously take us down the road of a CD30-positive lymphoproliferative disorder or CD138 positivity may convince us of a plasma cell neoplasm when in fact we are looking at a poorly differentiated carcinoma.

The entities discussed in the following pages are generally rare but not exceptional. Familiarity with the morphologic and (when necessary) immunophenotypic patterns will allow for confident recognition and diagnosis of these entities and will avoid the pitfall of erroneous workup for a lymphoproliferative process.

The chapter is divided into the following categories: Epithelial tumors, melanocytic tumors, and mesenchymal tumors, with a special emphasis on vascular lesions with a pronounced pseudolymphomatous infiltrate.

EPITHELIAL TUMORS

Cutaneous Lymphadenoma

Cutaneous lymphadenoma is a rare adnexal tumor originally described by Dr. Santa Cruz in 1991. Considered by many to be a variant of trichoblastoma, it has also been termed lymphotropic adamantinoid trichoblastoma, adamantinoid trichoblastoma, or lymphoepithelial tumor of skin. The tumor classically exhibits hints of follicular derivation as well as an invariable infiltrate of mature, small lymphocytes.

Clinical Features
The clinical features of cutaneous lymphadenoma are not specific. Asymptomatic, flesh-colored to erythematous papules or nodules with a domed surface involving the head, neck, or legs are most commonly reported. The tumor is typically diagnosed in young to middle-aged adults, possibly with a slight predominance in men.[1]

Histologic Features
Cutaneous lymphadenoma is composed of generally circumscribed but unencapsulated dermal nodules or islands of basaloid cells embedded in a fibrotic to desmoplastic stroma (Fig. 49-1). Epidermal connections are minimal, if present at all. The epithelial lobules are round or irregularly shaped and usually show peripherally located, palisaded basophilic cuboidal cells. Centrally, epithelial cells are larger with eosinophilic cytoplasm, vesicular nuclei, and occasional nucleoli.[1] The tumor lobules usually do not exhibit tumor-stroma clefting as would be seen in basal cell carcinoma. Focal follicular or sebaceous differentiation has been reported, suggesting pilosebaceous derivation, and is supported by the presence of occasional papillary mesenchymal bodies[2] and an immunohistochemical staining pattern similar to trichoblastoma.[3] However, ductal differentiation is also rarely reported,[4,5] although other authors have suggested that intratumoral ducts may represent entrapped normal structures.[6] The epithelial islands are invariably associated with a brisk lymphohistiocytic infiltrate. Plasma cells are not usually part of the infiltrate. Both within the epithelial and stromal components, small lymphocytes are seen, and within the paler central epithelial component there are frequently scattered large, sometimes multinucleated cells with prominent, eosinophilic nucleoli resembling the Reed-Sternberg cells of Hodgkin lymphoma (Fig. 49-2).[1] The lymphoid infiltrate has been reported to be heavier at the dermal-subcutaneous junction and at tumor lobules.[2,7] Spongiosis is often prominent within the epithelial nests.

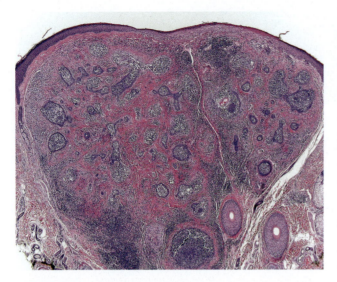

FIGURE 49-1. Cutaneous lymphadenoma. Low-power magnification shows an unencapsulated but circumscribed tumor composed of basaloid cells in nodules, embedded in a fibrotic stroma.

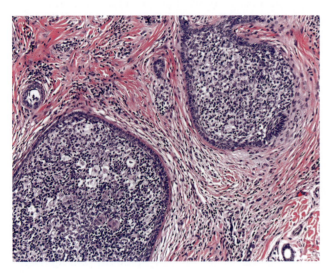

FIGURE 49-2. Cutaneous lymphadenoma. Close examination of the tumor islands discloses a peripheral rim of basaloid cells, central more eosinophilic epithelial cells, a "peppering" of lymphocytes, and scattered enlarged cells with prominent nucleoli.

The epithelial component of the tumor may be highlighted with cytokeratin immunohistochemical stains, although recognition of the epithelial nature is rarely problematic. The lymphoid infiltrate has previously been characterized. The lymphocytes are predominantly T cells, with B cells representing a minority of the infiltrate. Further analysis of T-cell subsets has suggested that they are memory and regulatory T cells.[8] A component of intraepithelial Langerhans cells (CD1a-positive and S100-positive) is also usually present. The large, Reed-Sternberg-like cells are decorated by CD30 and have been postulated variably to represent activated lymphocytes[6] or histiocytes.[3] Androgen receptor and PHLDA1 are diffusely positive in all cases of this tumor.

Differential Diagnosis

The differential diagnosis of cutaneous lymphadenoma includes clear cell basal cell carcinoma, clear cell syringoma, and lymphoepithelioma-like carcinoma. In spite of the consistent presence of a dense lymphoid infiltrate, the epithelial nature of the tumor is usually evident and consideration for lymphoma is rarely raised. Basal cell carcinoma may be distinguished from lymphadenoma by the presence of larger tumor cells, tumor-stroma clefting artifact, and brisk mitotic activity and the absence of a desmoplastic "follicular" stroma. CK17 has been reported to be highly sensitive in differentiating lymphadenomas from basal cell carcinomas, with basal cell carcinoma staining diffusely positive for CK17, while only the peripheral rim of tumor islands marks with CK17 in cutaneous lymphadenoma.[9] Clear cell syringoma demonstrates well-defined ductular differentiation, and, like clear cell basal cell carcinoma, usually lacks an associated prominent lymphoid infiltrate. Lymphoepithelioma-like carcinoma (discussed below) has a cytologically malignant epithelial component and lacks the CD30-positive Reed-Sternberg-like cells that may be seen in lymphadenoma.

Treatment

Although most regard cutaneous lymphadenoma to be a rare benign adnexal tumor, others have proposed it is best regarded as a variant of basal cell carcinoma.[10] Thus, the as-yet unclear histogenesis has prompted some authors to recommend complete surgical excision of these tumors.[11] Recurrence or aggressive clinical behavior is not reported after complete excision.

Spiradenoma With Dense Lymphoid Infiltrates

Spiradenoma is a benign adnexal tumor with differentiation toward the eccrine apparatus.

Clinical Features

Spiradenoma classically presents clinically as a painful dermal nodule. There is a predilection for occurrence on the trunk or head and neck, but it may be found on the extremities.

Histologic Features

While origin from the eccrine apparatus or apocrine derivation has not been conclusively settled, the dermal-based tumor typically exhibits clear areas of ductal differentiation. Composed classically of two epithelial cell types, a peripheral rim of small, dense, basaloid cells with hyperchromatic nuclei and central cells with larger, paler nuclei with vesicular chromatin pattern, spiradenomas are also invariably associated with an evenly dispersed infiltrate of inflammatory cells in the center of tumor lobules (Fig. 49-3). The reliability of such finding can be a diagnostic clue as lymphocytes are not classically associated in similar adnexal tumors such as cylindroma.[12]

The inflammatory cells associated with spiradenoma have been characterized immunohistochemically. CD3-positive T cells and Langerhans cells (S100 protein and CD1a positive) make up the inflammatory infiltrate, with approximately equally distributed numbers of CD8 and CD4 subsets distributed within the parenchyma of the tumor lobules.[13]

Differential Diagnosis

Should the inflammatory infiltrate overwhelm the epithelial elements, the low-power impression of a lobular aggregate of small blue cells could simulate a lymphomatous infiltrate

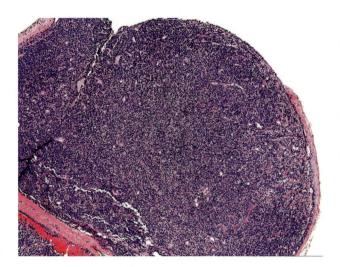

FIGURE 49-3. Spiradenoma. Conventional spiradenoma shows three cell types: peripheral basaloid cells; central cells with larger, paler nuclei and vesicular chromatin; and lymphocytes.

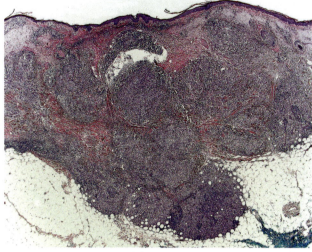

FIGURE 49-5. Cutaneous lymphoepithelial-like carcinoma. Low-power magnification demonstrates a dermal-based tumor with extension to the subcutis composed of a dense lymphoid infiltrate.

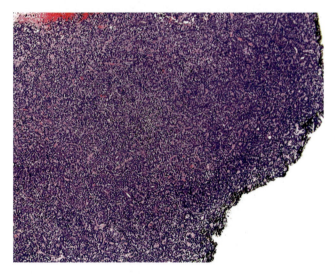

FIGURE 49-4. Spiradenoma. When the lymphocytes are prominent, the ductular differentiation and epithelial nature of the tumor may be somewhat obscured.

(Fig. 49-4). The unusual occurrence of malignant transformation of spiradenoma and its related hybrid tumor spiradenocylindroma has been described as histologically resembling lymphoepithelial carcinoma (discussed below).[14]

Treatment

As these lesions are benign, additional treatment following biopsy is not warranted.

Lymphoepithelioma-Like Carcinoma (Lymphoepithelial Carcinoma)

Lymphoepithelioma-like carcinoma (LELC) is an unusual cutaneous tumor exhibiting some histologic similarities, and also important differences, to its nasopharyngeal counterpart. In contrast to extracutaneous (including sinonasal and nasopharyngeal) tumors, cutaneous LELC is not associated with Epstein-Barr virus (EBV) infection,[15-19] save for one exceptional report.[20] Most commonly termed "lymphoepithelioma-like carcinoma of the skin" in the literature, the term lymphoepithelial carcinoma has been adopted by the World Health Organization (WHO) as preferred terminology for tumors in the oro- and nasopharynx.[21] Its dense associated lymphoid infiltrate results in histologic mimicry with a primary lymphoma, and identification of neoplastic epithelial cells within the inflammation is critical to arriving at the correct diagnosis.

Clinical Features

Cutaneous lymphoepithelioma-like carcinoma typically presents on the head and neck of older to elderly individuals as a slow-growing papule, plaque, or nodule. Tumors may be flesh colored or red and clinically mistaken for basal cell carcinoma, Merkel cell carcinoma, or squamous cell carcinoma.[22,23]

Histologic Features

On microscopic examination, LELC is usually a dermal-based tumor composed of lobules, small nests, or single cell clusters of cohesive, large, epithelioid but generally poorly differentiated cells (Fig. 49-5). Tumor cells are polygonal with large, chromatin-dense, and vesicular nuclei; prominent nucleoli; and often brisk mitotic activity. The epithelioid nature of the tumor cells may be obscured by a florid lymphoid infiltrate that permeates within and around tumor lobules (Fig. 49-6). Evidence of focal trichilemmal keratinization and ductal differentiation has been observed in some cases, leading to speculation that LELC may represent an adnexal tumor rather than a variant of squamous cell carcinoma, although this remains unproven.[15,22,24]

Concealed epithelioid tumor cells will be highlighted by epithelial markers such as cytokeratins, epithelial membrane antigen (EMA), p40 or p63 (Fig. 49-7). Some reports indicated staining with high-molecular-weight keratins,[25,26] providing some support for epidermal rather than adnexal derivation. The invariably associated lymphoid infiltrate is composed of a mix of B cells, T cells, and mature plasma cells. A single case report documents the concurrent

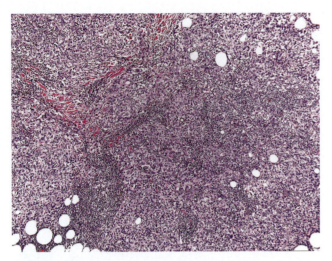

FIGURE 49-6. Cutaneous lymphoepithelial-like carcinoma. Even on higher magnification, the epithelial nature of the tumor cells can be difficult to appreciate.

Distinction of primary cutaneous LELC from metastatic lymphoepithelial carcinoma from another site may be accomplished by thorough clinical workup and by detection of EBV within the tumor. Polymerase chain reaction (PCR) or in situ hybridization studies for EBV-encoded RNA may be performed on paraffin-embedded tissue blocks.[16,17,19]

If the epithelial tumor cells are not appreciated on routine histologic sections, lymphoma and pseudolymphoma may enter the differential diagnosis.[23] Astute identification of epithelioid cells and utilization of cytokeratin immunohistochemical stains will facilitate the diagnosis.

Treatment

In contrast to its nasopharyngeal counterpart and despite its malignant cytologic features, cutaneous LELC generally displays low metastatic and malignant potential, although local recurrence is reported in cases of incomplete excision.[22,26,27] Regional lymph node involvement[27,28] and death from disease[29] are rarely reported. Complete excision is the recommended treatment modality, accomplished with wide local excision or Mohs micrographic surgery.[22,28,30]

MELANOCYTIC TUMORS

Halo Nevus and Regressing Melanoma

Melanocytic tumors, both benign and malignant, may incite a dense inflammatory reaction. Although the biologic behavior of these two entities is vastly different, the proposed purpose and function of the associated inflammatory infiltrate is thought to be related, a host immune response mounted against the melanocytic tumor. In both cases, such an infiltrate is associated with loss of tumor cells, possibly through cytotoxic-mediated cell death. The cellular components of the inflammatory infiltrate of both nevi and melanoma have been investigated, with important similarities and differences being elucidated. Both entities will be discussed together so that shared and contrasting elements may be highlighted.

Clinical Features

Halo nevi are melanocytic nevi surrounded clinically by a rim of depigmentation (a "halo"), which corresponds to spontaneous immune-mediated involution of the lesion. While possible at any age, halo nevi typically occur in children and adolescents. The nevi, prior to acquisition of the clinical halo, may be congenital or acquired and sometimes clinically atypical or of the Spitz type[31] but are generally small, evenly pigmented, and symmetric. Multiple halo nevi have been reported as occurring concurrent with or subsequent to the diagnosis of melanoma, posited to represent an immune response to melanoma resulting in cross-reactivity with benign melanocytes.[32] Similarly, patients with metastatic melanoma being treated with immune checkpoint inhibitors—therapies that stimulate the host immune response—have been reported to develop multiple halo nevi during the course of treatment.[33] If left alone, halo nevi typically result in an area of clinical depigmentation.[34]

In contrast, melanoma with features of regression usually has a markedly atypical clinical appearance. The lesion may be large, asymmetric and irregularly contoured, and

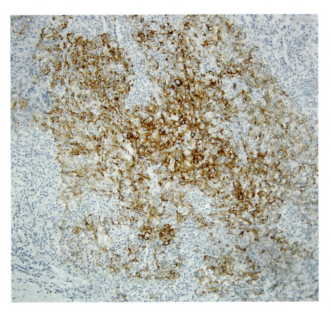

FIGURE 49-7. Cutaneous lymphoepithelial-like carcinoma. A pancytokeratin immunohistochemical stain is positive in the epithelial tumor cells.

diagnosis of LELC and cutaneous marginal zone lymphoma in the same specimen, as proven by the demonstration of light chain–restricted plasma cells and immunoglobulin heavy chain gene rearrangement. The authors hypothesized that the inflammatory infiltrate intrinsic to the LELC may have provided the chronic inflammatory stimuli necessary to induce the development of the low-grade B-cell lymphoma.[26]

Differential Diagnosis

Cutaneous lymphadenoma is a benign adnexal neoplasm exhibiting ductal differentiation. Although often associated with a similarly dense inflammatory infiltrate, the epithelial cells that comprise the tumor nests and lobules of lymphadenoma are typically better delineated, composed of small to medium lymphocytes that lack cytologic features of malignancy.[23] Malignant transformation of benign lymphadenoma and spiradenocylindroma has been said to resemble LELC.[1,14]

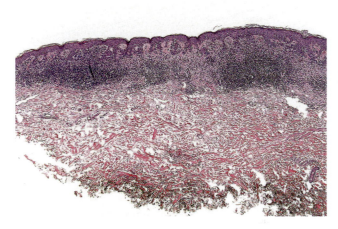

FIGURE 49-8. Melanoma with inflammatory regression. On scanning magnification, a lichenoid band of inflammation is seen, obscuring the melanocytic proliferation.

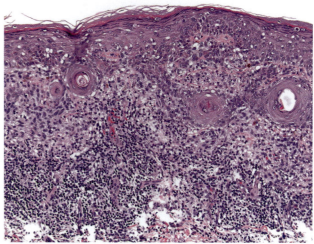

FIGURE 49-10. Melanoma with inflammatory regression. Prominent pagetoid extension and cytologic atypia of melanocytes classify this lesion as a melanoma.

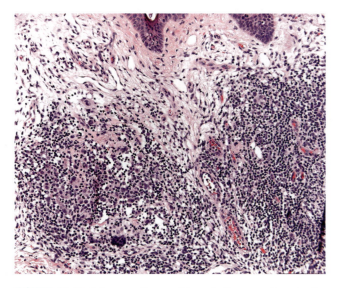

FIGURE 49-9. Halo nevus. Upon careful examination, nevomelanocytes displaying maturation may be seen among the dense lymphocytic infiltrate in this halo nevus.

variegated in color. Regression in particular is associated with a white to gray scar-like discoloration, often described as a "blue-white veil" on dermoscopic evaluation, or with blue to gray pepper-like granules.[35] Moreover, melanomas present in an older demographic than halo nevi, and incidence increases with age.

Histologic Features
Both halo nevi and regressing melanoma are characterized by melanocytic proliferations with sometimes obscuring lymphocytic inflammation (Fig. 49-8); however, the character of the melanocytic proliferation is different. Benign melanocytic nevi are symmetric, nested populations of melanocytes. Nests of melanocytes within the epidermis are most often found at the tips of rete-ridges, and confluent single cells along the junction or upward scatter of melanocytes are lacking. Nests of melanocytes in the dermis display "maturation"; that is, the nests and individual melanocytes decrease in size with further descent into the dermis (Fig. 49-9).

Cytologic atypia and mitotic figures are usually not apparent. Melanoma, on the other hand, tends toward a single cell over nested pattern of intraepidermal growth. Melanocytes classically extend above the basal layer in a Pagetoid manner (Fig. 49-10). Invasion into the dermis is characterized by expansile, sheet-like or large nests of cytologically atypical melanocytes. Large cells are present at the base of the lesion (an absence of maturation), and mitotic figures may be evident.

The inflammatory cells that are present in association with benign nevi are thought to account for the clinical halo phenomenon. These inflammatory cells have been found to be cytotoxic, CD8-positive lymphocytes, although it is interesting that apoptotic or dying melanocytes are seldom appreciated histologically in the evaluation of halo nevi.[34,36] By flow cytometry, a cytotoxic T-cell response has been found to be generated against the melanocytic antigens gp100 and Mart-1 in a regressing nevus.[32]

Similarly, an inflammatory infiltrate in melanoma typically comprises cytotoxic T cells. Interestingly, expression of major histocompatibility antigens HLA-A, B, and C on melanocytes is seen both in regressing melanoma and halo nevi, while this expression is absent in noninflamed nevi nests.[36,37] Specifically, the number of resting cytotoxic T cells, characterized by TIA-1 expression, is noted to be increased in melanoma compared with normal skin and benign nevi[38]; however, TIA-1-expressing lymphocytes appear to make up a smaller percentage of the inflammatory infiltrate with increasing tumor progression; halo nevi were not specifically examined.[39] Most recently, a more detailed analysis comparing the immunophenotype of the infiltrate in halo nevi and regressing melanoma was performed. In the largest size study of its kind to date, the inflammatory infiltrate of 62 melanomas undergoing regression (14 early, 48 late) and 15 halo nevi were characterized.[40] This study confirmed that the T cells with a cytotoxic phenotype are found in both halo nevi and regressing melanoma. Interestingly, expression of cytotoxic markers (granzyme and TIA-1) was found in a greater percentage of the infiltrate in halo nevi compared with regressing melanoma. Moreover, the presence of a higher percentage of PD-1-expressing lymphocytes in halo

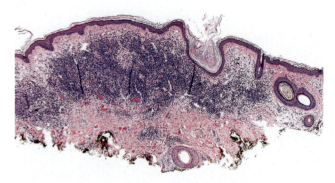

FIGURE 49-11. **Halo nevus.** On this low-power examination, the nevomelanocytes are nearly completely masked by the brisk lymphoid infiltrate.

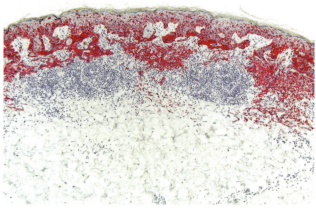

FIGURE 49-12. **Melanoma with inflammatory regression.** A Melan-A immunohistochemical stain highlights the melanocytic proliferation.

nevi compared with regressing melanoma was hypothesized to represent an equally strong *negative* regulator of cytotoxic activity in halo nevi, suggesting a balanced immune response in these lesions.[40] In contrast, regressing melanoma, particularly the early, inflammatory phase, demonstrated higher numbers of CD123-expressing plasmacytoid dendritic cells (implicated in induction of immune tolerance) than did halo nevi. Early regression was associated with more TIA-1 expressing lymphocytes than late regression, sharing some features of halo nevus, but the presence of a higher CD123 to TIA-1 ratio in melanoma suggested to the authors an overall less efficient immune response in regressing melanoma than in halo nevi.[40]

Differential Diagnosis
Halo nevi should be distinguished from inflammatory regression of melanoma using criteria as specified above. The clinical and cytologic attributes of the lesion typically are sufficient to allow for distinction, although the inflammatory cells may induce reactive cytologic atypia in otherwise benign halo nevi, particularly in variants like Spitz nevi that have a preexisting degree of cytologic atypia.[31]

On occasion, the associated inflammatory infiltrate may be so dense as to obscure the melanocytic nature of the lesion (Fig. 49-11). In these cases, the lymphohistiocytic infiltrate may be mistaken for an inflammatory dermatosis, cutaneous lymphoid hyperplasia, or even cutaneous lymphoma. Exocytosis of cytotoxic T cells may mimic the epidermotropism and Pautrier microabscesses of cutaneous T-cell lymphoma (mycosis fungoides).[41] Residual melanocytes may be mistaken for the large, CD30-positive lymphoid cells of lymphomatoid papulosis or less likely anaplastic large cell lymphoma or Hodgkin lymphoma.[41] In such cases, application of melanocytic-specific immunohistochemical stains (Mart-1, Melan-A, MiTF, HMB-45, Sox10, S100 protein) should allow for highlighting of residual melanocytes, leading to the correct diagnosis (Fig. 49-12).

Treatment
Halo nevi are benign and require no further treatment. Melanomas with inflammatory regression are treated with wide local excision, and, depending on the Breslow depth of the primary tumor, sentinel lymph node sampling. Radial growth phase and thin melanomas, generally considered to be less than 0.8 mm in depth, have an overall favorable prognosis, but life-long surveillance is necessary as recurrences can occur many years after primary diagnosis. The disease-free survival and overall survival decrease significantly with increasing tumor depth and regional or distant metastases.

MESENCHYMAL TUMORS

Epithelioid Hemangioma (Angiolymphoid Hyperplasia With Eosinophilia)
Epithelioid hemangioma is a vascular proliferation that presents as papules, plaques, or nodules. Given the invariable presence of a dense, mixed inflammatory infiltrate that characterizes this entity, the synonymous term of angiolymphoid hyperplasia with eosinophilia is preferred by many authors. The precise etiology and pathogenesis remain elusive, although a history of antecedent trauma can be elicited in a fraction of cases.[42]

Clinical Features
Epithelioid hemangioma most often presents clinically as red to brown papules, plaques, or nodules and may be single or multiple. A zosteriform distribution has also been reported.[43] The prototypic location is the head and neck, although extremities[44] and penis[45] are other frequently reported sites of occurrence. Extracutaneous lesions are even occasionally reported.[46] The lesions typically arise in adults with no definitive gender predilection and may clinically simulate cutaneous lymphoid hyperplasia, arthropod bite reactions, cutaneous lymphoma, or metastasis.[42]

Histologic Features
Epithelioid hemangioma is characterized by two dominant components: a vascular proliferation characterized by plump, histiocytic-appearing endothelial cells and a mixed inflammatory infiltrate that classically contains numerous eosinophils (Fig. 49-13). When the inflammatory component predominates, a lymphoproliferative process may be suspected, so careful attention to the detection of the background vascular component should be sought (Fig. 49-14). The vascular element is composed of a vaguely lobular to nodular proliferation of vessels lined by endothelial cells that

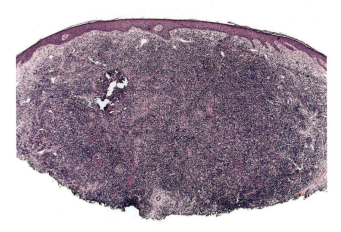

FIGURE 49-13. **Epithelioid hemangioma.** A dense mixed infiltrate is present in the dermis.

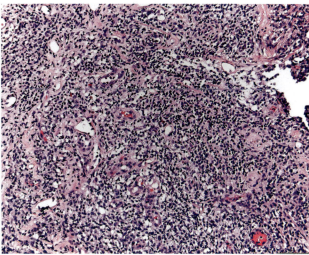

FIGURE 49-15. **Epithelioid hemangioma.** The vascular component is composed of well-formed vessels with plump endothelial cells and endothelial cells that sometimes protrude into the lumen ("hobnailing").

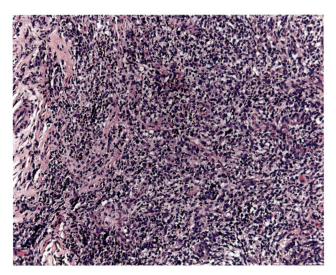

FIGURE 49-14. **Epithelioid hemangioma.** In areas, the mixed inflammation, including conspicuous eosinophils, overwhelms the vascular component.

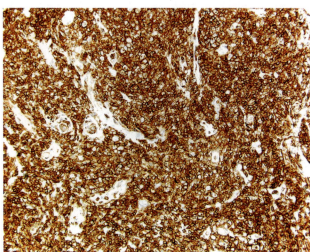

FIGURE 49-16. **Epithelioid hemangioma.** The lymphocytes in epithelioid hemangioma are classically CD4 predominant.

have variably been described as plump, histiocytoid, hobnailed, or epithelioid (Fig. 49-15). In some cases, a small muscular artery or vein demonstrating mural damage may be associated with the vascular proliferation, particularly when the lesions are more deeply seated in the subcutis, again suggesting a relationship to trauma in the development of this entity.[45] Intimately associated with the vascular component is a lymphohistiocytic infiltrate with eosinophils, scattered plasma cells, and, occasionally, large transformed/activated lymphocytes.[44] Exceptionally, giant cells with a granulomatous and fibrosing reaction pattern have been reported.[47] The inflammation tends to be perivascular and periadnexal and spans the dermis, with not infrequent extension to the subcutis. Lymphoid follicles with germinal center formation may be present, and the infiltrate may be more pronounced at the periphery of the lesion and/or at the junction of the dermis and subcutis.[44]

As would be expected, the vascular component of these lesions marks with endothelial markers. Focal aberrant immunoreactivity with cytokeratin has been reported,[45] but thankfully, the vascular nature of these lesions is usually appreciated without the use of immunohistochemistry and the prudent inclusion of a vascular marker when immunohistochemical studies are required will prove to be useful. The majority of lymphocytes are of T-cell lineage with an activated T-helper phenotype (CD4 positive) (Fig. 49-16), with aggregates of B cells comprising the areas resembling lymphoid follicles.[48] In some cases, CD30 expression may be detected in large, activated lymphocytes within the infiltrate (Fig. 49-17), resulting in a diagnostic pitfall of a CD30-positive lymphoproliferative disorder.[44]

Although most regard epithelioid hemangioma to represent a reactive vascular proliferation, several reports document the detection of T-cell clonality within the lymphoid population, thereby raising concern that it may be better classified as a low-grade lymphoproliferative disorder.[48,49] Follicular mucinosis has once been reported in association with epithelioid hemangioma.[50]

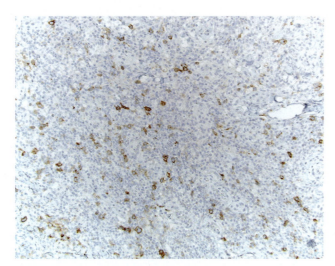

FIGURE 49-17. Epithelioid hemangioma. In some cases, large activated CD30-expressing lymphocytes may mimic a CD30-positive lymphoproliferative disorder.

Differential Diagnosis

In cases arising on nonclassic sites (such as the extremities), or in cases in which the inflammatory component predominates, epithelioid hemangioma may mimic a lymphoproliferative process. Lymphomatoid papulosis (particularly type A), a CD30-positive lymphoproliferative disorder, is characterized by multiple recurring crops of red-brown to violaceous papules. Microscopically, a mixed infiltrate with interspersed enlarged, CD30-positive immunoblasts is seen, resembling epithelioid hemangioma save for the prominent vascular proliferation. Recognition of this vascular component is critical for appropriate classification.

Epithelioid hemangioma also bears considerable histologic resemblance to Kimura disease; indeed, for some time it was unclear whether these were separate or identical entities, and some still regard them on a spectrum.[51] In contrast to epithelioid hemangioma, Kimura disease classically presents as larger, deeper, subcutaneous or salivary gland masses in Asian males. Regional lymphadenopathy, peripheral eosinophilia, and elevated IgE levels are common in Kimura disease but not seen in epithelioid hemangioma. On histopathologic examination, both entities show an exuberant lymphoeosinophilic infiltrate, but Kimura disease shows more frequent lymphoid follicles, more eosinophilic microabscesses, and less conspicuous and epithelioid vascular proliferation.[44,51,52]

Cutaneous manifestations of IgG4-related disease has been reported to have clinical and histologic similarity to Kimura disease and epithelioid hemangioma. The presence of a high proportion of IgG4-expressing plasma cells is essential for this diagnosis.[53,54]

Lastly, arthropod bite reactions may be considered within the histologic differential diagnosis of epithelioid hemangioma. Typically composed of a dense, superficial and deep perivascular to interstitial infiltrate with eosinophils, arthropod bite reactions lack the lobular arrangement of epithelioid vascular elements seen in epithelioid hemangioma.

Treatment

The treatment of epithelioid hemangioma typically requires surgical excision, although other treatment modalities, including cryotherapy, electrodessication, corticosteroids, and phototherapy have all been reported with variable success. Resistance to treatment is relatively common, and incomplete surgical excision is associated with recurrence in approximately one-third of cases.[52] Interferon alpha has been used in treatment-refractory cases, and its utility in this scenario has been used as an argument supporting the idea that this entity is actually a low-grade T-cell lymphoproliferative disorder.[48]

Acral Pseudolymphomatous Angiokeratoma of Children

In 1988 and again in 1990, Ramsay and colleagues first described five cases of a unilateral acral eruption affecting children.[55,56] Histologically, although thick-walled vessels were apparent, the overwhelming histopathologic feature was a dense lymphoid infiltrate spanning the entire dermis and extending to the subcutis. Composed of a mix of equal numbers of B and T cells, the lesions behaved in a benign manner and the term "Acral pseudolymphomatous angiokeratoma of children" (APACHE) was coined.[56] Following this initial description, additional cases were reported occurring in adults and at nonacral sites.[57-59] Moreover, determination of whether APACHE is better classified as a pseudolymphoma or a vascular lesion/malformation remains debated in the literature.[57,60,61] As a result, subsequent reports have proposed alternative names for the entity, including papular angiolymphoid hyperplasia, papular pseudolymphoma, acral angiokeratoma-like pseudolymphoma, and pseudolymphomatous angiokeratoma.[62,63]

Clinical Features

APACHE was first described in a group of five children ranging in age from 2 to 13 years. Composed clinically of clustered aggregates of bright red to violaceous papules to nodules with a keratotic surface, the clinical impression was of an angiokeratoma.[55,56] The lesions were all unilateral in distribution and affected the hands and feet. Subsequent case reports document similar lesions occurring in adulthood[57] and at nonacral sites, including upper arm, back, and legs.[57-59,64] A 2012 literature review suggests a female predominance, with roughly half of lesions arising on acral surfaces and approximately three-fourths of affected patients children.[61]

Histopathological Features

Under the microscope, APACHE demonstrates a dense lymphohistiocytic infiltrate occupying the entire dermis with variable infiltration into the subcutis. The infiltrate is composed of lymphocytes, histiocytes, scattered plasma cells and eosinophils, and occasional giant cells (Fig. 49-18). Interstitial and nodular patterns of growth are described, with formation of primary and secondary lymphoid follicles in some cases.[60] Within the infiltrate is a proliferation of blood vessels with thickened walls and plump endothelial cells (Fig. 49-19). The vascular changes have been likened to the "high endothelial venules" of the paracortical lymph node. Epidermal changes are variable, with some authors reporting hyperkeratosis[56] or vacuolar interface alterations,[61,65] while other reports note a normal epidermis. Epidermotropism has also been noted in rare case reports and is hypothesized to occur in more established lesions.[66]

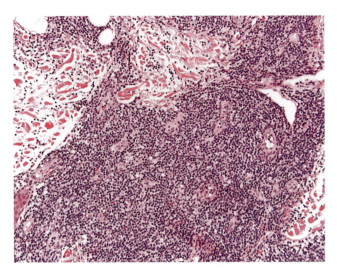

FIGURE 49-18. APACHE. There is a dense mixed lymphoid infiltrate composed of lymphocytes, histiocytes, plasma cells, and occasional eosinophils.

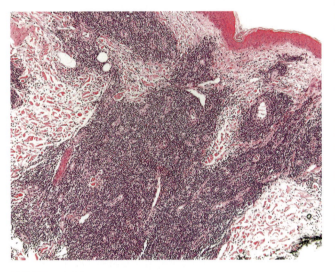

FIGURE 49-19. APACHE. Embedded within the lymphoid infiltrate are well-formed vessels mimicking the high endothelial venules of lymph nodes.

Immunohistochemical staining of the lymphoid infiltrate reveals a mixture of CD3-expressing T cells and CD20-expressing B cells. Interestingly, some reports suggest that B cells may be more prominent in younger patients, while T-cell infiltrates will predominate in adults with APACHE.[62] T cells generally demonstrate an approximately equal mixture of CD4 and CD8-expressing subsets, and B cells and plasma cells are typically polyclonal. CD30 is generally negative.[64] Gene rearrangements for T-cell receptor and immunoglobulin heavy chain, when performed, have usually been negative,[65] although one report classified as APACHE demonstrated IgH rearrangement.[67] Immunohistochemical staining of the prominent vasculature within APACHE has demonstrated expression of podoplanin and CD34, suggesting a lymphatic phenotype, which has been proposed as support for classification as a lymphovascular malformation rather than pseudolymphoma.[61]

Differential Diagnosis
APACHE shares many of the features of similar entities, including angiolymphoid hyperplasia with eosinophils (epithelioid hemangioma) and angioplasmacellular hyperplasia, as well as other rare pseudolymphomatous entities such as T-cell–rich angiomatoid polypoid pseudolymphoma and tibial lymphoplasmacytic plaque. Distinction from small/medium pleomorphic T-cell lymphoproliferative disorder, cutaneous marginal zone lymphoma, or other true lymphomatous infiltrates is imperative given the clinical implications and differing treatment and follow-up recommendations. The immunohistochemical staining pattern of APACHE suggests a reactive lymphoid infiltrate, and clonality studies, in contrast to true lymphomas, are usually negative in cases tested.[65] The vascular prominence that characterizes APACHE is also typically absent in most cutaneous lymphomas.

Epithelioid hemangioma, as discussed above, is distinguished from APACHE by the presence of a mixed inflammatory infiltrate that typically includes more eosinophils than are seen in APACHE. Moreover, the clinical site and distribution of lesions, as well as the age at presentation, serves to separate these entities, although their shared histologic features are acknowledged. Angioplasmacellular hyperplasia, discussed in more detail below, classically presents as a solitary lesion and demonstrates a greater proportion of polyclonal plasma cells within the infiltrate as well as proliferating vessels with characteristically vacuolated endothelial cells.[68]

T-cell-rich angiomatoid polypoid pseudolymphoma (TRAPP) is rarely described in the literature, with only 18 reported cases to date. Typically presenting as a solitary, small polypoid papule resembling a pyogenic granuloma (less than 1 cm), the lesions display a slight female predominance, present in young adulthood to middle age, and have been most commonly reported occurring on the head and neck. Histologically, a dense lymphohistiocytic infiltrate with occasional plasma cells is seen amid a background of prominent blood vessels lined by plump endothelial cells. In contrast to APACHE, the lymphoid infiltrate is T-cell predominant, with a mix of CD4 and CD8-expressing subsets.[69,70]

Tibial lymphoplasmacytic plaque (TLP) is a rarely described pseudolymphoma presenting in children as linear papules coalescing into red-brown to violaceous plaques specifically on the lower leg. Histologically, a mixed dermal infiltrate with a reactive vascular proliferation is observed. Authors acknowledge the close overlap with APACHE and suggest it may represent a clinical variant.[71]

More recently, there has been continued acknowledgment of the histologic similarities between APACHE, TRAPP, and TLP. These entities are all linked by the presence of vessels resembling high endothelial venules, and one study found immunohistochemical expression MECA-79, a marker of endothelial adherence molecules (peripheral node addressins) in all three of these entities while it was absent in cases of angioplasmacellular hyperplasia.[72] Some authors have now advocated for a unifying terminology of "inflammatory lobular hemangioma" to be used for vascular lesions with pseudolymphomatous infiltrates.[73]

Treatment
As these lesions are benign, additional treatment is not necessary, although the lesions may persist indefinitely and be of cosmetic consequence.[56] Topical or intralesional steroid treatment may lead to partial regression of the lesions, although recurrence after cessation of topical treatment has

been reported.[59,64] Complete destruction or excision appears to be curative, with no reported recurrences.

Angioplasmacellular Hyperplasia

A rare entity, angioplasmacellular hyperplasia refers to a unique reactive vascular proliferation surrounded by an infiltrate exclusively composed of polytypic plasma cells. The largest case series to date comprises 10 patients and is felt to represent a reactive inflammatory vascular hyperplasia.[68]

Clinical Features

Most commonly, angioplasmacellular hyperplasia has presented as a solitary papule or nodule with an inflammatory, erythematous rim and ulceration is not uncommon. The lesions occur in the head and neck region, as well as the trunk and legs. The clinical impression is usually of a hemangioma or pyogenic granuloma. Age at presentation ranges from young adult to elderly, with a mean age of 45 years. Men and women appear approximately equally affected. All patients were asymptomatic and without evidence of plasma cell dyscrasia at presentation or follow-up.[68] A lesion with the histopathologic features of angioplasmacellular hyperplasia has also been reported in the oral cavity and termed "plasma cell granuloma with angiokeratomatous features."[74]

Histopathologic Features

Microscopically, a vaguely polypoid lesion is seen with acanthosis of the epidermis and often an epidermal collarette. A perivascular to interstitial infiltrate of plasma cells comprises the majority of the infiltrate (up to 90% of the inflammatory cells), and the plasma cells may extend peripherally beyond the areas of vascular proliferation. Neutrophils and lymphocytes make up the remainder of the inflammatory cells. A proliferation of capillaries and small venules is typically seen in the center of the lesion, lacking the lobularity of a pyogenic granuloma. Endothelial cells are plump and vacuolization of endothelial cells is not uncommon, but atypia or mitotic activity is absent.[68] The plasma cells are polyclonal as demonstrated by equal numbers of kappa and lambda-expressing subsets. Angioplasmacellular hyperplasia lacked expression of high endothelial venule adhesion markers in one small study, setting it apart from APACHE, TRAPP, and TLP.[72]

Differential Diagnosis

The differential diagnosis of angioplasmacellular hyperplasia includes a variety of vascular, infectious, and hematolymphoid entities. Both angioplasmacellular hyperplasia and pyogenic granuloma have overlapping clinical features. However, pyogenic granuloma is characterized by a lobular vascular proliferation and more mixed inflammatory infiltrate, while angioplasmacellular hyperplasia shows scattered capillaries and venule expansion surrounded by a predominance of plasma cells.[68] Epithelioid hemangioma (angiolymphoid hyperplasia with eosinophils) and APACHE share the features of a vascular prominence with accompanying inflammatory infiltrate, although the clinical distribution of lesions and the composite of inflammatory cells will typically serve to distinguish and separate these entities.

Bacillary angiomatosis is a vascular proliferation due to *Bartonella* sp. infection occurring in immunocompromised patients. Silver-based stains (Warthin-Starry) or immunohistochemical stains will demonstrate the causative organisms, and clinical history will typically be different than for angioplasmacellular hyperplasia.[68] Other infectious entities may also need to be excluded. When occurring in the perigenital regions of immunocompromised patients, the pattern of angioplasmacellular hyperplasia has been recently reported as a clue to the diagnosis of chronic herpes simplex virus infection when classic keratinocyte viral inclusions may be lacking.[75]

Cutaneous plasmacytoma may be considered within the differential diagnosis; however, plasmacytoma typically lacks a characteristic vascular component and plasma cells will demonstrate light chain restriction.

Treatment

Complete surgical excision appears to be curative, with recurrences not noted.[68,76,77]

Angiosarcoma Variants

Angiosarcoma is an aggressive vascular neoplasm with high mortality and poor prognosis. Three predominant clinical subtypes of the malignancy are recognized: primary cutaneous angiosarcoma of the head and neck, angiosarcoma arising following radiation, and angiosarcoma associated with chronic lymphedema. Histologically, all subtypes are similar. Relatively recently, a pseudolymphomatous variant has been described in the literature, in which an inflammatory infiltrate obscures the vasoformative nature of the neoplasm, mimicking a lymphoma.[78,79] In addition, high-grade cutaneous lymphoma may also enter the differential diagnosis of the epithelioid variant of angiosarcoma, and accurate diagnosis may be further complicated by occasional shared immunoreactivity of CD30.[80]

Clinical Features

Angiosarcoma arising in the absence of prior radiation or lymphedema typically occurs on the head and neck region of elderly individuals without a specific sex predilection.[81] The lesions are typically violaceous and purpuric, with ill-defined borders that may simulate a hematoma. Facial edema with minimal erythema is an additionally reported presentation.[78] Angiosarcoma arising following radiation therapy classically demonstrates a long latency period and corresponds to sites of prior irradiation. The presence of long-standing, chronic lymphedema is also a risk factor for the development of angiosarcoma, and these tumors classically develop on the upper inner arm of women who have undergone radical mastectomy (Stewart-Treves syndrome). The clinical features of reported cases of the pseudolymphomatous variant of angiosarcoma have been similar to other angiosarcoma presentations, arising on the head and neck of elderly persons in five cases, and following irradiation of the chest wall in one case.[78,79]

Histologic Features

Angiosarcoma is characterized by a malignant proliferation of vascular spaces. Poor definition, infiltration, and irregularity define the architectural patterns of growth, and anastomosing vascular channels may be seen dissecting from the superficial dermis to the deep subcutis (Fig. 49-20).

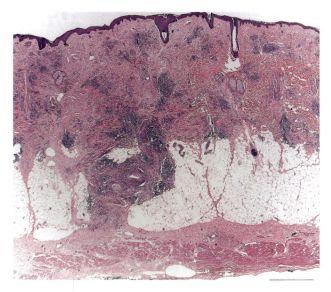

FIGURE 49-20. Angiosarcoma. Low-power magnification shows an ill-defined, deeply invasive tumor with extension to the subcutis.

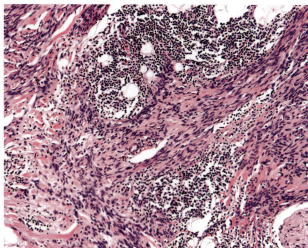

FIGURE 49-22. Angiosarcoma. Angiosarcoma may be associated with dense lymphoid infiltrates whereby the vasoformative regions may be difficult to appreciate.

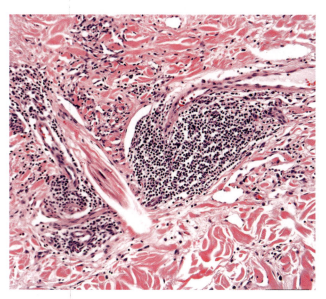

FIGURE 49-21. Angiosarcoma. Key to the diagnosis is the identification of vasoformative areas (upper left).

The identification of the vasoformative foci is critical to the accurate diagnosis. The malignant endothelial cells are hyperchromatic and pleomorphic, classically protruding into the lumens of the vascular spaces (termed "hobnailing"), particularly in more well-differentiated tumors (Fig. 49-21). The endothelial cells may also take on an epithelioid appearance, in which the cells are spindle to polygonal in shape with abundant, steel gray to amphophilic cytoplasm, vesicular nuclei, and prominent nucleoli.[82] The epithelioid variant tends to show sheeting of tumor cells, and the vasoformative areas may be difficult to appreciate. The presence of cytoplasmic vacuoles within neoplastic cells, thought to be abortive lumen formation, may be a helpful clue to diagnosis, as is the presence of extravasated erythrocytes.[83] Rarely, an obscuring lymphoid infiltrate may be present in and around the tumor, obscuring the vascular nature of the tumor (Fig. 49-22). This pseudolymphomatous variant was initially reported to be characterized by a diffuse, pan-dermal lymphoid infiltrate composed of small to medium lymphocytes (diffuse pattern) as well as the presence of numerous lymphoid follicles with germinal center formation (follicular pattern).[78]

The expression of lymphatic and endothelial cell-specific markers characterizes the immunohistochemical profile of angiosarcoma. CD31, CD34, factor VIII–related antigen (von Willebrand factor), FLI-1 protein, podoplanin, and ERG are all classically expressed by the malignant endothelial cells. ERG is one of the more recently characterized markers of endothelial derivation and has been proposed to exhibit superior sensitivity and specificity in the diagnosis of cutaneous angiosarcoma.[84] Exceptionally, cutaneous, postradiation angiosarcoma has been reported to mimic anaplastic large cell lymphoma due to aberrant CD30 expression.[80] The presence of *MYC* amplification (detected by in situ hybridization) or increased c-MYC expression by immunohistochemistry has emerged as a confirmatory diagnostic test in the diagnosis of secondary (and rarely primary cutaneous) angiosarcoma.[85,86]

The immunophenotype of the lymphoid infiltrate in the pseudolymphomatous variant of angiosarcoma has been described. The infiltrate is composed of T cells with a CD4 predominance over CD8 and no reported loss of T-cell antigens. When present, lymphoid follicles have stained with a reactive pattern, showing CD20 and Bcl-6 coexpression in germinal centers, along with CD21 expression, a high proliferative index, and expression of Bcl-2 in the mantle zone.[78] In one reported case, immunoglobulin heavy chain and T-cell gene rearrangements were polyclonal.[79]

Differential Diagnosis
As described above, angiosarcoma may occasionally simulate neoplasms of other derivation. The large, epithelioid and cytologically malignant cells of epithelioid angiosarcoma may mimic poorly differentiated carcinoma, particular carcinomas such a lymphoepithelial carcinoma or neuroendocrine carcinoma, melanoma, or large cell lymphoma.[82] Identification of vasoformation and selection of an appropriately broad panel of immunohistochemical stains should

allow for proper classification. The prominent lymphoid infiltrate in the pseudolymphomatous variant of angiosarcoma may be mistaken for cutaneous follicle center lymphoma (diffuse type or follicular) or primary cutaneous lymphoid hyperplasia. The reactive pattern of staining and negative gene rearrangement should be sufficient to exclude a primary lymphoma. However, once again, appreciation of subtle anastomosing vascular channels within the obscuring lymphoid infiltrate is essential to reaching the appropriate diagnosis.

Treatment

Angiosarcomas are typically treated with wide local excision, sometimes with subsequent radiation to the tumor bed. Angiosarcoma typically portends a poor prognosis, with 5-year survival only around 15%.[83] Younger patients, and those with truncal disease, may fare slightly better than elderly individuals.[81] Interestingly, the few reported cases of pseudolymphatous angiosarcoma or of angiosarcoma with a brisk lymphoid infiltrate with long-term follow-up suggest a possible survival advantage and increased intervals to recurrence.[78] However, given the rarity of such cases, additional study is warranted.

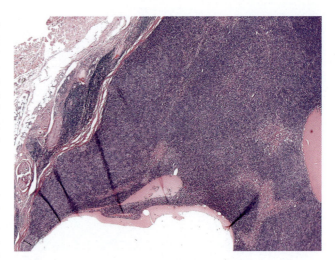

FIGURE 49-23. **Angiomatoid fibrous histiocytoma.** The subcutaneous mass is circumscribed and surrounded by a fibrous pseudocapsule with surrounding aggregates of lymphocytes and plasma cells.

Angiomatoid Fibrous Histiocytoma

Angiomatoid fibrous histiocytoma (AFH) is a soft tissue tumor most frequently arising on the extremities of adolescents and young adults. Not to be confused with the dermatofibroma (or fibrous histiocytoma) with aneurysmal change, which is an entirely benign variant of the common dermatofibroma, AFH is a fibrohistiocytic tumor of low-grade/intermediate malignancy, with a documented, albeit low, chance of metastasis and aggressive course. Typically harboring characteristic translocations that most frequently involve *EWSR1*, AFH is included in this chapter due to its low-power appearance that may simulate malignancy involving a lymph node.

Clinical Features

AFH usually presents as a soft tissue mass on the extremities of children, adolescents, and young adults. In some series, the median age is as young as 13 years,[87] although most patients are younger than 40 years.[88] Unusual sites of occurrences include the head and neck region and trunk,[89] but extracutaneous sites are also reported, including the lung, retroperitoneum, vulva, and mediastinum,[90] locations that may add to diagnostic confusion. There is a suggestion that patients outside of the classic age of presentation may also have a higher incidence of nonclassic sites of involvement.[89] The tumors are nodular, multinodular, or cystic and usually slow growing.[88] In one study of eight patients, the mean tumor size was 3 cm.[90] Most patients are asymptomatic; however, some patients present with constitutional symptoms due to the production of cytokines by the tumor.[88]

Histologic Features

AFH has a classic and fairly consistent histopathologic appearance. On low-power examination, the subcutaneous mass is circumscribed and surrounded by a fibrous pseudocapsule with surrounding aggregates of lymphocytes and plasma cells sometimes with germinal center formation

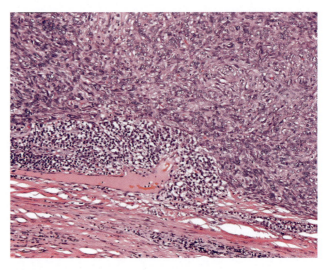

FIGURE 49-24. **Angiomatoid fibrous histiocytoma.** On higher power, tumor cells are histiocytoid with spindle to ovoid nuclei, growing in a solid to swirling growth pattern. Lymphocytes and plasma cells rim the tumor cells.

(Fig. 49-23). In one study, these two features were the most consistently observed features in the cases studied.[89] The tumor cells are usually cytologically innocuous and monotonous with a histiocytoid appearance with spindle to ovoid nuclei. The pattern of growth is variably solid, swirling, or storiform (Fig. 49-24). This encapsulated appearance with lymphocytes may mimic a lymph node replaced by a neoplasm, but astute examination will reveal the absence of a subcapsular or medullary sinuses.[88] The term "angiomatoid" derives from the typical presence of variably large cystic, blood-filled spaces that represent pseudovascular spaces rather than true vessels, present in many but not all cases, and often appreciated on gross examination of these tumors (Fig. 49-25).[88,89] Hemosiderin is often evident within tumor cells, and mitotic activity is low. Cytologic atypia, cellular pleomorphism, and osteoclast-like giant cells may be present in a subset of cases and does not seem to correlate with more aggressive behavior.[88,90] Sclerotic bands separating nodules

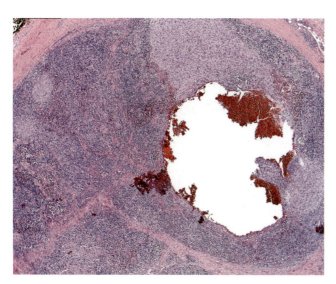

FIGURE 49-25. Angiomatoid fibrous histiocytoma. When present, blood filled cavities within the tumor is a helpful clue.

of tumor cells and myxoid background are other reported histologic features.[87,89] Myxoid change may be more commonly seen in tumors arising at nonclassic sites.[90]

Immunohistochemical stains have a limited role in the diagnosis of these tumors. Depending on the series, approximately half to slightly more than half of tumors will exhibit positivity for CD68, desmin, and EMA.[88,89] CD99 seems expressed in a higher percentage of tumors.[87,90] Perhaps more helpful are the negative stains in these tumors, namely, cytokeratins, S100 protein, CD31, and myogenin.[89] Recently reported ALK immunoreactivity in a subset of AFH may cause further confusion with a lymphoid process.[91,92] Interestingly, ALK expression is not linked to the presence of translocations involving the gene.

AFH typically has associated chromosomal translocations that can be detected through molecular techniques fluorescent in situ hybridization (FISH) or reverse transcription PCR, and these represent important diagnostic tools. The most commonly identified fusion gene is between *EWSR1* and *CREB1* genes t(2:22), although other partner genes have been described with *EWSR1*. FUS-ATF1 t(12:16) is also frequently identified. Detection using a break apart FISH assay allows for the detection of *EWSR* or *FUS* rearrangement, without requiring knowledge of the translocation partner.[89]

Differential Diagnosis

When the growth pattern is swirling, AFH can mimic a perineurioma. This misperception may be perpetuated by EMA positivity in AFH.[89] Some cases also demonstrate prominent eosinophils, which can occasionally give rise to histologic overlap with epithelioid hemangioma (angiolymphoid hyperplasia with eosinophilia). In these cases, search for the conventional features of AFH (fibrotic pseudocapsule, lymphoid aggregates, hemosiderin, hemorrhage, and pseudovascular spaces) will be helpful at arriving at the correct diagnosis. In histologically ambiguous cases, the detection of an *EWSR1* rearrangement through PCR or FISH may be useful.[89] An EWSR1-ATF translocation t(12,22) can be identified in clear cell sarcoma as well as AFH; however, the histologic features are sufficiently different generally to permit distinction of these two entities.[88]

Treatment

Complete surgical excision is the recommended treatment of choice. Most patients do well, but a subset of patients exhibit local recurrence and even metastatic disease.[89,90,93]

Myxoinflammatory Fibroblastic Sarcoma

Myxoinflammatory fibroblastic sarcoma is a low-grade sarcoma prone to recurrence that classically demonstrates a brisk accompanying mixed inflammatory infiltrate. Detection of the diagnostic viral-like neoplastic cells (which prompted the initial moniker of "inflammatory myxohyaline tumor of the distal extremities with virocyte or Reed-Sternberg-like cells") within the inflammatory infiltrate is necessary for correct identification of this tumor.

Clinical Features

The tumor most frequently arises on the distal extremities/acral sites in adults, with soft tissue of the hands and fingers representing the most commonly occurring site of involvement.[94] Nonacral sites are less common but not exceptional; increasing numbers of cases arising from nonacral sites prompted the WHO to remove the adjective "acral" from the tumor name in their most recent publication of tumor nomenclature.[95] The most common age group affected is those in the fourth and fifth decades of life. There is no sex predilection, and the tumors are typically slow growing and asymptomatic. Rarely, pain may be a presenting symptom, and in a subset of cases, injury or trauma is reported to precede tumor development.[88] The clinical impression is representative of the tumor location, with ganglion cyst, tenosynovitis, giant cell tumor, lipoma, or calcified bursa being included in the clinical differential diagnosis.[94] Given that the tumor is usually multinodular and poorly circumscribed, these tumors may be fragmented upon removal, with sizes averaging 3 to 4 cm. Grossly the tumors may have gelatinous to mucoid to rubbery consistency.[88,94]

Histologic Features

Myxoinflammatory fibroblastic sarcoma may be ill-defined and nodular or multinodular, with origination within the subcutis and extension along fascial planes or tendon sheaths, occasionally involving the dermis. The tumor is a biphasic one, composed of fibrohyaline and myxoid components (Fig. 49-26). Within the hypocellular myxoid regions, most cases have pools of mucin (Fig. 49-27). The more cellular, fibrohyaline zones are composed of a population of plump, spindled to epithelioid or histiocytoid cells with moderate pleomorphism with an admixed inflammatory infiltrate composed of lymphocytes and plasma cells and fewer eosinophils and neutrophils.[88] The amount of inflammation is variable, occasionally displaying germinal centers and resembling a lymph node with resultant obscuring of the tumor cells.[95] The characteristic and diagnostic cells of this tumor are bizarre stellate to polygonal epithelioid cells visible at low magnification, with macronucleoli resembling viral inclusions or smudgy chromatin (Fig. 49-28). Cells resembling lipoblasts may also be a component. Mitotic figures are usually relatively infrequent despite the marked cytologic pleomorphism, with mitotic counts averaging ~2 per 50 high-power fields, although the range may be considerably higher than

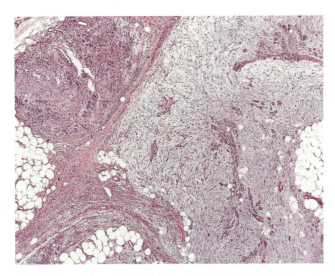

FIGURE 49-26. Myxoinflammatory fibroblastic sarcoma. On low-power examination, this is a biphasic tumor with myxoid and fibrohyaline components.

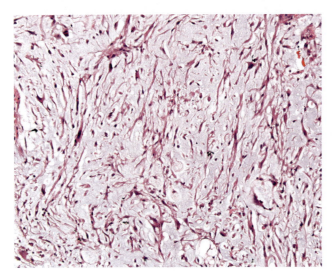

FIGURE 49-27. Myxoinflammatory fibroblastic sarcoma. Pleomorphic tumor cells are embedded in pools of mucinous material.

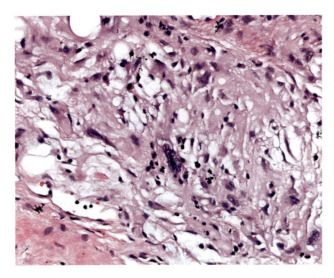

FIGURE 49-28. Myxoinflammatory fibroblastic sarcoma. The diagnostic cells are bizarrely shaped, with macronucleoli resembling viral inclusions.

this.[94] Necrosis is unusual. Atypical histologic features may be correlated with a higher risk for recurrence.[94]

Immunohistochemistry plays a minimal role in confirming the diagnosis. Although no specific markers are available, vimentin is consistently expressed in the tumor cells, while CD34, smooth muscle actin, and CD68 expression is variable.[88] Bcl-1, factor XIIIa, and CD10 have been shown to label the vast majority of these tumors.[96] More recently, reproducible translocations and complex molecular aberrations have been identified in myxoinflammatory fibroblastic sarcoma. A translocation t(1,10) that creates a fusion transcript between *TGFBR3* (chromosome 1p22) and *MGEA5* (chromosome 10q24) has been detected in a subset of these tumors. This translocation does not result in a functional fusion product gene but does give rise to a predictable upregulation of FGF8 levels.[95] In addition, myxoinflammatory fibroblastic sarcoma has been shown to have amplification of regions of chromosome 3p in an area encompassing the *VGLL3* locus, which is thought to function as a regulator of transcription.[95] DNA aneuploidy and DNA copy number changes on chromosome 7 have also been documented.[97]

Differential Diagnosis

The histologic differential diagnosis of myxoinflammatory fibroblastic sarcoma encompasses infectious, benign neoplastic, and malignant neoplastic processes. Despite the fact that the inflammatory infiltrate may sometimes be the predominant feature, its mixed nature does not often result in confusion with a lymphomatous process. However, on occasion, the inflammatory infiltrate will more likely obscure the diagnostic virocyte-like cells, thereby simulating an infectious etiology. Infectious processes may be easily excluded through negative microbial cultures, negative special stains for organisms, and careful histopathologic examination to identify the neoplastic sarcoma cells.

Proliferative fasciitis may be confused with myxoinflammatory fibroblastic sarcoma given the presence of large, ganglion-like cells present in the former entity, which mimic the virocyte-like cells of the latter entity. Although occurring in similar demographic groups with some overlapping clinical features, proliferative fasciitis is usually rapidly growing and tender with a history of antecedent trauma. Histologically, proliferative fasciitis is composed of bland myofibroblastic and fibroblastic spindle cells with interspersed, often clustered ganglion-like cells. The inflammatory infiltrate that characterized myxoinflammatory fibroblastic sarcoma is typically absent in proliferative fasciitis.[88]

Myxoinflammatory fibroblastic sarcoma should be distinguished from myxofibrosarcoma, a more aggressive and often high-grade sarcoma. Myxofibrosarcoma typically arises in axial (rather than acral) sites and histologically lacks the biphasic appearance and inflammatory infiltrate of myxoinflammatory fibroblastic sarcoma. The rich vascularity, with arcuate, arching vessels, has been stressed as a useful feature to identify myxofibrosarcoma. However, the two entities may be difficult to distinguish as they share the myxoid background, nodularity, and pseudolipoblasts.[95]

Treatment

Myxoinflammatory fibroblastic sarcoma has a propensity for local recurrence, occurring in up to 67% of cases of inadequate excision. Distant metastasis and death from disease are rare but reported. Complete re-excision followed by careful monitoring for recurrence or distant disease is recommended. Surgical amputation or radiation therapy may be necessary in cases of aggressive recurrence, while chemotherapy is reserved for metastatic disease.

CONCLUSION

In conclusion, a wide variety of neoplastic entities include a prominent inflammatory infiltrate. While infrequently prompting consideration of a lymphomatous process, careful histopathologic examination and familiarity with the entities discussed above will allow for proper classification and diagnosis.

References

1. Kazakov DV, Banik M, Kacerovska D, et al. A cutaneous adnexal neoplasm with features of adamantinoid trichoblastoma (lymphadenoma) in the benign component and lymphoepithelial-like carcinoma in the malignant component: a possible case of malignant transformation of a rare trichoblastoma variant. *Am J Dermatopathol*. 2011;33(7):729-732.
2. Yu R, Salama S, Alowami S. Cutaneous lymphadenoma: a rare case and brief review of a diagnostic pitfall. *Rare Tumors*. 2014;6(2):5358.
3. McNiff JM, Eisen RN, Glusac EJ. Immunohistochemical comparison of cutaneous lymphadenoma, trichoblastoma, and basal cell carcinoma: support for classification of lymphadenoma as a variant of trichoblastoma. *J Cutan Pathol*. 1999;26(3):119-124.
4. Requena L, Sanchez Yus E. Cutaneous lymphadenoma with ductal differentiation. *J Cutan Pathol*. 1992;19(5):429-433.
5. Tsang WY, Chan JK. So-called cutaneous lymphadenoma: a lymphotropic solid syringoma? *Histopathology*. 1991;19(4):382-385.
6. Rodriguez-Diaz E, Roman C, Yuste M, et al. Cutaneous lymphadenoma: an adnexal neoplasm with intralobular activated lymphoid cells. *Am J Dermatopathol*. 1998;20(1):74-78.
7. Alsadhan A, Taher M, Shokravi M. Cutaneous lymphadenoma. *J Am Acad Dermatol*. 2003;49(6):1115-1116.
8. Fujimura T, Itoigawa A, Haga T, et al. Cutaneous lymphadenoma: a case report and immunohistochemical study. *Case Rep Dermatol*. 2012;4(1):50-55.
9. Goyal A, Solus JF, Chan MP, et al. Cytokeratin 17 is highly sensitive in discriminating cutaneous lymphadenoma (a distinct trichoblastoma variant) from basal cell carcinoma. *J Cutan Pathol*. 2016;43(5):422-429.
10. Aloi F, Tomasini C, Pippione M. Cutaneous lymphadenoma. A basal cell carcinoma with unusual inflammatory reaction pattern? *Am J Dermatopathol*. 1993;15(4):353-357.
11. Allen JE, Lundin K, Erentaite D. Cutaneous lymphadenoma with unusual localization. *J Plast Reconstr Aesthet Surg*. 2013;66(9):1300-1302.
12. Michal M, Lamovec J, Mukensnabl P, et al. Spiradenocylindromas of the skin—tumors with morphological features of spiradenoma and cylindroma in the same lesion: report of 12 cases. *Pathol Int*. 1999;49(5):419-425.
13. Iida K, Iwai S, Hosaka H, et al. Immunohistochemical characterization of non-epithelial cells in spiradenoma. *J Dermatol*. 2013;40(11):896-900.
14. Chetty R, Perez-Ordonez B, Gilbert R, et al. Spiradenocarcinoma arising from a spiradenocylindroma: unusual case with lymphoepithelioma-like areas. *J Cutan Med Surg*. 2009;13(4):215-220.
15. Arsenovic N. Lymphoepithelioma-like carcinoma of the skin: new case of an exceedingly rare primary skin tumor. *Dermatol Online J*. 2008;14(8):12.
16. Carr KA, Bulengo-Ransby SM, Weiss LM, et al. Lymphoepitheliomalike carcinoma of the skin. A case report with immunophenotypic analysis and in situ hybridization for Epstein-Barr viral genome. *Am J Surg Pathol*. 1992;16(9):909-913.
17. Gillum PS, Morgan MB, Naylor MF, et al. Absence of Epstein-Barr virus in lymphoepitheliomalike carcinoma of the skin. Polymerase chain reaction evidence and review of five cases. *Am J Dermatopathol*. 1996;18(5):478-482.
18. Weiss LM, Movahed LA, Butler AE, et al. Analysis of lymphoepithelioma and lymphoepithelioma-like carcinomas for Epstein-Barr viral genomes by in situ hybridization. *Am J Surg Pathol*. 1989;13(8):625-631.
19. Ferlicot S, Plantier F, Rethers L, et al. Lymphoepithelioma-like carcinoma of the skin: a report of 3 Epstein-Barr virus (EBV)-negative additional cases. Immunohistochemical study of the stroma reaction. *J Cutan Pathol*. 2000;27(6):306-311.
20. Aoki R, Mitsui H, Harada K, et al. A case of lymphoepithelioma-like carcinoma of the skin associated with Epstein-Barr virus infection. *J Am Acad Dermatol*. 2010;62(4):681-684.
21. Barnes L, Eveson JW, Reichart P, Sidransky D, *WHO Classification of Tumors: Pathology and Genetics of Head and Neck Tumors*. 2nd ed. World Health Organization. IARC Press; 2007:430.
22. Lopez V, Martin JM, Santonja N, et al. Lymphoepithelioma-like carcinoma of the skin: report of three cases. *J Cutan Pathol*. 2011;38(1):54-58.
23. Sagatys E, Kirk JF, Morgan MB. Lymphoid lost and found. *Am J Dermatopathol*. 2003;25(2):159-161.
24. Wick MR, Swanson PE, LeBoit PE, et al. Lymphoepithelioma-like carcinoma of the skin with adnexal differentiation. *J Cutan Pathol*. 1991;18(2):93-102.
25. Morteza Abedi S, Salama S, Alowami S. Lymphoepithelioma-like carcinoma of the skin: case report and approach to surgical pathology sign out. *Rare Tumors*. 2013;5(3):e47.
26. Gebauer N, Merz H, Ottmann KW, et al. Lymphoepithelioma-like carcinoma and simultaneous marginal zone lymphoma of the skin: a case report. *Am J Dermatopathol*. 2014;36(2):e26-9.
27. Hall G, Duncan A, Azurdia R, et al. Lymphoepithelioma-like carcinoma of the skin: a case with lymph node metastases at presentation. *Am J Dermatopathol*. 2006;28(3):211-215.
28. Robins P, Perez MI. Lymphoepithelioma-like carcinoma of the skin treated by Mohs micrographic surgery. *J Am Acad Dermatol*. 1995;32(5 pt 1):814-816.
29. Swanson SA, Cooper PH, Mills SE, et al. Lymphoepithelioma-like carcinoma of the skin. *Mod Pathol*. 1988;1(5):359-365.
30. Jimenez F, Clark RE, Buchanan MD, et al. Lymphoepithelioma-like carcinoma of the skin treated with Mohs micrographic surgery in combination with immune staining for cytokeratins. *J Am Acad Dermatol*. 1995;32(5 pt 2):878-881.
31. Harvell JD, Meehan SA, LeBoit PE. Spitz's nevi with halo reaction: a histopathologic study of 17 cases. *J Cutan Pathol*. 1997;24(10):611-619.
32. Speeckaert R, van Geel N, Luiten RM, et al. Melanocyte-specific immune response in a patient with multiple regressing nevi and a history of melanoma. *Anticancer Res*. 2011;31(11):3697-3703.

33. Nicolétis-Lombart I, Kervarrec T, Zaragoza J, et al. Multiple "halo nevi" occurring during pembrolizumab treatment for metastatic melanoma. *Int J Dermatol*. 2019;58(6):739-741.
34. Zeff RA, Freitag A, Grin CM, et al. The immune response in halo nevi. *J Am Acad Dermatol*. 1997;37(4):620-624.
35. Lallas A, Apalla Z, Moscarella E, et al. Extensive regression in pigmented skin lesions: a dangerous confounding feature. *Dermatol Pract Concept*. 2012;2(2):202a08.
36. Bergman W, Willemze R, de Graaff-Reitsma C, et al. Analysis of major histocompatibility antigens and the mononuclear cell infiltrate in halo nevi. *J Invest Dermatol*. 1985;85(1):25-29.
37. Ruiter DJ, Bhan AK, Harrist TJ, et al. Major histocompatibility antigens and mononuclear inflammatory infiltrate in benign nevomelanocytic proliferations and malignant melanoma. *J Immunol*. 1982;129(6):2808-2815.
38. Hussein MR, Elsers DA, Fadel SA, et al. Immunohistological characterisation of tumour infiltrating lymphocytes in melanocytic skin lesions. *J Clin Pathol*. 2006;59(3):316-324.
39. Lyle S, Salhany KE, Elder DE. TIA-1 positive tumor-infiltrating lymphocytes in nevi and melanomas. *Mod Pathol*. 2000;13(1):52-55.
40. Botella-Estrada R, Kutzner H. Study of the immunophenotype of the inflammatory cells in melanomas with regression and halo nevi. *Am J Dermatopathol*. 2015;37:376-380.
41. Menasce LP, Shanks JH, Howarth VS, et al. Regressed cutaneous malignant melanoma mimicking lymphoma: a potential diagnostic pitfall. *Int J Surg Pathol*. 2005;13(3):281-284.
42. Stewart N, Zagarella S, Mann S. Angiolyphoid hyperplasia with eosinophilia occurring after venipuncture trauma. *J Dermatol*. 2013;40(5):393-395.
43. Kurihara Y, Inoue H, Kiryu H, et al. Epithelioid hemangioma (angiolymphoid hyperplasia with eosinophilia) in zosteriform distribution. *Indian J Dermatol*. 2012;57(5):401-403.
44. Cham E, Smoller BR, Lorber DA, et al. Epithelioid hemangioma (angiolymphoid hyperplasia with eosinophilia) arising on the extremities. *J Cutan Pathol*. 2010;37(10):1045-1052.
45. Fetsch JF, Sesterhenn IA, Miettinen M, et al. Epithelioid hemangioma of the penis: a clinicopathologic and immunohistochemical analysis of 19 cases, with special reference to exuberant examples often confused with epithelioid hemangioendothelioma and epithelioid angiosarcoma. *Am J Surg Pathol*. 2004;28(4):523-533.
46. Bui MM, Draper NL, Dessureault S, et al. Colonic angiolymphoid hyperplasia with eosinophilia masquerading as malignancy: a case report and review of the literature. *Clin Colorectal Cancer*. 2010;9(3):179-182.
47. Macarenco RS, do Canto AL, Gonzalez S. Angiolymphoid hyperplasia with eosinophilia showing prominent granulomatous and fibrotic reaction: a morphological and immunohistochemical study. *Am J Dermatopathol*. 2006;28(6):514-517.
48. Kempf W, Haeffner AC, Zepter K, et al. Angiolymphoid hyperplasia with eosinophilia: evidence for a T-cell lymphoproliferative origin. *Hum Pathol*. 2002;33(10):1023-1029.
49. Chen JF, Gao HW, Wu BY, et al. Angiolymphoid hyperplasia with eosinophilia affecting the scrotum: a rare case report with molecular evidence of T-cell clonality. *J Dermatol*. 2010;37(4):355-359.
50. Gutte R, Doshi B, Khopkar U. Angiolymphoid hyperplasia with eosinophilia with follicular mucinosis. *Indian J Dermatol*. 2013;58(2):159.
51. Liu XK, Ren J, Wang XH, et al. Angiolymphoid hyperplasia with eosinophilia and Kimura's disease coexisting in the same patient: evidence for a spectrum of disease. *Australas J Dermatol*. 2012;53(3):e47-50.
52. Zaraa I, Mlika M, Chouk S, et al. Angiolymphoid hyperplasia with eosinophilia: a study of 7 cases. *Dermatol Online J*. 2011;17(2):1.
53. Hamaguchi Y, Fujimoto M, Matsushita Y, et al. IgG4-related skin disease, a mimic of angiolymphoid hyperplasia with eosinophilia. *Dermatology*. 2011;223(4):301-305.
54. Hattori T, Miyanaga T, Tago O, et al. Isolated cutaneous manifestation of IgG4-related disease. *J Clin Pathol*. 2012;65(9):815-818.
55. Ramsay BDM, Malcolm AJ, Soyer HP, Wilson-Jones E. Acral Pseudolymphomatous angiokeratoma of children (APACHE). *Br J Dermatol*. 1988; 119(suppl 33):13.
56. Ramsay B, Dahl MC, Malcolm AJ, et al. Acral pseudolymphomatous angiokeratoma of children. *Arch Dermatol*. 1990;126(11):1524-1525.
57. Kaddu S, Cerroni L, Pilatti A, et al. Acral pseudolymphomatous angiokeratoma. A variant of the cutaneous pseudolymphomas. *Am J Dermatopathol*. 1994;16(2):130-133.
58. Okada M, Funayama M, Tanita M, et al. Acral angiokeratoma-like pseudolymphoma: one adolescent and two adults. *J Am Acad Dermatol*. 2001;45(6 suppl):S209-S211.
59. Kim Y, Dawes-Higgs E, Mann S, et al. Acral pseudolymphomatous angiokeratoma of children (APACHE). *Australas J Dermatol*. 2005;46(3):177-180.
60. Kiyohara T, Kumakiri M, Kawasaki T, et al. Linear acral pseudolymphomatous angiokeratoma of children (APACHE): further evidence that APACHE is a cutaneous pseudolymphoma. *J Am Acad Dermatol*. 2003;48(2 suppl):S15-S17.
61. Tokuda Y, Arakura F, Murata H, et al. Acral pseudolymphomatous angiokeratoma of children: a case report with immunohistochemical study of antipodoplanin antigen. *Am J Dermatopathol*. 2012;34(8):e128-132.
62. Lessa PP, Jorge JC, Ferreira FR, et al. Acral pseudolymphomatous angiokeratoma: case report and literature review. *An Bras Dermatol*. 2013;88(6 suppl 1):39-43.
63. Wagner G, Rose C, Sachse MM. Papular pseudolymphoma of adults as a variant of acral pseudolymphomatous angiokeratoma of children (APACHE). *J Dtsch Dermatol Ges*. 2014;12(5):423-424.
64. Okuyama R, Masu T, Mizuashi M, et al. Pseudolymphomatous angiokeratoma: report of three cases and an immunohistological study. *Clin Exp Dermatol*. 2009;34(2):161-165.
65. Hagari Y, Hagari S, Kambe N, et al. Acral pseudolymphomatous angiokeratoma of children: immunohistochemical and clonal analyses of the infiltrating cells. *J Cutan Pathol*. 2002;29(5):313-318.
66. Evans MS, Burkhart CN, Bowers EV, et al. Solitary plaque on the leg of a child: a report of two cases and a brief review of acral pseudolymphomatous angiokeratoma of children and unilesional mycosis fungoides. *Pediatr Dermatol*. 2019;36(1):e1-e5.
67. Lee MW, Choi JH, Sung KJ, et al. Acral pseudolymphomatous angiokeratoma of children (APACHE). *Pediatr Dermatol*. 2003;20(5):457-458.
68. Hsiao PF, Wu YH. Angioplasmocellular hyperplasia: a clinicopathologic study of 10 patients. *J Am Acad Dermatol*. 2011;64(3):542-547.
69. Dayrit JF, Wang WL, Goh SG, et al. T-cell-rich angiomatoid polypoid pseudolymphoma of the skin: a clinicopathologic study of 17 cases and a proposed nomenclature. *J Cutan Pathol*. 2011;38(6):475-482.

70. Sandhya V, Jayaraman A, Srinivas C. T-cell rich angiomatoid polypoid pseudolymphoma: a novel cutaneous pseudolymphoma. *Indian J Dermatol*. 2014;59(4):361-363.
71. Moulonguet I, Hadj-Rabia S, Gounod N, et al. Tibial lymphoplasmacytic plaque: a new, illustrative case of a recently and poorly recognized benign lesion in children. *Dermatology*. 2012;225(1):27-30.
72. Fernandez-Flores A, Suarez Peñaranda JM, De Toro G, et al. Expression of peripheral node addressins by plasmacytic plaque of children, APACHE, TRAPP, and primary cutaneous angioplasmacellular hyperplasia. *Appl Immunohistochem Mol Morphol*. 2018;26(6):411-419.
73. Santa Cruz D, Plaza JA, Wick MR, et al. Inflammatory lobular hemangioma: a vascular proliferation with a prominent lymphoid component. Review of a series of 19 cases. *J Cutan Pathol*. 2021;48:229-236.
74. Ide F, Shimoyama T, Horie N. Plasma cell granuloma of the oral mucosa with angiokeratomatous features: a possible analogue of cutaneous angioplasmocellular hyperplasia. *Oral Surg Oral Med Oral Pathol Oral Radiol Endod*. 2000;89(2):204-207.
75. Schimming TT, Griewank KG, Esser S, et al. Angioplasmacellular hyperplasia-a new histopathologic clue for anogenital herpes simplex recidivans in immunocompromised patients? *Am J Dermatopathol*. 2014;36(10):822-826.
76. Kumar S, Weedon D, De'Ambrosis B. Primary cutaneous angioplasmocellular hyperplasia. *Australas J Dermatol*. 2009;50(1):64-65.
77. Gonzalez S, Molgo M. Primary cutaneous angioplasmocellular hyperplasia. *Am J Dermatopathol*. 1995;17(3):307-311.
78. Requena L, Santonja C, Stutz N, et al. Pseudolymphomatous cutaneous angiosarcoma: a rare variant of cutaneous angiosarcoma readily mistaken for cutaneous lymphoma. *Am J Dermatopathol*. 2007;29(4):342-350.
79. Rongioletti F, Albertini AF, Fausti V, et al. Pseudolymphomatous cutaneous angiosarcoma: a report of 2 new cases arising in an unusual setting. *J Cutan Pathol*. 2013;40(9):848-854.
80. Weed BR, Folpe AL. Cutaneous CD30-positive epithelioid angiosarcoma following breast-conserving therapy and irradiation: a potential diagnostic pitfall. *Am J Dermatopathol*. 2008;30(4):370-372.
81. Albores-Saavedra J, Schwartz AM, Henson DE, et al. Cutaneous angiosarcoma. Analysis of 434 cases from the surveillance, epidemiology, and end results program, 1973-2007. *Ann Diagn Pathol*. 2011;15(2):93-97.
82. Bacchi CE, Silva TR, Zambrano E, et al. Epithelioid angiosarcoma of the skin: a study of 18 cases with emphasis on its clinicopathologic spectrum and unusual morphologic features. *Am J Surg Pathol*. 2010;34(9):1334-1343.
83. Requena L, and Sangueza OP. Cutaneous vascular proliferations. Part III. Malignant neoplasms, other cutaneous neoplasms with significant vascular component, and disorders erroneously considered as vascular neoplasms. *J Am Acad Dermatol*. 1998; 38(2 pt 1): 143-175; quiz 176-8.
84. McKay KM, Doyle LA, Lazar AJ, et al. Expression of ERG, an Ets family transcription factor, distinguishes cutaneous angiosarcoma from histological mimics. *Histopathology*. 2012;61(5):989-991.
85. Fernandez AP, Sun Y, Tubbs RR, et al. FISH for MYC amplification and anti-MYC immunohistochemistry: useful diagnostic tools in the assessment of secondary angiosarcoma and atypical vascular proliferations. *J Cutan Pathol*. 2012;39(2):234-242.
86. Ginter PS, Mosquera JM, MacDonald TY, et al. Diagnostic utility of MYC amplification and anti-MYC immunohistochemistry in atypical vascular lesions, primary or radiation-induced mammary angiosarcomas, and primary angiosarcomas of other sites. *Hum Pathol*. 2014;45(4):709-716.
87. Kao YC, Lan J, Tai HC, et al. Angiomatoid fibrous histiocytoma: clinicopathological and molecular characterisation with emphasis on variant histomorphology. *J Clin Pathol*. 2014;67(3):210-215.
88. Weiss SW, Goldblum JR, Enzinger FM. *Enzinger and Weiss's Soft Tissue Tumors*. 5th ed. Mosby; 2008:xiv, 1258.
89. Bohman SL, Goldblum JR, Rubin BP, et al. Angiomatoid fibrous histiocytoma: an expansion of the clinical and histological spectrum. *Pathology*. 2014;46(3):199-204.
90. Chen G, Folpe AL, Colby TV, et al. Angiomatoid fibrous histiocytoma: unusual sites and unusual morphology. *Mod Pathol*. 2011;24(12):1560-1570.
91. Cheah AL, Zou Y, Lanigan C, et al. ALK expression in angiomatoid fibrous histiocytoma: a potential diagnostic pitfall. *Am J Surg Pathol*. 2019;43(1):93-101.
92. De Noon S, Fleming A, Singh M. Angiomatoid fibrous histiocytoma with ALK expression in an unusual location and age group. *Am J Dermatopathol*. 2020;42(9):689-693.
93. Thway K, Stefanaki K, Papadakis V, et al. Metastatic angiomatoid fibrous histiocytoma of the scalp, with EWSR1-CREB1 gene fusions in primary tumor and nodal metastasis. *Hum Pathol*. 2013;44(2):289-293.
94. Laskin WB, Fetsch JF, Miettinen M. Myxoinflammatory fibroblastic sarcoma: a clinicopathologic analysis of 104 cases, with emphasis on predictors of outcome. *Am J Surg Pathol*. 2014;38(1):1-12.
95. Ieremia E, Thway K. Myxoinflammatory fibroblastic sarcoma: morphologic and genetic updates. *Arch Pathol Lab Med*. 2014;138(10):1406-1411.
96. Suster D, Michal M, Huang H, et al. Myxoinflammatory fibroblastic sarcoma: an immunohistochemical and molecular genetic study of 73 cases. *Mod Pathol*. 2020;33(12):2520-2533.
97. Baumhoer D, Glatz K, Schulten HJ, et al. Myxoinflammatory fibroblastic sarcoma: investigations by comparative genomic hybridization of two cases and review of the literature. *Virchows Arch*. 2007;451(5):923-928.

CHAPTER 50

Cutaneous lymphoid hyperplasia and related entities

Alejandro A. Gru

INTRODUCTION

Cutaneous lymphoid hyperplasia (CLH) refers to a heterogeneous group of "reactive" T- and B-cell processes that simulate cutaneous lymphomas both clinically and/or histologically.[1,2] Most CLHs consist of a mixture of reactive B and T cells along with macrophages and dendritic cells. B-cell-rich CLH exhibits unique clinical features; T-cell-rich cases can have a variety of different histologic patterns.[3-5] CLH may be idiopathic, or it may arise in response to a wide variety of foreign antigens, including arthropod bites,[6] stings, and infestations[7,8]; viral (herpes simplex virus [HSV], varicella zoster virus, molluscum), parasitic (leishmaniasis), or bacterial infections (*Borrelia*, syphilis, etc.); tattoos; vaccinations; photo-induced reactions (actinic reticuloid); trauma; contact allergens; injection of foreign substances; pierced ear jewelry; and drugs.[9,10] Since CLH often shows striking morphologic overlap with low-grade B-cell lymphomas, and sometimes with T-cell lymphoproliferations, a careful phenotypic and molecular characterization is mandatory to exclude lymphoid neoplasia. In this chapter, we will review the main forms of CLH and will also expand on a few related entities with unique clinicopathologic features (Table 50-1).

CUTANEOUS MIXED T- AND B-CELL HYPERPLASIA

Cutaneous mixed T- and B-cell hyperplasia (mixed T-B CLH) presents both in women and men, with an average age of 54 years at presentation (range 16-93 years). The lesions typically present as nodules, plaques, and papules. Most of the lesions are located in the head and neck region, followed by the trunk and extremities. Solitary lesions are much more common than multiple lesions.[1] Many different etiologic agents have been linked to CLH (Table 50-2).

CLH can develop because of scabies or arthropod bites (Fig. 50-1). Clinically, multiple pruritic firm erythematous to red-brown papules and nodules occur most commonly on the elbows, abdomen, genitalia, and axillae. Nodules following scabies may persist for many months after adequate anti-scabetic therapy. The cause of the persistent nodules is not known but is thought to be a delayed-type hypersensitivity reaction to a component of the mite. Scabies mites are seldom identified in scabetic nodules.[107-110]

CUTANEOUS B-CELL HYPERPLASIA

Other terms that had been used to describe this process include lymphadenosis cutis benigna (restricted to *Borrelia*-associated form, outdated); lymphocytoma cutis; benign lymphadenosis cutis; cutaneous B-cell pseudolymphoma.

Cutaneous B-cell hyperplasia (B-CLH) is characterized by flesh-colored to plum-red dermal and subcutaneous nodules and plaques similar to cutaneous B-cell lymphomas.[111] In idiopathic B-CLH, the most typical sites of involvement include the face (cheek, nose, ear lobe; 50%), chest (36%), and upper extremities (14%).[112-115] Lesions below the waist are infrequent.[112] The female-to-male ratio is 3:1. The disease predominantly affects white populations (white/black = 9:1). Two-thirds of patients are under the age of 40 years at initial biopsy. Approximately 8% of patients are under the age of 18 years. The *Borrelia*-associated form is found particularly in areas where *Borrelia* is endemic (eg, Northern America, Europe, Asia).[36] Other causes of B-CLH include medications,[1,116] antigen injection for allergy treatment[117,118] or vaccination,[74] tick bites,[33] arthropod bites, herpes zoster,[32] hair dyes, piercing, tattoo pigment,[79] and *Borrelia* species.[36,119] Many times the triggering factor cannot be identified.

Two clinical forms have been reported: the more common localized form (72%) and the less frequent generalized form (28%).[120,121] The localized form is usually seen as a single asymptomatic soft, doughy, or firm nodule or tumor measuring up to 4 cm in diameter; lesions may be aggregated in small clusters. The color varies from skin-colored to red to red-brown to red-purple. Scale and ulceration are generally absent. A miliarial type is characterized by multiple semitranslucent, small papules of few millimeters in diameter.[120,122-124]

TABLE 50-1 Cutaneous Lymphoid Hyperplasia and Related Entities

- Cutaneous lymphoid hyperplasia of B cells, T cells, and mixed T/B cells
- *Borrelia burgdorferi*–associated lymphocytoma cutis
- Atypical lymphoid hyperplasia
- Atypical marginal zone hyperplasia
- Lymphomatoid keratosis
- Syringolymphoid hyperplasia with alopecia

Histologically, the dermis shows top heavy infiltrates of small mature lymphocytes without epidermal involvement (Fig. 50-4). The infiltrate can be nodular,[125] nodular and diffuse, or predominantly diffuse (Figs. 50-5–50-7).[126-128] Germinal centers are typically seen with mantle zones forming well-defined follicles. The germinal centers contain a mixture of centrocytes (small cleaved lymphocytes) and centroblasts (large lymphocytes with prominent nucleoli). Polarization of the germinal centers can be seen in approximately 30% of cases. Most germinal centers also typically have tangible body macrophages and mitotic figures. Some cases can also show progressive transformation of germinal centers.[129] Plasmacytoid dendritic cells are found in 75% and closely approximate T cells and plasma cells.[130,131] The *Borrelia*-associated form often shows confluent large germinal centers with small or absent mantle zones and a lack of polarization in 82%. Tingible body macrophages are a consistent finding.[36] Plasma cell (99%) and eosinophils (84%) are very common. The miliarial type shows a more superficial and less dense infiltrate, with a diffuse, nodular, or follicle accentuated growth pattern.

Clonality studies reveal a polyclonal result in most cases for immunoglobulin heavy chain (IGH) and light chain (IGK) rearrangement. Nevertheless, clonality can be detected in about 10% to 20% of B-CLH.[115,132-134] Immunostains and in situ hybridization for kappa to lambda typically show a ratio of <5:1. RNA scope in situ hybridization has been proven to be an excellent technique that can evaluate for restriction in plasma cells and B cells.[1,122,135] On rare occasions, restricted plasma cells can be present.

CUTANEOUS T-CELL HYPERPLASIA

Other terms that have been used in the past and are not currently recommended include nodular T-cell pseudolymphoma, CD30+ T-cell pseudolymphoma, atypical lymphoid hyperplasia, T-cell dyscrasia, pseudolymphomatous folliculitis, lymphomatoid drug reaction, lymphomatoid contact dermatitis, actinic reticuloid, and benign atypical intravascular (CD30+) lymphoproliferation.

Three histologic patterns of cutaneous T-cell hyperplasia (T-CLH) have been described, although none of them are entirely specific for any particular etiology: (1) superficial diffuse (mimicking plaque-stage mycosis fungoides), (2) nodular, and (3) superficial and deep diffuse (arthropod-bite-like) patterns. Three additional patterns have also been proposed: (4) intravascular T-cell-rich lymphoid proliferation, (5) angiomatoid T-cell-rich lymphoid proliferation, and (6) subcutaneous T-cell-rich lymphoid proliferation.

The nodular T-CLH presents with a solitary reddish nonulcerated nodule.[130,136] Manifestations of other T-CLH forms include papules and small nodules (eg, CD30+ T-CLH), maculopapular eruptions or erythroderma (eg, in drug-induced lymphomatoid drug reaction, actinic reticuloid), as well as erythematous and scaly lesions (eg, lymphomatoid contact dermatitis).[126,137]

The etiology of T-CLH is multifactorial. Common associated conditions include medications[15,33,138-140]; arthropod bite; viral (HIV, herpes, molluscum contagiosum virus, ortho- and parapoxviruses),[141,142] bacterial (*Borrelia* sp., *Treponema pallidum*),[143] and parasitic (leishmania)

TABLE 50-2 Causes of CLH

1. **Medications:** oxaliplatin and 5-fluorouracil in advanced colon cancer[11]; simvastatin[12]; omeprazole; ranitidine[13]; aspirin; ramipril[12-14]; glyburide; alfuzosin; calcium channel blockers[12,15]; atenolol; metoprolol[15]; paroxetine; doxazosin mesylate[1]; fluoxetine and amytriptiline[16]; minoxidil[17]; antihistamtines[10]; benzodiazepines[12]; minocycline[12]; lupron injections[13]; carbamazepine[13]; isoflavin[13]; doxepin[13]; erythromycin[13]; sertraline[13]; losartan[18]; gabapentin[15]; phenytoin[19-30]; cefuroxime; cefepime[15]; terbinafine; levofloxacin[15]; gemcitabine[31]; leuprolide; hepatobiliary iminodiacetic acid (HIDA) scintigraphy.
2. **Infections:** Varicella-zoster-virus folliculitis promoted clonal cutaneous lymphoid hyperplasia[32]; tick bites[33]; zoster[34]; *B. burgdorferi*[3,35-40]; scabies[41]; secondary syphilis[42-50]; leishmaniasis[51]; HSV[52-54]; molluscum contagiosum[55-59]; *Helicobacter pylori*[60]; HIV[61-65]; HPV-related in common warts[66,67]; orf[68]; dermatophyte infections[69] (Fig. 50-2); *Mycobacterium tuberculosis*[70]; HTLV-1; hepatitis B/C; *Orientia tsutsugamushi*.
3. **Vaccinations**[71,72]: hepatitis B vaccine[72-74]; hepatitis A vaccine[74]; influenza vaccine.[75]
4. **Toxicologic/Traumatic:** venoms[7]; following feline scratches[76]; tattoos[77-81]; squaric acid[82]; following radiation therapy[83]; following a broken thermometer and presumptively secondary to mercury exposure.[84]
5. **Synchronous to other cutaneous disorders:** granuloma annulare[85]; melanocytic nevi[86]; scars mimicking subcutaneous panniculitis-like T-cell lymphoma[87,88]; folliculitis[89,90]; lymphomatoid contact dermatitis; lichen sclerosus (Fig. 50-3).
6. **Autoimmune disorders:** Sjögren syndrome[91]; lupus erythematosus.
7. **Neoplastic:** spiradenoma with dense lymphoid infiltrates[92]; lymphoepithelioma-like carcinoma[93-100]; halo nevus[101-104]; angiosarcoma[105,106]; myxoinflammatory fibroblastic sarcoma; angiomatoid fibrous histiocytoma; pyogenic granuloma/lobular capillary hemangioma.

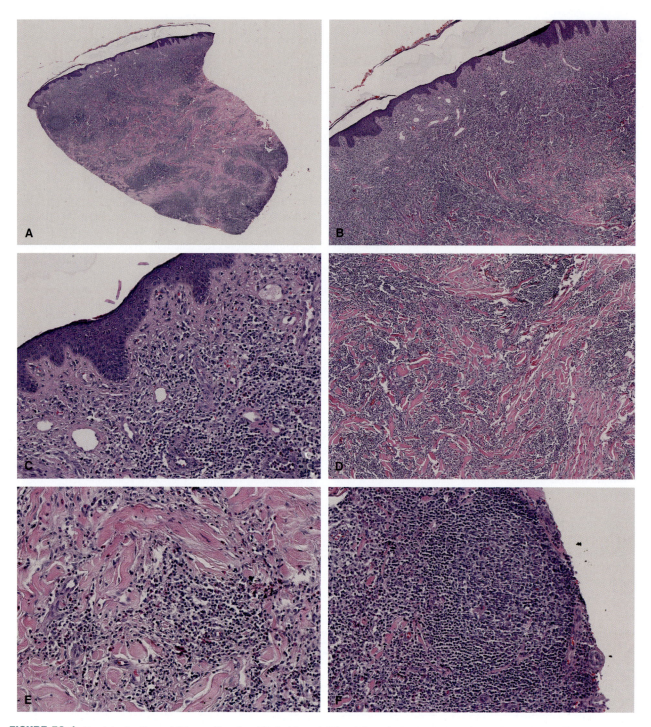

FIGURE 50-1. Persistent arthropod-bite reaction. A and **B.** Nodular and diffuse infiltrate in the dermis with sparing of the epidermis. The entire dermis is involved (20× and 100×, respectively). **C.** Grenz-zone and increased superficial dermal vascularity (200×). **D.** The infiltrate shows a diffuse pattern and extends within the collagen fibers (100×). **E.** Eosinophils are abundant in the infiltrate (200×). **F.** Germinal center formation can be identified (400×).

infections; vaccines; tattoo dyes[144,145]; contact allergens[146,147]; UV light (actinic reticuloid); and other inflammatory skin diseases or trauma.[148-150] All cases with an identifiable cause can formally be referred to as causative factor–associated T-CLH and thus be assigned to specific disorders (eg, T-cell-rich *Borrelia* infection). The term idiopathic T-CLH designates those cases in which a causative factor is cannot be identified.

In the superficial diffuse variant, T-CLH shows a superficial band-like infiltrate of mostly small T lymphocytes in the papillary dermis, with blurring of the dermoepidermal junction. A deep perivascular and periadnexal polymorphous infiltrate may be seen. The epidermal changes include variable acanthosis, minimal spongiosis, and variable epidermotropism of lymphocytes, with occasional Pautrier microabscess-like collections[12,14,19-23,112,151-155] (Figs. 50-8 and 50-9).

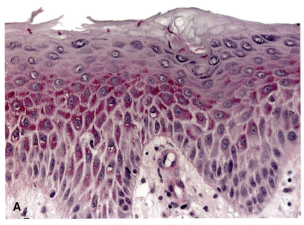
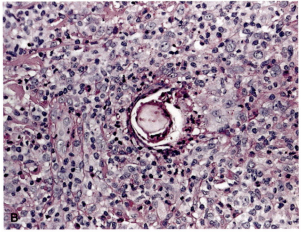

FIGURE 50-2. Cutaneous pseudolymphoma in association with a dermatophyte infection. A. Periodic acid-Schiff-positive hyphae and spores within the horny layer. **B.** Few periodic acid-Schiff-positive hyphae and spores within a hair follicle. (From Kash N, Ginter-Hanselmayer G, Cerroni L. Cutaneous mycotic infections with pseudolymphomatous infiltrates. *Am J Dermatopathol.* 2010;32:514-517, with permission.)

The nodular pattern consists mostly of small lymphocytes with a variable admixture of histiocytes, plasma cells, mast cells, and eosinophils (Fig. 50-10). Characteristically, the lymphocytes of this pattern reveal no or minimal cytologic atypia. Most lymphomatoid drug reactions show the mycosis fungoides (MF)-like pattern. Some lymphomatoid drug reactions can also have a more nodular appearance.[16,156] In the anticonvulsant-induced pseudolymphoma syndrome, the changes in lymph nodes include focal necrosis, an eosinophilic and histiocytic cell infiltrate that destroys the normal lymph node architecture, and an atypical lymphoid hyperplasia simulating lymphoma.[24-26,157,158] A "lymphomatous" infiltrate in the skin can sometimes be present (Fig. 50-11).

The arthropod-bite-like pattern shows variable epidermal acanthosis. The superficial and deep dermis reveal a moderate to dense perivascular and interstitial infiltrate composed of lymphocytes, histiocytes, plasma cells, and eosinophils. Large atypical mononuclear cells resembling Reed-Sternberg cells may be seen,[107-110,114] particularly in association with nodular lesions of scabies (Fig. 50-12). In this type of infiltrate, CD30 expression can be seen in the large cells, indicating a hyperplasia of immunoblasts. Cases with a histiocytic-rich pattern are composed of medium-sized and large lymphocytes with abundant CD68+ macrophages. Sometimes small epithelioid granulomas can be present.[1] A variable number of eosinophils and plasma cells are present. In this particular subtype, very frequent dermal dendritic cells (S100+) and Langerhans cells (CD1a+ and Langerin+) are seen. Some cases of CLH have been reclassified as lymphomas upon review of the original biopsies.[159]

The intravascular T-CLH is characterized by large blastoid cells with variable expression of CD30 in and around lymphatic vessels.[148-150] Rarely, T-CLH presents with subcutaneous infiltrates of small lymphocytes in a predominantly lobular pattern, for example, in *Borrelia* sp. infection.[160] Angiomatoid T-CLH has a prominent proliferation of capillaries or postcapillary venules.

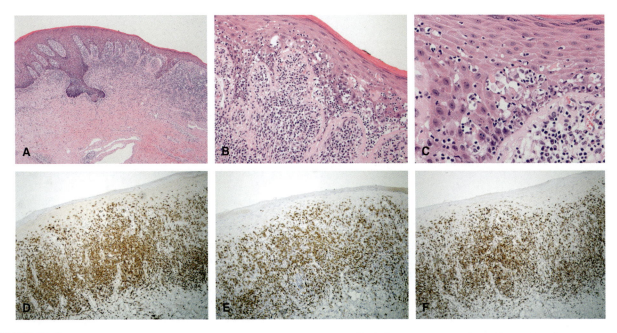

FIGURE 50-3. Cutaneous pseudolymphoma in association with lichen sclerosus. The findings were present in the excision specimen from a woman with squamous cell carcinoma of the vulva. **A.** Superficial band-like infiltrate with interface changes (20×). **B.** Prominent epidermotropism and marked interface changes (200×). **C.** The epidermotropic cells show no significant atypia (400×). **D.** CD3. **E.** CD8. The CD3:CD8 ratio is preserved. **F.** CD7 shows no significant loss among the T cells.

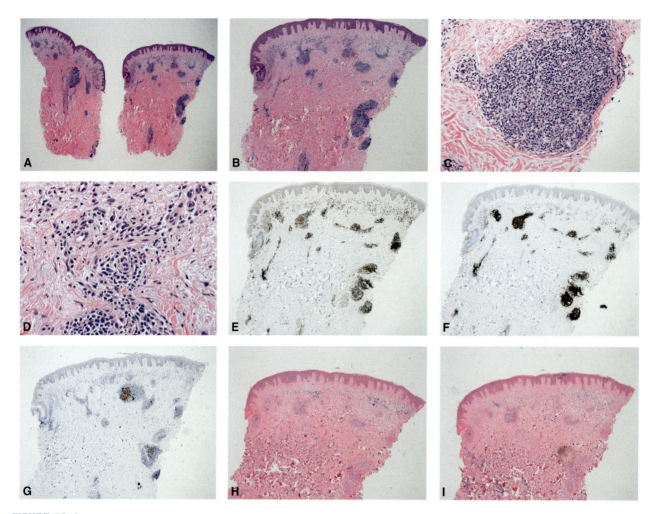

FIGURE 50-4. Cutaneous lymphoid hyperplasia of B cells. A and **B.** Nodular infiltrate in the dermis, top heavy (20× and 40×). **C.** Germinal center formation (200×). **D.** Frequent admixed plasma cells (400×). **E.** CD3. **F.** CD20. **G.** Ki67 shows very high (>90%) proliferation index in germinal centers. **H.** In situ hybridization κ. **I.** In situ hybridization λ. A polyclonal pattern among the plasma cells is noted.

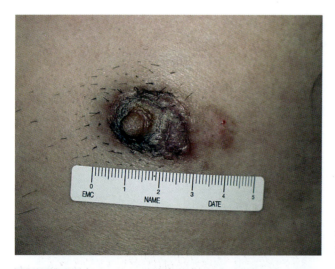

FIGURE 50-5. Cutaneous lymphoid hyperplasia of B cells in syphilis. A 2 × 1.5-cm nodular plaque with slight oozing at the left areola. (From Moon HS, Park K, Lee JH, et al. A nodular syphilid presenting as a pseudolymphoma: mimicking a cutaneous marginal zone B-cell lymphoma. *Am J Dermatopathol.* 2009;31:846-848, with permission.)

IMMUNOHISTOCHEMISTRY AND FLOW CYTOMETRY

Germinal centers are positive for CD20, CD10, HGAL, and BCL-6, while negative for BCL-2.[4,161-165] They typically show a very high proliferation index (>90%) as measured by Ki67 (MIB-1). The follicular dendritic networks can be demonstrated by CD21, CD23, D2-40, and CD35. Plasma cells show polytypic κ and λ light chains. In T-CLH, the CD4:CD8 ratio is <5:1, and CD7 expression is preserved.[166] The data on the discriminatory value of CD1a in B-CLH versus primary cutaneous marginal zone lymphoma are conflicting.[167,168] Flow cytometry on cutaneous lesions of CLH characteristically shows a polyclonal population of T cells and B cells, although monoclonal cases are not infrequent.[169] These data suggest that CLH represents a spectrum from polyclonal CLH to monoclonal CLH and monoclonal lymphoma. Because of the uncertainty of the biologic behavior of any CLH form, long-term clinical follow-up of patients is recommended.[126]

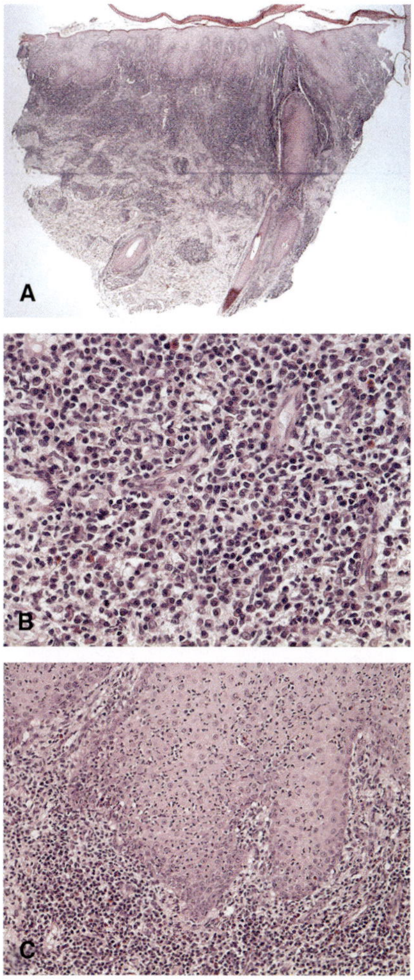

FIGURE 50-6. Cutaneous lymphoid hyperplasia of B cells in syphilis. **A.** Diffuse heavy infiltrate throughout the dermis (10×). **B.** Dense diffuse infiltrate composed of numerous lymphocytes, plasma cells, and eosinophils (400×). **C.** Epidermotropism and granulomatous inflammation were observed (200×). (From Moon HS, Park K, Lee JH, et al. A nodular syphilid presenting as a pseudolymphoma: mimicking a cutaneous marginal zone B-cell lymphoma. *Am J Dermatopathol.* 2009;31:846-848, with permission.)

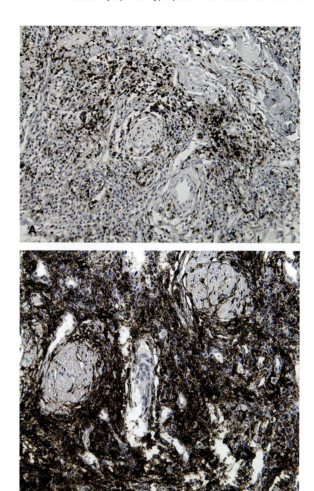

FIGURE 50-7. Cutaneous lymphoid hyperplasia of B cells in syphilis. Immunohistochemistry showed scattered CD3+ T cells **(A)**. In addition, there was an abundance of CD20+ B cells **(B)** in the dermal infiltrate. (From Moon HS, Park K, Lee JH, et al. A nodular syphilid presenting as a pseudolymphoma: mimicking a cutaneous marginal zone B-cell lymphoma. *Am J Dermatopathol.* 2009;31:846-848, with permission.)

MOLECULAR FINDINGS

The utility of gene rearrangement studies in the diagnosis of CLH is contradictory. While most "true" cases of CLH are polyclonal for T-cell receptor (TCR) and immunoglobulin gene rearrangement (IGH), many have documented the presence of clonal populations of T cells and B cells.[34,126,170] It is estimated that up to 10% to 20% of cases of CLH with a predominance of T cells can show a rearrangement of the TCR. A study of Nihal et al[171] has documented the presence of rare clonal bands using IGH gene rearrangement analysis of normal skin. Of 35 cases of B-CLH reported in five studies, approximately one-third (12 cases) had clonal immunoglobulin gene rearrangements.[5,170,172,173] Of these, long-term follow-up for 1 to 6 years showed that lymphoma developed in a few cases. Approximately 14% of patients with CLH (3 of 21 cases) had clonal TCR gene rearrangements, and one patient experienced the development of a CD30+ large-cell anaplastic T-cell lymphoma in an inguinal lymph node 1 year later.[174,175]

DIFFERENTIAL DIAGNOSIS

T-CLH: MF, lymphomatoid papulosis (LyP), cutaneous anaplastic large-cell lymphoma (C-ALCL), and primary cutaneous small to medium-sized CD4+ T-cell lymphoproliferative disorder (SMTCLPD). Features that are in favor of the diagnosis of MF over T-CLH include (1) focal sprinkling of lymphocytes in the epidermis associated with scant or no spongiosis, (2) lymphocytes arranged in solitary units aligned in the basal cell layer, (3) clear halos around the epidermotropic lymphocytes, (4) some lymphocytes in the epidermis being larger than lymphocytes in the dermis, (5) minute collections of lymphocytes situated in discrete foci within the epidermis, and (6) wiry bundles of collagen accompanied by a patchy infiltrate of

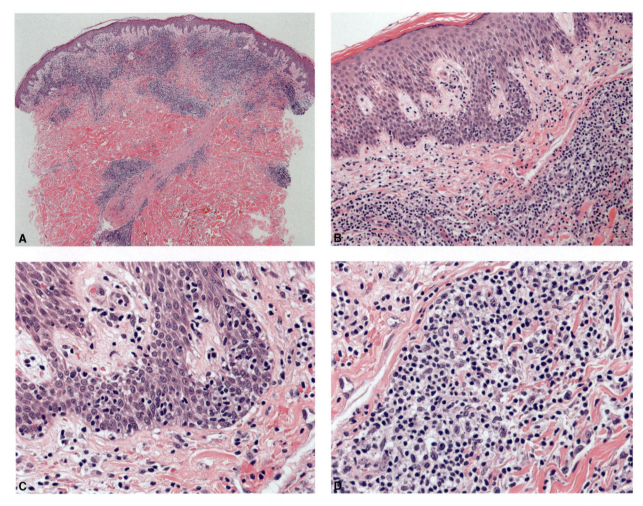

FIGURE 50-8. **Cutaneous lymphoid hyperplasia of T cells, MF-like pattern. A.** Band-like infiltrate in the superficial dermis with an additional deep perivascular component (20×). **B.** Acanthosis, mild spongiosis, and epidermotropism are noted. Note a lack of dermal fibrosis in the superficial papillary dermis (200×). **C.** The epidermotropic infiltrate shows tagging of cells along the dermal-epidermal junction and has associated perinuclear halos and mild hyperchromasia (400×). **D.** The dermal component in the surface also has similar histologic findings (400×).

lymphocytes in a thickened papillary dermis.[126] In addition, loss of CD7 and an abnormal CD4:CD8 ratio (typically >10:1) are characteristic of MF and not present in T-CLH. The presence of a clonal population of T cells is another argument in favor of MF. LyP and C-ALCL typically have a characteristic clinical presentation: papulonecrotic lesions with spontaneous resolution in LyP and large ulcerated tumors in C-ALCL that differ from T-CLH. In addition, the degree of expression of CD30 is larger in these lymphomas, and clonal populations of T cells are noted. SMTCLPD typically presents as a nodule in the head and neck region. Similarly to T-CLH, background eosinophils, plasma cells, and histiocytes are present. As opposed to T-CLH, large and pleomorphic cells are noted, the CD4:CD8 ratio is markedly altered, and the clonal populations of T cells show characteristically a follicular T-helper phenotype, with the expression of the germinal center markers (ICOS, BCL-6, and PD1). Expression of PD1 is typically sparse in CLH.[166]

B-CLH and mixed T-B CLH: primary cutaneous follicle center cell lymphoma (PCFCL) and primary cutaneous marginal zone B-cell lymphoma (PCMZBCL). The International Consensus Classification of lymphomas has recently proposed a change in the terminology of cutaneous marginal zone lymphomas to marginal B-cell lymphoproliferative disorders.[176]

The histologic features that favor CLH over B-cell lymphomas include (1) acanthosis, (2) a top heavy infiltrate, (3) a mixed cellular infiltrate, (4) presence of germinal centers, (5) presence of tingible bodies (fragmented basophilic nuclear debris of degenerated lymphoid cells), (6) vascular proliferation, (7) preservation of the adnexal structures, and (8) the appearance of the germinal centers.[151,177,178] PCFCL does not show distinctive germinal centers but follicles that lack tangible body macrophages. While BCL-2 is often negative in both PCFCL and CLH with germinal centers, the Ki67 is markedly elevated in reactive germinal centers and low or intermediate in PCFCL. In addition, some cases of PCFCL

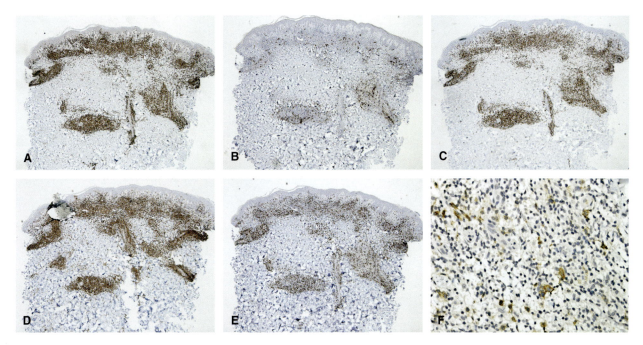

FIGURE 50-9. Cutaneous lymphoid hyperplasia of T cells, MF-like pattern, immunohistochemistry. A. CD3. **B.** CD20. **C.** CD7 (no significant loss of the antigen is noted). **D.** CD4. **E.** CD8. The CD4:CD8 ratio is relatively preserved (approximately 4:1). **F.** CD30 is positive in a few scattered cells.

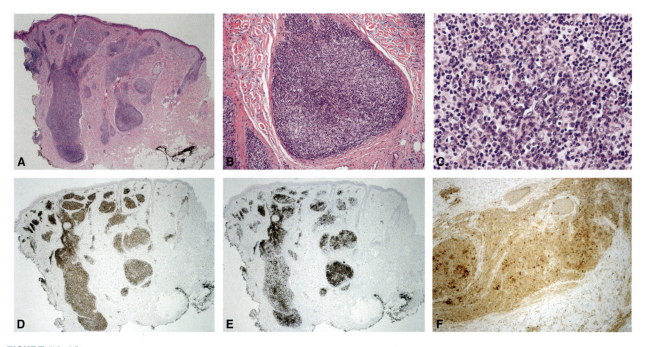

FIGURE 50-10. Cutaneous lymphoid hyperplasia of T cells, nodular pattern. A. Nodular infiltrate in the dermis, in both the superficial and deep portions of the biopsy (20×). **B.** Large nodular aggregate of small lymphocytes (200×). **C.** The infiltrate is composed of a heterogeneous population of cells, including many histiocytes (400×). **D.** CD3. **E.** CD20. Mixture of T cells and B cells. **F.** PD-1 immunostain in CLH. Scattered positive cells are seen, indicative of the presence of T cells with follicular helper phenotype.

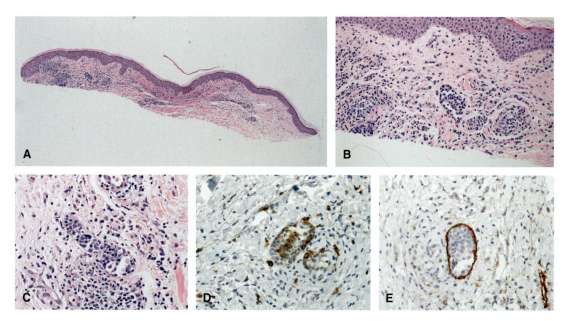

FIGURE 50-11. Cutaneous T-cell pseudolymphoma in association with phenytoin therapy. A. Shave biopsy of superficial dermal infiltrate (40×). **B** and **C.** The infiltrate shows an intravascular character and is composed of medium and large cells. Background eosinophils are noted (200× and 400×, respectively). **D.** CD30 is positive in many of the large cells. **E.** D2-40 shows staining in lymphatic channels.

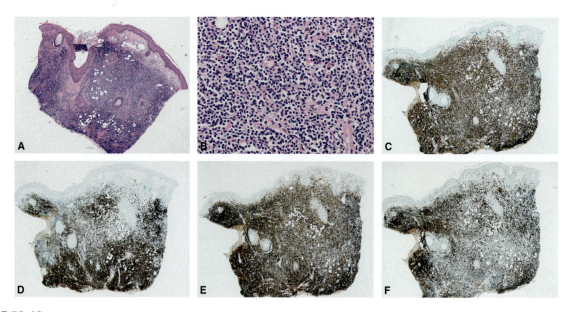

FIGURE 50-12. Cutaneous lymphoid hyperplasia of T cells, arthropod-like pattern. A. Diffuse dermal infiltrate in the superficial and deep portions of the biopsy with extension into the adipose tissue (40×). **B.** The infiltrate is composed of small lymphocytes and many admixed plasma cells (200×). **C.** CD3. **D.** CD20. **E.** CD4. **F.** CD8. There is an increased CD4:CD8 ratio among the T-cell infiltrate, a finding that should be interpreted cautiously.

are BCL-2 positive. PCFCL also shows a clonal population of B cells by IGH gene rearrangement, and sometimes by in situ hybridization. The malignant cells of PCFCL lack surface immunoglobulin light chain expression. Distinguishing PCMZBCL from B- or mixed T- and B-CLH is challenging particularly due to the presence of small and atrophic germinal centers in these lymphomas.[159] However, the presence of disrupted dendritic networks (by CD21, CD23, CD35), clonal plasma cells, and a background rich in IgG4+ cells are features in favor of PCMZBCL, over CLH.

CLH-RELATED ENTITIES

Borrelia burgdorferi–Associated Lymphocytoma Cutis

Borrelial lymphocytoma cutis is a rare manifestation of *B. burgdorferi* infection. In large series of patients with the clinical and/or serologic diagnosis of Lyme disease, the prevalence of borrelial lymphocytoma cutis has been reported to be 0.6% to 1.3%. It occurs most commonly in areas endemic for the

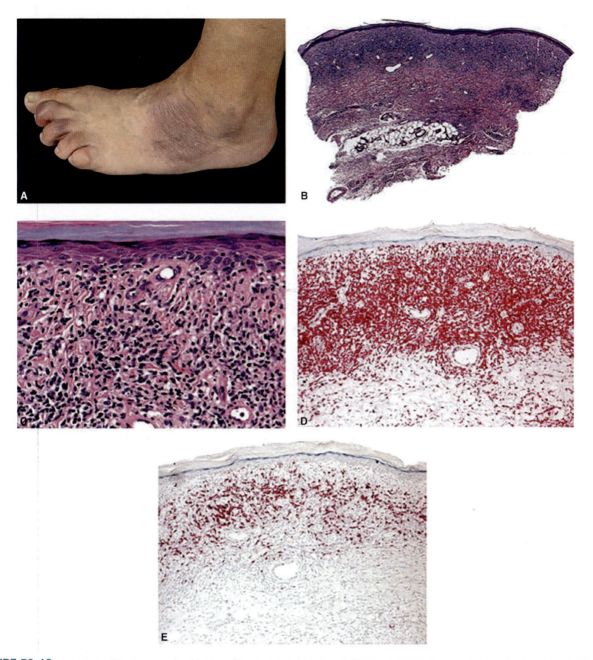

FIGURE 50-13. Acrodermatitis chronica atrophicans with pseudolymphomatous infiltrate. A. Infiltrated, reddish lesion on the dorsal aspect of the left foot. **B** and **C.** Dense, band-like infiltrate with several intraepidermal lymphocytes. **D.** Staining for CD3 and **E.** CD20 confirm that T lymphocytes predominate. (From Tee SI, Martinez-Escaname M, Zuriel D, et al. Acrodermatitis chronica atrophicans with pseudolymphomatous infiltrates. *Am J Dermatopathol.* 2013;35:338-342, with permission.)

Ixodes ricinus tick in Europe and is rare in North America. Borrelial lymphocytoma cutis (BLC) seems to be more common in children than in adults.[179-185] In this population, LC represents 21.6% of cases of cutaneous borreliosis.[186]

Clinically, BLC appears at the site of a tick bite or occurs close to the periphery of a large lesion of erythema chronicum migrans[179] (Fig. 50-13). Coexistence of both processes can also occur.[187] Rare cases can occur in patients with HIV.[180] Most patients are aware of having had a tick bite. In comparison with erythema chronicum migrans, BLC develops later and lasts longer.[35] The incubation period varies from a few weeks to 10 months.[180,181] Predilection sites include the ear lobe (17%), nipple and areola (59%), trunk (8%), axillary region and extremities (6%), nose (2%), and the scrotal area (8%), indicating that spirochetes may prefer regions with low skin temperature (Fig. 50-14). BLC usually has a blue-red plaque or nodule, 1 to 5 cm in diameter. Sometimes multiple discrete nodules may be within a localized area. There are usually no, or only slight, local symptoms, such as tenderness and itching. If treatment is not given, the lesion may persist for several months or more than a year. Regional lymphadenopathy is often found. Coexistence of BLC and acrodermatitis chronica atrophicans has been reported.[36] Only a small proportion of patients have constitutional symptoms or other late manifestations of Lyme disease. Serum antibodies to *B. burgdorferi* are elevated in 50% of cases.[188] The diagnosis is

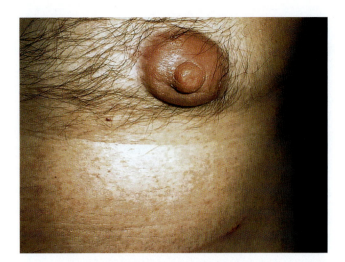

FIGURE 50-14. Cutaneous lymphoid hyperplasia of the nipple. Cutaneous lymphoid hyperplasia presenting as a circumscribed erythematous nodule of the nipple and areola of the left breast in a male patient. Many of these cases are associated with borrelial lymphocytoma cutis. (From Boudova L, Kazakov DV, Sima R, et al. Cutaneous lymphoid hyperplasia and other lymphoid infiltrates of the breast nipple: a retrospective clinicopathologic study of fifty-six patients. *Am J Dermatopathol.* 2005;27:375-386, with permission.)

typically made by (1) history of preceding erythema chronicum migrans or tick bite; (2) presence of blue-red nodule on the ear lobe or nipple, particularly in kids; (3) histologic findings compatible with LC; (4) elevated serum antibodies against *B. burgdorferi*; and (5) identification of the organism in the tissue by polymerase chain reaction (PCR) or immunohistochemistry. Cross-reactivity between *B. burgdorferi* and other treponemal organisms can be seen.[189]

Histologically, BLC shows a diffuse dermal infiltrate occupying the majority of the tissue biopsy (Fig. 50-15). Some cases can have a top or bottom-heavy distribution in the dermis. A grenz zone between the infiltrate and the epidermis is noted, but up to 10% of cases can show mild exocytosis of small lymphocytes. Germinal centers are present in >80% of cases. The germinal centers typically show a mixture of centroblasts, immunoblasts, and a low number of centrocytes with admixed tangible body macrophages. A normal mantle zone is present only in 12.2% of cases. Polarization of the GC can be seen in 20% of cases (Fig. 50-16). The background cells also include a mixture of histiocytes, eosinophils (84.2%), and plasma cells (99.9%).[36] Rare cases show an abundance of large cells and simulate large B-cell lymphoma.[37] Immunohistochemistry shows CD10+ and BCL-6+ germinal centers that are negative for BCL-2 and have a high proliferation index (>90%). Most cases are polyclonal using IGH gene rearrangement studies. Less than 5% of cases demonstrate clonality. Positive serology for IgM antibodies is present in 17% of cases, while elevated IgG antibodies are seen in 78.7% of cases. A positive PCR for *B. burgdorferi* DNA is noted in 67.5% of cases.[36]

The treatment of *B. burgdorferi* infections includes oral doxycycline, which is the mainstay of therapy of cutaneous borreliosis. Other first-line antibacterials are amoxicillin and cefuroxime axetil. Erythema migrans is treated for 2 weeks, lymphocytoma for 3 to 4 weeks, and acrodermatitis for at least 4 weeks.[35]

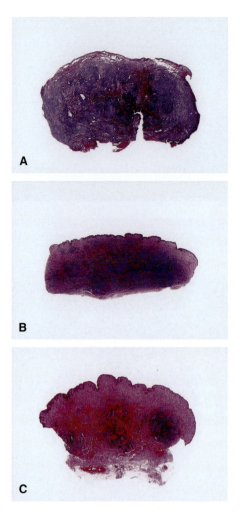

FIGURE 50-15. Cutaneous lymphoid hyperplasia of the nipple. A. Vaguely nodular cutaneous lymphoid hyperplasia composed of lymphoid follicles extending throughout the whole dermis. **B.** A dense diffuse lymphoid infiltrate of cutaneous lymphoid hyperplasia. **C.** A small, patchy infiltrate of cutaneous lymphoid hyperplasia is formed by several nodules consisting of coalescing follicles with germinal centers. (From Boudova L, Kazakov DV, Sima R, et al. Cutaneous lymphoid hyperplasia and other lymphoid infiltrates of the breast nipple: a retrospective clinicopathologic study of fifty-six patients. *Am J Dermatopathol.* 2005;27:375-386, with permission.)

Atypical Cutaneous Lymphoid Hyperplasia

Nihal et al[2] coined the term "atypical cutaneous lymphoid hyperplasia" (ACLH) to include a group of patients with CLH with associated clonal populations of B cells or T cells. Most of these patients had solitary lesions, and a subset (5%) had more widespread and disseminated lesions. Clonality was present in 61% of the samples. Approximately 30% showed a TCR rearrangement, 27% had an IGH rearrangement, and 4% had both B- and T-cell rearrangements. While most patients were disease-free after 36 months of follow-up, a few patients developed an overt cutaneous B-cell lymphoma, including a case where the IgH VDJ clones in the lymphoma and the antecedent lymphoid hyperplasia were identical (Figs. 50-17–50-20).

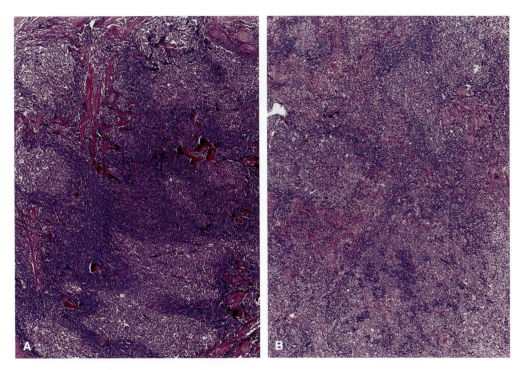

FIGURE 50-16. **Cutaneous lymphoid hyperplasia of the nipple. A.** Lymphoid follicles of cutaneous lymphoid hyperplasia with reactive germinal centers of various sizes and shapes. **B.** Lymphoid follicles in cutaneous lymphoid hyperplasia are closely packed and may coalesce. Mantle zones are markedly irregular and reduced. (From Boudova L, Kazakov DV, Sima R, et al. Cutaneous lymphoid hyperplasia and other lymphoid infiltrates of the breast nipple: a retrospective clinicopathologic study of fifty-six patients. *Am J Dermatopathol.* 2005;27:375-386, with permission.)

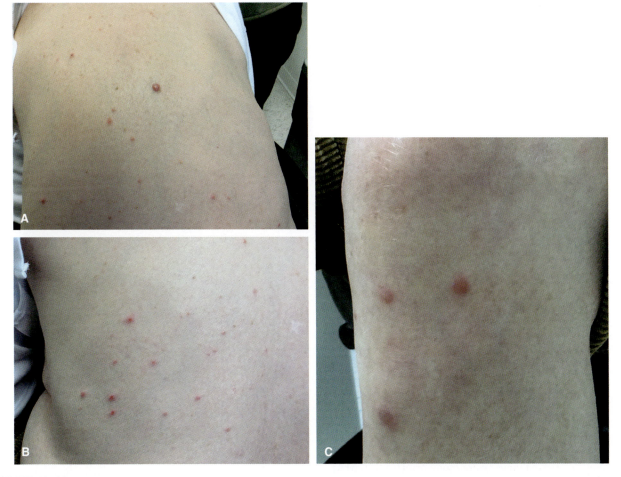

FIGURE 50-17. Papulonodular rash in the arm **(A)**, trunk **(B)**, and legs **(C)**. (Courtesy of Dr. Christopher Scott, Dermatology PLC and University of Virginia.)

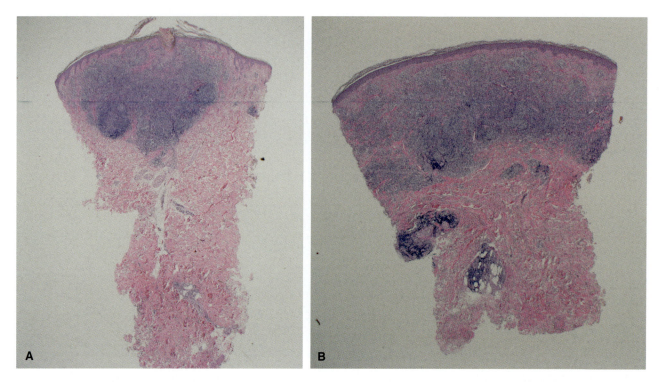

FIGURE 50-18. **Atypical lymphoid hyperplasia. A.** Perifollicular infiltrate (20×). **B.** Dense-band infiltrate in the superficial to mid-dermis (20×).

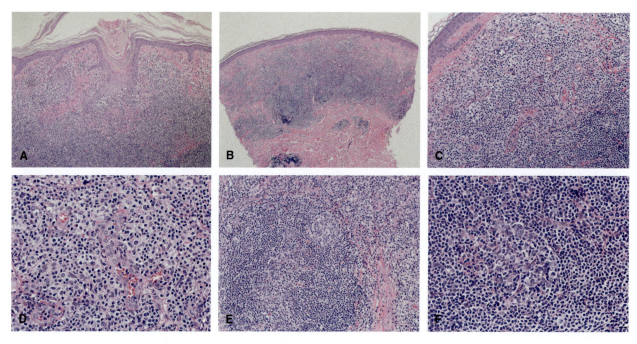

FIGURE 50-19. **Atypical lymphoid hyperplasia. A.** Perifollicular infiltrate (100×). **B.** Band-like infiltrate (100×). **C.** Increased vascularity in the superficial dermis and grenz zone of separation (200×). **D.** The infiltrate shows a prominent component of monocytoid atypical lymphocytes. Scattered mitotic figures are present (400×). **E.** Poorly formed and atrophic germinal centers are noted (200×). **F.** Small and atrophic germinal centers (400×).

Atypical Marginal Zone Hyperplasia

Attygalle et al[190] introduced the term atypical marginal zone hyperplasia (AMZH) to describe a series of six cases, affecting the tonsils and appendix of children, where the histopathologic changes were compatible with MALT lymphoma, with λ-light chain restriction by in situ hybridization, but polyclonal results with the use of PCR testing. Other cases of such atypical MZH were reported in the rectum and lymph nodes.[191,192] Guitart et al[193] presented a small series of two patients with AMZH in the skin. Similarly to the original series, both patients had λ-light chain restriction

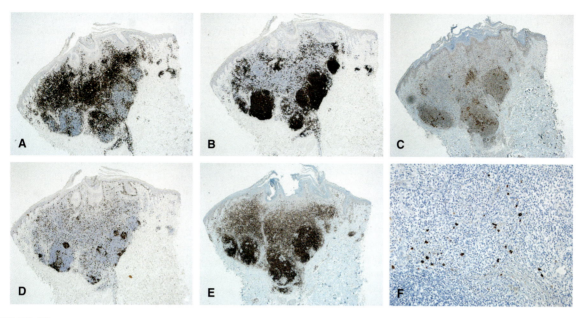

FIGURE 50-20. Atypical lymphoid hyperplasia—immunohistochemistry. A. CD3. **B.** CD20, many follicles are present. **C.** BCL-6 stains atropic germinal centers. **D.** Ki67 shows high proliferation in the germinal centers. **E.** BCL-2 is positive in T cells and negative in germinal centers. **F.** IgG4 highlights an increased number of plasma cells, an unusual finding in the setting of CLH.

and a polyclonal result using the BIOMED primers by PCR. Interestingly, Schmid et al[194] also published a series of ACLH with monotypic plasma cells in 20 patients. The latter series, though, included a mixture of κ or λ-light chain restricted plasma cells. The concept of ACLH was also recently emphasized by Guitart, claiming their precancerous significance.[195] In his model, a preexistent stimulus, external (eg, vaccine, tattoo, tick bite) or internal (eg, autoimmune, infectious, neoplastic), can lead to a "reactive" phase of hyperplasia, followed by early and late stages of MZL.

Lymphomatoid Keratosis

The term lymphomatoid keratosis (LyK) was originally proposed by Kossard[196] as a variant of benign lichenoid keratosis showing prominent lymphomatoid features. The term lymphomatoid indicates histologic simulation of MF, given the extent of exocytosis.[197] LyK is a pseudolymphoma or a form of CLH with a predominance of T cells.

Clinically, LyK presents in patients who range in age from 36 to 78 years, with a mean age of 59 years, and with a male:female ratio of 1:1. The size of the lesions ranges from 0.6 to 1.6 cm, with a mean of 0.85 cm. All cases reveal solitary scaly plaques, most commonly on the face, which is the most common location. Histologically, LyK resembles MF: there is hyperkeratosis, parakeratosis, acanthosis, and band-like lymphocytic infiltration. Epidermal exocytosis is prominent. Some cases can show Pautrier-like microabscesses and focal tagging of cells along the dermal-epidermal junction. There is no evidence of lymphocytic or keratinocytic atypia. Admixed plasma cells, eosinophils, and melanophages are characteristic.[196-199] The presence of solar lentigo or seborrheic keratosis adjacent to the lesion implies that LyK represents an exaggerated inflammatory host response in regressing solar lentigo or seborrheic keratoses.

As opposed to unilesional MF (pagetoid reticulosis), LyK exhibits a reactive T-cell population with normal CD4:CD8 ratio and a rich background of B cells and plasma cells, some of which exocytose into the epidermis. B cells are uncommon in lesions of MF, with the exception of cases with an associated T-helper phenotype. TCR rearrangement can be present in a small subset of cases (10%-20%).[197,200]

Syringolymphoid Hyperplasia With Alopecia

Syringolymphoid hyperplasia with alopecia (SLHA) is a term originally coined by Sarkany et al[201] to describe a distinctive form of CLH with specific clinical and histopathologic findings. Clinically, SLHA presents in adult men with well-circumscribed, erythematous or hypopigmented, hairless patches often with anhidrosis and follicular papules. Lesions develop over the course of several years, and systemic involvement is absent in all cases except for Sarkany patient, who eventually developed Hodgkin lymphoma.[201,202]

Biopsy specimens showed the distinctive findings of hypertrophy and hyperplasia of the eccrine glands and ducts, along with a surrounding dense lymphocytic infiltrate without significant atypia. Some speculate that SLHA is an early form of MF with syringotropic features.[203,204] Some cases can have associated follicular mucinosis.[203,205,206] Immunophenotypic evaluation reveals a CD4+ phenotype. T-cell rearrangement studies are positive in >50% of cases.[206-208] Close clinical follow-up is the mainstay of management.

References

1. Bergman R, Khamaysi K, Khamaysi Z, et al. A study of histologic and immunophenotypical staining patterns in cutaneous lymphoid hyperplasia. *J Am Acad Dermatol.* 2011;65:112-124.
2. Nihal M, Mikkola D, Horvath N, et al. Cutaneous lymphoid hyperplasia: a lymphoproliferative continuum with lymphomatous potential. *Hum Pathol.* 2003;34:617-622.
3. LeBoit PE, McNutt NS, Reed JA, et al. Primary cutaneous immunocytoma. A B-cell lymphoma that can easily be mistaken for cutaneous lymphoid hyperplasia. *Am J Surg Pathol.* 1994;18:969-978.
4. Medeiros LJ, Picker LJ, Abel EA, et al. Cutaneous lymphoid hyperplasia. Immunologic characteristics and assessment of criteria recently proposed as diagnostic of malignant lymphoma. *J Am Acad Dermatol.* 1989;21:929-942.
5. Wood GS, Ngan BY, Tung R, et al. Clonal rearrangements of immunoglobulin genes and progression to B cell lymphoma in cutaneous lymphoid hyperplasia. *Am J Pathol.* 1989;135:13-19.
6. Allen AC. Persistent insect bites (dermal eosinophilic granulomas) simulating lymphoblastomas, histiocytoses, and squamous cell carcinomas. *Am J Pathol.* 1948;24:367-387.
7. Barr-Nea L, Ishay J. Histopathological changes in mouse and rat skin injected with venom sac extracts of the oriental hornet (*Vespa orientalis*). *Toxicon.* 1977;15:301-306.
8. Sandbank M, Barr-Nea L, Ishay J. Pseudolymphoma of skin induced by oriental hornet (*Vespa orientalis*) venom ultrastructural study. *Arch Dermatol Res.* 1978;262:135-141.
9. Brady SP, Magro CM, Diaz-Cano SJ, et al. Analysis of clonality of atypical cutaneous lymphoid infiltrates associated with drug therapy by PCR/DGGE. *Hum Pathol.* 1999;30:130-136.
10. Magro CM, Crowson AN. Drugs with antihistaminic properties as a cause of atypical cutaneous lymphoid hyperplasia. *J Am Acad Dermatol.* 1995;32:419-428.
11. Addeo R, Montella L, Baldi A, et al. Atypical cutaneous lymphoid hyperplasia induced by chemotherapy in a patient with advanced colon carcinoma. *Clin Colorectal Cancer.* 2007;6:728-730.
12. Magro CM, Crowson AN. Drug-induced immune dysregulation as a cause of atypical cutaneous lymphoid infiltrates: a hypothesis. *Hum Pathol.* 1996;27:125-132.
13. Magro CM, Crowson AN, Kovatich AJ, et al. Drug-induced reversible lymphoid dyscrasia: a clonal lymphomatoid dermatitis of memory and activated T cells. *Hum Pathol.* 2003;34:119-129.
14. Furness PN, Goodfield MJ, MacLennan KA, et al. Severe cutaneous reactions to captopril and enalapril; histological study and comparison with early mycosis fungoides. *J Clin Pathol.* 1986;39:902-907.
15. Pulitzer MP, Nolan KA, Oshman RG, et al. CD30+ lymphomatoid drug reactions. *Am J Dermatopathol.* 2013;35:343-350.
16. Crowson AN, Magro CM. Antidepressant therapy. A possible cause of atypical cutaneous lymphoid hyperplasia. *Arch Dermatol.* 1995;131:925-929.
17. Garcia-Rodino S, Espasandin-Arias M, Suarez-Penaranda JM, et al. Persisting allergic patch test reaction to minoxidil manifested as cutaneous lymphoid hyperplasia. *Contact Dermatitis.* 2015;72:413-416.
18. Viraben R, Lamant L, Brousset P. Losartan-associated atypical cutaneous lymphoid hyperplasia. *Lancet.* 1997;350:1366.
19. Adams JD. Localized cutaneous pseudolymphoma associated with phenytoin therapy: a case report. *Australas J Dermatol.* 1981;22:28-29.
20. Rosenthal CJ, Noguera CA, Coppola A, et al. Pseudolymphoma with mycosis fungoides manifestations, hyperresponsiveness to diphenylhydantoin, and lymphocyte disregulation. *Cancer.* 1982;49:2305-2314.
21. D'Incan M, Souteyrand P, Bignon YJ, et al. Hydantoin-induced cutaneous pseudolymphoma with clinical, pathologic, and immunologic aspects of Sézary syndrome. *Arch Dermatol.* 1992;128:1371-1374.
22. Cooke LE, Hardin TC, Hendrickson DJ. Phenytoin-induced pseudolymphoma with mycosis fungoides manifestations. *Clin Pharm.* 1988;7:153-157.
23. Rijlaarsdam U, Scheffer E, Meijer CJ, et al. Mycosis fungoides-like lesions associated with phenytoin and carbamazepine therapy. *J Am Acad Dermatol.* 1991;24:216-220.
24. Harris DW, Ostlere L, Buckley C, et al. Phenytoin-induced pseudolymphoma. A report of a case and review of the literature. *Br J Dermatol.* 1992;127:403-406.
25. Braddock SW, Harrington D, Vose J. Generalized nodular cutaneous pseudolymphoma associated with phenytoin therapy. Use of T-cell receptor gene rearrangement in diagnosis and clinical review of cutaneous reactions to phenytoin. *J Am Acad Dermatol.* 1992;27:337-340.
26. Rosenfeld S, Swiller AI, Shenoy YM, et al. Syndrome simulating lymphosarcoma induced by diphenylhydantoin sodium. *JAMA.* 1961;176:491-493.
27. Charlesworth EN. Phenytoin-induced pseudolymphoma syndrome: an immunologic study. *Arch Dermatol.* 1977;113:477-480.
28. Gams RA, Neal JA, Conrad FG. Hydantoin-induced pseudo-pseudolymphoma. *Ann Intern Med.* 1968;69:557-568.
29. Isobe T, Horimatsu T, Fujita T, et al. Adult T-cell lymphoma following diphenylhydantoin therapy. *Nihon Ketsueki Gakkai Zasshi.* 1980;43:711-714.
30. Li FP, Willard DR, Goodman R, et al. Malignant lymphoma after diphenylhydantoin (dilantin) therapy. *Cancer.* 1975;36:1359-1362.
31. Marucci G, Sgarbanti E, Maestri A, et al. Gemcitabine-associated CD8+ CD30+ pseudolymphoma. *Br J Dermatol.* 2001;145:650-652.
32. Aram G, Rohwedder A, Nazeer T, et al. Varicella-zoster-virus folliculitis promoted clonal cutaneous lymphoid hyperplasia. *Am J Dermatopathol.* 2005;27:411-417.
33. Castelli E, Caputo V, Morello V, et al. Local reactions to tick bites. *Am J Dermatopathol.* 2008;30:241-248.
34. Gilliam AC, Wood GS. Cutaneous lymphoid hyperplasias. *Semin Cutan Med Surg.* 2000;19:133-141.
35. Mullegger RR, Glatz M. Skin manifestations of lyme borreliosis: diagnosis and management. *Am J Clin Dermatol.* 2008;9:355-368.
36. Colli C, Leinweber B, Mullegger R, et al. Borrelia burgdorferi-associated lymphocytoma cutis: clinicopathologic, immunophenotypic, and molecular study of 106 cases. *J Cutan Pathol.* 2004;31:232-240.
37. Grange F, Wechsler J, Guillaume JC, et al. Borrelia burgdorferi-associated lymphocytoma cutis simulating a primary cutaneous large B-cell lymphoma. *J Am Acad Dermatol.* 2002;47:530-534.
38. Eisendle K, Zelger B. The expanding spectrum of cutaneous borreliosis. *G Ital Dermatol Venereol.* 2009;144:157-171.

39. Tee SI, Martinez-Escaname M, Zuriel D, et al. Acrodermatitis chronica atrophicans with pseudolymphomatous infiltrates. *Am J Dermatopathol.* 2013;35:338-342.
40. Ziemer M, Eisendle K, Muller H, et al. Lymphocytic infiltration of the skin (Jessner–Kanof) but not reticular erythematous mucinosis occasionally represents clinical manifestations of Borrelia-associated pseudolymphoma. *Br J Dermatol.* 2009;161:583-590.
41. E Silva LG, Martins O. Persistent scabietic nodules with cutaneous lymphoplasia. [Article in Portuguese]. *Med Cutan Ibero Lat Am.* 1976;4:321-328.
42. McComb ME, Telang GH, Vonderheid EC. Secondary syphilis presenting as pseudolymphoma of the skin. *J Am Acad Dermatol.* 2003;49:S174-S176.
43. Duncan JR, Kaffenberger BH, Gru A. The necessity of clinicopathologic correlation: syphilis that could have been missed. . *J Cutan Pathol.* Published online 2015. doi:10.1111/cup.12629
44. Baum EW, Bernhardt M, Sams WM, Jr, et al. Secondary syphillis. Still the great imitator. *J Am Med Assoc.* 1983;249:3069-3070.
45. Cochran RE, Thomson J, Fleming KA, et al. Histology simulating reticulosis in secondary syphilis. *Br J Dermatol.* 1976;95:251-254.
46. Graham WR, Jr, Duvic M. Nodular secondary syphilis. *Arch Dermatol.* 1982;118:205-206.
47. Hodak E, David M, Rothem A, et al. Nodular secondary syphilis mimicking cutaneous lymphoreticular process. *J Am Acad Dermatol.* 1987;17:914-917.
48. Levin DL, Greenberg MH, Hasegawa J, et al. Secondary syphilis mimicking mycosis fungoides. *J Am Acad Dermatol.* 1980;3:92-94.
49. Moon HS, Park K, Lee JH, et al. A nodular syphilid presenting as a pseudolymphoma: mimicking a cutaneous marginal zone B-cell lymphoma. *Am J Dermatopathol.* 2009;31:846-848.
50. Tsai KY, Brenn T, Werchniak AE. Nodular presentation of secondary syphilis. *J Am Acad Dermatol.* 2007;57:S57-S58.
51. Recalcati S, Vezzoli P, Girgenti V, et al. Cutaneous lymphoid hyperplasia associated with Leishmania panamensis infection. *Acta Derm Venereol.* 2010;90:418-419.
52. Fukamachi S, Kimura T, Kobayashi M, et al. Palmar pseudolymphoma associated with herpes simplex infection. *J Cutan Pathol.* 2010;37:808-811.
53. Leinweber B, Kerl H, Cerroni L. Histopathologic features of cutaneous herpes virus infections (herpes simplex, herpes varicella/zoster): a broad spectrum of presentations with common pseudolymphomatous aspects. *Am J Surg Pathol.* 2006;30:50-58.
54. Lewin JM, Farley-Loftus R, Pomeranz MK. Herpes simplex virus-associated pseudolymphoma. *Cutis.* 2013;92:E1-E2.
55. Ackerman AB, Tanski EV. Pseudoleukemia cutis: report of a case in association with molluscum contagiosum. *Cancer.* 1977;40:813-817.
56. Cribier B, Scrivener Y, Grosshans E. Molluscum contagiosum: histologic patterns and associated lesions. A study of 578 cases. *Am J Dermatopathol.* 2001;23:99-103.
57. Del Boz Gonzalez J, Sanz A, Martin T, et al. Cutaneous pseudolymphoma associated with molluscum contagiosum: a case report. *Int J Dermatol.* 2008;47:502-504.
58. Guitart J, Hurt MA. Pleomorphic T-cell infiltrate associated with molluscum contagiosum. *Am J Dermatopathol.* 1999;21:178-180.
59. Moreno-Ramirez D, Garcia-Escudero A, Rios-Martin JJ, et al. Cutaneous pseudolymphoma in association with molluscum contagiosum in an elderly patient. *J Cutan Pathol.* 2003;30:473-475.
60. Mitani N, Nagatani T, Ikezawa Z, et al. A case of cutaneous T cell pseudolymphoma in a patient with *Helicobacter pylori* infection. *Dermatology.* 2006;213:156-158.
61. Bachelez H, Hadida F, Parizot C, et al. Oligoclonal expansion of HIV-specific cytotoxic CD8 T lymphocytes in the skin of HIV-1-infected patients with cutaneous pseudolymphoma. *J Clin Invest.* 1998;101:2506-2516.
62. Guitart J, Variakojis D, Kuzel T, et al. Cutaneous CD8 T cell infiltrates in advanced HIV infection. *J Am Acad Dermatol.* 1999;41:722-727.
63. Ingen-Housz-Oro S, Sbidian E, Ortonne N, et al. HIV-related CD8+ cutaneous pseudolymphoma: efficacy of methotrexate. *Dermatology.* 2013;226:15-18.
64. Schartz NE, De La Blanchardiere A, Alaoui S, et al. Regression of CD8+ pseudolymphoma after HIV antiviral triple therapy. *J Am Acad Dermatol.* 2003;49:139-141.
65. Zhang P, Chiriboga L, Jacobson M, et al. Mycosis fungoides-like T-cell cutaneous lymphoid infiltrates in patients with HIV infection. *Am J Dermatopathol.* 1995;17:29-35.
66. Cesinaro AM, Maiorana A. Verruca vulgaris with CD30-positive lymphoid infiltrate: a case report. *Am J Dermatopathol.* 2002;24:260-263.
67. Rose C, Starostik P, Brocker EB. Infection with parapoxvirus induces CD30-positive cutaneous infiltrates in humans. *J Cutan Pathol.* 1999;26:520-522.
68. Gonzalez LC, Murua MA, Perez RG, et al. CD30+ lymphoma simulating orf. *Int J Dermatol.* 2010;49:690-692.
69. Kash N, Ginter-Hanselmayer G, Cerroni L. Cutaneous mycotic infections with pseudolymphomatous infiltrates. *Am J Dermatopathol.* 2010;32:514-517.
70. Massi D, Trotta M, Franchi A, et al. Atypical CD30+ cutaneous lymphoid proliferation in a patient with tuberculosis infection. *Am J Dermatopathol.* 2004;26:234-236.
71. Lanzafame S, Micali G. Cutaneous lymphoid hyperplasia (pseudolymphoma) secondary to vaccination. [Article in Italian]. *Pathologica.* 1993;85:555-561.
72. Pham-Ledard A, Vergier B, Doutre MS, et al. Disseminated cutaneous lymphoid hyperplasia of 12 years' duration triggered by vaccination. *Dermatology.* 2010;220:176-179.
73. Atalar H, Sarifakioglu E, Dener C, et al. Cutaneous lymphoid hyperplasia and reactive lymphadenopathy induced by hepatitis B vaccination. *Eur J Dermatol.* 2008;18:188-189.
74. Maubec E, Pinquier L, Viguier M, et al. Vaccination-induced cutaneous pseudolymphoma. *J Am Acad Dermatol.* 2005;52:623-629.
75. May SA, Netto G, Domiati-Saad R, et al. Cutaneous lymphoid hyperplasia and marginal zone B-cell lymphoma following vaccination. *J Am Acad Dermatol.* 2005;53:512-516.
76. Madhogaria S, Carr RA, Gach JE. Childhood cutaneous lymphoid hyperplasia following feline scratches. *Pediatr Dermatol.* 2010;27:294-297.
77. Chiang C, Romero L. Cutaneous lymphoid hyperplasia (pseudolymphoma) in a tattoo after far infrared light. *Dermatol Surg.* 2009;35:1434-1438.
78. Gardair Bouchy C, Kerdraon R, Kluger N, et al. Cutaneous lymphoid hyperplasia (pseudolymphoma) on the red dye of a tattoo. [Article in French]. *Ann Pathol.* 2013;33:273-277.

79. Kluger N, Vermeulen C, Moguelet P, et al. Cutaneous lymphoid hyperplasia (pseudolymphoma) in tattoos: a case series of seven patients. *J Eur Acad Dermatol Venereol.* 2010;24:208-213.
80. Moulonguet I, Garcon N, Rivet J, et al. Nodule developing over a tattoo: challenge. Cutaneous lymphoid hyperplasia (pseudolymphoma). *Am J Dermatopathol.* 2014;36:88-89. 101-102.
81. Souza ES, Rocha Bde O, Batista Eda S, et al. T-cell-predominant lymphoid hyperplasia in a tattoo. *An Bras Dermatol.* 2014;89:1019-1021.
82. Millican EA, Conley JA, Sheinbein D. Cutaneous lymphoid hyperplasia related to squaric acid dibutyl ester. *J Am Acad Dermatol.* 2011;65:230-232.
83. Olson LE, Wilson JF, Cox JD. Cutaneous lymphoid hyperplasia: results of radiation therapy. *Radiology.* 1985;155:507-509.
84. Sau P, Solivan G, Johnson FB. Cutaneous reaction from a broken thermometer. *J Am Acad Dermatol.* 1991;25:915-919.
85. Cota C, Ferrara G, Cerroni L. Granuloma annulare with prominent lymphoid infiltrates ("pseudolymphomatous" granuloma annulare). *Am J Dermatopathol.* 2012;34:259-262.
86. Dadban A, Truchetet F. Cutaneous lymphoid hyperplasia on a preexistent melanocytic nevus. *Dermatology.* 2008;217:199-200.
87. Dargent JL, De Wolf-Peeters C. Subcutaneous lymphoid hyperplasia arising at site of ethnic scarifications and mimicking subcutaneous panniculitis-like T-cell lymphoma: a subcuticular T-cell lymphoid dyscrasia. *Virchows Arch.* 2004;444:395-396.
88. Dargent JL, Diedhiou A, Lothaire P, et al. Subcutaneous lymphoid hyperplasia arising at site of ethnic scarifications and mimicking subcutaneous panniculitis-like T-cell lymphoma. *Virchows Arch.* 2001;438:298-301.
89. Gutte RM. Pseudolymphomatous folliculitis: a distinctive cutaneous lymphoid hyperplasia. *Indian J Dermatol.* 2013;58:278-280.
90. Kakizaki A, Fujimura T, Numata I, et al. Pseudolymphomatous folliculitis on the nose. *Case Rep Dermatol.* 2012;4:27-30.
91. Horiuchi Y, Hakugawa J, Shimizu K, et al. Massive cutaneous follicular lymphoid hyperplasia in a patient with the Sjögren syndrome: 7-year follow-up and immunohistochemical study. *Rheumatol Int.* 2006;26:1044-1049.
92. Chetty R, Perez-Ordonez B, Gilbert R, et al. Spiradenocarcinoma arising from a spiradenocylindroma: unusual case with lymphoepithelioma-like areas. *J Cutan Med Surg.* 2009;13:215-220.
93. Arsenovic N. Lymphoepithelioma-like carcinoma of the skin: new case of an exceedingly rare primary skin tumor. *Dermatol Online J.* 2008;14:12.
94. Carr KA, Bulengo-Ransby SM, Weiss LM, et al. Lymphoepitheliomalike carcinoma of the skin. A case report with immunophenotypic analysis and in situ hybridization for Epstein–Barr viral genome. *Am J Surg Pathol.* 1992;16:909-913.
95. Ferlicot S, Plantier F, Rethers L, et al. Lymphoepithelioma-like carcinoma of the skin: a report of 3 Epstein–Barr virus (EBV)-negative additional cases. Immunohistochemical study of the stroma reaction. *J Cutan Pathol.* 2000;27:306-311.
96. Gillum PS, Morgan MB, Naylor MF, et al. Absence of Epstein–Barr virus in lymphoepitheliomalike carcinoma of the skin. Polymerase chain reaction evidence and review of five cases. *Am J Dermatopathol.* 1996;18:478-482.
97. Lopez V, Martin JM, Santonja N, et al. Lymphoepithelioma-like carcinoma of the skin: report of three cases. *J Cutan Pathol.* 2011;38:54-58.
98. Swanson SA, Cooper PH, Mills SE, et al. Lymphoepithelioma-like carcinoma of the skin. *Mod Pathol.* 1988;1:359-365.
99. Weiss LM, Movahed LA, Butler AE, et al. Analysis of lymphoepithelioma and lymphoepithelioma-like carcinomas for Epstein–Barr viral genomes by in situ hybridization. *Am J Surg Pathol.* 1989;13:625-631.
100. Wick MR, Swanson PE, LeBoit PE, et al. Lymphoepithelioma-like carcinoma of the skin with adnexal differentiation. *J Cutan Pathol.* 1991;18:93-102.
101. Botella-Estrada R, Kutzner H. Study of the immunophenotype of the inflammatory cells in melanomas with regression and halo nevi. *Am J Dermatopathol.* 2015;37:376-380.
102. Harvell JD, Meehan SA, LeBoit PE. Spitz's nevi with halo reaction: a histopathologic study of 17 cases. *J Cutan Pathol.* 1997;24:611-619.
103. Hussein MR, Elsers DA, Fadel SA, et al. Immunohistological characterisation of tumour infiltrating lymphocytes in melanocytic skin lesions. *J Clin Pathol.* 2006;59:316-324.
104. Zeff RA, Freitag A, Grin CM, et al. The immune response in halo nevi. *J Am Acad Dermatol.* 1997;37:620-624.
105. Requena L, Sangueza OP. Cutaneous vascular proliferations. Part III. Malignant neoplasms, other cutaneous neoplasms with significant vascular component, and disorders erroneously considered as vascular neoplasms. *J Am Acad Dermatol.* 1998;38:143-175. quiz 176-148.
106. Requena L, Santonja C, Stutz N, et al. Pseudolymphomatous cutaneous angiosarcoma: a rare variant of cutaneous angiosarcoma readily mistaken for cutaneous lymphoma. *Am J Dermatopathol.* 2007;29:342-350.
107. Fernandez N, Torres A, Ackerman AB. Pathologic findings in human scabies. *Arch Dermatol.* 1977;113:320-324.
108. Reunala T, Ranki A, Rantanen T, et al. Inflammatory cells in skin lesions of scabies. *Clin Exp Dermatol.* 1984;9:70-77.
109. Thomson J, Cochrane T, Cochran R, et al. Histology simulating reticulosis in persistent nodular scabies. *Br J Dermatol.* 1974;90:421-429.
110. Walton S, Bottomley WW, Wyatt EH, et al. Pseudo T-cell lymphoma due to scabies in a patient with Hodgkin's disease. *Br J Dermatol.* 1991;124:277-278.
111. Baldassano MF, Bailey EM, Ferry JA, et al. Cutaneous lymphoid hyperplasia and cutaneous marginal zone lymphoma: comparison of morphologic and immunophenotypic features. *Am J Surg Pathol.* 1999;23:88-96.
112. Brodell RT, Santa Cruz DJ. Cutaneous pseudolymphomas. *Dermatol Clin.* 1985;3:719-734.
113. Caro WA, Helwig HB. Cutaneous lymphoid hyperplasia. *Cancer.* 1969;24:487-502.
114. Kerl H, Ackerman AB. *Inflammatory Diseases that Simulate Lymphomas: Cutaneous Pseudolymphomas.* McGraw-Hill, Medical Pub. Division; 2003.
115. Boudova L, Kazakov DV, Sima R, et al. Cutaneous lymphoid hyperplasia and other lymphoid infiltrates of the breast nipple: a retrospective clinicopathologic study of fifty-six patients. *Am J Dermatopathol.* 2005;27(5):375-386. doi:10.1097/01.dad.0000179463.55129.8a
116. Goerdt S, Spieker T, Wölffer LU. Multiple cutaneous B-cell pseudolymphomas after allergen injections. *J Am Acad Dermatol.* 1996;34(6):1072-1074. doi:10.1016/s0190-9622(96)90289-3

117. Hernández I, Sanmartín O, Cardá C, Góme S, Alfaro A. B-cell pseudolymphoma caused by aluminium hydroxide following hyposensitization therapy. *Actas Dermosifiliogr.* 2008;99(3):213-216.
118. Cerroni L, Borroni RG, Massone C, Chott A, Kerl H. Cutaneous B-cell pseudolymphoma at the site of vaccination. *Am J Dermatopathol.* 2007;29(6):538-542. doi:10.1097/DAD.0b013e3181591bea
119. Arnež M, Ružić-Sabljić E. Borrelial lymphocytoma in children.*Pediatr Infect Dis J.* 2015;34(12):1319-1322. doi:10.1097/INF.0000000000000884
120. Moreno A, Curco N, Serrano T, et al. Disseminated, miliarial type lymphocytoma cutis. A report of two cases. *Acta Derm Venereol.* 1991;71:334-336.
121. Self SJ, Carter VH, Noojin RO. Disseminated lymphocytoma cutis. Case reports of miliarial and nodular types. *Arch Dermatol.* 1969;100:459-464.
122. Villalobos-Ayala RA, Espinoza-Gurrola AA, Guevara-Gutiérrez E, et al. Lymphocytoma cutis (cutaneous B-cell pseudolymphoma): study of 102 cases with emphasis on the histological characteristics and immunohistochemistry of the miliarial type. *Int J Dermatol.* 2022;61(3):316-323. doi:10.1111/ijd.15909
123. Moulonguet I, Ghnassia M, Molina T, Fraitag S. Miliarial-type perifollicular B-cell pseudolymphoma (Lymphocytoma cutis): a misleading eruption in two women. *J Cutan Pathol.* 2012;39:1016-1021.
124. Jauker P, Tittes J, Tanew A. Miliarial type perifollicular B-cell pseudolymphoma: an easily overlooked rare subtype of pseudolymphoma cutis manifesting as a centrofacial acneiform eruption. *J Eur Acad Dermatol Venereol.* 2021;35(12):e905-e906. doi:10.1111/jdv.175
125. Chirife AM, Bilbao ER, Gimenez L, et al. Cutaneous B cell processes with nodular pattern. [Article in Spanish]. *Medicina (B Aires).* 2006;66:307-312.
126. Ploysangam T, Breneman DL, Mutasim DF. Cutaneous pseudolymphomas. *J Am Acad Dermatol.* 1998;38:877-895. quiz 896-877.
127. Kerl H, Fink-Puches R, Cerroni L. Diagnostic criteria of primary cutaneous B-cell lymphomas and pseudolymphomas. *Keio J Med.* 2001;50(4):269-273. doi:10.2302/kjm.50.269
128. Mitteldorf C, Kempf W. Cutaneous pseudolymphoma-A review on the spectrum and a proposal for a new classification. *J Cutan Pathol.* 2020;47(1):76-97. doi:10.1111/cup.13532
129. Kojima M, Sakurai S, Shimizu K, et al. B-cell cutaneous lymphoid hyperplasia representing progressive transformation of germinal center: a report of 2 cases. *Int J Surg Pathol.* 2010;18:429-432.
130. Mitteldorf C, Kempf W. Cutaneous pseudolymphoma. *Surg Pathol Clin.* 2017;10(2):455-476.
131. Kutzner H, Kerl H, Pfaltz MC, Kempf W. CD123-positive plasmacytoid dendritic cells in primary cutaneous marginal zone B-cell lymphoma: diagnostic and pathogenetic implications. *Am J Surg Pathol.* 2009;33(9):1307-1313. doi:10.1097/pas.0b013e3181a6ae1e
132. Bouloc A, Delfau-Larue MH, Lenormand B, et al. Polymerase chain reaction analysis of immunoglobulin gene rearrangement in cutaneous lymphoid hyperplasias. French Study Group for Cutaneous Lymphomas. *Arch Dermatol.* 1999;135(2):168-172. doi:10.1001/archderm.135.2.168
133. Ritter JH, Wick MR, Adesokan PN, Fitzgibbon JF, Zhu X, Humphrey PA. Assessment of clonality in cutaneous lymphoid infiltrates by polymerase chain reaction analysis of immunoglobulin heavy chain gene rearrangement. *Am J Clin Pathol.* 1997;108(1):60-68.
134. Böer A, Tirumalae R, Bresch M, Falk TM. Pseudoclonality in cutaneous pseudolymphomas: a pitfall in interpretation of rearrangement studies. *Br J Dermatol.* 2008;159(2):394-402. doi:10.1111/j.1365-2133.2008.08670.x
135. Craddock AP, Kane WJ, Raghavan SS, Williams ES, Gru AA, Gradecki SE. Use of ultrasensitive RNA in situ hybridization for determining clonality in cutaneous B-cell lymphomas and lymphoid hyperplasia decreases subsequent use of molecular testing and is cost-effective. *Am J Surg Pathol.* 2022;46(7):956-962.
136. Bergman R, Khamaysi Z, Sahar D, et al. Cutaneous lymphoid hyperplasia presenting as a solitary facial nodule: clinical, histopathological, immunophenotypical, and molecular studies. *Arch Dermatol.* 2006;142(12):1561-1566.
137. Rijlaarsdam JU, Willemze R. Cutaneous pseudolymphomas: classification and differential diagnosis. *Semin Dermatol.* 1994;13(3):187-196.
138. Fukamachi S, Sugita K, Sawada Y, et al. Drug-induced CD30+ T cell pseudolymphoma. *Eur J Dermatol.* 2009;19(3):292-294.
139. Souteyrand P, d'Incan M. Drug-induced mycosis fungoides-like lesions. *Curr Probl Dermatol.* 1990;19:176-182.
140. Magro CM, Daniels BH, Crowson AN. Drug induced pseudolymphoma. *Semin Diagn Pathol.* 2018;35(4):247-259.
141. Mitteldorf C, Geissinger E, Pleimes M, et al. T-cell pseudolymphoma in recurrent herpes simplex virus infection. *J Cutan Pathol.* 2019;46(10):717-722.
142. Moreira E, Lisboa C, Azevedo F, et al. Postzoster cutaneous pseudolymphoma in a patient with B-cell chronic lymphocytic leukaemia. *J Eur Acad Dermatol Venereol.* 2007;21(8):1112-1114.
143. Mitteldorf C, Plumbaum H, Zutt M, et al. CD8-positive pseudolymphoma in lues maligna and human immunodeficiency virus with monoclonal T-cell receptor-beta rearrangement. *J Cutan Pathol.* 2019;46(3):204-210.
144. Portilla Maya N, Kempf W, Perez Muñoz N, et al. Histopathologic spectrum of findings associated with tattoos: multicenter study series of 230 cases. *Am J Dermatopathol.* 2021;43(8):543-553.
145. Miguel D, Peckruhn M, Elsner P. Treatment of cutaneous pseudolymphoma: a systematic review. *Acta Derm Venereol.* 2018;98(3):310-317.
146. Orbaneja JG, Diez LI, Lozano JL, et al. Lymphomatoid contact dermatitis: a syndrome produced by epicutaneous hypersensitivity with clinical features and a histopathologic picture similar to that of mycosis fungoides. *Contact Dermatitis.* 1976;2(3):139-143.
147. Coleman E, Bhawan J. Baby wet wipes: an unusual culprit of lymphomatoid contact dermatitis mimicking mycosis fungoides. *Am J Dermatopathol.* 2022;44(3):205-206.
148. Kempf W, Keller K, John H, et al. Benign atypical intravascular CD30+ T-cell proliferation – a recently described reactive lymphoproliferative process and simulator of intravascular lymphoma: report of a case associated with lichen sclerosus and review of the literature. *Am J Clin Pathol.* 2014;142(5):694-699.
149. Jang NR, Kim MK, Shin DH, et al. Benign atypical intralymphatic CD30+ T-cell proliferation: a case report and literature review. *Ann Dermatol.* 2019;31(1):108-110.
150. Calamaro P, Cerroni L. Intralymphatic proliferation of T-cell lymphoid blasts in the setting of hidradenitis suppurativa. *Am J Dermatopathol.* 2016;38(7):536-540.

151. Rijlaarsdam JU, Meijer CJ, Willemze R. Lymphadenosis benigna cutis versus primary cutaneous B-cell lymphomas of follicular center cell origin. *Curr Probl Dermatol.* 1990;19:189-195.
152. Wolf R, Kahane E, Sandbank M. Mycosis fungoides-like lesions associated with phenytoin therapy. *Arch Dermatol.* 1985;121:1181-1182.
153. Kerl H, Smolle J. Classification of cutaneous pseudolymphomas. *Curr Probl Dermatol.* 1990;19:167-175.
154. Smolle J, Torne R, Soyer HP, et al. Immunohistochemical classification of cutaneous pseudolymphomas: delineation of distinct patterns. *J Cutan Pathol.* 1990;17:149-159.
155. Ackerman AB, Breza TS, Capland L. Spongiotic simulants of mycosis fungoides. *Arch Dermatol.* 1974;109:218-220.
156. Kardaun SH, Scheffer E, Vermeer BJ. Drug-induced pseudolymphomatous skin reactions. *Br J Dermatol.* 1988;118:545-552.
157. Saltzstein SL, Ackerman LV. Lymphadenopathy induced by anticonvulsant drugs and mimicking clinically pathologically malignant lymphomas. *Cancer.* 1959;12:164-182.
158. Dorfman RF, Warnke R. Lymphadenopathy simulating the malignant lymphomas. *Hum Pathol.* 1974;5:519-550.
159. Arai E, Shimizu M, Hirose T. A review of 55 cases of cutaneous lymphoid hyperplasia: reassessment of the histopathologic findings leading to reclassification of 4 lesions as cutaneous marginal zone lymphoma and 19 as pseudolymphomatous folliculitis. *Hum Pathol.* 2005;36:505-511.
160. Kempf W, Kazakov DV, Kutzner H. Lobular panniculitis due to Borrelia burgdorferi infection mimicking subcutaneous panniculitis-like T-cell lymphoma. *Am J Dermatopathol.* 2013;35(2):e30-33.
161. Barr RJ, Sun NC, King DF. Immunoperoxidase staining of cytoplasmic immunoglobulins. A diagnostic aid in distinguishing cutaneous reactive lymphoid hyperplasia from malignant lymphoma. *J Am Acad Dermatol.* 1980;3:58-62.
162. Cerroni L, Kerl H. Immunoreactivity for bcl-2 protein in cutaneous lymphomas and lymphoid hyperplasias. *J Cutan Pathol.* 1995;22:476-478.
163. Chimenti S, Cerroni L, Zenahlik P, et al. The role of MT2 and anti-bcl-2 protein antibodies in the differentiation of benign from malignant cutaneous infiltrates of B-lymphocytes with germinal center formation. *J Cutan Pathol.* 1996;23:319-322.
164. Dummer R, Michie SA, Kell D, et al. Expression of bcl-2 protein and Ki-67 nuclear proliferation antigen in benign and malignant cutaneous T-cell infiltrates. *J Cutan Pathol.* 1995;22:11-17.
165. Kuo TT, Lo SK, Chan HL. Immunohistochemical analysis of dermal mononuclear cell infiltrates in cutaneous lupus erythematosus, polymorphous light eruption, lymphocytic infiltration of Jessner, and cutaneous lymphoid hyperplasia: a comparative differential study. *J Cutan Pathol.* 1994;21:430-436.
166. Hristov AC, Comfere NI, Vidal CI, Sundram U. Kappa and lambda immunohistochemistry and in situ hybridization in the evaluation of atypical cutaneous lymphoid infiltrates. *J Cutan Pathol.* 2020;47(11):1103-1110.
167. Goyal A, Moore JB, Gimbel D, et al. PD-1, S-100 and CD1a expression in pseudolymphomatous folliculitis, primary cutaneous marginal zone B-cell lymphoma (MALT lymphoma) and cutaneous lymphoid hyperplasia. *J Cutan Pathol.* 2015;42:6-15.
168. Shojiguchi N, Arai E, Anan T, Ansai S-I Tsuchida T, Yasuda M. Distribution of CD1a-positive cells is not different between pseudolymphomatous folliculitis and primary cutaneous marginal zone lymphoma. *J Dermatol.* 2021;48(4):464-469. doi:10.1111/1346-8138.15731.
169. Fan K, Kelly R, Kendrick V. Nonclonal lymphocytic proliferation in cutaneous lymphoid hyperplasia: a flow-cytometric and morphological analysis. *Dermatology.* 1992;185:113-119.
170. Hammer E, Sangueza O, Suwanjindar P, et al. Immunophenotypic and genotypic analysis in cutaneous lymphoid hyperplasias. *J Am Acad Dermatol.* 1993;28:426-433.
171. Nihal M, Mikkola D, Wood GS. Detection of clonally restricted immunoglobulin heavy chain gene rearrangements in normal and lesional skin: analysis of the B cell component of the skin-associated lymphoid tissue and implications for the molecular diagnosis of cutaneous B cell lymphomas. *J Mol Diagn.* 2000;2:5-10.
172. Nakayama F, Kurosu K, Yumoto N, et al. Immunoglobulin gene analysis of cutaneous pseudolymphoma by polymerase chain reaction. *J Dermatol.* 1995;22:403-410.
173. Rijlaarsdam U, Bakels V, van Oostveen JW, et al. Demonstration of clonal immunoglobulin gene rearrangements in cutaneous B-cell lymphomas and pseudo-B-cell lymphomas: differential diagnostic and pathogenetic aspects. *J Invest Dermatol.* 1992;99:749-754.
174. Griesser H, Feller AC, Sterry W. T-cell receptor and immunoglobulin gene rearrangements in cutaneous T-cell-rich pseudolymphomas. *J Invest Dermatol.* 1990;95:292-295.
175. Wechsler J, Bagot M. T-cell receptor and immunoglobulin gene rearrangements in cutaneous T-cell-rich pseudolymphomas. *J Invest Dermatol.* 1991;96:799.
176. Campo E, Jaffe ES, Cook JR, et al. The international consensus classification of mature lymphoid neoplasms: a report from the clinical advisory committee. *Blood.* Published online 2022. blood.2022015851.
177. Clark WH, Mihm MC, Jr, Reed RJ, et al. The lymphocytic infiltrates of the skin. *Hum Pathol.* 1974;5:25-43.
178. Connors RC, Ackerman AB. Histologic pseudomalignancies of the skin. *Arch Dermatol.* 1976;112:1767-1780.
179. Albrecht S, Hofstadter S, Artsob H, et al. Lymphadenosis benigna cutis resulting from Borrelia infection (Borrelia lymphocytoma). *J Am Acad Dermatol.* 1991;24:621-625.
180. Bratzke B, Stadler R, Gollnick H, et al. Borrelia burgdorferi-induced pseudolymphoma with pathogen cultivation in an HIV-1 positive patient. [Article in German]. *Hautarzt.* 1989;40:504-509.
181. Büchner SA, Fluckiger B, Rufli T. Infiltrating lymphadenosis benigna cutis as borreliosis of the skin. [Article in German]. *Hautarzt.* 1988;39:77-81.
182. Hovmark A. Role of Borrelia burgdorferi in lymphocytomas and sclerotic skin lesions. *Clin Dermatol.* 1993;11:363-367.
183. Hovmark A, Asbrink E, Olsson I. The spirochetal etiology of lymphadenosis benigna cutis solitaria. *Acta Derm Venereol.* 1986;66:479-484.
184. Stanek G, Wewalka G, Groh V, et al. Differences between Lyme disease and European arthropod-borne Borrelia infections. *Lancet.* 1985;1:401.
185. Weber K, Schierz G, Wilske B, et al. European erythema migrans disease and related disorders. *Yale J Biol Med.* 1984;57:463-471.
186. Glatz M, Resinger A, Semmelweis K, et al. Clinical spectrum of skin manifestations of Lyme borreliosis in 204 children in Austria. *Acta Derm Venereol.* 2015;95:565-571.

187. Maraspin V, Cimperman J, Lotric-Furlan S, et al. Solitary borrelial lymphocytoma in adult patients. *Wien Klin Wochenschr.* 2002;114:515-523.
188. Asbrink E, Hovmark A. *Lyme Borreliosis.* McGraw-Hill, Medical Pub. Division; 2003.
189. Quatresooz P, Pierard-Franchimont C, Pierard GE. Vulnerability of reactive skin to electric current perception—a pilot study implicating mast cells and the lymphatic microvasculature. *J Cosmet Dermatol.* 2009;8:186-189.
190. Attygalle AD, Liu H, Shirali S, et al. Atypical marginal zone hyperplasia of mucosa-associated lymphoid tissue: a reactive condition of childhood showing immunoglobulin lambda light-chain restriction. *Blood.* 2004;104:3343-3348.
191. Kojima M, Itoh H, Motegi A, et al. Localized lymphoid hyperplasia of the rectum resembling polypoid mucosa-associated lymphoid tissue lymphoma: a report of three cases. *Pathol Res Pract.* 2005;201:757-761.
192. Kojima M, Nakamura S, Tanaka H, et al. Massive hyperplasia of marginal zone B-cells with clear cytoplasm in the lymph node: a case report. *Pathol Res Pract.* 2003;199:625-628.
193. Guitart J, Gerami P. Is there a cutaneous variant of marginal zone hyperplasia? *Am J Dermatopathol.* 2008;30:494-496.
194. Schmid U, Eckert F, Griesser H, et al. Cutaneous follicular lymphoid hyperplasia with monotypic plasma cells. A clinicopathologic study of 18 patients. *Am J Surg Pathol.* 1995;19:12-20.
195. Guitart J. Rethinking primary cutaneous marginal zone lymphoma: shifting the focus to the cause of the infiltrate. *J Cutan Pathol.* 2015;42:600-603.
196. Kossard S. Unilesional mycosis fungoides or lymphomatoid keratosis? *Arch Dermatol.* 1997;133:1312-1313.
197. Arai E, Shimizu M, Tsuchida T, et al. Lymphomatoid keratosis – an epidermotropic type of cutaneous lymphoid hyperplasia: clinicopathological, immunohistochemical, and molecular biological study of 6 cases. *Arch Dermatol.* 2007;143:53-59.
198. Choi MJ, Kim HS, Kim HO, et al. A case of lymphomatoid keratosis. *Ann Dermatol.* 2010;22:219-222.
199. Evans LT, Mackey SL, Vidmar DA. An asymptomatic scaly plaque. Unilesional mycosis fungoides (MF). *Arch Dermatol.* 1997;133:231-234.
200. Al-Hoqail IA, Crawford RI. Benign lichenoid keratoses with histologic features of mycosis fungoides: clinicopathologic description of a clinically significant histologic pattern. *J Cutan Pathol.* 2002;29:291-294.
201. Sarkany I. Patchy alopecia, anhidrosis, eccrine gland wall hypertrophy and vasculitis. *Proc R Soc Med.* 1969;62:157-159.
202. Hobbs JL, Chaffins ML, Douglass MC. Syringolymphoid hyperplasia with alopecia: two case reports and review of the literature. *J Am Acad Dermatol.* 2003;49:1177-1180.
203. Burg G, Schmockel C. Syringolymphoid hyperplasia with alopecia—a syringotropic cutaneous T-cell lymphoma? *Dermatology.* 1992;184:306-307.
204. Zelger B, Sepp N, Weyrer K, et al. Syringotropic cutaneous T-cell lymphoma: a variant of mycosis fungoides? *Br J Dermatol.* 1994;130:765-769.
205. Tannous Z, Baldassano MF, Li VW, et al. Syringolymphoid hyperplasia and follicular mucinosis in a patient with cutaneous T-cell lymphoma. *J Am Acad Dermatol.* 1999;41:303-308.
206. Tomaszewski MM, Lupton GP, Krishnan J, et al. Syringolymphoid hyperplasia with alopecia. A case report. *J Cutan Pathol.* 1994;21:520-526.
207. Esche C, Sander CA, Zumdick M, et al. Further evidence that syringolymphoid hyperplasia with alopecia is a cutaneous T-cell lymphoma. *Arch Dermatol.* 1998;134:753-754.
208. Dubin DB, Hurowitz JC, Brettler D, et al. Adnexotropic T-cell lymphoma presenting with generalized anhidrosis, progressive alopecia, pruritus, and Sjögren's syndrome. *J Am Acad Dermatol.* 1998;38:493-497.

CHAPTER 51

Pseudolymphomas at sites of vaccination and in tattoos

Priyadharsini Nagarajan

INTRODUCTION

The introduction of extraneous materials in the form of tattoos and vaccines can induce a cutaneous inflammatory infiltrate that clinically and histologically invokes the possibility of a lymphoproliferative process.[1-3] It has been postulated that delayed hypersensitivity to specific components of the vaccine or tattoo ink may give raise to such immunologic reactions.

PSEUDOLYMPHOMAS ASSOCIATED WITH VACCINATION

The beneficial effects of vaccine-induced immunity outweigh the adverse effects in most people. Most of the local side effects such as pain, swelling, and redness are transient and usually last for a few days after vaccination.[4] In rare instances, papules or subcutaneous nodules may develop at the injection site and persist for months to years; such a response was first documented in 1974 by Bernstein et al in a patient receiving hyposensitization injections.[5]

Pseudolymphomas at vaccination sites have been reported more commonly in women.[6,7] The nodules usually develop as early as 1 month after vaccination or may be delayed up to 5 years.[7] Subcutaneous nodules are the most common presentation of vaccine-associated pseudolymphomas, followed by papules and indurated plaques. Single or multiple lesions may be present and are often accompanied by pruritus, pain, erythema, hyperpigmentation, and hypertrichosis.[8-13] A high degree of clinical suspicion with respect to anatomic site and history of immunization is essential for appropriate diagnosis and management.

Most of these lesions have developed after injection of vaccines or desensitization solutions that contain aluminum oxyhydroxide as an adjuvant,[14] such as hepatitis B, hepatitis A, Flavivirus-mediated early summer meningoencephalitis, varicella zoster, quadrivalent human papilloma virus, tetanus, and diphtheria/tetanus.[6,7,9,11,15,16] The development of a second pseudolymphoma in a patient with prior history after revaccination has been reported. Aluminum adjuvant from the vaccine is present in both the soluble (biologically reactive) form, which associates with antigens, antibodies, and other proteins and diffuses away from the injection site, and the insoluble (1-20 μm, particulate) form, which persists at the site of injection and functions as a constant source of soluble Al^{3+} ions and antigens.[17] The particulate form of aluminum is phagocytized by macrophages, functions as a constant source of immunologic activation and may lead to the development of pseudolymphomas in susceptible patients. Whether direct toxic effects of aluminum, a delayed hypersensitivity response through activation of Th-2-mediated response, or both could contribute to the development of pseudolymphomas is unknown.[18] Rare cases of T-lymphocytic pseudolymphomas have been reported at injection sites of antitumor vaccines.[19]

Histologically, a predominantly subcutaneous lymphocytic infiltrate is noted in all cases, with some involvement of deep dermis.[6] The infiltrate is dense and more often nodular than diffuse and is characterized by the presence of predominantly lymphocytes admixed with histiocytes as well as fewer numbers of polyclonal plasma cells and eosinophils (Fig. 51-1A,B). B-lymphocyte-predominant germinal centers are frequently seen with variable degree of interfollicular fibrosis and fat necrosis, which are also highlighted by CD10, CD20, CD79a, CD23, CD21, and Bcl6, while Bcl2 expression is restricted to the interfollicular T cells, which are also positive for CD3, CD5, CD7, and CD43. In addition, perivascular and periadnexal lymphohistiocytic infiltrate and, rarely, a lichenoid infiltrate may also be seen.[13] Molecular analysis reveals polyclonality in both the B and T lymphocytes.

In early lesions, histiocytes with abundant granular amphophilic cytoplasm may be prominent (Fig. 51-1C,D) and may palisade around necrotic debris.[6,7,20] These histiocytes also stain positive with diastase–periodic acid Schiff stain.[11] The presence of particulate aluminum with the histiocytes can be demonstrated rarely as fine, faintly polarizable material or by treating with hydrochloric acid to remove calcium from the tissue and then with Morin solution, followed by examination using a fluorescence microscope.[7,11] Electron microscopy demonstrates dense needle-shaped crystals within the histiocytes.[7,20] Energy-dispersive X-ray microanalysis can also be used to demonstrate the presence of inorganic aluminum in the tissues.[11,20]

vasculitis may be identified within the preserved myocyte fibers.[7]

Other injection site nodules include granulomatous reaction to vaccines such as varicella-zoster and bacilli Calmette-Guérin.[21,22] Deep granuloma annulare or rheumatoid nodule–like reactions with prominent necrobiosis and even lupus profundus–like patterns have been documented at vaccination sites.[20]

Spontaneous resolution of the subcutaneous nodules is not frequent. Intralesional steroid injections and surgical excisions are curative in most patients.[7] Local radiotherapy has also a role in controlling disease progression.[6] Topical high-potency steroids and systemic immunomodulators have also been tried. Future avoidance of the causative vaccinations and use of alternate vaccine preparations is also important, along with long-term follow-up.

PSEUDOLYMPHOMAS ASSOCIATED WITH TATTOOS

Tattooing has been a common tradition in many cultures throughout the world for several centuries[23] and in the recent times has also gained popularity for medical purposes.[24] Although tattoos are frequently innocent bystanders in patients with other skin diseases,[25] they can rarely be the primary cause of dermatologic complications including infections, allergic reactions, granulomas, and pseudolymphomas in up to 2% of subjects.[26,27] Pseudolymphomatous reaction in tattoos was first recognized more than a century ago by Ullmann.[28] Patients typically present with indurated, erythematous, and almost always nontender nodules or papules that may be pruritic.[29] The onset is usually within a few months to years after placement of the tattoo and may be triggered by exposure to ultraviolet or infrared light.[29,30]

Many of the exogenous pigments used in tattoos are capable of inducing an immunologic reaction. Tattoo pigments of red shades, which traditionally contained variable concentrations of mercuric sulfide, have been the most common offenders with respect to cutaneous disorders (Fig. 51-2A).[28,31] However, chromium (green), cobalt (blue), and carbon (black)[29,30] pigments have also been reported to induce dermal immunologic reactions.[26] Currently, organic Azo dyes are being used in tattoo inks, which may also produce similar reactions.

However, most people getting tattoos do not mount such a response, since much of the deposited pigment is frequently phagocytized by various cells including dermal histiocytes and fibroblasts sequestering them away from the immune system or the patient may be anergic to the pigment, or a combination of both.[32] Macrophages containing the tattoo pigment may process the pigments, giving raise to new epitopes, which might be more immunoreactive, explaining the frequently negative patch test results in patients who develop tattoo-associated reactions.[33] Exposure to ultraviolet light can lead to photolysis of the pigment, which may ultimately decrease the amount of pigment.[33] However, these altered pigments might be more immunogenic and/or even toxic than the parent compound.[30] In fact, a case of cutaneous lymphoid hyperplasia has been reported in a long-standing tattoo after exposure to infrared light in a sauna.[34]

Histologic examination reveals a dense diffuse or nodular or infrequently lichenoid mononuclear cell infiltrate, sometimes with a perivascular and rarely periadnexal accentuation.

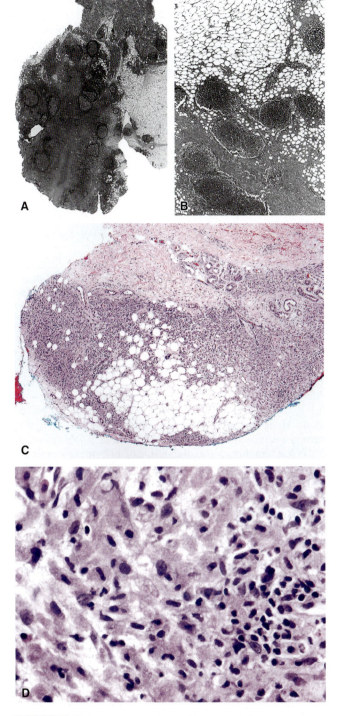

FIGURE 51-1. Pseudolymphoma at a vaccination site. Hematoxylin and eosin (H&E) sections show (**A** and **B**) prominent lymphohistiocytic infiltrate with germinal centers involving the subcutaneous fibroadipose tissue (modified from reference 5) and infiltration of histiocytes with granular cytoplasm admixed with small lymphocytes (**C**, magnification 40×), (**D**, magnification 600×). (From Cerroni L, Borroni RG, Massone C, Chott A, Kerl H. Cutaneous B-cell pseudolymphoma at the site of vaccination. Am J Dermatopathol. 2007;29(6):538-542.)

In most cases, a contiguous involvement of the underlying skeletal muscle has not been demonstrated. However, in patients with chronic fatigue syndrome and myalgia, macrophagic myofasciitis, a similar inflammatory infiltrate may be present in the perimuscular fat and focal lymphocytic

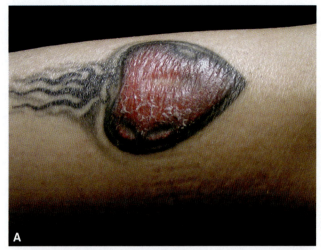
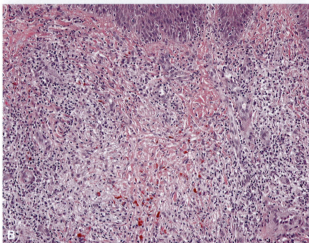
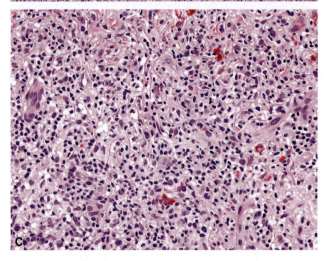

FIGURE 51-2. Pseudolymphoma at the site of red tattoo. Clinical presentation consists of swelling confined to the area containing the red pigment **(A)**. H&E sections show prominent lymphohistiocytic infiltrate admixed with macrophages containing tattoo pigment (**B**, lower magnification 100×, **C**, higher magnification 400×). (Contributed by Michael T. Tetzlaff, University of Texas MD Anderson Cancer Center.)

The cellular density is typically higher in the superficial dermis (top-heavy). In some cases, band-like infiltrates along the dermoepidermal junction have also been reported.[3,34] The inflammatory infiltrate is composed of predominantly small- to medium-sized lymphocytes without obvious atypical features, admixed with variable numbers of histiocytes, eosinophils, and a few plasma cells (Fig. 51-2B,C). Granular aggregates of exogenous pigment are seen free between the dermal collagen bundles or within epithelioid histiocytes. In older tattoos, the tattoo pigment may be difficult to identify and may be seen only within perivascular histiocytes. Formation of germinal centers is unusual.

A grenz zone often separates the dermal infiltrate from the overlying epidermis, which is usually acanthotic with hyper- or parakeratotic scale. Tattoo-associated cutaneous lymphoid hyperplasia is a CD3+ CD8+ cytotoxic T-lymphocyte-predominant process,[5,29,35] admixed with a small component of CD4+ T-helper cells and CD20+ B cells scattered through the infiltrate or in small aggregates. There is no loss of expression of T-cell markers such as CD2, CD5, and CD7.

T-cell receptor rearrangement and B-cell clonality studies reveal polytypic populations.

Electron microscopy, X-ray microanalysis, chemical analysis, and mass spectrometry have been used to identify the various components of a tattoo dye,[6,29,36] in an attempt to identify the immunogenic agent. However, the precise contributory elements may be difficult to pinpoint in many cases, especially since the manufacturers often do not disclose the proprietary compositions and the various dyes may be combined to achieve the desired hue for the tattoo.[7,37]

Lichenoid dermatoses, which are the most common delayed reactions seen in association with tattoos,[27,31,38,39] often develop within a few days to weeks of the tattoo placement. Histologically, there is a dense band-like infiltrate composed predominantly of CD8-positive, CD56-positive cytotoxic lymphocytes and scattered histiocytes; eosinophils may also be present.[40] Rare cases of generalized lichenoid dermatitis weeks after placement of tattoos have been reported[40,41]; whether these represent an "Id"-like reaction in response to the tattoo constituents is unclear. Lichenoid and pseudolymphomatous reactions have been reported to develop synchronously in response to different pigments within the same tattoo.[42,43] Granulomatous reactions of sarcoidal, allergic, or foreign body type have also been reported in tattoos.[26,37] Granulomas developing in tattoos are classically associated with pulmonary sarcoid.[44] When such lesions are identified in tattoos, it is essential to rule out infectious causes.[45] Necrobiotic granulomatous reactions and perforating granulomatous lesions have also been described in association with tattoos.[46,47] Components of invisible tattoo can also give raise to a granulomatous reaction.[48]

Cutaneous pseudolymphoma in general is a diagnosis of exclusion histologically. However, when the tattoo pigment is identified, the diagnosis is relatively straight forward. In older tattoos, the pigment may not be discerned easily; in such cases, clinical history is essential. A rare case of CD30-positive lymphoproliferative disorder has described, which raises the possibility of lymphomatoid papulosis associated with a tattoo.[50]

Rarely, patients may report spontaneous resolution of the lesions.[29,49,50] Commonly employed therapeutic options include intralesional steroid injections, systemic steroid therapy or immunomodulators, topical imiquimod, and topical steroids.[51,52] Oral antihistamines and sun protection also play an important role in mitigating hypersensitivity reactions in some patients.[30] In patients with persistent or resistant lesions, complete removal of the entire tattoo or the offending pigment might be the only option, which can be achieved by surgical excision[49,50] or laser therapy.[53] Other destructive therapies such as electrosurgery, cryotherapy, and dermabrasion have also been used; but, these methods may release and disperse sequestered pigment, increasing the risk for persistence of pseudolymphomatoid reactions and/or development of hypersensitivity.

Long-term follow-up is necessary for patients with tattoo- and vaccine-associated pseudolymphomas, since persistent immunologic activation may lead to malignant transformation over time.

References

1. Huynh TN, Jackson JD, Brodell RT. Tattoo and vaccination sites: possible nest for opportunistic infections, tumors, and dysimmune reactions. *Clin Dermatol.* 2014;32(5):678-684.
2. Ploysangam T, Breneman DL, Mutasim DF. Cutaneous pseudolymphomas. *J Am Acad Dermatol.* 1998;38(6 pt 1):877-895; quiz 896-877.
3. Mitteldorf C, Kempf W. Cutaneous pseudolymphoma-A review on the spectrum and a proposal for a new classification. *J Cutan Pathol.* 2020;47(1):76-97.
4. Nikkels AF, Nikkels-Tassoudji N, Pierard GE. Cutaneous adverse reactions following anti-infective vaccinations. *Am J Clin Dermatol.* 2005;6(2):79-87.
5. Bernstein H, Shupack J, Ackerman B. Cutaneous pseudolymphoma resulting from antigen injections. *Arch Dermatol.* 1974;110(5):756-757.
6. Cerroni L, Borroni RG, Massone C, Chott A, Kerl H. Cutaneous B-cell pseudolymphoma at the site of vaccination. *Am J Dermatopathol.* 2007;29(6):538-542.
7. Maubec E, Pinquier L, Viguier M, et al. Vaccination-induced cutaneous pseudolymphoma. *J Am Acad Dermatol.* 2005;52(4):623-629.
8. Atalar H, Sarifakioglu E, Dener C, Yanik B, Koktener A, Bayrak R. Cutaneous lymphoid hyperplasia and reactive lymphadenopathy induced by hepatitis B vaccination. *Eur J Dermatol.* 2008;18(2):188-189.
9. Avcin S, Jazbec J, Jancar J. Subcutaneous nodule after vaccination with an aluminum-containing vaccine. *Acta Dermatovenerol Alp Pannonica Adriat.* 2008;17(4):182-184.
10. Garcia-Patos V, Pujol RM, Alomar A, et al. Persistent subcutaneous nodules in patients hyposensitized with aluminum-containing allergen extracts. *Arch Dermatol.* 1995;131(12):1421-1424.
11. Guillard O, Fauconneau B, Pineau A, Marrauld A, Bellocq JP, Chenard MP. Aluminium overload after 5 years in skin biopsy following post-vaccination with subcutaneous pseudolymphoma. *J Trace Elem Med Biol.* 2012;26(4):291-293.
12. Pham-Ledard A, Vergier B, Doutre MS, Beylot-Barry M. Disseminated cutaneous lymphoid hyperplasia of 12 years' duration triggered by vaccination. *Dermatology.* 2010;220(2):176-179.
13. Stavrianeas NG, Katoulis AC, Kanelleas A, Hatziolou E, Georgala S. Papulonodular lichenoid and pseudolymphomatous reaction at the injection site of hepatitis B virus vaccination. *Dermatology.* 2002;205(2):166-168.
14. Kim H, Lim KY, Kang J, Park JW, Park SH. Macrophagic myofasciitis and subcutaneous pseudolymphoma caused by aluminium adjuvants. *Sci Rep.* 2020;10(1):11834.
15. Porto DA, Comfere NI, Myers LM, Abbott JJ. Pseudolymphomatous reaction to varicella zoster virus vaccination: role of viral in situ hybridization. *J Cutan Pathol.* 2010;37(10):1098-1102.
16. Ramos Pinheiro R, Duarte B, Joao A, Lencastre A. Cutaneous pseudolymphoma following quadrivalent human papillomavirus vaccination—a rare adverse event. *J Dtsch Dermatol Ges.* 2018;16(4):465-467.
17. Exley C, Siesjo P, Eriksson H. The immunobiology of aluminium adjuvants: how do they really work? *Trends Immunol.* 2010;31(3):103-109.
18. Brewer JM, Conacher M, Hunter CA, Mohrs M, Brombacher F, Alexander J. Aluminium hydroxide adjuvant initiates strong antigen-specific Th2 responses in the absence of IL-4- or IL-13-mediated signaling. *J Immunol.* 1999;163(12):6448-6454.
19. Staser K, Abner S, Anadkat M, Musiek A, Schaffer A. Injection-site cutaneous pseudolymphoma induced by a GM-CSF-producing tumor cell vaccine. *JAMA Dermatol.* 2017;153(4):332-334.
20. Chong H, Brady K, Metze D, Calonje E. Persistent nodules at injection sites (aluminium granuloma)—clinicopathological study of 14 cases with a diverse range of histological reaction patterns. *Histopathology.* 2006;48(2):182-188.
21. Keijsers RR, Bovenschen HJ, Seyger MM. Cutaneous complication after BCG vaccination: case report and review of the literature. *J Dermatol Treat.* 2011;22(6):315-318.
22. Wright NA, Torres-Cabala CA, Curry JL, Cutlan JE, Hymes SR. Post-varicella-zoster virus granulomatous dermatitis: a report of 2 cases. *Cutis.* 2014;93(1):50-54.
23. Sperry K. Tattoos and tattooing. Part I: history and methodology. *Am J Forensic Med Pathol.* 1991;12(4):313-319.
24. Glassy CM, Glassy MS, Aldasouqi S. Tattooing: medical uses and problems. *Cleve Clin J Med.* 2012;79(11):761-770.
25. Kluger N, Koljonen V. Tattoos, inks, and cancer. *Lancet Oncol.* 2012;13(4):e161-168.
26. Kazandjieva J, Tsankov N. Tattoos: dermatological complications. *Clin Dermatol.* 2007;25(4):375-382.
27. Bassi A, Campolmi P, Cannarozzo G, et al. Tattoo-associated skin reaction: the importance of an early diagnosis and proper treatment. *BioMed Res Int.* 2014;2014:354608.
28. Ullmann J. Über eigentümliche Geschwulstbildung in einer Tätowierungsmarken. *Monatsch prakt Dermatol.* 1903;37:49-52.
29. Kluger N, Vermeulen C, Moguelet P, et al. Cutaneous lymphoid hyperplasia (pseudolymphoma) in tattoos: a case series of seven patients. *J Eur Acad Dermatol Venereol.* 2010;24(2):208-213.
30. Jemec GB. Comment on: tattooing of skin results in transportation and light-induced decomposition of tattoo pigments. *Exp Dermatol.* 2010;19(1):61-62.
31. Mortimer NJ, Chave TA, Johnston GA. Red tattoo reactions. *Clin Exp Dermatol.* 2003;28(5):508-510.
32. Sperry K. Tattoos and tattooing. Part II: gross pathology, histopathology, medical complications, and applications. *Am J Forensic Med Pathol.* 1992;13(1):7-17.
33. Serup J, Hutton Carlsen K. Patch test study of 90 patients with tattoo reactions: negative outcome of allergy patch test to baseline batteries and culprit inks suggests allergen(s) are generated in the skin through haptenization. *Contact Dermatitis.* 2014;71(5):255-263.
34. King BJ, Lehman JS, Macon WR, Sciallis GF. Red tattoo-related mycosis fungoides-like CD8+ pseudolymphoma. *J Cutan Pathol.* 2018;45(3):226-228.

35. Marchesi A, Parodi PC, Brioschi M, et al. Tattoo ink-related cutaneous pseudolymphoma: a rare but significant complication. Case report and review of the literature. *Aesthetic Plast Surg.* 2014;38(2):471-478.
36. Slater DN, Durrant TE. Tattoos: light and transmission electron microscopy studies with X-ray microanalysis. *Clin Exp Dermatol.* 1984;9(2):167-173.
37. Kaur RR, Kirby W, Maibach H. Cutaneous allergic reactions to tattoo ink. *J Cosmet Dermatol.* 2009;8(4):295-300.
38. Sowden JM, Byrne JP, Smith AG, et al. Red tattoo reactions: X-ray microanalysis and patch-test studies. *Br J Dermatol.* 1991;124(6):576-580.
39. Cruz FA, Lage D, Frigerio RM, Zaniboni MC, Arruda LH. Reactions to the different pigments in tattoos: a report of two cases. *An Bras Dermatol.* 2010;85(5):708-711.
40. Jacks SK, Zirwas MJ, Mosser JL. A case of a generalized lichenoid tattoo reaction. *J Clin Aesthet Dermatol.* 2014;7(8):48-50.
41. Litak J, Ke MS, Gutierrez MA, Soriano T, Lask GP. Generalized lichenoid reaction from tattoo. *Dermatol Surg.* 2007;33(6):736-740.
42. Chave TA, Mortimer NJ, Johnston GA. Simultaneous pseudolymphomatous and lichenoid tattoo reactions triggered by re-tattooing. *Clin Exp Dermatol.* 2004;29(2):197-199.
43. Kuo WE, Richwine EE, Sheehan DJ. Pseudolymphomatous and lichenoid reaction to a red tattoo: a case report. *Cutis.* 2011;87(2):89-92.
44. Guerra JR, Alderuccio JP, Sandhu J, Chaudhari S. Granulomatous tattoo reaction in a young man. *Lancet.* 2013;382(9888):284.
45. Drage LA, Ecker PM, Orenstein R, Phillips PK, Edson RS. An outbreak of *Mycobacterium chelonae* infections in tattoos. *J Am Acad Dermatol.* 2010;62(3):501-506.
46. Wood A, Hamilton SA, Wallace WA, Biswas A. Necrobiotic granulomatous tattoo reaction: report of an unusual case showing features of both necrobiosis lipoidica and granuloma annulare patterns. *Am J Dermatopathol.* 2014;36(8):e152-155.
47. Sweeney SA, Hicks LD, Ranallo N, Snyder N, Soldano AC. Perforating granulomatous dermatitis reaction to exogenous tattoo pigment: a case report and review of the literature. *Am J Dermatopathol.* 2013;35(7):754-756.
48. Tsang M, Marsch A, Bassett K, High W, Fitzpatrick J, Prok L. A visible response to an invisible tattoo. *J Cutan Pathol.* 2012;39(9):877-880.
49. Munoz C, Guilabert A, Mascaro JM Jr, Lopez-Lerma I, Vilaplana J. An embossed tattoo. *Clin Exp Dermatol.* 2006;31(2):309-310.
50. Gutermuth J, Hein R, Fend F, Ring J, Jakob T. Cutaneous pseudolymphoma arising after tattoo placement. *J Eur Acad Dermatol Venereol: JEADV.* 2007;21(4):566-567.
51. Luebberding S, Alexiades-Armenakas M. New tattoo approaches in dermatology. *Dermatol Clin.* 2014;32(1):91-96.
52. Patrizi A, Raone B, Savoia F, et al. Tattoo-associated pseudolymphomatous reaction and its successful treatment with hydroxychloroquine. *Acta Derm Venereol.* 2009;89(3):327-328.
53. Campolmi P, Bassi A, Bonan P, et al. Cutaneous pseudolymphoma localized to black tattoo. *J Am Acad Dermatol.* 2011;65(5):e155-157.

CHAPTER 52

Lymphoid proliferations in association with viral and bacterial infections

Priyadharsini Nagarajan

INTRODUCTION

Host immune response to combat cutaneous infections depends primarily on the type of organism. For example, in case of pyogenic infections such as impetigo, the host mounts a neutrophilic inflammatory response and the diagnosis is usually straight forward, based on the clinical presentation and microbiology culture results and rarely necessitates a biopsy for a definitive answer. However, in some instances, the infection may be clinically atypical, with an indolent course and the infecting micro-organisms are often not cultured easily; the characteristic cytopathic effects may not be evident on histologic examination as well. Persistent, indolent infections may become constant source of antigens and induce a prolonged host immune response, which over time might result in lymphoid proliferations that resemble cutaneous lymphoproliferative processes.

LYMPHOID PROLIFERATIONS ASSOCIATED WITH VIRAL INFECTIONS

Latent viral infections are common causes of persistent host immune response, which may clinically and histologically resemble lymphomas. Herpes simplex viruses (HSV) 1 and 2, varicella zoster virus (VZV), molluscum contagiosum virus (MCV), human papilloma virus (HPV), and human immunodeficiency virus (HIV) are well-established causes of cutaneous pseudolymphomas.

Herpetic Viral Infections

Although herpes virus–associated pseudolymphoid proliferations are commonly linked to immunosuppression, they can be seen in immunocompetent subjects as well. The clinical presentation ranges from indurated erythematous plaques or nodules with or without accompanying vesicles to small discrete papules (folliculitis).[1-3] These lesions are usually asymptomatic but may be associated with pruritus, mild pain, or tenderness. The lesions may be clinically stable, progressively expand, or even wax and wane over time. In a review of 65 biopsies of cutaneous eruptions associated with herpes viruses, Leinweber et al identified that approximately a third exhibited dense superficial and deep perivascular and periadnexal and interstitial dermal lymphoid infiltrates (Fig. 52-1A). In several of these cases, the typical viral cytopathic effects including amphophilic or eosinophilic intranuclear viral inclusions with margination of host chromatin, multinucleation, molding of the multiple nuclei, and ballooning degeneration of keratinocytes were only focal, involving isolated epidermal or adnexal cells (Fig. 52-1B).

The dermal infiltrates were composed predominantly of $CD3^+$, $CD4^+$, or $CD8^+$ T lymphocytes and $CD20^+$ B cells were usually fewer in number.[4] In some cases, there may be an overt preponderant expression of CD4 over CD8, raising the possibility of a cutaneous lymphoproliferative disorder.[3] CD56 and TIA1 expression was also fairly common. Numerous atypical mononuclear cells with enlarged, hyperchromatic, convoluted nuclei were seen frequently, most of which were $CD30^+$. In cases of herpetic folliculitis, the formation of germinal centers can occur with the presence of large centroblast-like $CD20^+$ cells.[5] Molecular studies using polymerase chain reaction (PCR) for T-cell receptor-γ gene revealed polyclonal population in 50% and a monoclonal pattern in 25% of all tested cases, in which expression of HSV DNA was confirmed as well.[4]

Cutaneous lymphoid infiltrates have also been reported in the setting of varicella zoster inflammatory reactions, particularly in immunosuppressed patients.[6,7] In a case of post-zoster folliculitis, although monoclonal B- and T-lymphocytic proliferations were identified, there was prompt resolution of the lesions after antiviral therapy.[8] VZV DNA could be demonstrated in some of these cases by PCR or in situ hybridization.[7] In patients with HIV, anogenital HSV-2 infections often present as pseudolymphomas composed of dense dermal infiltrate composed predominately of polyclonal plasma cells as well as $CD8^+$ T lymphocytes and can be difficult to control even with antiviral therapy.[9]

Patients with chronic lymphocytic leukemia are prone to exaggerated cutaneous reactions and can rarely present

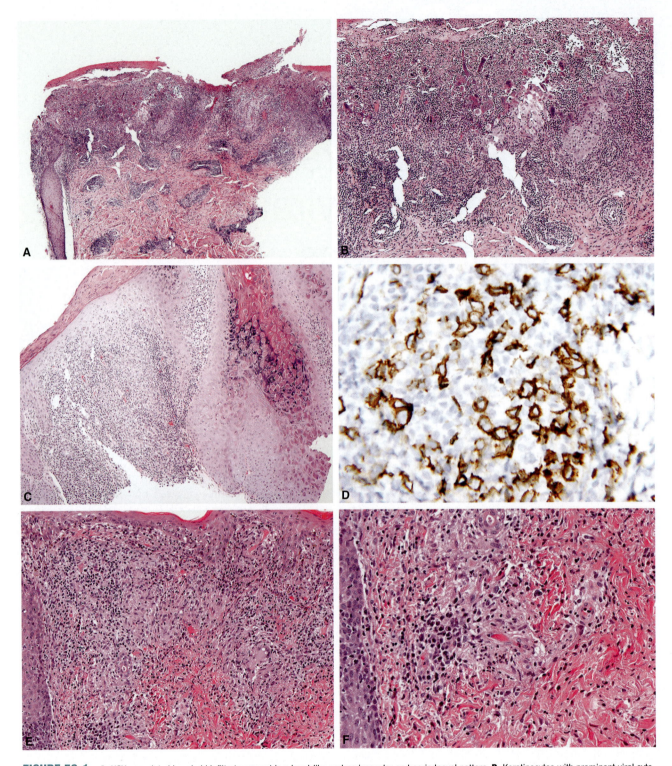

FIGURE 52-1. **A.** HSV-associated lymphoid infiltrate present in a band-like and perivascular and periadnexal pattern. **B.** Keratinocytes with prominent viral cytopathic effects are surrounded by a dense lymphohistiocytic infiltrate. **C.** Hyperplastic epidermis with viral cytopathic effects of MCV and lymphohistiocytic infiltrate. **D.** Several CD30+ large atypical lymphocytes are present. **E.** Inflammatory infiltrate in nodular secondary syphilis, composed of lymphocytes and (multinucleated) histiocytes. **F.** Plasma cells are prominent. (Images contributed by Alejandro A. Gru, MD.)

with erythematous papules or plaques at sites of prior herpes viral infections, representing an isomorphic phenomenon.[10] Histologically, there is a dense dermal and subcutaneous lymphoid infiltrate composed of CD20+ CD43+ neoplastic B lymphocytes, implicating cutaneous involvement of the patient's leukemic process and not a pseudolymphoid reaction.

Molluscum Contagiosum Infections

MCV typically induces self-limiting lesions, which are characterized histologically by hyperplastic epidermis composed of keratinocytes containing large intracytoplasmic inclusions that compress the nucleus against the cytoplasmic membrane (Henderson-Patterson bodies), with almost no immune response.[11] Cases of MCV folliculitis have also been described in the absence of epidermal involvement.[12] Rarely a dense dermal inflammatory infiltrate, composed of mononuclear cells, has been described in association with trauma to the lesion, which may lead to release of the viral particles into the dermis (Fig. 52-1C). Such an immune response may also be spontaneous and often precedes clinical clearance of the lesions and was first described in 1977.[13] The inflammatory infiltrate is composed predominantly of CD3+ CD8+ cytotoxic T cells admixed CD8+ CD56+ natural killer cells with a small fraction of B lymphocytes, rare plasma cells, and eosinophils.[14] CD30+ large atypical cells with vesicular nuclei and prominent nucleoli are also seen in variable numbers dispersed through the infiltrate or in clusters, resembling primary cutaneous anaplastic lymphoma[15-17] (Fig. 52-1D). In addition, CD123+ CD11c+ CD16+ plasmacytoid dendritic cells are also present.[18] Molecular studies reveal polyclonal populations of T and B lymphocytes.

Human Immunodeficiency Virus Infections

Patients with advanced HIV infection may present with generalized erythroderma or indurated plaques and nodules similar to mycosis fungoides.[19,20] In contrast to mycosis fungoides, the lesions tend to be photodistributed, commonly involving the extremities and face.[19] Histologically, the lesions are characterized by superficial and mid-dermal mononuclear infiltrate composed predominantly of small to medium-sized lymphocytes admixed with eosinophils and plasma cells. There is a predominance of CD3+ CD8+ lymphocytes that may have specific cytotoxicity against cells that express HIV1 Gag and Pol gene products.[21,22] In some cases, CD4+ cells may also be present in significant numbers. CD7 expression is usually preserved at least in a fraction of the cells. T-cell receptor rearrangements are not common. Recent reports have shown regression of these lesions after highly active antiretroviral therapy[23] or methotrexate therapy.[21] In addition, patients with HIV are also prone to development of cutaneous lymphoid infiltrates in association with other viral infections[9] and syphilis.[24]

Other Viral Infections

Verrucae are common skin lesions produced by infection of HPVs, some of which may exhibit an inflammatory infiltrate in the superficial dermis. This inflammatory response often precedes regression of the warts.[25] The inflammatory infiltrate is composed of CD3+ lymphocytes, a majority of which are also CD4+. Several large atypical CD3+ CD4+ CD30+ lymphocytes are also seen.[26,27] Similar cutaneous infiltrates are also seen in parapox infections (Orf).[28]

LYMPHOID PROLIFERATIONS ASSOCIATED WITH BACTERIAL INFECTIONS

Dense dermal lymphoid infiltrates are a rare phenomenon in cutaneous bacterial infections. However, certain bacteria such as spirochetes (*Borrelia*, *Treponema pallidum*) and mycobacteria can induce a predominantly lymphoid immune response and, thus, may lead to the development of cutaneous lymphoid hyperplasia, also known as lymphocytoma cutis.

Borrelial Infections

Borrelial lymphocytoma is the least common cutaneous manifestation of Lyme disease, constituting about 2% in adults and 5% in children.[29-31] Cases have been reported in Europe where Lyme disease is endemic and caused by *Borrelia afzelii* and *Borrelia garinii*, while it is rare in the United States where *Borrelia burgdorferi sensu strictu* is the main pathogen. Patients present with a solitary, well-demarcated, soft, and erythematous-violaceous plaque or nodule. It is slightly more common in women,[32] and nipples, areolae, and scrotum are common sites of involvement in adults, while ear lobes are favored in children. Infrequently trunk, extremities, and face may be affected.[32,33]

Histologically, borrelial lymphocytoma is characterized by a uniformly dense dermal lymphoid infiltrate.[32] The overlying epidermis is usually uninvolved but is frequently atrophic. Lymphoid follicles that often lack polarization and mantle zones are seen surrounding germinal center–like areas, composed of immunoblasts, centroblasts, tingible body macrophages, and centrocytes. Rarely, the lymphoid follicles may become confluent, raising the possibility of a lymphoproliferative disorder.[34] Histiocytes, plasma cells, and eosinophils are seen in the interfollicular regions. In some cases, the lymphoid infiltrate may be seen in a perivascular and periadnexal distribution.[35]

There was a predominance of CD20+ B lymphocytes within the follicles. Expression of CD21, CD10, and Bcl6 was restricted to the germinal centers, while Bcl2 was expressed only by the CD3+ T cells present in the interfollicular regions. Plasma cells always demonstrated polyclonality. Molecular analysis by PCR revealed polyclonal populations of B lymphocytes in most cases; rare monoclonal bands were seen. Most patients had demonstrable antiborrelial antibodies in their serum.

Rare cases of dense lymphoid infiltrates have been reported in association with lesions that are clinically consistent with acrodermatitis chronica atrophicans.[36] Most of these cases were characterized by a band-like lymphoid infiltrate of small CD3+ CD4+ CD8− T lymphocytes while B lymphocytes constituted only a minor fraction. In those cases that demonstrated a diffuse dermal infiltrate, there was a prominent polyclonal plasma cell population admixed with small lymphocytes and germinal centers were absent.

Treponemal Infections

Nodular lesions in secondary syphilis are extremely rare and such cases may be challenging to diagnose both on clinical and histologic grounds and requires a high degree of suspicion.[37-39] Most of the reported cases have been in adult men who present with multiple rubbery, nontender, erythematous or violaceous nodules of 1 to 6 months duration, commonly located on the face, upper trunk, and extremities.[24,40] Lymphadenopathy is frequently present but may not be prominent.[41,42] Histological examination reveals a vaguely wedge-shaped dense dermal infiltrate composed of small to medium lymphocytes, plasma cells, eosinophils, and rare histiocytes (Fig. 52-1E,F).[40] There is usually a predominance of B cells within the infiltrate; however, in some cases, there might be similar numbers of T and B lymphocytes[43,44] or rarely CD8 predominance.[24] Germinal centers are rare, but vasculitis and endarteritis are almost never seen. Monoclonality is not seen among B-cells or plasma cells. On rare occasions, monoclonal population of T-cells (even within separate biopsy sites with identical peaks) have been reported.[45] The overlying epidermis may be unremarkable or display irregular acanthosis and focal vacuolar changes. The prominence of plasma cells in the inflammatory infiltrate is often the tip off for the possibility of syphilis and is confirmed by serologic examination. Antibiotic treatment leads to complete resolution of the dermal nodules.

Other Bacterial Infections

Cutaneous lymphoid hyperplasia has been reported in association with other remote infections in an Id reaction–like response. Mitani et al described a case of widespread cutaneous plaques and nodules composed of polyclonal populations of lymphocytes and plasma cells admixed with histiocytes in an adult man with long-standing *Helicobacter pylori* infection.[46] The lesions cleared after combination anti-*H. pylori* antibiotic therapy. Pseudolymphomatous lesions involving the back, shoulder, and neck have been described in association with a chronic discharging sinus of the inguinal region, which regressed after treatment of the chronic wound.[47] Papular cutaneous eruptions composed of dense lymphoid infiltrates, containing predominantly of CD3+ T lymphocytes and CD30+ large pleomorphic atypical cells, was reported in a patient with *Mycobacterium tuberculosis* infection.[48] Although the cells were polyclonal, they persisted for about 12 months after starting antituberculosis multidrug regimen.

CONCLUSION

Diffuse dermal lymphoid infiltrates should always be investigated thoroughly, and only when all neoplastic processes have been ruled out should one entertain the possibility of reactive causes. Since prolonged antigenic stimulation may lead selective expansion of specific clones, every attempt should be made to identify the cause of a pseudolymphoid proliferation, especially since most infections can be controlled, if not cured. Also, long-term follow-up is also essential, to screen for potential lymphoproliferative processes.

References

1. Boer A, Herder N, Winter K, Falk T. Herpes folliculitis: clinical, histopathological, and molecular pathologic observations. *Br J Dermatol.* 2006;154(4):743-746.
2. Lewin JM, Farley-Loftus R, Pomeranz MK. Herpes simplex virus-associated pseudolymphoma. *Cutis.* 2013;92(6):E1-E2.
3. Ibarra BS, Huen A, Nagarajan P, Torres-Cabala CA, Prieto VG, Aung PP. From mycosis fungoides to herpetic folliculitis: the significance of deeper H&E tissue sections in dermatopathology. *J Cutan Pathol.* 2019;46(8):624-626.
4. Leinweber B, Kerl H, Cerroni L. Histopathologic features of cutaneous herpes virus infections (herpes simplex, herpes varicella/zoster): a broad spectrum of presentations with common pseudolymphomatous aspects. *Am J Surg Pathol.* 2006;30(1):50-58.
5. Fukamachi S, Kimura T, Kobayashi M, Hino R, Nakamura M, Tokura Y. Palmar pseudolymphoma associated with herpes simplex infection. *J Cutan Pathol.* 2010;37(7):808-811.
6. Requena L, Kutzner H, Escalonilla P, Ortiz S, Schaller J, Rohwedder A. Cutaneous reactions at sites of herpes zoster scars: an expanded spectrum. *Br J Dermatol.* 1998;138(1):161-168.
7. Porto DA, Comfere NI, Myers LM, Abbott JJ. Pseudolymphomatous reaction to varicella zoster virus vaccination: role of viral in situ hybridization. *J Cutan Pathol.* 2010;37(10):1098-1102.
8. Aram G, Rohwedder A, Nazeer T, Shoss R, Fisher A, Carlson JA. Varicella-zoster-virus folliculitis promoted clonal cutaneous lymphoid hyperplasia. *Am J Dermatopathol.* 2005;27(5):411-417.
9. Sbidian E, Battistella M, Legoff J, et al. Recalcitrant pseudotumoral anogenital herpes simplex virus type 2 in HIV-infected patients: evidence for predominant B-lymphoplasmocytic infiltration and immunomodulators as effective therapeutic strategy. *Clin Infect Dis.* 2013;57(11):1648-1655.
10. Cerroni L, Zenahlik P, Kerl H. Specific cutaneous infiltrates of B-cell chronic lymphocytic leukemia arising at the site of herpes zoster and herpes simplex scars. *Cancer.* 1995;76(1):26-31.
11. Cribier B, Scrivener Y, Grosshans E. Molluscum contagiosum: histologic patterns and associated lesions. A study of 578 cases. *Am J Dermatopathol.* 2001;23(2):99-103.
12. Jang KA, Kim SH, Choi JH, Sung KJ, Moon KC, Koh JK. Viral folliculitis on the face. *Br J Dermatol.* 2000;142(3):555-559.
13. Ackerman AB, Tanski EV. Pseudoleukemia cutis: report of a case in association with molluscum contagiosum. *Cancer.* 1977;40(2):813-817.
14. Moreno-Ramirez D, Garcia-Escudero A, Rios-Martin JJ, Herrera-Saval A, Camacho F. Cutaneous pseudolymphoma in association with molluscum contagiosum in an elderly patient. *J Cutan Pathol.* 2003;30(7):473-475.
15. Del Boz Gonzalez J, Sanz A, Martin T, Samaniego E, Martinez S, Crespo V. Cutaneous pseudolymphoma associated with molluscum contagiosum: a case report. *Int J Dermatol.* 2008;47(5):502-504.
16. Guitart J, Hurt MA. Pleomorphic T-cell infiltrate associated with molluscum contagiosum. *Am J Dermatopathol.* 1999;21(2):178-180.
17. Shalabi D, Ringe J, Lee JB, Nikbakht N. Molluscum contagiosum infection with features of primary cutaneous anaplastic large cell lymphoma. *Dermatol Online J.* 2019;25(11):13030/qt7vp863hz.
18. Vermi W, Fisogni S, Salogni L, et al. Spontaneous regression of highly immunogenic Molluscum Contagiosum Virus (MCV)-induced skin lesions is associated with plasmacytoid dendritic cells and IFN-DC infiltration. *J Invest Dermatol.* 2011;131(2):426-434.
19. Guitart J, Variakojis D, Kuzel T, Rosen S. Cutaneous CD8 T cell infiltrates in advanced HIV infection. *J Am Acad Dermatol.* 1999;41(5 pt 1):722-727.
20. Zhang P, Chiriboga L, Jacobson M, et al. Mycosis fungoides-like T-cell cutaneous lymphoid infiltrates in patients with HIV infection. *Am J Dermatopathol.* 1995;17(1):29-35.

21. Ingen-Housz-Oro S, Sbidian E, Ortonne N, et al. HIV-related CD8+ cutaneous pseudolymphoma: efficacy of methotrexate. *Dermatology.* 2013;226(1):15-18.
22. Bachelez H, Hadida F, Parizot C, et al. Oligoclonal expansion of HIV-specific cytotoxic CD8 T lymphocytes in the skin of HIV-1-infected patients with cutaneous pseudolymphoma. *J Clin Invest.* 1998;101(11):2506-2516.
23. Schartz NE, De La Blanchardiere A, Alaoui S, et al. Regression of CD8+ pseudolymphoma after HIV antiviral triple therapy. *J Am Acad Dermatol.* 2003;49(1):139-141.
24. Mitteldorf C, Plumbaum H, Zutt M, Schon MP, Kaune KM. CD8-positive pseudolymphoma in lues maligna and human immunodeficiency virus with monoclonal T-cell receptor-beta rearrangement. *J Cutan Pathol.* 2019;46(3):204-210.
25. Coleman N, Birley HD, Renton AM, et al. Immunological events in regressing genital warts. *Am J Clin Pathol.* 1994;102(6):768-774.
26. Cesinaro AM, Maiorana A. Verruca vulgaris with CD30-positive lymphoid infiltrate: a case report. *Am J Dermatopathol.* 2002;24(3):260-263.
27. Werner B, Massone C, Kerl H, Cerroni L. Large CD30-positive cells in benign, atypical lymphoid infiltrates of the skin. *J Cutan Pathol.* 2008;35(12):1100-1107.
28. Rose C, Starostik P, Brocker EB. Infection with parapoxvirus induces CD30-positive cutaneous infiltrates in humans. *J Cutan Pathol.* 1999;26(10):520-522.
29. Moniuszko A, Czupryna P, Pancewicz S, Kondrusik M, Penza P, Zajkowska J. Borrelial lymphocytoma--a case report of a pregnant woman. *Ticks Tick Borne Dis.* 2012;3(4):257-258.
30. Mullegger RR, Glatz M. Skin manifestations of lyme borreliosis: diagnosis and management. *Am J Clin Dermatol.* 2008;9(6):355-368.
31. Eisendle K, Zelger B. The expanding spectrum of cutaneous borreliosis. *G Ital Dermatol venereol Organo Uff Soc Ital Dermatol Sifilogr.* 2009;144(2):157-171.
32. Colli C, Leinweber B, Mullegger R, Chott A, Kerl H, Cerroni L. Borrelia burgdorferi-associated lymphocytoma cutis: clinicopathologic, immunophenotypic, and molecular study of 106 cases. *J Cutan Pathol.* 2004;31(3):232-240.
33. Amschler K, Schon MP, Mempel M, Zutt M. Atypical location of lymphocytoma cutis in a child. *Pediatr Dermatol.* 2013;30(5):628-629.
34. Grange F, Wechsler J, Guillaume JC, et al. Borrelia burgdorferi-associated lymphocytoma cutis simulating a primary cutaneous large B-cell lymphoma. *J Am Acad Dermatol.* 2002;47(4):530-534.
35. Ziemer M, Eisendle K, Muller H, Zelger B. Lymphocytic infiltration of the skin (Jessner-Kanof) but not reticular erythematous mucinosis occasionally represents clinical manifestations of Borrelia-associated pseudolymphoma. *Br J Dermatol.* 2009;161(3):583-590.
36. Tee SI, Martinez-Escaname M, Zuriel D, et al. Acrodermatitis chronica atrophicans with pseudolymphomatous infiltrates. *Am J Dermatopathol.* 2013;35(3):338-342.
37. Cochran RE, Thomson J, Fleming KA, Strong AM. Histology simulating reticulosis in secondary syphilis. *Br J Dermatol.* 1976;95(3):251-254.
38. Baum EW, Bernhardt M, Sams WM Jr, Alexander WJ, McLean GL. Secondary syphillis. Still the great imitator. *JAMA.* 1983;249(22):3069-3070.
39. Graham WR Jr, Duvic M. Nodular secondary syphilis. *Arch Dermatol.* 1982;118(3):205-206.
40. Tsai KY, Brenn T, Werchniak AE. Nodular presentation of secondary syphilis. *J Am Acad Dermatol.* 2007;57(2 suppl):S57-S58.
41. Levin DL, Greenberg MH, Hasegawa J, Roenigk HH Jr. Secondary syphilis mimicking mycosis fungoides. *J Am Acad Dermatol.* 1980;3(1):92-94.
42. Hodak E, David M, Rothem A, Bialowance M, Sandbank M. Nodular secondary syphilis mimicking cutaneous lymphoreticular process. *J Am Acad Dermatol.* 1987;17(5 pt 2):914-917.
43. McComb ME, Telang GH, Vonderheid EC. Secondary syphilis presenting as pseudolymphoma of the skin. *J Am Acad Dermatol.* 2003;49(2 suppl Case Reports):S174-S176.
44. Moon HS, Park K, Lee JH, Son SJ. A nodular syphilid presenting as a pseudolymphoma: mimicking a cutaneous marginal zone B-cell lymphoma. *Am J Dermatopathol.* 2009;31(8):846-848.
45. Raghavan SS, Wang JY, Gru AA, et al. Next-generation sequencing confirms T-cell clonality in a subset of pediatric pityriasis lichenoides. *J Cutan Pathol.* 2022;49(3):252-260. doi:10.1111/cup.14143
46. Mitani N, Nagatani T, Ikezawa Z, et al. A case of cutaneous T cell pseudolymphoma in a patient with *Helicobacter pylori* infection. *Dermatology.* 2006;213(2):156-158.
47. Sidwell RU, Doe PT, Sinett D, Francis N, Bunker CB. Lymphocytoma cutis and chronic infection. *Br J Dermatol.* 2000;143(4):909-910.
48. Massi D, Trotta M, Franchi A, Pimpinelli N, Santucci M. Atypical CD30+ cutaneous lymphoid proliferation in a patient with tuberculosis infection. *Am J Dermatopathol.* 2004;26(3):234-236.

CHAPTER 53

Cutaneous plasmacytosis

M. Yadira Hurley and Gillian Heinecke

INTRODUCTION

Cutaneous plasmacytosis is a rare entity consisting of a dermal infiltration of polyclonal plasma cells, with or without systemic manifestations including lymphadenopathy, fever, gammopathy, and in some cases infiltration of plasma cells into visceral organs. Given the frequency of extracutaneous manifestations of this disease, this entity is now preferentially referred to as cutaneous and systemic plasmacytosis (C/SP). In the past, cases without lymph node involvement have been termed "cutaneous plasmacytosis," and the term "systemic plasmacytosis" has been applied only to patients who also have lymphadenopathy. This disease was first described in 1976 by Yashiro,[1] as a "kind of plasmacytosis," and later in 1980 by Kitamura et al,[2] who defined "cutaneous plasmacytosis" as patients with skin lesions and polyclonal hypergammaglobulemia. In 1986, Watanabe et al[3] classified a group of patients as having "systemic plasmacytosis," noting characteristic skin findings, lymphadenopathy, and hypergammaglobulinemia. They postulated that the disease represented an overactive immune response to an unknown antigen. Given the rarity of this entity, and somewhat limited reports in the literature, much remains to be discovered regarding the pathogenesis, etiology, and management of this disorder.

EPIDEMIOLOGY

C/SP is a rare entity, with approximately 120 cases reported in the literature.[4,5] Onset most commonly occurs in middle age, with a median age at diagnosis reported to be 49 years.[6] This entity has also been rarely described in children, with cutaneous manifestations only and low risk of systemic progression. This particular presentation has been referred to as benign primary cutaneous plasmacytosis.[7-10] One case in the literature reported this disease as being present since birth, identifying the possibility of the congenital nature of this entity.[10] There is a slight male-to-female predominance, reported as 1.0:0.6 or 1.2:1.0.[11,12]

C/SP commonly affects individuals of Asian descent, particularly Japanese patients.[5,6,13-21] Much less common is this entity occurring in the Caucasian population. To date, around 10 patients of this subset have been documented.[7,8,22-28] There are also rare reports of it occurring in patients of Hispanic descent.[29]

ETIOLOGY

The etiology of C/SP is unknown; however, many speculations have been made regarding the pathogenesis of this condition. Several studies have demonstrated an increase in interleukin-6 (IL-6) levels, implicating the cytokine as an important player in the pathogenesis of this disease.[6,30,31] This is because a key function of IL-6 is the differentiation of B cells to immunoglobulin-producing cells, namely, plasma cells. One study showed that serum IL-6 levels parallel disease activity and that effective treatment, in turn, also lowers the serum IL-6 levels.[31] The underlying reason and mechanism for the elevated IL-6 levels remain unclear. Another study postulated a similar pathogenesis as primary cutaneous marginal zone B-cell lymphoma, in which stimulation by an unknown antigen or infectious agent is responsible for the perpetuation of the disease.[6] The authors of this study suggest that factors in the microenvironment of the skin or nearby lymph nodes stimulate IL-6 production, which in turn inhibits apoptosis of plasma cells and subsequently results in their proliferation.[6] The exact stimulus for this proposed mechanism has yet to be determined. These noted elevations in IL-6, coupled with similarities in clinical presentation, have led to the speculation of C/SP being closely related to or on a similar spectrum as cutaneous plasmacytic Castleman disease.[6,32] Other studies have showed that human herpesvirus 8 (HHV-8) is absent in patients with C/SP, in contrast to most cases of multicentric Castleman disease, revealing a key difference in the pathogenesis of these disorders.[33,34] Elevated IgG4 levels in the serum and plasma cell infiltrate of cutaneous plasmacytosis have also been identified, bringing into question the possible relationship of this disease to a T_H2-mediated hypersensitivity reaction or IgG4-related sclerosing disease.[35] The striking geographical predominance has prompted the theory of an environmental or infectious cause; however, studies have failed to identify a causative organism.[13,36] Further studies are needed to elucidate the underlying pathogenesis of this condition.

CLINICAL PRESENTATION AND PROGNOSIS

The cutaneous manifestations of C/SP classically include red-to-brown-to-black macules, papules, and plaques (Figs. 53-1–53-3). Lesions typically are evenly distributed and located on the face, trunk, and extremities, with sparing of acral surfaces.[4,17] A predilection for the axilla has been observed including a

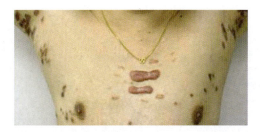

FIGURE 53-1. Firm, brown-to-black papules and plaques on chest. (Reprinted from Shadel BN, Frater JL, Gapp JDG, et al. Cutaneous and systemic plasmacytosis in an Asian male born in the North American continent: a controversial entity potentially related to multicentric Castleman disease. *J Cutan Pathol.* 2010;37(6):697-702, with permission.)

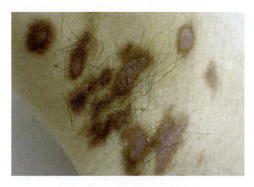

FIGURE 53-2. Firm, brown-to-black plaques on axilla. (Reprinted from Shadel BN, Frater JL, Gapp JDG, et al. Cutaneous and systemic plasmacytosis in an Asian male born in the North American continent: a controversial entity potentially related to multicentric Castleman disease. *J Cutan Pathol.* 2010;37(6):697–702, with permission.)

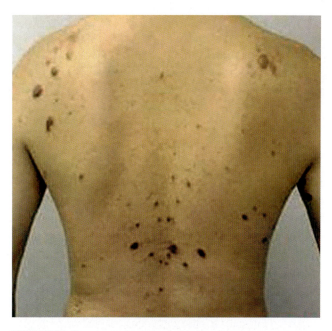

FIGURE 53-3. Firm, brown-to-black papules and plaques on the back. (Reprinted from Shadel BN, Frater JL, Gapp JDG, et al. Cutaneous and systemic plasmacytosis in an Asian male born in the North American continent: a controversial entity potentially related to multicentric Castleman disease. *J Cutan Pathol.* 2010;37(6):697–702, with permission.)

hidradenitis suppurativa-like presentation.[5,16,18] It has been noted in some cases that the lesions follow skin lines, or a "Christmas tree" pattern, similar to that seen in pityriasis rosea.[6,17] These lesions are often round or oval and occasionally infiltrative. There are also case reports of an indolent primary ulcerative presentation.[29,37] In general, the lesions are typically asymptomatic but may be pruritic in up to 40% of patients.[11,35]

The most frequently reported extracutaneous manifestation is superficial lymphadenopathy, which is often asymptomatic and has been reported as being present in up to 58% of patients.[11] The lymphadenopathy has been noted in the cervical, axillary, and inguinal lymph nodes and is typically multifocal and symmetric.[1] Some studies have demonstrated infiltration of plasma cells into lymph nodes, in the absence of palpable lymphadenopathy on examination, citing this observation as a reason to evaluate for systemic involvement in all patients with this condition.[12] On laboratory examination, hypergammaglobulinemia is the most frequently reported abnormality and has been noted in up to 80% to 90% of cases.[6,11] This gammopathy is typically polyclonal; however, monoclonal gammopathy is rarely reported.[6,11,36] Most commonly involved are elevations of IgG, over 80% reported, followed by IgA and IgM. Elevated levels of IgE have also been demonstrated.[6] Other commonly found laboratory abnormalities include elevated erythrocyte sedimentation rate and anemia.[6,11] Bone marrow infiltration of plasma cells as well as infiltration of visceral organs, resulting in hepatosplenomegaly, can also occur.[6,11,12]

Most patients with this condition follow a benign, stable course. However, complications, including renal disease in the form of interstitial nephritis, focal segmental glomerulosclerosis, renal amyloidosis or renal failure, myositis, interstitial pneumonia with respiratory failure, and anal and lung squamous cell carcinoma, have been reported.[3,6,11,17,21,26,38-40] Autoimmune hemolytic anemia (AIHA) has occurred in a patient with longstanding C/SP; AIHA has also been previously associated with other lymphoproliferative disorders including multicentric Castleman disease.[41] There is one case of T-cell lymphoma developing in a patient with C/SP.[42] Whether these observations are truly correlative is yet to be determined. Some studies have postulated that elevated levels of IgG (>5000 mg/dL) correspond with higher rates of extracutaneous findings and systemic complications.[6] Similarly, elevated plasma cells in the bone marrow (>6.9%) have portended a more complicated disease course.[6] Some researchers believe that these indices have value as prognostic indicators in this disease.[6]

HISTOLOGY

Histologically, this condition is characterized by a dermal infiltrate of plasma cells, admixed with lymphocytes and histiocytes. The epidermis is typically unaffected but may demonstrate mild acanthosis and basilar hyperpigmentation.[5,6] The plasmacytic infiltrate is most classically periadnexal and perivascular in the upper or mid-dermis but can be diffuse and involve the deep dermis and subcutis in some cases.[6,11,12,36] Less frequent observations include a perineural distribution of plasma cells, with intraneural plasma cells noted in a select number of cases.[36] The plasma cells in the infiltrate do not demonstrate cytologic atypia.[6,11,12,36] Also, frequently observed is the formation of lymphoid follicles with reactive germinal centers, surrounded by plasma cells[6,11,12,36] (Figs. 53-4–53-6). Mast cells, often

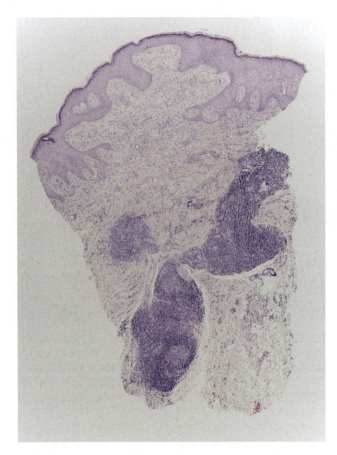

FIGURE 53-4. Punch biopsy, demonstrating germinal centers within the dermis surrounded by mature plasma cells (hematoxylin and eosin [H&E]; original magnification: 40×).

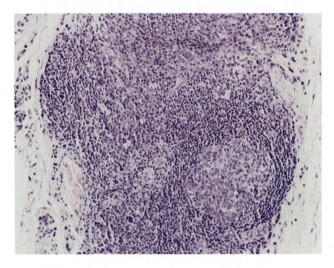

FIGURE 53-5. Reactive germinal centers surrounded by mature plasma cells (H&E; original magnification: 200×).

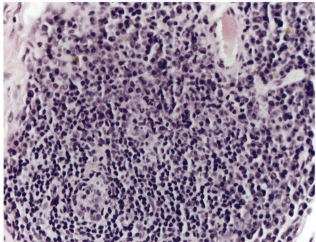

FIGURE 53-6. Infiltrate of mature plasma cells (H&E; original magnification: 400×).

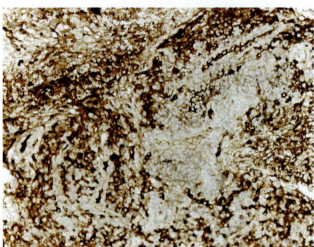

FIGURE 53-7. κ Antigen (in situ hybridization; original magnification: 200×).

large and globular, are also frequently seen in the dermal perivascular infiltrate, some with active degranulation.[5] Polyclonality of plasma cells by immunohistochemistry is observed in the vast majority of cases, with the presence of κ-chain- and λ-chain-positive cells[11,12,36] (Figs. 53-7 and 53-8). Immunoglobin heavy chain gene rearrangement studies were performed in a case series that found 8 of 12 cases to be polyclonal.[17] IgG-positive plasma cells typically predominate, but IgA- and IgM-positive plasma cells are also seen.[11] There can be an increased percentage of IgG4 to IgG in some cases.[43] Extracellular crystallized polyclonal immunoglobin deposition has also been reported in one case.[44]

Lymph node biopsies have revealed reactive germinal centers, with no atypical features, and an infiltration of mature, typical-appearing plasma cells in the perivascular zone in the paracortical area and medulla.[11,36] There has also been one case in which sarcoidal granulomas were visualized, where no underlying sarcoidosis was identified; thus, it was thought that the granuloma formation was secondary to the systemic plasmacytosis in that case.[36]

TREATMENT

Numerous treatment regimens have been attempted for this clinical entity, but there is no standard treatment for this rare disease. The evidence for treatment outcomes is limited to case reports and case series. Topical agents, including corticosteroids and calcineurin inhibitors, such as tacrolimus and pimecrolimus, have been met with overall poor results, with partial, if any, improvement.[5,7,15,45] Topical tacrolimus has been

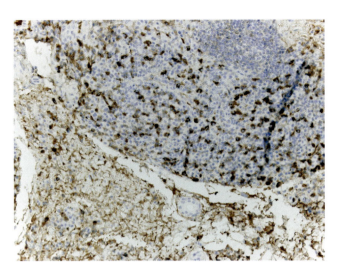

FIGURE 53-8. λ Antigen (in situ hybridization; original magnification: 200×).

shown to decrease the induration of the plaques in one patient, without any side effects.[46] Intralesional steroids have demonstrated improvement in the symptoms of pruritus and appearance of the cutaneous lesions in some cases[5,15,29,31]; however, they have been considered ineffective in others.[47] Systemic corticosteroids have also been used, with mixed results. Successful treatment with oral prednisone alone and in combination with intravenous immunoglobulin and pulse-dose cyclophosphamide has been reported.[22,45] Other reports of improvement of the appearance of the cutaneous lesions, without a change in the plasma cell infiltrate on histology, have questioned their effectiveness.[6] Furthermore, some studies have noted no improvement with the use of systemic corticosteroids for this condition.[3] Oral tetracyclines have not lead to improvement in this condition.[5] Treatment with light therapy, including narrowband ultraviolet light therapy and mask-bath and oral psoralen with ultraviolet A (PUVA) have shown mixed results with partial to most complete improvement in some case reports but lack of response in others.[6,15,16,20,31] Another case report found partial improvement including reduction of serum IL-6 levels with 308-nm excimer lamp.[19] Successful treatment, with improvement of the infiltrate on histology and clinical resolution of skin lesions, has been reported once, with photodynamic therapy, after failed attempts of treatment with PUVA and intralesional corticosteroids.[47] Improvement with thalidomide occurred in a patient with localized facial involvement.[48] Successful treatment with melphalan therapy and systemic chemotherapy (cyclophosphamide, doxorubicin, vinblastine, and prednisone) has also been reported in an atypical case of C/SP or multicentric plasmacytic Castleman disease (MPCD).[6,49] Treatment with rituximab has been unsuccessful.[13] IL-6 inhibitors, including tocilizumab and siltuximab, have been reported as successful in the cutaneous Castleman disease, which shares remarkable similarities with cutaneous plasmacytosis.[50,51] In summary, optimum treatment regimens for this condition have yet to be determined.

DIFFERENTIAL DIAGNOSIS

C/SP should be distinguished between other entities that can result in infiltration of plasma cells, including collagen disorders, in particular morphea and infectious causes, such as syphilis.[12,34,36] IgG4 disease can also have a polyclonal plasmacytic infiltrate, but the presence of storiform fibrosis and obliterative phlebitis in addition to increased IgG4 to IgG ratio can help distinguish this diagnosis. Other neoplastic conditions, including cutaneous plasmacytoma, marginal zone B-cell lymphoma (MZBCL), and lymphoplasmacytic leukemia, should also be considered; however, the plasma cell infiltrate would be monoclonal in these conditions.[34] Recent immunoglobin heavy chain gene rearrangement studies have found monoclonal expression in a minority of patients with an established diagnosis of C/SP highlighting the difficulty in differentiating C/SP from MZBCL in some cases.[17] As mentioned previously, many similarities exist between C/SP, HHV-8-negative MPCD, and idiopathic plasmacytic lymphadenopathy (IPL), all of which are polyclonal plasma cell proliferations of unknown etiology that predominantly affect Asian individuals.[32] The identification of HHV-8 allows for the diagnosis of MPCD to be made with certainty; however, in its absence, the diagnosis can be quite challenging. Classic multicentric Castleman disease typically exhibits systemic symptoms, along with a higher frequency of acquired immunodeficiency syndrome with its subsequent complications; however, cutaneous-only Castleman disease can follow a very indolent course and mimic C/SP.[32] Studies comparing C/SP, MPCD, and IPL have found remarkable consistencies and overlap between the entities, with few statistically significant differences, proposing that these diseases may occur on a spectrum.[6] Clinically, the differential diagnosis may also include acne, pityriasis rosea, parapsoriasis, lichen planus, postinflammatory hyperpigmentation, urticaria pigmentosa, hidradenitis suppurativa, and cutaneous lymphoma.[6,17,18,34]

References

1. Yashiro A. A kind of plasmacytosis: primary cutaneous plasmacytoma? [In Japanese]. *Jpn J Dermatol*. 1976;86:910.
2. Kitamura K, Tamura N, Hatano H, et al. A case of plasmacytosis with multiple peculiar eruptions. *J Dermatol*. 1980;7(5):341-349.
3. Watanabe S, Ohara K, Kukita A, et al. Systemic plasmacytosis. A syndrome of peculiar multiple skin eruptions, generalized lymphadenopathy, and polyclonal hypergammaglobulinemia. *Arch Dermatol*. 1986;122(11):1314-1320.
4. Wagner G, Rose C, Klapper W, et al. Cutaneous and systemic plasmacytosis. *J Dtsch Dermatol Ges*. 2013;11(12):1161-1167.
5. Han XD, Lee SSJ, Tan SH, et al. Cutaneous plasmacytosis: a clinicopathologic study of a series of cases and their treatment outcomes. *Am J Dermatopathol*. 2018;40(1):36-42.
6. Haque M, Hou JS, Hismichi K, et al. Cutaneous and systemic plasmacytosis vs. cutaneous plasmacytic Castleman disease: review and speculations about pathogenesis. *Clin Lymphoma Myeloma Leuk*. 2011;11(6):453-461.
7. González-López MA, González-Vela MC, Blanco R, et al. Cutaneous plasmacytosis limited to the extremities in a white patient: an unusual clinical picture. *Cutis*. 2010;86(3):143-147.
8. Gilliam AC, Mullen RH, Oviedo G, et al. Isolated benign primary cutaneous plasmacytosis in children: two illustrative cases. *Arch Dermatol*. 2009;145(3):299-302.
9. Shiba Y, Satoh T. Isolated benign primary cutaneous plasmacytosis. *Int J Dermatol*. 2014;53(9):397-398.
10. Song HS, Kim SK, Kim YC. Congenital form of isolated benign primary cutaneous plasmacytosis in a child. *Ann Dermatol*. 2014;26(1):121-122.
11. Uhara H, Saida T, Ikegawa S, et al. Primary cutaneous plasmacytosis: report of three cases and review of the literature. *Dermatology*. 1994;189(3):251-255.

12. Shimizu S, Tanaka M, Shimizu H, et al. Is cutaneous plasmacytosis a distinct clinical entity? *J Am Acad Dermatol.* 1997;36(5, pt 2):876-880.
13. Amin HM, McLaughlin P, Rutherford CJ, et al. Cutaneous and systemic plasmacytosis in a patient of Asian descent living in the United States. *Am J Dermatopathol.* 2002;24(3):241-245.
14. Ma HJ, Liu W, Li Y, et al. Cutaneous and systemic plasmacytosis: a Chinese case. *J Dermatol.* 2008;35(8):536-540.
15. Lee JS, Chiam L, Tan KB, et al. Extensive hyperpigmented plaques in a Chinese Singaporean woman: a case of cutaneous plasmacytosis. *Am J Dermatopathol.* 2011;33(5):498-503.
16. Mok ZR, Tan EST, Chong WS. Treatment of cutaneous plasmacytosis with mask bath PUVA: a therapeutic option. *Australas J Dermatol.* 2017;58(1):e1-e4.
17. Lu PE, Shih LY, Yang CH, et al. Cutaneous plasmacytosis: a clinicopathologic study of 12 cases in Taiwan revealing heterogeneous underlying causes. *Int J Dermatol.* 2015;54(10):1132-1137.
18. Goyal T, Varshney A, Zawar V, et al. Primary cutaneous plasmacytosis: marquerading as hidradenitis suppurativa. *Indian J Dermatol.* 2016;61(2):213-215.
19. Omura R, Sowa-Osako J, Fukai K, et al. Promising therapeutic option for cutaneous plasmacytosis: 308-nm excimer lamp. *J Dermatol.* 2018;45(8):e215-e216.
20. Yanaba K, Kajii T, Matsuzaki H, et al. Cutaneous plasmacytosis successfully treated with narrowband ultraviolet B irradiation therapy. *J Dermatol.* 2016;43(2):229-230.
21. Lee TG, Jeong WS, Moon SH, et al. Cutaneous and systemic plasmacytosis associated with renal amyloidosis. *Ann Dermatol.* 2015;27(6):759-762.
22. Carey WP, Rico MJ, Nierodzik M, et al. Systemic plasmacytosis with cutaneous manifestations in a white man: successful therapy with cyclophosphamide/prednisone. *J Am Acad Dermatol.* 1998;38(4):629-631.
23. López-Estebaranz JL, Rodriguez-Peralto JL, Ortiz Romero PL, et al. Cutaneous plasmacytosis: report of a case in a white man. *J Am Acad Dermatol.* 1994;31(5, pt 2):897-900.
24. Cerottini JP, Guillod J, Vion B, et al. Cutaneous plasmacytosis: an unusual presentation sharing features with POEMS syndrome? *Dermatology.* 2001;202(1):49-51.
25. Aricò M, Bongiorno MR. Primary cutaneous plasmacytosis in a child. Is this a new entity? *J Eur Acad Dermatol Venereol.* 2002;16(2):164-167.
26. Martín JM, Calduch L, Monteagudo C, et al. Cutaneous plasmacytosis associated with lung and anal carcinomas. *J Eur Acad Dermatol Venereol.* 2006;20(4):428-431.
27. Hafner C, Hohenleutner U, Babilas P, et al. Targeting T cells to hit B cells: successful treatment of cutaneous plasmacytosis with topical pimecrolimus. *Dermatology.* 2006;213(2):163-165.
28. Cannistraci C, Lesnoni La Parola I, Donati P, et al. Case of benign cutaneous plasmacytosis: immunohistochemical and flow cytometry study. *J Eur Acad Dermatol Venereol.* 2010;24(1):111-112.
29. Dautriche CN, Driessche FV, Chen L, et al. Ulcerative cutaneous plasmacytosis. *JAAD Case Rep.* 2019;5(6):540-554.
30. Kodama A, Tani M, Hori K, et al. Systemic and cutaneous plasmacytosis with multiple skin lesions and polyclonal hypergammaglobulinaemia: significant serum interleukin-6 levels. *Br J Dermatol.* 1992;127(1):49-53.
31. Yamamoto T, Soejima K, Katayama I, et al. Intralesional steroid-therapy-induced reduction of plasma interleukin-6 and improvement of cutaneous plasmacytosis. *Dermatology.* 1995;190(3):242-244.
32. Shadel BN, Frater JL, Gapp JDG, et al. Cutaneous and systemic plasmacytosis in an Asian male born in the North American continent: a controversial entity potentially related to multicentric castleman disease. *J Cutan Pathol.* 2010;37(6):697-702.
33. Okada H, Kano R, Watanabe S. Lack of evidence of human herpesvirus 8 DNA sequences in HIV-negative patients with systemic plasmacytosis. *Br J Dermatol.* 1999;141(5):942-943.
34. Jayaraman AG, Cesca C, Kohler S. Cutaneous plasmacytosis: a report of five cases with immunohistochemical evaluation for HHV-8 expression. *Am J Dermatopathol.* 2006;28(2):93-98.
35. Miyagawa-Hayashino A, Matsumura Y, Kawakami F. High ratio of IgG4-positive plasma cell infiltration in cutaneous plasmacytosis—is this a cutaneous manifestation of IgG4-related disease? *Hum Pathol.* 2009;40(9):1269-1277.
36. Honda R, Cerroni L, Tanikawa A, et al. Cutaneous plasmacytosis: report of 6 cases with or without systemic involvement. *J Am Acad Dermatol.* 2013;68(6):978-985.
37. Antonio AM, Alves JV, Coelho R, et al. Solitary ulcerated plaque on the face—an unusual presentation of cutaneous plasmacytosis? *An Bras Dermatol.* 2017;92(3):410-412.
38. Tada Y, Komine M, Suzuki S, et al. Plasmacytosis: systemic or cutaneous, are they distinct? *Acta Derm Venereol.* 2000;80(3):233-235.
39. Isobe S, Ohashi N, Katahashi N, et al. Focal segmental glomerulosclerosis associated with cutaneous and systemic plasmacytosis. *CEN Case Rep.* 2017;6(2):206-209.
40. Hatano T, Takanashi M, Tsuchihashi H, et al. Myalgia caused by chronic myositis associated with plasmacytosis: a case report. *BMC Neurol.* 2018;18(1):112.
41. Kiniwa Y, Matoba H, Hamano H, et al. Cutaneous plasmacytosis associated with autoimmune hemolytic anemia. *J Dermatol.* 2016;43(3):343-345.
42. Nitta Y. Case of malignant lymphoma associated with primary systemic plasmacytosis with polyclonal hypergammaglobulinemia. *Am J Dermatopathol.* 1997;19(3):289-293.
43. Takeoka S, Kamata M, Hau CS, et al. Evaluation of IgG4+ plasma cell infiltration in patients with systemic plasmacytosis and other plasma cell-infiltrating skin diseases. *Acta Derm Venereol.* 2018;98(5):506-511.
44. Ko JM, Jung KE, Choi CW, et al. Extracellular crystal deposition in cutaneous plasmacytosis. *JAMA Dermatol.* 2020;156(2):217-218.
45. Oka M, Kunisada M, Nishigori C. Cutaneous plasmacytosis in an 88-year-old woman successfully treated with low-dose oral corticosteroid. *Int J Dermatol.* 2013;52(11):1412-1414.
46. Miura H, Itami S, Yoshikawa K. Treatment of facial lesion of cutaneous plasmacytosis with tacrolimus ointment. *J Am Acad Dermatol.* 2003;49(6):1195-1196.
47. Tzung TY, Wu KH, Wu JC, et al. Primary cutaneous plasmacytosis successfully treated with topical photodynamic therapy. *Acta Derm Venereol.* 2005;85(6):542-543.
48. Fang S, Shan K, Chen AJ. Cutaneous and systemic plasmacytosis on the face: effective treatment of a case using thalidomide. *Oncol Lett.* 2016;11(3):1923-1925.
49. Lee DW, Choi SW, Park JW. Systemic plasmacytosis: a case which improved with melphalan. *J Dermatol.* 1995;22(3):205-209.
50. Ahmed B, Tschen JA, Cohen PR. Cutaneous Castleman's disease responds to anti–interleukin-6 treatment. *Mol Cancer Therapeut.* 2007;6(9):2386-2390.
51. Aita T, Hamaguchi S, Shimotani Y, et al. Idiopathic multicentric Castleman disease preceded by cutaneous plasmacytosis successfully treated by tocilizumab. *BMJ Case Rep.* 2020;13(11):e236283.

CHAPTER 54

Cutaneous IgG4-related disease

Alejandro A. Gru

DEFINITION

IgG4-related disease (IgG4-RD) is an immune-mediated histopathologic process that has been shown to underlie many disorders that were previously thought to be unrelated. IgG4-RD has been shown to affect nearly every organ system, including the skin. It is increasingly being recognized as an important mimic of many inflammatory and malignant conditions.[1,2]

EPIDEMIOLOGY

It tends to involve middle-aged to older men but can also occur in the pediatric age group. The exact incidence and prevalence in the skin is unclear. Most of the cases have been reported in Japan, with an estimated incidence of 0.28 to 1.08/100,000 population and 336 to 1300 new cases yearly.[3]

ETIOLOGY

IgG4-RD is an immune-mediated disease with the ability to affect nearly any organ system.[1,4,5] It has been recognized as a unifying pathogenic factor in many patients previously thought to have separate isolated single-organ system disease, such as type 1 autoimmune pancreatitis, Riedel thyroiditis, Mikulicz disease, interstitial pneumonitis, and inflammatory aortitis.[1,5] Reports of IgG4-related skin disease are limited. IgG4 is the least prevalent subclass of immunoglobulin G in the bloodstream and is also the least effective one in activating cells or complement due to its poor affinity for C1q or the Fc receptor.[6] Elevated IgG4 has been observed in a variety of conditions, such as allergic dermatitis (atopic dermatitis), blistering disorders (pemphigus foliaceus and vulgaris), and some parasitic infections.[7-9]

CLINICAL PRESENTATION AND PROGNOSIS

Most cases occur in middle-aged to older patients, and the condition has a clear male predominance. The most common symptoms of IgG4-RD are systemic complains such as fatigue, weight loss, and lymphadenopathy (present in 40% of cases).[3,10] However, system-based findings such as abdominal pain, diarrhea, sicca symptoms (dry eyes and dry mouth), respiratory problems, and pruritus can be present, and the specialty of the evaluating physician also influences the system-based symptoms reported in the case.[11] Elevated serum IgG4 is one of the hallmarks of the disease, and its extent correlates with the number of organs involved. Other laboratory abnormalities have been identified, which support a diagnosis of IgG4-RD: hypergammaglobulinemia, hypocomplementemia, peripheral blood eosinophilia, and elevated serum IgE.[12,13]

Like the systemic forms of IgG4-RD, IgG4-RD cutaneous disease is an entity of middle-aged to older patients with a clear male predilection. Cutaneous disease can occur as a primary process (without systemic manifestations)[14] or as a systemic disorder[15] where the skin is one of the affected organs.[2] One author estimated that around 6% of patients with IgG4-RD will have skin involvement.[16] Charrow et al[17] studied the skin lesions of IgG4-RD reported in the literature and found that the head and neck area is the most common area affected by cutaneous manifestations of IgG4-RD.[9] They reported that most of the lesions were papules, plaques, or nodules,[18,19] and the most common symptom was pruritus. Rare ulcers can be seen.[20] We have also encountered rare presentations with generalized erythroderma (in a patient with systemic IgG4-RD). Moreover, most of the patients had extracutaneous manifestations as well, affecting mainly the head and neck area. For example, most cases of IgG4-RD with skin involvement also suffered from dacryoadenitis or sialadenitis.[21] Some cases can also occur in the pediatric age group.[4,22] Indeed, we have reported a case of cutaneous IgG4-related skin disease in an adolescent 16-year-old girl (Fig. 54-1).[23] The median age of afflicted children is 13%, and 63% of patients are female, a feature that differs from adult patients.

HISTOLOGY AND IMMUNOPHENOTYPE

IgG4-RD is characterized by the infiltration of various tissues by IgG4+ plasma cells and is often accompanied by an elevated serum IgG4 level.[1,4,5] The general histopathologic picture of IgG4-RD is characterized by the three main hallmarks of a dense nonclonotypic lymphoplasmacytic infiltrate, storiform fibrosis, and obliterative phlebitis (Figs. 54-2 and 54-3). However, there is a significant variety in the histopathology of this entity in various organs.[3,23] For example and most relevant to our discussion, storiform fibrosis and obliterative phlebitis are rarely seen in cutaneous lesions of IgG4-RD.[3,23] Similarly, IgG4-RD lesions affecting the lungs, lymph nodes, and lacrimal glands often do not show those findings either. Even in cutaneous specimens with significant fibrosis, it does not show the cartwheel appearance of bands of fibrosis radiating from a center, a pattern that is defined as storiform. Furthermore, the presence of plasmablasts (immature precursors of plasma cells) in the peripheral blood is a unique finding that strongly supports diagnosis of IgG4-RD and has even been proposed as an excellent biomarker for monitoring disease activity.[24,25]

Common cutaneous pathologic manifestations include psoriasiform changes and a rich lymphoplasmacytic infiltrate.[3,15,23] Some cases can have spongiosis and more subtle inflammation in the dermis. The infiltrate can be centered in both the superficial and deep reticular dermis and subcutis. It has a perivascular, periadnexal, and perineural distribution. The plasma cells are polyclonal, and the lymphocytes are small to medium size, predominantly CD4+ T cells, intermixed with eosinophils, histiocytes, and scattered germinal centers (often reactive appearing). The plasma cells can be highlighted by a CD138, CD38, or CD79a immunostains.

In 2012, Umehara et al proposed the comprehensive diagnostic criteria of IgG4-RD, which consisted of three main criteria, one of which is the histopathologic analysis.[26] The histopathologic picture would need to show both (1) a marked lymphoplasmacytic infiltration and fibrosis and (2) an infiltration of IgG4+ plasma cells with a ratio of IgG4/IgG cells of more than 40% and more than 10 IgG4+ cells/high-power field (HPF) (Fig. 54-4). The clinical criteria include (1) presence of diffuse or localized swelling or a mass and (2) serum hematologic elevation of IgG4 >135 mg/dL. In the skin most suggest a number of >200 IgG4+ plasma cells/HPF as an appropriate criterion.[3]

PATHOGENESIS, GENETIC AND MOLECULAR FINDINGS

Recently, CD4+ cytotoxic T lymphocytes (CD4+ CTLs) appear to play a major role in understanding the IgG4-RD physiology. There is a clonal expansion of CD4+ CTLs detected using next-generation sequencing. These cells are thought to be the main drivers of the fibrosis seen in IgG4-RD. The expansion of this cell population was found in the lesions and in the peripheral

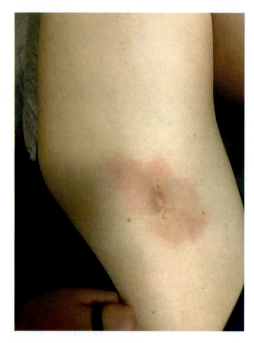

FIGURE 54-1. Erythematous nodule on the thigh. (From Shakeri A, Kindley KJ, Noland MM, Gru AA. IgG4-related skin disease presenting as a pseudolymphoma in a white adolescent girl. *Am J Dermatopathol.* 2019;41:675-679.)

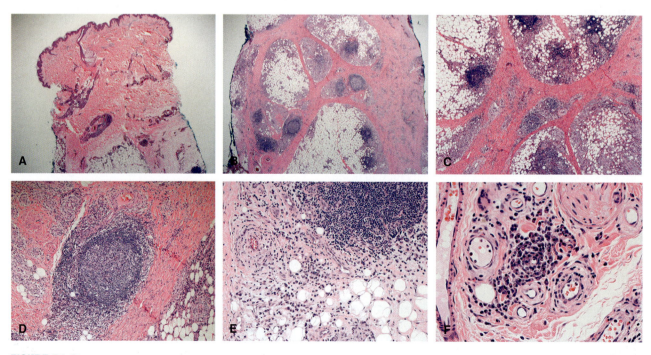

FIGURE 54-2. Skin biopsy. Mixed septal and lobular panniculitic infiltrate (**A** and **B**, ×20). A closer inspection shows small lymphoid follicles and septal/lobular fibrosis (**C**, ×40). Germinal centers are present (**D**, ×100). The septal and lobular inflammation contains small lymphocytes, numerous plasma cells, and scattered eosinophils (**E** and **F**, ×200 and ×400). (From Shakeri A, Kindley KJ, Noland MM, Gru AA. IgG4-related skin disease presenting as a pseudolymphoma in a white adolescent girl. *Am J Dermatopathol.* 2019;41:675-679.)

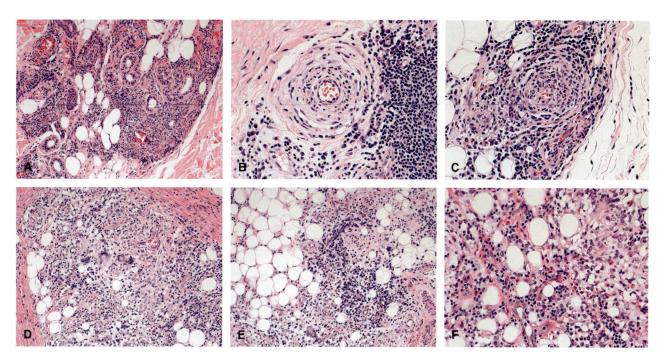

FIGURE 54-3. Skin biopsy. Specific features to support the diagnosis of IgG4-RD include the presence of phlebitis and mild perivascular fibrosis (**A–C**, ×200 and ×400). Other findings present in the biopsy include granulomatous inflammation with multinucleated giant cells (**D** and **E**, ×200). In some areas, the inflammation contains numerous eosinophils (**F**, ×400). (From Shakeri A, Kindley KJ, Noland MM, Gru AA. IgG4-related skin disease presenting as a pseudolymphoma in a white adolescent girl. *Am J Dermatopathol*. 2019;41:675-679.)

blood of affected individuals. These T cells produce granzyme B and perforin, IL-4, and IL-5 causing eosinophilia, transforming growth factor-beta, and interferon gamma, all of which are potentially important mediators of fibrosis and eosinophilia (present in many of the biopsies). Recent observations have also suggested that there is a significant increase in circulating PD-1+, CXCR5−, and CXCL13, which are ligands for CXCR5 in affected patients. Such study postulated its potential role in the initiation of the inflammation.[3]

DIFFERENTIAL DIAGNOSIS

Differential diagnostic considerations of IgG4-RD in the skin include reactive and neoplastic lymphoplasmacytic infiltrates. Cutaneous marginal zone lymphomas can also have a rich plasma cell infiltrate. In most cases, demonstration of clonality among the plasma cells by in situ hybridization or *IGH* gene rearrangement studies is sufficient to establish the diagnosis. Cutaneous marginal zone lymphoma can also have reactive germinal centers and is a dermal-based process. Similarly to IgG4-RD, a rich infiltrate of IgG4-positive plasma cells can be seen, particularly in cases with plasmacytic differentiation.[27] The follicular dendritic networks tend to show expansion and disruption. The cases of marginal zone lymphoma seen in Europe are often associated with *Borrelia burgdorferi* infection.

Lupus panniculitis is an autoimmune disorder and a variant of lupus erythematosus. Interface changes are frequently present. Like IgG4-RD, reactive appearing follicles are seen and the subcutis has fibrosis. However, a plasma cell IgG4-positive population is not typically seen, and dermal mucin can be easily demonstrated with the use of special stains. Although there is no definite agreement about serum IgG4 levels in lupus, a recent article compared this parameter between IgG4-RD and major rheumatologic disorders including Sjogren syndrome, rheumatoid arthritis, and lupus erythematosus.[28,29] This study found serum IgG4 to be significantly lower in major rheumatologic conditions compared with IgG4-RD.

Cutaneous plasmacytosis is a rare disorder seen in individuals from Japan. Pathologically, this entity shows dense, superficial, and deep lymphoplasmacytic infiltrates with or without follicles.[30] In some cases, IgG4-positive plasma cells can be seen, and most patients also have lymph node involvement. Some authors believe that this entity is closely linked to the plasma cell variant of Castleman disease. The latter is typically encountered in HIV-positive patients, often in association with HHV-8 infection.

Primary cutaneous Rosai-Dorfman-Destombes disease (RDD) is characterized by the presence of Rosai-Dorfman cells with emperipolesis in a background of lymphocytes and plasma cells, infiltrating dermal and subcutaneous tissue.[31,32] These cells are S-100 and CD68 positive and CD1a negative. Pathological features of RDD could overlap with IgG4-RD, such as light and dark areas, storiform sclerosis, and abundant Ig-G4 plasma cell. However, the presence of histiocytic cells S-100 positive with emperipolesis, the absence of obliterative phlebitis, and moderate count of IgG4 plasma cells can rule out the diagnosis of IgG4-RD. IgG4 plasma cells >200/HPF is suggestive of IgG4-RD in skin location.

Eosinophilic angiocentric fibrosis is a rare, indolent lesion that affects the mucosa of the upper respiratory tract, sinonasal cavity, and orbit. A previous history of allergy, surgery, or trauma in the same location is common. Histologic

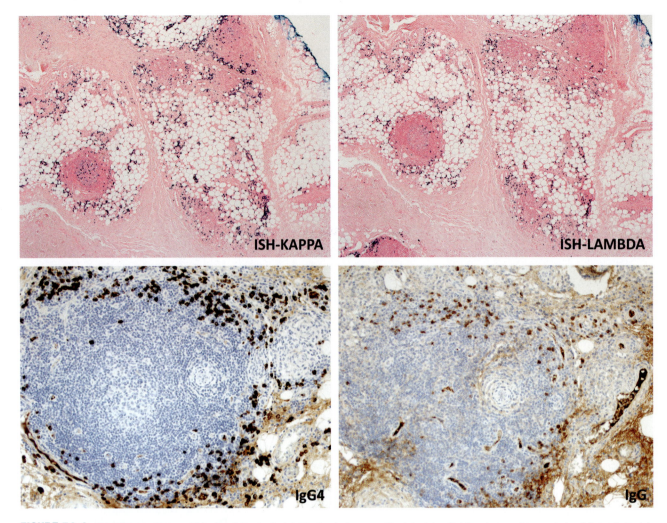

FIGURE 54-4. **Skin biopsy—immunohistochemistry.** In situ hybridization for kappa and lambda shows that the plasma cells are polyclonal (kappa to lambda ratio of 3-4:1). IgG4 stains most of the plasma cells, which in areas seem to represent >200 cells per high-power field. IgG stains a relatively smaller proportion of cells. The IgG4:IgG ratio is markedly elevated (>0.4:1). (From Shakeri A, Kindley KJ, Noland MM, Gru AA. IgG4-related skin disease presenting as a pseudolymphoma in a white adolescent girl. *Am J Dermatopathol.* 2019;41:675-679.)

examination shows a perivascular eosinophilic vasculitis with variable numbers of other inflammatory cells, such as plasma cells and lymphocytes. There are zones of "onion-skinning" fibrosis and an increased IgG4+/IgG ratio with high serum IgG4 levels. This might represent a localized mucosal form of IgG4-RD.[3]

Granuloma faciale (GF) and erythema elevatum diutinum (EED) are closely related disorders with a vasculitic component.[33] GF presents on the face and EED in the dorsum of joints. Both show a small vessel vasculitis. With the chronicity, onion-skinning fibrosis is evident. Both GF and EED shared a very rich plasma cell infiltrate, which can have a very large number of IgG4+ cells.

Cutaneous lymphoid hyperplasia (CLH) is not a specific entity but a pattern that is associated with multiple etiologic factors.[34] Arthropod bite reactions are one of the prototypic causes of CLH. In CLH, an abundance of eosinophils is present. A specific form of CLH seen in children, which is relevant to the differential diagnosis with the present case, is the so-called tibial lymphoplasmacytic plaque. It presents as well-demarcated, indolent, localized pink to violaceous papulonodular plaques. Histologically, a dense dermal lymphocytic infiltrate admixed with polyclonal plasma cells is seen.

CAPSULE SUMMARY

IgG4-related disease is an immune-mediated histopathologic process that can affect almost every organ and system, including the skin. Most cases occur in middle-aged to older patients, and the condition has a clear male predominance. Skin disease can occur as a primary form (in the absence of systemic symptoms) or as part of a systemic disorder involving other organs and systems. Most of the lesions were papules, plaques, or nodules, and the most common symptom was pruritus. Histopathologic findings include the presence of tissue infiltration by IgG4+ plasma cells, typically >200/HPF. Fibrosis and phlebitis are accompanying findings but could be missing in the skin.

References

1. Stone JH, Zen Y, Deshpande V. IgG4-related disease. *N Engl J Med*. 2012;366:539-551.
2. Shenoy A, Mohandas N, Gottlieb A. Cutaneous and systemic IgG4-related disease: a review for dermatologists. *Dermatol Online J*. 2019;25:13030/qt9w91m8dz.
3. Katerji R, Smoller BR. Immunoglobulin-G4-related skin disease. *Clin Dermatol*. 2021;39:283-290.
4. Karim F, Loeffen J, Bramer W, et al. IgG4-related disease: a systematic review of this unrecognized disease in pediatrics. *Pediatr Rheumatol Online J*. 2016;14:18.
5. Kempeneers D, Hauben E, De Haes P. IgG4-related skin lesions: case report and review of the literature. *Clin Exp Dermatol*. 2014;39:479-483.
6. Miyagawa-Hayashino A, Matsumura Y, Kawakami F, et al. High ratio of IgG4-positive plasma cell infiltration in cutaneous plasmacytosis--is this a cutaneous manifestation of IgG4-related disease? *Hum Pathol*. 2009;40:1269-1277.
7. Fernandez-Flores A. The role of IgG4 in cutaneous pathology. *Rom J Morphol Embryol*. 2012;53:221-231.
8. Sato Y, Takeuchi M, Takata K, et al. Clinicopathologic analysis of IgG4-related skin disease. *Mod Pathol*. 2013;26:523-532.
9. Takayama R, Ueno T, Saeki H. Immunoglobulin G4-related disease and its skin manifestations. *J Dermatol*. 2017;44:288-296.
10. Ebbo M, Daniel L, Pavic M, et al. IgG4-related systemic disease – features and treatment response in a French cohort: results of a multicenter registry. *Medicine (Baltimore)*. 2012;91:49-56.
11. Stone JH, Brito-Zeron P, Bosch X, Ramos-Casals M. Diagnostic approach to the complexity of IgG4-related disease. *Mayo Clin Proc*. 2015;90:927-939.
12. Kawano M, Saeki T, Nakashima H, et al. Proposal for diagnostic criteria for IgG4-related kidney disease. *Clin Exp Nephrol*. 2011;15:615-626.
13. Saeki T, Nishi S, Imai N, et al. Clinicopathological characteristics of patients with IgG4-related tubulointerstitial nephritis. *Kidney Int*. 2010;78:1016-1023.
14. Hegde P, Relhan V, Tomar R. IgG4-related disease: a rare case of isolated cutaneous involvement. *Clin Exp Dermatol*. 2021;46:343-345.
15. Komatsuzaki Y, Hayashi S, Saito F, Saito Y, Hamasaki Y, Igawa K. Immunoglobulin G4-related disease associated with asymptomatic aortic stenosis and diagnosed based on skin lesions. *J Dermatol*. 2020;47:e60-e61.
16. Yamada K, Hamaguchi Y, Saeki T, et al. Investigations of IgG4-related disease involving the skin. *Mod Rheumatol*. 2013;23:986-993.
17. Charrow A, Imadojemu S, Stephen S, Ogunleye T, Takeshita J, Lipoff JB. Cutaneous manifestations of IgG4-related disease (RD): a systematic review. *J Am Acad Dermatol*. 2016;75:197-202.
18. Akazawa T, Sekido M, Adachi K, Aihara Y, Myojo R. A tumor of IgG4-related skin disease on a forehead with relapse 3 years after resection. *JAAD Case Rep*. 2021;16:9-11.
19. Mizutani Y, Goto Y, Matsuyama K, Miyazaki T, Seishima M. A bulky tumor on the thigh diagnosed as IgG4-related skin disease. *J Dermatol*. 2021;48:e258-e9.
20. Gon J, Takemori C, Fujiwara S, Hirota S, Imayama S, Imai Y. A case of skin ulcer on the lower leg diagnosed as primary IgG4-related skin disease. *Eur J Dermatol*. 2021;31:669-671.
21. Arianayagam S, Ieremia E, Cooper SM, Matin RN. Case of the month: a case of IgG4-related skin disease. *Eur J Dermatol*. 2020;30:449-450.
22. Nastri MMF, Novak GV, Sallum AEM, Campos LMA, Teixeira RAP, Silva CA. Immunoglobulin G4-related disease with recurrent uveitis and kidney tumor mimicking childhood polyarteritis nodosa: a rare case report. *Acta Reumatol Port*. 2018;43:226-229.
23. Shakeri A, Kindley KJ, Noland MM, Gru AA. IgG4-related skin disease presenting as a pseudolymphoma in a white adolescent girl. *Am J Dermatopathol*. 2019;41:675-679.
24. Mattoo H, Mahajan VS, Della-Torre E, et al. De novo oligoclonal expansions of circulating plasmablasts in active and relapsing IgG4-related disease. *J Allergy Clin Immunol*. 2014;134:679-687.
25. Wallace ZS, Mattoo H, Carruthers M, et al. Plasmablasts as a biomarker for IgG4-related disease, independent of serum IgG4 concentrations. *Ann Rheum Dis*. 2015;74:190-195.
26. Umehara H, Okazaki K, Masaki Y, et al. Comprehensive diagnostic criteria for IgG4-related disease (IgG4-RD), 2011. *Mod Rheumatol*. 2012;22:21-30.
27. De Souza A, Ferry JA, Burghart DR, et al. IgG4 expression in primary cutaneous marginal zone lymphoma: a multicenter study. *Appl Immunohistochem Mol Morphol*. 2018;26:462-467.
28. Pan Q, Lan Q, Peng Y, et al. Nature, functions, and clinical implications of IgG4 autoantibodies in systemic lupus erythematosus and rheumatoid arthritis. *Discov Med*. 2017;23:169-174.
29. Wang L, Chu X, Ma Y, et al. A comparative analysis of serum IgG4 levels in patients with IgG4-related disease and other disorders. *Am J Med Sci*. 2017;354:252-256.
30. Hsiao PF, Wu YH. Characterization of cutaneous plasmacytosis at different disease stages. *Dermatology*. 2016;232:738-747.
31. Zghal M, Makni S, Saguem I, et al. Primary cutaneous Rosai-Dorfman-Destombes disease with features mimicking IgG4-related disease: a challenging case report and literature review. *Australas J Dermatol*. Published online 2022.
32. Zhang Y, Chen H, Jiang YQ, et al. Clinicopathological features of cutaneous Rosai-Dorfman disease and its relationship to IgG4-related disease: a retrospective study. *Br J Dermatol*. 2019;181:844-845.
33. Tran TA. Does a subset of localized chronic fibrosing vasculitis represent cutaneous manifestation of IgG4-related disease/a histologic pattern of IgG4-related skin disease? A reappraisal of an enigmatic pathologic entity. *Am J Dermatopathol*. 2020;42:683-688.
34. Kotani H, Ohtsuka T, Okada S, Kusama M, Taniguchi T. A case of IgG4-related disease presented with Kimura disease-like skin eruption, rheumatoid arthritis-like abnormality and interstitial pneumonia. *Clin Exp Dermatol*. 2020;45:733-734.

Lymphomatoid contact dermatitis

Caitlin M. Brumfiel, Meera H. Patel, Alejandro A. Gru, and Matthew J. Zirwas

DEFINITION

Lymphomatoid contact dermatitis (LCD) is a chronic, persistent allergic contact dermatitis that elicits a robust lymphocytic response to persistent antigenic stimulation, mimicking a cutaneous lymphoma. It was originally described by Gomez Orbaneja in 1976 in a series of patients originally diagnosed with mycosis fungoides (MF) but later found to have a lymphomatoid delayed hypersensitivity reaction caused by the striker on matchboxes.[1] Although the clinical and histopathologic appearance frequently simulates that of MF, most patients experience complete resolution of symptoms upon sustained avoidance of the allergen.

EPIDEMIOLOGY

There have been no formal epidemiologic studies to determine the incidence or gender predilection of LCD. It is an uncommon disease that affects both men and women, the majority of whom are more than 40 years of age as described in the literature. LCD has not yet been described in the pediatric population.

CLINICAL PRESENTATION AND PROGNOSIS

Patients with LCD classically exhibit erythematous plaques and papules associated with pruritus and periods of remission and exacerbation (Fig. 55-1).[2,3] Some patients experience an exfoliative erythroderma.[4,5] Dusky nodules and tumors, infiltration, and scaling have also been described, although these features seem to be less common.[3,6-8] Diagnosis can be difficult because it hinges on identifying the offending contact allergen, so a thorough history and comprehensive patch testing are essential. Many allergens have been implicated in LCD (Table 55-1). In most instances, complete avoidance of the contact allergen will result in lasting remission without significant sequelae.[2,3,27] Rare reports of indirect contact with allergens leading to the development of LCD have been documented, including systemic methylcobalamin (vitamin B12) administration[21] and airborne methylisothiazolinone exposure.[24]

Cases of persistent pseudolymphomatous contact dermatitis developing into a florid cutaneous lymphoma have been

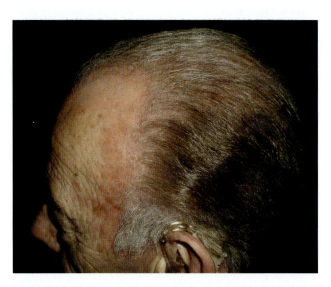

FIGURE 55-1. This patient had a yearlong history of pruritic rash on the scalp secondary to allergy to paraphenylenediamine in his hair dye. Pink-red erythematous patches and tumors were seen on physical examination. Skin biopsy showed changes consistent with LCD.

described, but it is possible that these patients had a lymphoproliferative disorder to begin with. This was described by Abraham et al[32] in a patient initially diagnosed with LCD induced by topical eye treatments who was, years later, found to have latent T-cell prolymphocytic leukemia. This patient most likely had cutaneous involvement as the herald symptom of his leukemia rather than LCD.[32] It is important to note that 45% of patients with cutaneous lymphoma and 38% of patients with all pseudolymphomas had positive patch testing, often to metals. Therefore, it is essential to stress that a positive patch test should not be interpreted as a marker of a benign inflammatory disorder.[23,33]

HISTOLOGY

The majority of allergen-induced pseudolymphomas show dense, perivascular, or band-like dermal T-cell infiltrates with exocytosis of lymphocytes reminiscent of MF (Figs. 55-2 and 55-3).[23,29,34] Differentiation can be made on the basis of spongiosis, intraepidermal vesiculation, and superficial papillary dermal edema, which favor a diagnosis of

TABLE 55-1 Allergens Implicated in LCD

Azo dyes[9]
Acrylate[10]
Baby wipes (methylchloroisothiazolinone and quaternium-15 preservatives)[11]
Benzydamine hydrochloride[12]
Cobalt naphthenate[13]
Ethylenediamine dihydrochloride[14]
Formaldehyde
Glutaraldehyde
Gold[8,15-17 a,b]
Isopropyl-diphenylenediamine[18]
Isopropylaminodiphenylamine[19]
Limonene hydroperoxides[20]
Mercaptobenzothiazole
Methylcobalamin[21 c]
Methylchloroisothiazolinone[11,22,23]
Methylisothiazolinone[22-24 d]
Nickel[25,26]
Para-phenylenediamine[2,3,27 a]
Para-tertyl-butyl phenol resin[28]
Tattoo ink
Phosphorus sesquisulfide[1]
Teak wood[29]
Textile dye[9,30,31]
Zinc[a]

[a]Reported to cause T- and/or B-cell LCD.
[b]Cutaneous exposure and subcutaneous implant.
[c]Systemic exposure.
[d]Cutaneous and airborne exposure.

LCD.[5,19,34] Moreover, the epidermis features nests that contain keratinocytes, Langerhans cells, and relatively few atypical lymphocytes. This is in contrast to MF, wherein focal abscess-like aggregations are formed primarily by atypical T lymphocytes.[34] There can be variable acanthosis and parakeratosis.[21,27,29] Cases of predominantly B-cell LCD have been reported in response to zinc, gold, and paraphenylenediamine.[3,16,17,35] The histology in those pseudolymphomas revealed dermal lymphoid, follicle-like structures with predominantly CD20+ cells (Figs. 55-4 and 55-5).[3,16,35]

IMMUNOPHENOTYPE

Most cases of LCD demonstrate a CD3, CD4, and/or CD30 T-lymphocyte predominance.[3,4,9,29,36] The few reported cases of a B-cell LCD featured an abundance of CD20+ B lymphocytes.[3,16,17,35] In the epidermis, staining for CD1a will highlight nests of Langerhans cells, which can help differentiate LCD from MF,[21,37] with the only caveat of contact dermatitis superimposed on a lesion of MF.[33]

GENETIC AND MOLECULAR FINDINGS

The majority of LCD case reports that detail T-cell rearrangement studies show a polyclonal expansion of T lymphocytes. Presence of a monoclonal lymphocytosis does not necessarily imply a true malignancy, as this has been shown to be present in biopsies of patients with positive patch tests and benign inflammatory disease.[36] Among a review of 11 cases of LCD with known results of T-cell receptor gene rearrangement studies, only one revealed a clonal population of T cells.[18,23]

DIFFERENTIAL DIAGNOSIS

A thorough history and comprehensive patch testing are usually necessary to differentiate LCD from MF. In a patient with a history and examination consistent with allergic contact dermatitis, positive patch tests, and histology resembling MF, a diagnosis of LCD should be entertained. Clearing of symptoms upon avoidance of the offending agent confirms the diagnosis. Other diagnostic considerations include conventional contact dermatitis, drug eruption, and the various other pseudolymphomatous dermatitides.

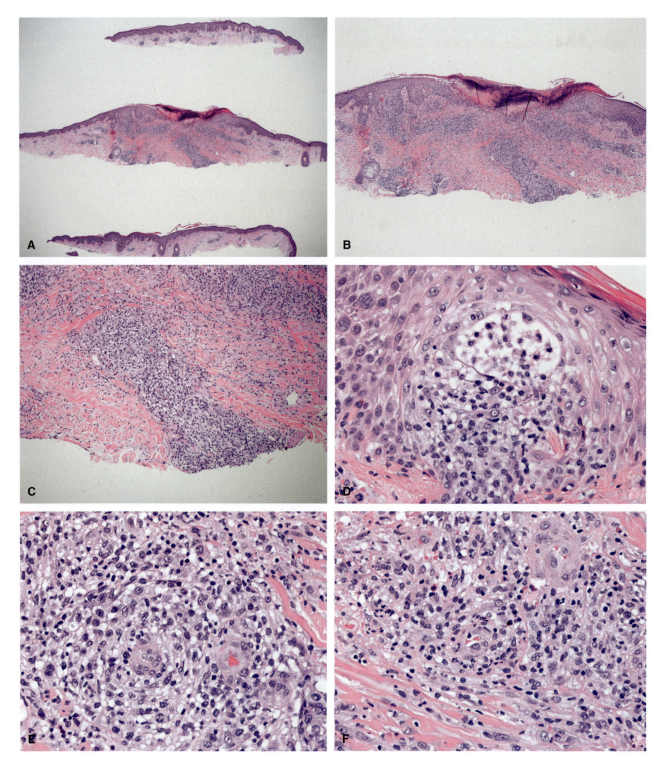

FIGURE 55-2. Right chest biopsy—LCD. This patient developed LCD to nickel. There is focal surface ulceration (**A** and **B**, low-power magnification). **C.** A dense infiltrate is seen in the dermis. **D.** Focal collections of Langerhans cells in the epidermis are noted. The infiltrate shows the admixture of large cells (**E**) and eosinophils (**F**).

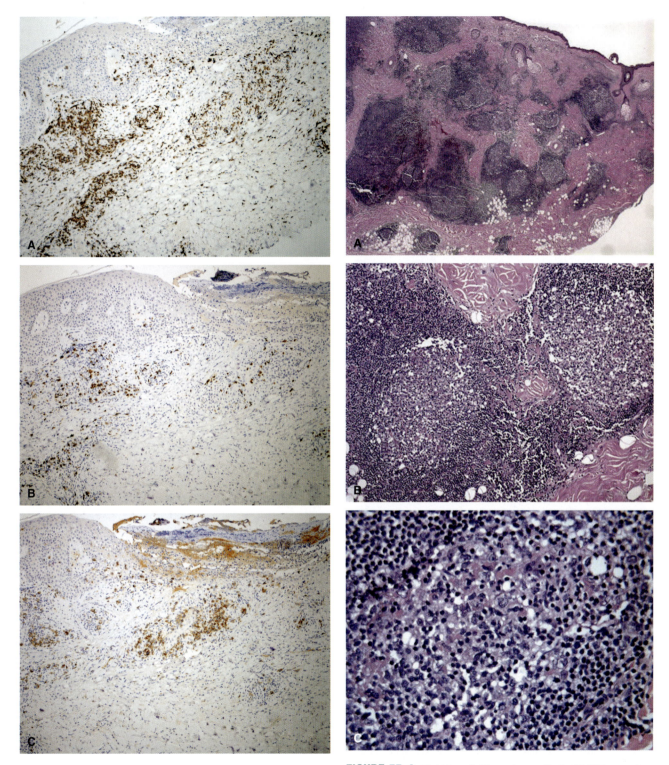

FIGURE 55-3. Right chest biopsy—immunohistochemistry. There is a predominance of CD4+ **(A)** T cells over CD8+ **(B)** cells and numerous CD30+ large cells **(C)**.

FIGURE 55-4. Right temple biopsy in a patient with LCD secondary to paraphenylenediamine revealed dense dermal lymphocytic infiltrate extending into subcutaneous adipose tissue and forming prominent germinal centers. Infiltrate is most pronounced in periadnexal and perineural regions. Increased eosinophils are noted. Overlying epidermis is not involved (H&E; original magnification: 2× **(A)**, close-up 10× **(B)**, and 40× **(C)**). (Reprinted from Paley K, Geskin LJ, Zirwas MJ. Cutaneous B-cell pseudolymphoma due to paraphenylenediamine. *Am J Dermatopathol.* 2006;28(5):438-441, with permission.)

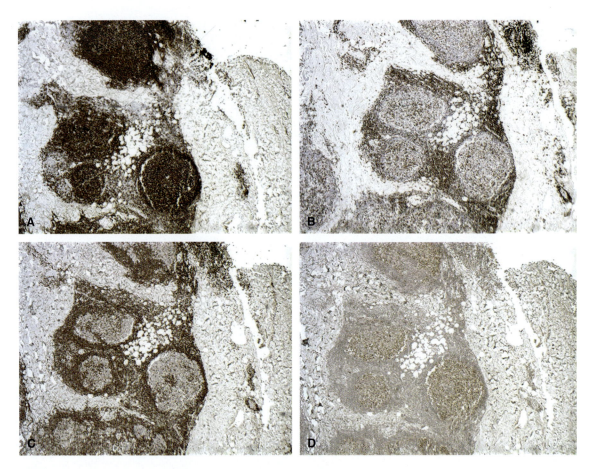

FIGURE 55-5. Immunohistochemistry for this patient with B-cell LCD shows abundance of CD20+ B cells within the germinal centers **(A)** and scattered CD3+ T cells **(B)**. BCL-2 staining is negative in the germinal center **(C)**, whereas BCL-6 staining highlights follicular center cells **(D)** (immunostain with hematoxylin counterstain; original magnification: 4×). (From Paley K, Geskin LJ, Zirwas MJ. Cutaneous B-cell pseudolymphoma due to paraphenylenediamine. *Am J Dermatopathol.* 2006;28(5):438-441, with permission.)

References

1. Orbaneja JG, Diez LI, Lozano JL, Salazar LC. Lymphomatoid contact dermatitis: a syndrome produced by epicutaneous hypersensitivity with clinical features and a histopathologic picture similar to that of mycosis fungoides. *Contact Dermatitis.* 1976;2(3):139-143.
2. Hospital V, Amarger S, Franck F, Ferrier Le Bouedec MC, Souteyrand P, D'Incan M. Proxy lymphomatoid contact dermatitis. [Article in French]. *Ann Dermatol Venereol.* 2011;138(4):315-318.
3. Paley K, Geskin LJ, Zirwas MJ. Cutaneous B-cell pseudolymphoma due to paraphenylenediamine. *Am J Dermatopathol.* 2006;28(5):438-441.
4. Marchesi A, Parodi PC, Brioschi M, et al. Tattoo ink-related cutaneous pseudolymphoma: a rare but significant complication. Case report and review of the literature. *Aesthetic Plast Surg.* 2014;38(2):471-478.
5. Ploysangam T, Breneman DL, Mutasim DF. Cutaneous pseudolymphomas. *J Am Acad Dermatol.* 1998;38(6 pt 1):877-895; quiz 96-97.
6. Kluger N, Vermeulen C, Moguelet P, et al. Cutaneous lymphoid hyperplasia (pseudolymphoma) in tattoos: a case series of seven patients. *J Eur Acad Dermatol Venereol.* 2010;24(2):208-213.
7. Laftah Z, Benton E, Bhargava K, et al. Two cases of bilateral earlobe cutaneous pseudolymphoma. *Br J Dermatol.* 2014;171(6):1567-1570.
8. Conde-Taboada A, Roson E, Fernandez-Redondo V, Garcia-Doval I, De La Torre C, Cruces M. Lymphomatoid contact dermatitis induced by gold earrings. *Contact Dermatitis.* 2007;56(3):179-181.
9. Narganes LM, Sambucety PS, Gonzalez IR, Rivas MO, Prieto MA. Lymphomatoid dermatitis caused by contact with textile dyes. *Contact Dermatitis.* 2013;68(1):62-64.
10. Fernandez-Canga P, Sanchez-Sambucety P, Valladares-Narganes LM, Varas-Meis E, Rodriguez-Prieto MA. Lymphomatoid contact dermatitis induced by acrylates mimicking lymphomatoid papulosis. *Dermatitis.* 2018;29(3):167-168.
11. Mendese G, Beckford A, Demierre MF. Lymphomatoid contact dermatitis to baby wipes. *Arch Dermatol.* 2010;146(8):934-935.
12. Alvarez-Garrido H, Sanz-Munoz C, Martinez-Garcia G, Miranda-Romero A. Lymphomatoid photocontact dermatitis to benzydamine hydrochloride. *Contact Dermatitis.* 2010;62(2):117-119.
13. Schena D, Rosina P, Chieregato C, Colombari R. Lymphomatoid-like contact dermatitis from cobalt naphthenate. *Contact Dermatitis.* 1995;33(3):197-198.
14. Wall LM. Lymphomatoid contact dermatitis due to ethylenediamine dihydrochloride. *Contact Dermatitis.* 1982;8(1):51-54.
15. Park YM, Kang H, Kim HO, Cho BK. Lymphomatoid eosinophilic reaction to gold earrings. *Contact Dermatitis.* 1999;40(4):216-217.

16. Fleming C, Burden D, Fallowfield M, Lever R. Lymphomatoid contact reaction to gold earrings. *Contact Dermatitis*. 1997;37(6):298-299.
17. Rodriguez-Villa Lario A, Medina-Montalvo S, Gomez-Zubiaur A, et al. Late cutaneous B-cell pseudolymphoma after an upper-eyelid gold weight implant. *Contact Dermatitis*. 2019;80(4):256-258.
18. Marliere V, Beylot-Barry M, Doutre MS, et al. Lymphomatoid contact dermatitis caused by isopropyl-diphenylenediamine: two cases. *J Allergy Clin Immunol*. 1998;102(1):152-153.
19. Martinez-Moran C, Sanz-Munoz C, Morales-Callaghan AM, Garrido-Rios AA, Torrero V, Miranda-Romero A. Lymphomatoid contact dermatitis. *Contact Dermatitis*. 2009;60(1):53-55.
20. Gatica-Ortega ME, Pastor-Nieto MA, Schoendorff-Ortega C, Mollejo-Villanueva M, Gimenez-Arnau A. Lymphomatoid contact dermatitis caused by limonene hydroperoxides confirmed by an exposure provocation test with the involved personal hygiene products. *Contact Dermatitis*. 2018;78(3):230-233.
21. Fujita Y, Mizukami T, Maya Y, et al. Vitamin B12 allergy manifesting as lymphomatoid contact dermatitis. *Eur J Dermatol*. 2020;30(3):304-305.
22. Smets K, Busschots A, Hauben E, Goossens A. B-cell lymphomatoid contact dermatitis caused by methylisothiazolinone and methylchloroisothiazolinone. *Eur J Dermatol*. 2018;28(1):91-93.
23. Knackstedt TJ, Zug KA. T cell lymphomatoid contact dermatitis: a challenging case and review of the literature. *Contact Dermatitis*. 2015;72(2):65-74.
24. Van Steenkiste E, Goossens A, Meert H, Apers S, Aerts O. Airborne-induced lymphomatoid contact dermatitis caused by methylisothiazolinone. *Contact Dermatitis*. 2015;72(4):237-240.
25. Houck HE, Wirth FA, Kauffman CL. Lymphomatoid contact dermatitis caused by nickel. *Am J Contact Dermat*. 1997;8(3):175-176.
26. Danese P, Bertazzoni MG. Lymphomatoid contact dermatitis due to nickel. *Contact Dermatitis*. 1995;33(4):268-269.
27. Calzavara-Pinton P, Capezzera R, Zane C, et al. Lymphomatoid allergic contact dermatitis from para-phenylenediamine. *Contact Dermatitis*. 2002;47(3):173-174.
28. Evans AV, Banerjee P, McFadden JP, Calonje E. Lymphomatoid contact dermatitis to para-tertyl-butyl phenol resin. *Clin Exp Dermatol*. 2003;28(3):272-273.
29. Ezzedine K, Rafii N, Heenen M. Lymphomatoid contact dermatitis to an exotic wood: a very harmful toilet seat. *Contact Dermatitis*. 2007;57(2):128-130.
30. Belhareth K, Korbi M, Kheder A, et al. Lymphomatoid contact dermatitis caused by textile dye arising on pre-existing vitiligo lesions. *Contact Dermatitis*. 2020;83(2):139-141.
31. Uzuncakmak TK, Akdeniz N, Ozkanli S, Turkoglu Z, Zemheri EI, Ka Radag AS. Lymphomatoid contact dermatitis associated with textile dye at an unusual location. *Indian Dermatol Online J*. 2015;6(suppl 1):S24-S26.
32. Abraham S, Braun RP, Matthes T, Saurat JH. A follow-up: previously reported apparent lymphomatoid contact dermatitis, now followed by T-cell prolymphocytic leukaemia. *Br J Dermatol*. 2006;155(3):633-634.
33. Khamaysi Z, Weltfriend S, Khamaysi K, Bergman R. Contact hypersensitivity in patients with primary cutaneous lymphoproliferative disorders. *Int J Dermatol*. 2011;50(4):423-427.
34. Bonamonte D, Foti C, Vestita M, Angelini G. Noneczematous contact dermatitis. *ISRN Allergy*. 2013;2013:361746.
35. Komatsu H, Aiba S, Mori S, Suzuki K, Tagami H. Lymphocytoma cutis involving the lower lip. *Contact Dermatitis*. 1997;36(3):167-169.
36. Kalimo K, Rasanen L, Aho H, Maki J, Mustikkamki UP, Rantala I. Persistent cutaneous pseudolymphoma after intradermal gold injection. *J Cutan Pathol*. 1996;23(4):328-334.
37. Kuo WE, Richwine EE, Sheehan DJ. Pseudolymphomatous and lichenoid reaction to a red tattoo: a case report. *Cutis*. 2011;87(2):89-92.

CHAPTER 56

Annular lichenoid dermatosis of youth

Alejandro A. Gru

DEFINITION

Annular lichenoid dermatosis of youth (ALDY) is a clinicopathologic entity originally described in children and young patients, which is clinically reminiscent of morphea, annular erythema, vitiligo, or mycosis fungoides (MF). ALDY is regarded as a form of pseudolymphoma.[1] More recently, some cases have been reported in adults.[2,3]

EPIDEMIOLOGY

ALDY was originally described by Annessi et al[4] in children and young adults (median age of 10 years). Because it can affect older patients,[1,5] renaming the entity to "annular lichenoid dermatosis" was proposed. ALDY lacks gender predilection. Most cases were described in individuals with Mediterranean descent, but cases from Japan, other areas in Europe, and the United States had been reported. ALDY has not been described in African Americans.

ETIOLOGY AND PATHOGENESIS

The pathogenesis of the disease is obscure. Autoimmunity, infections, and sensitization have been investigated.[1,4] Serologic studies for Lyme and parvovirus B19 and patch testing for various allergens were negative.[6-8] A single individual had been shown to be atopic.[1] Atopy and eczema were also noted in another case, in which ALDY occurred following hepatitis B vaccination.[9] Elevation of anti-streptolysin has been documented in three cases.[10] A study from Austria documented the presence of spirochetes in 11/14 cases of ALDY.[11]

A T cell–mediated cytotoxic immune reaction is favored as the main underlying pathogenesis. As such, ALDY can be considered an interface dermatitis, such as lichen planus, graft-versus-host disease, or lichen sclerosus et atrophicus (LSA).

CLINICAL PRESENTATION

The lesions consist of persistent asymptomatic erythematous macules and annular patches with raised red-brownish border and hypopigmented center.[12] The lesions are typically multiple, but cases with solitary lesions had been described. ALDY is usually located in the trunk, particularly on the flanks and abdomen (Fig. 56-1) and range from 3 to 10 cm in size. The axilla and neck are occasionally involved. Involvement of distal extremities, buttock, and face/scalp had not been reported. The duration of the clinical lesions prior to biopsy averages 1 to 15 months.[1] The clinical lesions can resemble morphea, MF, annular erythema, and vitiligo. A single case report described a hyperpigmented patch resembling ashy dermatosis (lichen planus pigmentosus/erythema dyschromicum perstans) adjacent to a hypopigmented lesion with erythematous border suggesting an overlapping spectrum with ALDY.[13]

TREATMENT

ALDY has been reported to respond partially to topical or systemic corticosteroids, ultraviolet (UV) A-1 light, or psoralen plus UVA (PUVA); however, the clinical course is more likely to be chronic with frequent failure of treatments and recurrence.[4,6,14]

HISTOLOGY

The histopathology varies depending on the age of the lesion and the site of the biopsy.[1,7,15,16] Early lesions show vacuolar changes of basal keratinocytes and a band-like lymphocytic infiltrate confined at the rete tips (Fig. 56-2). There is acanthosis with prominent thinning of the rete ridges. The lichenoid process ultimately obliterates the rete tips, resulting in a characteristic quadrangular-shaped or flat-bottomed rete, associated with collections of apoptotic keratinocytes (colloid bodies) at the base of the rete ridges. Colloid bodies

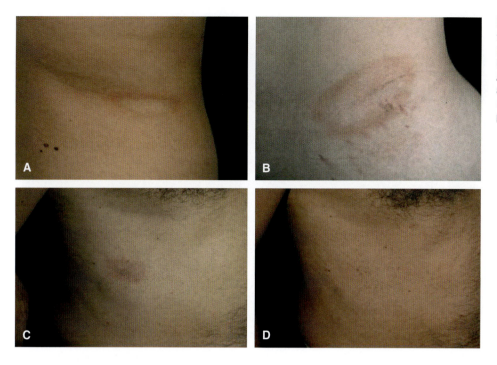

FIGURE 56-1. A–D. Annular erythematous plaques with central clearing and raised borders. (Reprinted from Cesinaro AM, Sighinolfi P, Greco A, et al. Annular lichenoid dermatosis of youth ... and beyond: a series of 6 cases. *Am J Dermatopathol.* 2009;31:263-267, with permission.)

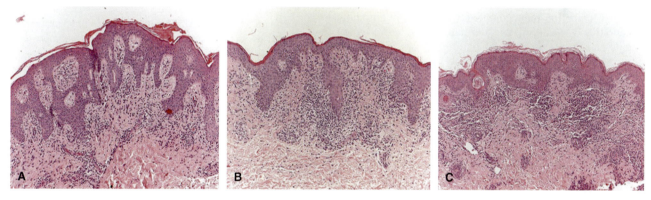

FIGURE 56-2. Lichenoid lymphocytic infiltrate with basal vacuolization in three different cases (**A–C**) (hematoxylin and eosin, 100×). (Reprinted from Cesinaro AM, Sighinolfi P, Greco A, et al. Annular lichenoid dermatosis of youth ... and beyond: a series of 6 cases. *Am J Dermatopathol.* 2009;31:263-267, with permission.)

are typical but usually not as numerous as in lichen planus. Intraepidermal lymphocytes lack cytologic atypia. Pautrier microabscesses are absent. Admixed dermal histiocytes and superficial dermal edema might be seen. Some cases can resemble lichen planus.[3]

IMMUNOHISTOCHEMISTRY

Both CD4- and CD8-predominant lichenoid infiltrates had been described.[1,4,7-9,12,14-16] CD8+ cases might express cytotoxic markers such as TIA-1 (Fig. 56-3). CD1a highlights aggregates of epidermal Langerhans cells. Expression of pan–T-cell antigens (CD2, CD3, CD5, and CD7) is preserved.

GENETICS/MOLECULAR FINDINGS

None of the cases revealed clonal rearrangement of the T-cell receptor (TCR) gene.[7]

DIFFERENTIAL DIAGNOSIS

Differentiation from hypopigmented MF and vitiligo can be challenging. In both entities, there is an infiltrate of CD8+ lymphoid cells, along with decreased number of melanocytes at the dermal-epidermal junction. It is believed that the cytotoxic effect of T cells results in a decrease in CD117 expression leading to dysfunction and loss of melanocytes.[17] Only few cases of "annular MF" have been reported in children.[18-20] Lymphocytes in MF exhibit cytologic and immunophenotypic atypia, tag along the dermal-epidermal junction, and show clonal TCR rearrangement, features that are absent in ALDY. In addition, papillary dermal fibroplasia is seen in 97% of adult and 42% of pediatric MF cases but not in ALDY.[21] Acanthosis is not characteristic for pediatric MF cases. More recently, Hodak et al[22] have shown that pediatric hypopigmented MF is typically accompanied by folliculotropism and keratosis pilaris–like lesions, features not seen in ALDY.

In vitiligo, the epidermis tends to be atrophic rather than acanthotic and the lichenoid infiltrate is diffuse along the

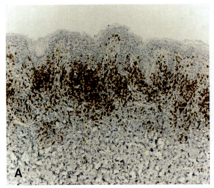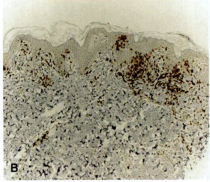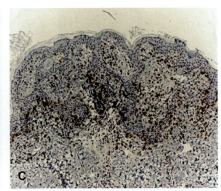

FIGURE 56-3. CD8+ lymphocytic infiltrate obscuring the dermal-epidermal junction in three different cases (**A–C**) of ALDY (100×). (Reprinted from Cesinaro AM, Sighinolfi P, Greco A, et al. Annular lichenoid dermatosis of youth ... and beyond: a series of 6 cases. *Am J Dermatopathol.* 2009;31:263-267, with permission.)

basal layer and not confined to the rete as seen in ALDY. Melanocytes are not affected in ALDY, whereas they are absent in vitiligo.

Histologic findings of thickened dermal collagen bundles are pathognomonic for morphea, a potential clinical mimic of ALDY. Early phase of LSA can also show prominent lichenoid infiltrates. The presence of plasma cells and predilection for genital skin help in differentiating LSA from ALDY. Medication-induced annular erythema might show lichenoid and granulomatous dermatitis.[23] Pediatric lichen planus can rarely show annular morphology.[24] Lichenoid infiltrates in lichen planus are diffusely distributed along the dermal-epidermal junction. Annular lesions in lichen planus actinicus, a variant of lichen planus,[25] often affect sun-exposed areas, typically the face and neck.[26-28] Its histologic features are similar to those of classic lichen planus including hypergranulosis, acanthosis with a sawtooth pattern, hyperorthokeratosis, and civatte bodies.

Other clinically annular lesions such as tinea, erythema annulare centrifugum, and erythema chronicum migrans should be readily distinguishable from ALDY by routine histology.

CAPSULE SUMMARY

- ALDY is a clinicopathologic entity originally described in children and young adults. Cases in older individuals had been reported.
- **Clinical:** The lesions present as asymptomatic erythematous macules and annular patches with a red-brownish border and central hypopigmentation, mostly distributed on the groin and flanks.
- **Histology:** Peculiar lichenoid pattern with
  - massive dyskeratosis limited to the tips of rete ridges.
  - lack of lymphocytic atypia, epidermotropism, or dermal sclerosis.
- **Immunohistochemistry:** CD4+ or CD8+ T cells with preserved pan–T-cell antigens; few B cells and macrophages.
- **Genetics/molecular findings**: Polyclonal T-cell rearrangement.
- **Differential diagnosis:** Morphea, MF, and annular erythema.

References

1. Cesinaro AM, Sighinolfi P, Greco A, et al. Annular lichenoid dermatitis of youth ... and beyond: a series of 6 cases. *Am J Dermatopathol.* 2009;31(3):263-267.
2. Mahmoudi H, Ghanadan A, Fahim S, Moghanlou S, Etesami I, Daneshpazhooh M. Annular lichenoid dermatitis of youth: report on two adult cases and one child. *J Dtsch Dermatol Ges.* 2019;17(11):1173-1176.
3. Cesinaro AM. Annular lichenoid dermatitis (of youth): report of a case with lichen planus-like features. *Am J Dermatopathol.* 2017;39(12):914-915.
4. Annessi G, Paradisi M, Angelo C, et al. Annular lichenoid dermatitis of youth. *J Am Acad Dermatol.* 2003;49(6):1029-1036.
5. Di Mercurio M, Gisondi P, Colato C, et al. Annular lichenoid dermatitis of youth: report of six new cases with review of the literature. *Dermatology.* 2015;231(3):195-200.
6. de la Torre C, Flórez A, Fernandez-Redondo V. Negative results of patch testing with standard and textile series in a case of annular lichenoid dermatitis of youth. *J Am Acad Dermatol.* 2005;53(1):172-173.
7. Kazlouskaya V, Trager JD, Junkins-Hopkins JM. Annular lichenoid dermatitis of youth: a separate entity or on the spectrum of mycosis fungoides? Case report and review of the literature. *J Cutan Pathol.* 2015;42(6):420-426.
8. Kleikamp S, Kutzner H, Frosch PJ. Annular lichenoid dermatitis of youth—a further case in a 12-year-old girl. *J Dtsch Dermatol Ges.* 2008;6(8):653-656.
9. Sans V, Leaute-Labreze C, Vergier B, et al. A further case of annular lichenoid dermatitis of youth: role of the anti-hepatitis B immunization? *Pediatr Dermatol.* 2008;25(5):577-579.
10. Annessi G, Annessi E. Annular lichenoid dermatitis (of youth). *Dermatopathology (Basel).* 2022;9(1):23-31. doi:10.3390/dermatopathology9010004
11. Wilk M, Zelger BG, Emberger M, Zelger B. Annular lichenoid dermatitis (of youth) immunohistochemical and serological evidence for another clinical presentation of Borrelia infection in patients of western Austria. *Am J Dermatopathol.* 2017;39(3):177-180. doi:10.1097/DAD.0000000000000621
12. Tsoitis G, Kanitakis J, Kyamidis K, et al. Annular lichenoid dermatosis of youth. *J Eur Acad Dermatol Venereol.* 2009;23(11):1339-1340.
13. Oiso N, Kawada A. Erythema dyschronicum perstans with both a macular lesion and a linear lesion following the lines of Blaschko. *J Dermatol.* 2013;40(2):127-128.

14. Durdu M, Akyilmaz M, Tuncer I. Annular lichenoid dermatitis of youth. *Pediatr Dermatol*. 2007;24(5):582-584.
15. Huh W, Kanitakis J. Annular lichenoid dermatosis of youth: report of the first Japanese case and published work review. *J Dermatol*. 2010;37(6):531-533.
16. Leger MC, Gonzalez ME, Meehan S, et al. Annular lichenoid dermatitis of youth in an American boy. *J Am Acad Dermatol*. 2013;68(5):e155-e156.
17. Singh ZN, Tretiakova MS, Shea CR, et al. Decreased CD117 expression in hypopigmented mycosis fungoides correlates with hypomelanosis: lessons learned from vitiligo. *Mod Pathol*. 2006;19(9):1255-1260.
18. Zackheim HS, McCalmont TH. Mycosis fungoides: the great imitator. *J Am Acad Dermatol*. 2002;47(6):914-918.
19. Crowley JJ, Nikko A, Varghese A, et al. Mycosis fungoides in young patients: clinical characteristics and outcome. *J Am Acad Dermatol*. 1998;38(5 pt 1):696-701.
20. Cogrel O, Boralevi F, Lepreux S, et al. Lymphomatoid annular erythema: a new form of juvenile mycosis fungoides. *Br J Dermatol*. 2005;152:565-566.
21. Castano E, Glick S, Wolgast L, et al. Hypopigmented mycosis fungoides in childhood and adolescence: a long-term retrospective study. *J Cutan Pathol*. 2013;40(11):924-934.
22. Hodak E, Amitay-Laish I, Feinmesser M, et al. Juvenile mycosis fungoides: cutaneous T-cell lymphoma with frequent follicular involvement. *J Am Acad Dermatol*. 2014;70(6):993-1001.
23. Magro CM, Crowson AN. Lichenoid and granulomatous dermatitis. *Int J Dermatol*. 2000;39(2):126-133.
24. Pandhi D, Singal A, Bhattacharya SN. Lichen planus in childhood: a series of 316 patients. *Pediatr Dermatol*. 2014;31(1):59-67.
25. Bouassida S, Boudaya S, Turki H, et al. Actinic lichen planus: 32 cases. [Article in French]. *Ann Dermatol Venereol*. 1998;125(6/7):408-413.
26. Salman SM, Kibbi AG, Zaynoun S. Actinic lichen planus. A clinicopathologic study of 16 patients. *J Am Acad Dermatol*. 1989;20(2 pt 1):226-231.
27. Dammak A, Masmoudi A, Boudaya S, et al. Childhood actinic lichen planus (6 cases) [Article in French]. *Arch Pediatr*. 2008;15(2):111-114.
28. Denguezli M, Nouira R, Jomaa B. Actinic lichen planus. An anatomoclinical study of 10 Tunisian cases. [Article in French]. *Ann Dermatol Venereol*. 1994;121(8):543-546.

CHAPTER 57

Eosinophilic dermatosis of hematologic malignancy

Joya Sahu and Jason B. Lee

INTRODUCTION

Eosinophilic dermatosis may be encountered in the setting of various hematologic malignancies and hematologic disorders, including blood dyscrasias and myelodysplastic syndromes. Eosinophilic dermatosis has been most frequently described in association with chronic lymphocytic leukemia (CLL). Previously designated as insect bite–like reaction and eosinophilic dermatosis of myeloproliferative disease, this rare and refractory dermatosis presents as a pruritic, papulovesicular eruption associated with an eosinophil-rich infiltrate on biopsy. Although clinical and histopathologic features may be indistinguishable from insect bites, affected patients often have no history of them. The rarity of this condition and the conditions that simulate eosinophilic dermatosis of hematologic malignancy (EDHM) present a diagnostic and therapeutic challenge.

A variety of cutaneous eruptions have been reported in CLL, one of the most common hematologic malignancies. These have been classified as either "specific" or "nonspecific" lesions. Cutaneous leukemic cell infiltration or leukemia cutis is a specific type of manifestation confirmed histologically and presents clinically as violaceous or reddish-brown papules or nodules in 8.3% of patients with CLL. Nonspecific refers to nonmetastatic, secondary lesions that can be of infectious, hemorrhagic, or hypersensitive origin.[1,2] Forty-five percent of patients with CLL will experience a nonspecific dermatosis, including petechiae, purpura, urticaria, erythema multiforme, exfoliative dermatitis, paraneoplastic pemphigus, vasculitis, and eosinophilic dermatosis.[1-5] EDHM or insect bite–like reaction is a rare cutaneous eruption reported most often in patients with CLL presenting as a papulovesicular eruption, clinically and histopathologically mimicking insect bites and other eosinophil-rich dermatoses.[3,5-7] EDHM has been described in other hematologic malignancies, primarily in patients with B-cell hematologic malignancies such as mantle cell lymphoma, acute lymphoblastic leukemia, and large cell lymphoma, as well as in acute monocytic leukemia and myelofibrosis.[3,8-11] It is now increasingly accepted that this entity can also be seen in patients with blood dyscrasias as well as myelodysplastic syndromes, and as such, EDHM remains a suitable, all-encompassing term.

HISTORICAL PERSPECTIVE

EDHM was first conceptualized by Weed[12] in 1965 as an insect bite–like reaction observed in patients with CLL. Although initially thought to be a specific hypersensitivity reaction to insect bites, particularly mosquitoes,[12-14] most patients with CLL deny a history of insect bites, and thus the term "insect bite–like reaction" was coined.[3] Byrd et al[15] further defined this process as "eosinophilic dermatosis of myeloproliferative disease" and proposed defining criteria: (a) pruritic papules, nodules, and/or vesiculobullous eruption refractory to standard treatment; (b) eosinophil-rich superficial and deep dermal lymphohistiocytic infiltrate on histopathology; (c) exclusion of other causes of tissue eosinophilia; and (d) diagnosis of hematologic malignancy. Although still believed to be underreported and underrecognized, EDHM is now increasingly recognized as over 200 cases have been reported in the literature.[7,16]

EPIDEMIOLOGY

Although limited, most case reports and series of EDHM generally corroborate these clinical, histopathologic, and immunologic criteria. Patients with CLL tend to present with EDHM in the fifth to seventh decade of life. Eruptions occur concurrently or months to years after CLL diagnosis, but on occasion EDHM can precede CLL diagnosis. EDHM most frequently presents as pruritic papules, nodules, and vesicles/bullae resembling insect bites occurring on both exposed and nonexposed areas of the body including the face, trunk, and extremities (Figs. 57-1–57-3). Lesions are often indurated, erythematous, and may be tender.[1,3,6-8,17-22] No discernible relationship with outdoor activity or seasonal changes can be identified, and a history of insect bites cannot be elicited.[3,6,7,17,19]

HISTOLOGY

In EDHM, increased numbers of eosinophils are seen in association with a superficial and/or deep perivascular lymphocytic infiltrate, which may have both a concurrent interstitial

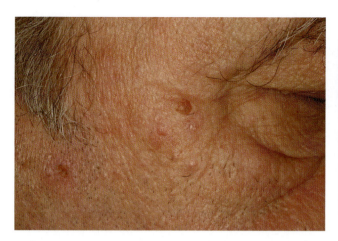

FIGURE 57-1. Excoriated, edematous, erythematous papules on the face.

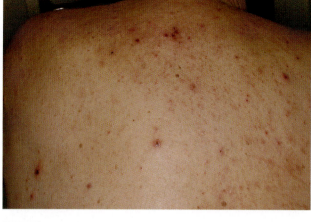

FIGURE 57-3. Numerous intact erythematous papules and excoriated papules on the upper back.

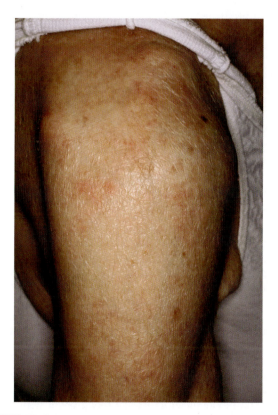

FIGURE 57-2. Multiple erythematous urticarial papules and plaques on the shoulder and arm.

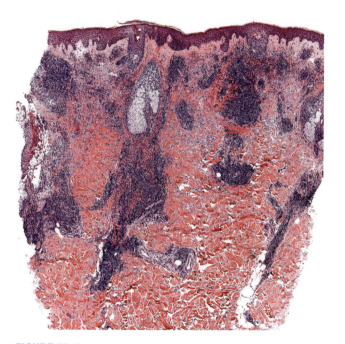

FIGURE 57-4. Dense perivascular and periadnexal and interstitial infiltrate of inflammatory cells with perifollicular involvement (40×).

lymphocytic component and prominent adnexal and hair follicle involvement (Figs. 57-4, 57-5). Papillary dermal edema, eosinophilic spongiosis, a wedge-shaped infiltrate, and follicular mucinosis of involved hair follicle units can commonly be found (Fig. 57-6). These features often lead to the misdiagnosis of insect bite reaction or eosinophilic folliculitis. The presence of excoriation or ulceration compounds diagnostic confusion owing to the additional presence of neutrophils.

Indicative of a reactive process, the often-dense lymphoid infiltrate in EDHM is composed of either mixed T and B cells[6] or largely T cells that are CD3+, CD43+, and CD45RO+. Recapitulation of germinal centers by these nodular lymphoid aggregates may be seen.[3,15,21] Immunohistochemical staining confirms an infiltrate of primarily reactive T cells and an absence of leukemic cells, demonstrating that EDHM is a hypersensitivity reaction rich in T cells and eosinophils.[2]

Both eosinophilic spongiosis and eosinophilic panniculitis have been reported.[3,6,7,19,23-25] Extensive intraepidermal or subepidermal edema may result in vesicles or bullae.[3,6,7,17,19,23,26] Some of the reported blistering dermatoses associated with CLL may indeed represent an actual exaggerated response to insect bites.[1,3,5,6]

DIFFERENTIAL DIAGNOSIS

EDHM is often a refractory diagnosis of exclusion. Clinical mimickers of EDHM include leukemia cutis, scabies, drug eruption, insect-bite reaction, papular urticaria, urticarial

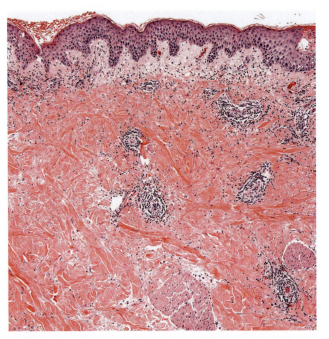

FIGURE 57-5. Papillary dermal edema, perivascular lymphocytes, and numerous eosinophils interstitially (100×).

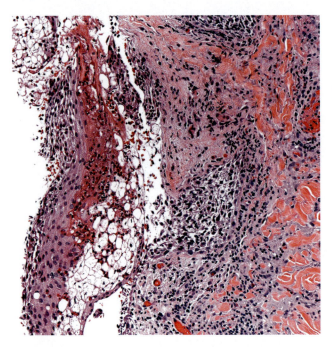

FIGURE 57-6. Numerous eosinophils infiltrating the follicular epithelium and sebaceous gland.

stage of bullous pemphigoid, dermatitis herpetiformis, eosinophilic folliculitis, and Wells syndrome requiring systematic exclusion. Leukemia cutis can be confirmed by immunohistochemical staining[3] and by the morphologic character of the immature infiltrate of blasts. Flow cytometry and immunoglobulin heavy chain (IgH) gene PCR analysis are useful adjunctive tests. Scabies infestation, drug eruption, insect bite reaction, and papular urticaria may be excluded clinically. Patients often receive treatment with courses of antiscabetic therapy or antibiotics prior to being diagnosed with EDHM. Drug eruptions are a common perceived culprit while bullous lesions may warrant elimination of autoimmune blistering disorders. In EDHM, occasional flame figures may be encountered, invoking Wells syndrome.[6,27]

When incidental follicle involvement is seen in EDHM, diagnostic difficulty abounds as identical histopathologic features are encountered in follicular mucinosis and eosinophilic folliculitis.[26,28] Often, the predisposition of lesions to present on the head and neck areas may clinically mimic eosinophilic folliculitis, acne, or rosacea. The presence of a dense perivascular, perieccrine, interstitial infiltrate in addition to follicle involvement is indicative of folliculitis being a secondary phenomenon, not a primary event. The clinical presence of nonfollicular lesions further supports the diagnosis of EDHM over other follicular-based diseases. Even in HIV-associated eosinophilic folliculitis, an analogous hypersensitivity phenomenon with a similar clinical presentation, it is unclear whether the folliculitis is the primary or an incidental event.[29-31] Diagnostic clues from the past medical history, disease course, and laboratory findings can be used to differentiate between the two entities. HIV-associated eosinophilic folliculitis is accompanied by a decreased $CD4^+$ T-cell count and lymphopenia associated with peripheral blood eosinophilia, and also tends to improve with highly active antiretroviral therapy.[29] In EDHM, these laboratory abnormalities are infrequent.[3,6,10,24] Diagnosis of EDHM ultimately depends on the correlation of clinical presentation, histopathological findings, laboratory results, and a high index of suspicion.

WORKUP

When considering EDHM, the authors recommend the following baseline workup and evaluation. After obtaining a detailed history of current illness, including presence of B symptoms, and medical history, a complete body skin examination including lymph node examination should be performed. A punch biopsy should be obtained from suspicious lesions, ideally in more than one representative site. To aid in evaluation of skin specimens, pertinent clinical history should accompany the biopsy specimen to allow an expert dermatopathologist to provide clinicopathologic correlation. Evaluation of the blood compartment with a baseline peripheral blood smear, complete blood count with differential, comprehensive metabolic panel, and flow cytometry of peripheral blood should be considered if a high index of clinical suspicion for an underlying hematologic malignancy exists. If any suspicious results are found, then referral to hematology-oncology is warranted. Serologic testing for HIV and bullous pemphigoid antigen may be indicated in certain situations.

TREATMENT

A variety of therapeutic modalities including antibiotics, topical and systemic steroids, antihistamines, dapsone, phototherapy, radiation, omalizumab, lenalidomide, interferon-α, intravenous immunoglobulin, rituximab, and even reinitiation of chemotherapy for the specific purpose of controlling the

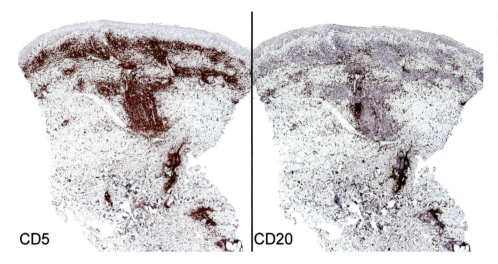

FIGURE 57-7. T cells (CD5+) make up the majority while B cells (CD20+) make up the minority of the infiltrate in EDHM.

eruption have been tried, often with dismal results.[3,6,7,23,32-35] Although there is an initial high response rate, particularly to systemic steroids, relapse is the usual course once the patient is off the medication.[7] Frequently, EDHM is extremely refractory, persistent, or recurrent despite clinical remission of the hematologic malignancy. This underscores the incomplete understanding regarding the pathogenesis of EDHM and the lack of targeted specific therapy. Dupilumab, IL-4 receptor antagonist, offers a promising therapeutic option for recalcitrant cases of EHDM as it inhibits IL-4 and IL-13 signaling pathway leading to the downregulation of the T_H2 immune response, including eosinophil-mediated inflammatory response.[36,37]

PROGNOSIS

EDHM may be associated with a more aggressive CLL-disease course. Review of the literature reveals reports of Richter transformation, malignant clone expansion, and other fatal complications in patients with CLL and EDHM eruptions.[3,6] Accelerated course with worse outcomes has not been consistently reported. In the largest series of patients with EDHM, the clinical course was no different than expected.[7] Patients with hematologic malignancies and other immunosuppressed states tend to present with atypical and recalcitrant cutaneous disorders, reflective of their immune status.[31] More outcome data are needed to determine whether patients with EDHM have a worse prognosis compared with those who do not.

PATHOGENESIS

The pathogenesis of EDHM in patients with CLL is poorly understood. An altered immunologic response has been ascribed to underlying malignancy,[38] resulting in an eosinophil-rich eruption that reflects a T_H2 chemokine milieu, with IL-5, the major eosinophil-recruiting cytokine, playing an important function in eosinophil recruitment. The role of underlying immune dysregulation in the pathogenesis of EDHM is further corroborated by reports of a similar papular eruption in patients with HIV.[39-41] Lesional eosinophils have been shown to survive longer in culture, suggestive of a predominance of cytokines upregulating eosinophilic function, including IL-3, IL-4, and IL-5.[6] Overproduction of IL-4 and IL-5 may concurrently promote proliferation of neoplastic B cells while stimulating eosinophils.[3,5] EDHM in patients with CLL is best characterized as a reactive process, but it is still possible that neoplastic B cells galvanize these eruptions.[3] Of note, most malignancies associated with a bite-like reaction are B-cell derived, indicating that similar immunologic alterations may directly augment both malignant B-cell proliferation and the insect bite–like hypersensitivity eruption.[3,42] The B cells present in the lesions of EDHM make up a small percentage of the infiltrate while the T cells make up the majority. It is believed that these B cells within the infiltrate, which are frequently the neoplastic leukemic cells, play a pathogenetic role in EDHM (Fig. 57-7).[43] While EDHM is considered to be a nonspecific eruption in patients with CLL, the consistent presence of leukemic B cells within the infiltrate lends support of reclassification of the eruption as a specific one.

The designation *EDHM* rather than *insect bite–like reaction* or *eosinophilic dermatosis of myeloproliferative disease* is a better descriptor of the pathologic process that encompasses the various hematologic malignancies and disorders. Additional nomenclature has been proposed and may change once the exact pathogenesis of the eruption is elucidated.[7,44] In the setting of hematologic malignancies, especially CLL, EDHM should be considered when patients present with clinical and histopathologic findings of an eosinophil-rich dermatitis that resembles insect bites, but with no history of them. Conversely, underlying hematologic disease should be appropriately excluded in patients who have clinical, laboratory, and biopsy findings suggestive of this process. Given the limited therapeutic options for EDHM, further investigation into more effective modalities is warranted.

References

1. Asakura K, Kizaki M, Ikeda Y. Exaggerated cutaneous response to mosquito bites in a patient with chronic lymphocytic leukemia. *Int J Hematol*. 2004;80(1):59-61.
2. Farber MJ, Forgia SL, Sahu J, et al. Eosinophilic dermatosis of hematologic malignancy. *J Cutan Pathol*. 2012;39(7):690-695.

3. Barzilai A, Shpiro D, Goldberg I, et al. Insect bite-like reaction in patients with hematologic malignant neoplasms. *Arch Dermatol.* 1999;135(12):1503-1507.
4. Epstein E, MacEachern K. Dermatologic manifestations of the lymphoblastoma-leukemia group. *Arch Intern Med.* 1937;60:867-875.
5. Robak E, Robak T. Skin lesions in chronic lymphocytic leukemia. *Leuk Lymphoma.* 2007;48(5):855-865.
6. Davis MD, Perniciaro C, Dahl PR, et al. Exaggerated arthropod-bite lesions in patients with chronic lymphocytic leukemia: a clinical, histopathologic, and immunopathologic study of eight patients. *J Am Acad Dermatol.* 1998;39(1):27-35.
7. Grandi V, Maglie R, Antiga E, et al. Eosinophilic dermatosis of hematologic malignancy: a retrospective cohort of 37 patients from an Italian center. *J Am Acad Dermatol.* 2019;81(1):246-249.
8. Khamayasi Z, Dodiuk-Gad RP, Weltfriend S, et al. Insect bite-like reaction associated with mantle cell lymphoma: clinicopathological, immunopathological, and molecular studies. *Am J Dermatopathol.* 2005;27(4):290-295.
9. Dodiuk-Gad RP, Dann EJ, Bergman R. Insect bite-like reaction associated with mantle cell lymphoma: a report of two cases and review of the literature. *Int J Dermatol.* 2004;43(10):754-758.
10. Kunitomi A, Konaka Y, Yagita M. Hypersensitivity to mosquito bites as a potential sign of mantle cell lymphoma. *Intern Med.* 2005;44(10):1097-1099.
11. Bottoni U, Mauro FR, Cozzani E, et al. Bullous lesions in chronic lymphocytic leukaemia: pemphigoid or insect bites? *Acta Derm Venerol.* 2006;86(1):74-76.
12. Weed RI. Exaggerated delayed hypersensitivity to mosquito bites in chronic lymphocytic leukemia. *Blood.* 1965;22:257-268.
13. Houston JG, Keene WR. Exaggerated delayed hypersensitivity to mosquito venom in association with lymphoproliferative disorders. *J Fla Med Assoc.* 1970;57(12):15-17.
14. Pederson J, Carganello J, Van-Der Weyden MB. Exaggerated reaction to insect bites in patients with chronic lymphocytic leukemia: clinical and histological findings. *Pathology.* 1990;22(3):141-143.
15. Byrd JA, Scherschun L, Chaffins ML, et al. Eosinophilic dermatosis of myeloproliferative disease: characterization of a unique eruption in patients with hematologic disorders. *Arch Dermatol.* 2001;137(10):1378-1380.
16. Cohen P. Hematologic-Related Malignancy-Induced Eosinophilic Dermatosis (He Remained): an eosinophilic dermatosis predominantly associated with chronic lymphocytic leukemia. *J Acad Am Acad Dermatol.* 2020;82(1):e13-e14.
17. Cocuroccia B, Gisondi P, Gubinelli E, et al. An itchy vesiculobullous eruption in a patient with chronic lymphocytic leukaemia. *Int J Clin Pract.* 2004;58(12):1177-1179.
18. Kolbusz RV, Micetich K, Armin AR, et al. Exaggerated response to insect bites: an unusual manifestation of chronic lymphocytic leukemia. *Int J Dermatol.* 1989;28(3):186-187.
19. Rosen LB, Frank BL, Rywlin AM. A characteristic vesiculobullous eruption in patients with chronic lymphocytic leukemia. *J Am Acad Dermatol.* 1986;15(5 pt 1):943-950.
20. Rodriguez-Lojo R, Almagro M, Pineyro F, et al. Eosinophilic panniculitis and insect bite-like eruption in a patient with chronic lymphocytic leukaemia: a spectrum of the same entity. *Dermatol Res Pract.* 2010;2010:263827.
21. Vassallo C, Passamonti F, Cananzi R, et al. Exaggerated insect bite-like reaction in patients affected by oncohaematological diseases. *Acta Derm Venereol.* 2005;85(1):76-77.
22. Walker F, Long D, James C, et al. Exaggerated insect bite reaction exacerbated by a pyogenic infection in a patient with chronic lymphocytic leukaemia. *Australas J Dermatol.* 2007;48(3):165-169.
23. Blum RR, Phelps RG, Wei H. Arthropod bites manifesting as recurrent bullae in a patient with chronic lymphocytic leukemia. *J Cutan Med Surg.* 2001;5:312-314.
24. Benmously R, Hammami H, Rouatbi M, et al. Insect bite-like reaction associated with the relapse of non-Hodgkin B-cell lymphoma. *Eur J Dermatol.* 2009;19(4):406-407.
25. Chassine AF, Dadban A, Charfi S, et al. Eosinophilic dermatosis associated with haematological disorders: a clinical, histopathological and immunohistochemical study of six observations. *Ann Dermatol Venerol.* 2010;137:181-188.
26. Rongioletti F, Rebora A. Follicular mucinosis in exaggerated arthropod-bite reactions of patients with chronic lymphocytic leukemia. *J Am Acad Dermatol.* 1999;41:500.
27. Melski JW. Wells' syndrome, insect bites, and eosinophils. *Dermatol Clin.* 1990;8:287-293.
28. Patrizi A, Chieregato C, Visani G, et al. Leukaemia-associated eosinophilic folliculitis (Ofuji's disease). *J Eur Acad Dermatol Venereol.* 2004;18:596-598.
29. Nervi SJ, Schwartz RA, Dmochowski M. Eosinophilic pustular folliculitis: a 40-year retrospect. *J Am Acad Dermatol.* 2006;55:285-289.
30. Basarab T, Jones RR. HIV-associated eosinophilic folliculitis: case report and review of the literature. *Br J Dermatol.* 1996;134:499-503.
31. Tschachler E, Bergstresser PR, Stingl G. HIV-related skin diseases. *Lancet.* 1996;348:659-663.
32. Ulmer A, Metzler G, Schanz S, et al. Dapsone in the management of "insect bite-like reaction" in a patient with chronic lymphocytic leukaemia. *Br J Dermatol.* 2007;156:172-174.
33. Lor M, Gates G, Yu Y. Eosinophilic dermatosis of hematologic malignancy effectively controlled with omalizumab maintenance therapy. *Dermatol Ther.* 2020;33(6):e14206.
34. Sato-Sano M, Teixeira SP, Vargas JC, et al. Lenalidomide in the management of eosinophilic dermatosis of hematological malignancy. *J Dermatol.* 2019;46(7):618-621.
35. Peringeth G, Sundaram S, Bogner P, Conroy E, Torka P. Successful use of venetoclax for treatment of eosinophilic dermatosis of myeloproliferative disease in a patient with chronic lymphocytic leukemia. *Ann Hematol.* 2020;99(5):1129-1131.
36. Jin A, Pousti BT, Savage KT, Mollanazar NK, Lee JB, Hsu S. Eosinophilic dermatosis of hematologic malignancy responding to dupilumab in a patient with chronic lymphocytic leukemia. *JAAD Case Rep.* 2019;5(9):815-817.
37. Goyal A, Lofgreen S, Mariash E, Bershow A, Gaddis KJ. Targeted inhibition of IL-4/13 with dupilumab is an effective treatment for eosinophilic dermatosis of hematologic malignancy. *Dermatol Ther.* 2020;33(4):e13725.
38. Agnew KL, Ruchlemer R, Catovsky D, et al. Cutaneous findings in chronic lymphocytic leukaemia. *Br J Dermatol.* 2004;150:1129-1135.
39. Hevia O, Jimenez-Acosta F, Ceballos PI, et al. Pruritic papular eruption of the acquired immunodeficiency syndrome: a clinicopathologic study. *J Am Acad Dermatol.* 1991;24:231-235.

40. Smith KJ, Skelton HGIII, Vogel P, et al. Exaggerated insect bite reactions in patients positive for HIV. *J Am Acad Dermatol*. 1993;29:269-272.
41. Sundharam JA. Pruritic skin eruption in the acquired immunodeficiency syndrome: arthropod bites [comment]? *Arch Dermatol*. 1990;126:539.
42. Mori T, Okamoto S, Kuramochi S, et al. An adult patient with hypersensitivity to mosquito bites developing mantle cell lymphoma. *Int J Hematol*. 2000;71:259-262.
43. Meiss F, Technau-Hafsi K, Kern JS, May AM. Eosinophilic dermatosis of hematologic malignancy: correlation of molecular characteristics of skin lesions and extracutaneous manifestations of hematologic malignancy. *J Cutan Pathol*. 2019;46(3):175-181.
44. Visseaux L, Durlach A, Barete S, et al. T-cell papulosis associated with B-cell malignancy: a distinctive clinicopathologic entity. *J Eur Acad Dermatol Venereol*. 2018;32(9):1469-1475.

PART IX: PRECURSOR LYMPHOID AND MYELOID NEOPLASMS

CHAPTER 58

Precursor B- and T-cell neoplasms

Alejandro A. Gru and Maxime Battistella

DEFINITION

Acute lymphoblastic leukemias/lymphomas (ALLs) are neoplasms of precursor lymphoid cells (lymphoblasts), committed to the B- or T-cell lineage (B-ALL or T-ALL). The main diagnostic criterion is the finding of at least 25% of leukemic small- to medium-sized blasts within the bone marrow or blood. Occasionally, the disease presents primarily in nodal or extra nodal sites, hence the term lymphoma.[1] Cases of T-ALL are frequently associated with a mediastinal mass (50%-65%).

EPIDEMIOLOGY

In the United States, the incidence of ALL is about 30 cases per million persons less than 20 years of age. The peak incidence occurs between the ages of 3 and 5 years. There is a slightly higher incidence in boys than in girls.[2] Approximately 80% to 85% of cases are B-ALL and 10% to 15%[3] are T-ALL.

ETIOLOGY

Although several genetic factors, including Down syndrome, are associated with increased risk of ALL,[2] most patients have no recognized inheritable factors. Genome-wide association studies have identified polymorphic variants in several genes (including *ARID5B*, *CEBPE*, *GATA3*, and *IKZF1*) that are associated with an increased risk of ALL or specific ALL subtypes.[4,5] Rare germline mutations in *PAX5*[6] and *ETV6*[7] are linked to familial ALL.[3] Few cases of B-ALL in the skin have been reported after COVID-19 infection. However, the overall prevalence of B-ALL has been shown to be lower since the start of the pandemic. Extramedullary blastic (B-ALL) transformation of chronic myeloid leukemia can occur with skin involvement.[8,9]

CLINICAL PRESENTATION AND PROGNOSIS

It is estimated that approximately 5% of B-ALL cases will have associated cutaneous dissemination. Over 100 cases of B-ALL have been reported in children with skin involvement.[10-13] Cutaneous extension by B-ALL does not appear to be associated with a worse prognosis.[14] The frequency of cutaneous involvement in T-ALL is less well documented. However, Lee et al reported an incidence of 4.3% in T-ALL and 15% in B-ALL.[15] Approximately 33% of patients with the lymphomatous variants had cutaneous involvement and only 1% in those with leukemic presentations. Cutaneous involvement by ALL presents as solitary (65%) or multiple (90%), firm, painless, and erythematous to bluish nodules with overlying telangiectasia. The lesions present typically in the head and neck (the scalp is the most common location), and sometimes in the trunk.[16,17] They range in size from 1 to 8 cm.[18] Millot et al[19] revealed cutaneous extension in 24 patients with ALL (*n* = 1359 children). In their study, 62% of patients had cutaneous lesions preceding the diagnosis of ALL. Bontoux et al only found that 31% of cases had cutaneous lesions preceding the hematologic diagnosis. Of interest, four patients had skin-limited disease. Multiple lesions were associated with high-risk ALL. Cutaneous aleukemic variants of ALL have been described,[20-25] including the presence of isolated forms confined to the skin without progression to systemic disease.[18-26]

Rare cutaneous presentations include generalized purpuric maculopapular eruption in association with T-ALL,[27,28] limited involvement in the breasts and skin in T-ALL,[23,29] facial nerve palsy,[30] numb chin syndrome in B-ALL,[31] a nodule at a site of a catheter insertion on a patient with a previous diagnosis of B-ALL,[32] and intraocular and cutaneous lesions.[33] Some cases of ALL with associated leukemia cutis could be congenital in nature.[34] We have also documented the occurrence of T-ALL presenting as a viral-exanthem-like rash[35] (Fig. 58.1).

The patient's age and initial white blood cell (WBC) count are predictive of outcome, with older age or a higher

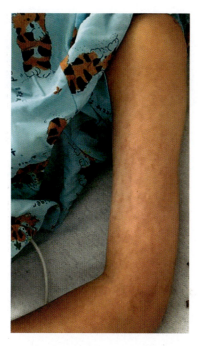

FIGURE 58-1. Lesions are also present in the proximal arm. (From Kwock JM, Kurpiel B, Gru AA. T-cell lymphoblastic lymphoma/leukemia presenting as a diffuse viral exanthem-like reaction: a clinical and histopathological challenge. *Am J Dermatopathol.* 2020;42(12):986-988.)

WBC count portending a worse prognosis. Another study found that age > 18 and cutaneous relapse were independent predictors of outcome. The current consensus defines "standard risk" (age 1-9.99 years and initial WBC < 50,000/mm³) and "high-risk" (age > 10, initial WBC > 50,000/mm³, or both) ALL subgroups comprising, respectively, two-thirds and one-third of children with B-ALL.[2] Supradiaphragmatic lymphadenopathy and involvement of the central nervous system and testis are also common. T-ALL patients, compared to those with B-ALL, are younger and have a higher rate of mediastinal tumors and bone marrow involvement. Patients are usually males in their teens to 20s and present with lymphadenopathy in cervical, supraclavicular, and axillary regions (50%), or with a mediastinal mass (50%-75%). In most patients, the mediastinal mass is anterior, bulky, and associated with pleural effusions, superior vena cava syndrome, tracheal obstruction, and pericardial effusions. Bone pain is also typical in cases with bone marrow involvement.

The prognosis in ALL has changed substantially over the last 30 to 40 years. With contemporary systemic chemotherapeutic regimens, CAR-T cell therapies, and the use of craniospinal or cranial irradiation and intrathecal chemotherapy,[2] the overall survival rates are 90% at 5 years.

HISTOPATHOLOGY

The histopathologic findings for both B- and T-ALL are identical.[13,18] There is a heavy nodular or diffuse monomorphous infiltrate in the dermis and adipose tissue that spares the epidermis with a grenz zone (Figs. 58-1–58-4). The infiltrate typically shows a "cobblestone" or "starry sky" pattern and is composed of small- to medium-sized mononuclear cells, with fine chromatin, scant cytoplasm, and variable nucleoli. Areas with a "single-file" pattern can also be seen, reminiscent to the findings present in lobular carcinomas of the breast. Mitotic figures and apoptotic cells are frequently seen. Skin ulceration has been reported rarely. Necrosis can also be present.[11] Focal infiltration of the skin adnexa, peripheral nerves, and adjacent muscles can be seen in some cases. In certain other cases, extensive crushed artifact and poor viability of the tumor cells can be seen, indicating the high turnover of the malignant cells.[36] The rare coexistence of ALL with a basal cell carcinoma[37] and kaposiform hemangioendothelioma[38] has been described.

IMMUNOPHENOTYPE

T-ALL (Figs. 58-4 and 58-5) blasts are positive for terminal deoxynucleotidyl transferase (TdT) with variable expression of CD45, CD34, CD1a, CD10, CD2, cCD3 (lineage specific), CD4, CD5, CD7, and CD8. CD4/CD8 coexpression is most frequently observed; however, coexpression is not necessarily a marker of an immature phenotype as cases of dual-positive mature T-cell lymphomas had been described. The most reliable markers to confirm an immature phenotype include TdT, CD1a, CD99, and CD34.[39] We have recently identified a case of T-ALL in association with a γδ phenotype of T-cell receptor (TCR), potentially mimicking a cutaneous γδ T-cell lymphoma (Fig. 58-6). According to the expression of specific markers, T-ALL can be subdivided into early or pro-T, pre-T, cortical-T, and medullary-T.

B-ALL is associated with expression of CD19, CD79a, CD22, PAX-5, TdT, CD10, BCL-2, and CD99. CD34 and CD20 show variable expression (see Fig. 58-2). CD45 is typically negative. Expression of surface immunoglobulins is usually absent, but the more mature stages can show expression of Ig.[1,3] Certain immunophenotypic findings are associated with characteristic cytogenetic aberrations. For example, expression of CD13, CD33, CD19, CD10, and most often CD34 is associated with rearrangement of the *TEL (ETV6)* gene, typically t(12; 21) (p13; q21) creating an *ETV6::RUNX1* fusion gene. Cases with *KMT2A* translocations, especially t(4; 11), usually display CD19⁺, CD10⁻, CD24⁻ (ie, pro-B immunophenotype), and are positive for CD15. Precursor B-ALLs with t(9; 22) (q34; q11.2) are typically CD10⁺, CD19⁺, and TdT⁺, and they frequently express myeloid antigens such as CD13 and CD33. In this subset, CD25 is highly associated, at least in adults.[3] Rare cases of biphenotypic ALL (CD3 and CD19⁺) have been described in the skin.[40]

Early T precursor lymphoblastic leukemia/lymphoma (ETP-ALL) is a neoplasm composed of blasts committed to the T-cell lineage with a unique immunophenotype that includes expression of stem cell markers and/or myeloid lineage markers. Patients typically present with bone marrow and peripheral blood involvement. Patients can present with lymph node involvement, a mediastinal mass, and sometimes CNS disease.[41-44] The ETP-ALL/LBL immunophenotype is defined as follows: (1) expression of cytoplasmic CD3; (2) absent (<5% positive blasts) CD1a and CD8 expression; (3) absent or dim (<75% positive blasts) CD5 expression; and (4) expression (≥25% positive blasts) of 1 or more myeloid (CD11b, CD13, CD33, CD65, CD117) and/or stem cell (CD34, HLA-DR) markers. The expression of CD123 has also been reported.[43,45,46]

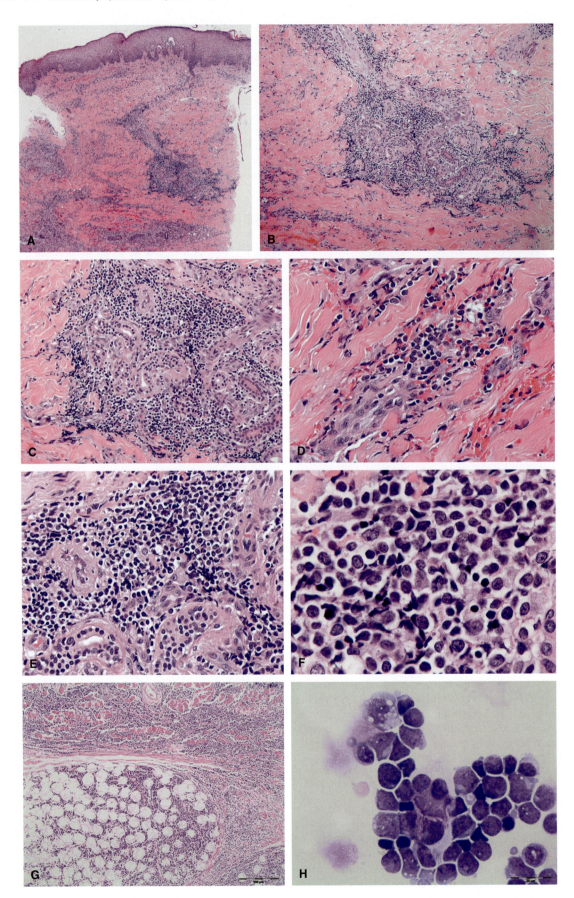

FIGURE 58-2. B-ALL. A. Diffuse dermal infiltrate sparing the epidermis (20×). **B** and **C.** Notable adnexotropism of the infiltrate is present (100× and 200×). **D.** Tumor cells dissect through the collagen fibers and form Indian files (400×). **E** and **F.** The malignant blasts are small to medium in size, and show fine nuclear chromatin (600× and 1000×). **G.** B-ALL with subcutaneous dissemination (100×). **H.** Touch preparation of B-ALL displaying the nuclear characteristics of the blasts. The cells have scant cytoplasm, prominent nucleoli, and occasional cytoplasmic vacuoles.

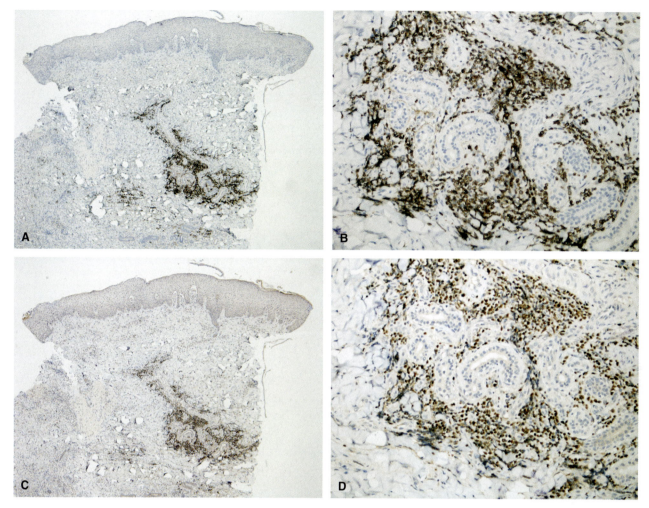

FIGURE 58-3. B-ALL—IHC. **A** and **B.** CD79a. **C** and **D.** TdT.

GENETIC AND MOLECULAR FINDINGS

In 25% to 30% of children with B-ALL, leukemic cells have hyperdiploidy (>50 chromosomes). This subtype is associated with excellent prognosis. Hypodiploidy (<44 chromosomes) occurs in 2% to 3% of children with B-ALL and is associated with a worse prognosis. Very low number of chromosomes is often a manifestation of Li-Fraumeni syndrome.[47]

Chromosomal translocations and intrachromosomal rearrangements are early, possibly initiating events in leukemogenesis. These are usually present in all the leukemic cells, are retained at relapse, and with additional genetic alterations can induce leukemia in experimental models.[2] Perhaps one of the most common translocations is the t(12; 21) (p13; q22) *ETV6::RUNX1* fusion, observed in about 25% of children with B-ALL. This translocation has a favorable prognosis with >90% survival at 5 years. The t(9; 22) (q34; q11.2) *BCR::ABL1* translocation is seen in 25% of adult B-ALL, but only 2% to 4% of pediatric ALLs. In both children and adults, the Philadelphia + B-ALL is the one associated with the worst prognosis of ALLs. In children, most cases are associated with the production of a bcr-abl protein of p190 kd. In adults, 50% of cases show the p190 kd and the other 50% the p210 kd, associated with cases of chronic myelogenous leukemia.[1] The p210 isoform is associated with responses to tyrosine kinase inhibitors (eg, imatinib, etc.), whereas the p190 isoform is more resistant to such agents. The third important group of B-ALL translocated is associated with rearrangements of the *KMT2A* gene. *KMT2A*-rearranged B-ALL represents the most common type of acute leukemia in individuals less than 1 year. More than 70 different translocations target *KMT2A*, creating fusion proteins that mediate aberrant self-renewal of hematopoietic progenitors. *KMT2A*-rearranged leukemias have very few additional somatic mutations, particularly in infants.[48,49] B-ALLs with *KMT2A* translocation have an aggressive clinical behavior. Additionally, rearrangements of the *IGH* heavy chain occur in most cases of B-ALL. *MYC* rearrangements can also occur, even in association with cutaneous dissemination.[50] More recently, mutations of the *PAX-5* (35%) and *IKZF1* (15%) have been described,[2] typically in association with a worse outcome.

Two provisional categories have been included in the updated WHO classification in 2018: BCR-ABL1-like and B-ALL with iAMP21.[51] The upcoming WHO provisionally recognizes a number of recently identified entities having distinct clinical, phenotypic, and/or prognostic features described together under "other defined genetic abnormalities." These include *DUX4*,[52,53] *MEF2D*,[54] *ZNF384*, *NUTM1*, *MYC*[55-59] rearranged B-ALL, and *PAX5alt* and *PAX5 P80R*[60]

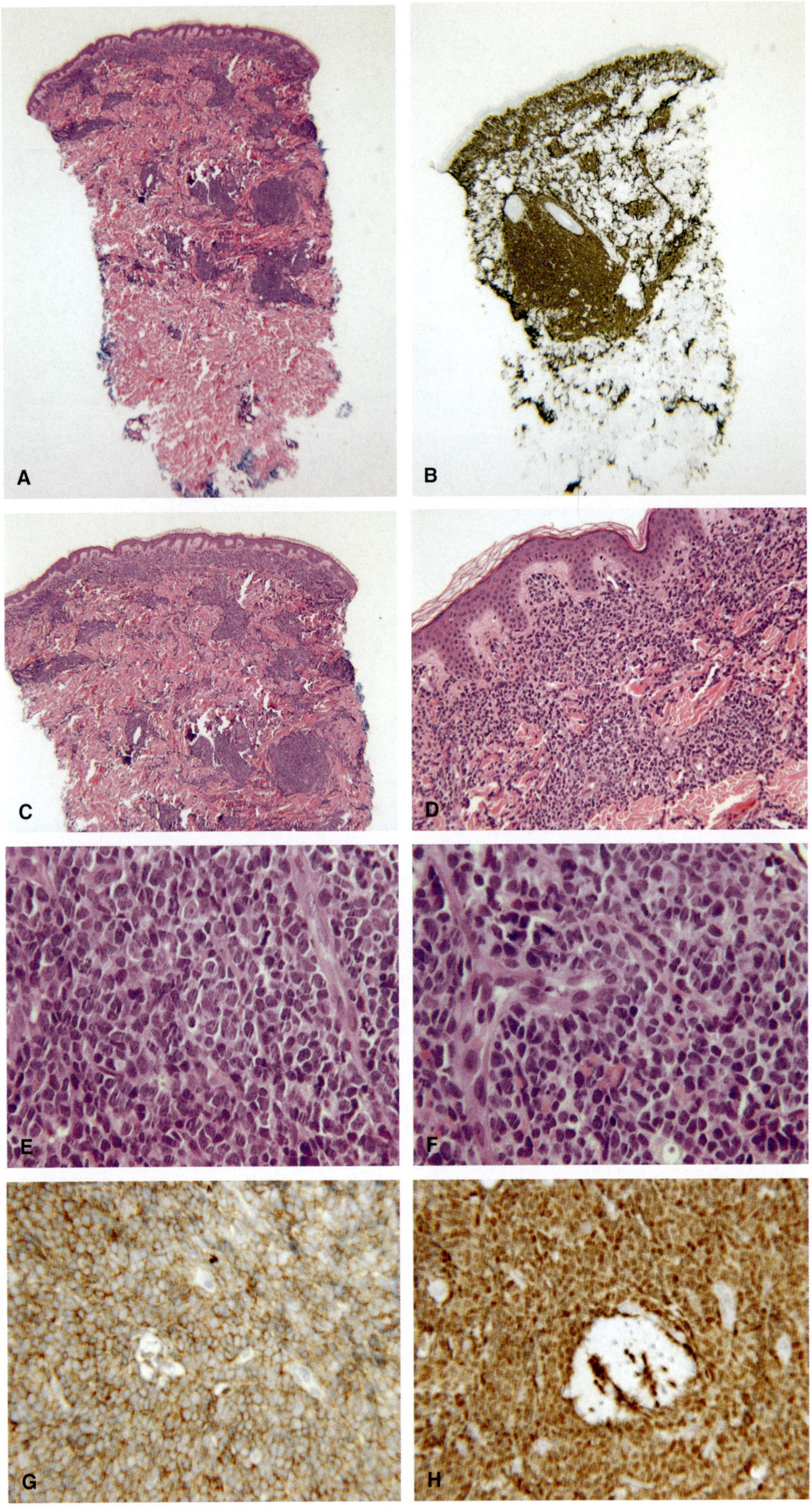

FIGURE 58-4. T-ALL. A. Nodular and diffuse infiltrate in the dermis (20×). **B.** The malignant cells are positive for CD3. **C** and **D.** A grenz zone is noted between the infiltrate and the epidermis (40× and 100×). **E** and **F.** The infiltrate is composed of small- to medium-sized blasts (400×). **G.** CD43. **H.** TdT.

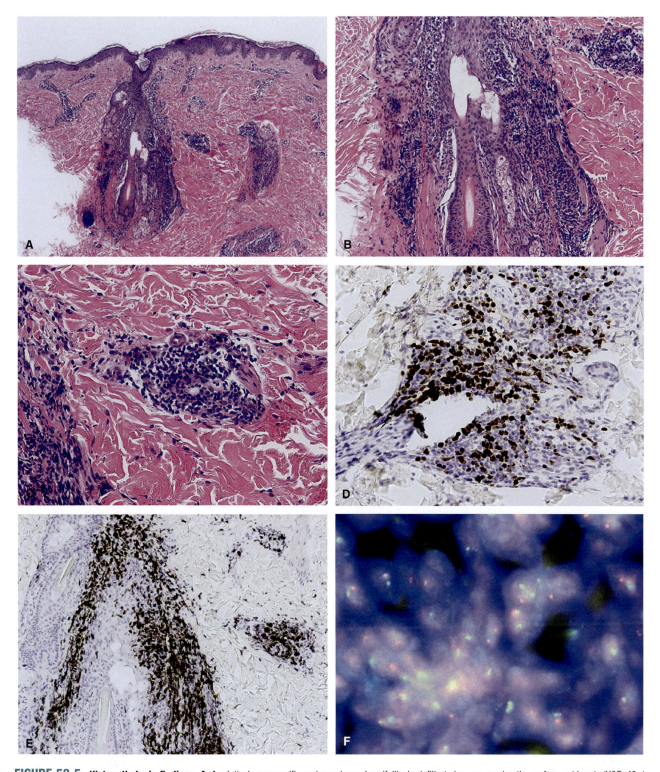

FIGURE 58-5. Histopathologic findings. A. A relatively nonspecific perivascular and perifollicular infiltrate is seen, sparing the surface epidermis (H&E, 40×); **(B)** a closer inspection shows some cells that appear to extend into the hair follicle epithelium (H&E, 200×); **(C)** the infiltrate shows extreme resemblance to "mature" lymphocytes, but crushed artifact is present at the edge of the image (H&E, 400×); the immature cells are positive for TdT **(D)** and CD3 **(E)**. **F.** Fluorescent in situ hybridization (FISH) studies using a double fusion probe for *BCR* (green) and *ABL* (red) genes display cells with loss of the *ABL* gene (red). The *NUP214* gene, similar to *ABL*, is located in the 9q34 region, a feature that can account for the findings seen by this molecular tool. (From Kwock JM, Kurpiel B, Gru AA. T-cell lymphoblastic lymphoma/leukemia presenting as a diffuse viral exanthem-like reaction: a clinical and histopathological challenge. *Am J Dermatopathol.* 2020;42(12):986-988.)

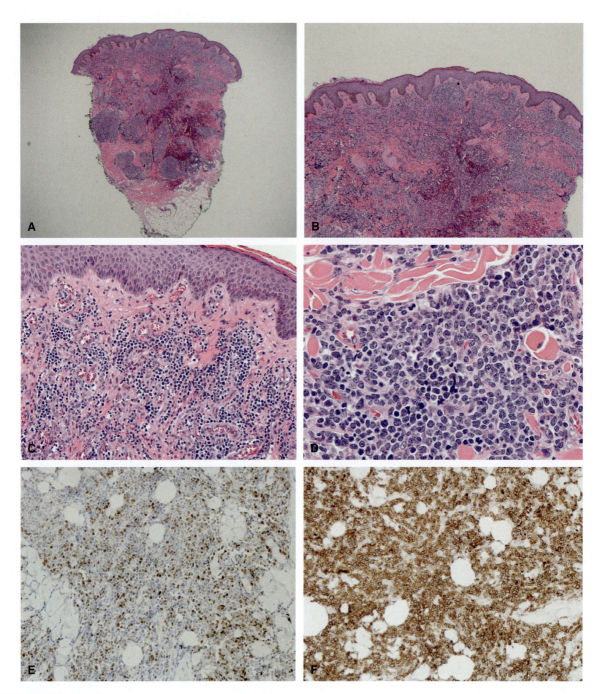

FIGURE 58-6. T-ALL with TCRγδ expression. **A** and **B.** Diffuse dermal-based infiltrate with a grenz zone sparing the epidermis (20× and 100×). **C** and **D.** Immature blasts are predominantly small, with fine chromatin and inconspicuous nucleoli. The cells show nuclear contour irregularities. The blasts are positive for TdT **(E)** and TCR-γ **(F)**.

abnormalities. The latter has a favorable outcome. A B-ALL with *ETV6::RUNX1*-like features is more frequent in childhood, representing 1% to 3% of B-ALL in this population, and uncommon in adults.[52,61]

The molecular background of T-ALL is less well understood. Cytogenetic abnormalities are frequent in T-ALL patients (50%-70%). The most common cytogenetic abnormalities involve 14q11 to 13 the site of TCRα/δ, including inv[16] (q11; q32) and deletions or translocations involving chromosomes 9, 10, and 11 corresponding to sites of TCR, α-, β-, and γ-subunit genes found in 47% of T-ALL. The most important is del(9p), resulting in loss of the tumor suppressor gene *CDKN2A* (an inhibitor of the cyclin-dependent kinase CDK4), which occurs at a frequency of about 30% by cytogenetics, and a greater frequency by molecular testing. Some cases can also present in association with myeloid hyperplasia, eosinophilia, and the t(8; 13) (p11; q11) aberration affecting the *FGFR1* gene. The latter has now been referred to as the 8p11 myeloproliferative disorder.[3,62] Similar to B-ALL, T-ALL is typically associated with rearrangements of the TCR. Activating mutations of the *NOTCH1* gene are present in more than 50% of cases.[63]

It has been proposed that T-ALL be divided into four distinct, nonoverlapping genetic subgroups based on specific translocations that lead to aberrant expression of (1) *TAL* or *LMO* genes, (2) *TLX1*, (3) *TLX3*, and (4) *HOXA* genes, resulting in arrest of T-cell maturation at distinct stages of thymocyte development.[64] The *TLX1* group appears to have a relatively favorable prognosis.[65] Another group, characterized by overexpression of *LYL1*, may correspond more closely to ETP-ALL.[64] More recently, eight subgroups of T-ALL were proposed based on genetic alterations and gene expression: *TAL1, TAL2, TLX1, TLX3, HOXA, LMO1/LMO2, LMO2/LYL1,* and *NKX2-1*.[66] In that study, the ETP-ALL cases commonly fit in the LMO2/LYL1 group.

POSTULATED CELL OF ORIGIN

B-ALL: Depending on the specific leukemia, B-ALL arises in a hematopoietic stem cell or immature precursor.
T-ALL: T-cell progenitor or thymic lymphocyte.

DIFFERENTIAL DIAGNOSIS

ALL is part of a spectrum of malignancies described as small, blue, round cell tumor. Because ALL is more typical in children than in adults, the differential diagnosis varies according to the age groups. In children, small, blue, round cell tumors include Ewing sarcoma/peripheral neuroectodermal tumor (EW/PNET), neuroblastoma, rhabdomyosarcoma, Wilm tumor, and lymphomas. Of particular importance is the distinction between EW/PNET and ALL. While CD99 was originally believed to be specific to EW, it was soon realized that the marker can be expressed in a wide variety of normal and neoplastic tissues.[67] Most cases of ALL are also positive for CD99.[68] In contrast to ALL cases, EW is negative for the lineage differentiation markers CD3, CD19, CD20, and CD79a. EW is also negative for the immaturity marker TdT. While very uncommon, cases of primary cutaneous EW have been reported.[69] Cutaneous rhabdomyosarcomas are easily distinguished on the basis of desmin, myogenin, muscle-specific actin, and MyoD1 expression. Additionally, rhabdomyosarcomas are negative for the lineage defining markers mentioned previously. Cutaneous neuroblastoma is also easily distinguished. A word of caution should be taken, given the fact that neuron-specific enolase expression (a marker typically positive in neuroblastoma) has been rarely reported in ALL.[11]

Similar to ALL, Burkitt lymphoma (BL) can frequently present in childhood. Histopathologically, both BL and ALL can show a "starry sky" pattern, typical of cases with high proliferation index. Although BL can rarely present in the skin, it is associated with a different immunophenotypic profile.[70,71] As opposed to ALL, BL lacks markers of immaturity (CD34, TdT, CD99, CD1a), shows strong expression of surface light chains, and is BCL-2 negative. Both ALL and BL can be CD10⁺. While *MYC* rearrangements are highly characteristic of BL, they have rarely been reported in ALL. The blastoid variant of mantle cell lymphoma (MCL) can also mimic a lymphoblastic process. However, MCL lacks the markers of immaturity and is CD5, cyclin D1, and SOX-11 positive. Another diagnostic category of lymphomas that can present in the skin of children is the ALK⁺ anaplastic large cell lymphoma (ALK⁺ ALCL). While most of them show high degrees of pleomorphism, the small cell variant can potentially mimic ALL. In counterpart, ALK⁺ ALCL is positive for CD30 and ALK1, while typically negative for the immaturity and lineage defining markers. Lastly, blastic plasmacytoid dendritic cell neoplasm (BPDCN) can also present in children and display a similar morphologic pattern. BPDCN shares with ALL the expression of TdT and sometimes CD123.[72,73] As opposed to ALL, BPDCN lacks expression of CD19, CD20, or CD3.

CAPSULE SUMMARY

- ALLs are neoplasms of precursor lymphoid cells (lymphoblasts), committed to the B- or T-cell lineage (B-ALL or T-ALL), and typically composed of small- to medium-sized blasts.
- It is estimated that 4.3% of T-ALL and 15% in B-ALL can show cutaneous dissemination. Approximately 33% of patients with the lymphomatous variants had cutaneous involvement and only 1% in those with leukemic presentations. Isolated cutaneous involvement can be the only manifestation of ALL.
- Most patients with T-ALL also have an accompanying mediastinal mass. Patients with B-ALL frequently have bone pain owing to bone marrow extension.
- It is important to recognize certain cytogenetic aberrations that are associated with worse prognosis, and those include the t(9; 22), MLL rearrangement, and hypodiploid variants.
- The histopathology of T- and B-ALL includes a heavy nodular or diffuse monomorphous infiltrate in the dermis and adipose tissue, which spares the epidermis with a grenz zone.
- Immunophenotypically, expression of the immaturity markers TdT and CD34 (B-ALL) and TdT, CD99, and CD1a (T-ALL) is characteristic of the disease.

References

1. Borowitz M, Chan JKC. *B Lymphoblastic Leukaemia/Lymphoma, Not Otherwise Specified*. International Agency for Research on Cancer; 2008.
2. Hunger SP, Mullighan CG. Acute lymphoblastic leukemia in children. *N Engl J Med.* 2015;373:1541-1552.
3. Cortelazzo S, Ponzoni M, Ferreri AJ, et al. Lymphoblastic lymphoma. *Crit Rev Oncol Hematol.* 2011;79:330-343.
4. Trevino LR, Yang W, French D, et al. Germline genomic variants associated with childhood acute lymphoblastic leukemia. *Nat Genet.* 2009;41:1001-1005.
5. Perez-Andreu V, Roberts KG, Harvey RC, et al. Inherited GATA3 variants are associated with Ph-like childhood acute lymphoblastic leukemia and risk of relapse. *Nat Genet.* 2013;45:1494-1498.
6. Shah S, Schrader KA, Waanders E, et al. A recurrent germline PAX5 mutation confers susceptibility to pre-B cell acute lymphoblastic leukemia. *Nat Genet.* 2013;45:1226-1231.
7. Zhang MY, Churpek JE, Keel SB, et al. Germline ETV6 mutations in familial thrombocytopenia and hematologic malignancy. *Nat Genet.* 2015;47:180-185.

8. Leclercq C, Toutain F, Baleydier F, et al. Pediatric acute B-cell lymphoblastic leukemia developing following recent SARS-CoV-2 infection. *J Pediatr Hematol Oncol.* 2021;43(8): e1177-e1180. doi:10.1097/MPH.0000000000002064
9. Mansoori H, Faraz M, Qadir H, Rashid A, Ali M. Precursor lymphoblastic lymphoma in the extramedullary tissue: a rare manifestation of chronic myeloid leukemia in blast crisis. *Cureus.* 2020;12(10):e11009. doi:10.7759/cureus.11009
10. Sander CA, Medeiros LJ, Abruzzo LV, et al. Lymphoblastic lymphoma presenting in cutaneous sites. A clinicopathologic analysis of six cases. *J Am Acad Dermatol.* 1991;25:1023-1031.
11. Kahwash SB, Qualman SJ. Cutaneous lymphoblastic lymphoma in children: report of six cases with precursor B-cell lineage. *Pediatr Dev Pathol.* 2002;5:45-53.
12. Boccara O, Blanche S, de Prost Y, et al. Cutaneous hematologic disorders in children. *Pediatr Blood Cancer.* 2012;58:226-232.
13. Boccara O, Laloum-Grynberg E, Jeudy G, et al. Cutaneous B-cell lymphoblastic lymphoma in children: a rare diagnosis. *J Am Acad Dermatol.* 2012;66:51-57.
14. Bontoux C, De Masson A, Boccara O, et al. Outcome and clinicophenotypical features of acute lymphoblastic leukemia/lymphoblastic lymphoma with cutaneous involvement: a multicenter case series. *J Am Acad Dermatol.* 2020;83(4):1166-1170. doi:10.1016/j.jaad.2020.01.058. Epub 2020 Jan 31.
15. Lee WJ, Moon HR, Won CH, et al. Precursor B- or T-lymphoblastic lymphoma presenting with cutaneous involvement: a series of 13 cases including 7 cases of cutaneous T-lymphoblastic lymphoma. *J Am Acad Dermatol.* 2014;70:318-325.
16. Anderson PC, Stotland MA, Dinulos JG, et al. Acute lymphocytic leukemia presenting as an isolated scalp nodule in an infant. *Ann Plast Surg.* 2010;64:251-253.
17. Siah TW, Windebank KP, Menon G, et al. A scalp nodule in a 4-year-old boy. Precursor B-cell lymphoblastic lymphoma. *Pediatr Dermatol.* 2013;30:135-136.
18. Muljono A, Graf NS, Arbuckle S. Primary cutaneous lymphoblastic lymphoma in children: series of eight cases with review of the literature. *Pathology.* 2009;41:223-228.
19. Millot F, Robert A, Bertrand Y, et al. Cutaneous involvement in children with acute lymphoblastic leukemia or lymphoblastic lymphoma. The children's leukemia cooperative group of the European Organization of Research and Treatment of Cancer (EORTC). *Pediatrics.* 1997;100:60-64.
20. Zengin N, Kars A, Ozisik Y, et al. Aleukemic leukemia cutis in a patient with acute lymphoblastic leukemia. *J Am Acad Dermatol.* 1998;38:620-621.
21. Kishimoto H, Furui Y, Nishioka K. Guess what. B-cell acute lymphoblastic leukemia with aleukemic leukemia cutis. *Eur J Dermatol.* 2001;11:151-152.
22. van Zuuren EJ, Wintzen M, Jansen PM, et al. Aleukaemic leukaemia cutis in a patient with acute T-cell lymphoblastic leukaemia. *Clin Exp Dermatol.* 2003;28:330-332.
23. Gallagher G, Chhanabhai M, Song KW, et al. Unusual presentation of precursor T-cell lymphoblastic lymphoma: involvement limited to breasts and skin. *Leuk Lymphoma.* 2007;48:428-430.
24. Najem N, Zadeh VB, Badawi M, et al. Aleukemic leukemia cutis in a child preceding T-cell acute lymphoblastic leukemia. *Pediatr Dermatol.* 2011;28:535-537.
25. Ansell LH, Mehta J, Cotliar J. Recurrent aleukemic leukemia cutis in a patient with pre-B-cell acute lymphoblastic leukemia. *J Clin Oncol.* 2013;31:e353-e355.
26. Kawakami T, Kimura S, Kinoshita A, et al. Precursor B-cell lymphoblastic lymphoma with only cutaneous involvement. *Acta Derm Venereol.* 2009;89:540-541.
27. Taniguchi S, Hamada T, Kutsuna H, et al. Lymphocytic aleukemic leukemia cutis. *J Am Acad Dermatol.* 1996;35:849-850.
28. Chao SC, Lee JY, Tsao CJ. Leukemia cutis in acute lymphocytic leukemia masquerading as viral exanthem. *J Dermatol.* 1999;26:216-219.
29. Stubert J, Hilgendorf I, Stengel B, et al. Bilateral breast enlargement and reddish skin macules as first signs of acute lymphoblastic T cell leukemia. *Onkologie.* 2011;34:384-387.
30. Gold HL, Grynspan D, Kanigsberg N. Leukemia cutis and facial nerve palsy as presenting symptoms of acute lymphoblastic leukemia. *Pediatr Dermatol.* 2014;31:393-395.
31. Kraigher-Krainer E, Lackner H, Sovinz P, et al. Numb chin syndrome as initial manifestation in a child with acute lymphoblastic leukemia. *Pediatr Blood Cancer.* 2008;51:426-428.
32. Lee JI, Park HJ, Oh ST, et al. A case of leukemia cutis at the site of a prior catheter insertion. *Ann Dermatol.* 2009;21:193-196.
33. Shinkuma S, Natsuga K, Akiyama M, et al. Precursor B-cell lymphoblastic lymphoma presented with intraocular involvement and unusual skin manifestations. *Ann Hematol.* 2008;87:677-679.
34. Frontanes A, Montalvo F, Valcarcel M. Congenital leukemia with leukemia cutis: a case report. *Bol Asoc Med P R.* 2012;104:52-54.
35. Kwock JM, Kurpiel B, Gru AA. T-cell lymphoblastic lymphoma/leukemia presenting as a diffuse viral exanthem-like Reaction: a clinical and histopathological challenge. *Am J Dermatopathol.* 2020;42(12):986-988.
36. Yaar R, Rothman K, Mahalingam M. When dead cells tell tales-cutaneous involvement by precursor T-cell acute lymphoblastic lymphoma with an uncommon phenotype. *Am J Dermatopathol.* 2010;32:183-186.
37. El Demellawy D, Sur M, Ross C, et al. Composite multifocal basal cell carcinoma and precursor B acute lymphoblastic leukemia: case report. *Diagn Pathol.* 2007;2:32.
38. Fichel F, Eschard C, Zachar D, et al. Kaposiform haemangioendothelioma associated with B-cell acute lymphoblastic leukemia. [Article in French]. *Ann Dermatol Venereol.* 2013;140:209-214.
39. Savage NM, Johnson RC, Natkunam Y. The spectrum of lymphoblastic, nodal and extranodal T-cell lymphomas: characteristic features and diagnostic dilemmas. *Hum Pathol.* 2013;44:451-471.
40. Lau LG, Tan LK, Koay ES, et al. Acute lymphoblastic leukemia with the phenotype of a putative B-cell/T-cell bipotential precursor. *Am J Hematol.* 2004;77:156-160.
41. Zhang Y, Qian JJ, Zhou YL, et al. Comparison of early T-cell precursor and non-ETP subtypes among 122 Chinese adults with acute lymphoblastic leukemia. *Front Oncol.* 2020;10:1423. doi:10.3389/fonc.2020.01423
42. Genescà E, Morgades M, Montesinos P, Barba P, et al. Unique clinico-biological, genetic and prognostic features of adult early T-cell precursor acute lymphoblastic leukemia. *Haematologica.* 2020;105(6):e294-e297. doi:10.3324/haematol.2019.225078
43. Jain N, Lamb AV, O'Brien S, et al. Early T-cell precursor acute lymphoblastic leukemia/lymphoma (ETP-ALL/LBL) in adolescents and adults: a high-risk subtype. *Blood.* 2016;127(15):1863-1869. doi:10.1182/blood-2015-08-661702

44. Neumann M, Heesch S, Gökbuget N, et al. Clinical and molecular characterization of early T-cell precursor leukemia: a high-risk subgroup in adult T-ALL with a high frequency of FLT3 mutations. *Blood Cancer J.* 2012;2(1):e55.
45. Angelova E, Audette C, Kovtun Y, et al. CD123 expression patterns and selective targeting with a CD123-targeted antibody-drug conjugate (IMGN632) in acute lymphoblastic leukemia. *Haematologica.* 2019;104(4):749-755. doi:10.3324/haematol.2018.205252
46. Coustan-Smith E, Mullighan CG, Onciu M, et al. Early T-cell precursor leukaemia: a subtype of very high-risk acute lymphoblastic leukaemia. *Lancet Oncol.* 2009;10(2):147-156.
47. Holmfeldt L, Wei L, Diaz-Flores E, et al. The genomic landscape of hypodiploid acute lymphoblastic leukemia. *Nat Genet.* 2013;45:242-252.
48. Meyer C, Hofmann J, Burmeister T, et al. The MLL recombinome of acute leukemias in 2013. *Leukemia.* 2013;27:2165-2176.
49. Andersson AK, Ma J, Wang J, et al. The landscape of somatic mutations in infant MLL-rearranged acute lymphoblastic leukemias. *Nat Genet.* 2015;47:330-337.
50. Shiratori S, Kondo T, Fujisawa S, et al. c-myc rearrangement in B-cell lymphoblastic lymphoma with the involvement of multiple extranodal lesions. *Leuk Lymphoma.* 2011;52:716-718.
51. Wenzinger C, Williams E, Gru AA. Updates in the pathology of precursor lymphoid neoplasms in the Revised fourth edition of the WHO classification of tumors of hematopoietic and lymphoid tissues. *Curr Hematol Malig Rep.* 2018;13(4):275-288. doi:10.1007/s11899-018-0456-8
52. Lilljebjörn H, Henningsson R, Hyrenius-Wittsten A, et al. Identification of ETV6-RUNX1-like and DUX4-rearranged subtypes in paediatric B-cell precursor acute lymphoblastic leukaemia. *Nat Commun.* 2016;7:11790. doi:10.1038/ncomms11790
53. Yasuda T, Tsuzuki S, Kawazu M, et al. Recurrent DUX4 fusions in B cell acute lymphoblastic leukemia of adolescents and young adults. *Nat Genet.* 2016;48(5):569-574. doi:10.1038/ng.3535
54. Gu Z, Churchman M, Roberts K, et al. Genomic analyses identify recurrent MEF2D fusions in acute lymphoblastic leukaemia. *Nat Commun.* 2016;7:13331. doi:10.1038/ncomms13331
55. Gu Z, Churchman ML, Roberts KG et al. PAX5-driven subtypes of B-progenitor acute lymphoblastic leukemia. *Nat Genet.* 2019;51(2):296-307. doi:10.1038/s41588-018-0315-5
56. Hirabayashi S, Ohki K, Nakabayashi K, et al. ZNF384-related fusion genes define a subgroup of childhood B-cell precursor acute lymphoblastic leukemia with a characteristic immunotype. *Haematologica.* 2017;102(1):118-129. doi:10.3324/haematol.2016.151035
57. Hormann FM, Hoogkamer AQ, Beverloo HB, et al. NUTM1 is a recurrent fusion gene partner in B-cell precursor acute lymphoblastic leukemia associated with increased expression of genes on chromosome band 10p12.31-12.2. *Haematologica.* 2019;104(10):e455-e459. doi:10.3324/haematol.2018.206961
58. Iacobucci I, Kimura S, Mullighan CG. Biologic and therapeutic implications of genomic alterations in acute lymphoblastic leukemia. *J Clin Med.* 2021;10(17):3792. doi:10.3390/jcm10173792
59. Wagener R, López C, Kleinheinz K, et al. IG-MYC+ neoplasms with precursor B-cell phenotype are molecularly distinct from Burkitt lymphomas. *Blood.* 2018;132(21):2280-2285.
60. Passet M, Boissel N, Sigaux F, et al; Group for Research on Adult ALL (GRAALL). PAX5 P80R mutation identifies a novel subtype of B-cell precursor acute lymphoblastic leukemia with favorable outcome. *Blood.* 2019;133(3):280-284. doi:10.1182/blood-2018-10-882142
61. Paietta E, Roberts KG, Wang V, et al. Molecular classification improves risk assessment in adult BCR-ABL1-negative B-ALL. *Blood.* 2021;138(11):948-958. doi:10.1182/blood.2020010144
62. Inhorn RC, Aster JC, Roach SA, et al. A syndrome of lymphoblastic lymphoma, eosinophilia, and myeloid hyperplasia/malignancy associated with t(8;13)(p11;q11): description of a distinctive clinicopathologic entity. *Blood.* 1995;85:1881-1887.
63. Weng AP, Ferrando AA, Lee W, et al. Activating mutations of NOTCH1 in human T cell acute lymphoblastic leukemia. *Science.* 2004;306:269-271.
64. Meijerink JP. Genetic rearrangements in relation to immunophenotype and outcome in T-cell acute lymphoblastic leukaemia. *Best Pract Res Clin Haematol.* 2010;23(3):307-318. doi:10.1016/j.beha.2010.08.002
65. Ferrando AA, Neuberg DS, Staunton J, et al. Gene expression signatures define novel oncogenic pathways in T cell acute lymphoblastic leukemia. *Cancer Cell.* 2002;1(1):75-87. doi:10.1016/s1535-6108(02)00018-1
66. Liu Y, Easton J, Shao Y, et al. The genomic landscape of pediatric and young adult T-lineage acute lymphoblastic leukemia. *Nat Genet.* 2017;49(8):1211-1218. doi:10.1038/ng.3909
67. Miettinen M, Chatten J, Paetau A, et al. Monoclonal antibody NB84 in the differential diagnosis of neuroblastoma and other small round cell tumors. *Am J Surg Pathol.* 1998;22:327-332.
68. Hsiao CH, Su IJ. Primary cutaneous pre-B lymphoblastic lymphoma immunohistologically mimics Ewing's sarcoma/primitive neuroectodermal tumor. *J Formos Med Assoc.* 2003;102:193-197.
69. Di Giannatale A, Frezza AM, Le Deley MC, et al. Primary cutaneous and subcutaneous Ewing sarcoma. *Pediatr Blood Cancer.* 2015;62:1555-1561.
70. Berk DR, Cheng A, Lind AC, et al. Burkitt lymphoma with cutaneous involvement. *Dermatol Online J.* 2008;14:14.
71. Leoncini L, Raphael M, Stein H, et al. *Burkitt Lymphoma.* International Agency for Research on Cancer; 2008.
72. Kong Y, Huang XJ, Hao L, et al. CD34(+)CD19(+) cells with CD123 overexpression are a novel prognostic marker in Ph chromosome-positive acute lymphoblastic leukemia [in Chinese]. *Zhongguo Shi Yan Xue Ye Xue Za Zhi.* 2014;22:6-10.
73. Shi Y, Wang E. Blastic plasmacytoid dendritic cell neoplasm: a clinicopathologic review. *Arch Pathol Lab Med.* 2014;138:564-569.

CHAPTER 59

Leukemia cutis/aleukemic leukemia cutis/myeloid sarcoma

Kari E. Sufficool and John L. Frater

INTRODUCTION

Acute leukemia may present in a variety of extramedullary tissues with or without bone marrow disease. Although rare, extramedullary involvement by acute leukemia is a clinically significant phenomenon. Leukemia cutis and myeloid sarcoma represent two well-known extramedullary manifestations of leukemia. This chapter summarizes the clinical and histologic features, illustrates the varying immunophenotypes, and offers an approach to the pathologic evaluation of these challenging lesions.

LEUKEMIA CUTIS/ALEUKEMIC LEUKEMIA CUTIS

Definition

Leukemia cutis is defined as infiltration by neoplastic leukocytes or their precursors (myeloid or lymphoid) into the epidermis, dermis, or subcutis, resulting in clinically identifiable skin lesions.[1] Cutaneous infiltrates have been described in patients with acute myeloid leukemia (AML), myelodysplastic syndromes (MDSs), and myeloproliferative disorders (MPDs). In individuals with prior MDSs and MPDs, leukemia cutis may represent transformation to an acute leukemia.[2] Skin involvement can occur subsequently to, concurrently with, or earlier than bone marrow or peripheral blood involvement.[3-5] Rarely, cutaneous infiltration is identified in patients who never develop systemic disease, which is termed *aleukemic leukemia cutis*.[3-6]

Epidemiology

Leukemia cutis occurs in 10% to 15% of patients with AML and less frequently in chronic MPDs.[7] Of note, the frequency of leukemia cutis varies on the basis of subtype of AML and can be seen in up to 50% of patients with acute monocytic and myelomonocytic types.[8,9] Cutaneous infiltrates can also be seen in patients with chronic myelomonocytic leukemia[10-13] but are exceedingly rare in acute erythroid leukemia.[14,15] In lymphocytic leukemias, skin involvement has been reported in 4% to 20% of chronic lymphocytic leukemia/small lymphocytic lymphoma (CLL/SLL).[16] In mature T-cell leukemia, the rate can range from 20% to 70%.[16] The frequency of disease is higher in children than in adults. Remarkably, 25% to 30% of infants with congenital leukemia subsequently develop skin involvement, usually related to a diagnosis of AML, but acute lymphoblastic leukemia (ALL) has also been implicated.[17,18]

Etiology

Etiology is the same as for acute and chronic leukemias as well as MDS and MPD.[2]

Clinical Presentation and Prognosis

Most patients present with single or multiple erythematous papules or nodules[19]; however, lesions can be violaceous, red-brown, or hemorrhagic and vary from papules to nodules to plaques.[19,20] The lesions of patients with an aleukemic presentation most frequently have a myeloid immunophenotype and are widespread in distribution with a papulonodular clinical appearance.[21-23] Children with congenital leukemia can also have cutaneous presentation, resulting in a "blueberry muffin" appearance (Fig. 59-1).[18] Most of these children have high leukemic tumor burden and concurrent hepatosplenomegaly.[18]

Other more unusual presentations of leukemia include oral petechiae or thickened gums, leonine faces, eczematous lesions, genital ulcers, and panniculitis.[20,24-26] A significant proportion of patients with leukemia cutis (90%) can also have involvement of other extramedullary sites, most commonly the meninges.[22]

In most cases, leukemia cutis is a local manifestation of an underlying acute leukemia, and treatment is aimed at eradicating the systemic disease usually via chemotherapy combined with local therapy. In general, the diagnosis of leukemia cutis portends a poorer prognosis, with many studies showing an aggressive course.[1] It has been reported that 88% of patients with leukemia cutis die within 1 year of the diagnosis.[21]

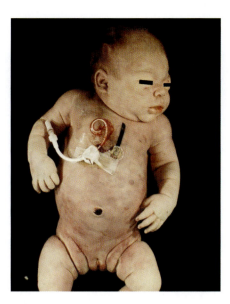

FIGURE 59-1. Clinical postmortem photograph of a patient with congenital leukemia with a cutaneous presentation resulting in a "blueberry muffin" appearance.

Histology

Diagnosis is based on the morphologic pattern of skin infiltration, cytologic features, and immunophenotype of the malignant cells. Correlation with clinical history, especially bone marrow and peripheral blood findings, is imperative. Typically, leukemia cutis shows a perivascular and/or periadnexal pattern of involvement at low-power magnification.[2] It can also have a dense diffuse/interstitial or nodular deep infiltrate involving the dermis and subcutis with sparing of the papillary dermis (grenz zone; Fig. 59-2).[1] Stromal fibrosis is common, and when tumor cells invade between collagen bundles, the cells can resemble a single file pattern similar to that seen in lobular carcinoma of the breast (Fig. 59-3).[2] Rarely, sparse interstitial infiltrates can also be the first presentation of disease, and care should be taken to recognize these subtle findings.

Numerous subtypes of leukemia can infiltrate the skin (Table 59-1). In acute myeloblastic leukemia (FAB-M1 and FAB-M2), the cells are predominately myeloblasts and myelocytes, characterized as medium to large mononuclear cells with scant cytoplasm and slightly basophilic, eccentrically placed nucleus with central prominent nucleolus (Fig. 59-4).[2] Acute myelomonocytic and monoblastic/monocytic leukemias (FAB-M4 and FAB-M5) are characterized by medium-sized atypical oval monocytoid cells with kidney-shaped nuclei.[2] Conversely, the infiltrate of chronic myeloid leukemia is more pleomorphic with both immature and mature granulocytes (myelocytes, metamyelocytes, segmented neutrophils).[27] Tumor cells with large eosinophilic granules are a helpful clue that the cutaneous infiltrate is of myeloid origin (Fig. 59-5).[2] Mitoses and apoptotic bodies are often present.

Immunophenotype

A diagnosis of leukemia cutis alone is nonspecific. Thus, elucidation of an immunophenotype is critical in providing clinically useful information. For myeloid infiltrates,

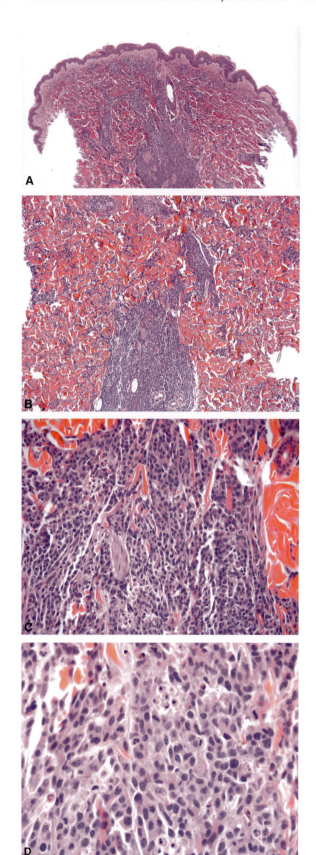

FIGURE 59-2. Hematoxylin-and-eosin–stained sections of a representative myeloid leukemia cutis case showing a nodular mid-dermal aggregate of large mononuclear cells with sparing of the papillary dermis (grenz zone) at low-power magnification (**A**, 4×; **B**, 10×); the perivascular and periadnexal infiltrate is composed of immature mononuclear cells with eosinophilic cytoplasm, finely stippled chromatin, and central prominent nucleoli (**C**, 20×); readily identifiable mitoses and apoptotic cells can be seen (**D**, 40×).

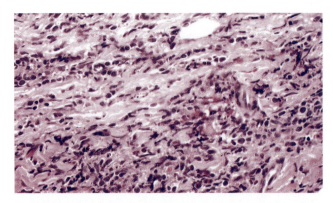

FIGURE 59-3. Tumor cells can percolate between collagen bundles resembling a single file pattern that can mimic lobular carcinoma of the breast in this hematoxylin-and-eosin–stained section (40×). Negative cytokeratin staining is sufficient to exclude the possibility of carcinoma in the differential diagnosis.

TABLE 59-1 Subtypes of Leukemia Presenting as Leukemia Cutis

Myeloid/Monocytic Disorders
- Acute myeloid leukemia
- Acute myelomonocytic leukemia
- Acute monocytic leukemia
- Chronic myelogenous leukemia
- Chronic myelomonocytic leukemia (transformation)
- Myelodysplastic syndromes (transformation)

T-Cell Leukemia/Lymphoma
- Precursor T-cell ALL
- Adult T-cell leukemia/lymphoma
- T-cell prolymphocytic leukemia
- Sézary syndrome

B-Cell Leukemia/Lymphoma
- Precursor B-cell ALL
- Chronic lymphocytic leukemia/small lymphocytic lymphoma

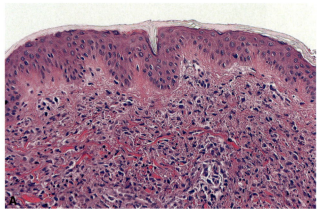

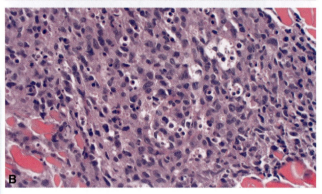

FIGURE 59-4. In this hematoxylin-and-eosin–stained case example of acute myeloblastic leukemia cutis, there is a dense and diffuse infiltration of relatively monotonous round-to-oval cells (**A**, 20×); the atypical myeloblasts display scant cytoplasm and slightly basophilic, eccentrically placed nuclei with central prominent nucleoli; numerous apoptotic bodies can be seen, along with scattered background necrosis (**B**, 40×).

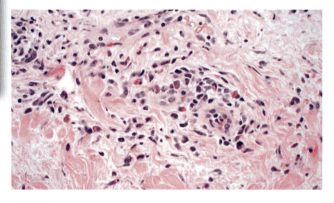

FIGURE 59-5. In this hematoxylin-and-eosin–stained section, tumor cells with large eosinophilic granules are a helpful clue that the cutaneous infiltrate is of myeloid origin (40×).

CD68 and lysozyme are the most sensitive markers but are not lineage-specific.[2] Myeloperoxidase, CD45, HLA-DR, and CD43 are also useful markers.[27] Other markers that may be present are CD34, CD123, CD56, and CD117 (Fig. 59-6).[2]

ERG (erythroblast transformation specific regulated gene-1) overexpression has been reported in a variety of hematopoietic disorders, and a recent study suggests that ERG is a potentially useful immunostain to distinguish cases of leukemia cutis from those of reactive myeloid infiltrates in the skin.[28] In this study, the authors suggest that a moderate-to-strong nuclear staining pattern of ERG in a dermal leukemic/leukocytic infiltrate comparable with that seen in resident endothelial cells, which serve as an internal control, could be a useful clue toward the diagnosis of leukemia cutis when incorporated into the diagnostic workup of particularly challenging cases.[28]

In mature B-cell neoplasms, such as CLL/SLL, the neoplastic lymphocytes will show positive immunoreactivity for CD5, CD20, CD23, and CD43 but will be negative for CD10.[1] The combination of PAX-5 and TdT positivity are useful in the identification of precursor B-cell acute lymphoblastic leukemia/lymphoma (Pre-B-ALL).[1] CD10, CD19, and CD79a are also positive in most cases of Pre-B-ALL, although CD45 expression may be absent.[1,27]

The tumor cells in adult T-cell leukemia/lymphoma will be positive for CD2, CD3, CD4, and CD5 but often show decreased CD7 expression; there is lack of expression of TIA-1, granzyme B, CD1a, and TdT.[1,27] Combined

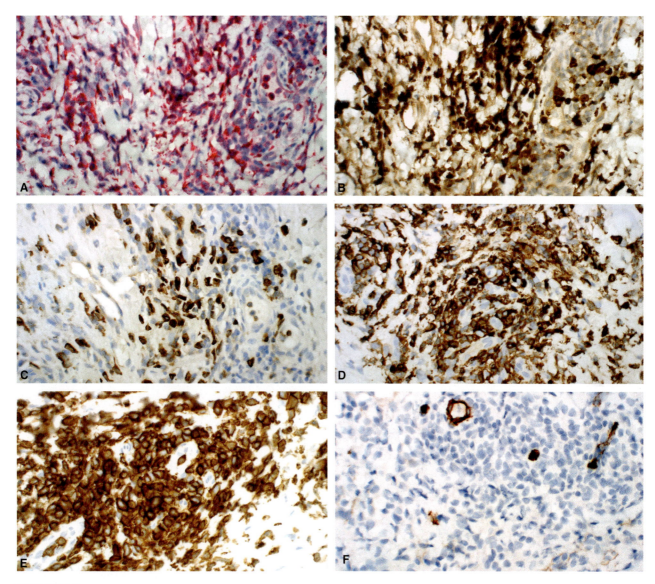

FIGURE 59-6. Immunochemical findings in a representative leukemia cutis case with myeloid differentiation and bone marrow diagnosis of transformed myelodysplastic/myeloproliferative neoplasm showing positivity for CD68 **(A)**, lysozyme **(B)**, myeloperoxidase **(C)**, CD45 **(D)**, and CD43 **(E)**, and negativity for CD34 (**F**, 40×). FISH performed on the concurrent bone marrow identified *MLL* (11q) rearrangement.

immunopositivity for CD3 with TdT and/or CD1a is the most specific indicator of precursor T-cell acute lymphoblastic leukemia/lymphoma (P-T-ALL).[1] Other T-cell markers, CD2, CD3, CD4, CD5, and CD8, are also useful in the diagnosis of T-cell leukemia.[2,27]

Most cases of T-cell prolymphocytic leukemia are positive for CD3, CD4, CD45RO, and T-cell leukemia 1 (TCL1) and negative for CD1a, CD34, and TdT.[1] Finally, Sézary syndrome will be positive for CD3, CD4, CD25, and CD45RO, typically with diminished or absent expression of CD7 and CD26.[29,30]

Patients with leukemia of ambiguous lineage (including biphenotypic acute leukemia) may also present with cutaneous involvement. Identification of some combination of B-cell-, T-cell-, and myeloid-associated antigens is necessary (Fig. 59-7).

Genetic and Molecular Findings

Many chromosomal abnormalities have been reported in patients with AML-related leukemia cutis; however, aberrations in chromosome 8 are most commonly seen.[6,7,22] In other subtypes of cutaneous leukemic infiltrates, the molecular genetics are less defined. Yet, the migration of leukemic cells to the skin is thought to be related to the expression of various chemokine receptors and adhesion molecules, which has been borne out in recent studies.[31-37]

Postulated Cell of Origin

Hematopoietic stem cell.

Differential Diagnosis

The differential diagnosis for leukemia cutis is vast and includes extramedullary hematopoiesis, lymphoid hyperplasia (pseudolymphoma), lymphomatoid drug reactions, pseudolymphomatous folliculitis, Jessner lymphocytic infiltrate, acral pseudolymphomatous angiokeratoma, cutaneous

CD8+ T-cell infiltrates in patients with HIV/AIDS, and posttransplant lymphoproliferative disorders.[2] Other considerations are infiltrates composed of reactive neutrophils such as neutrophilic dermatoses, infection, or traumatic inflammatory infiltrates.[28] Neutrophil-rich infiltrates such as these may potentially pose a diagnostic challenge, particularly if there is a prominent left shift.[28]

Capsule Summary

- Leukemia cutis is defined as infiltration by neoplastic leukocytes or their precursors into the epidermis, dermis, or subcutis, resulting in clinically identifiable skin lesions that can occur subsequently to, concurrently with, or earlier than bone marrow or peripheral blood involvement.

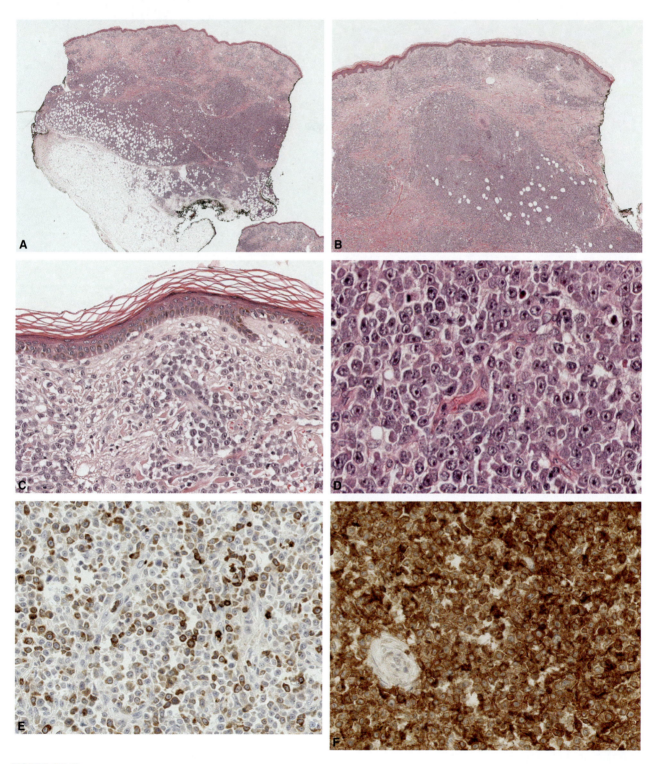

FIGURE 59-7. Hematoxylin-and-eosin–stained sections of a skin lesion from a patient with biphenotypic (T/myeloid) acute leukemia (A–D), demonstrating an immature-appearing mononuclear cell infiltrate in the superficial and deep dermis (**A**, 2×; **B**, 40×; **C**, 100×; **D**, 400×). The malignant cells express CD3 **(E)**, CD4 **(F)**, CD7 **(G)**, CD33 **(H)**, and CD45 **(I)**.

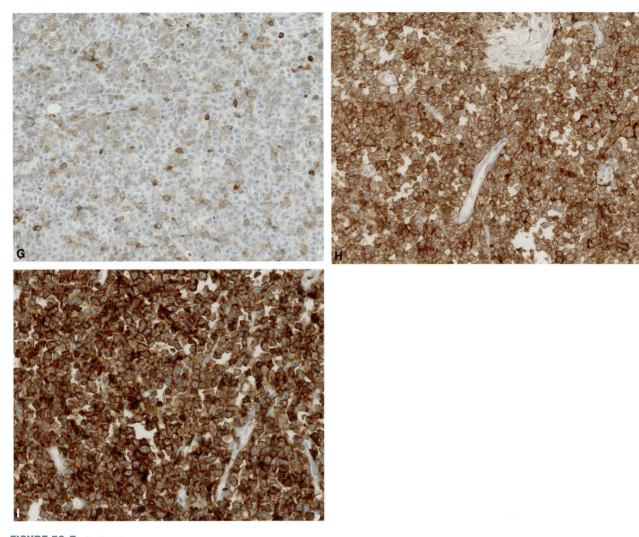

FIGURE 59-7. Continued

- Rarely, cutaneous infiltration is identified in patients who never develop systemic disease (aleukemic leukemia cutis).
- A term of leukemia cutis is nonspecific, and the immunophenotype depends on the subtype of leukemic infiltrate present in the skin.
- To be clinically impactful, a panel of immunostains should be performed when the amount of tissue is sufficient to allow for immunohistochemical workup.
- Notwithstanding, clinical correlation, especially with bone marrow and peripheral blood findings, is critical in arriving at the correct diagnosis.

MYELOID SARCOMA

Definition

In contrast to leukemia cutis, the World Health Organization (WHO) recognizes myeloid sarcoma as a specific entity whereby there is an extramedullary proliferation of immature myeloid cells (blasts) that partially or completely effaces the architecture of their sites of involvement.[24,38] These tumors have also been referred to as granulocytic/monoblastic sarcomas or extramedullary myeloid tumors and historically were termed chloromas because of the green color they imparted on the gross specimen owing to myeloperoxidase production.[39] Currently, any extramedullary manifestation of AML can be termed a granulocytic sarcoma. Specific terms that can overlap with granulocytic sarcoma include leukemia cutis, a term describing infiltration of the skin by leukemic cells, which is also referred to as cutaneous granulocytic sarcoma, and meningeal leukemia, in which there is invasion of the subarachnoid space by leukemic cells. In recent years, the term myeloid sarcoma has been favored for extramedullary involvement by immature myeloid cells.[40] Importantly, restraint must be exercised when applying the term myeloid sarcoma, because infiltrates by myeloid blasts in leukemic patients are *not* classified as myeloid sarcoma unless they present as a tumor that effaces the tissue architecture.[27]

Epidemiology

Myeloid sarcomas have a predilection for males, with a male-to-female ratio of 1.2:1, and usually present in the last decades of life.[27] The median age is 56 years, with an age range spanning from 1 month to 89 years.[41,42]

Etiology

The etiology is the same as for AML and myeloproliferative neoplasms.[27]

Clinical Presentation and Prognosis

Myeloid sarcomas have been reported at nearly every anatomic site but are most frequently encountered in the skin and soft tissues, lymph nodes, and gastrointestinal tract.[43] The associated symptoms are largely dependent on the location of involvement. In the skin, lesions commonly present as multiple papules, plaques, or nodules. The torso is the most common region of involvement, although the head and neck as well as the extremities are also involved in many cases. Although there is a large age distribution as previously mentioned, studies have shown that myeloid sarcomas appear to be more common in pediatric patients with an incidence of up to 30% of pediatric AML versus 2% to 5% in adults.[43] Although myeloid sarcoma typically presents concurrently with a new diagnosis of AML or as evidence of disease recurrence,[44] a significant subset of myeloid sarcomas will present de novo.[42] It is this subset of cases that can be most diagnostically challenging, as the morphologic appearance can easily be confused with other hematologic malignancies, such as aggressive B-cell lymphomas, or even nonhematolymphoid tumors.[45,46]

Myeloid sarcomas may occur in the presence or absence of bone marrow disease. The presence of myeloid sarcoma is sufficient to establish a clinical diagnosis of AML. Studies have suggested that bone marrow involvement will become evident in nearly all patients who initially present with an isolated myeloid sarcoma, with a mean interval of 10 months.[47] Furthermore, isolated myeloid sarcoma appears to be more common at relapse in patients who have undergone allogeneic stem cell transplantation, with one study reporting rates of 8% to 20% of transplanted patients.[48] The reasons for this are currently unclear. As this is a rare diagnosis, outcome studies and response to treatment data are limited. Therapeutic modalities often include local radiation, systemic chemotherapy, immunotherapy, and donor lymphocyte infusions.[48] Overall, outcomes are typically poor but tend to be slightly better than those of primary or relapsed AML without extramedullary involvement.[48-50] Allogeneic or autologous bone marrow transplantation seems to provide higher probability of prolonged survival or cure.[27]

Histology

Morphologically, myeloid sarcomas are proliferations of immature hematopoietic cells that efface the surrounding tissue architecture (Fig. 59-8). The cellular infiltrate may

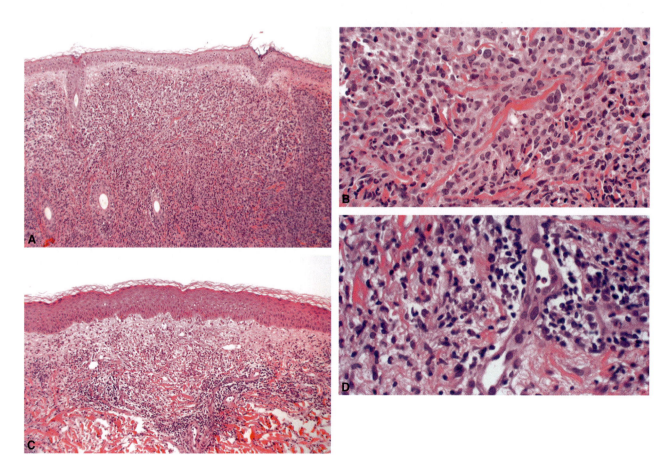

FIGURE 59-8. Hematoxylin-and-eosin–stained sections of a representative cutaneous myeloid sarcoma case showing a dense and diffuse interstitial infiltrate, extensively involving the dermis (**A**, 10×; **B**, 50×), and a cutaneous myeloid sarcoma case showing a minimal perivascular leukemic infiltrate (**C**, 10×; **D**, 50×).

be composed of myeloblasts, monoblasts/promonocytes, or less commonly promyelocytes.[27] Necrosis may be present, as well as numerous mitotic figures and tingible-body macrophages, owing to the aggressive nature of the disease.[51] The pattern of infiltration is dependent on the type of tissue involved. Leukemic blasts will diffusely infiltrate tissue within extranodal sites and can appear cohesive in areas with dense fibroconnective tissue or prominent stromal reaction where it can mimic metastatic carcinoma.[51] Within lymph nodes, the infiltrate may be confined to the paracortex or sinuses with occasional residual germinal centers or it may obliterate the entire nodal architecture.[51] In patients with AML, especially those with high blood tumor burden, small clusters of blasts may be present in extramedullary sites; however, a diagnosis of myeloid sarcoma should *not* be established in these cases.[27]

Usually myeloblasts, or blast equivalents such as promonocytes, are the predominant cell population; however, varying degrees of myeloid maturation may be present.[52] Myelomonocytic forms, similar to acute myelomonocytic leukemia, are also common. Rarely, myeloid sarcomas with erythroid and megakaryoblastic differentiation have been reported[53]; and, while exceedingly rare, extramedullary cases of acute promyelocytic leukemia have been published, with the majority occurring at relapse with a preference for central nervous system involvement.[53]

Immunophenotype

Immunohistochemically, CD43 and lysozyme are considered the most sensitive markers, as they are expressed in nearly 100% of myeloid sarcoma cases in most studies[42,53-56]; however, neither is specific. Tumor cells frequently express CD68 and myeloperoxidase, a myeloid lineage–defining antigen.[57] CD34 positivity is not a consistent finding[42,58] and is often negative in tumors demonstrating monocytic differentiation.[58] HLA-DR has been found to be more sensitive than CD34.[55] Expression of CD45 (leukocyte common antigen) can be variable.[46] Other widely utilized myeloid markers are CD33[59] and CD117 (c-kit), which is considered to be a marker of myeloid cells as well as immaturity (Fig. 59-9).[56]

Myeloid sarcomas with monocytic differentiation can be negative for many of the aforementioned markers, particularly CD34 and/or CD117.[60] Myeloperoxidase (MPO) is classically negative, but positivity for myeloperoxidase is not sufficient to exclude monocytic differentiation.[55] Other positive markers include CD68, CD43, CD33, and lysozyme. CD163 can be positive in cases with monocytic differentiation,[61] as can CD56 (N-CAM).[62] CD4 is commonly expressed but lacks specificity. CD14 and Krüppel-like factor (KLF4) may be useful in monocytic leukemias (Fig. 59-10).[63] Lastly, myelomonocytic myeloid sarcomas demonstrate mixed immunoreactivity for the previously mentioned myeloid and monocytic markers.

Rare cases of erythroid differentiation can be highlighted with glycophorin A, hemoglobin, or CD71 (transferrin receptor); notably, these markers may show variable immunoreactivity.[64-66] In cases with megakaryocytic differentiation, CD61 (platelet glycoprotein IIIa), CD41 (platelet glycoprotein IIB), vWF (factor VIII–related antigen), or CD31 can be useful.[67]

Genetic and Molecular Findings

By fluorescence in situ hybridization (FISH) and/or cytogenetics, chromosomal aberrations are found in ~55% of cases,[27] including monosomy 7, trisomy 8, *MLL* rearrangement, inv(16), trisomy 4, monosomy 16, 16q-, 5q-, 20q-, and trisomy 11.[42] Myeloid sarcomas of the orbital region of children are often associated with *AML1-ETO (RUNX1-RUNX1T1)* translocations [t(8; 21)(q22; q22)],[68] whereas those with inv(16) have high incidence in the breast or gastrointestinal tract of adults.[42,56] There also appears to be an increase of cutaneous myeloid sarcoma with trisomy 8, although owing to the low rate of cytogenetic analysis in cutaneous disease, the significance of this finding is uncertain.[69] Patients with myeloid and lymphoid neoplasms with *FGFR1* abnormalities/8p11 syndrome have been noted to have lymph node involvement by myeloid sarcoma.[70] Also reported are cases of *FIP1L1-PDGFRA*-associated myeloid sarcomas,[71] and particular attention should be given to the histomorphology in these cases as *PDGFR*-rearranged myeloid neoplasms frequently present with increased local and peripheral eosinophils; this diagnosis is of large clinical importance, as these tumors are exquisitely sensitive to tyrosine kinase inhibitors such as imatinib. Lastly, about 15% of cases show evidence of *NPM1* mutations as shown by aberrant cytoplasmic NPM (nucleophosmin) expression.[72]

Postulated Cell of Origin

Hematopoietic stem cell.

Differential Diagnosis

There is a broad differential diagnosis for myeloid sarcoma. Diagnosis is often influenced by clinical history, especially age and history of prior/concurrent myeloid neoplasm. For optimal diagnosis, fresh material should be sent for flow cytometric analysis and molecular studies. The most common differential diagnosis is non-Hodgkin lymphoma,[46] but in contrast to B-cell lymphomas, myeloid sarcomas are unlikely to express CD20 or CD79a.[46,53] Differentiation from a mature T-cell lymphoma is more challenging in that expression of CD4 (especially monocytic leukemias), CD7, CD43, and CD45 can be seen in both entities. While increased eosinophils can be seen within the background of both tumor types, immature eosinophils are highly suggestive of a myeloid process. Furthermore, the expression of myeloperoxidase, lysozyme, and CD68 in myeloid sarcomas should be sufficient to avoid misdiagnosis.

The presence of a CD4+/CD56+ infiltrate within a cutaneous site may raise the possibility of a blastic plasmacytoid dendritic cell neoplasm (BPDCN). A broad immunohistochemical (IHC) panel is suggested in these cases and should include lysozyme and myeloperoxidase, which are not expressed in BPDCN.[50] CD123 and CD43 are uniformly positive in BPDCN, but CD33 is typically not expressed. T-cell leukemia 1 (TCL1), a plasmacytoid dendritic cell antigen, shows higher frequency of expression in BPDCN than in myelomonocytic leukemia cutis.[35,73] In addition, BPDCN usually displays a dot-like, peri-Golgi pattern of immunoreactivity for CD68 (Fig. 59-11).[73] More recently, it has been

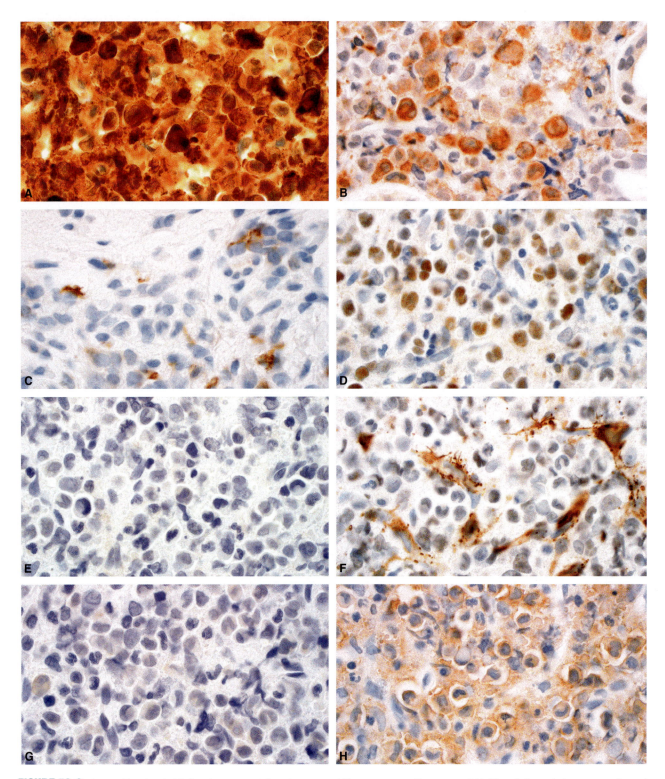

FIGURE 59-9. Immunohistochemical findings in a representative cutaneous myeloid sarcoma case with nonmonocytoid differentiation and a bone marrow diagnosis of AML (FAB-M2) showing positivity for lysozyme **(A)**, myeloperoxidase **(B)**, CD117 **(D)**, and CD33 **(H)** and negativity for the remaining markers (**C**, CD163; **E**, CD14; **F**, CD34; **G**, KLF-4, 100×).

shown that most cases of BPDCN are positive for TCF-4, a marker that is consistently negative in AML.

Histiocytic sarcomas are rare tumors that also occur in extranodal sites, including the skin, and can be a confounding diagnosis owing to overlapping clinical and immunomorphologic features. Monocytic markers are positive—CD68, CD163, and lysozyme—in addition to CD45, HLA-DR, and frequently CD4.[38,61,74] Other entities that may also enter the differential diagnosis include malignant melanoma and/or poorly differentiated carcinoma. S100, SOX10, Melan-A, HMB-45, and cytokeratin AE1/AE3 are usually adequate to exclude these diagnoses. If

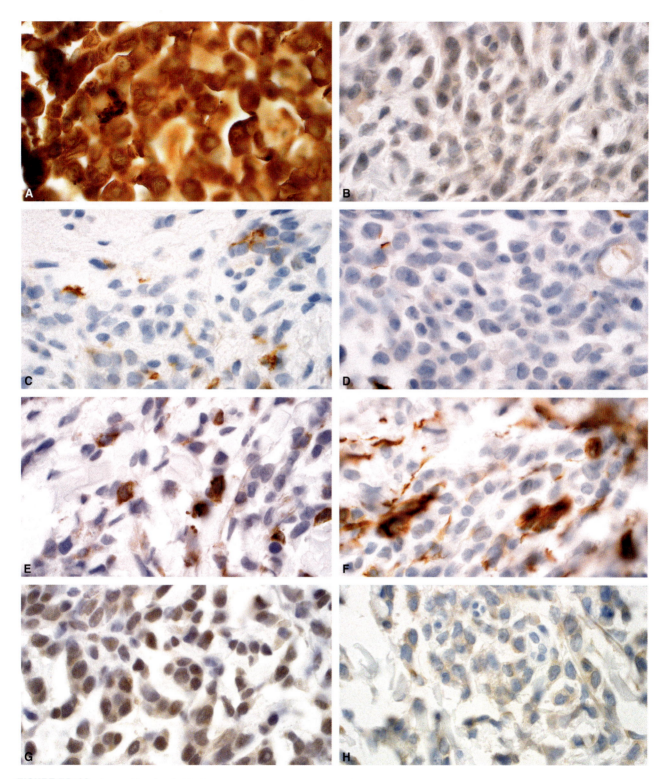

FIGURE 59-10. Immunohistochemical findings in a representative cutaneous myeloid sarcoma case with monocytic differentiation and a bone marrow diagnosis of acute myelomonocytic leukemia (FAB-M4) showing positivity for lysozyme (**A**), CD14 (**E**), and KLF-4 (nuclear) (**G**), and negativity for the remaining markers (**B**, myeloperoxidase; **C**, CD163; **D**, CD117; **F**, CD34; **H**, CD33, 100×).

the tumor is identified in a pediatric patient, one must also exclude small round cell tumors such as Ewing sarcoma/primitive neuroectodermal tumor, and medulloblastoma, but caution should be exercised when interpreting CD99, as a percentage of nonmonocytic myeloid sarcomas show CD99 immunoreactivity.[75]

It is suggested that a minimum panel of IHC stains should include CD43 and lysozyme (as a lack of immunoreactivity for either would be inconsistent with a diagnosis of myeloid sarcoma) as well as CD33, myeloperoxidase, CD34, and CD117 to define the lesion as myeloid and exclude non-Hodgkin lymphomas.[51] The IHC panel could be expanded

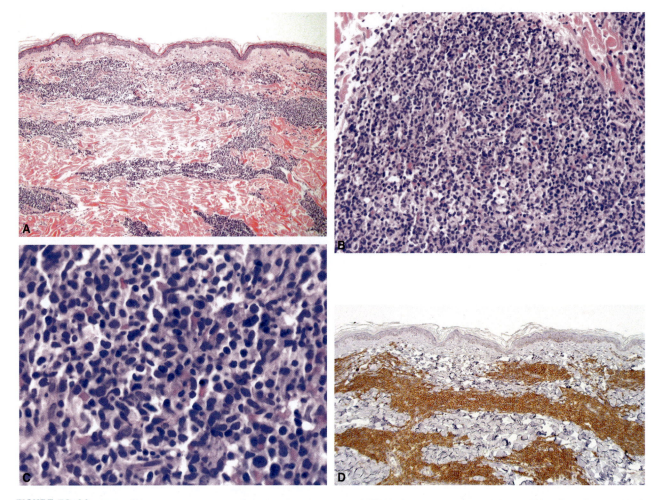

FIGURE 59-11. Hematoxylin-and-eosin–stained sections of a representative case of BPDCN showing a monotonous infiltrate of blast-like cells located in the superficial-to-deep dermis in a predominantly perivascular pattern (**A**, 10×); the epidermis is notably spared (grenz zone). At higher magnification, the tumor cells are round to oval with an increased nuclear:cytoplasmic ratio, irregular nuclear contours, fine immature chromatin, and inconspicuous nucleoli (**B**, 40×; **C**, 100×). Importantly, tumor cells show strong and diffuse staining for CD123 (**D**, 20×).

as dictated by the morphologic impression and/or clinical history.

Capsule Summary

- Myeloid sarcoma is a proliferation of immature hematopoietic cells occurring at an anatomical site other than the bone marrow that effaces the surrounding tissue architecture.
- Myeloid sarcoma may present before, simultaneously, or after systemic acute leukemia.
- Histologically, myeloid sarcoma may be composed of myeloblasts, monoblasts/promonocytes, or less commonly promyelocytes.
- Immunohistochemistry is important to minimize the risk of misdiagnosis: CD43, CD69, and lysozyme have the highest sensitivity for AML but are nonspecific and should be used in concert with other confirmatory immunostains such as CD33, myeloperoxidase, and CD117.
- When possible, flow cytometric analysis and cytogenetic studies should be performed to identify an AML-specific phenotype or AML-associated genetic abnormality.
- Correlation with past medical history is paramount as many patients have concurrent or antecedent AML, simplifying the diagnosis of extramedullary disease.
- Concurrent bone marrow biopsy is recommended to compare the morphologic features and immunophenotype as well as to determine the extent of disease.

References

1. Cho-Vega JH, Medeiros LJ, Prieto VG, et al. Leukemia cutis. *Am J Clin Pathol.* 2008;129:130-142.
2. Weedon D. *Cutaneous infiltrates: lymphomatous and leukemic.* In: *Skin Pathology.* 3rd ed. Churchill Livingstone; 2010:999-1000.
3. Benet C, Gomez A, Aguilar C, et al. Histologic and immunohistologic characterization of skin localization of myeloid disorders: a study of 173 cases. *Am J Clin Pathol.* 2011;135:278-290.
4. Hurley MY, Ghahramani GK, Frisch S, et al. Cutaneous myeloid sarcoma: natural history and biology of an uncommon manifestation of acute myeloid leukemia. *Acta Derm Venereol.* 2013;93(3):319-324.
5. Amador-Ortiz C, Hurley MY, Ghahramani GK, et al. Use of classic and novel immunohistochemical markers in the diagnosis of cutaneous myeloid sarcoma. *J Cutan Pathol.* 2011;28:945-953.

6. Gru AA, Coughlin CC, Schapiro ML, et al. Pediatric leukemia cutis: report of 3 cases and review of the literature. *Am J Dermatopathol.* 2015;37(6):477-484.
7. Agis H, Weltermann A, Fonatsch C, et al. A comparative study on demographic, hematological, and cytogenetic findings and prognosis in acute myeloid leukemia with and without leukemia cutis. *Ann Hematol.* 2002;81:90-95.
8. Kaddu S, Zenahlik P, Beham-Schmid C, et al. Specific cutaneous infiltrates in patients with myelogenous leukemia: a clinicopathologic study of 26 patients with assessment of diagnostic criteria. *J Am Acad Dermatol.* 1999;40:966-978.
9. Horlick HP, Silvers DN, Knobler EH, et al. Acute meylomonocytic leukemia presenting as a benign-appearing cutaneous eruption. *Arch Dermatol.* 1990;126:653-656.
10. Dyachenko P, Rozenman D, Bennett M. Unusual skin and testicular lesions in a patient with CMML. *Eur J Intern Med.* 2006;17:290-291.
11. Copplestone JA, Oscier DG, Mufti GJ, et al. Monocytic skin infiltration in chronic myelomonocytic leukaemia. *Clin Lab Haematol.* 1986;8:115-119.
12. Braga D, Manganoni AM, Boccaletti V, et al. Specific skin infiltration as first sign of chronic myelomonocytic leukemia with an unusual phenotype. *J Am Acad Dermatol.* 1996;35:804-807.
13. Elenitoba-Johnson K, Hodges GF, King TC, et al. Extramedullary myeloid cell tumors arising in the setting of chronic myelomonocytes leukemia: a report of two cases. *Arch Pathol Lab Med.* 1996;120:62-67.
14. Shaklai M, Nir M, Feuerman E, et al. Cutaneous involvement in erythroleukemia: report of a case. *Dermatol.* 1974;149:385-387.
15. Janier M, Raynaud E, Blanche P, et al. Leukemia cutis and erythroleukemia. *Br J Dermatol.* 1999;141:372-373.
16. Siegel RS, Gartenhaus RB, Kuzel TM. Human T-cell lymphotropic-1-associated leukemia/lymphoma. *Curr Treat Options Oncol.* 2001;2:291-300.
17. Zhang IH, Zane LT, Braun BS, et al. Congenital leukemia cutis with subsequent development of leukemia. *J Am Acad Dermatol.* 2006;54(2 suppl):S22-S27.
18. Resnik KS, Brod BB. Leukemia cutis in congenital leukemia: analysis and review of the world literature with report of an additional case. *Arch Dermatol.* 1993;129:1301-1306.
19. Watson KM, Mufti G, Salisbury JR, et al. Spectrum of clinical presentation, treatment and prognosis in a series of eight patients with leukaemia cutis. *Clin Exp Dermatol.* 2006;31:218-221.
20. Su WP, Buechner SA, Li CY. Clincopathology correlations in leukemia cutis. *J Am Acad Dermatol.* 1984;11:121-128.
21. Su WP. Clinical, histopathologic, and immunohistochemical correlations in leukemia cutis. *Semin Dermatol.* 1994;13:223-230.
22. Baer MR, Barcos M, Farrell H, et al. Acute myelogenous leukemia with leukemia cutis; eighteen cases seen between 1969 and 1986. *Cancer.* 1989;63:2192-2200.
23. Tomasini C, Quaglino P, Novelli M, et al. "Aleukemic" granulomatous leukemia cutis. *Am J Dermatopathol.* 1998;20:417-421.
24. O'Connell DM, Fagan WA, Skinner SM, et al. Cutaneous involvement in chronic myelomonocytic leukemia. *Int J Dermatol.* 1994;33:628-631.
25. Zax RH, Kulp-Shorten CL, Callen JP. Leukemia cutis presenting as a scrotal ulcer. *J Am Acad Dermatol.* 1989;21:410-413.
26. Sumaya CV, Babu S, Reed RJ. Erythema nodosum-like lesions of leukemia. *Arch Dematol.* 1974;110:415-418.
27. Swerdlow SH, Campo E, Harris NL, et al. *WHO Classification of Haematopoietic and Lymphoid Tissue.* IARC Press; 2008.
28. Xu B, Naughton D, Busam K, et al. ERG is a useful immunohistochemical marker to distinguish leukemia cutis from nonneoplastic infiltrates of the skin. *Am J Dermatopathol.* 2016;38(9):672-677.
29. Herling M, Khoury JD, Washington LT, et al. A systematic approach to diagnosis of mature T-cell leukemias reveals heterogeneity among WHO categories. *Blood.* 2004;104:328-335.
30. Diwan AH, Prieto VG, Herling M, et al. Primary Sézary syndrome commonly shows low-grade cytologic atypia and an absence of epidermotropism. *Am J Clin Pathol.* 2005;123:510-515.
31. Campbell JJ, Haraldsen G, Pan J, et al. The chemokine receptor CCR4 in vascular recognition by cutaneous but not intestinal memory T cells. *Nature.* 1999;400:776-780.
32. Ferenczi K, Fuhlbrigge RC, Pinkus J, et al. Increased CCR4 expression in cutaneous T cell lymphoma. *J Invest Dermatol.* 2002;119:1405-1410.
33. Kantele A, Savilahti E, Tiimonen H, et al. Cutaneous lymphocyte antigen expression on human effector B cells depends on the site and on the nature of antigen encounter. *Eur J Immunol.* 2003;33:3275-3283.
34. Picker LJ, Michle SA, Rott LS, et al. A unique phenotypes of skin-associated lymphocytes in humans: preferential expression of the HECA-452 epitope by benign and malignant T cells at cutaneous sites. *Am J Pathol.* 1990;135:1053-1068.
35. Petrella T, Meijer CJ, Dalac S, et al. TCL1 and CLA expression in agranular CD4/CD56 hematodermic neoplasms (blastic NK-cell lymphomas) and leukemia cutis. *Am J Clin Pathol.* 2004;122:307-313.
36. Yoshie O. Expression of CCR4 in adult T-cell leukemia. *Leuk Lymphoma.* 2005;46:185-190.
37. Wolf-Henning B. *Lymphocyte Homing to the Skin.* Informa Health Care; 2005:53-79.
38. Jaffe ES, Harris NL, Stein H, et al. *World Health Organization classification of tumours.* In: *Pathology and Genetics of Tumours of the Haematopoietic and Lymphoid Tissues.* IARC Press; 2001.
39. King A. A case of chloroma. *Mon J Med Soc.* 1853;17:17.
40. Chevallier P, Mohty M, Lioure B, et al. Allogeneic hematopoietic stem-cell transplantation for myeloid sarcoma: a retrospective study from the SFGM-TC. *J Clin Oncol.* 2008;26(30):4940-4943.
41. Falini B, Lenze D, Hasserjian R, et al. Cytoplasmic mutated nucleophosmin (NPM) defines the molecular status of a significant fraction of myeloid sarcomas. *Leukemia.* 2007;21:1566-1570.
42. Pileri SA, Ascani S, Cox MC, et al. Myeloid sarcoma: clinicopathologic, phenotypic and cytogenetic analysis of 92 adult patients. *Leukemia.* 2007;21:340-350.
43. Byrd JC, Edenfield WJ, Shields DJ, et al. Extramedullary myeloid cell tumors in acute nonlymphocytic leukemia: a clinical review. *J Clin Oncol.* 1995;13:1800-1816.
44. Koc Y, Miller KB, Schenkein DP, et al. Extramedullary tumors of myeloid blasts in adults as a pattern of relapse following allogeneic bone marrow transplantation. *Cancer.* 1999;85:608-615.

45. Trawek ST, Arber DA, Rappaport H, et al. Extramedullary myeloid cell tumors: an immunohistochemical and morphologic study of 28 cases. *Am J Surg Pathol.* 1993;17:1011-1019.
46. Menasce LP, Banerjee SS, Beckett E, et al. Extra-medullary myeloid tumor (granulocytic sarcoma) is often misdiagnosed: a study of 26 cases. *Histopathology.* 1999;34:391-398.
47. Neiman RS, Barcos M, Berard C, et al. Granulocytic sarcoma: a clinicopathologic study of 61 biopsied cases. *Cancer.* 1981;48:1426-1437.
48. Clark WB, Strickland SA, Barrett AJ, et al. Extramedullary relapses after allogeneic stem cell transplantation for acute myeloid leukemia and myelodysplastic syndrome. *Haematologica.* 2010;95:860-863.
49. Tsimberidou AM, Kantarjan HM, Wen S, et al. Myeloid sarcoma is associated with superior event-free survival and overall survival compared with acute myeloid leukemia. *Cancer.* 2008;113:1370-1378.
50. Lan TY, Lin DT, Tien HF, et al. Prognostic factors of treatment outcomes in patients with granulocytic sarcoma. *Acta Haematol.* 2009;122:238-246.
51. Klco JM, Welch JS, Nguyen TT, et al. State of the art in myeloid sarcoma. *Int J Lab Hematol.* 2011;33(6):555-565.
52. Hirose Y, Masaki Y, Shimoyama K, et al. Granulocytic sarcoma of megakaryoblastic differentiation in the lymph nodes terminating as acute megakaryoblastic leukemia in a case of chronic idiopathic myelofibrosis persisting for 16 years. *Eur J Haematol.* 2001;67:194-198.
53. Vega-Ruiz A, Faderi S, Estrov Z, et al. Incidence of extramedullary disease in patients with acute promyelocytic leukemia: a single-institution experience. *Int J Hematol.* 2009;89:489-496.
54. Quintanilla-Martinez L, Zukerberg LR, Ferry JA, et al. Extramedullary tumors of lymphoid or myeloid blasts. The role of immunohistology in diagnosis and classification. *Am J Clin Pathol.* 1995;104:431-443.
55. Chang CC, Eshoa C, Kampalath B, et al. Immunophenotypic profile of myeloid cells in granulocytic sarcoma by immunohistochemistry. Correlation with blast differentiation in bone marrow. *Am J Clin Pathol.* 2000;114:807-811.
56. Alexiev BA, Wang W, Ning Y, et al. Myeloid sarcomas: a histologic, immunohistochemical, and cytogenetic study. *Diagn Pathol.* 2007;2:42.
57. Lau SK, Chu PG, Weiss LM. CD163: a specific marker of macrophages in paraffin-embedded tissue samples. *Am J Clin Pathol.* 2004;122:794-801.
58. Chang H, Brandwein J, Yi QL, et al. Extramedullary infiltrates of AML are associated with CD56 expression, 11q23 abnormalities and inferior clinical outcome. *Leuk Res.* 2004;28:1007-1011.
59. Hoyer JD, Grogg KL, Hanson CA, et al. CD33 detection by immunohistochemistry in paraffin-embedded tissues: a new antibody shows excellent specificity and sensitivity for cells of myelomonocytic lineage. *Am J Clin Pathol.* 2008;129:316-323.
60. Dunphy CH, O'Malley DP, Perkins SL, et al. Analysis of immunohistochemical markers in bone marrow sections to evaluate for myelodysplastic syndromes and acute myeloid leukemias. *Appl Immunohistochem Mol Morphol.* 2007;15:154-159.
61. Nguyen TT, Schwartz EJ, West RB, et al. Expression of CD163 (hemoglobin scavenger receptor) in normal tissues, lymphomas, carcinomas, and sarcomas is largely restricted to the monocyte/macrophage lineage. *Am J Surg Pathol.* 2005;29:617-624.
62. Yang DH, Lee JJ, Mun YC, et al. Predictable prognostic factor of CD56 expression in patients with acute myeloid leukemia with t(8;21) after high dose cytarabine or allogeneic hematopoietic stem cell transplantation. *Am J Hematol.* 2007;82:1-5.
63. Klco JM, Kulkarni S, Kreisel FH, et al. Immunohistochemical analysis of monocytic leukemias: usefulness of CD14 and Kruppel-like factor, a novel monocyte marker. *Am J Clin Pathol.* 2011;135:720-730.
64. Marsee DK, Pinkus GS, Yu H. CD71 (transferring receptor): an effective marker for erythroid precursors in bone marrow biopsy specimens. *Am J Clin Pathol.* 2010;134:429-435.
65. Zuo Z, Polski JM, Kasyan A, et al. Acute erythroid leukemia. *Arch Pathol Lab Med.* 2010;134:1261-1270.
66. Dong HY, Wilkes S, Yang H. CD71 is selectively and ubiquitously expressed at high levels in erythroid precursors of all maturation stages: a comparative immunochemical study with glycophorin A and hemoglobin A. *Am J Surg Pathol.* 2011;35:723-732.
67. Olsen RJ, Chang CC, Herrick JL, et al. Acute leukemia immunohistochemistry: a systematic diagnostic approach. *Arch Pathol Lab Med.* 2008;132:462-475.
68. Bonig H, Gobel U, Nurnberger W. Bilateral exopthalmus due to retro-orbital chloromas in a boy with t(8;21)-positive acute myeloblastic acute leukemia. *Pediatr Hematol Oncol.* 2002;19:597-600.
69. Sen F, Zhang XX, Prieto VG, et al. Increased incidence of trisomy 8 in acute myeloid leukemia with skin infiltration (leukemia cutis). *Diagn Mol Pathol.* 2000;9:190-194.
70. Jackson CC, Medeiros LJ, Miranda RN. 8p11 Myeloproliferative syndrome: a review. *Hum Pathol.* 2010;41:461-476.
71. Vedy D, Muehlematter D, Rausch T, et al. Acute myeloid leukemia with myeloid sarcoma and eosinophilia: prolonged remission and molecular response to imatinib. *J Clin Oncol.* 2010;28:e33-e35.
72. Falini B, Mecucci C, Tiacci E, et al. Cytoplasmic nucleophosmin in acute myelogenous leukemia with a normal karyotype. *N Engl J Med.* 2005;352:254-266.
73. Petrella T, Bagot M, Willemze R, et al. Blastic NK-cell lymphomas (agranular CD4+CD56+ hematodermic neoplasms): a review. *Am J Clin Pathol.* 2005;123:662-675.
74. Pileri SA, Grogan TM, Harris NL, et al. Tumours of histiocytes and accessory dendritic cells: an immunohistochemical approach to classification from the International Lymphoma Study Group based on 61 cases. *Histopathology.* 2002;41:1-29.
75. Haresh KP, Joshi N, Gupta C, et al. Granulocytic sarcoma masquerading as Ewing's sarcoma: a diagnostic dilemma. *J Cancer Res Therapeut.* 2008;4:137-139.

CHAPTER 60

Cutaneous manifestations of myeloproliferative neoplasms

Richard Danialan and Carlos A. Torres-Cabala

INTRODUCTION

Myeloproliferative neoplasms (MPNs) are a group of hematopoietic disorders characterized by the clonal proliferation of cells in the myeloid lineage (granulocytes, erythrocytes, megakaryocytes). The 2016 World Health Organization (WHO) classification expanded this group of diseases to include seven entities: essential thrombocythemia (ET), primary myelofibrosis (PMF), polycythemia rubra vera (PRV) (these three associated with *JAK2/CALR/MPL* mutations), chronic myeloid leukemia (CML), chronic neutrophilic leukemia, chronic eosinophilic leukemia-not otherwise specified, and MPN, unclassifiable (MPN-U). [1] We will discuss the cutaneous manifestations (CMs) present in the most common MPNs (Table 60-1). MPNs that will not be discussed in this chapter include chronic neutrophilic leukemia, chronic eosinophilic leukemia, and MPN-U. In the majority of cases, MPNs affect adults in the fifth to seventh decade, but cases occurring in pediatric patients have been described. Organomegaly, in particular splenomegaly, is a common finding in all MPNs, along with nonspecific symptoms such as fever, weight loss, and fatigue. MPNs are relatively rare, occurring in about 6 to 10 patients per 100,000 persons. Survival depends on the type: ET has the best overall survival, and CML has the worst. Almost any MPN can progress to a fibrotic phase, characterized by a hypocellular bone marrow with increased reticulin or collagen fibrosis. In addition, any MPN can transform into a more aggressive blast phase, with PRV and ET having a 4% to 8% risk, while PMF shows a greater tendency of blastic transformation at 23%.[1] CMs of MPNs can either precede the diagnosis of an MPN or occur during the disease, and, according to one study, were found in about 10% of patients with ET at diagnosis.[2] They can be categorized into disease-related or treatment-related CMs. The disease-related CMs are those that are directly associated with the MPN, and this group includes specific disease manifestations, paraneoplastic lesions, and cutaneous infections. The treatment-related group consists of CMs occurring secondary to drug therapy, such as hydroxyurea (HU), tyrosine kinase inhibitor (TKI), or Janus kinase inhibitor therapy.[3]

DISEASE-RELATED CUTANEOUS MANIFESTATIONS

Polycythemia Rubra Vera

PRV is an MPN characterized by the clonal production of red blood cells (RBCs) that is almost always associated with the *JAK2* V617F mutation. Patients often develop a concomitant increase in granulocytes and megakaryocytes (panmyelosis) in the early to middle stages of the disease, followed by cytopenias in the late stage or fibrotic phase. Affected patients are in their 60s, with a greater frequency in males than females. They may present with hepatosplenomegaly, headaches, dizziness, or signs of arterial or venous thrombosis. Gout may occur secondary to the increased cell turnover. Erythromelalgia, which is painful redness of the hands after heat exposure, is a common cutaneous finding.[1,3] Ichthyosis is a cutaneous disorder in which the skin becomes dry and hyperkeratotic, and its acquired form has been described in PRV as well as other inflammatory and neoplastic conditions.[4] PRV patients often develop vascular thrombosis, thought to be due to increased red cell mass causing vascular stasis and tissue hypoxia. As such, patients may present with leg pain thought to be due to peripheral vascular disease. A livedo-reticularis type of skin reaction may be seen in patients presenting with cyanosis.[5] Similarly, an acute myocardial infarction may be the initial presentation of PRV. A complete blood count showing increased RBC indices and *JAK2* molecular assays may be helpful in reaching a diagnosis.[6]

Cutaneous infections occur in PRV and other MPNs under the rubric of neutrophilic dermatoses (NDs) such as pyoderma gangrenosum (PG) and acute febrile ND (also termed Sweet syndrome [SS]). However, the underlying hematologic disorder of NDs most commonly is an acute leukemia. Patients with PG have solitary or multiple large, necrotic, and painful ulcers that present on the lower extremities, although the trunk, face, and arms may also be affected. SS, on the other hand, presents as multiple circumscribed painful red plaques or nodules. It may present on the extremities as well as the head and neck region. Histologically, both entities are characterized by dermal and subcutaneous neutrophilic infiltrates. One hypothesis for the appearance of pustular dermatosis is a defect in neutrophil superoxide anion (O_2^-) generation. Support for this hypothesis stems from the fact that ND resolves after neutrophil function is improved via treatment with dapsone.[7] Magro et al[8] also explored the possibility that PG and SS are characterized by clonally restricted neutrophilic infiltrates that develop secondary to an underlying hematologic disease, most often myeloid dyscrasias. Using human androgen receptor assays, they found that 20% to 40% of cases of PG and SS cases contained clonally restricted neutrophils and that this restriction either preceded or occurred subsequent to an underlying hematologic disease. However, after systemic workup, they also found cases that were not associated with hematologic disease. Nevertheless, a diagnosis of SS and PG should alert the clinician to rule out any underlying hematologic condition. An important entity to consider in the differential diagnosis of NDs is that of rheumatoid neutrophilic dermatitis, which presents as nodules and plaques on the extensor aspects of the upper and lower extremities. Histologically, it is identical to other NDs; the key distinguishing characteristic is positive serology for rheumatoid factor.[9]

Patients with PRV also have variable degrees of pruritus, which can precede the disease by years. Dermatologic examination may often reveal no grossly visible lesion, in which case it is attributed to an *invisible dermatosis*. Pruritus may occur at any time, but is often exacerbated after exposure to warm water (aquagenic pruritus) and sometimes may mimic eczematous dermatitis.[10] One study showed that the degree of epidermal and papillary dermal infiltration by mononuclear cells (including eosinophils) was higher in PRV patients exposed to warm water than in healthy control patients and PRV patients exposed to room temperature water. The degree of mononuclear and eosinophil infiltration correlated with the severity of pruritus, but the infiltrate itself was deemed to be reactive in nature.[11]

PRV may present with urticarial vasculitis, a condition that is seen in other entities such as viral infections (eg, hepatitis B), collagen vascular diseases (eg, systemic lupus erythematosus), and hematologic conditions (eg, Hodgkin lymphoma). It is characterized clinically by painful, recurrent episodes of pruritic papules or wheals that last longer than 24 hours, which is different from other urticarial presentations. Histologically, urticarial vasculitis is characterized by endothelial cell swelling, extravasated RBCs, and perivascular neutrophilic infiltrate. Direct immunofluorescence may reveal immunoglobulin and C3 deposits within the walls of the blood vessels and at the dermal–epidermal junction. Treatment of the underlying PRV may resolve the vasculitis.[12]

An increased occurrence of nonmelanoma skin cancers has been reported in patients with PRV and ET, possibly in association with HU or JAK inhibitors therapy.[13]

Essential Thrombocythemia

ET is characterized by a clonal proliferation of megakaryocytes as evidenced by persistent thrombocytosis (ie., platelet count higher than 450×10^9/L) in the peripheral blood. It occurs in patients in their 50s and 60s, although it has been reported in younger individuals. Men and women are equally affected. Causes of reactive thrombocytosis must first be excluded before a diagnosis of ET is considered, although demonstration of a *JAK2* V617F mutation in the presence of isolated thrombocytosis is highly suggestive of ET. A *BCR::ABL1* gene fusion is not detected. Bone marrow examination usually reveals increased atypical megakaryocytes with hyperchromatic, irregular nuclei imparting a "stag-horn" morphology.[1] Rarely, ET may transform into acute leukemia.[14]

CMs of ET show some overlap with those of PRV. Patients often present with signs of thrombosis and/or hemorrhage, which may accompany pain (erythromelalgia), especially in the upper and lower extremities and following heat exposure or exercise. Raynaud phenomenon, necrotizing vasculitis, urticaria, acrocyanosis, superficial

TABLE 60-1 Most Common Clinical/Histologic Findings in Myeloproliferative Disorders

Myeloproliferative neoplasm	Extramedullary Hematopoiesis	Neutrophilic Dermatosis	Thrombosis	Erythromelalgia	Livedo Reticularis	Urticarial Vasculitis	Aquagenic Pruritus
Polycythemia rubra vera	−	+	++	++	++	++	++
Essential thrombocythemia	−	+	++	++	++	+/−	+/−
Primary myelofibrosis	++	+	+	+	+	−	−
Chronic myelogenous leukemia	−	++ (especially in blast phase)	+	+	+	−	−

thrombophlebitis, pruritus, livedo reticularis, ischemic gangrene, leg ulcers, hematomas, petechiae, ecchymoses, and purpura have all been described in patients with ET.[2,15,16] Livedo racemosa, with obstruction and recanalization of blood vessels in the deep dermis in the absence of fibrinoid necrosis or inflammation, has been found to be frequent in Japanese patients.[17] Acquired angioedema as the presenting feature of ET has been recently reported in one patient.[18] A hemorrhagic diathesis, although rare, occurs from altered function of von Willebrand factor when platelet levels are very high.[19]

Histologically, small-vessel thrombosis and endothelial hyperplasia are most often noted in the acute setting, with nonspecific findings in the chronic/resolved phase. The pathophysiology behind thrombosis is clonally stimulated dysfunctional thrombocytes with an increased affinity for aggregation and thus thrombosis. The workup of ET includes the exclusion of other causes of coagulopathy such as factor V Leiden deficiency. Treatment is aimed at reducing the number of platelets via cryoreductive agents such as HU, interferon α, pegylated interferon, and anagrelide, as well as preventing aggregation via aspirin.

Primary Myelofibrosis

PMF is a rare, clonal MPN characterized by the proliferation of atypical megakaryocytes and granulocytes in the bone marrow and is divided into a prefibrotic (cellular) phase and a fibrotic (paucicellular) phase. The fibrotic phase is characterized by bone marrow reticulin or collagen fibrosis, which often results in few, if any, bone marrow elements during aspiration ("dry-tap"). Any MPN can become fibrotic in the latter stages of the disease process and therefore may resemble PMF. It affects approximately 1 per 100,000 persons and occurs in the sixth to the seventh decade of life with an equal sex distribution. The hallmark of PMF is the presence of extramedullary hematopoiesis (EMH), the formation and development of blood cells in sites other than the bone marrow. It most often involves the liver, spleen, and lymph nodes.[1,20,21] It is rarely found in the skin[22] and occurs in approximately 0.4% of PMF cases.[23] PMF is characterized by infiltration of the bone marrow by atypical megakaryocytes with hyperlobated, "cloud-like" nuclei that are often localized to the sinusoidal spaces. The distinction of PMF from CML is important, as PMF demonstrates a *JAK2* V617F or *MPL* W515K and W515L mutation, whereas CML has a characteristic *BCR::ABL1* fusion.[1] More recently, *JAK2*-negative cases of MPN (including PMF) have been shown to harbor mutations of the calreticulin gene.[24]

EMH is a normal physiologic phenomenon in the early fetal development up to the fifth month of gestation where dermal mesenchymal cells still have the ability to undergo hematopoietic differentiation.[23] In the postnatal period, however, it is pathologic and associated with TORCH infections (toxoplasmosis, other agents, rubella/German measles, cytomegalovirus, and herpes simplex), twin transfusion syndrome, and rhesus hemolytic disease. Pediatric patients often present with a red- or magenta-colored maculopapular rash due to persistent dermal hematopoiesis, often referred to as "blueberry muffin syndrome."[25] In adults, EMH may be reactive and seen in conditions leading to acquired or functional hyposplenism such as sickle cell disease, hereditary spherocytosis, immune thrombocytopenic purpura, and myelophthisic processes such as metastatic carcinoma involving bone marrow.[21] However, EMH in adults is most often associated with an underlying MPN.[26] Clinically, patients with cutaneous EMH may present with multiple red–purple nodules, papules, bullae, erythema, rash, and ulcers and thus may mimic inflammatory disorders and leukemia cutis (LC).[27] Histologically, EMH is characterized by a nodular dermal or subcutaneous, predominantly intravascular infiltrate of atypical megakaryocytes with typical or atypical mitotic figures as well as a mixture of mature and immature myeloid cells and erythroid precursors. Occasional blasts may be present, but when the predominant cell is a blast, a leukemic transformation must be considered. Immunohistochemical studies may be useful in the distinction of the latter. Blasts are usually CD34, CD117, or TdT positive, whereas megakaryocytes are CD61 and CD42b positive and CD34, CD117, and TdT negative. O'Malley et al[21] have argued that the term "cutaneous EMH" is misleading and favored the term "neoplastic myeloid proliferations" when EMH is associated with an underlying hematologic disorder. Hoss and McNutt recommended the use of the term "cutaneous myelofibrosis" (CMF) as a more accurate term to describe cutaneous EMH associated with an underlying PMF in comparison to cutaneous EMH of a reactive nature. Support for CMF is provided by the fact that the same clonal population has been identified in both the skin and the bone marrow. They postulated that the atypical megakaryocytes travel from the bone marrow to the skin via the vasculature and that this finding accounts for their intravascular location.[20] Distinguishing reactive cutaneous EMH from CMF may be difficult (Table 60-2), yet of paramount significance as the latter finding may portend an aggressive clinical course of the underlying hematologic disease.[22] CMF clinically presents as multiple firm dermal/subcutaneous nodules, similar to metastases, while reactive cutaneous EMH usually presents as mildly elevated papules. In addition, while CMF implies the presence of predominantly atypical megakaryocytes and immature myeloid/erythroid elements in a background of fibrosis, reactive cutaneous EMH is associated with a predominance of mature myeloid/erythroid elements in a nonfibrotic background. While lesions of reactive cutaneous EMH spontaneously resolve, those of CMF rarely do, and as such portend an aggressive clinical course with median survivals of only a few months. Lastly, CMF may demonstrate a *JAK2* mutation, while reactive cutaneous EMH does not (Figs. 60-1 and 60-2).[28,29] Similarly, splenic "EMH" in patients with MPNs has been demonstrated to harbor *JAK2* mutations, further supporting that these lesions are neoplastic and likely represent involvement by the disease in extramedullary sites[30]

Dermal fibrosis, as in the bone marrow, may be present secondary to excess platelet-derived growth factor, transforming growth factor-B, calmodulin, and vascular endothelial growth factor production by the neoplastic megakaryocytes.[31]

TABLE 60-2 Clinical and Histologic Features in the Distinction of Reactive Extramedullary Hematopoiesis From Myelofibrosis-Associated Extramedullary Hematopoiesis

Clinical/Histologic Features	Reactive Extramedullary Hematopoiesis	Extramedullary Hematopoiesis Associated With Myelofibrosis
Clinical appearance	Mildly raised papules	Multiple firm dermal/subcutaneous nodules
Clinical course	Spontaneously resolve	Persistent
Concurrent systemic/bone marrow neoplastic hematologic disorder	Absent	Present
Predominant cell types	Mature erythroid/myeloid elements	Immature myeloid/erythroid elements with occasional blasts
Dysplastic megakaryocytes with mitotic figures	Absent	Present
Associated fibrosis	Absent	Present
JAK2 mutation	Absent	Present

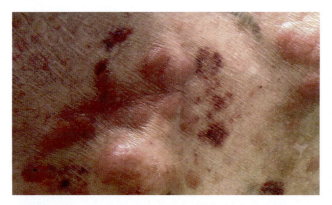

FIGURE 60-1. Cutaneous nodules associated with myelofibrosis. (From Fraga GR, Caughron SK. Cutaneous myelofibrosis with JAK2 V627F mutation: metastasis, not merely extramedullary hematopoiesis. *Am J Dermatopathol.* 2010;32:727-730, with permission.)

Type III collagen is the main type of collagen that is produced, although other collagen types are also found. In early fibrotic lesions, a reticulin stain may be necessary as hematoxylin and eosin and trichrome stains may not highlight fibrosis.[28]

Rarely, reactive cutaneous EMH may occur following granulocyte colony-stimulating factor (G-CSF) therapy secondary to neutropenia in cases of myelodysplastic syndrome. The reactive nature of this phenomenon is evident when, upon cessation of G-CSF therapy, the EMH resolves.[32,33] Thrombosis, NDs, and cutaneous vasculitis may also be found in PMF as in other MPNs.[34,35] Moreover, patients with PMF may present with paraneoplastic syndromes characterized by dermatomyositis[36] and scleroderma-like skin changes that may predate the diagnosis of PMF by years.[37] Paraneoplastic syndromes seen in patients with blastic transformation of PMF include unilateral lower extremity swelling with an inflammatory dermal and subcutaneous infiltrate[38] and septal/paraseptal panniculitis accompanied by a mixed inflammatory infiltrate with vasculitis.[39] Secondary erythromelalgia that histopathologically showed marked perivascular and intramural mucin deposition has been reported in a patient with PMF.[40]

Chronic Myeloid Leukemia

CML is an MPN characterized by the clonal proliferation of the granulocytic lineages in various stages of development and occurs in 1.0 to 1.5 per 100,000 people.[41] Its hallmark molecular profile consists of a t(9; 22) (q34; q11.2) translocation which leads to a fusion between the *BCR* and *ABL1* genes on chromosomes 22 and 9, respectively. This fusion creates the Philadelphia chromosome, which has increased tyrosine kinase activity and is implicated in the clonal proliferation of the granulocytic lineage. CML, like the aforementioned MPNs, may either present with or progress to a fibrotic stage within the bone marrow. Also, CML may progress from the indolent chronic phase to an accelerated phase and a blast phase, depending on the number of blasts in the bone marrow and peripheral smear. Progression of CML is associated with additional mutations such as isochromosome 17q, trisomies 8 and 18, and an extra Philadelphia chromosome.[1]

Patients with CML present with visible cutaneous lesions when their disease has transformed into blast crisis, or LC, which occurs in 2% to 8% of treated CML.[42] Clinically, LC is characterized by red–brown, violaceous papules, nodules, or plaques, most commonly found in the legs, but any site including the head may be affected.[43] LC may rarely present as vitiligo[44] or occur in association with a bullous variant of SS.[45] Therefore, a high index of suspicion for LC must be maintained in any CML patient presenting with NDs and new skin lesions.[45]

LC is infrequently observed in ET, PRV, and PMF, but heralds a more aggressive course of disease when present. It is not a term specific to the blast form of CML and can

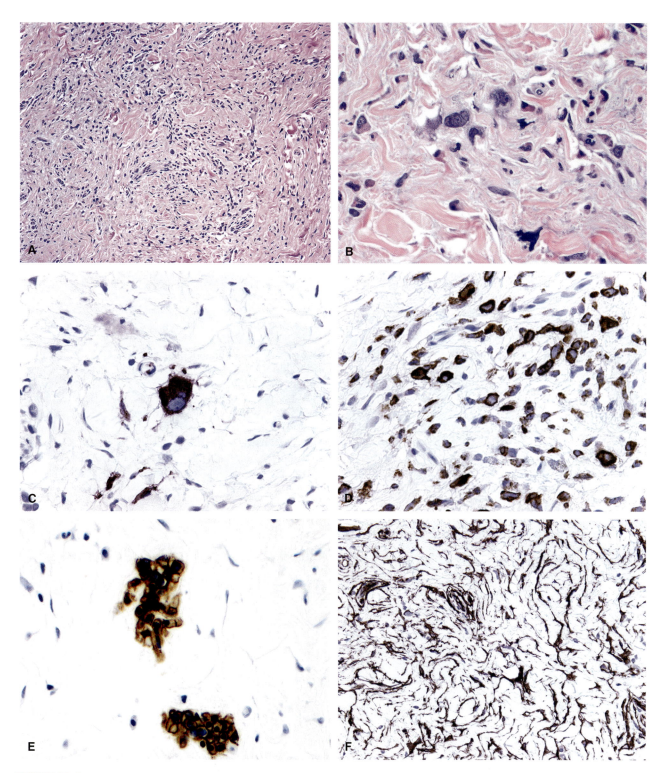

FIGURE 60-2. **Cutaneous involvement by primary myelofibrosis, as "neoplastic extramedullary hematopoiesis." A.** An interstitial polymorphous infiltrate associated with dense collagen fibers is seen involving the dermis (H&E, ×40). **B.** At higher magnification, dysmorphic large cells consistent with megakaryocytes along with mononuclear myeloid cells are seen. Clusters of round cells, consistent with erythroid cells, were also present (not shown) (H&E, ×400). **C.** By immunohistochemistry, the abnormal megakaryocytes are demonstrated to express CD61 (×400). **D.** The mononuclear cells are positive for myeloperoxidase by immunohistochemistry (×400). **E.** An immunohistochemical study for glycophorin A highlights clusters of mononucleated cells, confirming erythroid cells in the dermis (×400). **F.** A CD34 immunohistochemical study decorates dermal fibroblasts and is negative in the interstitial infiltrate (×40).

be seen in cutaneous involvement by T-cell and B-cell leukemias/lymphomas as well as other nonmyeloid leukemias, usually after systemic disease has manifested. Rarely, LC may be the initial presentation of an MPN. Granulocytic sarcoma/chloromas is also a term used to denote the CM of the blast phase of CML.[46] Histologically, the main findings in LC are leukemic infiltrates that have superficial and deep, perivascular and periadnexal involvement with a grenz zone in the upper dermis, but less frequently, sparse leukemic cells may be noted instead. The tumor cells are generally large with blastic-appearing nuclei with fine chromatin, although the morphology may depend on the particular leukemia or lymphoma. Immunophenotyping is important because myeloid cells express myeloperoxidase (MPO), CD33, lysozyme, and various levels of immature blast markers, CD34 and CD117. Establishing blast lineage can best be accomplished via flow cytometry.[47-49] Very rarely, involvement of the skin by CML manifests as EMH-like lesions, similar to other MPNs.[50]

Chronic Myelomonocytic Leukemia

Chronic myelomonocytic leukemia (CMML) is a chronic hematologic disorder that displays features of both a myeloproliferative and a myelodysplastic syndrome. It is characterized by a persistent monocytosis (>1 × 10^9/L) in the absence of any reactive cause of monocytosis. The myelodysplastic component may involve one or more myeloid lineages. Per WHO guidelines, a *BCR::ABL1* fusion or *PDGFRA/PDGFRB* rearrangements must be absent and blasts and their equivalents (promonocytes) must number less than 20% in the peripheral blood or bone marrow. While the peripheral blood and bone marrow are always involved, the most common sites of extramedullary involvement include the spleen, liver, skin, and lymph nodes.[1] CMML rarely involves the skin (~10% of cases); when it occurs, it usually happens in elderly males. The clinical presentation varies from solitary ulcers to multiple erythematous and violaceous papules, nodules, as well as erysipelas-like eruption.[51] Cutaneous involvement may occur in the setting of CMML-1 (blasts, including promonocytes number <5% in the peripheral blood, <10% in the bone marrow), CMML-2 (blasts, including promonocytes number 5%-19% in the peripheral blood and 10%-19% in the bone marrow), or when CMML has transformed to frank acute myeloid leukemia. Cutaneous involvement may at times be the sole presentation of a yet undiagnosed CMML or concurrent with or after a diagnosis of CMML has been established.[52] Multiple studies have shown that cutaneous involvement is a poor overall prognostic indicator with overall survival measured in months.[52-55] Vitte et al[51] studied 42 cases of CMML with cutaneous involvement in a retrospective study. They found that CMML could histologically present in four different ways in the skin. They established four distinct groups using histopathologic and immunophenotypic profiles and assessed for differences in overall survival between the four groups, which were as follows:

1. Myelomonocytic cell tumors with a majority of medium-sized blasts (CD4$^{+/-}$, CD45$^{+/-}$, CD68$^+$, MPO$^+$, CD33$^+$, CD13$^+$, S100$^-$, CD1a$^-$, Langerin$^-$) (Fig. 60-3)

2. Mature plasmacytoid dendritic cell proliferations (MPDCPs) composed of medium-sized cells with round or oval nuclei and absent nucleoli (CD4$^+$, CD13$^+$, CD33$^+$, CD56$^-$, CD123$^+$, CD303$^+$, TCL1$^+$, granzyme B$^+$, Langerin$^-$). A case masquerading as lupus erythematosus has been reported[56] (Fig. 60-4)

3. Blastic plasmacytoid dendritic cell neoplasms containing medium-sized blast cells with irregular nuclei and small nucleoli (CD68$^+$, MPO$^-$, CD13$^-$, CD33$^-$, CD4$^+$, CD56$^+$, CD1a$^-$, CD123$^+$, TCL1$^+$, granzyme B$^-$) (Fig. 60-5)

4. Blastic indeterminate dendritic cell tumors (BIDCTs) featuring large blast cells with round, oval nuclei and prominent nucleoli (CD4$^+$, CD13$^+$, CD33$^+$, CD56$^+$, CD68$^+$, CD1a$^+$, S100$^+$, Langerin$^-$)[57,58] (Fig. 60-6)

Overall survival from the time of the skin lesions to patient death/last follow-up was different among the four groups, although the findings were not statistically significant. The MPDCP group had the best overall survival (23 months), whereas the BIDCT group had the worst (6.8 months).[51] Cutaneous lesions showing unusual immunophenotypes may not be rare, as exemplified in a case with mixed histiocytic and Langerhans cell differentiation[59] and a patient with T-cell large granular lymphocytic leukemia and CMML presenting with multiple arthropod bite-like papules that showed myelomonocytic (CD4$^+$, CD1a$^+$) differentiation.[60]

While the aforementioned scheme suggested by Vitte et al[51] has not yet transitioned to standard medical practice in the setting of cutaneous involvement by CMML, patients should be closely followed by a dermatologist for any signs of cutaneous involvement. A biopsy may be necessary to establish a diagnosis in cases of ambiguous cutaneous presentations of CMML, such as in those mimicking a dermatitis. Cutaneous lesions should be managed promptly and aggressively, as they are associated with an adverse prognosis and disease progression.[53,54,61]

Idiopathic Hypereosinophilic Syndrome

Hypereosinophilic syndrome (HES) was originally defined by Chusid et al[62] as persistent unexplained peripheral blood eosinophilia (≥1.5 × 10^9 for at least 6 months with symptoms of end-organ damage (ie., myocarditis, GI disturbances, neurologic symptoms) secondary to increased eosinophils and their degranulation products. Reactive causes of eosinophilia including collagen vascular disease, other hematologic neoplasms with secondary eosinophils, drugs, allergic diseases, Churg–Strauss syndrome, and parasitic infestation need to be ruled out. Importantly, the eosinophils are nonclonal in nature and increased myeloblasts are not seen in the peripheral blood or bone marrow, which allows separation from chronic eosinophilic leukemia. No *BCR::ABL1* fusion is identified. The most common sites of organ involvement include the lungs, GI tract, central nervous system, and the heart, which can lead to endomyocardial fibrosis and restrictive cardiomegaly.[1] HES is further subdivided into myeloproliferative and lymphocytic variants. The myeloproliferative variant shows clonal expansion of eosinophils, dysplastic myeloid precursors, normal serum IgE levels, a higher tendency for organ involvement, but a lower tendency to involve skin. Commonly, the myeloproliferative variant is characterized by a *FIPL1-and-PDGFRA* fusion, leading to activation of *PDGFRA*. Recognition of this variant is important, as it

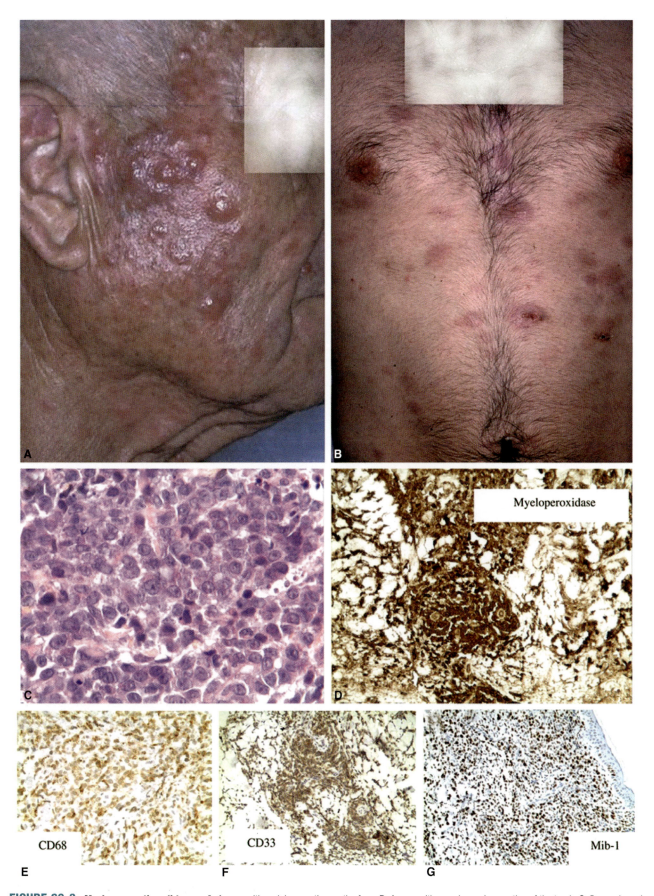

FIGURE 60-3. Myelomonocytic cell tumor. A. A case with nodular eruption on the face. **B.** A case with maculopapular eruption of the trunk. **C.** Dense dermal infiltrate of large blast cells (H&E). **D.** Immunostaining for MPO. 13% of MMCTs were positive for MPO. **E.** Immunostaining for CD68; 98% of MMCTs were positive for CD68. **F.** Immunostaining for CD33; 13% of MMCTs were positive for CD33. **G.** Immunostaining for Mib-1; intermediate positivity (34%-66%). (From Vitte F, Fabiani B, Benet C, et al. Specific skin lesions in chronic myelomonocytic leukemia: a spectrum of myelomonocytic and dendritic cell proliferations. a study of 42 cases. *Am J Surg Pathol.* 2012;36(9):1302-1316, with permission.)

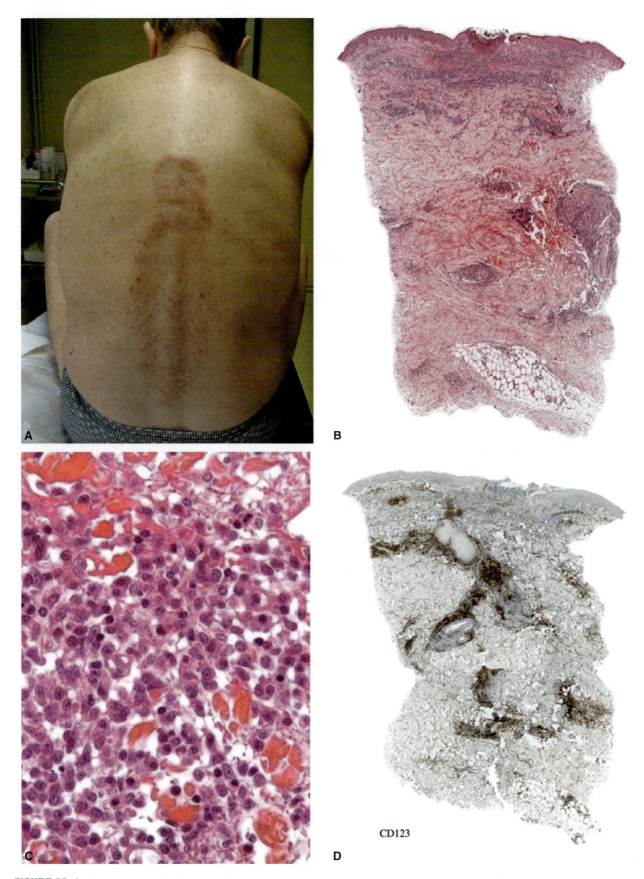

FIGURE 60-4. **Mature plasmacytoid dendritic cell proliferation. A.** Itchy erythemato-macular eruption of the back. **B.** Nodular dermal infiltrate with epidermal scratching excoriation (H&E). **C.** Cluster of PDC intermixed with small lymphocytes (H&E). **D.** Immunostaining for CD123 showing large and confluent clusters of PDC at low magnification. (From Vitte F, Fabiani B, Benet C, et al. Specific skin lesions in chronic myelomonocytic leukemia: a spectrum of myelomonocytic and dendritic cell proliferations. a study of 42 cases. *Am J Surg Pathol.* 2012;36(9):1302-1316, with permission.)

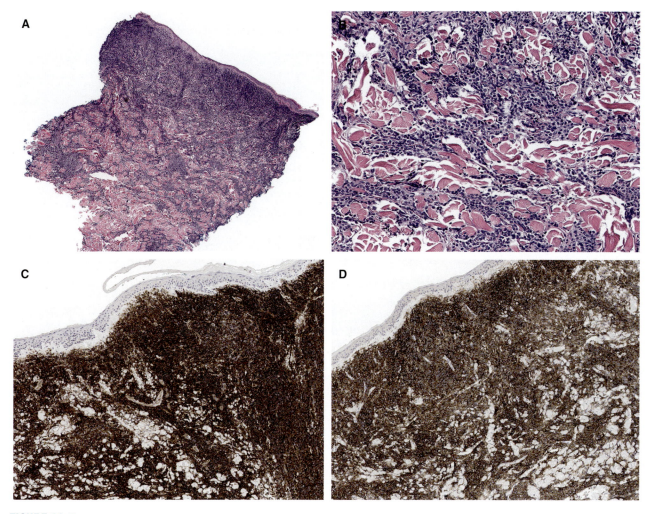

FIGURE 60-5. Blastic plasmacytoid dendritic cell neoplasm. A. Diffuse infiltration of the dermis by mononuclear cells is seen (H&E, ×20). **B.** The cells reveal blastoid appearance (H&E, ×100). **C.** By immunohistochemistry, diffuse expression of CD123 is detected in the tumor cells (×40). **D.** The tumor cells are also strongly and diffusely positive for CD56 by immunohistochemistry (×40).

responds to treatment with imatinib. The lymphocytic variant of HES is characterized by nonmalignant clonal expansion of T-cells that produce cytokines via activation of IL-4 and IL-5, which subsequently leads to hypereosinophilia. Patients have increased serum IgE levels, fewer organopathic changes and myocardial fibrosis, and more common cutaneous involvement in the form of erythroderma, eczema, atopic dermatitis, and other nonspecific dermatitides.[63]

Cutaneous involvement by HES has been documented to occur as high as 56% and usually presents concurrently at the time of diagnosis. Rarely, skin involvement occurs as the sole presentation of HES. Raynaud phenomenon, livedo reticularis, pruritus, palmoplantar hyperkeratosis, mucosal ulcerations, angioedema, and intraepidermal bullous lesions[64] have all been demonstrated to represent CMs of HES. As such, HES should always be included in the differential diagnosis of an unexplained erythroderma.[65]

The histopathology of HES may be nonspecific and mimic Wells syndrome, although HES and Wells syndrome may form a continuum. HES may present histologically as a chronic spongiotic dermatitis with a mixed dermal inflammatory infiltrate of variable intensity. Flame figures are not commonly seen in HES. In contrast, Wells syndrome features a dermal-based, predominantly eosinophilic infiltrate with flame figures and granulomatous inflammation with possible collagen necrobiosis, depending on the age of the lesions.[66]

Since prompt treatment is necessary to prevent fatal or irreversible outcomes of end-organ damage, Simon et al[63] argued that the arbitrary criteria for diagnosis of HES set forth by Chusid et al may be too rigid and deprive patients of much needed early treatment. They suggested that treatment should commence when there is any marked eosinophilia with symptoms of organ involvement, irrespective of eosinophil counts or duration of symptoms. Conversely, patients with a long history of elevated eosinophil counts but no systemic symptoms should be followed clinically as they may develop end-organ damage in the future.

Juvenile Myelomonocytic Leukemia

Juvenile myelomonocytic leukemia (JMML) is, although rare, the most common myeloproliferative syndrome in young children. JMML is an aggressive clonal disorder of the granulocytic and monocytic lineages which, like CMML, also contains features of myelodysplastic syndrome. Blasts, including blast equivalents, number less than 20% in the

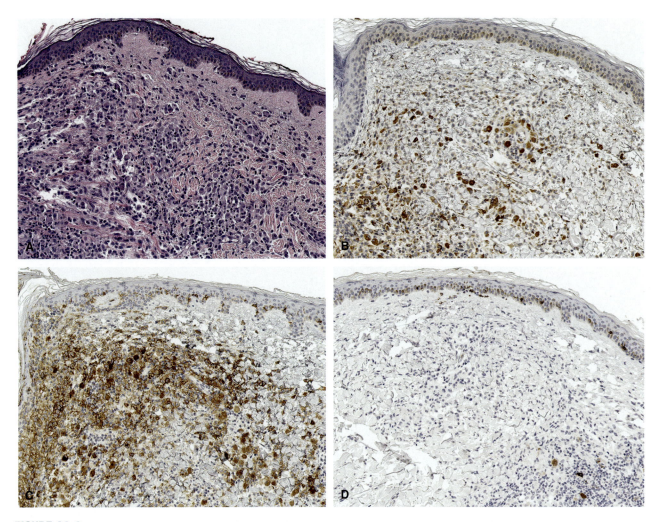

FIGURE 60-6. Blastic indeterminate dendritic cell tumor. A. The skin biopsy reveals dermal infiltration by cells of histiocytic appearance and large nuclei (H&E, ×200). **B.** The tumor cells are variably positive for CD68 by immunohistochemistry (×200). **C.** The tumor cells express CD1a by immunohistochemistry (×200). **D.** Langerin is negative in the tumor cells (×200).

peripheral blood or bone marrow. A *BCR::ABL1* fusion is not detected although *NRAS, KRAS,* and *PTPN11* mutations, among others, may be seen, and the condition is considered a RASopathy syndrome.[67] Children affected with JMML have higher than normal hemoglobin F levels. As the name suggests, younger patients are affected, with ages ranging from 0 to 14 years and predominance of boys over girls.[1,68] There is an association with neurofibromatosis type 1, juvenile xanthogranulomas,[69] and Noonan's syndrome. While the peripheral blood and bone marrow are always involved, extramedullary sites such as the spleen, lymph node, respiratory tract, and skin can be affected. Cutaneous involvement may precede a diagnosis of JMML. Clinically, they may present as several indurated erythematous lesions or other nonspecific rashes, which may not be biopsied.[70] However, concurrent lymphadenopathy and/or hepatosplenomegaly may alert the clinician to perform a biopsy to determine if the skin rash is related to the systemic symptoms. Histopathologically, dermal involvement demonstrates atypical monocytes which stain positive for CD45, CD68, MPO, and lysozyme, while being negative for CD3 and CD20. The prognosis of JMML is often poor with frequent relapse despite bone marrow transplantation.[71]

TREATMENT-RELATED CUTANEOUS MANIFESTATIONS

Hydroxyurea

Patients treated for MPN are often administered HU which acts as a chemotherapeutic agent by preventing the conversion of ribonucleotides into deoxyribonucleotides through the inhibition of the M2 subunit of ribonucleotide reductase. The result is diminished DNA synthesis and cell death in the S-phase of the cell cycle.[72] HU has been successfully used in the treatment of MPN, psoriasis, and sickle cell disease. Patients, especially those receiving long-term HU therapy, may complain of painful skin ulcers, typically in older women who have received HU for at least 1 year (Table 60-3). The ulcers are commonly found at areas of leg and foot trauma, such as the malleoli.[73,74] Some patients displayed paraneoplastic syndromes consisting of dermatomyositis-like skin changes on the hands with purple gottron-like papules on the interphalangeal joints as well as a violaceous facial rash and widespread telangiectasias. However, muscle weakness or positive autoantibody screens are not detected, in contrast

TABLE 60-3 Dermatologic Findings Associated With Chronic Hydroxyurea Therapy

Anatomic Site	Findings
Hair	Alopecia
General skin	Hyperpigmentation, xerosis, skin atrophy, poikiloderma, secondary ichthyosis, actinic keratosis, squamous cell carcinoma, invisible dermatosis (pruritus)
Nails	Melanonychia, onycholysis
Extremities	Ulcers, dermatomyositis-like changes, scleroderma-like changes
Mucous membranes	Ulcers, hyperpigmentation

TABLE 60-4 Most Common Dermatologic Findings Associated With Tyrosine Kinase Inhibitor Therapy

Anatomic Site	Findings
General skin	Nonspecific pruritic rash, maculopapular dermatitis, lichenoid dermatitis, xerosis, keratosis pilaris, hypopigmentation, hyperpigmentation, acute generalized exanthematous pustulosis (AGEP), drug reaction with eosinophilia and systemic symptoms (DRESS), Stevens–Johnson syndrome, pseudoporphyria, pityriasis rubra pilaris-like reaction, pityriasis rosea-like eruption, ichthyosiform eruptions
Hair	Depigmentation, alopecia
Head and neck	Periorbital edema/purpura
Extremities	Acral lividosis

with dermatomyositis.[75] The etiology of the leg ulcers is not entirely known, although some researchers have postulated that the ulcers occur as a result of the toxic effects of HU on basal keratinocytes. Another possible explanation is that the RBCs become larger secondary to HU treatment, preventing them from easily passing through the blood vessels, eventually leading to anoxia. Other effects of long-term HU therapy include diffuse hyperpigmentation of the skin, nails, or mucosa, xerosis, skin atrophy, melanonychia, palmoplantar keratoderma, stomatitis, aphthoid ulcers, alopecia, and poikiloderma.[72,76] Hyperpigmentation has been thought to occur secondary to the direct effect of melanocyte activation by the drug. African American patients and those with sickle cell disease are at increased risk of hyperpigmentation. Patients have also been known to develop nonmelanoma skin cancers and premalignant lesions, such as actinic keratoses and squamous cell carcinomas.[77] A rare case of sclerodermoid changes in the skin of the lower extremities in association with a 12-year history of HU treatment for an MPN was described. Once HU was discontinued, the lesions resolved.[78] HU treatment is associated with nonspecific histologic findings such as vacuolar interface dermatitis, which may mimic other differential diagnoses including dermatomyositis. Some researchers have postulated that these dermatomyositis-like skin changes are secondary to DNA synthesis inhibition in the basal keratinocytes.[79]

Tyrosine Kinase and Janus Kinase Inhibitors

With the advent of TKIs, the prognosis of CML has drastically improved. Before TKI therapy, most cases of CML progressed to blast phase, but that number has decreased to about 5% with TKIs.[49] Imatinib (Gleevec) prevents the neoplastic proliferation of immature myeloid cells by displacing ATP from its binding site on the BCR–ABL1 fusion protein. However, various drug reactions have been reported with imatinib and other second- and third-generation TKIs (Table 60-4), including maculopapular dermatitis, lichenoid dermatitis,[80] an increased risk of cutaneous malignancies,[81,82] leukotrichia,[83,84] periorbital purpura,[85] Stevens–Johnson syndrome,[86] pityriasis rosea-like eruption,[87] pityriasis rubra pilaris-like reaction,[88] pseudoporphyria,[89] diffuse hyperpigmentation of oral mucosa, skin, and nails,[90] ichthyosiform eruptions,[80] and others. Knowledge of the CM of TKI therapy is important in the overall management of patients with MPNs.[91] Ruxolitinib, a small molecule JAK2 inhibitor, has been associated with SS, solitary foot ulcer, and erythematous lesions with necrotic centers in lower extremities.[92]

75. Nofal A, El-Din ES. Hydroxyurea-induced dermatomyositis: true amyopathic dermatomyositis or dermatomyositis-like eruption?. *Int J Dermatol*. 2012;51:535-541.
76. Bulte CA, Hoegler KM, Kutlu Ö, Khachemoune A. Hydroxyurea: a reappraisal of its cutaneous side effects and their management. *Int J Dermatol*. 2021;60(7):810-817.
77. Criado PR, Moure ERD, Junior JAS. Adverse mucocutaneous reactions related to chemotherapeutic agents—part II. *An Bras Dermatol*. 2010;85:591-608.
78. Garcia-Martinez FJ, Garcia-Gavin J, Alvarez-Perez A, et al. Scleroderma-like syndrome due to hydroxyurea. *Clin Exp Dermatol*. 2012;37:755-758.
79. Haniffa MA, Speight EL. Painful leg ulcers and a rash in a patient with polycythaemia rubra vera. Diagnosis: hydroxyurea-induced leg ulceration and dermatomyositis-like skin changes. *Clin Exp Dermatol*. 2006;31:733-734.
80. Ransohoff JD, Kwong BY. Cutaneous adverse events of targeted therapies for hematolymphoid malignancies. *Clin Lymphoma Myeloma Leuk*. 2017;17(12):834-851.
81. Campione E, Diluvio L, Paterno EJ, et al. Kaposi's sarcoma in a patient treated with imatinib mesylate for chronic myeloid leukemia. *Clin Ther*. 2009;21:2565-2569.
82. Verma D, Kantarjian H, Strom SS, et al. Malignancies occurring during therapy with tyrosine kinase inhibitors (TKIs) for chronic myeloid leukemia (CML) and other hematologic malignancies. *Blood*. 2011;118:4353-4358.
83. Samimi S, Chu E, Seykora J, et al. Dasatinib-induced leukotrichia in a patient with chronic myelogenous leukemia. *Jama Dermatol*. 2013;149:637-639.
84. Wang Y, Zhao Y, Liu L, et al. Inhibitory effects of imatinib mesylate on human epidermal melanocytes. *Clin Exp Dermatol*. 2014;39:202-208.
85. Anzalone CL, Cohen PR, Kurzrock R, et al. Imatinib-induced postoperative periorbital purpura: GASP (gleevec-associated surgical purpura) in women with imatinib-treated chronic myelogenous leukemia. *Dermatol Online J*. 2014;20:1-7.
86. Jha P, Himanshu D, Jain N, et al. Imatinib-induced Stevens-Johnsons syndrome. *BMJ Case Rep*. 2013;2013:1-3.
87. Brazzelli V, Prestinari F, Roveda E, et al. Pityriasis rosea-like eruption during treatment with imatinib mesylate: description of 3 cases. *J Am Acad Dermatol*. 2005;53:S240-S243.
88. Plana A, Carrascosa JM, Vilavella M, et al. Pityriasis rubra pilaris-like reaction induced by imatinib. *Clin Exp Dermatol*. 2013;38:520-522.
89. Mahon C, Purvis D, Laughton S, et al. Imatinib mesylate-induced pseudoporphyria in two children. *Pediatr Dermatol*. 2014;31:603-607.
90. Di Tullio F, Mandel VD, Scotti R, et al. Imatinib-induced diffuse hyperpigmentation of the oral mucosa, the skin, and the nails in a patient affected by chronic myeloid leukemia: report of a case and review of the literature. *Int J Dermatol*. 2018;57(7):784-790.
91. Delgado L, Giraudier S, Ortonne N, et al. Adverse cutaneous reactions to the new second-generation tyrosine kinase inhibitors (dasatinib, nilotinib) in chronic myeloid leukemia. *J Am Acad Dermatol*. 2013;69:839-840.
92. Dasanu CA. Erythematous skin lesions with necrotic centers on lower extremities due to the use of ruxolitinib for primary myelofibrosis. *J Oncol Pharm Pract*. 2019;25(4):990-992.

Cutaneous extramedullary hematopoiesis

Shadi Khalil and András Schaffer

DEFINITION

Hematopoiesis, the process by which hematopoietic stem cells (HSCs) differentiate into mature circulating blood cells, occurs in the bone marrow beginning in the 16th week of embryogenesis.[1] Hematopoiesis is closely coupled to mature blood needs of the body, and HSCs can be rapidly mobilized to generate additional lineages of lymphoid and myeloid cells. Extramedullary hematopoiesis (EMH) occurs when proliferating HSCs exit the bone marrow, often to the splenic red pulp and liver sinusoids, where they continue to generate blood. This is frequently observed in association with diseases of marrow insufficiency or neoplasm, including myelofibrosis, myelodysplastic syndrome, and myeloid metaplasia.[2] The skin, which is also recognized as a site of fetal hematopoiesis in normal physiology, is infrequently observed to house hematopoiesis in the process termed cutaneous EMH. Two categories of cutaneous EMH can be distinguished on the basis of pathogenesis, clinical presentation, and histopathology: neonatal and adult cutaneous EMH. In neonatal cutaneous EMH, intrauterine insult results in transient dermal hematopoiesis. Adult cutaneous EMH is best regarded as a neoplastic or paraneoplastic phenomenon associated with compromised bone marrow hematopoiesis secondary to primary myelofibrosis (PMF), or other forms of chronic myeloproliferative disease.

EPIDEMIOLOGY

PMF has an incidence of 0.5 to 1.5 per 100,000 patients per year.[3] Cutaneous EMH most commonly presents in neonates and in adults in the sixth and seventh decades of life. It rarely presents in children.[4] Both sexes are equally affected.

ETIOLOGY

Fetal hematopoiesis under normal physiology occurs in the yolk sac, liver, spleen, and skin. Dermal hematopoiesis is recognized to occur physiologically through month 5 of gestation.[5-7] The liver, spleen, and skin are frequently observed sites of EMH, likely due to hospitable biochemical profiles of the tissues that allow for development of new HSC niches.[2] HSC proliferation is reported closely coupled to end-organ needs of mature blood through various cytokines including IFN-a and IFN-g.[8-10] Circulation and mobilization to other organs can be appreciated in these circumstances.[11-13] Neonatal cutaneous EMH, commonly referred to as a "blueberry muffin rash," was first noted in 1925. While historically cutaneous EMH is recognized as a fetal process that occurs secondary to gestational insult, numerous cases of adult cutaneous EMH have also been described.

Neonatal cutaneous EMH is traditionally associated with TORCH syndrome complex gestational infections, which include rubella virus, *Toxoplasma gondii*, and cytomegalovirus.[14-16] However, various noninfectious gestational insults associated with hematologic insufficiency have been described in association with neonatal cutaneous EMH. These include ABO incompatibility,[17] Rh incompatibility,[18] twin-twin transfusion syndrome,[19] maternal anemia,[20] and hereditary spherocytosis.[5]

In adults, cutaneous EMH is strongly associated with primary idiopathic myelofibrosis. Patients often demonstrate hepatosplenic EMH in conjunction with dermal hematopoiesis.[21,22] Cutaneous EMH is a sign of severe disease associated with high mortality.[23] Often, cutaneous EMH can be observed in patients following splenectomy, suggesting that cutaneous EMH may be an adaptive response when hepatosplenic EMH is insufficient.[24,25] Less commonly, adult EMH is seen in association with polycythemia vera and chronic myelogenous leukemia as a neoplastic or paraneoplastic phenomena.[26,27] About 50% of patients with PMF carry the *JAK2 V617F* mutation.[28] *JAK2* mutation can also be detected in dermal EMH confirming clonal relatedness.[29] Approximately 5% of adult patients exhibit mutation of *MPL*, such as *MPL W515L/K*.[30]

CLINICAL PRESENTATION/PROGNOSIS/TREATMENT

The hallmark clinical feature of neonatal cutaneous EMH is the blueberry muffin rash, which consists of nonblanching violaceous macules and firm dome-shaped papules of the trunk, head, and neck. The lesions are transient and spontaneously resolve by 3 to 6 weeks after birth with light-brown macular discoloration. Extramedullary erythropoiesis can be treated with frequent blood transfusions to limit the hematopoietic stimulus.[31] In addition, hydroxyurea therapy has been reported to decrease the size of masses of hematopoietic cells and to relieve spinal cord compression, as well as to reduce the size of cutaneous masses.[32,33]

Adult cutaneous EMH clinically presents as focally clustered nonblanching painless pink, red, or violaceous macules, papules, and nodules of the head and neck (Fig. 61-1). Lesions can demonstrate locus minoris resistenciae phenomena in sites of previous scars or other compromised skin.[34,35] Bullae formation, hemorrhage, and ulcerations have also been observed.[36,37] No clear treatment guidelines exist for adult EMH, but rare reports on visceral and dermal EMH in PMF described the use of radiotherapy.[38]

HISTOPATHOLOGY

Neonatal cutaneous EMH is characterized histopathologically by erythroblastic islands of similar morphology to those seen in the bone marrow.[15] Myeloid and megakaryocytic elements may or may not be present. In contrast with blueberry muffin rashes seen in neonates, adult cutaneous EMH is often skewed toward megakaryocyte lineages and not erythropoietic lineages.[39] Megakaryocytes can be the most dominant component of the infiltrate and may show cytologic atypia.[32] The dermis may have fibrosis similar to that seen in the bone marrow.

IMMUNOPHENOTYPE

CD61, factor VIII-related antigen (VIIIRA), factor VIII-von Willebrand activity (VIIIVWF), and CD31 can be used to demonstrate the megakaryocytes, glycophorin A, or hemoglobin for erythroid precursors, and CD34, CD117, and TdT for blasts. Megakaryocytes can be small and hypolobulated and might be missed without CD61 staining.

DIFFERENTIAL DIAGNOSIS

The differential diagnosis of blueberry muffin appearance includes congenital leukemia cutis, Langerhans cells histiocytosis, congenital vascular malformations such as multifocal hemangiomas, and lymphangioendotheliomatosis, glomangiomas, and blue rubber bleb nevus syndrome.[40]

CAPSULE SUMMARY

Adult and neonatal cutaneous EMH forms are recognized.

- Adult cutaneous EMH:
  - Regarded as metastatic or paraneoplastic disease, often associated with PMF
  - Cutaneous EMH is rare, and a poor prognostic indicator of PMF
  - Skin findings include focally clustered violaceous macules, papules, and nodules
  - Histology shows trilineage hematopoiesis, often with atypical megakaryocytes and dermal fibrosis (cutaneous myelofibrosis)
- Neonatal cutaneous EMH:
  - Likely represents persistent dermal hematopoiesis, a normal part of early to middle gestation
  - Associated with intrauterine infections (TORCH syndrome) and other gestational insults
  - Morphologically presents as a blueberry muffin baby
  - Histology shows dermal erythroblasts (nucleated precursors) without myeloid and megakaryocytic elements or fibrosis

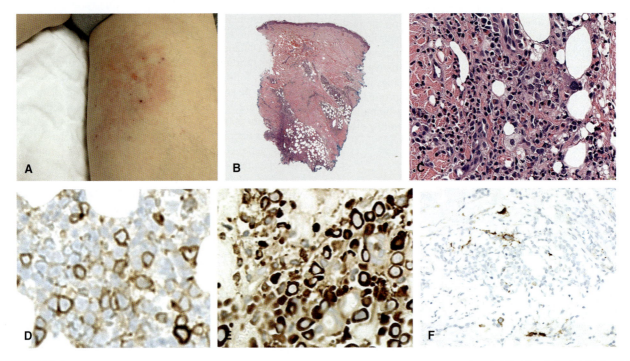

FIGURE 61-1. **A.** EMH presenting as pink, erythematous patch (photo courtesy of Urvi Patel, MD, Washington University School of Medicine, St. Louis, MO). **B** and **C.** Dermal perivascular infiltrates stained with hematoxylin and eosin show scattered blasts, immature myeloid forms, eosinophils, erythroid elements, and dysmorphic hypolobulated megakaryocytes. **D.** Megakaryocytes are decorated by CD61. **E.** Scattered blasts express C-Kit. **F.** Immature myeloid cells are highlighted by myeloperoxidase.

References

1. Pahal GS, Jauniaux E, Kinnon C, Thrasher AJ, Rodeck CH. Normal development of human fetal hematopoiesis between eight and seventeen weeks' gestation. *Am J Obstet Gynecol*. 2000;183(4):1029-1034.
2. Johns JL, Christopher MM. Extramedullary hematopoiesis: a new look at the underlying stem cell niche, theories of development, and occurrence in animals. *Vet Pathol*. 2012;49(3):508-523.
3. Tefferi A. Myelofibrosis with myeloid metaplasia. *N Engl J Med*. 2000;342(17):1255-1265.
4. Cervantes F, Barosi G, Demory JL, et al. Myelofibrosis with myeloid metaplasia in young individuals: disease characteristics, prognostic factors and identification of risk groups. *Br J Haematol*. 1998;102(3):684-690.
5. Argyle JC, Zone JJ. Dermal erythropoiesis in a neonate. *Arch Dermatol*. 1981;117:492-494.
6. Mehta V, Balachandran C, Lonikar V. Blueberry muffin baby: a pictoral differential diagnosis. *Dermatol Online J*. 2008;14:8.
7. Taj FTS, Sarin V. Blueberry muffin baby (dermal erythropoiesis) with non-ketotic hyperglycinemia. *Indian J Paediatr Dermatol*. 2013;14(1):30.
8. Raaijmakers MHGP, Mukherjee S, Guo S, et al. Bone progenitor dysfunction induces myelodysplasia and secondary leukaemia. *Nature*. 2010;464:852-857.
9. Essers MA, Offner S, Blanco-Bose WE, et al. IFNalpha activates dormant haematopoietic stem cells in vivo. *Nature*. 2009;458:904-908.
10. Baldridge MT, King KY, Boles NC, Weksberg DC, Goodell MA. Quiescent haematopoietic stem cells are activated by IFN-gamma in response to chronic infection. *Nature*. 2010;465:793-797.
11. Heissig B, Hattori K, Dias S, et al. Recruitment of stem and progenitor cells from the bone marrow niche requires MMP-9 mediated release of kit-ligand. *Cell*. 2002;109:625-637.
12. Spiegel A, Shivtiel S, Kalinkovich A, et al. Catecholaminergic neurotransmitters regulate migration and repopulation of immature human CD34+ cells through Wnt signaling. *Nat Immunol*. 2007;8(10):1123-1131.
13. Asakura A, Rudnicki MA. Side population cells from diverse adult tissues are capable of in vitro hematopoietic differentiation. *Exp Hematol*. 2002;30(11):1339.
14. Blackburn S. *Maternal, Fetal, Neonatal Physiology*. 4th ed. Saunders; 2012.
15. Hödl S, Auböck L, Reiterer F, Soyer HP, Muller WD. Blueberry muffin baby: the pathogenesis of cutaneous extramedullary hematopoiesis. *Hautarzt*. 2001;52(11):1035-1042.
16. Epps RE, Pittelkow MR, Su WP. TORCH syndrome. *Semin Dermatol*. 1995;14(2):179-186.
17. Bowden JB, Hebert AA, Rapini RP. Dermal hematopoiesis in neonates: report of five cases. *J Am Acad Dermatol*. 1989;20(6):1104-1110.
18. Hebert AA, Esterly NB, Gardner TH. Dermal erythropoiesis in Rh hemolytic disease of the newborn. *J Pediatr*. 1985;107:799-801.
19. Schwartz JL, Maniscalco WM, Lane AT, Currao WJ. Twin transfusion syndrome causing cutaneous erythropoiesis. *Pediatrics*. 1984;74:527-529.
20. De Carolis MP, Salvi S, Bersani I, Lacerenza S, Romagnoli C, De Carolis S. Fetal hypoxia secondary to severe maternal anemia as a causative link between blueberry muffin baby and erythroblastosis: a case report. *J Med Case Rep*. 2016;10(1):155.
21. Loewy G, Mathew A, Distenfeld A. Skin manifestation of agnogenic myeloid metaplasia. *Am J Hematol*. 1994;45(2):167-170.
22. Pecci A, Croci G, Balduini CL, Boveri E. Cutaneous involvement by post-polycythemia vera myelofibrosis. *Am J Hematol*. 2014;89:448.
23. Yoshida M, Horiuchi M, Ueda H, et al. Cutaneous extramedullary hematopoiesis associated with myelodysplastic/myeloproliferative neoplasm, unclassifiable. *Rinsho Ketsueki*. 2015;56:911-914.
24. Sarma DP. Extramedullary hemopoiesis of the skin. *Arch Dermatol*. 1981;117(1):58.
25. Green LK, Klima M, Burns TR. Extramedullary hematopoiesis occurring in a hemangioma of the skin. *Arch Dermatol*. 1988;124(11):1720.
26. Collie AM, Uchin JM, Bergfeld WF, Billings SD. Cutaneous intravascular extramedullary hematopoiesis in a patient with post-polycythemia vera myelofibrosis. *J Cutan Pathol*. 2013;40:615-620.
27. Tanaka M, Kanamori H, Yamaji S, et al. Subcutaneous extramedullary hematopoiesis in a patient with secondary myelofibrosis following polycythemia vera. *Leuk Lymphoma*. 2001;40:437-440.
28. Jones AV, Kreil S, Zoi K, et al. Widespread occurrence of the JAK2 V617F mutation in chronic myeloproliferative disorders. *Blood*. 2005;106(6):2162-2168.
29. Fraga GR, Caughron SK. Cutaneous myelofibrosis with JAK2 V617F mutation: metastasis, not merely extramedullary hematopoiesis! *Am J Dermatopathol*. 2010;32(7):727-730.
30. Pardanani AD, Levine RL, Lasho T, et al. MPL515 mutations in myeloproliferative and other myeloid disorders: a study of 1182 patients. *Blood*. 2006;108(10):3472-3476.
31. Krouwels FH, Bresser P, von dem Borne AE. Extramedullary hematopoiesis: breathtaking and hair-raising. *N Engl J Med*. 1999;341(22):1702-1704.
32. Schofield JK, Shun JL, Cerio R, et al. Cutaneous extramedullary hematopoiesis with a preponderance of atypical megakaryocytes in myelofibrosis. *J Am Acad Dermatol*. 1990;22(2 Pt 2):334-337.
33. Konstantopoulos K, Vagiopoulos G, Kantouni R, et al. A case of spinal cord compression by extramedullary haemopoiesis in a thalassaemic patient: a putative role for hydroxyurea? *Haematologica*. 1992;77(4):352-354.
34. Hocking WG, Lazar GS, Lipsett JA, Busuttil RW. Cutaneous extramedullary hematopoiesis following splenectomy for idiopathic myelofibrosis. *Am J Med*. 1984;76:956.
35. Patel BM, Su WP, Perniciaro C, Gertz MA. Cutaneous extramedullary hematopoiesis. *J Am Acad Dermatol*. 1995;32(5 Pt 1):805.
36. Mizoguchi M, Kawa Y, Minami T, et al. Cutaneous extramedullary hematopoiesis in myelofibrosis. *J Am Acad Dermatol*. 1990;22(2 Pt 2):351-355.
37. Kuo T. Cutaneous extramedullary hematopoiesis presenting as leg ulcers. *J Am Acad Dermatol*. 1981;4(5):592-596.
38. Lee CM, Salzman KL, Blumenthal DT, et al. Intracranial extramedullary hematopoiesis: brief review of response to radiation therapy. *Am J Hematol*. 2005;78(2):151-152.
39. Penalver A, Garcia V, Pocurull E, Borrull F, Marce RM. Stir bar sorptive extraction and large volume injection gas chromatography to determine a group of endocrine disrupters in water samples. *J Chromatogr A*. 2003;1007(1-2):1.
40. Khalil S, Ariel Gru A, Saavedra AP. Cutaneous extramedullary haematopoiesis: implications in human disease and treatment. *Exp Dermatol*. 2019;28(11):1201-1209.

CHAPTER 62

Blastic plasmacytoid dendritic cell neoplasm

M. Yadira Hurley, Joseph D. Khoury, Alejandro A. Gru, Tony Petrella, and Martin Dittmer

DEFINITION

Blastic plasmacytoid dendritic cell neoplasm (BPDCN) is a distinct neoplasm of plasmacytoid dendritic cells (PDCs) that often manifests with cutaneous lesions at presentation. Previously, it has been referred to as blastic natural killer (NK)-cell leukemia/lymphoma[1] and CD4+CD56+ hematodermic neoplasm[2] but is now known to be derived from a PDC progenitor.[3]

EPIDEMIOLOGY

BPDCN is a rare disease that comprises <1% of all cutaneous hematologic malignancies. Elderly patients are most commonly affected (mean age 60-70 years), but it can occur at any age, including in infants.[4-7] A bimodal distribution has been demonstrated (<20 and >60 years).[8] There is a male predominance with a reported male:female ratio of approximately 4:1.[4,9] No difference in predisposition based on race or ethnicity has been reported.[8,9]

CLINICAL PRESENTATION AND PROGNOSIS

Cutaneous lesions are the hallmark of the disease and are the primary presentation in around 90% of the cases (range 60%-100%),[4,9,10] and about half of the cases have isolated cutaneous involvement at presentation[11] which precedes bone marrow infiltration by 2 to 3 months in 45% of the cases.[12] Skin lesions can be multiple (>60% of the time) or single. The lesions range from tumors and nodules to plaques and patches that are brown, erythematous, or violaceous. A characteristic clinical finding is that the lesions are bruise-like or hemorrhagic in appearance. They may be found anywhere on the body, especially the scalp, face, trunk, and extremities (Fig. 62-1). The head and neck area is particularly more commonly affected. Clinically, the skin lesions can simulate other entities including vascular neoplasms, vasculitis, and traumatic bruises.[4,10,13]

Bone marrow and peripheral blood involvement eventually develop in nearly all cases but are often absent or present at very low levels initially.[6,10,14] Thrombocytopenia and other cytopenias are common at the time of presentation, but B symptoms are unusual.[6] Around 10% to 20% of cases have associated chronic myelomonocytic leukemia at the time of presentation.[15] Some cases are associated with myelodysplastic syndromes.[4,10,14] Lymph node involvement also occurs in 40% to 50% of cases.[4,14] The spleen, liver, mucosal surfaces, and the central nervous system (in order of decreasing frequency) may also be involved.[14]

Although around 65% of the patients has an Eastern Cooperative Oncology Group 0 to 1 score at diagnosis, BPDCN is an aggressive neoplasm of poor prognosis with a median of overall survival between 14 months[2] and 18 months.[9] Patients with disease limited to the skin at presentation do not have a better prognosis than those presenting with bone marrow dissemination.[16] Therefore, aggressive therapy should be employed even in the setting of isolated cutaneous involvement.[2] Chemotherapy remains an effective treatment option for BPDCN in fit patients who may be eligible for hematopoietic stem cell transplant (HSCT), and until now, aggressive chemotherapy options are recommended.[17] Regimens used for lymphoblastic leukemia tend to give better outcomes than therapies used for acute myeloid leukemia, despite the apparent closer relationship that PDCs have to the myeloid lineage.[6,11,16] Most patients initially achieve complete remission with several different chemotherapy regimens. However, >80% of patients have systemic relapse with cutaneous and extracutaneous dissemination usually in less than 2 years and often with bone marrow involvement.[2,4,6] Of the few patients who achieve sustained clinical remission, most have received acute leukemia regimens and allogeneic stem cell transplantation.[6,16,18] Age seems to be a significant prognostic factor,[16] with the best outcomes occurring in children.[19,20]

However, increased understanding of the pathogenesis and development of targeted therapy brings new perspectives in the treatment of the disease. Ubiquitous overexpression of CD123 in BPDCN was the basis of investigating of tagraxofusp (SL-401), a CD123-targeted diphtheria toxin conjugate which was approved by the Food and Drug Administration in 2018. A pilot study of tagraxofusp in monotherapy in adults demonstrated response rates as high as 90% in frontline-treated patients,[21-23] including remission permitting bridging to HSCT. In view of mechanisms of

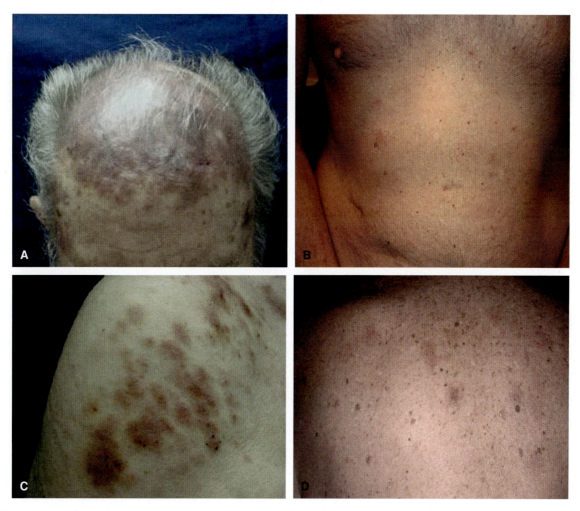

FIGURE 62-1. BPDCN—Clinical manifestations. The four clinical images show plaques and nodules with a violaceous appearance in the **(A)** scalp, **(B)** trunk, **(C)** extremities, and the **(D)** back.

tagraxofusp resistance,[24] future combinations with BCL2 inhibitors (venetoclax) and other antiapoptotic agents could be investigated.[25] Lenalidomide and bortezomib are also promising agents to be explored.[26,27] Azacitidine, a DNA methyltransferase inhibitor, may be used by restoring lost activity in the diphthamide synthesis pathway.[24] Furthermore, multiple phase 1 clinical trials targeting CD123 using chimeric antigen receptor T cell (CD123-CARTs) are under active development for patients with relapsed/refractory BPDCN.[28,29]

HISTOLOGY

Cutaneous lesions of BPDCN are characterized by a dermal infiltrate composed of sheets of neoplastic cells (Fig. 62-2). The infiltrate is typically diffuse, but can often show an accentuated periadnexal or perivascular distribution (Fig. 62-3). The epidermis is characteristically spared with an underlying Grenz zone.[13] The cells are typically intermediate to large with high nucleus-to-cytoplasm ratio and finely dispersed chromatin reminiscent of lymphoblasts or myeloblasts (Fig. 62-4). Nuclear contours are irregular and may be notched, folded, or occasionally show moderate pleomorphism. Nucleoli are usually inconspicuous, but one to several prominent nucleoli can be present.[10,13,30] With hematoxylin and eosin staining, the cytoplasm is pale to eosinophilic, agranular, and usually scant, but can be moderate to abundant in some cases.[6,14] There may also be significant erythrocyte extravasation, but little or no inflammatory response.[14] The erythrocyte extravasation accounts for the clinical bruise-like or hemorrhagic appearance. Necrosis is generally absent.[11] Cells of an "immunoblastoid" variant manifest single large nucleoli centered within vesicular nuclei. This cytomorphology has been associated with MYC expression and recurrent 8q24 rearrangements[31] (Fig. 62-5). On rare occurrences, the infiltrate can be very sparse and a potential mimicker of an inflammatory process (Fig. 62-6).

Involved lymph nodes may show effaced architecture but more frequently demonstrate paracortical, focal interfollicular, medullary, and/or intrasinusoidal deposition of malignant cells.[10,14] Likewise, involvement of the marrow may show inconspicuous interstitial clusters or complete architectural

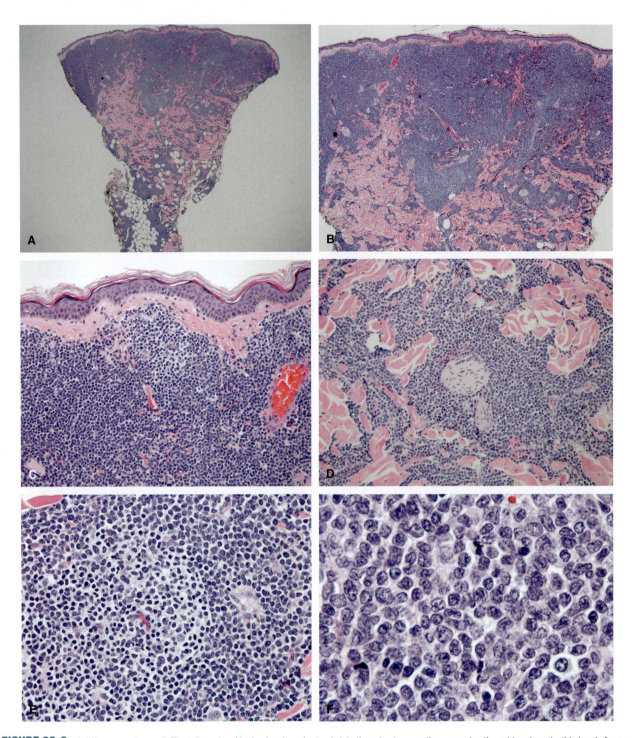

FIGURE 62-2. A diffuse, monotonous infiltrate is centered in the dermis and extends into the subcutaneous tissue, sparing the epidermis and a thin band of superficial dermis ("Grenz zone") (**A–C**). The infiltrate dissects through collagen bundles, surrounding nerves, and blood vessels (**D**). The cells of BPDCN have predominantly round nuclei with notching and folding of the nuclear contours with little or no pleomorphism. Nucleoli are generally inconspicuous, but can be identified in some cells (**E** and **F**).

effacement (Fig. 62-7). In 5% to 10% of cases, there is background myelodysplasia.[6,10] Evidence of clonal hematopoiesis with multiple genes mutated at high variant allele frequency may be seen in the marrow of patients with apparently skin-limited disease, calling into question the notion that malignant transformation occurs in the periphery.[32] On Wright-Giemsa–stained preparations of marrow aspirates or of the peripheral blood, the BPDCN cells have gray-blue cytoplasm often with characteristic cytoplasmic extensions (pseudopodia) with cytoplasmic vacuoles of varying sizes which are described as resembling a string of pearls[6] (Fig. 62-8).

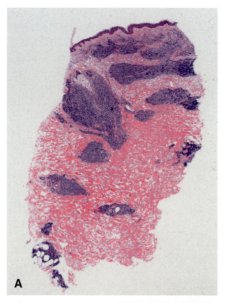
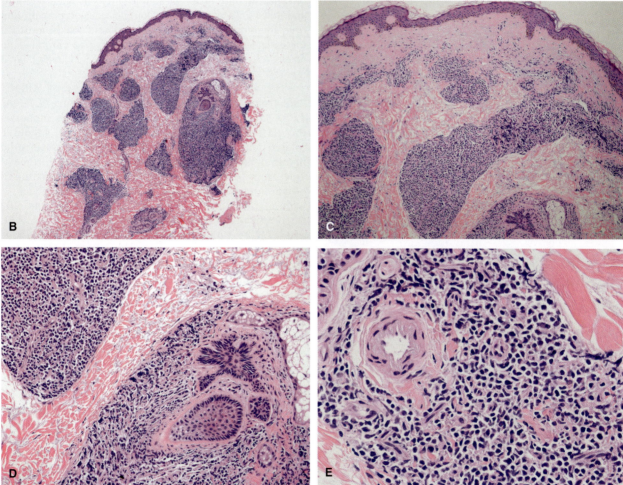

FIGURE 62-3. This case shows a more nodular infiltrate of neoplastic cells with a pronounced periadnexal and perivascular distribution. The epidermis and superficial dermis are also spared (**A–E**).

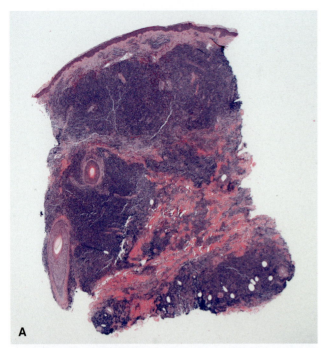

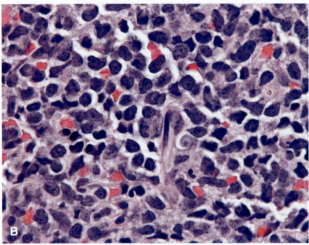

FIGURE 62-4. A sheet-like infiltrate throughout the dermis surrounds hair follicles and dissects dermal collagen bundles **(A)**. The infiltrate is composed of neoplastic cells with notched and folded nuclei with occasional, small nucleoli. The chromatin is fine and evenly dispersed, imparting a "blastic" quality **(B)**.

IMMUNOPHENOTYPE

Immunophenotyping by immunohistochemistry and/or flow cytometry is essential for the diagnosis of BPDCN. Tumor cells are characteristically positive for CD123, CD4, CD56, and TCL1[27] (Fig. 62-9). CD123 (interleukin-3 α chain receptor) expression is an obligatory finding for making the diagnosis of BPDCN (Fig. 62-10). TCF4 is a transcription factor that is required for PDC programming.[33] Sukswai et al demonstrated that coexpression of TCF4 and CD123 by immunohistochemistry is highly sensitive and specific for BPDCN[34] (Fig. 62-11). Of note, some BPDCN cases lack CD4, CD56, or TCL1. BPDCN is also usually positive for BDCA-2/CD303, CD43, CD45RA, CLA, and MxA.[3,35] Tumor cells may be variably positive for TdT, CD2, CD7, CD33, CD36, CD38, and CD117.[36,37] By definition, the diagnosis of BPDCN requires absence of lineage-specific markers of myeloid, monocytic, B-cell, and T-cell differentiation; namely, detection of myeloperoxidase, lysozyme, PAX5, CD3, or CD19 precludes a diagnosis of BPDCN. BPDCN is negative for Epstein-Barr virus (EBV).[3,14] In general, the immunophenotype of BPDCN overlaps with that of normal PDCs, with the exception of CD56 and TdT expression[38] (Figs. 62-10 and 62-12). In rare cases, however, heterogeneous CD56 expression may be detected in reactive PDC proliferations.[36]

GENETIC AND MOLECULAR FINDINGS

No specific chromosomal abnormality has been identified and up to 75% cases have a complex karyotype with multiple abnormalities (three or more). These consist mostly of losses and seem to most frequently involve chromosomes 5q21 or 5q32 (72%), 12p13 (64%), 13q13-21 (64%), 6q23-qter (50%), 15q43 (43%), and 9 (28%).[30,39-41]

The first work on genetic mutations of BPDCN date from 2011[42] when mutations involving *TET2* and *TP53* have been identified, which lent some support to the classification of BPDCN as a precursor myeloid–related malignancy, as these are also present in other myeloid leukemias and myelodysplastic syndromes.[43] One study of 33 cases identified mutually exclusive point mutations in *NRAS*, *KRAS*, and *ATM* genes, as well as mutations in *MET*, *IDH2*, *KIT*, *APC*, and *RB1*. Recurrent mutations were found in *NRAS*, *IDH2*, *APC*, and *ATM*.[44] Mutations in other genes common in acute myeloid leukemias, such as *FLT3*, *NPM1*, *IDH1*, *JAK2*, and *EZH2*, have not been identified.[44] More recently, using a whole exome sequencing/targeted sequencing technique to study 14 cases of BPDCN, Sapienza et al observed a large number of mutated genes (*ARID1A, CHD8, SMARCA5, SMARCAD1, TET2, IDH2, ASH1L, ASXL1, ASXL3, MLL2, MLL3, MLL4, SETMAR, SUZ12, KDM4D, PHF2, EP300, EP400, MYST3, MYST4, PHC1, PHC2, EYA2, SRCAP, NRAS, KRAS, BRCA1, ATM, ATR, RAD52, ZRSR2, RET, MAPK1, BRAF, RUNX2, SYK, WNT10, WNT7B, BCL9L, WNT3*).[45] The authors showed that 25 epigenetic pathway genes were mutated, controlling either chromatin accessibility, DNA methylation, or histone posttranscriptional modifications. Besides the epigenetic pathway, mutations affecting programs common to either myeloid malignancies were also identified.[46] The epigenetic modifier mutations seem to have a clinical impact with significant reduction of the overall survival of patients mutated in any of the DNA methylation genes (*TET2, IDH1/2, DNMT3A*).[47] All these genetic abnormalities open promising and exciting new strategies to match each patient with the most appropriate epigenetic-targeted therapy.

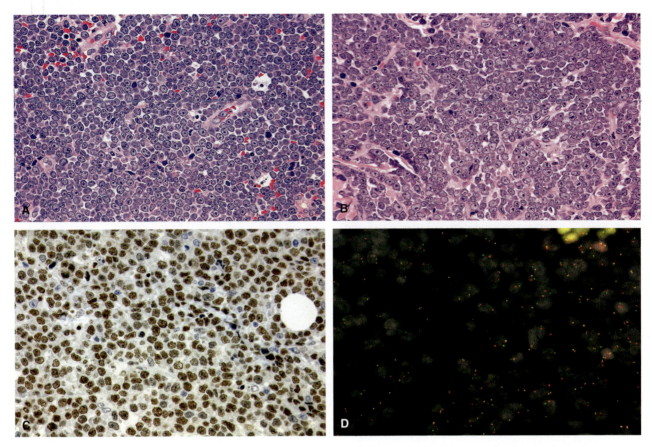

FIGURE 62-5. **This variant of BPDCN is characterized by the presence of malignant cells with an immunoblastoid morphology.** The cell shows eccentric nuclei and prominent nucleoli (**A** and **B**). The malignant cells are positive for MYC (**C**), and show a translocation involving the gene (**D**). (Images courtesy of Dr. Kengo Takeuchi.)

POSTULATED CELL OF ORIGIN

Genetic and immunohistochemical features point to the precursor of benign resting PDCs as the counterpart of the malignant cells of BPDCN.[48] PDCs are specialized immune cells that are distinguished by high production of α-interferon.[14,38,49] They have previously been referred to as plasmacytoid monocytes and interferon-I-producing cells. They constitute <0.1% of circulating monocytes. They have been shown to be capable of differentiating into dendritic cells in vitro and may play a role in antigen presentation. Like the cells of BPDCN, they express CD4, CD123, CD68, TCL1, CLA, and BDCA-2. They are usually negative for CD56 aiding in the distinction between BPDCN and other tumoral PDC collections, but a small proportion of normal PDCs are CD56+.[14]

The PDC has been the accepted normal analog to BPDCN cells for nearly a decade, but our understanding of PDC lineage continues to evolve. Mounting transcriptional evidence in mice including single-cell messenger RNA sequencing data has shown previously unappreciated heterogeneity of the normal PDC pool, historically classified within the myeloid compartment. This recent work supports a lymphoid derivation for most PDCs, with only a minor subset populated from myeloid dendritic cell progenitors ("PDC-like cells").[50] In contrast, BPDCN remains classified as a unique myeloid neoplasm in the 2016 WHO classification based in part on myeloid precursor gene expression in a large international series.[48,51] The precise subset of PDCs acting center stage in BPDCN tumorigenesis may be clarified with future study.

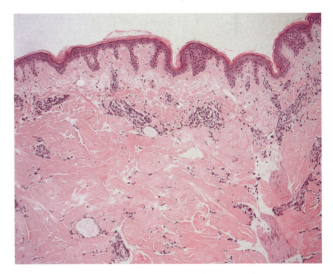

FIGURE 62-6. **This case of BPDCN is characterized by a very subtle perivascular infiltrate of atypical mononuclear cells.** The sparse character of the infiltrate can potentially mimic a diagnosis of a reactive inflammatory process.

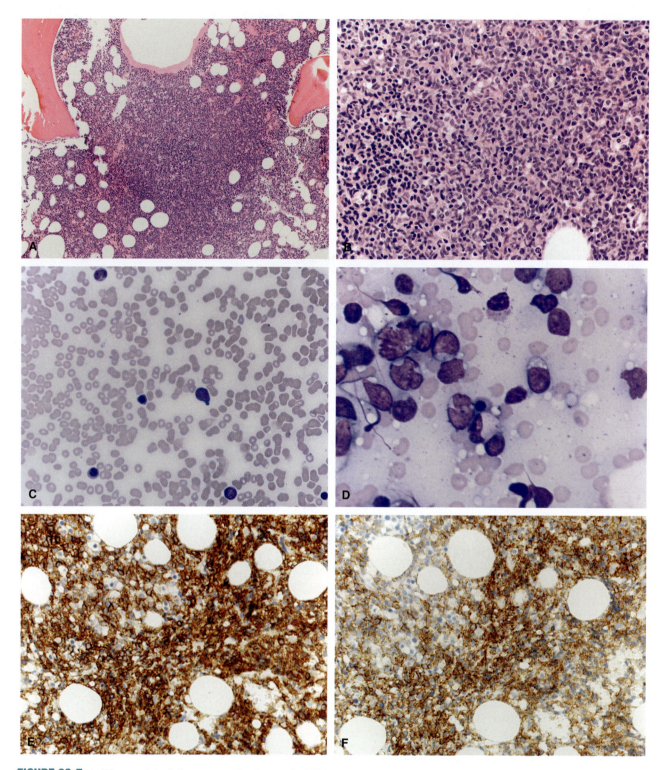

FIGURE 62-7. In this case, there is bone marrow involvement by BPDCN. The infiltrate shows a diffuse and nodular appearance (**A** and **B**). The blasts in the circulation show the presence of pseudopods (**C**). In the bone marrow aspirate, the blasts show the presence of cytoplasmic vacuoles (**D**). The blasts are positive for CD123 (**E**) and CD56 (**F**).

DIFFERENTIAL DIAGNOSIS

The most closely related lesions that mimic BPDCN are the clonal, tumoral proliferations of PDCs that can occur in the skin, lymph nodes, bone marrow, and spleen secondary to a variety of myeloid neoplasms with monocytic differentiation. Tumoral PDC proliferations can most reliably be distinguished from BPDCN by a Ki-67 index (usually <10% in PDC proliferations and >30% in BPDCN). When positive, TdT is also helpful in excluding a tumoral PDC proliferation, because these are uniformly negative.[14,52] CD56 is valuable, but as mentioned previously, rare mature PDCs may show faint expression, and CD56-negative BPDCN cases occur.[14] Not only do PDC proliferations accompanying myeloid neoplasms mimic BPDCN, but myeloid neoplasms with monocytic differentiation themselves (especially myelomonocytic leukemia) frequently have significant cutaneous localization.

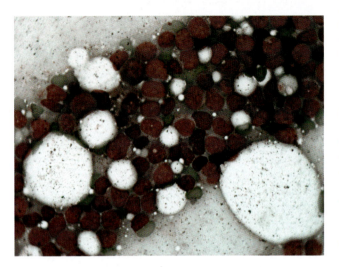

FIGURE 62-8. BPDCN, bone marrow aspirate (Wright-Giemsa–stained smear). The cells are intermediate in size, with fine chromatin and variable nucleoli.

These are also often positive for CD4, CD56, and CD123, making their distinction from BPDCN even more difficult. Thorough cytochemical analysis and immunophenotyping is necessary for definitive classification. If available, Wright-Giemsa–stained cytologic preparations will often show cytoplasmic granules. When granules are present, myeloperoxidase and/or lysozyme will usually be positive, excluding BPDCN from the differential. Less mature myeloid neoplasms may lack cytoplasmic granules but will be positive for CD13, CD34, and/or CD117, excluding BPDCN. CD68 is positive in both BPDCN and other myeloid neoplasms, but shows distinctive dot-like cytoplasmic positivity in BPDCN as opposed to the diffuse cytoplasmic staining seen in other lesions.[10,11,53] Other potentially useful markers include MxA and BDCA-2, which are more specific for BPDCN.[10,53] Generally, the difficulties in distinguishing myelomonocytic or monoblastic leukemia from a BPDCN can be avoided by careful assessment of clinical history.

The expression of CD4, other T-cell antigens, TdT, and cutaneous infiltration raises the possibility of a cutaneous T-cell leukemia/lymphoma. Absence of CD3, CD5, CD8, and the absence of a *TCR* gene rearrangement supports BPDCN.[10,11,54]

NK-cell leukemia also needs to be included in the differential of BPDCN. Both entities express CD56, but NK-cell leukemia often shows distinctive areas of angiodestruction and necrosis. NK-cell leukemia will also be positive for

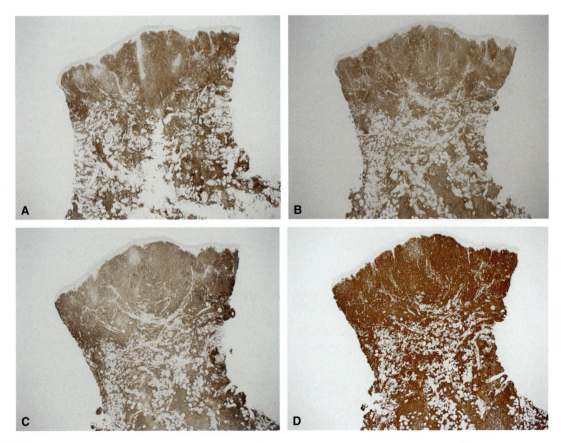

FIGURE 62-9. The cells are usually diffusely and strongly positive for CD4, CD56, CD43, and TCL1 (**A–D**).

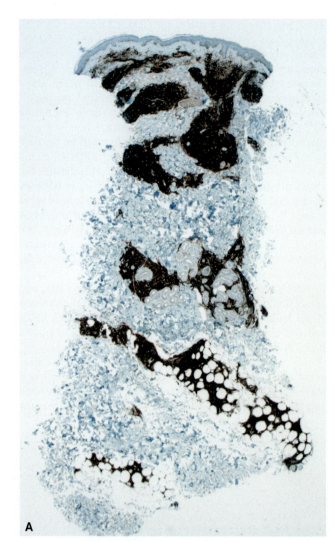

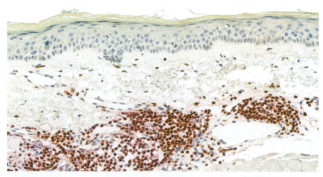

FIGURE 62-11. Characteristic pattern of dual expression of CD123 (red) and TCF-4 (brown) on immunohistochemistry.

EBV studies and will express cytoplasmic CD3 and granzyme B by immunohistochemistry, both of which are absent in BPDCN.[10,11]

Many other entities can mimic the morphologic features of BPDCN, including other lymphomas, Merkel cell carcinoma, and melanoma, but these can be clearly distinguished based on clinical and immunophenotypic grounds.

CAPSULE SUMMARY

BPDCN is a distinct neoplasm of PDCs. It is characterized by early, often isolated skin lesions that almost inevitably progress to systemic and bone marrow involvement with a poor prognosis. The skin lesions have a characteristic bruise-like or hemorrhagic appearance. The diagnosis requires thorough immunophenotyping to exclude a number of other pathologies with similar clinical and histomorphologic features.

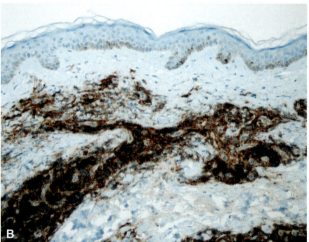

FIGURE 62-10. The cells of BPDCN are diffusely positive for CD123 (**A** and **B**).

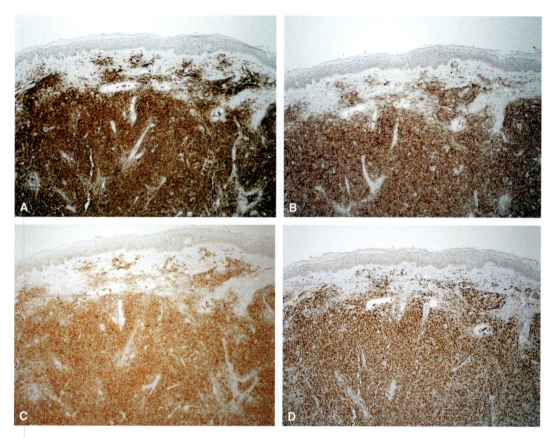

FIGURE 62-12. The cells show diffuse and strong positivity for CD45 **(A)**, CD56 **(B)**, CD4 **(C)**, and TdT **(D)**.

References

1. Jaffe E, Harris N, Stein H, Vardiman JE. *Blastic NK-cell lymphoma. World Health Organization Classification of Tumors: Pathology and Genetics of Tumours of Hematopoietic and Lymphoid Tissues.* IARC Press; 2001.
2. Willemze R, Jaffe ES, Burg G, et al. WHO-EORTC classification for cutaneous lymphomas. *Blood.* 2005;105(10):3768-3785.
3. Facchetti F, Jones DM, Petrella T. Blastic plasmacytoid dendritic cell neoplasm. In: Swerdlow SH, Campo E, Hazzis NL, et al, eds. 4th ed. *WHO Classification of Tumors of Haematopoietic and Lymphoid Tissues.* IARC press; 2008:145-147.
4. Gera S, Dekmezian MS, Duvic M, et al. Blastic plasmacytoid dendritic cell neoplasm: evolving insights in an aggressive hematopoietic malignancy with a predilection of skin involvement. *Am J Dermatopathol.* 2014;36(3):244-251.
5. Julia F, Petrella T, Beylot-Barry M, et al. Blastic plasmacytoid dendritic cell neoplasm: clinical features in 90 patients. *Br J Dermatol.* 2013;169(3):579-586.
6. Feuillard J, Jacob MC, Valensi F, et al. Clinical and Biologic features of CD4+CD56+ malignancies. *Blood.* 2002;99:1556-1563.
7. Hu SC, Tsai KB, Chen GS, et al. Infantile CD4+/CD56+ hematodermic neoplasm. *Haematologica.* 2007;92(9):e91-e93.
8. Guru Murthy GS, Pemmaraju N, Atallah E. Epidemiology and survival of blastic plasmacytoid dendritic cell neoplasm. *Leuk Res.* 2018;73:21-23.
9. Laribi K, Baugier de Materre A, Sobh M, et al. Blastic plasmacytoid dendritic cell neoplasms: results of an international survey on 398 adult patients. *Blood Adv.* 2020;4:4838-4848.
10. Herling M, Jones D. CD4+/CD56+ hematodermic tumor: the features of an evolving entity and its relationship to dendritic cells. *Am J Clin Pathol.* 2007;127(5):687-700.
11. Petrella T, Bagot M, Willemze R, et al. Blastic NK-cell lymphomas (agranular CD4+CD56+ hematodermic neoplasms): a review. *Am J Clin Pathol.* 2005;123:662-675.
12. Garnache-Ottou F, Vidal C, Biichle S, et al. How should we diagnose and treat blastic plasmacytoid dendritic cell neoplasm patients? *Blood Adv.* 2019;3:4238-4251.
13. Cota C, Vale E, Viana I, et al. Cutaneous manifestations of blastic plasmacytoid dendritic cell neoplasm-morphologic and phenotypic variability in a series of 33 patients. *Am J Surg Pathol.* 2010;34(1):75-87.
14. Jegalian AG, Facchetti F, Jaffe ES. Plasmacytoid dendritic cells: physiologic roles and pathologic states. *Adv Anat Pathol.* 2009;16:393-404.
15. Vitte F, Fabiani B, Benet C, et al. Specific skin lesions in chronic myelomonocytic leukemia: a spectrum of myelomonocytic and dendritic cell proliferations – a study of 42 cases. *Am J Surg Pathol.* 2012;36:1302-1316.
16. Reimer P, Rudiger T, Kraemer D, et al. What is CD4+CD56+ malignancy and how should it be treated? *Bone Marrow Transplant.* 2003;32:637-646.
17. Haddadin M, Taylor J. Chemotherapy options for blastic plasmacytoid dendritic cell neoplasm. *Hematol Oncol Clin North Am.* 2020;34:539-552.

18. Ham JC, Janssen JJ, Boers JE, et al. Allogeneic stem-cell transplantation for blastic plasmacytoid dendritic cell neoplasm. *J Clin Oncol.* 2012;30:e102-e103.
19. Jegalian AG, Buxbaum NP, Facchetti F, et al. Blastic plasmacytoid dendritic cell neoplasm in children: diagnostic features and clinical implications. *Haematologica.* 2010;95:1873-1879.
20. Rossi JG, Felice MS, Bernasconi AR, et al. Acute leukemia of dendritic cell lineage in childhood: incidence, biological characteristics and outcome. *Leuk Lymphoma.* 2006;47:715-725.
21. Hammond D, Pemmaraju N. Tagraxofusp for blastic plasmacytoid dendritic cell neoplasm. *Hematol Oncol Clin North Am.* 2020;34:565-574.
22. Pemmaraju N, Konopleva M. Approval of tagraxofusp-erzs for blastic plasmacytoid dendritic cell neoplasm. *Blood Adv.* 2020;4:4020-4027.
23. Pemmaraju N, Lane AA, Sweet KL, et al. Tagraxofusp in blastic plasmacytoid dendritic-cell neoplasm. *N Engl J Med.* 2019;380:1628-1637.
24. Togami K, Pastika T, Stephansky J, et al. DNA methyltransferase inhibition overcomes diphthamide pathway deficiencies underlying CD123-targeted treatment resistance. *J Clin Invest.* 2019;129:5005-5019.
25. Montero J, Stephansky J, Cai T, et al. Blastic plasmacytoid dendritic cell neoplasm is dependent on BCL2 and sensitive to venetoclax. *Cancer Discov.* 2017;7:156-164.
26. Lane AA. Novel therapies for blastic plasmacytoid dendritic cell neoplasm. *Hematol Oncol Clin North Am.* 2020;34:589-600.
27. Khoury JD. Blastic plasmacytoid dendritic cell neoplasm. *Curr Hematol Malig Rep.* 2018;13(6):477-483.
28. Xue T, Budde LE. Immunotherapies targeting CD123 for blastic plasmacytoid dendritic cell neoplasm. *Hematol Oncol Clin North Am.* 2020;34:575-587.
29. Bole-Richard E, Fredon M, Biichle S, et al. CD28/4-1BB CD123 CAR T cells in blastic plasmacytoid dendritic cell neoplasm. *Leukemia.* 2020;34:3228-3241.
30. Reichard KK, Burks EJ, Foucar MK, et al. CD4+CD56+ lineage-negative malignancies are rare tumors of plasmacytoid dendritic cells. *Am J Surg Pathol.* 2005;29(10):1274-1283.
31. Sakamoto K, Katayama R, Asaka R, et al. Recurrent 8q24 rearrangement in blastic plasmacytoid dendritic cell neoplasm: association with immunoblastoid cytomorphology, MYC expression, and drug response. *Leukemia.* 2018;32(12):2590-2603. doi: 10.1038/s41375-018-0154-5
32. Griffin GK, Togami K, Morgan EA, Lane AA. Developmental ontogeny of blastic plasmacytoid dendritic cell neoplasm (BPDCN) revealed by recurrent high Burden clonal hematopoiesis, including in "Skin-Only" disease. *Blood.* 2018;132(suppl 1):2755. doi: 10.1182/blood-2018-99-119945
33. Cerebelli M, Hou ZE, Kelly ZE, et al. A druggable TCF4- and BRD4-dependent transcriptional network sustains malignancy in blastic plasmacytoid dendritic cell neoplasm. *Cancer Cell.* 2016;30(5):764-778.
34. Sukswai M, Hou ZE, Kelly ZE, et al. Dual expression of TCF4 and CD123 is highly sensitive and specific for blastic plasmacytoid dendritic cell neoplasm. *Am J Surg Pathol.* 2019;43(10):1429-1437.
35. Julia F, Dalle S, Duru G, et al. Blastic plasmacytoid dendritic cell neoplasms: clinico-immunohistochemical correlations in a series of 91 patients. *Am J Surg Pathol.* 2014;38(5):673-680.
36. Wang W, Khoury JD, Miranda RN, et al. Immunophenotypic characterization of reactive and neoplastic plasmacytoid dendritic cells permits establishment of a 10-color flow cytometric panel for initial workup and residual disease evaluation of blastic plasmacytoid dendritic cell neoplasm. *Haematologica.* 2021;106(4):1047-1055.
37. Alayed K, Patel KP, Konoplev S, et al. TET2 mutations, myelodysplastic features, and a distinct immunoprofile characterize blastic plasmacytoid dendritic cell neoplasm in the bone marrow. *Am J Hematol.* 2013;88(12):1055-1061.
38. Facchetti F, Vermi W, Mason D, et al. The plasmacytoid monocyte/interferon producing cells. *Virchows Arch.* 2003;443(6):703-717.
39. Leroux D, Mugneret F, Callanan M, et al. CD4+, CD56+ DC2 acute leukemia is characterized by recurrent clonal chromosomal changes affecting 6 major targets: a study of 21 cases by the Groupe Français de Cytogénétique Hématologique. *Blood.* 2002;99(11):4154-4159.
40. Petrella T, Dalac S, Maynadié M, et al. CD4+CD56+ cutaneous neoplasms: a distinct hematological entity? Groupe Français d'Etude des Lymphomes Cutanés (GFELC). *Am J Surg Pathol.* 1999;23(2):137-146.
41. Sapienza MR, Pileri A, Derenzini E, et al. Blastic plasmacytoid dendritic cell neoplasm: state of the art and prospects. *Cancers.* 2019;11.
42. Lindsley RC, Ebert BL. The biology and clinical impact of genetic lesions in myeloid malignancies. *Blood.* 2013;122(23):3741-3748.
43. Jardin F, Ruminy P, Parmentier F, et al. TET2 and TP53 mutations are frequently observed in blastic plasmacytoid dendritic cell neoplasm. *Br J Haematol.* 2011;153(3):413-416.
44. Stenzinger A, Endris V, Pfarr N, et al. Targeted ultra-deep sequencing reveals recurrent and mutually exclusive mutations of cancer genes in blastic plasmacytoid dendritic cell neoplasm. *Oncotarget.* 2014;5(15):6404-6413.
45. Sapienza MR, Abate F, Melle F, et al. Blastic plasmacytoid dendritic cell neoplasm: genomics mark epigenetic dysregulation as a primary therapeutic target. *Haematologica.* 2019;104:729-737.
46. Sapienza MR, Pileri S. Molecular features of blastic plasmacytoid dendritic cell neoplasm: DNA mutations and epigenetics. *Hematol Oncol Clin North Am.* 2020;34:511-521.
47. Menezes J, Acquadro F, Wiseman M, et al. Exome sequencing reveals novel and recurrent mutations with clinical impact in blastic plasmacytoid dendritic cell neoplasm. *Leukemia.* 2014;28:823-829.
48. Sapienza MR, Fuligni F, Agostinelli C, et al. Molecular profiling of blastic plasmacytoid dendritic cell neoplasm reveals a unique pattern and suggests selective sensitivity to NF-kB pathway inhibition. *Leukemia.* 2014;28(8):1606-1616.
49. Cella M, Jarrossay D, Facchetti F, et al. Plasmacytoid monocytes migrate to inflamed lymph nodes and produce large amounts of type I interferon. *Nat Med.* 1999;5(8):919-923.
50. Rodrigues PF, Tussiwand R. Novel concepts in plasmacytoid dendritic cell (pDC) development and differentiation. *Mol Immunol.* 2020;126:25-30. doi: 10.1016/j.molimm.2020.07.006
51. Swerdlow S, Campo E, Jaffe E, et al. *WHO Classification of Tumours of Haematopoietic and Lymphoid Tissues.* Revised 4th ed. International Agency for Research on Cancer; 2017.
52. Vermi W, Facchetti F, Rosati S, et al. Nodal and extranodal tumor-forming accumulation of plasmacytoid monocytes/

interferon-producing cells associated with myeloid disorders. *Am J Surg Pathol.* 2004;28(5):585-595.

53. Shi Y, Wang E. Blastic plasmacytoid dendritic cell neoplasm: a clinicopathologic review. *Arch Pathol Lab Med.* 2014;138(4):564-569.

54. Pilichowska ME, Fleming MD, Pinkus JL, et al. CD4+/CD56+ hematodermic neoplasm ("blastic natural killer cell lymphoma"): neoplastic cells express the immature dendritic cell marker BDCA-2 and produce interferon. *Am J Clin Pathol.* 2007;128(3):445-453.

PART X — CUTANEOUS MAST CELL PROLIFERATIONS

CHAPTER 63

Mast cell neoplasms

Clive E. Grattan and Hans-Peter Horny

INTRODUCTION

Cutaneous mastocytosis (CM) is, by definition, one of the two major subvariants of mastocytosis, in which, there is no evidence of systemic disease (systemic mastocytosis [SM]). CM is primarily a disease of children before puberty and unusually encountered in adults. Patients may show evidence of mast cell clonality in peripheral blood (mutations in KIT) without fulfilling the diagnostic criteria for SM. SM in children (confirmed by bone marrow biopsy) is rare but, theoretically, may go unrecognized in those with the common D816V mutation who do not have a bone marrow examination.

The main subtypes of CM are (WHO, 2017)[1]

1. Mastocytoma
2. Maculopapular CM (syn. urticaria pigmentosa)
    a. Monomorphic ("adult") subtype
    b. Polymorphic ("juvenile") subtype
3. Diffuse ("erythrodermic") CM
4. Mast cell sarcoma (MCS)

Since the major form of SM, namely, indolent SM, almost always affects the skin with maculopapular lesions, it is strongly recommended that clinicians and pathologists recognizing cutaneous involvement by mastocytosis should use the preliminary and descriptive term "mastocytosis in the skin (MIS)" in adults to reflect that it could be cutaneous or systemic. This helps to avoid terminological errors that might occur before the clinical investigation is completed. While mastocytoma and maculopapular CM and diffuse CM have an excellent prognosis regarding life expectancy, MCS is a life-threatening disease and is not confined to skin. The monomorphic type of maculopapular CM, significantly and chronically elevated serum tryptase levels, and presence of the activating point mutation D816V of KIT almost exclude the diagnosis of "pure" CM favoring SM, in particular its indolent subvariant. Skin involvement is frequent in indolent or smoldering SM but less common in other subtypes of SM (aggressive, leukemic, and SM-AHN).

CRITERIA FOR CM THAT ARE USUALLY PRESENT[2]

Major criterion: typical macroscopic (clinical) skin lesions, associated with the Darier sign.

Minor criteria:

1. Increased mast cell (MC) numbers in lesional skin
2. Activating point mutation of KIT in lesional skin

Histopathology

For a proper recognition of MC, the application of basic histochemical dyes like Giemsa is strongly recommended. Hereby, the metachromatic intracytoplasmic MC granules can easily be detected. However, enumeration of MC is much better facilitated when appropriate immunostains are used. For diagnostic purposes, antibodies against tryptase and CD117 (KIT) yield the best results. The MC antigen tryptase is highly specific and sensitive. The antigen CD117 is also extremely sensitive (a cell not expressing CD117 cannot be a MC) but much less specific since a variety of other cell types including hematopoietic stem cells are also CD117 positive. Coexpression of tryptase and CD117 define the mature immunophenotype of MC seen in reactive and neoplastic states. Aberrant expression of antigens not seen on normal/reactive MC therefore may help to recognize MIS. Here, CD25 and CD30 are of utmost diagnostic importance but immunophenotypical aberrancies are only detected in a minority of CM lesions. Detection of CD30-positive tumor cells may lead to wrong diagnoses harmful to the patient, in particular when the correct diagnosis of mastocytosis is not considered.

Considering the first minor criterion of the WHO definition of CM/MIS, it should be the first step in the pathologist's diagnostic approach to confirm the presence of a significantly increased number of intradermal MCs by use of appropriate immunostains (anti-tryptase and/or CD117). The reported MC numbers in the normal skin are generally low or very low (published data seem somewhat confusing, however). It should be emphasized that it is easy to recognize MIS immunohistochemically since numbers of loosely scattered MCs are markedly increased, even at first glance and at lower magnification. In most cases, a minor proportion of MC is spindle shaped but this does not serve as a minor diagnostic criterion like in SM. The presence of exclusively round hypergranular-appearing MC is typical for a well-differentiated mastocytosis, which is not a special subtype of mastocytosis but rather a phenotypical variant occurring in all types of CM and SM. MCs tend to accumulate around small vessels and adnexae forming groups and small aggregates, but compact infiltrates consisting of >15 MCs in skin lesions of maculopapular cutaneous mastocytosis (MPCM) (the only major criterion of SM) are rarely encountered. Most MCs are seen in the upper dermis but epidermotropism is absent. Larger, even transdermal, MC infiltrates are seen only in mastocytoma and MCS.

MASTOCYTOMA

Definition

A form of cutaneous mastocytosis characterized by the presence of up to three solitary cutaneous tumors composed of numerous mast cells without systemic involvement.[1,2]

Epidemiology

Solitary mastocytomas usually present in infants and children under 2 years of age, with the highest prevalence in the first month of life.[2] True solitary mastocytomas (isolated lesions without systemic disease) are only very rarely seen in adults and children over the age of 16 years, with only a handful of cases reported in the literature.[3,4] Solitary mastocytomas account for approximately 20% of cutaneous mastocytosis cases (with the remaining 80% of cases representing MPCM [syn. urticaria pigmentosa, UP] and diffuse cutaneous mastocytosis [DCM]).[5,6]

Etiology

Although their etiology is not fully understood, mastocytomas may show activating mutations in the KIT gene.[7] KIT is a receptor tyrosine kinase and proto-oncogene that is expressed by mast cells and some hemopoietic lineages, including leukemic blast cells.[8] *KIT* activating mutations are key molecular carcinogenic events in gastrointestinal stromal tumors, as well as some melanomas and acute myeloid leukemias.[7] KIT mutations may be seen in childhood as well as adult mastocytosis.[9-11] One small study reported *KIT* mutations, including D816V and exon 9 in 67% of solitary mastocytomas.[7]

Clinical Presentation/Prognosis

Mastocytomas are skin-colored, brown, or yellow-brown nodules. The lesions are most commonly distributed on the trunk but may occur on the face and limbs.[12] Typically, solitary mastocytomas are at least 1 cm in diameter.[2] The surface of the lesions may be smooth or may have a characteristic orange peel (peau d'orange) appearance. Rubbing the lesions causes mast cell degranulation, resulting in localized itchy wheal and flare formation (referred to as the Darier sign). Extralesional symptoms such as generalized flushing, pruritus, nausea, vomiting, and headaches may occur in a small subset of patients with mastocytomas and are due to the release of mast cell mediators into the circulation.[13]

Patients with solitary mastocytomas have an excellent prognosis. The majority of mastocytomas will resolve spontaneously—in most cases within 4 to 10 years, and often by the time the patient reaches puberty.[2,3,12] Adult-onset mastocytomas are less likely to involute spontaneously than the typical pediatric mastocytomas.[3] Malignant transformation of solitary mastocytomas to primary MCS would be exceptional, but has been described in one adult case.[14]

Treatment

Most patients with mastocytomas do not require treatment as the lesions often resolve spontaneously and do not cause significant systemic symptoms.[15] For patients with cosmetic concerns, topical or intralesional corticosteroids may be effective treatments.[15] Systemic symptoms related to mast cell mediator release into the circulation (such as flushing, itching, and gastrointestinal complaints) are usually treated with H1 antihistamines or mast cell stabilizers, although surgical excision of solitary lesions may be feasible.[15]

Histology

Histological sections of mastocytomas show a dense, nodular aggregate of mature mast cells in the dermis (Fig. 63-1), with occasional extension into the deeper levels of the dermis and subcutaneous tissues.[16] Mast cells are ovoid to round and often contain an abundance of metachromatic granules containing tryptase, histamine, and heparin.

Solitary mastocytomas of the skin do not pose problems for the histopathologist and are easily recognizable (even in the absence of immunostains) when Giemsa staining is used. The intra- or transdermal tumors are sharply demarcated, and mast cell numbers are not significantly increased in nonlesional skin.

The rare mastocytomas seen in adults usually exhibit marked cytological atypia and a significantly increased proliferative activity, especially when immunostaining with the antibody Ki-67 (MIB1) is used. These cases are at least borderline to an overt MCS that also may arise primarily in the skin.

Immunophenotype

Mastocytomas express normal mast cell markers such as CD33, CD5, CD68, CD117, tryptase, and chymase.[17,18] Mast cells also express CD45 (common leukocyte antigen).[17] Histochemical stains such as toluidine blue, Giemsa, and chloroacetate esterase (the Leder stain) may also be used to highlight mast cells.[1,17] Anti-CD117 is the most sensitive marker for mast cells but is not entirely specific. Conversely, chymase is highly specific for mast cells but less sensitive.[17] Childhood mastocytoses very rarely express aberrant

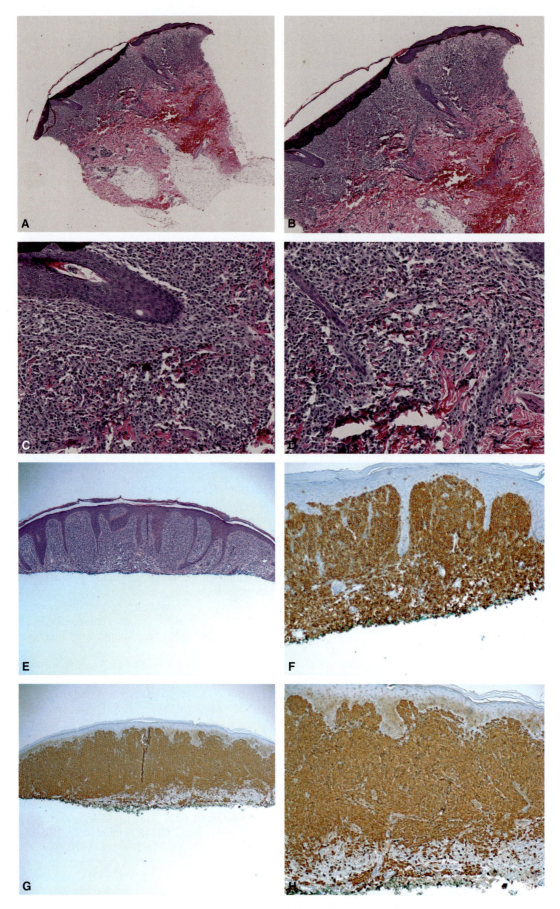

FIGURE 63-1. Mastocytoma. There is a diffuse dermal and band-like infiltrate in the dermis, with sparing of the surface epidermis (**A** and **B**, 20× and 40×). The infiltrate is composed of polygonal-shaped cells with slightly basophilic and granular cytoplasm (**C** and **D**, 100× and 200×). Shave biopsy of similar histologic process (**E**, 20×). The lesional cells are positive for CD117 (**F**) and mast cell tryptase (**G** and **H**).

immunohistochemical markers such as CD25 or CD2, with very few reported cases in the literature.[19] Limited cutaneous mastocytoses (including solitary mastocytomas) express aberrant CD25 much less often than the cutaneous lesions of SM.[20]

Genetic and Molecular Findings

The genetic and molecular findings of solitary mastocytomas are not well characterized. In one small study, 67% of solitary mastocytomas had mutations in *KIT*.[7]

Differential Diagnosis

Mast cells typically have a characteristic histological appearance with amphophilic cytoplasmic granules that are uncommonly seen in other cell types. Nevertheless, in certain cases, mast cells may bear resemblance to melanocytes, histiocytes, and Langerhans cells.[21] Langerhans cell histiocytosis (LCH) also frequently presents as a cutaneous tumor in infants and young children.[22] However, histologically, Langerhans cells are pale histiocytes devoid of cytoplasmic granules and often demonstrate characteristic folded (or reniform) nuclei. Langerhans cells are positive for S100 and CD1a (Langerin), whereas mast cells are negative for these markers.[19,21,22] An eosinophilic infiltrate is common in lesions of LCH,[22] but this feature has also rarely been described in cases of mastocytoma.[23,24] Histologically, mastocytomas may also bear resemblance to melanocytic nevi. Rare instances of mastocytomas combined with melanocytic nevi have even been reported (Fig. 63-2).[25] Unlike junctional melanocytic nevi, mastocytomas involve only the dermis and do not typically involve or extend into the epidermis.[21] Furthermore, mastocytomas do not generally show the nesting pattern that is characteristic of most melanocytic nevi and instead are generally composed of a single dense aggregate of cells.[21] Immunohistochemical stains for S100 protein, CD117, and melanocyte-specific markers may be used if the distinction cannot be made on histologic examination alone.

In an adult with a presumed solitary cutaneous mastocytoma, cutaneous involvement by SM should also be considered. Aberrant CD25 expression is more commonly seen in cases of SM, and this marker may be useful for identifying patients with cutaneous mastocytosis who are more likely to have systemic disease and may require further workup.[20]

Variants

Rare cases of mastocytomas with dense eosinophilic infiltrates have been described.[23,24] A histiocyte-rich pleomorphic mastocytoma has also been described. This lesion was characterized by a rich histiocytic infiltrate with enlarged, bilobed, and multinucleated mast cells.[19] A child with CM and disseminated juvenile xanthogranuloma has been reported.[26]

Capsule Summary

- Mastocytomas are solitary tumors composed of mast cells. Solitary mastocytomas by definition have no systemic involvement.
- Mastocytomas are most commonly seen in infants and children under the age of 2 years. Adult-onset solitary mastocytomas are extremely rare.
- Most solitary mastocytomas resolve spontaneously within a few years or by the time the child reaches puberty and do not require treatment.
- Solitary mastocytomas may have mutations in *KIT*.
- Routine skin biopsies of mastocytomas in children are not required but should be considered for atypical lesions, especially in adults.

MACULOPAPULAR CUTANEOUS MASTOCYTOSIS

Definition

A clinical presentation of mastocytosis characterized by discrete cutaneous lesions (usually macules, papules, nodules, or plaques) with abnormal mast cell infiltrates that may be monomorphic (usually adults) or polymorphic (usually children).[2]

For practical purposes, the terms MPCM and UP can be used synonymously. UP is easier to remember and has a long heritage since the original description by Sangster in 1878[27] and may therefore be preferred.

The original description of telangiectasia macularis eruptiva perstans (TMEP)[28] implies that the erythematous (telangiectatic) presentation of UP seen in some adults is part of a spectrum rather than a separate subtype,[29] which is the rationale for combining the two terms under the umbrella diagnosis of MPCM in the WHO classification. It has been proposed that fixed patches of telangiectatic erythema that do not urticate on rubbing or show an obvious excess of mast cells on histology should be regarded as subtype of TMEP.[30] Further studies involving molecular genetics, potential comorbidities, and long-term prognosis are required. In practical terms, patients with MPCM may present with typical UP, nonpigmented patches, or both. TMEP may still be

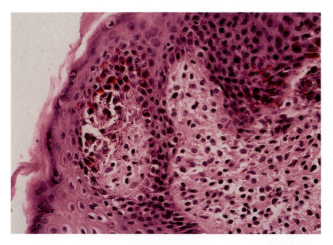

FIGURE 63-2. Coexistence of mastocytoma and junctional melanocytic nevus. (Reproduced from Northcutt AD, Tschen JA. Combined mastocytoma-junctional nevus. *Am J Dermatopathol.* 2004;26(6):478-481, with permission.)

a useful descriptive term for red patches but should not be regarded as a special subtype of MPCM in terms of risk of systemic involvement, management, or prognosis.

Epidemiology

UP is the most common clinical presentation of cutaneous mastocytosis, representing 75% to 80% of all cases.[5,6] As with other forms of cutaneous mastocytosis, UP most commonly occurs in infants and children, with 80% of cases occurring within the first year of life.[2,31] Adult patients presenting with UP frequently show systemic disease, and these patients should be classified as MIS until SM has been confirmed. Thereafter, they should be classified as SM with cutaneous involvement[31] denoted as SM+. Those without skin lesions can be designated SM−. However, rare cases of adults with pure cutaneous UP have been described.[2,32] How many of them show evidence of clonality on PB KIT mutation is currently unclear. Studies have shown an equal sex predilection to slight male predominance.[6,31]

Etiology

As with other forms of cutaneous mastocytosis, both sporadic and germline activating mutations in the KIT proto-oncogene have been demonstrated in UP. Although the disease is usually sporadic, familial forms of UP with a variety of germline mutations in KIT have been described.[33-38] A minority of cases of cutaneous mastocytosis are KIT mutation-negative on skin biopsy.[10] In these cases, it has been suggested that the aetiologic agent is the abnormal expression of mast cell growth factors.[33]

Clinical Presentation/Prognosis

The lesions of UP are usually red or brown, oval, and typically vary in size.[2] Most of the lesions are larger than 0.5 mm and may be macules or papules. Nodules or plaques may also be seen in children.[2] The lesions may be sharply demarcated or have indistinct borders (Fig. 63-3).[2] Typically, they are symmetrically distributed on the head, neck, and extremities.[2,11] Rubbing or scratching the lesions results in localized itch, wheal, or blister formation (Darier sign) in children and some adults due to mast cell degranulation.[2] Generalized itching is a reported symptom in about half of patients.[11] Patients with cutaneous mastocytosis generally have lower serum tryptase levels than those with SM.[39] In children with UP, serum tryptase levels are usually within the normal range,[2,39] which is consistent with the observation that UP in children is frequently a skin-limited process.

The rash regresses by the time the patient reaches adolescence in most children with the polymorphic pattern of UP but in those with the monomorphic pattern and raised tryptase may persist into adulthood.[2] Adults with UP are likely to have persistent disease and systemic involvement.[2]

Treatment

As with other forms of isolated cutaneous mastocytosis, often no treatment is necessary in UP as the lesions often resolve.[15] In children with cosmetic concerns, topical corticosteroids with occlusive dressings may be effective.[15] For generalized itching and other histamine-related symptoms, antihistamines (both H1 and H2 blockers) may provide relief, although topical calcineurin inhibitors, for example, pimecrolimus, have been reported to be effective at improving the appearance of skin lesions in children.[40] Improvement of skin lesions has been reported in adults with advanced SM treated with the tyrosine kinase inhibitor midostaurin[41] and the nucleotide analogue cladribine.[42] Early reports from clinical trials of novel tyrosine kinase inhibitors for highly symptomatic ISM suggest that clearance or substantial reduction of skin lesions may occur.

Histology

Biopsies of UP lesions show an increase in dermal mast cells that is 4 to 8 times higher than that seen in normal skin and 2 to 3 times higher than that seen in inflamed skin.[2] The mast cells may be spindled or ovoid and show characteristic amphophilic cytoplasmic granules similar to the mast cells seen in other cutaneous mastocytoses.[2,11] The number of dermal mast cells identified histologically can vary significantly from patient to patient.[2] Taking biopsies from lesional and perilesional skin for mast cell counts may be helpful to demonstrate a difference when lesions are

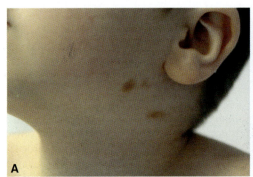
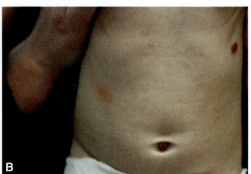

FIGURE 63-3. **Urticaria pigmentosa in a young child. A.** Red-to-brown, oval patches and plaques on the neck. **B.** An erythematous plaque on the chest illustrates the Darier sign. (Courtesy of Dr. Patricia Witman, Nationwide Children's Hospital, Columbus, OH.)

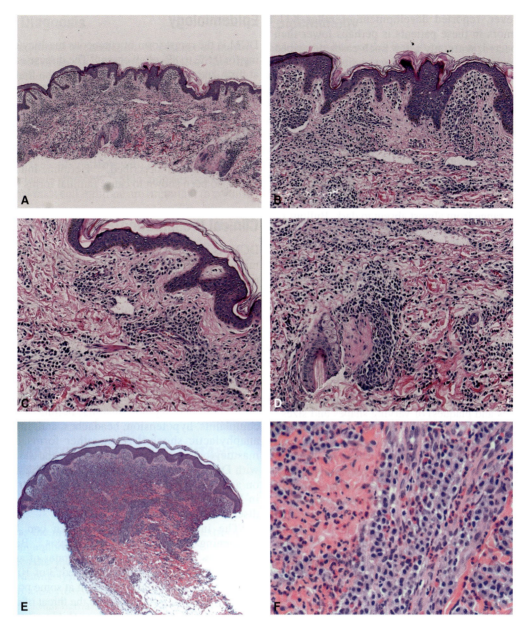

FIGURE 63-4. Urticaria pigmentosa—histopathology. Dense superficial and deep infiltrate in the dermis with a notable perivascular accentuation (**A** and **B**, 20× and 100×). The infiltrate is composed of epithelioid cells, which also extend and infiltrate adnexal structures (**C** and **D**, 200× and 400×). Another example of UP with a brisk eosinophilic infiltrate (**E** and **F**, 20× and 400×).

indistinct. The infiltrate is predominantly in the upper third of the dermis, at times in proximity to the dermoepidermal junction (Fig. 63-4).[39]

Immunophenotype

Mast cells express CD33, CD5, CD68, CD117, tryptase, and chymase, as well as CD45 (leukocyte common antigen).[18,20] Toluidine blue, Giemsa, and chloroacetate esterase (the Leder stain) can also be used to highlight mast cells.[1,18] CD117 is the most sensitive marker for mast cells but is not entirely specific. Conversely, chymase positivity is highly specific for mast cells but less sensitive.[18] Tryptase has been recommended as the standard immunohistochemical marker for the identification and quantification of mast cells in mastocytosis.[2]

Genetic and Molecular Findings

Both childhood and adult forms of mastocytosis show mutations in the KIT proto-oncogene.[2] Over 90% of adults with mastocytosis show a specific KIT mutation: D816V in exon 17.[2] By contrast, only 35% of childhood mastocytosis cases (most of which are UP) have D816V KIT mutations.[2] Children with cutaneous mastocytosis more commonly exhibit activating KIT mutations involving exons other than exon 17 (40% of cases) or have no KIT mutations whatsoever (25% of cases).[2,10] Most KIT mutations are sporadic, although familial forms of UP with a variety of germline mutations in KIT have been described.[33-38] The majority of these familial cases follow an autosomal dominant pattern of inheritance. Some patients with germline KIT mutations are also prone to developing gastrointestinal stromal of symptoms such as irritability, fatigue, poor attention span, and depression.[51] The bone marrow is commonly involved in adult patients with mastocytosis (Fig. 63-6). Lymphadenopathy can occur in advanced disease with or without hepatosplenomegaly ("B" findings). Involvement of the gastrointestinal tract is frequent, and symptoms such as abdominal pain, diarrhea, nausea, and vomiting may occur. Persistent abnormal liver function tests (alkaline phosphatase) without an alternative cause is a "C" finding.

Prognosis

The prognosis of SM also depends on the subtype. Patients with ISM have a normal life expectancy and only 1% to 5% of patients will progress to more severe forms of SM such as SM-AHN.[51] The prognosis of SM-AHN largely depends on the associated hematologic disease, but the overall survival is poor with a median survival of 2 to 4.4 years.[49,50,54] The median survival of ASM is 3.5 to 7 years.[49,50,55] MCL carries the worst prognosis, with a median survival time of less than 6 months[56] prior to the introduction of midostaurin. Other mutations have been identified in advanced SM, including CBL, RUNX1, TET2, ASXL1, and SRSF2.[51] These additional mutations appear to be associated with more aggressive disease and a worse prognosis.[47] The prognosis for advanced disease has improved with the advent of novel tyrosine kinase inhibitors.

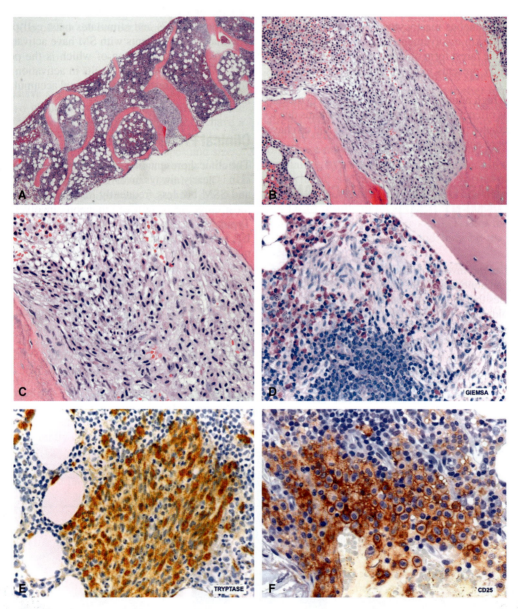

FIGURE 63-6. Systemic mastocytosis—bone marrow findings. Nodular paratrabecular and nonparatrabecular aggregates of spindle-shaped mast cells are present with associated fibrosis (**A–C**, 20×, 100× and 400×). The aggregates are positive for Giemsa (**D**), tryptase (**E**), and CD25 (**F**).

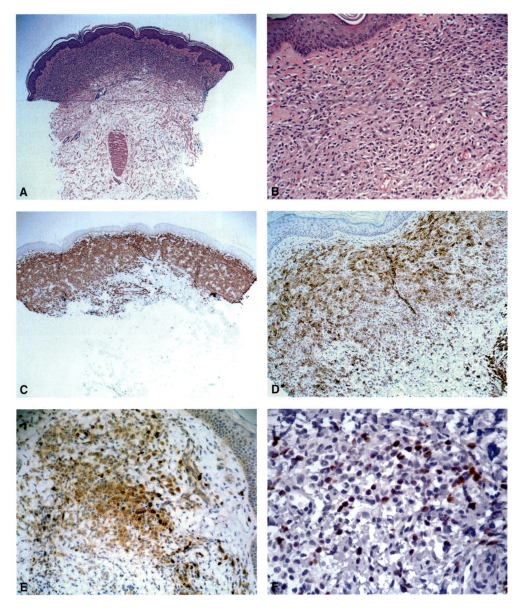

FIGURE 63-7. Systemic mastocytosis—histopathology. Diffuse band-like infiltrate in the superficial dermis, sparing the epidermis (**A**, 20×). The infiltrate is composed of spindle cells (**B**, 200×). Abnormal mast cells are positive for CD117 (**C**), CD30 (**D**), CD25 (**E**), and CD2 (**F**).

Skin Histopathology of Systemic Mastocytosis

The histologic appearance of cutaneous involvement by SM can be identical to that of patients with isolated cutaneous mastocytosis. In patients with UP lesions, histologic sections show an increase in dermal mast cells 4 to 8 times higher than that seen in normal skin[2] (Fig. 63-7).

Treatment

In patients with ISM, the treatment is generally aimed at controlling symptoms. Avoidance of agents that trigger mast cell degranulation is an important aspect of treatment.[51] These include alcohol, exercise, extremely hot or extremely cold temperatures, and certain medications (such as nonsteroidal anti-inflammatory drugs and aspirin).[15] Second-generation H1 antihistamines and mast cell stabilizers (such as sodium cromoglycate) may also be helpful in controlling symptoms. Tyrosine kinase inhibitors have also been shown to reduce symptoms in some patients with advanced disease, although imatinib is not effective in patients with the KIT D816V mutation, which is present in most patients with ISM.[51] Trials of other tyrosine kinase inhibitors (avapritinib and masitinib) are ongoing for symptomatic ISM at the time of publication. The more aggressive forms of SM (SM-AHN, ASM, and MCL) may require treatment with cytotoxic chemotherapy and regulate the MEK-ERK signaling cascade of the MAPK pathway (Fig. 64-2). Of the RAF kinases, BRAF has a high frequency of mutations in many human cancers with the *BRAF*-V600E mutation accounting for nearly 90% of activating BRAF mutations in human neoplasia, including a high prevalence in the histiocytoses, leading to constitutive kinase activation.[22,28] In tissue sections, the clustered, mutant lesional histiocytes are often surrounded by a robust secondary reactive inflammatory population; thus, isolating and accurately detecting the percentage of mutant cells for molecular testing requires sensitive testing techniques, along with well-validated mutation-specific immunohistochemistry (ie, BRAF VE1 and pERK stains) for paired analysis. The mutant-specific BRAF-VE1 antibody will express moderate to strong cytoplasmic granular staining in lesional cells as a correlate to the *BRAF*-V600E-mutant protein (Fig. 64-3); however, false-positive staining in cilia, anterior pituitary cells, plasma cells, smooth muscle, and background glial tissue must all be taken into consideration.[29,30] The pERK stain is a delicate stain to interpret, as the quality of the fixation plays an important role along with high background staining of nonneoplastic tissue (eg, endothelium of blood vessels, reactive fibroblastic proliferations, smooth muscle, nerves, variable squamous staining). While it is known that there are elevated levels of pERK expression across all the histiocytic lesions, the tissue stain can be difficult to interpret, if not focused on a discrete lesional cell population. The robust staining of the blood vessels serves as an internal control on the quality of tissue fixation, and pERK immunostaining should not be interpreted if there is complete absence of vascular staining (Fig. 64-3).

In LCH and ECD, the cell of origin appears closely related to a hematopoietic precursor with myeloid dendritic cell lineage,[5,6,31] in which phenotypic differences of disease presentation may result from both the timing of somatic mutations at critical stages of myeloid cell differentiation toward dendritic and monocyte development, along with local cytokine milieu. A theory of the misguided myeloid differentiation model in LCH, in which activating MAPK mutations at either the pluripotent hematopoietic, tissue-restricted, or local precursor level, may also explain the different clinical phenotypes in LCH, including high-risk multisystem, multifocal low-risk, or unifocal LCH disease, respectively, as this model has been exemplified in the context of LCH murine models.[12,32] Furthermore, while kinase activating mutations, especially *BRAF*-V600E, appear to confer tissue growth advantage via disrupted cell migration and inhibition of apoptosis,[11] both LCH and ECD have rather low proliferation, unlike their malignant counterpart. Thus, the link between *BRAF*-V600E pathogenesis and disease presentation may be best understood in terms of oncogene-induced senescence, in which an acquired *BRAF*-V600E mutation in multipotent hematopoietic progenitor cells leads to growth arrest, apoptosis resistance, and a senescence-associated secretory phenotype that in turn leads to skewing toward the mononuclear phagocyte (MNP) lineage, ultimately leading

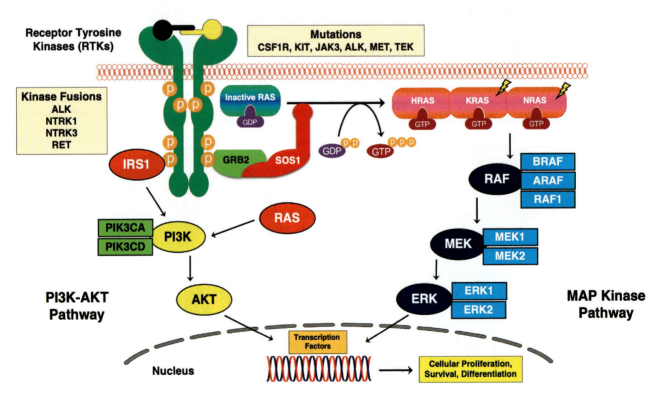

FIGURE 64-2. Overview of the biochemical signaling pathways key to the molecular pathogenesis of histiocytic neoplasms. Diagram of the components of the mitogen-activated protein kinase (MAPK), PI3K-AKT, and receptor tyrosine kinase (RTK) signaling pathways with description of the activation of the RAS proteins (HRAS, KRAS, and NRAS) with the signaling proteins affected by genetic alterations in the histiocytic neoplasms. ("Copyright Dr. Jennifer Picarsic and Dr. Benjamin Durham.")

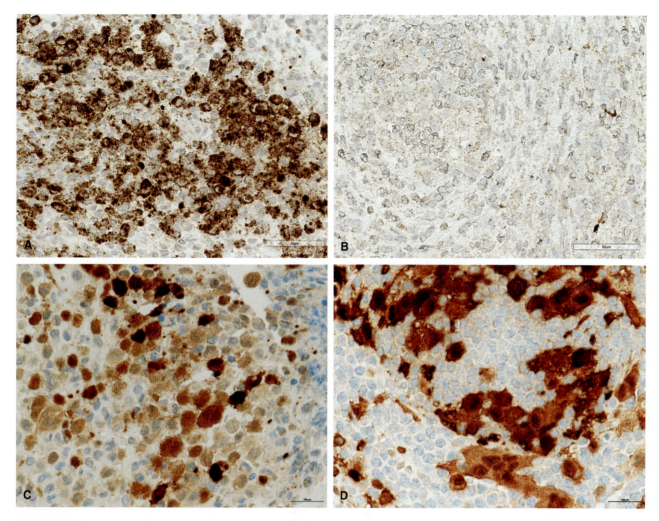

FIGURE 64-3. Mutant-specific immunohistochemistry. A positive BRAF VE1 antibody correlating with the BRAF-V600E mutation should show a moderate to strong cytoplasmic staining in lesional histiocytes (**A**, LCH, BRAF VE1 Immunostain, digital scanned image, original objective magnification 40×) as compared to weak punctate granular staining of a negative BRAF VE1 that is correlated with wild type status (**B**, LCH, BRAF VE1 Immunostain, digital scanned image, original objective magnification 40×). Phosphorylated ERK antibody (pERK) stain will highlight the lesional histiocytes both in the (**C**) presence and (**D**) absence of BRAF-V600E mutation (C LCH with BRAF-V600E mutation, pERK immunostain, original objective magnification 40×; D LCH, BRAF wild type, pERK immunostain original objective magnification 40×). Caution should be taken in interpretation of pERK immunostain as both fixation/processing time can affect staining, thus a strong staining of the endothelium of the blood vessels serves as a useful internal control for adequate tissue staining quality. ("Copyright Dr. Jennifer Picarsic and Dr. Benjamin Durham".)

to the accumulation of senescent MNPs in tissue and the formation of LCH lesions.[13] It may then be extrapolated, at least in LCH, that the permanent tissue consequences are related to the small collection of clonal histiocytes inciting persistent inflammation and resultant fibrosis in older children (ie, biliary cirrhosis in the liver, neurodegeneration/gliosis in the brain) or in turn activating a hyperinflammatory pathway with macrophage activation pathways in the youngest patients.[33-35] A similar process may likely also be happening in the other related histiocytic lesions with similar kinase activating mutations, for which further investigations are ongoing.

Clinical Implications

Clinically, worse outcomes in LCH also appear related to BRAF-V600E status, although the data is variable.[12,36,37] In general, mortality has been restricted in pediatric LCH to the high-risk multisystem category (see also Chapter 67, risk organs include the liver, spleen, and bone marrow), comprising about 20% of cases, characterized by fevers, hepatosplenomegaly, hematopoietic failure, and liver dysfunction.[38] The French cohort has provided evidence that such a subgroup of children tends to have higher incidence of BRAF-V600E with permanent consequences and often fail standard LCH-based chemotherapy.[36] It is still to be determined, but this initial cohort study also suggested that the so-called "CNS-risk" patients, including those with specific skull base and facial bone involvement (ie, mastoid, sphenoid, orbit, clivus, or temporal bone), which have been variably associated with a high likelihood of diabetes insipidus and increased risk for a late CNS neurodegenerative cerebellar disease,[39-41] also appear enriched with the BRAF-V600E mutation.[36] Such studies and accumulating case reports[35] suggest that this group may best benefit from upfront BRAF or MEK inhibitor therapy, given that about 30% of patients will relapse after completing 1 year of standard chemotherapy, and 15% to 20% of patients do not respond to current standard therapies at all, which is even higher (up to 49% treatment failure) for the risk organ (RO+) MS-LCH patients.[36,38] Thus, the identification of BRAF-V600E with sensitive testing is becoming the standard of care in histiocytosis for helping decide prognostic significance and treatment decisions, especially in children with MS-LCH RO+ that fail standard therapy[42] and in adults with ECD for which FDA-approval for vemurafenib and breakthrough therapy designation to cobimetinib for MEK inhibition in histiocytic neoplasm has been granted, based on a series of published studies.[43,44]

BRAF INSERTION/DELETIONS IN HISTIOCYTIC NEOPLASMS

After the landmark discovery of *BRAF*-V600E in the majority of LCH and ECD patients, recent studies have uncovered important in-frame insertion/deletion (indels) mutations in the BRAF kinase domain. For example, a 2012 study identified *BRAF*-V600insDLAT involving the activation segment of the BRAF kinase domain[45]; and although this in-frame insertion has not been functionally evaluated, the *BRAF*-V600insDLAT insertion should constitutively activate BRAF kinase activity in a similar fashion to *BRAF*-V600E.[45] Furthermore, recurrent in-frame deletions involving exon 12 of *BRAF*, which encodes the β3-αC loop (coordinates the movements of two structural elements critical for the activation of the BRAF kinase), have been functionally shown to activate BRAF.[4,46,47] These in-frame *BRAF* exon 12 deletions are the third most frequent group of driver alteration in LCH, but they also occur at a lower frequency in ECD and have not been described in other subtypes of histiocytic neoplasms at present (see Fig. 64-1).[4,46,47]

OTHER BRAF AND RAF MUTATIONS IN HISTIOCYTIC NEOPLASMS

While much less frequent in the histiocytoses, LCH, in particular, may harbor other non-*BRAF*-V600E mutations.[45-50] It should be noted that the mutant-specific BRAF VE1 immunostain will be negative in such cases, but pERK staining should highlight the lesional cells. The malignant histiocytoses may have additional cooperating mutations including variant BRAF and RAS mutations.[51] Readers are referred to in-depth reviews.[22,52]

The *ARAF* mutations are infrequent in LCH,[53] with higher frequency found in non-LCH, with one study showing 21% of ECD cases, 18% of JXG, and 12.5% of RDD harboring the mutation with mutual exclusivity in ECD and RDD but cooccurring with *RAS* mutations in JXG.[54] Further functional studies are needed to investigate if such mutations have similar impact on pathogenesis as in *BRAF*-V600E cases, but most appear to cause pERK upregulation and would likely respond to MEK inhibition.

MAP2K1, MAP3K1, and Other Related Mutations in Histiocytic Neoplasms

The second most frequent group of MAPK pathway mutations in the L-group histiocytoses (including LCH and ECD) are mutations in the *MAP2K1* gene, which appear to be mutually exclusive to *BRAF*-V600E.[4,54,55] JXG and RDD also harbor this mutation with increased frequency (see Fig. 64-1). The mutations described in histiocytoses appear to cluster in the N-terminal negative regulatory domain (exon 2) and the N-terminal catalytic core of the kinase domain (exon 3). The expression of pERK is noted in cases (see Fig. 64-3), but rare examples have shown resistance to MEK inhibition, one characterized by a *MAP2K1* p.L98_K104 > Q deletion.[56] Histiocytic neoplasms with mutations in *MAP3K1* theoretically should lead to phosphorylation of MEK1 in the MAPK cascade,[57] but in the rare reports in LCH, such mutations have been difficult to prove, as one manifested as a frameshift mutation leading to loss of function, one was associated with a *BRAF*-V600E mutation, and another as a missense variant that was likely germline given its high allelic fraction.[55] In ECD, a *MAP3K1* amplification was noted, but functional activity was not reported.[47] In more recent, larger cohort studies, *MAP3K1* mutations were not identified, but two ECD patients harbored an *MAP3K19* and *MAP3K10* associated with a *BRAF*-V600E and a *MAP2K1* mutation, respectively.[4]

RAS Mutations in Histiocytic Neoplasms

The *NRAS*, *KRAS*, and *HRAS* genes, which encode small GTPases that regulate the MAPK and PI3K-AKT signaling pathways,[28] have been identified in the histiocytic neoplasms, with higher frequency in non-LCH cases and predominately as the exclusive MAPK pathway mutation.[2-4] However, rare examples have shown cooccurring RAS mutations with other *BRAF* and *MAP2K1* mutations including exceptional cases of LCH (*KRAS* and *NRAS* with *BRAF*-V600E),[4] rare cases of JXG (*NRAS* with *ARAF*),[54] and rare malignant histiocytic neoplasms of histiocytic sarcoma phenotype (*KRAS* with *MAP2K1*; *HRAS* with *BRAF*-F595L).[4,51] In most protein expression data, pERK is present with such RAS mutations, but further functional investigation is needed with larger cohorts.[3]

Mutations of the PI3K Isoforms in the Histiocytic Neoplasms

The genes that encode subunits of PI3K (phosphatidylinositol-4,5-bisphosphate 3 kinase, catalytic subunit α and phosphatidylinositol-4,5-bisphosphate 3 kinase, catalytic subunit δ) have been implicated in histiocytic neoplasms (namely ECD and LCH with rare reports in JXG) (see Fig. 64-1). These PI3K isoforms belongs to a family of lipid kinases whose cellular functions include cell proliferation and survival and are part of the PI3K-AKT signaling pathway[4,54,58-60]; however, further functional data are needed to better understand the role of such mutations in the pathogenesis of histiocytic neoplasms.

Mutations of CSF1R in the Histiocytic Neoplasms

The most recent molecular discovery in histiocytic neoplasms is the in-frame deletions of the *CSF1R* gene that has been found with increased frequency in JXG family lesions with both localized cutaneous presentations, along with more systemic involvement, including monozygotic twins[4] with subsequent cases found in young children with deeply infiltrative periorbital and tongue involvement (*JP 2021, personal communications*). It remains clinically unknown if systemic lesions with such mutations also respond favorably to targeted MEK inhibitor therapies, but at least in vitro data suggest that these deletions increase levels of MEK1/2 and ERK1/2 expression.[4]

STRUCTURAL GENE REARRANGEMENTS

ALK Rearrangement in Histiocytic Neoplasms Including the ALK-Positive Histiocytosis

While the majority of somatic genetic alterations in the histiocytic neoplasms are mutations, a significant subset also harbor kinase gene rearrangements that lead to upregulation of the MAPK pathway with subsequent ERK activation. The most notable and distinct of these is the ALK gene rearrangement that has led to the distinction of ALK-positive histiocytosis, which is emerging as a distinct entity from its current grouping in the L-group histiocytosis designation under ECD.[1] In nearly all cases, the ALK-positive histiocytosis is a non-LCH with an immunophenotype closely overlapping with the JXG family but with clinical–pathological distinctions. The original descriptions were limited to neonatal/infantile cases with hematopoietic and liver involvement overlapping with clinical features of a storage disease; however, this disease group tended to slowly resolve with supportive therapy or systemic treatment as needed.[61-63] As more cases are reported, the spectrum of ALK-positive histiocytosis has increased to include older children and adults with both multifocal, systemic disease involvement and single-system disease, with the CNS being a prevalent site.[4,47,63-74] We have described cases in the skin with an infiltrative growth pattern, dissecting through the dermal collagen without a classical xanthogranuloma appearance (ie, no Touton giant cells or xanthomatous cells) but rather composed of a monomorphic collection of histiocytes with a JXG immunophenotype and punctate granular cytoplasmic ALK expression (Fig. 64-4). In addition, light S100 staining, along with pERK expression, was noted in the majority of histiocytes.[4,74] These cases demonstrate a *KIF5B-ALK* rearrangement (Fig. 64-5). The partner gene *KIF5B* (Kinesin Family Member 5B), involving exons 1 to 24 fused with either exons 19 to 29 or exons 20 to 29 of the *ALK* gene, is the most common fusion in the ALK-positive histiocytoses.[64,66,68,74,75] The fusion of the N-terminal coiled-coil domain of KIF5B to the intact kinase domain of ALK results in the inappropriate expression and constitutive activation of ALK, for which ALK inhibitor–based therapy has been effective in cases of *ALK*-rearranged, nonmalignant histiocytoses cases.[64,68-70,74] Other fusion partners with *ALK* include *TPM3* in an infant with systemic disease,[61] *COL1A2* in a teenager

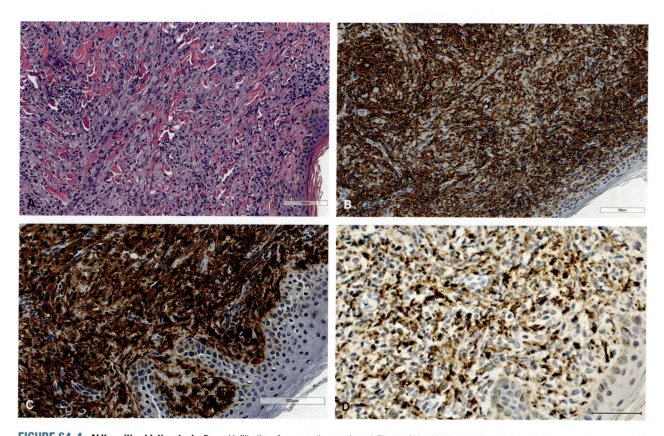

FIGURE 64-4. ALK positive histiocytosis. Dermal infiltration of a nonxanthogranuloma infiltrate of bland histiocytes (**A**, H&E stain, digital scanned image, original objective magnification 20×) with diffuse CD163 (**B**, CD163 Immunostain, digital scanned image, original objective magnification 20×) and Factor XIIIa staining (**C**, Factor XIIIa Immunostain, digital scanned image, original objective magnification 20×) and punctate cytoplasmic ALK expression (**D**, ALK Immunostain, original objective magnification 40×) which correlated with ALK rearrangement by FISH. ("Copyright Dr. Jennifer Picarsic and Dr. Benjamin Durham.")

with a foot skin/soft tissue lesion,[64] and *EML4* in two adult patients, one with a solitary lung nodule[72] and another with an anterior mediastinal mass.[73] A rare report of fusion partner *TRIM33* in a young adult with a large mesenteric mass[71] may better represent an atypical ALK-rearrangement case with a histiocyte-rich background, given that the CD68+ histiocytes appeared more spindled as compared to the diffuse ALK immunostain expression. While most ALK-positive histiocytoses are described in the context of low-grade histiocytic lesions with a cutaneous or systemic JXG or ECD-like involvement, a rare report of a malignant histiocytic neoplasm with histiocytic sarcoma phenotype found in an adult female with lymph node and subcutaneous nodule involvement has been described with the *CLTC-ALK* rearrangement and later died of progressive disease.[69]

NTRK1 Rearrangements in Histiocytic Neoplasms

Another activating kinase fusion in both the MAPK and PI3K-AKT pathways that has shown variable frequency in JXG and ECD are the *NTRK1* gene rearrangements involving exons 12 to 17. Various 5′ gene partners have been found including the first discovered in 2015 with the partner genes *LMNA*, an in-frame fusion involving exons 1 to 5 of *LMNA*[54] and later in 2017 with *TPR* (Translocated Promoter Region, Nuclear Basket Protein) involving exons 1 to 10, in an ECD and non-LCH , not otherwise specified, respectively.[47] Both fusions result in the fusion of the N-terminal coiled-coil domains of partner genes to the intact kinase domain of NTRK1 resulting in the inappropriate expression and constitutive activation of NTRK1 (see Fig. 64-5). Since those initial discoveries, we have found a clustered frequency of *NTRK1* rearrangements in otherwise indolent, cutaneous JXG lesions with deep infiltration into the dermis with an epithelioid appearance, including partners *IRF2BP2*, *TPM3*, and *SQSTM1*,[4] all with pan-TRK expression by immunohistochemistry.

ETV3-NCOA2 Rearrangement in the Histiocytic Neoplasms

The recurrent gene rearrangement *ETV3-NCOA2* (ETS Variant 3 and Nuclear Receptor Coactivator 2) almost exclusively involves a subset of histiocytic neoplasms within the ICH category (see also Chapter 67) in which the cells have variable Langerhans cell features, including nuclear grooves along with CD1a and S100 expression, but lack Birbeck granules

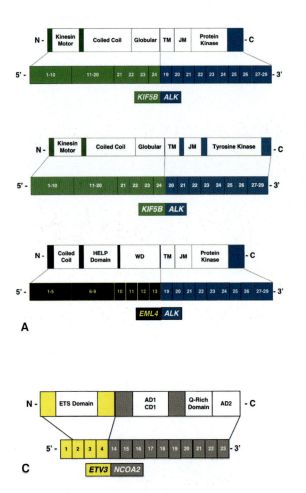

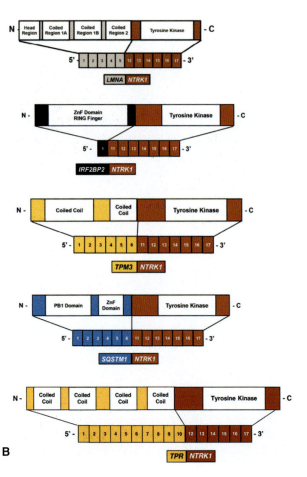

FIGURE 64-5. Summary of selected kinase fusions in histiocytic neoplasms. A. Illustrations of recurrent *ALK* fusions described in ALK-positive histiocytoses and other non-Langerhans cell histiocytic neoplasms. **B.** Illustrations of the recurrent *NTRK1* fusions uncovered in non-Langerhans cell histiocytoses. **C.** Illustration of the recurrent *ETV3-NCOA2* fusion discovered in both Langerhans cell histiocytosis and indeterminate cell histiocytosis. ("Copyright Dr. Jennifer Picarsic and Dr. Benjamin Durham.")

by ultrastructural analysis and thus lack Langerin/CD207 expression.[76] One adult patient with LCH was also noted to harbor the same fusion.[47] While the functional role of the *ETV3-NCOA2* fusion in the pathogenesis of histiocytic neoplasms is still warranted, the described fusion of the NCOA2 C-terminal transcriptional activation domains (AD1, CID, and AD2 involving exons 14-23) to the N-terminal ETS domain of ETV3 (exons 1-4), which is a winged helix-turn-helix DNA-binding domain, is similarly described in other human cancers.[22]

FOLLICULAR DENDRITIC CELL SARCOMAS AND FIBROBLASTIC RETICULAR CELL TUMOR

Both the 5th edition WHO and the Histiocyte Society revised classification specifically exclude follicular dendritic cell sarcomas (FDCS) and fibroblastic reticular cell tumor within the histiocytic/dendritic cell category, as these two entities are now recognized as mesenchymal-derived neoplasms with historical "dendritic cell" terminology.[1,77] Nevertheless, rare examples of FDCS have shown *BRAF*-V600E, although skin involvement is exceptional.[78] Fibroblastic reticular cell tumor is a mesenchymal-derived tumor with tissue cells thought to be derived from common progenitors located in the perivascular space, similar to FDCS but located in T-cell zones[79] and with an immunophenotype more like myofibroblasts (including vimentin, smooth muscle actin, desmin) and variable keratin expression but lack of CD45 and CD31 expression.[80,81] The other key phenotypic differentiation from the hematopoietic-derived dendritic cell lesions is their consistent lack of the Langerhans (CD1a, Langerin), interdigitating (S100, fascin), and follicular (CD21, CD23, and CD35) phenotypes, and despite variable expression of CD68, these lesions are negative for more specific macrophage/monocyte markers, including CD163 and CD14.

References

1. Emile JF, Abla O, Fraitag S, et al. Revised classification of histiocytoses and neoplasms of the macrophage-dendritic cell lineages. *Blood*. 2016;127(22):2672-2681.
2. Abla O, Jacobsen E, Picarsic J, et al. Consensus recommendations for the diagnosis and clinical management of Rosai-Dorfman-Destombes disease. *Blood*. 2018;131(26):2877-2890.
3. Garces S, Medeiros LJ, Patel KP, et al. Mutually exclusive recurrent KRAS and MAP2K1 mutations in Rosai-Dorfman disease. *Mod Pathol*. 2017;30(10):1367-1377.
4. Durham BH, Lopez Rodrigo E, Picarsic J, et al. Activating mutations in CSF1R and additional receptor tyrosine kinases in histiocytic neoplasms. *Nat Med*. 2019;25(12):1839-1842.
5. Milne P, Bigley V, Bacon CM, et al. Hematopoietic origin of Langerhans cell histiocytosis and Erdheim Chester disease in adults. *Blood*. 2017;130(2):167-175.
6. Durham BH, Roos-Weil D, Baillou C, et al. Functional evidence for derivation of systemic histiocytic neoplasms from hematopoietic stem/progenitor cells. *Blood*. 2017;130(2):176-180.
7. Xiao Y, van Halteren AG, Lei X, et al. Bone marrow-derived myeloid progenitors as driver mutation carriers in high-and low-risk Langerhans cell histiocytosis. *Blood*. 2020;136(19):2188-2199.
8. Lim KPH, Milne P, Poidinger M, et al. Circulating CD1c+ myeloid dendritic cells are potential precursors to LCH lesion CD1a+CD207+ cells. *Blood Adv*. 2020;4(1):87-99.
9. Allen CE, Merad M, McClain KL. Langerhans-cell histiocytosis. *N Engl J Med*. 2018;379(9):856-868.
10. Goyal G, Heaney ML, Collin M, et al. Erdheim-Chester disease: consensus recommendations for evaluation, diagnosis, and treatment in the molecular era. *Blood*. 2020;135(22):1929-1945.
11. Hogstad B, Berres ML, Chakraborty R, et al. RAF/MEK/extracellular signal-related kinase pathway suppresses dendritic cell migration and traps dendritic cells in Langerhans cell histiocytosis lesions. *J Exp Med*. 2018;215(1):319-336.
12. Berres ML, Lim KP, Peters T, et al. BRAF-V600E expression in precursor versus differentiated dendritic cells defines clinically distinct LCH risk groups. *J Exp Med*. 2014;211(4):669-683.
13. Bigenwald C, Le Berichel J, Wilk CM, et al. BRAF(V600E)-induced senescence drives Langerhans cell histiocytosis pathophysiology. *Nat Med*. 2021;27(5):851-861.
14. Ruhland MK, Coussens LM, Stewart SA. Senescence and cancer: an evolving inflammatory paradox. *Biochim Biophys Acta*. 2016;1865(1):14-22.
15. Cangi MG, Biavasco R, Cavalli G, et al. BRAFV600E-mutation is invariably present and associated to oncogene-induced senescence in Erdheim-Chester disease. *Ann Rheum Dis*. 2015;74(8):1596-1602.
16. Egan C, Lack J, Skarshaug S, et al. The mutational landscape of histiocytic sarcoma associated with lymphoid malignancy. *Mod Pathol*. 2021;34(2):336-347.
17. Castro EC, Blazquez C, Boyd J, et al. Clinicopathologic features of histiocytic lesions following ALL, with a review of the literature. *Pediatr Dev Pathol*. 2010;13(3):225-237.
18. Willman CL. Detection of clonal histiocytes in Langerhans cell histiocytosis: biology and clinical significance. *Br J Cancer Suppl*. 1994;23:S29-S33.
19. Chetritt J, Paradis V, Dargere D, et al. Chester-Erdheim disease: a neoplastic disorder. *Hum Pathol*. 1999;30(9):1093-1096.
20. Badalian-Very G, Vergilio JA, Degar BA, et al. Recurrent BRAF mutations in Langerhans cell histiocytosis. *Blood*. 2010;116(11):1919-1923.
21. Haroche J, Charlotte F, Arnaud L, et al. High prevalence of BRAF V600E mutations in Erdheim-Chester disease but not in other non-Langerhans cell histiocytoses. *Blood*. 2012;120(13):2700-2703.
22. Durham BH. Molecular characterization of the histiocytoses: neoplasia of dendritic cells and macrophages. *Semin Cell Dev Biol*. 2019;86:62-76.
23. Picarsic J, Pysher T, Zhou H, et al. BRAF V600E mutation in Juvenile Xanthogranuloma family neoplasms of the central nervous system (CNS-JXG): a revised diagnostic algorithm to include pediatric Erdheim-Chester disease. *Acta Neuropathol Commun*. 2019;7(1):168.
24. Techavichit P, Sosothikul D, Chaichana T, Teerapakpinyo C, Thorner PS, Shuangshoti S. BRAF V600E mutation in pediatric intracranial and cranial juvenile xanthogranuloma. *Hum Pathol*. 2017;69:118-122.
25. Fatobene G, Haroche J, Helias-Rodzwicz Z, et al. BRAF V600E mutation detected in a case of Rosai-Dorfman disease. *Haematologica*. 2018;103(8):e377-e379.
26. Mastropolo R, Close A, Allen SW, McClain KL, Maurer S, Picarsic J. BRAF-V600E-mutated Rosai-Dorfman-Destombes disease and Langerhans cell histiocytosis with response to BRAF inhibitor. *Blood Adv*. 2019;3(12):1848-1853.

27. O'Malley DP, Agrawal R, Grimm KE, et al. Evidence of BRAF V600E in indeterminate cell tumor and interdigitating dendritic cell sarcoma. *Ann Diagn Pathol.* 2015;19(3):113-116.
28. Wellbrock C, Karasarides M, Marais R. The RAF proteins take centre stage. *Nat Rev Mol Cell Biol.* 2004;5(11):875-885.
29. Ballester LY, Cantu MD, Lim KPH, et al. The use of BRAF V600E mutation-specific immunohistochemistry in pediatric Langerhans cell histiocytosis. *Hematol Oncol.* 2018;36(1):307-315.
30. Dvorak K, Aggeler B, Palting J, McKelvie P, Ruszkiewicz A, Waring P. Immunohistochemistry with the anti-BRAF V600E (VE1) antibody: impact of pre-analytical conditions and concordance with DNA sequencing in colorectal and papillary thyroid carcinoma. *Pathology.* 2014;46(6):509-517.
31. Allen CE, Li L, Peters TL, et al. Cell-specific gene expression in Langerhans cell histiocytosis lesions reveals a distinct profile compared with epidermal Langerhans cells. *J Immunol.* 2010;184(8):4557-4567.
32. Berres ML, Merad M, Allen CE. Progress in understanding the pathogenesis of Langerhans cell histiocytosis: back to Histiocytosis X? *Br J Haematol.* 2015;169(1):3-13.
33. Favara BE, Jaffe R, Egeler RM. Macrophage activation and hemophagocytic syndrome in langerhans cell histiocytosis: report of 30 cases. *Pediatr Dev Pathol.* 2002;5(2):130-140.
34. Chellapandian D, Hines MR, Zhang R, et al. A multicenter study of patients with multisystem Langerhans cell histiocytosis who develop secondary hemophagocytic lymphohistiocytosis. *Cancer.* 2019;125(6):963-971.
35. Lee LH, Krupski C, Clark J, et al. High-risk LCH in infants is serially transplantable in a xenograft model but responds durably to targeted therapy. *Blood Adv.* 2020;4(4):717-727.
36. Heritier S, Emile JF, Barkaoui MA, et al. BRAF mutation correlates with high-risk langerhans cell histiocytosis and increased resistance to first-line therapy. *J Clin Oncol.* 2016;34(25):3023-3030.
37. Goyal G, Acosta-Medina AA, Hu M, et al. Phenotypes and prognostic factors in adults with Langerhans cell histiocytosis. *J Clin Oncol.* 2021;39(15_suppl):7049.
38. Gadner H, Minkov M, Grois N, et al. Therapy prolongation improves outcome in multisystem Langerhans cell histiocytosis. *Blood.* 2013;121(25):5006-5014.
39. Haupt R, Minkov M, Astigarraga I, et al. Langerhans cell histiocytosis (LCH): guidelines for diagnosis, clinical work-up, and treatment for patients till the age of 18 years. *Pediatr Blood Cancer.* 2013;60(2):175-184.
40. Allen CE, Ladisch S, McClain KL. How I treat Langerhans cell histiocytosis. *Blood.* 2015;126(1):26-35.
41. Grois N, Potschger U, Prosch H, et al. Risk factors for diabetes insipidus in langerhans cell histiocytosis. *Pediatr Blood Cancer.* 2006;46(2):228-233.
42. Eckstein OS, Visser J, Rodriguez-Galindo C, Allen CE. Clinical responses and persistent BRAFV600E+ blood cells in children with LCH treated with MAPK pathway inhibition. *Blood.* 2019:133(15):1691-1694.
43. Diamond EL, Durham BH, Ulaner GA, et al. Efficacy of MEK inhibition in patients with histiocytic neoplasms. *Nature.* 2019;567(7749):521-524.
44. Diamond EL, Subbiah V, Lockhart AC, et al. Vemurafenib for BRAF V600-mutant Erdheim-Chester disease and langerhans cell histiocytosis: analysis of data from the histology-independent, phase 2, open-label VE-BASKET study. *JAMA Oncol.* 2018;4(3):384-388.
45. Satoh T, Smith A, Sarde A, et al. B-RAF mutant alleles associated with Langerhans cell histiocytosis, a granulomatous pediatric disease. *PLoS One.* 2012;7(4):e33891.
46. Chakraborty R, Burke TM, Hampton OA, et al. Alternative genetic mechanisms of BRAF activation in Langerhans cell histiocytosis. *Blood.* 2016;128(21):2533-2537.
47. Lee LH, Gasilina A, Roychoudhury J, et al. Real-time genomic profiling of histiocytoses identifies early-kinase domain BRAF alterations while improving treatment outcomes. *JCI insight.* 2017;2(3):e89473.
48. Kansal R, Quintanilla-Martinez L, Datta V, Lopategui J, Garshfield G, Nathwani BN. Identification of the V600D mutation in Exon 15 of the BRAF oncogene in congenital, benign langerhans cell histiocytosis. *Gene Chromosome Cancer.* 2013;52(1):99-106.
49. Héritier S, Hélias-Rodzewicz Z, Chakraborty R, et al. New somatic BRAF splicing mutation in Langerhans cell histiocytosis. *Mol Cancer.* 2017;16(1):1-5.
50. Messinger YH, Bostrom BC, Olson DR, Gossai NP, Miller LH, Richards MK. Langerhans cell histiocytosis with BRAF p.N486_P490del or MAP2K1 p.K57_G61del treated by the MEK inhibitor trametinib. *Pediatr Blood Cancer.* 2020;67(12):e28712.
51. Kordes M, Roring M, Heining C, et al. Cooperation of BRAF(F595L) and mutant HRAS in histiocytic sarcoma provides new insights into oncogenic BRAF signaling. *Leukemia.* 2016;30(4):937-946.
52. Chakraborty R, Abdel-Wahab O, Durham BH. MAP-kinase-driven hematopoietic neoplasms: a decade of progress in the molecular age. *Cold Spring Harb Perspect Med.* 2021;11(5):a034892.
53. Nelson DS, Quispel W, Badalian-Very G, et al. Somatic activating ARAF mutations in Langerhans cell histiocytosis. *Blood.* 2014;123(20):3152-3155.
54. Diamond EL, Durham BH, Haroche J, et al. Diverse and targetable kinase alterations drive histiocytic neoplasms. *Cancer Discov.* 2016;6(2):154-165.
55. Nelson DS, van Halteren A, Quispel WT, et al. MAP2K1 and MAP3K1 mutations in langerhans cell histiocytosis. *Gene Chromosome Cancer.* 2015;54(6):361-368.
56. Azorsa DO, Lee DW, Wai DH, et al. Clinical resistance associated with a novel MAP2K1 mutation in a patient with Langerhans cell histiocytosis. *Pediatr Blood Cancer.* 2018;65(9):e27237.
57. Lange-Carter CA, Pleiman CM, Gardner AM, Blumer KJ, Johnson GL. A divergence in the MAP kinase regulatory network defined by MEK kinase and Raf. *Science.* 1993;260(5106):315-319.
58. Emile JF, Diamond EL, Helias-Rodzewicz Z, et al. Recurrent RAS and PIK3CA mutations in Erdheim-Chester disease. *Blood.* 2014;124(19):3016-3019.
59. Héritier S, Saffroy R, Radosevic-Robin N, et al. Common cancer-associated PIK3CA activating mutations rarely occur in Langerhans cell histiocytosis. Blood. *J Am Soc Hematol.* 2015;125(15):2448-2449.
60. Chakraborty R, Hampton OA, Shen X, et al. Mutually exclusive recurrent somatic mutations in MAP2K1 and BRAF support a central role for ERK activation in LCH pathogenesis. *Blood.* 2014;124(19):3007-3015.
61. Chan JK, Lamant L, Algar E, et al. ALK+ histiocytosis: a novel type of systemic histiocytic proliferative disorder of early infancy. *Blood.* 2008;112(7):2965-2968.
62. Huang H, Gheorghe G, North PE, Suchi M. Expanding the phenotype of ALK-positive histiocytosis: a report of 2 cases. *Pediatr Dev Pathol.* 2018;21(5):449-455.

63. Xu J, Huang X, Wen Y, et al. Systemic juvenile xanthogranuloma has a higher frequency of ALK translocations than BRAFV600E mutations. *J Am Acad Dermatol*. 2020. 18:S0190-9622(20)32445-2. doi:10.1016/j.jaad.2020.08.053
64. Chang KTE, Tay AZE, Kuick CH, et al. ALK-positive histiocytosis: an expanded clinicopathologic spectrum and frequent presence of KIF5B-ALK fusion. *Mod Pathol*. 2019;32(5):598-608.
65. Cuviello A, Rice J, Cohen B, Zambidis ET. Infant with a skin lesion and respiratory distress. *BMJ Case Rep*. 2018;2018:bcr-2018-224506.
66. Lucas CHG, Gilani A, Solomon DA, et al. ALK-positive histiocytosis with KIF5B-ALK fusion in the central nervous system. *Acta Neuropathol*. 2019;138(2):335-337.
67. Rossi S, Gessi M, Barresi S, Tamburrini G, Giovannoni I, Ruggiero A, et al. ALK-rearranged histiocytosis: report of two cases with involvement of the central nervous system. *Neuropathol Appl Neurobiol*. 2021;47(6):878-881.
68. Kashima J, Yoshida M, Jimbo K, et al. ALK-positive histiocytosis of the breast: a clinicopathologic study highlighting spindle cell histology. *Am J Surg Pathol*. 2021;45(3):347-355.
69. Takeyasu Y, Okuma HS, Kojima Y, et al. Impact of ALK inhibitors in patients with ALK-rearranged nonlung solid tumors. *JCO Precis Oncol*. 2021;5:PO.20.00383.
70. Ross JS, Ali SM, Fasan O, et al. ALK fusions in a wide variety of tumor types respond to anti-ALK targeted therapy. *Oncologist*. 2017;22(12):1444-1450.
71. Tran TAN, Chang KTE, Kuick CH, Goh JY, Chang CC. Local ALK-positive histiocytosis with unusual morphology and novel TRIM33-ALK gene fusion. *Int J Surg Pathol*. 2020;29(5):543-549. doi:10.1177/1066896920976862
72. Bai Y, Sun W, Niu D, et al. Localized ALK-positive histiocytosis in a Chinese woman: report of a case in the lung with a novel EML4-ALK rearrangement. *Virchows Arch*. 2021;479:1-5.
73. Mehta J, Borges A. ALK positive histiocytosis in an adult female with an EML4-ALK RNA fusion. *Hum Pathol Case Rep*. 2020;21:200404.
74. Kemps PG, Picarsic J, Durham BH, et al. ALK-positive histiocytosis: a new clinicopathologic spectrum highlighting neurologic involvement and responses to ALK inhibition. *Blood*. 2022;139(2):256-280.
75. Gupta GK, Xi L, Pack SD, et al. ALK-positive histiocytosis with KIF5B-ALK fusion in an adult female. *Haematologica*. 2019;104(11):e534.
76. Brown RA, Kwong BY, McCalmont TH, et al. ETV3-NCOA2 in indeterminate cell histiocytosis: clonal translocation supports sui generis. *Blood*. 2015;126(20):2344-2345.
77. Khoury JD, Solary E, Abla O, et al. The 5th edition of the World Health Organization classification of haematolymphoid tumours: Myeloid and histiocytic/dendritic neoplasms. *Leukemia*. 2022. doi:10.1038/s41375-022-01613-1
78. Go H, Jeon YK, Huh J, et al. Frequent detection of BRAF(V)(600E) mutations in histiocytic and dendritic cell neoplasms. *Histopathology*. 2014;65(2):261-272.
79. Aguzzi A, Kranich J, Krautler NJ. Follicular dendritic cells: origin, phenotype, and function in health and disease. *Trends Immunol*. 2014;35(3):105-113.
80. Andriko JW, Kaldjian EP, Tsokos M, Abbondanzo SL, Jaffe ES. Reticulum cell neoplasms of lymph nodes: a clinicopathologic study of 11 cases with recognition of a new subtype derived from fibroblastic reticular cells. *Am J Surg Pathol*. 1998;22(9):1048-1058.
81. Fletcher AL, Acton SE, Knoblich K. Lymph node fibroblastic reticular cells in health and disease. *Nat Rev Immunol*. 2015;15(6):350-361.

CHAPTER 65

Langerhans cell proliferations and related disorders ("L" group)

Jacob R. Bledsoe, Jennifer Picarsic, Louis P. Dehner, and Rosalynn M. Nazarian

LANGERHANS CELL HISTIOCYTOSIS

Langerhans cell histiocytosis (LCH) is a clinically heterogeneous disorder characterized by a clonal proliferation of bone marrow–derived Langerhans cells (LCs) at one or more body sites. In the recent reclassification of histiocytoses and neoplasms of macrophage/dendritic cell lineages, in addition to LCH in the "L group," Erdheim–Chester disease (ECD), mixed ECD-LCH and indeterminant cell histiocytosis are also included.[1] Cutaneous or mucocutaneous involvement by LCH is present in 25% to 35% of all cases,[2,3] typically in the context of multisystem disease. Isolated cutaneous LCH occurs less frequently with published estimates of skin-limited disease making up <5% of all cases. LCH should be differentiated from LC hyperplasia and Langerhans cell sarcoma (LCS). Congenital self-healing reticulohistiocytosis (or self-healing skin only LCH) is another uncommon manifestation. Juvenile xanthogranuloma is also a consideration in the differential diagnosis since there are some overlapping microscopic features with LCH.

Pathogenesis

LCs are bone marrow–derived dendritic cells that normally function as an immunologic barrier to cutaneous and mucosal insults by foreign antigens (see Chapter 4).[4,5] In normal skin, LCs have long dendritic processes that form a meshwork throughout the epidermis, being particularly numerous in the stratum spinosum. Following exposure to a foreign antigen, LCs migrate through dermal lymphatics to regional lymph nodes where they localize to the T-cell–rich paracortex, upregulate costimulatory molecules, and prime T-cells through antigen presentation.[5-8] LCs characteristically express CD1a and langerin (CD207), the latter of which is associated with the presence of Birbeck granules.[9]

Historically, there has been some contention over whether LCH represents a neoplastic or reactive process; it is currently regarded as clonal proliferations of LCs.[10-15] With the identification of *BRAF V600E* and *MAP2K1* (*MEK1*) mutations (see Genetics below), these perturbations of the MAPK signaling pathway support the neoplastic pathogenesis of LCH. Mutation-targeted therapies are directed toward the RAS/RAF/MEK/ERK pathway.[16,17]

One of the more perplexing presentations of LCH is in the lung where it presents as isolated disease in young and middle-aged smokers, but also in children usually with multisystem disease.[18] It was thought that the former was a reactive proliferation of LCs, but it appears that isolated pulmonary LCH is also a clonal process with *BRAF* or concurrent mutations in *BRAF* and *NRAS*.[19,20]

Epidemiology

The overall incidence of LCH based on large epidemiologic studies is approximately 4 cases per million per year, with an incidence approaching 10 per million per year in those <1 year of age.[21-23] The approximate median age at diagnosis is 3.5 to 5 years and the male:female ratio is 1.2 to 1.5:1.[21,22] The most frequent sites of involvement include the bone (77%), skin (39%), and lymph nodes (19%), followed by the liver, spleen, and bone marrow.[1] Multisystem disease is seen in 30% to 70% of cases whereas the most common single site is the bone.[2,3,24,25] The median age at diagnosis is approximately 5 to 7 years for single system disease, 3 years for multisystem disease without risk-organ involvement (liver, spleen, or bone marrow; discussed below), and 0.7 to 1.4 years of age for multisystem disease with risk organ involvement.[21,26]

Skin involvement occurs in 25% to 40% of all cases and in approximately 50% of cases with multisystem disease.[2,3,24] It is highest in the <1-year age group (55% in one study) and gradually decreases with increasing age.[26] Among children who present with cutaneous LCH, age >18 months has been associated with multisystem disease.[27] In cases of LCH with skin involvement and coexisting disease elsewhere, the commonest extracutaneous sites are the bone (64%), hypothalamic–pituitary axis (32%), lung (25%), and lymph node (17%).[3] Isolated skin involvement is seen infrequently with published rates of <5% of total cases; many of these cases are congenital self-healing LCH in infants, also termed LC histiocytoma by some authors on the basis of the spontaneous resolution of lesions without evidence of systemic involvement upon clinical follow-up.[3,24,28,29]

Clinical Presentation

The clinical presentation of LCH is variable. Acute or infantile disseminated LCH with progressive organ dysfunction has an unfavorable outcome in 40% or more of cases.[30] A more indolent clinical course is manifested in those children with multisystem disease without appreciable organ dysfunction despite involvement in these sites. The bone, skin, pituitary (diabetes insipidus), orbit, and middle ear are the more commonly affected sites. Isolated osseous LCH (formerly eosinophilic granuloma) is the least clinically aggressive of the classical presentations. Approximately 70% of children with bone involvement have single site disease and the remainder have multisystem LCH.[31] There is a preference for craniofacial sites (70%-80%) followed by the femur or rib. The lesion(s) present as one or multiple lytic bone lesions without extraskeletal involvement.

The skin lesions are quite variable and any disseminated rash in an infant or young child should include LCH in the differential diagnosis. Cutaneous involvement is one of the most common manifestations (75%-90% of cases) in disseminated multisystem disease in infants and children followed by fever, hepatosplenomegaly, bone, and lung lesions.[23,26] In multisystem disease, the skin lesions are erythematous and maculopapular (Fig. 65-1) or nodular, sometimes with ulceration; the scalp, intertriginous areas, and trunk are the sites of predilection, but involvement of the perineal, perianal, and perivulvar regions is not uncommon with a resemblance to so-called diaper rash.[2,23,32,33] The skin lesions can sometimes resemble seborrheic dermatitis or eczema.[27] Petechiae may be seen in the involved skin (Fig. 65-1).[34] Involvement of the scalp may mimic seborrheic dermatitis ("cradle cap"), with irritation, scaling, and crusting.[34] In some cases in the neonate, the lesions present with the blueberry muffin appearance. One study documented mucosal involvement—most frequently the oral or genital mucosa—in 21% of cases with otherwise isolated skin LCH.[3,35] Skin-limited LCH occurs in the form of one or multiple, often asymptomatic lesions but occasionally erosive, papules or nodules with surrounding erythema,[33,36] rarely forming tumor-like masses with or without ulceration.[37]

Occasionally, LCH may occur synchronously or asynchronously with another malignancy, including lymphoma, leukemia, myelodysplasia, and solid tumors.[38,39] It has been observed that an adult with cutaneous LCH should be evaluated for a hematologic malignancy.[40] Interestingly, several studies have documented identical T-cell receptor or *IGH* gene rearrangements in LCH arising in patients with prior or concurrent T-cell acute lymphoblastic lymphoma, chronic lymphocytic leukemia, and follicular lymphoma, suggesting that these cases of LCH arose through transdifferentiation of a lymphoid or leukemic clone or precursor.[41-44] On the other hand, a putative case of LCH with a lymphoma may represent LC hyperplasia.[45]

Histopathology

Regardless of site, the histopathology of LCH is characterized by clusters, aggregates, or a more diffuse infiltrate of LCs at the dermo-epidermal interface. LCH cells demonstrate abundant pale eosinophilic cytoplasm and elongated or reniform nuclei, often with a longitudinal groove (Fig. 65-2). Nucleoli are inconspicuous, but mitotic figures may be apparent. Unlike normal epidermal LCs, the cells of LCH do not have dendritic processes, instead appearing as epithelioid cells with ill-defined cytoplasmic borders. Binucleate and multinucleate forms may be seen.[46] A background inflammatory infiltrate is variably conspicuous and may or may not be dominated by eosinophils (Fig. 65-2). Eosinophils are particularly prevalent in unifocal osseous LCH. In disseminated and multifocal forms of LCH, eosinophils may be less conspicuous and the diagnosis often depends on recognition of the cytomorphologic features of the clonal LCHs. Plump LCs arranged in a diffuse, sheet-like pattern rather than a perivascular distribution of spindled LCs are the most helpful clue to the diagnosis of LCH since LC hyperplasia tends to be more perivascular with dendritic processes as compared to LCH, while in the lymph node it has a paracortical expansion rather than an exclusive sinus involvement as in LCH. Occasional background small lymphocytes, eosinophils, plasma cells, and neutrophils are variably present. Petechial lesions also show red blood cell extravasation (Fig. 65-2). Cytologic atypia is generally minimal, but a subset of cases may show a moderate degree of nuclear pleomorphism and/or prominent nucleoli.[46] Atypical mitotic figures or marked cytologic atypia should raise concern for LCS (see below).[47] Small foci of necrosis may be present and are often associated with eosinophilic microabscesses in LCH.[47]

Cutaneous LCH has several patterns from a superficial, variably dense infiltrate within the papillary dermis to a more dense infiltrate with extension into the reticular dermis and beyond in the extreme cases with a nodular or tumefactive appearance.[37] The overlying epidermis may be unremarkable, hyperplastic, spongiotic, with or without basal vacuolar changes, bullous or eroded/ulcerated.[48,49] The dermal–epidermal junction is often distorted by the infiltrate and epidermotropism of the LCs individually and in microabscesses can be seen.[34] Within the epidermis, the LCs retain their rounded appearance without dendritic processes, a feature that may be useful in distinguishing LCH from the LC hyperplasia seen in certain dermatoses (discussed below). The admixed inflammatory infiltrate may

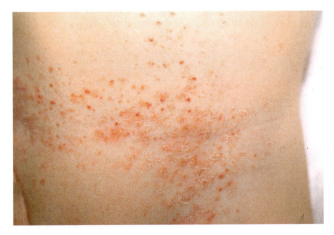

FIGURE 65-1. Langerhans cell histiocytosis. Skin findings are variable. The most common manifestations are those of a persistent erythematous maculopapular rash with subtle petechiae. In infants, presentation on the scalp and groin folds is typical and often simulates "cradle cap" or diaper dermatitis, respectively.

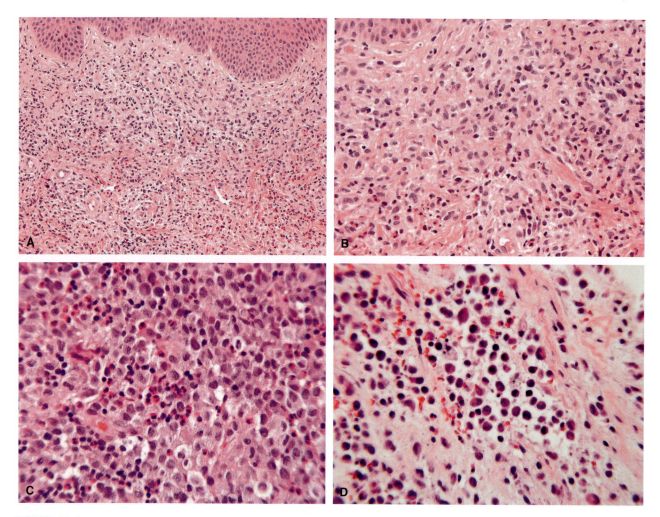

FIGURE 65-2. Langerhans cell histiocytosis. At low power, there is a dermal proliferation of pale spindle-shaped to epithelioid cells in a mixed inflammatory background with numerous eosinophils **(A)**. The Langerhans cells occur in dermal clusters and have ovoid to grooved nuclei, some with the characteristic "coffee bean" appearance and abundant pale eosinophilic cytoplasm **(B)**. Eosinophils **(C)** and red blood cell extravasation **(D)** are frequent findings.

predominate in LCH, resulting in underrecognition of the lesional LCs. Similarly, there may be overlying epidermal erosion or ulceration associated with marked acute inflammation. Fibrosis may be present in older lesions, and periadnexal spread is frequent, particularly in adults.[50]

Immunohistochemistry and Ancillary Studies

LCs are positive for CD68 (cytoplasmic dot-like staining), S100, CD1a, and langerin (CD207); the latter two markers are highly specific for LCH (Fig. 65-3).[9,46] In general, a histiocytic lesion with CD1a and/or langerin expression is diagnostic of LCH or LCS in cases with high-grade atypia.[46] Langerin functions as a cell surface transmembrane lectin receptor that upon binding undergoes endocytosis and is associated with Birbeck granules and has cytoplasmic granular staining.[51] Given the specialized function of langerin, its high specificity and sensitivity for LCH is not surprising, and studies have demonstrated that the specificity of langerin for LCs and LCH approaches 100%.[9,52] However, focal nonspecific staining has been documented in CD1a− histiocytic sarcomas.[52] CD1a expression in a histiocytic neoplasm is also highly specific for LCH, but extremely rare CD1a+ langerin tumors termed indeterminate cell histiocytosis (ICH) (dendritic cell tumor), which may represent tumors of LC precursors, should be considered.[53] Importantly, both CD1a and langerin also stain nonneoplastic LCs. Immunohistochemistry against the JL1 epitope of CD43 may be useful as a marker of immature or neoplastic LCs,[54] but the antibody is not widely available and its diagnostic utility has not been extensively studied. Cyclin D1 expression can be seen in LCH, is not significantly expressed in nonneoplastic LCs, and may be a useful marker to distinguish neoplastic from reactive LC proliferation.[55]

A *BRAF V600E* mutation is a consistent finding in LCH, is not entirely specific, but is present in approximately 65% of cases.[56] Immunohistochemistry with a BRAF VE1 mutant-specific antibody with dark cytoplasmic staining of LCs is highly concordant with the presence of *BRAF* mutation (Fig. 65-4).[57] An unequivocally positive BRAF VE1 immunostain is supportive of a diagnosis of LCH over LC hyperplasia, but caution should be taken to rule out nonspecific light granular staining.[58] Interestingly, the *BRAF V600E* mutation has recently been identified in cases of ICH and interdigitating dendritic cell sarcoma[59]; this finding suggests that dual langerin and CD1a immunohistochemical positivity is the most reliable marker of LCH.

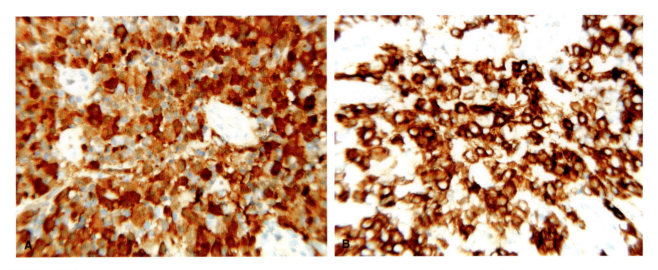

FIGURE 65-3. Langerhans cell histiocytosis. The lesional cells are positive for S100 **(A)** and CD1a **(B)** by immunohistochemistry.

LCs are characterized by the presence of cytoplasmic Birbeck granules, which ultrastructurally appear as pentalamellar structures with a "tennis racket" appearance (Fig. 65-5), and are thought to be involved in routing of internalized antigens.[51] Birbeck granules are specific for LCs but not diagnostic of LCH given their presence in both reactive LCs and in the cells of LCH. Interpretation of electron microscopy should therefore be in the context of histomorphology, since reactive LC proliferations may be present in the background of inflammatory conditions and mimic LCH. In LCH, Birbeck granules are identified by electron microscopy in the majority of cases.[46]

Genetics

BRAF V600E mutations are identified in approximately 65% of LCH cases. Children younger than 2 years more often have mutation-positive LCH which has been correlated with a higher relapse rate.[60] Whole exome sequencing subsequently identified the presence of *MAP2K1* (*MEK1*) mutations in 33% of cases of LCH with wild-type *BRAF* and in none of 20 *BRAF V600E* mutant cases.[61] These studies implicate aberrations of the MAPK signaling pathway in the pathogenesis of LCH.

In patients with high-risk LCH, *BRAF V600E* mutations have been identified in circulating peripheral blood mononuclear cells (PBMCs) and bone marrow hematopoietic stem cells, whereas *BRAF* mutations are typically not detected in PBMCs in patients with low-risk LCH.[62] Similar findings have been described in children with cutaneous LCH, where *BRAF* mutation was not detected in PBMCs in those with skin-limited disease, but were frequently detected in multisystem LCH with skin lesions.[27] These studies support the so-called "misguided myeloid differentiation model" of LCH wherein disease extent and severity correlate with the differentiation of the cell in which the *BRAF* mutation arises.

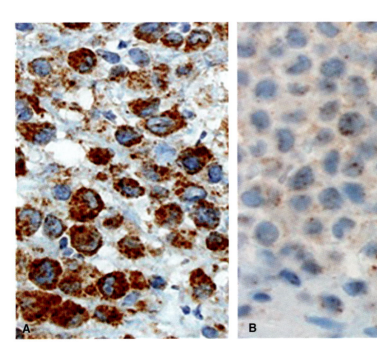

FIGURE 65-4. Langerhans cell histiocytosis. BRAF VE1 mutant specific antibody with positive cytoplasmic staining correlating with *BRAF V600E* mutation **(A)**. Negative BRAF VE1 immunohistochemical staining pattern lacks association with *BRAF V600E* mutation **(B)**.

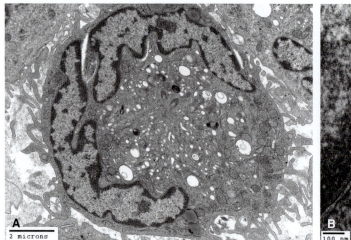
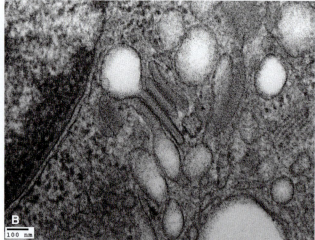

FIGURE 65-5. Langerhans cell histiocytosis. Ultrastructurally, Langerhans cells demonstrate grooved to irregular nuclei, abundant cytoplasm, and numerous surface filopodia **(A)**. Birbeck granules are pentalaminar rod or "tennis racket"–shaped cytoplasmic structures that are specific for Langerhans cells **(B)**.

Differential Diagnosis

LCS (also referred to as malignant histiocytosis/M-group)[1] is a high-grade malignant neoplasm with marked cytologic atypia and nuclear pleomorphism, a high mitotic rate of typically >50 mitoses/10 HPF, and a nonspecific morphologic features of a high-grade round cell or undifferentiated pleomorphic sarcoma.[46] Other cytologic features that are often present include prominent nucleoli, occasional nuclear grooves, and eccentric placement of the nucleus with a resemblance to an INI1-deficient sarcoma or malignant rhabdoid tumor.[46,63] In comparison to LCH, cutaneous LCS is more likely to involve the deep dermis and subcutis.[63] One review disclosed an age range of 10 to 81 years with a 1:1 male:female ratio, and 9 of 31 cases presenting with cutaneous involvement.[63] Compared with LCH, LCS patients are typically older, have higher-stage disease, and have a higher rate of death.[46,64]

LCS is a poorly differentiated malignancy and is generally not recognizable as being derived from LCs on the basis of morphology alone. This determination instead relies on the demonstration of S100+/CD1a+/langerin+ or the finding of Birbeck granules on electron microscopy.[46] In one study of nine cases of LCS, S100 and CD1a were positive in all cases, but CD1a demonstrated variable staining ranging from rare positive cells to weak positivity to staining of just a subset of malignant cells.[46] Two of these nine cases presented with skin nodules.[46] In another report of four cases of cutaneous LCS, CD1a expression varied from weak to strong, and langerin expression ranged from absent to strong.[63] These studies suggest that expression of the classical LC markers may be muted or even absent in LCS. In the setting of expression of CD1a without langerin, a diagnosis of indeterminate dendritic cell sarcoma should be considered as an alternative interpretation.[53]

The differential diagnosis of LCS includes other malignant neoplasms including histiocytic sarcoma, dendritic cell sarcomas, myeloid sarcoma, and melanoma. Immunohistochemical staining for CD1a and langerin separates LCS from these processes. Histiocytic sarcoma is typically positive for CD68 and lysozyme. Follicular dendritic cell sarcoma is defined by the expression of CD21 and/or CD35. Useful markers for myeloid sarcoma include CD68, lysozyme, CD43, myeloperoxidase, and CD117.

Congenital self-healing LCH (CSHLCH, Hashimoto–Pritzker disease, LCHoma) occurs transiently in the neonatal-early infancy period with the development of multiple small red-brown, often firm, papules or nodules distributed over the trunk, extremities, face, and scalp.[28,29,65-67] Erosion and ulceration are common. Rarely CSHLCH may present as a solitary lesion.[68] The cells are LCs with eosinophils in the background in many cases, as well as multinucleated cells.[68] Immunohistochemically, the cells are positive for S100, CD1a, and langerin, and Birbeck granules can be seen by electron microscopy, consistent with LC origin.[68,69] Some also suggest that the lesion can have a spectrum of histiocytic phenotypes within the same lesion including those with an LCH (CD1a+/langerin+), indeterminate (CD1a+/langerin−), and macrophage line of differentiation (CD163+/CD1a-/langerin−).[29] CSHLCH is a self-limited disease and typically regresses in weeks to months[68]; however, careful clinical follow-up is necessary to be assured that the disease is not in fact a more aggressive form of LCH. Recommended workup for children who present with cutaneous LCH includes radiographic skeletal survey and skull series, chest radiography, bone scan, complete blood count, liver function tests, and additional imaging based on clinical presentation or the results of prior studies.[27] One study showed that 40% of patients referred for presumed skin-limited LCH were found to have multisystem disease, including risk organ disease in 20%.[27]

LC hyperplasia occurs in various inflammatory and reactive dermatoses such as eczematous dermatitis, including contact dermatitis, lichen planus, scabies infestation, pityriasis lichenoides et varioliformis acuta, and pityriasis lichenoides chronica.[70,71] Occasionally, the degree of LC hyperplasia can be impressive to the point of an interpretation of LCH or as ICH as there is often low to negative langerin staining.[72] However, common features of LC hyperplasia in the setting of a spongiotic dermatitis is the perivascular distribution of LC and presence of small or large clusters of LCs in intraepidermal spongiotic vesicles.[71] Dendritic cytomorphology with cellular processes may be appreciable and favors hyperplasia over LCH—in LCH, the

LCs are epithelioid without processes. LC hyperplasia in the setting of scabies infestation is characterized by a prominent superficial dermal perivascular and interstitial mixed inflammatory infiltrate with frequent eosinophils and many dermal and intraepidermal CD1a+ LCs.[73] LC hyperplasias, or "LCH-like lesions," have also been reported in association with various lymphoproliferative processes including T-cell lymphoblastic leukemia, cutaneous T-cell lymphoma, lymphomatoid papulosis (Fig. 65-6), Hodgkin lymphoma, and cutaneous B-cell pseudolymphoma.[74] In these cases, the LC proliferations are closely associated with the lymphoproliferative disorder, with the two processes often contiguous or intermixed in contrast to the absence of a mixed inflammatory infiltrate in LCH.[74]

Prognosis and Therapy

The prognosis for LCH has shown a substantial improvement over the past 20 years or so with refinements in staging and an appreciation of the natural history based upon extent of disease including the recognition of "risk organ" involvement with or without dysfunction in the latter.[75] The risk organs include the liver, spleen, and bone marrow and their response to initial therapy is significant to clinical outcome.[27] The definition of risk organ involvement is reviewed elsewhere.[56] LCH is clinically classified into multisystem involvement (12%-15% of cases), single system (65%-70% of cases) with or without multiple sites (eg, solitary or multiple bony lesions), lung only (5% of cases), and central nervous system (CNS) with tumefactive or neurodegenerative manifestations.[75] The 5-year overall survival rates in children with single system LCH, multisystem disease without risk-organ involvement, and multisystem disease with risk-organ involvement are reported as 99.8%, 98.4%, and 77%, respectively.[26] Furthermore, multisystem involvement is a risk factor for relapse after treatment.[26] Concomitant osseous and mucocutaneous disease had a particularly high rate of recurrent disease in one study.[3] Age ≤ 2 years, multisystem disease, and disease reactivation after initial therapy are associated with an increased morbidity including orthopedic defects, diabetes insipidus, and pituitary dysfunction.[26] Involvement of the craniofacial skeleton, eyes, or oral cavity, the so-called "CNS risk areas," is associated with CNS involvement and diabetes insipidus.[2]

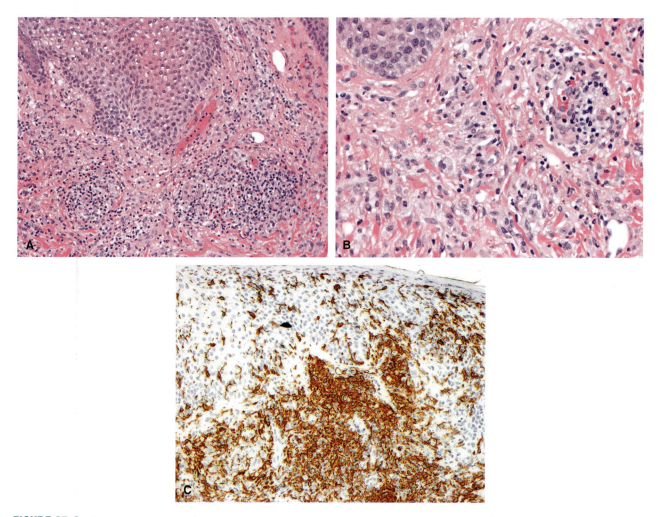

FIGURE 65-6. **Marked Langerhans cell hyperplasia in a patient with lymphomatoid papulosis.** Langerhans cell hyperplasia can be pronounced in cutaneous inflammatory and neoplastic processes. In this case of lymphomatoid papulosis, there was a marked dermal proliferation of spindle-shaped to epithelioid cells with pale cytoplasm and irregular nuclei with a reniform shape, occurring in a mixed inflammatory cell background (**A** and **B**). An immunostain for CD1a is strikingly positive **(C)**.

Skin-limited LCH has a high likelihood of spontaneous resolution.[27] Because of the rarity of such cases, there is no standard initial therapy for skin-limited LCH, and reported management strategies include observation, topical or systemic steroids, surgical excision, phototherapy, and various chemotherapeutic regimens, among other therapies.[27] In one study of 14 patients with isolated cutaneous LCH, 2 had spontaneous remission and 6 achieved remission following local excision.[3] The 3-year progression-free survival after therapy was 89% in this cohort.[27] In contrast, in cases of the skin and multisystem disease, the progression-free survival was 44% following initial treatment with vinblastine/prednisone.[27] However, the overall survival of both of these groups approached 100% due to the ability to treat relapsed or refractory disease successfully with other therapeutic modalities.[27]

Solitary bone lesions may be treated with excision/curettage and/or radiation therapy.[3] About 97% of patients with isolated bone lesions remain disease free after treatment.[3] Most cases of pulmonary LCH in adults abate with cessation of smoking. Initial therapy for multisystem LCH is with chemotherapeutic regimens, often vinblastine plus prednisone/prednisolone.[27] LCS is treated as other high-grade sarcomas with excision followed by chemotherapy and/or radiation therapy.

INDETERMINATE CELL HISTIOCYTOSIS

ICH or dendritic cell tumor is included among the "L group" since its morphologic and immunophenotypic features overlap with LCH.[76-78] A dense and diffuse or vaguely nodular dermal infiltrate of LC-like cells with few eosinophils is the histologic feature.[53] Two cases showed extension into subcutaneous fat and minimal epidermotropism. Like LCs of LCH, the cells of ICH are CD1a/S100/CD68 positive, but CD207 negative. S100 protein may also be negative. *BRAF* mutations or *ETV3-NCOA2* fusion are detected in some cases.[53]

ERDHEIM–CHESTER DISEASE

ECD, long considered a non-LCH, is included with LCH in the "L group" of histiocytosis.[1] One must acknowledge that the linkage of ECD with LCH is not through the LC since the histiocyte in ECD has xanthomatous features and lacks Birbeck granules but is rather through common activating kinase mutations in MAPK and PI3K-AKT pathways.[79] There are also examples of concurrent ECD-LCH in overlap mixed histiocytosis with *BRAF V600E* mutation.[80] Another example is LCH, ECD, and Rosai–Dorfman disease with a *MAP2K1* mutation in a patient who progressed to acute myeloid leukemia.[81] In terms of ECD, its pathologic features of a xanthogranulomatous family lesion with variable foamy histiocytes and Touton giant cells have a shared morphology with juvenile xanthogranuloma, but has a clinical-radiographic distinctive presentation, along with a unique molecular profile with frequent *BRAF V600E* mutations, which is only rarely found in juvenile xanthogranuloma lesions except for those limited to the CNS.[82,83] One can appreciate from these introductory comments that several of the histiocytic disorders, thought distinctive in terms of pathologic and immunophenotypic attributes, have found considerable common ground at the molecular genetic level. Whether the pathologic features are those of LCH, ICH, or ECD, these disorders represent a spectrum of hematopoietic neoplasms of monohistiocytic-myeloid lineage.

ECD is a multisystem disorder in most cases, presents in adults and rarely in children, and is less common than LCH. The incidence of this rare disorder is unknown and it typically occurs in individuals over 40 years of age with a male predilection.[84] Bilateral cortical osteosclerosis of lower extremities (distal femur, proximal tibia, and fibula) present as bone pain in 90% or more of cases, unlike the usual circumscribed osteolytic defect of LCH. Systemic, constitutional symptoms and signs are relatively common. Virtually all major organ systems may be affected as well as the pituitary with diabetes insipidus, orbital pseudotumor, and obstructive uropathy with retroperitoneal fibrosis-like features with a xanthogranuloma-like appearance.[85] It is estimated that approximately 10% of cases develop a myeloid malignancy.[86]

Skin involvement occurs in 25% to 30% of cases with xanthelasma-like, yellowish papules on the eyelids, elsewhere on the face and neck and inguinal region.[87,88] The dermis contains a diffuse or a more nodular infiltrate with or without an interstitial infiltrative pattern which is composed of finely vacuolated, xanthomatized histiocytes with or without similar-appearing multinucleated cells. These latter cells may have the features of Touton giant cells associated with JXG and for that reason ECD was once considered by some as a variant of JXG. In addition to this typical xanthoma-like appearance, the histiocytes may be more subtly distributed through the interstitial collagen. Scattered eosinophils, neutrophilic microabscesses, interstitial necrobiosis, and perivascular lymphocytic infiltrates are some of the less specific features. Unlike LCH, the overlying epidermis is generally undisturbed. Immunohistochemically, lesional cells are reactive for CD163, CD68, and BRAF VE1 mutant-specific antibody (cytoplasmic) but only pale, variable S100 positivity. ALK is positive in cases associated with ALK fusion.[89] *BRAF V600E*, *MAP2K1*, or *RAS* isoforms are present in approximately 50%, 20%, and 10%, respectively.[79] It is reported that a *BRAF V600E* mutation is identified more often in those cases with cutaneous involvement.[87]

CAPSULE SUMMARY

- LCH is a clinically heterogeneous disorder characterized by a clonal proliferation of bone marrow–derived LCs at one or more body sites.
- Cutaneous involvement is most common in disseminated multisystem disease in infants and children, although bone is the most frequently involved site overall. Cutaneous involvement may also represent a self-resolving form in isolation, although this diagnosis can only be made retrospectively.
- Skin lesions are variable, and include erythematous, maculopapules or nodules, with involvement of the scalp, intertriginous areas, and trunk.

- Clonal LCs in LCH often present with diffuse infiltration of the papillary dermis, possess characteristic nuclear grooves imparting a "coffee bean" appearance, lack cytoplasmic dendritic processes, and usually have an associated inflammatory infiltrate with a variable component of eosinophils.
- Immunohistochemically, LCs are positive for CD68, S100, CD1a, and langerin; the latter two are highly specific, and ultrastructurally demonstrate "tennis racket"–shaped cytoplasmic Birbeck granules.
- *BRAF V600E* mutations are identified in 60% or more of cases.
- ECD, though regarded as a non-LCH morphologically, is classified with LCH as an L-group lesion because of its related BRAF status and possible presentation in the same patient.
- The prognosis of LCH depends on the extent of disease, "risk organ" involvement including the liver, spleen, and bone marrow, and response to initial therapy.

ACKNOWLEDGMENTS

We would like to thank Martin Selig, Massachusetts General Hospital electron microscopy unit, for providing the ultrastructural photomicrographs.

References

1. Emile JF, Abla O, Fraitag S, et al; Histiocyte Society. Revised classification of histiocytoses and neoplasms of the macrophage-dendritic cell lineages. *Blood*. 2016;127(22):2672-2681.
2. Grois N, Pötschger U, Prosch H, et al. Risk factors for diabetes insipidus in Langerhans cell histiocytosis. *Pediatr Blood Cancer*. 2006;46:228-233.
3. Howarth DM, Gilchrist GS, Mullan BP, et al. Langerhans cell histiocytosis: diagnosis, natural history, management, and outcome. *Cancer*. 1999;85:2278-2290.
4. Stingl G, Tamaki K, Katz SI. Origin and function of epidermal Langerhans cells. *Immunol Rev*. 1980;53:149-174.
5. Kissenpfennig A, Henri S, Dubois B, et al. Dynamics and function of Langerhans cells in vivo: dermal dendritic cells colonize lymph node areas distinct from slower migrating Langerhans cells. *Immunity*. 2005;22:643-654.
6. Merad M, Ginhoux F, Collin M. Origin, homeostasis and function of Langerhans cells and other langerin-expressing dendritic cells. *Nat Rev Immunol*. 2008;8:935-947.
7. Kashem SW, Haniffa M, Kaplan DH. Antigen-presenting cells in the skin. *Annu Rev Immunol*. 2017;35:469-499.
8. Otsuka M, Egawa G, Kabashima K. Uncovering the mysteries of langerhans cells, inflammatory dendritic epidermal cells, and monocyte-derived langerhans cell-like cells in the epidermis. *Front Immunol*. 2018;9:1768.
9. Chikwava K, Jaffe R. Langerin (CD207) staining in normal pediatric tissues, reactive lymph nodes, and childhood histiocytic disorders. *Pediatr Dev Pathol*. 2004;7:607-614.
10. Willman CL, Busque L, Griffith BB, et al. Langerhans'-cell histiocytosis (histiocytosis X)—a clonal proliferative disease. *N Engl J Med*. 1994;331:154-160.
11. Yu RC, Chu C, Buluwela L, et al. Clonal proliferation of Langerhans cells in Langerhans cell histiocytosis. *Lancet*. 1994;343:767-768.
12. Badalian-Very G, Vergilio JA, Fleming M, Rollins BJ. Pathogenesis of Langerhans cell histiocytosis. *Annu Rev Pathol*. 2013;8:1-20.
13. Milne P, Bigley V, Bacon CM, et al. Hematopoietic origin of Langerhans cell histiocytosis and Erdheim-Chester disease in adults. *Blood*. 2017;130(2):167-175.
14. Allen CE, Li L, Peters TL, et al. Cell-specific gene expression in Langerhans cell histiocytosis lesions reveals a distinct profile compared with epidermal Langerhans cells. *J Immunol*. 2010;184(8):4557-4567.
15. Lim KPH, Milne P, Poidinger M, et al. Circulating CD1c+ myeloid dendritic cells are potential precursors to LCH lesion CD1a+CD207+ cells. *Blood Adv*. 2020;4(1):87-99.
16. Tran G, Huynh TN, Paller AS. Langerhans cell histiocytosis: a neoplastic disorder driven by Ras-ERK pathway mutations. *J Am Acad Dermatol*. 2018;78(3):579-590.e4.
17. Abla O, Rollins B, Ladisch S. Langerhans cell histiocytosis: progress and controversies. *Br J Haematol*. 2019;187(5):559-562.
18. Radzikowska E. Update on pulmonary langerhans cell histiocytosis. *Front Med (Lausanne)*. 2021;7:582581.
19. Mourah S, How-Kit A, Meignin V, et al. Recurrent NRAS mutations in pulmonary Langerhans cell histiocytosis. *Eur Respir J*. 2016;47(6):1785-1796.
20. Liu H, Osterburg AR, Flury J, et al. MAPK mutations and cigarette smoke promote the pathogenesis of pulmonary Langerhans cell histiocytosis. *JCI Insight*. 2020;5(4):e132048.
21. Salotti JA, Nanduri V, Pearce MS, et al. Incidence and clinical features of Langerhans cell histiocytosis in the UK and Ireland. *Arch Dis Child*. 2009;94:376-380.
22. Guyot-Goubin A, Donadieu J, Barkaoui M, et al. Descriptive epidemiology of childhood Langerhans cell histiocytosis in France, 2000-2004. *Pediatr Blood Cancer*. 2008;51:71-75.
23. Krooks J, Minkov M, Weatherall AG. Langerhans cell histiocytosis in children: history, classification, pathobiology, clinical manifestations, and prognosis. *J Am Acad Dermatol*. 2018;78(6):1035-1044.
24. Arico M, Girschikofsky M, Généreau T, et al. Langerhans cell histiocytosis in adults. Report from the international registry of the histiocyte society. *Eur J Cancer*. 2003;39:2341-2348.
25. Braier J, Latella A, Balancini B, et al. Outcome in children with pulmonary Langerhans cell histiocytosis. *Pediatr Blood Cancer*. 2004;43:765-769.
26. Kim BE, Koh KN, Suh JK, et al. Clinical features and treatment outcomes of Langerhans cell histiocytosis: a nationwide survey from Korea histiocytosis working party. *J Pediatr Hematol Oncol*. 2014;36:125-133.
27. Simko SJ, Garmezy B, Abhyankar H, et al. Differentiating skin-limited and multisystem Langerhans cell histiocytosis. *J Pediatr*. 2014;165:990-996.
28. Schwartz Z, Bender A, Magro CM. Solitary congenital Langerhans cell histiocytoma: a pattern of benign, spontaneous regression in patients with single lesion disease. *Pediatr Dermatol*. 2020;37(6):1009-1013.
29. Dupeux M, Boccara O, Frassati-Biaggi A, et al. Langerhans cell histiocytoma: a benign histiocytic neoplasm of diverse lines of terminal differentiation. *Am J Dermatopathol*. 2019;41(1):29-36.
30. Monsereenusorn C, Rodriguez-Galindo C. Clinical characteristics and treatment of langerhans cell histiocytosis. *Hematol Oncol Clin North Am*. 2015;29(5):853-873.

31. Abdelaal AHK, Sedky M, Gohar S, et al. Skeletal involvement in children with Langerhans cell histiocytosis: healing, complications, and functional outcome. *SICOT J*. 2020;6:28.
32. Morren MA, Vanden Broecke K, Vangeebergen L, et al. Diverse cutaneous presentations of langerhans cell histiocytosis in children: a retrospective cohort study. *Pediatr Blood Cancer*. 2016;63(3):486-492.
33. Lieberman PH, Jones CR, Steinman RM, et al. Langerhans cell (eosinophilic) granulomatosis. A clinicopathologic study encompassing 50 years. *Am J Surg Pathol*. 1996;20:519-552.
34. Chu T. Langerhans cell histiocytosis. *Australas J Dermatol*. 2001;42:237-242.
35. AbdullGaffar B, Awadhi F. Oral manifestations of Langerhans cell histiocytosis with unusual histomorphologic features. *Ann Diagn Pathol*. 2020;47:151536.
36. Avram MM, Gobel V, Sepehr A. Case records of the Massachusetts General Hospital. Case 30-2007. A newborn girl with skin lesions. *N Engl J Med*. 2007;357:1327-1335.
37. Gerbig AW, Zala L, Hunziker T. Tumorlike eosinophilic granuloma of the skin. *Am J Dermatopathol*. 2000;22:75-78.
38. Egeler RM, Neglia JP, Puccetti DM, et al. Association of Langerhans cell histiocytosis with malignant neoplasms. *Cancer*. 1993;71:865-873.
39. Kiavash K, Malone JC. Langerhans cell histiocytosis associated with underlying hematolymphoid disorders in adults: report of 2 cases and review of the literature. *Am J Dermatopathol*. 2018;40(8):588-593.
40. Edelbroek JR, Vermeer MH, Jansen PM, et al. Langerhans cell histiocytosis first presenting in the skin in adults: frequent association with a second haematological malignancy. *Br J Dermatol*. 2012;167(6):1287-1294.
41. Feldman AL, Berthold F, Arceci RJ, et al. Clonal relationship between precursor T-lymphoblastic leukaemia/lymphoma and Langerhans-cell histiocytosis. *Lancet Oncol*. 2005;6:435-437.
42. Shao H, Xi L, Raffeld M, et al. Clonally related histiocytic/dendritic cell sarcoma and chronic lymphocytic leukemia/small lymphocytic lymphoma: a study of seven cases. *Mod Pathol*. 2011;24:1421-1432.
43. West DS, Dogan A, Quint PS, et al. Clonally related follicular lymphomas and Langerhans cell neoplasms: expanding the spectrum of transdifferentiation. *Am J Surg Pathol*. 2013;37:978-986.
44. Castro EC, Blazquez C, Boyd J, et al. Clinicopathologic features of histiocytic lesions following ALL, with a review of the literature. *Pediatr Dev Pathol*. 2010;13(3):225-237.
45. Pina-Oviedo S, Medeiros LJ, Li S, et al. Langerhans cell histiocytosis associated with lymphoma: an incidental finding that is not associated with BRAF or MAP2K1 mutations. *Mod Pathol*. 2017;30(5):734-744.
46. Pileri SA, Grogan TM, Harris NL, et al. Tumours of histiocytes and accessory dendritic cells: an immunohistochemical approach to classification from the International Lymphoma Study Group based on 61 cases. *Histopathology*. 2002;41:1-29.
47. El Demellawy D, Young JL, de Nanassy J, et al. Langerhans cell histiocytosis. *Pathology*. 2015;47:294-301.
48. Chan MMH, Tan DJA, Koh MJ, et al. Blistering Langerhans cell histiocytosis. *Lancet Oncol*. 2018;19(9):e500.
49. St Claire K, Bunney R, Ashack KA, et al. Langerhans cell histiocytosis: a great imitator. *Clin Dermatol*. 2020;38(2):223-234.
50. Helm KF, Lookingbill DP, Marks JG. A clinical and pathologic study of histiocytosis X in adults. *J Am Acad Dermatol*. 1993;29:166-170.
51. Valladeau J, Ravel O, Dezutter-Dambuyant C, et al. Langerin, a novel C-type lectin specific to Langerhans cells, is an endocytic receptor that induces the formation of Birbeck granules. *Immunity*. 2000;12:71-81.
52. Lau SK, Chu PG, Weiss LM. Immunohistochemical expression of langerin in Langerhans cell histiocytosis and non-Langerhans cell histiocytic disorders. *Am J Surg Pathol*. 2008;32:615-619.
53. Rezk SA, Spagnolo DV, Brynes RK, et al. Indeterminate cell tumor: a rare dendritic neoplasm. *Am J Surg Pathol*. 2008;32:1868-1876.
54. Park HJ, Jeon YK, Lee AH, et al. Use of the JL1 epitope, which encompasses the nonglycosylation site of CD43, as a marker of immature/neoplastic Langerhans cells. *Am J Surg Pathol*. 2012;36:1150-1157.
55. Shanmugam V, Craig JW, Hornick JL, et al. Cyclin D1 is expressed in neoplastic cells of Langerhans cell histiocytosis but not reactive Langerhans cell proliferations. *Am J Surg Pathol*. 2017;41:1390-1396.
56. Rodriguez-Galindo C, Allen CE. Langerhans cell histiocytosis. *Blood*. 2020;135(16):1319-1331.
57. Roden AC, Hu X, Kip S, et al. BRAF V600E expression in Langerhans cell histiocytosis: clinical and immunohistochemical study on 25 pulmonary and 54 extrapulmonary cases. *Am J Surg Pathol*. 2014;38:548-551.
58. Ballester LY, Cantu MD, Lim KPH, et al. The use of BRAF V600E mutation-specific immunohistochemistry in pediatric Langerhans cell histiocytosis. *Hematol Oncol*. 2018;36(1):307-315.
59. O'Malley DP, Agrawal R, Grimm KE, et al. Evidence of BRAF V600E in indeterminate cell tumor and interdigitating dendritic cell sarcoma. *Ann Diagn Pathol*. 2015;19:113-116.
60. Nann D, Schneckenburger P, Steinhilber J, et al. Pediatric Langerhans cell histiocytosis: the impact of mutational profile on clinical progression and late sequelae. *Ann Hematol*. 2019;98(7):1617-1626.
61. Chakraborty R, Hampton OA, Shen X, et al. Mutually exclusive recurrent somatic mutations in MAP2K1 and BRAF support a central role for ERK activation in LCH pathogenesis. *Blood*. 2014;124:3007-3015.
62. Berres ML, Lim KP, Peters T, et al. BRAF-V600E expression in precursor versus differentiated dendritic cells defines clinically distinct LCH risk groups. *J Exp Med*. 2104;211:669-683.
63. Sagransky MJ, Deng AC, Magro CM. Primary cutaneous Langerhans cell sarcoma: a report of four cases and review of the literature. *Am J Dermatopathol*. 2013;35:196-204.
64. Howard JE, Dwivedi RC, Masterson L, et al. Langerhans cell sarcoma: a systematic review. *Cancer Treat Rev*. 2015;41(4):320-331.
65. Alexis JB, Poppiti RJ, Turbat-Herrera E, et al. Congenital self-healing reticulohistiocytosis. Report of a case with 7-year follow-up and a review of the literature. *Am J Dermatopathol*. 1991;13:189-194.
66. Yu J, Rubin AI, Castelo-Soccio L, et al. Congenital self-healing langerhans cell histiocytosis. *J Pediatr*. 2017;184:232-232.e1.
67. Pan Y, Zeng X, Ge J, et al. Congenital self-healing langerhans cell histiocytosis: clinical and pathological characteristics. *Int J Clin Exp Pathol*. 2019;12(6):2275-2278.

68. Kapur P, Erickson C, Rakheja D, et al. Congenital self-healing reticulohistiocytosis (Hashimoto–Pritzker disease): ten-year experience at dallas children's medical center. *J Am Acad Dermatol.* 2007;56:290-294.
69. Ballin JS, Green BP, Gehris R, et al. A congenital, erythematous eruption. *Dermatol Online J.* 2010;16:15.
70. Deguchi M, Aiba S, Ohtani H, et al. Comparison of the distribution and numbers of antigen-presenting cells among T-lymphocyte-mediated dermatoses: CD1a+, factor XIIIa+, and CD68+ cells in eczematous dermatitis, psoriasis, lichen planus and graft-versus-host disease. *Arch Dermatol Res.* 2002;294:297-302.
71. Drut R, Peral CG, Garone A, et al. Langerhans cell hyperplasia of the skin mimicking Langerhans cell histiocytosis: a report of two cases in children not associated with scabies. *Fetal Pediatr Pathol.* 2010;29:231-238.
72. Picarsic J, Jaffe R. Nosology and pathology of langerhans cell histiocytosis. *Hematol Oncol Clin North Am.* 2015;29(5):799-823.
73. Bhattacharjee P, Glusac EJ. Langerhans cell hyperplasia in scabies: a mimic of Langerhans cell histiocytosis. *J Cutan Pathol.* 2007;34:716-720.
74. Christie LJ, Evans AT, Bray SE, et al. Lesions resembling Langerhans cell histiocytosis in association with other lymphoproliferative disorders: a reactive or neoplastic phenomenon? *Hum Pathol.* 2006;37:32-39.
75. Rigaud C, Barkaoui MA, Thomas C, et al. Langerhans cell histiocytosis: therapeutic strategy and outcome in a 30-year nationwide cohort of 1478 patients under 18 years of age. *Br J Haematol.* 2016;174(6):887-898.
76. Xu XL, Bu WB, Zong WK, et al. Indeterminate cell histiocytosis: a case series and review of the literature. *Eur J Dermatol.* 2017;27(5):559-561.
77. Amin S, Jamerson J, Tee RG, et al. A case of S-100-negative CD1a-positive indeterminate cell histiocytosis. *J Cutan Pathol.* 2019;46(12):945-948.
78. Kong FW, Read J, Pitney L, et al. S100-negative indeterminate cell histiocytosis: in an eight-month-old boy. *Australas J Dermatol.* 2021;62(1):e124-e127.
79. Goyal G, Heaney ML, Collin M, et al. Erdheim-Chester disease: consensus recommendations for evaluation, diagnosis, and treatment in the molecular era. *Blood.* 2020;135(22):1929-1945.
80. Ocak S, Bayramoglu Z, Tugcu D, et al. Mixed langerhans cell histiocytosis and Erdheim-chester disease in a girl: a rare and puzzling diagnosis. *J Pediatr Hematol Oncol.* 2021;43(3):e375-e379.
81. Bonometti A, Ferrario G, Parafioriti A, et al. MAP2K1-driven mixed Langerhans cell histiocytosis, Rosai-Dorfman-Destombes disease and Erdheim-Chester disease, clonally related to acute myeloid leukemia. *J Cutan Pathol.* 2021;48(5):637-643.
82. Techavichit P, Sosothikul D, Chaichana T, et al. BRAF V600E mutation in pediatric intracranial and cranial juvenile xanthogranuloma. *Hum Pathol.* 2017;69:118-122.
83. Picarsic J, Pysher T, Zhou H, et al. BRAF V600E mutation in Juvenile Xanthogranuloma family neoplasms of the central nervous system (CNS-JXG): a revised diagnostic algorithm to include pediatric Erdheim-Chester disease. *Acta Neuropathol Commun.* 2019;7(1):168.
84. Starkebaum G, Hendrie P. Erdheim-Chester disease. *Best Pract Res Clin Rheumatol.* 2020;34(4):101510.
85. Ozkaya N, Rosenblum MK, Durham BH, et al. The histopathology of Erdheim-Chester disease: a comprehensive review of a molecularly characterized cohort. *Mod Pathol.* 2018;31(4):581-597.
86. Cohen AF, Roos-Weil D, Armand M, et al. High frequency of clonal hematopoiesis in Erdheim-Chester disease. *Blood.* 2021;28;137(4):485-492.
87. Chasset F, Barete S, Charlotte F, et al. Cutaneous manifestations of Erdheim-Chester disease (ECD): clinical, pathological, and molecular features in a monocentric series of 40 patients. *J Am Acad Dermatol.* 2016;74(3):513-520.
88. Kobic A, Shah KK, Schmitt AR, et al. Erdheim-Chester disease: expanding the spectrum of cutaneous manifestations. *Br J Dermatol.* 2020;182(2):405-409.
89. Estrada-Veras JI, O'Brien KJ, Boyd LC, et al. The clinical spectrum of Erdheim-Chester disease: an observational cohort study. *Blood Adv.* 2017;1(6):357-366.

CHAPTER 66

Rosai–Dorfman disease

Kristin C. Smith and M. Yadira Hurley

DEFINITION

Rosai–Dorfman disease (RDD), also referred to as Rosai–Dorfman–Destombes syndrome, is a benign proliferative disorder of histiocytes. RDD is also termed "sinus histiocytosis with massive lymphadenopathy," although this phrase does not appropriately reflect the extranodal manifestations of the disease. Extranodal sites of involvement most frequently include the skin, nasal cavity, bone, soft tissue, and retroorbital tissue.[1] RDD was previously classified by the Working Group of the Histiocyte Society of 1987 as a non-Langerhans cell histiocytosis (LCH); however, in 2016, this society reclassified RDD as part of the "R group" of histiocytoses, including familial, classical (nodal), extranodal (noncutaneous), and neoplasia-associated RDD.[1] Systemic RDD (SRDD) most commonly presents with fever and massive, painless, bilateral, and cervical lymphadenopathy with or without fever, night sweats, fatigue, and weight loss. Other nodal locations may be involved as well. Usual laboratory abnormalities include anemia, elevated erythrocyte sedimentation rate (ESR), neutrophilia, and polyclonal hypergammaglobulinemia. Cutaneous lesions occur in conjunction with severe systemic disease. Rosai and Dorfman first described the cutaneous manifestations of RDD among 10 patients, 7 of whom were children.[2] Rarely, RDD can present solely with cutaneous lesions without systemic findings, nodal, or additional extranodal involvement; this is known as cutaneous RDD (CRDD).[1,3,4] Due to the unique epidemiological and clinical features of CRDD, it is now considered a separate entity from RDD and is part of the "C group" of histiocytoses in the revised histiocytosis society classification.[1,5]

EPIDEMIOLOGY

RDD is uncommon, with a prevalence of 1:200,000 and an estimated 100 new cases per year in the United States.[6] It is most common in the West Indies, though it has spanned many geographical regions. About 80% of cases develop in the first 2 decades of life.[4] SRDD with cutaneous manifestations occurs in one-third of patients.[7] CRDD (disease without any other manifestations) is extremely rare.[8] SRDD favors young adult men and male children[3] with a mean age of 20.6 years[9]; however, CRDD favors older white and Asian women, with a reported mean age group of 43.5 to 45.2 years and a female:male ratio of approximately 2:1.[3-5,8,9]

ETIOLOGY

The etiology of RDD is not fully understood. The association with histiocytosis and reactive proliferation of Langerhans cells may play a role in its development.[4] It has also been suggested that the histiocytes in CRDD may be derived from circulating monocytes that are stimulated by macrophage colony-stimulating factor.[10,11]

The detection of human herpes virus 6 (HHV-6) in the lymph nodes of affected patients suggests a possible viral etiology. However, HHV-6 has also been found in lymph nodes of patients with many other reactive disorders; thus, there is no definite correlation between this virus and the disease.[3,12] Parvovirus B19 has also been proposed as an etiology because of recent studies reporting parvovirus-related antigens in the tissue of affected individuals. Additional viral associations that have been implicated include Epstein–Barr virus, human immunodeficiency virus, and herpes simplex virus; however, a definitive link has not yet been established.[6,9]

IgG4-related disease, which includes autoimmune pancreatitis and various extrapancreatic sclerosing lesions, has shown an increased number of IgG4+ plasma cells in the lesions and is associated with tissue sclerosis and elevated serum IgG4 concentrations. It has been proposed that type 2 T helper cells and regulatory T-cells regulate IgG4 expression. RDD lesions are often accompanied by a significant population of IgG4+ plasma cells, and recent evidence shows possible overlap with IgG4-related disease, although this is controversial.[5] One study demonstrated that a proportion of both nodal and extranodal RDD may have features of IgG4-related disease, which may correlate with disease progression, recurrent disease, and sclerosis.[13]

CLINICAL PRESENTATION AND PROGNOSIS

SRDD is benign and self-limited, but can run a long course with multiple exacerbations and remissions. It most commonly presents with fever and massive, nontender, bilateral cervical lymph node enlargement. However, lymphadenopathy may be unilateral or nonexistent. Over 40% of patients will have extranodal involvement, the most common locations being the skin, nasal cavity, bone, soft tissue, and retroorbital tissue.[1] There has been one case of a 10-year-old girl in India who presented with bilateral eyelid swelling consistent with ocular involvement.[14] Intrathoracic manifestations

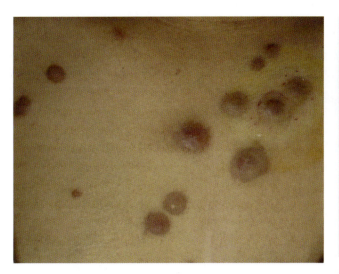

FIGURE 66-1. Brown to violaceous dermal nodules on the trunk.

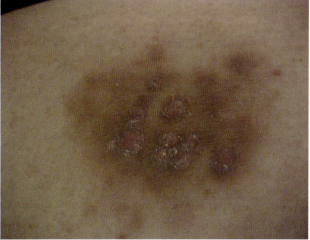

FIGURE 66-3. Hyperpigmented indurated plaque with overlying papules.

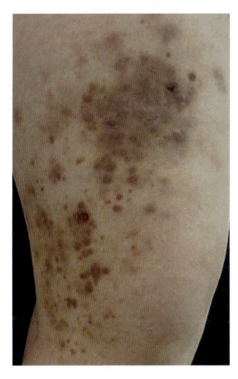

FIGURE 66-2. Brown to violaceous papules coalescing into plaques.

of SRDD are also relatively common and present as mediastinal lymphadenopathy, airway disease, pleural effusion, cystic lung disease, and interstitial lung disease. These usually have a good prognosis.[15] Central nervous system involvement may also occur. There has been one rare case of cerebellar extranodal involvement that responded well to suboccipital craniotomy.[16] Involvement of the lower respiratory tract, liver, and kidney portends a poor prognosis.[3] Some patients can present with bone pain. Rare cases of RDD coexisting with LCH and marginal zone lymphoma have been reported.[10,17]

Immunologic features are associated with 15% of patients with SRDD. These commonly include autoimmune hemolytic anemia and neutrophilia.[18] Laboratory analysis of the hemolytic anemia reveals normal mean corpuscular hemoglobin volume with increased reticulocytosis. Patients may also present with elevated ESR, anti-red blood cell antibodies, and polyclonal hypergammaglobulinemia. Immune disease is a sign of poor prognosis.[3,19-21] Although RDD is usually benign, it may run a protracted course that can result in significant morbidity and mortality. Death can be a result of multiorgan infiltration or immunologic disturbances.[3]

Cutaneous lesions associated with SRDD usually present on the eyelids and malar region. These are often nonspecific and appear as multiple, focal, erythematous, brown, or xanthomatous macules, papules, pustules, nodules, or plaques. Some of these lesions can be as large as 4 cm in diameter. There is reportedly a higher proportion with multifocal cutaneous disease, increased ESR, and serum globulins in these patients as compared to pure CRDD.[10]

In the rare cases of CRDD, the clinical findings are variable but most commonly present as a central plaque or nodule with satellite papules or as multiple papules and nodules that coalesce into plaques[19,20] (Figs. 66-1–66-3). Some studies have shown that there is no specific site predilection for the cutaneous lesions,[21] although recent studies found frequent involvement of the face[10] and extremities.[22] Its clinical presentation has been divided into three subtypes. The most common is the papulonodular subtype, representing 80% of cases (Fig. 66-1). Following this are the indurated plaque type and the tumor type[23] (Figs. 66-2 and 66-3). The disease process in these patients tends to remain indolent and localized despite long-term follow-up.[5]

HISTOLOGY

Although the clinical manifestations of RDD are varied and nonspecific in many cases, the histology of this disease is fairly characteristic.

Lymph nodes will show dilated sinuses containing neutrophils, lymphocytes, plasma cells, and histiocytes with an abundant cytoplasm and large vesicular nuclei. Occasionally, lymph nodes may have dilated lymphatics, thick-walled venules, lymphoid aggregates, and fibrosis.[3]

CRDD is typically a nodular and poorly circumscribed dermal-based lesion that occasionally extends into the subcutaneous tissue. Epidermal collarette, overlying acanthosis,

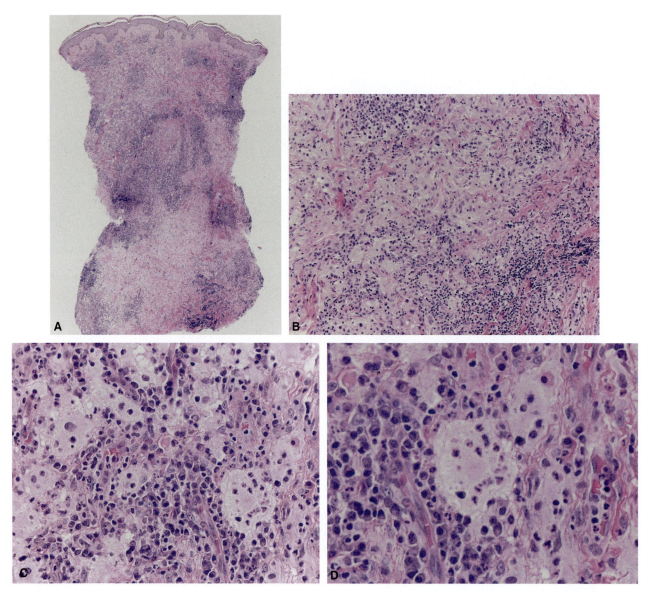

FIGURE 66-4. **A.** Scanning view of CRDD showing a dense multinodular cellular infiltrate with lymphoid aggregates (H&E, 4×). **B.** Large polygonal histiocytes, neutrophils, plasma cells, and scattered lymphocytes are densely packed in the dermis (H&E, 20×). **C.** Emperipolesis (intracytoplasmic inflammatory cells contained within histiocytes), a characteristic feature of CRDD (H&E, 40×). **D.** Emperipolesis (H&E, 60×).

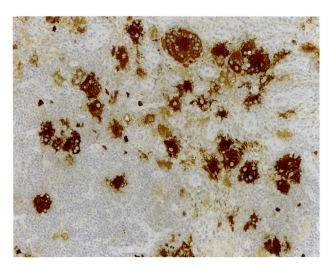

FIGURE 66-5. The histiocytes of CRDD are positive with S-100 (H&E, 203).

increased pigmentation of the epidermal basal keratinocytes, or ulceration may be seen. Lesions are composed of densely packed histiocytes with neutrophils, plasma cells, and scattered lymphocytes (Fig. 66-4A,B). The histiocytes are polygonal and characteristically have an abundant, foamy, lightly eosinophilic cytoplasm with feathery borders and large vesicular nuclei and small nucleoli.[3] Emperipolesis (inflammatory cells and cell fragments engulfed within histiocytes) is a very important feature that characterizes RDD (Fig. 66-4C,D). The histiocytes are characteristically positive for S-100 and negative for CD1a[24] (Fig. 66-5) and Langerin (CD207). There are often abundant IgG4-positive plasma cells present, and the 2016 working group of the Histiocyte Society now recommends that all cases of RDD be evaluated for IgG4-positive plasma cells.[1] Although the plasma cells may be of the IgG4 subset, RDD is not considered part of the spectrum of IgG4 sclerosing disease.[10] Multinucleated histiocytes may present as aggregates in Touton-like giant cell formation. In

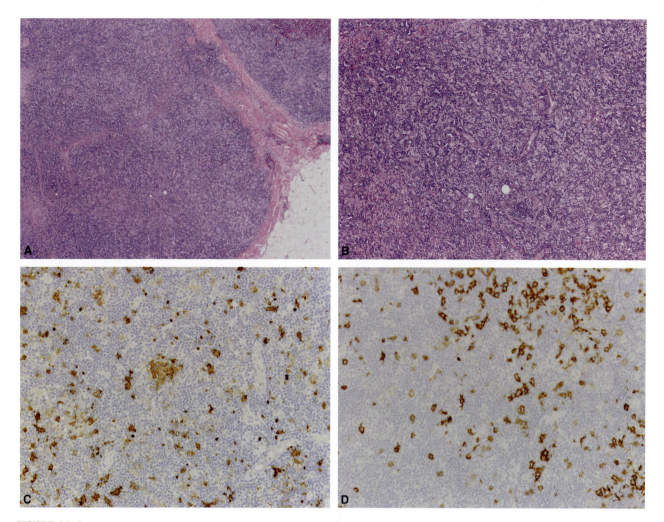

FIGURE 66-6. CRDD presenting concurrently with LCH. **A.** Dense multinodular cellular infiltrate in the dermis (H&E, 4×). **B.** The infiltrate is composed of large polygonal histiocytes with admixed lymphocytes (H&E, 10×). **C.** The large polygonal histiocytes stain positively with S-100 (H&E, 20×). **D.** In addition, there are aggregates of Langerhans cells (CD1a+, 20×).

the cutaneous lesions, plasma cells may contain Russell bodies and present with associated xanthoma cells, fibrosis, and necrosis. CRDD differs histologically from nodal disease in that there is a greater degree of fibrosis, fewer histiocytes, and less emperipolesis. Thus, CRDD can be overlooked if the index of suspicion for the disease is low, perhaps contributing to its rare diagnosis.[14] The histology may also demonstrate a mixed septal and lobular panniculitis.[4]

IMMUNOPHENOTYPE

Histiocytes in RDD stain positive for α_1-antitrypsin, CD11c, CD14, CD163, CD68, laminin 5, lysozyme, Mac387, S-100, and stabilin 1 (a marker of non-LCH). Factor XIIIa (a dendrocyte marker) has been occasionally positive. CD1a and Langerin should be negative.[3,4] Histopathologic samples that are suspicious for RDD or another form of histiocytosis are stained with S-100, CD163, CD68, and CD1a. Positive staining of histiocytes with S-100 and CD68 with a negative CD1a stain suggests RDD. Positivity of all three stains suggests LCH or other histiocytic proliferations. More recently, OCT-2 and cyclin D1 were reported in 97% of cases of RDD. In contrast, Erdheim–Chester disease can also be positive for cyclin D1, but is usually negative for OCT-2.

GENETIC AND MOLECULAR FINDINGS

RDD is predominantly sporadic; however, inherited cases can occur. Germline mutations in *SLC29A3* have been reported in familial RDD and constitute the SLC29A3 disease spectrum, including H syndrome, Faisalabad histiocytosis, and pigmented hypertrichotic dermatosis with insulin-dependent diabetes.[1,6] In two families reported to have hereditary RDD, biallelic germline mutations in *SLC29A3* have been found with phenotypic expression in the central nervous system, eye, inner ear, and epithelial tissues. SLC29A3 encodes an intracellular equilibrate nucleoside transporter (hENT3).[25] FAS deficiency or autoimmune lymphoproliferative syndrome–related RDD type Ia has been shown to be associated with TNFRSF6 heterozygous germline mutations that affect the gene-encoding FAS.[1,3,26] Although the clinical manifestations in these patients tend to be more aggressive, the RDD-like features are usually self-limited.[6] Familial RDD usually overlaps with other familial histiocytoses, which can be caused by mutations in perforin genes (*PRF1* and *PRF2*), mammalian uncoordinated 13-4, and syntaxin 11.[27] Mutations and large deletions of greater than 50 base pairs in mitochondrial DNA have rarely been identified in tissue samples of CRDD.[28] Kinase mutations have recently been reported in nodal and extranodal (noncutaneous) RDD, including mutations in *ARAF*, *MAP2K1*, *NRAS*, and *KRAS*.[5]

POSTULATED CELL OF ORIGIN

This is a polyclonal disorder of macrophage origin.

DIFFERENTIAL DIAGNOSIS

The differential diagnosis of SRDD includes diseases that present with massive lymphadenopathy: Hodgkin and non-Hodgkin lymphomas and infectious diseases. Other histiocytoses present similarly; Kikuchi disease is a necrotizing lymphadenitis that afflicts young Asian women. This disease, however, exhibits few to no plasma cells and neutrophils on histology, has a high rate of apoptosis of the lymphocytes and histiocytes, and shows positive immunostaining with monoclonal antibody Ki-M1P. Infectious processes, infiltrative disorders, and sarcoidosis should also be considered.[3]

The differential diagnosis of CRDD includes eruptive xanthoma, LCH, reticulohistiocytoma, juvenile xanthogranuloma, Hodgkin lymphoma, malignant histiocytosis, inflammatory pseudotumor, and IgG4-related sclerosing disease.[29]

Classical Hodgkin lymphoma, which is very rare in the skin, is distinguished by the presence of Reed–Sternberg cells and mononuclear variants, which are large malignant cells with eosinophilic macronucleoli. The malignant cells of classical Hodgkin lymphoma react positively for CD15 and CD30 antibodies (with a membranous pattern with Golgi accentuation) and are weakly positive for nuclear Pax-5 and negative for CD45 antibodies. The background population of inflammatory cells includes more eosinophils and neutrophils than those identified in the inflammatory background of RDD.

Coexistence of localized LCH and CRDD is uncommon but has been reported (Fig. 66-6). One group found only one such patient in their series of 25 cases of CRDD.[22] Furthermore, another group describes a 10-year-old boy with concomitant LCH of the right parietal scalp bone and RDD of the overlying skin. This patient initially presented with right scalp swelling characteristic of bony LCH, was started on prednisone and vinblastine, then subsequently developed diffuse papules revealed to be CRDD. Both were ameliorated with continued therapy.[30]

Because CRDD follows a benign course, it is important to differentiate it from other benign and malignant lesions. Recognition of its wide clinical spectrum and histologic features combined with the characteristic S-100-positive histiocytes can help to establish the correct diagnosis.

TREATMENT

The major challenge in the management of patients with this entity is to differentiate CRDD from SRDD, which can be more aggressive. A complete physical examination and imaging are important to determine the presence of extracutaneous disease, with emphasis on evaluation for lymphadenopathy.

Focal cutaneous disease requires no treatment if the lesions are asymptomatic and self-limited. If the patient desires removal of the skin lesions, effective options include simple excision, radiotherapy, and intralesional steroid injection.[22] Sirolimus has been suggested as possible treatment modality as it is involved in the control of proliferation and cytokine production from immune cells due to its involvement with the mammalian target of rapamycin and its pathway.[6,31] It was found to be beneficial in a child with resistant RDD and recurrent autoimmune cytopenias.[6] For disseminated, refractory, or relapsed disease, various chemotherapy agents and modalities have been reported with some success. These include methotrexate,[32] systemic retinoids, systemic corticosteroids, alkylating agents, and immunomodulatory therapy such as TNF-alpha inhibitors, thalidomide, lenalidomide, and rituximab. High-dose thalidomide at 300 mg per day may be effective in controlling extensive cutaneous disease.[19] Some have had success with lower doses.[33]

CAPSULE SUMMARY

- RDD is a rare clonal histiocytic proliferation.
- SRDD clinically presents with fever and massive, painless, bilateral, cervical lymphadenopathy and is part of the "R" group of histiocytoses.
- Common extranodal sites of involvement include the skin, oral and nasal cavities, respiratory tract, eyelid, and periorbital area.
- CRDD refers to the disease that is limited to the skin without nodal or systemic involvement; this presents with plaques, nodules, or tumors and is part of the "C" group of histiocytoses.
- The etiology is not fully understood, but there may be an association with histiocytosis and reactive proliferation of Langerhans cells.
- This is usually a benign, self-limited disease.
- The defining cutaneous histologic feature is the emperipolesis—inflammatory cells engulfed in histiocyte cytoplasm.
- The large histiocytes are positive for S-100 and negative for CD1a.

References

1. Emile JF, Abla O, Fraitag S, et al; Histiocyte Society. Revised classification of histiocytoses and neoplasms of the macrophage-dendritic cell lineages. *Blood*. 2016;127(22):2672-2681. doi:10.1182/blood-2016-01-690636
2. Thawerani H, Sanchez RL, Rosai J, et al. The cutaneous manifestations of sinus histiocytosis with massive lymphadenopathy. *Arch Dermatol*. 1978;114(2):191-197.

3. Goodman WT, Barrett TL. Disorders of Langerhans cells and macrophages. In: Bolognia JL, Jorrizzo JL, Schaffer JV, eds. *Dermatology*. 3rd ed. Elsevier Saunders; 2012:1542-1544.
4. Weedon D. Cutaneous infiltrates—non-lymphoid. In: Weedon D, ed. *Skin Pathology*. 3rd ed. Churchill Livingstone: Elsevier; 2010:959-960.
5. Bruce-Brand C, Schneider JW, Schubert P. Rosai-Dorfman disease: an overview. *J Clin Pathol*. 2020;73(11):697-705. doi:10.1136/jclinpath-2020-206733. Epub 2020 Jun 26. PMID: 32591351
6. Abla O, Jacobsen E, Picarsic J, et al. Consensus recommendations for the diagnosis and clinical management of Rosai-Dorfman-Destombes disease. *Blood*. 2018;131(26):2877-2890. doi:10.1182/blood-2018-03-839753
7. Chappell JA, Burkemper NM, Frater JL, et al. Cutaneous Rosai–Dorfman disease and morphea: coincidence or association? *Am J Dermatopathol*. 2009;31(5):487-489.
8. Frater JL, Maddox JS, Obadiah JM, et al. Cutaneous Rosai–Dorfman disease: comprehensive review of cases reported in the medical literature since 1990 and presentation of an illustrative case. *J Cutan Med Surg*. 2006;10(6):281-290.
9. Weitzman S, Jaffe R. Uncommon histiocytic disorders: the non-Langerhans cell histiocytoses. *Pediatr Blood Cancer*. 2005;45(3):256-264. doi:10.1002/pbc.20246
10. Ahmed A, Crowson N, Magro CM. A comprehensive assessment of cutaneous Rosai-Dorfman disease. *Ann Diagn Pathol*. 2019;40:166-173. doi:10.1016/j.anndiagpath.2019.02.004
11. Jadus MR, Sekhon S, Barton BE, et al. Macrophage colony stimulatory factor-activated bone marrow macrophages suppress lymphocytic responses through phagocytosis; a tentative in vitro model of Rosai-Dorfman disease. *J Leukoc Biol*. 1995;57(6):936-942.
12. Levine PH, Jahan N, Murari P, et al. Detection of human herpes virus 6 in tissues involved by sinus histiocytosis with massive lymphadenopathy (Rosai–Dorfman disease). *J Infect Dis*. 1992;166(2):291-295.
13. Zhang X, Hyjek E, Vardiman J. A subset of Rosai–Dorfman disease exhibits features of IgG4-related disease. *Am J Clin Pathol*. 2013;139(5):622-632.
14. Kala C, Agarwal A, Kala S. Extranodal manifestation of Rosai–Dorfman disease with bilateral ocular involvement. *J Cytol*. 2011;28(3):131-133.
15. Cartin-Ceba R, Golbin JM, Yi ES, et al. Intrathoracic manifestations of Rosai–Dorfman disease. *Respir Med*. 2010;104(9):1344-1349.
16. Gaetani P, Tancioni F, Di Rocco M, et al. Isolated cerebellar involvement in Rosai–Dorfman disease: case report. *Neurosurgery*. 2000;46(2):479-481.
17. Machan S, Medina C, Rodriguez-Pinilla SM, et al. Primary cutaneous marginal IgG4 lymphoma and Rosai-Dorfman's disease coexisting in several lesions of the same patient. *Am J Dermatopathol*. 2015;37(5):413-418.
18. Grabczynska SA, Toh CT, Francis N, et al. Rosai–Dorfman disease complicated by autoimmune haemolytic anaemia: case report and review of a multisystem disease with cutaneous infiltrates. *Br J Dermatol*. 2001;145(2):323-326.
19. Lu CI, Kuo TT, Wong WR, et al. Clinical and histopathologic spectrum of cutaneous Rosai–Dorfman disease in Taiwan. *J Am Acad Dermatol*. 2004;51(6):931-939.
20. Kong YY, Lu HF, Zhu XZ, et al. Cutaneous Rosai–Dorfvman disease [in Chinese]. *Zhonghua Bing Li Xue Za Zhi*. 2005;34(3):133-136.
21. Wang KH, Chen WY, Liu HN, et al. Cutaneous Rosai–Dorfman disease: clinicopathological profiles, spectrum and evolution of 21 lesions in six patients. *Br J Dermatol*. 2006;154(2):277-286.
22. Kong YY, Kong JC, Shi DR, et al. Cutaneous Rosai–Dorfman disease: a clinical and histopathologic study of 25 cases in China. *Am J Surg Pathol*. 2007;31(3):341-350.
23. Fernandez-Vega I, Santos-Juanes J, Ramsay A. Cutaneous Rosai–Dorfman disease following a classical Hodgkin lymphoma, nodular sclerosis subtype. *Am J Dermatopathol*. 2014;36(3):280-281.
24. Chu P, LeBoit PE. Histologic features of cutaneous sinus histiocytosis (Rosai–Dorfman disease): study of cases both with and without systemic involvement. *J Cutan Pathol*. 1992;19(3):201-206.
25. Morgan NV, Morris MR, Cangul H, et al. Mutations in SLC29A3, encoding an equilibrative nucleoside transporter ENT3, cause a familial histiocytosis syndrome (Faisalabad histiocytosis) and familial Rosai–Dorfman disease. *PLoS Genet*. 2010;6(2):e1000833.
26. Maric I, Pittaluga S, Dale JK, et al. Histologic features of sinus histiocytosis with massive lymphadenopathy in patients with autoimmune lymphoproliferative syndrome. *Am J Surg Pathol*. 2005;29(7):903-911.
27. Zur Stadt U, Beutel K, Kolberg S, et al. Mutation spectrum in children with primary hemophagocytic lymphohistiocytosis: molecular and functional analyses of PRF1, UNC13D, STX11, and RAB27A. *Hum Mutat*. 2006;27(1):62-68.
28. Zheng M, Bi R, Li W, et al. Generalized pure cutaneous Rosai–Dorfman disease: a link between inflammation and cancer not associated with mitochondrial DNA and SLC29A3 gene mutation? *Discov Med*. 2013;16(89):193-200.
29. Foucar E, Rosai J, Dorfman R. Sinus histiocytosis with massive lymphadenopathy (Rosai–Dorfman disease): review of the entity. *Semin Diagn Pathol*. 1990;7(1):19-73.
30. Cohen-Barak E, Rozenman D, Schafer J, et al. An unusual co-occurrence of Langerhans cell histiocytosis and Rosai–Dorfman disease: report of a case and review of the literature. *Int J Dermatol*. 2014;53(5):558-563.
31. Vandersee S, Rowert-Huber HJ, Wohner S, et al. Cutaneous Rosai–Dorfman syndrome. Successful therapy with intralesion-al corticosteroids. [Article in German]. *Hautarzt*. 2014;65(8):725-727.
32. Sun NZ, Galvin J, Cooper KD. Cutaneous Rosai–Dorfman disease successfully treated with low-dose methotrexate. *JAMA Dermatol*. 2014;150(7):787-788.
33. Wang F, Zhou H, Luo DQ. Dermatoscopic findings in cutaneous Rosai–Dorfman disease and response to low-dose thalidomide. *J Dtsch Dermatol Ges*. 2014;12(4):350-352.

CHAPTER 67

Non-Langerhans cell histiocytoses (C and H groups)

Andrea P. Moy, Jacob R. Bledsoe, Louis P. Dehner, and Rosalynn M. Nazarian

INTRODUCTION

Non-Langerhans cell histiocytosis (NLCH) still maintains some currency in the literature, but as discussed in Chapter 67, the contemporary approach to histiocytic disorders has been largely reconceptualized on the basis of molecular genetic findings. However, the clinical and pathologic bases of these various conditions serves as the framework for understanding the natural history, management, and outcome.

The classification of histiocytic disorders has undergone any number of revisions over the years, but its basis in some respects remains Langerhans cell histiocytosis (LCH) and NLCH, with the latter category presently consisting of the "C group" (xanthomatous granuloma including juvenile and adult xanthogranulomas [JXG, AXG], benign cephalic histiocytosis, generalized eruptive histiocytosis, and solitary reticulohistiocytoma, among others).[1] The C group also includes systemic JXG and multicentric reticulohistiocytoma. "R group" is represented by Rosai-Dorfman disease (RDD) with its varied clinical and pathologic manifestation (Chapter 66).[2] "M group" comprises malignant histiocytosis, which included at one time anaplastic large cell lymphoma until it was defined as a separate histogenetic entity.[3] Primary and secondary hemophagocytic histiocytoses are inherited or acquired disorders as the representatives of "H group." Although this classification is comprehensive, it is not entirely inclusive as in the case of ALK+ histiocytosis and other difficult-to-classify histiocytic disorders that may or may not qualify as a C group histiocytosis.

JUVENILE AND ADULT XANTHOGRANULOMA

Juvenile and adult xanthogranuloma (JXG-AXG) are presumably the same entity presenting in children and adults as a proliferation of non-Langerhans histiocytes. As noted above, this disorder(s) is classified in the C group with purely cutaneous, multiple-site, or systemic manifestations.[1] It was appreciated in some of the earlier reports about its congenital and multifocal presentation and its systemic potentially lethal outcome.[4-6] It was later proposed that JXG was an appropriate designation for this group of NLCHs.[6,7]

Epidemiology

JXG is the most common NLCH, although the exact incidence is unknown since many cases are diagnosed based upon clinical findings and without histologic confirmation. One study reported that JXG represented 1.5% of almost 25,000 pediatric tumors.[8] In one pediatric skin biopsy experience, approximately 1% of cases were JXGs, compared with less than 1% in the case of LCH.[9] The majority of cases are diagnosed in infants and young children, most often in the first year of life but are seen in older children and adolescents.[8,10,11] Males may be slightly more affected than females, especially when lesions are multiple.[10,12] Adults are also affected, without an apparent gender predilection; in such instances, the diagnosis of JXG-like or adult xanthogranuloma (AXG) is rendered.[13,14]

Clinical Features

In the skin, JXG presents as a well-demarcated, firm, round to oval dermal nodule with a predilection for the head and neck region, but it also occurs on the trunk or upper limbs (Fig. 67-1).[8,10] Less common locations include the genitalia, sole, and fingers.[8] The shape of the lesions can vary greatly, as it may have a keratotic, pedunculated, linear, flat, or plaque-like appearance. The papules and/or nodules are usually 5 to 10 mm in diameter but can measure up to several centimeters. Initially, the lesion is a raised, pink to red nodule but over time becomes yellow-brown and may flatten with xanthomatization and regression (Fig. 67-1). The lesion in the skin often spontaneously regresses within months to years and may be followed by hyperpigmentation, atrophy, or anetoderma. Telangiectatic blood vessels or ulceration may be seen overlying the larger lesion. On dermoscopy, the lesion has an orange-yellow coloration with an erythematous border.[15] Most cases are asymptomatic but some are pruritic or painful. Approximately 65% to 70% of cases occur as a solitary cutaneous lesion.[10] Multifocal skin lesions are seen in 10% to 25% of cases and are more often congenital in presentation than the solitary JXG and without extracutaneous sites of involvement in about 40% of cases. However, the remaining cases are accompanied by one or more extracutaneous sites.[8,10,12,16]

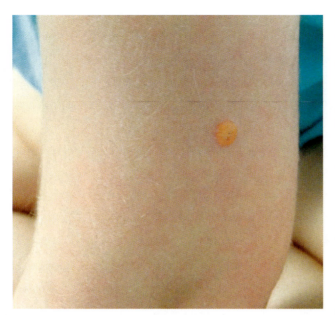

FIGURE 67-1. Juvenile xanthogranuloma. Dome shaped, smooth, yellowish papule on the arm of a 3-year-old girl. (Photo courtesy of Dr. Carrie C. Coughlin, Washington University in Saint Louis.)

While JXG is typically limited to the skin, it may arise in extracutaneous sites with or without skin involvement. The most common extracutaneous site is the subcutaneous or deep soft tissue, which occurs in about 15% of cases.[10] Several other extracutaneous sites of JXG are present in 3% to 5% of all cases and are typically found in the eye, liver, spleen, kidney, lung, testis, and central nervous system.[10,12] In the case of congenital JXG, the liver and lung are particular sites of predilection. Spontaneous regression is generally the natural history of systemic JXG, but hepatic involvement with diffuse infiltration can result in liver failure with a background of giant cell (infantile) hepatitis.[10] Ocular JXG occurs in less than 1% of children with multiple JXGs, typically in young children, and presents without cutaneous involvement in about 60% of cases.[17,18] Ocular lesions most commonly involve the iris, manifest with hyphema, and can cause secondary unilateral glaucoma.[19] Spontaneous regression is very uncommon with ocular involvement.

JXG presenting in an individual over 20 years of age is often preferred to as "adult" xanthogranuloma. There is the question whether the distinction between AXG and JXG is clinically relevant. The clinical presentation is a solidary cutaneous lesion or multiple lesions in a minority of cases.[13,14,20] Like JXG, they are known to undergo spontaneous regression. There is a report of an AXG with a small BRAF+ population of Langerhans cells (LCs).[21] Also like JXG, cases of orbital and periorbital disease are reported.[22,23] AXGs may occur in the context of a hematologic disorder or malignancy, such as essential thrombocytosis, chronic lymphocytic leukemia, large B-cell lymphoma, and monoclonal gammopathy.[24]

Pathogenesis

JXG-AXG was thought to arise from dermal/interstitial dendritic histiocytes. All histiocytes, including dermal dendritic histiocytes, arise from CD34-positive hematopoietic stem cells.[25] However, dermal dendritic histiocytes mature along a different line of differentiation than LCs. While LCs are CD14-negative histiocytes, dermal dendrocytes are CD14 positive. One immunohistochemical study has suggested that JXGs arise from the plasmacytoid monocyte, a specific type of dendritic cell precursor of the monocyte/macrophage lineage.[26] However, the answer to the question about the histogenesis of JXG may exist in plain sight with the example of those cases of LCH preceding the development of JXG or the case of multiple cutaneous lesions in a 10-year-old man with a mixed population of LCs and non-LCs with the features of JXG.[27,28] It is interesting that those cases of JXG developed after treatment for LCH.[29,30] The argument could be made that relapsed LCH reactivates as JXG rather than as LCH as a reflection of a common progenitor; the latter hypothesis is supported by BRAF V600E expression in a post-LCH JXG.[31] Yet another example of the coalescence of a histiocytic disorder arising from a myelomonocytic progenitor is MAP2K1-driven mixed LCH, Erdheim-Chester disease (ECD), and RDD, which progressed to acute myeloid leukemia.[32] Earlier observations on clonality in JXG have reported some positive results.[33,34] BRAF V600E mutations in JXG, other than the previously cited examples, have been reported in intracranial/cranial lesions.[35,36] ARAF and MAP2K1 mutations are present in NLCH, but it is not clear whether these cases are JXG.[37] There is some sense at this point in our understanding that morphologic and immunophenotypic variations occur beyond the cell of origin in the various types of NLCH.

Genetic studies of JXG have supported that it is a clonal, presumably neoplastic disorder. The genetic landscape has demonstrated a loss of heterozygosity in 5q and 3p and trisomy 5 and 17 in selected cases.[38]

JXG has been associated with neurofibromatosis type 1 (NF1) and juvenile myelomonocytic leukemia (JMML).[39] Approximately 3% to 10% of all NF1 cases and up to 30% of those less than 2 years of age are reported to have JXG.[40] The association between JXG, NF1, and JMML, while well described, is not well understood, but the linkage is likely through the activation of the RAS-MAPK pathway.[41-44] Yet another RASopathy, Noonan syndrome, has a reported association with JXG.[45]

Histopathology

The challenge in the pathologic diagnosis of JXG is the morphologic variability in any one particular lesion that is reflected in the clinical appearance as noted above. Although not particularly well documented, the histologic variations may reflect the evolutionary aspects of a lesion from its onset to the eventual stage of spontaneous resolution. The classic microscopic feature is the dense infiltrate of uniform mononuclear cells within the dermis (Fig. 67-2A); the smaller lesion demonstrates an infiltrate that is limited to the superficial dermis, but a larger lesion fills the dermis with extension into the subcutis. The dermal stroma may be entirely replaced or has an infiltrative, interstitial pattern. Despite the infiltrative appearance, the margins are often well demarcated. There is usually flattening of the epidermis with loss of the rete ridges (Fig. 67-2B); however, the epidermis and adnexa are spared. The infiltrate is composed of rounded

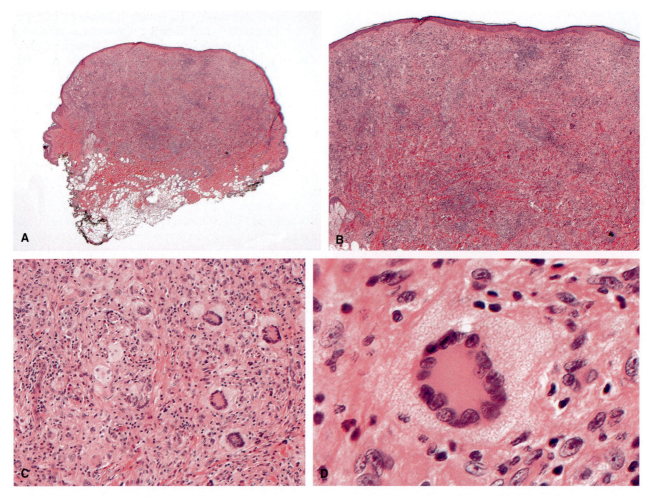

FIGURE 67-2. Juvenile xanthogranuloma. A. There is a well-demarcated cellular infiltrate filling the papillary and reticular dermis. The infiltrate may extend into the deep dermis as well as the superficial subcutaneous tissue (hematoxylin and eosin [H&E], 20×). **B.** The infiltrate abuts the overlying epidermis, which is flattened with loss of the rete ridges (H&E, 200×). **C.** The dermal infiltrate is composed of both small, mononuclear histiocytes and multinucleated giant cells. Admixed lymphocytes, eosinophils, plasma cells, neutrophils, and/or mast cells are often present (H&E, 200×). **D.** Touton giant cells are multinucleated histiocytes characterized by a ring or wreath of nuclei surrounded by a rim of foamy xanthomatous cytoplasm. The presence of these cells can be highly suggestive of JXG, but they are not always present (H&E, 400×).

mononuclear cells with a variable number of multinucleated cells with and without the classic Touton morphology. Some lesions contain numerous giant cells and others have few, if any. Lymphocytes, eosinophils, plasma cells, neutrophils, and mast cells are scattered throughout the infiltrate in variable numbers (Fig. 67-2C). The morphology of the histiocytes can vary depending on the age of the lesion.[8,46] Early lesions have a predominantly monomorphic appearance with abundant eosinophilic and minimally vacuolated cytoplasm. More "mature" lesions contain histiocytes that have finely vacuolated cytoplasm with a "lipidized" or xanthomatous appearance. Touton giant cells, which are characterized by a ring or wreath of nuclei surrounded by a rim of foamy cytoplasm, are found in this phase, but not in all cases (Fig. 67-2D). Scalloped histiocytes with an angulated or jagged border and spindled histiocytes may also be seen. Mitotic figures may be seen, but atypical mitotic figures are absent.

A presumed transitional phase is characterized by an accompanying spindle cell pattern, which may be interdigitated among the mononuclear cells. The spindle cell population may entirely replace the mononuclear cells whose features resemble a dermatofibroma-fibrous histiocytoma.[8,10,47]

Immunophenotype

Unlike LCH with a specific immunophenotype of CD1a and CD207 reactivity, JXG is characterized by various more generic histiocytic markers, including CD68, CD163, CD4, CD14, Factor XIIIa, HLA-DR, fascin, vimentin, and lysozyme. The histiocytes may show patchy S-100 protein positivity or none at all. Lipid vacuoles, lysosomes, cholesterol clefts, comma-shaped bodies, and myeloid bodies are the ultrastructural features of the lipidized histiocytes. No Birbeck granules are present.[48]

Differential Diagnosis

The differential diagnosis of the biopsy in JXG is generally a limited one with a dermal mononuclear round cell infiltrate whose features focus upon a hematolymphoid proliferation, but one with low-grade cytomorphologic features and without the dermal distinctive pattern of a leukemia or lymphoma. In addition to a histiocytic process, mast cell proliferation (mastocytosis-mastocytoma), epithelioid melanocytic lesion, dermatofibroma-fibrous histiocytoma, and other NLCH lesions are other considerations.

In general, JXG is differentiated from LCH with an absence of CD1a and CD207 (langerin) expression, but the distinction between the mononuclear cells in JXG and LCs is also facilitated by the often xanthomatized cytoplasm of the histiocytes, multinucleated cells, and a spindle cell component in the case of JXG in contrast to LCH. Like LCH, JXG may have a substantial infiltrate of eosinophils.

In some instances, there may be histologic overlap between JXG and dermatofibroma (DF). In general, DF is not seen in early childhood and has a predilection for the extremities and trunk unlike the head and neck region in JXG. However, the lipidized variant of DF contains numerous large, foamy cells and even Touton-like giant cells (Fig. 67-3A,B). However, foci of spindle cells with a whorled or storiform pattern may be present and collagen trapping is seen at the periphery of a DF (Fig. 67-3C). Furthermore, DFs often have epidermal inductive changes, such as acanthosis, hyperpigmentation of epidermal basal cells, folliculosebaceous induction, and basaloid proliferation with a resemblance to basal cell carcinoma, as well as hemosiderin deposition in the background. Both lesions can be positive for factor XIIIa, but DFs are usually negative or only weakly positive for CD68.[11]

Reticulohistiocytoma also presents clinically as a solitary, firm, dermal lesion (often less than 1 cm in diameter) on the trunk or extremity. This lesion is characterized by enlarged round cells with densely eosinophilic "ground glass" or "oncocytic" cytoplasm unlike JXG. However, immunohistochemically both lesions express CD68 and CD163, but JXG is more often factor XIIIa reactive.

Intradermal epithelioid and spindle-cell (Spitz) nevi may clinically resemble JXG as a single, pink-red papule on the face or extremities of children. A symmetrical proliferation of epithelioid and spindled melanocytes is seen, and those cells may have a histiocytoid appearance. Notably, cases of

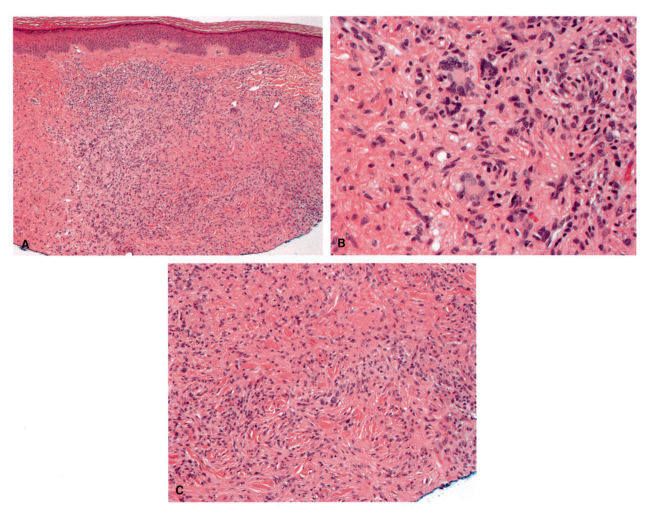

FIGURE 67-3. Dermatofibroma. A. There is a dermal proliferation of spindled to epithelioid histiocytes with admixed lymphocytes that is separated from the epidermis by a grenz zone. In this case, the overlying epidermis shows mild epidermal hyperplasia (H&E, 200×). **B.** Occasional admixed multinucleated giant cells, some with features reminiscent of Touton giant cells can be seen (H&E, 400×). **C.** Classically, the periphery of dermatofibromas shows entrapment of collagen between the histiocytic cells (H&E, 200×).

JXG that express S-100 may be confused histopathologically with a Spitz nevus. However, the identification of an intraepidermal melanocytic component as well as the use of other melanocytic markers (eg, Melan-A) and CD68 immunostains can help make this distinction.

Mastocytoma presents as a red-golden brown papule or plaque with urtication upon rubbing or scratching the skin (Darier sign). The mononuclear cell infiltrate of JXG can resemble a mast cell infiltrate, but the uniform nuclear density, the finely granular amphophilic cytoplasm, and interspersed spindle cells in some cases are features of mast cells. CD117 and tryptase immunostaining of mast cells differentiates a mastocytoma from JXG.

Xanthogranuloma can be distinguished generally from a xanthoma on a clinical and pathologic basis. Most xanthomas occur in the setting of hyperlipidemia in contrast to JXG-AXG. Tuberous xanthomas are firm, red-yellow asymptomatic nodules that occur at pressure points in those with elevated cholesterol and low-density lipoprotein. Tuberous xanthomas typically lack an associated inflammatory infiltrate and multinucleated giant cells, such as Touton cells. Eruptive xanthomas occur in the clinical setting of those with hypertriglyceridemia as crops of small, yellow-red papules with underlying erythema on the trunk and extensor surfaces of the extremities; facial and oral involvement may also be present. Histologically, there is a dermal infiltrate of histiocytes, lymphocytes, and neutrophils with scattered small foamy cells (Fig. 67-4).

Management

Since JXG is often self-limited, treatment is not required in most cases; a lesion may be removed for cosmetic reasons or to confirm the diagnosis. Ocular involvement often requires treatment; topical steroids can be used for lesions involving the iris but excision may be necessary for those in other parts of the eye.[17] Other extracutaneous sites can be monitored until spontaneous resolution unless normal function is impacted due to mass effect. In such instances, various approaches to therapeutic intervention may be considered.[10,49,50] Since lesions spontaneously regress, response to therapy can be difficult to assess.

Rare systemic cases with involvement of vital organs may require aggressive management with clinical deterioration. In a series of JXGs that included eight systemic cases, two patients died of hepatic failure and another of hypercalcemia.[10] Additional fatal cases have also reported hepatic failure and central nervous system involvement.[51,52]

Xanthomatous Granuloma Family

Other disorders presumably related to JXG are included in C group with distinctive clinical manifestations, more so than the histopathologic features that overlap with typical JXG.[1] Various hypotheses and speculations have been proposed over the years in an attempt to account for the varied clinical manifestations of a disorder presumably arising from a single cell type.[11,53,54] for example, JXG, benign cephalic histiocytosis (BCH), and generalized eruptive histiocytosis (GEH) may arise from relatively "immature" histiocytes and usually resolve spontaneously; a blinded histologic study of these clinical disorders revealed minimal distinction to differentiate one from the other to support the proposition that they are part of a disease spectrum.[55] Xanthoma disseminatum (XD) and progressive nodular histiocytosis (PNH) are thought to represent lesions of "mature" histiocytes; XD resolves slowly while PNH is progressive and resistant to therapy. Other reported solitary lesions in the JXG family, such as the spindle cell xanthogranuloma and scalloped cell xanthogranuloma, are possibly histologic variants of JXG in which one morphologic type of histiocyte predominates; however, they may also represent solitary variants of PNH and XD, respectively. While these concepts may be helpful when thinking about these clinical entities, they remain in the realm of speculation.

DISORDERS THAT PRIMARILY INVOLVE THE SKIN

Benign Cephalic Histiocytosis

BCH is a rare disorder that is localized to the skin, with its onset in the first 3 years of life, usually before 1 year of age.

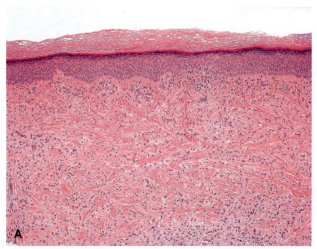
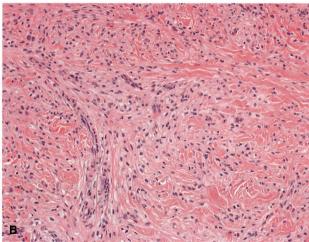

FIGURE 67-4. Eruptive xanthoma. A. There is a dermal infiltrate of histiocytes with sparse admixed inflammation and lack of giant cells (H&E, 100×). **B.** Both foamy and nonfoamy histiocytes are present, with admixed scattered lymphocytes (H&E, 200×).

Multiple, even hundreds of small (up to 5 mm) maculopapular lesions develop in the head and neck region and proximal extremities and trunk. The reddish-tan to yellowish-brown, dome-shaped papules have a similarity to JXG.[56,57] Like JXG, the lesions eventually resolve spontaneously. There is a diffuse dermal infiltrate of monotonous mononuclear cells with pale cytoplasm without lipidized features, but later lesions with the yellowish-brown appearance are composed of finely vacuolated, xanthomatized histiocytes with indistinguishable features from JXG.

Generalized Eruptive Histiocytosis

GEH is an uncommon disorder to the point that there are many uncertainties as to its relationship to JXG. Unlike BCH, the pathologic features are dominated by non-xanthomatized histiocytes. Both children and adults are afflicted by recurrent crops of numerous small, red papules symmetrically distributed on the trunk and extensor surfaces of the extremities.[58,59] Visceral involvement does not occur. Lesions develop over a short period of time and tend to resolve spontaneously with no residual findings or slight hyperpigmentation.[60] Some may appear several weeks after a bacterial or viral illness. In adults, GEH may be associated with an underlying myeloid malignancy.[61-63] A LMNA-NTRK1 fusion has been reported in one case.[64] Numerous histiocytes, including spindled forms, are present within the upper to mid dermis; these cells may be present with a perivascular distribution. Scattered lymphocytes may be seen, but foamy cells or giant cells are absent. The disease course is unpredictable as some cases resolve entirely and others progress to PNH or XD.[65]

Progressive Nodular Histiocytosis

PNH is an example of an NLCH whose pathologic features are indistinguishable from those of JXG in its various stages from a purely mononuclear and multinucleated Touton cells phase to the later spindle cell pattern.[66] The onset generally occurs in later childhood into adulthood with the presence of two types of skin lesions: multiple small, superficial yellow-brown papules and larger subcutaneous nodules.[67,68] The papules measure up to 5 mm in diameter and are asymmetrically distributed over the body, although often sparing flexural areas. These lesions can become larger with time, have a truncal localization, may ulcerate, and become painful; they often do not regress and may be progressive and deforming unlike the behavior of typical JXG. Mucosal lesions may be present. Like JXG and GEH, PNH may be complicated by a myeloid malignancy or a hypothalamic tumor.[69-71] A dermal infiltrate of histiocytes, predominantly spindle-shaped forms, and xanthomatized cells (including Touton cells) are the features in a biopsy. The infiltrate is present within a fibrous stroma, especially in older lesions, and, in some areas, a storiform pattern may be observed.[72] It has been proposed that spindle cell xanthogranuloma is the solitary counterpart of PNH.

There are still many unanswered questions about these various xanthomatous granuloma disorders with their overlapping clinical and histopathologic features, but the age and clinical context are important in the ascertainment of the particular diagnostic category and it is not surprising that nosologic ambiguity persists in some cases.

DISORDERS THAT INVOLVE THE SKIN AND HAVE A SYSTEMIC COMPONENT

Xanthoma Disseminatum

Another rare disease in the JXG family typically presents in young adults with a male to female ratio of 2:1. There is no associated hyperlipidemia. Numerous red-brown papules, nodules, and plaques are symmetrically distributed on the trunk and upper extremities, including flexural sites; lesions may become yellow and coalesce with time. Mucocutaneous sites, such as the oropharynx, larynx, conjunctiva, and cornea, are involved in up to 50% of cases.[73,74] Diabetes insipidus is reported in almost 50% of cases; pituitary stalk involvement can also lead to hyperprolactinemia and hypopituitarism.[46,71,75] Other central nervous system manifestations may occur. Histologic findings are very similar to those of JXG and other JXG-related disorders with a predominance of histiocytes in early lesions with the subsequent accumulation of foam cells, scalloped and spindled cells, Touton giant cells, and other inflammatory cells. However, these lesions can have features of a xanthoma without obvious JXG-like features. The natural history of the XD is variable: some lesions resolve spontaneously with areas of cutaneous scarring or atrophy, some achieve a partial remission, and others have persistent or progressive disease.[76]

So-called scalloped cell xanthogranulomas have been rarely described as 5- to 10-mm yellow-red papules presenting on the back, head, or neck of young adults. The histopathologic features are similar to those seen in XD, suggesting that it may represent a solitary variant of XD.[77]

Necrobiotic Xanthogranuloma

Necrobiotic xanthogranuloma (NXG) is classified among the C group histiocytoses, but it is not included with JXG and the other xanthomatous granulomas.[1] It is a chronic, progressive disorder that occurs in association with an underlying paraproteinemia, (typically monoclonal IgG kappa), monoclonal gammopathy of undetermined significant (MGUS), multiple myeloma, or Waldenstrom macroglobulinemia.[78] Other associated hematologic disorders include Hodgkin and non-Hodgkin lymphoma, chronic lymphocytic leukemia, myelodysplastic syndrome, cryoglobulinemia, and amyloidosis. It is regarded among the various paraneoplastic cutaneous conditions.[79]

Given the association of NXG with paraproteinemia and lymphoid malignancies, it is typically diagnosed in patients over 50 years of age with no gender predilection.[80,81]

Clinical Features

Violaceous red to yellow indurated papules, nodules, and plaques, some with ulceration, typically involving periorbital skin (>80%) as well as other sites, are the clinical features.[79] Skin lesions are usually asymptomatic, although some may be pruritic. The respiratory tract and heart are the most common extracutaneous sites of involvement, but not to the exclusion of other organ systems.[82] An underlying paraproteinemia, most commonly of the monoclonal IgG kappa subtype; elevated erythrocyte sedimentation rate; decreased C4 levels; and leukopenia are the various abnormalities.[81,82] An assessment for an underlying hematological disorder such as MGUS and multiple myeloma is advisable. Long-term clinical follow-up should be prompted with a diagnosis of NXG since a paraproteinemia may occur before, after, or concurrently with NXG.[78]

Histopathology
Palisading granulomatous infiltrates composed of histiocytes, admixed multinucleated giant cells with "foamy" cytoplasm surround zones of collagen necrobiosis and cholesterol clefts, and lymphoid follicles involve the mid-lower dermis and subcutis. Touton and foreign body–type giant cells are commonly present. There is a resemblance to necrobiosis lipoidica (NL), although there is a difference in the distribution of the lesions with an upper vs lower body dichotomy. While cholesterol clefts are a useful histopathologic clue to the diagnosis of NXG, they are also present infrequently in NL.

ALK-Positive Histiocytosis

ALK-positive histiocytosis is one of the more recent additions to the clinical category of NLCHs, and like LCH and JXG it has a predilection for infants less than 6 months old but may be seen in older children and infrequently in adults.[83] In infants, it is a multisystem disease much like LCH and JXG, but it may also have isolated cutaneous and central nervous system involvement.[84] The histopathologic features are those of a mononuclear population of cells with clefted to lobulated nuclei like those of LCH, uniform eosinophilic cytoplasm, and also finely vacuolated or xanthomatized, multinucleated cells with or without a central array of nuclei like JXG or ECD, emperipolesis like RDD, and a variable background of neutrophils and some hemosiderin. CD68, CD163, and factor XIII are consistently immunopositive with patchy S-100 protein reactivity. CD1a, langerin, and BRAF V600E are all nonreactivity, but ALK displays cytoplasmic positivity to reflect the KIF5B-ALK, TPM3-ALK, or COL1A2-ALK gene fusions.[83] In addition to the hybrid morphology of other similar-appearing histiocytic disorders, the lesion may have a spindle cell pattern like some cases of JXG or ECD.

Multicentric Reticulohistiocytosis

Multicentric reticulohistiocytosis (MRH) is a C-group NLCH. Although MRH and solitary reticulohistiocytoma have similar histopathologic features, it is difficult to be certain about their pathogenetic relationship, if any. MRH is a disorder of adults, usually between 45 and 55 years with a female preponderance and a clinical onset with polyarthropathy.[85-87] Unlike several of the other histiocytic disorders, it is infrequently seen in children with the exceptional case study.[88,89]

Clinical Features
The initial manifestation of MRH is polyarthritis in 70% or more of cases, which is followed by a cutaneous eruption months to years later.[90] Approximately 20% of cases initially present with cutaneous disease, and a similar proportion present with simultaneous skin and joint disease.[90,91] Mucosal membranes with nodules occur in 25% or more of cases. Cutaneous involvement consists of red to yellow-brown, often pruritic, papules and nodules ranging in size from 1 mm to several centimeters.[90,92] The skin of the face and dorsal hands is most frequently involved, with over 90% of cases demonstrating nodules at these sites.[90,91] Facial disease can be extensive and disfiguring. Involvement of the ears or scalp occurs in the majority of cases.[90] Periungual nodularity is characteristic, resulting in the classical "coral band" appearance,[90] and lesions at mucocutaneous junctions such as the corner of the mouth and nasal alae are common.[92] Other less common sites include the chest, back, abdomen, and extremities. The nodular lesions may be preceded by an erythematous rash resembling dermatomyositis in a minority of cases.[91,93] Overlying ulceration of the nodules is infrequent.[90] Mucosal nodules are similar to cutaneous nodules in gross appearance.

Joint involvement is polyarticular, typically symmetric, and rapidly progressive and involves the distal and proximal interphalangeal joints in most cases.[90,92] Large joints including the shoulders, elbow, knees, and ankles are also affected with spinal involvement in about 50% of cases.[90,92] The most severe involvement is the interphalangeal joints. Progressive, erosive arthropathy with destruction of articular cartilage and bone and shortening of fingers result in deformation of the hands. There is often waxing and waning of disease activity including arthritis and associated skin lesions.[90] Case reports have described involvement of sites other than the skin and joints, including liver, lungs, thyroid, salivary glands, and bone marrow.[94,95] An elevated erythrocyte sedimentation rate is present in 50% of cases with infrequent anemia and hyperlipidemia.[90,91,94] There is an apparent increased incidence of xanthelasma.[90]

Approximately 30% of cases have an autoimmune disease, most commonly rheumatoid arthritis and dermatomyositis as well as other immune disorders.[94,96] Despite cutaneous findings that resemble Gottron papules and the facial rash of dermatomyositis, the presence of joint disease and distinctive histopathologic findings of the cutaneous nodules allow distinction of MRH from dermatomyositis with its subtle interface dermatitis.[93] Celiac disease and vasculitis are also reported.[94]

MRH is associated with a malignancy in as many as 30% of cases, which may develop before an underlying malignancy, persist after treatment of a malignancy, or resolve in the face of ongoing malignancy.[91,94,97,98] However, cases of MRH have been diagnosed concurrently with, or shortly after, a malignancy, and it is now regarded as a paraneoplastic process in a subset of cases.[79,97,98] Unlike some of the other histiocytic disorders, there is no preference for hematologic malignancies, but rather a mixture of carcinomas, sarcomas, and melanoma.[97,98]

Histopathology
MRH and reticulohistiocytoma (RH) have similar if not identical histologic features: a well-defined dermal infiltrate of plump epithelioid histiocytes (Figs. 67-5 and 67-6) with abundant pink, granular cytoplasm with a ground glass quality and round to ovoid nuclei with peripheral condensation of vesicular chromatin and prominent nucleoli (Figs. 67-7 and 67-8). Multinucleated giant cells are common, particularly in older lesions, and include forms with both central and peripherally placed nuclei. Giant cells resembling Touton giant cells with a circular ring of peripheral nuclei may be infrequently seen.[93] Occasional mitotic figures—0 to 4 per 10 HPF (high-power fields) in one study—and cells with slight nuclear atypia can be seen.[99] Atypical mitoses are not seen.

The histiocytes often have an infiltrative pattern and may surround fine strands of collagen and reticulin fibrosis (Fig. 67-8).[90,99] The overlying epidermis is usually separated from the proliferation by a thin grenz zone but may show changes including loss of rete ridges and epidermal thinning or hyperplasia; erosion and ulceration are uncommon.[90,99] Occasional cases may demonstrate infiltration of the histiocytes into the subcutis or epidermis. A mixed inflammatory infiltrate in the background is often present, and acute inflammation may be more prominent in early lesions and in solitary RH than MRH (Figs. 67-9 and 67-10).[90] Other changes described in solitary RH include the presence of focal spindling of the histiocytes and cytoplasmic vacuolization.[93,99] In MRH, similar histiocytic infiltrates are present within the synovium (histiocytic synovitis) of affected joints and have been documented in visceral organs.[90]

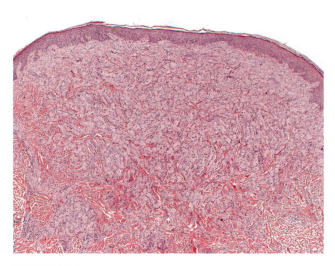

FIGURE 67-5. **Solitary reticulohistiocytoma.** This forms a circumscribed dermal nodule of infiltrative appearing pale eosinophilic epithelioid cells (H&E, 40×).

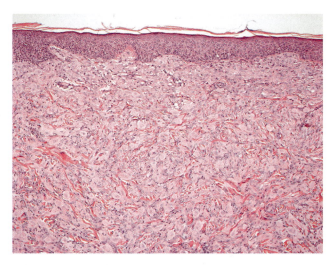

FIGURE 67-6. **Solitary reticulohistiocytoma.** The lesional cells are plump eosinophilic histiocytes with abundant cytoplasm that occur in small clusters, often separated by thin bands of dermal collagen (H&E, 100×).

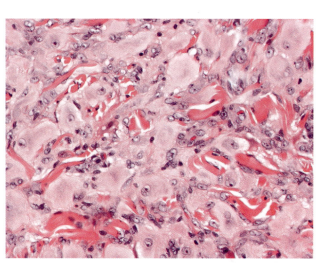

FIGURE 67-8. **Solitary reticulohistiocytoma.** The nuclei are ovoid with vesicular to clear chromatin, and large prominent nucleoli. The cytoplasm is dense and eosinophilic, with a so-called ground glass appearance (H&E, 400×).

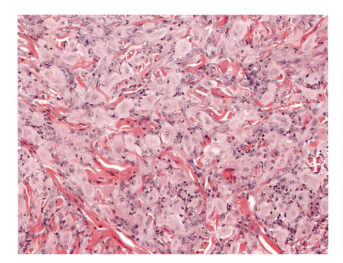

FIGURE 67-7. **Solitary reticulohistiocytoma.** The histiocytes are large epithelioid cells with ovoid nuclei and prominent nucleoli. Thin intervening collagen bands are often conspicuous (H&E, 200×).

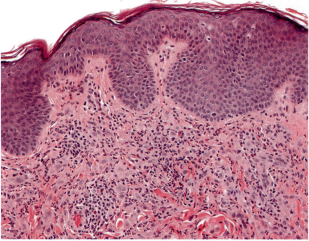

FIGURE 67-9. **Cutaneous lesion from a patient with multicentric reticulohistiocytosis.** There is a dermal infiltrate of plump epithelioid cells accompanied by a mixed inflammatory cell infiltrate (H&E, 100×).

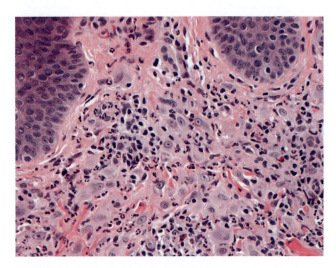

FIGURE 67-10. Multicentric reticulohistiocytosis. The epithelioid histiocytes have cytomorphologic features identical to those of solitary RH with large ovoid nuclei, pale chromatin, prominent nucleoli, and abundant dense eosinophilic cytoplasm. A mixed inflammatory infiltrate is often seen (H&E, 400×).

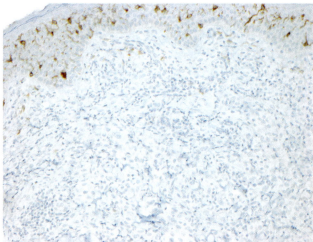

FIGURE 67-12. Multicentric reticulohistiocytosis. The lesional cells are negative for CD1a immunostain (IHC, 100×).

Differential Diagnosis

The differential diagnosis of MRH and RH includes cutaneous histiocytic and granulomatous processes as well as other dermal proliferations of epithelioid cells. In general, when histiocytic proliferations are present in the dermis, the presence of the characteristic arthropathy described above generally corroborates the suspected diagnosis of MRH.

RH may show some degree of morphologic overlap with JXG, and the cutaneous lesions of MRH may clinically and morphologically resemble other members of the xanthomatous granuloma or JXG family such as generalized eruptive histiocytosis, progressive nodular histiocytosis, or xanthoma disseminatum. In contrast to the JXG family, MRH and RH are rarely characterized by the presence of xanthomatized cells and rather display dense eosinophilic granular cytoplasm, and although multinucleated cells are present, they are not the characteristic Touton giant cells.

Cutaneous granular cell tumor (GCT) presents as a dermal nodule of plump epithelioid cells with eosinophilic cytoplasm. Clues to the diagnosis include a granular eosinophilic cytoplasm in GCT than in RH, with overlying pseudoepitheliomatous hyperplasia seen in a subset of cases of GCT. GCT is diffusely and strongly positive for S-100 and also for CD68.

RDD can have similar features to those of RH and MRH and is similarly accompanied by a mixed inflammatory cell infiltrate. Distinctive features of RH and MRH include dense granular cytoplasm and lack of the emperipolesis that is characteristic of RDD. Unlike RH and MRH, the histiocytes of RDD stain for S-100 protein.

Melanocytic lesions may have an epithelioid appearance similar to RH, but the latter typically does not exhibit the tight clustering seen in melanocytic lesions. A minor subset of histiocytes in RH can stain for S-100 and MiTF but should not be diffusely positive for these stains; RH does not stain for HMB-45.[99]

Dermal sarcomas including undifferentiated pleomorphic sarcoma, epithelioid sarcoma, and histiocytic sarcoma, as well as atypical fibroxanthoma, may contain giant cells. The marked cellular atypia and pleomorphism, necrosis, and high mitotic rate seen in these lesions are features not present in RH or MRH.

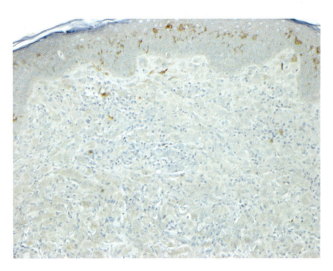

FIGURE 67-11. Multicentric reticulohistiocytosis. The lesional cells are negative for S100 immunostain (immunohistochemistry [IHC], 100×).

Immunophenotype

The histiocytes of MRH and RH stain for CD68, CD163, lysozyme, CD14, and CD11b. Like the other NLCHs, patchy S-100 protein immunopositivity may be seen (Figs. 67-11 and 67-12). Similarly, MiTF positivity can be seen in a small percentage (0%-30%) of the histiocytes, but HMB-45 expression is not seen.[99]

Solitary Reticulohistiocytoma

Clinical Features

Solitary RH typically presents as an asymptomatic smooth cutaneous red-brown nodule, typically <1 cm in size, usually on the trunk, abdomen, back, head, neck, or extremities.[94,99] Unlike MHR, there is no predisposition for a specific anatomic site, and involvement of digits is infrequent.[99] Solitary RH occasionally involves mucosal sites including the buccal mucosa, nasal mucosa, and tongue.[99]

Prognosis

Although the cutaneous manifestations of MRH can be severe and disfiguring, the morbidity is related to the joint disease with a waxing and waning course or is more often rapidly progressive with marked deformity and substantial disability. In most cases of MRH, there is a gradual decrease in disease activity over years, followed by eventual abatement of new symptoms.[90] In such cases, the patients usually have evidence of prior MRH including deformed hands and disfigured faces[90] but are free from further disease progression. Owing to the rarity of MRH, there is no standard therapy.

Pathogenesis

Although substantial speculation and some studies have attempted to elucidate the pathogenesis of MRH over the years, recent reports have seemingly aligned the disorders with other similar-appearing histiocytic proliferations, each with their unique and overlapping clinical manifestations, with activating mutations in TET2 and MAP2K1 in MRH.[100] A BRAF V600E mutation has been reported in a case of disseminated RH; this finding among others points to the merging pathogenesis of the various histiocytic disorders.

References

1. Emile JF, Abla O, Fraitag S, et al. Revised classification of histiocytoses and neoplasms of the macrophage-dendritic cell lineages. *Blood*. 2016;127(22):2672-2681.
2. Abla O, Jacobsen E, Picarsic J, et al. Consensus recommendations for the diagnosis and clinical management of Rosai-Dorfman-Destombes disease. *Blood*. 2018;131(26):2877-2890.
3. Pletneva MA, Smith LB. Anaplastic large cell lymphoma: features presenting diagnostic challenges. *Arch Pathol Lab Med*. 2014;138(10):1290-1294.
4. Adamson HG. Society intelligence: the dermatological society of London. *Br J Dermatol*. 1905;17:222.
5. McDonagh JER. A contribution to our knowledge of the naevoxantho-endotheliomata. *Br J Dermatol*. 1912;24:85-99.
6. Helwig EB, Hackney VC. Juvenile xanthogranuloma (nevoxanthoendothelioma). *Am J Pathol*. 1954;30:625-626.
7. Zelger BW, Cerio R. Xanthogranuloma is the archetype of non-Langerhans cell histiocytoses. *Br J Dermatol*. 2001;145:369-371.
8. Janssen D, Harms D. Juvenile xanthogranuloma in childhood and adolescence: a clinicopathologic study of 129 patients from the Kiel pediatric tumor registry. *Am J Surg Pathol*. 2005;29:21-28.
9. Dehner LP, Gru AA. Nonepithelial tumors and tumor-like lesions of the skin and subcutis in children. *Pediatr Dev Pathol*. 2018;21(2):150-207.
10. Dehner LP. Juvenile xanthogranulomas in the first two decades of life: a clinicopathologic study of 174 cases with cutaneous and extracutaneous manifestations. *Am J Surg Pathol*. 2003;27:579-593.
11. Marrogi AJ, Dehner LP, Coffin CM, Wick MR. Benign cutaneous histiocytic tumors in childhood and adolescence, excluding Langerhans' cell proliferations: a clinicopathologic and immunohistochemical analysis. *Am J Dermatopathol*. 1992;14:8-18.
12. So N, Liu R, Hogeling M. Juvenile xanthogranulomas: Examining single, multiple, and extracutaneous presentations. *Pediatr Dermatol*. 2020;37(4):637-644.
13. Rodríguez J, Ackerman AB. Xanthogranuloma in adults. *Arch Dermatol*. 1976;112:43-44.
14. Whitmore SE. Multiple xanthogranulomas in an adult: case report and literature review. *Br J Dermatol*. 1992;127:177-181.
15. Pretel M, Irarrazaval I, Lera M, Aguado L, Idoate MA. Dermoscopic "setting sun" pattern of juvenile xanthogranuloma. *J Am Acad Dermatol*. 2015;72:S73-S75.
16. Samuelov L, Kinori M, Chamlin SL, et al. Risk of intraocular and other extracutaneous involvement in patients with cutaneous juvenile xanthogranuloma. *Pediatr Dermatol*. 2018;35(3):329-335.
17. Kontos G, Borooah S, Khan A, Fleck BW, Coupland SE. The epidemiology, clinical characteristics, histopathology and management of juvenile- and adult-onset corneoscleral limbus xanthogranuloma. *Graefes Arch Clin Exp Ophthalmol*. 2016;254(3):413-420.
18. Hernández-San Martín MJ, Vargas-Mora P, Aranibar L. Juvenile Xanthogranuloma: an entity with a wide clinical spectrum. *Actas Dermosifiliogr (Engl Ed)*. 2020;111(9):725-733.
19. Vendal Z, Walton D, Chen T. Glaucoma in juvenile xanthogranuloma. *Semin Ophthalmol*. 2006;21(3):191-194.
20. Saad N, Skowron F, Dalle S, Forestier JY, Balme B, Thomas L. Multiple adult xanthogranuloma: case report and literature review. *Dermatology*. 2006;212:73-76.
21. Ishikawa M, Endo Y, Uehara A, et al. Cutaneous adult xanthogranuloma with a small portion of BRAF[V600E] mutated Langerhans cell histiocytosis populations: a case report and the review of published work. *J Dermatol*. 2019;46(2):161-165.
22. Ortiz Salvador JM, Subiabre Ferrer D, Pérez Ferriols A. Adult xanthogranulomatous disease of the orbit: clinical presentations, evaluation, and management. *Actas Dermosifiliogr*. 2017;108(5):400-406.
23. Andron AA, Nair AG, Della Rocca D, Della Rocca RC, Reddy HS. Concomitant adult onset xanthogranuloma and IgG4-related orbital disease: a rare occurrence. *Orbit*. 2020;26:1-4.
24. Shoo BA, Shinkai K, McCalmont TH, Fox LP. Xanthogranulomas associated with hematologic malignancy in adulthood. *J Am Acad Dermatol*. 2008;59:488-493.
25. Sidney LE, Branch MJ, Dunphy SE, Dua HS, Hopkinson A. Concise review: evidence for CD34 as a common marker for diverse progenitors. *Stem Cell*. 2014;32(6):1380-1389.
26. Kraus MD, Haley JC, Ruiz R, et al. "Juvenile" xanthogranuloma: an immunophenotypic study with a reappraisal of histogenesis. *Am J Dermatopathol*. 2001;23:104-111.
27. Bains A, Parham DM. Langerhans cell histiocytosis preceding the development of juvenile xanthogranuloma: a case and review of recent developments. *Pediatr Dev Pathol*. 2011;14(6):480-484.
28. Martín JM, Jordá E, Martín-Gorgojo A, Beteta G, Monteagudo C. Histiocytosis with mixed cell populations. *J Cutan Pathol*. 2016;43(5):456-460.
29. Strehl JD, Stachel KD, Hartmann A, Agaimy A. Juvenile xanthogranuloma developing after treatment of Langerhans cell histiocytosis: case report and literature review. *Int J Clin Exp Pathol*. 2012;5(7):720-725.
30. Lee TK, Jung TY, Baek HJ, Kim SK, Lee KH, Yun SJ. Disseminated juvenile xanthogranuloma occurring after treatment of Langerhans cell histiocytosis: a case report. *Childs Nerv Syst*. 2018;34(4):765-770.
31. Bellinato F, Maurelli M, Colato C, Balter R, Girolomoni G, Schena D. BRAF V600E expression in juvenile xanthogranuloma occurring after Langerhans cell histiocytosis. *Br J Dermatol*. 2019;180(4):933-934.

32. Bonometti A, Ferrario G, Parafioriti A, et al. MAP2K1-driven mixed Langerhans cell histiocytosis, Rosai-Dorfman-Destombes disease and Erdheim-Chester disease, clonally related to acute myeloid leukemia. *J Cutan Pathol.* 2021;48(5):637-643.
33. Janssen D, Folster-Holst R, Harms D, et al. Clonality in juvenile xanthogranuloma. *Am J Surg Pathol.* 2007;31:812-813.
34. Perez-Becker R, Szczepanowshi M, Leuschner I, et al. An aggressive systemic juvenile xanthogranuloma clonally related to a preceding T-cell acute lymphoblastic leukemia. *Pediatr Blood Cancer.* 2011;56:859-862.
35. Techavichit P, Sosothikul D, Chaichana T, Teerapakpinyo C, Thorner PS, Shuangshoti S. BRAF V600E mutation in pediatric intracranial and cranial juvenile xanthogranuloma. *Hum Pathol.* 2017;69:118-122.
36. Picarsic J, Pysher T, Zhou H, et al. BRAF V600E mutation in Juvenile Xanthogranuloma family neoplasms of the central nervous system (CNS-JXG): a revised diagnostic algorithm to include pediatric Erdheim-Chester disease. *Acta Neuropathol Commun.* 2019;7(1):168.
37. Diamond EL, Durham BH, Haroche J, et al. Diverse and targetable kinase alterations drive histiocytic neoplasms. *Cancer Discov.* 2016;6(2):154-165.
38. Paxton CN, O'Malley DP, Bellizzi AM, et al. Genetic evaluation of juvenile xanthogranuloma: genomic abnormalities are uncommon in solitary lesions, advanced cases may show more complexity. *Mod Pathol.* 2017;30(9):1234-1240.
39. Maly E, Przyborska M, Rybczynska A, et al. Juvenile xanthogranuloma with clonal proliferation in the bone marrow. *J Pediatr Hematol Oncol.* 2012;34:222-225.
40. Miraglia E, Moliterni E, Iacovino C, et al. Cutaneous manifestations in neurofibromatosis type 1. *Clin Ter.* 2020;171(5):e371-e377.
41. Fenot M, Stadler JF, Barbarot S. Juvenile xanthogranulomas are highly prevalent but transient in young children with neurofibromatosis type 1. *J Am Acad Dermatol.* 2014;71:389-390.
42. Newman B, Weimen H, Nigro K, et al. Aggressive histiocytic disorders that can involve the skin. *J Am Acad Dermatol.* 2007;56:302-316.
43. Paulus S, Koronowska S, Fölster-Holst R. Association between juvenile myelomonocytic leukemia, juvenile xanthogranulomas and neurofibromatosis type 1: case report and review of the literature. *Pediatr Dermatol.* 2017;34(2):114-118.
44. Bátai B, Krizsán S, Gángó A, et al. Juvenile myelomonocytic leukaemia presentation after preceding juvenile xanthogranuloma harbouring an identical somatic PTPN11 mutation. *Pediatr Blood Cancer.* 2020;67(9):e28368.
45. Ali MM, Gilliam AE, Ruben BS, Tidyman WE, Rauen KA. Juvenile xanthogranuloma in Noonan syndrome. *Am J Med Genet A.* Published online 2021. doi:10.1002/ajmg.a.62353
46. Sonoda T, Hashimoto H, Enjoji M. Juvenile xanthogranuloma. Clinicopathologic analysis and immunohistochemical study of 57 patients. *Cancer.* 1985;56(9):2280-2286.
47. Pan Z, Xu ML. Histiocytic and dendritic cell neoplasms. *Surg Pathol Clin.* 2019;12(3):805-829.
48. Esterly NB, Sahihi T, Medenica M. Juvenile xanthogranuloma. An atypical case with study of ultrastructure. *Arch Dermatol.* 1972;105(1):99-102.
49. Stover DG, Alapati S, Regueira O, et al. Treatment of juvenile xanthogranuloma. *Pediatr Blood Cancer.* 2008;51:130.
50. DePaula AM, Andre N, Fernandez C, et al. Solitary, extracutaneous, skull-based juvenile xanthogranuloma. *Pediatr Blood Cancer.* 2010;55:380-382.
51. Hu WK, Gilliam AC, Wiersma SR, Dahms BB. Fatal congenital systemic juvenile xanthogranuloma with liver failure. *Pediatr Dev Pathol.* 2004;7:71-76.
52. Flach DB, Winkelmann RK. Juvenile xanthogranuloma with central nervous system lesions. *J Am Acad Dermatol.* 1986;14:405-411.
53. Cozzutto C, Carbone A. The xanthogranulomatous process. Xanthogranulomatous inflammation. *Pathol Res Pract.* 1988;183(4):395-402.
54. Weitzman S, Jaffe R. Uncommon histiocytic disorders: the non-Langerhans cell histiocytoses. *Pediatr Blood Cancer.* 2005;45(3):256-264.
55. Gianotti R, Alessi E, Caputo R. Benign cephalic histiocytosis: a distinct entity or a part of a wide spectrum of histiocytic proliferative disorders of children? A histopathological study. *Am J Dermatopathol.* 1993;15:315-319.
56. Patsatsi A, Kyriakou A, Sotiriadis D. Benign cephalic histiocytosis: case report and review of the literature. *Pediatr Dermatol.* 2014;31:547-550.
57. Polat Ekinci A, Buyukbabani N, Baykal C. Novel clinical observations on benign cephalic histiocytosis in a large series. *Pediatr Dermatol.* 2017;34(4):392-397.
58. Seward JL, Malone JC, Callen JP. Generalized eruptive histiocytosis. *J Am Acad Dermatol.* 2004;50(1):116-120.
59. Dobrosavljevic D, Majstorovic J, Bosic M. Dermoscopy of generalized eruptive histiocytosis: case report and brief review of the literature. *Dermatol Pract Concept.* 2020;10(3):e2020057.
60. Caputo R, Marzano AV, Passoni E, Berti E. Unusual variants of non-Langerhans cell histiocytoses. *J Am Acad Dermatol.* 2007;57(6):1031-1045.
61. Klemke CD, Dippel E, Geilen CC, et al. Atypical generalized eruptive histiocytosis associated with acute monocytic leukemia. *J Am Acad Dermatol.* 2003;49:S233-S236.
62. Shon W, Peters MS, Reed KB, Ketterling RP, Dogan A, Gibson LE. Atypical generalized eruptive histiocytosis clonally related to chronic myelomonocytic leukemia with loss of Y chromosome. *J Cutan Pathol.* 2013;40(8):725-729.
63. Ziegler B, Peitsch WK, Reiter A, Marx A, Goerdt S, Géraud C. Generalized eruptive histiocytosis associated with FIP1L1-PDGFRA-positive chronic eosinophilic leukemia. *JAMA Dermatol.* 2015;151(7):766-769.
64. Pinney SS, Jahan-Tigh RR, Chon S. Generalized eruptive histiocytosis associated with a novel fusion in LMNA-NTRK1. *Dermatol Online J.* 2016;22(8):13030/qt07d3f2xk.
65. Tamiya H, Tsuruta D, Takeda E, Moriwaki K, Kobayash H, Ishii M. Generalized eruptive histiocytoma with rapid progression and resolution following exanthema subitum. *Clin Exp Dermatol.* 2005;30:300-301.
66. Guidolin L, Noguera-Morel L, Hernández-Martín A, Fernández-Llaca H, Rodríguez-Peralto JL, Torrelo A. A case with juvenile xanthogranuloma and progressive nodular histiocytosis overlap. *Pediatr Dermatol.* 2017;34(2):e102-e103. doi:10.1111/pde.13073
67. Glavin FL, Chhatwall H, Karimi K. Progressive nodular histiocytosis: a case report with literature review, and discussion of differential diagnosis and classification. *J Cutan Pathol.* 2009;36(12):1286-1292.
68. Chapman LW, Hsiao JL, Sarantopoulous P, Chiu MV. Reddish-brown nodules and papules in an elderly man. Progressive nodular histiocytosis. *JAMA Dermatol.* 2013;149:1229-1230.

69. Gonzalez Ruiz A, Bernal Ruiz AI, Aragoneses FH, Peral Martinez I, Garcia Munoz M. Progressive nodular histiocytosis accompanied by systemic disorders. *Br J Dermatol.* 2000;143:628-631.
70. Beswick SJ, Kirk M, Bradshaw K, Sanders DS, Moss C. Progressive nodular histiocytosis in a child with a hypothalamic tumor. *Br J Dermatol.* 2002;146:138-140.
71. Woollons A, Darley CR. Xanthoma disseminatum: a case with hepatic involvement, diabetes insipidus and type IIb hyperlipidaemia. *Clin Exp Dermatol.* 1998;23:277-280.
72. Zelger BW, Staudacher C, Orchard G, et al. Solitary and generalized variants of spindle cell xanthogranuloma (progressive nodular histiocytosis). *Histopathology.* 1995;27:11-19.
73. Yang GZ, Li J, Wang LP. Disseminated intracranial xanthoma disseminatum: a rare case report and review of literature. *Diagn Pathol.* 2016;11(1):78.
74. Bonometti A, Gliozzo J, Moltrasio C, et al. Disfiguring nodular cephalic xanthoma disseminatum: an exceptional variant of a forgotten entity. *Acta Derm Venereol.* 2019;99(4):450-451.
75. Pinto ME, Escalaya GR, Escalaya ME, et al. Xanthoma disseminatum: case report and literature review. *Endocr Pract.* 2010;16:1003-1006.
76. Park HY, Cho DH, Kang HC, Yun SJ. A case of xanthoma disseminatum with spontaneous resolution over 10 years: review of the literature on long-term follow-up. *Dermatology.* 2011;222:236-243.
77. Zelger BG, Orchard G, Rudolph P, et al. Scalloped cell xanthogranuloma. *Histopathology.* 1998;32:368-374.
78. Nelson CA, Zhong CS, Hashemi DA, et al. A multicenter cross-sectional study and systematic review of necrobiotic xanthogranuloma with proposed diagnostic criteria. *JAMA Dermatol.* 2020;156(3):270-279.
79. Wick MR, Patterson JW. Cutaneous paraneoplastic syndromes. *Semin Diagn Pathol.* 2019;36(4):211-228.
80. Miguel D, Lukacs J, Illing T, Elsner P. Treatment of necrobiotic xanthogranuloma - a systematic review. *J Eur Acad Dermatol Venereol.* 2017;31(2):221-235.
81. Hilal T, DiCaudo DJ, Connolly SM, Reeder CB. Necrobiotic xanthogranuloma: a 30-year single-center experience. *Ann Hematol.* 2018;97(8):1471-1479.
82. Spicknall KE, Mehregan DA. Necrobiotic xanthogranuloma. *Int J Dermatol.* 2009;48(1):1-10.
83. Chang KTE, Tay AZE, Kuick CH, et al. ALK-positive histiocytosis: an expanded clinicopathologic spectrum and frequent presence of KIF5B-ALK fusion. *Mod Pathol.* 2019;32(5):598-608.
84. Lucas CG, Gilani A, Solomon DA, et al. ALK-positive histiocytosis with KIF5B-ALK fusion in the central nervous system. *Acta Neuropathol.* 2019;138(2):335-337.
85. Selmi C, Greenspan A, Huntley A, Gershwin ME. Multicentric reticulohistiocytosis: a critical review. *Curr Rheumatol Rep.* 2015;17(6):511.
86. Toz B, Büyükbabani N, İnanç M. Multicentric reticulohistiocytosis: rheumatology perspective. *Best Pract Res Clin Rheumatol.* 2016;30(2):250-260.
87. Sanchez-Alvarez C, Sandhu AS, Crowson CS, et al. Multicentric reticulohistiocytosis: the mayo clinic experience (1980-2017). *Rheumatology (Oxford).* 2020;59(8):1898-1905.
88. Jha VK, Kumar R, Kunwar A, et al. Efficacy of vinblastine and prednisone in multicentric reticulohistiocytosis with onset in infancy. *Pediatrics.* 2016;137(6):e20152118.
89. de Leon D, Chiu Y, Co D, Sokumbi O. Multicentric reticulohistiocytosis in a 5-year-old girl. *J Pediatr.* 2016;177:328-328.e1.
90. Zelger B, Cerio R, Soyer HP, et al. Reticulohistiocytoma and multicentric reticulohistiocytosis. Histopathologic and immunophenotypic distinct entities. *Am J Dermatopathol.* 1994;16:577-584.
91. Oliver GF, Umbert I, Winkelmann RK, et al. Reticulohistiocytoma cutis—review of 15 cases and an association with systemic vasculitis in two cases. *Clin Exp Dermatol.* 1990;15:1-6.
92. McKenna DB, Mooney EE, Young MM, et al. Multiple cutaneous reticulohistiocytosis. *Br J Dermatol.* 1998;139:544-546.
93. Hsiung SH, Chan EF, Elenitsas R, et al. Multicentric reticulohistiocytosis presenting with clinical features of dermatomyositis. *J Am Acad Dermatol.* 2003;48:S11-S14.
94. Yang HJ, Ding YQ, Deng YJ. Multicentric reticulohistiocytosis with lungs and liver involved. *Clin Exp Dermatol.* 2009;34:183-185.
95. Rapini RP. Multicentric reticulohistiocytosis. *Clin Dermatol.* 1993;11:107-111.
96. Shrader ME, Burrack HJ, Pfeiffer DG. Effects of interspecific Larval competition on developmental parameters in nutrient sources between Drosophila suzukii (Diptera: drosophilidae) and *Zaprionus indianus*. *J Econ Entomol.* 2020;113(1):230-238.
97. Snow JL, Muller SA. Malignancy-associated multicentric reticulohistiocytosis: a clinical, histological and immunophenotypic study. *Br J Dermatol.* 1995;133:71-76.
98. Catarall MD, White JE. Multicentric reticulohistiocytosis and malignant disease. *Br J Dermatol.* 1978;98:221-224.
99. Miettinen M, Fetsch JF. Reticulohistiocytoma (solitary epithelioid histiocytoma): a clinicopathologic and immunohistochemical study of 44 cases. *Am J Surg Pathol.* 2006;30:521-528.
100. Yoshimi A, Trippett TM, Zhang N, et al. Genetic basis for iMCD-TAFRO. *Oncogene.* 2020;39(15):3218-3225.

Histiocytic and dendritic cell sarcomas

Archana Shenoy and Louis P. Dehner

INTRODUCTION

Mononuclear phagocytes (MPs) comprise a category of bone marrow–derived cells with a myeloid lineage with the morphology and functional attributes of "effectors and regulators of inflammation and immune response."[1] The cell types in the MP system are histiocytes, not otherwise specified, dendritic cells, Langerhans cells (LCs), and plasmacytoid cells; each of these cell types has a specialized function beyond the scope of this discussion.[2] In the broadest terms, the designation of "histiocytosis" has been applied to benign and malignant proliferations and has been classified into five morphologic categories with a range of somatic mutations in the MAPK-ERK signaling pathway.[3] The "M" group includes primary and secondary malignant histiocytosis with histiocytic, interdigitating, Langerhans and indeterminate cell subtypes. As an immunophenotypic generalization, the neoplastic cells express CD68, CD163, CD4, and lysozyme with dendritic type cells expressing additional markers including CD1a, CD207, CD21, and CD35.

The advent of molecular and genetic testing has resulted in the revision of previous cases that were interpreted as "malignant histiocytosis" in the past; an example is anaplastic large cell lymphoma and another is "histiocytic medullary reticulosis" which is primary or secondary hemophagocytic lymphohistiocytosis in "H" group.

A mass lesion in the skin, lymph node, bone, and brain in addition to other single sites is the presentation of histiocytic or dendritic cell sarcoma (DCS) in contrast to multi-system disease which is more typical of LC histiocytosis, especially in children 5 years or less and Erdheim–Chester disease.

Malignant histiocytosis can be subclassified based on morphologic, immunophenotypic, and ultrastructural characteristics.[3-5] Five distinct diagnostic subtypes are discussed here: (i) histiocytic sarcoma (HS); (ii) follicular dendritic cell sarcoma (FDCS); (iii) interdigitating dendritic cell sarcoma (IDCS); (iv) indeterminate dendritic cell tumor (INDCT) (Table 68-1); and (v) blastic plasmacytoid dendritic cell neoplasm (BPDCN). LC sarcoma is discussed in Chapter 67.

HISTIOCYTIC SARCOMA

Definition

HS is defined as a malignancy with morphologic and immunophenotypic features that resemble those of mature tissue histiocytes and is differentiated from myeloid sarcoma with a monohistiocytic phenotype (M5).[6] This highly aggressive neoplasm presents across a broad age range from childhood into later adulthood, as a primary neoplasm or secondary to a prior hematologic malignancy.[7] Two age peaks have been reported in association with secondary HS; the first occurs between 0 and 29 years and the second between 50 and 69 years.[8] The smaller initial peak corresponds to the cases associated with pre–B-cell and T-cell leukemia/lymphoma; the second peak is reported in those cases associated with B-cell lymphoma.[8,9] It has been suggested that the latter cases are transdifferentiation of the original lymphoid neoplasm with retention of the translocation of the precursor lymphoma.[10]

Solitary or multiple lesions involving lymph nodes or extranodal sites are the presenting manifestations with a solitary mass more common than disseminated disease and a rare leukemic variant.[5,8,11] The skin is one of the most common sites of extranodal involvement with solitary or multiple lesions or as a rash. A punch or excisional biopsy is the usual approach, and in a patient with a previous history of a lymphoma or other malignancy, the inquiry is one of local recurrence or metastasis.

Histopathology

The dermis is occupied by a dense mononuclear and/or spindle cell population with diffuse or nodular pattern of high-grade malignant cells. Scattered small lymphocytes and eosinophils are present in some cases. The individual tumor cells have rounded contours with an epithelioid appearance in the presence of eosinophilic cytoplasm or a vacuolated or lipidized cytoplasm. Phagocytosis is present in scattered tumor cells. Pleomorphism and nuclear hyperchromatism with readily identified mitotic figures are additional features (Fig. 68-1A). The overlying epidermis is generally

TABLE 68-1 Salient Features of Histiocytic and Dendritic Cell Sarcoma

	HS	FDCS	IDCS	INDCT
Clinical findings	Solitary or multiple cutaneous lesions	Asymptomatic lymph node lesion, solitary or multiple		Papules, nodules, and plaques on skin
	Skin rash			Rare cutaneous involvement
Morphology	Discohesive epithelioid–spindle cells	Spindle to epithelioid cells with whorls		Epithelioid cells with nuclear grooves and clefts
Immunophenotype				
CD68	+	+/−	+/−	+/−
CD163	+	N/A	N/A	−
Lysozyme	+	−	+/−	+/−
CD1a	−/+	−	−	+
S100	−/+	+/−	+	+
CD21	−	+	−	−
CD23	−	+	−	−
CD35	−	+	−	−
CD4	Cytoplasmic	−	−	+/−
Ultrastructural characteristics				
Cytoplasmic processes	Absent	Numerous, slender	Interdigitating, complex	Interdigitating, complex
Desmosomes	Absent	Mature	Absent	Absent
Birbeck granules	Absent	Absent	Absent	Absent
Lysosomes	Abundant	Sparse	Scattered	Unknown

FDCS, follicular dendritic cell sarcoma; HS, histiocytic sarcoma; IDCS, interdigitating dendritic cell sarcoma; INDCT, indeterminate dendritic cell tumor.
Adapted with modifications from Dalia S, Shao H, Sagatys E, et al. Dendritic cell and histiocytic neoplasms: biology, diagnosis, and treatment. *Cancer Control.* 2014;21(4):290–300. Republished with permission by *Cancer Control: Journal of the Moffitt Cancer Center.*

unremarkable, often with an underlying grenz zone. Direct extension into the subcutis is common.

There are few difficulties encountered in the decision about the malignant nature of the infiltrate, but the type of tumor is the challenge so that the initial approach should be a comprehensive one with the differential diagnosis to include carcinoma or melanoma when the tumor cells have epithelioid appearances (CAM 5.2, vimentin, SOX10), hematolymphoid neoplasm (CD45, CD43, CD30), and sarcoma or melanoma with a spindle cell pattern (vimentin, SOX10). In the presence of CD45 positivity, the panel is expanded to B- and T-cell and myeloid (CD34, CD117, CD43, MPO) markers. The latter markers are relevant since myeloid sarcoma with monocytic differentiation is CD68, CD163, and lysozyme positive. A cautionary note is that HS may show CD1a positivity, but less likely CD207 immunoreactivity so that LC sarcoma becomes less likely once the "histiocytic" phenotype has been established with CD68, CD163, lysozyme, CD11c, and CD4 positivity (Fig. 68-1B,C).[12] Both CD21 and CD35, dendritic cell markers, are nonreactive.

In keeping with the various other nonmalignant histiocytoses, mutations have been detected in the MAPK/RAS/ERK pathway.[13,14] Some of the mutations are seemingly unique to primary HS, but are usually not present in secondary examples.

DENDRITIC CELL TUMOR SARCOMA

Definition

DCS is an inclusive designation for a category of neoplasms with three principal defined subtypes, FDCS, IDCS, and INDCT.[15] BPDCN and inflammatory pseudotumor-like variant of FDCS generally occupy their niche because of

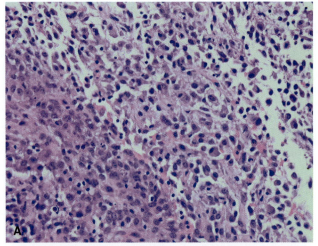
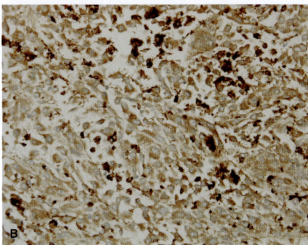
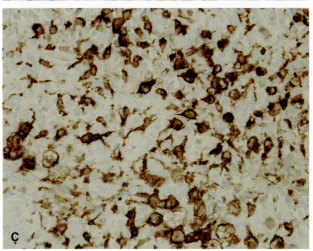

FIGURE 68-1. Histiocytic sarcoma shows discohesive epithelioid to spindle cells with abundant cytoplasm and ovoid irregular hyperchromatic nuclei **(A)** positive CD68 **(B)** and CD163 **(C)** immunohistochemical stains.

their leukemic or organ-specific manifestations. The differentiated counterpart, not its progenitor, is the dendritic cell whose role in adaptive and innate immunity is one of initiation and regulation of the immune response through antigen presentation to T-cells and cytokines.[2]

FDCS and IDCS present across a wide age range, but are predominantly seen in adults with a mean age of 53 years, but a somewhat younger age (49 years) for FDCS than IDCS (64 years).[16] Both nodal (solitary or generalized) and extranodal presentations have a predilection for the head and neck and abdominal sites.[17] Among 462 cases of DCS in the literature, cutaneous involvement occurred in 5% or less of all cases.[17] One or more skin nodules measuring 2-3 cm is the more common mode of presentation in the skin, but paraneoplastic pemphigus is the other example in a subset of cases with FDCS in the absence of neoplastic skin lesions.[18] Another association with FDCS is the hyaline vascular variant of Castleman disease; however, the pathologic findings without the benefit of immunohistochemistry can be challenging since the histologic features overlap with each other.[19,20] Inflammatory pseudotumor-like FDCS, an Epstein–Barr–associated tumor, has been reported in the liver and spleen and presently has not been reported in the skin.[21,22]

Histopathology

FDCS and IDCS have some overlapping histologic features so that the differential aspects reside in their respective immunophenotypes. Both tumors have a nodal predilection although FDCS is somewhat better documented in the skin, although about 30% of cases of FDCS have other sites of extranodal presentation.[12,15,23]

Nodular, fascicular, storiform, and diffuse patterns accompany a predominantly uniform spindle to a less frequent epithelioid cell proliferation in FDCS; the tumor cells tend to have low-grade ovoid to more elongated nuclei and pale eosinophilic to clear cytoplasm (Fig. 68-2A,B). Mitotic figures are typically sparing in numbers. A scattered background of small lymphocytes in the absence of plasma cells is commonly observed.

An IDCS is contrasted from FDCS by a tumor cell population with pleomorphic and epithelioid cellular features.[12] A nested and nodular pattern of epithelioid cells may initially suggest the possibility of melanoma and various other epithelial and mesenchymal neoplasms.

FDCS demonstrates positive staining for the follicular dendritic cell markers including CD21, CD23, CD35, D2-40, and fascin, while IDCS does not express any of the latter markers, but is reactive for S-100 protein, CD45, CD163, and lysozyme, and is nonreactive for CD1a and CD207. However, SOX-10 is reportedly immunopositive in some cases to create obvious consternation.[12] The combination of positive histiocytic markers and absence of melan-A reactivity should assist in the resolution of the dilemma.[24,25]

INDCT is seemingly the least common and most indolent of the dendritic cell neoplasms, but one with almost exclusive cutaneous manifestations.[15] A solitary or a more generalized presentation of a cutaneous nodule(s) shows a diffuse dermal and subcutaneous infiltrate of mononuclear cells with typical LC features in the biopsy. Like LCs, S-100 protein and CD1a are reactive, but CD207 is negative to differentiate it from LCH.[26] BRAF V600E mutations are present in these lesions, like LCH.[27]

BPDCN, known previously as CD4+/CD56+ hematodermic neoplasm or CD56+/TdT+ blastic NK cell tumor, is a myeloid neoplasm whose differentiated counterpart, the plasmacytoid DC (pDC), is a copious producer of type I interferon.[28,29] One or more brownish to deeply maroon

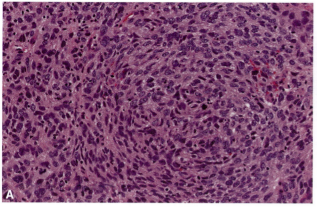
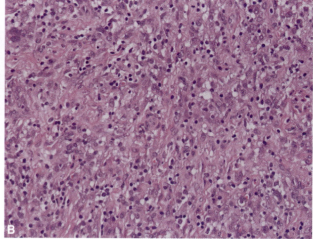

FIGURE 68-2. **A.** Follicular dendritic cell sarcoma shows a storiform to whorled pattern of spindled and epithelioid cells. **B.** Interdigitating dendritic cell sarcoma shows a diffuse sheet-like pattern with scattered giant cells.

cutaneous plaques or nodules are the most common presenting manifestations with synchronous or metachronous bone marrow, nodal, or leukemic involvement.[30] A diffuse dermal and subcutaneous infiltrate consists of monotonous, small to medium sized tumor cells with finely dispersed or more vesicular chromatin pattern.[31] The dermal infiltration readily suggests a hematolymphoid neoplasm with the necessary immunophenotypic evaluation. CD4 and CD56 are expressed in virtually all cases, in addition to TdT (70% of cases); the specific pDC markers include CD123, CD303, and TCL1. Less than 5% of cases are MPO positive to exclude myeloid sarcoma.

DIFFERENTIAL DIAGNOSIS

For each of these lesions, there is a need to distinguish them from other hematologic, myofibroblastic, and nerve sheath neoplasms (Table 68-2). This task is accomplished by a panel of immunohistochemical stains outlined in Table 68-1. ALCL can variably express CD68, but is usually positive for CD30, ALK, and T-cell markers (CD2, CD43, CD4, TIA-1, granzyme B, and CD5). Melanoma is positive for HMB-45, melan-A, and/or SOX-10. Myofibroblastic tumors express CD34 and smooth muscle actin whereas peripheral nerve sheath tumors are positive for S-100 and SOX-10; both tumor categories are typically negative for histiocytic and dendritic cell markers. However, EBER in situ hybridization should be performed to exclude inflammatory pseudotumor-like follicular/fibroblastic DCS.[32] Other considerations in the differential diagnosis include poorly differentiated carcinomas, which are usually keratin positive, and other lymphoid neoplasms which are positive for markers of their cell lineage (T- or B-cells).

MOLECULAR ALTERATIONS

The molecular landscape of histiocytic neoplasms has substantially altered the pathogenetic perspective with the demonstration of somatic mutations in the RAS-MAPK signaling pathway in LC histiocytosis, LC sarcoma, and

TABLE 68-2 Differential Diagnosis of Histiocytic/Dendritic Cell Sarcoma.

HS	FDCS and IDCS	INDCT
Anaplastic large cell lymphoma	Anaplastic large cell lymphoma	Langerhans cell histiocytosis
Diffuse, large B-cell lymphoma	Inflammatory pseudotumors	T-cell lymphomas
Hemophagocytic lymphohistiocytosis	Myofibroblastic tumors	
Langerhans cell histiocytosis	Langerhans cell histiocytosis	
Metastatic carcinoma or melanoma	Non-Hodgkin lymphoma	
	True histiocytic lymphomas	

FDCS, follicular dendritic cell sarcoma; HS, histiocytic sarcoma; IDCS, interdigitating dendritic cell sarcoma, INDCT, indeterminate dendritic cell tumor.
Adapted with modifications from Dalia S, Shao H, Sagatys E, et al. Dendritic cell and histiocytic neoplasms: biology, diagnosis, and treatment. *Cancer Control.* 2014;21(4):290–300.
Republished with permission by *Cancer Control: Journal of the Moffitt Cancer Center.*

Erdheim–Chester disease to include the more malignant end of their spectrum.[33] Several translocations have also been detected in FDCS.[34] In cases of HS associated with follicular lymphoma (synchronous and metachronous), identical *Bcl2* gene rearrangements have been demonstrated.[35] The identification of these molecular alterations has provided opportunities for targeted therapy.

THERAPY, PROGNOSIS, AND OUTCOME

HS and IDCS are aggressive neoplasms with a poor outcome, while FDCS has an indolent clinical course and INDCT has a variable outcome. FDCS with pronounced cellular atypia, necrosis, and increased mitotic rate has been associated with a worse prognosis.[17] Treatment involves multimodal therapy that includes surgical excision and chemoradiation.[5] Localized surgically resectable disease has been reported to have a better outcome in contrast to widespread disease. There are rare examples of less dismal outcomes in the case of HS and IDCS, with a report of the latter showing complete response to ABVD (adriamycin, bleomycin, vinblastine, and dacarbazine) chemotherapy.[36-38] The clinical course in INDCT is variable and not clearly known thus far because of the paucity of well-documented cases.

CAPSULE SUMMARY

- HS, FDCS, IDCS, and INDCT represent malignant cutaneous neoplasms of the macrophage lineage.
- Diagnosis is based on histology and a panel of immunohistochemical markers performed to confirm histiocytic and dendritic cell lineage: CD4, CD68, CD163, and lysozyme (histiocytes); CD21, CD23, CD35, and S100 (dendritic cells).
- Ultrastructure can serve as a valuable adjunct in diagnosis.
- HS and IDCS have poor prognosis, while FDCS has an indolent clinical course; localized disease has a better outcome.

References

1. Geissmann F, Manz MG, Jung S, Sieweke MH, Merad M, Ley K. Development of monocytes, macrophages, and dendritic cells. *Science*. 2010;327(5966):656-661. doi:10.1126/science.1178331
2. Cabeza-Cabrerizo M, Cardoso A, Minutti CM, Pereira da Costa M, Reis e Sousa C. Dendritic cells revisited. *Annu Rev Immunol*. 2021;39(1):131-166. doi:10.1146/annurev-immunol-061020-053707
3. Emile JF, Abla O, Fraitag S, et al. Revised classification of histiocytoses and neoplasms of the macrophage-dendritic cell lineages. *Blood*. 2016;127(22):2672-2681. doi:10.1182/blood-2016-01-690636
4. Pileri SA, Grogan TM, Harris NL, et al. Tumours of histiocytes and accessory dendritic cells: an immunohistochemical approach to classification from the International Lymphoma Study Group based on 61 cases. *Histopathology*. 2002;41(1):1-29. doi:10.1046/j.1365-2559.2002.01418.x
5. Dalia S, Shao H, Sagatys E, Cualing H, Sokol L. Dendritic cell and histiocytic neoplasms: biology, diagnosis, and treatment. *Cancer Control*. 2014;21(4):290-300. doi:10.1177/107327481402100405
6. Weiss LM, Pileri SA, Chan JKC. Histiocytic sarcoma. In: Swerdlow SH et al., ed. *WHO Classification of Tumours of Haematopoietic and Lymphoid Tissues*. International Agency for Research on Cancer; 2017:468-470.
7. Skala SL, Lucas DR, Dewar R. Histiocytic sarcoma: review, discussion of transformation from B-cell lymphoma, and differential diagnosis. *Arch Pathol Lab Med*. 2018;142(11):1322-1329. doi:10.5858/arpa.2018-0220-RA
8. Takahashi E, Nakamura S. Histiocytic sarcoma: an updated literature review based on the 2008 WHO classification. *J Clin Exp Hematop*. 2013;53(1):1-8. doi:10.3960/jslrt.53.1
9. Castro ECC, Blazquez C, Boyd J, et al. Clinicopathologic features of histiocytic lesions following ALL, with a review of the literature. *Pediatr Dev Pathol*. 2010;13(3):225-237. doi:10.2350/09-03-0622-OA.1
10. Zeng W, Meck J, Cheson BD, Ozdemirli M. Histiocytic sarcoma transdifferentiated from follicular lymphoma presenting as a cutaneous tumor. *J Cutan Pathol*. 2011;38(12):999-1003. doi:10.1111/j.1600-0560.2011.01769.x
11. Hofstetter L, Aranovich D, Bernstine H, et al. Leukemic phase of histiocytic sarcoma of the digestive system: a rare manifestation of a rare disease. *Acta Haematol*. 2021;144(2):229-235. doi:10.1159/000509723
12. Magro CM, Kazi N, Sisinger AE. Primary cutaneous histiocytic sarcoma: a report of five cases with primary cutaneous involvement and review of the literature. *Ann Diagn Pathol*. 2018;32:56-62. doi:10.1016/j.anndiagpath.2017.10.004
13. Egan C, Nicolae A, Lack J, et al. Genomic profiling of primary histiocytic sarcoma reveals two molecular subgroups. *Haematologica*. 2020;105(4):951-960. doi:10.3324/haematol.2019.230375
14. Egan C, Lack J, Skarshaug S, et al. The mutational landscape of histiocytic sarcoma associated with lymphoid malignancy. *Mod Pathol*. 2021;34(2):336-347. doi:10.1038/s41379-020-00673-x
15. Pan Z, Xu ML. Histiocytic and dendritic cell neoplasms. *Surg Pathol Clin*. 2019;12(3):805-829. doi:10.1016/j.path.2019.03.013
16. Perkins SM, Shinohara ET. Interdigitating and follicular dendritic cell sarcomas. *Am J Clin Oncol*. 2013;36(4):395-398. doi:10.1097/COC.0b013e31824be22b
17. Saygin C, Uzunaslan D, Ozguroglu M, Senocak M, Tuzuner N. Dendritic cell sarcoma: a pooled analysis including 462 cases with presentation of our case series. *Crit Rev Oncol Hematol*. 2013;88(2):253-271. doi:10.1016/j.critrevonc.2013.05.006
18. Akel R, Fakhri G, Salem R, Boulos F, Habib K, Tfayli A. Paraneoplastic pemphigus as a first manifestation of an intra-abdominal follicular dendritic cell sarcoma: rare case and review of the literature. *Case Rep Oncol*. 2018;11(2):353-359. doi:10.1159/000489602
19. Kazakov DV, Morrisson C, Plaza JA, Michal M, Suster S. Sarcoma arising in hyaline-vascular castleman disease of skin and subcutis. *Am J Dermatopathol*. 2005;27(4):327-332. doi:10.1097/01.dad.0000171606.55810.86
20. Viola P, Vroobel KM, Devaraj A, et al. Follicular dendritic cell tumour/sarcoma: a commonly misdiagnosed tumour in the thorax. *Histopathology*. 2016;69(5):752-761. doi:10.1111/his.12998
21. Bruehl FK, Azzato E, Durkin L, Farkas DH, Hsi ED, Ondrejka SL. Inflammatory pseudotumor-like follicular/

fibroblastic dendritic cell sarcomas of the spleen are EBV-associated and lack other commonly identifiable molecular alterations. *Int J Surg Pathol*. 2021;29(4):443-446. doi:10.1177/1066896920949675

22. Cheuk W, Chan JKC, Shek TWH, et al. Inflammatory pseudotumor-like follicular dendritic cell tumor. *Am J Surg Pathol*. 2001;25(6):721-731. doi:10.1097/00000478-200106000-00003

23. Nguyen CM, Cassarino D. Primary cutaneous interdigitating dendritic cell sarcoma: a case report and review of the literature. *Am J Dermatopathol*. 2016;38(8):628-631. doi:10.1097/DAD.0000000000000618

24. Weiss LM, Chan JKC. *Interdigitating dendritic cell sarcoma.* In: *WHO Classification of Tumours of Haematopoietic and Lymphoid Tissues*. International Agency for Research on Cancer; 2017:475-476.

25. Chan JKC, Pileri SA, Fletcher CDM, Weiss LM, Grogg KL. *Follicular dendritic cell sarcoma.* In: *WHO Classification of Tumours of Haematopoietic and Lymphoid Tissues*. International Agency for Research on Cancer; 2017:476-478.

26. Liu J, Zheng S, Li J-H, et al. Indeterminate dendritic cell sarcoma in a patient with myelodysplastic syndrome. *Am J Dermatopathol*. 2019;41(2):164-166. doi:10.1097/DAD.0000000000001073

27. O'Malley DP, Agrawal R, Grimm KE, et al. Evidence of BRAF V600E in indeterminate cell tumor and interdigitating dendritic cell sarcoma. *Ann Diagn Pathol*. 2015;19(3):113-116. doi:10.1016/j.anndiagpath.2015.02.008

28. Mitchell D, Chintala S, Dey M. Plasmacytoid dendritic cell in immunity and cancer. *J Neuroimmunol*. 2018;322:63-73. doi:10.1016/j.jneuroim.2018.06.012

29. Suzuki Y, Kato S, Kohno K, et al. Clinicopathological analysis of 46 cases with CD4 + and/or CD56 + immature haematolymphoid malignancy: reappraisal of blastic plasmacytoid dendritic cell and related neoplasms. *Histopathology*. 2017;71(6):972-984. doi:10.1111/his.13340

30. Hirner JP, O'Malley JT, LeBoeuf NR. Blastic plasmacytoid dendritic cell neoplasm. *Hematol Oncol Clin North Am*. 2020;34(3):501-509. doi:10.1016/j.hoc.2020.01.001

31. Shi Y, Wang E. Blastic plasmacytoid dendritic cell neoplasm: a clinicopathologic review. *Arch Pathol Lab Med*. 2014;138(4):564-569. doi:10.5858/arpa.2013-0101-RS

32. Van Baeten C, Van Dorpe J. Splenic Epstein-Barr virus–associated inflammatory pseudotumor. *Arch Pathol Lab Med*. 2017;141(5):722-727. doi:10.5858/arpa.2016-0283-RS

33. Shanmugam V, Griffin GK, Jacobsen ED, Fletcher CDM, Sholl LM, Hornick JL. Identification of diverse activating mutations of the RAS-MAPK pathway in histiocytic sarcoma. *Mod Pathol*. 2019;32(6):830-843. doi:10.1038/s41379-018-0200-x

34. Facchetti F, Simbeni M, Lorenzi L. Follicular dendritic cell sarcoma. *Pathologica*. 2021;113(5):316-329. doi:10.32074/1591-951X-331

35. Feldman AL, Arber DA, Pittaluga S, et al. Clonally related follicular lymphomas and histiocytic/dendritic cell sarcomas: evidence for transdifferentiation of the follicular lymphoma clone. *Blood*. 2008;111(12):5433-5439. doi:10.1182/blood-2007-11-124792

36. Hornick JL, Jaffe ES, Fletcher CDM. Extranodal histiocytic sarcoma: clinicopathologic analysis of 14 cases of a rare epithelioid malignancy. *Am J Surg Pathol*. 2004. 28. doi:10.1097/01.pas.0000131541.95394.23

37. Olnes MJ, Nicol T, Duncan M, Bohlman M, Erlich R. Interdigitating dendritic cell sarcoma: a rare malignancy responsive to ABVD chemotherapy. *Leuk Lymphoma*. 2002;43(4):0817-0821. doi:10.1080/10428190290016944

38. Kyogoku C, Seki M, Ogawa S, et al. Complete remission in systemic skin interdigitating dendritic cell sarcoma after ABVD chemotherapy. *J Clin Exp Hematop*. 2015;55(1):33-37. doi:10.3960/jslrt.55.33

CHAPTER 69

Intralymphatic histiocytosis and Melkersson–Rosenthal syndrome

Andrea P. Moy, Louis P. Dehner, and Rosalynn M. Nazarian

These seemingly disparate disorders are included together since Melkersson–Rosenthal syndrome (MRS) may have intralymphatic histiocytosis (ILH) as a microscopic finding in a skin biopsy.[1] They may also share a common pathogenetic mechanism through autoimmunity.

INTRALYMPHATIC HISTIOCYTOSIS

Definition

ILH is a rare disorder that is characterized by aggregates of histiocytes within the lumen of dermal lymphatic vessels. Although the understanding of this disorder has evolved over time, the etiopathogenesis still remains unclear. It is not included among the other better defined histiocytic disorders.[2]

Pathogenesis

The disorder was initially reported in a 77-year-old woman with a nontender, erythematous rash on her lower extremities with a skin biopsy revealing dilated dermal vessels containing CD68+ macrophages and was designated "intravascular histiocytosis."[3] A subsequent report of two cases was initially thought to represent reactive angioendotheliomatosis (RAE), but additional studies revealed the histiocytic nature of the intraluminal proliferation.[4]

In 2000, Pruim et al[5] reported two patients with rheumatoid arthritis (RA) with intravascular histiocytes manifesting as erythematous plaques on the upper extremities; based on histopathologic findings, the authors suggested that the involved vessels were lymphatic channels. Takiwaki et al[6] proposed the terminology "rheumatoid intravascular or intralymphatic histiocytosis of the skin" as the nature of the vessels remained unclear at the time. However, Okazaki et al[7] used immunohistochemistry for D2-40 to show that the implicated vessels were, in fact, lymphatics. In the largest series published, Requena et al[8] confirmed that the vessels are lymphatic in nature and suggested that, as such, ILH and intravascular RAE are distinct disorders. Few examples of histiocytic aggregates present within cutaneous blood vessels have been reported; some also have features of hemophagocytosis, suggesting that rarely blood vessels rather than lymphatics may be involved.[9-11]

ILH likely represents a nonspecific inflammatory reaction pattern, and it has been associated with several clinical conditions. Multiple reports have demonstrated an association with RA, such that about 50% of cases occur in this setting.[6,8,12-15] Rare cases have been reported in association with tonsillitis,[16] vulvar necrosis,[10] Crohn disease,[17] and healing cellulitis.[18] Other cases have been associated with orthopedic surgical procedures, in particular those involving metallic prostheses,[19-23] or surgery in the setting of malignancy, such as breast carcinoma, colonic carcinoma, melanoma in situ, and Merkel cell carcinoma.[8,24] ILH has been recently reported on the trunk of a patient with a history of lung adenocarcinoma after treatment with pembrolizumab as another possible manifestation of checkpoint inhibitors.[25] Despite the multiple associations, ILH has also been reported in a subset of patients without any known underlying inflammatory condition.[17]

It is thought that the histiocytes within the vascular spaces have drained via lymphatics around joints involved by an inflammatory process. Lymphatic obstruction secondary to abnormal vessel formation or damage from inflammation, infection, trauma, or surgery may cause lymphangiectasia, blockage, and lymph stasis.[5,8] Requena et al[8] hypothesized that lymph stasis can lead to poor antigen clearance, subsequent localized immune dysfunction, and persistent inflammation with intraluminal accumulation of histiocytes. Okamoto et al[26] implicated the release of cytokines, including tumor necrosis factor-alpha (TNF-α), from inflamed joints, such as in RA, with the aggregation of histiocytes. Clinical response following treatment with the TNF-α inhibitor, infliximab, supports this hypothesis.[27] TNF-α levels were found to be elevated in the patient who developed ILH after pembrolizumab treatment,[25] possibly providing additional evidence for this hypothesis that TNF-α has a role in the pathogenesis of ILH. Although the activity of skin disease in ILH does not seem to directly correlate with severity of RA, the treatment of known associated conditions may lead to regression of skin lesions.[8,17] The role of M1 versus M2-polarized macrophages in the pathogenesis has been investigated; however, underlying disease mechanisms remain to be fully elucidated.[28,29]

Epidemiology

ILH is rare with few cases reported in the literature. It is more common in females than males and typically affects middle-aged to elderly individuals, with a mean age of 62–70 years in two studies.[8,17] One reported case, associated with tonsillitis and scrotal lesions, occurred in an adolescent.[16]

Clinical Features

Skin lesions are ill-defined, erythematous, or violaceous patches or plaques and may have a livedo reticularis-like appearance. The extremities are usually involved, and skin near an inflamed joint is often affected in the cases associated with RA.[7,8,14,15] Less commonly, the trunk or head and neck is involved.[6] One case involving the vulva has been reported.[10] Most recently, a case involving the oral mucosa, clinically mimicking oral lymphangioma circumscriptum, and rare cases of laryngeal involvement presenting as breathing difficulties in patients without any evidence of systemic disease have been reported.[30-32]

Histopathology

The biopsy shows dilated, irregularly shaped, thin-walled lymphatic vessels within the reticular dermis (Fig. 69-1). Variably cohesive aggregates of epithelioid mononuclear histiocytes with pale, finely granular cytoplasm, and vesicular, oval, and uniform nuclei are present within the vascular spaces (Figs. 69-2–69-4). Cytologic atypia or mitotic figures are absent.[8,13,17] The vascular channels are lined by a single layer of flat endothelial cells without atypical features (Fig. 69-5). In some cases, the endothelial cells may be hyperplastic with tufting into the luminal space. Intraluminal lymphocytes and/or neutrophils may be present.[8] Thrombosis or vasculitis is typically not seen; however, vessel thrombosis was reported in one case involving the scrotum.[16] The surrounding dermis may contain a patchy mixed inflammatory infiltrate composed of lymphocytes, histiocytes, plasma cells, and/or neutrophils. The overlying epidermis and papillary dermis are unremarkable.

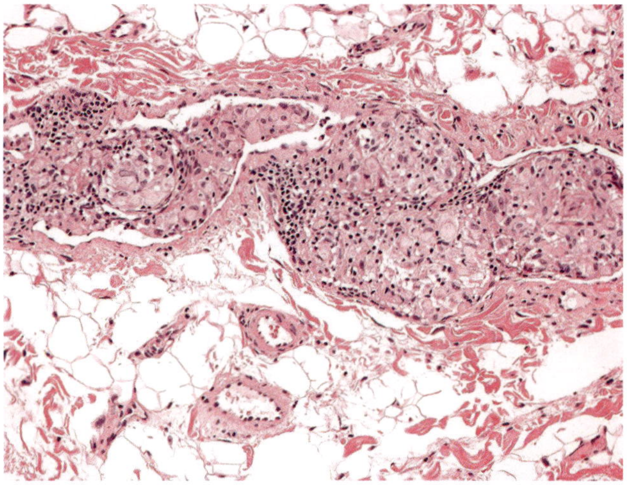

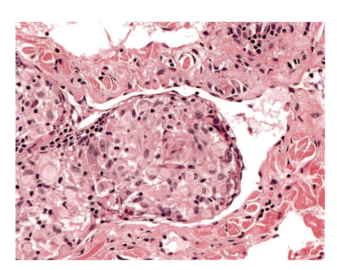

FIGURE 69-2. Multiple lymphatic spaces are dilated by aggregates of epithelioid mononuclear histiocytes. Scattered lymphocytes may be associated with the histiocytes (H&E, 200×).

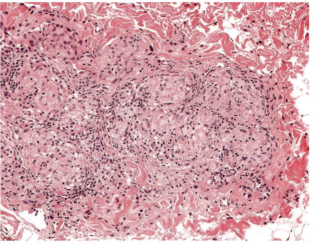

FIGURE 69-3. The luminal epithelioid histiocytes have abundant pale and finely granular cytoplasm and oval, vesicular nuclei (H&E, 400×).

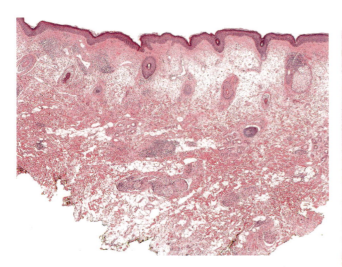

FIGURE 69-1. In intralymphatic histiocytosis, the superficial and deep dermis contains dilated, thin-walled vessels and a patchy perivascular mixed inflammatory infiltrate (H&E, 40×).

FIGURE 69-4. Some vessels are distended and occluded by the dense intraluminal histiocytic infiltrate (H&E, 200×).

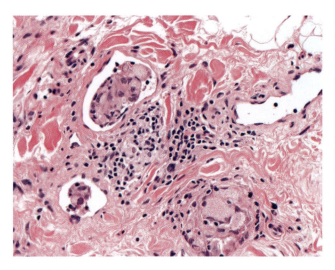

FIGURE 69-5. Free-floating, variably cohesive aggregates are present within vascular spaces that are lined by a single layer of flat endothelial cells without nuclear pleomorphism (H&E, 400×).

Immunophenotype

The endothelial lining cells are positive for D2-40, Lyve-1, and Prox-1. The intravascular lesional cells express CD68, CD163, PGM-1, Mac387, and HLA-DR and are negative for S100 and CD1a (Fig. 69-6)[17]; they may occasionally be positive for myeloperoxidase, podoplanin, and CD31.[8] It should be pointed out that CD31 is also a monohistiocytic marker. The Ki67 proliferative index of the histiocytes is low. Few admixed CD3+ T-cells may be seen within the lymphatic lumina. CD3+ T-cells, CD20+ B-cells, and CD79a+ plasma cells may be present as an associated dermal inflammatory infiltrate.

Differential Diagnosis

RAE and ILH have been proposed as part of a continuous spectrum in the absence of a consensus on this point.[4,11,33] Angioendotheliomatosis was initially thought to be a neoplastic proliferation of endothelial cells.[34] However, subsequent reports described two subtypes of angioendotheliomatosis,

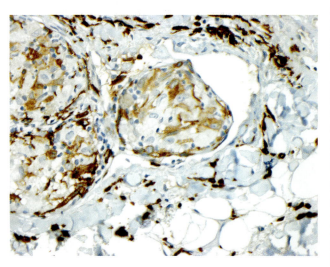

FIGURE 69-6. The intraluminal histiocytes have surface expression for CD163 (H&E, 400×).

a benign (or hyperplastic) form and a malignant form; these entities are now regarded as entirely different diseases as further studies have demonstrated that so-called malignant angioendotheliomatosis is intravascular large B-cell or less often NK/T-cell lymphoma.[35-37]

RAE is a benign, self-limited proliferation of endothelial cells within previously formed blood vessels. This proliferation may occlude the vascular lumen and result in the formation of new vascular channels. While the etiology of RAE is unknown, it has been described in association with many other disorders, including systemic infections (eg, tuberculosis, subacute bacterial endocarditis),[38-42] microvascular occlusive disorders (eg, cryoglobulinemia, antiphospholipid syndrome),[43-46] vascular diseases (eg, peripheral vascular disease, hypertensive portal gastropathy),[47,48] and hematologic disorders (eg, Castleman disease).[49] Additionally, RAE has also been associated with RA as a link to ILH.[11,50] Some have suggested that the organization of microthrombi within vascular spaces can lead to the accumulation of intraluminal histiocytes and subsequent proliferation of endothelial cells manifesting as ILH or angioendotheliomatosis.[4] Clinically, there is significant overlap between these two conditions in the range of clinical findings.[51] One report has described the presence of both ILH and RAE in a wide reexcision for malignant melanoma; these concurrent findings suggested that these entities are related phenomena.[52] However, other authors believe that these are distinctly different entities—one occurring within blood vessels and the other within lymphatic vessels.[8] There is also some morphologic overlap between RAE and intravascular papillary endothelial hyperplasia (Masson lesion) as well as glomeruloid hemangioma.[53] It is also reported as a type of drug reaction.[54]

Intravascular lymphoma (IVL) is a consideration in the differential diagnosis of ILH.[55-57] IVL is a rare, aggressive type of lymphoma with widespread dissemination in extranodal sites, including the bone marrow and most other organs including the skin.[58-60] Neoplastic cells are occasionally present within the peripheral blood, but lymph nodes are usually not involved.[61] Atypical lymphocytes fill dilated vascular spaces at all levels of the dermis and subcutis. However, only an isolated vascular space may contain a few neoplastic cells. The tumor cells are large with prominent nucleoli and mitotic figures may be observed. Immunohistochemistry can help distinguish IVL from ILH as the cells present in IVL are CD20+ B-cells.[56] Rare cases of intravascular NK/T-cell lymphomas have also been reported.[62-66]

The differential diagnosis may also include intralymphatic CD30+ T-cell proliferations. It has been shown that intralymphatic neoplastic CD30+ cells can be seen in primary cutaneous anaplastic large cell lymphoma, secondary cutaneous involvement by systemic ALCL, and lymphomatoid papulosis,[67,68] and does not have implications regarding prognosis or clinical course. Additionally, enlarged CD30+ T-cells may rarely be identified within lymphatics incidentally as a reactive process. This has been described in association with trauma,[69] benign vascular lesions,[70,71] lichen sclerosus,[72] keratoacanthoma,[73] hidradenitis suppurative,[74] DRESS syndrome,[75] and seborrheic dermatitis with ruptured folliculitis.[76] Immunohistochemistry can help differentiate intralymphatic CD30+ T-cell proliferations from intralymphatic histiocytic aggregates; T-cell receptor gene rearrangement studies may also help in some cases.

Lymphovascular invasion by carcinoma or melanoma[52] should be readily distinguishable from ILH using melanocyte and/or keratin-specific stains.

Management and Prognosis

Since ILH is a reactive condition, there is no specific treatment. The clinical course is characteristically indolent but chronic so that various approaches to management have been proposed.[3,4,11,13] Pressure bandages have been reported to produce positive results, supporting the hypothesis that lymph stasis may play a role in the pathogenesis.[77] One case treated with topical tacrolimus has been reported.[78] Additionally, treatment of the underlying disease, such as RA, can result in resolution of cutaneous manifestation. For example, anti-TNF-α blockade, such as with infliximab, or humanized anti-IL6, tocilizumab, has been shown to improve skin lesions in cases associated with RA.[27,79]

MELKERSSON–ROSENTHAL SYNDROME

MRS is a rare condition involving the skin with intralymphatic collections of histiocytes. The triad of chronic orofacial swelling, recurrent facial nerve palsy, and a fissured tongue are the typical clinical manifestations; however, the full triad is present in only a minority of cases.[80-82] Most patients present with a monosymptomatic or oligosymptomatic form. Facial swelling involving the lips is the most common clinical presentation. Orofacial granulomatosis is the generic designation for this spectrum of disease to include not only MRS, but also granulomatous cheilitis, or Miescher cheilitis, which is now regarded as a monosymptomatic form of MRS.[83-85] Localized eyelid edema is another manifestation.[1,86,87] The average age at presentation is between 20 and 40 years,[81,83] although rare cases have been reported in children and adolescents in 8%–10% of cases.[81,83,88-94] Some studies suggest that women are more often affected than men.[81]

Etiology

The etiology of MRS is unknown. Some cases are believed to be a manifestation of Crohn disease or sarcoidosis,[83] and others have been associated with psoriasis.[95] However, the syndrome has been described in a number of cases without an underlying systemic granulomatous disease; proposed etiologies in these cases have included an allergic reaction, chronic infection, and immune dysregulation as well as a genetic predisposition.[96-98] One report noted the presence of Demodex infestation and associated follicular dilation and perifolliculitis in skin biopsies from patients with a diagnosis of MRS. It has been suggested that rosacea may play a role in the pathogenesis.[1]

Therapy

Management is a challenge with the one principal goal of ameliorating the facial swelling and paralysis. Symptoms may spontaneously remit or persist. Treatment with corticosteroids or nerve compression has been successful.[96,99,100] Granulomatous cheilitis has been treated with clofazimine, thalidomide, and infliximab.[101-103] Triamcinolone injections with or without dapsone have also been shown to provide some relief.[104-107] Surgery may be necessary for persistent symptoms.[108,109]

Pathologic Features

Those biopsies from the region of orofacial edema show the presence of noncaseating granulomatous inflammation with an accompanying mixed inflammatory reaction unlike the more inactive epithelioid granulomas of typical sarcoid (Fig. 69-7). There is often dermal edema with a perivascular and interstitial mixed inflammatory infiltrate composed of lymphocytes, plasma cells, and histiocytes. Tuberculoid granulomas or isolated multinucleated giant cells may also be seen within the inflammatory infiltrate. Many ectatic and dilated vascular channels are present within the dermis and intralymphatic collections of epithelioid histiocytes or granulomas are typically present (Figs. 69-8–69-13).[1,87,97]

Immunophenotype

Immunohistochemistry studies have demonstrated that the vessels with collections of epithelioid histiocytes are lined by D2-40 and CD34 positive endothelial cells. The intraluminal

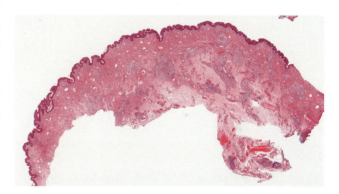

FIGURE 69-7. In Melkersson–Rosenthal syndrome (MRS), there is noncaseating granulomatous inflammation in the dermis with dilated and ectatic lymphatic channels (H&E, 20×).

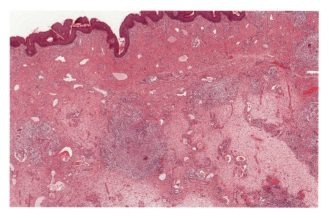

FIGURE 69-8. Dilated lymphatic channels and nodular clusters of multinucleated giant cells and epithelioid histiocytes (H&E, 40×).

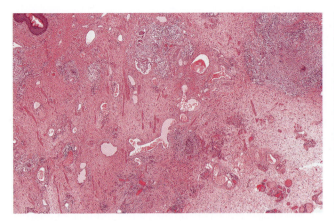

FIGURE 69-9. Many of the granulomas have an intralymphatic distribution (H&E, 100×).

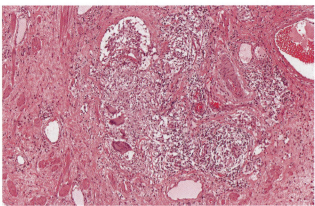

FIGURE 69-12. Intralymphatic granulomata are present on higher magnification (H&E, 200×).

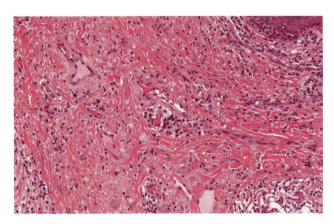

FIGURE 69-10. Lymphocytes and abundant plasma cells are seen (H&E, 200×).

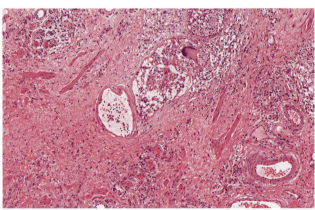

FIGURE 69-13. Intralymphatic granulomata are present on higher magnification (H&E, 200×).

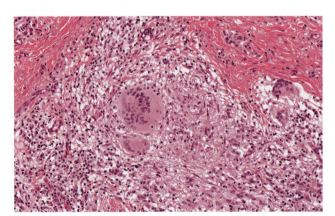

FIGURE 69-11. Very large multinucleated giant cells and epithelioid histiocytes are the constituents of the granulomata (H&E, 200×).

epithelioid cells are positive for CD68 and CD163 as in the case of ILH; some studies have reported scattered positivity for CD1a within the intraluminal proliferation.[87] An associated lymphocytic infiltrate is mainly composed of CD3+ T-cells with a mixture of CD4+ and CD8+ cells and rare CD20+ B-cells; in some cases, a decreased CD4:CD8 ratio has been noted.[87,97,110,111] One study showed that in the complete form or triad of the syndrome, the inflammatory infiltrate was composed predominantly of CD20+ B-cells, which were located within the center of the granulomatous infiltrate, with surrounding CD3+ T-cells; these are features of a reactive lymphoid follicle.[97] Given the granulomatous character of the infiltrate, special stains for microorganisms are needed and should be negative.

Differential Diagnosis

The differential diagnosis of MRS on the basis of the skin biopsy includes Crohn disease, sarcoidosis, tuberculosis, leprosy, rosacea, Ascher syndrome (eyelid and lip swelling and euthyroid goiter), allergic angioedema, RAE, IVL, and lymphovascular invasion of malignancy (ie, carcinoma or melanoma). Morbihan disease (MD) may also be a diagnostic consideration in some cases, since it is characterized clinically by periorbital erythema and edema and associated with rosacea.[112] The histopathologic features of MD may include perivascular and intravascular histiocytes or granulomas, whose features overlap with MRS.[113-115] Thus, the diagnosis of MRS requires correlation with the clinical history and findings on clinical examination as well as other ancillary tests as needed.

References

1. Emanuel PO, Lewis I, Gaskin B, Rosser P, Angelo N. Periocular intralymphatic histiocytosis or localized Melkersson-Rosenthal syndrome? *J Cutan Pathol*. 2015;42(4):289-294.
2. Pan Z, Xu ML. Histiocytic and dendritic cell neoplasms. *Surg Pathol Clin*. 2019;12(3):805-829.
3. O'Grady JT, Shahidullah H, Doherty VR, et al. Intravascular histiocytosis. *Histopathology*. 1994;24:265-268.
4. Rieger E, Soyer HP, Leboit PE, et al. Reactive angioendotheliomatosis or intravascular histiocytosis? An immunohistochemical and ultrastructural study in two cases of intravascular histiocytic cell proliferation. *Br J Dermatol*. 1999;140:497-504.
5. Pruim B, Strutton G, Congdon S, et al. Cutaneous histiocytic lymphangitis: an unusual manifestation of rheumatoid arthritis. *Australas J Dermatol*. 2000;41:101-105.
6. Takiwaki H, Adachi A, Kohno H, et al. Intravascular or intralymphatic histiocytosis associated with rheumatoid arthritis: a report of 4 cases. *J Am Acad Dermatol*. 2004;50:585-590.
7. Okazaki A, Asada H, Nhzeki H, et al. Intravascular histiocytosis associated with rheumatoid arthritis: report of a case with lymphatic endothelial proliferation. *Br J Dermatol*. 2005;152:1385-1387.
8. Requena L, El-Shabrawi-Caelen L, Walsh SN, et al. Intralymphatic histiocytosis: a clinicopathologic study of 16 cases. *Am J Dermatopthol*. 2009;31:140-151.
9. Fernandez-Figueras MR, Martin-Urda MT, Plana A, et al. Intravascular (blood vessel) histiocytosis with haemophagocytosis. *Histopathology*. 2016;69:1077-1081.
10. Pouryazdanparast P, Yu L, Dalton NK, et al. Intravascular histiocytosis presenting with extensive vulvar necrosis. *J Cutan Pathol*. 2009;36S:1-7.
11. Mensing CH, Krengel S, Tronnier M, et al. Reactive angioendotheliomatosis: is it 'intravascular histiocytosis'?. *J Eur Acad Dermatol Venereol*. 2005;19:216-219.
12. Magro CM, Crowson AN. The spectrum of cutaneous lesions in rheumatoid arthritis: a clinical and pathological study of 43 patients. *J Cutan Pathol*. 2003;30:1-10.
13. Catalina-Fernández I, Alvárez AC, Martin FC, et al. Cutaneous intralymphatic histiocytosis associated with rheumatoid arthritis: report of a case and review of the literature. *Am J Dermatopathol*. 2007;29:165-168.
14. Nishie W, Sawamura D, Litoyo M, et al. Intravascular histiocytosis associated with rheumatoid arthritis. *Dermatology*. 2008;217:144-145.
15. Huang HY, Liang CW, Hu SL, et al. Cutaneous intravascular histiocytosis associated with rheumatoid arthritis: a case report and review of the literature. *Clin Exp Dermatol*. 2009;34:e302-e303.
16. Asagoe K, Torigeo R, Ofuji R, et al. Reactive intravascular histiocytosis associated with tonsillitis. *Br J Dermatol*. 2006;154:560-562.
17. Bakr F, Webber N, Fassihi H, et al. Primary and secondary intralymphatic histiocytosis. *J Am Acad Dermatol*. 2014;70:927-933.
18. Goldsmith JF, Tahan SR. Intralymphatic histiocytosis in healing cellulitis: case report and review of the literature. *J Cutan Pathol*. 2020;47:960-966.
19. Watanabe T, Yamada N, Yoshida Y, et al. Intralymphatic histiocytosis with granuloma formation associated with orthopedic metal implants. *Br J Dermatol*. 2008;158:402-404.
20. Grekin S, Mesfin M, Kang S, et al. Intralymphatic histiocytosis following placement of a metal implant. *J Cutan Pathol*. 2011;38:351-353.
21. Rossari S, Scatena C, Gori A, et al. Intralymphatic histiocytosis: cutaneous nodules and metal implants. *J Cutan Pathol*. 2011;38:534-535.
22. Saggar S, Lee B, Krivo J, et al. Intralymphatic histiocytosis associated with orthopedic implants. *J Drugs Dermatol*. 2011;10:1208-1209.
23. de Unamuno Bustos B, Garcia Rabasco A, Ballester Sanchez R, et al. Erythematous indurated plaque on the right upper limb. Intralymphatic histiocytosis (IH) associated with orthopedic metal implant. *Int J Dermatol*. 2013;52:547-549.
24. Echeverria-Garcia B, Botella-Estrada R, Requena C, et al. Intralymphatic histiocytosis and cancer of the colon. *Actas Dermosifiliogr*. 2010;101:257-262.
25. Sugano T, Seike M, Funasaka Y, et al. Intralymphatic histiocytosis in a patient with lung adenocarcinoma treated with pembrolizumab: a case report. *J Immunother Cancer*. 2019;7:59.
26. Okamoto N, Tanioka M, Yamamoto T, et al. Intralymphatic histiocytosis associated with rheumatoid arthritis. *Clin Exp Dermatol*. 2008;3:516-518.
27. Sakaguchi M, Nagai H, Tsuji G, et al. Effectiveness of infliximab for intralymphatic histiocytosis with rheumatoid arthritis. *Arch Dermatol*. 2011;147:131-133.
28. Fujimoto N, Nakanishi G, Manabe T, et al. Intralymphatic histiocytosis comprises M2 macrophages in superficial dermal lymphatics with or without smooth muscles. *J Cutan Pathl*. 2016;43:898-902.
29. Iwasaki M, Kamiya K, Murata S, et al. Involvement of M1/M2 macrophages in the pathomechanisms of intralymphatic histiocytosis associated with rheumatoid arthritis. *J Dermatol*. 2019;46:e42-e43.
30. Park YJ, Kwon JE, Han JH, et al. Intralymphatic histiocytosis mimicking oral lymphoangioma circumscriptum. *Am J Dermatopathol*. 2014;36:759-761.
31. Reznitsky M, Daugaard S, Charabi BW. Two rare cases of laryngeal intralymphatic histiocytosis. *Eur Arch Otorhinolayngol*. 2016;273:783-788.
32. Kemps PG, Buijs J, Verdijk RM, Ledeboer QCP, Baatenburg de Jong RJ, van Laar JAM. Persistent laryngeal swelling caused by primary intralymphatic histiocytosis. *JAMA Otolaryngol Head Neck Surg*. 2020;146:675-677.
33. Mazloom SE, Stallings A, Kyei A. Differentiating intralymphatic histiocytosis, invascular histiocytosis, and subtypes of reactive angioendotheliomatosis: review of clinical and histologic features of all cases reported to date. *Am J Dermatopathol*. 2017;39:33-39.
34. Tappeiner J, Pfleger L. Angioendotheliomatosis proliferans systematisata. A clinically and pathohistologically new disease picture [in German]. *Hautarzt*. 1963;14:67-70.
35. Wick MR, Rocamora A. Reactive and malignant "angioendotheliomatosis": a discriminant clinicopathological study. *J Cutan Pathol*. 1988;15:260-271.
36. Ponzoni M, Campo E, Nakamura S. Intravascular large B-cell lymphoma: a chameleon with multiple faces and many masks. *Blood*. 2018;132(15):1561-1567.
37. Matsue K, Abe Y, Narita K, et al. Diagnosis of intravascular large B cell lymphoma: novel insights into clinicopathological features from 42 patients at a single institution over 20 years. *Br J Haematol*. 2019;187(3):328-336.
38. Ruiter M, Mandema E. New cutaneous syndrome in subacute bacterial endocarditis. *Arch Intern Med*. 1964;113:175-182.

39. Fievez M, Fievez C, Hustin J. Proliferating systematized angioendotheliomatosis. *Arch Dermatol*. 1971;104:320-324.
40. Pasyk K, Depowski M. Proliferating systematized angioendotheliomatosis of a 5-month-old infant. *Arch Dermatol*. 1978;114:1512-1515.
41. Martin S, Pitcher D, Tschen J, et al. Reactive angioendotheliomatosis. *J Am Acad Dermatol*. 1980;2:117-123.
42. Person JR. Systemic angioendotheliomatosis: a possible disorder of a circulating angiogenic factor. *Br J Dermatol*. 1997;96:329-331.
43. Cohen SJ, Pittelkow MR, Su WPD. Cutaneous manifestations of cryoglobulinemia: clinical and histopathologic study of seventy two patients. *J Am Acad Dermatol*. 1991;25:21-27.
44. LeBoit PE, Solomon AR, Santa Cruz DJ, et al. Angiomatosis with luminal cryoprotein deposition. *J Am Acad Dermatol*. 1992;27:969-973.
45. Lazova R, Slater C, Scott G. Reactive angioendotheliomatosis. Case report and review of the literature. *Am J Dermatopathol*. 1996;18:63-69.
46. Creamer D, Black MM, Calonje E. Reactive angioendotheliomatosis in association with the antiphospholipid syndrome. *J Am Acad Dermatol*. 2000;42(pt. 2):903-906.
47. Krell JM, Sanchez RL, Solomon AR. Diffuse dermal angiomatosis: a variant of reactive cutaneous angioendotheliomatosis. *J Cutan Pathol*. 1994;21:363-370.
48. Quinn TR, Alora MB, Momtaz KT, et al. Reactive angioendotheliomatosis with underlying hepatopathy and hypertensive portal gastropathy. *Int J Dermatol*. 1998;37:382-385.
49. Judge MR, McGibbon DH, Thompson RP. Angioendotheliomatosis associated with Castleman's lymphoma and POEMS syndrome. *Clin Exp Dermatol*. 1993;18:360-362.
50. Tomasini C, Soro E, Pippione M. Angioendotheliomatosis in a woman with rheumatoid arthritis. *Am J Dermatopathol*. 2000;22:334-338.
51. McMenamin ME, Fletcher CD. Reactive angioendotheliomatosis: a study of 15 cases demonstrating a wide clinicopathologic spectrum. *Am J Surg Pathol*. 2002;26:685-697.
52. Aung PP, Ballester LY, Goldberg LJ, et al. Incidental simultaneous finding of intravascular histiocytosis and reactive angioendotheliomatosis: a case report. *Am J Dermatopathol*. 2015;37:401-404.
53. Chen XF, Ong NWR, Tang PY, Pang SM, Sittampalam K. Glomeruloid haemangioma pattern in reactive angioendotheliomatosis leading to the diagnosis of POEMS syndrome. *Pathology*. 2021;53(2):273-276.
54. Di Filippo Y, Cardot-Leccia N, Long-Mira E, et al. Reactive angioendotheliomatosis revealing a glomerulopathy secondary to a monoclonal gammopathy successfully treated with lenalidomide. *J Eur Acad Dermatol Venereol*. 2021;35(2):e115-e118. doi:10.1111/jdv.16840. Epub 2020 Aug 17. PMID: 32735354.
55. Wick MR, Mills SE, Scheithauer BW, et al. Reassessment of malignant angioendotheliomatosis: evidence in favour of its reclassification as "intravascular lymphomatosis.". *Am J Surg Pathol*. 1986;10:112-123.
56. Ferry JA, Harris NL, Picker LJ, et al. Intravascular lymphomatosis (malignant angioendotheliomatosis). A B-cell neoplasm expressing surface homing receptors. *Mod Pathol*. 1988;1:444-452.
57. Molina A, Lombard C, Donlon T, et al. Immunohistochemical and cytogenetic studies indicate that malignant angioendotheliomatosis is a primary intravascular (angiotropic) lymphoma. *Cancer*. 1990;66:474-479.
58. Goyal A, LeBlanc RE, Carter JB. Cutaneous B-cell lymphoma. *Hematol Oncol Clin N Am*. 2019;33(1):149-161.
59. Grimm KE, O'Malley DP. Aggressive B cell lymphomas in the 2017 revised WHO classification of tumors of hematopoietic and lymphoid tissues. *Ann Diagn Pathol*. 2019;38:6-10.
60. Hope CB, Pincus LB. Primary cutaneous B-cell lymphomas with large cell predominance-primary cutaneous follicle center lymphoma, diffuse large B-cell lymphoma, leg type and intravascular large B-cell lymphoma. *Semin Diagn Pathol*. 2017;34(1):85-98.
61. Nakamura S, Ponzoni M, Campo E. Intravascular large B-cell lymphoma. In: Swerdlow SH, Campo E, Harris NL, et al., eds. *WHO Classification of Tumours of Haematopoietic and Lymphoid Tissues*. 4th ed. International Agency for Research on Cancer; 2008:296-298.
62. Sepp N, Schuler G, Romani N, et al. "Intravascular lymphomatosis" (angioendotheliomatosis): evidence for a T-cell origin of two cases. *Hum Pathol*. 1990;21:1051-1058.
63. Shimokawa I, Higami Y, Sakai H, et al. Intravascular malignant lymphomatosis: a case of T cell lymphoma probably associated with human T cell lymphotropic virus. *Hum Pathol*. 1991;22:200-202.
64. Sangueza OP, Hyder DM, Sangueza P. Intravascular lymphomatosis: report of an unusual case with T cell phenotype occurring in an adolescent male. *J Cutan Pathol*. 1992;19:226-231.
65. Cerroni L, Massone C, Kutzner H, et al. Intravascular large T-cell or NKcell lymphoma. A rare variant of intravascular large cell lymphoma with frequent cytotoxic phenotype and association with Epstein–Barr virus infection. *Am J Surg Pathol*. 2008;32:891-898.
66. Fujikura K, Yoshida M, Uesaka K. Transcriptome complexity in intravascular NK/T-cell lymphoma. *J Clin Pathol*. 2020;73(10):671-675. doi:10.1136/jclinpath-2020-206461. Epub 2020 Mar 18. PMID: 32188628.
67. Samols MA, Su A, Ra S, et al. Intralymphatic cutaneous anaplastic large cell lymphoma/lymphomatoid papulosis: expanding the spectrum of CD30-positive lymphoproliferative disorders. *Am J Surg Pathol*. 2014;38(9):1203-1211.
68. Ferrara G, Ena L, Cota C, Cerroni L. Intralymphatic spread is a common finding in cutaneous CD30+ lymphoproliferative disorders. *Am J Surg Pathol*. 2015;39(11):1511-1517.
69. Baum CL, Stone MS, Liu V. Atypical intravascular CD30+ T-cell proliferation following trauma in a healthy 17-year-old male: first reported case of a potential diagnostic pitfall and literature review. *J Cutan Pathol*. 2009;36(3):350-354.
70. Ardighieri L, Lonardi S, Vermi W, Medicina D, Cerroni L, Facchetti F. Intralymphatic atypical T-cell proliferation in a cutaneous hemangioma. *J Cutan Pathol*. 2010;37(4):497-503.
71. Riveiro-Falkenbach E, Fernández-Figueras MT, Rodríguez-Peralto JL. Benign atypical intravascular CD30(+) T-cell proliferation: a reactive condition mimicking intravascular lymphoma. *Am J Dermatopathol*. 2013;35(2):143-150.
72. Kempf W, Keller K, John H, Dommann-Scherrer C. Benign atypical intravascular CD30+ T-cell proliferation: a recently described reactive lymphoproliferative process and simulator of intravascular lymphoma – report of a case associated with lichen sclerosus and review of the literature. *Am J Clin Pathol*. 2014;142(5):694-699.
73. Kailas A, Elston DM, Crater SE, Cerruto CA. Cutaneous intravascular CD30+ T-cell pseudolymphoma occurring in a regressing keratoacanthoma. *J Cutan Pathol*. 2018;45(4):296-298.

74. Calamaro P, Cerroni L. Intralymphatic proliferation of T-cell lymphoid blasts in the setting of hidradenitis suppurativa. *Am J Dermatopathol.* 2016;38(7):536-540.
75. Weingertner N, Mitcov M, Chenard MP, Cribier B. Intralymphatic CD30+ T-cell proliferation during DRESS: a mimic of intravascular lymphoma. *J Cutan Pathol.* 2016;43(11):1036-1040.
76. Gralewski J, Post GR. Cutaneous intralymphatic CD30+ pseudolymphoma: a reactive condition mimicking lymphoma. *Blood.* 2018;132(17):1859.
77. Washio K, Nakata K, Nakamura A, et al. Pressure bandage as an effective treatment for intralymphatic histiocytosis associated with rheumatoid arthritis. *Dermatology.* 2011;223:20-24.
78. Tsujiawki M, Hata H, Miyauchi T, et al. Warty intralymphatic histiocytosis successfully treated with topical tacrolimus. *J Eur Acad Dermatol Venereol.* 2015;29(11):2267-2269.
79. Nakajima T, Kawabata D, Nakabo S, et al. Successful treatment with tocilizumab in a case of intralymphatic histiocytosis associated with rheumatoid arthritis. *Intern Med.* 2014;53:2255-2258.
80. Kanerva M, Moilanen K, Virolainen S, et al.. Melkersson–Rosenthal syndrome. *Otolaryngol Head Neck Surg.* 2008;138:245-251.
81. Elias MK, Mateen FJ, Weiler CR. The Melkersson–Rosenthal syndrome: a retrospective study of biopsied cases. *J Neurol.* 2013;260:138-142.
82. Liu R, Yu S. Melkersson–Rosenthal syndrome: a review of seven patients. *J Clin Neurosci.* 2013;20:993-995.
83. Wiesenfeld D, Ferguson MM, Mitchell DN, et al. Oro-facial granulomatosis—a clinical and pathological analysis. *Q J Med.* 1985;54:101-113.
84. Rogers RSIII. Melkersson–Rosenthal syndrome and orofacial granulomatosis. *Dermatol Clin.* 1996;14:371-379.
85. Wehl G, Rauchenzauner M. A systematic review of the literature of the three related disease entities cheilitis granulomatosa, orofacial granulomatosis and Melkersson–Rosenthal syndrome. *Curr Pediatr Rev.* 2018;14(3):196-203.
86. Rawlings NG, Valenzuela AA, Allen LH, et al. Isolated eyelid edema in Melkersson–Rosenthal syndrome: a case series. *Eye.* 2012;26:163-166.
87. Chen X, Jakobiec FA, Yadav P, Werdich XQ, Fay A. Melkersson-Rosenthal syndrome with isolated unilateral eyelid edema: an immunopathologic study. *Ophthalmic Plast Reconstr Surg.* 2015;31(3):e70-7. doi:10.1097/IOP.0000000000000088. PMID: 24853119.
88. Roseman B, Fryns JP, Van DBC. Melkersson–Rosenthal syndrome in a 7-year-old girl. *Pediatrics.* 1975;61:490-491.
89. Yuzuk S, Trau H, Levy A, et al. Melkersson–Rosenthal syndrome. *Int J Dermatol.* 1985;24:456-457.
90. Cohen HA, Cohen Z, Ashkenasi A, et al. Melkersson–Rosenthal syndrome. *Cutis.* 1994;54:327-328.
91. Bohra S, Kariya PB, Bargale SD, et al. Clinicopathological significance of Melkersson–Rosenthal syndrome. *BMJ Case Rep.* 2015; pii: bcr2015210138. doi:10.1136/bcr-2015-210138
92. Gavioli CF, Florezi GP, Lourenço SV, Nico MM. Clinical profile of Melkersson–Rosenthal syndrome/orofacial granulomatosis: a review of 51 patients. *J Cutan Med Surg.* 2021:1203475421995132. doi:10.1177/1203475421995132. Epub ahead of print. PMID: 33573395.
93. Bakshi SS. Melkersson–Rosenthal syndrome. *J Allergy Clin Immunol Pract.* 2017;5(2):471-472.
94. Savasta S, Rossi A, Foiadelli T, et al. Melkersson–Rosenthal syndrome in childhood: report of three paediatric cases and a review of the literature. *Int J Environ Res Publ Health.* 2019;16(7):1289.
95. Halevy S, Shalom G, Trattner A, et al. Melkersson–Rosenthal syndrome: a possible association with psoriasis. *J Am Acad Dermatol.* 2012;67:795-796.
96. Hornstein OP. Melkersson–Rosenthal syndrome: a neuro-muco-cutaneus disease of complex origin. *Curr Probl Dermatol.* 1973;5:117-156.
97. Kamainagakura E, Jorge J. Melkersson–Rosenthal syndrome: a histopathologic mystery and dermatologic challenge. *J Cutan Pathol.* 2011;38:241-245.
98. Pei Y, Beaman GM, Mansfield D, Clayton-Smith J, Stewart M, Newman WG. Clinical and genetic heterogeneity in Melkersson–Rosenthal syndrome. *Eur J Med Genet.* 2019;62(6):103536.
99. Green RM, Rogers RSIII. Melkersson–Rosenthal syndrome: a review of 36 patients. *J Am Acad Dermatol.* 1989;21:1263-1270.
100. Orlando MR, Atkjns JS Jr. Melkersson–Rosenthal syndrome. *Arch Otolaryngol Head Neck Surg.* 1990;116:728-729.
101. Thomas P, Walchner M, Ghoreschi K, et al. Successful treatment of granulomatous cheilitis with thalidomide. *Arch Dermatol.* 2003;139:136-138.
102. Barry O, Barry J, Langan S, et al. Treatment of granulomatous cheilitis with infliximab. *Arch Dermatol.* 2005;141:1080-1082.
103. Ratzinger G, Sepp N, Vogetseder W, et al. Cheilitis granulomatosa and Melkersson–Rosenthal syndrome: evaluation of gastrointestinal involvement and therapeutic regimens in a series of 14 patients. *J Eur Acad Dermatol Venereol.* 2007;21:1065-1070.
104. Camacho F, García-Bravo B, Carrizosa A. Treatment of Miescher's cheilitis granulomatosa in Melkersson–Rosenthal syndrome. *J Eur Acad Dermatol Venereol.* 2001;15:546-549.
105. Mignogna MD, Fedele S, Lo Russo L, et al. Effectiveness of small-volume, intralesional, delayed-release triamcinolone injections in orofacial granulomatosis: a pilot study. *J Am Acad Dermatol.* 2004;51:265-268.
106. Ratzinger G, Sepp N. Dapsone in combination with topical triamcinolone as a therapeutic option for cheilitis granulomatosa and Melkersson–Rosenthal disease?. *J Eur Acad Dermatol Venereol.* 2008;22:1027-1028.
107. Sobjanek M, Włodarkiewicz A, Z´elazny I, et al. Successful treatment of Melkersson–Rosenthal syndrome with dapsone and triamcinolone injections. *J Eur Acad Dermatol Venereol.* 2008;22:1028-1030.
108. Oliver DW, Scott MJ. Lip reduction cheiloplasty for Miescher's granulomatous macrocheilitis (cheilitis granulomatosa) in childhood. *Clin Exp Dermatol.* 2002;27:129-131.
109. Kruse-Lösler B, Presser D, Metze D, et al. Surgical treatment of persistent macrocheilia in patients with Melkersson–Rosenthal syndrome and cheilitis granulomatosa. *Arch Dermatol.* 2005;141:1085-1091.
110. Henry CH. Orofacial granulomatosis: report of a case with decreased CD4/CD8 ratio. *J Oral Maxillofac Surg.* 1994;52:317.
111. Facchetti F, Signorini S, Majorana A, et al. Non-specific influx of T-cell receptor alpha/beta and gamma/delta lymphocytes in mucosal biopsies from a patient with orofacial granulomatosis. *J Oral Pathol Med.* 2000;29:519.

112. Boparai RS, Levin AM, Lelli GJ Jr. Morbihan disease treatment: two case reports and a systematic literature review. *Ophthalmic Plast Reconstr Surg*. 2019;35:126-132.
113. Nagasaka T, Koyama T, Matsumura K, et al. Persistent lymphedema in Morbihan disease: formation of perilymphatic epithelioid cell granulomas as a possible pathogenesis. *Clin Exp Dermatol*. 2008;33:764-767.
114. Ramirez-Bellver JL, Perez-Gonzalez YC, Chen KR, et al. Clinicopathologic and immunohistochemical study of 14 cases of Morbihan disease: an insight into its pathogenesis. *Am J Dermatopathol*. 2019;41:701-710.
115. Belousova IE, Kastnerova L, Khairutdinov VR, et al. Unilateral periocular intralymphatic histiocytosis, associated with rosacea (Morbihan disease). *Am J Dermatopathol*. 2020;42:452-454.

PART XII — LYMPHOID PROLIFERATIONS OF SPECIAL SITES/SPECIAL POPULATIONS

CHAPTER 70

Oral lymphoproliferative disorders

Kristin K. McNamara

INTRODUCTION

Lymphoproliferative diseases (LPDs) that affect the oral region are incredibly diverse. The clinicopathologic spectrum ranges from reactive lymphoid hyperplasia to relentlessly aggressive forms of lymphoma. Although relatively uncommon, lymphoid malignancies are ranked third in incidence of oral malignant disease, following squamous cell carcinoma and salivary gland neoplasms. This chapter will explore a selection of the most common and significant LPDs affecting the oral soft and hard tissues. Important elements of clinical presentation, histopathologic findings, and patient management will be discussed, with emphasis on oral cavity manifestations of these disease processes.

LEUKEMIA

Leukemia represents a group of disorders that result from the uncontrolled proliferation of a clone of hematopoietic stem cells, initially occupying bone marrow and eventually overflowing into the peripheral blood. The disease is generally classified according to histogenetic origin (myeloid or lymphoid) and clinical behavior (acute or chronic). Thus, the four primary categories of leukemia are *acute myeloid leukemia* (*AML*), *acute lymphoblastic leukemia* (*ALL*), *chronic myeloid leukemia* (*CML*), and *chronic lymphocytic leukemia* (*CLL*), although multiple subclassifications are recognized within this diagnostic framework.[1,2]

The annual incidence of leukemia in the United States is over 60,000, representing ~3% of the overall cancer burden.[3] Although the acute leukemias are diagnosed across a broad age range, ALL is generally a childhood disease and AML is more often seen in adults. Chronic leukemia is primarily seen in adults, and CLL, the most common type of leukemia, is typically diagnosed in men over 50 years of age.[1,2] If untreated, acute leukemia is expected to follow an aggressive clinical course resulting in death in a matter of months, but chronic leukemia is typically more indolent and expected to slowly progress over many years. The clinical course, however, is quite variable.

The etiology of leukemia is uncertain, although both environmental and genetic factors seem to contribute. Viral infection, ionizing radiation, and chemical exposure to benzene and pesticides have been associated with increased risk.[1,2] Multiple genetic syndromes, such as Down syndrome, Bloom syndrome, neurofibromatosis type I, and Fanconi anemia, are also known risk factors.[1] A variety of specific cytogenetic abnormalities have been linked with most forms of leukemia, with the Philadelphia chromosome associated with CML being the first chromosomal abnormality detected.[4] Early genetic alterations in hematopoietic stem cells may lead to *myelodysplastic syndrome*, a rare group of hematologic disorders thought to represent a precursor stage in the evolution of AML.[5,6]

Given the diverse and complex nature of leukemias, as well as the varied treatment approaches and prognoses associated with each of the many subclassifications, this discussion is limited to aspects of the disease that relate to the oral cavity and head and neck region.

The presenting signs and symptoms of an acute leukemia are generally related to bone marrow suppression. Malignant leukemic cells replace normal hematopoietic cells in the marrow, causing *myelophthisic anemia*. Resultant pancytopenia may manifest as fatigue, dyspnea, easy bruising/bleeding, and infection. Patients may also experience flu-like symptoms with bone and/or joint pain secondary to the bone marrow infiltration.[1,2] The development of a chronic leukemia is typically more insidious and ~50% of patients will be diagnosed incidentally on the basis of blood studies performed for unrelated purposes.[1] Although constitutional symptoms are uncommon in this group, hepatosplenomegaly and lymphadenopathy may be found on physical examination.

Oral manifestations are more often observed in association with acute forms of leukemia, but may also arise in the setting of a chronic leukemia. The most common oral manifestations include petechiae and spontaneous gingival hemorrhage, which may be accompanied by gingival enlargement.[6,7] Oral mucosal ulcerations, secondary to neutropenia or local infection, may also be seen.[6] Oral candidiasis and herpetic infections are common. Herpetic infections typically represent reactivation of the latent virus and may involve any oral mucosa surface, which contrasts with the clinical distribution of lesions in immunocompetent individuals that are limited to keratinized surfaces of the hard palate and attached gingiva. Leukemic infiltration of salivary glands, tonsils, and lymph nodes may lead to clinical enlargement of these structures, a manifestation most often seen with CLL[7] (Fig. 70-1). This infiltrate may be referred to as *small lymphocytic lymphoma (SLL)*, particularly in the absence of a known leukemic (CLL) setting. Given identical morphologic and immunophenotypic profiles, SLL and CLL are thought to represent different manifestations of the same disease process. SLL/CLL may also occasionally result in palatal enlargement.[7] Leukemic infiltration of the oral mucosa is *most often* seen in association with the monocytic subtype of AML. This generally results in diffuse, boggy, nontender gingival enlargement.[6,8] Occasionally, a solitary tumor-like growth will develop and this is referred to as *myeloid sarcoma (MS)* (previously termed *granulocytic sarcoma*). Historically, this has been called "chloroma" owing to a greenish color observed on the freshly cut surface of the tumor.[9]

MS is an extramedullary collection of malignant myeloid cells that clinically forms a mass and is strongly associated with myeloid leukemia. It can occur in virtually any anatomic region, but most commonly involves subperiosteal bone and soft tissues, skin, lymph nodes, and the gastrointestinal tract.[9,10] While intraoral involvement is rare, it is strongly associated with AML and may be the initial manifestation of the disease.[10,11] A few cases of intraoral MS have been reported in association with CML.[12] Oral mucosal sites include the gingiva, palate, buccal mucosa, tongue, and lips. The typical clinical presentation is a solitary, possibly ulcerated, mass that ranges in color from normal (pink) to red, purple, or bluish-black[13-15] (Fig. 70-2). Bony involvement of the mandible and maxilla may occur, which has been reported in the setting of nonhealing extraction sites or mimicking periapical inflammatory disease.[13,14]

Histopathologic assessment of tissues infiltrated by a leukemic cell population reveals destruction of normal tissue architecture by a diffuse proliferation of immature cells with either myeloid or lymphoid features (Figs. 70-3 and 70-4). Classifying the type of leukemia requires immunophenotyping, performed on solid tissue and/or flow cytometry (Fig. 70-5). Cytogenetic testing and molecular testing also play an increasingly vital role from a diagnostic and risk stratification standpoint.

Patient management and prognosis are highly variable and dependent on multiple factors, including patient age and presence of comorbid conditions, type of leukemia, and associated cytogenetic alterations. Treatment strategies may include various forms of chemotherapy, monoclonal antibodies, tyrosine kinase inhibitors, and other targeted therapeutics, as well as radiation or hematopoietic stem cell transplantation (HSCT). One of the major success stories in cancer management is related to the treatment of ALL of childhood. While this condition used to be uniformly fatal, cure rates for children and adolescents are now approaching 90%.[16] In contrast, AML is still associated with significant morbidity and mortality.[17] Recent introduction of tyrosine kinase inhibitors in therapeutic management of CML has been associated with dramatic improvement in 5-year survival rates, with most centers reporting up to 87% long-term survival.[4] Despite dramatic advancements in treatment strategies, CLL remains an incurable disease outside the setting of hematologic stem cell transplantation. The clinical course is highly variable, with median survival at diagnosis ranging between 1 and more than 10 years.[18] A prognostic index has been developed using a weighted grading of independent risk factors, which separates CLL patients into 4 risk groups with overall 5-year survival rates ranging from 18% to 95%.[19]

Oral mucosal treatment-related complications often arise secondary to myeloablative therapy. *Oral mucositis* may develop a few days after the start of chemotherapy and slowly resolve within 2 to 3 weeks following cessation of the cytotoxic drugs. Sites of involvement typically include nonkeratinized surfaces, such as the labial mucosa, buccal mucosa, ventrolateral tongue, soft palate, and floor of mouth. Lesions clinically present as patchy areas of erythema and atrophy that evolve to form ulcerations. Neutropenic ulcerations and oral infections may also occur secondary to treatment-related myelosuppression. The significance of

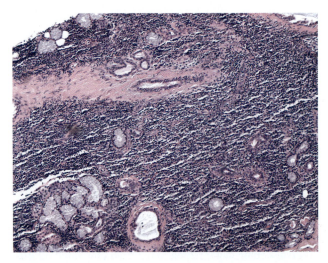

FIGURE 70-1. Chronic lymphocytic leukemia/small lymphocytic lymphoma. An 86-year-old man with a history of CLL exhibits a monotonous population of small lymphocytes infiltrating an accessory salivary gland, resulting in effacement of the glandular architecture (H&E, 100×).

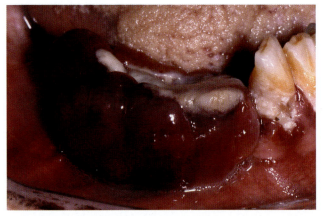

FIGURE 70-2. Myeloid sarcoma. The ulcerated soft tissue mass of the mandibular gingiva represents an extramedullary collection of malignant myeloid cells.

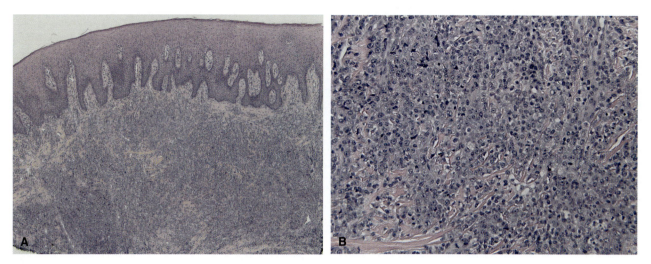

FIGURE 70-3. Myeloid sarcoma. A diffuse malignant mononuclear infiltrate presenting in the gingiva of a 100-year-old woman, consistent with MS (**A** and **B**, H&E; 100× and 200×).

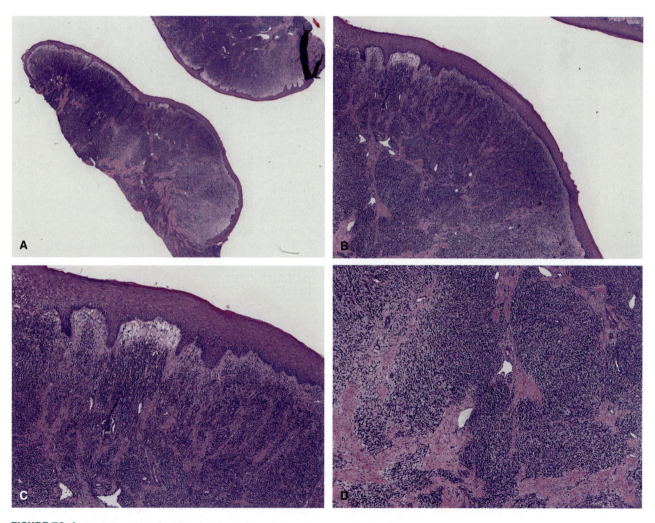

FIGURE 70-4. Myeloid sarcoma. A diffuse malignant infiltrate in the submucosa is present with a grenz zone between the overlying squamous mucosa (**A** and **B**, H&E; 10× and 40×). The infiltrate dissects through the collagen fibers (**C** and **D**, H&E; 100× and 200×). High magnifications show that the infiltrate is composed of medium-sized cells with fine chromatin and no distinctive nucleoli. The cells show a monocytoid appearance (**E** and **F**, H&E; 200× and 400×).

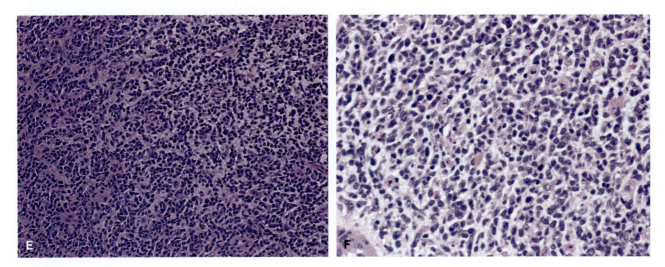

FIGURE 70-4. (continued)

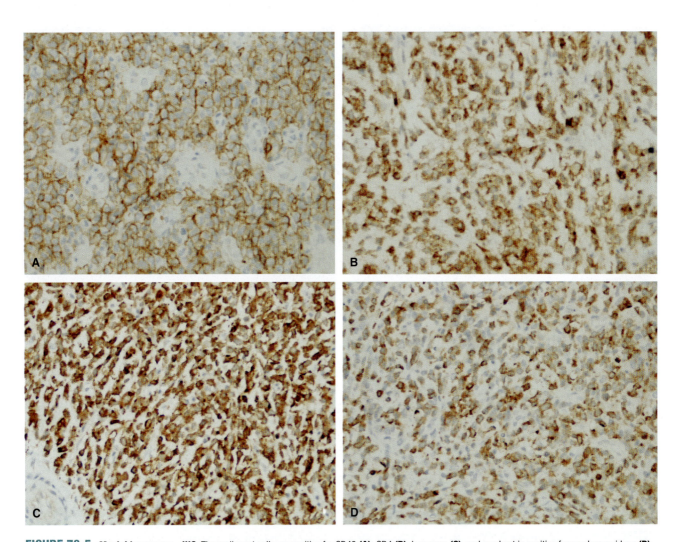

FIGURE 70-5. Myeloid sarcoma—IHC. The malignant cells are positive for CD43 **(A)**, CD4 **(B)**, lysozyme **(C)**, and a subset is positive for myeloperoxidase **(D)**.

such lesions, in addition to causing considerable pain and discomfort, is that breakdown in the mucosal barrier may allow entryway for systemic bacterial, fungal, and viral infections. Additionally, the presence of severe oral lesions may significantly delay or alter the designed treatment regimen, thus impacting cancer control and overall prognosis. Meticulous oral hygiene, antimicrobials, and systemic antibiotics are of paramount importance, which may be used in conjunction with systemic analgesics and topical agents for palliative care. In addition to topical anesthetics, various bioadherent oral rinses are available to coat, hydrate, and lubricate the oral mucosa. Prophylactic cryotherapy is also frequently used. Numerous novel agents, such as keratinocyte growth factor-1, fibroblast growth factor-7, transforming growth factor-β3, granulocyte–macrophage colony-stimulating factor, and interleukin-11, are also being evaluated for their protective properties.[20,21] Additionally, patients who have undergone allogenic bone marrow transplantation will be at risk for development of lichenoid oral mucosal lesions and oral ulcerations associated with *graft-versus-host disease*. These lesions clinically mimic lichen planus and are associated with increased risk for development of oral epithelial dysplasia and oral squamous cell carcinoma.[22]

LANGERHANS CELL HISTIOCYTOSIS

Synonyms: Histiocytosis X, Langerhans cell disease, idiopathic histiocytosis, and eosinophilic granuloma.

Langerhans cell histiocytosis (LCH) is a rare group of disorders characterized by proliferation of histiocytic cells phenotypically similar to Langerhans cells. It has long been debated whether LCH is a malignant or reactive condition, but clonality studies have shown the proliferation to be monoclonal, consistent with a neoplastic process. Nonetheless, the natural history of the disease ranges from rapidly progressive and fatal, to chronic and relapsing, to spontaneously regressing.[23] The clinical presentation is also quite variable, and LCH has been classified into three distinct forms: single-system single site, single-system multisite, and multisystem types. Single-organ system disease is most common and typically presents as solitary or multifocal osteolytic bone lesions ("eosinophilic granuloma"); however, lungs, soft tissues (skin and mucosa), and the central nervous system are also common sites of involvement.[24] This disease is generally seen in older children and young adults, with the majority of patients diagnosed before age 20.[23] Multiorgan system disease is less common and has traditionally been designated as *Letterer–Siwe disease* (acute disseminated histiocytosis), occurring in infants, and *Hand–Schüller–Christian disease* (chronic disseminated histiocytosis), occurring in children. However, it is now understood that significant clinical overlap exists between these multisystem designations and the classification has largely been dismissed. In addition to bone, multisystem disease often involves skin as an eczematous exanthem, with possible visceral sites to include the liver, lungs, pituitary, spleen, lymph nodes, and bone marrow.[23,24] Visceral involvement is uncommon in adult patients, but when present is a sign of poor prognosis.[24,25] LCH can involve virtually any bone; however, the skull, ribs, vertebrae, and mandible are most often affected.[23,26]

Oral and maxillofacial lesions are frequently encountered in LCH, particularly in adult patients, with involvement of the jaws in up to 77% of cases.[27] In addition, oral manifestations may be the initial or only sign of disease. Pain or tenderness is often the initial clinical finding; however, bone lesions may also be discovered incidentally on dental radiographs taken for routine dental care. The condition typically presents with punched-out radiolucencies that lack a corticated rim, although they may also be ill defined. The posterior mandible is most commonly affected, and lesions have classically been described as appearing "scooped out" with "teeth floating in air" owing to the tendency for superficial alveolar bone destruction.[23,28,29] This disease pattern and resultant loosening of teeth may clinically mimic severe periodontitis (Fig. 70-6). Lesions occurring within the body of the mandible or maxilla may also radiographically resemble periapical inflammatory disease. Ulcerative or exophytic lesions of the overlying oral mucosa may occur if the disease breaks out of bone, but occasionally LCH may be limited to oral soft tissues.[30]

The histopathologic features of LCH consist of a diffuse infiltrate of large, pale-staining mononuclear cells with abundant eosinophilic to amphophilic cytoplasm and indistinct borders, resembling histiocytes. Vesicular nuclei appear rounded to reniform, with deep indentations or grooves. The presence of eosinophils is characteristic, but varies from a prominent infiltrate to sparse or even absent. Lymphocytes, plasma cells, and occasional multinucleated giant cells may also be observed (Fig. 70-7). Hemorrhage and necrosis within this lesion are not unusual; however, mitotic activity tends to be low to moderate and without atypical mitoses.[23,25] The gold standard for diagnosis has traditionally been electron microscopic identification of rod-shaped cytoplasmic structures known as Birbeck granules, which differentiate Langerhans cells from other mononuclear cells. Although this technique may still prove helpful in difficult-to-characterize tumors, it is rarely necessary today.[23] Immunohistochemistry (IHC) is generally used to identify lesional Langerhans cells on the basis of their reactivity to antibodies directed against either CD1a or CD207 (langerin), the latter being quite sensitive and specific for Langerhans cells. Lesional cells will also show affinity for antibodies directed against S100 protein; however, this marker shows less specificity

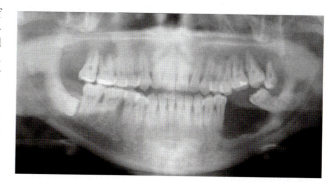

FIGURE 70-6. Langerhans cell histiocytosis. Panoramic radiograph demonstrates severe alveolar bone loss of the right and left posterior maxilla and left posterior mandible, resulting in a "floating-in-air" appearance of the posterior maxillary teeth and a "scooped out" appearance of the mandible.

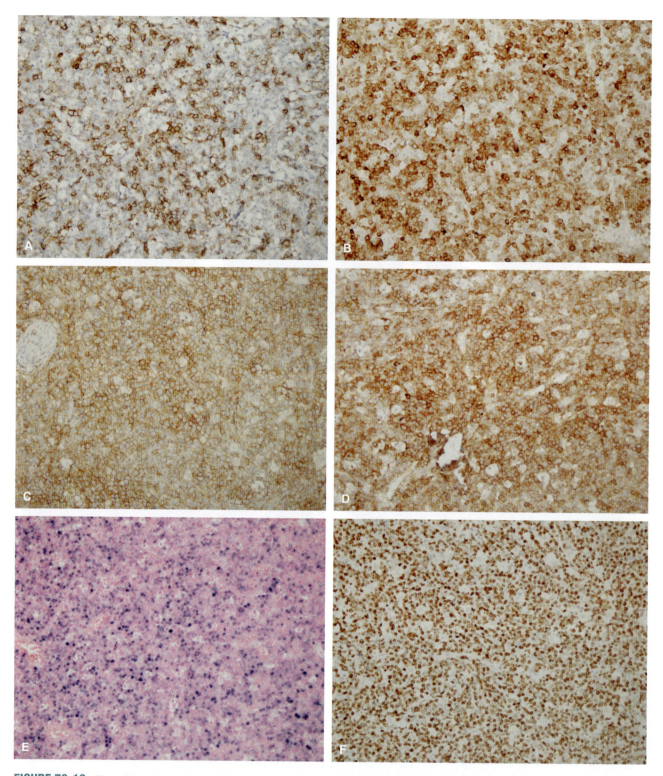

FIGURE 70-13. Plasmablastic lymphoma—IHC. The malignant cells are positive for CD79a **(B)**, CD44 **(C)**, EMA **(D)**, whereas they are predominantly negative for CD20 **(A)**. EBER is diffusely positive in the cells **(E)**. Ki-67 shows an extraordinary high (>95%) proliferation index **(F)**.

occurring in the oral cavity are quite rare.[44] Histopathologic features include small lymphocytes that resemble centrocytes admixed with a smaller population of larger cells resembling centroblasts. A prominent nodular growth pattern is characteristic, recapitulating poorly formed follicles. Tumor cells typically express B-cell markers and CD10. BCL-2 is also frequently overexpressed in these tumors, reflective of the characteristic BCL-2 gene translocation t(14; 18) (q32; q21).[39,44] FL is generally considered an indolent and incurable malignancy, although the possibility for transformation to DLBCL exists and is associated with poor prognosis.[42,44]

Extranodal Marginal Zone B-Cell Lymphoma

Extranodal marginal zone B-cell lymphoma represents a group of B-cell neoplasms that are composed of cells that resemble lymphocytes of the normal marginal zone. When arising in areas containing mucosa-associated lymphatic tissue, these are termed *mucosa-associated lymphoid tissue (MALT) lymphoma*. These tumors typically arise in areas of chronic inflammation and most commonly occur in the gastrointestinal tract in association with *H. pylori*. Oral mucosal lesions are well described and often associated with Sjögren syndrome or other autoimmune diseases such as lupus erythematosus or rheumatoid arthritis.[44,48] Patients with Sjögren syndrome or lymphoepithelial sialadenitis have a 44-fold increased risk of developing lymphoma, and the vast majority of these tumors will be of the MALT subtype.[39] MALT lymphoma of the oral cavity generally presents as a painless soft tissue swelling, frequently in association with minor salivary glands of the palate; however, other anatomic sites harboring salivary tissue, such as the labial or buccal mucosa, may also be affected.[52,53] Histopathologically, MALT lymphomas exhibit cytologic heterogeneity. Tumor cells are small- to medium-sized and are typically seen surrounding reactive B-cell follicles, but may evolve into a more sheet-like growth pattern (Figs. 70-14–70-16). The neoplastic cells often exhibit slightly irregular nuclei and abundant cytoplasm, resembling centrocytes, although plasmacytic differentiation is also frequently encountered. Lesional cells may occasionally resemble small lymphocytes, making histologic distinction from a reactive lymphoid infiltrate difficult. When glandular tissues are involved, so-called *lymphoepithelial lesions* may develop because of infiltration of the epithelium. Neoplastic cells typically express CD21 and CD35 in addition to pan–B-cell markers. Immunoglobulin light-chain restriction is also characteristic. Lack of expression of CD5, cyclin D1, and CD10 is helpful in ruling out the other small-cell lymphomas, such as SLL, mantle cell lymphoma (MCL), and FL, respectively (Fig. 70-17).[39,53] Up to half of cases will show a characteristic t(11; 18) (q21; q21) chromosomal translocation.[44] MALT lymphoma characteristically follows an indolent course, is slow to disseminate, and demonstrates a high response rate to conventional therapies, such as surgical excision, radiotherapy, and rituximab with or without combination chemotherapy. Recent investigations have focused on less aggressive, chemotherapy-free approaches using immunomodulators and targeted therapies for tumor control without acute and chronic toxicity.[54] Transformation to DLBCL is possible and confers a poorer prognosis.[39]

Small Lymphocytic Lymphoma

SLL is defined as a soft tissue neoplasm of small monomorphic B lymphocytes that infiltrate and destroy normal tissue architecture and typically coexpress CD5 and CD23. The neoplastic cells are morphologically and phenotypically identical to those of CLL; thus, these entities are believed to represent different manifestations of the same disease process.[39,44] Whereas the oral cavity is occasionally affected, oral mucosal involvement in a nonleukemic setting is uncommon. SLL/CLL is typically an indolent but incurable disease, with a 2%-8% chance for transformation to a more aggressive DLBCL.[39]

Mantle Cell Lymphoma

MCL is a rare small-to-medium–sized B-cell neoplasm arising from the mantle zone of lymphoid follicles. Lymph nodes, bone marrow, and spleen are most commonly involved, with few reported cases of primary MCL arising within the oral cavity.[55] A small series of oral cases reported a male predominance with mean age of 71 years. Sites of involvement include the palate, floor of mouth, and tongue.[55] Histopathologic evaluation shows a monomorphic CD20+ B-cell population arranged in solid sheets or vague nodules, with coexpression of CD5 and CD43. The characteristic translocation t(11; 14) (q13; q32) results in overexpression of CCND1. The vast majority of cases are positive for SOX-11. CD10 and CD23 are generally negative, which help differentiate MCL from FL and SSL/CLL, respectively.[44] Best practices in therapeutic management of MCL are currently not known. While aggressive treatment approaches, such as high-dose chemotherapy with autologous stem cell transplantation, continue to be emphasized, a better understanding of MCL biology has led to promising new therapeutic strategies utilizing induction immuno-chemotherapy.[56] In addition, while an aggressive clinical course is typical, more indolent variants are now well recognized. Risk stratification based on clinical parameters categorizes patients as low- or high risk, with 5-year overall survival rates ranging from 84% to 34%, respectively.[56,57]

Burkitt Lymphoma

BL is a high-grade B-cell neoplasm associated with reciprocal chromosomal translocations resulting in C-MYC overexpression. This entity was first described in the jaws of young children living in sub-Saharan Africa. An association with malaria and EBV infection is recognized, and the disease is now termed *endemic BL*. Tumors exhibiting similar histomorphology have rarely been observed in the United States and other regions of the world. Cases diagnosed outside endemic areas are termed *sporadic BL* and those associated with HIV infection are termed *immunodeficiency-associated*

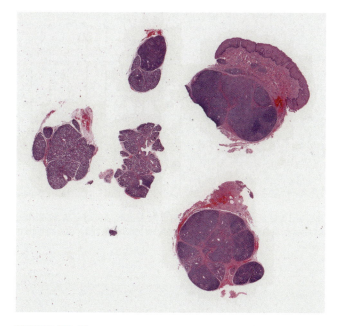

FIGURE 70-14. **Extranodal marginal zone B-cell (MALT) lymphoma.** This low-magnification image reveals a dense nodular deep submucosal infiltrate that involves minor salivary gland tissue.

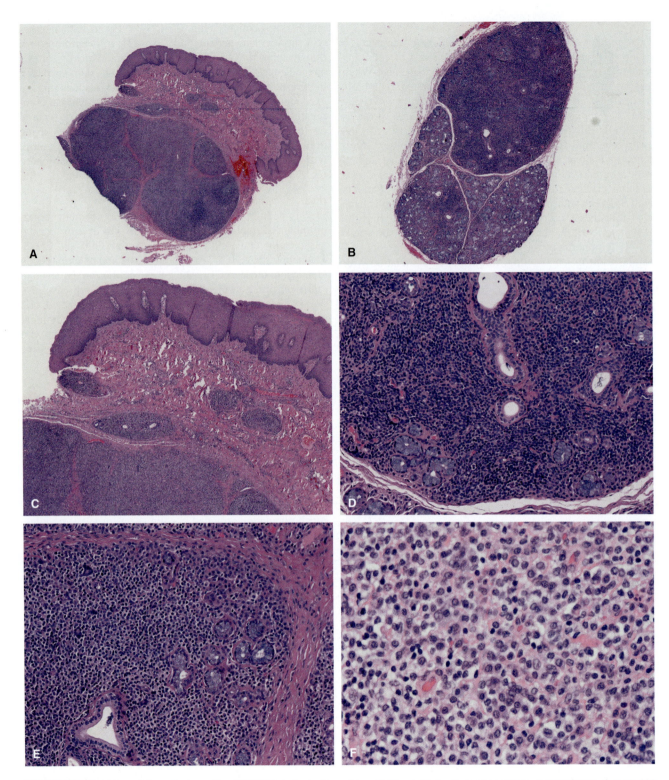

FIGURE 70-15. Extranodal marginal zone B-cell (MALT) lymphoma. The nodular and diffuse infiltrate shows sparing of the superficial mucosa (**A** and **B**, H&E; 20×; **C**, 40×). The infiltrate partially effaces the parenchyma of accessory salivary gland lobules, but does not have lymphoepithelial lesions (**D**, 200×). The infiltrate is composed of medium-sized cells with a plasmacytoid appearance (**E** and **F**, 200× and 400×).

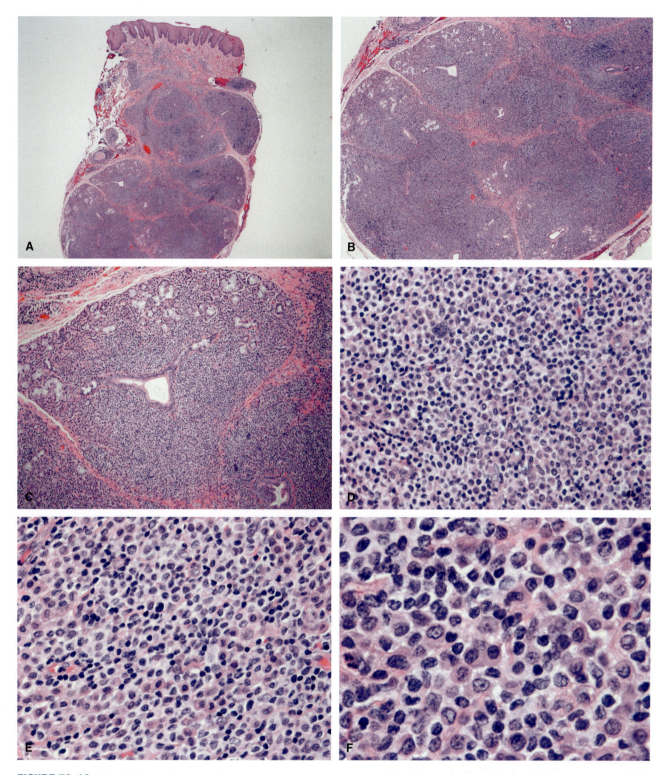

FIGURE 70-16. Extranodal marginal zone B-cell (MALT) lymphoma. This is a different case of a MALT lymphoma in the oral cavity. The infiltrate also shows a nodular and diffuse appearance (**A** and **B**, H&E; 20× and 40×). Partial effacement of the salivary gland parenchyma is present (**C**, 100×). Cytologically, this case is composed of a mixture of monocytoid cells and plasmacytoid lymphocytes (**D** and **E**, 400×; **F**, 600×).

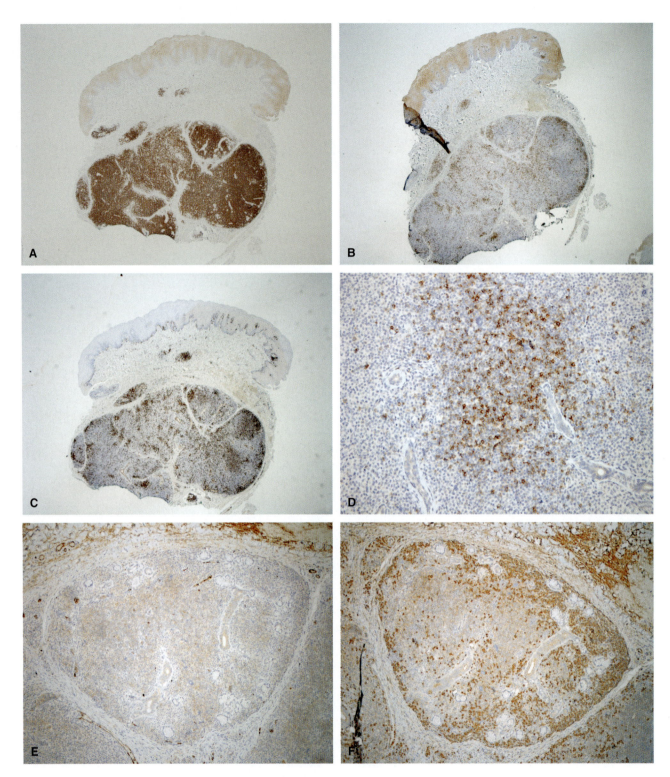

FIGURE 70-17. Extranodal marginal zone B-cell (MALT) lymphoma—IHC. The lymphoma cells are positive for CD20 **(A)**, but negative for CD3 **(B)** and CD5 **(C)**. CD23 **(D)** shows disruption of the follicular dendritic networks. κ **(E)** and λ **(F)** immunostains show λ restriction in the mature plasma cells.

BL. EBV infection is almost always associated with endemic cases, but EBV is only detected in up to 30% and 40% of sporadic and immunodeficiency-associated cases, respectively.[39,44,58] Sporadic BL primarily affects children and young adults, and it most commonly arises in the abdomen.[48] Very few reports of primary sporadic BL arising in the oral cavity have been reported.[59] The gingiva and alveolar processes are most commonly affected, with rapid swelling and aggressive destruction of the bone. The histopathology consists of a diffuse proliferation of monotonous medium-sized lymphoid cells exhibiting dark round nuclei, sparse cytoplasm, frequent mitotic figures, apoptotic cells, and tingible body macrophages, resulting in the characteristic "starry-sky" pattern on low-power magnification. Lesional cells express

CD20, CD10, and BCL-6, but are negative for BCL-2 and CD5. Ki-67 shows a proliferation index of greater than 95%, and fluorescence in situ hybridization is used to identify the *MYC* translocation, which is present in over 90% of cases.[39] Overlapping histomorphologic and immunophenotypic features with DLBCL are occasionally observed, making diagnosis challenging. The more recent WHO classification has incorporated the category of "high-grade B-cell lymphoma," to include those cases that have intermediate features between BL and DLBCL. This diagnostic distinction is important to ensure appropriate management, with BL requiring more intensive chemotherapeutic regimens.[39,59] Overall, BL is a highly aggressive but potentially curable disease, particularly in children. Intensive combination chemotherapy results in 70% to 90% overall survival for pediatric BL.[39,58]

T-Cell Lymphomas

Anaplastic Large-Cell Lymphoma

Anaplastic large-cell lymphoma (ALCL) is a form of T-cell lymphoma that is CD30$^+$ and frequently harbors the t(2; 5)(p23; q35) translocation, resulting in overexpression of anaplastic lymphoma kinase (ALK). *ALK$^+$* tumors generally occur in children and young adults, are chemoresponsive, and are associated with a good prognosis. In contrast, the *ALK−* tumors are typically diagnosed in an elderly population and confer a less favorable prognosis.[39,60] Regardless of subtype, ALCL often arises within lymph nodes; however, extranodal disease is also frequently observed, and bone, soft tissues, lung, liver, and skin may be affected.[48] Primary ALCL of the oral cavity has rarely been reported. Most cases are ALK− and involve the gingiva, hard palate, or lip.[60,61] Characteristic histopathologic features include a proliferation of large atypical cells exhibiting irregular nuclei, which often demonstrate a horseshoe shape and perinuclear eosinophilic region. These "hallmark cells" are admixed with a variably prominent population of nonneoplastic mixed inflammatory cells (Fig. 70-18). The malignant cells are strongly positive for CD30, with variable reactivity to EMA, granzyme B, and T-cell markers. A case series by Sciallis et al[60] highlighted the importance of clinical history and staging to differentiate primary from secondary oral ALCL. In their small series, cases in which clinical staging indicated disease limited to the oral mucosa ("primary oral ALCL") showed an indolent clinical course more similar to primary cutaneous ALCL than to systemic ALCL. In contrast, when clinical staging revealed mucosal lesions that were a component of systemic ALCL ("secondary oral ALCL"), these patients had a negative outcome, similar to secondary cutaneous ALCL. This behavior is reflective of the generally poor prognosis of systemic ALK− tumors, which exhibit a 49% overall 5-year survival. Nonetheless, mucosal involvement by ALCL is unfortunately not as well documented as primary or secondary cutaneous ALCL, and analyses of larger series would be necessary to better characterize this entity.

Primary cutaneous CD30$^+$ LPDs are discussed in detail in Chapter 15. These diseases show a broad range of clinicopathologic presentations, from lymphomatoid papulosis to cutaneous ALCL. This spectrum has recently been described in oral mucosal lesions. It has been suggested that the oral mucosal condition referred to as *traumatic ulcerative granuloma (TUG)*, also termed *traumatic ulcerative granuloma with stromal eosinophilia, traumatic eosinophilic granuloma, eosinophilic ulcer of the oral mucosa,* or *Riga–Fede disease* in infants, may be an oral counterpart on this spectrum. However, this comparison is somewhat confusing, as the designation of TUG has been applied to various lesions, not all of which contain CD30$^+$ cells. Although gene rearrangement studies have shown that some cases of TUG may contain a clonal T-cell population, the lack of well-defined diagnostic criteria suggests the possibility that lesions designated as TUG represent a heterogeneous group.[62] TUG has been best described in the oral and maxillofacial pathology literature. Salisbury et al[63] reported a series of 37 TUG cases and found that, in the absence of histopathologic or clinical evidence of lymphoma, T-cell clonality or CD30 positivity was not indicative of a malignant clinical course in these lesions. Thus, TUG is generally considered a chronic, benign, reactive process. Trauma is thought to play an important etiologic role; however, the exact pathogenesis is unknown. The tongue is most commonly involved and clinically presents with surface

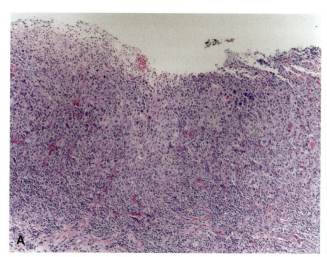
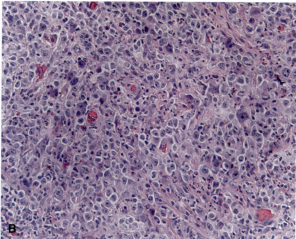

FIGURE 70-18. Anaplastic large-cell lymphoma. Proliferation of large pleomorphic cells, with prominent nucleoli and frequent atypical mitotic figures, set in a background of nonneoplastic mixed inflammatory cells (**A** and **B**, H&E; 100× and 200×).

ulceration exhibiting raised, rolled borders that are often somewhat firm on palpation, a clinical presentation mimicking oral squamous cell carcinoma and necessitating biopsy. Histopathologic findings show a diffuse, polymorphous infiltrate with variable numbers of eosinophils and scattered large pale-staining mononuclear cells resembling histiocytes, which may or may not express CD30. The inflammatory infiltrate extends deeply into the submucosa and is characteristically seen infiltrating between superficial fascicles of skeletal muscle. Spontaneous resolution is almost universal following incisional biopsy, although multiple episodes of recurrent, self-healing oral ulcerations are not uncommon.[64]

Mycosis Fungoides

Mycosis fungoides (MF) and its leukemic variant, Sézary syndrome, are the most common cutaneous T-cell lymphomas, which are characterized by malignant proliferation of CD4+, and less commonly CD8+, T lymphocytes. Although lymph nodes and viscera may be involved, by definition, MF is largely confined to the skin at diagnosis. Invasion of the epidermis is due to a property called epidermotropism, which infrequently may also result in involvement of oral epithelium. MF is discussed in detail in Chapter 13; thus, the focus of this section is limited to oral mucosal manifestations.

Reports of oral cavity involvement of MF are rare, with fewer than 60 published cases in the literature since the first case report in 1914.[65,66] Sirois et al[67] reported the largest series of 8 patients, which represented a less than 1% prevalence of oral lesions in 824 patients with MF over a 25-year period. Autopsy studies, however, have found a greater prevalence of oral lesions, with Long and Mihm[68] reporting oral manifestations in 13% (2/15) of MF patients.[68]

The average age at diagnosis of oral MF is 60 years.[66] While cutaneous MF generally precedes oral involvement by an average of 6-7 years, oral alterations may be the initial manifestation of disease.[66] Oral lesions may be solitary or multifocal and vary from erythematous plaques to ulcerated tumors. Any oral mucosal surface may be affected, but the tongue, palate, and gingiva are most frequently involved[66,67,69] (Fig. 70-19). The clinical differential diagnosis is highly variable depending on the clinical presentation and distribution of lesions. Extracutaneous lesions indicate systemic disease progression, and oral involvement has generally been associated with a poor prognosis with most patients succumbing to disease-related complications within 1-2 years of developing oral lesions.[67] More recently, a trend toward improved prognosis has been recognized, with some patients experiencing prolonged disease-free survival, a trend undoubtedly related to improved therapeutic options.[66]

The histopathologic findings, therapeutic management, and overall prognosis of MF are discussed in Chapter 12. A representative case is also presented (Fig. 70-20).

Extranodal NK/T-Cell Lymphoma, Nasal Type

Extranodal NK/T-cell lymphoma, nasal type (ENKTCL) is a rare, aggressive form of NHL that is associated with EBV and most commonly occurs in East Asia, Central and South America, but with increasing incidence in the United States.[70,71] For many decades, the pathophysiology of this disease was unknown, which is reflected in the various terms used to describe the process, including *angiocentric T-cell lymphoma, midline lethal granuloma, idiopathic midline destructive disease, polymorphic reticulosis, midline malignant reticulosis, angiocentric immunoproliferative lesion, malignant granuloma, and lethal granulomatous ulceration.* ENKTCL is discussed in detail in Chapter 19; thus, the focus of this section is limited to oral cavity manifestations of the disease.

ENKTCL is characterized by swelling, ulceration, and aggressive destruction of the midface region (Fig. 70-21). Although the oral cavity may be affected, only rarely is it the initial site of involvement.[72] Oral manifestations more often result from direct extension of disease from the nasal fossa or paranasal sinuses. Swelling of the hard and soft palate, usually occupying a midline position, often precedes the formation of a deep, necrotic ulceration that can eventually destroy the palatal hard and soft tissues, resulting in oroantral fistula[70,72] (Fig. 70-21). ENKTCL can involve the maxillary gingiva, causing pain, necrotic ulceration, bony destruction, and tooth mobility.[70,73] Rarely, an ulcerated, necrotic mass of the posterior tongue may be seen.[74] Regardless of the oral mucosal site of involvement, the necrotic lesions typically result in a fetid oral malodor.[73]

In addition to ENKTCL, destructive palatal lesions can also be seen in association with immunologic (granulomatosis with polyangiitis, formerly known as Wegener granulomatosis) or infectious (tertiary syphilis; deep fungal infections; necrotizing ulcerative stomatitis) etiologies, as well as secondary to recreational drug abuse (nasal insufflation). Thus, thorough diagnostic evaluation, including biopsy and culture, is necessary to make a definitive diagnosis. The histopathologic features, treatment strategies, and prognosis of ENKTCL are discussed in Chapter 23.

EBV-ASSOCIATED LYMPHOID PROLIFERATIONS

EBV is a herpesvirus that is one of the most common viruses in humans, infecting over 90%-95% of adults worldwide.[75] Primary EBV infection is often asymptomatic, or may present as infectious mononucleosis, and will subsequently establish latency in host B-cells. Latent infection and periodic reactivation of the virus are primarily controlled by an EBV-specific cytotoxic T-cell response. When the immune system is debilitated, however, proliferation of the latently infected B-cells may occur.[76,77]

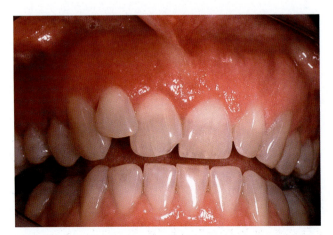

FIGURE 70-19. Mycosis fungoides. Diffuse erythema of the right maxillary gingiva in a 49-year-old female represents an example of rare oral involvement by MF.

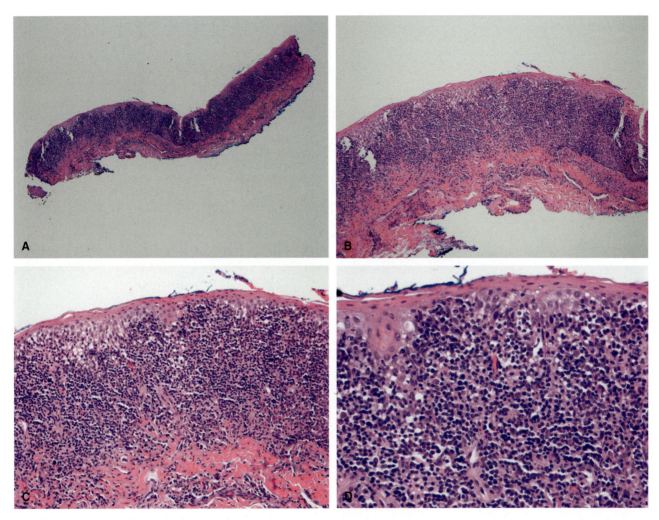

FIGURE 70-20. Mycosis fungoides. There is a band-like infiltrate in the mucosa with significant epidermotropism (**A** and **B**, H&E; 40× and 100×). The infiltrate shows tagging along the mucosal–submucosal junction and epidermotropism in a similar way to how it presents in the skin. Cytologically, the cells are small to medium in size, with hyperchromatic nuclei, perinuclear halos, and irregular nuclear borders (**C** and **D**, 200× and 400×).

It has long been reported that *EBV-driven B-cell LPDs* may arise in the clinical setting of primary immune deficiency, HIV infection, or iatrogenic posttransplantation immunosuppression. More recently, the spectrum of immunosuppressive etiologies has expanded to include additional iatrogenic causes, primarily methotrexate (MTX) and tumor necrosis factor-α antagonists, which may be prescribed for management of various autoimmune diseases, such as rheumatoid arthritis, psoriasis, dermatomyositis, and inflammatory bowel disease.[78,79] The newest recognized risk factor is age-related immunologic impairment, termed *immunosenescence*, which is thought to be a physiologic deterioration of the immune system that is part of the aging process.[80,81]

A broad clinical and histopathologic spectrum exists for EBV-driven B-cell LPD, which commonly involves extranodal sites and ranges from reactive lymphoid hyperplasia or mucocutaneous ulcerations to malignant polymorphic or monomorphic lymphoid proliferations. Despite improvements in classification, significant overlap exists, and diagnosis and management are often challenging.[77,82]

Posttransplant LPD (PT-LPD) results from potent antirejection immunosuppressive therapy following HSCT or SOT. Most cases associated with HSCT arise from donor B cells and develop within the first 6 months following transplantation. In contrast, cases associated with SOT generally arise from recipient B-cells and are diagnosed within the first year following transplantation; however, some may arise multiple years later.[76] PT-LPD are diagnosed across a broad age range, with a median age of ~43 years.[78] Extranodal disease is common, with lungs and gastrointestinal tract commonly involved. From a histopathologic perspective, these lesions represent a heterogeneous group and are thought to evolve from a polyclonal disorder to a more aggressive monoclonal variant. A polymorphic cell population often makes it difficult to predict a benign or malignant clinical course.[76,78]

Iatrogenic LPDs arising in a *nontransplantation setting* have most commonly been associated with MTX therapy used for treatment of rheumatoid arthritis. Thus, the terms *MTX-related EBV-associated LPD* or *MTX-associated LPD (MTX-LPD)* are frequently used. Additional immunosuppressive agents that have been implicated include tumor necrosis factor-α antagonists, cyclosporine, azathioprine, mycophenolate mofetil, and corticosteroids.[78,83] Cases typically arises in middle-aged to elderly females with a 5.2-year mean duration of MTX therapy.[84] However, the relationship between the duration of treatment or total

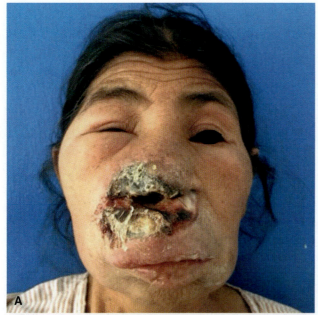
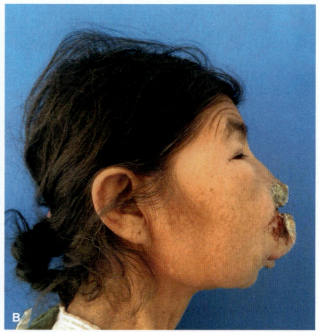
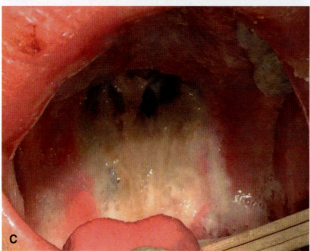

FIGURE 70-21. Extranodal NK/T-cell lymphoma, nasal type. This 60-year-old Guatemalan female exhibited dramatic swelling of the midface region, with deep necrotic ulceration (**A** and **B**) and a destructive palatal lesion (**C**), which proved to be a NK/T-cell lymphoma. (Photographs courtesy of Dr. Román Carlos.)

dose received and the occurrence of MTX-LPD is somewhat controversial. Approximately 40% of cases occur in extranodal sites, including the skin, gastrointestinal tract, lung, kidney, and soft tissues.[85] Oral mucosal involvement is rare; however, the overall incidence of this disease may be rising owing to the increasing number of patients on immunomodulatory therapy. The typical oral presentation is an ulcerated lesion, possibly associated with a mass. In addition to the tongue and palatal mucosa, the gingiva is frequently involved and may result in exposure of underlying necrotic bone.[84] When lesions clinically present as a well-circumscribed, solitary ulceration of the skin or mucosal surface, the designation *EBV-positive mucocutaneous ulcer* (EBVMCU) may be applied.[82] This provisional entity was added to the WHO 2017 Classification of Tumours of Haematopoietic and Lymphoid Tissues and has been reported to arise in the setting of age-related immunosenescence in addition to iatrogenic immunosuppression.[39] No evidence of systemic lymphadenopathy, hepatosplenomegaly or bone marrow involvement is seen. Although considered biologically indolent, the histopathologic features of EBVMCU ulcer frequently resemble DLBCL and many also exhibit Hodgkin-like features. Variable numbers of large pleomorphic B-cells, reminiscent of HRS cells, set in a background of reactive lymphocytes, plasma cells, histiocytes, and eosinophils are observed.[84] The HRS-like B-cells typically show reactivity to antibodies directed against CD20, CD79a, CD30, PAX5, and LMP1. In situ hybridization for EBER will show localization within the atypical B-cells.

MTX-LPD should be distinguished from *MTX-related ulcerative stomatitis*, which occurs in ~14% of patients treated with MTX.[86] Stomatitis may arise at any time in the course of treatment and it is believed to be attributable to a toxic/metabolic effect of the medication, rather than LPD. These shallow ulcerations may be large and painful, but are not as deep or destructive as MTX-LPD and they will gradually resolve upon withdrawal of the MTX.[84,86]

EBV+ diffuse large B-cell lymphoma, not otherwise specific (EBV+ DLBCL, NOS) is a clinicopathologic entity recognized by the 2017 WHO lymphoma classification.[39] This clonal B-cell proliferation typically occurs in elderly individuals and is associated with short survival. Synonyms for this entity include *senile EBV-associated B-cell LPD*, *age-related EBV+ B-cell LPD*, and *EBV-associated B-cell LPD of the elderly*. The median age at diagnosis is 71 years, with up to 25% of cases occurring in individuals over the age of 90 years.[39] While most affected patients are over the age of 50, occurrence in younger individuals without immunosuppression is occasionally seen; thus, additional factors may play a role in pathogenesis.[75] About 70% of patients present with extranodal disease, with or without lymph node involvement, and commonly affected sites include the skin, lung, tonsil, and stomach.[39,79] Oral cavity involvement is extremely rare, but may present as a nonhealing mucosal ulcer or lytic bone lesion.[81] Histopathologic features include effacement of normal tissue architecture, often accompanied by necrosis, with a diffuse or polymorphic proliferation of large B-cells. Some of the neoplastic cells may exhibit HRS-like features, which may be associated with varying numbers of reactive lymphocytes, plasma cells, histiocytes, and epithelioid cells (Fig. 70-22).

Thus, overlapping features with DLBCL and classic HL are observed. Lesional cells are typically positive for antibodies directed against CD20, CD79a, and LMP1, with variable CD30 positivity and no reactivity to CD15. Most cases have an activated B-cell phenotype, expressing MUM1/IRF4, and are negative for CD10 and BCL6.[75] In situ hybridization for EBER is universally positive, although the degree of positivity is variable and ranges from 10%-50% of large neoplastic B-cells (Fig. 70-23).[75,79,81] EBV+ DLBCL, NOS typically demonstrates an aggressive clinical course and less favorable prognosis than EBV-negative DLBCL. Outcomes appear somewhat better with chemoimmunotherapy than chemotherapy alone; however, 5-year overall survival is still only 54%-64%.[75,81]

Regardless of immunosuppressive etiology, significant histopathologic overlap exists among the EBV-driven B-cell LPDs, and pathologic assessment often provides limited insight into the biologic potential of a given lesion. Some cases demonstrate complete regression with decreased immunosuppression, whereas others require active treatment. The lack of clear diagnostic distinction and prognostic features leads to treatment decisions that are often empirically

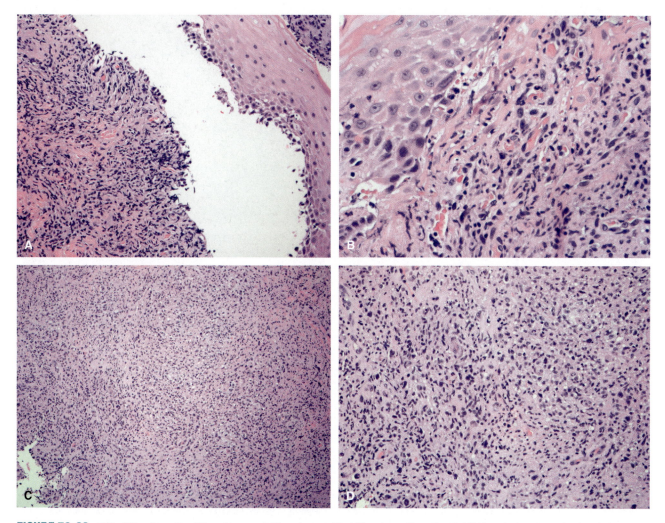

FIGURE 70-22. EBV+ **diffuse large B-cell lymphoma, not otherwise specified.** There is a malignant lymphoid infiltrate in the submucosa with relative sparing of the overlying mucosal surface (**A** and **B**, H&E; 100× and 200×). The infiltrate has a diffuse appearance and shows numerous background histiocytes (**C** and **D**, 100× and 200×). Cytologically, the malignant cells are medium to large, with a vague spindle-cell appearance and prominent nucleoli (**E** and **F,** 400× each).

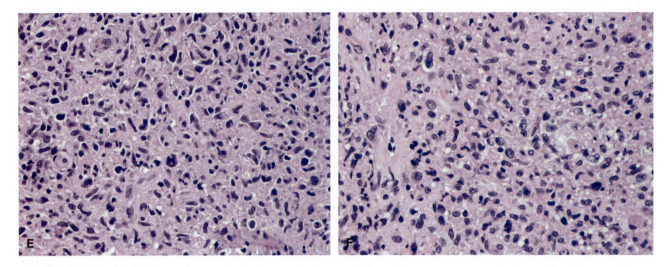

FIGURE 70-22. (continued)

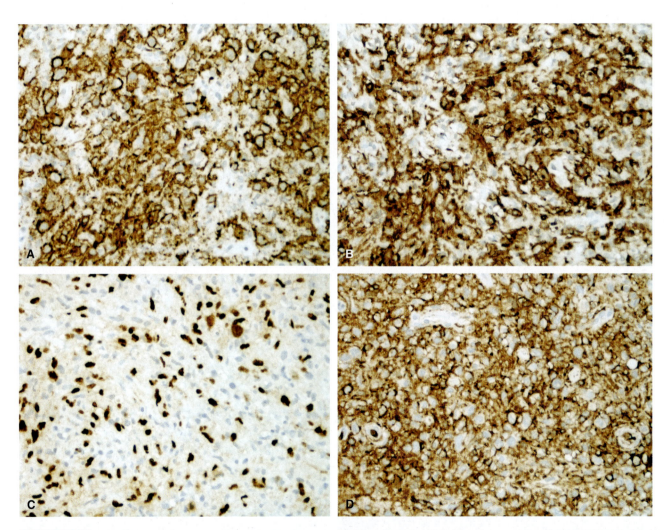

FIGURE 70-23. EBV⁺ diffuse large B-cell lymphoma, not otherwise specified—IHC. The neoplastic cells are positive for CD20 **(A)** and show diffuse staining for CD30 **(B)**. Contrary to classic Hodgkin disease, the cells show strong immunoreactivity for PAX5 **(C)** and CD45 **(D)**. EBER **(E)** is positive in the malignant cells, as well as the EBV antigen LMP1 **(F)**.

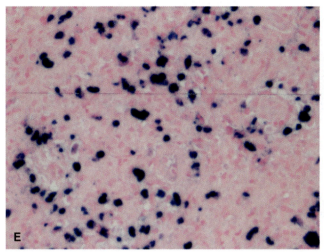
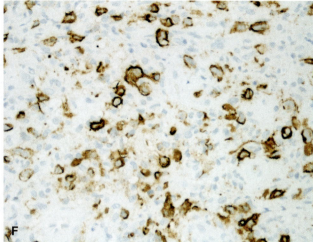

FIGURE 70-23. (continued)

driven and strongly influenced by clinical parameters.[77,82] When immunosuppression is iatrogenic, the first step in management is typically reduction of the immunosuppressive therapy when feasible. Spontaneous regression is seen in approximately half of cases upon MTX withdrawal.[84] If active therapy becomes necessary, one treatment strategy is to eliminate EBV-infected B-cells using antibody therapy that targets specific surface antigens. Rituximab, a chimeric murine/human monoclonal anti-CD20 antibody, has been the most commonly used first-line therapy.[76,77] When patients fail to respond to immunosuppression reduction or rituximab, chemotherapy with protocols commonly used in lymphoma treatment, such as CHOP (cyclophosphamide, doxorubicin, vincristine, and prednisone) or R-CHOP (rituximab and CHOP), is often employed and response rates between 50%-100% have been reported.[75,76,87] Radiation and/or surgery may also be effective in controlling local disease.[76,87] The prognosis for EBV-driven B-cell LPD is highly variable, with many lesions demonstrating an indolent behavior with spontaneous regression, others characterized by a relapsing and remitting pattern, and a small subset following an aggressive clinical course.[76,78]

Patients with underlying immune deficiency are also at increased risk for developing *lymphomatoid granulomatosis (LYG)*, a rare angiocentric, angiodestructive EBV-associated B-cell lymphoproliferative disorder. LYG is most commonly diagnosed in middle-aged adults during the fourth to sixth decades of life. It exhibits a male predilection and has been associated with a spectrum of biologic behavior.[88,89] The lungs are characteristically involved; however, extranodal sites, such as the central nervous system, skin, kidney, and liver, may also be affected.[39,89] LYG of the oral cavity is extremely rare and generally represents spread of pulmonary disease.[90,91] Two oral cases presenting in individuals with no known underlying immunodeficiency have recently been reported, presumably secondary to immunosenescence.[88,92] Most common oral sites of involvement include the gingiva and hard palate, with the clinical presentation of a destructive necrotic ulceration[91] (Figs. 70-24–70-27). Diagnostic considerations, treatment strategies, and prognosis of LYG are discussed in Chapter 34.

MULTIPLE MYELOMA

Synonyms: Plasma cell myeloma, myelomatosis, Kahler disease.

Multiple myeloma (MM) is a multicentric neoplastic proliferation of plasma cells that develops within bone marrow and results in accumulation of myeloma protein (M-protein) in serum and/or urine. The development of MM may be preceded by a diagnosis of solitary *plasmacytoma*; however, most cases evolve from an asymptomatic premalignant stage termed *monoclonal gammopathy of undetermined significance* or from a more advanced

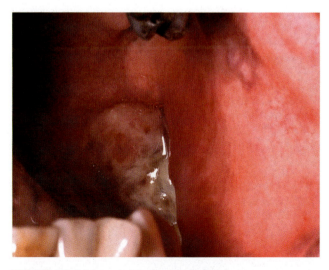

FIGURE 70-24. Lymphomatoid granulomatosis. An 82-year-old male with an ulcerated lesion of the left posterior mandibular ridge represents a rare example of oral mucosal involvement by LYG.

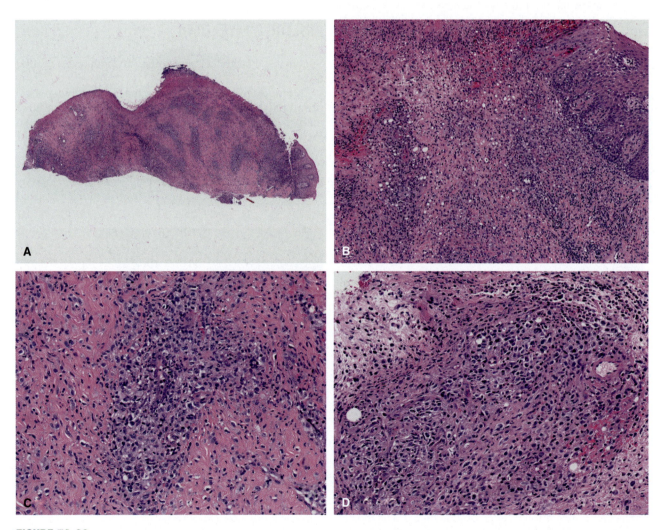

FIGURE 70-25. Lymphomatoid granulomatosis. This is the biopsy taken from the ulcerated lesion on the mandibular ridge. The mucosa is acanthotic and shows a dense submucosal infiltrate with a perivascular distribution (**A** and **B**: H&E; 10× and 20×).

FIGURE 70-26. Lymphomatoid granulomatosis. The biopsy shows an ulcer with a dense perivascular infiltrate that at these magnifications suggest the possibility of a vasculitic process (**A** and **B**, H&E; 40× and 100×). The closer view of the infiltrate shows a dense perivascular population of medium and large cells with fibrinoid changes of the vessel walls (**C** and **D,** 200×; **E** and **F**, 400×).

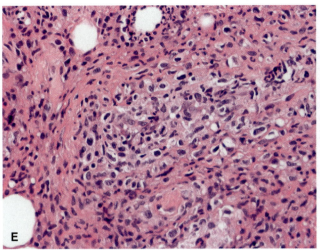
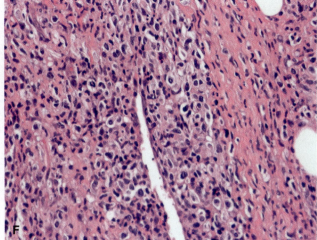

FIGURE 70-26. (continued)

premalignant stage called *smoldering myeloma*.[93] As the precursor phase is typically asymptomatic, it is thought that the majority of patients may have had the condition for over a decade prior to diagnosis.

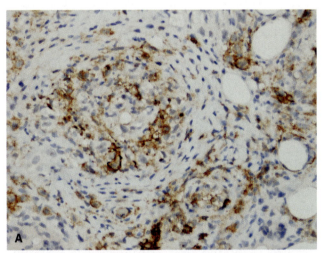
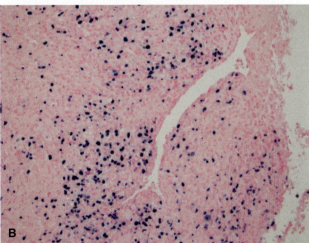

FIGURE 70-27. Lymphomatoid granulomatosis. The large cells are positive for CD20 **(A)** and EBER **(B)**. Grading of LYG is typically based on the number of EBER+ cells, and in this case, the number of cells corresponds to a grade III.

MM comprises ~1% of all malignancies and 10%-15% of hematologic malignancies.[93] Over 24,000 cases are diagnosed annually in the United States, and when metastatic disease is excluded, myeloma accounts for over 50% of all malignancies that involve bone.[3] MM generally affects an older population, with a median age of 66-70 years at diagnosis and 63% of cases occurring after age 65. Only 2% of cases present in individuals under age 40.[94] There is a slight male predilection and the condition occurs twice as frequently in African Americans compared to Caucasians.[93,94] Individuals who have a first-degree relative with the disease are at a 2.9-fold increased risk for developing MM.[93]

Signs and symptoms of MM develop secondary to the accumulation of the malignant cells in bone marrow and/or the accumulation of their protein products in serum and urine. As neoplastic plasma cells replace bone marrow, symptoms of myelophthisic anemia may develop and are frequently the presenting sign of MM, seen in ~73% of patients at diagnosis.[94,95] Fatigue, petechial hemorrhage of the skin and oral mucosa, fever, and increased susceptibility to infection may be present. Bone pain, secondary to lytic bone lesions, is a common presenting symptom in up to 70% of cases.[95] The lumbar spine is frequently involved, with the possibility for vertebral compression fractures. Pathologic fracture of long bones may also be seen, which can be the first sign of disease.[94,95] Radiographically, multiple well-defined "punched-out" radiolucent lesions are characteristic; however, ragged or ill-defined lytic lesions may also be observed. Bone lesions are often visualized on skull films; however, skeletal survey, PET-CT, and low-dose CT are all valid methods for detection of lytic bone lesions.[96] Any bone may be affected and the mandible is a common site, with involvement in up to 15% of cases[95,97] (Fig. 70-28). The lytic bone lesions contain tumor cells that release cytokines causing increased osteoclast activity and decreased osteoblast function. This myeloma-related osteolysis may result in generalized osteopenia and hypercalcemia, with the possibility for development of metastatic calcifications in soft tissues.[95]

Similar to a normal plasma cell, the clonal neoplastic plasma cells continue to produce immunoglobulin, albeit abnormal and nonfunctional. Accumulation of light-chain products in the urine is referred to as *Bence Jones proteins*,

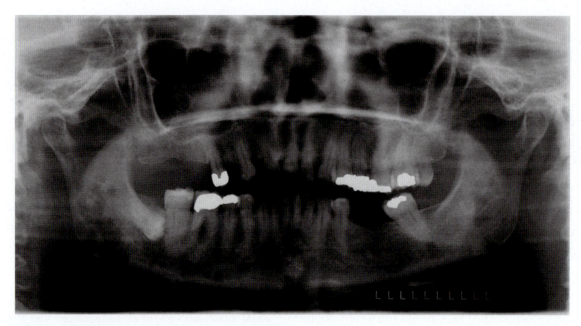

FIGURE 70-28. Multiple myeloma. Numerous punched-out radiolucencies of the mandible.

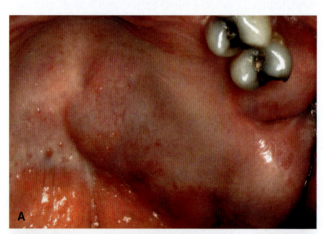

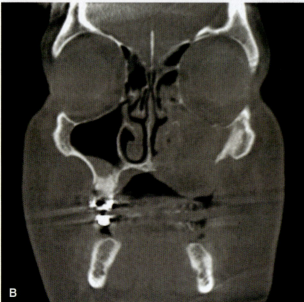

FIGURE 70-29. Plasmacytoma. A, Palatal swelling in a 61-year-old male. **B,** Cone beam computed tomography (CBCT) scan of the same patient shows involvement of the left maxilla and paranasal sinuses, which proved to be plasmacytoma.

named after the British physician who first described them. The etiology of renal impairment, which is seen in up to half of myeloma patients, is primarily due to overburdening of tubular reabsorption associated with the excessive amount of circulating light-chain components.[94,95]

Amyloidosis may also be a sign of MM and is seen in ~10% of patients.[95] Amyloid deposits are composed of monoclonal light-chain immunoglobulins and commonly affect the head and neck region. This may result in diffuse enlargement or increased firmness of the tongue. Nodules on the dorsal tongue, hard palate, and buccal or labial mucosa can also be seen and may be ulcerated.[98] The periorbital skin is frequently affected, resulting in waxy, firm, plaque-like deposits.[98]

The diagnosis of MM is made by identifying clonal plasmacytosis occupying at least 10% of bone marrow or a biopsy-proven plasmacytoma plus one or more myeloma-defining events, including hypercalcemia, renal insufficiency, anemia, lytic bone lesions, or serum free light chain ratio ≥100.[99] Histopathologic evaluation of lesional tissue reveals diffuse sheets of plasmacytoid cells exhibiting eccentric nuclei and clumped nuclear chromatin. These variably differentiated plasma cells generally show cytologic atypia and mitotic activity. Immunohistochemical analysis demonstrates lesional cell positivity to antibodies directed against CD138, CD38, and CD79 A, similar to normal plasma cells. Additionally, up to 79% of myeloma cells aberrantly express CD56. Expression of CD117, CD20, CD52, and CD10 may also be seen in decreasing order of frequency. Some cases are cyclin D1 positive.[39] Clonality can be ascertained using antibodies directed against κ and λ light-chain proteins by IHC or in situ hybridization. A monoclonal neoplastic proliferation will demonstrate a restriction of either κ or λ light chains, which contrasts with a reactive plasma cell infiltrate that will show a mixture of reactivity to both immunoglobulin components. Amyloid production may occasionally be seen in association with the neoplastic proliferation. This material presents as a homogeneous "glassy" extracellular eosinophilic substance that shows affinity for Congo red, demonstrating apple-green birefringence when viewed with polarized light.[98]

Therapeutic advances over the past decade have resulted in significant improvement in patient prognosis, with most newly diagnosed MM patients experiencing over 10 years overall survival. A corticosteroid (prednisone or dexamethasone) in conjunction with an alkylating agent (cyclophosphamide or melphalan) has long been used in combination drug therapy.[93,95] However, the recent introduction of bortezomib (a proteasome inhibitor) and thalidomide and lenalidomide (immunomodulators) has dramatically improved therapeutic responses. These drugs have become the mainstay of treatment and generally result in a period of disease stability. Nonetheless, MM is characterized by relapses and remissions; each remission typically lasts less than the previous and becomes increasingly difficult to control until recalcitrant end-stage disease ensues.[93,95,99] Younger patients with aggressive disease may receive high-dose chemotherapy with autologous stem cell transplantation. Older patients, however, generally are deemed ineligible for transplantation and receive combination chemotherapy only.[93-95,99] Although novel therapeutic approaches have transformed the outlook for many myeloma patients, the disease is heterogenous and specific genetic signatures are associated with worse prognosis. Risk stratification, based on cytogenetic findings, can help predict disease aggressiveness and be useful for both counseling and therapeutic decision-making.[93]

Adjuvant treatment with bisphosphonate medications, such as zolendronate, pamidronate, or ibandronate, or the RANK ligand inhibitor, denosumab, has been shown to minimize bone pain and significantly reduce risk for myeloma-related fracture.[100] Bisphosphonates and denosumab, however, are associated with an increased risk for osteonecrosis of the jaw. Several terms have been used to define this process and include *bisphosphonate-related osteonecrosis of the jaw*, *antiresorptive agent–related osteonecrosis of the jaw*, and *medication-related osteonecrosis of the jaw*. Although only a small number of patients will experience this complication, complete dental examination with preventative dental care is crucial in minimizing risk and should be completed prior to commencing antiresorptive treatment.

PLASMACYTOMA

The *plasmacytoma* is a monoclonal proliferation of plasma cells that presents as a localized process, but has an identical cytologic and immunophenotypic profile as MM. It typically arises within bone but may occur in soft tissues as an extramedullary plasmacytoma. Plasmacytoma is generally considered to be on the least aggressive end of a continuum with MM, as the majority of patients with solitary plasmacytomas of bone will eventually develop into myeloma.[101,102]

The peak incidence of plasmacytoma is in the sixth decade of life, and a male predominance is seen, with a nearly 3:1 male-to-female ratio.[103] The spine, long bones, and skull are the most common sites of involvement. Although relatively uncommon in the maxillofacial region, the mandible may rarely be affected, particularly in the marrow-rich posterior areas.[104] Bone pain and swelling, paresthesia, tooth mobility, hemorrhage, or pathologic fracture are the most common presenting symptoms of jaw involvement; however, bone lesions may also be incidentally identified on routine radiographic examination. The radiographic findings consist of a "punched-out" unilocular or multilocular lytic lesion that lacks a sclerotic border and occasionally appears ragged. The extramedullary plasmacytoma generally presents as a well-defined soft tissue mass, with ~80% occurring in the head and neck region, with a predilection for the nasal cavity, nasopharynx, and paranasal sinuses[105] (Fig. 70-29). Approximately 24% of head and neck plasmacytomas arise within the oral cavity and pharynx.[101] Reports of parotid gland involvement are also well documented.[106]

Histopathologically identical to MM, plasmacytoma exhibits a diffuse proliferation of monoclonal plasma cells exhibiting variable degrees of differentiation. Lesional cells are positive for antibodies directed against CD138, CD38, and CD79A and show a light-chain (κ or λ) restriction by IHC or in situ hybridization (Fig. 70-30). To exclude the possibility of MM, the diagnostic criteria for plasmacytoma also include a normal bone marrow and no distant lesions identified on skeletal survey. Blood studies should rule out anemia, hypercalcemia, renal impairment, and presence of serum or urine paraproteins, which would suggest a diagnosis of MM.[103,105]

Plasmacytomas are highly radiosensitive and are, therefore, typically treated with primary radiation therapy. However, the optimal radiation dose has been a subject of debate, and a recent study showed improved outcomes with doses ≥40 Gy.[101] In some cohorts, surgical treatment, either alone or in conjunction with radiotherapy, has been associated with improved mortality than either monotherapy.[101] Chemotherapy has not been shown to improve outcome, and thus is reserved for advanced cases showing progression to MM.[102,103] Additionally, there has been recent interest in novel therapeutic agents, such as monoclonal antibodies, immunomodulatory agents, and proteasome inhibitors.[102]

Long-term follow-up is recommended following treatment for plasmacytoma, as greater than 75% of patients with plasmacytoma of bone will progress to MM.[101] The extramedullary plasmacytoma is treated similarly; however, it carries a much better prognosis, with less than 30% of patients progressing to MM and up to a 90% 5-year survival rate.[101] Five-year survival rate for plasmacytoma of bone is more favorable for individuals diagnosed before age 60, with 5-year overall survival rate of 70% and 5-year disease-free survival of 46%.[101,105]

BENIGN LYMPHOID PROLIFERATIONS

A variety of benign lymphoid proliferations may occur within the oral cavity. *Lymphoid hyperplasia* is frequently seen in association with normal anatomy of the lymphoid-rich tissues of Waldeyer ring. Multiple discrete lymphoid aggregates may present in the floor of mouth, ventral tongue, or tonsillar pillar area. The foliate papillae (lingual tonsils)

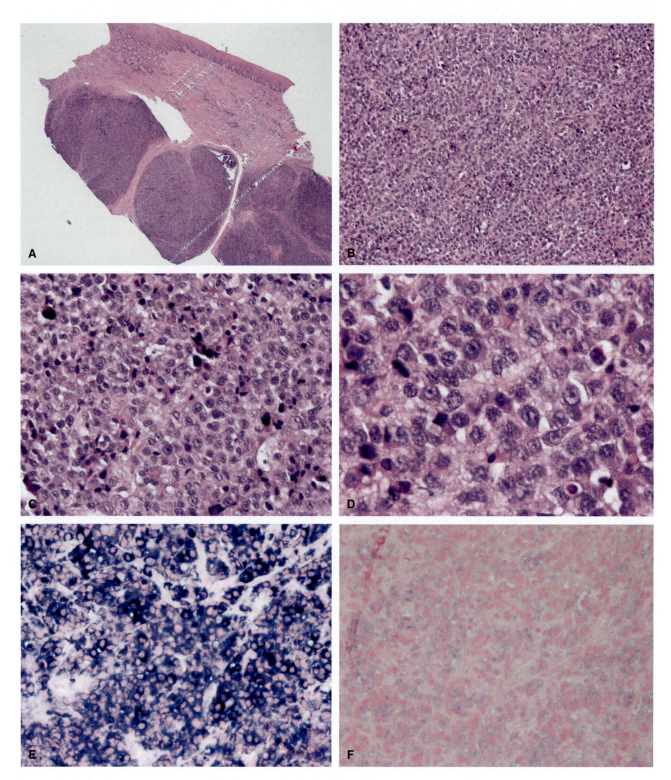

FIGURE 70-30. Plasmacytoma. A dense nodular infiltrate in the submucosa is present (**A,** H&E; 10×). Sheets of plasma cells are present, many of which contain a distinctive nucleoli (**B–D,** 100×, 400×, and 600×). In situ hybridization for κ (**E**) and λ (**F**) highlights that the plasma cells are κ restricted.

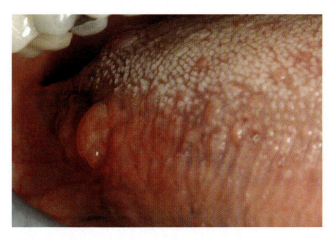

FIGURE 70-31. Lymphoid hyperplasia. This smooth-surfaced nodule of the right posterior lateral tongue represents an enlarged lymphoid aggregate associated with the foliate papilla.

are often affected, and this process presents clinically as a smooth-surfaced or bosselated nodule of the posterior lateral tongue, which represent enlarged lymphoid aggregates (Figs. 70-31 and 70-32). Bilateral symmetry generally helps to clinically differentiate this benign process from malignancy.

Hypersensitivity to dental amalgam (silver fillings) can result in a band-like lymphocytic interface reaction of the superficial lamina propria, consistent with a *lichenoid amalgam reaction* (lichenoid contact reaction). Clinically, these lesions present as interlacing keratotic striae, with variable degrees of erythema, localized to a mucosal surface in direct contact with the dental material. On histopathologic examination, the chronic lymphocytic infiltrate may become remarkably dense and develop prominent well-demarcated tertiary germinal center formations (Fig. 70-33).

An idiopathic *follicular lymphoid hyperplasia* infrequently involves the palate. This condition typically occurs

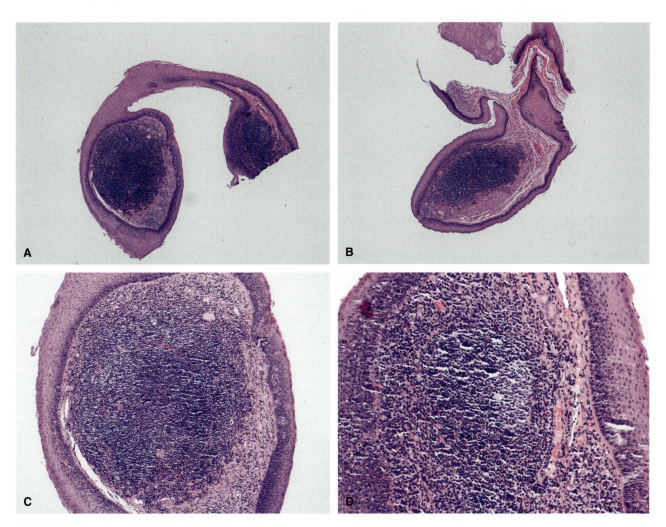

FIGURE 70-32. Lymphoid hyperplasia—histologic findings. Histopathologic features demonstrate benign lymphoid hyperplasia composed of well-differentiated small lymphocytes, which may occasionally form germinal centers. (**A–D,** H&E; 20×, 20×, 100×, and 200×).

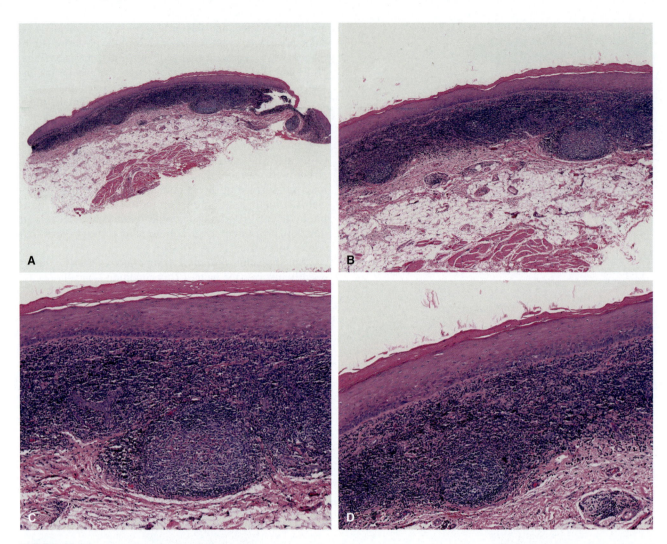

FIGURE 70-33. Lichenoid amalgam reaction. Oral mucosa demonstrating significant interface reaction, with a prominent band-like lymphocytic infiltrate and germinal center formation (**A,** H&E; 10×; **B,** 40×; **C** and **D,** 200×).

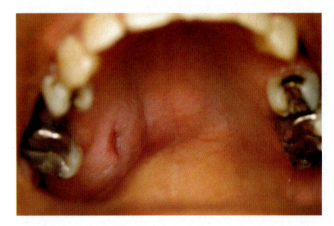

FIGURE 70-34. Idiopathic lymphoid hyperplasia. Soft tissue swelling of the posterior lateral hard palate, with a central depression representing recent biopsy site.

in older patients, with a female predilection. It generally presents as a slow-growing, nontender, boggy enlargement of the posterior lateral hard palate, clinically mimicking an extranodal lymphoma and thus requiring biopsy[107] (Fig. 70-34). Histopathologic examination reveals a proliferation of small well-differentiated lymphocytes that form variably sized sharply defined germinal centers (Fig. 70-35). Immunohistochemical analysis will substantiate the reactive nature of this lesion, with antibodies directed against CD3 and CD5 showing the characteristic orientation of T-cells in the parafollicular areas. Lymphoid follicles exhibit reactivity to CD10, CD21, and BCL-6, but are negative to antibodies directed against BCL-2. Confirmation of a polyclonal population can be achieved by polymerase chain reaction analysis for immunoglobulin heavy chain. Surgical excision is considered curative for these lesions, and long-term follow-up has not shown evidence of malignant transformation.[107]

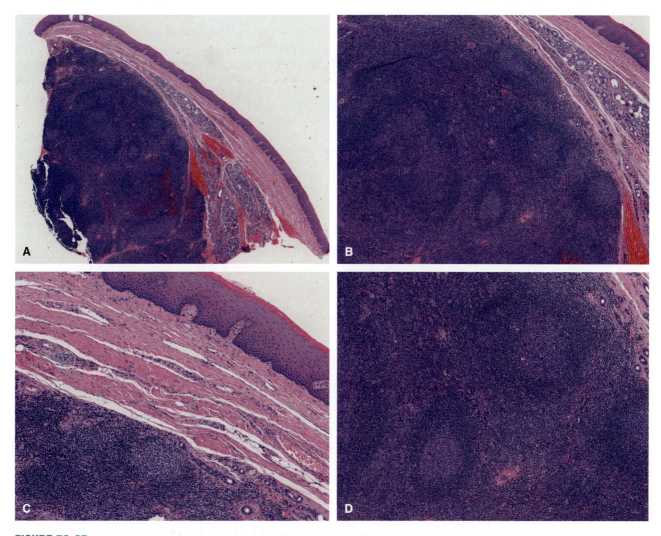

FIGURE 70-35. Idiopathic lymphoid hyperplasia—histologic findings. Dense submucosal infiltrate that shows sparing of the overlying mucosa. Numerous reactive-appearing germinal centers are present with frequent mitotic figures and tingible body macrophages (**A**, H&E; 10×; **B**, 100×, **C** and **D**, 200×).

References

1. Davis AS, Viera AJ, Mead MD. Leukemia: an overview for primary care. *Am Fam Physician*. 2014;89(9):731-738.
2. Widick P., Winer ES. Leukocytosis and leukemia. *Prim Care Clin Off Pract*. 2016;43(4):575-587.
3. Siegel RL, Miller KD, Jemal A. Cancer statistics, 2020. *CA Cancer J Clin*. 2020;70(7):7-30.
4. Apperley JF. Chronic myeloid leukaemia. *Lancet*. 2015;385(9976):1447-1459.
5. Kennedy JA, Ebert BL. Clinical implications of genetic mutations in myelodysplastic syndrome. *J Clin Oncol*. 2017;35(9):968-974.
6. Cammarata-Scalisi F, Girardi K, Strocchio L, et al. Oral manifestations and complications in childhood acute myeloid leukemia. *Cancers*. 2020;19(12):1634. doi:10.3390/cancers12061634
7. Vibhute P, Carneiro E, Genden E, et al. Palatal enlargement in chronic lymphocytic leukemia. *Am J Neuroradiol*. 2006;27(8):1649-1650.
8. Vural F, Ozcan MA, Ozsan GH, et al. Gingival involvement in a patient with CD56+ chronic myelomonocytic leukemia. *Leuk Lymphoma*. 2004;45(2):415-418.
9. Almond LM, Charalampakis M, Ford SJ, et al. Myeloid sarcoma: presentation, diagnosis, and treatment. *Clin Lymphoma Myeloma Keuk*. 2017;17(5):263-267.
10. Zhou J, Bell D, Medeiros LJ. Myeloid sarcoma of the head and neck region. *Arch Pathol Lab Med*. 2013;137(11):1560-1568.
11. da Silva Santos PS, Fontes A, de Andrade F, et al. Gingival leukemic infiltration as the first manifestation of acute myeloid leukemia. *Otolaryngol Head Neck Surg*. 2010;143(3):465-466.
12. Xie Z, Zhang F, Song E, et al. Intraoral granulocytic sarcoma presenting as multiple maxillary and mandibular masses: a case report and literature review. *Oral Surg Oral Med Oral Pathol Oral Radiol Endod*. 2007;103(6):e44-e48.
13. Pau M, Beham-schmid C, Semann W, et al. Intraoral granulocytic sarcoma: a case report and review of the literature. *J Oral Maxillofac Surg*. 2010;68(10):2569-2574.

14. Ponnam SR, Srivastava G, Jampani N, et al. A fatal case of rapid gingival enlargement: case report with brief review. *J Oral Maxillofac Pathol.* 2014;18(1):121-126.
15. Srinivasan B, Ethunandan M, Anand R, et al. Granulocytic sarcoma of the lips: report of an unusual case. *Oral Surg Oral Med Oral Pathol Oral Radiol Endod.* 2008;105(1):e34-e36.
16. Man LM, Morris AL, Keng M. New therapeutic stragegies in acute lymphocytic leukemia. *Curr Hematol Malig Reg.* 2107;12(3):197-206.
17. De Kouchkovsky I, Abdul-Hay M. Acute myeloid leukemia: a comprehensive review and 2016 update. *Blood Cancer J.* 2016;6(7):e441.
18. Ladyzynski P, Molik M, Foltynski P. A network meta-analysis of progression free survival and overall survival in first-line treatment of chronic lymphocytic leukemia. *Cancer Treat Rev.* 2015;41(2):77-93.
19. Nabhan C, Raca G, Wang UL. Predicting prognosis in CLL in the contemporary era. *JAMA Oncol.* 2015;1(7);965-974.).
20. Campos MI, Campos CN, Aarestrup FM, et al. Oral mucositis in cancer treatment: natural history, prevention and treatment. *Mol Clin Oncol.* 2014;2(3):337-340.
21. Riley P, Glenny AM, Worthington HV, et al. Interventions for preventing oral mucositis in patients with cancer receiving treatment: cytokines and growth factors. *Cochran Database Syst Rev.* 2017;(11):Art No:CD011990.
22. Kuten-Shorrer M, Woo SB, Treister NS. Oral graft-versus-host disease. *Dent Clin North Am.* 2014;58(2):351-368.
23. Hicks J, Flaitz CM. Langerhans cell histiocytosis: current insights in a molecular age with emphasis on clinical oral and maxillofacial pathology practice. *Oral Surg Oral Med Oral Pathol Oral Radiol Endod.* 2005;100(2 suppl):S42-S66.
24. Krooks J, Minkov M, Weatherall AG, et al. Langerhans cell histiocytosis in children: diagnosis, differential diagnosis, treatment, sequelae, and standardized follow-up. *J Am Acad Dermatol.* 2018;78(6):1047-1056.
25. Satter EK, High WA. Langerhans cell histiocytosis: a review of the current recommendations of the Histiocyte Society. *Pediatr Dermatol.* 2008;25(3):291-295.
26. Stull MA, Kransdorf MJ, Devaney KO. Langerhans cell histiocytosis of bone. *Radiographics.* 1992;12(4):801-823.
27. Xhang C, Gao J, He J, et al. Regulatory T-cell expansion in oral and maxillofacial Langerhans cell histiocytosis. *Oral Surg oral Med Oral Pathol Oral Radiol.* 2020;130(5);547-556.
28. Dagenais M, Pharoah MJ, Sikorski PA. The radiographic characteristics of histiocytosis X: a study of 29 cases that involve the jaws. *Oral Surg Oral Med Oral Pathol.* 1992;74(2):230-236.
29. Annibali S, Cristalli MP, Solidani M, et al. Langerhans cell histiocytosis: oral/periodontal involvement in adult patients. *Oral Dis.* 2009;15(8):596-601.
30. Cleveland DB, Goldberg KM, Greenspan JS, et al. Langerhans' cell histiocytosis: report of three cases with unusual oral soft tissue involvement. *Oral Surg Oral Med Oral Pathol Oral Radiol Endod.* 1996;82(5):541-548.
31. Abla O, Egeler RM, Weitzman S. Langerhans cell histiocytosis: current concepts and treatments. *Cancer Treat Rev.* 2010;36(4):354-359.
32. Ng-Cheng-Hin B, O'Hanlon-Brown C, Alifrangis C, et al. Langerhans cell histiocytosis: old disease new treatment. *QJM.* 2011;104(2):89-96.
33. Piris MA, Medeiros LJ, Chang KC. Hodgkin lymphoma: a review of pathological features and recent advances in pathogenesis. *Pathology.* 2020;52(1):154-165.
34. Ansell SM. Hodgkin lymphoma: 2018 update on diagnosis, risk stratification, and management. *Am J Hematol.* 2018;9:704-715.
35. Iyengar P, Mazloom A, Shihadeh F, et al. Hodgkin lymphoma involving extranodal and nodal head and neck sites: characteristics and outcomes. *Cancer.* 2010;116(16):3825-3829.
36. Darling MR, Cuddy KK, Rizkalla K. Hodgkin lymphoma of the oral mucosa. *Head Neck Pathol.* 2012;6(4):507-510.
37. Whitt JC, Dunlap CL, Martin KF. Oral Hodgkin lymphoma: a wolf in wolf's clothing. *Oral Surg Oral Med Oral Pathol Oral Radiol Endod.* 2007;104(5):e45-e51.
38. Yencha MW. Primary parotid gland Hodgkin's lymphoma. *Ann Otol Rhinol Laryngol.* 2002;111(4):338-342.
39. Swerdlow SH, Campo E, Harris NL, et al. eds. *WHO Classification of Tumours of Haematopoietic and Lymphoid Tissues.* Revised 4th ed.. Stylus Publishing; 2017.
40. Borchmann P, Eichenauer DA, Engert A. State of the art in the treatment of Hodgkin lymphoma. *Nat Rev Clin Oncol.* 2012;9(8):450-459.
41. Zapater E, Bagan JV, Carbonell F, et al. Malignant lymphoma of the head and neck. *Oral Dis.* 2010;16(2):119-128.
42. Shankland KR, Armitage JO, Hancock BW. Non-Hodgkin lymphoma. *Lancet.* 2012;380(9844):848-857.
43. Scherfler S, Freier K, Seeberger R, et al. Cranio-maxillofacial non-Hodgkin's lymphoma: clinical and histological presentation. *J Cranio-Maxillo-Fac Surg.* 2012;40(7):e211-e213.
44. Kemp S, Gallagher G, Kabani S, et al. Oral non-Hodgkin's lymphoma: review of the literature and World Health Organization classification with reference to 40 cases. *Oral Surg Oral Med Oral Pathol Oral Radiol Endod.* 2008;105(2):194-201.
45. Kusuke N, Custodio M, Sousa S. Oral Lesions as the primary diagnosis of non-hodgkin's lymphoma: a 20-year experience. *Eur Arch Oto-Rhino-Laryngol.* 2019;276:2873-2879.
46. Li S, Young KH, Medeiros LJ. Diffuse large B-cell lymphoma. *Pathology.* 2018;50(1):74-87.
47. Bhattacharyya I, Chehal HK, Cohen DM, et al. Primary diffuse large B-cell lymphoma of the oral cavity: germinal center classification. *Head Neck Pathol.* 2010;4(3):181-191.
48. Wright DH. Pathology of extra-nodal non Hodgkin lymphomas. *Clin Oncol.* 2012;24(5):319-328.
49. Cultrera JL, Dalia SM. Diffuse large B-cell lymphoma: current strategies and future directions. *Cancer Control.* 2012;19(3):204-213.
50. Rodrigues-Fernandes CI, de Souza LL, dos Santos-Costa SF, et al. Clinicopathologic analysis of oral plasmablastic lymphoma: a systemiatic review. *Oral Pathol Med.* 2018;47(10):915-922.
51. Medel N, Hamao-Sakamoto A. A case of oral plasmablastic lymphoma and review of current trends in oral manifestations associated with human immunodeficiency virus infection. *J Oral Maxillofac Surg.* 2014;72(9):1729-1735.
52. Gerami P. Oral mucosal MALT lymphoma clinically simulating oral facial granulomatosis. *Int J Dermatol.* 2007;46(8):868-871.
53. Manveen JK, Subramanyam R, Harshaminder G, et al. Primary B-cell MALT lymphoma of the palate: a case report and distinction from benign lymphoid hyperplasia (pseudolymphoma). *J Oral Maxillofac Pathol.* 2012;16(1):97-102.
54. Ferreri AJM, Sassone M, Kiesewetter B, et al. High-dose clarithromycin is an active monotherapy for patients with relapsed/refractory extranodal marginal zone lymphoma of mucosa-associated lymphoid tissue (MALT): the HD-K phase II trial. *Ann Oncol.* 2015;28(8):1760-1765.

55. Guggisberg K, Jordan RC. Mantle cell lymphoma of the oral cavity: case series and comprehensive review of the literature. *Oral Surg Oral Med Oral Pathol Oral Radiol Endod*. 2010;109(1):98-104.
56. Schieber M, Gordon LI, Karmali R. Current overview and treatment of mantle cell lymphoma. *F1000Res*. 2018;7:F1000. Faculty/Rev-1136.
57. Williams ME, Dreyling M, Winter J, et al. Management of mantle cell lymphoma: key challenges and next steps. *Clin Lymphoma Myeloma Leuk*. 2010;10(5):336-346.
58. Rodrigues-Fernandes CI, de-Oliveira MEP, Arboleda LPA, et al. Clinicopathological analysis of oral Burkitt's lymphoma in pediatric patients: a systematic review. *Int J Pediatr Otorhinolaryngol*. 2020;134:110033.
59. Kikuchi K, Inoue H, Miyazaki Y, et al. Adult sporadic Burkitt lymphoma of the oral cavity: a case report and literature review. *J Oral Maxillofac Surg*. 2012;70(12):2936-2943.
60. Sciallis AP, Law ME, Inwards DJ, et al. Mucosal CD30-positive T-cell lymphoproliferations of the head and neck show a clinicopathologic spectrum similar to cutaneous CD30-positive T-cell lymphoproliferative disorders. *Mod Pathol*. 2012;25(7):983-992.
61. Matsumoto N, Ohki H, Mukae S, et al. Anaplastic large cell lymphoma in gingiva: case report and literature review. *Oral Surg Oral Med Oral Pathol Oral Radiol Endod*. 2008;106(4):e29-e34.
62. Alobeid B, Pan LX, Milligan L, et al. Eosinophil-rich CD30+ lymphoproliferative disorder of the oral mucosa: a form of "traumatic eosinophilic granuloma". *Am J Clin Pathol*. 2004;121(1):43-50.
63. Salisbury CL, Budnick SD, Li S. T-cell receptor gene rearrangement and CD30 immunoreactivity in traumatic ulcerative granuloma with stromal eosinophilia of the oral cavity. *Am J Clin Pathol*. 2009;132(5):722-727.
64. Hirshberg A, Amariglio N, Akrish S, et al. Traumatic ulcerative granuloma with stromal eosinophilia: a reactive lesion of the oral mucosa. *Am J Clin Pathol*. 2006;126(4):522-529.
65. Goldsmith SM, Seo BL, Kumara de Silva R, et al. Oral mycosis fungoides: report with immune profile. *Oral Surg Oral Med Oral Pathol Oral Radiol*. 2014;118(2):e48-e52.
66. Rosebush MS, Allen CM, Accurso BT, et al. Oral mycosis fungoides: a report of three cases and review of the literature. *Head Neck Pathol*. 2019;13(3):492-499.
67. Sirois DA, Miller AS, Harwick RD, et al. Oral manifestations of cutaneous T-cell lymphoma: a report of eight cases. *Oral Surg Oral Med Oral Pathol*. 1993;75(6):700-705.
68. Long JC, Mihm MC. Mycosis fungoides with extracutaneous dissemination: a distinct clinicopathologic entity. *Cancer*. 1974;34(5):1745-1755.
69. Chua MS, Veness MJ. Mycosis fungoides involving the oral cavity. *Australas Radiol*. 2002;46(3):336-339.
70. Al-Hakeem DA, Fedele S, Carlos R, et al. Extranodal NK/T-cell lymphoma, nasal type. *Oral Oncol*. 2007;43(1):4-14.
71. Haverkos BM, Pan Z, Gru A, et al. Extranodal NK/T-cell lymphoma, nasal type (ENKTL-NT): an update on epidemiology, clinical presentation, and natural history in North American and European cases. *Curr Hematol Malig Rep*. 2016;11(6):514-527.
72. Yin HF, Jamlikhanova V, Okada N, et al. Primary natural killer/T-cell lymphomas of the oral cavity are aggressive neoplasms. *Virchows Arch*. 1999;435(4):400-406.
73. Sanches-Romero C, de Almeida OP, Henao JR, Carlos R. Extranodal NK/T-Cell lymphoma, nasal type in Guatemala: an 86-cases series emphasizing clinical presentation and microscopic characteristis. *Head Neck Pathol*. 2019;13(4):624-634.
74. Cho KJ, Cho SG, Lee DH. Natural killer T-cell lymphoma of the tongue. *Ann Otol Rhinol Laryngol*. 2005;114(1 pt. 1):55-57.
75. Beltran BE, Castro D, Paredes, et al. EBV-Positive diffuse large B-cell lymphoma, not otherwise specified: 2020 update on diagnosis, risk stratification and management. *Am J Hemtol*. 2020;95(4):435-445.
76. Heslop HE. How I treat EBV lymphoproliferation. *Blood*. 2009;114(19):4002-4008.
77. Hatton O, Martinez OM, Esquivel CO. Emerging therapeutic strategies for Epstein–Barr virus+ post-transplant lymphoproliferative disorder. *Pediatr Transplant*. 2012;16(3):220-229.
78. Knowles DM. Immunodeficiency-associated lymphoproliferative disorders. *Mod Pathol*. 1999;12(2):200-217.
79. Dojcinov SD, Venkataraman G, Pittaluga S, et al. Age-related EBV-associated lymphoproliferative disorders in the Western population: a spectrum of reactive lymphoid hyperplasia and lymphoma. *Blood*. 2011;117(18):4726-4735.
80. Oyama T, Yamamoto K, Asano N, et al. Age-related EBV-associated B-cell lymphoproliferative disorders constitute a distinct clinicopathologic group: a study of 96 patients. *Clin Cancer Res*. 2007;13(17):5124-5132.
81. Kikuchi K, Fukunaga S, Inoue H, et al. A case of age-related Epstein–Barr virus (EBV)-associated B cell lymphoproliferative disorder, so-called polymorphous subtype, of the mandible, with a review of the literature. *Head Neck Pathol*. 2013;7(2):178-187.
82. Dojcinov SD, Venkataraman G, Raffeld M, et al. EBV positive mucocutaneous ulcer—a study of 26 cases associated with various sources of immunosuppression. *Am J Surg Pathol*. 2010;34(3):405-417.
83. Adams B, Lazarchick J, Medina AM, et al. Iatrogenic immunodeficiency-associated lymphoproliferative disease of the Hodgkin lymphoma-like variant in a patient treated with mycophenolate mofetil for autoimmune hepatitis. *Am J Hematol*. 2010;85(8):627-629.
84. Horie N, Kawano R, Kaneko T, et al. Methotrexate-related lymphoproliferative disorder arising in the gingiva of a patient with rheumatoid arthritis. *Aust Dent J*. 2015;60(3):408-411. doi:10.1111/adj.12235
85. Kikuchi K, Miyazaki Y, Tanaka A, et al. Methotrexate-related Epstein–Barr Virus (EBV)-associated lymphoproliferative disorder—so-called "Hodgkin-like lesion"—of the oral cavity in a patient with rheumatoid arthritis. *Head Neck Pathol*. 2010;4(4):305-311.
86. Kalantzis A, Marshman Z, Falconer DT, et al. Oral effects of low-dose methotrexate treatment. *Oral Surg Oral Med Oral Pathol Oral Radiol Endod*. 2005;100(1):52-62.
87. Trappe R, Oertel S, Leblond V, et al. Sequential treatment with rituximab followed by CHOP chemotherapy in adult B-cell post-transplant lymphoproliferative disorder (PTLD): the prospective international multicentre phase 2 PTLD-1 trial. *Lancet Oncol*. 2012;13(2):196-206.
88. Alinari L, Pant S, McNamara K, et al. Lymphomatoid granulomatosis presenting with gingival involvement in an immune competent elderly male. *Head Neck Pathol*. 2012;6(4):496-501.
89. Melani C, Jaffe ES, Wilson WH. Pathobiology and treatment of lymphomatoid granulomatosis, a rare EBV-driven disorder. *Blood*. 2020;135(16):1344-1352.
90. Jaffe ES. Lymphoid lesions of the head and neck: a model of lymphocyte homing and lymphomagenesis. *Mod Pathol*. 2002;15(3):255-263.

91. Pereira AAC, Ferreira CB, Hanemann JAC, et al. Oral manifestations of lymphomatoid granulomatosis. *Head Neck Pathol*. 2019;13(2):270-276.
92. Cargini P, Civica M, Sollima L, et al. Oral lymphomatoid granulomatosis, the first sign of a "rare disease": a case report. *J Med Case Rep*. 2014;8:152.
93. Kazandjian D. Multiple myeloma epidemiology and survival: a unique malignancy. *Semin Oncol*. 2016;43(6):676-681.
94. Smith D, Yong K. Multiple myeloma. *BMJ*. 2013;346:f3863.
95. Pingali SR, Haddad RY, Saad A. Current concepts of clinical management of multiple myeloma. *Dis Mon*. 2012;58(4):195-207.
96. Landgren O, Rajkumar SV. New development in diagnosis, prognosis and assessment of response in multiple myeloma. *Clin Cancer Res*. 2016;22(22):5428-5433.
97. Hogan MC, Lee A, Solberg LA, et al. Unusual presentation of multiple myeloma with unilateral visual loss and numb chin syndrome in a young adult. *Am J Hematol*. 2002;70(1):55-59.
98. Gouvea AF, Ribeiro AC, Leon JE, et al. Head and neck amyloidosis: clinicopathological features and immunohistochemical analysis of 14 cases. *J Oral Pathol Med*. 2012;41(2):178-185.
99. Rajkumar SV, Kumar S. Multiple myeloma: diagnosis and treatment. *Mayo Clin Proc*. 2016;91(1):101-119.
100. Ruggiero SL, Dodson TB, Fantasia J, et al. American Association of Oral and Maxillofacial Surgeons position paper on medication-related osteonecrosis of the jaw – 2014 Update. *J Oral Maxillofac Surg*. 2014;72:1938-1956.
101. Goyal G, Bartley AC, Funni S, et al. Treatment approaches and outcomes in plasmacytomas: analysis using a national dataset. *Leukemia*. 2018;32(6):1414-1420.
102. Caers J, Piava B, Zamagni E, et al. Diagnosis, treatment and response assessment in solitary plasmacytoma: updated recommendations from a European Expert Panel. *J Hematol Oncol*. 2018;11(1):10. doi:10.1186/s13045-017-0549-1
103. Kilciksiz S, Karakoyun-Celik O, Agaoglu FY, et al. A review for solitary plasmacytoma of bone and extramedullary plasmacytoma. *Sci World J*. 2012;2012:895765.
104. Chittemsetti S, Guttikonda VR, Sravya T, Manchikatla PK. Solitary plasmacytoma of mandible: a rare entity. *J Oral Maxillofac Pathol*. 2019;23(1):136-139.
105. Alwan H, Moor JW, Wright D, et al. Extramedullary plasmacytoma of the tongue base: a case report and clinical review of head and neck plasmacytoma. *Ear Nose Throat J*. 2010;89(8):369-373.
106. Rothfield RE, Johnson JT, Stavrides A. Extramedullary plasmacytoma of the parotid. *Head Neck*. 1990;12(4):352-354.
107. Jham BC, Binmadi NO, Scheper MA, et al. Follicular lymphoid hyperplasia of the palate: case report and literature review. *J Cranio-Maxillo-Fac Surg*. 2009;37(2):79-82.

CHAPTER 71

Ocular lymphoproliferative disorders

Carolina M. Gentile and Paola de la Iglesia Niveyro

INTRODUCTION

The "ocular adnexum" is the comprehensive name for those tissues that sustain and give strength to the globe, including the conjunctiva, the lids, and the orbital soft tissues and bones. It holds the lacrimal gland and is extended on the lacrimal drainage and lacrimal sac. Ocular adnexal lymphomas (OALs) involve the orbit in approximately 45% of cases, the lacrimal gland in 26% of cases, the conjunctiva in 25% of cases, the eyelid in 8% to 9% of cases, and are relatively rare in the lacrimal sac.[1-3] Ocular lymphomas can occur at any age. They most commonly develop in patients in the fifth to seventh decades of life and are slightly more prevalent in women.[4] Ocular adnexal lymphoid tumors are very rare in children.[5] About 80% to 90% of primary OALs are extranodal marginal zone B-cell lymphomas of mucosa-associated lymphoid tissue (MALT lymphomas).[3,4] Although specific lymphoma subtypes are particularly linked to certain outcomes, location, unilateral or bilateral disease, and extension into the deep soft tissues, other clinical signs can also provide valuable information for the risk of relapse and disease-specific survival.[6-8] This chapter will review the epidemiology, etiology, clinical presentation, management, and outcomes for OAL.

ANATOMICAL BASIS

The globe, excluding the cornea and limbal rim, and the external surface of the superior and inferior eyelids, is covered with a mucous membrane, the conjunctiva. The surface is layered by a nonkeratinizing squamous epithelium with a variable number of goblet cells. The conjunctiva may be divided into the bulbar conjunctiva that is freely movable and delicate, the tarsal or palpebral conjunctiva that is firmly attached to the inner surface of the inferior and superior eyelids, and the forniceal-orbital where the conjunctival tissue is redundant and loose.[9] Two other references of the ocular surface are the plica semilunaris and the caruncle. The first is a nasal fold of redundant conjunctiva. The caruncle is a fleshy mass lying at the median interpalpebral inner canthus composed of the conjunctiva and lid tissues.

The lids have four layers: (1) the outer skin with elastic and baggy scant subcutaneous tissue, (2) the orbicularis striated muscle, (3) the dense fibrous tarsal plate holding the meibomian glands, and (4) the inner adherent tarsal conjunctiva layer. The lymphatic drainage of the lateral portion of the lid goes to the preauricular and intraparotid lymph nodes, and the medial lymphatic drainage goes to the submental and submandibular nodes. A clinically important landmark is the insertion of the levator palpebrae superioris. This structure attaches to the medial orbital rims and terminates in the upper lid penetrating the orbital septum. The ligaments are reinforced by orbital fibrous connective tissue and fascia expansion of the extraocular rectus muscles.

Each orbit has a volume of about 30 mm³ bounded by several bones. It contains a wide variety of tissues: neural, adipose, muscle, vascular excluding lymphatics, connective, and cartilage. The bony orbital walls contact with the paranasal sinuses. The lacrimal gland is accommodated in a shallow lacrimal fossa located in the anterosuperolateral orbit and measures 20 × 12 × 5 mm. It is split in a larger orbital lobe and a smaller palpebral lobe. Fluid from the main and accessory lacrimal gland is drained by the lacrimal canaliculi into the lacrimal sac and then into the nasal cavity. Unlike the parotid gland, the lacrimal gland does not possess lymph nodes. However, the parenchyma of the lobules contains dispersed lymphocytes and plasma cells. The glands drain into the superficial parotid lymph nodes.

EYE-ASSOCIATED LYMPHOID TISSUE

The eye-associated lymphoid tissue (EALT), which comprehensively forms the immune system of the eye, is recognized as a component of the MALT found in different organs of the body.[10,11] MALT is composed of lymphoid cells situated in and closely underneath the epithelium. These cells detect antigens and induce an immune response. EALT includes the lacrimal gland, the conjunctiva-associated lymphoid tissue (CALT), and the lacrimal drainage-associated lymphoid tissue.[9]

In normal conditions, the eye and orbit are devoid of native lymphoid tissue. The surface of the eye is covered by an immune system, providing detection and response to external antigens.[10] From birth to 3 or 4 years of age, the ocular surface is usually devoid of CALT.[12] The lymphatic tissue develops after antigen stimulation and plasma cells secrete IgA, an important molecule present in the tears with activity against individual pathogens. This associated lymphoid tissue comprises the lacrimal gland and the lacrimal sac. Lymphocytes are present in the lamina propia (misleadingly called adenoid layer) and within the epithelium. Local immune responses also include the formation of lymphocytic aggregates and high endothelial venules. Chronic antigen stimulation initiates a reactive lymphoid infiltrate with polyclonality in the conjunctival tissues. The locations of lymphoid follicles are the upper and lower tarsal conjunctiva and fornix. These locations are concordant with the most common sites of conjunctival lymphomas (CLs).

ETIOLOGY

Lymphomas are neoplasms derived from clonal proliferations of lymphocytes and comprise a diverse group of diseases with different subtypes. OALs constitute 2% of all extranodal lymphomas, and 25% to 30% of all OALs are located in the conjunctiva.[7]

Extranodal marginal zone lymphomas (EMZLs) of the conjunctiva and orbit are often preceded by chronic inflammation and reactive lymphoid hyperplasia (RLH) at the site of lymphoma development. The etiology is usually unknown.[13] The current hypothesis of lymphomagenesis of extranodal marginal zone B-cell lymphoma of MALT type includes the following steps: antigenic-driven RLH, clonal expansion and proliferation of B-cells, genetic alterations, and sustained growth of abnormal populations of B-cells that develop specific gene mutations that ultimately lead to continued proliferation and immortality. According to this hypothesis, histologically suspicious lymphoid infiltrates should be studied for B-cell or plasma cell clonality using various methods, including immunohistochemistry, flow cytometry, in situ hybridization, and/or molecular gene rearrangement methods (usually PCR-based) for the immunoglobulin heavy (*IGH*) gene.

Because of the clinicopathologic similarities between conjunctival and gastric MALT lymphomas, several studies have evaluated for the presence and role of infectious organisms in the pathogenesis of the disease: *Helicobacter pylori* (*H. pylori*),[14-17] *Chlamydophila psittaci* (*C. psittaci*), *Chlamydophila pneumoniae*,[18-22] hepatitis C virus (HCV),[23] and herpes virus have been studied in OALs. In one study including 31 patients with ocular adnexa MALT lymphoma, 10 (32%) had gastric *H. pylori* and three of them were also positive for *C. psittaci*.[16] The patients with ocular adnexal MALT lymphoma showed no response to helicobacter eradication therapy. The same group reported that 80% of 40 patients carried *C. psittaci*. Interestingly, most of the lymphomas were MALT subtype and regressed following antibiotic treatment with doxycycline.[19,20] Another series revealed no evidence of *H. pylori*, *C. psittaci*, or *C. pneumoniae*.[24-26] A link between HCV infection, liver cancer, and B-cell lymphomas has been clearly documented; a study of ocular adnexal MALT lymphoma revealed that 13% of 55 patients had HCV seropositivity.[23] Furthermore, the authors claimed that HCV is associated with aggressive behavior.[23]

The variability of these results among different patient cohorts has been interpreted as due to geographic variations in the prevalence of infectious agents and variability of used methods to identify the organism. In the absence of well-controlled and randomized studies, the relationship of infectious agents and OALs should be taken cautiously.[27] Rare associations were observed between Epstein–Barr virus and natural killer/T-cell lymphomas. Interestingly, evolving diffuse large B-cell lymphoma from low-grade OAL has been reported in the setting of Ig4 chronic dacryoadenitis, coexistent with autoimmune conditions such as Sjögren disease, Hashimoto thyroiditis, myasthenia gravis, Graves' disease, rheumatoid arthritis, discoid lupus, mucous membrane pemphigoid, and autoimmune diseases unclassified.[28,29]

Also, Asao et al recently suggested that conjunctival dysbiosis may play a role in the genesis of MALT lymphoma as different microbiota was found in MALT lymphoma patients compared to healthy controls.[30]

EPIDEMIOLOGY

Extraocular lymphoproliferative lesions and lymphomas may occur in the orbit, conjunctiva, lacrimal gland, lacrimal sac, and rarely in the eyelid skin. OALs represent 1% to 2.5% of all lymphomas and approximately 5% to 15% of extranodal lymphomas.[31-33] With very few exceptions, intraocular and adnexal lymphomas are non-Hodgkin B-cell lymphomas representing 10% to 15% of orbital, conjunctival, eyelid, and lacrimal sac tumors.[33] Most lymphomas involving the ocular adnexa are primary (78%-92%) and the rest are secondary (8%-22%).[31-35] An estimated 5% of non-Hodgkin lymphoma patients develop OAL during the course of their disease.[36] The vast majority of adnexal lymphomas are low-grade marginal zone lymphomas (MZLs). According to the World Health Organization (WHO) classification of lymphoid tissues, MZL of the ocular adnexa is designated as EMZL of MALT.[36] Nevertheless, since the behavior of OAL varies, it is convenient to use EMZL for primary lymphomas in the orbit and restrict the term MALT to the conjunctiva lacrimal gland and lacrimal sac.[37] A noncomprehensive list of lymphomas affecting the OAL is summarized in Table 71-1. Because many of these studies have not separated conjunctiva, orbit, and lacrimal gland lesions from those of other origins, it is difficult to track the incidence and characteristics of the lymphomas in specific periocular sites.

Intraocular lymphomas, although exceedingly rare, encompass highly aggressive primary central nervous system lymphomas (PCNSL) (so-called primary vitreoretinal lymphoma), primary choroidal lymphomas, and secondary disseminated lymphomas. Statistical data disclosed a rapid and increasing incidence of ocular and adnexal non-Hodgkin lymphoma between 1975 and 2001.[33] The diagnosis of OAL is commonly a challenge for the pathologist. Because of location and complexity of the ocular tissues, biopsies are generally very small and artifacts frequently make difficult the cytologic and architectural characteristics required to distinguish between malignant and RLH. In the past, histologically indeterminate lymphoproliferative lesions were designated as atypical lymphoid hyperplasia (ALH) of the ocular adnexa. The reported incidence was 3% to 12% of

TABLE 71-1 Lymphoma Types in the Ocular Adnexa

- Extranodal marginal zone lymphoma
- Marginal zone lymphoma of mucosa-associated lymphoid tissue (MALT lymphoma)
- Follicular lymphoma
- Diffuse large B-cell lymphoma
- Mantle cell lymphoma
- Chronic lymphocytic leukemia/small lymphocytic lymphoma
- Lymphoplasmacytic lymphoma
- Precursor B-cell lymphoblastic lymphoma
- Splenic marginal zone lymphoma
- B-lymphoblastic leukemia/lymphoma
- Low-grade B-cell, NOS[a]
- Plasma cell neoplasms
- T- and NK-cell lymphomas[b]
- Peripheral T-cell lymphoma[b]
- Hodgkin lymphoma[c]

[a]Not otherwise specified.
[b]Rare.
[c]Extremely rare.

OAL.[3,38] Curiously, those lesions showed recurrences and may progress to low-grade lymphomas.[39] Currently, these cases are mostly absorbed into the EMZL.[4]

Benign reactive lymphoid hyperplasia (BLRH) of the conjunctiva is a rare, lymphoproliferative process that belongs to the broad spectrum of ocular adnexal lymphocytic infiltrative disorders. It exhibits a polyclonal proliferation and presents in three different histologic types: follicular, diffuse, and sheet-like. The exact etiology and pathogenesis of BRLH remains unknown. However, BRLH is thought to result from a chronic inflammatory response of lymphoid cells to antigenic stimulation.[40]

GENETICS

IGH and light chain gene and clonality rearrangements have demonstrated IgH rearrangement in as many as 80% of the reported cases of OAL (MALT).[31,35,36,41] All chromosomal alterations affect a common signaling pathway, resulting in activation of the nuclear factor-κB complex, leading to transcription of several genes contributing to lymphomatous transformation, cell proliferation, and survival. High-resolution single nucleotide polymorphism array is a useful method to discriminate OALs from benign lymphoproliferative diseases.

Translocations which have been found to be important for the pathogenesis of EMZL in the ocular adnexal region are t(11; 18) (q21; q21) involving API2 and MALT1, t(14; 18) (q32; q21) involving IGH and MALT1, t(3; 14) (p14; q32) involving FOXP1 and IGH, and t(1; 14) (p22; q32) involving Bcl-10 and IGH.[42] The t(11; 18) (q21; q21) translocation is present in approximately 20% of conjunctival EMZLs and is related to oxidative damage induced by genotoxic factors.[43] The t(14; 18) (q32; q21) translocation is found in around 15% to 20% of ocular adnexal EMZLs and is described in the conjunctiva in particular.[44-46] Another 15% to 20% of ocular adnexal EMZL patients carry the t(3; 14) (p14; q32) translocation, whereas t(1; 14) (p22; q32) occurs in approximately 10% of these.[44,45,47] Trisomy of chromosomes 3 and 18 is another cytogenetic abnormality associated with EMZL.[48-50] Gains of chromosome 3 are rarely found in EMZL of the conjunctiva, whereas trisomy 18 is very common in conjunctival EMZL, found in as many as 67% of patients.[50,51] Trisomy of these chromosomes is often associated with the t(14; 18) (q32; q21) and t(3; 14) (p14; q32) translocations.[44,52] The t(14; 18) (q32.3; q21.3) translocation is present in approximately 85% of follicular lymphomas (FLs), including ocular adnexal FLs, and has also been found in conjunctival FL. This translocation involves BCL2 and IGH gene. As for MCL, the t(11; 14) (q13; q32) translocation occurs in more than 95% of MCL cases, including ocular adnexal mantle cell lymphoma (MCL), and has also been found in conjunctival MCL. This chromosomal translocation involves cyclin D-1 (CCND1) and IGH.

IMMUNOPHENOTYPE OF OALS

Extranodal Marginal Zone Lymphoma of Mucosa-Associated Lymphoid Tissue (MALT lymphoma): sIG^+ (IGM or IGA or IGG), $sIGD^-$, $cIG^{-/+}$, pan B-cell markers (CD20, PAX-5, CD19, CD79a), $CD5^-$, $CD10^-$, $CD23^-$, $CD43^{-/+}$; IGH and IGL gene rearrangements, BCL1 and BCL2 germline, trisomy 3, or t(11; 18) (q21; q21) may be seen.

Follicular Lymphoma: sIG^+ (usually $IGM^{+/-}$ IGD, IGG, IGA), pan B^+, $CD10^{+/-}$, $CD5^{-/+}$, $CD23^{-/+}$, $CD43^-$, $CD11c^-$, $CD25^-$; overexpression of $BCL2^+$ (useful to distinguish from reactive follicles), $BCL6^+$; IGH and IGL gene rearrangements, t(14; 18) (q32; q21) with rearranged BCL2 gene (70%-95% in adults).

Diffuse Large B-Cell Lymphoma (DLBCL), NOS: Pan B^+, surface or cytoplasmic $IGM > IGG > IGA$, $CD45^{+/-}$, $CD5^{-/+}$, $CD10^{+/-}$, $BCL6^{+/-}$, 3q27 region abnormalities involving BCL6 seen in 30% of cases, t(14; 18) involving BCL2 seen in 20% to 30% of cases, and MYC rearrangement seen in 10% of cases. A series of 20 cases of DLBCL revealed that most cases had a germinal center phenotype ($BCL6^+/MUM1^-$ or $CD10^+$) according to the Hans or Choi algorithm and a smaller percentage was of nongerminal center origin ($BCL6^+/MUM1^+$ or $MUM1^+/CD10^-$).[43]

Mantle Cell Lymphoma: $sIGM^+$, $sIGD^+$, lambda > kappa, $PanB^+$, $CD5^+$, $CD10^{-/+}$, $CD23^-$, $CD43^+$, $CD11c^-$, $CD25^-$, cyclin $D1^+$; IGH and IGL gene rearrangements, t(11; 14) (q13; q32); BCL1 gene rearrangements (CCND1/cyclinD1) are typical.

Lymphoplasmacytic Lymphoma: sIGM⁺, sIGD⁻ᐟ⁺, cIG⁺, pan B⁺, CD19⁺, CD20⁺, CD138⁺ (in plasma cells), CD79a⁺, CD5⁻, CD10⁻, CD43⁺ᐟ⁻, CD25⁻ᐟ⁺; *IGH* and *IGL* gene rearrangements, no specific cytogenetic findings.

Extraosseous Plasmacytoma: *cIG*⁺ (*IGG*, *IGA*, rare *IGD*, *IGM*, or *IGE* or light chain only), pan B-(CD19⁻, CD20⁻, CD22⁻), CD79a⁺ᐟ⁻, CD45⁻ᐟ⁺, HLA-DR⁻ᐟ⁺, CD38⁺, CD56⁺ᐟ⁻, CD138⁺, EMA⁻ᐟ⁺, CD43⁺ᐟ⁻, cyclin D1⁺; *IGH* and *IGL* gene rearrangements; deletions, most commonly 13q, and occasional translocations, in particular t(11; 14) (q13; q32).

Chronic Lymphocytic Leukemia/Lymphocytic Lymphoma: *IgM/IgD*, CD20⁺ᐟ⁻, CD22⁺ᐟ⁻, CD5⁺ᐟ⁻, CD19⁺ᐟ⁻, CD79a⁺ᐟ⁻, CD23⁺ᐟ⁻, CD43⁺ᐟ⁻, CD11c⁺ᐟ⁻, CD10⁻, FMC7⁻, CD79b⁻, cyclin D1⁻; mutated tyrosine kinase ZAP-70 expression, *IGHV* unmutated, micro-RNA genes miR-16-1 and miR15a expression.

CLINICAL PRESENTATION AND PROGNOSIS

OAL can present as a single, localized tumor or it can be multifocal. It may affect unilateral or bilateral ocular adnexal structures. Disseminated disease involving regional, central, and peripheral lymph nodes, as well as other distant extranodal sites, is also observed.

ORBITAL LYMPHOMAS

The orbit is the most frequent site of OAL. Orbital lymphomas (OLs) are the most common neoplasms in the adult population, and represent 34% to 55% of orbital malignancies.[53] The age of the patients ranges from 2 to 95 years (mean 64 years).[39,54] In general, they appear to be slightly more frequent in women than in men, with few exceptions in relation to certain specific locations. Ocular lymphoma is rare in children and patients under 21 years of age.[5] Lymphoproliferative tumors of the ocular adnexa may not be noted by the patients for months or years. The specific clinical presentation varies according to the location of the tumor. The most frequent presenting symptoms include the presence of a palpable mass, proptosis, exophthalmos, swelling, tearing, diplopia, ptosis, and rarely pain or irritation (Fig. 71-1). Other unusual signs and symptoms include visual changes, nasolacrimal gland obstruction, and intraocular hypertension. The physical examination usually reveals palpable masses, proptosis, motility disturbances, blepharoptosis, and periorbital edema.

Two-thirds of the patients have unilateral orbital lesions. There is no difference between right or left sides for the frequency of tumor location. The anterior location within the orbit is more often affected than the posterior site. Imaging studies disclose a diffuse infiltrating mass. Computed tomography (CT) or magnetic resonance imaging (MRI) should be considered in patients with proptosis, especially unilateral proptosis, since it is the most common symptom of orbital B-cell lymphoma.[55]

Well-circumscribed lesions are less frequently observed. Lymphoproliferative lesions restricted to the lacrimal gland disclose an antero-posterior oval mass. Secondary lymphomas may involve extraocular muscles. Bone destruction is unusual and may be seen in aggressive lymphomas.

Ocular adnexal lymphoid proliferations have been grouped into RLHs and lymphomas (Fig. 71-2).[56] In the past, the term ALH was used for indeterminate lesions with diffuse infiltrates of small lymphocytes with large hyperchromatic nuclei and which were found to be polyclonal for immunoglobulin (Ig) light or heavy chains. Lymphoproliferative lesions must be distinguished from reactive, nongranulomatous, polymorphic, hypocellular, and fibrotic disorders of the orbit referred to as idiopathic orbital inflammatory disease, entities that may mimic lymphomas including infectious diseases, Kimura disease, Castleman disease, and IgG4-related disease.[57,58]

In one study of 160 lymphoproliferative lesions of the orbit, 9% were RLH, 13% were ALH, and the remaining 78% lymphomas.[59] The most frequent subtypes of B-cell lymphoma include EMZL, FL, small lymphocytic lymphoma,

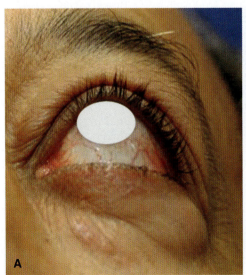
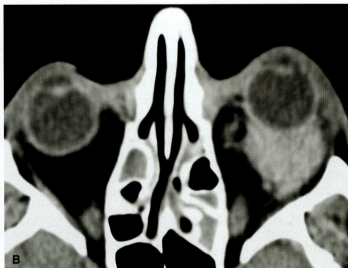

FIGURE 71-1. **Orbital lymphoma in the left eye.** Signs included proptosis, ptosis, and edema **(A)**. CT scan revealed a homogeneous retro-ocular mass infiltrating the orbit **(B)**.

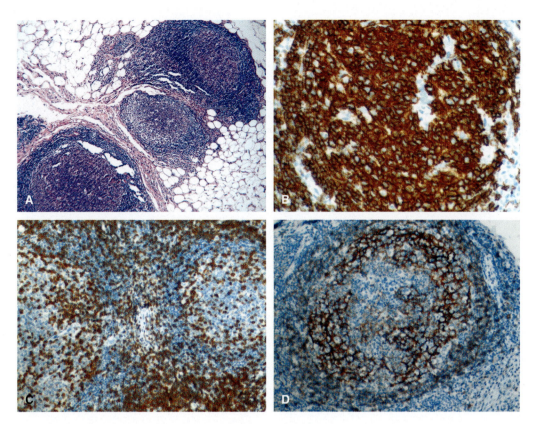

FIGURE 71-2. Reactive lymphoid hyperplasia of the ocular adnexa. Note multiple lymphoid follicles within the adipose tissue **(A)**. The follicles contained CD20+ B cells **(B)** and surrounding CD3+ T cells **(C)** Follicular dendritic cells are highlighted by CD23+ **(D)**.

diffuse large B-cell lymphoma, lymphoplasmacytic lymphoma, and MCL. Some patients may have a history of systemic lymphoma in other locations (25%), such as the head and neck lymph nodes. The systemic disease may be present at the time of diagnosis (9%) or develop after local therapy (17%).[59]

An epidemiological study of OL in the United States also demonstrated that MALT lymphoma conferred the best prognosis (10-year cancer-specific survival 90.2%) and DLBCL conferred the worst prognosis (10-year CSS 68.6%) Older age, male sex, no radiation, and DLBCL histology were significant predictors of worse overall survival.[60]

Four lymphoma subtypes were primarily found in patients with OL: EMZL, DLBCL, FL, and MCL. The histologic subtype was found to be the main predictor for outcome, with EMZL and FL patients having a markedly better prognosis than DLBCL and MCL.[61] It has been observed that the various histologic subtypes of OL confer different overall survival rates. In the largest study reporting the effect of histologic subtype of OL on survival, Olsen et al found extranodal marginal zone B-cell lymphoma to confer the best prognosis and MCL to confer the worst prognosis in a cohort of 797 patients from seven international cancer centers.[55,60,61]

CONJUNCTIVAL LYMPHOMAS

Most CLs appear to be more indolent than those lymphomas arising in the orbit.[62-64] In a retrospective study, Kirkegaard et al found that the great majority of CL were low-grade B-cell lymphomas, with 68% of EMLZ subtypes and 16.3% of FL. Also, in more than half of the patients, they correspond to primary lymphomas. On the other hand, more aggressive types of lymphoma such as DLBCL and ML represent less than 12% of CL and are more frequently secondary infiltration of systemic lymphomas.[7] The mean age at presentation is approximately 60 years (range 20-90 years).[64,65] Males and females are virtually equally affected. However, some lymphoma subtypes occur more often in a particular gender. Conjunctival EMZL occurs somewhat more frequently in women than in men, whereas the high-grade DLBCL and MCL have a predilection for male gender.[66-68]

Patients usually are unaware of the lesion for several months before consultation. Short durations are associated with aggressive lymphomas.[69,70] Most conjunctival EMZLs are unilateral. Bilateral and systemic disease is mostly related to higher grades.[71-73] Coexisting systemic disease is seen in FL, DLBCL, MCL, T-cell NHL, myeloma, and lymphomatoid granulomatosis.[74-79]

The most frequent locations are the superior and inferior conjunctival quadrants usually buried in the fornix under the eyelid, bulbar conjunctiva, and the caruncle/plica semilunaris (Figs. 71-3 to 71-7). Curiously, the rarer T-cell lymphomas involve the corneal lymbus and present signs of episcleritis, scleritis, and symblepharon.[80-82]

Symptoms included mass, chemosis, hyperemia, dryness, irritation, epiphora, ptosis, blurred vision, and symblepharon. The most conspicuous sign is a nonscleral adhered salmon-color vascularized mass that may or may not have a nodular or follicular finely smooth surface. The color varies from red to pink, yellow, and gray. Multiplicity of lesions within

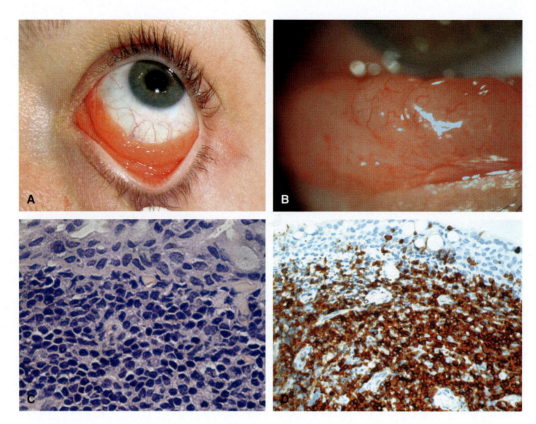

FIGURE 71-3. Conjunctival lymphoma. Smooth, salmon-red-colored lesions with vascularization (**A** and **B**). Histology revealed intermediate-sized (**C**), moderately irregular-shaped CD20+ (**D**) lymphocytes, and mild involvement of the surface epithelium diagnosed as extranodal marginal zone B-cell lymphoma of mucosa-associated lymphoid tissue (MALT).

a unilateral site is common. Some tumors may be masked by the upper eyelid and compromise the levator palpebral and Muller muscles. The differential diagnosis of conjunctiva lymphoma includes inflammatory diseases, follicular conjunctivitis, chronic conjunctivitis, amyloidosis, scleritis, foreign bodies, extraocular extension of uveal lymphoma, and nonpigmented melanocytic nevi, BLRH among others. Concurrent sites in other adnexal locations included the eyelid, orbit, and intraocular (choroid and vitreous). In a study of 117 lymphoproliferative tumors of the conjunctiva, the proportion of lesions was RLH, 17%; ALH, 22%; and lymphoma, 56%.[62]

In the multicentric retrospective study by Kirkegaard and colleagues, disease recurrence was observed in 37.9% of patients with conjunctival EMZL, with a median of 24 months.[7]

In this study of 263 patients with CL, the authors found the following 5-year survival rates: EMZL 97.0%, FL 82.0%, DLBCL 55.0%, and MCL 9.0%. Most patients with localized disease were treated with EBRT with or without chemotherapy.[7]

Lesions restricted to the conjunctiva, unilateral disease, and low Ki-67 proliferation index are indicators of good prognosis. Bilateral presentations have more risk of systemic disease than unilateral cases (47% vs 17%). Systemic disease occurs in 20% to 30% of cases before or after diagnosis and therapy with a mean interval of 51 and 21 months. The most frequent secondary locations are the lymph nodes, abdomen, bone marrow, brain, and lung. The risk of systemic disease development at 1, 5, and 10 years was 7%, 15%, and 28%, respectively.[62]

LACRIMAL GLAND LYMPHOMAS

Approximately 20% of OALs arise in the lacrimal gland and nearly half of the tumors developing in the lacrimal fossa correspond to lymphomas.[83] Lymphomas are more common than benign RLH. Along with the increased proportion of OAL, lacrimal gland lymphomas have steadily increased between 1973 and 1990. The patients are commonly females in their mid-60s. The disease-specific and general survival rates at 10 years' follow-up were 79.1% and 55.1%, correspondingly. Lacrimal gland lymphomas most commonly spread to the lymph nodes (43%). Signs and symptoms include oblong painless enlargement of the lacrimal gland. Bilateral involvement is seen in less than 30% of the lymphomas.

In a retrospective multicenter study, Stine Dahl Vest and colleagues reported that the major NHL subtypes of lacrimal gland are extranodal marginal zone B-cell lymphoma (68%), FL (10%), diffuse large B-cell lymphoma LBCL (10%), and MCL (7%), which resemble the distribution of lymphoma subtypes in the ocular adnexa rather than that of the salivary glands as previously assumed. The prognosis of lacrimal gland lymphoma was good with a 5-year overall survival of 73.8% and a 5-year disease-specific survival of 87.5%. Lymphoma subtype was a significant predictor in explaining

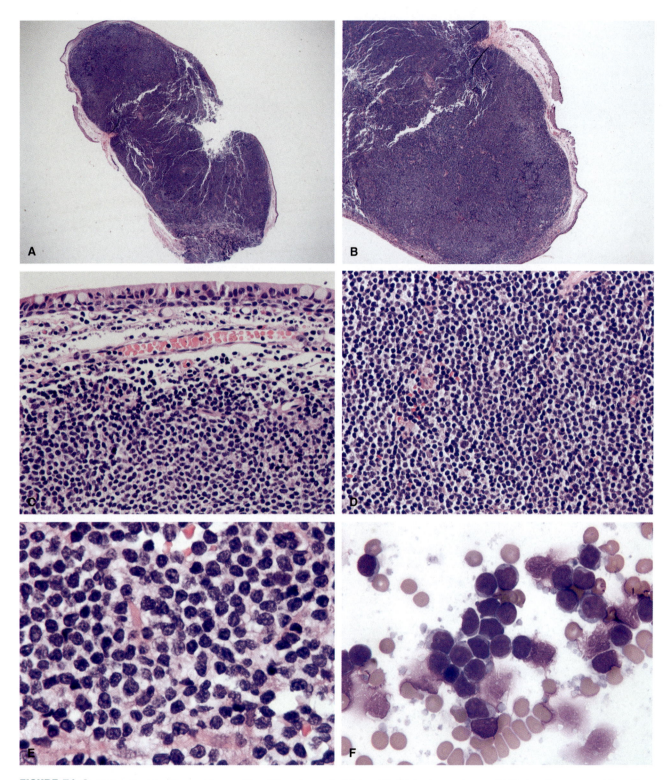

FIGURE 71-4. Conjunctival involvement by mantle cell lymphoma. A. (20×) and **B.** (40×)—dense submucosal infiltrate with a vague nodular pattern. **C.** (100×)—the infiltrate spares the mucosal surface. **D.** (200×) and **E.** (400×)—the infiltrate is composed of medium-sized lymphocytes with irregular nuclear borders. **F.** (600×)—touch imprint of the malignant lymphocytes.

the difference in disease-specific mortality with EMZL having the best prognosis and DLBCL having the worst.[84]

Lymphoproliferative lesions of the lacrimal gland may masquerade as chronic dacryoadenitis, sarcoidosis, Sjögren syndrome, and amyloidosis among many other conditions.

The secretion from the main lacrimal gland and accessory lacrimal glands located in the eyelids drains to the lacrimal sac. Lymphomas of the lacrimal sac are rare; however, in one demographic study, 55% of lacrimal sac tumors were lymphoproliferative lesions.[85] Clinical presentations are nonspecific, such as epiphora, duct obstruction, and palpable mass or swelling. Before the diagnosis takes place, the patients usually undergo dacryocystorinostomy. A comprehensive study of lacrimal sac lymphomas revealed five

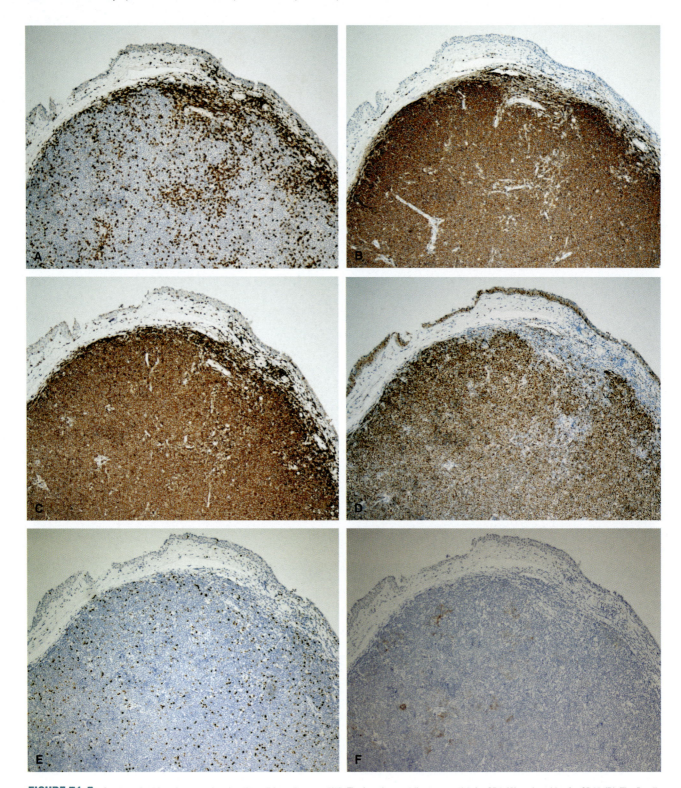

FIGURE 71-5. Conjunctival involvement by mantle cell lymphoma—IHC. The lymphoma cells are negative for CD3 **(A)** and positive for CD20 **(B)**. The B cells show coexpression of CD5 **(C)** and cyclin D1 **(D)**. Ki67 proliferation index is low **(E)**. No definitive follicular dendritic networks are present by CD23 **(F)**.

diffuse large B-cell lymphomas, five extranodal marginal zone B-cell lymphoma of MALT lymphoma, three were classified as "transitional MALT lymphoma," being in transition from MALT lymphoma to DLBCL, and two were unclassified B-cell lymphomas. The average patient age was 70 years, and except one, they were in stage 1.[86] The 5-year overall survival was 65%. Clinicians should consider a primary malignant lymphoma in the differential diagnosis in patients with chronic dacryocystitis.[87] Selective biopsy of the lacrimal sac during external dacryocystorhinostomy is indicated if there is suspicion other than chronic inflammation, to allow early diagnosis and management.

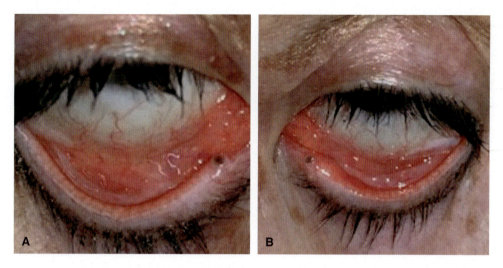

FIGURE 71.6. Conjunctival follicular lymphoma in both eyes presenting as chronic follicular conjunctivitis in both eyes right (A) and left (B).

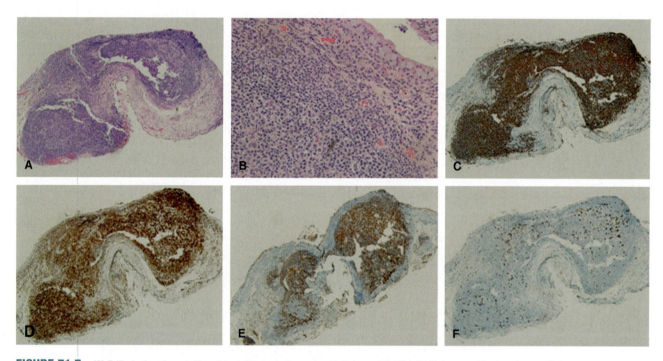

FIGURE 71.7. **(A)** Follicular lymphoma with nodular infiltrates in the conjunctival stroma (HE 20×) **(B)** Higher magnification of subepithelial infiltrates with occasional centroblasts (HE 40×). **(C)** Positivity for CD20 stain. **(D)** Abnormal expression of BCL2 protein. **(E)** Positivity for germinal center marker CD10 **(F)** Low proliferation index Ki-67.

EYELID LYMPHOMAS

The incidence of eyelid lymphomas among OAL is quite variable (0%-44%, mean approximately 10%). Eyelid lymphomas have varied histologic subtypes (Table 71-2) and a poor prognosis.[88] The spectrum of subtypes of B-cell lymphoma subtypes was the same as for other ocular adnexal region lymphomas, whereas T-cell lymphoma is very rare in other ocular adnexal structures. T-cell lymphomas, particularly mycosis fungoides, have a predilection for the skin, and therefore, T-cell lymphomas have a higher incidence in the eyelid region compared to the rest of the eye region.[89]

They have the highest rate of prior systemic lymphoma history, concurrent local extension, and systemic lymphoma at diagnosis (Fig. 71-8). Systemic lymphoma is associated with eyelid lymphoma in 67% and 75% to 100% in two different series.[4,6] The patients with eyelid non-Hodgkin lymphoma (including chronic lymphocytic leukemia) have a high risk of developing aggressive eyelid carcinomas (melanoma and squamous cell carcinoma).

TABLE 71-2 Lymphoma Types Arising From Eyelid and Conjunctiva

Lymphocytic lymphoma
Extranodal marginal zone B-cell lymphoma
MALT lymphoma
Follicular lymphoma
Lymphoplasmacytic lymphoma
Mantle cell lymphoma
Diffuse large cell lymphoma
Anaplastic large cell lymphoma
CD30+ lymphoid proliferations
Extranodal natural killer/T-cell lymphoma
Pleomorphic T-cell lymphoma
Angioimmunoblastic T-cell lymphoma
Diffuse large T-cell lymphoma
T-cell lymphomas NOS (not otherwise specified)
Nonclassical mycosis fungoides
Hodgkin lymphoma
Plasmacytoma
Myeloma

The most frequent presentation of eyelid lymphomas is cutaneous edema. Other clinical presentations include papules, single or multiple nodules, and ulcers. T-cell lymphomas can present with ulceration and ectropion. Lymphomas of the eyelid should be differentiated from causes of periocular swelling, inflammatory diseases, basal cell carcinoma, keratoacanthoma, squamous cell carcinoma, sebaceous carcinoma, melanoma, and vascular tumors such as Kaposi sarcoma.

INTRAOCULAR LYMPHOMAS

Primary intraocular lymphomas (PIOLs) and secondary systemic intraocular lymphomas are rare. Two distinctive types of PIOL exist and include vitreoretinal and uveal lymphomas. Vitreoretinal lymphoma is considered a subset of PCNSL. The vast majority of cases are diffuse large B-cell lymphoma.[90,91] T-cell lymphomas are exceptional. An increased incidence has been associated with both immunocompromised and immunocompetent populations. Malignancy often masquerades as infectious and noninfectious uveitis. The diagnosis is based on cytology of the vitreous fluid, immunohistochemistry and flow cytometry, the use of interleukin IL10:IL ratio >1, and polymerase chain reaction amplification for clonality.[92,93] Molecular analysis with microdissection and polymerase chain reaction is used to detect Ig^H gene rearrangements in B-cell lymphoma and T-cell receptor gene rearrangements in T-cell lymphoma. The limitations of molecular testing, particularly with the small samples available from the eye, can give a false-positive result or a false-negative result. Diffuse large B-cell lymphoma arising in immune-privileged sites as well as vitreoretinal lymphomas shows a high frequency of MYD88 mutations, especially L265P.[94] The detection significantly improves the diagnostic

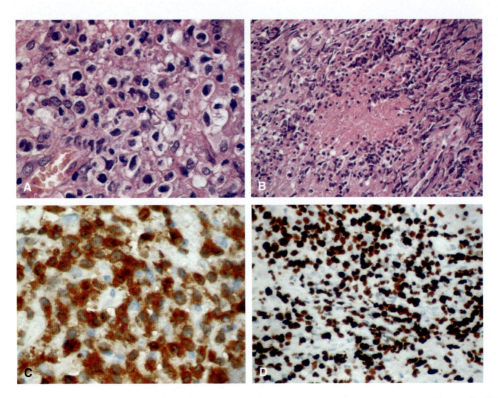

FIGURE 71-8. **Eyelid involvement by peripheral T-cell lymphoma not otherwise specified.** Tumor cells are composed of large cells with irregular vesicular nuclei (**A** and **B**). There is focal necrosis. Immunohistochemistry disclosed CD3+ cells (**C**) and high Ki-67 labeling (**D**).

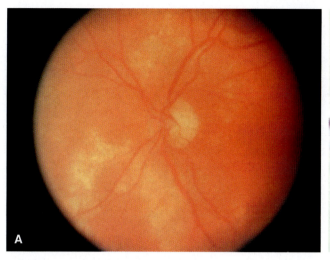 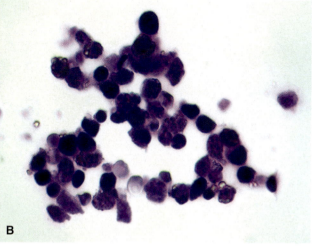

FIGURE 71-9. **Vitreoretinal intraocular lymphoma (primary diffuse large B-cell lymphoma of the central nervous system).** A 67-year-old man presented with loss and blurred vision. Fundus examination revealed vitritis with mild vitreous haze and multiple yellow infiltrates deep to the retina and retinal pigment epithelium **(A)**. Cellular sample obtained from fine needle aspiration of the vitreous through the pars plana and stained with Diff-Quik showed large cells with scanty basophilic cytoplasm, bean-shaped nuclei, and multiple large nucleoli **(B)**. The atypical cells expressed CD20 (not shown).

yields of very small vitrectomy specimens. Most cases have a post germinal center immunophenotype with positivity for CD79a, CD20, PAX5, BCL2, BCL6, IgM, and MUM-1.[95]

Specimens for diagnosis are obtained by vitreous aspiration or diagnostic vitrectomy procedure (Fig. 71-9). Because of the rapid cell degradation, the samples should be transported in appropriate media. Previous use of corticosteroid treatment may alter cell viability and make difficult the morphology. Systemic corticosteroid should be discontinued at least 2 weeks before surgery.

Clinically, vitreous and fundus examinations reveal moderate or dense vitritis and yellow creamed deposits beneath the retina or subretinal pigment epithelium (RPE). Other findings include retinal lesions with "leopard-skin" appearance and RPE atrophy. Severe vitreous infiltration without macular edema is the most likely presentation.[96]

The optic nerve and papilla may be affected. Although unilateral involvement may be the initial presentation, bilateral disease occurs in 60% to 80% of cases. Despite apparent intraocular location, approximately 15% to 25% of PCNSL patients develop ocular manifestations, and 65% to 90% of PIOL patients develop neurologic disease.[96] Several therapeutic procedures are available including ocular irradiation, systemic chemotherapy, intraocular methotrexate, and intravitreal rituximab.[97] The prognosis of patients with PCNSL is poor.

In the past, choroidal (uveal) lymphomas were subsumed under different names, such as lymphoid hyperplasia of the uveal tract, inflammatory pseudotumor of the uveal tract, RLH, lymphoid infiltration, lymphoid tumor, and uveal lymphoid neoplasia.[98] A study by Coupland et al established that most (60%-80%) of the lymphoproliferative lesions were extranodal marginal zone B-cell lymphomas.[99] Patients are usually asymptomatic, and the main symptom is loss of vision. These tumors mainly involved the choroid without vitritis and frequently have extrascleral extension. Fundus examination, fluorescein angiography, optical coherence tomography, and ultrasonography display multifocal patches or diffuse confluent areas of orange pigment, choroidal thickness, vascular anomalies, choroidal folds without dispersed subretinal fluid, and retinal detachment (Fig. 71-10). Reddish extrascleral nodules are seen beneath the conjunctiva. Diagnosis requires a sample of the choroid or epibulbar nodules if present. Common therapeutic modalities include observation, radiotherapy, and systemic chemotherapy with rituximab.[100] Remission is completely achieved in 80% of cases. Systemic disease develops in less than 10% of the patients.[101]

Secondary uveal lymphomas clearly differ from PIOL. A comparison between patients with primary and secondary uveal lymphomas showed that patients with secondary lymphomas are more frequently symptomatic, have greater visual loss, are more likely bilateral, have higher involvement of iris and ciliary body, have vitreous opacity, and usually are high-grade lymphomas.[102]

THERAPY AND MANAGEMENT

Treatment depends on the lymphoma subtype, location, presence or absence of systemic disease, age, and status (Table 71-3). The biopsy procedures vary according to the ocular adnexa location of the lesion as well as the obtained specimen. Intraoperative pathology control of the sample is indicated in lesions of the orbit. Although the majority of the procedures are biopsies, complete excision may be achieved in circumscribed and encapsulated lesion of the conjunctiva.[100,101]

Since the majority of CLs are EMZL–MALT, therapy after biopsy confirmation includes external-beam radiotherapy (EBRT) excision, immunotherapy with rituximab or interferon-α, and chemotherapy.[77,103-116] Since in geographic areas there is a strong correlation with specific microorganisms and viruses, clarithromycin and doxycycline have been used alone or in association with other therapies.[111,112] However, the indication of antibiotics in cases of EMZL is still controversial.

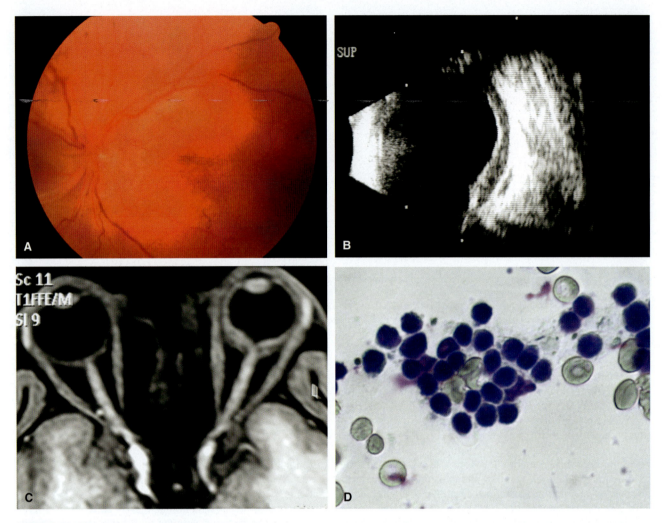

FIGURE 71-10. Primary uveal lymphoma. A 41-year-old woman with loss of vision in the left eye. Fundus examination revealed yellow choroidal patches and retinochoroidal folds **(A)**. B-scan ultrasonography showed diffuse thickening of the choroid **(B)** and a posterior episcleral lesion (not shown). MRI clearly differentiated the normal contour of the right eye from the thickened left eye **(C)**. Fine needle intraocular choroidal aspiration revealed numerous small hyperchromatic lymphocytes **(D)**.

A few cases of spontaneous regression without treatment have been published; however, the patients are exposed to higher risk of recurrences and progression.[77] Patients with primary OAL, Stage IE, usually receive 25 to 30 Gy in several fractions.[103] Twenty-seven studies were reviewed with respect to available treatments and outcomes; local control rate of MALT lymphomas with treatments involving radiotherapy averaged 95.9%.[117]

Phoenix and colleagues reported a review of 22 patients who underwent ultralow-dose EBRT, 4 Gy delivered to the orbit(s) in two 2-Gy fractions on two consecutive days. They observed complete response rate of 86%, but more extensive follow-up is required.[118]

Ophthalmologic complications in patients treated with radiotherapy include dry eyes, cataracts, keratitis, and blepharitis. The most frequent complaint is dryness, followed by cataracts corrected by cataract extraction. Less frequent complications include radiation retinopathy, tearing, and nasolacrimal duct obstruction. Chemotherapy has been used either in combination with other treatments or alone in restricted cases.[77,103-116,119]

Patients having OAL should undergo a multidisciplinary therapeutic approach (ocular oncologist, clinical oncologist, and hematologist), ophthalmologic evaluation, and careful physical examination with palpation of head and neck lymph nodes. A systemic imaging workup includes positron emission tomography (PET)-CT, CT or MRI (of the head, chest, abdomen, and pelvis), complete blood count, serum protein electrophoresis, liver and kidney function tests (serum lactate dehydrogenase [LDH] and β2-microglobulin), bone marrow biopsy, performance status, and evaluation for the presence of B-symptoms (fever, night sweats, and weight loss). FDG-PET is an important part of initial staging but is less sensitive than CT and MRI and is helpful in further identifying disease. Lymphoma risk factors include advanced-stage disease, age greater than 60, presence of B-symptoms, nodal involvement, and elevated serum LDH level. PET is a valuable study for staging OALs and evaluating their response to therapy and recurrences.[120-123]

Generally, CLs have a good prognosis, reaching 90% of patients without recurrence at 1 year. Progression depends

TABLE 71-3 Protocol for the Examination of Specimens From Patients With Hematopoietic Neoplasms of the Ocular Adnexa

American Joint Committee on Cancer (AJCC) 7th Edition, tumor-node-metastasis (TNM) clinical staging system for OAL
Protocol applies to primary hematopoietic neoplasms of the conjunctiva, orbital soft tissue, lacrimal gland, lacrimal drainage apparatus, and eyelid. Intraocular lymphomas and secondary hematopoietic neoplasms are not included.

Ocular Adnexa (Checklist)

Specimen

___ Conjunctiva

___ Orbital soft tissue (orbit)

___ Lacrimal gland

___ Lacrimal sac or nasolacrimal duct (lacrimal drainage apparatus)

___ Eyelid

___ Other (specify): _____

___ Not specified

Procedure

___ Biopsy

___ Resection

___ Other (specify): _____

___ Not specified

Lymph Node Sampling (Select All That Apply)

___ Not applicable

___ Regional lymph node(s) (preauricular/parotid, submandibular, or cervical)

___ Central lymph node(s) (lymph nodes from the trunk, e.g., mediastinal, para-aortic)

___ Peripheral lymph node(s) (lymph nodes from distant sites other than central)

___ Other (specify): _____

___ Not specified

Tumor Size (May Be Determined From Radiographic Studies)

Greatest dimension: ___ cm

Additional dimensions: ___ × ___ cm

___ Cannot be determined

Histologic Type (Based on the 2008 World Health Organization [WHO] Classification)

___ Extranodal marginal zone lymphoma of mucosa-associated lymphoid tissue (MALT lymphoma)

___ Follicular lymphoma

___ Diffuse large B-cell lymphoma, not otherwise specified (NOS)

___ Mantle cell lymphoma

___ Chronic lymphocytic leukemia/small lymphocytic lymphoma

___ Lymphoplasmacytic lymphoma

___ Other (specify): _____

(Continued)

TABLE 71-3 Protocol for the Examination of Specimens From Patients With Hematopoietic Neoplasms of the Ocular Adnexa (Continued)

Pathologic Staging (pTNM)

TNM Descriptors

___ b (bilateral)

___ m (multiple)

___ r (recurrent)

___ y (posttreatment)

Primary Tumor (pT)

___ pTX: Lymphoma extent not specified

___ pT0: No evidence of primary tumor

pT1: Lymphoma involving the conjunctiva alone without orbital involvement

___ pT1a: Bulbar conjunctiva involvement only

___ pT1b: Palpebral conjunctiva involvement (with or without fornix or caruncle involvement)

___ pT1c: Extensive conjunctival involvement (ie, both bulbar and nonbulbar conjunctiva involvement)

pT2: Lymphoma with orbital involvement with or without conjunctival involvement

___ pT2a: Anterior orbital involvement, but no lacrimal gland involvement (with or without conjunctival involvement)

___ pT2b: Anterior orbital involvement with lacrimal gland involvement (with or without conjunctival involvement)

___ pT2c: Posterior orbital involvement (with or without anterior orbital involvement; with or without conjunctival involvement; with or without extraocular muscle involvement)

___ pT2d: Nasolacrimal drainage system involvement (with or without conjunctival involvement, but not involving nasopharynx)

pT3: Lymphoma with preseptal eyelid involvement (with or without orbital or conjunctival involvement)

pT4: Lymphoma extends beyond orbit to involve adjacent structures (e.g., bone, brain)

___ pT4a: Involvement of nasopharynx

___ pT4b: Osseous involvement (including periosteum)

___ pT4c: Involvement of maxillofacial, ethmoidal, and/or frontal sinuses

___ pT4d: Intracranial spread

Lymph Node Involvement (pN)

___ pNX: Involvement of lymph nodes not assessed

___ pN0: No evidence of lymph node involvement

___ pN1: Involvement of ipsilateral regional lymph nodes (preauricular/parotid, submandibular, or cervical)

___ pN2: Involvement of contralateral or bilateral regional lymph nodes (preauricular/parotid, submandibular, or cervical)

___ pN3: Involvement of peripheral lymph nodes not draining ocular adnexal region

___ pN4: Involvement of central lymph nodes

Specify: Number examined: ___

Number involved: ___

TABLE 71-3 Protocol for the Examination of Specimens From Patients With Hematopoietic Neoplasms of the Ocular Adnexa (Continued)

Distant Metastasis (pM)

___ Not applicable

___ pM1a: Noncontiguous involvement of tissues or organs external to the ocular adnexa (e.g., salivary glands, lung, liver)

Specify site(s), if known: _____

___ pM1b: Bone marrow involvement

___ pM1c: Both pM1a and pM1b involvement

Additional Pathologic Findings

Specify: _____

Immunophenotyping (Flow Cytometry and/or Immunohistochemistry)

___ Performed, see separate report: _____

___ Performed

Specify method(s) and results: _____

___ Not performed

Cytogenetic Studies (Note F)

___ Performed, see separate report: _____

___ Performed

Specify method(s) and results: _____

___ Not performed

Molecular Genetic Studies (Note G)

___ Performed, see separate report: _____

___ Performed

Specify method(s) and results: _____

___ Not performed

Comment(s) _____

From Bradley KT, Arber DA, Brown MSet al. *Protocol for the examination of specimens from patients with hematopoietic neoplasms of the ocular adnexa*. College of American Pathologists, Cancer Protocol Templates. 2010. Accessed December 1, 2015. Reproduced with permission from the College of American Pathologists. Visit www.cap.org for the most recent protocols. Reprinted by permission from Springer: Springer. TNM Staging from Ocular Adnexal Lymphoma. In: Edge SB, Byrd DR, Compton CC, eds. *AJCC Cancer Staging Manual*. 7th ed. Springer, 2010.

on the subtype of lymphoma. Isolated cases of low-grade EMZL and FL are associated with the best outcome after treatment.[77,103-117]

Studies that included data on multiple histologic subtypes of lymphoma or non-MALT lymphomas (988 patients) reported local control rates to be 93.1%; 5-year and 10-year disease-free survival rates to be 75.7% and 71.0%, respectively; and 5-year and 10-year overall survival rates to be 78.9% and 73.5%, respectively.[117]

Various studies have assessed the usefulness of the correlation with prognosis of TNM (tumor [T], node [N], and metastasis [M]) staging.[124-127] A recent study of 63 patients with OAL (median follow-up: 27.9 months) included 60.3% cases from the orbit, 42.9% from the conjunctiva, and 4.8% from the eyelid; 80% had an EMZL.[127] The TNM system for primary OAL was a useful and precise characterization for the extent of local disease. N1 and M1 correlated with less favorable survival.[127] The T stage was not associated with relapse (see Protocol).

SUMMARY

- OAL has been recognized as the most frequent orbital malignancy in adults.
- The vast majority of OAL are low-grade lymphomas, including extranodal marginal zone, MALT lymphoma, and follicular center cell lymphoma (grade 1).

- Primary OAL is usually associated with good prognosis. The overall 5-year survival rates are 90% to 95%.
- Local and systemic studies are required for staging.
- The treatment of localized OAL includes EBRT, rituximab, or both. Chemotherapy is indicated for secondary involvement or for high-grade histologic subtypes.

References

1. Coupland SE, Krause L, Delecluse HJ, et al. Lymphoproliferative lesions of the ocular adnexa. Analysis of 112 cases. *Ophthalmol*. 1998;105:1430-1441.
2. Cahill M, Barnes C, Moriarty P, et al. Ocular adnexal lymphoma-comparison of MALT lymphoma with other histological types. *Br J Ophthalmol*. 1999;83:742-747.
3. Jenkins C, Rose G, Bunce C, et al. Histological features of ocular adnexal lymphoma (REAL classification) and their association with patient morbidity and survival. *Br J Ophthalmol*. 2000;84:907-913.
4. Ferry JA, Fung CY, Zukerberg L, et al. Lymphoma of the ocular adnexa: a study of 353 cases. *Am J Surg Pathol*. 2007;31:170-184.
5. Beykin G, Pe'er J, Amir J, et al. Paediatric and adolescent elevated conjunctival lesions in the plical area: lymphoma or reactive lymphoid hyperplasia? *Br J Ophthalmol*. 2014;98:645-650.
6. Chung H, Son J. Ocular adnexal lymphoma: an updated review of pathogenesis, diagnosis, and treatment. *J Yeungnam Med Sci*. 2021;39(1):3-11.
7. Kirkegaard M, Rasmussen P, Coupland S, Esmaeli B, Finger F, et al. l.Conjunctival lymphoma—an international multicenter retrospective study. *JAMA Ophthalmol*. 2016;134(4):406-414. doi:10.1001/jamaophthalmol.2015.6122
8. Coupland SE, Hummel M, Stein H. Ocular adnexal lymphomas: five case presentations and a review of the literature. *Surv Ophthalmol*. 2002;47:470-490.
9. Knop N, Knop N. Conjunctiva-associated lymphoid tissue in the human eye. *Invest Ophthalmol Vis Sci*. 2000;41:1270-1279.
10. Knop E, Knop N. The role of eye-associated lymphoid tissue in corneal immune protection. *J Anat*. 2005;206:271-285.
11. Steven P, Gebert A. Conjunctiva-associated lymphoid tissue—current knowledge, animal models and experimental prospects. *Ophthalmic Res*. 2009;42:2-8.
12. Knop E, Knop N. Eye-associated lymphoid tissue (EALT) is continuously spread throughout the ocular surface from the lacrimal gland to the lacrimal drainage system [in German]. *Ophthalmologe*. 2003;100:929-942.
13. Verma V, Shen D, Sieving PC, et al. The role of infectious agents in the etiology of ocular adnexal neoplasia. *Surv Ophthalmol*. 2008;53:312-331.
14. Chan CC, Smith JA, Shen DF, et al. *Helicobacter pylori* (*H. pylori*) molecular signature in conjunctival mucosa-associated lymphoid tissue (MALT) lymphoma. *Histol Histopathol*. 2004;19:1219-1226.
15. Lee SB, Yang JW, Kim CS. The association between conjunctival MALT lymphoma and *Helicobacter pylori*. *Br J Ophthalmol*. 2008;92:534-536.
16. Ferreri AJ, Ponzoni M, Viale E, et al. Association between *Helicobacter pylori* infection and MALT-type lymphoma of the ocular adnexa: clinical and therapeutic implications. *Hematol Oncol*. 2006;24:33-37.
17. Sjö NC, Foegh P, Juhl BR, et al. Role of *Helicobacter pylori* in conjunctival mucosa-associated lymphoid tissue lymphoma. *Ophthalmol*. 2007;114:182-186.
18. Ferreri AJ, Guidoboni M, Ponzoni M, et al. Evidence for an association between Chlamydia psittaci and ocular adnexal lymphoma. *J Natl Cancer Inst*. 2004;96:586-594.
19. Ferreri AJ, Ponzoni M, Guidoboni M, et al. Regression of ocular adnexal lymphoma after Chlamydia psittaci-eradicating antibiotic therapy. *J Clin Oncol*. 2005;23:5067-5073.
20. Grunberger B, Hauff W, Lukas J, et al. "Blind" antibiotic treatment targeting Chlamydia is not effective in patients with MALT lymphoma of the ocular adnexa. *Ann Oncol*. 2006;17:484-487.
21. Ponzoni M, Ferreri AJ, Guidoboni M, et al. Chlamydia infection and lymphomas: association beyond ocular adnexal lymphomas highlighted by multiple detection methods. *Clin Cancer Res*. 2008;14:5794-5800.
22. Ferreri AJ, Dolcetti R, Magnino S, et al. Chlamydial infection: the link with ocular adnexal lymphomas. *Nat Rev Clin Oncol*. 2009;6:658-669.
23. Ferreri AJ, Viale E, Guidoboni M, et al. Clinical implications of hepatitis C virus infection in MALT-type lymphoma of the ocular adnexa. *Ann Oncol*. 2006;17:769-772.
24. Chanudet E, Zhou Y, Bacon CM, et al. Chlamydia psittaci is variably associated with ocular adnexal MALT lymphoma in different geographical regions. *J Pathol*. 2006;209:344-351.
25. De Cremoux P, Subtil A, Ferreri AJ, et al. Low prevalence of Chlamydia psittaci infection in French patients with ocular adnexal lymphomas. *J Natl Cancer Inst*. 2006;98:365-366.
26. Van Maldegem F, Wormhoudt TA, Mulder MM, et al. Chlamydia psittaci-negative ocular adnexal marginal zone B-cell lymphomas have biased VH4-34 immunoglobulin gene expression and proliferate in a distinct inflammatory environment. *Leukemia*. 2012;26:1647-1653.
27. Ferreri AJ, Govi S, Pasini E, et al. Chlamydophila psittaci eradication with doxycycline as first-line targeted therapy for ocular adnexae lymphoma: final results of an international phase II trial. *J Clin Oncol*. 2012;30:2988-2994.
28. Tonami H, Matoba M, Yokota H, et al. Mucosa-associated lymphoid tissue lymphoma in Sjögren's syndrome: initial and follow-up imaging features. *AJR Am J Roentgenol*. 2002;179:485-489.
29. Cheuk W, Yuen HK, Chan AC, et al. Ocular adnexal lymphoma associated with IgG4-chronic sclerosing dacryoadenitis: a previously undescribed complication of IgG4-related sclerosing disease. *Am J Surg Pathol*. 2008;32:1159-1167.
30. Kazunobu Asao K, Hashida N, Ando S, et al. Conjunctival dysbiosis in mucosa-associated lymphoid tissue lymphoma. *Sci Rep*. 2019;9(1):8424.
31. Stefanovic A, Lossos IS. Extranodal marginal zone lymphoma of the ocular adnexa. *Blood*. 2009;114:501-510.
32. Ponzoni M, Govi S, Licata G, et al. A reappraisal of the diagnostic and therapeutic management of uncommon histologies of primary ocular adnexal lymphoma. *Oncol*. 2013;18(7):876-884.
33. Moslehi R, Devesa SS, Schairer C, et al. Rapidly increasing incidence of ocular non-Hodgkin lymphoma. *J Natl Cancer Inst*. 2006;98:936-939.
34. Sjö LD. Ophthalmic lymphoma: epidemiology and pathogenesis. *Acta Opthalmol*. 2009;87 Thesis 1:120.
35. Sjö LD, Heegaard S, Prause JU, et al. Extranodal marginal zone lymphoma in the ocular region: clinical, immunophenotypical, and cytogenetical characteristics. *Invest Ophthalmol Vis Sci*. 2009;50:516-522.

36. Fung CY, Tarbell NJ, Lucarelli MJ, et al. Ocular adnexal lymphoma: clinical behavior of distinct World Health Organization classification subtypes. *Int J Radiat Oncol Biol Phys*. 2003;57:1382-1391.
37. Jakobiec F. Ocular adnexal lymphoid tumors: progress in need clarification. *Am J Ophthalmol*. 2008;145:941-950.
38. Sullivan TJ, Whitehead K, Williamson R, et al. Lymphoproliferative disease of the ocular adnexa: a clinical and pathologic study with statistical analysis of 69 patients. *Ophthalmic Plast Reconstr Surg*. 2005;21:177-184.
39. Polito E, Galieni P, Leccisotti A. Clinical and radiological presentation of 95 orbital lymphoid tumors. *Graefes Arch Clin Exp Ophthalmol*. 1996;234:504-509.
40. Klavdianou O; Kondylis G. Bilateral benign reactive lymphoid hyperplasia of the conjunctiva: a case treated with oral doxycycline and review of the literature. *Eye and Vision* 2019;6:26.
41. Chen PN, Chiou TJ, Yu IT, et al. Molecular analysis of mucosa-associated lymphoid tissue (MALT) lymphoma of ocular adnexa. *Leuk Lymphoma*. 2001;42(1/2):207-214.
42. Inagaki H. Mucosa-associated lymphoid tissue lymphoma: molecular pathogenesis and clinicopathological significance. *Pathol Int*. 2007;57:474-484.
43. Ye H, Liu H, Attygalle A, et al. Variable frequencies of t(11;18)(q21;q21) in MALT lymphomas of different sites: significant association with CagA strains of H pylori in gastric MALT lymphoma. *Blood*. 2003;102:1012-1018.
44. Cerrone M, Collina F, De Chiara A, et al. BCL10 expression and localization in ocular adnexa MALT lymphomas: a comparative cytogenetic and immunohistochemical study. *Histol Histopathol*. 2014;29:77-87.
45. Coupland SE. Molecular pathology of lymphoma. *Eye*. 2013;27:180-189.
46. Murga Penas EM, Hinz K, Biller L, et al. Frequency of chromosomal aneuploidies and deletions of the RB and TP53 genes in MALT lymphomas harboring the t(14;18)(q32;q21). *Cancer Genet Cytogenet*. 2006;164:81-83.
47. Streubel B, Vinatzer U, Lamprecht A, et al. T(3;14)(p14.1;q32) involving IGH and FOXP1 is a novel recurrent chromosomal aberration in MALT lymphoma. *Leukemia*. 2005;19:652-658.
48. Matteucci C, Galieni P, Leoncini L, et al. Typical genomic imbalances in primary MALT lymphoma of the orbit. *J Pathol*. 2003;200:656-660.
49. Schiby G, Polak-Charcon S, Mardoukh C, et al. Orbital marginal zone lymphomas: an immunohistochemical, polymerase chain reaction, and fluorescence in situ hybridization study. *Hum Pathol*. 2007;38:435-442.
50. Tanimoto K, Sekiguchi N, Yokota Y, et al. Fluorescence in situ hybridization (FISH) analysis of primary ocular adnexal MALT lymphoma. *BMC Cancer*. 2006;6:249.
51. Ruiz A, Reischl U, Swerdlow SH, et al. Extranodal marginal zone B-cell lymphomas of the ocular adnexa: multiparameter analysis of 34 cases including interphase molecular cytogenetics and PCR for Chlamydia psittaci. *Am J Surg Pathol*. 2007;31:792-802.
52. Streubel B, Lamprecht A, Dierlamm J, et al. T(14;18)(q32;q21) involving IGH and MALT1 is a frequent chromosomal aberration in MALT lymphoma. *Blood*. 2003;101:2335-2339.
53. Stacy RC, Jakobiec FA, Herwig MC, et al. Diffuse large B-cell lymphoma of the orbit: clinicopathologic, immunohistochemical, and prognostic features of 20 cases. *Am J Ophthalmol*. 2012;154:87-98.
54. Shields JA, Shields CL, Scartozzi R. Survey of 1264 patients with orbital tumors and simulating lesions: the 2002 Montgomery Lecture, part 1. *Ophthalmol*. 2004;111:997-1008.
55. Olsen TG, Heegaard S. Orbital lymphoma. *Surv Ophthalmol* 2019;64(1):45-66.
56. Stacy RC, Jakobiec FA, Schoenfield L, et al. Unifocal and multifocal reactive lymphoid hyperplasia vs follicular lymphoma of the ocular adnexa. *Am J Ophthalmol*. 2010;150:412-426.
57. Thakral B, Zhou J, Medeiros LJ. Extranodal hematopoietic neoplasms and mimics in the head and neck: an update. *Hum Pathol*. 2015;46:1079-1100.
58. Li K, Xu M, Wu X, et al. The expression of IgG and IgG4 in orbital MALT lymphoma: the similarities and differences of IgG4-related diseases. *OncoTargets Ther*. 2020;13:5755-5761.
59. Demirci H, Shields CL, Karatza EC, et al. Orbital lymphoproliferative tumors: analysis of clinical features and systemic involvement in 160 cases. *Ophthalmol*. 2008;115:1626-1631.
60. Ahmed O; Ma A; Ahmed T, et al. Epidemiology, outcomes, and prognostic factors of orbital lymphoma in the United States. *Orbit*. 2020;39(6):397-402.
61. Olsen T, Holm F, Mikkelsen L, et al. Orbital lymphoma—an international multicenter retrospective study. *Am journal of ophthalmology*. 2019;199:P44-P57.
62. Shields CL, Shields JA, Carvalho C, et al. Conjunctival lymphoid tumors: clinical analysis of 117 cases and relationship to systemic lymphoma. *Ophthalmol*. 2001;108:979-984.
63. Meunier J, Lumbroso-Le Rouïc L, Dendale R, et al. Conjunctival low-grade non-Hodgkin's lymphoma: a large single-center study of initial characteristics, natural history and prognostic factors. *Leuk Lymphoma*. 2006;47:1295-1305.
64. Kirkegaard MM, Coupland SE, Prause JU, et al. Malignant lymphoma of the conjunctiva. *Surv Ophthalmol*. 2015;60:444-458.
65. Khanlari M, Bagheri B, Vojdani R, et al. Conjunctival mass as an initial presentation of mantle cell lymphoma: a case report. *BMC Res Notes*. 2012;5:671.
66. Kim NJ, Khwarg SI. Primary diffuse large B-cell lymphoma of the palpebral conjunctiva. *Can J Ophthalmol*. 2007;42:630-631.
67. Takada S, Yoshino T, Taniwaki M, et al. Involvement of the chromosomal translocation t(11;18) in some mucosa-associated lymphoid tissue lymphomas and diffuse large B-cell lymphomas of the ocular adnexa: evidence from multiplex reverse transcriptase-polymerase chain reaction and fluorescence in situ hybridization on using formalin- fixed, paraffin-embedded specimens. *Mod Pathol*. 2003;16:445-452.
68. Al-Muammar A, Hodge WG, Farmer J. Conjunctival T-cell lymphoma: a clinicopathologic case report. *Ophthalmol*. 2006;113:459-461.
69. Mannami T, Yoshino T, Oshima K, et al. Clinical, histopathological, and immunogenetic analysis of ocular adnexal lymphoproliferative disorders: characterization of malt lymphoma and reactive lymphoid hyperplasia. *Mod Pathol*. 2001;14:641-649.
70. Rasmussen P, Sjo LD, Prause JU, et al. Mantle cell lymphoma in the orbital and adnexal region. *Br J Ophthalmol*. 2009;93:1047-1051.
71. Isola V, Mazzacane D, Defelice N, et al. Malignant conjunctival T cell lymphoma diagnosed by punch biopsy as a primary manifestation of systemic cancer. *Clin Ophthalmol*. 2012;6:777-780.
72. Kirn TJ, Levy NB, Gosselin JJ, et al. Peripheral T-cell lymphoma presenting as sclerouveitis. *Cornea*. 2012;26:1147-1149.

73. Masir N, Campbell LJ, Goff LK, et al. BCL2 protein expression in follicular lymphomas with t(14;18) chromosomal translocations. *Br J Haematol.* 2009;144:716-725.
74. Jaffe ES, Harris NL, Stein H, et al. *World Health organization classification of tumours.* In: *Pathology and Genetics of Tumours of Haematopoietic and Lymphoid Tissues.* IARC Press; 2001.
75. Jiang J, Liu Y, Wang F, et al. An unusual occurrence of solitary extramedullary plasmacytoma in the conjunctiva. *Oncol Lett.* 2012;4:245-246.
76. Lugassy G, Rozenbaum D, Lifshitz L, et al. Primary lymphoplasmacytoma of the conjunctiva. *Eye.* 1992;6(pt. 3):326-327.
77. Matsuo T, Ichimura K, Yoshino T. Spontaneous regression of bilateral conjunctival extranodal marginal zone B-cell lymphoma of mucosa-associated lymphoid tissue. *J Clin Exp Hematop.* 2007;47:79-81.
78. Orii K, Kobayashi H, Ueno M, et al. Mantle cell lymphoma with multiple extranodal involvement [in Japanese]. *Rinsho Ketsueki.* 1997;38:520-525.
79. Taghipour Z, Miratashi S, Nazemian M, et al. Primary follicular lymphoma of the conjunctiva in a 12 year-old male. *Iran J Ped Hematol Oncol.* 2013;3:83-85.
80. Buggage RR, Smith JA, Shen D, et al. Conjunctival T-cell lymphoma caused by human T-cell lymphotrophic virus infection. *Am J Ophthalmol.* 2001;131:381-383.
81. Coupland SE, Foss HD, Assaf C, et al. T-cell and T/natural killer-cell lymphomas involving ocular and ocular adnexal tissues: a clinicopathologic, immunohistochemical, and molecular study of seven cases. *Ophthalmol.* 1999;106:2109-2120.
82. Abd Al-Kader L, Sato Y, Takata K, et al. A case of conjunctival follicular lymphoma mimicking mucosa-associated lymphoid tissue lymphoma. *J Clin Exp Hematop.* 2013;53:49-52.
83. Shields CL, Shields JA, Eagle RC, et al. Clinicopathologic review of 142 cases of lacrimal gland lesions. *Ophthalmol.* 1989;96:431-435.
84. Dahl Vest S, Mikkelsen LH, Holm F, et al. Lymphoma of the lacrimal gland—an international multicenter retrospective study. *Am J Ophthalmol.* November 2020;219:107-120.
85. Guo P, Fei Y, Cheng T, et al. Imaging and histopathological findings of lacrimal sac lymphoma. *Chin Med J.* 2014;127:120-124.
86. Sjö LD, Ralfkiaer E, Juhl BR, et al. Primary lymphoma of the lacrimal sac: an EORTC ophthalmic oncology task force study. *Br J Ophthalmol.* 2006;90:10041009.
87. de Palma P, Ravalli L, Modestino R, et al. Primary lacrimal sac Bcell immunoblastic lymphoma simulating an acute dacryocystitis *Orbit.* 2003;22:171-175.
88. Shome D, Bell D, Esmaeli B. Eyelid carcinoma in patients with systemic lymphoma. *J Ophthalmic Vis Res.* 2010;5:38-43.
89. Svendsen F, Rasmussen P, Coupland S, et al. Lymphoma of the eyelid—an international multicenter retrospective study. *Am J Ophthalmol.* 2017;177:58-68.
90. Chan CC, Wallace DJ. Intraocular lymphoma: update on diagnosis and management. *Cancer Control.* 2004;11:285-295.
91. Coupland SE, Bechrakis NE, Anastassiou G, et al. Evaluation of vitrectomy specimens and chorioretinal biopsies in the diagnosis of primary intraocular lymphoma in patients with Masquerade syndrome. *Graefes Arch Clin Exp Ophthalmol.* 2003;241:860-870.
92. Cassoux N, Giron A, Bodaghi B, et al. IL-10 measurement in aqueous humor for screening patients with suspicion of primary intraocular lymphoma. *Invest Ophthalmol Vis Sci.* 2007;48:3253-3259.
93. Coupland SE, Heimann H, Bechrakis NE. Primary intraocular lymphoma: a review of the clinical, histopathological and molecular biological features. *Graefe's Arch Clin Exp Ophthalmol.* 2004;242:901-913.
94. Bonzheim l, Giese S, Deuter C, et al. High frequency of MYD88 mutations in vitreoretinal B-cell lymphoma: a valuable tool to improve diagnostic yield of vitreous aspirates. *Blood.* 2015;126:76-79.
95. Coupland S, Loddenkemper C, Smith J, et al. Expression of immunoglobulin transcription factors in primary intraocular lymphoma and primary central nervous system lymphoma. *Invest Ophthalmol Vis Sci.* 2005;46(11):3957-3964.
96. Grimm SA, Pulido JS, Jahnke K, et al. Primary intraocular lymphoma: an international primary central nervous system lymphoma collaborative group report. *Ann Oncol.* 2007;18:1851-1855.
97. Raval V, Vinclay E, Aronow M, et al. Primary central nervous system lymphoma - ocular variant: an interdisciplinary review on management. *Surv Ophthalmol.* 2021;66(6):1009-1020.
98. Cockerham GC, Hidayat AA, Bijwaard KE, et al. Reevaluation of "reactive lymphoid hyperplasia of the uvea": an immunohistochemical and molecular analysis of 10 cases. *Ophthalmol.* 2000;107:151-158.
99. Coupland SE, Joussen A, Anastassiou G, et al. Diagnosis of a primary uveal extranodal marginal zone B-cell lymphoma by chorioretinal biopsy: case report. *Graefes Arch Clin Exp Ophthalmol.* 2005;243:482-486.
100. Aronow M, Portell CA, Sweetenham JW, et al. Uveal lymphoma: clinical features, diagnostic studies, treatment selection, and outcomes. *Ophthalmol.* 2014;121:334-341.
101. Mashayekhi A, Shukla SY, Shields JA, et al. Choroidal lymphoma clinical features and association with systemic lymphoma. *Ophthalmol.* 2014;121:342-351.
102. Valenzuela J, Yeaney G, Hsi E, et al. Large B-cell lymphoma of the uvea: histopathologic variants and clinicopathologic correlation. *Surv Ophthalmol.* 2020;65(3):361-370.
103. Tenenbaum R, Galor A; Dubovy S, Karp C. Classification, diagnosis and management of conjunctival lymphoma. *Eye and Vision*:2019:6:22. doi:10.1186/s40662-019-0146-1
104. Hashimoto N, Sasaki R, Nishimura H, et al. Long-term outcome and patterns of failure in primary ocular adnexal mucosa-associated lymphoid tissue lymphoma treated with radiotherapy. *Int J Radiat Oncol Biol Phys.* 2012;82:1509-1514.
105. Harada K, Murakami N, Kitaguchi M, et al. Localized ocular adnexal mucosa-associated lymphoid tissue lymphoma treated with radiation therapy: a long-term outcome in 86 patients with 104 treated eyes. *Int J Radiation Oncol Biol Phys.* 2014;88:650-654.
106. Ohga S, Nakanura K, Shioyama Y, et al. Treatment outcome of radiotherapy for localized primary ocular adnexal MALT lymphoma. Prognostic effect of the AJCC tumor-node-metastasis clinical staging system. *Anticancer Res.* 2015;35:3591-3597.
107. Woolf SK, Kuhan H, Shoffren O, et al. Outcomes of primary lymphoma on the ocular adnexa (orbital lymphoma) treated with radiotherapy. *Clin Oncol.* 2015;27:153-159.
108. Russell W, Herskovic A, Gessert D, et al. Ocular adnexal MALTomas: case series of patients treated with primary radiation. *Clin Adv Hematol Oncol.* 2013;11:209-214.

109. Ferreri AJ, Govi S, Colucci A, et al. Intralesional rituximab: a new therapeutic approach for patients with conjunctival lymphomas. *Ophthalmol*. 2011;118:24-28.
110. Animali O, Chiodi F, Sarlo C, et al. Rituximab as single agent in primary MALT lymphoma of the ocular adnexa. *BioMed Res Int*. 2015;2015:895105. doi:10.1155/2015/895105
111. Ferreri AJ, Sassone M, Kiesewetter B, et al. High-dose clarithromycin is an active monotherapy for patients with relapsed/refractory extranodal marginal zone lymphoma of mucosa-associated lymphoid tissue (MALT): the HD-K phase II trial. *Ann Oncol*. 2015;26:1760-1765.
112. Han JJ, Kim TM, Jeon YK, et al. Long-term outcomes of first-line treatment with doxycycline in patients with previously untreated ocular adnexal marginal zone B-cell lymphoma. *Ann Hematol*. 2015;94:575-581.
113. Foster LH, Portell CA. The role of infectious agents, antibiotics, and antiviral therapy in the treatment of extranodal marginal zone lymphoma and other low-grade lymphomas. *Curr Treat Options Oncol*. 2015;16:28.
114. Martinet S, Ozsahin M, Belkacemi Y, et al. Outcome and prognostic factors in orbital lymphoma: a rare cancer network study on 90 consecutive patients treated with radiotherapy. *Int J Radiat Oncol Biol Phys*. 2003;55:892-898.
115. Kiesewetter B, Lukas J, Kuchar A, Mayerhoefer ME, Müllauer L, Raderer M. Clarithromycin leading to complete remission in the first-line treatment of ocular adnexal mucosa-associated lymphoid tissue lymphoma. *J Clin Oncol*. 2015;33(35):e130-2.
116. Ma WL, Yao M, Liao SL, et al. Chemotherapy alone is an alternative treatment in treating localized primary ocular adnexal lymphomas. *Oncotarget*. 2017;8(46):81329-81342.
117. Yen M, Bilyk J, Wladis E. Treatments of ocular adnexal lymphoma. A report by the American academy of ophthalmology. *Ophthalmology*. 2018;125(1):127-136.
118. Pinnix CC, Dabaja BS, Milgrom SA, et al. Ultra-low-dose radiotherapy for definitive management of ocular adnexal Bcell lymphoma. *Head Neck*. 2017;39(6):1095-1100.
119. Frenkel S, Hendler K, Siegal T, et al. Intravitreal methotrexate for treating vitreoretinal lymphoma: 10 years of experience. *Br J Ophthalmol*. 2008;92:383-388.
120. English JF, Sullivan TJ. The role of FDG-PET in the diagnosis and staging of ocular adnexal lymphoproliferative disease. *Orbit*. 2015;34:284-291.
121. Gayed I, Eskandari MF, McLaughlin P, et al. Value of positron emission tomography in staging ocular adnexal lymphomas and evaluating their response to therapy. *Ophthalmic Surg Lasers Imaging*. 2007;38:319-325.
122. Matsuo T, Ichimura K, Tanaka T, et al. Conjunctival lymphoma can be detected by FDG PET. *Clin Nucl Med*. 2012;37:516-519.
123. Zanni M, Moulin-Romsee G, Servois V, et al. Value of 18FDG PET scan in staging of ocular adnexal lymphomas: a large single-center experience. *Hematology*. 2012;17:76-84.
124. Lee SE, Paik JS, Cho WK, et al. Feasibility of the TNM-based staging system of ocular adnexal. *Am J Hematol*. 2011;86:262-266.
125. Coupland SE, White V, Rootman S, et al. TNM staging of ocular adnexal lymphomas. In: Edge SB, Byrd DR, Compton CA, et al., eds. *AJCC Cancer Staging Manual*. 7th ed. Springer; 2009:583-589.
126. Graue GF, Finger PT, Maher E, et al. Ocular adnexal lymphoma staging and treatment: American joint committee on cancer versus ann arbor. *Eur J Ophthalmol*. 2013;23:344-355.
127. Aronow ME, Portell CA, Rybicki LA, et al. Ocular adnexal lymphoma: assessment of a tumor-node-metastasis staging system. *Ophthalmol*. 2013;120:1915-1919.

CHAPTER 72

Cutaneous hematolymphoid proliferations in children

Julia Scarisbrick, Louis P. Dehner, and Alejandro A. Gru

INTRODUCTION

Primary cutaneous lymphomas are rare cutaneous neoplasms with varied clinical presentation and course. Initial examination must differentiate between primary cutaneous lymphomatoid diseases and secondary involvement of the skin by systemic lymphoma. Systemic lymphomas and leukemias are more common than primary cutaneous lymphoma in children and may present in the skin. Children may require full staging investigations to include a bone marrow biopsy and imaging to ensure a correct diagnosis of a primary cutaneous lymphoma. The clinical course of primary cutaneous lymphomas differs from their systemic counterparts and they require different management. A careful team-based approach that involves hematologists, dermatologists, and other specialists allows for an adequate and careful approach to the diagnosis of these neoplasms. A rapid morphologic interpretation of some of these tumors involves the use of cytologic touch-preparations, flow cytometry, FISH, and conventional cytogenetics. It is capital to make a careful morphologic decision that can help decide what panel of immunohistochemistry or molecular tools to use. This is of paramount importance as treatments vary from expectant/watchful wait approach to aggressive chemotherapy regimens and possible autologous bone marrow transplantation depending on histologic subtype of the skin lymphoma.

Four major histologic subtypes account for most non-Hodgkin lymphomas (NHL) in the pediatric setting: Burkitt lymphoma (39%), diffuse large B-cell lymphoma (DLBCL) (16%), lymphoblastic lymphoma (28%), and anaplastic large cell lymphoma (ALCL; 10%).[1] Approximately 7% of pediatric NHL includes more unusual histologic subtypes, including cutaneous lymphomas. The epidemiologic aspects of cutaneous hematopoietic tumors in children are poorly studied, as most of them are derived from small case series that are highly biased by private consultation material from single institutions.[2] In the series by Fink-Puches et al[3] ($n = 69$), ~35% of pediatric cutaneous lymphomas were accounted by mycosis fungoides (MF), another ~35% by CD30+ lymphoproliferative disorders (ALCL and lymphomatoid papulosis [LyP]), and 20% included marginal zone lymphomas (MZLs) and B-lymphoblastic lymphomas. The pediatric series by Boccara et al[4] in France ($n = 51$) showed that nearly half of these tumors (47%) were composed by LyP, 27% by lymphoblastic lymphomas/leukemias and leukemic infiltrates by acute myeloid leukemia (AML), and approximately 10% included cases of EBV+ lymphoproliferative neoplasms and MF.

Most cutaneous lymphomas present similarly in children and adults but some differences in disease characteristics have been described. While MF is the most common skin lymphoma in adults and children, a disproportionate number of the lesions in children have a particular clinical and immunophenotypic profile: Hypopigmented lesions are much more prevalent in the pediatric setting.[5] Most of the hypopigmented forms have a CD8+ phenotype. Invariably, all cases in children have a very indolent behavior. Similarly, leukemic infiltrates by lymphoblastic and myeloid leukemias are overrepresented in this age group, as the diseases occur with relatively frequency in the pediatric age group. Histiocytoses with cutaneous presentation are more frequent in children as compared to adults.

MATURE T-CELL AND NK-CELL LYMPHOMAS

Primary Cutaneous ALCL, ALK-Negative

Definition and Epidemiology
PC-ALCL is a primary cutaneous lymphoma composed of large and pleomorphic cells (indistinguishable from anaplastic lymphoma kinase-positive [ALK+] ALCL) with diffuse expression of CD30 in the tumor cells (greater than 75%).[6,7] The diagnosis is limited to those cases without a history of LyP or MF.[8,9] Unlike ALK+ ALCL, PC-ALCL is very rare in children compared to adults[10-15] and a diagnosis of LyP (Type A or C) should first be considered. In some cases of PC-ALCL in childhood, an association with HIV infection has been documented.[10]

Clinical Findings
Rapidly growing, asymptomatic, solitary, or multiple skin nodules/tumors with a tendency to ulcerate (Fig. 72-1) are the characteristic clinical presentations.[13,16] Similar to adults, pediatric patients can also be treated with radiotherapy.[17,18]

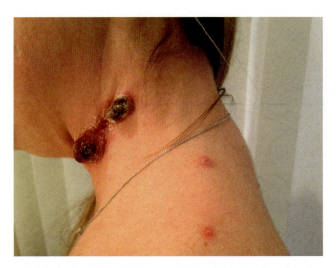

FIGURE 72-1. Cutaneous anaplastic large cell lymphoma of the neck, in a girl with coexisting lymphomatoid papulosis. Large ulcerated necrotic tumors on the neck. (From Gru AA. *Pediatric Dermatopathology and Dermatology.* 2018; Wolters Kluwer Health. Fig. 27.1.)

Histologic Features

Microscopically, ALCL has diffuse, cohesive sheets of large pleomorphic tumor cells, strongly CD30+, similar to ALK+ ALCL (Figs. 72-2 and 72-3). Even among the conventional variants, a rich inflammatory infiltrate is present, which can lead to a misdiagnosis of an inflammatory process in the skin.[19] The neutrophilic variant (pyogenic) of PC-ALCL contains a neutrophilic-rich infiltrate (Fig. 72-4). Although the conventional variant does not have a predilection for immunocompromised individuals, the pyogenic variant is seen in those with HIV,[20] transplant recipients,[21] and hematologic malignancies including young individuals.[11,22]

The tumors are frequently CD4+ and show expression of cytotoxic markers (TIA-1, perforin, granzyme B) (Fig. 72-3). There is variable loss of T-cell antigens and, as opposed to systemic ALK+ ALCL, PC-ALCL is usually negative for epithelial membrane antigen.[23] CD99 can also be positive.[10] The pyogenic variant can have a higher rate of CD8 and EMA (57%) expression, compared to the conventional form.[11,24] CD56 expression is more common in ALK+ ALCL.[25] T-cell clonality is proven in the vast majority of cases by conventional T-cell receptor (TCR) studies. We have encountered an isolated case of ALK+ ALCL with aberrant myeloperoxidase expression.[26] ALK− ALCL has shown convergent mutations and kinase fusions that lead to constitutive activation of the JAK/STAT3 pathway, and a subset with rearrangements at the locus containing *DUSP22 and IRF4* in chromosome 6p25 tends to be relatively monomorphic, usually lacks cytotoxic granules, and has been reported to have a superior prognosis, whereas a small subset with *TP63* rearrangements is very aggressive.[27-29] A dim intraepidermal CD30 staining pattern, with stronger staining in the dermis, is present in *DUSP22*-rearranged tumors.

Differential Diagnosis

The clinical differential diagnosis for the pyogenic variant of PC-ALCL includes pyoderma gangrenosum, pyoderma faciale (rosacea fulminans), Sweet syndrome, leishmaniasis, deep fungal infection, or pyogenic granuloma. Bacterial cellulitis has also been described as another differential diagnostic consideration. Among the neoplastic conditions, the main considerations include LyP, which is not uncommon to present in children (see discussion below), and tumor stage MF which typically presents in the fifth to sixth decade and is exceedingly rare in kids; the latter two disorders are best distinguished on a clinical background. Those with transformed MF have had a long-standing history of the disease and present with multiple tumors, whereas LyP has a history of self-remitting papules. ALK staining and CD30 are useful to rule out the possibility of cutaneous involvement by systemic ALK+ ALCL.[11]

Capsule Summary

PC-ALCL is a primary cutaneous lymphoma composed of large and pleomorphic cells (indistinguishable from ALK+ ALCL) with diffuse expression of CD30 in the tumor cells (greater than 75%). The tumor cells show variable loss of T-cell antigens and cytotoxic marker expression. Rapidly growing, asymptomatic, solitary, or multiple skin nodules/tumors with a tendency to ulcerate are the characteristic clinical presentations.

Mycosis Fungoides

Definition and Epidemiology

MF is the most common form of cutaneous T-cell lymphoma in both adults[30,31] and children.[4,32-35] It accounts for approximately 4% of pediatric NHL, and 4% to 5% of all MF cases.[36] MF in children has a characteristic clinical appearance of hypopigmented patches (Fig. 72-5) and plaques that generally do not progress to the tumoral phase and has a CD8+ phenotype.[37] It has been reported in children as young as 3 years of age.[3,5,33,38-40] It more typically begins around the age of 6 to 8, and is usually diagnosed between 6 and 9 years of age, highlighting (similar to adult cases) a significant delay in the diagnosis. The male-to-female ratio is nearly equal in the pediatric setting.[33,38,40,41] Fink-Puches et al showed that MF represented almost 35% of all cutaneous lymphomas in individuals younger than 20 years.[3,42] Pediatric MF has been reported in few cases to be associated with pityriasis lichenoides (PL),[43] atopic dermatitis,[44] immunodeficiencies (eg, DOCK8),[45] LyP, Wiskott-Aldrich syndrome, follicular mucinosis, and other malignancies.[36,46] A rare case in association with *BRCA2* mutation has been reported.[47]

Etiology

Advances have been published recently in relationship to the mutational landscape of MF and Sézary syndrome (SS), in addition to the discovery of specific molecular rearrangements.[48-52] Choi et al[48] found frequent deletions in chromatin-modifying genes (*ARID1A* [62.5%], *CTCF* [12.5%], and *DNMT3A* [42.5%]). *RB1* was deleted in 25% of samples. *CARD11* and *JAK2* amplification were seen in 22.5% and 12.5% of cases, respectively. *MYC* amplification was noted in 42.5% of samples. Da Silva Almeida et al[49] identified a median of 21 copy number alterations per sample (range of 0-56) in SS, with characteristic recurrent gains in chromosome 7 (5/25, 20%), 8q (13/25, 52%), and 17q (2/25, 8%), as well as recurrent deletions involving tumor-suppressor genes in 17p13.1 (TP53; 13/25, 52%), 13q14.2 (RB1; 4/25, 16%), 10q23.3 (PTEN, 5/25; 20%), and 12p13.1 (CDKN1B; 5/25, 20%). Kiel et al[50] showed numerous (*n* = 42) fusion genes

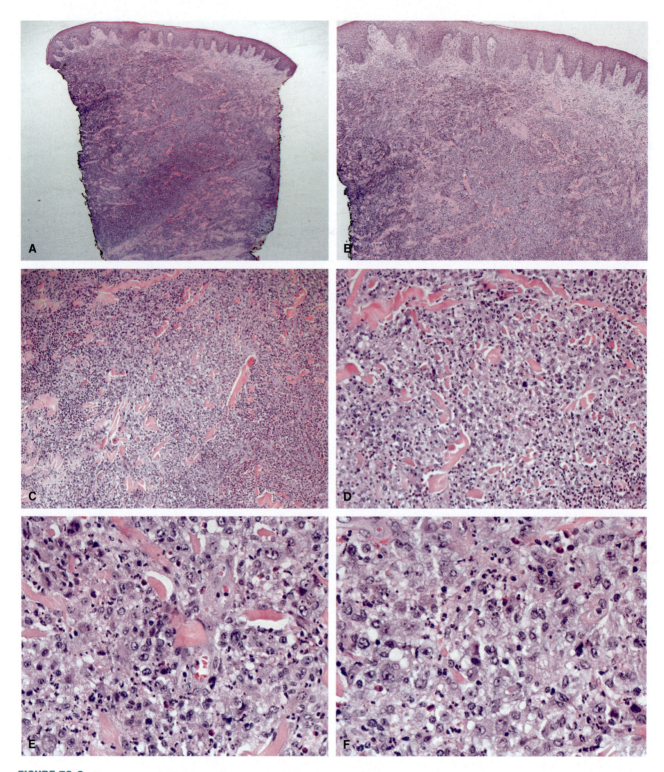

FIGURE 72-2. Cutaneous anaplastic large cell lymphoma—histopathologic findings. Diffuse dermal infiltrate sparing the surface epidermis (**A** and **B**). The malignant infiltrate dissects through the collagen bundles (**C**). There is a rich admixed neutrophilic inflammatory infiltrate (**D**). The infiltrate is composed of malignant appearing large cells with many "hallmark" cells. Eosinophils are also seen (**E** and **F**). (From Gru AA. *Pediatric Dermatopathology and Dermatology*. 2018; Wolters Kluwer Health. Fig. 27.2.)

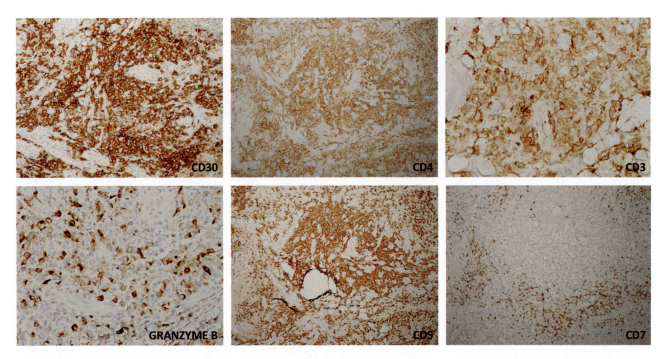

FIGURE 72-3. Cutaneous anaplastic large cell lymphoma—immunohistochemistry. The malignant cells are strong and diffusely positive for CD30 (>75%), CD4, and CD3 and have patchy positivity for granzyme B. They have retained expression of CD5, while marked loss of CD7. (From Gru AA. *Pediatric Dermatopathology and Dermatology.* 2018; Wolters Kluwer Health. Fig. 27.3.)

including TPR-MET, MYBL1-TOX, DNAJC15-ZMYM2, and EZH2-FOXP1, which, albeit not recurrent, could contribute to the pathogenesis of SS. Khavari et al[51] found structural variation events (excluding copy number gains) in pathways related to T-cell survival and proliferation in 11% of patients with MF or SS. Interestingly, the structural variants were largely mutually exclusive with the TNFR2 alterations. The structural variants included NFKB2 gene truncations in 5% (4/73) of cases with the deletion of a region whose loss is known to generate a truncated p100 protein with predicted proteasome-independent NF-κB2 nuclear localization, as well as a deletion involving TRAF3 that would also be expected to increase noncanonical NF-κB signaling. A recurrent CTLA4-CD28 fusion was also discovered.

Clinical Findings

Clinically, pediatric and adult MF may be difficult to diagnose partially because they can potentially mimic numerous benign inflammatory dermatoses (Fig. 72-6).[25,53] In fact, a delay in the diagnosis is common and may take several years and numerous biopsies are often required to eventually establish or consider the diagnosis before clonality studies are performed. Ackerman raised concerns about the diagnosis of MF in the pediatric setting in the past: in their review of 106 cases, it was claimed that only 23 cases had information "sufficient" for a diagnosis of hypopigmented MF.[54] Indeed in 83 of those cases there was no significant clinicopathologic correlation to confidently establish the diagnosis. MF also enters into the differential diagnosis of psoriasis, tinea corporis, PL, lichen aureus, atopic dermatitis, and the various hypopigmented dermatoses.

Vitiligo and pityriasis alba are the two most frequent misdiagnoses in children.[55,56] A case series from Castano et al reported that all cases (100%, n = 69) in children presented at the patch stage; almost all cases had hypopigmented lesions and most of these occurred in African-American children.[32] The more frequent lesions in adults that consist of sharply demarcated patches with atrophy, and a cigarette paper appearance, are less common in children (Figs. 72-7 and 72-8). An earlier study by Crowley et al of 58 patients with MF (younger than 35 years) showed that 17% presented with the tumor stage, and approximately 4% had generalized erythroderma.[33] In another series of 46 cases, Heng et al reported that over 90% of cases had hypopigmented MF.[57] A recent study from Iran showed a small increased number of cases presenting as pigmented pupura.[58] The most common locations of presentation included the buttocks, trunk, and extremities (sun-protected areas). About 6% of patients have solitary lesions. Rare cases of MF can present following organ transplantation.[59] Folliculotropic MF (FMF) presents with follicular papules occasionally with an erythematous base and follicular plugging and/or alopecia; this is the second most common clinical variant and seemingly occurs more frequently in individuals younger than 40 years (Fig. 72-9) (8% of all variants).[60-64] In FMF, the lesions are usually located in the head and neck region, with the presentation of plaques and/or tumors and intense pruritus. FMF has been associated with a worse outcome in adults and children unlike the more indolent and common patch/plaque lesions without FMF.[60] A more recent publication by Reiter et al reported a case series of 71 patients, all of which (except for 2) have early stage disease.[42] Hypopigmented (55%), folliculotropic (42%),

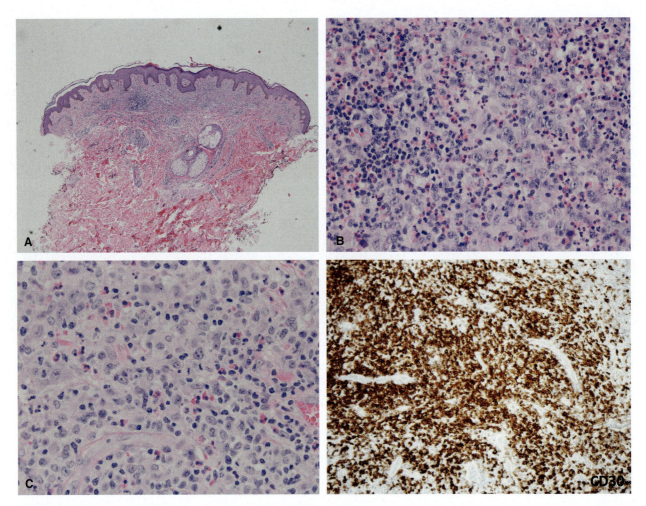

FIGURE 72-4. Cutaneous anaplastic large cell lymphoma, pyogenic variant. The very dense infiltrate is obscured by a rich acute inflammatory infiltrate with neutrophils and numerous eosinophils (**A-C**). The malignant cells are unmasked by a CD30 stain. (From Gru AA. *Pediatric Dermatopathology and Dermatology*. 2018; Wolters Kluwer Health.)

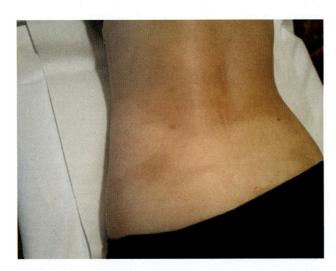

FIGURE 72-5. Mycosis fungoides in an adolescent. Characteristic hypopigmented patches on the upper torso. (From Gru AA. *Pediatric Dermatopathology and Dermatology*. 2018; Wolters Kluwer Health.)

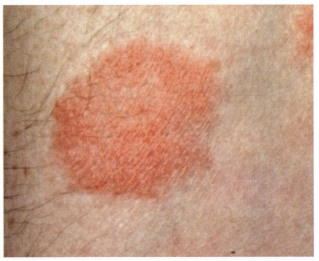

FIGURE 72-6. A patch of MF may be similar to other more common childhood dermatoses such as eczema or psoriasis. (From Gru AA. *Pediatric Dermatopathology and Dermatology*. 2018; Wolters Kluwer Health.)

and classical MF (39%), alone or in combination, were the most common clinical forms.[42] Less common clinical variants in the pediatric population include "granulomatous slack skin" or granulomatous MF (GMF),[65-69] characterized by the development of areas of pendulous, lax skin in the major skin folds (especially axillae and groins).[70] Localized pagetoid reticulosis (PR) (Woringer-Kolopp disease) presents as a solitary, slowly growing erythematous and verrucous plaque on the extremities; rare cases have been reported in children.[71-73] SS is a distinctive erythrodermic cutaneous T-cell lymphoma, characterized by pruritic erythroderma, generalized lymphadenopathy, and circulating malignant cells with cerebriform nuclei. It is a disease of adults, with only rare cases in the pediatric population.[74-76] A rare clinical presentation of palmo-plantar keratoderma has also been described in children.[77]

Histologic Features

Morphologically, pediatric MF is histologically indistinguishable from that seen in adults (Figs. 72-10 through 72-13). According to the series from Castano el al, the most frequent histologic findings include the following: lymphocytes in clusters, patchy lichenoid infiltrates, perivascular/periadnexal infiltrates, psoriasiform hyperplasia, papillary dermal fibroplasia, dermal melanophages, and Pautrier microabscesses. The infiltrate shows epidermotropism with tagging of cells along the dermal-epidermal junction.[78] The atypical lymphocytes show nuclear hyperchromasia and irregular and sometimes cerebriform nuclei. Distinctive perinuclear halos are seen surrounding the intraepidermal lesional cells. Admixed histiocytes, plasma cells, and eosinophils can be present. As the lesions progress clinically, so does the extent of the infiltrate. Large cell transformation is defined as the presence of large cells (at least four times the size of a small lymphocyte) comprising >25% of the infiltrate or nodular aggregates. Only rarely has such a phenomenon been described in lesions in children.[79,80] In FMF, there is infiltration of the hair follicle epithelium with or without epidermotropism (epidermotropism is more frequently seen). The infiltrate involves the infundibulum of the hair follicle and at times deeper portions of the follicle. Follicular mucinosis may be an accompanying feature that can be better demonstrated by colloidal iron or Alcian blue stains. Additionally, FMF is often accompanied by a syringotropic infiltrate.[60] However, a Dutch study revealed that interfollicular epidermotropism is actually rare.[64] FMF is not usually accompanied by intraepidermal Pautrier microabscesses.[81] Dermal eosinophilia can be prominent, particularly during the progression of the disease, and might be a manifestation of an autoimmune response to the keratin of the hair shafts in the dermis. In GMF, dense nodular and diffuse granulomas are present in the dermis, with or without epidermotropism and with destruction of elastic fibers and elastophagocytosis. In the PR variant of MF, prominent pagetoid epidermotropism is noted (Fig. 72-14). Such cases show a very impressive clinical response to radiation treatment.

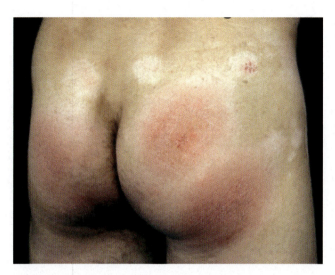

FIGURE 72-7. Distribution of patches of MF is more common in the "bathing suit" area. (From Gru AA. *Pediatric Dermatopathology and Dermatology*. 2018; Wolters Kluwer Health.)

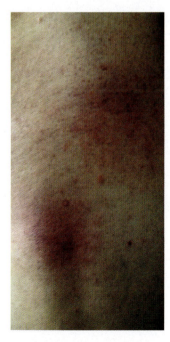

FIGURE 72-8. Patches of MF may show poikilodermatous skin change with atrophy, telangiectasia, and dyspigmentation. (From Gru AA. *Pediatric Dermatopathology and Dermatology*. 2018; Wolters Kluwer Health.)

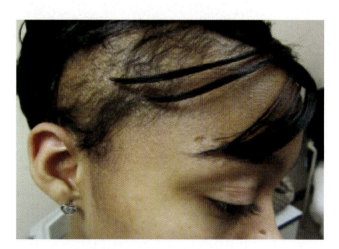

FIGURE 72-9. MF, folliculotropic form. Patches of alopecia in an adolescent girl. (From Gru AA. *Pediatric Dermatopathology and Dermatology*. 2018; Wolters Kluwer Health.)

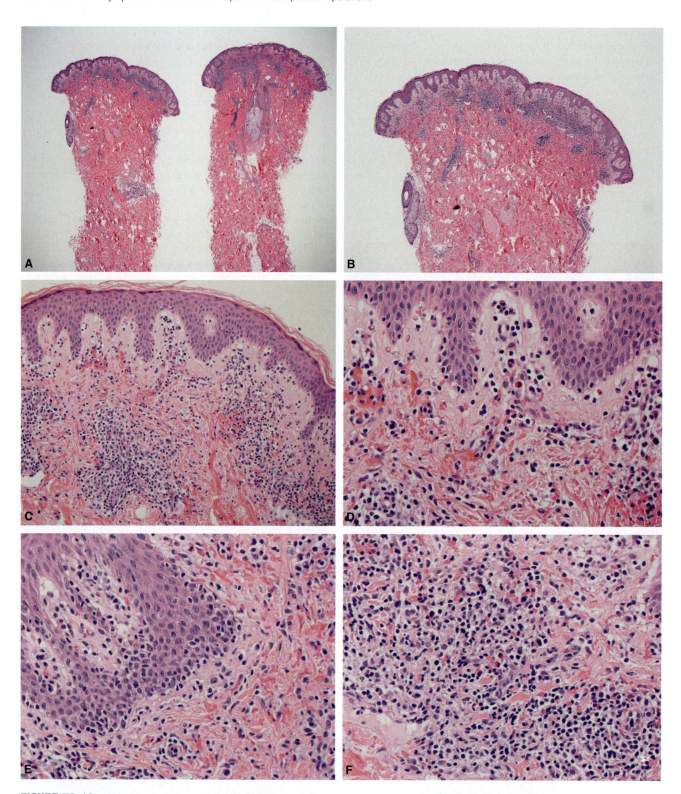

FIGURE 72-10. Pediatric hypopigmented mycosis fungoides. (**A** and **B**, low magnification—20× and 40×). There is a superficial dermal band-like infiltrate. (**C** and **D**, intermediate magnification, 100× and 200×). The infiltrate is associated with extravasation of red blood cells. There is tagging of lymphoid cells at the dermal-epidermal junction. (**E** and **F**, high magnification, 400× each). The infiltrate is composed of small to medium sized lymphocytes, with hyperchromasia, and irregular nuclear borders. The epidermotropic cells do not reveal definitive intraepidermal collections of lymphocytes in the form of Pautrier microabscesses.

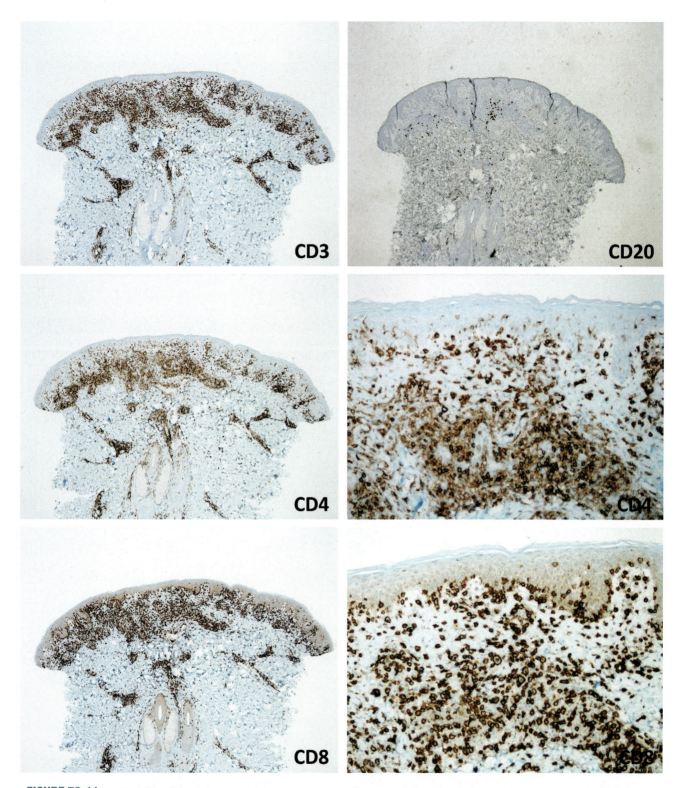

FIGURE 72-11. Pediatric hypopigmented mycosis fungoides—Immunohistochemistry. CD3 is positive in the majority of the dermal and epidermal lymphocytes. CD20 is predominantly negative. CD4 shows positive staining in many of the T-cells and the dermal lymphocytes. However, the vast majority of the T-cells in the epidermis are negative for CD4 and positive for CD8, which reveals extensive epidermotropism and tagging of cells along the dermal-epidermal junction.

The immunophenotype of pediatric MF is different from most of the adult forms (Figs. 72-11 and 72-13): hypopigmented MF is a CD8+ cytotoxic T-cell lymphoma (whereas most cases in adults are CD4+).[3,32-35,38,39,54,55,57,60,82-89] Another study showed CD4 expression in non-FMF cases in ~26% of cases. Also, CD30 expression is usually negative or reacts with only a few scattered cells (80% of cases are entirely nonreactive). Decreased expression of both CD4 and CD8 can also be seen in some cases of hypopigmented MF.[90,91] Similarly to adult MF, there is usually preserved expression of CD2 and CD5 with loss of CD7. Rare cases with coexpression of CD56 have been reported with an associated indolent clinical course.[92,93] In FMF, the infiltrate usually shows a predominance of CD4+ cells like the adult cases.[60]

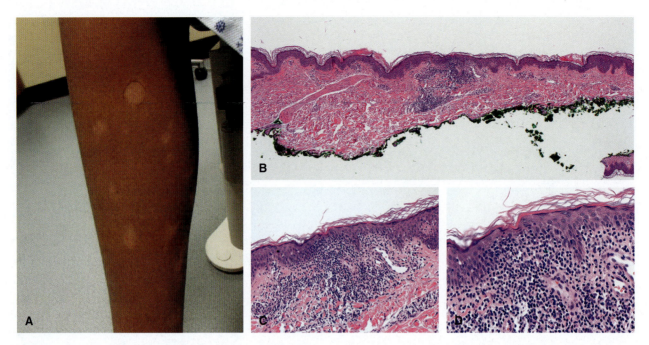

FIGURE 72-12. **Pediatric mycosis fungoides, hypopigmented variant.** Ill-defined hypopigmented patches are present in the leg **(A)**. Histopathologically, there is an atypical lymphoid infiltrate with epidermotropism (**B**, 40×). Tagging of lymphocytes along the dermal-epidermal junction is seen (**C**, 100×). The lymphocytes are small, with hyperchromasia, irregular nuclear borders, and perinuclear halos (**D**, 200×). (Obtained with permission. Gru A, Dehner LP. Cutaneous hematolymphoid and histiocytic proliferations in children. *Pediatr Dev Pathol.* 2018;21(2):208-251. Reprinted by Permission of SAGE Publications.)

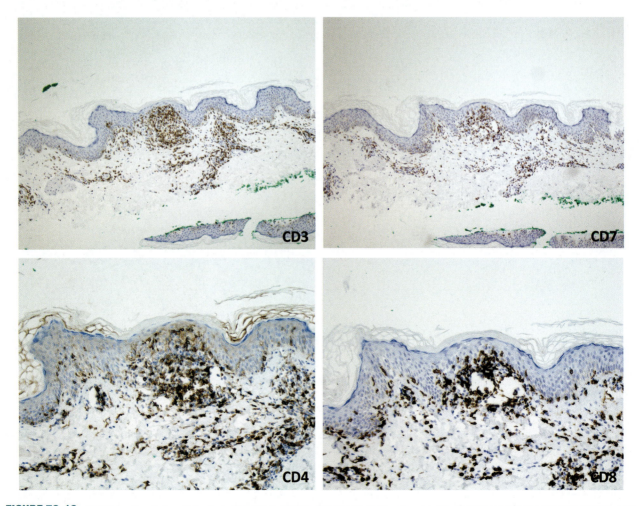

FIGURE 72-13. **Pediatric mycosis fungoides, hypopigmented variant—IHC.** The neoplastic cells are positive for CD3 and CD8. The CD4:CD8 ratio is inverted. There is aberrant loss of CD7. (Gru A, Dehner LP. Cutaneous hematolymphoid and histiocytic proliferations in children. *Pediatr Dev Pathol.* 2018;21(2):208-251. Reprinted by Permission of SAGE Publications.)

GMF is also a disease of CD4+ T-cells. The genetics of MF and SS is less well understood in the context of the pediatric cases when compared to adult MF. When T-cell gene rearrangement studies have been performed in pediatric MF, TCR clonality was proven in approximately 64% of cases, and a polyclonal result was obtained in 16% of cases. These numbers appear to be lower when compared to the adult experience of 80% clonality which may reflect a relatively lower number of neoplastic cells in skin biopsies from children. However, sensitivity for TCR is lower in early lesions of MF (up to 60%).[94] Hodak et al revealed that monoclonality was demonstrated in only 43% of cases.[36,60]

Differential Diagnosis

The differential diagnosis of MF includes a number of inflammatory dermatoses: Pityriasis alba usually presents with hypopigmented macules and patches, situated in the face, but may also affect the trunk and limbs. Histologically, there are very sparse lymphoid infiltrates, with very slight spongiosis, and without the dermal fibrosis seen in MF; vitiligo consists of depigmented macules and patches in localized, segmental, or widespread distribution. The lesions are usually on the face and distal extremities. Histologically, the findings are minimal, and if present, there is a subtle perivascular infiltrate of lymphocytes with minimal epidermal involvement. As lesions evolve, there is a decrease in the numbers of melanocytes at the dermal-epidermal junction, which can be proven with the use of a MART-1 immunostain. Acral pseudolymphomatous angiokeratoma of children (APACHE) can also mimic PR. A dense lymphoid infiltrate beneath the epidermis and thick wall vessels are seen.[95] Pityriasis lichenoides chronica and varioliformis acuta (PLC/PLEVA) can also share histomorphologic features. A lymphocytic vasculitis and interface changes are present in both conditions.

As opposed to MF, loss of T-cell antigens (CD7) is not typical. Molecular studies (TCR rearrangement) should not be used to distinguish between both conditions, particularly if using the BIOMED primers, as PLC and PLEVA can have positive clonality studies in up to 25% of cases. More recently, next-generation sequencing has been shown to accurately distinguish between inflammatory dermatoses with clonal populations of cells and cutaneous T-cell lymphomas.[96] However, this technique is currently expensive and unlikely to replace TCR gene analysis in the current clinical setting. Spongiotic dermatoses (eczema, contact dermatitis, etc) can also enter the differential. The latter typically lack significant cytologic atypia of the lymphoid population or aberrant antigenic loss. If the infiltrate is positive for CD30, other CD30+ lymphoproliferative disorders (LPDs) can enter the differential diagnosis (LyP and PC-ALCL). The clinical presentation is capital to distinguish between MF and those. In children, Langerhans cell histiocytosis is also accompanied by extensive pagetoid epidermotropism of the histiocytic cells. As opposed to MF, LCH is positive with histiocytic markers (CD68, S100, CD1a, and Langerin), while negative for T-cell antigens. A word of caution should be made with LCH, as many cases can have clonal rearrangements of the TCR.

Capsule Summary

MF is the most common form of cutaneous T-cell lymphoma in both adults and children. MF in children has a characteristic clinical appearance of hypopigmented patches and plaques that generally do not progress to the tumoral phase and more frequently has a CD8+ phenotype. More recently, folliculotropic forms have been reported with a high prevalence in this population, but without an association with a more aggressive clinical course. Loss of T-cell antigens (CD7) is common. Differential diagnosis, particularly in the

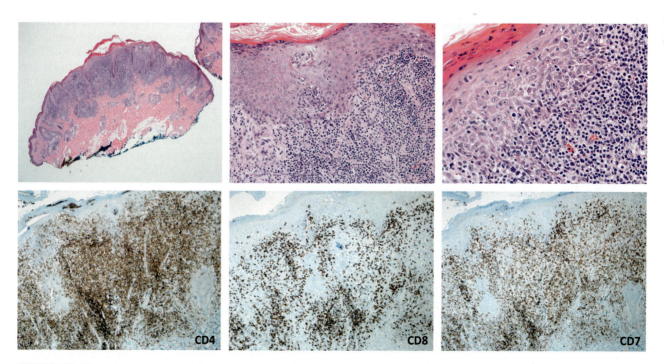

FIGURE 72-14. Pediatric mycosis fungoides, pagetoid reticulosis variant. In this case, the infiltrate shows very extensive pagetoid epidermotropism. Lymphoma cells are CD4 positive, CD8 negative, and have loss of CD7. (Gru A, Dehner LP. Cutaneous hematolymphoid and histiocytic proliferations in children. *Pediatr Dev Pathol*. 2018;21(2):208-251. Reprinted by Permission of SAGE Publications.)

Lymphomatoid Papulosis

Definition and Epidemiology
Lymphomatoid papulosis is a CD30+ T-cell lymphoproliferative disorder characterized by recurrent crops of papulonecrotic lesions that usually prevail for 3 and 8 weeks and then resolve spontaneously.[97] The lesions are clinically "benign" appearing, but the histologic features suggest otherwise. However, lesions may frequently heal with atrophic scarring which may be disfiguring. LyP is the third most common type of cutaneous lymphoproliferative disorder in children.[3,98] Boys are reported to have an earlier onset of LyP compared to girls. It is estimated that between 5% and 20% of those with LyP can develop a subsequent lymphoma, usually MF, Hodgkin lymphoma, or ALCL; this proportion appears to be smaller in the pediatric setting (approximately 9%).[98-103] The frequency of LyP ranges from 16% to 47% of all skin lymphomas in children, across different case series.[2-4] Rare examples in association with B lymphoblastic leukemia have occurred.[104]

Etiology
Karai et al reported for the first time a group of patients with LyP and associated rearrangements of the *IRF4-DUSP22* locus on 6p25.3.[105] These cases show some unusual histologic findings, including PR-like epidermal changes with a proliferating dermal tumor. A consistent histologic finding also included a typical periadnexal infiltrate and hallmark-like cells.

Clinical Findings
Clinically, LyP presents with erythematous papules and nodules that become hemorrhagic and necrotic after a few days with resolution as a depigmented scar.[4,8,85,97-102,106-109] Lesions at different stages of evolution are characteristically present (Fig. 72-15). A recent series of nine cases in Italy showed that six of the cases presented with ulcerated nodules.[110] In children, there is a clinical resemblance to PL, the most important disease in the differential diagnosis. The sites of predilection are the trunk and extremities, but other locations have been reported.[109] Regional LyP with crops of lesions located in a single anatomic region is seemingly more common in children.[108,109] Nearly 50% of cases in children have more than 50 lesions at one point during their clinical course.

LyP is a clinical diagnosis of self-resolving papulonecrotic lesions; while most are CD30 positive, the histology may be varied and indistinguishable from transformed CD30+ MF, popular MF, or PC-ALCL in some cases.

Histologic Features
Several histologic variants have now been described in LyP: types A, B, C, D, E, and F. None of the histologic subtypes have any prognostic significance. The importance in differentiating the various subtypes is related to the differential diagnosis that each subtype entails. Many of these lesions have substantial histopathologic overlap: type A LyP has a wedge-shaped dermal infiltrate composed of medium to large and pleomorphic cells scattered throughout the infiltrate or arranged in clusters (Fig. 72-16). The malignant cells can show features of Hodgkin-like cells and there is a rich background of inflammatory cells. Ulceration, edema of the dermis, and focal vasculitic changes may be present; type B LyP is characterized by an epidermotropic infiltrate reminiscent of MF; and type C LyP has features identical histologically to PC-ALCL, and clearly the clinical distinction is more important in a sense than the histologic findings. Cerroni et al showed that most cases in children represented types A and C, with no examples of type B. In another pediatric series of 250 cases of LyP in children, most cases were type A.[103] Type D LyP mimics aggressive epidermotropic CD8+ T-cell lymphoma histologically[111]; this variant expresses other cytotoxic markers such as granzyme and TIA-1. In the latter study, four of the nine original patients were less than 25 years of age. Type E LyP is characterized by an angioinvasive and angiodestructive CD8+ cytotoxic T-cell infiltrate with CD30 coexpression; 2 of the 16 original patients were children.[112] Another study of 14 children with LyP revealed that 10 cases had a CD8+ cytotoxic phenotype; most cases were considered either type A or type C. Pierard et al introduced the term follicular LyP (type F) to describe a subtype with a predominant perifollicular pattern of infiltration.[113,114] A few cases of LyP (type F) have been reported in children.[115-117]

The immunophenotype of types A and C is very similar with a uniform population of CD30+ cells, with frequent CD3 and CD4 coexpression. Typically, CD8 and CD56 are negative. CD15 is usually negative, but cytotoxic molecules (TIA-1 and granzyme) are positive.[118-120] Types D and E have a CD8+ phenotype. MUM1 is frequently expressed in all cases of LyP (but also in MF and PC-ALCL). Some cases of LyP can also have a *DUSP22* translocation.[105]

Differential Diagnosis
Arthropod bite reactions should be particularly considered in the differential diagnosis. Arthropod bites tend to be more itchy, and do not heal with scarring. Those can also have a wedge-shaped pattern histologically of inflammation as seen in type A LyP. As opposed to LyP cases, arthropod bites never have the number of CD30+ cells, or the aberrant loss of T-cell antigens. Pseudolymphomas should also be distinguished from LyP. While the density of the infiltrate can be similar, the number of CD30+ cells is lower in pseudolymphomas, and they also lack T-cell antigenic loss. PC-ALCL can also be seen in children, and the main distinction appears to be clinical, rather than a pathologic one. PC-ALCL tends

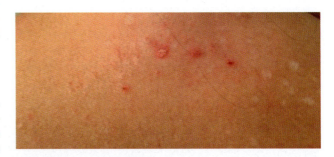

FIGURE 72-15. Lymphomatoid papulosis. Lesions of LyP often appear in crops; they mature from red papules and may ulcerate and tend to heal with atrophic hypopigmented scars. (From Gru AA. *Pediatric Dermatopathology and Dermatology.* 2018; Wolters Kluwer Health.)

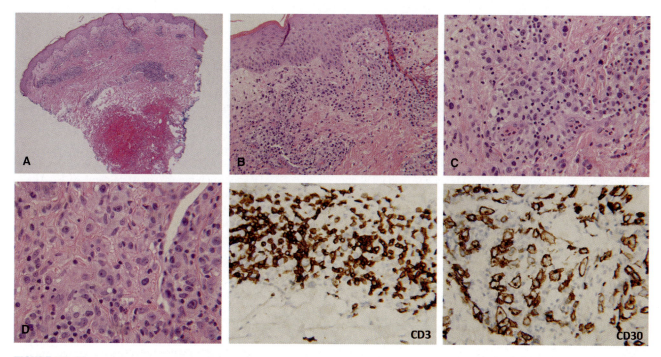

FIGURE 72-16. Lymphomatoid papulosis (LyP), type A. In LyP, there is a wedge-shaped infiltrate with only partial epidermal involvement (**A** and **B**). Malignant large and pleomorphic cells are present with a rich acute inflammatory (**C** and **D**) background. The lesional cells are positive for CD30 and have significant loss of CD3. (From Gru AA. *Pediatric Dermatopathology and Dermatology*. 2018; Wolters Kluwer Health.)

to be more solitary, persists for a longer period of time, and less frequently shows spontaneous resolution. At the molecular level, both can have the *DUSP22* translocation.

Capsule Summary

LyP is a CD30+ T-cell lymphoproliferative disorder characterized by recurrent crops of papular lesions that usually prevail for 3 to 8 weeks and then resolve spontaneously, leaving an atrophic scar. Several histologic variants have now been described in LyP: types A, B, C, D, E, and F. None of the histologic subtypes have any prognostic significance. The first three types are CD4+, whereas types D and E are CD8+. A higher prevalence of CD8+ cases have been reported in children.

Anaplastic Large Cell Lymphoma, ALK-Positive

Definition and Epidemiology

ALK+ ALCL represents approximately 10% to 30% of childhood lymphomas and is more frequent in the first three decades of life. There is a slight male predominance and the majority of patients (70%) present with stage III or IV disease and B-symptoms. The skin is the most frequent extranodal site of involvement (present in 26% of cases). Other extranodal sites include the bone, soft tissues, lung, and liver.[121-124] ALK+ ALCL has a good prognosis with 5-year survival rate of 70% to 80% in contrast to 49% and 32% 5-year survival rates for ALK− ALCL and PTCL-NOS (peripheral T-cell lymphoma, not otherwise specified), respectively.[125,126]

Etiology

ALK+ ALCL has rearrangements of the *ALK* gene on 2p23 with various partner genes, most typically the nucleophosmin (*NPM*) on 5q35.[127,128] Some translocations can be cryptic by conventional cytogenetic methods. Other translocation partners include nonmuscle tropomyosin (*TPM3*, 1q25 and TPM4, 19p13.1); amino-terminus of 5-aminoimidazole-4-carboxamide ribonucleotide formyltransferase/IMP cyclohydrolase gene (*ATIC*, 2q35); TRK-fused gene (*TFG*, 3q21); clathrin heavy polypeptide gene (*CLTC*, 17q23); moesin gene (*MSN*, Xq11-12); myosin heavy chain 9 gene (*MYH9*, 22q11.2); and ALK lymphoma oligomerization partner on chromosome 17 (*ALO17*, 17q25).[123,129]

Clinical Findings

Most cases of ALK+ ALCL present with lymphadenopathy. The most common extranodal site is the skin (26%).[130-133] Other affected sites include the bone, lung, liver, and soft tissues.[123] A leukemic presentation is rare but more frequent in the small cell variant.[134] The bone marrow is affected in a small percentage (10%-30%) of cases.[135]

The cutaneous manifestation of ALCL, ALK+ can be precipitated by insect bites.[136,137] Lesions resemble typical arthropod bite reactions without clinical resolution. Most patients with ALCL, ALK+ or ALK− have pink papulonodular lesions.[138-140] The lesions are more frequently solitary and rarely multiple. Rare cases of isolated cutaneous ALCL, ALK+ have been reported.[141] Some uncommon clinical appearances include generalized erythroderma,[142] orbital lesions,[143] and ichthyosis.[144]

Histologic Features

ALK+ ALCL has a variety of morphologic presentations. All cases show a malignant population of large cells with eccentric horseshoe or kidney-shaped nuclei with an eosinophilic region near the nucleus, referred to as "hallmark" cells. In some variants, the hallmark cells can be small. Occasionally, the malignant cells can mimic Reed-Sternberg cells or their variants. There are five distinctive variants of ALK⁺ ALCL: common, small cell variant, Hodgkin-like pattern, lymphohistiocytic pattern, and combined forms.[129,141,145-147] Any of these patterns may present in the skin (Figs. 72-17 and 72-18). The immunophenotype of ALK⁺ ALCL includes CD30 and ALK expression; the pattern of CD30 expression is both Golgi and cytoplasmic. Most cases are positive for EMA, TIA-1, granzyme B, and perforin and most show loss of T-cell antigens such as CD3, CD5, and CD7. Some cases can be null for all T-cell markers. CD43, CD2, and CD4 are more frequently positive.

The cellular localization of the ALK expression correlates with the pattern of translocation: the *NPM/ALK* fusion leads to both nuclear and cytoplasmic ALK staining. The ALK staining patterns in less common translocation variants include diffuse cytoplasmic (eg, *TPM3, ATIC, TFG, TPM4, MYH9, ALO17*), granular cytoplasmic (*CLTC*) (Fig. 72-18), or membranous (*MSN*). ALCL, ALK⁻ shows strong and diffuse expression of CD30. The pattern can be membranous, Golgi, and/or cytoplasmic. The strong and diffuse character is often a helpful clue to distinguish ALCL, ALK⁻ from PTCL-NOS. Lack of multiple pan T-cell antigens and the expression of cytotoxic markers are characteristic. EMA and clusterin can be positive, but less frequently than in ALCL, ALK⁺.[126]

Lamant et al suggested a possible relationship between insect bites and the development of ALK⁺ ALCL[136]; this series of five patients had recent arthropod bites and developed nodal disease in the area of the skin lesions. Two of the skin biopsies revealed the presence of ALK⁺ cells. A complete remission was obtained after chemotherapy in all but one case who developed progressive disease and died. More recently, Oschlies et al[141] described a series of 6 children, within the context of 487 patients enrolled in the Anaplastic Large Cell Lymphoma-99 trial with disease limited to the skin; these patients had complete remissions on follow-up, and most were treated with surgical excision only. In all cases but one, the pattern of ALK staining was nuclear and cytoplasmic, and FISH was positive for the ALK-NPM translocation. Clinically, in 5/6 cases lesions were solitary (maculopapules or nodules) and one patient had multiple lesions. Previous isolated case reports of cutaneous presentations of ALK⁺ ALCL have been described.[131,148,149] Despite such reports, most cases of ALK⁺ ALCL have associated systemic disease and require full staging. A more recent series by Mulcher et al reported a total of six cases of ALK⁺ ALCL, four of which did not have extracutaneous disease, including one pediatric patient.[150]

Differential Diagnosis

From the diagnostic perspective, a diagnosis of ALK⁺ ALCL implies the presence of a systemic lymphoma "until proven otherwise." The rare isolated cutaneous forms are very infrequent. All patients should invariably undergo extensive staging procedures. The presence of ALK⁺ distinguishes this process from PC-ALCL. More recently, molecular studies have proven that systemic ALK⁻ ALCL with the presence of *DUSP22* translocations has a similar clinical outcome to cases of ALK⁺ ALCL. Inflammatory myofibroblastic tumors in children can also be ALK⁺. As opposed to ALK⁺ ALCL, such tumors are only positive for histiocytic markers and lack the cellular pleomorphism that is typical of ALCL cases. An interesting association of the existence of both an ALK⁺ Spitz nevus and ALK⁺ ALCL with the exact same fusion has been reported in the literature.[151]

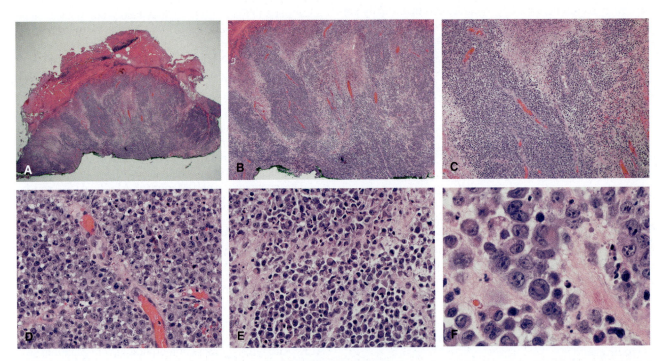

FIGURE 72-17. ALK⁺ Anaplastic large cell lymphoma with initial skin presentation. A dense malignant infiltrate in the dermis with surface ulceration, but sparing of the epidermis (**A** and **B**). The infiltrate shows angiotropism (**C** and **D**). It is composed of malignant large cells with frequent hallmark forms (**E** and **F**). (From Gru AA, Voorhess PJ. A case of ALK⁺ anaplastic large-cell lymphoma with aberrant myeloperoxidase expression and initial cutaneous presentation. *Am J Dermatopathol.* 2018;40(7):519-522.)

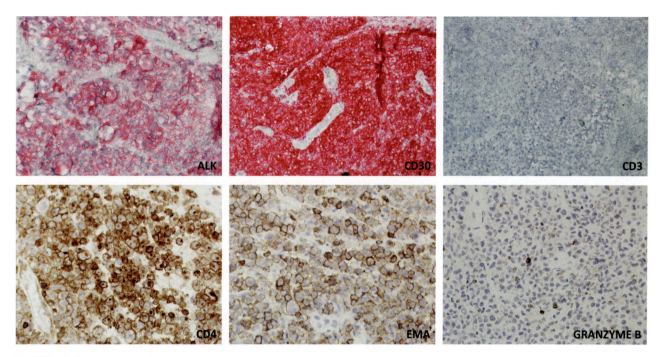

FIGURE 72-18. ALK+ anaplastic large cell lymphoma with initial skin presentation. The large cells are positive for ALK (cytoplasmic granular staining), CD30, CD4, EMA and weakly for granzyme B. They are negative for CD3. (From Gru AA, Voorhess PJ. A case of ALK+ anaplastic large-cell lymphoma with aberrant myeloperoxidase expression and initial cutaneous presentation. *Am J Dermatopathol.* 2018;40(7):519-522.)

Capsule Summary

ALK+ ALCL represents approximately 10% to 30% of childhood lymphomas and is more frequent in the first three decades of life. The skin is the most frequent extranodal site of involvement (present in 26% of cases). ALK+ ALCL has a variety of morphologic presentations. All cases show a malignant population of large cells with eccentric horseshoe- or kidney-shaped nuclei with an eosinophilic region near the nucleus, referred to as "hallmark" cells. Rare examples of ALK+ ALCL isolated to the skin have been reported. The cellular localization of the ALK expression correlates with the pattern of translocation: the NPM/ALK fusion leads to both nuclear and cytoplasmic ALK staining.

Subcutaneous Panniculitis–Like T-Cell Lymphoma

Definition and Epidemiology

Subcutaneous panniculitis–like T-cell lymphoma (SPTCL) is a mature T-cell lymphoma of the skin with TCRαβ expression, subcutaneous involvement, and sparing of the epidermis. In a review study of 143 cases of nonanaplastic T-cell lymphomas in children and adolescents, SPTCL accounted for 15% of cases.[152] It most commonly involves the extremities, occurs at different age groups (including children), and has an indolent clinical behavior.[153] Rare cases have occurred in children less than 1 year of age.[154] SPTCL with the expression of γδ TCR has distinct clinicopathological features and is classified under the γδ T-cell lymphomas.[155] It is more common in women and has a predilection for younger individuals. The median age at presentation is 36 years (range 1-79). Approximately 50% of cases occurred in individuals of 21 to 40 years of age and 19% of cases are in 20-year-old or younger patients.[156] Numerous cases have now been reported in children.[152,156-160] A subsequent study of cutaneous lymphomas in children noted that SPTCL was rare with only 3.4% of cases in this age group.[85]

Etiology

The etiology of SPTCL remains unknown. It has been reported that nearly 19% of cases of SPTCL have associated autoimmune disorders. Those included systemic lupus erythematosus, juvenile rheumatoid arthritis, Sjögren disease, type 1 diabetes mellitus, idiopathic thrombocytopenia, multiple sclerosis, Raynaud disease, and Kikuchi disease.[156] A study by Yi et al[161] showed a series of 11 cases of SPTCL initially diagnosed as autoimmune disorders; the authors divided the original diagnoses in three separate groups: (1) a group with a preceding diagnosis of erythema nodosum, pyoderma gangrenosum, and lupus profundus; (2) vasculitis; and (3) inflammatory myopathy-like lesions. The authors speculated that cases with inflammatory myositis and/or Behcet represented paraneoplastic manifestations of SPTCL. Some of these cases (2/11) had an elevation of antinuclear antibodies in the serum, anti-DS DNA antibody, and one case had an elevated ANCA (antineutrophil cytoplasmic antibody). A study from the Mayo clinic on a series of 23 patients revealed preceding diagnoses of autoimmune disorders in approximately 57% of cases including lupus panniculitis, erythema nodosum, venous stasis, Weber-Christian disease, cellulitis, and granulomatous panniculitis of unknown etiology. The association between SPTCL and lupus erythematosus profundus (LEP) has led to the hypothesis that perhaps the two entities represent two ends of the same spectrum.[162,163] It should be noted that some cases of lobular panniculitis with a CD8+ phenotype can occur in children in association with clonal populations of T-cells in the setting of congenital immune deficiency syndromes. Rare cases in association with HIV[164] and sarcoidosis have also been documented.[165] The association between certain medications and development of SPTCL has been described in patients receiving anti-TNFα therapy (etanercept)[166] and following rituximab and cyclophosphamide.[167] More unusual presentations have been reported in patients with Down syndrome,[168] cervical cancer,[169] during pregnancy,[170] and neurofibromatosis type 1.[171]

More recently, molecular characterization of cases of SPTCL has reported the presence of *HAVCR2* mutations in cases of SPTCL associated with hemophagocytosis (HPS).[172,173] Notoriously, homozygous mutations of the gene have been encountered in familial cases of SPTCL from Vietnamese origin.[174] A similar report has come from a little girl from China, with a homozygous mutation.[175] Germline mutations of the gene have been seen in association with sporadic cases.[172] HAVCR2 encodes the TIM-3 protein, which is a negative checkpoint and critical regulator of innate immunity and inflammatory responses. It suppresses effector T cell (the TH1 subset of helper T cells) responses by decreasing interferon-γ-driven inflammation, and defects in its function may thus account for the hemophagocytic lymphohistiocytosis (HLH) manifestations seen in TIM-3-mutant SPTCL.

Clinical Findings

The typical lesions consist of nodules/tumors or skin plaques, which can vary in diameter from 1 to 20 cm or more and are frequently multifocal (78%). Sometimes the nodules leave areas of lipoatrophy after resolution. Ulceration is rare (6%). The lesions present in the extremities (legs, arms) and less frequently the trunk and face. Facial lesions can present with extraocular muscle palsy.[176] Rare cases in the breast have been reported.[177,178] The skin lesions often simulate other causes of panniculitis, such as erythema nodosum[179] and lupus panniculitis. Other rare clinical presentations might simulate dermatomyositis,[180,181] morphea,[182] cellulitis,[183] facial edema,[184] venous stasis-like ulceration,[185] lipomembranous panniculitis,[186] eschar-like crusting,[187] erythromelalgia,[188] and alopecia.[189] The delay from the onset of symptoms to the diagnosis of SPTCL can range from 3 weeks to 10 years.[190] Systemic symptoms occur in 40% to 50% of cases, including fever, chills, night sweats, and weight loss. Cytopenias and alterations in liver enzymes often occur. HPS is seen in 17% of cases[156] and is associated with high mortality (46% at 5 years). HPS is more prevalent in subcutaneous panniculitic T-cell lymphomas with γδ phenotype (45%).[191,192] Less common clinical manifestations include lymphadenopathy, hepatosplenomegaly, pleural effusions, and bone marrow involvement.[193,194] Systemic workup for involvement by SPTCL is usually negative for extracutaneous disease.[195,196] Transmission of the disease has been documented after allogeneic bone marrow transplantation[166] and cardiac transplantation.[197] Some cases show spontaneous resolution.[158,198,199]

The prognosis of SPTCL in general is excellent. Approximately 60% of patients achieve complete remission, and about 12% die of the disease. Most deaths are due to hemophagocytic syndrome, which usually develops late in the disease course.[156] Five-year overall survival is >80%.[191] The development of HPS is associated with a survival of approximately 46% at 5 years.[156,191] The largest series of SPTCL in the pediatric age group revealed a slightly higher rate of recurrences (>50%), but overall low mortality.[157] A fatal case with overlap features of lupus and HPS had been reported.[200]

Histologic Features

A dense, nodular, interstitial, or combined lymphoid infiltrate showing adipotropism with a predilection of the subcutaneous lobule mimicking a lobular panniculitis is seen in virtually all cases (Fig. 72-19).[4,85,157,158,168,201-212] Septal involvement is typically mild or absent. Extension of the infiltrate into the reticular dermis, surrounding and occasionally infiltrating sweat glands, hair follicles, and sebaceous glands can be seen.[213] Infiltration of the superficial epidermis and/or dermis is exceedingly rare and, if present, should raise the diagnostic consideration of MF with a secondary panniculitic presentation or γδ T-cell lymphoma. Rimming of neoplastic cells around adipocytes is characteristic but not pathognomonic. This pattern can be also seen in lupus panniculitis and in association with other lymphoproliferative disorders such as tumor stage MF, aggressive epidermotropic CD8+ T-cell lymphoma, extranodal NK/T-cell lymphoma (ENKTL), γδ T-cell lymphoma, blastic plasmacytoid dendritic cell neoplasm (BPDCN), secondary DLBCL, and leukemia cutis (LC).[214] Intravascular thrombi adjacent to tissue necrosis are not uncommon, whereas angiotropism and angiodestruction are exceedingly rare. Necrosis and karyorrhexis along with nonneoplastic inflammatory infiltrates (histiocytes, small lymphocytes, and neutrophils) are often prominent, and may mask the underlying neoplastic process. In such scenarios, the presence of ghost cells (necrotic malignant lymphocytes) could be useful in identifying the atypical population. Later stages might show collections of epithelioid histiocytes, granulomas, or lipomembranous changes.[186] Eosinophils and plasma cells are uncommon; however, the presence of plasma cells should raise the differential diagnosis of LEP or LEP/SPTCL overlap.[162,215-222] In cases where the presence of intralobular histiocytes with phagocytosed red blood cells or apoptotic elements is present, workup for hemophagocytic syndrome is warranted.[223] Similar to the skin findings, bone marrow infiltration by SPTCL also shows adipocyte rimming.[193]

The immunophenotype reveals CD3+, BF1+, CD8+, and cytotoxic molecules, such as TIA-1, perforin, and granzyme B. CD56 and CD30 are typically negative. Ki67 is moderately high (>50%)[224] (Fig. 72-20). Loss of CD2, CD5, and/or CD7 is seen in 10%, 50%, and 44% of cases, respectively.[156] CD45RO is usually positive and CD45RA is negative. Epstein-Barr virus (EBV) has been rarely documented in patients from Asian descent.[225-229]

Differential Diagnosis

An important differential diagnosis of SPTCL is lupus panniculitis which can present in children.[222] In contrast to SPTCL, lupus panniculitis presents with subcutaneous fibrosis, frequent clusters of plasmacytoid dendritic cells (CD123+), reactive germinal centers, and absence of the phenotype of SPTCL. A study from Liau et al has shown that the most useful criteria to distinguish LP from SPTCL include the cytologic atypia of the lymphoid cells (low in the former), presence of dermal mucin, and follicles of B-cells with the formation of germinal centers. Those three features are more typical of LP and not seen in cases of SPTCL. Additionally, their study showed that clusters of plasmacytoid dendritic cells (intrinsically linked to the pathogenesis of LE), as detected by CD123 immunostain, are typically seen in LP, but not or only minimally present in SPTCL.[219] Ki67-increased proliferation is also more typical of SPTCL.[230] Pincus et al[163] have shown a

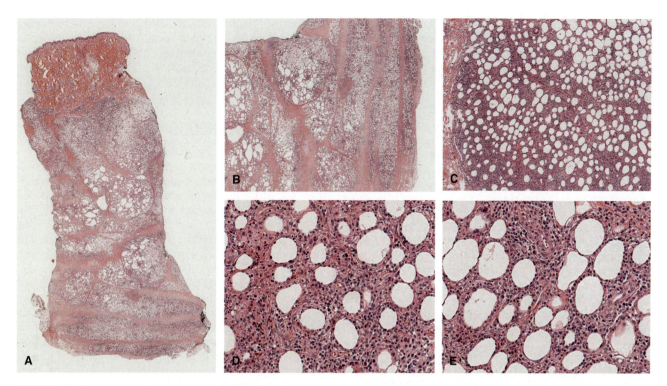

FIGURE 72-19. Subcutaneous panniculitis–like T-cell lymphoma. There is a mostly lobular panniculitis with dermal and epidermal sparing (**A** and **B**). A very dense lymphoid infiltrate in the subcutaneous lobule is seen (**C**). The atypical lymphocyte population shows prominent adipocyte "rimming" (**D** and **E**). (From Gru AA. *Pediatric Dermatopathology and Dermatology*. 2018; Wolters Kluwer Health.)

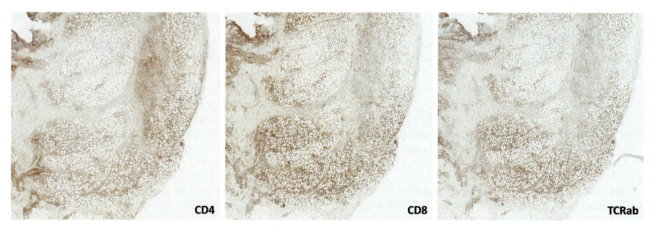

FIGURE 72-20. Subcutaneous panniculitis–like T-cell lymphoma—IHC. The malignant infiltrate is positive for CD3, CD8, and TCRαβ, while negative for CD4. (Adapted and obtained with permission. Gru AA et al. Hematopathology of the skin. LWW.)

series of five cases of biopsies of patients who meet criteria for LE and SPTCL. They proposed that some cases show histologic overlap. Those biopsies revealed the presence of dermal mucin, admixed atypical lymphocytes, interface changes, and rimming of adipocytes. Clusters of CD123+ cells were seen in the biopsies within the areas of lupus. Ki67 was elevated in all cases, and one of the cases also had a positive direct immunofluorescent study. All cases have clonal T-cell populations by T-cell gene rearrangement studies.

Another "reactive" panniculitis with overlap features with SPTCL and some cases with coexistence between the two represents the so-called cytophagic histiocytic panniculitis, a disease typically seen in children.[202,203,209,231-234] The original series of five cases[235] described patients originally believed to have Weber-Christian disease, with a chronic, intermittent course and HPS.[236] The clinical manifestations included fever, hepatosplenomegaly, ulcers, and serosal effusions. Pancytopenia, liver failure, and intravascular coagulation developed in all cases. Erythrophagocytosis or cytophagocytosis of nonerythroid cells can be seen in different organs. Marzano et al presented a series of seven cases of cytophagic panniculitis, of which four patients had SPCTL (although two of them will be categorized as γδ T-cell lymphoma by current criteria). Five of the seven patients died because of HPS. But two of the cases had a more indolent course over several years. Although most authors will regard cytophagic panniculitis as a possible subtype of lymphoma, cases without over clonality and aggressive course are seen, and the term should be perhaps preserved in some of these cases.[237] Cytophagic panniculitis can be associated with systemic macrophage activation syndrome and occurs isolated, and in association with viral infections, connective tissue disorders, as well as malignancies.[203] Some cases occur in association with mutations of the perforin gene.[231]

Capsule Summary

SPTCL is a mature T-cell lymphoma of the skin with TCRαβ expression, subcutaneous involvement, and sparing of the epidermis. It most commonly involves the extremities, occurs at different age groups (including children), and has a variable clinical behavior (worse in patients with HPS). The typical lesions consist of nodules/tumors or skin plaques, which can vary in diameter from 1 to 20 cm or more, and are frequently multifocal. It has been reported that nearly 19% of cases of SPTCL have associated autoimmune disorders. A dense, nodular, interstitial, or combined lymphoid infiltrate showing adipotropism with a predilection of the subcutaneous lobule mimicking a lobular panniculitis is seen in virtually all cases. The immunophenotype reveals $CD3^+$, $BF1^+$, $CD8^+$, and cytotoxic molecules, such as TIA-1, perforin, and granzyme B. HAVCR2 mutations are associated with HPS and can occur sporadically or in a familial manner.

PRIMARY CUTANEOUS CD4⁺ SMALL TO MEDIUM T-CELL LYMPHOPROLIFERATIVE DISORDER

Primary cutaneous $CD4^+$ small to medium T-cell LPD (SMPTCL) is exceedingly rare (incidence <1 per million) but has been known to present in children in a minority of cases.[238] This lymphoproliferative disorder remains in a provisional category in the WHO classification.[239] The terminology in the revised classification has been modified from "lymphoma" to "LPD" to reflect this uncertain malignant potential, designating these cases as primary cutaneous $CD4^+$ SMPTCL. The clinical behavior is almost always indolent, with most patients presenting with localized disease. Systemic disease is rare, and conservative local management is sufficient in most patients. It has been suggested that this may represent a limited clonal response to an unknown stimulus, not fulfilling criteria for malignancy.[29,240,241]

All cases presenting to date in children have a solitary lesion, usually a papule, nodule, or plaque in the head and neck region. The infiltrate consists of a nodular, diffuse, and interstitial infiltrate of lymphoid cells with sparing of the epidermis (Fig. 72-21). There is expression of CD4, but a rich background of B-cells is also encountered with the expression of germinal center markers (BCL-6, CD10, PD1, ICOS).[146,242,243] CD30 is usually negative (Fig. 72-22).

AGGRESSIVE CD8-POSITIVE EPIDERMOTROPIC T-CELL LYMPHOMA (BERTI LYMPHOMA)

The original series of primary cutaneous epidermotropic $CD8^+$ T-cell lymphoma had a single case in a child.[244] Kikuchi et al[245] subsequently described a second case in a 6-year-old girl with disseminated lesions. A multicenter study of 30 cases included 2 cases in individuals younger than 25 years. The median survival is approximately 12 months.[246] Papulonecrotic lesions in the extremities are usual presentation. Morphologically, these lesions typically reveal an acanthotic epidermis with prominent epidermotropism and keratinocytic necrosis. The immunophenotype includes TCRβ, TIA-1, and CD8 expression.

PRIMARY CUTANEOUS γδ T-CELL LYMPHOMA

This extraordinarily rare disorder has been reported in children, but it is basically an adult condition.[4,233,247-251] Merrill et al reported the occurrence of CGDTCL in three individuals before the age of 25, including a 1-year-old child.[252] The lesions are usually found on the extremities and trunk. The malignant infiltrate is accompanied by epidermal necrosis with frequent involvement of the subcutis. Vasculitis and ulceration can be seen, and HPS is also present. The most common immunophenotype includes $CD3^+$, $CD4^-$, $CD8^-$, and $CD56^{+/-}$ (Fig. 72-23). The identifying feature is the presence of TCRγ expression. An important differential diagnostic consideration is LyP since some cases in children can have TCRγ expression. The distinction between LyP and CGDTCL is an important one since the former is an indolent disease and the latter requires systemic chemotherapy and bone marrow transplant. The previously reported cases of SPTCL with a γδ phenotype have now been reclassified as CGDTCL.[192]

Systemic Chronic Active EBV Disease of T-Cell or NK-Cell Type

Definition and Epidemiology

This rare systemic EBV^+ polyclonal, oligoclonal, or monoclonal T-cell or NK-cell lymphoproliferative disorder manifests with variable clinical severity. It was originally defined as a severe illness with a duration of more than 6 months, after a primary EBV infection with continued high titers to EBV and evidence of major organ involvement (pneumonia, bone marrow aplasia, uveitis, lymphadenitis, hepatitis, splenomegaly). EBV by in situ hybridization (EBER) expression has been used to document EBV in the infected tissues.[253] The updated criteria also allow for the diagnosis in the presence of symptoms that last for longer than 3 months (infectious mononucleosis-like) and have high levels of EBV viremia and/or tissue infiltration by EBV^+ T- or NK-cells.[29,254,255] While the affected cells are typically T- or NK-cells, rare cases of B-cell derivation can occur.[256]

The disease has a strong predilection for individuals of Asian or South American descent, and most notably occurs in children and adolescents.[257-260] Less frequently, CAEBV can occur in middle-aged or older adults with prolonged fevers, hepatosplenomegaly, anemia, thrombocytopenia, lymphadenopathy, and cutaneous manifestations. The latter are typically in the form of mosquito bite allergy (33%), rash (26%), and HV-like manifestations. Most patients have high antibody titers (EBV VCA IgG, EBNA), as well as high EBV viremia.[254,256,259-261]

Clinical and Histologic Findings

The cutaneous findings will be discussed with the hydroa vacciniforme (HV)-like LPD and severe mosquito bite

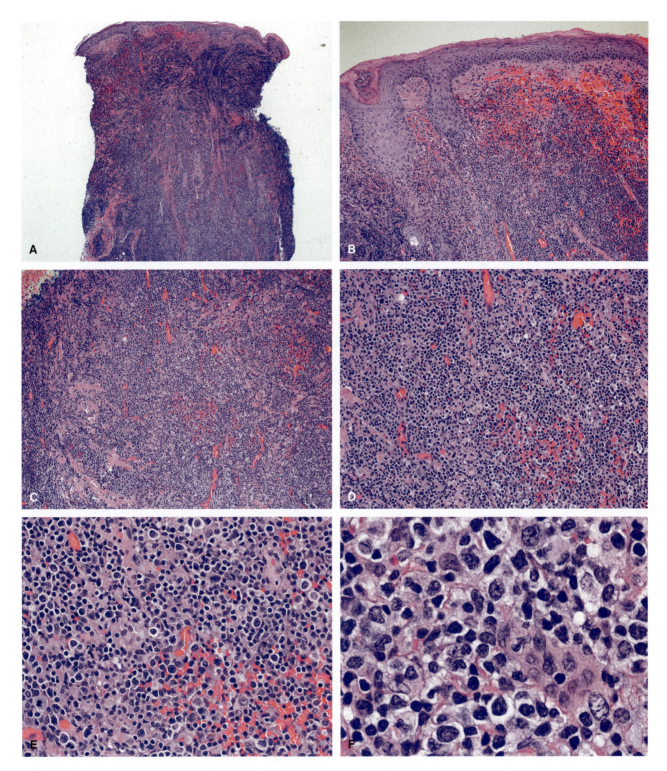

FIGURE 72-21. Primary cutaneous CD4+ small to medium T-cell lymphoproliferative disorder. There is a dense and vaguely nodule dermal infiltrate with sparing of the epidermis, and extending very deep into the bottom of the biopsy (**A** and **B**). The infiltrate shows a monotonous appearance (**C**). Scattered larger cells are seen (**D**). The infiltrate is composed of a mixture of small, medium, and large pleomorphic cells (**E** and **F**). (Adapted and obtained with permission. Gru A, Dehner LP. Cutaneous hematolymphoid and histiocytic proliferations in children. *Pediatr Dev Pathol.* 2018;21(2):208-251. Reprinted by Permission of SAGE Publications.)

allergy (SMBA) (which are considered cutaneous forms of CAEBV). In other sites, such as the lymph nodes, CAEBV is characterized by paracortical hyperplasia, a polymorphous infiltrate, and a rich background of inflammatory cells that include plasma cells and granulomas at times. Some cases are accompanied by associated HLH, best demonstrated in BW, lymph node, and liver biopsies.[259,262] Numerous EBV+ cells are seen. When monotonous sheets of EBV+ tumor cells are noted, such cases are best classified as systemic EBV+ T-cell lymphoma of childhood (ENKTL) or aggressive NK-cell leukemia (ANKL).[263] Somatic mutations in driver genes including *DDX3X* are detected in

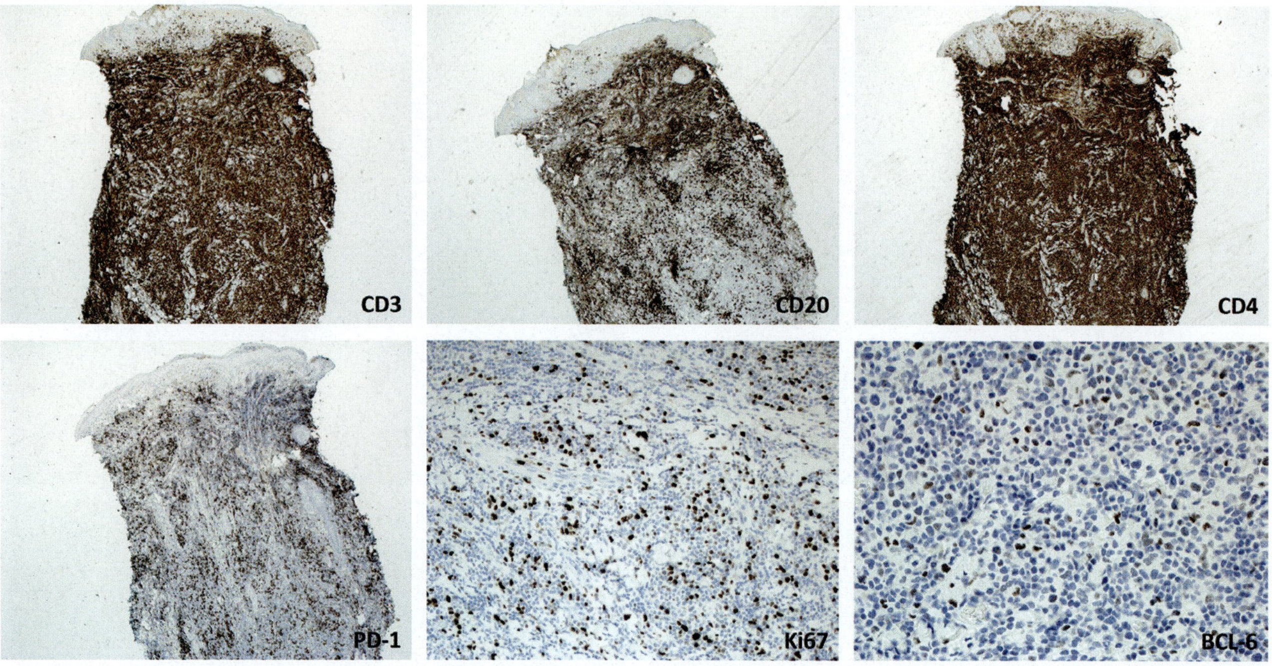

FIGURE 72-22. Primary cutaneous CD4+ small to medium T-cell lymphoproliferative disorder—IHC. The infiltrate is diffusely positive for CD3 and CD4. CD20 shows a background very rich in B-cells. PD-1 and BCL-6 are positive in a significant proportion of T-cells, indicating a T_{FH} phenotype. Ki67 is overall low (10%). (Adapted and obtained with permission. Gru A, Dehner LP. Cutaneous hematolymphoid and histiocytic proliferations in children. *Pediatr Dev Pathol*. 2018;21(2):208-251. Reprinted by Permission of SAGE Publications.)

EBV-positive cells. These cells expand and may evolve to overt leukemia or lymphoma. The EBV genome harbors frequent intragenic deletions (27 of 77 cases), suggesting a unique role of these mutations in the development of the disease.[264]

The prognosis of CAEBV is variable, with some patients experiencing a relatively indolent clinical course, while others succumb to the disease, especially in the presence of HLH. The median survival is approximately 70 to 78 months, and adverse markers of clinical outcome include late onset (>8 years of age), thrombocytopenia, and T-cell infection (5-year survival is approximately 60% for T-cell disease and 87% for NK-cell disease).[254,256,262] T-cell clonality is sometimes associated with a more aggressive clinical course.[259]

Capsule Summary

It is defined as a severe illness with a duration of more than 3 months, after a primary EBV infection with continued high titers to EBV and evidence of major organ involvement (pneumonia, bone marrow aplasia, uveitis, lymphadenitis, hepatitis, splenomegaly).

SEVERE MOSQUITO BITE ALLERGY

The cutaneous manifestations of CAEBV infection may be precipitated by mosquito bites or vaccination.[265,266] SMBA is very uncommon, and most cases occur in individuals from Asia and Mexico.[267-275] This disorder is not a hypersensitive reaction in the classic sense, but is rather a cutaneous manifestation of CAEBV of NK-cell lineage, with oligoclonal or monoclonal populations of NK-cells.[276]

Most patients are less than 20 years of age, with a median age of 6.7.[276] Erythematous papules, macules, and plaques can subsequently evolve into bullae with ulceration and eventual scarring. Systemic symptoms are also common, and include fever, lymphadenopathy, and liver dysfunction.[277,278] Recovery occurs when the systemic symptoms resolve until the next mosquito bite. Vaccinations can also sometimes elicit a similar reaction.[279] High levels of IgE, high EBV viremia, and NK-cell lymphocytosis (80%) are present in SMBA.[265] The skin shows epidermal necrosis with ulceration. Marked dermal edema and infiltration by neutrophils and a dense lymphoid infiltrate are noted. Vasculitis is present in the center with karyorrhectic debris, and extravasated red blood cells in the dermis. The lymphoid infiltrate is composed of a mixture of CD4+, CD8+ T-cells and NK-cells. EBV-positive cells represent a minority of the infiltrate (<10%). Those patients with persistent systemic symptoms for over 3 months should be best classified as systemic CAEBV.

The prognosis is variable: some patients have an indolent course, with chronic protracted cutaneous manifestations, while others may develop fulminant HLH or progress to lymphoma, such as ANKL.[279] Somatic mutations including *DDX3X* are detected in EBV-positive cells indicating that this is a neoplastic disease.[264]

Hydroa Vacciniforme Lymphoproliferative Disease

Definition and Epidemiology

This chronic cutaneous form of EBV+ LPD of childhood (CAEBV) has a risk of progression to a systemic

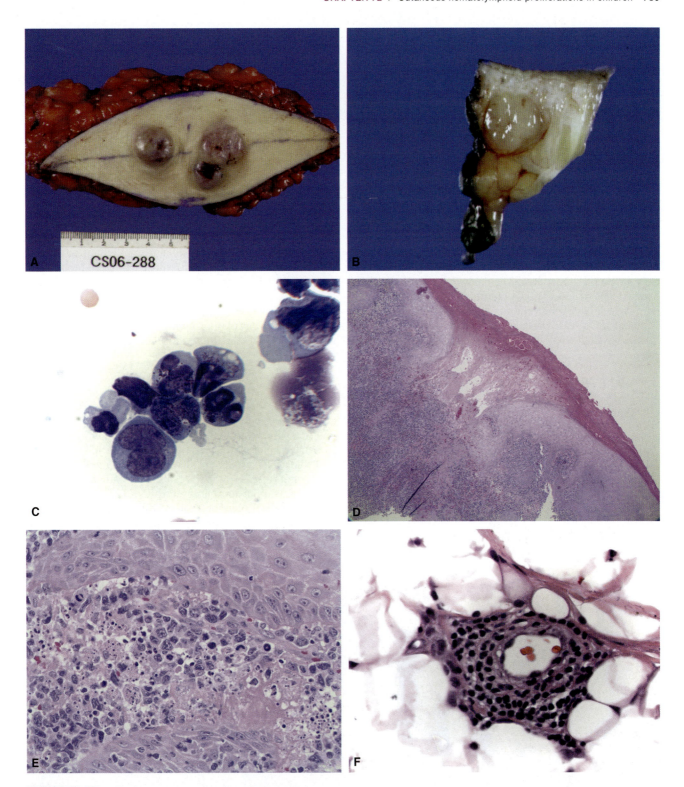

FIGURE 72-23. Primary cutaneous γδ T-cell lymphoma. A and **B.** Gross specimen from excisional biopsy. There is a dermal nodule with surface ulceration. **C** (touch imprint—1000×). The malignant cells are medium to large, with pleomorphic nuclei with abnormal lobation, and numerous cytoplasmic granules. **D** (low magnification—40×). The tumor is ulcerated. **E** and **F** (high magnification—400×). The infiltrate is close to the epidermis and composed of very pleomorphic cells. Focal necrosis is noted. The infiltrate shows prominent angiotropism.

lymphoma.[255] Classic HV is a rare, intermittent ultraviolet light–induced vesiculopapular and scarring eruption that typically remits after adolescence.[280-282] Systemic symptoms are not usually present in HV. The estimated prevalence of HV is approximately 0.34 cases/100.000.[280] In some cases, the lesions can occur in sun-unexposed areas. Later studies have shown an association between HV and clonal proliferations of T-cells; the term HV-like lymphoma (HVLL) was introduced in the WHO classification in 2008.[283] However, because of the inability to predict which patients will have an indolent course, and which ones will develop overt lymphoma, the term hydroa vacciniforme lymphoproliferative disease (HV-LPD) is now the preferred one in the new edition of the WHO monograph.[29] This diagnostic category is considered under the EBV-positive T-cell and NK-cell lymphoid proliferations and lymphomas of childhood. Other terms that have applied to describe HVLL in the past included edematous scarring vasculitic panniculitis, angiocentric cutaneous T-cell lymphoma of childhood, hydroa-like cutaneous T-cell lymphoma, and severe HV.

Most cases of HV-LPD are seen in children and adolescents from Asia, Native Americans from central and south America (Peru, Guatemala, and Bolivia), and Mexico and rarely occur in adults.[281,284-292] In the Peruvian studies, approximately 50% of cases are found in the southern region of the country, correlating with a higher prevalence of early EBV infection in that area. The median age at diagnosis is 8 years. The male-to-female ratio is 2.3:1. Males with HV may have a later onset and longer duration than females. Although the disease presents in children, some patients can have persistent symptoms into adulthood.

Etiology
It has been proposed that certain populations (eg, Asian and South American) have a risk for development of lymphoma, while in others (North American and European) the disease has an indolent course.[280,290] Recent clinical studies suggest that HV-LPD can be successfully treated with immunomodulators (thalidomide,[293] antivirals,[294] interferon,[295] etc) rather than systemic chemotherapy, as the latter has been associated with a higher mortality among these patients.[284]

Clinical Findings
Classical HV is characterized by a sporadic, itchy erythematous eruption in sun-exposed areas that occurs shortly (minutes to hours) after sun exposure. The eruption progresses through different stages: papules, vesicles, crusts, and eventually vacciniform (pox-like) scars after several weeks (Fig. 72-24). Severe forms of the disease can have conjunctival and corneal ulceration and scarring. Marked facial edema is common in the more aggressive forms, associated with unilateral or bilateral eyelid compromise. Periorbital swelling can be the first manifestation of the disease.[280,281,286] The lesions can become chronic (lasting months to years) and are prone to recurrence, often characterized by temporal heterogeneity, from papules with crusts to well-formed scars in the same area.[280] Clinical progression to lymphoma is heralded by a lack of improvement with photoprotection, severe facial and lip swelling, and systemic complications. Some cases can coexist with SMBA. When extracutaneous involvement occurs (hepatosplenomegaly, lymphadenopathy, bone marrow infiltration), those cases are best classified as EBV+ T-cell lymphoma of childhood. Fever, weight loss, and asthenia can be present. Elevations of LDH and liver enzymes are noted in one-third of patients.[284,296,297] Expansion of circulating gamma-delta T-cells is seen in the blood, usually with the morphology of large granular lymphocytes.

Histologic Features
In HV-LPD, the lymphoid infiltrate is composed of small to medium-sized hyperchromatic cells centered in the dermis with a perivascular/periadnexal distribution and with associated epidermal necrosis (Fig. 72-25). Spongiosis and intraepidermal vesicles are also seen. In the more aggressive forms of the disease, the cells can show significant atypia and somewhat similar morphology to ENKTL. Mitotic figures are infrequent. Epidermotropism without Pautrier microabscesses is a common feature. Fully developed lesions are deeply infiltrative into the adipose tissue, but without significant rimming of the adipocytes as seen in SPTCL.

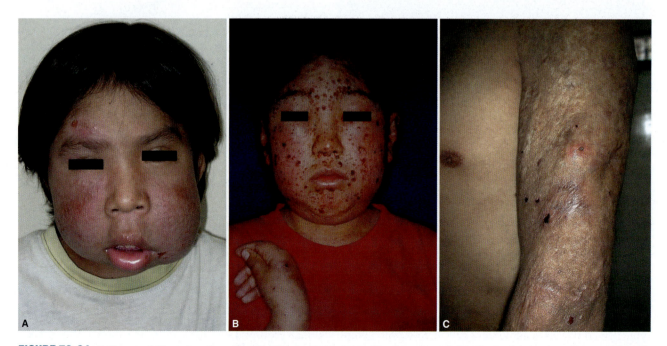

FIGURE 72-24. **Hydroa vacciniforme lymphoproliferative disorder.** Facial edema with erythematous and ulcerative-crusty lesions in an 11-year-old child **(A)**. Numerous vesicular hemorrhagic lesions on the face are present **(B)**, with many lesions showing severe scarring **(C)**.

Angiotropism with or without angionecrosis and fibrinoid changes can be seen.[284,287,289-291]

The EBV-infected cells are cytotoxic T-cells (CD3+, CD8+, TIA-1+, granzyme B+, perforin+) or NK-cells (CD56+).[284,287,290,291] A minority of cases can be CD4+ or CD4+/CD8+,[298-302] particularly in patients from China. The latter are cases with common subcutaneous involvement which can mimic SPTCL.[290,292,302,303] CD30 is occasionally positive, but LMP-1 is negative. The number of EBV+ cells is variable (Fig. 72-26). The Ki-67 index is variable and is very low in some cases, or as high as 50% in others. Expression of CD5, CD7, CD43, and CD25 is variable. CD57 is negative. The T-cells can be positive for either TCR$\alpha\beta$ or TCR$\gamma\delta$. Clonal rearrangements of the TCR are almost always demonstrated. Deletion of the long arm of chromosome 6 has been documented.[304] The genomic landscape is otherwise poorly understood.[305]

Differential Diagnosis

The differential diagnosis includes other NK/T-cell LPD, such as ANKL and ENKTL. In the latter entities, diffuse sheets of atypical CD56+, EBER+ cells are noted. Some cases of ANKL can also show skin involvement.[306] SPTCL can have overlap in the immunophenotype, being composed of CD8+ cells. However, SPTCL is negative for CD56 and lacks epidermotropism and EBV expression. Primary cutaneous $\gamma\delta$ T-cell lymphoma (PCGDL) can also be CD56+, but is more typically negative for EBV, presents in older adults, and the location is more typically truncal and in the extremities.

Capsule Summary

Classic HV is a rare, intermittent ultraviolet light–induced vesiculopapular and scarring eruption, that typically remits after adolescence. Because of the inability to predict which patients will have an indolent course, and which ones will develop overt lymphoma, the term HV-LPD has been accepted in the new edition of the WHO monograph. In HV-LPD, the lymphoid infiltrate is composed of small to medium-sized hyperchromatic cells centered in the dermis with a perivascular/periadnexal distribution, and with associated epidermal necrosis. Spongiosis and intraepidermal vesicles are also seen.

Extranodal NK/T-Cell Lymphoma

Definition and Epidemiology

ENKTL, nasal type, is a mature NHL derived by NK-cells (more frequently) and sometimes T-cells with extranodal (frequently upper aerodigestive) infiltration by EBV-infected cytotoxic lymphocytes with angioinvasion and necrosis.[255] In the United States, ENKTL is very rare, accounting for less than 1% of NHL. The disease is more prevalent in the areas of Mexico, South and Central America, and Asia where it represents nearly 6% of all NHL, and in certain areas, up to 22% to 44% of all NHL.[307,308] Overall, approximately 150 cases of ENKTL have been reported in children.[152,309,310] The median age of presentation is 13, with a male to female ratio of 3.25:1.

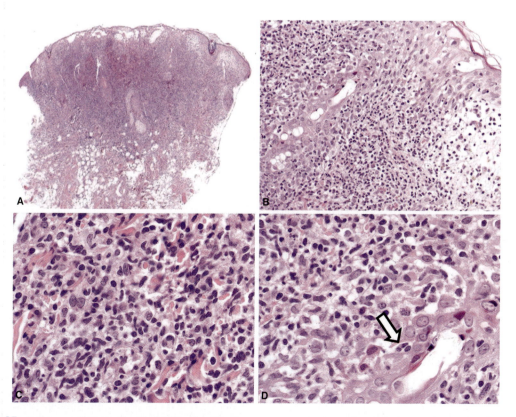

FIGURE 72-25. Hydroa vacciniforme lymphoproliferative disorder. A. Lymphoid infiltrates extend from the epidermis to the subcutaneous tissue. Intraepidermal vesicles are evident. **B.** Prominent epidermotropism. **C.** Medium-sized neoplastic cells with hyperchromatic nuclei and irregular nuclear contours. **D.** Infiltration of an eccrine duct (arrow).

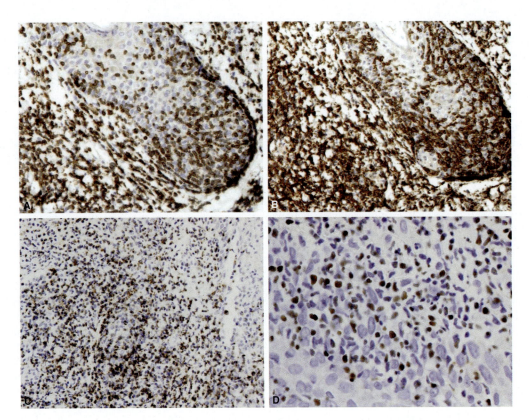

FIGURE 72-26. Immunophenotypic features of HVLL. Epidermotropic neoplastic cells with diffuse CD3 **(A)**, CD8 **(B)**, and granzyme B **(C)** expressions. **D.** EBER highlights EBV-infected malignant cells.

Etiology

ENKTL shows a strong association with EBV infection, irrespective of the patient's origin, which supports a direct pathogenic role of the virus in lymphomagenesis.

Clinical Findings

The disease presents in extranodal sites, most often in the upper aerodigestive tract (70%), including the nasal cavity (by far the most frequent site), orbital soft tissue, paranasal sinuses, and palate. Some cases can present in extra nasal cavity sites, but lymph node involvement is uncommon. Most often, there are signs of local tumor infiltration: ulceration, perforation of the nasal septum (in the past, many of these cases were called midline lethal granuloma[311]), and epistaxis are frequently seen.[255] B-symptoms, such as fever, weight loss, malaise, and night sweats, are also common (65%-77% of pediatric cases)[312] and are the second most common clinical presentation of ENKTL in children. ENKTL can also be associated with HPS which worsens the prognosis.[313] Dissemination to the skin, gastrointestinal tract, testis, or cervical lymph nodes can also be present, while bone marrow involvement is relatively uncommon. Skin involvement is present in 10% of cases of ENKTL and manifests as nodules that ulcerate and often have a necrotic center, erythematous maculopapules, cellulitis, and abscess-like swelling (Fig. 72-27).

The survival rate is 30% to 40%[314,315] but in recent years has improved with more intensive therapy including upfront radiotherapy and the SMILE regimen.[316] Unfavorable prognostic factors include advanced stage (III or IV), bone marrow or skin involvement, and high levels of EBV DNA in the serum.[314,317] Cases with extranasal presentations have a more aggressive clinical behavior, compared to the nasal ones,[318] and those with primary skin disease (and without systemic dissemination) appear to have a better prognosis.[314,315,317] Higher EBV viral load correlates with a worse outcome and disease activity.[319,320]

Histologic Features

ENKTL has an angiocentric and angiodestructive growth pattern with coagulative necrosis, admixed apoptotic bodies, and fibrinoid change in blood vessels, even in the absence of angioinvasion (Fig. 72-28).[321,322] Pseudoepitheliomatous changes are present in some cases. The tumor cells can exhibit a marked range in cell size. The nuclei are round or folded, have coarse or vesicular chromatin, and small inconspicuous nucleoli. Mitotic figures are frequently seen, in addition to apoptosis and karyorrhectic debris. Cytoplasmic granules are seen in some cases. Areas of geographic necrosis can also be present. Background inflammatory cells are variable, and include plasma cells, histiocytes, and neutrophils. In the skin, focal epidermotropism is seen on occasion. When the adipose tissue is affected, necrosis and rimming of the adipocytes by the malignant cells is noted, which can mimic the findings present in primary CGDTCL and SPTCL. Permeation of the tumor cells into the skeletal muscle with associated myonecrosis can also be present.[255,306]

ENKTL originates from T- or NK-cells with a cytotoxic phenotype and[323-326] expression of cytotoxic granules (granzyme B, TIA-1, and perforin); however, most cases are derived from NK-cells, are CD56-positive, and negative for surface CD3 expression yet positive for cytoplasmic CD3 subunits including CD3ε and CD3ζ. As such, ENKTL is positive for CD3 when polyclonal anti-CD3 antibodies are applied. Most cases are positive for CD2, CD43, CD45RO, HLA-DR, CD25, CD7, and FAS (CD95) and negative for CD4, CD5, CD8, TCRγ, βF1, CD16, and CD57.[327,328] CD30 is positive in 20% to 40% of cases, particularly in cases with a rich large cell component.[309] The Ki-67 proliferation index is typically very high (>50%), even in the presence of small cell–predominant tumors. *In situ* hybridization studies for EBV-encoded RNA (EBER) are positive in virtually all cases.

The TCR and immunoglobulin heavy chain (IGH) genes are in germline configuration in ENKTL derived from NK-cells. Clonal rearrangements of the TCR genes are detected in 10% to 40% of cases, particularly in those of T-cell origin.[329,330] Recent studies have demonstrated activation of the JAK-STAT signaling pathway in ENKTL.[255] A recent study of ENKTL in children showed high mutation frequencies detected in *KMT2C* (5/5), *MST1* (5/5), *HLA-A* (3/5), and *BCL11A* (3/5), which involved in modifications, tumor suppression, and immune surveillance.[312]

Differential Diagnosis

The differential diagnosis of ENKTL in the skin includes other aggressive types of cutaneous lymphoma. PCGDL is often CD56+, but usually lacks expression of CD5, CD4, and CD8. As opposed to ENTKL, epidermotropism is more frequently found, and the lesions show strong expression of TCRγ. Rare cases are double positive for βF1, and some cases of PCGDL are TCR silent. EBER is only rarely expressed (<5% of cases).[248] MF can rarely be CD56+[331,332] and, as opposed to ENTKL, shows more prominent epidermotropism and frequent formation of Pautrier microabscesses. Most cases of MF are positive for βF1, and more typically CD4 positive. Other entities included in the differential diagnosis are other EBV-associated T-cell or NK-cell lymphoproliferative disorders such as EBV+ PTCL-NOS, CAEBV infection, systemic EBV+ T-cell lymphoproliferative disease of childhood, and HV-like lymphoproliferative disorder, which also occurs predominantly in children. ANKL can

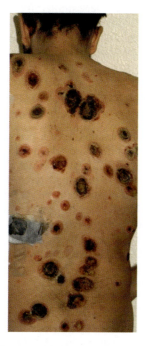

FIGURE 72-27. Extranodal NK/T-cell lymphoma. Such tumors frequently have an aggressive clinical course with numerous necrotic plaques. (From Gru AA. Pediatric Dermatopathology and Dermatology. 2018; Wolters Kluwer Health.)

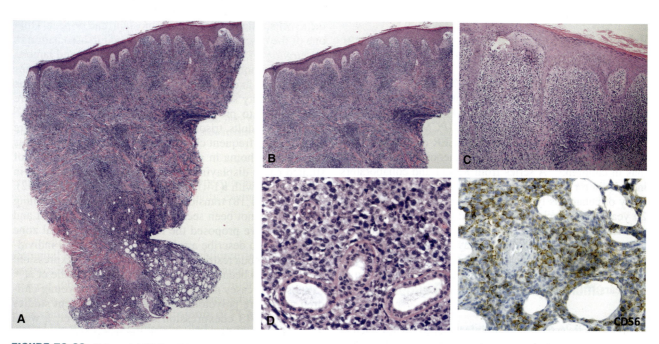

FIGURE 72-28. Extranodal NK/T-cell lymphoma. There is a dermal-based malignant lymphoid infiltrate with angiotropism and epidermal sparing **(A-C)**. The infiltrate is composed of medium-sized cells with abundant granular cytoplasm **(D)**. The infiltrate is diffusely positive for CD56. (From Gru AA. Pediatric Dermatopathology and Dermatology. 2018; Wolters Kluwer Health.)

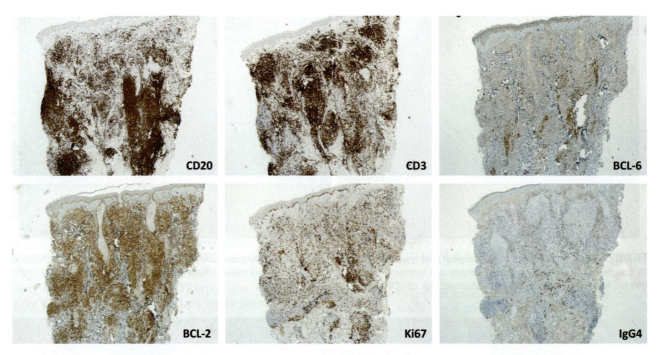

FIGURE 72-31. Cutaneous marginal zone lymphoma—IHC. The lymphoma cells are positive for CD20. CD3 shows a rich background of T-cells. The atrophic germinal centers are positive for BCL-6, while negative for BCL-2. They have a high Ki67. IgG4 is positive in abundant plasma cells. (From Gru AA. *Pediatric Dermatopathology and Dermatology.* 2018; Wolters Kluwer Health.)

but extraordinarily rare in children.[359] By definition, PC-FCL is limited to the skin at the time of diagnosis, without evidence of systemic or nodal involvement, and is a distinct entity separate from systemic or nodal follicular lymphoma (FL). Armitay-Laish reported the occurrence of a spindle cell variant of PC-FCL in a 17-year-old girl.[344] Condarco et al reported a case of PC-FCL in the scalp of an 8-year-old boy.[360] In the large series ($n = 69$) of pediatric cutaneous NHL from Gratz, a single case of a PC-FCL on a 20-year-old individual has been reported.[3] A case of PC-FCL in the setting of the rare congenital immunodeficiency WHIM syndrome (warts, hypogammaglobulinemia, infections, and myelokathexis) has been described.[361] Another case was reported in a 16-year-old boy of PC-FCL arising in the nose and extending into the maxillary sinus and soft palate.[362] We have also reported a case of a PC-FCL in a 16-year-old girl with a lesion on her arm.[363]

Clinical and Histologic Findings

It typically presents as a solitary or clustered smooth, erythematous to violaceous infiltrative papules, plaques, nodules, or tumors, in the head and neck or upper trunk (Fig. 72-32).[364] Histologically, PC-FCL has a nodular, nodular and diffuse, or diffuse growth patterns in the dermis with sparing of the surface epidermis (a Grenz zone separating the infiltrate from the epidermis is invariably present)[365] (Fig. 72-33). The infiltrate can extend into the adipose tissue. As opposed to systemic FL, grading has no prognostic significance as all cases of PC-FCL show an indolent course. The areas with abnormal follicles lack the tangible body macrophages present in reactive germinal centers (Fig. 72-13). The neoplastic cells are composed of small cleaved centrocytes and larger centroblasts.[366-368] The lesions with a diffuse growth pattern show a predominance of centroblasts and can be potential mimickers for large B-cell lymphomas. There is a variant composed largely of spindle cells (sarcomatoid form), originally referred to as "reticulohistiocytoma dorsi" or "Crosti lymphoma."[369,370] In such, fascicles of spindle cells admixed with areas of atypical centroblasts and centrocytes are present. One of the reported pediatric cases showed the spindle cell cytology.

By immunohistochemistry, PC-FCL is positive for CD19, PAX-5, CD20, CD79a, and BCL-6. CD10 is variably positive, depending on the pattern of growth (nodular growth is more typically positive, whereas diffuse growth is negative). BCL-2 is positive in approximately 50% of cases. The follicular dendritic networks can be highlighted by a CD21, CD23, and D2-40 immunostains. Clonality studies can be used to demonstrate a rearrangement of the IGH gene. In situ hybridization can also show on occasions in a clonal population of B-cells. Translocations of the IGH-BCL2 genes t(14;18) can be present in 18% to 41% of PC-FCL.[371,372]

Differential Diagnosis

Differential diagnostic considerations with PC-FCL include reactive lymphoid hyperplasias, PCMZL, cutaneous involvement by systemic FL, and DLBCLs (particularly the so-called leg-type lymphoma). PCMZL differs in the lack of germinal center markers. While PCMZL can show atrophic germinal centers, those typically have a very high proliferation and are rather small, in counterpart with the neoplastic follicles of PC-FCL that have a lower Ki67. In situ hybridization can help highlight a clonal population of plasma cells. Some cases of PCZML can also show a high proportion of IgG4+ plasma cells. Cutaneous involvement by systemic FL has never been documented in the pediatric setting as systemic FL is a disease of older individuals and systemic pediatric FL is a more localized disease. DLBCL leg type has never been documented in the pediatric age and is a

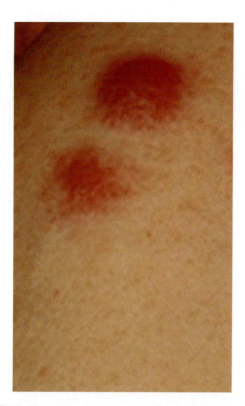

FIGURE 72-32. Primary cutaneous follicle center lymphoma. Lesions typically present as small dermal tumors and may be grouped. (From Gru AA. *Pediatric Dermatopathology and Dermatology.* 2018; Wolters Kluwer Health.)

disease of older adults. In counterpart, DLBCL-LT presents clinically in the legs and has a nongerminal center profile (MUM1 strongly positive).

Capsule Summary

PC-FCL is an indolent neoplastic proliferation of B-cells with a germinal center phenotype. While this is a disorder of middle-aged individuals, rare cases in children have been described. It typically presents as a solitary or clustered smooth, erythematous to violaceous infiltrative papules, plaques, nodules, or tumors, in the head and neck or upper trunk. Histologically, PC-FCL has a nodular, nodular and diffuse, or diffuse growth pattern in the dermis with sparing of the surface epidermis. The neoplastic cells are composed of small cleaved centrocytes and larger centroblasts, the latter being more frequent in the diffuse variants. By immunohistochemistry, PC-FCL is positive for CD19, PAX-5, CD20, CD79a, and BCL-6. CD10 is variably positive. BCL-2 is positive in approximately 50% of cases.

Precursor T-/B-Cell Lymphoblastic Leukemias/Lymphomas

Definition and Epidemiology

Acute lymphoblastic leukemia/lymphoma (ALL) is the most common type of leukemia in childhood, representing 80% of cases.[373] In the United States, the incidence of ALL is about 30 cases per million persons younger than 20 years. The peak incidence occurs between the ages of 3 to 5. There is a slightly higher incidence of ALL in boys than girls.[374] Approximately 80% to 85% of cases are B-ALL and 10% to 15% T-ALL.[375] Although the etiology of the disease is still largely unknown, certain genetic disorders have a greater predisposition for the development of ALL, including trisomy 21 and ataxia-telangiectasia. Some cases are associated with *MLL* gene rearrangements and might be secondary to chemotherapy.

Between 5% and 20% to 30% of patients develop cutaneous dissemination. Nearly 50 to 60 cases of B-ALL have been reported in children with skin involvement.[4,375-377] The frequency of cutaneous involvement in T-ALL is less well documented. However, Lee et al[378] reported an incidence of 4.3% in T-ALL and 15% in B-ALL. Approximately 33% of patients with the lymphomatous variants had cutaneous involvement, and only 1% in those with leukemic presentations.

Clinical Findings

The lesions present as erythematous or violaceous nodules, tumors, or plaques (sometimes can be multiple). The distribution of the lesions is typically the head and neck, upper trunk, and abdomen (Fig. 72-34). In a series of six cases,[376] most presented between the ages of 5 to 15 years and all occurred in girls. Occasional cases of aleukemic forms have been reported.[375,379-381] A single case with a congenital presentation has also been described in association with an *MLL* rearrangement.[382] Cases of T-ALL are frequently associated with a mediastinal mass (50%-65%). Many cases of ALL present in neonates with multiple blue/purple plaques or nodules on the skin, hence the term "blueberry muffin syndrome."

Histologic Features

The histopathologic findings for both B-ALL and T-ALL are identical.[377,383] There is a diffuse and dense dermal infiltrate with extension into the subcutaneous tissue[4,344,375,376,380-382,384] (Fig. 72-35). A Grenz zone is typically present with epidermal sparing. Cytologically, the infiltrate consists of small lymphoblasts with scant cytoplasm, fine nuclear chromatin, irregular nuclei, and inconspicuous nucleoli. Linear arrangements of lymphoblasts forming linear files can be noted. Infiltration of the skin adnexae is also frequently seen, as well as nerves and piloerector muscles. Mitotic activity is typically brisk.

By immunohistochemistry, the blasts of B-ALL express CD19, PAX5, CD79a, and CD43. TdT and CD34 are often expressed in the malignant cells, and CD99 can be seen in >50% of cases. Expression of CD45 is dim or negative, and most cases are negative for CD20, but CD10 is present in most, but not all cases. B-ALL with *MLL* rearrangement is typically CD15 positive and CD10 negative. Those cases of B-ALL with the t(12;21) translocation (Philadelphia chromosome) have a worse prognosis and are associated with CD10 coexpression.

The immunophenotype of cells in T-ALL usually includes positivity for TdT with variable expression of CD45, CD34, CD1a, CD10, CD2, cCD3 (lineage specific), CD4, CD5, CD7, and CD8. CD4/CD8 coexpression is most frequently observed; however, coexpression is not necessarily a marker of an immature phenotype because cases of mature T-cell lymphomas have been described with dual positivity. More reliable markers to confirm an immature phenotype include TdT, CD1a, CD99, and CD34.[385]

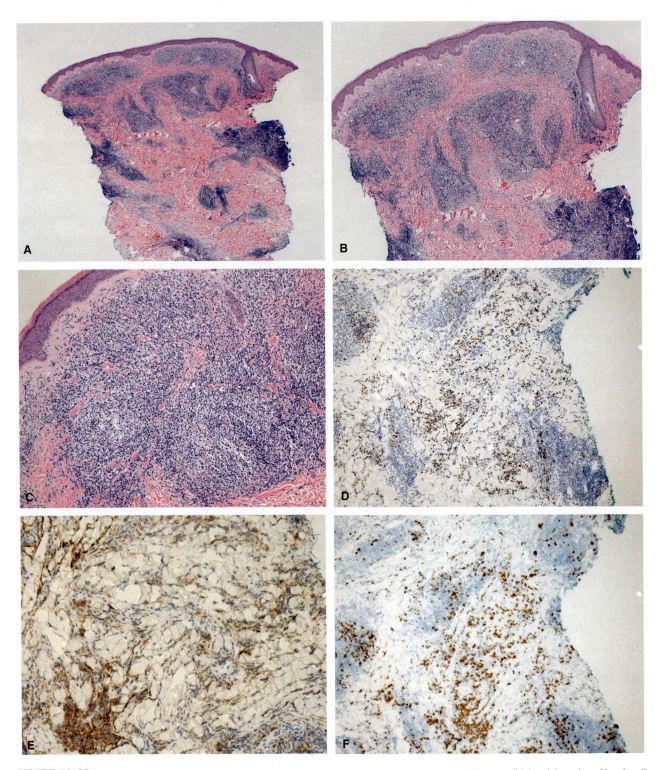

FIGURE 72-33. Primary cutaneous follicle center lymphoma in a pediatric patient. There is a vaguely nodular, superficial, and deep, dermal lymphocytic infiltrate (**A** and **B**, 20× and 400×). Poorly formed follicles are present (**C**, 200×). The atypical cells are positive for BCL-6 **(D)**, CD10 **(E)**, and show lambda-restriction by RNA scope in situ hybridization **(F)**.

According to the expression of specific markers, T-ALL can be subdivided into early or pro-T, pre-T, cortical-T, and medullary-T. The molecular background of T-ALL is less well understood. Cytogenetic abnormalities are frequent in T-ALL patients (50%-70%). The most common cytogenetic abnormalities involve 14q11 to 13 the site of TCR alpha/delta, including inv(14)(q11;q32) and deletions or translocations involving chromosomes 9, 10, and 11 corresponding to sites of TCR alpha, beta, and gamma-subunit genes found in 47% of T-ALL. Some cases can also present in association with myeloid hyperplasia, eosinophilia, and the t(8;13)(p11;q11) aberration affecting the *FGFR1* gene. The

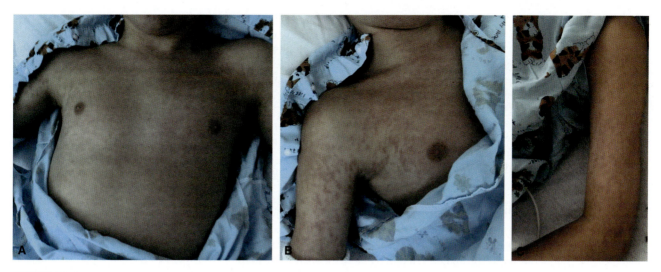

FIGURE 72-34. Acute lymphoblastic leukemia presenting as a viral exanthem **(A-C)**. (From Gru AA. *Pediatric Dermatopathology and Dermatology.* 2018; Wolters Kluwer Health.)

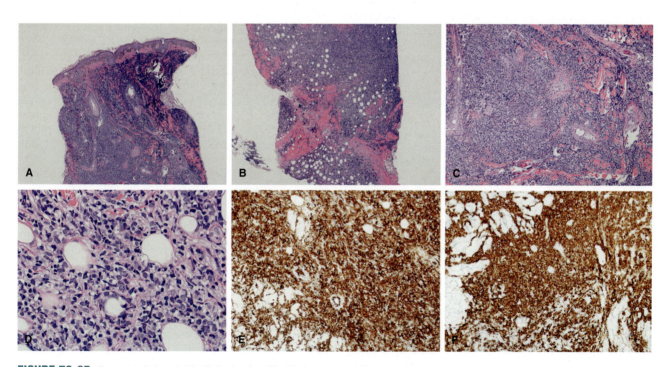

FIGURE 72-35. Precursor B-lymphoblastic leukemia with skin involvement. There is a diffuse dermal infiltrate with a Grenz zone (**A** and **B**). The infiltrate extends and dissect through the collagen fibers **(C)**. It is composed of small to medium-sized lymphoblasts **(D)** which are positive for CD34 **(E)** and CD10 **(F)**. (From Gru AA. *Pediatric Dermatopathology and Dermatology.* 2018; Wolters Kluwer Health.)

latter has now been referred to as the 8p11 myeloproliferative disorder.[386,387] Similarly to B-ALL, T-ALL is typically associated with rearrangements of the TCR.

Differential Diagnosis

The differential diagnosis can be challenging in the primary lymphomatous lesions, or its aleukemic forms. The differential diagnosis in "blue-berry muffin" syndrome includes neuroblastoma, myeloid leukemia, rhabdoid tumor, and rhabdomyosarcoma. In fact, a case originally diagnosed as Ewing sarcoma (EWS), represented an example of B-ALL with CD99 coexpression.[380] However, EWS does not express B-cell antigens. Indeed, CD99, CD34, and TdT in B-ALL are useful in the differentiation from mature B-cell lymphomas in the skin, which, overall, are extraordinarily uncommon. In the differential diagnosis, Merkel cell carcinoma may rarely present in children[388,389] and show CD99 expression similar to B-ALL. CK20 and neuron-specific enolase can help in the distinction between the two. Cutaneous involvement by neuroblastoma is also rare and might be a pitfall, but CD99 is negative in the latter.[390,391] However, CD99 expression is more typically cytoplasmic, rather than the crisp staining seen in EWS.[392] Neuroblastomas are also positive for neuroendocrine markers. Other small round cell sarcomas can be distinguished with the presence of specific markers (myogenin, desmin, etc).

Capsule Summary
ALL is the most common type of leukemia in childhood, representing 80% of cases. Approximately 80% to 85% of cases are B-ALL and 10% to 15% T-ALL. Between 5% and 20% to 30% of patients develop cutaneous dissemination: erythematous or violaceous nodules, tumors, or plaques (sometimes can be multiple). Patients with T-ALL often have a mediastinal mass. There is a diffuse and dense dermal infiltrate with extension into the subcutaneous tissue. Linear arrangement of small lymphoblasts is seen. Expression of immature markers is typical (CD34, TdT, CD99, CD1a).

Cutaneous Myeloid Neoplasms

Definition and Epidemiology
LC is manifested by a cutaneous infiltration of neoplastic myeloid cells, lymphoid blasts, or mature lymphoma cells. AML, particularly in those with monocytic or myelomonocytic differentiation, occurs as LC.[393] However, LC is seen in association with chronic myelogenous leukemia, myelodysplastic syndromes (MDS), and acute lymphoblastic leukemias (T-ALL and B-ALL).[394-397] Myeloid sarcoma, extramedullary myeloid tumor, granulocytic sarcoma, and monocytic sarcoma are often termed LC when occurring in the skin, but many now prefer the term "myeloid sarcoma" when there is a nodular infiltrate of immature blasts in the dermis.[398] In contrast, LC is the preferred term when the malignant infiltrate shows a diffuse, interstitial pattern through the dermis with the clinical appearance of a rash. LC in children may present at or soon after birth.

Rarely, cutaneous involvement by a leukemic infiltrate can occur in the absence of bone marrow or peripheral blood involvement by acute leukemia; this then is referred to as aleukemic leukemia cutis (ALC)[379,399-407] or aleukemic myeloid sarcoma.[393,408] Byrd et al[398] proposed using aleukemic to describe those cases of extramedullary involvement in the absence of blood and bone marrow disease for at least 1 month. The literature also includes cases described as aleukemic despite concomitant bone marrow disease in patients who do not have circulating peripheral blasts.[409,410] An adverse prognosis has been associated with, while others have proposed that ALC is a heterogeneous condition that can even result in spontaneous resolution without the need for aggressive chemotherapy.[345,398,411-413] We have recently published a series of cases of ALC including some with spontaneous resolution, and in two cases there was the presence of *MLL* rearrangements.[414] ALC can also be seen in association with pre-B-cell ALL[379,406,409] and in rare cases of T-cell ALL.[381,415] A monocytic phenotype and certain cytogenetic aberrations, such as t(8;21) or inv(16), are found in a disproportionate number of cases. In addition, the expression of T-cell markers and CD56 are more frequent in extramedullary myeloid blast cells.[398,416] Otsubo et al reported the development of an acute promyelocytic leukemia following ALC in association with *NPM-RARA* fusion transcript in a child.[417] Agrawal et al reported ALC in siblings at birth.[411] Interestingly, 11q23 abnormalities have been detected by FISH in some cases of congenital LC, which strongly raises the likelihood of abnormalities in the *MLL* gene.[418,419] Torrelo et al described a very aggressive clinical presentation of ALC in a newborn, clinically manifested as "blueberry muffin" skin lesions.[420] Transient abnormal myelopoiesis (TAM) is an entity characterized by the presence of blasts in the blood of children with trisomy 21, which in many cases can be reversible. Cutaneous lesions with blast infiltration have been reported in children with TAM.[421-423]

Clinical Findings
Cutaneous interstitial deposits of immature blasts present as papules, nodules, or plaques and are found in 2% to 12% of AML cases (Fig. 72-36). Newborns can present with blueberry muffin appearance (Fig. 72-37). Although less common, LC occurs in the setting of lymphoblastic leukemias, with an estimated incidence of 1% to 3%.[424] The diagnosis of ALC is a challenging one not only because of its infrequency but also due to the absence of concomitant blood or bone marrow involvement. The diagnosis can also be elusive because the infiltrate can adopt a very sparse perivascular and periadnexal distribution.[425]

Histologic Features
Morphologically, the leukemic cells are centered in the dermis and may extend into the subcutaneous tissue[426] (Fig. 72-38). Epidermotropism is usually not seen. The malignant cells can disrupt the vessels and adnexal structures, and a "leukemic vasculitis" can also occur.[427] The vasculitis is thought to represent direct endothelial injury by the leukemic cells.[428] A diagnosis of LC is invariably corroborated by immunohistochemistry. Because of the frequent monocytic lineage, CD34, TdT, and CD117 are often not helpful in identifying immature blasts, but Cibull et al found that CD68 and lysozyme were additionally helpful in the diagnosis.[426] The CD68 KP1 clone appears to be more specific and reliable to identify the myeloid origin of the cells.[429] On the other hand, Cronin et al suggested that the combination of CD43 and CD68 was more reliable (Fig. 72-39).[430] Amador-Ortiz et al, with a panel including CD117, CD33, and lysozyme, confirmed most cases of cutaneous myeloid sarcoma. The addition of CD14 and KLF-4 was also useful in achieving a greater degree of sensitivity and specificity in those lesions of monocytic lineage.[431] ERG is a more recent marker that has been used with success to help in the diagnosis of LC.[432] However, a problem with the use of immunostains is that numerous histiocytic disorders (benign and malignant) in cutaneous sites have a similar phenotype. In fact, some LCs have been masked by the presence of a prominent granulomatous reaction in the dermis, as reported by Tomasini et al.[410] Ideally, correlation with the bone marrow immunophenotypic findings of the immature blasts could be helpful. Interestingly, discrepancies in the phenotype of the immature cells in the skin and the bone marrow have been documented, a feature that can complicate the diagnosis further.[430,431] Other molecular tools can sometimes be helpful in establishing a diagnosis, such as *MLL* rearrangements (Fig. 72-40) by FISH or *NPM1* and *FLT3-ITD* mutations by PCR analysis.

Differential Diagnosis
In the setting of a clinical context and history of AML, the findings of an immature infiltrate in the dermis are strongly suggestive of a diagnosis of LC. However, one should be aware of the possibility that patients with AML or MDS can develop Sweet syndrome, particularly the histiocytoid

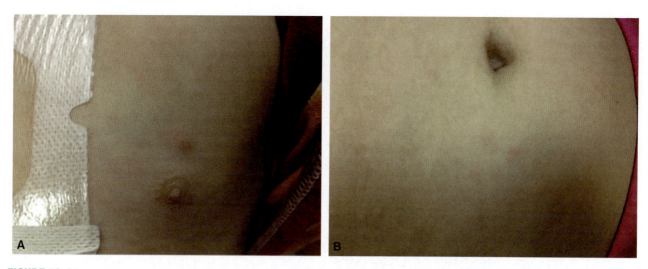

FIGURE 72-36. Small red papules and nodules on the upper chest and lower abdomen in a case of aleukemic leukemia cutis (**A** and **B**). (Obtained with permission. Gru AA et al. Pediatric aleukemic leukemia cutis: report of 3 cases and review of the literature. *Am J Dermatopathol*. 2015;37(6):477-484.)

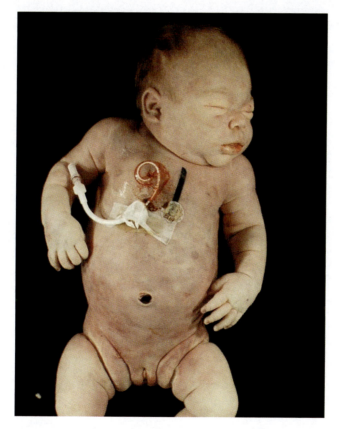

FIGURE 72-37. Clinical postmortem photograph of a patient with congenital leukemia with a cutaneous presentation resulting in a "blueberry muffin" appearance. (From Gru AA. *Pediatric Dermatopathology and Dermatology*. 2018; Wolters Kluwer Health. Fig. 27.39B.)

variant. The latter can be associated with a somewhat immature infiltrate in the dermis, lacks expression of immature markers (CD34, CD123, CD117), and has myeloperoxidase positivity. Many have argued that a diagnosis of histiocytoid Sweet syndrome reflects an "immature myeloid infiltrate" in the skin. Other diagnostic considerations that can mimic LC, particularly in newborns and small infants, are cutaneous deposits of extramedullary hematopoiesis (EMH). As opposed to LC, most EMH deposits have a predominance of erythroid precursors. Rare megakaryocytes can be seen. In many occasions, an etiologic cause for EMH (viral infection—CMV, HSV, etc) can be encountered in children.

Capsule Summary

LC is manifested by a cutaneous infiltration of neoplastic myeloid cells, lymphoid blasts, or mature lymphoma cells.

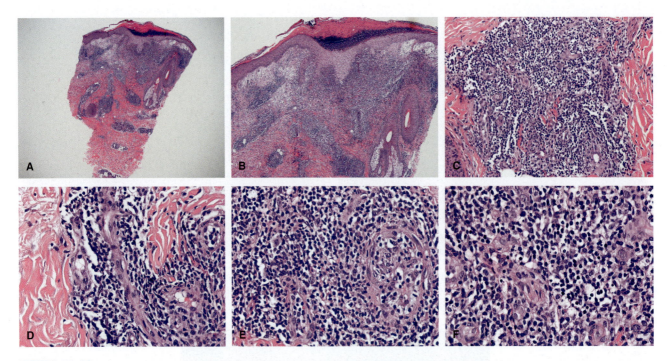

FIGURE 72-38. A leukemic infiltrate is present in the dermis with a focus of acute folliculitis (**A** and **B**). The infiltrate shows an interstitial and perivascular distribution (**C** and **D**). It is composed of medium-sized cells, with fine chromatin and variable nucleoli (**E** and **F**). (From Gru AA. *Pediatric Dermatopathology and Dermatology.* 2018; Wolters Kluwer Health.)

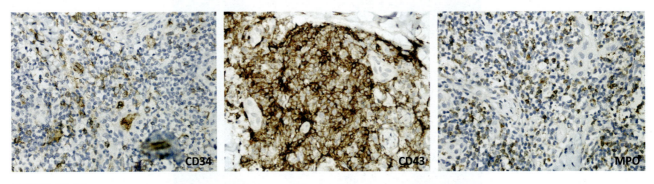

FIGURE 72-39. Leukemia cutis—IHC. The infiltrate is weakly positive for CD34, but more diffusely positive for MPO and CD43. (From Gru AA. *Pediatric Dermatopathology and Dermatology.* 2018; Wolters Kluwer Health.)

AMLs, particularly those with monocytic or myelomonocytic differentiation, may present as LC. Myeloid sarcoma, extramedullary myeloid tumor, granulocytic sarcoma, and monocytic sarcoma are often termed LC when occurring in the skin, but many now prefer the term "myeloid sarcoma" when there is a nodular infiltrate of immature blasts in the dermis. Aleukemic LC occurs in the absence of bone marrow involvement by leukemia. Cutaneous interstitial deposits of immature blasts present as papules, nodules, or plaques and are found in 2% to 12% of AML cases. Morphologically, the leukemic cells are centered in the dermis and may extend into the subcutaneous tissue. Because of the frequent monocytic differentiation of the malignant cells, often the immature markers (CD34, CD117, and TdT) are negative in the cells.

Blastic Plasmacytoid Dendritic Cell Neoplasm

Definition and Epidemiology

BPDCN is an extremely rare subtype of acute leukemia and was formerly known as blastic natural killer (NK)-cell lymphoma or CD4+/CD56+ hematodermic neoplasm.[433-436] Once postulated to originate from NK-lineage precursors, accumulating phenotypic, functional, and genetic evidence has pointed to its derivation from hematopoietic precursors with commitment to the plasmacytoid dendritic cell lineage, cells which are positive for CD123.[435,437-441] BPDCN is rare in children[334,433,442-445] and the largest series from BPDCN in the pediatric setting was reported by Jegalian et al.[335]

Clinical Findings

Clinically, most cases have cutaneous lesions at diagnosis in adults (85%), but the opposite has been found in children: 7 of the 29 cases (24%) lacked cutaneous disease at presentation, with disease confined to the bone marrow, peripheral blood, lymph nodes, spleen, and/or liver.[335] Skin lesions can be multiple (>60% of the time) or single. The lesions range from tumors and nodules to plaques and patches that are brown, erythematous, or violaceous (Fig. 72-41). A characteristic clinical finding is that the lesions are bruise-like or hemorrhagic in appearance. They may be found anywhere on the body, especially the scalp, face, trunk, and extremities. Those without cutaneous disease at presentation had 100% survival at 60 months follow-up. Most adults relapsed within the first year of diagnosis with bone marrow and central nervous system involvement (approximately 33% of cases). The disease has an overall survival of approximately 74% in children.[335]

Histologic Features

Morphologically, BPDCN in children tends to have smaller sized cells and a lymphoblast-like appearance of the blasts. In adults, BPDCN has a more pleomorphic appearance (Fig. 72-42). Cutaneous lesions of BPDCN are characterized by a dermal infiltrate composed of sheets of neoplastic cells. The infiltrate is typically diffuse but can often show an accentuated periadnexal or perivascular distribution. The epidermis is characteristically spared with an underlying Grenz zone. The cells are typically intermediate to large with round nuclei and finely dispersed "blastic" chromatin. Nuclear contours are irregular and may be notched, folded, or occasionally show moderate pleomorphism. Nucleoli are usually inconspicuous but one to several prominent nucleoli can be present. With hematoxylin and eosin staining, the cytoplasm is pale to eosinophilic, agranular, and usually scant, but can be moderate to abundant in some cases.

CD123, CD4, and CD56 positivity, the most common BPDCN immunophenotypic profile, is not specific since these markers are also expressed in both AML and ALL (Figs. 72-42 and 72-43).[444] Virtually all cases are positive for TCF-4. myeloperoxidase and lysozyme must be negative. However, cases without cutaneous involvement also expressed other BPDCN markers, including BDCA-4, CD303/BDCA-2, CD2AP, and TCL1. CD68 (KP1) is generally negative, but focal punctate staining is seen in a minority of cases. Strong staining for CD68 should raise the suspicion of acute or chronic myeloid leukemia with monocytic differentiation.[335] Myeloid cell nuclear differentiation antigen can be used effectively to distinguish between LC and BPDCN, since only LC is positive.[446] Additionally, S100 expression is seen in approximately 75% of pediatric cases, compared to only 25% of cases in the adult population.[447] The genetics of this disease is poorly understood, but recently one case was reported with *EWSR* gene rearrangement, an important diagnostic consideration in the pediatric population.[448] *TET2* is the most common mutated gene (36%-80%)[449]; other recurrent somatic mutations include

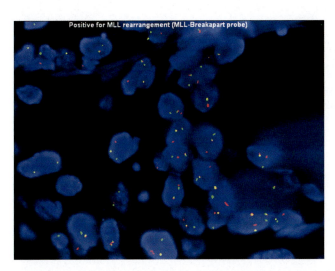

FIGURE 72-40. *MLL* **rearrangement in a case of aleukemic leukemia cutis arising in a myeloid neoplasm after treatment for osteosarcoma.** A break-apart probe was used. (From Gru AA. *Pediatric Dermatopathology and Dermatology.* 2018; Wolters Kluwer Health.)

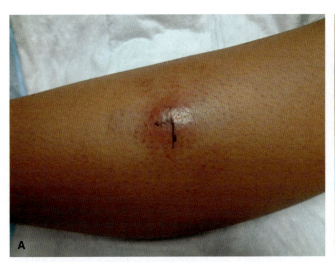
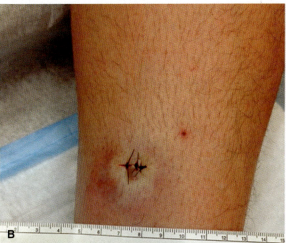

FIGURE 72-41. **Blastic plasmacytoid dendritic cell neoplasm.** Solitary 2.1 cm indurated red-brown nodule with smaller violaceous macules at the periphery **(A)**. Single bruise-like subcutaneous nodule **(B)**. (Adapted and obtained with permission. Nguyen CM et al. Blastic plasmacytoid dendritic cell neoplasm in the pediatric population: a case series and review of the literature. *Am J Dermatopathol.* 2015;37(12):924-928.)

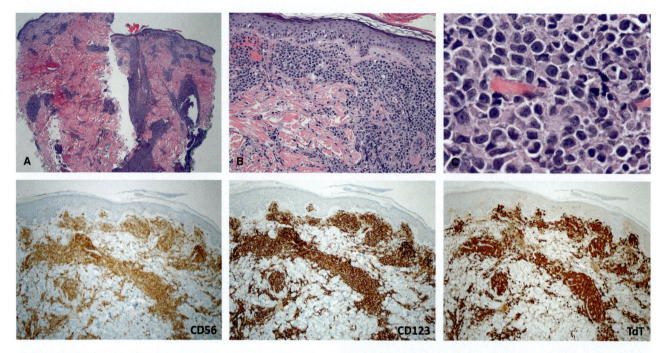

FIGURE 72-42. **Blastic plasmacytoid dendritic cell neoplasm.** Diffuse adnexotropic dermal infiltrate (**A** and **B**). The infiltrate is composed of blastic cells with variable pleomorphism (**C**). The infiltrate is positive for CD56, CD123, and TdT. (From Gru AA. *Pediatric Dermatopathology and Dermatology*. 2018; Wolters Kluwer Health.)

IKZF3 and *ZEB2* (12%-16%),[449] *ASXL1* (32%), *NPM1* (10%), and *RAS* (9%-27%).[450] Gene expression profiling has demonstrated a unique signature, distinct from AML and ALL.[451] Compared with normal plasmacytoid dendritic cells, BPDCN has shown increased expression of genes involved in Notch signaling and NFKB activation.

Differential Diagnosis
The most closely related lesions that mimic BPDCN are the clonal, tumoral proliferations of plasmacytoid dendritic cells that can occur in the skin, lymph nodes, bone marrow, and spleen secondary to a variety of myeloid neoplasms with monocytic differentiation. Tumoral PDC proliferations can most reliably be distinguished from BPDCN by a Ki-67 index (usually <10% in PDC proliferations and >30% in BPDCN). When positive, TdT is also helpful in excluding a tumoral PDC proliferation, because these are uniformly negative.

Acute monocytic leukemias, myelomonocytic leukemia, and juvenile myelomonocytic leukemia frequently have significant cutaneous localization. These are also often positive for CD4, CD56, and CD123, making their distinction from BPDCN even more difficult. Thorough cytochemical analysis and immunophenotyping is necessary for definitive classification. If available, Wright-Giemsa–stained cytologic preparations will often show cytoplasmic granules. When granules are present, myeloperoxidase and/or lysozyme will usually be positive, excluding BPDCN from the differential. Less mature myeloid neoplasms may lack cytoplasmic granules but will be positive for CD13, CD34, and/or CD117, excluding BPDCN. CD68 is positive in both BPDCN and other myeloid neoplasms but shows distinctive dot-like cytoplasmic positivity in BPDCN as opposed to the diffuse cytoplasmic staining seen in other lesions.

The expression of CD4, other T-cell antigens, TdT, and cutaneous infiltration raise the possibility of a cutaneous T-cell leukemia/lymphoma. Absence of CD3, CD5, CD8 and the absence of a TCR gene rearrangement support BPDCN. NK-cell leukemia also needs to be included in the differential of BPDCN. Both entities express CD56, but NK-cell leukemia often shows distinctive areas of angiodestruction and necrosis. NK-cell leukemia will also be positive for EBV studies and will express cytoplasmic CD3 and granzyme B by immunohistochemistry, both of which are absent in BPDCN.

Capsule Summary
BPDCN is a rare, distinct form of myeloid precursor neoplasm differentiated toward plasmacytoid dendritic cells. It is characterized by early, often isolated skin lesions that almost inevitably progresses to systemic and bone marrow involvement with a poor prognosis. The skin lesions have a characteristic bruise-like or hemorrhagic appearance. The diagnosis requires thorough immunophenotyping to exclude a number of other pathologies with similar clinical and histomorphologic features.

Extramedullary Hematopoiesis

Definition and Epidemiology
EMH is defined as nonneoplastic extramedullary erythropoiesis that is typically seen secondary to intrauterine infections and hemoglobinopathies. The most common sites for EMH are the spleen and liver, but almost any organ can be involved. Skin involvement is an extremely rare manifestation.[452]

Etiology
The original TORCH syndrome complex includes intrauterine infections by *Toxoplasma gondii*, rubella virus, cytomegalovirus, and herpes simplex virus, types 1 and 2. Dermal erythropoiesis is mostly associated with toxoplasma, CMV

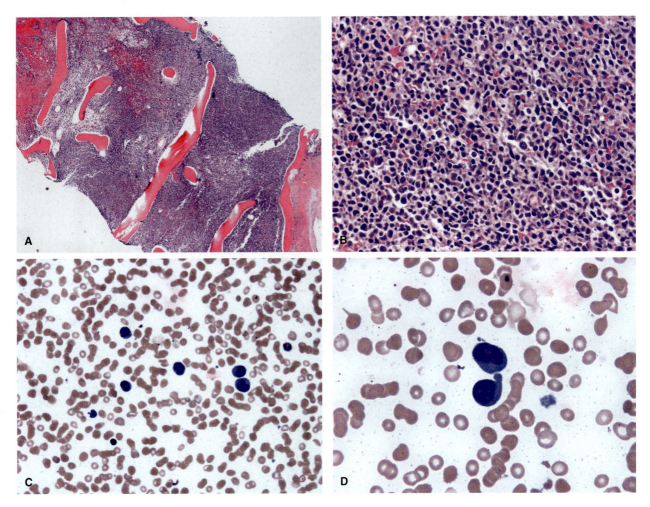

FIGURE 72-43. Bone marrow dissemination. The marrow space is diffusely replaced by blasts (**A** and **B**). A smear shows a plasmacytoid appearance of the malignant cells (**C** and **D**). (From Gru AA. *Pediatric Dermatopathology and Dermatology.* 2018; Wolters Kluwer Health.)

and rubella infections.[453] The commonest hematological etiologies causing reactive erythropoiesis include erythroblastosis fetalis, hereditary spherocytosis, and twin-twin transfusion syndrome.[454]

Clinical Findings
The clinical presentation of EMH is similar to those of other cutaneous metastases, such as the presence of pink or red-violaceous macules, papules, and nodules, typically on the trunk. Bulla formation, hemorrhage, and ulcerations had been also observed.[455,456] The clinical features of blueberry muffin baby include nonblanching, violaceous macules or firm, dome-shaped papules (<1 cm). The lesions are mostly generalized with preference to the trunk, head, and neck. The lesions typically resolve by 3 to 6 weeks after birth and often leave light brown macular discoloration.

Histologic Features
Histopathologically, there are clusters of normoblastic erythropoiesis with nucleated red blood cell precursors in the dermis (Fig. 72-44). Myeloid and megakaryocytic elements as well as dermal fibrosis are not typically present. CD61, Factor VIIIra, and CD31 can be used to demonstrate the megakaryocytes, glycophorin A, or hemoglobin for erythroid precursors, and CD34, CD117, and TdT for blasts. Megakaryocytes can be small and hypolobulated and might be missed without CD61 staining.

Differential Diagnosis
The differential diagnosis of blueberry muffin appearance includes congenital LC, Langerhans cells histiocytosis, congenital vascular malformations such as multifocal hemangiomas and lymphangioendotheliomatosis, glomangiomas, and blue rubber bleb nevus syndrome.

Capsule Summary
EMH is defined as nonneoplastic extramedullary erythropoiesis that is typically seen secondary to intrauterine infections and hemoglobinopathies. Skin involvement is an extremely rare manifestation. The clinical presentation of EMH is similar to those of other cutaneous metastases, such as the presence of pink or red-violaceous macules, papules, and nodules, typically on the trunk, or as "blueberry muffin." Histopathologically, there are clusters of normoblastic erythropoiesis with nucleated red blood cell precursors in the dermis.

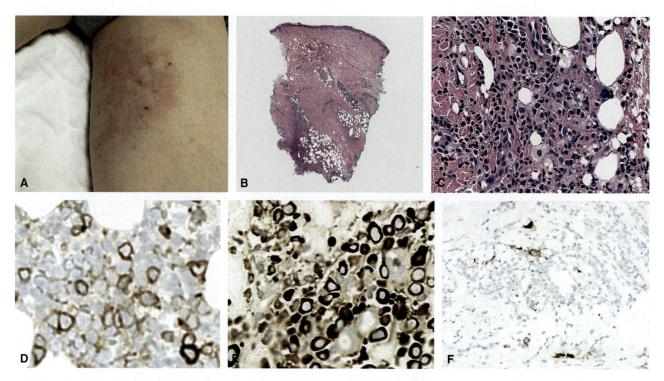

FIGURE 72-44. Extramedullary hematopoiesis. (A) Extramedullary hematopoiesis presenting as pink, erythematous patch. **(B and C)** Dermal perivascular infiltrates stained with hematoxylin and eosin show scattered blasts, immature myeloid forms, eosinophils, erythroid elements, and dysmorphic hypolobulated megakaryocytes. **(D)** Megakaryocytes are decorated by CD61. **(E)** Scattered blasts express C-Kit. **(F)** Immature myeloid cells are highlighted by myeloperoxidase. (**A**, Photo courtesy of Urvi Patel, MD, Washington University School of Medicine in St. Louis.)

References

1. O'Suoji C, Welch JJ, Perkins SL, et al. Rare pediatric non-Hodgkin lymphomas: a report from children's oncology group study ANHL 04B1. *Pediatr Blood Cancer.* 2016;63(5):794-800.
2. Kempf W, Kazakov DV, Belousova IE, Mitteldorf C, Kerl K. Paediatric cutaneous lymphomas: a review and comparison with adult counterparts. *J Eur Acad Dermatol Venereol.* 2015;29(9):1696-1709.
3. Fink-Puches R, Chott A, Ardigo M, et al. The spectrum of cutaneous lymphomas in patients less than 20 years of age. *Pediatr Dermatol.* 2004;21(5):525-533.
4. Boccara O, Blanche S, de Prost Y, Brousse N, Bodemer C, Fraitag S. Cutaneous hematologic disorders in children. *Pediatr Blood Cancer.* 2012;58(2):226-232.
5. Wain EM, Orchard GE, Whittaker SJ, Spittle MSMF, Russell-Jones R. Outcome in 34 patients with juvenile-onset mycosis fungoides: a clinical, immunophenotypic, and molecular study. *Cancer.* 2003;98(10):2282-2290.
6. Beljaards RC, Kaudewitz P, Berti E, et al. Primary cutaneous CD30-positive large cell lymphoma: definition of a new type of cutaneous lymphoma with a favorable prognosis. A European Multicenter Study of 47 patients. *Cancer.* 1993;71(6):2097-2104.
7. Ralfkiaer E, Willemze R, Paulli M, Kadin ME. *CD30-positive T-Cell Lymphoproliferative Disorders.* 4th ed. International Agency for Research on Cancer; 2008.
8. Willemze R, Beljaards RC. Spectrum of primary cutaneous CD30 (Ki-1)-positive lymphoproliferative disorders. A proposal for classification and guidelines for management and treatment. *J Am Acad Dermatol.* 1993;28(6):973-980.
9. Kempf W. CD30+ lymphoproliferative disorders: histopathology, differential diagnosis, new variants, and simulators. *J Cutan Pathol.* 2006;33(suppl 1):58-70.
10. Kumar S, Pittaluga S, Raffeld M, Guerrera M, Seibel NL, Jaffe ES. Primary cutaneous CD30-positive anaplastic large cell lymphoma in childhood: report of 4 cases and review of the literature. *Pediatr Dev Pathol.* 2005;8(1):52-60.
11. Papalas JA, Van Mater D, Wang E. Pyogenic variant of primary cutaneous anaplastic large-cell lymphoma: a lymphoproliferative disorder with a predilection for the immunocompromised and the young. *Am J Dermatopathol.* 2010;32(8):821-827.
12. Sciallis AP, Law ME, Inwards DJ, et al. Mucosal CD30-positive T-cell lymphoproliferations of the head and neck show a clinicopathologic spectrum similar to cutaneous CD30-positive T-cell lymphoproliferative disorders. *Mod Pathol.* 2012;25(7):983-992.
13. Tomaszewski MM, Moad JC, Lupton GP. Primary cutaneous Ki-1(CD30) positive anaplastic large cell lymphoma in childhood. *J Am Acad Dermatol.* 1999;40(5 pt 2):857-861.
14. Vaid R, Cohen B. Primary cutaneous CD30 positive anaplastic large cell lymphoma in an adolescent. *Pediatr Dermatol.* 2009;26(6):721-724.
15. Mahajan VK, Jindal R. Primary cutaneous anaplastic large cell lymphoma in a child simulating primary cutaneous Hodgkin's disease. *Indian J Dermatol Venereol Leprol.* 2016;82(1):98-101.
16. Capo A, Cinalli S, Angelucci D, Amerio P. Primary cutaneous anaplastic large cell lymphoma in a 5-year-old child: a diagnostic challenge. *Dermatol Ther.* 2020;33(6):e14195.
17. Linggonegoro DW, McCormack L, Grenier PO, Vrooman LM, Devlin PM, Huang JT. Pediatric

17. primary cutaneousanaplasticlargecelllymphoma treated with brachytherapy. *Pediatr Dermatol.* 2021;38(3):712-713.
18. Piccinno R, Damiani G, Rossi LC, Berti E. Radiotherapy of primary cutaneous anaplastic large cell lymphoma: our experience in 30 cases. *Int J Dermatol.* 2020;59(4):469-473.
19. Camisa C, Helm TN, Sexton C, Tuthill R. Ki-1-positive anaplastic large-cell lymphoma can mimic benign dermatoses. *J Am Acad Dermatol.* 1993;29(5 pt 1):696-700.
20. Jhala DN, Medeiros LJ, Lopez-Terrada D, Jhala NC, Krishnan B, Shahab I. Neutrophil-rich anaplastic large cell lymphoma of T-cell lineage. A report of two cases arising in HIV-positive patients. *Am J Clin Pathol.* 2000;114(3):478-482.
21. Salama S. Primary "cutaneous" T-cell anaplastic large cell lymphoma, CD30+, neutrophil-rich variant with subcutaneous panniculitic lesions, in a post-renal transplant patient: report of unusual case and literature review. *Am J Dermatopathol.* 2005;27(3):217-223.
22. Kong YY, Dai B, Kong JC, Lu HF, Shi DR. Neutrophil/eosinophil-rich type of primary cutaneous anaplastic large cell lymphoma: a clinicopathological, immunophenotypic and molecular study of nine cases. *Histopathology.* 2009;55(2):189-196.
23. de Bruin PC, Beljaards RC, van Heerde P, et al. Differences in clinical behaviour and immunophenotype between primary cutaneous and primary nodal anaplastic large cell lymphoma of T-cell or null cell phenotype. *Histopathology.* 1993;23(2):127-135.
24. Plaza JA, Feldman AL, Magro C. Cutaneous CD30-positive lymphoproliferative disorders with CD8 expression: a clinicopathologic study of 21 cases. *J Cutan Pathol.* 2013;40(2): 236-247.
25. Valencia Ocampo OJ, Julio L, Zapata V, et al. Mycosis fungoides in children and adolescents: a series of 23 cases. *Actas Dermosifiliogr (Engl Ed).* 2020;111(2):149-156.
26. Gru AA, Voorhess PJ. A case of ALK+ anaplastic large-cell lymphoma with aberrant myeloperoxidase expression and initial cutaneous presentation. *Am J Dermatopathol.* 2018;40(7):519-522.
27. Wang X, Boddicker RL, Dasari S, et al. Expression of p63 protein in anaplastic large cell lymphoma: implications for genetic subtyping. *Hum Pathol.* 2017;64:19-27.
28. Onaindia A, Montes-Moreno S, Rodriguez-Pinilla SM, et al. Primary cutaneous anaplastic large cell lymphomas with 6p25.3 rearrangement exhibit particular histological features. *Histopathology.* 2015;66(6):846-855.
29. Swerdlow SH, Campo E, Pileri SA, et al. The 2016 revision of the World Health Organization classification of lymphoid neoplasms. *Blood.* 2016;127(20):2375-2390.
30. Burg G, Kempf W, Cozzio A, et al. WHO/EORTC classification of cutaneous lymphomas 2005: histological and molecular aspects. *J Cutan Pathol.* 2005;32(10):647-674.
31. Willemze R, Jaffe ES, Burg G, et al. WHO-EORTC classification for cutaneous lymphomas. *Blood.* 2005;105(10):3768-3785.
32. Castano E, Glick S, Wolgast L, et al. Hypopigmented mycosis fungoides in childhood and adolescence: a long-term retrospective study. *J Cutan Pathol.* 2013;40(11):924-934.
33. Crowley JJ, Nikko A, Varghese A, Hoppe RT, Kim YH. Mycosis fungoides in young patients: clinical characteristics and outcome. *J Am Acad Dermatol.* 1998;38(5 pt 1):696-701.
34. El-Shabrawi-Caelen L, Cerroni L, Medeiros LJ, McCalmont TH. Hypopigmented mycosis fungoides: frequent expression of a CD8+ T-cell phenotype. *Am J Surg Pathol.* 2002;26(4):450-457.
35. Pope E, Weitzman S, Ngan B, et al. Mycosis fungoides in the pediatric population: report from an international childhood registry of cutaneous lymphoma. *J Cutan Med Surg.* 2010;14(1):1-6.
36. Kothari R, Szepietowski JC, Bagot M, et al. Mycosis fungoides in pediatric population: comprehensive review on epidemiology, clinical presentation, and management. *Int J Dermatol.* Published online 2022. doi:10.1111/ijd.16098
37. Cervini AB, Torres-Huamani AN, Sanchez-La-Rosa C, et al. Mycosis fungoides: experience in a pediatric hospital. *Actas Dermosifiliogr.* 2017;108(6):564-570.
38. Koch SE, Zackheim HS, Williams ML, Fletcher V, LeBoit PE. Mycosis fungoides beginning in childhood and adolescence. *J Am Acad Dermatol.* 1987;17(4):563-570.
39. Peters MS, Thibodeau SN, White JW, Jr, Winkelmann RK. Mycosis fungoides in children and adolescents. *J Am Acad Dermatol.* 1990;22(6 pt 1):1011-1018.
40. Zackheim HS, McCalmont TH, Deanovic FW, Odom RB. Mycosis fungoides with onset before 20 years of age. *J Am Acad Dermatol.* 1997;36(4):557-562.
41. Tan E, Tay YK, Giam YC. Profile and outcome of childhood mycosis fungoides in Singapore. *Pediatr Dermatol.* 2000;17(5):352-356.
42. Reiter O, Amitay-Laish I, Oren-Shabtai M, Feinmesser M, Ben-Amitai D, Hodak E. Paediatric mycosis fungoides - characteristics, management and outcomes with particular focus on the folliculotropic variant. *J Eur Acad Dermatol Venereol.* 2022;36(5):671-679. Epub 2022 Mar 2. doi:10.1111/jdv.17971
43. Lowe E, Jacobsen JR, Taylor S, Miller R, Price HN, Andrews ID. Mycosis fungoides preceding pityriasis lichenoides et varioliformis acuta by twelve years in a pediatric patient. *Am J Dermatopathol.* 2021;43(12):e259-e262.
44. Young GJ, Luu M, Izadi N. Mycosis fungoides in 2 pediatric patients with atopic dermatitis. *J Allergy Clin Immunol Pract.* 2021;9(5):2068-2069.
45. Rubio-Gonzalez B, Frieden IJ, McCalmont TH, Dorsey M, Funk T, Pincus LB. Folliculotropic mycosis fungoides driven by DOCK8 immunodeficiency syndrome. *Pediatr Dermatol.* 2021;38(1):229-232.
46. Purnak S, Lawrence AM. Pediatric mycosis fungoides: retrospective analysis of a series with CD8+ profile and female predominance. *J Pediatr Hematol Oncol.* Published online 2021. doi:10.1097/MPH.0000000000002354
47. Gross AM, Turner J, Kirkorian AY, et al. A pediatric case of transformed mycosis fungoides in a BRCA2 positive patient. *J Pediatr Hematol Oncol.* 2020;42(5):e361-e364.
48. Choi J, Goh G, Walradt T, et al. Genomic landscape of cutaneous T cell lymphoma. *Nat Genet.* 2015;47(9):1011-1019.
49. da Silva Almeida AC, Abate F, Khiabanian H, et al. The mutational landscape of cutaneous T cell lymphoma and Sezary syndrome. *Nat Genet.* 2015;47(12):1465-1470.
50. Kiel MJ, Sahasrabuddhe AA, Rolland DC, et al. Genomic analyses reveal recurrent mutations in epigenetic modifiers and the JAK-STAT pathway in Sezary syndrome. *Nat Commun.* 2015;6:8470.
51. Ungewickell A, Bhaduri A, Rios E, et al. Genomic analysis of mycosis fungoides and Sezary syndrome identifies recurrent alterations in TNFR2. *Nat Genet.* 2015;47(9):1056-1060.
52. Wang L, Ni X, Covington KR, et al. Genomic profiling of Sezary syndrome identifies alterations of key T cell signaling and differentiation genes. *Nat Genet.* 2015;47(12): 1426-1434.

53. Saleem MD, Oussedik E, Picardo M, Schoch JJ. Acquired disorders with hypopigmentation: a clinical approach to diagnosis and treatment. *J Am Acad Dermatol*. 2019;80(5):1233-1250.e10.
54. Werner B, Brown S, Ackerman AB. "Hypopigmented mycosis fungoides" is not always mycosis fungoides!. *Am J Dermatopathol*. 2005;27(1):56-67.
55. Ngo JT, Trotter MJ, Haber RM. Juvenile-onset hypopigmented mycosis fungoides mimicking vitiligo. *J Cutan Med Surg*. 2009;13(4):230-233.
56. Zackheim HS, McCalmont TH. Mycosis fungoides: the great imitator. *J Am Acad Dermatol*. 2002;47(6):914-918.
57. Heng YK, Koh MJ, Giam YC, Tang MB, Chong WS, Tan SH. Pediatric mycosis fungoides in Singapore: a series of 46 children. *Pediatr Dermatol*. 2014;31(4):477-482.
58. Nasimi M, Kamyab K, Aghahi T, Fahim S, Ghandi N. Childhood mycosis fungoides: a clinicopathologic study of 30 cases from Iran. *Australas J Dermatol*. 2020;61(2):e259-e261.
59. Amin A, Burkhart C, Groben P, Morrell DS. Primary cutaneous T-cell lymphoma following organ transplantation in a 16-year-old boy. *Pediatr Dermatol*. 2009;26(1):112-113.
60. Hodak E, Amitay-Laish I, Feinmesser M, et al. Juvenile mycosis fungoides: cutaneous T-cell lymphoma with frequent follicular involvement. *J Am Acad Dermatol*. 2014;70(6):993-1001.
61. Alikhan A, Griffin J, Nguyen N, Davis DM, Gibson LE. Pediatric follicular mucinosis: presentation, histopathology, molecular genetics, treatment, and outcomes over an 11-year period at the mayo clinic. *Pediatr Dermatol*. 2013;30(2):192-198.
62. Hess Schmid M, Dummer R, Kempf W, Hilty N, Burg G. Mycosis fungoides with mucinosis follicularis in childhood. *Dermatology*. 1999;198(3):284-287.
63. Santos-Briz A, Canueto J, Garcia-Dorado J, Alonso MT, Balanzategui A, Gonzalez-Diaz M. Pediatric primary follicular mucinosis: further evidence of its relationship with mycosis fungoides. *Pediatr Dermatol*. 2013;30(6):e218-220.
64. van Doorn R, Scheffer E, Willemze R. Follicular mycosis fungoides, a distinct disease entity with or without associated follicular mucinosis: a clinicopathologic and follow-up study of 51 patients. *Arch Dermatol*. 2002;138(2):191-198.
65. Convit J, Kerdel F, Goihman M, Rondon AJ, Soto JM. Progressive, atrophying, chronic granulomatous dermohypodermitis. Autoimmune disease? *Arch Dermatol*. 1973;107(2):271-274.
66. Helm KF, Cerio R, Winkelmann RK. Granulomatous slack skin: a clinicopathological and immunohistochemical study of three cases. *Br J Dermatol*. 1992;126(2):142-147.
67. LeBoit PE, Beckstead JH, Bond B, Epstein WL, Frieden IJ, Parslow TG. Granulomatous slack skin: clonal rearrangement of the T-cell receptor beta gene is evidence for the lymphoproliferative nature of a cutaneous elastolytic disorder. *J Invest Dermatol*. 1987;89(2):183-186.
68. Noto G, Pravata G, Miceli S, Arico M. Granulomatous slack skin: report of a case associated with Hodgkin's disease and a review of the literature. *Br J Dermatol*. 1994;131(2):275-279.
69. Wieser I, Wohlmuth C, Duvic M. Granulomatous mycosis fungoides in an adolescent-A rare encounter and review of the literature. *Pediatr Dermatol*. 2016;33(5):e296-298.
70. Camacho FM, Burg G, Moreno JC, Campora RG, Villar JL. Granulomatous slack skin in childhood. *Pediatr Dermatol*. 1997;14(3):204-208.
71. Matsuzaki Y, Kimura K, Nakano H, Hanada K, Sawamura D. Localized pagetoid reticulosis (Woringer-Kolopp disease) in early childhood. *J Am Acad Dermatol*. 2009;61(1):120-123.
72. Mendese GW, Beckford A, Krejci N, Mahalingam M, Goldberg L, Gilchrest BA. Pagetoid reticulosis in a prepubescent boy successfully treated with photodynamic therapy. *Clin Exp Dermatol*. 2012;37(7):759-761.
73. Miedler JD, Kristjansson AK, Gould J, Tamburro J, Gilliam AC. Pagetoid reticulosis in a 5-year-old boy. *J Am Acad Dermatol*. 2008;58(4):679-681.
74. Ai WZ, Keegan TH, Press DJ, et al. Outcomes after diagnosis of mycosis fungoides and Sezary syndrome before 30 years of age: a population-based study. *JAMA Dermatol*. 2014;150(7):709-715.
75. LeBoit PE, Abel EA, Cleary ML, et al. Clonal rearrangement of the T cell receptor beta gene in the circulating lymphocytes of erythrodermic follicular mucinosis. *Blood*. 1988;71(5):1329-1333.
76. Meister L, Duarte AM, Davis J, Perez JL, Schachner LA. Sezary syndrome in an 11-year-old girl. *J Am Acad Dermatol*. 1993;28(1):93-95.
77. Magro CM, Nguyen GH. Keratoderma-like T cell dyscrasia: a report of 13 cases and its distinction from mycosis fungoides palmaris et plantaris. *Indian J Dermatol Venereol Leprol*. 2016;82(4):395-403.
78. Smoller BR, Santucci M, Wood GS, Whittaker SJ. Histopathology and genetics of cutaneous T-cell lymphoma. *Hematol Oncol Clin N Am*. 2003;17(6):1277-1311.
79. Romero M, Haney M, Desantis E, Zlotoff B. Mycosis fungoides with focal CD 30 transformation in an adolescent. *Pediatr Dermatol*. 2008;25(5):565-568.
80. Carrie E, Buzyn A, Fraitag S, Hermine O, Bodemer C. Transformed juvenile-onset mycosis fungoides: treatment by bone marrow transplantation with graft-versus-lymphoma effect. *Ann Dermatol Venereol*. 2007;134(5 pt 1):471-476.
81. Gerami P, Guitart J. The spectrum of histopathologic and immunohistochemical findings in folliculotropic mycosis fungoides. *Am J Surg Pathol*. 2007;31(9):1430-1438.
82. Ben-Amitai D, Michael D, Feinmesser M, Hodak E. Juvenile mycosis fungoides diagnosed before 18 years of age. *Acta Derm Venereol*. 2003;83(6):451-456.
83. Hanna S, Walsh N, D'Intino Y, Langley RG. Mycosis fungoides presenting as pigmented purpuric dermatitis. *Pediatr Dermatol*. 2006;23(4):350-354.
84. Lu D, Patel KA, Duvic M, Jones D. Clinical and pathological spectrum of CD8-positive cutaneous T-cell lymphomas. *J Cutan Pathol*. 2002;29(8):465-472.
85. Moon HR, Lee WJ, Won CH, et al. Paediatric cutaneous lymphoma in Korea: a retrospective study at a single institution. *J Eur Acad Dermatol Venereol*. 2014;28(12):1798-1804.
86. Neuhaus IM, Ramos-Caro FA, Hassanein AM. Hypopigmented mycosis fungoides in childhood and adolescence. *Pediatr Dermatol*. 2000;17(5):403-406.
87. Quaglino P, Zaccagna A, Verrone A, Dardano F, Bernengo MG. Mycosis fungoides in patients under 20 years of age: report of 7 cases, review of the literature and study of the clinical course. *Dermatology*. 1999;199(1):8-14.
88. Wang T, Liu YH, Zheng HY, et al. Hypopigmented mycosis fungoides in children: a clinicopathological study of 6 cases. *Zhonghua Yixue Zazhi*. 2010;90(46):3287-3290.
89. Whittam LR, Calonje E, Orchard G, Fraser-Andrews EA, Woolford A, Russell-Jones R. CD8-positive

89. juvenile onset mycosis fungoides: an immunohistochemical and genotypic analysis of six cases. *Br J Dermatol.* 2000;143(6):1199-1204.
90. Singh ZN, Tretiakova MS, Shea CR, Petronic-Rosic VM. Decreased CD117 expression in hypopigmented mycosis fungoides correlates with hypomelanosis: lessons learned from vitiligo. *Mod Pathol.* 2006;19(9):1255-1260.
91. Hodak E, David M, Maron L, Aviram A, Kaganovsky E, Feinmesser M. CD4/CD8 double-negative epidermotropic cutaneous T-cell lymphoma: an immunohistochemical variant of mycosis fungoides. *J Am Acad Dermatol.* 2006;55(2):276-284.
92. Wain EM, Orchard GE, Mayou S, Atherton DJ, Misch KJ, Russell-Jones R. Mycosis fungoides with a CD56+ immunophenotype. *J Am Acad Dermatol.* 2005;53(1):158-163.
93. Rovaris M, Colato C, Girolomoni G. Pediatric CD8+/CD56+ mycosis fungoides with cytotoxic marker expression: a variant with indolent course. *J Cutan Pathol.* 2018;45(10):782-785.
94. Pimpinelli N, Olsen EA, Santucci M, et al. Defining early mycosis fungoides. *J Am Acad Dermatol.* 2005;53(6):1053-1063.
95. Ramsay B, Dahl MC, Malcolm AJ, Wilson-Jones E. Acral pseudolymphomatous angiokeratoma of children. *Arch Dermatol.* 1990;126(11):1524-1525.
96. Kirsch IR, Watanabe R, O'Malley JT, et al. TCR sequencing facilitates diagnosis and identifies mature T cells as the cell of origin in CTCL. *Sci Transl Med.* 2015;7(308):308ra158.
97. Macaulay WL. Lymphomatoid papulosis. A continuing self-healing eruption, clinically benign--histologically malignant. *Arch Dermatol.* 1968;97(1):23-30.
98. Nijsten T, Curiel-Lewandrowski C, Kadin ME. Lymphomatoid papulosis in children: a retrospective cohort study of 35 cases. *Arch Dermatol.* 2004;140(3):306-312.
99. Kunishige JH, McDonald H, Alvarez G, Johnson M, Prieto V, Duvic M. Lymphomatoid papulosis and associated lymphomas: a retrospective case series of 84 patients. *Clin Exp Dermatol.* 2009;34(5):576-581.
100. Zackheim HS, Jones C, Leboit PE, Kashani-Sabet M, McCalmont TH, Zehnder J. Lymphomatoid papulosis associated with mycosis fungoides: a study of 21 patients including analyses for clonality. *J Am Acad Dermatol.* 2003;49(4):620-623.
101. Miquel J, Fraitag S, Hamel-Teillac D, et al. Lymphomatoid papulosis in children: a series of 25 cases. *Br J Dermatol.* 2014;171(5):1138-1146.
102. Martorell-Calatayud A, Hernandez-Martin A, Colmenero I, et al. Lymphomatoid papulosis in children: report of 9 cases and review of the literature. *Actas Dermosifiliogr.* 2010;101(8):693-701.
103. Wieser I, Wohlmuth C, Nunez CA, Duvic M. Lymphomatoid papulosis in children and adolescents: a systematic review. *Am J Clin Dermatol.* 2016;17(4):319-327.
104. Oura K, Sato T, Iguchi A, Toriumi N, Sarashina T. Lymphomatoid papulosis development in acute lymphoblastic leukemia. *J Med Cases.* 2021;12(8):306-309.
105. Karai LJ, Kadin ME, Hsi ED, et al. Chromosomal rearrangements of 6p25.3 define a new subtype of lymphomatoid papulosis. *Am J Surg Pathol.* 2013;37(8):1173-1181.
106. Bekkenk MW, Geelen FA, van Voorst Vader PC, et al. Primary and secondary cutaneous CD30(+) lymphoproliferative disorders: a report from the Dutch Cutaneous Lymphoma Group on the long-term follow-up data of 219 patients and guidelines for diagnosis and treatment. *Blood.* 2000;95(12):3653-3661.
107. de Souza A, Camilleri MJ, Wada DA, Appert DL, Gibson LE, el-Azhary RA. Clinical, histopathologic, and immunophenotypic features of lymphomatoid papulosis with CD8 predominance in 14 pediatric patients. *J Am Acad Dermatol.* 2009;61(6):993-1000.
108. Scarisbrick JJ, Evans AV, Woolford AJ, Black MM, Russell-Jones R. Regional lymphomatoid papulosis: a report of four cases. *Br J Dermatol.* 1999;141(6):1125-1128.
109. Thomas GJ, Conejo-Mir JS, Ruiz AP, Linares Barrios M, Navarrete M. Lymphomatoid papulosis in childhood with exclusive acral involvement. *Pediatr Dermatol.* 1998;15(2):146-147.
110. Bassi A, Piccolo V, Filippeschi C, et al. Clinical and dermoscopic features of pediatric lymphomatoid papulosis: an Italian multicenter study. *Int J Dermatol.* 2020;59(8):e294-e296.
111. Saggini A, Gulia A, Argenyi Z, et al. A variant of lymphomatoid papulosis simulating primary cutaneous aggressive epidermotropic CD8+ cytotoxic T-cell lymphoma. Description of 9 cases. *Am J Surg Pathol.* 2010;34(8):1168-1175.
112. Kempf W, Kazakov DV, Scharer L, et al. Angioinvasive lymphomatoid papulosis: a new variant simulating aggressive lymphomas. *Am J Surg Pathol.* 2013;37(1):1-13.
113. Pierard GE. A reappraisal of lymphomatoid papulosis and of its follicular variant. *Am J Dermatopathol.* 1981;3(2):179-181.
114. Pierard GE, Ackerman AB, Lapiere CM. Follicular lymphomatoid papulosis. *Am J Dermatopathol.* 1980;2(2):173-180.
115. Kempf W, Kazakov DV, Baumgartner HP, Kutzner H. Follicular lymphomatoid papulosis revisited: a study of 11 cases, with new histopathological findings. *J Am Acad Dermatol.* 2013;68(5):809-816.
116. Ross NA, Truong H, Keller MS, Mulholland JK, Lee JB, Sahu J. Follicular lymphomatoid papulosis: an eosinophilic-rich follicular subtype masquerading as folliculitis clinically and histologically. *Am J Dermatopathol.* 2016;38(1):e1-10.
117. Georgesen C, Magro C. Lymphomatoid papulosis in children and adolescents: a clinical and histopathologic retrospective cohort. *Ann Diagn Pathol.* 2020;46:151486.
118. Kummer JA, Vermeer MH, Dukers D, Meijer CJ, Willemze R. Most primary cutaneous CD30-positive lymphoproliferative disorders have a CD4-positive cytotoxic T-cell phenotype. *J Invest Dermatol.* 1997;109(5):636-640.
119. Kadin ME. Common activated helper-T-cell origin for lymphomatoid papulosis, mycosis fungoides, and some types of Hodgkin's disease. *Lancet.* 1985;2(8460):864-865.
120. Kaudewitz P, Burg G, Stein H, Klepzig K, Mason DY, Braun-Falco O. Monoclonal antibody patterns in lymphomatoid papulosis. *Dermatol Clin.* 1985;3(4):749-757.
121. Benharroch D, Meguerian-Bedoyan Z, Lamant L, et al. ALK-positive lymphoma: a single disease with a broad spectrum of morphology. *Blood.* 1998;91(6):2076-2084.
122. Criscione VD, Weinstock MA. Incidence of cutaneous T-cell lymphoma in the United States, 1973-2002. *Arch Dermatol.* 2007;143(7):854-859.
123. Delsol G, Falini B, Muller-Hermelink HK, et al. *Anaplastic Large Cell Lymphoma (ALCL), ALK-Positive.* 4th ed. International Agency for Research on Cancer; 2008.
124. Falini B, Pileri S, Zinzani PL, et al. ALK+ lymphoma: clinico-pathological findings and outcome. *Blood.* 1999;93(8):2697-2706.

125. Bajor-Dattilo EB, Pittaluga S, Jaffe ES. Pathobiology of T-cell and NK-cell lymphomas. *Best Pract Res Clin Haematol.* 2013;26(1):75-87.
126. Savage KJ, Harris NL, Vose JM, et al. ALK- anaplastic large-cell lymphoma is clinically and immunophenotypically different from both ALK+ ALCL and peripheral T-cell lymphoma, not otherwise specified: report from the International Peripheral T-Cell Lymphoma Project. *Blood.* 2008;111(12):5496-5504.
127. de Leval L. Molecular classification of ganglionic T cell lymphomas. pathological and diagnostic implications. *Bull Mem Acad R Med Belg.* 2010;165(1-2):99.
128. de Leval L, Bisig B, Thielen C, Boniver J, Gaulard P. Molecular classification of T-cell lymphomas. *Crit Rev Oncol-Hematol.* 2009;72(2):125-143.
129. Kinney MC, Higgins RA, Medina EA. Anaplastic large cell lymphoma: twenty-five years of discovery. *Arch Pathol Lab Med.* 2011;135(1):19-43.
130. Ando K, Tamada Y, Shimizu K, et al. ALK-positive primary systemic anaplastic large cell lymphoma with extensive cutaneous manifestation. *Acta Derm Venereol.* 2010;90(2):198-200.
131. Chan DV, Summers P, Tuttle M, et al. Anaplastic lymphoma kinase expression in a recurrent primary cutaneous anaplastic large cell lymphoma with eventual systemic involvement. *J Am Acad Dermatol.* 2011;65(3):671-673.
132. Hosoi M, Ichikawa M, Imai Y, Kurokawa M. A case of anaplastic large cell lymphoma, ALK positive, primary presented in the skin and relapsed with systemic involvement and leukocytosis after years of follow-up period. *Int J Hematol.* 2010;92(4):667-668.
133. Ogunrinade O, Lin O, Steinhertz P, Pulitzer M. ALK-positive (2p23 rearranged) anaplastic large cell lymphoma with localization to the skin in a pediatric patient. *J Cutan Pathol.* 2015;42(3):182-187.
134. Bayle C, Charpentier A, Duchayne E, et al. Leukaemic presentation of small cell variant anaplastic large cell lymphoma: report of four cases. *Br J Haematol.* 1999;104(4):680-688.
135. Fraga M, Brousset P, Schlaifer D, et al. Bone marrow involvement in anaplastic large cell lymphoma. Immunohistochemical detection of minimal disease and its prognostic significance. *Am J Clin Pathol.* 1995;103(1):82-89.
136. Lamant L, Pileri S, Sabattini E, Brugieres L, Jaffe ES, Delsol G. Cutaneous presentation of ALK-positive anaplastic large cell lymphoma following insect bites: evidence for an association in five cases. *Haematologica.* 2010;95(3):449-455.
137. Piccaluga PP, Ascani S, Fraternali Orcioni G, et al. Anaplastic lymphoma kinase expression as a marker of malignancy. Application to a case of anaplastic large cell lymphoma with huge granulomatous reaction. *Haematologica.* 2000;85(9):978-981.
138. Hoshina D, Arita K, Mizuno O, et al. Skin involvement in ALK-negative systemic anaplastic large-cell lymphoma. *J Am Acad Dermatol.* 2012;67(4):e159-160.
139. Marschalko M, Eros N, Hollo P, et al. Secondary ALK negative anaplastic large cell lymphoma in a patient with lymphomatoid papulosis of 40 years duration. *Am J Dermatopathol.* 2010;32(7):708-712.
140. Querfeld C, Khan I, Mahon B, Nelson BP, Rosen ST, Evens AM. Primary cutaneous and systemic anaplastic large cell lymphoma: clinicopathologic aspects and therapeutic options. *Oncology.* 2010;24(7):574-587.
141. Oschlies I, Lisfeld J, Lamant L, et al. ALK-positive anaplastic large cell lymphoma limited to the skin: clinical, histopathological and molecular analysis of 6 pediatric cases. A report from the ALCL99 study. *Haematologica.* 2013;98(1):50-56.
142. Hanafusa T, Igawa K, Takagawa S, et al. Erythroderma as a paraneoplastic cutaneous disorder in systemic anaplastic large cell lymphoma. *J Eur Acad Dermatol Venereol.* 2012;26(6):710-713.
143. Mencia-Gutierrez E, Gutierrez-Diaz E, Salamanca J, Martinez-Gonzalez MA. Cutaneous presentation on the eyelid of primary, systemic, CD30+, anaplastic lymphoma kinase (ALK)-negative, anaplastic large-cell lymphoma (ALCL). *Int J Dermatol.* 2006;45(6):766-769.
144. Rodis DG, Liatsos GD, Moulakakis A, Pirounaki M, Tasidou A. Paraneoplastic cerebellar degeneration: initial presentation in a patient with anaplastic T-cell lymphoma, associated with ichthyosiform cutaneous lesions. *Leuk Lymphoma.* 2009;50(8):1369-1371.
145. Ferreri AJ, Govi S, Pileri SA, Savage KJ. Anaplastic large cell lymphoma, ALK-positive. *Crit Rev Oncol Hematol.* 2012;83(2):293-302.
146. Jaffe ES, Nicolae A, Pittaluga S. Peripheral T-cell and NK-cell lymphomas in the WHO classification: pearls and pitfalls. *Mod Pathol.* 2013;26(suppl 1):S71-S87.
147. Vassallo J, Lamant L, Brugieres L, et al. ALK-positive anaplastic large cell lymphoma mimicking nodular sclerosis Hodgkin's lymphoma: report of 10 cases. *Am J Surg Pathol.* 2006;30(2):223-229.
148. Beylot-Barry M, Groppi A, Vergier B, Pulford K, Merlio JP. Characterization of t(2;5) reciprocal transcripts and genomic breakpoints in CD30+ cutaneous lymphoproliferations. *Blood.* 1998;91(12):4668-4676.
149. Kadin ME, Pinkus JL, Pinkus GS, et al. Primary cutaneous ALCL with phosphorylated/activated cytoplasmic ALK and novel phenotype: EMA/MUC1+, cutaneous lymphocyte antigen negative. *Am J Surg Pathol.* 2008;32(9):1421-1426.
150. Melchers RC, Willemze R, van de Loo M, et al. Clinical, histologic, and molecular characteristics of anaplastic lymphoma kinase-positive primary cutaneous anaplastic large cell lymphoma. *Am J Surg Pathol.* 2020;44(6):776-781. doi:10.1097/PAS.0000000000001449
151. Melchers RC, Willemze R, van Doorn R, et al. Corresponding anaplastic lymphoma kinase-tropomyosin 3 (ALK-TPM3) fusion in a patient with a primary cutaneous anaplastic large-cell lymphoma and a Spitz nevus. *JAAD Case Rep.* 2019;5(11):970-972. eCollection 2019 Nov. doi:10.1016/j.jdcr.2019.09.021
152. Mellgren K, Attarbaschi A, Abla O, et al. Non-anaplastic peripheral T cell lymphoma in children and adolescents-an international review of 143 cases. *Ann Hematol.* 2016;95(8):1295-1305.
153. Jaffe ES, Gaulard P, Ralfiaer E. *Subcutaneous Panniculitis-like T-Cell Lymphoma.* 4th ed. International Agency for Research on Cancer; 2008.
154. Gizewska-Kacprzak K, Karpinska-Kaczmarczyk K, Ociepa T. Subcutaneous panniculitis-like T-cell lymphoma presenting as a local inflammation of a thigh in an 8-month-old child. *Eur J Pediatr Surg Rep.* 2017;5(1):e68-e70.
155. Slater DN. The new World Health Organization-European Organization for Research and Treatment of Cancer classification for cutaneous lymphomas: a practical marriage of two giants. *Br J Dermatol.* 2005;153(5):874-880.
156. Willemze R, Jansen PM, Cerroni L, et al. Subcutaneous panniculitis-like T-cell lymphoma: definition, classification,

and prognostic factors – an EORTC Cutaneous Lymphoma Group Study of 83 cases. *Blood.* 2008;111(2):838-845.
157. Huppmann AR, Xi L, Raffeld M, Pittaluga S, Jaffe ES. Subcutaneous panniculitis-like T-cell lymphoma in the pediatric age group: a lymphoma of low malignant potential. *Pediatr Blood Cancer.* 2013;60(7):1165-1170.
158. Kawachi Y, Furuta J, Fujisawa Y, Nakamura Y, Ishii Y, Otsuka F. Indolent subcutaneous panniculitis-like T cell lymphoma in a 1-year-old child. *Pediatr Dermatol.* 2012;29(3): 374-377.
159. Gupta V, Arava S, Bakhshi S, Vashisht KR, Reddy R, Gupta S. Subcutaneous panniculitis-like T-cell lymphoma with hemophagocytic syndrome in a child. *Pediatr Dermatol.* 2016;33(2):e72-76.
160. Johnston EE, LeBlanc RE, Kim J, et al. Subcutaneous panniculitis-like T-cell lymphoma: pediatric case series demonstrating heterogeneous presentation and option for watchful waiting. *Pediatr Blood Cancer.* 2015;62(11): 2025-2028.
161. Yi L, Qun S, Wenjie Z, et al. The presenting manifestations of subcutaneous panniculitis-like T-cell lymphoma and T-cell lymphoma and cutaneous gammadelta T-cell lymphoma may mimic those of rheumatic diseases: a report of 11 cases. *Clin Rheumatol.* 2013;32(8):1169-1175.
162. Bosisio F, Boi S, Caputo V, et al. *Lobular Panniculitic Infiltrates with Overlapping Histopathologic Features of Lupus Panniculitis (Lupus Profundus) and Subcutaneous T-Cell Lymphoma: A Conceptual and Practical Dilemma.* Am J Surg Pathol. 2015;39(2):206-211.
163. Pincus LB, LeBoit PE, McCalmont TH, et al. Subcutaneous panniculitis-like T-cell lymphoma with overlapping clinicopathologic features of lupus erythematosus: coexistence of 2 entities? *Am J Dermatopathol.* 2009;31(6):520-526.
164. Joseph LD, Panicker VK, Prathiba D, Damodharan J. Subcutaneous panniculitis-like T cell lymphoma in a HIV positive patient. *J Assoc Phys India.* 2005;53:314-316.
165. Iqbal K, Bott J, Greenblatt D, et al. Subcutaneous panniculitis-like T-cell lymphoma in association with sarcoidosis. *Clin Exp Dermatol.* 2011;36(6):677-679.
166. Michot C, Costes V, Gerard-Dran D, Guillot B, Combes B, Dereure O. Subcutaneous panniculitis-like T-cell lymphoma in a patient receiving etanercept for rheumatoid arthritis. *Br J Dermatol.* 2009;160(4):889-890.
167. Schmutz JL, Trechot P. Subcutaneous panniculitis-like T-cell lymphoma following treatment with rituximab and cyclophosphamide. *Annales de dermatologie et de venereologie.* 2013;140(3):246-247.
168. Mixon B, Drach L, Monforte H, Barbosa J. Subcutaneous panniculitis-like T-cell lymphoma in a child with trisomy 21. *Fetal Pediatr Pathol.* 2010;29(6):380-384.
169. Swain M, Swarnalata G, Bhandari T. Subcutaneous panniculitis-like T-cell lymphoma in a case of carcinoma cervix. *Indian J Med Paediatr Oncol.* 2013;34(2):104-106.
170. Reimer P, Rudiger T, Muller J, Rose C, Wilhelm M, Weissinger F. Subcutaneous panniculitis-like T-cell lymphoma during pregnancy with successful autologous stem cell transplantation. *Ann Hematol.* 2003;82(5):305-309.
171. Reich A, Butrym A, Mazur G, et al. Subcutaneous panniculitis-like T-cell lymphoma in type 1 neurofibromatosis: a case report. *Acta Dermatovenerol Croat.* 2014;22(2):145-149.
172. Polprasert C, Takeuchi Y, Kakiuchi N, et al. Frequent germline mutations of HAVCR2 in sporadic subcutaneous panniculitis-like T-cell lymphoma. *Blood Adv;*3(4) 2019:588-595. PMID: 30792187. doi:10.1182/bloodadvances.2018028340.
173. Gayden T, Sepulveda FE, Khuong-Quang DA, et al. Germline HAVCR2 mutations altering TIM-3 characterize subcutaneous panniculitis-like T cell lymphomas with hemophagocytic lymphohistiocytic syndrome. *Nat Genet.* 2018;50(12):1650-1657. Epub 2018 Oct 29. PMID: 30374066. doi:10.1038/s41588-018-0251-4
174. Nguyen MC, Nguyen V, Le H, et al. Subcutaneous panniculitis-like T-cell lymphomas with homozygous inheritance of HAVCR2 mutations in Vietnamese pedigrees. *Pediatr Blood Cancer.* 2021;68(12):e29292.
175. Frederiks AJ, Spagnolo DV, Ramachandran S, Brand R. Subcutaneous panniculitis-like T-cell lymphoma in a 14-year-old female homozygous for HAVCR2 mutation. *Australas J Dermatol.* 2021;62(4):e576-e579. Epub 2021 Aug 16. doi:10.1111/ajd.13684
176. Leonard GD, Hegde U, Butman J, Jaffe ES, Wilson WH. Extraoular muscle palsies in subcutaneous panniculitis-like T-cell lymphoma. *J Clin Oncol.* 2003;21(15):2993-2995.
177. Gualco G, Chioato L, Harrington WJ, Jr, Weiss LM, Bacchi CE. Primary and secondary T-cell lymphomas of the breast: clinico-pathologic features of 11 cases. *Appl Immunohistochem Mol Morphol.* 2009;17(4):301-306.
178. Jeong SI, Lim HS, Choi YR, et al. Subcutaneous panniculitis-like T-cell lymphoma of the breast. *Korean J Radiol.* 2013;14(3):391-394.
179. Risulo M, Rubegni P, Sbano P, et al. Subcutaneous panniculitis lymphoma: erythema nodosum-like. *Clinical Lymphoma Myeloma.* 2006;7(3):239-241.
180. Chiu HY, He GY, Chen JS, Hsiao PF, Hsiao CH, Tsai TF. Subcutaneous panniculitis-like T-cell lymphoma presenting with clinicopathologic features of dermatomyositis. *J Am Acad Dermatol.* 2011;64(6):e121-123.
181. Kaieda S, Idemoto A, Yoshida N, Ida H. A subcutaneous panniculitis-like T-cell lymphoma mimicking dermatomyositis. *Intern Med.* 2014;53(13):1455.
182. Troskot N, Lugovic L, Situm M, Vucic M. From circumscribed scleroderma (morphea) to subcutaneous panniculitis-like T-cell lymphoma: case report. *Acta Dermatovenerol Croat.* 2004;12(4):289-293.
183. Tzeng HE, Teng CL, Yang Y, Young JH, Chou G. Occult subcutaneous panniculitis-like T-cell lymphoma with initial presentations of cellulitis-like skin lesion and fulminant hemophagocytosis. *J Formos Med Assoc.* 2007;106(2 suppl):S55-S59.
184. Velez NF, Ishizawar RC, Dellaripa PF, et al. Full facial edema: a novel presentation of subcutaneous panniculitis-like T-cell lymphoma. *J Clin Oncol.* 2012;30(25):e233-236.
185. Weenig RH, Daniel Su WP. Subcutaneous panniculitis-like T-cell lymphoma presenting as venous stasis ulceration. *Int J Dermatol.* 2006;45(9):1083-1085.
186. Weenig RH, Ng CS, Perniciaro C. Subcutaneous panniculitis-like T-cell lymphoma: an elusive case presenting as lipomembranous panniculitis and a review of 72 cases in the literature. *Am J Dermatopathol.* 2001;23(3):206-215.
187. Ghosh SK, Roy D, Mondal P, Bhunia D, Dutta DP. Subcutaneous panniculitis-like T-cell lymphoma with unusual eschar-like crusting. *Dermatol Online J.* 2014;20(2):doj_21535.
188. Thomas J, Maramattom BV, Kuruvilla PM, Varghese J. Subcutaneous panniculitis like T cell lymphoma associated

with erythromelalgia. *J Postgrad Med.* 2014;60(3): 335-337.
189. Torok L, Gurbity TP, Kirschner A, Krenacs L. Panniculitis-like T-cell lymphoma clinically manifested as alopecia. *Br J Dermatol.* 2002;147(4):785-788.
190. Hahtola S, Burghart E, Jeskanen L, et al. Clinicopathological characterization and genomic aberrations in subcutaneous panniculitis-like T-cell lymphoma. *J Invest Dermatol.* 2008;128(9):2304-2309.
191. Koh MJ, Sadarangani SP, Chan YC, et al. Aggressive subcutaneous panniculitis-like T-cell lymphoma with hemophagocytosis in two children (subcutaneous panniculitis-like T-cell lymphoma). *J Am Acad Dermatol.* 2009;61(5):875-881.
192. Parveen Z, Thompson K. Subcutaneous panniculitis-like T-cell lymphoma: redefinition of diagnostic criteria in the recent World Health Organization-European Organization for Research and Treatment of Cancer classification for cutaneous lymphomas. *Arch Pathol Lab Med.* 2009;133(2):303-308.
193. Gao J, Gauerke SJ, Martinez-Escala ME, et al. Bone marrow involvement by subcutaneous panniculitis-like T-cell lymphoma: a report of three cases. *Mod Pathol.* 2014;27(6):800-807.
194. Ghobrial IM, Weenig RH, Pittlekow MR, et al. Clinical outcome of patients with subcutaneous panniculitis-like T-cell lymphoma. *Leuk Lymphoma.* 2005;46(5):703-708.
195. Babb A, Zerizer I, Naresh KN, Macdonald D. Subcutaneous panniculitis-like T-cell lymphoma with extracutaneous dissemination demonstrated on FDG PET/CT. *Am J Hematol.* 2011;86(4):375-376.
196. Huang CT, Yang WC, Lin SF. Positron-emission tomography findings indicating the involvement of the whole body skin in subcutaneous panniculitis-like T cell lymphoma. *Ann Hematol.* 2011;90(7):853-854.
197. Berg KD, Brinster NK, Huhn KM, et al. Transmission of a T-cell lymphoma by allogeneic bone marrow transplantation. *N Engl J Med.* 2001;345(20):1458-1463.
198. Hathaway T, Subtil A, Kuo P, Foss F. Efficacy of denileukin diftitox in subcutaneous panniculitis-like T-cell lymphoma. *Clin Lymphoma Myeloma.* 2007;7(8):541-545.
199. Messeguer F, Gimeno E, Agusti-Mejias A, San Juan J. Primary cutaneous CD4+ small- to medium-sized pleomorphic T-cell lymphoma: report of a case with spontaneous resolution. Article in Spanish. *Actas Dermo-Sifiliográficas.* 2011;102(8):636-638.
200. Ma L, Bandarchi B, Glusac EJ. Fatal subcutaneous panniculitis-like T-cell lymphoma with interface change and dermal mucin, a dead ringer for lupus erythematosus. *J Cutan Pathol.* 2005;32(5):360-365.
201. Acree SC, Tovar JP, Pattengale PK, et al. Subcutaneous panniculitis-like T-cell lymphoma in two pediatric patients: an HIV-positive adolescent and a 4-month-old infant. *Fetal Pediatr Pathol.* 2013;32(3):175-183.
202. Ali SK, Othman NM, Tagoe AB, Tulba AA. Subcutaneous panniculitic T cell lymphoma mimicking histiocytic cytophagic panniculitis in a child. *Saudi Med J.* 2000;21(11):1074-1077.
203. Bader-Meunier B, Fraitag S, Janssen C, et al. Clonal cytophagic histiocytic panniculitis in children may be cured by cyclosporine A. *Pediatrics.* 2013;132(2):e545-549.
204. Bittencourt AL, Vieira M, Carvalho EG, Cunha C, Araujo I. Subcutaneous Panniculitis-Like T-Cell Lymphoma (SPTL) in a child with spontaneous resolution. *Case Rep Oncol Med.* 2011;2011:639240.
205. Grassi S, Borroni RG, Brazzelli V. Panniculitis in children. *G Ital Dermatol Venereol.* 2013;148(4):371-385.
206. Kobayashi R, Yamato K, Tanaka F, et al. Retrospective analysis of non-anaplastic peripheral T-cell lymphoma in pediatric patients in Japan. *Pediatr Blood Cancer.* 2010;54(2):212-215.
207. Lim GY, Hahn ST, Chung NG, Kim HK. Subcutaneous panniculitis-like T-cell lymphoma in a child: whole-body MRI in the initial and follow-up evaluations. *Pediatr Radiol.* 2009;39(1):57-61.
208. Merritt BY, Curry JL, Duvic M, Vega F, Sheehan AM, Curry CV. Pediatric subcutaneous panniculitis-like T-cell lymphoma with features of hemophagocytic syndrome. *Pediatr Blood Cancer.* 2013;60(11):1916-1917.
209. Moraes AJ, Soares PM, Zapata AL, Lotito AP, Sallum AM, Silva CA. Panniculitis in childhood and adolescence. *Pediatr Int.* 2006;48(1):48-53.
210. Nagai K, Nakano N, Iwai T, et al. Pediatric subcutaneous panniculitis-like T-cell lymphoma with favorable result by immunosuppressive therapy: a report of two cases. *Pediatr Hematol Oncol.* 2014;31(6):528-533.
211. Rajic L, Bilic E, Femenic R, et al. Subcutaneous panniculitis-like T-cell lymphoma in a 19 month-old boy: a case report. *Coll Antropol.* 2010;34(2):679-682.
212. Yim JH, Kim MY, Kim HO, Cho B, Chung NG, Park YM. Subcutaneous panniculitis-like T-cell lymphoma in a 26-month-old child with a review of the literature. *Pediatr Dermatol.* 2006;23(6):537-540.
213. Hoque SR, Child FJ, Whittaker SJ, et al. Subcutaneous panniculitis-like T-cell lymphoma: a clinicopathological, immunophenotypic and molecular analysis of six patients. *Br J Dermatol.* 2003;148(3):516-525.
214. Lozzi GP, Massone C, Citarella L, Kerl H, Cerroni L. Rimming of adipocytes by neoplastic lymphocytes: a histopathologic feature not restricted to subcutaneous T-cell lymphoma. *Am J Dermatopathol.* 2006;28(1):9-12.
215. Cassis TB, Fearneyhough PK, Callen JP. Subcutaneous panniculitis-like T-cell lymphoma with vacuolar interface dermatitis resembling lupus erythematosus panniculitis. *J Am Acad Dermatol.* 2004;50(3):465-469.
216. Fraga J, Garcia-Diez A. Lupus erythematosus panniculitis. *Dermatol Clin.* 2008;26(4):453-463, vi.
217. Gonzalez EG, Selvi E, Lorenzini S, et al. Subcutaneous panniculitis-like T-cell lymphoma misdiagnosed as lupus erythematosus panniculitis. *Clin Rheumatol.* 2007;26(2):244-246.
218. Li JY, Liu HJ, Wang L. Subcutaneous panniculitis-like T-cell lymphoma accompanied with discoid lupus erythematosus. *Chin Med J.* 2013;126(18):3590.
219. Liau JY, Chuang SS, Chu CY, Ku WH, Tsai JH, Shih TF. The presence of clusters of plasmacytoid dendritic cells is a helpful feature for differentiating lupus panniculitis from subcutaneous panniculitis-like T-cell lymphoma. *Histopathology.* 2013;62(7):1057-1066.
220. Massone C, Kodama K, Salmhofer W, et al. Lupus erythematosus panniculitis (lupus profundus): clinical, histopathological, and molecular analysis of nine cases. *J Cutan Pathol.* 2005;32(6):396-404.
221. Rose C, Leverkus M, Fleischer M, Shimanovich I. Histopathology of panniculitis--aspects of biopsy

techniques and difficulties in diagnosis. *J Dtsch Dermatol Ges*. 2012;10(6):421-425.
222. Weingartner JS, Zedek DC, Burkhart CN, Morrell DS. Lupus erythematosus panniculitis in children: report of three cases and review of previously reported cases. *Pediatr Dermatol*. 2012;29(2):169-176.
223. Ikeda E, Endo M, Uchigasaki S, et al. Phagocytized apoptotic cells in subcutaneous panniculitis-like T-cell lymphoma. *J Eur Acad Dermatol Venereol*. 2001;15(2):159-162.
224. Sen F, Rassidakis GZ, Jones D, Medeiros LJ. Apoptosis and proliferation in subcutaneous panniculitis-like T-cell lymphoma. *Mod Pathol*. 2002;15(6):625-631.
225. Go RS, Wester SM. Immunophenotypic and molecular features, clinical outcomes, treatments, and prognostic factors associated with subcutaneous panniculitis-like T-cell lymphoma: a systematic analysis of 156 patients reported in the literature. *Cancer*. 2004;101(6):1404-1413.
226. Kong YY, Dai B, Kong JC, et al. Subcutaneous panniculitis-like T-cell lymphoma: a clinicopathologic, immunophenotypic, and molecular study of 22 Asian cases according to WHO-EORTC classification. *Am J Surg Pathol*. 2008;32(10):1495-1502.
227. Nemoto Y, Taniguchi A, Kamioka M, et al. Epstein-Barr virus-infected subcutaneous panniculitis-like T-cell lymphoma associated with methotrexate treatment. *Int J Hematol*. 2010;92(2):364-368.
228. Soylu S, Gul U, Kilic A, Heper AO, Kuzu I, Minareci BG. A case with an indolent course of subcutaneous panniculitis-like T-cell lymphoma demonstrating Epstein-Barr virus positivity and simulating dermatitis artefacta. *Am J Clin Dermatol*. 2010;11(2):147-150.
229. Wang L, Yang Y, Liu W, et al. Subcutaneous panniculitis-like T-cell lymphoma: expression of cytotoxic-granule-associated protein TIA-1 and its relation with Epstein-Barr virus infection. Article in Chinese. *Zhonghua Bing Li xue za zhi*. 2000;29(2):103-106.
230. LeBlanc RE, Tavallaee M, Kim YH, Kim J. Useful parameters for distinguishing subcutaneous panniculitis-like T-cell lymphoma from lupus erythematosus panniculitis. *Am J Surg Pathol*. 2016;40(6):745-754.
231. Chen RL, Hsu YH, Ueda I, et al. Cytophagic histiocytic panniculitis with fatal haemophagocytic lymphohistiocytosis in a paediatric patient with perforin gene mutation. *J Clin Pathol*. 2007;60(10):1168-1169.
232. Li MT, Zeng XF, Zhang FC, Tang FL. Cytophagic histiocytic panniculitis: a report of 6 cases with literature review. *Zhonghua Nei Ke Za Zhi*. 2004;43(8):576-579.
233. Marzano AV, Berti E, Paulli M, Caputo R. Cytophagic histiocytic panniculitis and subcutaneous panniculitis-like T-cell lymphoma: report of 7 cases. *Arch Dermatol*. 2000;136(7):889-896.
234. Pasqualini C, Jorini M, Carloni I, et al. Cytophagic histiocytic panniculitis, hemophagocytic lymphohistiocytosis and undetermined autoimmune disorder: reconciling the puzzle. *Ital J Pediatr*. 2014;40(1):17.
235. Crotty CP, Winkelmann RK. Cytophagic histiocytic panniculitis with fever, cytopenia, liver failure, and terminal hemorrhagic diathesis. *J Am Acad Dermatol*. 1981;4(2):181-194.
236. Raciborska A, Gadomski A, Wypych A, Maldyk J, Gutowska-Grzegorczyk G. 5- year old boy with Weber-Christian Syndrome or histiocytic cytophagic panniculitis? Diagnostic difficulties. Case presentation. *Med Wieku Rozwoj*. 2004;8(2 pt 1):201-208.
237. Fardet L, Galicier L, Vignon-Pennamen MD, et al. Frequency, clinical features and prognosis of cutaneous manifestations in adult patients with reactive haemophagocytic syndrome. *Br J Dermatol*. 2010;162(3):547-553.
238. Alberti-Violetti S, Torres-Cabala CA, Talpur R, et al. Clinicopathological and molecular study of primary cutaneous CD4+ small/medium-sized pleomorphic T-cell lymphoma. *J Cutan Pathol*. 2016;43(12):1121-1130.
239. Baum CL, Link BK, Neppalli VT, Swick BL, Liu V. Reappraisal of the provisional entity primary cutaneous CD4+ small/medium pleomorphic T-cell lymphoma: a series of 10 adult and pediatric patients and review of the literature. *J Am Acad Dermatol*. 2011;65(4):739-748.
240. Garcia-Herrera A, Colomo L, Camos M, et al. Primary cutaneous small/medium CD4+ T-cell lymphomas: a heterogeneous group of tumors with different clinicopathologic features and outcome. *J Clin Oncol*. 2008;26(20):3364-3371.
241. Grogg KL, Jung S, Erickson LA, McClure RF, Dogan A. Primary cutaneous CD4-positive small/medium-sized pleomorphic T-cell lymphoma: a clonal T-cell lymphoproliferative disorder with indolent behavior. *Mod Pathol*. 2008;21(6):708-715.
242. Beltraminelli H, Leinweber B, Kerl H, Cerroni L. Primary cutaneous CD4+ small-/medium-sized pleomorphic T-cell lymphoma: a cutaneous nodular proliferation of pleomorphic T lymphocytes of undetermined significance? A study of 136 cases. *Am J Dermatopathol*. 2009;31(4):317-322.
243. Volks N, Oschlies I, Cario G, Weichenthal M, Folster-Holst R. Primary cutaneous CD4+ small to medium-size pleomorphic T-cell lymphoma in a 12-year-old girl. *Pediatr Dermatol*. 2013;30(5):595-599.
244. Berti E, Tomasini D, Vermeer MH, Meijer CJ, Alessi E, Willemze R. Primary cutaneous CD8-positive epidermotropic cytotoxic T cell lymphomas. A distinct clinicopathological entity with an aggressive clinical behavior. *Am J Pathol*. 1999;155(2):483-492.
245. Kikuchi Y, Kashii Y, Gunji Y, et al. Six-year-old girl with primary cutaneous aggressive epidermotropic CD8+ T-cell lymphoma. *Pediatr Int*. 2011;53(3):393-396.
246. Guitart J, Martinez-Escala ME, Subtil A, et al. Primary cutaneous aggressive epidermotropic cytotoxic T-cell lymphomas: reappraisal of a provisional entity in the 2016 WHO classification of cutaneous lymphomas. *Mod Pathol*. 2017;30(5):761-772.
247. Garcia-Herrera A, Song JY, Chuang SS, et al. Nonhepatosplenic gammadelta T-cell lymphomas represent a spectrum of aggressive cytotoxic T-cell lymphomas with a mainly extranodal presentation. *Am J Surg Pathol*. 2011;35(8):1214-1225.
248. Guitart J, Weisenburger DD, Subtil A, et al. Cutaneous gammadelta T-cell lymphomas: a spectrum of presentations with overlap with other cytotoxic lymphomas. *Am J Surg Pathol*. 2012;36(11):1656-1665.
249. Magro CM, Wang X. Indolent primary cutaneous gamma/delta T-cell lymphoma localized to the subcutaneous panniculus and its association with atypical lymphocytic lobular panniculitis. *Am J Clin Pathol*. 2012;138(1):50-56.
250. Tripodo C, Iannitto E, Florena AM, et al. Gamma-delta T-cell lymphomas. *Nat Rev Clin Oncol*. 2009;6(12):707-717.
251. Kerbout M, Mekouar F, Bahadi N, et al. A rare pediatric case of cutaneous gamma/delta T-cell lymphoma. *Ann Biol Clin*. 2014;72(4):483-485.
252. Merrill ED, Agbay R, Miranda RN, et al. Primary cutaneous T-cell lymphomas showing gamma-delta (gammadelta)

phenotype and predominantly epidermotropic pattern are clinicopathologically distinct from classic primary cutaneous gammadelta T-cell lymphomas. *Am J Surg Pathol.* 2017;41(2):204-215.
253. Straus SE. The chronic mononucleosis syndrome. *J Infect Dis.* 1988;157(3):405-412.
254. Kimura H, Morishima T, Kanegane H, et al. Prognostic factors for chronic active Epstein-Barr virus infection. *J Infect Dis.* 2003;187(4):527-533.
255. Ko YH, Chan JKC, Quintanilla-Martinez L. Virally associated T-cell and NK-cell neoplasms. In: Jaffe ES, Arber DA, Campo E, Harris NL, Quintanilla-Martinez L, eds. *Hematopathology.* 2nd ed. 2016. https://www.clinicalkey.com/dura/browse/bookChapter/3-s2.0-C20120027822
256. Kimura H, Hoshino Y, Kanegane H, et al. Clinical and virologic characteristics of chronic active Epstein-Barr virus infection. *Blood.* 2001;98(2):280-286.
257. Cho EY, Kim KH, Kim WS, Yoo KH, Koo HH, Ko YH. The spectrum of Epstein-Barr virus-associated lymphoproliferative disease in Korea: incidence of disease entities by age groups. *J Kor Med Sci.* 2008;23(2):185-192.
258. Hong M, Ko YH, Yoo KH, et al. EBV-positive T/NK-cell lymphoproliferative disease of childhood. *Korean J Pathol.* 2013;47(2):137-147.
259. Ohshima K, Kimura H, Yoshino T, et al. Proposed categorization of pathological states of EBV-associated T/natural killer-cell lymphoproliferative disorder (LPD) in children and young adults: overlap with chronic active EBV infection and infantile fulminant EBV T-LPD. *Pathol Int.* 2008;58(4):209-217.
260. Okano M, Matsumoto S, Osato T, Sakiyama Y, Thiele GM, Purtilo DT. Severe chronic active Epstein-Barr virus infection syndrome. *Clin Microbiol Rev.* 1991;4(1):129-135.
261. Cohen JI, Kimura H, Nakamura S, Ko YH, Jaffe ES. Epstein-Barr virus-associated lymphoproliferative disease in non-immunocompromised hosts: a status report and summary of an international meeting, 8-9 September 2008. *Ann Oncol.* 2009;20(9):1472-1482.
262. Kimura H, Hoshino Y, Hara S, et al. Differences between T cell-type and natural killer cell-type chronic active Epstein-Barr virus infection. *J Infect Dis.* 2005;191(4):531-539.
263. Gru AA, Jaffe ES. Cutaneous EBV-related lymphoproliferative disorders. *Semin Diagn Pathol.* 2017;34(1):60-75.
264. Okuno Y, Murata T, Sato Y, et al. Defective Epstein-Barr virus in chronic active infection and haematological malignancy. *Nat Microbiol.* 2019;4(3):404-413. Epub 2019 Jan 21. doi:10.1038/s41564-018-0334-0
265. Ishihara S, Ohshima K, Tokura Y, et al. Hypersensitivity to mosquito bites conceals clonal lymphoproliferation of Epstein-Barr viral DNA-positive natural killer cells. *Jpn J Cancer Res.* 1997;88(1):82-87.
266. Kawa K, Okamura T, Yagi K, Takeuchi M, Nakayama M, Inoue M. Mosquito allergy and Epstein-Barr virus-associated T/natural killer-cell lymphoproliferative disease. *Blood.* 2001;98(10):3173-3174.
267. Cho JH, Kim HS, Ko YH, Park CS. Epstein-Barr virus infected natural killer cell lymphoma in a patient with hypersensitivity to mosquito bite. *J Infect.* 2006;52(6):e173-176.
268. Chung JS, Shin HJ, Lee EY, Cho GJ. Hypersensitivity to mosquito bites associated with natural killer cell-derived large granular lymphocyte lymphocytosis: a case report in Korea. *Korean J Intern Med (Korean Ed).* 2003;18(1):50-52.
269. Fan PC, Chang HN. Hypersensitivity to mosquito bite: a case report. *Gaoxiong Yi Xue Ke Xue Za Zhi.* 1995;11(7):420-424.
270. Hidano A, Kawakami M, Yago A. Hypersensitivity to mosquito bite and malignant histocytosis. *Jpn J Exp Med.* 1982;52(6):303-306.
271. Ishihara S, Okada S, Wakiguchi H, Kurashige T, Hirai K, Kawa-Ha K. Clonal lymphoproliferation following chronic active Epstein-Barr virus infection and hypersensitivity to mosquito bites. *Am J Hematol.* 1997;54(4):276-281.
272. Ishihara S, Okada S, Wakiguchi H, Kurashige T, Morishima T, Kawa-Ha K. Chronic active Epstein-Barr virus infection in children in Japan. *Acta Paediatr.* 1995;84(11):1271-1275.
273. Ohsawa T, Morimura T, Hagari Y, et al. A case of exaggerated mosquito-bite hypersensitivity with Epstein-Barr virus-positive inflammatory cells in the bite lesion. *Acta Derm Venereol.* 2001;81(5):360-363.
274. Tokura Y, Tamura Y, Takigawa M, et al. Severe hypersensitivity to mosquito bites associated with natural killer cell lymphocytosis. *Arch Dermatol.* 1990;126(3):362-368.
275. Tsai WC, Luo SF, Liaw SJ, Kuo TT. Mosquito bite allergies terminating as hemophagocytic histiocytosis: report of a case. *Taiwan Yi Xue Hui Za Zhi.* 1989;88(6):639629-639642.
276. Ishihara S, Yabuta R, Tokura Y, Ohshima K, Tagawa S. Hypersensitivity to mosquito bites is not an allergic disease, but an Epstein-Barr virus-associated lymphoproliferative disease. *Int J Hematol.* 2000;72(2):223-228.
277. Asada H, Saito-Katsuragi M, Niizeki H, et al. Mosquito salivary gland extracts induce EBV-infected NK cell oncogenesis via CD4 T cells in patients with hypersensitivity to mosquito bites. *J Invest Dermatol.* 2005;125(5):956-961.
278. Tokura Y, Matsuoka H, Koga C, et al. Enhanced T-cell response to mosquito extracts by NK cells in hypersensitivity to mosquito bites associated with EBV infection and NK cell lymphocytosis. *Cancer Sci.* 2005;96(8):519-526.
279. Tokura Y, Ishihara S, Tagawa S, Seo N, Ohshima K, Takigawa M. Hypersensitivity to mosquito bites as the primary clinical manifestation of a juvenile type of Epstein-Barr virus-associated natural killer cell leukemia/lymphoma. *J Am Acad Dermatol.* 2001;45(4):569-578.
280. Gupta G, Man I, Kemmett D. Hydroa vacciniforme: a clinical and follow-up study of 17 cases. *J Am Acad Dermatol.* 2000;42(2 pt 1):208-213.
281. Iwatsuki K, Satoh M, Yamamoto T, et al. Pathogenic link between hydroa vacciniforme and Epstein-Barr virus-associated hematologic disorders. *Arch Dermatol.* 2006;142(5):587-595.
282. Iwatsuki K, Yamamoto T, Tsuji K. Hypersensitivity to mosquito bites and hydroa vacciniforme. *Nihon Rinsho.* 2006;64(suppl 3):657-661.
283. Quintanilla-Martinez L, Kimura H, Jaffe ES. *EBV+ T-Cell Lymphoproliferative Disorders of Childhood.* 4th ed. International Agency for Research on Cancer; 2008.
284. Barrionuevo C, Anderson VM, Zevallos-Giampietri E, et al. Hydroa-like cutaneous T-cell lymphoma: a clinicopathologic and molecular genetic study of 16 pediatric cases from Peru. *Appl Immunohistochem Mol Morphol.* 2002;10(1):7-14.
285. Boddu D, George R, Nair S, Bindra M, Mathew LG. Hydroa vacciniforme-like lymphoma: a case report from India. *J Pediatr Hematol Oncol.* 2015;37(4):e223-226.
286. Iwatsuki K, Ohtsuka M, Akiba H, Kaneko F. Atypical hydroa vacciniforme in childhood: from a smoldering stage to Epstein-Barr virus-associated lymphoid malignancy. *J Am Acad Dermatol.* 1999;40(2 pt 1):283-284.

287. Magana M, Sangueza P, Gil-Beristain J, et al. Angiocentric cutaneous T-cell lymphoma of childhood (hydroa-like lymphoma): a distinctive type of cutaneous T-cell lymphoma. *J Am Acad Dermatol.* 1998;38(4):574-579.
288. Oono T, Arata J, Masuda T, Ohtsuki Y. Coexistence of hydroa vacciniforme and malignant lymphoma. *Arch Dermatol.* 1986;122(11):1306-1309.
289. Plaza JA, Sangueza M. Hydroa vacciniforme-like lymphoma with primarily periorbital swelling: 7 cases of an atypical clinical manifestation of this rare cutaneous T-cell lymphoma. *Am J Dermatopathol.* 2015;37(1):20-25.
290. Quintanilla-Martinez L, Ridaura C, Nagl F, et al. Hydroa vacciniforme-like lymphoma: a chronic EBV+ lymphoproliferative disorder with risk to develop a systemic lymphoma. *Blood.* 2013;122(18):3101-3110.
291. Rodriguez-Pinilla SM, Barrionuevo C, Garcia J, et al. EBV-associated cutaneous NK/T-cell lymphoma: review of a series of 14 cases from Peru in children and young adults. *Am J Surg Pathol.* 2010;34(12):1773-1782.
292. Sangueza M, Plaza JA. Hydroa vacciniforme-like cutaneous T-cell lymphoma: clinicopathologic and immunohistochemical study of 12 cases. *J Am Acad Dermatol.* 2013;69(1):112-119.
293. Beltran BE, Maza I, Moises-Alfaro CB, et al. Thalidomide for the treatment of hydroa vacciniforme-like lymphoma: report of four pediatric cases from Peru. *Am J Hematol.* 2014;89(12):1160-1161.
294. Lysell J, Wiegleb Edstrom D, Linde A, et al. Antiviral therapy in children with hydroa vacciniforme. *Acta Derm Venereol.* 2009;89(4):393-397.
295. Gambichler T, Al-Muhammadi R, Boms S. Immunologically mediated photodermatoses: diagnosis and treatment. *Am J Clin Dermatol.* 2009;10(3):169-180.
296. Chen HH, Hsiao CH, Chiu HC. Hydroa vacciniforme-like primary cutaneous CD8-positive T-cell lymphoma. *Br J Dermatol.* 2002;147(3):587-591.
297. Wu YH, Chen HC, Hsiao PF, Tu MI, Lin YC, Wang TY. Hydroa vacciniforme-like Epstein-Barr virus-associated monoclonal T-lymphoproliferative disorder in a child. *Int J Dermatol.* 2007;46(10):1081-1086.
298. Cho KH, Lee SH, Kim CW, et al. Epstein-Barr virus-associated lymphoproliferative lesions presenting as a hydroa vacciniforme-like eruption: an analysis of six cases. *Br J Dermatol.* 2004;151(2):372-380.
299. Demachi A, Nagata H, Morio T, et al. Characterization of Epstein-Barr virus (EBV)-positive NK cells isolated from hydroa vacciniforme-like eruptions. *Microbiol Immunol.* 2003;47(7):543-552.
300. Morizane S, Suzuki D, Tsuji K, Oono T, Iwatsuki K. The role of CD4 and CD8 cytotoxic T lymphocytes in the formation of viral vesicles. *Br J Dermatol.* 2005;153(5):981-986.
301. Guo N, Chen Y, Wang Y, et al. Clinicopathological categorization of hydroa vacciniforme-like lymphoproliferative disorder: an analysis of prognostic implications and treatment based on 19 cases. *Diagn Pathol.* 2019;14(1):82. doi:10.1186/s13000-019-0859-4
302. Liu Y, Ma C, Wang G, Wang L. Hydroa vacciniforme-like lymphoproliferative disorder: clinicopathologic study of 41 cases. *J Am Acad Dermatol.* 2019;81(2):534-540.
303. Iwatsuki K, Miyake T, Hirai Y, Yamamoto T. Hydroa vacciniforme: a distinctive form of Epstein-Barr virus-associated T-cell lymphoproliferative disorders. *Eur J Dermatol.* 2019;29(1):21-28. doi:10.1684/ejd.2018.3490
304. Zhang Y, Nagata H, Ikeuchi T, et al. Common cytological and cytogenetic features of Epstein-Barr virus (EBV)-positive natural killer (NK) cells and cell lines derived from patients with nasal T/NK-cell lymphomas, chronic active EBV infection and hydroa vacciniforme-like eruptions. *Br J Haematol.* 2003;121(5):805-814.
305. Cohen JI, Manoli I, Dowdell K, et al. *Blood.* Hydroa vacciniforme-like lymphoproliferative disorder: an EBV disease with a low risk of systemic illness in whites. 2019;133(26):2753-2764.
306. Chan JK, Quintanilla-Martinez L, Ferry JA, Peh SC. *Extranodal NK/T-Cell Lymphoma, Nasal Type.* 4th ed. International Agency for Research on Cancer; 2008.
307. Greer JP, Mosse CA. Natural killer-cell neoplasms. *Curr Hematol Malig Rep.* 2009;4(4):245-252.
308. Lima M. Aggressive mature natural killer cell neoplasms: from epidemiology to diagnosis. *Orphanet J Rare Dis.* 2013;8:95.
309. Termuhlen AM. Natural killer/T-cell lymphomas in pediatric and adolescent patients. *Clin Adv Hematol Oncol.* 2017;15(3):200-209.
310. Huang Y, Xie J, Ding Y, Zhou X. Extranodal natural killer/T-cell lymphoma in children and adolescents: a report of 17 cases in China. *Am J Clin Pathol.* 2016;145(1):46-54.
311. Dickson RJ. Radiotherapy of lethal mid-line granuloma. *J Chron Dis.* 1960;12:417-427.
312. Wang G-N, Zhao W-G, Zhang X-D, et al. A retrospective study on the clinicopathological and molecular features of 22 cases of natural killer/T-cell lymphoma in children and adolescents. *Sci Rep.* 2022;12(1):7118. doi:10.1038/s41598-022-11247-z
313. Chan JK, Sin VC, Wong KF, et al. Nonnasal lymphoma expressing the natural killer cell marker CD56: a clinicopathologic study of 49 cases of an uncommon aggressive neoplasm. *Blood.* 1997;89(12):4501-4513.
314. Chim CS, Ma SY, Au WY, et al. Primary nasal natural killer cell lymphoma: long-term treatment outcome and relationship with the International Prognostic Index. *Blood.* 2004;103(1):216-221.
315. Barrionuevo C, Zaharia M, Martinez MT, et al. Extranodal NK/T-cell lymphoma, nasal type: study of clinicopathologic and prognosis factors in a series of 78 cases from Peru. *Appl Immunohistochem Mol Morphol.* 2007;15(1):38-44.
316. Yamaguchi M, Suzuki R, Kwong YL, et al. Phase I study of dexamethasone, methotrexate, ifosfamide, L-asparaginase, and etoposide (SMILE) chemotherapy for advanced-stage, relapsed or refractory extranodal natural killer (NK)/T-cell lymphoma and leukemia. *Cancer Sci.* 2008;99(5):1016-1020.
317. Huang WT, Chang KC, Huang GC, et al. Bone marrow that is positive for Epstein-Barr virus encoded RNA-1 by in situ hybridization is related with a poor prognosis in patients with extranodal natural killer/T-cell lymphoma, nasal type. *Haematologica.* 2005;90(8):1063-1069.
318. Au WY, Weisenburger DD, Intragumtornchai T, et al. Clinical differences between nasal and extranasal natural killer/T-cell lymphoma: a study of 136 cases from the International Peripheral T-Cell Lymphoma Project. *Blood.* 2009;113(17):3931-3937.
319. Wang XM, Xu CG. Diagnostic value of serum levels of BamHI-W, LMP-1 and BZLF1 in NK/T-cell lymphoma. *Zhonghua Xue Ye Xue Za Zhi.* 2013;34(1):36-40.
320. Wang ZY, Liu QF, Wang H, et al. Clinical implications of plasma Epstein-Barr virus DNA in early-stage extranodal

nasal-type NK/T-cell lymphoma patients receiving primary radiotherapy. *Blood.* 2012;120(10):2003-2010.
321. Chan JK. Natural killer cell neoplasms. *Anat Pathol (Chic IL).* 1998;3:77-145.
322. Liang X, Graham DK. Natural killer cell neoplasms. *Cancer.* 2008;112(7):1425-1436.
323. Ohshima K, Suzumiya J, Shimazaki K, et al. Nasal T/NK cell lymphomas commonly express perforin and Fas ligand: important mediators of tissue damage. *Histopathology.* 1997;31(5):444-450.
324. Nagata H, Konno A, Kimura N, et al. Characterization of novel natural killer (NK)-cell and gammadelta T-cell lines established from primary lesions of nasal T/NK-cell lymphomas associated with the Epstein-Barr virus. *Blood.* 2001;97(3):708-713.
325. Kanavaros P, Lescs MC, Briere J, et al. Nasal T-cell lymphoma: a clinicopathologic entity associated with peculiar phenotype and with Epstein-Barr virus. *Blood.* 1993;81(10):2688-2695.
326. Cuadra-Garcia I, Proulx GM, Wu CL, et al. Sinonasal lymphoma: a clinicopathologic analysis of 58 cases from the Massachusetts General Hospital. *Am J Surg Pathol.* 1999;23(11):1356-1369.
327. Hasserjian RP, Harris NL. NK-cell lymphomas and leukemias: a spectrum of tumors with variable manifestations and immunophenotype. *Am J Clin Pathol.* 2007;127(6):860-868.
328. Kuo TT, Shih LY, Tsang NM. Nasal NK/T cell lymphoma in Taiwan: a clinicopathologic study of 22 cases, with analysis of histologic subtypes, Epstein-Barr virus LMP-1 gene association, and treatment modalities. *Int J Surg Pathol.* 2004;12(4):375-387.
329. Swerdlow SH, Jaffe ES, Brousset P, et al. Cytotoxic T-cell and NK-cell lymphomas: current questions and controversies. *Am J Surg Pathol.* 2014;38(10):e60-71.
330. Jhuang JY, Chang ST, Weng SF, et al. Extranodal natural killer/T-cell lymphoma, nasal type in Taiwan: a relatively higher frequency of T-cell lineage and poor survival for extranasal tumors. *Hum Pathol.* 2015;46(2):313-321.
331. Kempf W, Kazakov DV, Broekaert SM, Metze D. Pediatric CD8(+)CD56(+) non-poikilodermatous mycosis fungoides: case report and review of the literature. *Am J Dermatopathol.* 2014;36(7):598-602.
332. Poppe H, Kerstan A, Bockers M, et al. Childhood mycosis fungoides with a CD8+ CD56+ cytotoxic immunophenotype. *J Cutan Pathol.* 2015;42(4):258-264.
333. Nicolae A, Ganapathi KA, Pham TH, et al. EBV-negative aggressive NK-cell leukemia/lymphoma: clinical, pathologic, and genetic features. *Am J Surg Pathol.* 2017;41(1):67-74.
334. Ferrandiz-Pulido C, Lopez-Lerma I, Sabado C, Ferrer B, Pisa S, Garcia-Patos V. Blastic plasmacytoid dendritic cell neoplasm in a child. *J Am Acad Dermatol.* 2012;66(6):e238-240.
335. Jegalian AG, Buxbaum NP, Facchetti F, et al. Blastic plasmacytoid dendritic cell neoplasm in children: diagnostic features and clinical implications. *Haematologica.* 2010;95(11):1873-1879.
336. Isaacson PG, Chott A, Nakamura S, et al. *Extranodal Marginal Zone Lymphoma of Mucosa-Associated Lymphoid Tissue (MALT Lymphoma).* 4th ed. International Agency for Research on Cancer; 2008.
337. Taddesse-Heath L, Pittaluga S, Sorbara L, Bussey M, Raffeld M, Jaffe ES. Marginal zone B-cell lymphoma in children and young adults. *Am J Surg Pathol.* 2003;27(4):522-531.
338. Bomze D, Sprecher E, Goldberg I, Samuelov L, Geller S. Primary cutaneous B-cell lymphomas in children and adolescents: a SEER population-based study. *Clin Lymphoma Myeloma Leuk.* 2021;21(12):e1000-e1005.
339. Kempf W, Kazakov DV, Buechner SA, et al. Primary cutaneous marginal zone lymphoma in children: a report of 3 cases and review of the literature. *Am J Dermatopathol.* 2014;36(8):661-666.
340. Sharon V, Mecca PS, Steinherz PG, Trippett TM, Myskowski PL. Two pediatric cases of primary cutaneous B-cell lymphoma and review of the literature. *Pediatr Dermatol.* 2009;26(1):34-39.
341. Park MY, Jung HJ, Park JE, Kim YC. Pediatric primary cutaneous marginal zone B-cell lymphoma treated with intralesional rituximab. *Eur J Dermatol.* 2010;20(4):533-534.
342. Sroa N, Magro CM. Pediatric primary cutaneous marginal zone lymphoma: in association with chronic antihistamine use. *J Cutan Pathol.* 2006;33 Suppl 2:1-5.
343. Zambrano E, Mejia-Mejia O, Bifulco C, Shin J, Reyes-Mugica M. Extranodal marginal zone B-cell lymphoma/maltoma of the lip in a child: case report and review of cutaneous lymphoid proliferations in childhood. *Int J Surg Pathol.* 2006;14(2):163-169.
344. Amitay-Laish I, Feinmesser M, Ben-Amitai D, et al. Juvenile onset of primary low-grade cutaneous B-cell lymphoma. *Br J Dermatol.* 2009;161(1):140-147.
345. Amitay-Laish I, Tavallaee M, Kim J, et al. Paediatric primary cutaneous marginal zone B-cell lymphoma: does it differ from its adult counterpart?. *Br J Dermatol.* 2017;176(4):1010-1020.
346. Brenner I, Roth S, Puppe B, Wobser M, Rosenwald A, Geissinger E. Primary cutaneous marginal zone lymphomas with plasmacytic differentiation show frequent IgG4 expression. *Mod Pathol.* 2013;26(12):1568-1576.
347. Ghatalia P, Porter J, Wroblewski D, Carlson JA. Primary cutaneous marginal zone lymphoma associated with juxta-articular fibrotic nodules in a teenager. *J Cutan Pathol.* 2013;40(5):477-484.
348. Salama S. Primary cutaneous B-cell lymphoma and lymphoproliferative disorders of skin: current status of pathology and classification. *Am J Clin Pathol.* 2000;114(suppl):S104-S128.
349. De Souza A, Ferry JA, Burghart DR, et al. IgG4 expression in primary cutaneous marginal zone lymphoma: a multicenter study. *Appl Immunohistochem Mol Morphol.* 2018;26(7):462-467.
350. Swerdlow SH. Cutaneous marginal zone lymphomas. *Semin Diagn Pathol.* 2017;34(1):76-84.
351. Streubel B, Lamprecht A, Dierlamm J, et al. T(14;18)(q32;q21) involving IGH and MALT1 is a frequent chromosomal aberration in MALT lymphoma. *Blood.* 2003;101(6):2335-2339.
352. Streubel B, Simonitsch-Klupp I, Mullauer L, et al. Variable frequencies of MALT lymphoma-associated genetic aberrations in MALT lymphomas of different sites. *Leukemia.* 2004;18(10):1722-1726.
353. Streubel B, Vinatzer U, Lamprecht A, Raderer M, Chott A. T(3;14)(p14.1;q32) involving IGH and FOXP1 is a novel recurrent chromosomal aberration in MALT lymphoma. *Leukemia.* 2005;19(4):652-658.
354. Guitart J, Gerami P. Is there a cutaneous variant of marginal zone hyperplasia? *Am J Dermatopathol.* 2008;30(5):494-496.
355. Attygalle AD, Liu H, Shirali S, et al. Atypical marginal zone hyperplasia of mucosa-associated lymphoid tissue: a reactive condition of childhood showing immunoglobulin lambda light-chain restriction. *Blood.* 2004;104(10):3343-3348.
356. Swerdlow SH, Quintanilla-Martinez L, Willemze R, Kinney MC. Cutaneous B-cell lymphoproliferative disorders: report

of the 2011 Society for Hematopathology/European association for Haematopathology workshop. *Am J Clin Pathol.* 2013;139(4):515-535.
357. Boudova L, Kazakov DV, Sima R, et al. Cutaneous lymphoid hyperplasia and other lymphoid infiltrates of the breast nipple: a retrospective clinicopathologic study of fifty-six patients. *Am J Dermatopathol.* 2005;27(5):375-386.
358. Moulonguet I, Hadj-Rabia S, Gounod N, Bodemer C, Fraitag S. Tibial lymphoplasmacytic plaque: a new, illustrative case of a recently and poorly recognized benign lesion in children. *Dermatology.* 2012;225(1):27-30.
359. Senff NJ, Hoefnagel JJ, Jansen PM, et al. Reclassification of 300 primary cutaneous B-Cell lymphomas according to the new WHO-EORTC classification for cutaneous lymphomas: comparison with previous classifications and identification of prognostic markers. *J Clin Oncol.* 2007;25(12):1581-1587.
360. Condarco T, Sagatys E, Prakash AV, Rezania D, Cualing H. Primary cutaneous B-cell lymphoma in a child. *Fetal Pediatr Pathol.* 2008;27(4-5):206-214.
361. Yoshii Y, Kato T, Ono K, et al. Primary cutaneous follicle center lymphoma in a patient with WHIM syndrome. *J Eur Acad Dermatol Venereol.* 2016;30(3):529-530.
362. Ghislanzoni M, Gambini D, Perrone T, Alessi E, Berti E. Primary cutaneous follicular center cell lymphoma of the nose with maxillary sinus involvement in a pediatric patient. *J Am Acad Dermatol.* 2005;52(5 suppl 1):S73-S75.
363. Edmonds N, Hernández-Pérez M, Holsinger M, Gru AA. Primary cutaneous follicle center lymphoma in a 16-year-old girl. *J Cutan Pathol.* 2021;48(5):663-668.
364. Senff NJ, Noordijk EM, Kim YH, et al. European organization for research and treatment of cancer and international Society for cutaneous lymphoma consensus recommendations for the management of cutaneous B-cell lymphomas. *Blood.* 2008;112(5):1600-1609.
365. Bergman R, Kurtin PJ, Gibson LE, Hull PR, Kimlinger TK, Schroeter AL. Clinicopathologic, immunophenotypic, and molecular characterization of primary cutaneous follicular B-cell lymphoma. *Arch Dermatol.* 2001;137(4):432-439.
366. Cerroni L, Arzberger E, Putz B, et al. Primary cutaneous follicle center cell lymphoma with follicular growth pattern. *Blood.* 2000;95(12):3922-3928.
367. Cerroni L, Kerl H. Primary cutaneous follicle center cell lymphoma. *Leuk Lymphoma.* 2001;42(5):891-900.
368. Cerroni L, Kerl H. Cutaneous follicle center cell lymphoma, follicular type. *Am J Dermatopathol.* 2001;23(4):370-373.
369. Berti E, Alessi E, Caputo R. Reticulohistiocytoma of the dorsum (Crosti's disease) and other B-cell lymphomas. *Semin Diagn Pathol.* 1991;8(2):82-90.
370. Berti E, Alessi E, Caputo R, Gianotti R, Delia D, Vezzoni P. Reticulohistiocytoma of the dorsum. *J Am Acad Dermatol.* 1988;19(2 pt 1):259-272.
371. Abdul-Wahab A, Tang SY, Robson A, et al. Chromosomal anomalies in primary cutaneous follicle center cell lymphoma do not portend a poor prognosis. *J Am Acad Dermatol.* 2014;70(6):1010-1020.
372. Streubel B, Scheucher B, Valencak J, et al. Molecular cytogenetic evidence of t(14;18)(IGH;BCL2) in a substantial proportion of primary cutaneous follicle center lymphomas. *Am J Surg Pathol.* 2006;30(4):529-536.
373. Borowitz M, Chan CH. *B Lymphoblastic Leukaemia/lymphoma, Not Otherwise Specified.* 4th ed. International Agency for Research on Cancer; 2008.
374. Hunger SP, Mullighan CG. Acute lymphoblastic leukemia in children. *N Engl J Med.* 2015;373(16):1541-1552.
375. Sander CA, Medeiros LJ, Abruzzo LV, Horak ID, Jaffe ES. Lymphoblastic lymphoma presenting in cutaneous sites. A clinicopathologic analysis of six cases. *J Am Acad Dermatol.* 1991;25(6 pt 1):1023-1031.
376. Kahwash SB, Qualman SJ. Cutaneous lymphoblastic lymphoma in children: report of six cases with precursor B-cell lineage. *Pediatr Dev Pathol.* 2002;5(1):45-53.
377. Boccara O, Laloum-Grynberg E, Jeudy G, et al. Cutaneous B-cell lymphoblastic lymphoma in children: a rare diagnosis. *J Am Acad Dermatol.* 2012;66(1):51-57.
378. Lee WJ, Moon HR, Won CH, et al. Precursor B- or T-lymphoblastic lymphoma presenting with cutaneous involvement: a series of 13 cases including 7 cases of cutaneous T-lymphoblastic lymphoma. *J Am Acad Dermatol.* 2014;70(2):318-325.
379. Ansell LH, Mehta J, Cotliar J. Recurrent aleukemic leukemia cutis in a patient with pre-B-cell acute lymphoblastic leukemia. *J Clin Oncol.* 2013;31(20):e353-355.
380. Hsiao CH, Su IJ. Primary cutaneous pre-B lymphoblastic lymphoma immunohistologically mimics Ewing's sarcoma/primitive neuroectodermal tumor. *J Formos Med Assoc.* 2003;102(3):193-197.
381. Taniguchi S, Hamada T, Kutsuna H, Ishii M. Lymphocytic aleukemic leukemia cutis. *J Am Acad Dermatol.* 1996;35(5 pt 2):849-850.
382. Frontanes A, Montalvo F, Valcarcel M. Congenital leukemia with leukemia cutis: a case report. *Bol Asoc Med P R.* 2012;104(1):52-54.
383. Muljono A, Graf NS, Arbuckle S. Primary cutaneous lymphoblastic lymphoma in children: series of eight cases with review of the literature. *Pathology.* 2009;41(3):223-228.
384. Yang CC, Chen YA, Tsai YL, Shih IH, Chen W. Neoplastic skin lesions of the scalp in children: a retrospective study of 265 cases in Taiwan. *Eur J Dermatol.* 2014;24(1):70-75.
385. Savage NM, Johnson RC, Natkunam Y. The spectrum of lymphoblastic, nodal and extranodal T-cell lymphomas: characteristic features and diagnostic dilemmas. *Hum Pathol.* 2013;44(4):451-471.
386. Inhorn RC, Aster JC, Roach SA, et al. A syndrome of lymphoblastic lymphoma, eosinophilia, and myeloid hyperplasia/malignancy associated with t(8;13)(p11;q11): description of a distinctive clinicopathologic entity. *Blood.* 1995;85(7):1881-1887.
387. Cortelazzo S, Ponzoni M, Ferreri AJ, Hoelzer D. Lymphoblastic lymphoma. *Crit Rev Oncol Hematol.* 2011;79(3):330-343.
388. Koksal Y, Toy H, Talim B, Unal E, Akcoren Z, Cengiz M. Merkel cell carcinoma in a child. *J Pediatr Hematol Oncol.* 2009;31(5):359-361.
389. Marzban S, Geramizadeh B, Farzaneh MR. Merkel cell carcinoma in a 17-year-old boy, report of a highly aggressive fatal case and review of the literature. *Rare Tumors.* 2011;3(3):e34.
390. Isaacs H, Jr. Cutaneous metastases in neonates: a review. *Pediatr Dermatol.* 2011;28(2):85-93.
391. Vanchinathan V, Marinelli EC, Kartha RV, Uzieblo A, Ranchod M, Sundram UN. A malignant cutaneous neuroendocrine tumor with features of Merkel cell carcinoma and differentiating neuroblastoma. *Am J Dermatopathol.* 2009;31(2):193-196.
392. Magro G, Longo FR, Angelico G, Spadola S, Amore FF, Salvatorelli L. Immunohistochemistry as potential diagnostic

pitfall in the most common solid tumors of children and adolescents. *Acta Histochem*. 2015;117(4-5):397-414.
393. Aboutalebi A, Korman JB, Sohani AR, et al. Aleukemic cutaneous myeloid sarcoma. *J Cutan Pathol*. 2013;40(12):996-1005.
394. Desch JK, Smoller BR. The spectrum of cutaneous disease in leukemias. *J Cutan Pathol*. 1993;20(5):407-410.
395. Kaiserling E, Horny HP, Geerts ML, Schmid U. Skin involvement in myelogenous leukemia: morphologic and immunophenotypic heterogeneity of skin infiltrates. *Mod Pathol*. 1994;7(7):771-779.
396. Cho-Vega JH, Medeiros LJ, Prieto VG, Vega F. Leukemia cutis. *Am J Clin Pathol*. 2008;129(1):130-142.
397. Su WP, Buechner SA, Li CY. Clinicopathologic correlations in leukemia cutis. *J Am Acad Dermatol*. 1984;11(1):121-128.
398. Byrd JC, Edenfield WJ, Shields DJ, Dawson NA. Extramedullary myeloid cell tumors in acute nonlymphocytic leukemia: a clinical review. *J Clin Oncol*. 1995;13(7):1800-1816.
399. Bachmeyer C, Turc Y, Fraitag S, Delmer A, Aractingi S. Aleukemic monoblastic leukemia cutis. *Ann Dermatol Venereol*. 2003;130(8-9 pt 1):773-775.
400. Barzilai A, Lyakhovitsky A, Goldberg I, Meytes D, Trau H. Aleukemic monocytic leukemia cutis. *Cutis*. 2002;69(4):301-304.
401. Daoud MS, Snow JL, Gibson LE, Daoud S. Aleukemic monocytic leukemia cutis. *Mayo Clin Proc*. 1996;71(2):166-168.
402. Gil-Mateo MP, Miquel FJ, Piris MA, Sanchez M, Martin-Aragones G. Aleukemic "leukemia cutis" of monocytic lineage. *J Am Acad Dermatol*. 1997;36(5 pt 2):837-840.
403. Hejmadi RK, Thompson D, Shah F, Naresh KN. Cutaneous presentation of aleukemic monoblastic leukemia cutis - a case report and review of literature with focus on immunohistochemistry. *J Cutan Pathol*. 2008;35(suppl 1):46-49.
404. Heskel NS, White CR, Fryberger S, Neerhout RC, Spraker M, Hanifin JM. Aleukemic leukemia cutis: juvenile chronic granulocytic leukemia presenting with figurate cutaneous lesions. *J Am Acad Dermatol*. 1983;9(3):423-427.
405. Imanaka K, Fujiwara K, Satoh K, et al. A case of aleukemic monocytic leukemia cutis treated with total body electron therapy. *Radiat Med*. 1988;6(5):229-231.
406. Kishimoto H, Furui Y, Nishioka K. Guess what. B-cell acute lymphoblastic leukemia with aleukemic leukemia cutis. *Eur J Dermatol*. 2001;11(2):151-152.
407. Iliadis A, Koletsa T, Georgiou E, Patsatsi A, Sotiriadis D, Kostopoulos I. Bilateral aleukemic myeloid sarcoma of the eyelids with indolent course. *Am J Dermatopathol*. 2016;38(4):312-314.
408. Jung HD, Kim HS, Park YM, Kim HO, Lee JY. Multiple granulocytic sarcomas in a patient with longstanding complete remission of acute myelogenous leukemia. *Ann Dermatol*. 2011;23(suppl 2):S270-S273.
409. Zengin N, Kars A, Ozisik Y, Canpinar H, Turker A, Ruacan S. Aleukemic leukemia cutis in a patient with acute lymphoblastic leukemia. *J Am Acad Dermatol*. 1998;38(4):620-621.
410. Tomasini C, Quaglino P, Novelli M, Fierro MT. "Aleukemic" granulomatous leukemia cutis. *Am J Dermatopathol*. 1998;20(4):417-421.
411. Agrawal AK, Guo H, Golden C. Siblings presenting with progressive congenital aleukemic leukemia cutis. *Pediatr Blood Cancer*. 2011;57(2):338-340.
412. Kanegane H, Nomura K, Abe A, et al. Spontaneous regression of aleukemic leukemia cutis harboring a NPM/RARA fusion gene in an infant with cutaneous mastocytosis. *Int J Hematol*. 2009;89(1):86-90.
413. Landers MC, Malempati S, Tilford D, Gatter K, White C, Schroeder TL. Spontaneous regression of aleukemia congenital leukemia cutis. *Pediatr Dermatol*. 2005;22(1):26-30.
414. Gru AA, Coughlin CC, Schapiro ML, et al. Pediatric aleukemic leukemia cutis: report of 3 cases and review of the literature. *Am J Dermatopathol*. 2015;37(6):477-484.
415. Najem N, Zadeh VB, Badawi M, Kumar R, Al-Otaibi S, Al-Abdulrazzaq A. Aleukemic leukemia cutis in a child preceding T-cell acute lymphoblastic leukemia. *Pediatr Dermatol*. 2011;28(5):535-537.
416. Zebisch A, Cerroni L, Beham-Schmid C, Sill H. Therapy-related leukemia cutis: case study of an aggressive disorder. *Ann Hematol*. 2003;82(11):705-707.
417. Otsubo K, Horie S, Nomura K, Miyawaki T, Abe A, Kanegane H. Acute promyelocytic leukemia following aleukemic leukemia cutis harboring NPM/RARA fusion gene. *Pediatr Blood Cancer*. 2012;59(5):959-960.
418. Monpoux F, Lacour JP, Hatchuel Y, et al. Congenital leukemia cutis preceding monoblastic leukemia by 3 months. *Pediatr Dermatol*. 1996;13(6):472-476.
419. Monpoux F, Sirvent N, Sudaka I, Mariani R. Acute congenital monoblastic leukemia and 9;11 translocation: a case. *Pediatrie*. 1992;47(10):691-694.
420. Torrelo A, Madero L, Mediero IG, Bano A, Zambrano A. Aleukemic congenital leukemia cutis. *Pediatr Dermatol*. 2004;21(4):458-461.
421. Bidet A, Dulucq S, Aladjidi N. Transient abnormal myelopoiesis (TAM) in a neonate without Down syndrome. *Br J Haematol*. 2015;168(1):2.
422. Krawczyk J, McDermott M, Irvine AD, O'Marcaigh A, Storey L, Smith O. Skin involvement in down syndrome transient abnormal myelopoiesis. *Br J Haematol*. 2012;157(3):280.
423. Winckworth LC, Chonat S, Uthaya S. Cutaneous lesions in transient abnormal myelopoiesis. *J Paediatr Child Health*. 2012;48(2):184-185.
424. Boggs DR, Wintrobe MM, Cartwright GE. The acute leukemias. Analysis of 322 cases and review of the literature. *Medicine (Baltim)*. 1962;41:163-225.
425. Martinez-Escaname M, Zuriel D, Tee SI, Fried I, Massone C, Cerroni L. Cutaneous infiltrates of acute myelogenous leukemia simulating inflammatory dermatoses. *Am J Dermatopathol*. 2013;35(4):419-424.
426. Cibull TL, Thomas AB, O'Malley DP, Billings SD. Myeloid leukemia cutis: a histologic and immunohistochemical review. *J Cutan Pathol*. 2008;35(2):180-185.
427. Jones D, Dorfman DM, Barnhill RL, Granter SR. Leukemic vasculitis: a feature of leukemia cutis in some patients. *Am J Clin Pathol*. 1997;107(6):637-642.
428. Seckin D, Senol A, Gurbuz O, Demirkesen C. Leukemic vasculitis: an unusual manifestation of leukemia cutis. *J Am Acad Dermatol*. 2009;61(3):519-521.
429. Harris NL, Demirjian Z. Plasmacytoid T-zone cell proliferation in a patient with chronic myelomonocytic leukemia. Histologic and immunohistologic characterization. *Am J Surg Pathol*. 1991;15(1):87-95.
430. Cronin DM, George TI, Sundram UN. An updated approach to the diagnosis of myeloid leukemia cutis. *Am J Clin Pathol*. 2009;132(1):101-110.
431. Amador-Ortiz C, Hurley MY, Ghahramani GK, et al. Use of classic and novel immunohistochemical markers in the

432. Xu B, Naughton D, Busam K, Pulitzer M. ERG is a useful immunohistochemical marker to distinguish leukemia cutis from nonneoplastic leukocytic infiltrates in the skin. *Am J Dermatopathol*. 2016;38(9):672-677.
433. Feuillard J, Jacob MC, Valensi F, et al. Clinical and biologic features of CD4(+)CD56(+) malignancies. *Blood*. 2002;99(5):1556-1563.
434. Meyer N, Petrella T, Poszepczynska-Guigne E, et al. CD4+ CD56+ blastic tumor cells express CD101 molecules. *J Invest Dermatol*. 2005;124(3):668-669.
435. Petrella T, Bagot M, Willemze R, et al. Blastic NK-cell lymphomas (agranular CD4+CD56+ hematodermic neoplasms): a review. *Am J Clin Pathol*. 2005;123(5):662-675.
436. Facchetti F, Jones D, Petrella T. *Blastic Plasmacytoid Dendritic Cell Neoplasm*. 4th ed. International Agency for Research on Cancer; 2008.
437. Chaperot L, Bendriss N, Manches O, et al. Identification of a leukemic counterpart of the plasmacytoid dendritic cells. *Blood*. 2001;97(10):3210-3217.
438. Chaperot L, Perrot I, Jacob MC, et al. Leukemic plasmacytoid dendritic cells share phenotypic and functional features with their normal counterparts. *Eur J Immunol*. 2004;34(2):418-426.
439. Dijkman R, van Doorn R, Szuhai K, Willemze R, Vermeer MH, Tensen CP. Gene-expression profiling and array-based CGH classify CD4+CD56+ hematodermic neoplasm and cutaneous myelomonocytic leukemia as distinct disease entities. *Blood*. 2007;109(4):1720-1727.
440. Marafioti T, Paterson JC, Ballabio E, et al. Novel markers of normal and neoplastic human plasmacytoid dendritic cells. *Blood*. 2008;111(7):3778-3792.
441. Petrella T, Comeau MR, Maynadie M, et al. 'Agranular CD4+ CD56+ hematodermic neoplasm' (blastic NK-cell lymphoma) originates from a population of CD56+ precursor cells related to plasmacytoid monocytes. *Am J Surg Pathol*. 2002;26(7):852-862.
442. Chang SE, Choi HJ, Huh J, et al. A case of primary cutaneous CD56+, TdT+, CD4+, blastic NK-cell lymphoma in a 19-year-old woman. *Am J Dermatopathol*. 2002;24(1):72-75.
443. Eguaras AV, Lo RW, Veloso JD, Tan VG, Enriquez ML, Del Rosario ML. CD4+/CD56+ hematodermic neoplasm – blastic NK cell lymphoma in a 6-year-old child: report of a case and review of literature. *J Pediatr Hematol Oncol*. 2007;29(11):766-769.
444. Julia F, Dalle S, Duru G, et al. Blastic plasmacytoid dendritic cell neoplasms: clinico-immunohistochemical correlations in a series of 91 patients. *Am J Surg Pathol*. 2014;38(5):673-680.
445. Rossi JG, Felice MS, Bernasconi AR, et al. Acute leukemia of dendritic cell lineage in childhood: incidence, biological characteristics and outcome. *Leuk Lymphoma*. 2006;47(4):715-725.
446. Johnson RC, Kim J, Natkunam Y, et al. Myeloid cell nuclear differentiation antigen (MNDA) expression distinguishes extramedullary presentations of myeloid leukemia from blastic plasmacytoid dendritic cell neoplasm. *Am J Surg Pathol*. 2016;40(4):502-509.
447. Jegalian AG, Facchetti F, Jaffe ES. Plasmacytoid dendritic cells: physiologic roles and pathologic states. *Adv Anat Pathol*. 2009;16(6):392-404.
448. Cao Q, Liu F, Niu G, Xue L, Han A. Blastic plasmacytoid dendritic cell neoplasm with EWSR1 gene rearrangement. *J Clin Pathol*. 2014;67(1):90-92.
449. Menezes J, Acquadro F, Wiseman M, et al. Exome sequencing reveals novel and recurrent mutations with clinical impact in blastic plasmacytoid dendritic cell neoplasm. *Leukemia*. 2014;28(4):823-829.
450. Stenzinger A, Endris V, Pfarr N, et al. Targeted ultra-deep sequencing reveals recurrent and mutually exclusive mutations of cancer genes in blastic plasmacytoid dendritic cell neoplasm. *Oncotarget*. 2014;5(15):6404-6413.
451. Sapienza MR, Fuligni F, Agostinelli C, et al. Molecular profiling of blastic plasmacytoid dendritic cell neoplasm reveals a unique pattern and suggests selective sensitivity to NF-kB pathway inhibition. *Leukemia*. 2014;28(8):1606-1616.
452. Fraga GR, Caughron SK. Cutaneous myelofibrosis with JAK2 V617F mutation: metastasis, not merely extramedullary hematopoiesis. *Am J Dermatopathol*. 2010;32(7):727-730.
453. Epps RE, Pittelkow MR, Su WP. TORCH syndrome. *Semin Dermatol*. 1995;14(2):179-186.
454. Hoss DM, McNutt NS. Cutaneous myelofibrosis. *J Cutan Pathol*. 1992;19(3):221-225.
455. Kuo T. Cutaneous extramedullary hematopoiesis presenting as leg ulcers. *J Am Acad Dermatol*. 1981;4(5):592-596.
456. Mizoguchi M, Kawa Y, Minami T, Nakayama H, Mizoguchi H. Cutaneous extramedullary hematopoiesis in myelofibrosis. *J Am Acad Dermatol*. 1990;22(2 pt 2):351-355.

CHAPTER 73

Alopecia in lymphoproliferative disorders

Allen F. Shih, Ali Al-Haseni, and Lynne J. Goldberg

INTRODUCTION

Alopecia is an uncommon presentation in patients with cutaneous lymphoproliferative disorders. If present, it can provide clinicians with insight into the subtype and biology of disease. Several types of alopecia in such patients have been reported (Table 73-1). While patients dealing with cutaneous lymphomas may have debilitating pruritus and disfiguring lesions, it is important to realize that alopecia can be equally disturbing and lead to reduced quality of life.[1]

Here, we review the types of alopecia that can occur in lymphoproliferative diseases, whether primary (due to the disease process itself) or secondary, for example, due to therapeutic interventions. Histopathologic features are included whenever possible, but unfortunately, they are not always reported.

ALOPECIA IN CUTANEOUS T-CELL LYMPHOMA

Mycosis Fungoides and Its Variants

Folliculotropic Mycosis Fungoides

Of all the subsets of mycosis fungoides (MF), alopecia is most commonly observed in folliculotropic mycosis fungoides (FMF). Multiple case series have observed alopecia in anywhere from 33% to 81% of patients with FMF.[2-7] It is commonly appreciated as infiltrated pruritic plaques on the scalp (Fig. 73-1); however, alopecic FMF lesions have been observed in all hair-bearing regions including the eyebrows (Fig. 73-2) and eyelashes,[8] the trunk, and the upper and lower extremities including the axillae.[9] Clinically, hair-bearing areas may be replaced by noninflammatory alopecia areata-like (AA-like) hair loss,[10,11] grouped follicular papules, inflammatory alopecic patches or plaques, or acneiform lesions with comedones and epidermal cysts (Figs. 73-2 and 73-3). In pediatric patients, as in adults, alopecia is a prominent finding in FMF lesions. However, it can be subtle to absent in very young patients.[4]

Histologically, both inflammatory and AA-like alopecia in FMF exhibit perifollicular inflammation with variable infiltration of follicular epithelium by neoplastic lymphocytes (Fig. 73-4). Most lesions show mucin deposition within the follicular epithelium, referred to as follicular mucinosis (FM) (Fig. 73-5).[8,10] A case series of 51 patients with FMF found that 96% had evidence of FM, ranging from focal deposition to lakes of mucin; however, the degree of mucin did not correlate with number of folliculotropic atypical lymphocytes.[8] During disease progression, these patients exhibited a denser dermal infiltrate with complete effacement of hair follicles. Gerami and Guitart[12] described additional histologic patterns of FMF including granulomatous inflammation, cystic and comedonal changes (Fig. 73-6), eosinophilic folliculitis, basaloid folliculolymphoid hyperplasia, pustular changes, interface dermatitis, and an interstitial dermatitis-like pattern.

The alopecia is caused by the destruction of the hair follicle from either mucinous degeneration or dense inflammatory infiltrate.[8] However, not all patients with folliculotropic infiltrates on histology develop alopecia.

Syringotropic Mycosis Fungoides

Syringotropic mycosis fungoides (SMF), considered by the World Health Organization–European Organization for Research and Treatment of Cancer (WHO-EORTC) to be a rare histologic subtype of FMF characterized by prominent perieccrine infiltration with varying degrees of eccrine hyperplasia and folliculotropism (Figs. 73-7 and 73-8), can also present with alopecia (Figs. 73-9 and 73-10).[13] Clinically, lesions of SMF are more commonly found on the trunk and extremities, unlike the predominant head and neck distribution of FMF. Lesions of SMF may present as inflammatory scaly patches and plaques with prominent alopecia,[14] as well as alopecic hypopigmented patches composed of follicular erythematous papules.[15] Marked hypohidrosis has been observed in cases of SMF.[16] Histologically, there is significant overlap between SMF and FMF. The largest case series of SMF reviewed a total of 19 patients and found that 63% had clinical alopecia, and 68% exhibited folliculotropism histologically.[17]

The histological findings in SMF were originally thought to represent a benign inflammatory dermatosis called "syringolymphoid hyperplasia" or "syringolymphoid hyperplasia with alopecia."[15] It is now appreciated that these early cases in the literature are syringotropic variants of MF. However,

TABLE 73-1 Clinical Presentations of Hair Loss in Lymphoproliferative Disorders

Alopecia Areata-like

Mycosis fungoides (MF)
Folliculotropic MF
Subcutaneous panniculitis–like T-cell lymphoma

Inflammatory lesions (patches, plaques, tumors, nodules)

Mycosis fungoides
Erythrodermic MF
Sézary syndrome
Lymphomatoid papulosis
B-cell lymphoma

Follicular papules

Hypopigmented MF
Folliculotropic MF
Syringotropic MF

Alopecia universalis-like

Erythrodermic MF
Sézary syndrome
Ichthyosiform MF

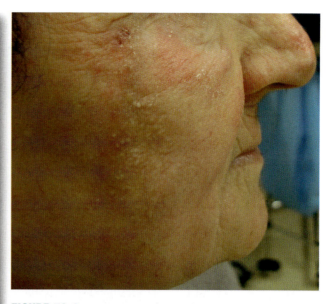

FIGURE 73-2. Scaly plaques, milia, and eyebrow loss in the same patient as in Figure 73-1.

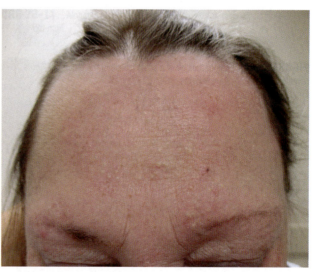

FIGURE 73-3. Eyebrow loss and forehead milia in a 57-year-old woman with follicular mycosis fungoides.

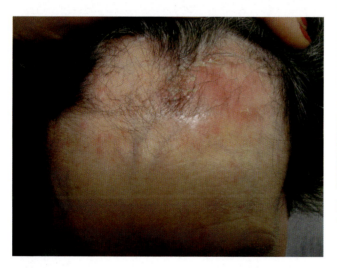

FIGURE 73-1. Scalp alopecia in a 72-year-old woman with follicular mycosis fungoides.

there are isolated case reports of syringolymphoid hyperplasia presenting with similar alopecic patches that are felt to have no histological evidence of cutaneous lymphoma.[18,19] The authors in these cases, and others, have proposed that this entity is a syringotropic variant of FM.[19,20]

Patch, Plaque, and Tumor Stage Mycosis Fungoides

Two patterns of alopecia have been described in patients with MF. Alopecia may be limited to clinically overt patches, plaques, or tumors (Fig. 73-11) or may appear as AA-like patches of hair loss in areas clinically devoid of inflammatory skin changes.[10]

The incidence of alopecia in patch or plaque lesions of MF is unknown. A large retrospective review of 1550 patients by Bi et al, including patients with MF, follicular MF, and Sézary syndrome (SS), identified only six patients with alopecia in patches or plaques in the absence of histological evidence of folliculotropism.[10] Another review of 157 MF patients demonstrated 5 patients with alopecia whose MF was between stage IB and IIB.[21] When MF evolves from patches and plaques to tumors, there is often a loss of epidermotropism and a denser dermal infiltrate with complete effacement of hair follicles.[8,13] Thus, it is reasonable to conclude that alopecia in tumor stage MF is a result of follicular destruction by the lymphocytic infiltrate (Fig. 73-12). The histological findings in alopecic patch and plaque stage MF are not sufficiently characterized to address the mechanism of alopecia in these early stages.

most commonly the result of metastatic breast cancer,[22] one case report identified MF as the cause of alopecia prior to the observation of MF lesions elsewhere.[23]

Erythrodermic Cutaneous T-Cell Lymphoma

Erythrodermic cutaneous T-cell lymphoma consists of three subtypes: SS, erythrodermic MF, and erythrodermic cutaneous T-cell lymphoma, not otherwise defined.[24] Despite their similar histology, alopecia appears to be more common in SS (Fig. 73-13). Small case series have indicated that between 16.5% and 21% of SS patients have alopecia.[25,26] Erythrodermic MF, in the presence or absence of SS, can exhibit patchy alopecia[27,28] or diffuse hair loss with an alopecia universalis-like presentation.[29] Miteva et al described dermatoscopic findings in patients with this pattern of hair loss, which included perifollicular or diffuse scaling, a reduction in follicular orifices, and follicular openings with short, broken hairs or keratotic horny spines.[29] Histologically, these patients had decreased follicular density, absent sebaceous glands, an interface-like epidermotropic lymphoid infiltrate of the follicular epithelium with focal giant cells and FM. Hair follicles were predominately in telogen phase and miniaturized. Several follicular infundibula showed lamellar hyperkeratosis surrounding vellus hairs. The alopecia in these patients may be directly related to the presence of an atypical lymphocytic infiltrate, secondary to FM, or indirectly related, as erythroderma in the absence of cutaneous lymphoma (eg., from pityriasis rubra pilaris) can lead to patchy or diffuse but reversible alopecia.[30,31] In these cases, alopecia may be caused by the effect of the inflammatory cytokine milieu on cycling hair follicles, which triggers anagen hair loss with dystrophic hairs in the acute stage and follicular miniaturization in the chronic stages.[29]

Hypopigmented MF

Hypopigmented MF is a clinical variant of MF that most commonly presents in the pediatric population.[32] Interestingly, alopecia has been observed in a subset of these patients.[33] Clinically, this presents as follicular papules within alopecic lesions of hypopigmented MF (Fig. 73-14). Folliculotropism is seen histologically (Fig. 73-15).[4]

Ichthyosiform MF

Very rarely, patients may present with a diffuse or localized ichthyosiform eruption overlying MF lesions. This uncommon secondary change, reported in less than 20 patients, predominately occurs in folliculotropic MF,[34-36] but has also been reported to occur in patients with patch and plaque MF,[37-40] granulomatous MF,[41] lymphomatoid papulosis (LyP),[42] and anaplastic large cell lymphoma (ALCL).[43,44] Four patients have been reported to have alopecia developed in ichthyosiform MF. Three patients with a diffuse ichthyosiform eruption in the setting of FMF presented with a moth-eaten pattern of patchy alopecia of the scalp and sparse body hair.[35,36,45] In these patients, skin biopsies revealed focal parakeratosis, hyperkeratosis, acanthosis, and a thinned granular layer consistent with ichthyosis, with an underlying atypical lymphocytic infiltrate. The lymphocytic infiltrate displayed folliculotropism in a pattern consistent with FMF. A fourth patient with ichthyosis and granulomatous MF presented with alopecia universalis. Interestingly, his skin biopsy had evidence of folliculotropism along with granulomatous inflammation.[41] It is unclear if this represents FMF with granulomatous change.

Follicular Mucinosis

FM is a controversial disease entity that presents with alopecia in the setting of grouped or coalescing follicular papules forming erythematous, eczematous, or hypopigmented plaques.[46] While FM is defined as an epithelial reaction

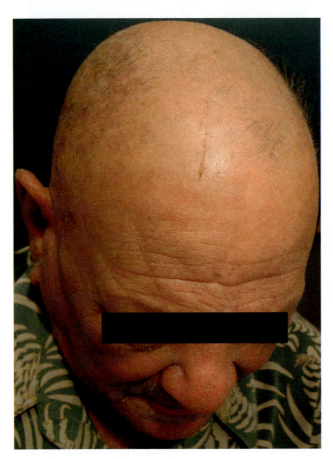

FIGURE 73-13. Scalp and eyebrow loss in a 70-year-old man with Sezary syndrome.

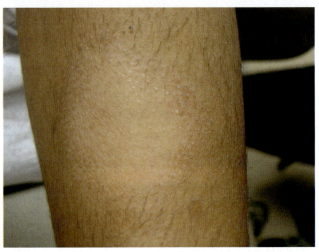

FIGURE 73-14. Hair loss on the leg in a 7-year-old girl with hypopigmented mycosis fungoides.

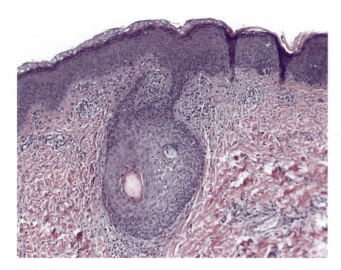

FIGURE 73-15. Histopathology of the patient in Figure 73-14. Careful inspection revealed focal follicular mucinosis (H&E 100×).

TABLE 73-2 Follicular Mucinosis in Lymphoproliferative Disorders

Follicular Mucinosis in Cutaneous Lymphomas and Lymphoproliferative Disorders	Follicular Mucinosis in Systemic Lymphoproliferative Disorders
Follicular mycosis fungoides	Acute lymphoblastic leukemia
Anaplastic large cell lymphoma	Acute myelogenous leukemia
Adult T-cell leukemia/lymphoma	Chronic lymphocytic leukemia
Cutaneous B-cell lymphoma	Chronic myelogenous leukemia
Lymphomatoid papulosis	Chronic myelomonocytic leukemia
	Hodgkin's lymphoma

pattern characterized by the accumulation of mucin within hair follicles,[47] it is included here because it occurs in the setting of two distinct diagnostic entities: a benign idiopathic form and a lymphoma-associated form.[48] Idiopathic FM is commonly observed as a solitary lesion with hair loss. Initially termed alopecia mucinosa, it usually occurs in the head and neck area in pediatric patients and young adults. Lymphoma-associated FM usually presents as multifocal lesions with alopecia in older adults with histologic evidence of MF. A review of patients diagnosed with idiopathic FM and lymphoma-associated FM has identified several overlapping clinical, histologic, and molecular features.[46,48,49] Some hypothesize that idiopathic FM may lie on a clinical spectrum with lymphoma-associated FM and that it represents a solitary variant of MF with a relatively benign course.[50] As such, several reports have demonstrated that idiopathic FM may progress into a cutaneous T-cell lymphoma.

It should be noted that FM can also be found histologically in lesions of folliculotropic MF, in other primary cutaneous lymphomas including adult T-cell leukemia/lymphoma (ATLL),[51-54] in ALCL,[55,56] in LyP,[57] in cutaneous B-cell lymphoma,[58,59] in cutaneous infiltrates of chronic lymphocytic leukemia (CLL),[60] in nonmalignant inflammatory dermatoses (eg, insect bite),[61] and in systemic lymphoproliferative disorders. A list of lymphoproliferative disorders reported to be associated with FM can be found in Table 73-2. Morphologically, patients present with follicular papules or erythematous macules, papules, or nodules.[54] The presence of alopecia within affected lesions in these case reports is poorly characterized.

Interestingly, several reports have identified papular eruptions with histological evidence of FM in the setting of a systemic lymphoma or leukemia, independent of a malignant cutaneous infiltrate. Case reports have described FM in acute myeloblastic leukemia,[62] acute lymphoblastic leukemia,[63] CLL,[64] chronic myelomonocytic leukemia,[65] and Hodgkin's lymphoma (HL).[66-68] In these patients, skin lesions consisted of erythematous follicular papules or erythematous papules, nodules, and plaques on glabrous skin. In contrast to FM associated with MF, alopecia is uncommon in cases associated with non-CTCL malignancies.[33] However, two patients with HL were reported to have patchy hair loss within skin lesions. One patient presented with alopecic scaling plaques with follicular hyperkeratosis on the trunk and extremities.[66] Histologically, the plaques had a moderate lymphocytic infiltrate involving spongiotic hair follicles with associated FM. Another patient had extensive indurated plaques, ulcerated nodules, and "follicular lesions" coalescing to form plaques, similar to lichen spinulosus.[68] This patient had patchy infiltrate composed of histiocytes and eosinophils with ruptured hair follicles, some with FM, and dermal mucinosis, in the absence of a malignant cutaneous infiltrate.

ALOPECIA IN OTHER T-CELL LYMPHOMAS

Other Cutaneous T-Cell Lymphomas

There are several rare types of cutaneous T-cell lymphomas identified by the WHO-EORTC[13] in which alopecia has not been reported (Table 73-3). It is reasonable to consider that inflammatory nodules or tumor stage disease in these entities may have secondary alopecia if lesions occur in hair-bearing areas; however, the presence or absence of alopecia is rarely mentioned in case reports or series. The few reports where alopecia is specifically noted in malignant cutaneous lesions are discussed below.

Subcutaneous Panniculitis–Like T-Cell Lymphoma

Subcutaneous panniculitis–like T-cell lymphoma (SPLTCL) is a rare variant of lymphoma that, as the name suggests, resembles panniculitis. A patient with SPLTCL presented with multifocal erythematous patches of alopecia in the scalp, which resembled alopecia areata, except for the apparent inflammation.[69] Histologically, there was nonspecific "chronic dermal inflammation" and confluent lobular subcutaneous necrosis leading to fibrinoid necrosis of a hair follicle. A second biopsy obtained 1 year later showed a granulomatous panniculitis with confluent necrosis affecting and surrounding hair follicles. The hair loss did not resolve with intralesional steroids. A 3-year-old boy with SPTCL presented with fever, diffuse edema, and rapid-onset total alopecia.[33]

CD30+ Lymphoproliferative Disorders

Many variants of LyP have been described, some of which involve the hair follicle.[57,70] However, clinically most

TABLE 73-3 Cutaneous Lymphomas Not Known to Present With Alopecia

Blastic plasmacytoid dendritic cell neoplasm
Extranodal NK/T-cell lymphoma, nasal type
Primary cutaneous peripheral T-cell lymphoma, unspecified
Primary cutaneous aggressive epidermotropic CD8+ T-cell lymphoma (provisional)
Cutaneous γ/δ T-cell lymphoma (provisional)
Cutaneous B-cell lymphoblastic lymphoma[a]
Cutaneous T-cell lymphoblastic lymphoma[a]

[a]Lymphoblastic lymphoma is not included in the current WHO-EORTC cutaneous lymphoma classification. The World Health Organization classification of tumors of hematopoietic and lymphoid tissue considers it as a secondary tumor involving the skin.

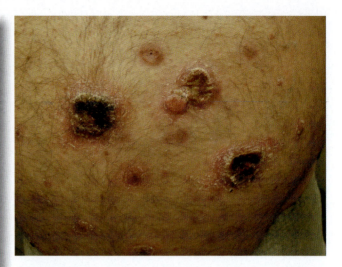

FIGURE 73-16. Hair loss on the abdomen in a 51-year-old man with lymphomatoid papulosis who developed primary cutaneous anaplastic large cell lymphoma.

affected patients do not exhibit alopecia due to the mild nature of folliculotropism in this disorder. A retrospective histologic study identified 11 of 113 patients with LyP with follicular involvement.[57] These patients clinically presented with widespread papules and nodules or a localized nodule (regional LyP). Four were histologic type A (Hodgkin's-like) and six type C (ALCL-like), all with perifollicular infiltrates of CD30+ atypical lymphocytes with variable degree of folliculotropism, FM, and intrafollicular neutrophils. The authors found that LyP lesions in the hair-bearing areas of the face usually present as folliculitis, acneiform papules, follicular pustules, or very rarely appeared as friable, alopecic erythematous papules or nodules. Some have proposed that the follicular variant of LyP be referred to as LyP type F.[71]

Primary cutaneous ALCL may present in hair-bearing regions (Fig. 73-16). In one patient who presented with a nodule on the face, there was histological evidence of folliculotropism and FM associated with follicular disruption.[55]

Adult T-Cell Leukemia/Lymphoma

Patients with ATLL may present with polymorphous skin findings. Several reviews on the cutaneous manifestations of ATLL do not note alopecia despite the fact that histologic studies have found both folliculotropism and FM.[72,73] However, a recent case reports describes alopecia areata in a patient with smoldering ATLL.[74] A histological review of ATLL skin lesions found that 65% displayed folliculotropism and 10% had evidence of FM,[73] which has also been reported in several other case reports.[52-54] In two such cases, patients had erythematous follicular papules on the scalp[54] and on the face and neck.[53] In a Japanese cohort of 124 cases of ATLL, the first skin manifestation in one patient with lymphoma-type ATLL was alopecia; another patient with acute type ATLL first presented with folliculitis.[75]

Primary Cutaneous CD4+ Small to Medium T-Cell Lymphoproliferative Disorder

There are few reports of alopecia associated with primary cutaneous CD4+ small to medium T-cell lymphoproliferative disorder. A 12-year-old girl presented with eyebrow alopecia.[76] Additionally, the authors had one patient with this type of tumor who presented with a large warm, smooth, indurated erythematous plaque on the abdomen that was accompanied by patchy areas of alopecia (Fig. 73-17).

Hepatosplenic T-Cell Lymphoma

There is a single case report of a male patient who was ultimately diagnosed with hepatosplenic T-cell lymphoma who presented with alopecia areata. His hair loss started on the parietotemporal areas of the scalp then progressed rapidly to alopecia universalis within 3 months. It was associated with onychodystrophy of all 20 nails (onycholysis, onychorrhexis, and leukonychia), fever, severe pancytopenia, and hepatosplenomegaly. Skin biopsy from the alopecic patch on the scalp revealed histopathological changes that were consistent with AA.[77]

ALOPECIA IN B-CELL LYMPHOMA

Cutaneous B-Cell Lymphoma

The two most common primary cutaneous B-cell lymphomas, primary cutaneous follicle center lymphoma (PCFCL),

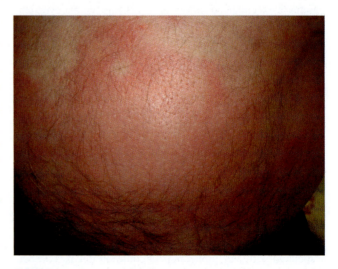

FIGURE 73-17. Hair loss on the abdomen of a patient with primary cutaneous CD4+ small to medium T-cell lymphoproliferative disorder.

and cutaneous marginal zone lymphoma (MZL), can both exhibit hair loss within lesions. Lesions of PCFCL are often located on the scalp, and while MZL has a predilection for the trunk and extremities, lesions also occur in the head and neck.[78] The mechanism of alopecia in these patients is unclear, as the histology of the alopecia is not well characterized. There are four case reports of cutaneous B-cell lymphoma presenting with alopecia. Two were in patients with PCFCL presenting with an AA-like patch,[79-81] one of which appeared following the regression of a PCFCL scalp nodule.[80] The third was in a patient with male pattern hair loss that preceded frontal scalp itching and erythema by 1.5 years. Sequential biopsies showed an inflammatory scarring alopecia with a mixed infiltrate of plasma cells and neutrophils initially and later a proliferation of atypical lymphocytes.[81] The fourth patient had an unspecified cutaneous B-cell lymphoma presenting with an inflammatory alopecic plaque involving the eyebrow.[58] Histologically, this patient had a follicular T-cell infiltrate with FM. As T-cell infiltrates are commonly found in cutaneous B-cell lymphomas, the authors concluded that the follicular infiltrate was composed of reactive T cells.

Seven patients with PCFCL presented with alopecia along with unusual lesions such as erythematous macules. All patients required histology and IgH clonality studies for the diagnosis of lymphoma, which was inapparent clinically. Two patients developed a scarring alopecia.[82]

Systemic B-Cell Lymphoma

Hair loss in patients with systemic B-cell lymphoma (prior to treatment) is extremely rare. Hair loss has been reported to present as FM or as alopecia areata, and could conceivably present within cutaneous metastases of lymphoma.

There are several reports of alopecia areata developing in the setting of HL.[83-88] Patients were young to middle-aged adults and presented with well-circumscribed, round alopecic patches on the scalp or diffuse alopecia in the absence of inflammation. The alopecia started either up to 13 months prior to, or simultaneously with, the development of B symptoms: fever, malaise, and weight loss.[83,84,87] One patient developed alopecia universalis in the setting of polyglandular autoimmune syndrome 3 years after diagnosis and treatment for HL.[86] In these patients, the alopecia areata is likely related to the HL given its temporal association. Another case report described alopecia in a 4-month-old infant with high-grade B cell lymphoma, but did not specify the type of alopecia.[88]

Patients necessitating treatment with multiagent chemotherapy had complete resolution of alopecia. It is unclear whether the alopecia resolved secondary to the immunosuppressive treatment or due to remission of the lymphoma. In one case report, the appearance of AA-like lesions in an ophiasis pattern (band-like hair loss at the posterior scalp margin) appeared 3 months following the completion of multidrug therapy with rituximab, cyclophosphamide, doxorubicin, vincristine, and prednisone (R-CHOP) for the treatment of non-HL. The authors attributed the onset of hair loss to completion of R-CHOP and discontinuing prednisone, which they suspected to be suppressing alopecia areata.[77]

ALOPECIA IN LEUKEMIA

Alopecia secondary to leukemic cutaneous infiltrates is extremely rare and restricted to isolated case reports. One patient with a history of CLL had diffuse erythema, scaling, and near total alopecia of the scalp with sparse patchy areas of hair growth. These findings were thought to be secondary to the leukemic infiltration of the skin and resolved with radiation therapy (RT).[89]

Several patients with CLL have presented with folliculocentric erythematous alopecic papules with clusters of malignant B cells accompanied by an indolent polyclonal folliculotropic T-cell infiltrate on histology.[90] Many have had associated FM. These patients were felt to have pseudo-MF. It is unclear whether the cutaneous neoplastic B-cell infiltrates were present in the skin prior to the development of a folliculotropic infiltrate or if the neoplastic B cells were attracted to the follicular lesions as a result of a "Koebner-like phenomenon."

SECONDARY CAUSES OF ALOPECIA IN LYMPHOPROLIFERATIVE DISORDERS

Alopecia From Treatment of Lymphoproliferative Disease

Chemotherapy

Treatment regimens for lymphoproliferative diseases vary widely, depending on the disease, stage, host factors, and institution, to name just a few variables. Chemotherapeutic agents are often used, and because alopecia is among the most dreaded complications of chemotherapy, a few words about this side effect are in order.

Much of what we know about the mechanisms of chemotherapy-induced alopecia (CIA) comes from animal models.[91-93] It is known that hair matrix keratinocytes have a high proliferation rate and are very sensitive to toxins and drugs. Follicular stem cells and telogen hair follicles are less sensitive due to enhanced DNA repair, expression of inhibitors of apoptosis, and mechanisms to promote transport of drugs out of the cell.[94]

There are two known pathways of CIA in mice.[92] In one, mild-to-moderate damage to the hair follicle induces a "dystrophic anagen" state, whereby the hair shaft is shed and the hair follicle remains in anagen, but there is a long latency until full recovery. In the other pathway, more severe damage to the hair follicle results in "dystrophic catagen," where the hair shaft is likewise shed but the hair follicle cycles into a shortened catagen stage, resulting in a shorter recovery period. Telogen hair shafts have been observed in CIA in humans.[95] Molecular mechanisms of CIA are unknown, but in mice increased levels of proapoptotic proteins (Bax, p53, Fas, c-kit) likely play a role.[96-99]

The estimated incidence of CIA is 65%. It typically begins days to weeks after the onset of chemotherapy, and is complete by 2 to 3 months. The hair loss is often diffuse but can be patchy and is not limited to the scalp. Eyebrows, axillary, and pubic hair can also be affected. On trichoscopy, black dots, yellow dots, exclamation mark hairs, and color and thickness changes along the hair shaft can be present.[100] Biopsies are often not performed because the hair loss is expected and typically temporary, with full regrowth occurring within 6 months after chemotherapy is stopped.[100,101] Patients with persistent or "permanent chemotherapy–induced alopecia (PCIA)," often due to conditioning regimens for bone marrow transplantation and more recently for breast carcinoma, are being increasingly reported.

One study found that CIA was the most common side effect of cancer chemotherapy, and this was more commonly associated with platinum compounds followed by anticancer antibiotic agents, alkylating agents, and taxanes in decreasing order.[102] Another study reported the highest rate with paclitaxel (>80%), followed by doxorubicin (60%-100%), and cyclophosphamide (>60%).[103]

PCIA was described in 1991 in patients with hematologic malignancies who received conditioning chemotherapy regimens prior to bone marrow transplantation.[104] They all received a regimen containing high doses of busulfan and cyclophosphamide. Since then, many additional cases of permanent CIA have been reported, both prior to bone marrow or stem cell transplantation[105-110] and, more recently, with use of taxanes for breast cancer, where 30% of survivors developed persistent alopecia.[100,111-115]

The histopathology of PCIA seen in patients with breast cancer or leukemia resembles nonscarring alopecia. Findings are similar to androgenetic alopecia with reduction in hair density, increase in vellus hair, increase in telogen hairs, retention of sebaceous glands, and absence of significant inflammation or scarring.[111,112,115-118] Changes resembling alopecia areata have been reported with a reduction of terminal hairs and a peribulbar lymphocytic infiltrate.[111,112,118] Perivascular inflammation can occur.[115] The degree of hair loss is variable; a mild decrease in follicular number may be hard to appreciate without the clinical history.

The management of alopecia induced by anticancer therapy is divided into preventive and reactive measures, and is mostly being studied for breast carcinoma and other solid organ tumors. Preventive measures include the use topical minoxidil 2% solution, scalp cooling devices,[100] and recently calcitriol.[119] A randomized trial of 22 patients receiving chemotherapy for breast cancer showed a 50 day reduction in the duration of complete alopecia when topical minoxidil 2% solution was compared with placebo.[120] Scalp cooling devices are the most widely used method for prevention of CIA in solid organ tumors. It is hypothesized that cooling leads to vasoconstriction, reduced drug delivery, decreased follicular uptake of drug, and decreased follicular metabolic activity, all preventing damage to the hair follicle.[100] There is 39% to 66% "hair preservation," with differences between devices likely related to operator experience and types of chemotherapy regimens. However, the use of these devices remains limited due to lack of insurance coverage (as of now they are FDA approved for solid organ tumors only)[100] and resources needed to administer the device during infusion. Topical calcipotriol has shown benefit in a phase I trial.[120] Reactive measures include the use of topical bimatoprost solution 0.03% for the treatment of CIA of eyelashes.[100]

Radiation Therapy

Cutaneous lymphomas, notably MF, are among the most radiosensitive tumors, and as such, ionizing RT is arguably one of the most effective single agent therapies.[121] Radiation-induced alopecia (RIA) is a common complication when the scalp is within the treatment field and is characterized by an anagen effluvium caused by acute damage to actively dividing follicular matrix cells. This can occur during total skin irradiation, total scalp irradiation, or when a local tumor on the scalp is targeted. The development of alopecia is related to the dose of the radiation administered; higher doses of radiation are more likely to cause alopecia. For cutaneous lymphoma, patients often receive a total dose between 20 and 30 Gy, delivered in 1.5 to 2 Gy fractions.[121] Use of higher doses is limited by acute toxicities, including erythema, desquamation, skin edema, bullae, ulceration, hypohidrosis, alopecia, skin pain, nail dystrophy and loss, and agranulocytosis.[121-124] In general, alopecia is reversible if the scalp dose is limited to 25 Gy.[121,122]

Evaluation of acute toxicities of total skin electron beam therapy at 20 Gy found that 100% of patients experienced partial alopecia of the scalp and 20% had alopecia of the eyebrows and eyelashes.[121] Another study found that at 36 Gy, 66% of patients had total scalp alopecia and 56% experienced alopecia of the eyebrows and eyelashes.[122] The alopecia tends to be irreversible when doses of radiation exceed 25 Gy.[125]

Newer techniques pioneered for total scalp irradiation have been achieved by the use of hybrid electron and photon intensity-modulated radiotherapy (IMRT)[123] or brachytherapy.[89] IMRT allows RT to more precisely conform to three-dimensional objects. In a small case series of total scalp irradiation using photon IMRT, two patients with lymphoma, one with MF, and one with cutaneous B cell lymphoma, treatment with a total of 30 Gy caused total scalp alopecia by posttreatment week 4.[123] Treatment-induced alopecia was reversible with full hair regrowth noted 3 months post-treatment. In the patient with cutaneous B-cell lymphoma, a small patch of irreversible hair loss remained, but this was felt to be secondary to the lymphoma and less likely a result of treatment.

The management of RIA includes the use of topical minoxidil 5% solution (after resolution of acute radiation dermatitis).[100] The topical gel APC-400 (Tempol), a nitric oxide radioprotector for the prevention of radiation dermatitis, is in phase Ib trials for evaluation of its efficacy in preventing RIA. Full scalp retention was noted in three of five patients when Tempol gel was applied 15 minutes prior to the RT.[126]

Targeted Therapy

With the advancement of cancer therapeutics and the emergence of many targeted medications, new cutaneous medication side effects are being reported. Among patients receiving such treatment, the calculated incidence of all-grade alopecia is approximately 15%. The underlying mechanism of alopecia is unclear, but it is likely due to blockage of cell growth and survival pathways. It has been shown that dysregulation of the epidermal growth factor receptor (EGFR)-RAS-RAF pathway results in abnormal hair follicle morphogenesis in mice.[100]

Tyrosine kinase inhibitors (TKIs) have been reported to cause diffuse nonscarring or scarring hair loss, resembling alopecia areata and lichen planopilaris, respectively. The most common TKIs associated with alopecia are imatinib and nilotinib; the latter has an alopecia incidence ranging between 8% and 20% after 1-year follow-up. Variable degrees of inflammation are present on biopsy, with histopathologic changes ranging from anagen effluvium to those resembling lichen planopilaris.[101] The long-term toxicity profile of the new TKIs (eg, bosutinib and ponatinib) has not been fully characterized, and therefore, their risk of alopecia is yet to be determined.

Other new targeted medications are associated with alopecia. These include hedgehog pathway inhibitors, BRAF inhibitors, and MEK inhibitors (glasdegib, vemurafenib, and binimetinib, respectively), all being studied in trials for the treatment of various lymphoproliferative diseases. The risk of alopecia is estimated to be 57% in patients on hedgehog pathway inhibitors, 24% with BRAF inhibitors, and 13.3% with MEK inhibitors.[101,127-130] The hair loss in these cases is typically described as diffuse and nonscarring, with a median onset of 3 to 4 months in hedgehog pathway inhibitors, and 3 months in BRAF inhibitors. Histopathology reveals a noninflammatory alopecia with an increased number of telogen and catagen hair follicles.[131]

EGFR inhibitors have been associated mostly with nonscarring hair loss that is similar clinically to androgenetic alopecia, although scarring alopecia has been reported.[100] Biopsies of nonscarring alopecia showed near-equal number of anagen and catagen/telogen hairs, with a superficial and deep perivascular lymphoplasmacytic infiltrate.[132] Scarring alopecia can occur and is likely proportionate to the severity of the perifollicular inflammatory reaction. A biopsy of scarring alopecia in a patient taking the EGFR inhibitor erlotinib showed a mixed perifollicular inflammatory cells infiltrate of neutrophils, lymphocytes, and plasma cells suggestive of erosive pustular dermatosis of the scalp,[133] while another revealed of acute suppurative and destructive folliculitis consistent with folliculitis decalvans.[134] The anti-CD30 monoclonal antibody brentuximab vedotin is associated with diffuse nonscarring alopecia in 14% of patients. Unfortunately, histopathologic findings were not reported.[101,135]

Check-Point Inhibitors (Immunotherapy)

Hair loss presenting as alopecia areata, alopecia universalis, or diffuse nonscarring hair thinning is estimated to affect 1% to 2% of patients receiving immunotherapy.[100,127] This is hypothesized to be secondary to programmed death ligand-1 expression on hair follicle dermal papilla and dermal sheath cup cells, with subsequent activation of the inflammatory response against follicular antigens. Histopathological examination reveals nonscarring alopecia with a periinfundibular lymphocytic infiltrate suggestive of alopecia areata. Treatment of this type of hair loss is mostly reactive and includes the use of topical or intralesional steroids.[100,136,137] Discontinuation of immunotherapy is rarely needed due to hair loss, but it was reported to cause resolution of alopecia in one patient.[137]

Alopecia is a common, dreaded and distressing side effect of therapy for lymphoreticular and other malignancies.[138] As more patients receive targeted and immunotherapy with favorable response, quality of life will play an increased role when making therapeutic decisions. The authors anticipate that the clinical classification and description of histopathologic findings in therapy associated hair loss will take on increasing importance moving forward.

ACKNOWLEDGMENTS

The authors would like to acknowledge Dr. Cecilia Larocca, who coauthored the original chapter on which this chapter is based, and Drs. Debjani Sahni and Dean George for their assistance in obtaining the clinical images.

References

1. Molloy K, Jonak C, Woei-A-Jin FJSH, et al. Characteristics associated with significantly worse quality of life in mycosis fungoides/Sézary syndrome from the prospective cutaneous lymphoma international prognostic index study. *Br J Dermatol*. 2020;182(3):770-779. doi:10.1111/bjd.18089
2. Lehman JS, Cook-Norris RH, Weed BR, et al. Folliculotropic mycosis fungoides: single-center study and systematic review. *Arch Dermatol*. 2010;146:607-613.
3. Gerami P, Rosen S, Kuzel T, et al. Folliculotropic mycosis fungoides: an aggressive variant of cutaneous T-cell lymphoma. *Arch Dermatol*. 2008;144:738-746.
4. Hodak E, Amitay-Laish I, Feinmesser M, et al. Juvenile mycosis fungoides: cutaneous T-cell lymphoma with frequent follicular involvement. *J Am Acad Dermatol*. 2014;70(6):993-1001.
5. Vergier B, Beylot-Barry M, Beylot C, et al. Pilotropic cutaneous T-cell lymphoma without mucinosis. A variant of mycosis fungoides? French Study Group of Cutaneous Lymphomas. *Arch Dermatol*. 1996;132:683-687. doi:10.1001/archderm.132.6.683
6. Wieser I, Wang C, Alberti-Violetti S, et al. Clinical characteristics, risk factors and long-term outcome of 114 patients with folliculotropic mycosis fungoides. *Arch Dermatol Res*. 2017;309(6):453-459. doi:10.1007/s00403-017-1744-1
7. Van Santen S, Roach REJ, Van Doorn R, et al. Clinical staging and prognostic factors in folliculotropic mycosis fungoides. *JAMA Dermatol*. 2016;152(9):992-1000. doi:10.1001/jamadermatol.2016.1597
8. van Doorn R, Scheffer E, Willemze R. Follicular mycosis fungoides, a distinct disease entity with or without associated follicular mucinosis: a clinicopathologic and follow-up study of 51 patients. *Arch Dermatol*. 2002;138(2):191-198.
9. Bakar O, Seçkin D, Demirkesen C, et al. Two clinically unusual cases of folliculotropic mycosis fungoides: one with and the other without syringotropism. *Ann Dermatol*. 2014;26(3):385-391.
10. Bi MY, Curry JL, Christiano AM, et al. The spectrum of hair loss in patients with mycosis fungoides and Sézary syndrome. *J Am Acad Dermatol*. 2011;64(1):53-63.
11. Iorizzo M, El Shabrawi-Caelen L, Vincenzi C, et al. Folliculotropic mycosis fungoides masquerading as alopecia areata. *J Am Acad Dermatol*. 2010;63(2):e50-2.
12. Gerami P, Guitart J. The spectrum of histopathologic and immunohistochemical findings in folliculotropic mycosis fungoides. *Am J Surg Pathol*. 2007;31(9):1430-1438.
13. Willemze R, Jaffe ES, Burg G, et al. WHO-EORTC classification for cutaneous lymphomas. *Blood*. 2005;105:3768-3785.
14. Yost JM, Do TT, Kovalszki K, et al. Two cases of syringotropic cutaneous T-cell lymphoma and review of the literature. *J Am Acad Dermatol*. 2009;61(1):133-138.
15. Jacob R, Scala M, Fung MA. A case of syringotropic cutaneous T-cell lymphoma treated with local radiotherapy. *J Am Acad Dermatol*. 2009;60(1):152-154.

16. Kakizaki A, Fujimura T, Mizuashi M, Watabe A, Kambayashi Y, Aiba S. Successful treatment of syringotropic CD8+ mycosis fungoides accompanied by hypohidrosis with vorinostat and retinoids. *Australas J Dermatol.* 2013;54(4):e82-e84. doi:10.1111/j.1440-0960.2012.00944.x
17. de Masson A, Battistella M, Vignon-Pennamen MD, et al. Syringotropic mycosis fungoides: clinical and histologic features, response to treatment, and outcome in 19 patients. *J Am Acad Dermatol.* 2014;71(5):926-934.
18. Hobbs JL, Chaffins ML, Douglass MC. Syringolymphoid hyperplasia with alopecia: two case reports and review of the literature. *J Am Acad Dermatol.* 2003;49(6):1177-1180.
19. Haller A, Elzubi E, Petzelbauer P. Localized syringolymphoid hyperplasia with alopecia and anhidrosis. *J Am Acad Dermatol.* 2001;45(1):127-130.
20. Echols KF, Bressler L, Armeson K, Maize JC. Syringotropic mycosis fungoides. *Am J Dermatopathol.* 2019;41(11):807-809. doi:10.1097/DAD.0000000000001403
21. Ehsani A, Azizpour A, Noormohammadpoor P, et al. Folliculotropic mycosis fungoides: clinical and histologic features in five patients. *Indian J Dermatol.* 2016;61(5):554-558. doi:10.4103/0019-5154.190124
22. Scheinfeld N. Review of scalp alopecia due to a clinically unapparent or minimally apparent neoplasm (SACUMAN). *Acta Derm Venereol.* 2006;86(5):387-392.
23. Kossard S, White A, Killingsworth M. Basaloid folliculolymphoid hyperplasia with alopecia as an expression of mycosis fungoides (CTCL). *J Cutan Pathol.* 1995;22(5):466-471.
24. Olsen E, Vonderheid E, Pimpinelli N, et al. Revisions to the staging and classification of mycosis fungoides and Sezary syndrome: a proposal of the International Society for Cutaneous Lymphomas (ISCL) and the cutaneous lymphoma task force of the European Organization of Research and Treatment of Cancer (EORTC). *Blood.* 2007;110(6):1713-1722.
25. Kubica AW, Davis MD, Weaver AL, et al. Sézary syndrome: a study of 176 patients at Mayo Clinic. *J Am Acad Dermatol.* 2012;67(6):1189-1199.
26. Booken N, Nicolay JP, Weiss C, et al. Cutaneous tumor cell load correlates with survival in patients with Sézary syndrome. *J Dtsch Dermatol Ges.* 2013;11(1):67-79.
27. Goyal T, Varshney A. A rare presentation of erythrodermic mycosis fungoides. *Cutis* 2012;89(5):229-232, 236.
28. Ah-Weng A, Howatson SR, Goodlad JR, et al. Erythrodermic syringotropic cutaneous T-cell lymphoma. *Br J Dermatol.* 2003;148(2):349-352.
29. Miteva M, El Shabrawi-Caelen L, Fink-Puches R, et al. Alopecia universalis associated with cutaneous T cell lymphoma. *Dermatology.* 2014;229(2):65-69.
30. Pal S, Haroon TS. Erythroderma: a clinico-etiologic study of 90 cases. *Int J Dermatol.* 1998;37(2):104-107.
31. Sigurdsson V, Toonstra J, Hezemans-Boer M, et al. Erythroderma. A clinical and follow-up study of 102 patients, with special emphasis on survival. *J Am Acad Dermatol.* 1996;35(1):53-57.
32. Boulos S, Vaid R, Aladily TN, et al. Clinical presentation, immunopathology, and treatment of juvenile-onset mycosis fungoides: a case series of 34 patients. *J Am Acad Dermatol.* 2014;71(6):1117-1126.
33. Amin SM, Tan T, Guitart J, Colavincenzo M, Gerami P, Yazdan P. CD8+ mycosis fungoides clinically masquerading as alopecia areata. *J Cutan Pathol* 2016;43(12):1179-1182. doi:10.1111/cup.12805
34. Hodak E, Feinmesser M, Segal T, et al. Follicular cutaneous T-cell lymphoma: a clinicopathological study of nine cases. *Br J Dermatol.* 1999;141:315-322.
35. Ryan C, Whittaker S, D'Arcy C, et al. Juvenile folliculotropic and ichthyosiform mycosis fungoides. *Clin Exp Dermatol.* 2009;34(5):e160-162.
36. Zhou Q, Zhu K, Yu H, et al. Ichthyosiform mycosis fungoides with alopecia and atypical membranous nephropathy. *Indian J Dermatol Venereol Leprol.* 2011;77(2):180-183.
37. Hodak E, Amitay L, Feinmesser M, et al. Icthyosiform mycosis fungoides: an atypical variant of cutaneous T cell lymphoma. *J Am Acad Dermatol.* 2004;50:368-374.
38. Marzano AV, Borghi A, Facchetti M, et al. Ichthyosiform mycosis fungoides. *Dermatology.* 2002;204:124-129.
39. Badawy E, D'Incan M, Majjaoui SE, et al. Ichthyosiform mycosis fungoides. *Eur J Dermatol.* 2002;12:594-596.
40. Kütting B, Metze D, Luger TA, et al. Mycosis fungoides presenting as an acquired ichthyosis. *J Am Acad Dermatol.* 1996;34(5 pt 2):887-889.
41. Eisman S, O'Toole EA, Jones A, et al. Granulomatous mycosis fungoides presenting as an acquired ichthyosis. *Clin Exp Dermatol.* 2003;28(2):174-176.
42. Yokote R, Iwatsuki K, Hashizume H, et al. Lymphomatoid papulosis associated with acquired ichthyosis. *J Am Acad Dermatol.* 1994;30(5 pt 2):889-892.
43. Kato N, Yasukawa K, Kimura K, et al. Anaplastic large-cell lymphoma associated with acquired ichthyosis. *J Am Acad Dermatol.* 2000;42(5 pt 2):914-920.
44. Morizane S, Setsu N, Yamamoto T, et al. Ichthyosiform eruptions in association with primary cutaneous T-cell lymphomas. *Br J Dermatol.* 2009;161(1):115-120.
45. Sato M, Sohara M, Kitamura Y, et al. Ichthyosiform mycosis fungoides: report of a case associated with IgA nephropathy. *Dermatology.* 2005;210(4):324-328.
46. Alikhan A, Griffin J, Nguyen N, et al. Pediatric follicular mucinosis: presentation, histopathology, molecular genetics, treatment, and outcomes over an 11-year period at the Mayo Clinic. *Pediatr Dermatol.* 2013;30(2):192-198.
47. Hempstead RW, Ackerman AB. Follicular mucinosis. A reaction pattern in follicular epithelium. *Am J Dermatopathol.* 1985;7(3):245-257.
48. Cerroni L, Fink-Puches R, Bäck B, et al. Follicular mucinosis: a critical reappraisal of clinicopathologic features and association with mycosis fungoides and Sézary syndrome. *Arch Dermatol.* 2002;138(2):182-189.
49. Zvulunov A, Shkalim V, Ben-Amitai D, et al. Clinical and histopathologic spectrum of alopecia mucinosa/follicular mucinosis and its natural history in children. *J Am Acad Dermatol.* 2012;67(6):1174-1181.
50. Santos-Briz A, Cañueto J, García-Dorado J, et al. Pediatric primary follicular mucinosis: further evidence of its relationship with mycosis fungoides. *Pediatr Dermatol.* 2013;30(6):e218-e220.
51. Ballester LY, Cowen EW, Lee CC. Adult T-cell leukemia-lymphoma associated with follicular mucinosis. *Am J Dermatopathol.* 2014;36(11):901-903.
52. Ishida M, Iwai M, Yoshida K, et al. Adult T-cell leukemia/lymphoma accompanying follicular mucinosis: a case report with review of the literature. *Int J Clin Exp Pathol* 2013;6(12):3014-3018. eCollection 2013.
53. Wada T, Yoshinaga E, Oiso N, et al. Adult T-cell leukemia-lymphoma associated with follicular mucinosis. *J Dermatol.* 2009;36(12):638-642.

54. Camp B, Horwitz S, Pulitzer MP. Adult T-cell leukemia/lymphoma with follicular mucinosis: an unusual histopathological finding and a commentary. *J Cutan Pathol.* 2012;39(9):861-865.
55. Bittencourt AL, de Oliveira RF, Santos JB. Primary cutaneous folliculotropic and lymphohistiocytic anaplastic large cell lymphoma. *J Cutan Med Surg.* 2011;15(3):172-176.
56. Kacerovska D, Michal M, Kazakov DV. Pediatric case of primary cutaneous eosinophil-rich CD30⁺ anaplastic large-cell lymphoma with follicular mucinosis. *Am J Dermatopathol.* 2014;36(3):e78-80.
57. Kempf W, Kazakov DV, Baumgartner HP, et al. Follicular lymphomatoid papulosis revisited: a study of 11 cases, with new histopathological findings. *J Am Acad Dermatol.* 2013;68(5):809-816.
58. Benchikhi H, Wechsler J, Rethers L, et al. Cutaneous B-cell lymphoma associated with follicular mucinosis. *J Am Acad Dermatol.* 1995;33(4):673-675.
59. Garrido MC, Riveiro-Falkenbach E, Rodriguez-Peralto JL. Primary cutaneous follicle center lymphoma with follicular mucinosis. *JAMA Dermatol.* 2014;150(8):906-907.
60. di Meo N, Stinco G, Trevisan G. Cutaneous B-cell chronic lymphocytic leukaemia resembling a granulomatous rosacea. *Dermatol Online J.* 2013;19(10):20033.
61. Mir-Bonafé JM, Cañueto J, Fernández-López E, et al. Follicular mucinosis associated with nonlymphoid skin conditions. *Am J Dermatopathol.* 2014;36(9):705-709.
62. Sumner WT, Grichnik JM, Shea CR, et al. Follicular mucinosis as a presenting sign of acute myeloblastic leukemia. *J Am Acad Dermatol.* 1998;38(5 pt 2):803-805.
63. Lee KK, Lee JY, Tsai YM, et al. Follicular mucinosis occurring after bone marrow transplantation in a patient with acute lymphoblastic leukemia. *J Formos Med Assoc.* 2004;103(1):63-66.
64. Rongioletti F, Rebora A. Follicular mucinosis in exaggerated arthropod-bite reactions of patients with chronic lymphocytic leukemia. *J Am Acad Dermatol.* 1999;41(3 pt 1):500.
65. Rashid R, Hymes S. Folliculitis, follicular mucinosis, and papular mucinosis as a presentation of chronic myelomonocytic leukemia. *Dermatol Online J.* 2009;15(5):16.
66. Ramon D, Jorda E, Molina I, et al. Follicular mucinosis and Hodgkin's disease. *Int J Dermatol.* 1992;31(11):791-792.
67. Stewart M, Smoller BR. Follicular mucinosis in Hodgkin's disease: a poor prognostic sign?. *J Am Acad Dermatol.* 1991;24(5 pt 1):784-785.
68. Stankler L, Ewen SW. Hodgkin's disease in a patient with follicular and dermal mucinosis and spontaneous ooze of mucin (mucinorrhoea). *Br J Dermatol.* 1975;93(5):581-586.
69. Török L, Gurbity TP, Kirschner A, et al. Panniculitis-like T-cell lymphoma clinically manifested as alopecia. *Br J Dermatol.* 2002;147(4):785-788.
70. Kato N, Matsue K. Follicular lymphomatoid papulosis. *Am J Dermatopathol.* 1997;19(2):189-196.
71. Kempf W, Kazakov DV, Baumgartner HP, Kutzner H. Follicular lymphomatoid papulosis revisited: a study of 11 cases, with new histopathological findings. *J Am Acad Dermatol.* 2013;68(5):809-816. doi:10.1016/j.jaad.2012.12.952
72. Tokura Y, Sawada Y, Shimauchi T. Skin manifestations of adult T-cell leukemia/lymphoma: clinical, cytological and immunological features. *J Dermatol.* 2014;41(1):19-25.
73. Marchetti MA, Pulitzer MP, Myskowski PL, et al. Cutaneous manifestations of human T-cell lymphotrophic virus type-1-associated adult T-cell leukemia/lymphoma: a single-center, retrospective study. *J Am Acad Dermatol.* 2014;S0190-9622(14)02025-8. doi:10.1016/j.jaad.2014.10.006
74. Takahashi N, Sugaya M, Oka T, Miyagaki T, Sato S. Alopecia areata, thyroiditis and vitiligo vulgaris in a Japanese patient with smoldering type adult T-cell leukemia/lymphoma. *J Dermatol.* 2017;44(4):e79-e80. doi:10.1111/1346-8138.13582
75. Setoyama M, Katahira Y, Kanzaki T. Clinicopathologic analysis of 124 cases of adult T-cell leukemia/lymphoma with cutaneous manifestations: the smouldering type with skin manifestations has a poorer prognosis than previously thought. *J Dermatol.* 1999;26(12):785-790.
76. Volks N, Oschlies I, Cario G, Weichenthal M, Fölster-Holst R. Primary cutaneous CD4⁺ small to medium-size pleomorphic T-cell lymphoma in a 12-year-old girl. *Pediatr Dermatol.* 2013;30(5):595-599. doi:10.1111/pde.12168
77. Ramot Y, Gural A, Zlotogorski A. Alopecia areata as a manifestation of systemic lymphoma: report of two cases. *Ski Appendage Disord.* 2016;2(1-2):63-66. doi:10.1159/000448379
78. Suárez AL, Pulitzer M, Horwitz S, et al. Primary cutaneous B-cell lymphomas: part I. Clinical features, diagnosis, and classification. *J Am Acad Dermatol.* 2013;69(3):329.e1-13.
79. Richmond HM, Lozano A, Jones D, et al. Primary cutaneous follicle center lymphoma associated with alopecia areata. *Clin Lymphoma Myeloma.* 2008;8(2):121-124.
80. Ahmed AA, Almohanna H, Griggs J, Tosti A. Unusual clinical presentation of a primary cutaneous follicle center lymphoma on the scalp of a middle-Aged female: case report and review of the literature. *Skin Appendage Disord.* 2019;5(6):379-385. doi:10.1159/000501174
81. McCrary WJ, Hurst MD, Hiatt KM, Singh ZN, Wirges ML. Acute alopecia with underlying pruritic erythema. *J Am Acad Dermatol.* 2015;73(5):893-894. doi:10.1016/j.jaad.2012.09.021
82. Massone C, Fink-Puches R, Cerroni L. Atypical clinical presentation of primary and secondary cutaneous follicle center lymphoma (FCL) on the head characterized by macular lesions. *J Am Acad Dermatol.* 2016;75(5):1000-1006. doi:10.1016/j.jaad.2016.05.039
83. Garg S, Mishra S, Tondon R, et al. Hodgkin's lymphoma presenting as alopecia. *Int J Trichol.* 2012;4:169-171.
84. Chan PD, Berk MA, Kucuk O, et al. Simultaneously occurring alopecia areata and Hodgkin's lymphoma: complete remission of both diseases with MOPP/ABV chemotherapy. *Med Pediatr Oncol.* 1992;20(4):345-348.
85. Mlczoch L, Attarbaschi A, Dworzak M, et al. Alopecia areata and multifocal bone involvement in a young adult with Hodgkin's disease. *Leuk Lymphoma.* 2005;46(4):623-627.
86. Quintyne KI, Barratt N, O'Donoghue L, et al. Alopecia universalis, hypothyroidism and pituitary hyperplasia: polyglandular autoimmune syndrome III in a patient in remission from treated Hodgkin lymphoma. *BMJ Case Rep.* 2010;2010:bcr1020092335. doi:10.1136/bcr.10.2009.2335
87. Gong J, Lim SW. Alopecia areata as a paraneoplastic syndrome of Hodgkin's lymphoma: a case report. *Mol Clin Oncol.* 2014;2(4):596-598.
88. Albar R, Mahdi M, Alkeraithe F, Almufarriji KN. Epstein-Barr virus associated with high-grade B-cell lymphoma in nude severe combined immunodeficiency. *BMJ Case Rep.* 2019;12(5):e227715. doi:10.1136/bcr-2018-227715
89. Liebmann A, Pohlmann S, Heinicke F, et al. Helmet mold-based surface brachytherapy for homogeneous scalp treatment: a case report. *Strahlenther Onkol.* 2007;183(4):211-214.

90. Ingen-Housz-Oro S, Franck N, Beneton N, et al. Folliculotropic T-cell infiltrates associated with B-cell chronic lymphocytic leukaemia or MALT lymphoma may reveal either true mycosis fungoides or pseudolymphomatous reaction: seven cases and review of the literature. *J Eur Acad Dermatol Venereol.* 2015;29(1):77-85.

91. Hussein AM. Chemotherapy-induced alopecia: new developments. *South Med J.* 1993;86(5):489-496.

92. Paus R, Handjiski B, Eichmuller S, et al. Chemotherapy-induced alopecia in mice. Induction by cyclophosphamide, inhibition by cyclosporine A, and modulation by dexamethasone. *Am J Pathol.* 1994;144:719-734.

93. Hendrix S, Handjiski B, Peters EMJ, et al. A guide to assessing damage response pathways of the hair follicle: lessons from cyclophosphamide-induced alopecia in mice. *J Invest Dermatol.* 2005;125:42-51.

94. Paus R, Haslam IA, Sharov AA, et al. Pathobiology of chemotherapy-induced hair loss. *Lancet Oncol.* 2013;14:e50-59.

95. Bleiker TO, Nicolaou J, Traulsen J, et al. "Atrophic telogen effluvium" from cytotoxic drugs and a randomized controlled trial to investigate the possible protective effect of pretreatment with a topical vitamin D3 analogue in humans. *Br J Dermatol.* 2001;153:103-112.

96. Lindner G, Botchkarev VA, Botchkareva NV, et al. Analysis of apoptosis during hair follicle regression (catagen). *Am J Pathol.* 1997;151:1601-1617.

97. Botchkarev VA, Lomarova RA, Siebenhaar F, et al. p53 is essential for chemotherapy-induced hair loss. *Cancer Res.* 2000;60:5002-5006.

98. Sharov AA, Siebenhaar F, Sharova TY, et al. Fas signaling is involved in the control of hair follicle response to chemotherapy. *Cancer Res.* 2004;62:6266-6270.

99. Sharov AA, Li GZ, Palkina TN, et al. Fas and c-kit are involved in the control of hair follicle melanocyte apoptosis and migration in chemotherapy-induced hair loss. *J Invest Dermatol.* 2003;120:27-35.

100. Freites-Martinez A, Shapiro J, Goldfarb S, et al. Hair disorders in patients with cancer. *J Am Acad Dermatol.* 2019;80(5):1179-1196. doi:10.1016/j.jaad.2018.03.055

101. Belum VR, Marulanda K, Ensslin C, et al. Alopecia in patients treated with molecularly targeted anticancer therapies. *Ann Oncol.* 2015;26(12):2496-2502. doi:10.1093/annonc/mdv390

102. Kaur K, Sood M, Bhagat S, et al. Spontaneous adverse drug reaction monitoring in oncology: our experience. *Indian J Cancer.* 2015;52(3):467. doi:10.4103/0019-509X.176713

103. Salzmann M, Marmé F, Hassel JC. Prophylaxis and management of skin toxicities. *Breast Care.* 2019;14(2):72-77. doi:10.1159/000497232

104. Baker BW, Wilson CL, Davis AL, et al. Busulphan/cyclophosphamide conditioning for bone marrow transplantation may lead to failure of hair regrowth. *Bone Marrow Transplant.* 1991;7:43-47.

105. Ljungman P, Hassan M, Bekassy AN, et al. Busulfan concentration in relation to permanent alopecia in recipients of bone marrow transplants. *Bone Marrow Transplant.* 1995;15:869-871.

106. Tran D, Sinclair RD, Schwarer AP, et al. Permanent alopecia following chemotherapy and bone marrow transplantation. *Australas J Dermatol.* 2000;41:106-108.

107. Tosti A, Piraccini BM, Vincenzi C, et al. Permanent alopecia after busulphan chemotherapy. *Br J Dermatol.* 2005;152:1056-1058.

108. Machado M, Moreb JS, Khan SA. Six cases of permanent alopecia after various conditioning regimens commonly used in hematopoietic stem cell transplantation. *Bone Marrow Transplant.* 2007;40:979-982.

109. Haider M, Hamadah I, Almutawa A. Radiation- and chemotherapy-induced permanent alopecia: case series. *J Cutan Med Surg.* 2013;17(1):55-61.

110. Choi M, Kim MS, Park SY, et al. Clinical characteristics of chemotherapy-induced alopecia in childhood. *J Am Acad Dermatol.* 2014;70(3):499-505.

111. Prevezas C, Matard B, Pinquier L, et al. Irreversible and severe alopecia following docetaxel or paclitaxel cytotoxic therapy for breast cancer. *Br J Dermatol* 2009;160(4):883-885. doi:10.1111/j.1365-2133.2009.09043.x

112. Tallon B, Blanchard E, Goldberg LJ. Permanent chemotherapy-induced alopecia: case report and review of the literature. *J Am Acad Dermatol* 2010;63(2):333-336. doi:10.1016/j.jaad.2009.06.063

113. Palamaras I, Misciali C, Vincenzi C, et al. Permanent chemotherapy-induced alopecia: a review. *J Am Acad Dermatol* 2011;64(3):604-606. doi:10.1016/j.jaad.2010.03.020

114. Miteva M, Misciali C, Fanti PA, et al. Permanent alopecia after systemic chemotherapy: a clinicopathologic study of 10 cases. *Am J Dermatopathol.* 2011;33(4):2011.

115. Kluger N, Jacot W, Frouin E, et al. Permanent scalp alopecia related to breasts cancer chemotherapy by sequential fluorouracil/epirubicin/cyclophosphamide (FEC) and docetaxel: a prospective study of 20 patients. *Ann Oncol* 2012;23(11):2879-2884. doi:10.1093/annonc/mds095

116. Palamaras I, Misciali C, Vincenzi C, Robles WS, Tosti A. Permanent chemotherapy-induced alopecia: a review. *J Am Acad Dermatol.* 2011;64(3):604-606. doi:10.1016/j.jaad.2010.03.020

117. Miteva M, Misciali C, Fanti PA, Vincenzi C, Romanelli P, Tosti A. Permanent alopecia after systemic chemotherapy: a clinicopathological study of 10 cases. *Am J Dermatopathol.* 2011;33(4):345-350. doi:10.1097/DAD.0b013e3181fcfc25

118. Fonia A, Cota C, Setterfield JF, Goldberg LJ, Fenton DA, Stefanato CM. Permanent alopecia in patients with breast cancer after taxane chemotherapy and adjuvant hormonal therapy: clinicopathologic findings in a cohort of 10 patients. *J Am Acad Dermatol.* 2017;76(5):948-957. doi:10.1016/j.jaad.2016.12.027

119. Lacouture ME, Dion H, Ravipaty S, et al. A phase I safety study of topical calcitriol (BPM31543) for the prevention of chemotherapy-induced alopecia. *Breast Cancer Res Treat.* 2020. doi:10.1007/s10549-020-06005-6

120. Duvic M, Lemak NA, Valero V, et al. A randomized trial of minoxidil in chemotherapy-induced alopecia. *J Am Acad Dermatol.* 1996;35(1):74-78. doi:10.1016/S0190-9622(96)90500-9

121. Hoppe RT. Mycosis fungoides: radiation therapy. *Dermatol Ther.* 2003;16(4):347-354.

122. Desai KR, Pezner RD, Lipsett JA, et al. Total skin electron irradiation for mycosis fungoides: relationship between acute toxicities and measured dose at different anatomic sites. *Int J Radiat Oncol Biol Phys.* 1988;15(3):641-645.

123. Ostheimer C, Janich M, Hübsch P, et al. The treatment of extensive scalp lesions using coplanar and non-coplanar photon IMRT: a single institution experience. *Radiat Oncol.* 2014;9:82.

124. Lloyd S, Chen Z, Foss FM, et al. Acute toxicity and risk of infection during total skin electron beam therapy for mycosis fungoides. *J Am Acad Dermatol.* 2013;69(4):537-543.

125. Chowdhary M, Chhabra AM, Kharod S, Marwaha G. Total skin electron beam therapy in the treatment of mycosis fungoides: a review of conventional and low-dose regimens. *Clin Lymphoma, Myeloma & Leukemia.* 2016;16(12):662-671. doi:10.1016/j.clml.2016.08.019
126. Metz JM, Smith D, Mick R, et al. A phase I study of topical tempol for the prevention of alopecia induced by whole brain radiotherapy. *Clin Cancer Res.* 2004;10(19):6411-6417. doi:10.1158/1078-0432.CCR-04-0658
127. Lacouture M, Sibaud V. Toxic side effects of targeted therapies and immunotherapies affecting the skin, oral mucosa, hair, and nails. *Am J Clin Dermatol.* 2018;19(Suppl 1):31-39. doi:10.1007/s40257-018-0384-3
128. Couban S, Benevolo G, Donnellan W, et al. A phase Ib study to assess the efficacy and safety of vismodegib in combination with ruxolitinib in patients with intermediate- or high-risk myelofibrosis. *J Hematol Oncol.* 2018;11(1). doi:10.1186/s13045-018-0661-x
129. Gerds AT, Tauchi T, Ritchie E, et al. Phase 1/2 trial of glasdegib in patients with primary or secondary myelofibrosis previously treated with ruxolitinib. *Leuk Res.* 2019;79:38-44. doi:10.1016/j.leukres.2019.02.012
130. Marconato L, Aresu L, Stefanello D, et al. Opportunities and challenges of active immunotherapy in dogs with B-cell lymphoma: a 5-year experience in two veterinary oncology centers. *J Immunother Cancer.* 2019;7. doi:10.1186/s40425-019-0624-y
131. Piraccini BM, Patrizi A, Fanti PA, et al. RASopathic alopecia: hair changes associated with vemurafenib therapy. *J Am Acad Dermatol.* 2015;72(4):738-741. doi:10.1016/j.jaad.2015.01.011
132. Pongpudpunth M, Demierre MF, Goldberg LJ. A case report of inflammatory nonscarring alopecia associated with the epidermal growth factor receptor inhibitor erlotinib. *J Cutan Pathol.* 2009;36(12):1303-1307. doi:10.1111/j.1600-0560.2009.01275.x
133. Toda N, Fujimoto N, Kato T, et al. Erosive pustular dermatosis of the scalp-like eruption due to gefitinib: case report and review of the literature of alopecia associated with EGFR inhibitors. *Dermatology.* 2012;225(1):18-21. doi:10.1159/000341528
134. Dervout C, Chiappa AM, Fleuret C, Plantin P, Acquitter M. Erlotinib-induced scarring alopecia with a folliculitis decalvans-like presentation. *Ann Dermatol Venereol.* 2020;147(12):848-852. doi:10.1016/j.annder.2020.08.043
135. Pileri A, Starace M, Alessandrini A, Casadei B, Zinzani PL, Piraccini BM. New therapies and old side-effects in mycosis fungoides treatment: brentuximab vedotin-induced alopecia. *Br J Dermatol.* 2019;180(6):1535-1536. doi:10.1111/bjd.17533
136. Wang X, Marr AK, Breitkopf T, et al. Hair follicle mesenchyme-associated PD-L1 regulates T-cell activation induced apoptosis: a potential mechanism of immune privilege. *J Invest Dermatol.* 2014;134(3):736-745. doi:10.1038/jid.2013.368
137. Zarbo A, Belum VR, Sibaud V, et al. Immune-related alopecia (areata and universalis) in cancer patients receiving immune checkpoint inhibitors. *Br J Dermatol.* 2017;176(6):1649-1652. doi:10.1111/bjd.15237
138. Chon SY, Champion RW, Geddes ER, et al. Chemotherapy-induced alopecia. *J Am Acad Dermatol.* 2012;67:e37-47.

CHAPTER 74

Cutaneous adverse reactions to chemotherapeutic agents

Jacob Nosewicz, Brittany O. Dulmage, Jose A. Plaza, and Benjamin H. Kaffenberger

REACTIONS TO CHEMOTHERAPEUTIC REGIMENS

Advances in cancer therapy have given rise to a multitude of treatment-related self-limiting or life-threatening mucocutaneous side effects, which can mimic unrelated cutaneous disorders. Knowledge of the clinical presentation, histopathology, and therapy for these reactions is essential in their management, especially when aiming to provide uninterrupted care. A wide variety of chemotherapy drugs are used to target hematologic malignancies. The most common regimens and their mucocutaneous adverse reactions are discussed in this chapter, and they are organized by the disease treated.

ACUTE LEUKEMIAS

Acute lymphoblastic leukemias (ALLs) are the most common malignancy in children, making up about 30% of neoplasms in this age group.[1] ALL presents about five times more often than its counterpart, acute myeloid leukemia (AML). These malignancies are also well represented in the adolescent age group, making up about 12% of new cancer cases per year,[1] although incidence rate of AML tends to increase with age, while ALL peaks in early childhood.[2]

In the treatment of these disorders, antileukemic therapies target rapidly dividing cells. As a result, other rapidly dividing areas, such as the skin and mucosa, are also commonly affected. This section reviews targeted and cytotoxic therapies by class, commonly used in the induction, consolidation, and maintenance phases of these diseases.

Anthracyclines

Anthracyclines have been widely utilized as antineoplastic agents for systemic malignancy since their isolation from the *Streptomyces* genus in the 1960s. These drugs work by intercalating between base pairs during DNA replication, ceasing further mitotic activity, as well as producing cytotoxic free oxygen radicals that disrupt cell membranes and other vital structures. In the treatment of ALL and AML, daunorubicin, doxorubicin, and idarubicin are commonly used, especially in the induction and consolidation phases. The polyethylene glycol–coated (pegylated) liposomal form of doxorubicin appears to be associated with a lower incidence of significant side effects, such as cardiotoxicity,[3] as it concentrates in tumor tissue.[4]

Liposomal doxorubicin has increased longevity in the circulation, which enhances its cutaneous deposition and side effects.[5,6] Two such reactions include the clinically similar but morphologically and regionally distinct palmar–plantar erythrodysesthesia (PPE) syndrome and malignant intertrigo (Fig. 74-1). These syndromes may represent a host-versus-altered-host reaction, as natural killer (NK) cells and cytotoxic T cells are less susceptible to anthracyclines, and implementation of such regimens may result in an increased number of typically suppressed autoreactive lymphocytes.[7] Furthermore, the locations of involvement suggest that the damage may be more prevalent in areas with high sweat duct density (palms and soles) or areas where occluded sweat cannot evaporate efficiently, such as in the skin folds.

PPE has an incidence between 20%[8] and 29%[9] in patients taking liposomal doxorubicin. PPE displays vacuolar necrosis of basal keratinocytes with mild spongiosis and scattered dyskeratotic keratinocytes.[10] Intertrigo-like eruptions, on the other hand, are typically associated with bacterial[11] or fungal[12] infiltrate with neutrophils, as well as an interface dermatitis and dysmaturation of the overlying epidermis. Ischemia of the eccrine coils may trigger squamous syringometaplasia (Fig. 74-2).[11,13] The microbial component is often secondary to maceration. Treatment is generally supportive, although application of ice packs has been proven as an efficacious strategy for the treatment or prophylaxis of PPE.[14] Short-term corticosteroids with topical corticosteroids[15] and pyridoxine supplementation with antioxidant vitamins[12,16] have also been useful in reducing the severity of both PPE and intertrigo-like erosions.

Doxorubicin is well known for causing a vesicant chemical cellulitis, occurring in 2%[17] to 5%[18] of patients. This presents initially with erythematous, burning lesions that progress to vesicles about intravenous or other access sites. Histopathology demonstrates epidermal hyperplasia and ulceration with ischemic changes in the epidermis and dermis that may spread to deeper structures. Focal lymphocytic

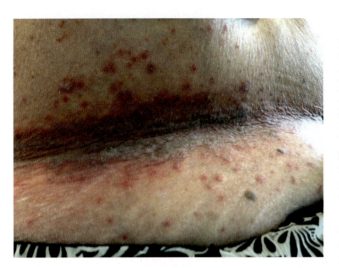

FIGURE 74-1. Malignant intertrigo in the setting of induction chemotherapy using doxorubicin. There is an erythematous maculopapular eruption in the intertriginous areas.

satellitosis may also be present.[19] Areas of necrosis are typically debrided, while rescue therapy includes dexrazoxane.[20] Intralesional granulocyte–macrophage colony-stimulating factor has also shown potential benefits in recovery after extravasation injuries,[20] while cold compresses and corticosteroids may be added to doxorubicin recovery but are contraindicated with vinca alkaloid extravasations.[21]

Anagen effluvium is another toxicity commonly associated with the anthracyclines, and doxorubicin in particular. It typically occurs about 5 to 30 days after initiation of therapy.[17,22-24] In animal models, alopecia is preceded by reduction in size of sebocytes with depleted secretory granules. Increased apoptosis of sebocytes leads to apoptosis of connective tissue sheath and matrix cells.[22] Also, dose-related stomatitis presents after 1 to 2 weeks of treatment[25] in 11% to 70% of cases.[18,23,26] Both of these conditions are self-limiting, reversible, and typically treated with supportive therapy. No reduction in dosage is usually required. The patient may also experience acute hypersensitivity reactions, typically type I, which require discontinuation of therapy.[27,28]

Neutrophilic eccrine hidradenitis (NEH) is another rare side effect of these medications, which may trigger subsequent reduction or cessation of dosing.[29,30] NEH is characterized by neutrophilic infiltration around eccrine glands in the dermis leading to necrosis of the eccrine cells (Figs. 74-3 and 74-4). In some cases, there is direct extension of the neutrophils to the sweat gland epithelium.

Chromonychia with transverse bands of white and brown coloring due to dysfunction of the nail plate[31] is also associated with anthracyclines. Onycholysis with associated pain has also been seen in conjunction with doxorubicin therapy.[32-34] It appeared to be reversible with cessation of successful chemotherapy,[32] and it may correlate with zinc deficiency.[33]

Radiation recall dermatitis presenting with erythematous desquamation at sites of prior radiotherapy can be also seen

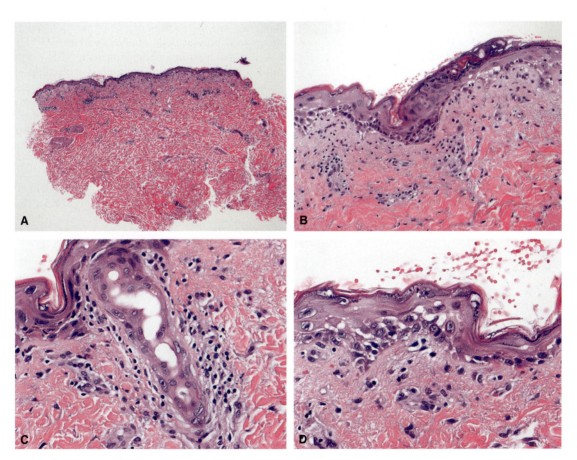

FIGURE 74-2. Malignant intertrigo. A–D. Vacuolar interface changes with dyskeratotic cells and focal squamous syringometaplasia (400×).

in patients receiving doxorubicin. The histopathology often overlaps with acute radiation dermatitis. Other features might include interface reaction (lymphocytic exocytosis, basal vacuolization, apoptotic or necrotic keratinocytes), psoriasiform acanthosis, or follicular hyperkeratosis. At times, the vacuolar degeneration is so conspicuous that a subepidermal vesiculation can be seen. Inflammatory cells are typically mixed populations of neutrophils, lymphocytes, eosinophils, and plasma cells in a perivascular and interstitial distribution. The dermis might show vascular dilatation and endothelial atypia. The subcutis is typically unaffected.[35] Treatment is generally supportive without any need for corticosteroids, and the lesion tends to resolve over a month's time.[35,36]

Oral cavity squamous cell carcinomas (SCCs) also seem to be correlated with a history of prolonged pegylated liposomal doxorubicin use, notably in middle-aged patients with no history of alcohol or tobacco exposure.[37-40] This may be secondary to an increased exposure of the mucous membranes to the chemotherapeutic agent because of its increased duration within the vasculature.[41] Treatment includes excision and subsequent routine oral examinations.

Hyperpigmentation, generalized or on the digits and nail beds, is also commonly associated with doxorubicin.[42] The mechanism seems to be secondary to an undiscovered direct stimulation of melanocytes themselves[43] rather than excessive melanocyte-stimulating hormone from the pituitary.[44] The nails may appear diffusely discolored with some longitudinal banding, and this abnormal nail pigmentation appears to be more common in the black population.[45] There have been reported cases of discoloration of mucosal surfaces during treatment as well.[42,46] Histopathologically, these lesions have an increase in melanophages in the lamina propria with increased melanin throughout the mucosal epithelium.[42] The hyperpigmentation does not require additional therapy, and it tends to subside after the therapy has been discontinued.

Antimetabolites

Antimetabolites block DNA synthesis as nucleoside analogs. They include cytarabine, a drug used for consolidation therapy in AML and ALL, as well as 6-mercaptopurine (6MP) and methotrexate (MTX), which are often used simultaneously as a maintenance therapy in ALL. MTX is occasionally used for consolidation therapy as well.

Cytarabine

Cytarabine, a purine analog, has cutaneous side effects that are dose dependent and become more prevalent with an increased duration of therapy.[47,48] In one study, 53% of patients treated with high-dose cytarabine demonstrated cutaneous eruptions in response to the therapy, most commonly either a mild acral erythema or transient morbilliform eruption in about 40% of cases.[47] It should be noted that moderate-to-severe cases of cytarabine-induced acral erythema may present with a bullous variant.[47,49-53] Cytarabine has also had a strong association with NEH.[54-56] NEH and mild acral erythema may be treated with supportive care without any alterations in therapy, as they should resolve spontaneously,[55] while severe acral erythema may need a dose reduction for the patient's benefit.[57] Cytarabine may also cause inflamed seborrheic keratoses termed the pseudosign of Leser–Trelat,[58,59] as well as hypersensitivity reactions.[60] It has also rarely been mentioned with toxic epidermal necrolysis (TEN),[61] evident by a necrotic epidermis.

Another important dermatologic side effect of cytarabine therapy is papular purpuric eruption (Fig. 74-5). Thrombotic

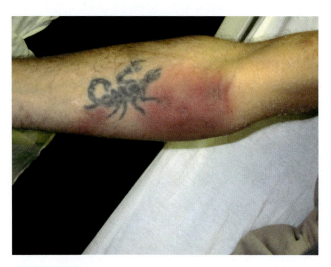

FIGURE 74-3. NEH secondary to doxorubicin manifested by a prominent erythematous plaque on the forearm.

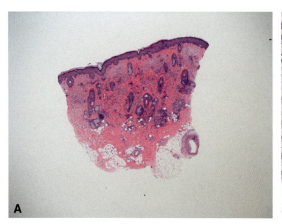
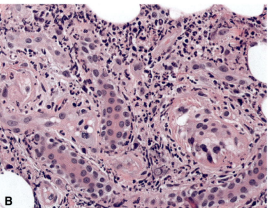

FIGURE 74-4. **NEH secondary to doxorubicin. A.** Perivascular and periadnexal inflammatory infiltrate in the superficial and deep reticular dermis. **B.** Neutrophils extend into and around adnexal structures. Focal necrosis within the eccrine duct epithelium is present.

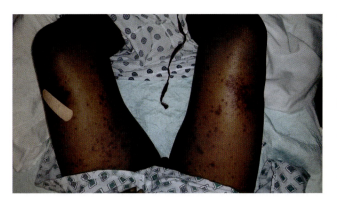

FIGURE 74-5. Papular purpuric eruption from cytarabine.

thrombocytopenic purpura has been reported in connection to intense consolidation therapy for AML. Cytarabine likely damages the vascular endothelium causing blockage with eosinophilic material and swelling of the endothelium[62] along with fibrinoid necrosis of the vessel walls with perivascular myxoid degeneration.[63] This results in petechiae and sometimes palpable purpura of the skin (Fig. 74-6). Despite the palpable purpura, the papular purpuric eruption is not a leukocytoclastic vasculitis (LCV). Treatment of these skin lesions consists of steroids, plasma exchange, and rituximab, but interestingly, future use of cytarabine is not contraindicated. Conversely, cytarabine can also cause palpable purpura in conjunction with other manifestations of Henoch–Schönlein purpura. The purpura results from vasculitis that histologically shows superficial perivascular neutrophils with prominent leukocytoclasia along with fibrinoid necrosis of the involved venules.[64] If these lesions occur, cytarabine will likely have to be discontinued, and the vasculitis can be treated with corticosteroids.

Methotrexate/6-Mercaptopurine

This regimen is most commonly associated with mucositis as a side effect.[65-68] 6MP is less commonly associated with acral erythema,[69] enhancement of radiation therapy,[70] and photo-onycholysis associated with chemotherapy-induced pellagra, which typically presents two or more weeks after initiation of 6MP treatment.[71,72]

Methotrexate

MTX, due to its role as an irreversible dihydrofolate reductase inhibitor, affects all rapidly proliferating cells, causing an array of clinical side effects in a dose-dependent manner.[73] Its toxicity also seems to arise from a long elimination half-life.[74] Progressive alopecia[75] and mucositis[74,76,77] top the list of appreciable cutaneous disorders. An uncommon but significant finding with MTX chemotherapy is the reactivation of previous solar erythema,[78-80] which typically presents 48 hours after receiving MTX.[78] The prior solar burns are usually recent, and leucovorin rescue has not been found to ameliorate the issue.[80] In patients with recent solar burns, it is recommended that MTX therapy be started about 1 week after the effects subside.[78] Its use should be reconsidered if paired concomitantly with either recreational or therapeutic ultraviolet (UV) light exposure.[79]

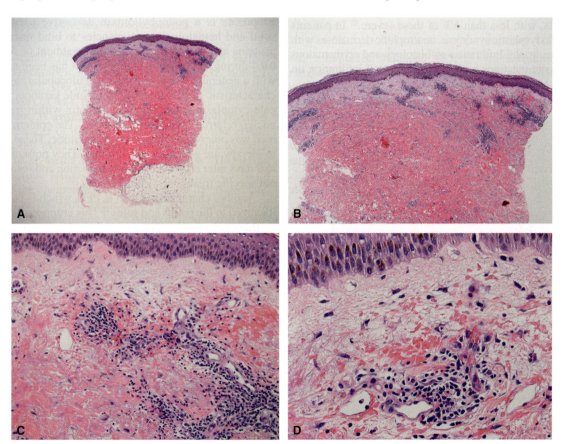

FIGURE 74-6. Papular purpuric eruption from cytarabine. A and **B.** Superficial perivascular lymphocytic infiltrates. **C** and **D.** Red blood cell extravasation in the superficial dermis without definitive vasculitis.

These ulcerations should be distinguished from acute febrile neutrophilic dermatosis, or Sweet syndrome (Figs. 74-9 and 74-10), which may also be induced by ATRA. The classic triad of Sweet syndrome includes tender, erythematous plaques or papular vesicles, fever, and leukocytosis with neutrophilia.[131] Histology shows dermal neutrophilic infiltrates and papillary dermal edema without vasculitis.[132,133] Exclusion of infectious agents by histopathology and tissue culture is a prerequisite for final diagnosis. The pathogenesis of Sweet syndrome is not well understood, although it is believed to be secondary to exogenous induction of cytokine production with a resultant promotion of neutrophilic activation and invasion.[134] Dexamethasone or prednisone therapy results in rapid resolution of lesions.[132,133] Repeat ATRA treatments in AML patients with prior reactions do not seem to induce recurrences of Sweet syndrome.[135]

Cheilitis is one of the more common mucocutaneous toxicities of ATRA treatment, presenting in 73%[136] to 93%[137] of patients, although it is typically minor in severity and treated symptomatically. One study described the rare progression to gangrenous cheilitis, presenting as painful black eschars about the lips.[138] It appears to be secondary to the infiltration of tissue destructive neutrophils, similar to what is seen in scrotal ulcerations. The histologic features exhibit neutrophilic infiltrates with or without vasculitis, as well as a lack of microbial etiology. This condition tends to heal slowly over months and typically does not necessitate cessation of ATRA therapy.[138]

Targeted Inhibitors

Glasdegib

Glasdegib is a small molecule inhibitor of the smoothened receptor in the hedgehog signaling pathway. Glasdegib, in combination with low-dose cytarabine (LDAC), improves overall survival in AML patients not suitable for intensive chemotherapy.[139] Exposure to hedgehog pathway inhibitors is associated with rash and diffuse hair shedding which can persist after cessation of therapy.[139-143]

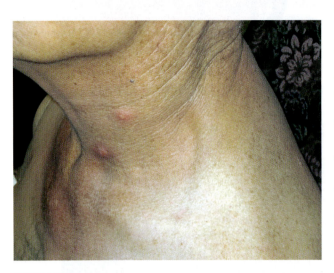

FIGURE 74-9. **ATRA-induced Sweet syndrome.** Dermal inflamed nodules in the neck and the trunk in a patient undergoing induction chemotherapy for APL.

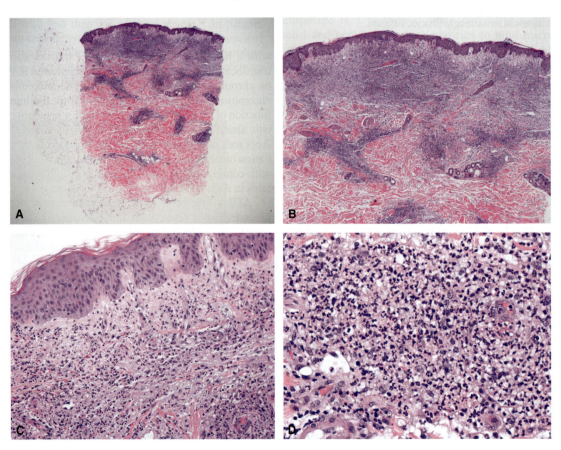

FIGURE 74-10. **ATRA-induced Sweet syndrome.** Diffuse dermal infiltrate composed of neutrophils and leukocytoclastic nuclear debris. Prominent superficial dermal edema is also noted (**A–D**).

Venetoclax

Venetoclax is a small molecule inhibitor of the B-cell chronic lymphocytic leukemia (CLL)/lymphoma 2 (BCL-2) family of proteins. BCL-2 proteins bind proapoptotic proteins; inhibition of BCL-2 by venetoclax displaces proapoptotic proteins and induces apoptosis.[144] Combination therapy with venetoclax and LDAC increases overall survival in AML patients ineligible for induction chemotherapy.[145,146] Cutaneous adverse events in patients with CLL include rash and disseminated herpes zoster.[147,148]

Ivosidenib

Ivosidenib is a small molecule inhibitor of isocitrate-dehydrogenase 1 (IDH1). The IDH1 enzyme catalyzes the oxidative decarboxylation of isocitrate to a-ketoglutarate (a-KG) in the Krebs cycle. The mutant *IDH1* gene is found in 6% to 16% of patients with AML and confers a worse prognosis compared to AML patients with wild type *IDH1*.[149,150] Mutant IDH1 enzymes harbor a gain-of-function ability to reduce a-KG to 2-hydroxyglutarate (2HG). In turn, increased cellular levels of 2HG inhibit a-KG-dependent enzymes required for proper DNA methylation and differentiation.[150] Ivosidenib is efficacious in elderly adult patients with relapsed/refractory AML and *IDH1* mutations and adult patients with newly diagnosed AML and *IDH1* mutations.[151,152] Drug rash is reported in 26% of patients exposed to ivosidenib.[153]

Duvelisib

Duvelisib is an oral small molecule inhibitor of the gamma and delta isoforms of phosphoinositide 3-kinase (PI3K). PI3K signaling promotes B-cell growth and survival in hematologic malignancies.[154] Duvelisib increases progression-free survival in patients with relapsed/refractory CLL/small lymphocytic lymphoma compared with ofatumumab.[154] Cutaneous adverse events associated with duvelisib exposure include erythematous or maculopapular rash, exfoliative dermatitis, toxic skin eruption, and allergic dermatitis.[155] Drug rash has been reported in 41% of patients exposed to combination therapy duvelisib with either rituximab or rituximab and bendamustine.[156]

Multi-Targeted Protein Kinase Inhibitors

Midostaurin

Midostaurin is a first in class multitargeted protein kinase inhibitor that targets the fms-related tyrosine kinase 3 (FLT3) protein. FLT3 is a cytokine receptor tyrosine kinase that regulates the proliferation and differentiation of early hematopoietic progenitor and stem cells.[157] The addition of midostaurin to standard chemotherapy prolongs overall survival in patients with AML and an *FLT3* mutation.[158] Midostaurin exposure in patients with *FLT3*-mutated AML is associated with severe rash or desquamation.[158]

Small Molecule Tyrosine Kinase Inhibitors

Gilteritinib

Gilteritinib is an oral small molecule tyrosine kinase inhibitor (TKI) with selectivity for FLT3 and AXL tyrosine kinases. Gilteritinib may increase survival in patients with relapsed or refractory *FLT3*-mutated AML compared to conventional salvage chemotherapy.[159] Various neutrophilic dermatoses have been reported following initiation of gilteritinib.[160] Cutaneous reactions may manifest as red, tender, subcutaneous nodules or pustulonodules on the cheeks, ears, and scalp.[161] Histopathologic analysis reveals neutrophil predominant lobular panniculitis or interstitial neutrophilic infiltrate. Sweet syndrome has also been described in a neutropenic patient exposed to gilteritinib.[162] Here, the rash was characterized as violaceus, macular, papular, and nodular distributed across the bilateral upper and lower extremities. Histopathology demonstrated neutrophilic infiltration of the dermis, with superficial dermal edema and epidermal spongiosis. Altogether, gilteritinib may induce a differentiation-like syndrome manifesting as neutrophilic dermatoses in AML patients with *FLT3* mutations. Other FLT3 inhibitors, including quizartinib and sorafenib, are also reported to induce neutrophilic dermatoses.[163]

Enasidenib

Enasidenib is a small molecule TKI that targets mutant isocitrate dehydrogenase 2 (*IDH2*). IDH2 mutations occur in approximately 8% to 19% of patients with AML.[164] Enasidenib is efficacious in patients with relapsed or refractory AML and *IDH2* mutations.[165] Enasidenib is associated with low-grade rash in multiple early-stage clinical trials.[165,166]

CHRONIC LEUKEMIAS

Chronic leukemias most commonly present in adulthood. Their incidence increases with age.[2] The incidence of CLL among new leukemia cases per year in the United States is higher than that of chronic myeloid leukemia (CML) (30% vs 11%, respectively).[167] Hairy cell leukemia (HCL) presents as a rare form of chronic leukemia, making up about 2% of leukemias each year. Chronic leukemia has a tendency to affect males more than females with a ratio of nearly 2:1 overall, with HCL in particular affecting approximately four times more males than females.[2] The mainstays of therapy currently for CLL include rituximab and fludarabine and TKIs for CML. The dermatologic effects of these drugs and others are discussed later.

Monoclonal Antibodies

Monoclonal antibodies (MAbs) are engineered against cell-surface markers implicated in various malignancies. In the treatment of CLL, MAbs have introduced a wide array of new therapeutics in the treatment of refractory patients. These MAbs in CLL include alemtuzumab, ofatumumab, and rituximab.

Alemtuzumab is a recombinant DNA-encoded humanized immunoglobulin G1 MAb that targets the cell-surface protein CD52, which is highly expressed on normal and abnormal mature lymphocytes, both of T- and B-cell origin, but not on hematopoietic stem cells.[168] Both ofatumumab[169] and rituximab[170] target CD20, which is widely expressed on B lineage cells. These MAbs are typically associated with rash, urticaria, and infusion-related reactions upon initial infusion, typically of grade 1 to 2 severity. These usually subside after the first week of therapy.[168,169,171-175]

Alemtuzumab has recently been shown to have a better safety profile when administered subcutaneously, while sustaining prior efficacy standards seen in infusion studies.[168,171,172,176] This should be started after an initial week of infusion therapy, as subcutaneous alemtuzumab has had a greater rate of injection site skin reactions, as well as a prolonged dose escalation, when administered as the introductory therapy. Areas of erythema up to 30 cm were seen in some patients under this subcutaneous dosing.[171] An effective route for lessening the prevalence of infusion-related toxicities is to premedicate the patient with 50 mg of diphenhydramine about 30 minutes before the initial infusion.[176]

Additionally, the inclusion of alemtuzumab with total body irradiation (TBI) and cyclophosphamide (Cy) in a conditioning dose for the patient with CLL before autologous stem cell transplantation causes a marked increase in the incidence rate of autologous graft-versus-host disease (auto-GVHD).[177] Twelve of 16 patients on this therapy developed unexplained skin rashes, while seven of them were clinically diagnosed with auto-GVHD. Comparatively, 11 patients treated preemptively with TBI/Cy alone had no evidence of GVHD or other mucocutaneous conditions. Five patients with the clinical diagnosis of auto-GVHD were biopsied, which demonstrated apoptotic figures in the epidermal basal layer with vacuolar interface changes and superficial perivascular lymphocytic infiltrates. Thus, the addition of alemtuzumab to TBI/Cy therapy should be evaluated through a risk-versus-benefit analysis, as the depletion of T-regulatory cells may predispose toward auto-GVHD.[177]

Rituximab has been associated with severe mucocutaneous reactions. It has been reported to induce Stevens–Johnson syndrome (SJS) in some patients.[178,179] An association with paraneoplastic pemphigus when used in combination therapy with bendamustine had also been noted.[180] Paraneoplastic pemphigus demonstrates suprabasal acantholysis and intercellular and linear basement membrane deposition of IgG and C3 in the epidermis. It should be noted that CLL and NHL are the most commonly associated predisposing conditions for paraneoplastic pemphigus.

Rituximab has some association with serum sickness in the classic type III hypersensitivity pattern approximately 1 to 2 weeks after initial infusion,[181-184] secondary to host IgG antibodies targeted against the murine Fab fragments of rituximab.[185] Serum sickness usually presents in a febrile patient complaining of arthralgias and a pruritic purpuric eruption. Laboratory findings include decreased C3 and C4 markers with increased erythrocyte sedimentation rates and C-reactive protein (CRP) levels.[186] As the classic triad of symptoms allows for clinical diagnosis, the rash in this condition is rarely biopsied; however, it should reveal an LCV. Treatment involves intravenous methylprednisolone with favorable outcomes. Mild cases of serum sickness, after resolution of symptoms, have been followed with reintroduction of rituximab without recurrence.[187]

Purine Analogs

Fludarabine, cladribine, and pentostatin are used in oncology as agents that resemble the compounds adenosine and deoxyadenosine, although their mechanisms for induction of cytotoxicity differ significantly. Notably, these chemotherapeutics show a propensity for reducing the CD4/CD8 ratio[188] and increasing the susceptibility to opportunistic infections. Fludarabine is used in the treatment of CLL, while cladribine and pentostatin are frequently used in HCL.

There are multiple reports of fludarabine inducing paraneoplastic pemphigus in CLL patients within weeks of induction therapy, presenting as a maculopapular eruption with extensive oral erosions.[189-191] One case developed into pemphigus vegetans, confirmed by histopathologic findings of acanthosis and suprabasal acantholysis.[189] The mucocutaneous eruptions of paraneoplastic pemphigus show marked improvement after discontinuation of the pulsed fludarabine treatments.[190,191]

Pentostatin has also been linked to cutaneous reactions, most commonly a minor skin reaction seen in 90% of patients[192] that may appear erythematous, papular, or vesiculobullous. Higher-grade skin toxicities, including those resulting in termination of therapeutic regimen, and both low- and high-grade stomatitis have also been frequently observed.[193,194] Severe, biopsied reactions appear rare, although it should be noted that a clinically diagnosed fatal erythroderma has been attributed to pentostatin injection.[195]

Some authors have also suggested elevated surveillance when administering purine analogs. Fludarabine[196] and cladribine[197] when given with nonirradiated donor red blood cells and platelets have been implicated in the development of transfusion-associated GVHD. These two medications are also believed to facilitate aggressive epithelial growth, a side effect likely secondary to the lymphocytic depletion. Accelerated SCC infiltration has been noted, and rapid recurrence and metastasis have been seen in these cases.[198-200]

Tyrosine Kinase Inhibitors

TKIs target the tyrosine kinase receptor, which functions to phosphorylate various downstream signaling proteins involved in malignant transformation. They have become a mainstay of therapy in the treatment of B-cell receptor (BCR)–ABL tyrosine kinase protein–positive diseases. Imatinib is used as a first-line therapy against the BCR-ABL receptor, whereas nilotinib and dasatinib are used in refractory or resistant disease. Ibrutinib is also actively used against the Bruton tyrosine kinase (BTK) receptor in CLL.

Imatinib is an inhibitor of the BCR-ABL receptor, and thus used as a first-line drug in the treatment of Philadelphia chromosome–positive (Ph+) CML and Ph+ ALL. It has been observed that between 10% and 67%[201-203] of patients will experience a cutaneous adverse event while receiving this medication, the majority of which are dose dependent,[204] mild,[201] and self-limiting.[203] These typically include edema, particularly localized to the eyelids, and skin rashes, which have been estimated to occur 60% and 32% of the time, respectively.[205] Other mild reactions have included photosensitization, believed to be secondary to cumulative dosing of the medication,[206] as well as hypopigmentation,[207,208] histopathologically showing scant melanin pigmentation secondary to inadequate melanocytes at the basal layer.[209]

Imatinib has also been implicated in the onset of pseudoporphyria, presenting clinically with hemorrhagic bullae and erosions most commonly on the dorsal and lateral aspects of the hands. A biopsy of the area demonstrated subepidermal vesicles and bullae, with minimal cellular inflammation.[210,211] Therapy may be continued despite the presence of these bullae, although clearance generally occurs concomitantly with cessation of imatinib.[211] Prevention of trauma is needed if therapy is continued. Imatinib has also been associated with exacerbations of underlying psoriasis, which may become refractory to topical corticosteroids. Cessation of the therapy was required.[212]

Although most of these reactions are mild to moderate and self-limiting, imatinib has been associated with more severe cutaneous eruptions including Sweet syndrome. Clearance of the plaques can be achieved with discontinuation of imatinib.[213] Other severe reactions include erythema multiforme (EM)[214] and SJS/TEN.[215-217] Imatinib can also cause acute generalized pustulosis, clinically presenting with a febrile rash with pustules and papules located diffusely, albeit sparing the palms and soles. Biopsies demonstrate subcorneal pustules with accompanying parakeratosis and an abundance of neutrophils.[218] Control of severe, recurrent eruptions may be viably achieved through once-weekly dosing or providing predose and adjuvant administrations of corticosteroids with imatinib.[219]

Dasatinib and nilotinib are structurally similar to imatinib, and serve as alternates in imatinib-refractory CML. They have generally been recorded with fewer side effects than imatinib, although less reported data may be a contributing factor.[204] The vast majority of cutaneous reactions reported tend to be grade 1 or 2 rashes, pruritus, and xeroderma.[204,220] Rarer but more severe side effects have also been reported. Nilotinib has been found to induce bullous Sweet syndrome, demonstrating subepidermal edema owing to extreme papillary dermal edema and infiltration by neutrophils and atypical CD68+ monocytoid cells. Bullous lesions disappeared with prednisolone and antibiotics, and nilotinib therapy was continued without recurrence.[221] Dasatinib, in turn, has been linked to two cases of lobular panniculitis during CML therapy. These cases presented with painful nodules with overlying erythema, which were microscopically shown to have massive subcutaneous infiltration by neutrophils. These lesions resolved with discontinuation of dasatinib.[222]

Ibrutinib, a BTK inhibitor, plays a key role in neutralizing the constitutive BCR signaling seen in CLL. This medication has been largely efficacious with little toxicity.[223,224] Cutaneous and mucocutaneous eruptions are seldom seen with only 8% of patients present with a rash during their course and 11% demonstrate stomatitis believed to be therapy related. Conversely, petechiae attributed to ibrutinib use does seem to be more substantial than other medications used for CLL, as it presents in about 14% of cases.[224] The main cutaneous side effect other than petechiae is a mixed septal and lobular panniculitis, which can be accompanied by neutrophilia, lymphocytosis, leukocytoclasis, and granulomatous features (Figs. 74-11 and 74-12).

Alkylating Agents

Alkylating agents are classically used in chemotherapeutics for the disruption of DNA synthesis by the addition of

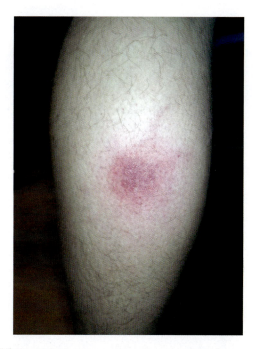

FIGURE 74-11. Panniculitis in association with the TKI ibrutinib in a patient undergoing treatment for CLL.

an alkyl group to the guanine bases of DNA. In CLL, the mainstay of alkylating treatment includes bendamustine and chlorambucil, both of which are associated with cutaneous reactions. Busulfan is frequently used in CML as a palliative treatment.

Bendamustine

Bendamustine combines the effects of the alkylating agent mechlorethamine and the purine metabolite benzimidazole.[225] Although it has demonstrated a high-efficacy profile with manageable toxicities,[225-227] bendamustine might produce minor pruritic cutaneous reactions. A large study of 161 patients undergoing bendamustine therapy demonstrated that 15 (9.3%) developed a rash with the majority of grade 2 or less. Nine of these patients were discontinued from further therapy.[225] Histologically, skin findings showed scant mononuclear cells and collagen deposition around adnexal structures.[228] Symptomatic therapy using oral antihistamines and topical emollient creams seems to be most appropriate, as drug dose alteration does not seem to be necessary in most cases.[228]

More severe side effects had also been observed during bendamustine therapy, especially when it was used in combination with other chemotherapies. Concomitant use with rituximab[179,229] and allopurinol[179] has resulted in SJS/TEN. Additionally, a case study describes a patient who developed SJS while on bendamustine without the parallel infusion of either rituximab or allopurinol, although coadministered antibiotics may have played a synergistic role in the precipitation of this condition.[230]

Bendamustine-induced severe skin reactions in the form of purpuric exanthema with hemorrhagic bullae, desquamating rash, and drug reaction with eosinophilia and systemic symptoms (DRESS) syndrome have also been reported.[230-232] These cases responded well to corticosteroids. Treatment of DRESS syndrome involves immediate withdrawal of the

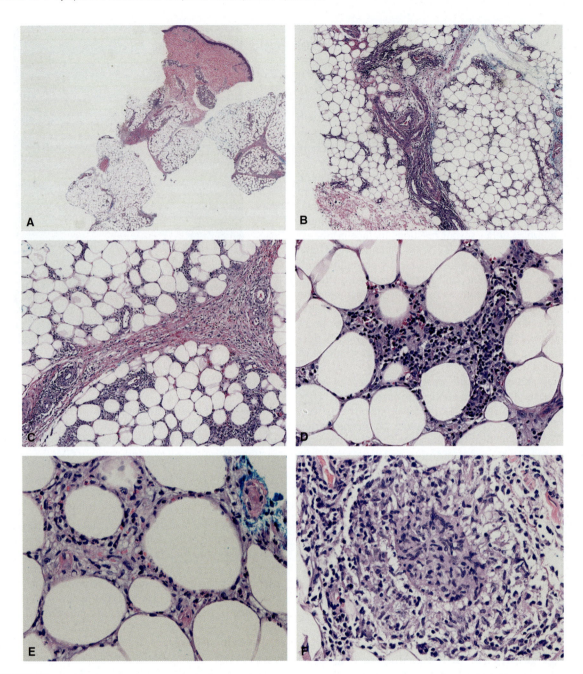

FIGURE 74-12. Panniculitis in association with the TKI ibrutinib. (**A** and **B**). Mixed lobular and septal panniculitis with predominance of lymphocytes. **C** and **D.** Adipocyte rimming by lymphocytes. **E.** A case rich in neutrophils with leukocytoclasis. **F.** A granulomatous focus mimicking Miescher radial granuloma seen in erythema nodosum.

offending agent with systemic corticosteroids, as this condition frequently involves extracutaneous organs, most commonly the liver.

Chlorambucil

Chlorambucil is a classic alkylating agent previously used as a first-line therapy for CLL.[176] It has a slightly lower rate of medication-induced rash and pruritus than bendamustine,[225] but its association with life-threatening conditions such as TEN[233] and DRESS[234] syndrome should alert the clinician when cutaneous eruptions present. Delayed-type skin hypersensitivity to the medication in the form of diffuse urticarial erythema had also been described.[235,236]

Busulfan

Busulfan was the first-line therapy for CML before the introduction of imatinib. Long-term administration had been associated with diffuse, dusky brown hyperpigmentation in 5% to 10% of patients.[237] Symptoms of fatigue and wasting could mimic Addison disease, but there is a lack of mucosal involvement and workup for adrenal insufficiency is negative.[238,239]

Busulfan has also been related to toxic erythema of chemotherapy (TEC), especially when used in conjunction with fludarabine.[240] It presents with burning areas of desquamation and erosion, especially at intertriginous areas. Scrotal involvement is a frequent presentation. Intertriginous TEC is likely an irritant reaction to sweat-excreted busulfan. Biopsies may display keratinocyte atypia with vacuolar degeneration of the basal layer and eccrine squamous syringometaplasia.[240,241] These lesions will resolve with time, and no specific therapy is indicated. Busulfan-related permanent alopecia has also been reported.[242]

Antimetabolites

Hydroxyurea

Hydroxyurea (HU) is an alternate therapy for CML and it inhibits synthesis of DNA by blocking ribonucleoside diphosphate reductase.[243] Although less frequently used in CML, it is still a treatment of choice for sickle cell disease and essential thrombocythemia. Approximately 13% of patients on long-term HU therapy develop cutaneous or mucosal side effects,[244] which most commonly manifest as leg ulcerations around the malleoli.[245-248] Leg ulcers typically occur spontaneously after 6 to 13 years of continuous chemotherapy,[248] and they heal quickly with cessation of the medication.[247] These lesions may be caused by cutaneous anoxia secondary to a HU-induced reduction in red blood cell susceptibility to deformation via megaloblastic changes.[248] Skin biopsies of these ulcerations typically show epidermal atrophy with dermal fibrosis and minimal to no inflammatory cell infiltration.[248-250]

HU has also been implicated in producing dermatomyositis-like eruptions when used in long-term therapy. These typically present on the dorsum of the hands,[244] and improvement is achieved with discontinuation of the drug.[251] Histology shows epidermal atrophy and vacuolar interface dermatitis with cytoid bodies.[244,252,253] Lichenoid eruptions are also commonly seen, distributed on the hands and feet. This presents as pink, speckled, flat-topped papules with atrophy, along with variable epidermal atrophy and occasional areas of parakeratosis, epidermal hyperplasia, hypergranulosis, and a saw-toothed epidermis, resembling lichen planus.[254]

Otherwise, HU had also been associated with the development of SCC, basal cell carcinoma (BCC), and actinic keratoses (AKs) on sun-exposed areas,[255,256] as well as acral erythema,[257,258] mucocutaneous hyperpigmentation,[259] and transverse melanonychia.[260,261] Microscopic evaluations of the nail clippings show a keratinized layer with disorganized brownish granules, positive for melanin staining and negative for iron staining.[262] One study has also shown a rare HU-induced scleroderma-like syndrome with shiny and flat skin with a loss of hair follicles throughout the skin.[263] Histopathologically, this presents with collagen bundle thickening throughout the reticular dermis and subcutaneous tissue, as well as apoptotic keratinocytes in the epidermis. The fibrosis is hypothesized to be induced by activation of fibroblasts through inflammatory signaling.[263] HU should be discontinued and replaced with an appropriate alternative in such cases.

BRAF Inhibitors

HCL is a rare chronic LPD with circulating neoplastic B lymphocytes exhibiting ruffled, hair-like cytoplasmic projections.[264] Because a *BRAF V600 E* mutation appears to be a pathogenic driver mutation, BRAF inhibitors (BRAFi) including vemurafenib and dabrafenib hold great promise in HCL therapy.[265-268]

A broad range of benign and neoplastic cutaneous side effects have been described with BRAFi. These include inflammatory skin reactions such as photosensitivity, morbilliform eruptions, folliculitis, keratosis pilaris, alopecia, curly hair, and hand–foot syndrome.[269] Cutaneous SCCs, keratoacanthomas (KAs) (Figs. 74-13 and 74-14), and verrucous keratoses (Fig. 74-15) are seen following the acquisition of the RAS mutation during treatment.[269,270] BRAFi-associated KAs are indistinguishable from those seen in the general population. They are characterized by crateriform, endophytic growth of well-differentiated keratinocytes with glassy, eosinophilic cytoplasm and abrupt keratinization.[271] BRAFi-associated verrucous keratoses show histologic resemblance to typical warts without the viral cytopathic changes. Recent studies have shown that trametinib, an inhibitor of MEK, substantially decreases the risk of these cutaneous squamous proliferations.[272] Rare cases of BRAFi-associated TEN have also been reported.[273]

CUTANEOUS T-CELL LYMPHOMA

Cutaneous T-cell lymphoma (CTCL) is an extranodal NHL confined to the skin. Its incidence has gradually increased over the past 40 years, rising from 2.8 cases per million in 1973 to 1977 to 9.6 cases per million in 1998 to 2002.[274] No distinct chromosomal abnormalities have yet been discovered for CTCL, although constitutive or cytokine-stimulated JunD expression may play a role in the progression of the disease.[275] Human T-lymphotropic virus 1 is directly associated with adult T-leukemia/lymphoma, a malignant process that often has associated cutaneous manifestations that can pathologically mimic mycosis fungoides (MF).[276]

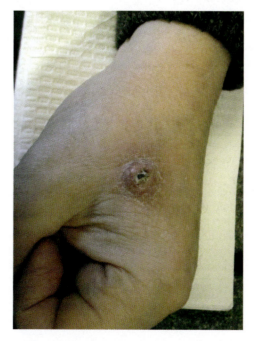

FIGURE 74-13. Keratoacanthoma-like squamous cell carcinoma on the dorsum of the hand in a patient with HCL treated with BRAF inhibitor.

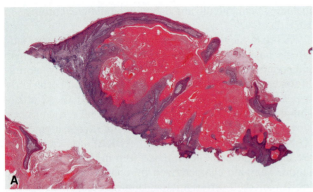
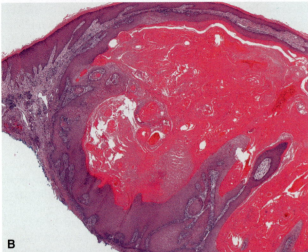
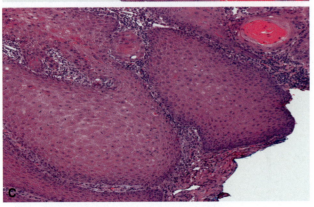

FIGURE 74-14. Keratoacanthoma-like squamous cell carcinoma on the dorsum of the hand in a patient with HCL treated with BRAF inhibitor. **A–C**. A crateriform squamous proliferation with invasive carcinoma in the dermis and parakeratosis (20×–100× and 400×).

The treatment regimens for MF, as well as the leukemic Sézary syndrome (SS) subtype, depend on the clinical stage (see Chapters 12 and 13) and range from topical therapies, including corticosteroids, mechlorethamine, carmustine, and retinoids, to systemic modalities, including interferons, retinoids, and chemotherapeutics, to photochemotherapy and radiotherapy. The main medications and their cutaneous side effects are explored in the following sections.

Corticosteroids

Topical corticosteroids may be used alone or in conjunction with other medications for stage IA MF. Side effects from long-term use may include acne, telangiectasias due to stimulation of dermal microvascular endothelial cells,[277] and dermal atrophy secondary to decreased collagen synthesis.[278] Another long-term sequela is striae formation, classically presenting diffusely on the abdomen, chest, and extremities.[279] The most ominous sequela of long-term high-potency topical steroid use is iatrogenic Cushing syndrome with weight gain and fat redistribution.[280,281] Skin histology shows superficial perivascular lymphocytic infiltrates, mild spongiosis, and extensive suprabasal mitoses.[281]

Alkylating Agents

Alkylating agents cross-link DNA to prevent DNA replication. In the treatment of early-stage MF, two topical alkylating agents, mechlorethamine and carmustine, are commonly used with a high degree of success. Topical mechlorethamine has shown complete response in stage I disease for 73% to 78% of cases, although relapses after discontinuation tend to be common.[282-285] Topical carmustine, in turn, has complete remission rates around 86%[286,287] of patients with stage I disease. Recurrence-free survival of stage I MF appears to be longer in carmustine-treated patients.[286,288]

Topical mechlorethamine is a nitrogen mustard derivative with a more efficacious response when used as a 0.02% gel compared to its use as an ointment, without differences in adverse events.[289] Most commonly, mechlorethamine may cause a contact dermatitis in about 65% of patients at the area of application, presenting with erythema and itching, which may progress to blistering and ulceration.[285] The incidence of this contact dermatitis has drastically decreased with a change from aqueous preparations.[290] An upregulation of collagenase activity, especially matrix metalloproteases, is seen in this dermatitis.[291] If severe, this reaction can be contained with application of povidone–iodine, as this medication directly oxidizes the sulfhydryl functional groups of the proteases responsible, in addition to other inhibitory actions.[291,292] Desensitization may be used to overcome the allergic reaction in affected patients, as well.[293] Immediate hypersensitivity reactions with urticaria may also occur, although this seems less common.[294]

Topical nitrogen mustards can be also associated with atypical epidermal dysmaturation, which is usually seen in patients treated with systemic chemotherapeutic agents such as etoposide, busulfan, and bleomycin.[295] The histology shows slight epidermal hyperplasia, atypical keratinocytes with large nuclei in the lower epidermis, suprabasal mitotic figures, hypergranulosis, orthokeratosis, focal vacuolar alteration of the basal layer, and foci of flat rete ridges. Cytologic atypia is also appreciated in junctional melanocytes and dermal endothelial cells and fibroblasts.[295]

Other cutaneous inflammatory reactions to topical mechlorethamine include allergic contact dermatitis, EM-like dermatitis, SJS,[296] and postinflammatory hyperpigmentation.[297] Although the development of secondary malignancy with topical chemotherapies is of significant concern, studies have shown conflicting reports of mechlorethamine-associated secondary squamoproliferative lesions. Long-term studies have shown both negligible[284] and mild (5%)[285] relationships of this drug with the development of secondary malignancies, typically BCC.[285]

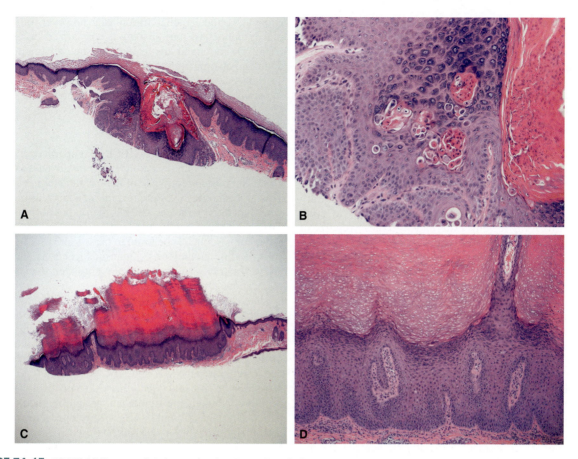

FIGURE 74-15. BRAF inhibitor–associated verrucous keratoses. **A** and **B.** Cup-shaped, benign keratosis with focal acantholytic dyskeratosis reminiscent of warty dyskeratoma. **C** and **D.** Benign verrucous keratosis resembling verruca vulgaris. There is acanthosis, papillomatosis, columns of parakeratosis, hypergranulosis, and vascular ectasia.

Topical carmustine, another alkylating agent, is less frequently used to treat early-stage CTCL because of the risk of systemic absorption and resultant leukopenia.[298] The main cutaneous manifestation of carmustine application is erythema, which may present as hyperpigmentation in patients with darker complexion. These erythematous lesions are often followed or accompanied by tenderness and telangiectasias without any signs of desquamation. The biopsy typically shows superficial telangiectasias that tend to persist for years after treatment has ended.[298] In contrast to mechlorethamine, carmustine tends to induce less severe contact dermatitis and does not appear to be associated with secondary skin cancers.[298]

Histone Deacetylase Inhibitors

Histone deacetylase (HDAC) inhibitors target the epigenome, which regulates gene expression. Romidepsin, a bicyclic peptide derived from *Chromobacterium violaceum*, and vorinostat, a hydroxamic acid derivative, are novel HDAC inhibitors used in the treatment of CTCL and SS. Like most HDAC inhibitors, drug-related cutaneous adverse events appeared exceedingly rare in clinical trials.[299-301]

Fusion Proteins

Denileukin diftitox is a fusion protein composed of interleukin-2 (IL-2) and the diphtheria toxin, aimed at targeting IL-2 receptor–expressing cells and inhibiting protein synthesis. It aids in the treatment of stage IB to IVA CTCL with persistent CD25 expression on IL-2 receptors. Denileukin trials have shown a response rate of 30%[302] to 40%,[303] as well as an absence of notable cutaneous side effects during therapy.

Nucleoside Analogs

Gemcitabine hydrochloride is a pyrimidine nucleoside analog that disrupts DNA replication. It has shown to be effective in patients with advanced and refractory CTCL. Generally, a well-tolerated chemotherapeutic medication, gemcitabine rarely presents with cutaneous toxicities,[304,305] although one study noted several cases of diffuse hyperpigmentation and one case of radiation recall ulceration.[306]

Monoclonal Antibodies

Mogamulizumab is a humanized MAb directed against C-C chemokine receptor 4, which is highly expressed in CTCL.[307] Mogamulizumab treatment prolongs progression free-survival in CTCL patients compared with vorinostat treatment.[308] Patients with CTCL exposed to mogamulizumab frequently experience drug rash, the most common adverse event cited for treatment discontinuation.[308] Patients exposed to mogamulizumab may experience a cutaneous granulomatous drug eruption (CGDE) that resembles MF.[309] The lesions appear after a median treatment time of 4.6 months and have been described as erythematous macules distributed to photoprotective areas that may progress into scaly, erythematous plaques. Patients with mogamulizumab-induced CGDE may have increased progression free survival compared to mogamulizumab exposure without development of CGDE. The development of this MFs-like CGDE may signal durable mogamulizumab response. Treatments for mogamulizumab drug rash include topical steroid ointments.[308,309] Other reported cutaneous adverse events are cellulitis and alopecia.

Simultaneous mogamulizumab and narrowband UVB phototherapy may also be associated with phototoxicity.[310] Histopathologic analysis of these phototoxic lesions may reveal a lichenoid reaction with predominant CD8+ infiltrates and decreased Foxp3+ regulatory T-cells in comparison to CTCL lesions. Alternatively, these reports of mogamulizumab-associated phototoxicity may represent flares of cutaneous lymphoma induced by phototherapy.[311]

Mogamulizumab treatment prior to allogenic hematopoietic stem cell transplantation (allo-HSCT) may be associated with an increased risk of GVHD. A short treatment interval between last mogamulizumab administration and subsequent regulatory T-cell depletion may be risk factors for acute GVHD following allo-HSCT.[312,313]

The histologic findings of mogamulizumab-associated rash are diverse. Three major histopathologic patterns identified in mogamulizumab-associated rash include spongiotic/psoriasiform dermatitis, granulomatous dermatitis, and interface dermatitis (Fig. 74-16 A–D).[314] Lesions commonly display at least two of the three major histologic patterns. The presence of eosinophils is variable. In some cases, one can observe features mimicking MF, including lymphocyte exocytosis and lamellar fibroplasia; however, intraepidermal lymphocytes may display a normalized or decreased CD4:CD8 ratio, and this feature may help distinguish mogamulizumab drug eruptions from CTCL.[309,314] Lastly, SJS and TEN have been associated with exposure to mogamulizumab in patients with adult T-cell leukemia/lymphoma.[315]

Photochemotherapies

Extracorporeal photophoresis (ECP) was approved by the U.S. Food and Drug Administration (FDA) for advanced CTCL in 1987, and it is currently one of the frontline regimens for SS. This procedure involves pretreating mononuclear blood cells with 8-methoxypsoralen, which is then exposed to UVA light. The cells are then reinfused into the patient, and the activated 8-methoxypsoralen is believed to cross-link DNA in exposed cells, leading to apoptosis. Cutaneous reactions during ECP are very rarely seen, and generally attributed to concomitant medications if they do arise.[316]

Psoralen plus UVA (PUVA), a first-line therapy in early-stage plaque MF, similarly involves UVA exposure after photosensitization. The photosensitizer, psoralen, is administered either topically or systemically with subsequent exposure of the patient to UVA irradiation. PUVA has shown excellent results in stages IA and IB CTCL, showing complete responses in 79% and 59% of cases, respectively. The rates of relapse, though, are significant, as approximately 60% of patients in stages IA and IB CTCL developed a recurrence of their malignancy.[317] As PUVA is photosensitizing, the patient should be instructed to wear protective clothing and/or sunscreen about sun-exposed areas.

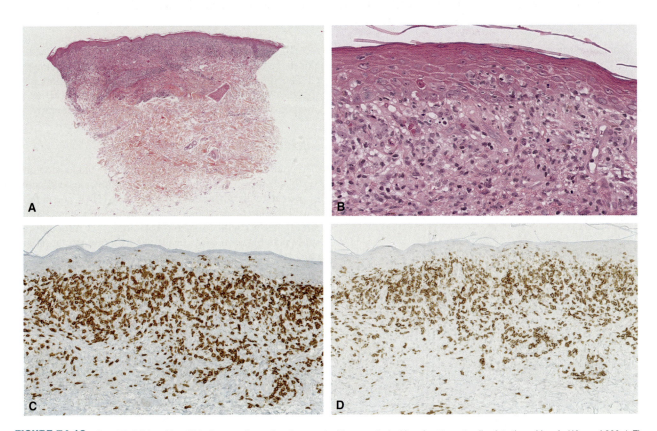

FIGURE 74.16. **A** and **B.** A lichenoid and interface reaction pattern is present with some atypical lymphocytes extending into the epidermis (40× and 200×). The atypical cells are positive for CD3 (**C**) and CD8 (**D**). Most of the T-cells show a CD8+ phenotype (pictures courtesy of Dr. Maxime Battistella, Hospital St. Louis, Paris).

Long-term PUVA treatment has been associated with secondary nonmelanocytic, melanocytic, and dermal malignancies, likely secondary to direct carcinogenic DNA damage. In one study, AKs were observed in 16% of PUVA-treated patients.[318] Thirty-fold increase in the number of SCCs and a 5-fold increase in BCCs have been reported in a long-term study.[319] Dermatologists should be particularly cognizant of scrotal and genital nonmelanoma skin cancers as a result of PUVA. Additionally, the incidence of melanoma is about sevenfold in PUVA-treated patients when compared to nontreated Caucasians in the United States.[320]

PUVA may also be associated with various other non-specific skin reactions, including erythema and pruritus. Hyperpigmentation has also been noted, including acquired dermal melanocytosis and PUVA lentigines. This presents with blue-brown macules and displaying spindle-shaped dendritic cells composed of melanin granules distributed throughout the mid- to upper dermis.[321]

Narrowband UVB light has also shown efficacy in suppressing neoplastic T-cell function and proliferation. This treatment might be associated with erythematous rashes, phototoxicity, and pruritus, although these symptoms tend to be self-limiting.[322,323] It is generally used more often than PUVA for early-stage MF owing to a lower side effect profile, including no association with cutaneous carcinomas, and comparable efficacy.[322-326]

Radiotherapy

Total skin electron beam therapy (TSEBT) provides a shallow penetrating ionizing radiation to the entire skin. It is especially effective in CTCL, as the neoplastic T-cells of MF, as well as normal lymphocytes, are especially radiosensitive. TSEBT can be used for any stage of CTCL. Although there are conflicting reports of its efficacy as a monotherapy in SS,[327,328] combining TSEBT with ECP has shown promising results in patients with stage IV MF.[329]

The most common acute side effects of TSEBT are dose dependent and include erythema, desquamation, and hyperpigmentation.[330] These acute radiation responses can be seen during or immediately after treatments, and they can be accompanied by bulla formation or ulceration at higher radiation doses. Late features of chronic dermatitis include epidermal atrophy with upper dermal edema, capillary ectasia, and melanophage deposition in the upper dermis.[331] The extent of damage throughout the epithelium is significantly correlated with the amount of radiation given during therapy.[331] Low-dose radiation (10 Gy) is generally considered efficacious with a reduction in associated side effects.[332] Other side effects of TSEBT include alopecia, onychodystrophy, and mild distal edematous changes in the extremities.[330]

Retinoids

Bexarotene is a synthetic retinoid that selectively activates the retinoid X receptor, inducing cell differentiation and apoptosis.[333] It is pregnancy category X. The FDA approved topical bexarotene 1% gel in 2000 for refractory early-stage CTCL (IA–IB). The FDA had earlier approved oral bexarotene for all stages of CTCL in 1999.

Topical bexarotene has shown overall response rates ranging from 44%[334] to 63%[335] and complete clinical responses ranging from 2%[334] to 21%[335] when treating patients with early-stage CTCL. Bexarotene is generally well tolerated, although most patients developed a cutaneous reaction presenting as a dose-related irritant dermatitis at the application site, as well as occasional pruritus and burning sensation. These symptoms are generally self-limiting and can be controlled with interruptions or decreased dosing, in addition to emollients or topical corticosteroids.[334,335]

Systemic bexarotene as a monotherapy is used in all stages of refractory CTCL and it has shown overall response rates of 45% to 54%.[336-338] It is most effective and safe at 300 mg/m^2/day.[336] Approximately 13% of patients achieve a complete response.[337] This medication is well tolerated with most reactions presenting as dose-dependent skin peeling, rash, or pruritus that are self-limiting.[336,337] These side effects may worsen in rare cases, as a patient with SS treated with oral bexarotene developed generalized exfoliative erythroderma with diffuse fissuring and edema, as well as intense hyperkeratosis about the palms, soles, and gluteal area. Cessation of bexarotene greatly improved symptoms in this case. The mechanism of this injury is unclear, although the concomitant SS is believed to play a key role in its development.[339]

Interferon-α

Interferon-α2b is an antiviral drug utilized in CTCL, HCL, and metastatic melanoma. Interferon's success as an antineoplastic is likely attributed to its role in enhancing the number and function of NK cells, the main cellular effectors of antitumoral cytotoxicity.[340] It also promotes cytotoxic T-cell–mediated tumor lysis by enhancing the cell surface expression of adhesion molecules CD11a and CD54.[341]

Livedo reticularis is a characteristic side effect of interferon treatment, and it can develop from 2 weeks[342] to 3 months[343] after initiation of therapy. The lesions present as mottled, lacy reddish-purple rash with geometric reticulations. Histology shows scant perivascular infiltrates and superficial dermal vascular ectasia without any signs of vasculitis.[342,343] Serologies for antiphospholipid antibody syndrome or systemic lupus erythematosus are negative. Although the exact mechanism of livedo reticularis remains unclear, it is hypothesized to be related to deoxygenation of the blood in the dermal microvasculature owing to decreased arteriolar flow.[344] The central area with normal skin is the site of a constricted cutaneous arteriole, whereas the periphery is the edge of the arteriolar unit. Interferon's role is believed to involve ischemic insult through vasospasm,[345] inhibition of angiogenesis,[346] promotion of endothelial cell apoptosis,[347] and downregulation of endothelial urokinase type plasminogen activator with a resultant increase in microthrombi.[348] This side effect tends to disappear with discontinuation of interferon.[342]

Raynaud phenomenon can be also precipitated by interferon-induced vasospasm.[349-352] Progression to distal necrosis is rare.[351] Addition of a calcium channel blocker may improve vasospasm and prevent dose alteration. In severe cases, dose alteration or cessation of therapy may be indicated.

Injection site reactions may also occur and include initial erythema, which may progress to a necrotic ulcer with associated fever and pain within weeks.[353-355] Alternating the position of subcutaneous injection with each administration may prevent these ulcerations. Histology exhibits necrosis of the epidermis and superficial dermis. Panniculitis with neutrophils[353] and venous thrombosis within the dermis and subcutaneous fat may also be present.[355] Lastly, interferon may precipitate or worsen classic psoriasis owing to an upregulation of the psoriasis cytokine cascade.[356]

MULTIPLE MYELOMA

Multiple myeloma (MM) is a neoplastic proliferation of monoclonal plasma cells with a uniform immunoglobulin. It accounts for about 1% of newly diagnosed malignancies every year, as well as 2% of malignancy-related deaths per year.[167] Although historically considered a terminal malignancy, MM has begun to be regarded as curable with the institution of recent, novel chemotherapeutic regimens over the past decade.[357] Median survival times have increased,[358-360] and the 10-year survival rate of patients diagnosed and treated before the age of 50 is approximately 41%.[360] Treatment of MM starts with specific chemotherapy regimens followed by autologous hematopoietic cell transplantation for eligible patients. Some of these medications and their cutaneous side effects are reviewed in the following sections.

Proteasome Inhibitors

Bortezomib was FDA-approved for the treatment of MM in 2003. It reversibly inhibits the 26S proteasome, which degrades ubiquitinated proteins. This allows the inhibitor protein IκB to persist, disallowing activation of the transcription factor nuclear factor κB (NF-κB). Cutaneous side effects are commonly seen with its use, although they are typically ill defined.

A Sweet syndrome–like presentation has been seen with bortezomib, initially presenting with erythematous and edematous lesions that can be painful or pruritic. This clinical eruption most commonly occurs after the first cycle of bortezomib administration,[361-363] although it may present later.[364] Some cases appear to be in line with a classic Sweet syndrome, displaying papillary dermal edema, numerous dermal neutrophils, and leukocytoclasia.[364-366] In these cases, bortezomib seems to upregulate proinflammatory cytokines, resulting in neutrophilic immigration into the dermis.[363] Cases of Sweet syndrome with mononuclear/histiocytic infiltrates rather than neutrophils[361-363] have also been described and termed "histiocytoid Sweet syndrome."[367] These histiocytes appear to correspond to immature myeloid precursors (CD68+, lysozyme+, and myeloperoxidase+).[361,363,367] Patients tend to respond well to topical corticosteroids, although systemic corticosteroids are often administered with bortezomib cycles.[367]

Bortezomib has also induced lupus erythematosus tumidus, which presents as evanescent, erythematous plaques often in an arcuate appearance. This rare form of chronic, cutaneous lupus displays perivascular and periadnexal lymphocytic infiltrates without an interface reaction, along with a characteristic deposition of dermal mucin.[368,369] This condition may be caused by bortezomib-mediated inhibition of NF-κB, which triggers apoptosis,[369] a known provoker of lupus. Cessation of bortezomib may alleviate this condition along with introduction of topical corticosteroids and hydroxychloroquine sulfate.[369] Generally, only severe reactions should prompt the discontinuation of this medication.[368]

Additionally, bortezomib has been associated with an LCV, presenting as palpable purpura. Biopsies have demonstrated an accumulation of neutrophils and leukocytoclastic nuclear debris around superficial capillaries along with fibrinoid vessel changes and extravasation of erythrocytes.[370,371] In one study, a patient with LCV had elevated IL-6, tumor necrosis factor (TNF)-α, and CRP levels, consistent with a bortezomib-induced overproduction of proinflammatory cytokines.[371] Although dose reduction or cessation is a viable option in resolving this condition, continuation of bortezomib cyclical infusions appears to lack significant adverse effects. Intriguingly, patients who continued therapy despite the development of LCV showed a fourfold increase in clinical response.[372] Thus, cutaneous LCV may serve as a surrogate marker of bortezomib response.

Ixazomib

Ixazomib is an oral proteasome inhibitor approved in combination with lenalidomide and dexamethasone for treatment of adult patients with relapsed or refractory MM.[373] Patients exposed to ixazomib commonly experience rash. The majority of rashes are low grade and self-limiting. Medical management, when necessary, includes antihistamines or topical glucocorticoids.[373]

Cutaneous necrotizing vasculitis is scarcely reported in patients exposed to ixazomib.[373,374] These necrotizing lesions are described as fixed, indurated, urticarial-like plaques and may be distributed to the cheeks, neck, chest, and back. Histopathologic findings include neutrophilic dermal and pannicular infiltrates in conjunction with necrotizing vasculitis. Treatment options include discontinuing ixazomib and dexamethasone.[375]

Cyclophosphamide and Melphalan

Alkylating agents, such as cyclophosphamide and melphalan, cross-link DNA strands, preventing DNA synthesis and progression of the cell cycle. Cyclophosphamide is commonly used for a wide range of conditions, including oncology-related issues, minimal change disease, various autoimmune disorders, and vasculitides. Its systemic complications, including bone marrow suppression and hemorrhagic cystitis, have been well explored in the literature, but it also presents with certain skin manifestations that the practicing physician should be aware of prior to treatment.

A characteristic finding of cyclophosphamide treatment is chromonychia, either presenting with darkened longitudinal bands or diffuse gray pigmentation. This seems to correlate with a dosage range of 0.7 to 2.475 g with a duration of cyclophosphamide infusion from 10 to 60 days.[376] The lesions tend to originate proximally in the lunula and progress distally, which implicates dysfunction of the nail matrix.[377] Cessation of the medication tends to resolve this condition, in the same proximal to distal manner in which it arose.

Rarely, skin hyperpigmentation in a diffuse reticulated pattern has also been seen in conjunction with cyclophosphamide therapy. On biopsy, the lesions show diffuse epidermal necrosis and melanin deposition in the superficial dermis.[378] Melanin can be confirmed by positive Masson–Fontana and negative Perl stainings.[379] Resolution of clinical findings has been described after cessation of therapy.[378]

Cyclophosphamide-associated radiation recall dermatitis has been reported.[380] This condition may occur months to years after radiotherapy, and it is treated with discontinuation of the cytotoxic therapy. Painful, erythematous-violaceous patches might appear at the site of prior irradiation, immediately following cyclophosphamide treatment. Histology will show changes within the deep dermis, subcutaneous fat, and underlying myofascia, including thickening of the connective tissue, replacement of adipose lobules with sclerosis, and coarse collagen fibers with fibroblasts. Blood and lymphatic vessels can be decreased.

Melanonychia secondary to melphalan cutaneous toxicity presents as darkened striations of the nail plate and should resolve several months after stopping melphalan.[381] When melphalan is given systemically, extravasation might precipitate cutaneous lesions reminiscent of reticular morphea showing white reticular sclerotic bands.[382] Histologically, there are thickened, eosinophilic collagen bundles in the dermis with slight thickening of dermal capillaries. The mechanism of injury appears to be drug-induced cytotoxicity of the endothelium. Treatment includes hydrocolloid dressings and topical antibiotics. Topical corticosteroids may be added if needed.[382]

Antiangiogenic Agents

Thalidomide and its analogs have antiinflammatory and antiangiogenic effects by inhibiting TNF-α mRNA, while also inducing apoptosis within tumor-associated neovasculature.[383,384] Thalidomide and lenalidomide were FDA approved in combination therapies with dexamethasone for the treatment of refractory MM in 2006.

Approximately 20% to 25% of patients undergoing thalidomide treatment experience rash with a minor degree of exfoliation.[385] Rarely, it has been shown to progress to TEN when combined with dexamethasone, displaying evidence of interface reaction and full-thickness epidermal necrosis on biopsy.[386,387] This increased degree of toxicity is believed to be secondary to dexamethasone affecting the nonenzymatic cleavage of thalidomide. Drug discontinuation is critical in the treatment of this disorder.[386]

Thalidomide as a TNF-α inhibitor has been explored in the treatment of TEN,[388] as TNF-α has been connected with its pathogenesis.[389,390] However, this study was halted owing to increase in the incidence of TEN and mortality, likely because of a paradoxical increase in TNF-α levels. Thalidomide had also been associated with increase in de novo psoriasis[391] or exacerbation of preexisting psoriasis during treatment for EM[392] and Behçet disease.[393]

Lenalidomide is an orally available analog of thalidomide. It is used with dexamethasone for the treatment of MM among other hematologic diseases. Unlike thalidomide, cutaneous toxicity appears to be much higher and affect nearly 30% of patients treated, regardless of use of dexamethasone. Cutaneous toxicities are usually low grade and do not necessitate dose adjustment or therapeutic termination.[394] Morbilliform and urticarial reactions are the most common cutaneous side effects,[395] but Sweet syndrome, pustular pyoderma gangrenosum, and epidermal dysmaturation can also be seen.[396]

Monoclonal Antibodies

Elotuzumab is an MAb directed against signaling lymphocytic activation molecule F7 and is approved in combination with pomalidomide and dexamethasone or lenalidomide and dexamethasone for treatment of adult patients with relapsed or refractory MM. Drug rash has been reported in 10% of patients exposed to elotuzumab; however, this was not significantly different from the control group, indicating the eruption could be attributable to pomalidomide coadministration.[397]

Daratumumab is a human IgGκ MAb directed against CD38 and is approved for both intravenous and subcutaneous administration. Combination therapy with daratumumab, bortezomib, and dexamethasone prolongs progression-free survival in patients with relapsed/refractory MM compared to bortezomib and dexamethasone.[398] Subcutaneous injection of daratumumab with hyaluronidase-fihj is also approved for patients with relapsed/refractory MM and patients with newly diagnosed MM.[399] Daratumumab is also approved in combination with bortezomib, melphalan, and prednisone or lenalidomide and dexamethasone in patients with newly diagnosed MM who are ineligible for autologous stem cell transplant.[400,401] Monotherapy daratumumab is approved for patients who have received at least three lines of therapy including a proteasome inhibitor and immunomodulatory agent.[402] Infusion reactions commonly occur in patients exposed to daratumumab, with the majority of reactions occurring during the first infusion.[398] Cutaneous manifestations of these infusion reactions are limited, but include pruritus and rash.[398] Antihistamines, antipyretics, and corticosteroids should be administered prior to infusion. Subcutaneous daratumumab is associated with a significantly decreased reaction rate compared to intravenous daratumumab.[399]

HODGKIN LYMPHOMA

The first-line treatment of HL is the ABVD regimen (doxorubicin, bleomycin, vinblastine, dacarbazine). Other regimens more commonly used in advanced disease include Stanford V (doxorubicin, vinblastine, mechlorethamine, vincristine, bleomycin, etoposide, prednisone) and BEACOPP (bleomycin, etoposide, doxorubicin, cyclophosphamide, vincristine, procarbazine, prednisone).

Alkylating Agents

Dacarbazine introduces double-strand breaks during DNA replication, which causes apoptosis of cancer cells. Cutaneous side effects include phototoxicity,[403] violaceous discoloration at injection site,[404] and vitiligo-like hypopigmentation.[405]

Anthracyclines

Doxorubicin is an anthracycline antibiotic used in combination therapy of HL. It is also used in breast cancer and various disseminated neoplastic conditions such as acute leukemia. A more detailed discussion of the cutaneous side effects of anthracyclines is described previously in the section Acute Leukemias. Anthracyclines may be associated with cutaneous manifestations including PPE, an intertrigo-like eruption, anagen effluvium, NEH, chromonychia, onycholysis, radiation recall dermatitis, SCC, and hyperpigmentation.

Antimicrotubules

Vinblastine and vincristine inhibit the M and S phases of the cell cycle, while also interfering with glutamic acid utilization to suppress cell proliferation.[406] Vinblastine has been associated with radiation recall, notably in an immunosuppressed patient,[407] as well as with Raynaud syndrome when given with bleomycin.[408] These side effects are self-limiting. Vincristine has been most commonly associated with anagen effluvium and nail pigmentation. Urticarial reactions and PPE were also reported.[409]

Glycopeptide Antibiotics

Bleomycin, a glycopeptide derived from *Streptomyces verticillus*, has numerous actions on cell replication. It blocks G2 of the cell cycle, degrades DNA and RNA, and produces free radicals to initiate apoptosis.

Bleomycin has been shown to induce a scleroderma-like skin fibrosis through the upregulation of TGF-β1 mRNA in human fibroblasts.[410] Clinically, patients present with infiltrated nodules and plaques on the hands.[411] TGF-β will, in turn, cause fibroblast proliferation with a rise in the production of extracellular proteins,[410] as well as suppression of adipocyte generation, which are believed to produce antifibrotic factors.[412] Histopathologic examination of the affected areas shows morphologic changes consistent with scleroderma, including dermal thickening and sclerosis, thickened and coarse collagen bundles, and subtle lymphoplasmacytic infiltrates.[413,414] Various therapeutic regimens are being explored for bleomycin-induced systemic sclerosis, including ghrelin as an antifibrotic and antiinflammatory agent,[415] as well as N-acetylcysteine to prevent skin fibrosis, as it has shown reductions in oxidative stress in the mouse model.[416] Simple cessation of bleomycin, though, appears to resolve the sclerotic changes in most patients.[414]

Bleomycin is also classically associated with a dose-related flagellate hyperpigmentation. Up to 20% of patients taking this medication,[417] especially at doses of 90 to 285 mg, tend to develop this linear hyperpigmentation between 24 hours and 9 weeks after initial administration.[418] Bleomycin is believed to amass under the skin owing to a lack of hydrolase in this area, preventing cutaneous inactivation.[419,420] It preferably affects pressure points and areas of prior irritation, most commonly fingers, elbows, and knees, although it may appear diffusely.[421] The increased mechanical pressure is thought to result in hyperperfusion, which additionally increases the local concentration of bleomycin.[421] Under light microscopy, these lesions present with epidermal atrophy, loss of epidermal appendages, homogeneous deposition of collagen, and an increased number of dermal fibroblasts without inflammatory infiltrates.[422] Electron microscopy shows an increased number of melanosomes in the basal keratinocytes. Clinically indistinguishable flagellate hyperpigmentation has also been observed in Cushing syndrome[423] and Shiitake mushroom ingestion.[424] Cessation or alteration of therapy is typically not needed.

Bleomycin-induced NEH (see Figs. 74-3 and 74-4) might present as nodules, plaques, and macules. The histopathologic findings show neutrophilic infiltrates around eccrine glands with eccrine gland necrosis and sparing of coiled and straight dermal ducts.[425] Direct epithelial cytotoxicity of the excreted drug had been postulated in the pathogenesis.[426] Typically, the lesions are self-limiting, but they may recur. Dapsone, given at 100 mg daily, has proven promising in controlling this side effect.[427]

Raynaud's phenomenon is common in patients treated with combination bleomycin and vinblastine.[427] The pathomechanism is likely driven by sympathetically mediated digital vasoconstriction. This is supported by the therapeutic effect of dihydropyridine calcium channel blockers and dorsal sympathectomy.[428] Severe cases may progress to acral gangrene,[408,429] which appears unresponsive to calcium channel blockers.[429] Drug discontinuation will typically result in resolution.

NON-HODGKIN LYMPHOMA

NHL is a diverse group of malignancies. About 85% to 90% are caused by B lymphocytes and the rest come from T lymphocytes or NK cells.[430] NHL accounts for about 4% of new cancers each year in the United States.[167] The subtypes of NHL include precursor B-cell, mature B-cell, B-cell proliferation of uncertain malignant potential, precursor T-cell, extranodal mature T-cell and NK-cell, and nodal mature T-cell and NK-cell lymphomas. NHL typically starts in lymph nodes but can occur in any organ. The gastrointestinal tract is the most common site of extranodal involvement.[430] The overall 5-year survival rate was 71% from 2003 to 2009,[167] but survival is quite variable considering the range of malignancies from indolent follicular lymphoma to aggressive diffuse large B-cell lymphoma (DLBCL) and Burkitt lymphoma. Common medication regimens are discussed in the following section in relationship to the predominant subtypes. As these medications have been previously explored, please refer to their relevant prior sections for mucocutaneous side effects.

Diffuse Large B-Cell Lymphoma

DLBCL, the most common type of NHL, is typically treated with the R-CHOP (rituximab, cyclophosphamide, doxorubicin, vincristine, prednisone) regimen. Other regimens are more commonly used for relapsed or refractory disease.

Polatuzumab vedotin-piiq, an MAb targeting CD79b, is approved in combination with bendamustine and rituximab for treatment of adult patients with relapsed/refractory DLBCL after at least two prior therapies. Alopecia, hyperhidrosis, and pruritus have been reported in patients exposed to polatuzumab.[431]

Follicular Lymphoma

The BR (bendamustine, rituximab) regimen is the first-line therapy for follicular lymphoma, the second most common type of NHL. Other regimens, such as R-CHOP and R-CVP (rituximab, cyclophosphamide, vincristine, prednisone) may be used as well. Infarcted skin tags in the setting of ifosfamide treatment for follicular lymphoma might occur.

Copanlisib is a pan-class 1 PI3K inhibitor approved for treatment of adult patients with follicular lymphoma who have received at least two prior systemic therapies. Cutaneous adverse events associated with copanlisib include maculopapular rash.[432]

Small-Cell Lymphocytic Lymphoma

Small-cell lymphocytic lymphoma (SCLL) is the lymphatic form of CLL, and as such is treated in the same way as CLL. Typical regimens include fludarabine and rituximab; fludarabine, rituximab, and cyclophosphamide; chlorambucil and ofatumumab; and bendamustine and rituximab.

Duvelisib, a first in class oral inhibitor of PI3K-δ, γ, is approved for use in patients with relapsed or refractory SCLL. Cutaneous adverse events seen in SCLL patients include generalized rash, DRESS syndrome, and TEN.[433] Duvelisib-associated drug rash in patients with SCLL may manifest as a photoaccentuated psoriasiform eruption or pityriasisiform reaction. Histopathologic findings include spongiotic dermatitis and dermal lymphocytic and eosinophilic infiltrates.[434]

Mantle-Cell Lymphoma

Mantle-cell lymphoma (MCL) is usually an aggressive disease and treated with the BR regimen. Other regimens commonly used include R-CHOP, R-CVP, and VcR-CAP (bortezomib, rituximab, cyclophosphamide, doxorubicin, prednisone). Zanubrutinib is a selective inhibitor of BTK approved for treatment of adult patients with MCL who have received at least one prior therapy. Exposure to zanubrutinib is commonly associated with low-grade rash.[435]

Marginal-Zone Lymphoma

There are three major types of marginal-zone lymphoma: mucosa-associated lymphoid tissue (MALT), nodal, and splenic. *Helicobacter pylori* eradication treats gastric MALT, and rituximab may be added to the antibiotic regimen. Nongastric MALT can be treated in the same way as follicular lymphoma. Unfortunately, there is no consensus on treatment of the nodal form and usually the regimens for follicular lymphoma are used. Rituximab as single-agent therapy is typically used for the splenic type with or without splenectomy.

Burkitt Lymphoma

Burkitt lymphoma is a very aggressive disease and as such requires aggressive chemotherapy regimens. The chemotherapy regimens include R-CODOX-M (rituximab, cyclophosphamide, vincristine, doxorubicin, high-dose MTX) with IVAC (ifosfamide, cytarabine, etoposide, intrathecal MTX) and CALGB 9251 (cyclophosphamide, prednisone, ifosfamide, high-dose MTX, vincristine, dexamethasone, doxorubicin or etoposide/cytarabine, intrathecal MTX, intrathecal cytarabine, intrathecal hydrocortisone). These regimens typically require extended hospitalizations. Other options include R-Hyper-CVAD (rituximab, hyperfractionated cyclophosphamide, vincristine, doxorubicin, dexamethasone) and EPOCH (etoposide, vincristine, doxorubicin, prednisone, cyclophosphamide).

T-Cell Lymphomas

T-cell lymphomas mostly arise from mature T-cells and therefore are considered peripheral T-cell lymphomas (PTCLs). The four main subtypes are cutaneous, anaplastic large cell, angioimmunoblastic, and PTCL not otherwise specified. PTCLs other than CTCL and primary cutaneous anaplastic large-cell lymphoma are treated with CHOP or EPOCH (CHOP plus etoposide). Treatment of the cutaneous group utilizes specific immunotherapies, retinoids, and skin-directed therapies, which are addressed in the CTCL section. Sorafenib, an inhibitor of the VEGFR and PDGFR pathways, has been used with success in cutaneous and systemic T-cell NHL and has a variety of toxic effects in the skin (Fig. 74-17).

CONCLUSION

Mucocutaneous reactions are common side effects of chemotherapeutic agents used in the treatment of hematologic malignancies. Their clinical presentation is wide-ranging from benign and self-limiting to the life threatening and rapidly fatal. Clinicopathologic correlation between oncologists, dermatologists, and dermatopathologists is critical to recognize and appropriately treat these adverse reactions.

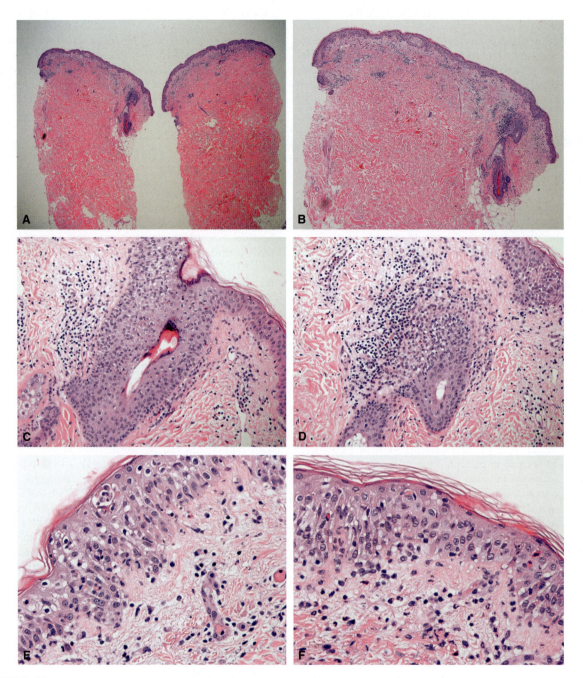

FIGURE 74-17. Drug toxicities from sorafenib. A and **B.** Superficial and perivascular inflammatory infiltrates. **C** and **D.** Folliculitis with intrafollicular eosinophils. **E** and **F.** Mixed-pattern dermatitis with spongiosis and interface changes. Dyskeratotic keratinocytes and dermal eosinophils are present.

References

1. Ward E, DeSantis C, Robbins A, et al. Childhood and adolescent cancer statistics. *CA Cancer J Clin*. 2014. 2014;64(2):83-103.
2. Yamamoto JF, Goodman MT. Patterns of leukemia incidence in the United States by subtype and demographic characteristics, 1997-2002. *Cancer Causes Control*. 2008;19(4):379-390.
3. O'Brien M, Wigler N, Inbar M, et al. Reduced cardiotoxicity and comparable efficacy in a phase III trial of pegylated liposomal doxorubicin HCl (CAELYX/Doxil) versus conventional doxorubicin for first-line treatment of metastatic breast cancer. *Ann Oncol*. 2004;15(3):440-449.
4. Gabizon A, Shmeeda H, Barenholz Y. Pharmacokinetics of pegylated liposomal doxorubicin: review of animal and human studies. *Clin Pharmacokinet*. 2003;42(5):419-436.
5. Lyass O, Uziely B, Ben-Yosef R, et al. Correlation of toxicity with pharmacokinetics of pegylated liposomal doxorubicin (Doxil) in metastatic breast carcinoma. *Cancer*. 2000;89(5):1037-1047.
6. Waterhouse DN, Tardi PG, Mayer LD, et al. A comparison of liposomal formulations of doxorubicin with drug administered in free form: changing toxicity profiles. *Drug Saf*. 2001;24(12):903-920.
7. Skelton H, Linstrum J, Smith K. Host-vs.-altered-host eruptions in patients on liposomal doxorubicin. *J Cutan Pathol*. 2002;29(3):148-153.

8. Uziely B, Jeffers S, Isacson R, et al. Liposomal doxorubicin: antitumor activity and unique toxicities during two complementary phase i studies. *J Clin Oncol.* 1995;13(7):1777-1785.
9. Muggia F, Hainsworth J, Jeffers S, et al. Phase II study of liposomal doxorubicin in refractory ovarian cancer: antitumor activity and toxicity modification by liposomal encapsulation. *J Clin Oncol.* 1997;15(3):987-993.
10. Nagore E, Insa A, Sanmartín O. Antineoplastic therapy-induced palmar plantar erythrodysesthesia ('hand-foot') syndrome: incidence, recognition and management. *Am J Clin Dermatol.* 2000;1(4):225-234.
11. Korver GE, Harris R, Petersen MJ. An intertrigo-like eruption from pegylated liposomal doxorubicin. *J Drugs Dermatol JDD.* 2006;5(9):901-902.
12. Henarejos P, Martínez S, Zafra G, et al. Intertrigo-like eruption caused by pegylated liposomal doxorubicin (PLD). *Clin Transl Oncol.* 2009;11(7):486-487.
13. Garcia-Navarro X, Puig L, Fernández-Figueras M, et al. Eccrine squamous syringometaplasia secondary to pegylated liposomal doxorubicin. *Arch Dermatol.* 2008;144(10):1402-1403.
14. Mangili G, Petrone M, Gentile C, et al. Prevention strategies in palmar-plantar erythrodysesthesia onset: the role of regional cooling. *Gynecol Oncol.* 2008;108(2):332-335.
15. Najem A, Deregnaucourt D, Ramdane S, et al. Intertrigo-like dermatitis with pegylated liposomal doxorubicin: diagnosis and management. *J Clin Oncol.* 2014;32(31):e104-e106.
16. Korać B, Buzadžić B. Doxorubicin toxicity to the skin: possibility of protection with antioxidants enriched yeast. *J Dermatol Sci.* 2001;25:45-52.
17. Tan C, Etcubanas E, Wollner N, et al. Adriamycin—an antitumor antibiotic in the treatment of neoplastic diseases. *Cancer.* 1973;32(1):9-17.
18. Wang J, Cortes E, Sinks L, et al. Therapeutic effect and toxicity of adriamycin in patients with neoplastic disease. *Cancer.* 1971;28(4):837-843.
19. Bhawan J, Petry J, Rybak M. Histologic changes induced in skin by extravasation of doxorubicin (adriamycin). *J Cutan Pathol.* 1989;16(3):158-163.
20. Saghir N, Otrock Z, Mufarrij A, et al. Dexrazoxane for anthracycline extravasation and GM-CSF for skin ulceration and wound healing. *Lancet Oncol.* 2004;5:320-321.
21. Maslovsky I. Extravasation injury as a result of VAD chemotherapy. *J Wound, Ostomy Cont Nurs.* 2007;34(3):297-298.
22. Selleri S, Seltmann H, Gariboldi S, et al. Doxorubicin-induced alopecia is associated with sebaceous gland degeneration. *J Invest Dermatol.* 2006;126:711-720.
23. Middleman E, Luce J, Frei E. Clinical trials with adriamycin. *Cancer.* 1971;28(4):844-850.
24. Spiegel R. The acute toxicities of chemotherapy. *Cancer Treat Rev.* 1981;8(3):197-207.
25. Hortobagyi GN. Anthracyclines in the treatment of cancer: an overview. *Drugs.* 1997;54(suppl 4):1-7.
26. Gardner R. Substitution with doxorubicin for daunorubicin during induction for high risk pediatric acute lymphoblastic leukemia results in increased toxicity. *Pediatr Blood Cancer.* 2013;60:338-339.
27. Crowther D, Powles RL, Bateman CJ, et al. Management of adult acute myelogenous leukaemia. *Br Med J.* 1973;1(5846):131-137.
28. Vietti T, Starling K, Wilbur J, et al. Vincristine, prednisone, and daunomycin in acute leukemia of childhood. *Cancer.* 1971;27(3):602-607.
29. Katsanis E, Luke K, Hsu E, et al. Neutrophilic eccrine hidradenitis in acute myelomonocytic leukemia. *J Pediatr Hematol Oncol.* 1987;9(3):204-208.
30. Beutner K, Packman C, Markowitch W. Neutrophilic eccrine hidradenitis associated with Hodgkin's disease and chemotherapy: a case report. *Arch Dermatol.* 1986;122(7):809-811.
31. Lopes M, Jordão C, Grynszpan R, et al. Chromonychia secondary to chemotherapy. *Case Rep Dermatol.* 2013;5(2):163-167.
32. Curran CF. Onycholysis in doxorubicin-treated patients. *Arch Dermatol.* 1990;126(9):1244.
33. Cunningham D, Gilchrist N, Forrest G, et al. Onycholysis associated with cytotoxic drugs. *Br Med J.* 1985;290:675-676.
34. Manalo FB, Marks A, Davis HL. Doxorubicin toxicity: onycholysis, plantar callus formation, and epidermolysis. *JAMA.* 1975;233(1):56-57.
35. Gzell CE, Carroll SL, Suchowerska N, et al. Radiation recall dermatitis after pre-sensitization with pegylated liposomal doxorubicin. *Cancer Invest.* 2009;27:397-401.
36. Haas RL, de Klerk G. An illustrated case of doxorubicin-induced radiation recall dermatitis and a review of the literature. *Neth J Med.* 2011;69(2):72-75.
37. Muggia F, Cannon T, Safra T, et al. Delayed neoplastic and renal complications in women receiving long-term chemotherapy for recurrent ovarian cancer. *J Natl Cancer Inst.* 2011;103(2):160-161.
38. Gu P, Wu J, Sheu M, et al. Aggressive squamous cell carcinoma of the oral tongue in a woman with metastatic giant cell tumor treated with pegylated liposomal doxorubicin. *Oncol.* 2012;17(12):1596-1597.
39. Bonomi MR, Misiukiewicz K, Posner M, et al. Squamous cell carcinoma of the oral tongue in two patients previously exposed to long-term pegylated liposomal doxorubicin. *Oncol.* 2012;17(12):1594-1595.
40. Cannon TL, Lai DW, Hirsch D, et al. Squamous cell carcinoma of the oral cavity in nonsmoking women: a new and unusual complication of chemotherapy for recurrent ovarian cancer? *Oncol.* 2012;17(12):1541-1546.
41. Harrington K, Mohammadtaghi S, Uster P, et al. Effective targeting of solid tumors in patients with locally advanced cancers by radiolabeled pegylated liposomes. *Clin Cancer Res.* 2001;7(2):243-254.
42. Alagaratnam TT, Choi TK, Ong GB. Doxorubicin and hyperpigmentation. *Aust N Z J Surg.* 1982;52(5):531-533.
43. Kew M, Mzamane D, Smith A, et al. Melanocyte-stimulating-hormone levels in doxorubicin-induced hyperpigmentation. *Lancet.* 1977;1(8015):811.
44. Priestman T, James K. Adriamycin and longitudinal pigmented banding of fingernails [Letter]. *Lancet.* 1975;1(7920):1337-1338.
45. Giacobetti R, Esterly NB, Morgan E. Nail hyperpigmentation secondary to therapy with doxorubicin. *Am J Dis Child.* 1981;135(4):317-318.
46. Blaya M, Saba N. Images in clinical medicine. Chemotherapy-induced hyperpigmentation of the tongue. *N Engl J Med.* 2011;365(10):e20.
47. Cetkovská P, Pizinger K, Cetkovský P. High-dose cytosine arabinoside-induced cutaneous reactions. *J Eur Acad Dermatol Venereol.* 2002;16(5):481-485.
48. Herzig R, Wolff S, Lazarus H, et al. High-dose cytosine arabinoside therapy for refractory leukemia. *Blood.* 1983;62(2):361-369.
49. Waltzer J, Flowers F. Bullous variant of chemotherapy-induced acral erythema. *Arch Dermatol.* 1993;129:43-45.

50. Özkaya-Bayazit E, Diz-Küçükkaya R, Akasya E, et al. Bullous acral erythema and concomitant pigmentation on the face and occluded skin. *J Eur Acad Dermatol Venereol.* 2000;14(2):139-145.
51. Azurdia RM, Clark RE, Friedmann PS. Chemotherapy-induced acral erythema (CIAE) with bullous reaction. *Clin Exp Dermatol.* 1999;24(2):64-66.
52. Burgdorf WH, Gilmore WA, Ganick RG. Peculiar acral erythema secondary to high-dose chemotherapy for acute myelogenous leukemia. *Ann Intern Med.* 1982;97(1):61-62.
53. Crawford JH, Eikelboom JW, McQuillan A. Recurrent palmar-plantar erythrodysaesthesia following high-dose cytarabine treatment for acute lymphoblastic leukemia. *Eur J Haematol.* 2002;69:315-317.
54. Wong GC, Lee LH, Chong YY. A case report of neutrophilic eccrine hidradenitis in a patient receiving chemotherapy for acute myeloid leukaemia. *Ann Acad Med Singapore.* 1998;27(6):860-863.
55. Thorisdottir K, Tomecki KJ, Bergfeld WF, et al. Neutrophilic eccrine hidradenitis. *J Am Acad Dermatol.* 1993;28(5):775-777.
56. Payne AS, James WD, Weiss RB. Dermatologic toxicity of chemotherapeutic agents. *Semin Oncol.* 2006;33(1):86-97.
57. Von Moos R, Thuerlimann BJ, Aapro M, et al. Pegylated liposomal doxorubicin-associated hand-foot syndrome: recommendations of an international panel of experts. *Eur J Cancer.* 2008;44(6):781-790.
58. Patton T, Zirwas M, Nieland-Fisher N, et al. Inflammation of seborrheic keratoses caused by cytarabine: a pseudo sign of Leser-Trelat. *J Drugs Dermatol JDD.* 2004;3(5):565-566.
59. Williams JV, Helm KF, Long D. Chemotherapy-induced inflammation in seborrheic keratoses mimicking disseminated herpes zoster. *J Am Acad Dermatol.* 1999;40(4):643-644.
60. Rassiga A, Schwartz H, Forman W, et al. Cytarabine-induced anaphylaxis: demonstration of antibody and successful desensitization. *Arch Intern Med.* 1980;140:425-426.
61. Ozkan A, Apak H, Celkan T, et al. Toxic epidermal necrolysis after the use of high-dose cytosine arabinoside. *Pediatr Dermatol.* 2001;18(1):38-40.
62. Byrnes J, Baquerizo H, Gonzalez M, et al. Thrombotic thrombocytopenic purpura subsequent to acute myelogenous leukemia chemotherapy. *Am J Hematol.* 1986;21:299-304.
63. Regragui S, Amelal S, Astati S, et al. Thrombotic microangiopathy with skin localization secondary to cytarabine-daunorubicin association: report of a case. *Case Rep Hematol.* 2012;2012:806476.
64. Aktas B, Topcuoglu P, Kurt OK, et al. Severe Henoch-Schönlein purpura induced by cytarabine. *Ann Pharmacother.* 2009;43(4):792-793.
65. Winter SS, Holdsworth MT, Devidas M, et al. Antimetabolite-based therapy in childhood T-cell acute lymphoblastic leukemia: a report of POG Study 9296. *Pediatr Blood Cancer.* 2006;46(2):179-186.
66. Ogden A, Pollock B, Bernstein M, et al. Intermediate-dose methotrexate and intravenous 6-mercaptopurine chemotherapy for children with acute lymphoblastic leukemia who did not respond to initial induction therapy. *J Pediatr Hematol Oncol.* 2002;24(3):182-187.
67. Camitta B, Leventhal B, Lauer S, et al. Intermediate-dose intravenous methotrexate and mercaptopurine therapy for non-T, non-B acute lymphocytic leukemia of childhood: a pediatric oncology group study. *J Clin Oncol.* 1989;7(10):1539-1544.
68. Frandsen TL, Abrahamsson J, Lausen B, et al. Individualized toxicity-titrated 6-mercaptopurine increments during high-dose methotrexate consolidation treatment of lower risk childhood acute lymphoblastic leukaemia. A Nordic Society of Paediatric Haematology and Oncology (NOPHO) pilot study. *Br J Haematol.* 2011;155(2):244-247.
69. Cox GJ, Robertson DB. Toxic erythema of palms and soles associated with high-dose mercaptopurine chemotherapy. *Arch Dermatol.* 1986;122(12):1413-1414.
70. Phillips TL, Fu KK. Quantification of combined radiation therapy and chemotherapy effects on critical normal tissues. *Cancer.* 1976;37(2):1186-1200.
71. Gould J, Mercurio M, Elmets C. Cutaneous photosensitivity diseases induced by exogenous agents. *J Am Acad Dermatol.* 1995;33(4):551-573.
72. Oliveira A, Sanches M, Selores M. Azathioprine-induced pellagra. *J Dermatol.* 2011;38(10):1035-1037.
73. Troeltzsch M, von Blohn G, Kriegelstein S, et al. Oral mucositis in patients receiving low-dose methotrexate therapy for rheumatoid arthritis: report of 2 cases and literature review. *Oral Surg Oral Med Oral Pathol Oral Radiol.* 2013;115(5):e28-e33.
74. Olsen EA. The pharmacology of methotrexate. *J Am Acad Dermatol.* 1991;25(2):306-318.
75. Vogler W, Huguley C, Kerr W. Toxicity and antitumor effect of divided doses of methotrexate. *Arch Intern Med.* 1965;115:285-293.
76. Moe P, Seip M. High dose methotrexate in acute lymphocytic leukemia in childhood. *Acta Paediatr Scand.* 1978;67(3):265-268.
77. Vogler WR, Jacobs J. Toxic and therapeutic effects of methotrexate-folinic acid (leucovorin) in advanced cancer and leukemia. *Cancer.* 1971;28(4):894-901.
78. Mallory S, Berry D. Severe reactivation of sunburn following methotrexate use. *Pediatrics.* 1986;78(3):514-515.
79. Armstrong R, Poh-Fitzpatrick M. Methotrexate and ultraviolet radiation. *Arch Dermatol.* 1982;118(3):177-178.
80. Corder M, Stone W. Failure of leucovorin rescue to prevent reactivation of a solar burn after high dose methotrexate. *Cancer.* 1976;37(4):1660-1662.
81. Naidu A, Kessler HP, Pavelka MA. Epstein–Barr virus-positive oral ulceration simulating Hodgkin lymphoma in a patient treated with methotrexate: case report and review of the literature. *J Oral Maxillofac Surg.* 2014;72(4):724-729.
82. Sadasivam N, Johnson RJ, Owen RG. Resolution of methotrexate-induced Epstein–Barr virus-associated mucocutaneous ulcer. *Br J Haematol.* 2014;165(5):584.
83. Hanakawa H, Orita Y, Sato Y, et al. Large ulceration of the oropharynx induced by methotrexate-associated lymphoproliferative disorders. *Acta Med Okayama.* 2013;67(4):265-269.
84. Hatanaka K, Nakamura N, Kojima M, et al. Methotrexate-associated lymphoproliferative disorders mimicking angioimmunoblastic T-cell lymphoma. *Pathol Res Pract.* 2010;206:9-13.
85. Varela CR, McNamara J, Antaya RJ. Acral erythema with oral methotrexate in a child. *Pediatr Dermatol.* 2007;24(5):541-546.
86. Doyle L, Berg C, Bottino G, et al. Erythema and desquamation after high-dose methotrexate. *Ann Intern Med.* 1983;98(5):611-612.
87. Millot F, Auriol F, Brecheteau P, et al. Acral erythema in children receiving high-dose methotrexate. *Pediatr Dermatol.* 1999;16(5):398-400.

88. Hellier I, Bessis D, Sotto A, et al. High-dose methotrexate-induced bullous variant of acral erythema. *Arch Dermatol.* 1996;132:590-591.
89. Zils K, Wilhelm M, Reeh T, et al. Bullous variant of acral erythema in a child after high-dose methotrexate. *Pediatr Hematol Oncol.* 2012;29(4):378-379.
90. Kuruvila S, Dalal M, Sivanesan B. Bullous variant of acral erythema due to methotrexate. *Indian J Dermatol Venereol Leprol.* 2006;72(6):440-443.
91. Aytaç S, Gümrük F, Cetin M, et al. Acral erythema with bullous formation: a side effect of chemotherapy in a child with acute lymphoblastic leukemia. *Turk J Pediatr.* 2010;52(2):211-214.
92. Wheeland RG, Burgdorf WH, Humphrey GB. The flag sign of chemotherapy. *Cancer.* 1983;51(8):1356-1358.
93. Goldberg NH, Romolo JL, Austin EH. Anaphylactoid type reactions in two patients receiving high dose intravenous methotrexate. *Cancer.* 1978;41(1):52-55.
94. Gogia A, Pathania S, Das P, et al. Methotrexate-induced toxic epidermal necrolysis in a child. *Indian J Dermatol.* 2013;58(2):161.
95. Primka EJ, Camisa C. Methotrexate-induced toxic epidermal necrolysis in a patient with psoriasis. *J Am Acad Dermatol.* 1997;36(5, pt. 2):815-818.
96. Yang C, Yang L, Jaing T, et al. Toxic epidermal necrolysis following combination of methotrexate and trimethoprim-sulfamethoxazole. *Int J Dermatol.* 2000;39(8):621-623.
97. Schuh AC, Döhner H, Pleyer L, Seymour JF, Fenaux P, Dombret H. Azacitidine in adult patients with acute myeloid leukemia. *Crit Rev Oncol Hematol.* 2017;116:159-177.
98. Ravandi F, Alattar ML, Grunwald MR, et al. Phase 2 study of azacytidine plus sorafenib in patients with acute myeloid leukemia and FLT-3 internal tandem duplication mutation. *Blood.* 2013;121(23):4655-4662.
99. Ohanian M, Garcia-Manero G, Levis M, et al. Sorafenib combined with 5-azacytidine in older patients with untreated FLT3-ITD mutated acute myeloid leukemia. *Am J Hematol.* 2018;93(9):1136-1141.
100. Dombret H, Seymour JF, Butrym A, et al. International phase 3 study of azacitidine vs conventional care regimens in older patients with newly diagnosed AML with >30% blasts. *Blood.* 2015;126(3):291-299.
101. Wei AH, Döhner H, Pocock C, et al. The QUAZAR AML-001 maintenance trial: results of a phase III international, randomized, double-blind, placebo-controlled study of CC-486 (oral formulation of azacitidine) in patients with acute myeloid leukemia (AML) in first remission. *Blood.* 2019;134(supplement_2):LBA-3-LBA-3.
102. Shimoda-Komatsu Y, Mizukawa Y, Takayama N, Ohyama M. Cutaneous adverse events induced by azacitidine in myelodysplastic syndrome patients: case reports and a lesson from published work review. *J Dermatol.* 2020;47(4):363-368.
103. Evans W, Tsiatis A, Rivera G, et al. Anaphylactoid reactions to *Escherichia coli* and Erwinia asparaginase in children with leukemia and lymphoma. *Cancer.* 1982;49(7):1378-1383.
104. Ettinger L, Kurtzberg J, Voûte P, et al. An open-label, multicenter study of polyethylene glycol-l-asparaginase for the treatment of acute lymphoblastic leukemia. *Cancer.* 1995;75(5):1176-1181.
105. Haas N, Hermes B, Henz BM. Adhesion molecules and cellular infiltrate: histology of urticaria. *J Invest Dermatol Symp Proc.* 2001;6(2):137-138.
106. Weiss R, Baker J. Hypersensitivity reactions from antineoplastic agents. *Cancer Metastasis Rev.* 1987;6(3):413-432.
107. Silverman L, Gelber R, Dalton V, et al. Improved outcome for children with acute lymphoblastic leukemia: results of Dana-Farber Consortium Protocol 91-01. *Blood.* 2001;97(5):1211-1218.
108. Rytting M. Peg-asparaginase for acute lymphoblastic leukemia. *Expet Opin Biol Ther.* 2010;10(5):833-839.
109. Panosyan E, Seibel N. Asparaginase antibody and asparaginase activity in children with higher-risk acute lymphoblastic leukemia: children's Cancer Group Study CCG-1961. *J Pediatr Hematol Oncol.* 2004;26(4):217-226.
110. Zalewska-Szewczyk B, Andrzejewski W, Bodalski J. Development of anti-asparaginase antibodies in childhood acute lymphoblastic leukemia. *Pediatr Blood Cancer.* 2004;43(5):600-602.
111. Yokel B, Friedman K, Farmer E, et al. Cutaneous pathology following etoposide therapy. *J Cutan Pathol.* 1987;14(6):326-330.
112. Murphy C, Harden E, Herzig R. Dose-related cutaneous toxicities with etoposide. *Cancer.* 1993;71(10):3153-3155.
113. Williams BJ, Roth DJ, Callen JP. Ultraviolet recall associated with etoposide and cyclophosphamide therapy. *Clin Exp Dermatol.* 1993;18(5):452-453.
114. Kellie SJ, Crist WM, Pui CH, et al. Hypersensitivity reactions to epipodophyllotoxins in children with acute lymphoblastic leukemia. *Cancer.* 1991;67(4):1070-1075.
115. Starks D, Prinz D, Armstrong A, et al. Management of a type I hypersensitivity reaction to IV etoposide in a woman with a yolk sac tumor: a case report. *Case Rep Obstet Gynecol.* 2011;2011:837160.
116. Dorr RT, Alberts DS. Vinca alkaloid skin toxicity: antidote and drug disposition studies in the mouse. *J Natl Cancer Inst.* 1985;74:113-120.
117. Kesik V, Kurt B, Tunc T, et al. Adrenomedullin worsens skin necrosis in rats subjected to vincristine-induced extravasation. *Clin Exp Dermatol.* 2010;35(8):897-901.
118. De Thé H, Chomienne C, Lanotte M, et al. The t(15;17) translocation of acute promyelocytic leukaemia fuses the retinoic acid receptor α gene to a novel transcribed locus. *Nature.* 1990;347(6293):558-561.
119. Alcalay M, Zangrilli D, Pandolfi P, et al. Translocation breakpoint of acute promyelocytic leukemia lies within the retinoic acid receptor alpha locus. *Proc Natl Acad Sci USA.* 1991;88:1977-1981.
120. Chang K, Stass S, Chu D, et al. Characterization of a fusion cDNA (RARA/myl) transcribed from the t(15;17) translocation breakpoint in acute promyelocytic leukemia. *Mol Cell Biol.* 1992;12(2):800-810.
121. Hillestad LK. Acute promyelocytic leukemia. *Acta Med Scand.* 1957;159(3):189-194.
122. Breitman TR, Selonick SE, Collins SJ. Induction of differentiation of the human promyelocytic leukemia cell line (HL-60) by retinoic acid. *Proc Natl Acad Sci U S A.* 1980;77(5):2936-2940.
123. Da Costa Moraes CA, Trompieri NM, Cavalcante Felix FH. Pediatric acute promyelocytic leukemia: all-transretinoic acid therapy in a Brazilian Pediatric Hospital. *J Pediatr Hematol Oncol.* 2008;30(5):387-390.
124. Tazi I, Rachid M, Quessar A, et al. Scrotal ulceration following all-trans retinoic acid therapy for acute promyelocytic leukemia. *Indian J Dermatol.* 2011;56(5):561-563.
125. Lee H, Ang A, Lim L, et al. All-trans retinoic acid-induced scrotal ulcer in a patient with acute promyelocytic leukaemia. *Clin Exp Dermatol.* 2010;35:91-92.

126. Drago M, Kim B, Bennett D, et al. All-trans-retinoic acid-induced scrotal ulcers in a patient with acute promyelocytic leukemia. *Cutis*. 2013;91(5):246-247.
127. Shimizu D, Nomura K, Matsuyama R, et al. Scrotal ulcers arising during treatment with all-trans retinoic acid for acute promyelocytic leukemia. *Intern Med*. 2005;44(5):480-483.
128. Mourad YA, Jabr F, Salem Z. Scrotal ulceration induced by all-trans retinoic acid in a patient with acute promyelocytic leukemia. *Int J Dermatol*. 2005;44:68-69.
129. Ramzi J, Hend BN, Lamia A, et al. Scrotal ulcerations during all-transretinoic acid therapy for acute promyelocytic leukemia. *Ann Hematol*. 2007;86(4):289-290.
130. Al-Saad K, Khanani M, Naqvi A, et al. Sweet syndrome developing during treatment with all-trans retinoic acid in a child with acute myelogenous leukemia. *J Pediatr Hematol Oncol*. 2004;26(3):197-199.
131. Park CJ, Bae YB, Choi JY, et al. Sweet's syndrome during the treatment of acute promyelocytic leukemia with all-trans retinoic acid. *Korean J Intern Med*. 2001;16(3):218-221.
132. Shirono K, Kiyofuji C, Tsuda H. Sweet's syndrome in a patient with acute promyelocytic leukemia during treatment with all-trans retinoic acid. *Int J Hematol*. 1995;62(3):183-187.
133. Voelter-Mahlknecht S, Bauer J, Metzler G, et al. Bullous variant of Sweet's syndrome. *Int J Dermatol*. 2005;44:946-947.
134. Astudillo L, Loche F, Reynish W, et al. Sweet's syndrome associated with retinoic acid syndrome in a patient with promyelocytic leukemia. *Ann Hematol*. 2002;81(2):111-114.
135. Phuphanich S, Scott C, Fischbach A, et al. All-trans-retinoic acid: a phase II radiation therapy oncology group study (RTOG 91-13) in patients with recurrent malignant astrocytoma. *J Neuro Oncol*. 1997;34(2):193-200.
136. Lee J, Newman R, Lippman S, et al. Phase I evaluation of all-trans-retinoic acid in adults with solid tumors. *J Clin Oncol*. 1993;11(5):959-966.
137. Tanaka M, Fukushima N, Itamura H, et al. Gangrenous cheilitis associated with all-trans retinoic acid therapy for acute promyelocytic leukemia. *Int J Hematol*. 2010;91:132-135.
138. Siegel R, Ma J, Zou Z, et al. Cancer statistics, 2014. *CA Cancer J Clin*. 2014;64:9-29.
139. Cortes JE, Heidel FH, Hellmann A, et al. Randomized comparison of low dose cytarabine with or without glasdegib in patients with newly diagnosed acute myeloid leukemia or high-risk myelodysplastic syndrome. *Leukemia*. 2019;33(2):379-389.
140. Ferguson JS, Hannam S, Toholka R, Chong AH, Magee J, Foley P. Hair loss and Hedgehog inhibitors: a class effect? *Br J Dermatol*. 2015;173(1):262-264.
141. Martinelli G, Oehler VG, Papayannidis C, et al. Treatment with PF-04449913, an oral smoothened antagonist, in patients with myeloid malignancies: a phase 1 safety and pharmacokinetics study. *Lancet Haematol*. 2015;2(8):e339-e346.
142. Minami Y, Minami H, Miyamoto T, et al. Phase I study of glasdegib (PF-04449913), an oral smoothened inhibitor, in Japanese patients with select hematologic malignancies. *Cancer Sci*. 2017;108(8):1628-1633.
143. Wagner AJ, Messersmith WA, Shaik MN, et al. A phase I study of PF-04449913, an oral hedgehog inhibitor, in patients with advanced solid tumors. *Clin Cancer Res*. 2015;21(5):1044-1051.
144. Souers AJ, Leverson JD, Boghaert ER, et al. ABT-199, a potent and selective BCL-2 inhibitor, achieves antitumor activity while sparing platelets. *Nat Med*. 2013;19(2):202-208.
145. DiNardo CD, Jonas BA, Pullarkat V, et al. Azacitidine and venetoclax in previously untreated acute myeloid leukemia. *N Engl J Med*. 2020;383(7):617-629.
146. Wei AH, Montesinos P, Ivanov V, et al. Venetoclax plus LDAC for newly diagnosed AML ineligible for intensive chemotherapy: a phase 3 randomized placebo-controlled trial. *Blood*. 2020;135(24):2137-2145.
147. Zandvakili I, Lloyd JW, Giridhar KV. Hepatitis, pancreatitis and rash in a patient with chronic lymphocytic leukemia. *Gastroenterology*. 2019;157(4):e8-e9.
148. Coutre S, Choi M, Furman RR, et al. Venetoclax for patients with chronic lymphocytic leukemia who progressed during or after idelalisib therapy. *Blood, Am Soc Hemat*. 2018;131:1704-1711.
149. Im AP, Sehgal AR, Carroll MP, et al. DNMT3A and IDH mutations in acute myeloid leukemia and other myeloid malignancies: associations with prognosis and potential treatment strategies. *Leukemia*. 2014;28(9):1774-1783.
150. Xu Q, Li Y, Lv N, et al. *Biology of Human Tumors Correlation between Isocitrate Dehydrogenase Gene Aberrations and Prognosis of Patients with Acute Myeloid Leukemia: A Systematic Review and Meta-Analysis*. 2017.
151. DiNardo CD, Stein EM, de Botton S, et al. Durable remissions with ivosidenib in IDH1-mutated relapsed or refractory AML. *N Engl J Med*. 2018;378(25):2386-2398.
152. Roboz GJ, DiNardo CD, Stein EM, et al. Ivosidenib induces deep durable remissions in patients with newly diagnosed IDH1-mutant acute myeloid leukemia. *Blood*. 2020;135(7):463-471.
153. Norsworthy KJ, Luo L, Hsu V, et al. FDA approval summary: ivosidenib for relapsed or refractory acute myeloid leukemia with an isocitrate dehydrogenase-1 mutation. *Clin Cancer Res*. 2019;25(11):3205-3209.
154. Flinn IW, Hillmen P, Montillo M, et al. The phase 3 DUO trial: duvelisib vs ofatumumab in relapsed and refractory CLL/SLL. *Blood*. 2018;132(23):2446-2455.
155. *A Phase 3 Study of Duvelisib Versus Ofatumumab in Patients With Relapsed or Refractory CLL/SLL (DUO) - Study Results - ClinicalTrials.gov*. Accessed December 21, 2020. https://clinicaltrials.gov/ct2/show/results/NCT02004522
156. Flinn IW, Cherry MA, Maris MB, Matous JV, Berdeja JG, Patel M. Combination trial of duvelisib (IPI-145) with rituximab or bendamustine/rituximab in patients with non-Hodgkin lymphoma or chronic lymphocytic leukemia. *Am J Hematol*. 2019;94(12):1325-1334.
157. Small D, Levenstein M, Kim E, et al. STK-1, the human homolog of Flk-2/Flt-3, is selectively expressed in CD34+ human bone marrow cells and is involved in the proliferation of early progenitor/stem cells. *Proc Natl Acad Sci U S A*. 1994;91(2):459-463.
158. Stone RM, Mandrekar SJ, Sanford BL, et al. Midostaurin plus chemotherapy for acute myeloid leukemia with a FLT3 mutation. *N Engl J Med*. 2017;377(5):454-464.
159. Perl AE, Martinelli G, Cortes JE, et al. Gilteritinib or chemotherapy for relapsed or refractory FLT3-mutated AML. *N Engl J Med*. 2019;381(18):1728-1740.
160. McMahon CM, Canaani J, Rea B, et al. Gilteritinib induces differentiation in relapsed and refractory FLT3-mutated acute myeloid leukemia. *Blood Adv*. 2019;3(10):1581-1585.
161. Varadarajan N, Boni A, Elder DE, et al. FLT3 inhibitor-associated neutrophilic dermatoses. *JAMA Dermatology*. 2016;152(4):480-482.
162. Paudel A, Dhital R, Areoye G, Basnet S, Tachamo N. Sweet's syndrome in a granulocytopenic patient with acute myeloid leukemia on FLT3 inhibitor. *J Community Hosp Intern Med Perspect*. 2020;10(3):275-278.

163. Fathi AT, Le L, Hasserjian RP, Sadrzadeh H, Levis M, Chen YB. FLT3 inhibitor-induced neutrophilic dermatosis. *Blood.* 2013;122(2):239-242.
164. Döhner H, Weisdorf DJ, Bloomfield CD. Acute myeloid leukemia. Longo DL, ed. *N Engl J Med.* 2015;373(12):1136-1152.
165. Stein EM, DiNardo CD, Fathi AT, et al. Molecular remission and response patterns in patients with mutant-IDH2 acute myeloid leukemia treated with enasidenib. *Blood.* 2019;133(7):676-687.
166. Pollyea DA, Tallman MS, de Botton S, et al. Enasidenib, an inhibitor of mutant IDH2 proteins, induces durable remissions in older patients with newly diagnosed acute myeloid leukemia. *Leukemia.* 2019;33(11):2575-2584.
167. Hillmen P, Skotnicki AB, Robak T, et al. Alemtuzumab compared with chlorambucil as first-line therapy for chronic lymphocytic leukemia. *J Clin Oncol.* 2007;25(35):5616-5623.
168. Wierda WG, Kipps TJ, Mayer J, et al. Ofatumumab as single-agent CD20 immunotherapy in fludarabine-refractory chronic lymphocytic leukemia. *J Clin Oncol.* 2010;28(10):1749-1755.
169. Bryan J, Borthakur G. Role of rituximab in first-line treatment of chronic lymphocytic leukemia. *Therapeut Clin Risk Manag.* 2010;7:1-11.
170. Lundin J, Kimby E, Bjorkholm M, et al. Phase II trial of subcutaneous anti-CD52 monoclonal antibody alemtuzumab (Campath-1H) as first-line treatment for patients with B-cell chronic lymphocytic leukemia (B-CLL). *Blood.* 2002;100(3):768-773.
171. Keating MJ, Flinn I, Jain V, et al. Therapeutic role of alemtuzumab (Campath-1H) in patients who have failed fludarabine: results of a large international study. *Blood.* 2002;99(10):3554-3561.
172. Ogawa Y, Ogura M, Suzuki T, et al. A phase I/II study of ofatumumab (GSK1841157) in Japanese and Korean patients with relapsed or refractory B-cell chronic lymphocytic leukemia. *Int J Hematol.* 2013;98(2):164-170.
173. Barth MJ, Czuczman MS. Ofatumumab: a novel, fully human anti-CD20 monoclonal antibody for the treatment of chronic lymphocytic leukemia. *Future Oncol.* 2013;9(12):1829-1839.
174. McLaughlin P, Grillo-López A, Link B, et al. Rituximab chimeric anti-CD20 monoclonal antibody therapy for relapsed indolent lymphoma: half of patients respond to a four-dose treatment program. *J Clin Oncol.* 1998;16(8):2825-2833.
175. Robak T. Alemtuzumab in the treatment of chronic lymphocytic leukemia. *BioDrugs.* 2005;19(1):9-22.
176. Zenz T, Ritgen M, Dreger P, et al. Autologous graft-versus-host disease–like syndrome after an alemtuzumab-containing conditioning regimen and autologous stem cell transplantation for chronic lymphocytic leukemia. *Blood.* 2006;108(6):2127-2130.
177. Lowndes S, Darby A, Mead G, et al. Stevens–Johnson syndrome after treatment with rituximab. *Ann Oncol.* 2002;13(12):1948-1950.
178. Fallon MJ, Heck JN. Fatal Stevens–Johnson syndrome/toxic epidermal necrolysis induced by allopurinol–rituximab–bendamustine therapy. *J Oncol Pharm Pract.* 2015;21(5):388-392.
179. Higo T, Miyagaki T, Nakamura F, et al. Paraneoplastic pemphigus occurring after bendamustine and rituximab therapy for relapsed follicular lymphoma. *Ann Hematol.* 2015;94(4):683-685.
180. Ungprasert P, Srivali N, Kittanamongkolchai W, et al. Rituximab-induced serum sickness in overlapping syndrome between Sjögren syndrome and systemic lupus erythematosus. *J Clin Rheumatol.* 2013;19(6):360.
181. Le Guenno G, Ruivard M, Charra L, et al. Rituximab-induced serum sickness in refractory immune thrombocytopenic purpura. *Intern Med J.* 2011;41(2):202-205.
182. Hellerstedt B, Ahmed A. Delayed-type hypersensitivity reaction or serum sickness after rituximab treatment. *Ann Oncol.* 2003;14(12):1792.
183. Herishanu Y. Rituximab-induced serum sickness. *Am J Hematol.* 2002;70(4):329.
184. D'Arcy C, Mannik M. Serum sickness secondary to treatment with the murine–human chimeric antibody IDEC-C2B8 (rituximab). *Arthritis Rheum.* 2001;44(7):1717-1718.
185. Todd DJ, Helfgott SM. Serum sickness following treatment with rituximab. *J Rheumatol.* 2007;34(2):430-433.
186. Mehsen N, Yvon C, Richez C, et al. Serum sickness following a first rituximab infusion with no recurrence after the second one. *Clin Exp Rheumatol.* 2008;26(5):967.
187. Seymour J, Kurzrock R, Freireich E, et al. 2-Chlorodeoxyadenosine induces durable remissions and prolonged suppression of CD4+ lymphocyte counts in patients with hairy cell leukemia. *Blood.* 1994;83(10):2906-2911.
188. Powell A, Albert S, Oyama N, et al. Paraneoplastic pemphigus secondary to fludarabine evolving into unusual oral pemphigus vegetans. *J Eur Acad Dermatol Venereol.* 2004;18(3):360-364.
189. Gooptu C, Littlewood TJ, Frith P, et al. Paraneoplastic pemphigus: an association with fludarabine? *Br J Dermatol.* 2001;144(6):1255-1261.
190. Yildiz O, Ozguroglu M, Yanmaz MT, et al. Paraneoplastic pemphigus associated with fludarabine use. *Med Oncol.* 2007;24(1):115-118.
191. Ho A, Suciu S, Stryckmans P, et al. Pentostatin in T-cell malignancies—a phase II trial of the EORTC. *Ann Oncol.* 1999;10:1493-1498.
192. Kay NE, Wu W, Kabat B, et al. Pentostatin and rituximab therapy for previously untreated patients with B-cell chronic lymphocytic leukemia. *Cancer.* 2010;116(9):2180-2187.
193. Dillman RO, Mick R, McIntyre OR. Pentostatin in chronic lymphocytic leukemia: a phase II trial of cancer and leukemia group B. *J Clin Oncol.* 1989;7(4):433-438.
194. Ghura H, Carmichael A, Bairstow D, et al. Fatal erythroderma associated with pentostatin. *Br Med J.* 1999;319(7209):549.
195. Leitman S, Tisdale J, Bolan C, et al. Transfusion-associated GVHD after fludarabine therapy in a patient with systemic lupus erythematosus. *Transfusion.* 2003;43(12):1667-1671.
196. Zulian GB, Roux E, Tiercy JM, et al. Transfusion-associated graft-versus-host disease in a patient treated with cladribine (2-chlorodeoxyadenosine): demonstration of exogenous DNA in various tissue extracts by PCR analysis. *Br J Haematol.* 1995;89:83-89.
197. Larsen CR, Hansen PB, Clausen NT. Aggressive growth of epithelial carcinomas following treatment with nucleoside analogues. *Am J Hematol.* 2002;70:48-50.
198. Rashid K, Ng R, Mastan A, et al. Accelerated growth of skin carcinoma following fludarabine therapy for chronic lymphocytic leukemia. *Leuk Lymphoma.* 2005;46(7):1051-1055.
199. Herr D, Borelli S, Kempf W, et al. Fludarabine: risk factor for aggressive behaviour of squamous cell carcinoma of the skin? *Ann Oncol.* 2005;16(3):515-516.
200. Kantarjian H, Cortes J, O'Brien S, et al. Imatinib mesylate (STI571) therapy for Philadelphia chromosome-positive chronic myelogenous leukemia in blast phase. *Blood.* 2002;99(10):3547-3553.

201. Valeyrie L, Bastuji-Garin S, Revuz J, et al. Adverse cutaneous reactions to imatinib (STI571) in Philadelphia chromosome-positive leukemias: a prospective study of 54 patients. *J Am Acad Dermatol*. 2003;48(2):201-206.
202. Breccia M, Carmosino I, Russo E, et al. Early and tardive skin adverse events in chronic myeloid leukaemia patients treated with imatinib. *Eur J Haematol*. 2005;74(2):121-123.
203. Amitay-Laish I, Stemmer SM, Lacouture ME. Adverse cutaneous reactions secondary to tyrosine kinase inhibitors including imatinib mesylate, nilotinib, and dasatinib. *Dermatol Ther*. 2011;24(4):386-395.
204. Kantarjian H, Sawyers C, Hochhaus A, et al. Hematologic and cytogenetic responses to imatinib mesylate in chronic myelogenous leukemia. *N Engl J Med*. 2002;346(9):645-652.
205. Rousselot P, Larghero J, Raffoux E, et al. Photosensitization in chronic myelogenous leukaemia patients treated with imatinib mesylate. *Br J Haematol*. 2003;120:1091-1092.
206. Arora B, Kumar L, Sharma A, et al. Pigmentary changes in chronic myeloid leukemia patients treated with imatinib mesylate. *Ann Oncol*. 2004;15(2):358-359.
207. Tsao AS, Kantarjian H, Cortes J, et al. Imatinib mesylate causes hypopigmentation in the skin. *Cancer*. 2003;98(11):2483-2487.
208. Campbell T, Felsten L, Moore J. Disappearance of lentigines in a patient receiving imatinib treatment for familial gastrointestinal stromal tumor syndrome. *Arch Dermatol*. 2009;145(11):1313-1316.
209. Pérez N, Esturo S, Viladomiu Edel A, et al. Pseudoporphyria induced by imatinib mesylate. *Int J Dermatol*. 2014;53(2):e143-e144.
210. Mahon C, Purvis D, Laughton S, et al. Imatinib mesylate-induced pseudoporphyria in two children. *Pediatr Dermatol*. 2014;31(5):603-607.
211. Woo SM, Huh CH, Park KC, et al. Exacerbation of psoriasis in a chronic myelogenous leukemia patient treated with imatinib. *J Dermatol*. 2007;34(10):724-726.
212. Ayirookuzhi SJ, Ma L, Ramshesh P, et al. Imatinib-induced sweet syndrome in a patient with chronic myeloid leukemia. *Arch Dermatol*. 2005;141(3):368-370.
213. Sanchez-Gonzalez B, Pascual-Ramirez J, Fernandez-Abellan P, et al. Severe skin reaction to imatinib in a case of Philadelphia-positive acute lymphoblastic leukemia. *Blood*. 2003;101(6):2446.
214. Bois E, Holle LM, Farooq U. Late onset imatinib-induced Stevens–Johnson syndrome. *J Oncol Pharm Pract*. 2014;20(6):476-478.
215. Schaich M, Schäkel K, Illmer T, et al. Severe epidermal necrolysis after treatment with imatinib and consecutive allogeneic hematopoietic stem cell transplantation. *Ann Hematol*. 2003;82(5):303-304.
216. Mahapatra M, Mishra P, Kumar R. Imatinib-induced Stevens–Johnson syndrome: recurrence after re-challenge with a lower dose. *Ann Hematol*. 2007;86(7):537-538.
217. Schwarz M, Kreuzer KA, Baskaynak G, et al. Imatinib-induced acute generalized exanthematous pustulosis (AGEP) in two patients with chronic myeloid leukemia. *Eur J Haematol*. 2002;69(4):254-256.
218. Tanvetyanon T, Nand S. Overcoming recurrent cutaneous reactions from imatinib using once-weekly dosing. *Ann Pharmacother*. 2003;37(12):1818-1820.
219. Kantarjian H, Giles F, Wunderle L, et al. Nilotinib in imatinib-resistant CML and Philadelphia chromosome-positive ALL. *N Engl J Med*. 2006;354(24):2542-2551.
220. Kaune K, Baumgart M, Gesk S, et al. Bullous Sweet syndrome in a patient with t(9;22)(q34;q11)-positive chronic myeloid leukemia treated with the tyrosine kinase inhibitor nilotinib: interphase cytogenetic detection of BCR-ABL-positive lesional cells. *Arch Dermatol*. 2008;144(3):361-364.
221. Assouline S, Laneuville P, Gambacorti-Passerini C. Panniculitis during dasatinib therapy for imatinib-resistant chronic myelogenous leukemia. *N Engl J Med*. 2006;354(24):2623-2624.
222. Hutchinson CV, Dyer MJ. Breaking good: the inexorable rise of BTK inhibitors in the treatment of chronic lymphocytic leukaemia. *Br J Haematol*. 2014;166:12-22.
223. Byrd JC, Brown JR, O'Brien S, et al. Ibrutinib versus ofatumumab in previously treated chronic lymphoid leukemia. *N Engl J Med*. 2014;371(3):213-223.
224. Knauf WU, Lissichkov T, Aldaoud A, et al. Phase III randomized study of bendamustine compared with chlorambucil in previously untreated patients with chronic lymphocytic leukemia. *J Clin Oncol*. 2009;27(26):4378-4384.
225. Kolibaba KS, Sterchele JA, Joshi AD, et al. Demographics, treatment patterns, safety, and real-world effectiveness in patients aged 70 years and over with chronic lymphocytic leukemia receiving bendamustine with or without rituximab: a retrospective study. *Ther Adv Hematol*. 2013;4(3):157-171.
226. Tadmor T, Polliack A. Optimal management of older patients with chronic lymphocytic leukemia: some facts and principles guiding therapeutic choices. *Blood Rev*. 2012;26:15-23.
227. Malipatil B, Ganesan P, Sundersingh S, et al. Preliminary experience with the use of bendamustine: a peculiar skin rash as the commonest side effect. *Hematol Oncol Stem Cell Ther*. 2011;4(4):157-160.
228. Lambertini M, Del Mastro L, Gardin G, et al. Stevens–Johnson syndrome after treatment with bendamustine. *Leuk Res*. 2012;36(7):e153-e154.
229. Carilli A, Favis G, Sundharkrishnan L, et al. Severe dermatologic reactions with bendamustine: a case series. *Case Rep Oncol*. 2014;7(2):465-470.
230. Gavini A, Telang GH, Olszewski AJ. Generalized purpuric drug exanthem with hemorrhagic plaques following bendamustine chemotherapy in a patient with B-prolymphocytic leukemia. *Int J Hematol*. 2012;95(3):311-314.
231. Alamdari HS, Pinter-Brown L, Cassarino DS, et al. Severe cutaneous interface drug eruption associated with bendamustine. *Dermatol Online J*. 2010;16(7).
232. Pietrantonio F, Moriconi L, Torino F, et al. Unusual reaction to chlorambucil: a case report. *Cancer Lett*. 1990;54(3):109-111.
233. Vaida I, Roszkiewicz F, Gruson B, et al. Drug rash with eosinophilia and systemic symptoms after chlorambucil treatment in chronic lymphocytic leukaemia. *Pharmacology*. 2009;83(3):148-149.
234. Millard L, Rajah S. Cutaneous reaction to chlorambucil. *Arch Dermatol*. 1977;113(9):1298.
235. Knisley RE, Settipane GA, Albala MM. Unusual reaction to chlorambucil in a patient with chronic lymphocytic leukemia. *Arch Dermatol*. 1971;104:77-79.
236. Möller H. Pigmentary disturbances due to drugs. *Acta Derm Venereol*. 1966;46(5):423-431.
237. Harrold BP. Syndrome resembling Addison's disease following prolonged treatment with busulphan. *Br Med J*. 1966;1(5485):463-464.
238. Feingold M, Koss L. Effects of long-term administration of busulfan: report of a patient with generalized nuclear

abnormalities, carcinoma of vulva, and pulmonary fibrosis. *Arch Intern Med.* 1969;124:66-71.
239. Parker TL, Cooper DL, Seropian SE, et al. Toxic erythema of chemotherapy following IV BU plus fludarabine for allogeneic PBSC transplant. *Bone Marrow Transplant.* 2013;48(5):646-650.
240. Valks R, Fraga J, Porras-Luque J, et al. Chemotherapy-induced eccrine squamous syringometaplasia: a distinctive eruption in patients receiving hematopoietic progenitor cells. *Arch Dermatol.* 1997;133(7):873-878.
241. Palamaras I, Misciali C, Vincenzi C, et al. Permanent chemotherapy-induced alopecia: a review. *J Am Acad Dermatol.* 2011;64(3):604-606.
242. Young CW, Schochetman G, Karnofsky DA. Hydroxyurea-induced inhibition of deoxyribonucleotide synthesis: studies in intact cells. *Cancer Res.* 1967;27(3):526-534.
243. Vassallo C, Passamonti F, Merante S, et al. Muco-cutaneous changes during long-term therapy with hydroxyurea in chronic myeloid leukaemia. *Clin Exp Dermatol.* 2001;26(2):141-148.
244. Best P, Daoud M, Pittelkow M, et al. Hydroxyurea-induced leg ulceration in 14 patients. *Ann Intern Med.* 1998;128(1):29-32.
245. Weinlich G, Schuler G, Greil R, et al. Leg ulcers associated with long-term hydroxyurea therapy. *J Am Acad Dermatol.* 1998;39(2):372-374.
246. Dissemond J, Körber A. Hydroxyurea-induced ulcers on the leg. *Can Med Assoc J.* 2009;180(11):1132.
247. Sirieix ME, Debure C, Baudot N, et al. Leg ulcers and hydroxyurea. *Arch Dermatol.* 1999;135:818-820.
248. Crittenden SC, Gilbert JE, Callen JP. Hydroxyurea-induced leg ulceration in a patient with a homozygous MTHFR polymorphism misdiagnosed as pyoderma gangrenosum. *JAMA Dermatol.* 2014;150(7):780-781.
249. Quattrone F, Dini V, Barbanera S, et al. Cutaneous ulcers associated with hydroxyurea therapy. *J Tissue Viability.* 2013;22(4):112-121.
250. Daoud MS, Gibson LE, Pittelkow MR. Hydroxyurea dermopathy: a unique lichenoid eruption complicating long-term therapy with hydroxyurea. *J Am Acad Dermatol.* 1997;36(2):178-182.
251. Elliott R, Davies M, Harmse D. Dermatomyositis-like eruption with long-term hydroxyurea. *J Dermatol Treat.* 2006;17:59-60.
252. Senet P, Aractingi S, Porneuf M, et al. Hydroxyurea-induced dermatomyositis-like eruption. *Br J Dermatol.* 1995;133(3):455-459.
253. Kennedy BJ, Smith LR, Goltz RW. Skin changes secondary to hydroxyurea therapy. *Arch Dermatol.* 1975;111:183-187.
254. Papi M, Didona B, DePità O, et al. Multiple skin tumors on light-exposed areas during long-term treatment with hydroxyurea. *J Am Acad Dermatol.* 1993;28(3):485-486.
255. Baskaynak G, Kreuzer KA, Schwarz M, et al. Squamous cutaneous epithelial cell carcinoma in two CML patients with progressive disease under imatinib treatment. *Eur J Haematol.* 2003;70(4):231-234.
256. Butler D, Nambudiri VE, Nandi T. Hydroxyurea-associated acral erythema in a patient with polycythemia vera. *Am J Hematol.* 2014;89(9):931-932.
257. Silver FS, Espinoza LR, Hartmann RC. Acral erythema and hydroxyurea. *Ann Intern Med.* 1983;98(5, pt. 1):675.
258. Hendrix J, Greer K. Cutaneous hyperpigmentation caused by systemic drugs. *Int J Dermatol.* 1992;31(7):458-466.
259. Aste N, Fumo G, Contu F, et al. Nail pigmentation caused by hydroxyurea: report of 9 cases. *J Am Acad Dermatol.* 2002;47(1):146-147.
260. Cakir B, Sucak G, Haznedar R. Longitudinal pigmented nail bands during hydroxyurea therapy. *Int J Dermatol.* 1997;36:236-237.
261. Gropper CA, Don PC, Sadjadi MM. Nail and skin hyperpigmentation associated with hydroxyurea therapy for polycythemia vera. *Int J Dermatol.* 1993;32(10):731-733.
262. García-Martínez FJ, García-Gavín J, Alvarez-Pérez A, et al. Scleroderma-like syndrome due to hydroxyurea. *Clin Exp Dermatol.* 2012;37(7):755-758.
263. Golomb HM, Braylan R, Polliack A. "Hairy" cell leukaemia (leukaemic reticuloendotheliosis): a scanning electron microscopic study of eight cases. *Br J Haematol.* 1975;29(3):455-460.
264. Dietrich S, Glimm H, Andrulis M, et al. BRAF inhibition in refractory hairy-cell leukemia. *N Engl J Med.* 2012;366(21):2038-2040.
265. Samuel J, Macip S, Dyer MJ. Efficacy of vemurafenib in hairy-cell leukemia. *N Engl J Med.* 2014;370(3):286-288.
266. Vergote V, Dierickx D, Janssens A, et al. Rapid and complete hematological response of refractory hairy cell leukemia to the BRAF inhibitor dabrafenib. *Ann Hematol.* 2014;93(12):2087-2089.
267. Tiacci E, Trifonov V, Schiavoni G, et al. BRAF mutations in hairy-cell leukemia. *N Engl J Med.* 2011;364(24):2305-2315.
268. Rinderknecht JD, Goldinger SM, Rozati S, et al. RASopathic skin eruptions during vemurafenib therapy. *PLoS One.* 2013;8(3).
269. Su F, Viros A, Milagre C, et al. RAS mutations in cutaneous squamous-cell carcinomas in patients treated with BRAF inhibitors. *N Engl J Med.* 2012;366(3):207-215.
270. Harvey NT, Millward M, Wood BA. Squamoproliferative lesions arising in the setting of BRAF inhibition. *Am J Dermatopathol.* 2012;34(8):822-826.
271. Flaherty KT, Infante JR, Daud A, et al. Combined BRAF and MEK inhibition in melanoma with BRAF V600 mutations. *N Engl J Med.* 2012;367(18):1694-1703.
272. Jeudy G, Dalac-Rat S, Bonniaud B, et al. Successful switch to dabrafenib after vemurafenib-induced toxic epidermal necrolysis. *Br J Dermatol.* 2015;172(5):1454-1455.
273. Criscione V, Weinstock M. Incidence of cutaneous T-cell lymphoma in the United States, 1973-2002. *Arch Dermatol.* 2007;143(7):854-859.
274. Qin J, Dummer R, Burg G, et al. Constitutive and interleukin-7/interleukin-15 stimulated DNA binding of Myc, Jun, and novel Myc-like proteins in cutaneous T-cell lymphoma cells. *Blood.* 1999;93(1):260-267.
275. Poiesz B, Ruscetti F, Gazdar A, et al. Detection and isolation of type C retrovirus particles from fresh and cultured lymphocytes of a patient with cutaneous T-cell lymphoma. *Proc Natl Acad Sci U S A.* 1980;77(12):7415-7419.
276. Hettmannsperger U, Tenorio S, Orfanos C, et al. Corticosteroids induce proliferation but do not influence TNF-or IL-1β-induced ICAM-1 expression of human dermal microvascular endothelial cells in vitro. *Arch Dermatol Res.* 1993;285:347-351.
277. Lavker R, Schechter N, Lazarus G. Effects of topical corticosteroids on human dermis. *Br J Dermatol.* 1986;115(suppl 31):101-107.
278. Rogalski C, Haustein U, Glander H, et al. Extensive striae distensae as a result of topical corticosteroid therapy in psoriasis vulgaris. *Acta Derm Venereol.* 2003;83:54-55.
279. Ermis B, Ors R, Tastekin A, et al. Cushing's syndrome secondary to topical corticosteroids abuse. *Clin Endocrinol.* 2003;58:795-796.

280. Joe EK. Cushing syndrome secondary to topical glucocorticoids. *Dermatol Online J.* 2003;9(4):16.
281. Ramsay D, Halperin P, Zeleniuch-Jacquotte A. Topical mechlorethamine therapy for early stage mycosis fungoides. *J Am Acad Dermatol.* 1988;19(4):684-691.
282. Kim Y, Jensen R, Watanabe G, et al. Clinical stage IA (limited patch and plaque) mycosis fungoides: a long-term outcome analysis. *Arch Dermatol.* 1996;132:1309-1313.
283. Kim Y, Martinez G, Varghese A, et al. Topical nitrogen mustard in the management of mycosis fungoides: update of the Stanford experience. *Arch Dermatol.* 2003;139:165-173.
284. Lindahl LM, Fenger-Gron M, Iversen L. Topical nitrogen mustard therapy in patients with mycosis fungoides or parapsoriasis. *J Eur Acad Dermatol Venereol.* 2013;27(2):163-168.
285. Zackheim HS. Topical carmustine (BCNU) in the treatment of mycosis fungoides. *Dermatol Ther.* 2003;16:299-302.
286. Zackheim HS, Epstein EH. Treatment of mycosis fungoides with topical nitrosourea compounds: further studies. *Arch Dermatol.* 1975;11:1564-1570.
287. Zackheim HS, Epstein EH, McNutt NS, et al. Topical carmustine (BCNU) for mycosis fungoides and related disorders: a 10-year experience. *J Am Acad Dermatol.* 1983;9(3):363-374.
288. Lessin SR, Duvic M, Guitart J, et al. Topical chemotherapy in cutaneous T-cell lymphoma: positive results of a randomized, controlled, multi-center trial testing the efficacy and safety of a novel 0.02% mechlorethamine gel in mycosis fungoides. *JAMA Dermatol.* 2013;149(1):25-32.
289. Price N, Hoppe R, Deneau D. Ointment-based mechlorethamine treatment for mycosis fungoides. *Cancer.* 1983;52(12):2214-2219.
290. Wormser U, Brodsky B, Reich R. Topical treatment with povidone iodine reduces nitrogen mustard-induced skin collagenolytic activity. *Arch Toxicol.* 2002;76(2):119-121.
291. Wormser U, Brodsky B, Green B, et al. Protective effect of povidone-iodine ointment against skin lesions induced by sulphur and nitrogen mustards and by non-mustard vesicants. *Arch Toxicol.* 1997;71:165-170.
292. Constantine V, Fuks Z, Farber E. Mechlorethamine desensitization in therapy for mycosis fungoides: topical desensitization to mechlorethamine (nitrogen mustard) contact hypersensitivity. *Arch Dermatol.* 1975;111:484-488.
293. Daughters D, Zackheim H, Maibach H. Urticaria and anaphylactoid reactions: after topical application of mechlorethamine. *Arch Dermatol.* 1973;107(3):429-430.
294. Reddy VB, Ramsay D, Garcia JA, et al. Atypical cutaneous changes after topical treatment with nitrogen mustard in patients with mycosis fungoides. *Am J Dermatopathol.* 1996;18(1):19-23.
295. Newman JM, Rindler JM, Bergfeld WF, et al. Stevens–Johnson syndrome associated with topical nitrogen mustard therapy. *J Am Acad Dermatol.* 1997;36(1):112-114.
296. Flaxman B, Sosis A, Van Scott E. Changes in melanosome distribution in Caucasoid skin following topical application of nitrogen mustard. *J Invest Dermatol.* 1973;60(5):321-326.
297. Zackheim HS, Epstein EH, Crain WR. Topical carmustine (BCNU) for cutaneous T cell lymphoma: a 15-year experience in 143 patients. *J Am Acad Dermatol.* 1990;22(5):802-810.
298. Whittaker SJ, Demierre MF, Kim EJ, et al. Final results from a multicenter, international, pivotal study of romidepsin in refractory cutaneous T-cell lymphoma. *J Clin Oncol.* 2010;28(29):4485-4491.
299. Poligone B, Lin J, Chung C. Romidepsin: evidence for its potential use to manage previously treated cutaneous T cell lymphoma. *Core Evid.* 2011;6:1-12.
300. Duvic M, Olsen EA, Breneman D, et al. Evaluation of the long-term tolerability and clinical benefit of vorinostat in patients with advanced cutaneous T-cell lymphoma. *Clin Lymphoma Myeloma.* 2009;9(6):412-416.
301. Olsen E, Duvic M, Frankel A, et al. Pivotal phase III trial of two dose levels of denileukin diftitox for the treatment of cutaneous T-cell lymphoma. *J Clin Oncol.* 2001;19(2):376-388.
302. Duvic M, Geskin L, Prince HM. Duration of response in cutaneous T-cell lymphoma patients treated with Denileukin Diftitox: results from 3 phase III studies. *Clin Lymphoma, Myeloma & Leukemia.* 2013;13(4):377-384.
303. Marchi E, Alinari L, Tani M, et al. Gemcitabine as frontline treatment for cutaneous T-cell lymphoma: phase II study of 32 patients. *Cancer.* 2005;104(11):2437-2441.
304. Jidar K, Ingen-Housz-Oro S, Beylot-Barry M, et al. Gemcitabine treatment in cutaneous T-cell lymphoma: a multicentre study of 23 cases. *Br J Dermatol.* 2009;161(3):660-663.
305. Duvic M, Talpur R, Wen S, et al. Phase II evaluation of gemcitabine monotherapy for cutaneous T-cell lymphoma. *Clin Lymphoma Myeloma.* 2006;7(1):51-58.
306. Quaglino P, Knobler R, Fierro MT, et al. Extracorporeal photopheresis for the treatment of erythrodermic cutaneous T-cell lymphoma: a single center clinical experience with long-term follow-up data and a brief overview of the literature. *Int J Dermatol.* 2013;52(11):1308-1318.
307. Ferenczi K, Fuhlbrigge RC, Pinkus JL, Pinkus GS, Kupper TS. Increased CCR4 expression in cutaneous T cell lymphoma. *J Invest Dermatol.* 2002;119(6):1405-1410.
308. Kim YH, Bagot M, Pinter-Brown L, et al. Mogamulizumab versus vorinostat in previously treated cutaneous T-cell lymphoma (MAVORIC): an international, open-label, randomised, controlled phase 3 trial. *Lancet Oncol.* 2018;19(9):1192-1204.
309. Chen L, Carson KR, Staser KW, et al. Mogamulizumab-associated cutaneous granulomatous drug eruption mimicking mycosis fungoides but possibly indicating durable clinical response. *JAMA Dermatology.* 2019;155(8):968-971.
310. Masuda Y, Tatsuno K, Kitano S, et al. Mogamulizumab-induced photosensitivity in patients with mycosis fungoides and other T-cell neoplasms. *J Eur Acad Dermatol Venereol.* 2018;32(9):1456-1460.
311. Hönigsmann H. Commentary to "Mogamulizumab-induced photosensitivity in patients with mycosis fungoides and other T-cell neoplasms" by Y. Masuda et al. *J Eur Acad Dermatol Venereol.* 2018;32(10):1626.
312. Kawano N, Kuriyama T, Yoshida S, et al. The impact of a humanized CCR4 antibody (mogamulizumab) on patients with aggressive-type Adult T-cell leukemia-lymphoma treated with allogeneic hematopoietic stem cell transplantation. *J Clin Exp Hematop.* 2017;56(3):135-144.
313. Dai J, Almazan TH, Hong EK, et al. Potential association of anti-CCR4 antibody mogamulizumab and graft-vs-host disease in patientswithmycosis fungoides and sézary syndrome. *JAMA Dermatology.* 2018;154(6):728-730.
314. Wang JY, Hirotsu KE, Neal TM, et al. Histopathologic characterization of mogamulizumab-associated rash. *Am J Surg Pathol.* 2020;44(12):1666-1676.
315. Honda T, Hishizawa M, Kataoka TR, et al. Stevens-Johnson syndrome associated with mogamulizumab-induced

deficiency of regulatory T cells in an adult T-cell leukaemia patient. *Acta Derm Venereol.* May 1, 2015;95(5):606-607.
316. Herrmann J, Roenigk H, Hurria A, et al. Treatment of mycosis fungoides with photochemotherapy (PUVA): long-term follow-up. *J Am Acad Dermatol.* 1995;33(2):234-242.
317. Abel EA, Cox AJ, Farber EM. Epidermal dystrophy and actinic keratoses in psoriasis patients following oral psoralen photochemotherapy (PUVA). *J Am Acad Dermatol.* 1982;7(3):333-340.
318. Stern RS. The risk of squamous cell and basal cell cancer associated with psoralen and ultraviolet A therapy: a 30-year prospective study. *J Am Acad Dermatol.* 2012;66(4):553-562.
319. Stern RS. The risk of melanoma in association with long-term exposure to PUVA. *J Am Acad Dermatol.* 2001;44(5):755-761.
320. Nagase K, Hirashima N, Koba S, et al. Acquired dermal melanocytosis induced by psoralen plus ultraviolet A therapy. *Acta Derm Venereol.* 2012;92(6):691-692.
321. Brazzelli V, Antoninetti M, Palazzini F, et al. Narrow-band ultraviolet therapy in early-stage mycosis fungoides: study on 20 patients. *Photodermatol Photoimmunol Photomed.* 2007;23:229-233.
322. Boztepe G, Sahin S, Ayhan M, et al. Narrowband ultraviolet B phototherapy to clear and maintain clearance in patients with mycosis fungoides. *J Am Acad Dermatol.* 2005;53(2):242-246.
323. Man I, Crombie IK, Dawe RS, et al. The photocarcinogenic risk of narrowband UVB (TL-01) phototherapy: early follow-up data. *Br J Dermatol.* 2005;152(4):755-757.
324. Black RJ, Gavin AT. Photocarcinogenic risk of narrowband ultraviolet B (TL-01) phototherapy: early follow-up data. *Br J Dermatol.* 2006;154(3):566-567.
325. Weischer M, Blum A, Eberhard F, et al. No evidence for increased skin cancer risk in psoriasis patients treated with broadband or narrowband UVB phototherapy: a first retrospective study. *Acta Derm Venereol.* 2004;84(5):370-374.
326. Jones GW, Rosenthal D, Wilson LD. Total skin electron radiation for patients with erythrodermic cutaneous T-cell lymphoma (mycosis fungoides and the Sézary syndrome). *Cancer.* 1999;85(9):1985-1995.
327. Introcaso CE, Micaily B, Richardson SK, et al. Total skin electron beam therapy may be associated with improvement of peripheral blood disease in Sézary syndrome. *J Am Acad Dermatol.* 2008;58(4):592-595.
328. Wilson LD, Jones GW, Kim D, et al. Experience with total skin electron beam therapy in combination with extracorporeal photopheresis in the management of patients with erythrodermic (T4) mycosis fungoides. *J Am Acad Dermatol.* 2000;43(1):54-60.
329. Desai K, Pezner R, Lipsett J, et al. Total skin electron irradiation for mycosis fungoides: relationship between acute toxicities and measured dose at different anatomic sites. *Int J Radiat Oncol Biol Phys.* 1988;15(3):641-645.
330. Price NM. Radiation dermatitis following electron beam therapy: an evaluation of patients ten years after total skin irradiation for mycosis fungoides. *Arch Dermatol.* 1978;114:63-66.
331. Harrison C, Young J, Navi D, et al. Revisiting low-dose total skin electron beam therapy in mycosis fungoides. *Int J Radiat Oncol Biol Phys.* 2011;81(4):e651-e657.
332. Dawson MI, Xia Z. The retinoid X receptors and their ligands. *Biochim Biophys Acta.* 2012;1821(1):21-56.
333. Heald P, Mehlmauer M, Martin A, et al. Topical bexarotene therapy for patients with refractory or persistent early-stage cutaneous T-cell lymphoma: results of the phase III clinical trial. *J Am Acad Dermatol.* 2003;49(5):801-815.
334. Breneman D, Duvic M, Kuzel T, et al. Phase 1 and 2 trial of bexarotene gel for skin-directed treatment of patients with cutaneous T-cell lymphoma. *Arch Dermatol.* 2002;138(3):325-332.
335. Duvic M, Martin AG, Kim Y, et al. Phase 2 and 3 clinical trial of oral Bexarotene (Targretin capsules) for the treatment of refractory or persistent early-stage cutaneous T-cell lymphoma. *Arch Dermatol.* 2001;137(5):581-593.
336. Duvic M, Hymes K, Heald P, et al. Bexarotene is effective and safe for treatment of refractory advanced-stage cutaneous T-cell lymphoma: multinational phase II–III trial results. *J Clin Oncol.* 2001;19(9):2456-2471.
337. Talpur R, Ward S, Apisarnthanarax N, et al. Optimizing bexarotene therapy for cutaneous T-cell lymphoma. *J Am Acad Dermatol.* 2002;47(5):672-684.
338. Bagazgoitia L, Perez-Carmona L, Rios L, et al. Acute hyperkeratotic and desquamative reaction in a patient with Sézary syndrome treated with bexarotene. *J Eur Acad Dermatol Venereol.* 2008;22(3):389-390.
339. Shimoda S, Sumida K, Iwasaka S, et al. Interferon-α-induced changes to natural killer cells are associated with the treatment outcomes in patients with HCV infections. *Hepat Res Treat.* 2013;2013:374196.
340. Jansen JH, van der Harst D, Wientjens GJ, et al. Induction of CD11a/leukocyte function antigen-1 and CD54/intercellular adhesion molecule-1 on hairy cell leukemia cells is accompanied by enhanced susceptibility to T-cell but not lymphokine-activated killer-cell cytotoxicity. *Blood.* 1992;80(2):478-483.
341. Ruiz-Genao DP, García-F-Villalta MJ, Hernández-Núñez A, et al. Livedo reticularis associated with interferon α therapy in two melanoma patients. *J Eur Acad Dermatol Venereol.* 2005;19(2):252-254.
342. Fox M, Tahan S, Kim CC. Livedo reticularis: a side effect of interferon therapy in a pediatric patient with melanoma. *Pediatr Dermatol.* 2012;29(3):333-335.
343. Gibbs MB, English JC, Zirwas MJ. Livedo reticularis: an update. *J Am Acad Dermatol.* 2005;52(6):1009-1019.
344. Zeidman A, Dicker D, Mittelman M. Interferon-induced vasospasm in chronic myeloid leukaemia. *Acta Haematol.* 1998;100(2):94-96.
345. Sidky Y, Borden E. Inhibition of angiogenesis by interferons: effects on tumor-and lymphocyte-induced vascular responses. *Cancer Res.* 1987;47(19):5155-5161.
346. Sgonc R, Fuerhapter C, Boeck G, et al. Induction of apoptosis in human dermal microvascular endothelial cells and infantile hemangiomas by interferon-α. *Int Arch Allergy Immunol.* 1998;117(3):209-214.
347. Pepper M, Vassalli J, Wilks J, et al. Modulation of bovine microvascular endothelial cell proteolytic properties by inhibitors of angiogenesis. *J Cell Biochem.* 1994;55(4):419-434.
348. Creutzig A, Caspary L, Freund M. The Raynaud phenomenon and interferon therapy. *Ann Intern Med.* 1996;125(5):423.
349. Roy V, Newland AC. Raynaud's phenomenon and cryoglobulinaemia associated with the use of recombinant human alpha-interferon. *Lancet.* 1988;1(8591):944-945.
350. Bachmeyer C, Farge D, Gluckman E, et al. Raynaud's phenomenon and digital necrosis induced by interferon-alpha. *Br J Dermatol.* 1996;135(3):481-483.
351. Kruit WH, Eggermont AM, Stoter G. Interferon-α induced Raynaud's syndrome. *Ann Oncol.* 2000;11(11):1501-1502.
352. Oeda E, Shinohara K. Cutaneous necrosis caused by injection of α-interferon therapy in a patient with chronic myelogenous leukemia. *Am J Hematol.* 1993;44:213-214.

353. Orlow SJ, Friedman-Kien AE. Cutaneous ulcerations secondary to interferon alfa therapy of Kaposi's sarcoma. *Arch Dermatol.* 1992;128(4):566.
354. Cnudde F, Gharakhanian S, Luboinski J, et al. Cutaneous local necrosis following interferon injections. *Int J Dermatol.* 1991;30(2):147.
355. Quesada J, Gutterman J. Psoriasis and alpha-interferon. *Lancet.* 1986;1(8496):1466-1468.
356. Barlogie B, Mitchell A, van Rhee F, et al. Curing myeloma at last: defining criteria and providing the evidence. *Blood.* 2014;124(20):3043-3051.
357. Ludwig H, Durie BG, Bolejack V, et al. Myeloma in patients younger than age 50 years presents with more favorable features and shows better survival: an analysis of 10 549 patients from the International Myeloma Working Group. *Blood.* 2008;111(8):4039-4047.
358. Kumar SK, Rajkumar SV, Dispenzieri A, et al. Improved survival in multiple myeloma and the impact of novel therapies. *Blood.* 2008;111(5):2516-2520.
359. Brenner H, Gondos A, Pulte D. Recent major improvement in long-term survival of younger patients with multiple myeloma. *Blood.* 2008;111(5):2521-2526.
360. Kim J, Roh H, Lee J, et al. Distinct variant of Sweet's syndrome: bortezomib-induced histiocytoid Sweet's syndrome in a patient with multiple myeloma. *Int J Dermatol.* 2012;51(12):1491-1493.
361. Truchuelo M, Bagazgoitia L, Alcántara J, et al. Sweet-like lesions induced by bortezomib: a review of the literature and a report of 2 cases. *Actas Dermosifiliogr.* 2012;103(9):829-844.
362. Kolb-Mäurer A, Kneitz H, Goebeler M. Sweet-like syndrome induced by bortezomib. *J Dtsch Dermatol Ges.* 2013;11(12):1200-1202.
363. Zobniw CM, Saad SA, Kostoff D, et al. Bortezomib-induced sweet's syndrome confirmed by rechallenge. *Pharmacotherapy.* 2014;34(4):e18-e21.
364. Van Regenmortel N, Van de Voorde K, De Raeve H, et al. Bortezomib-induced sweet's syndrome. *Br J Haematol.* 2005;90(12):e116-e117.
365. Knoops L, Jacquemain A, Tennstedt D, et al. Bortezomib-induced sweet syndrome. *Br J Haematol.* 2005;131(2):142.
366. Murase JE, Wu JJ, Theate I, et al. Bortezomib-induced histiocytoid Sweet syndrome. *J Am Acad Dermatol.* 2009;60(3):496-497.
367. Aguayo-Leiva I, Vano-Galvan S, Carrillo-Gijon R, et al. Lupus tumidus induced by bortezomib not requiring discontinuation of the drug. *J Eur Acad Dermatol Venereol.* 2010;24(11):1363-1364.
368. Böckle BC, Baltaci M, Weyrer W, et al. Bortezomib-induced lupus erythematosus tumidus. *Oncol.* 2009;14(6):637-639.
369. Garcia-Navarro X, Puig L, Fernández-Figueras M, et al. Bortezomib-associated cutaneous vasculitis. *Br J Dermatol.* 2007;157(4):799-801.
370. Min CK, Lee S, Kim YJ, et al. Cutaneous leucoclastic vasculitis (LV) following bortezomib therapy in a myeloma patient; association with pro-inflammatory cytokines. *Eur J Haematol.* 2006;76(3):265-268.
371. Gerecitano J, Goy A, Wright J, et al. Drug-induced cutaneous vasculitis in patients with non-Hodgkin lymphoma treated with the novel proteasome inhibitor bortezomib: a possible surrogate marker of response? *Br J Haematol.* 2006;134(4):391-398.
372. Ranawaka R. Patterns of chromonychia during chemotherapy in patients with skin type V and outcome after 1 year of follow-up. *Clin Exp Dermatol.* 2009;34(8):e920-e926.
373. Moreau P, Masszi T, Grzasko N, et al. Oral ixazomib, lenalidomide, and dexamethasone for multiple myeloma. *N Engl J Med.* 2016;374(17):1621-1634.
374. Katz H, Shenouda M, Dahshan D, Sonnier G, Lebowicz Y. A rare case of ixazomib-induced cutaneous necrotizing vasculitis in a patient with relapsed myeloma. *Case Rep Hematol.* 2019;2019:1-4.
375. Alloo A, Khosravi H, Granter SR, et al. Ixazomib-induced cutaneous necrotizing vasculitis. *Support Care Cancer.* 2018;26(7):2247-2250.
376. Srikanth M, Van Veen J, Raithatha A, et al. Cyclophosphamide-induced nail pigmentation. *Br J Haematol.* 2002;117(1):2.
377. Youssef M, Mokni S, Belhadjali H, et al. Cyclophosphamide-induced generalised reticulated skin pigmentation: a rare presentation. *Int J Clin Pharm.* 2013;35(3):309-312.
378. Chittari K, Tagboto S, Tan BB. Cyclophosphamide-induced nail discoloration and skin hyperpigmentation: a rare presentation. *Clin Exp Dermatol.* 2009;34(3):405-406.
379. Borroni G, Vassallo C, Brazzelli V, et al. Radiation recall dermatitis, panniculitis, and myositis following cyclophosphamide therapy: histopathologic findings of a patient affected by multiple myeloma. *Am J Dermatopathol.* 2004;26(3):213-216.
380. Malacarne P, Zavagli G. Melphalan-induced melanonychia striata. *Arch Dermatol Res.* 1977;258:81-83.
381. Landau M, Brenner S, Gat A, et al. Reticulate scleroderma after isolated limb perfusion with melphalan. *J Am Acad Dermatol.* 1998;39(6):1011-1012.
382. D'Amato R, Loughnan M, Flynn E, et al. Thalidomide is an inhibitor of angiogenesis. *Proc Natl Acad Sci U S A.* 1994;91(9):4082-4085.
383. Kenyon B, Browne F, D'amato R. Effects of thalidomide and related metabolites in a mouse corneal model of neovascularization. *Exp Eye Res.* 1997;64(6):971-978.
384. Singhal S, Mehta J, Desikan R, et al. Antitumor activity of thalidomide in refractory multiple myeloma. *N Engl J Med.* 1999;341(21):1565-1571.
385. Rajkumar SV, Gertz MA, Witzig TE. Life-threatening toxic epidermal necrolysis with thalidomide therapy for myeloma. *N Engl J Med.* 2000;343(13):972-973.
386. Horowitz S, Stirling A. thalidomide-induced toxic epidermal necrolysis. *Pharmacotherapy.* 1999;19(10):1177-1180.
387. Wolkenstein P, Latarjet J, Roujeau J, et al. Randomised comparison of thalidomide versus placebo in toxic epidermal necrolysis. *Lancet.* 1998;352(9140):1586-1589.
388. Paul C, Wolkenstein P, Adle H, et al. Apoptosis as a mechanism of keratinocyte death in toxic epidermal necrolysis. *Br J Dermatol.* 1996;134(4):710-714.
389. Heng MC, Allen SG. Efficacy of cyclophosphamide in toxic epidermal necrolysis: clinical and pathophysiologic aspects. *J Am Acad Dermatol.* 1991;25(5):778-786.
390. Ferrazzi A, Zambello R, Russo I, et al. Psoriasis induced by thalidomide in a patient with multiple myeloma. *BMJ Case Rep.* 2014;2014.
391. Varma K, Finlay A. Exacerbation of psoriasis by thalidomide in a patient with erythema multiforme. *Br J Dermatol.* 2006;154(4):789-790.
392. Dobson C, Parslew R. Exacerbation of psoriasis by thalidomide in Behçet's syndrome. *Br J Dermatol.* 2003;149(2):432-433.
393. Nardone B, Wu S, Garden BC, et al. Risk of rash associated with lenalidomide in cancer patients: a systematic review of the literature and meta-analysis. *Clin Lymphoma, Myeloma & Leukemia.* 2013;13(4):424-429.

394. Sviggum H, Davis M, Rajkumar S, et al. Dermatologic adverse effects of lenalidomide therapy for amyloidosis and multiple myeloma. *Arch Dermatol.* 2006;142(10):1298-1302.
395. Thieu KP, Rosenbach M, Xu X, et al. Neutrophilic dermatosis complicating lenalidomide therapy. *J Am Acad Dermatol.* 2009;61(4):709-710.
396. Treudler R, Georgieva J, Geilen CC, et al. Dacarbazine but not temozolomide induces phototoxic dermatitis in patients with malignant melanoma. *J Am Acad Dermatol.* 2004;50(5):783-785.
397. Dimopoulos MA, Dytfeld D, Grosicki S, et al. Elotuzumab plus pomalidomide and dexamethasone for Multiple Myeloma. *N Engl J Med.* 2018;379(19):1811-1822.
398. Palumbo A, Chanan-Khan A, Weisel K, et al. Daratumumab, bortezomib, and dexamethasone for multiple myeloma. *N Engl J Med.* 2016;375(8):754-766.
399. Mateos MV, Nahi H, Legiec W, et al. Subcutaneous versus intravenous daratumumab in patients with relapsed or refractory multiple myeloma (COLUMBA): a multicentre, open-label, non-inferiority, randomised, phase 3 trial. *Lancet Haematol.* 2020;7(5):e370-e380.
400. Mateos M-V, Dimopoulos MA, Cavo M, et al. Daratumumab plus bortezomib, melphalan, and prednisone for untreated myeloma. *N Engl J Med.* 2018;378(6):518-528.
401. Facon T, Kumar S, Plesner T, et al. Daratumumab plus lenalidomide and dexamethasone for untreated myeloma. *N Engl J Med.* 2019;380(22):2104-2115.
402. *Daratumumab Prescribing Information.* Accessed December 23, 2020. https://www.accessdata.fda.gov/drugsatfda_docs/label/2018/761036s013lbl.pdf
403. Koehn G, Balizet L. Unusual local cutaneous reaction to Dacarbazine. *Arch Dermatol.* 1982;118(12):1018-1019.
404. Roider E, Schneider J. Hypopigmentation in the sites of regressed melanoma metastases after successful dacarbazine therapy. *Int J Dermatol.* 2012;51(9):1142-1144.
405. Rzeski W, Turski L, Ikonomidou C. Glutamate antagonists limit tumor growth. *Proc Natl Acad Sci U S A.* 2001;98(11):6372-6377.
406. Nemechek P, Corder M. Radiation recall associated with Vinblastine in a patient treated for Kaposi sarcoma related to acquired immune deficiency syndrome. *Cancer.* 1992;70(6):1605-1606.
407. Reiser M, Bruns C, Hartmann P, et al. Raynaud's phenomenon and acral necrosis after chemotherapy for AIDS-related Kaposi's sarcoma. *Eur J Clin Microbiol Infect Dis.* 1998;17:58-60.
408. Kamil N, Ahmed SP, Kamil S, et al. Vincristine induced dermal toxicities. *Pakistan J Pharmacol.* 2008;25(1):53-60.
409. Yamamoto T, Eckes B, Krieg T. Bleomycin increases steady-state levels of type I collagen, fibronectin and decorin mRNAs in human skin fibroblasts. *Arch Dermatol Res.* 2000;292(11):556-561.
410. Cohen I, Mosher M, O'Keefe E, et al. Cutaneous toxicity of Bleomycin therapy. *Arch Dermatol.* 1973;107(4):553-555.
411. Ohgo S, Hasegawa S, Hasebe Y, et al. Bleomycin inhibits adipogenesis and accelerates fibrosis in the subcutaneous adipose layer through TGF-β1. *Exp Dermatol.* 2013;22(11):769-771.
412. Yamamoto T. Animal model of systemic sclerosis. *J Dermatol.* 2010;37:26-41.
413. Inaoki M, Kawabata C, Nishijima C, et al. Case of bleomycin-induced scleroderma. *J Dermatol.* 2012;39(5):482-484.
414. Koca SS, Ozgen M, Sarikaya M, et al. Ghrelin prevents the development of dermal fibrosis in bleomycin-induced scleroderma. *Clin Exp Dermatol.* 2014;39(2):176-181.
415. Zhou C, Yu J, Zhang J, et al. *N*-acetylcysteine attenuates subcutaneous administration of bleomycin-induced skin fibrosis and oxidative stress in a mouse model of scleroderma. *Clin Exp Dermatol.* 2013;38(4):403-409.
416. Blum R, Carter S, Agre K. A Clinical review of Bleomycin—a new antineoplastic agent. *Cancer.* 1973;31(4):903-914.
417. Kumar R, Pai V. Bleomycin induced flagellate pigmentation. *Indian Pediatr.* 2006;43:74-75.
418. Lindae M, Hu C, Nickoloff B. Pruritic erythematous linear plaques on the neck and back. *Arch Dermatol.* 1987;123(3):397-398.
419. Kamata Y, Yamamoto M, Kawakami F, et al. Bleomycin hydrolase is regulated biphasically in a differentiation- and cytokine-dependent manner: relevance to atopic dermatitis. *J Biol Chem.* 2011;286(10):8204-8212.
420. Lowitz BB. Streaking with bleomycin. *N Engl J Med.* 1975;292(24):1300-1301.
421. Mountz J, Minor M, Turner R, et al. Bleomycin-induced cutaneous toxicity in the rat: analysis of histopathology and ultrastructure compared with progressive systemic sclerosis (scleroderma). *Br J Dermatol.* 1983;108(6):679-686.
422. Tsuji T, Sawabe M. Hyperpigmentation in striae distensae after bleomycin treatment. *J Am Acad Dermatol.* 1993;28(3):503-505.
423. Czarnecka A, Kreft B, Marsch W. Flagellate dermatitis after consumption of Shiitake mushrooms. *Postep Dermatol Alergol.* 2014;31(3):187-190.
424. Flynn TC, Harrist TJ, Murphy GF, et al. Neutrophilic eccrine hidradenitis: a distinctive rash associated with cytarabine therapy and acute leukemia. *J Am Acad Dermatol.* 1984;11(4):584-590.
425. Scallan P, Kettler A, Levy M, et al. Neutrophilic eccrine hidradenitis: evidence implicating Bleomycin as a causative agent. *Cancer.* 1988;62(12):2532-2536.
426. Shear NH, Knowles SR, Shapiro L, et al. Dapsone in prevention of recurrent neutrophilic eccrine hidradenitis. *J Am Acad Dermatol.* 1996;35(5):819-822.
427. Vogelzang NJ, Bosl GJ, Johnson K, et al. Raynaud's phenomenon: a common toxicity after combination chemotherapy for testicular cancer. *Ann Intern Med.* 1981;95(3):288-292.
428. MacLeod P, Tyrrell C, Bliss B. Raynaud's phenomenon following cytotoxic chemotherapy successfully managed by dorsal sympathectomy. *Eur J Surg Oncol.* 1989;15(1):79-81.
429. Fertakos R, Mintzer D. Digital gangrene following chemotherapy for AIDS-related Kaposi's sarcoma. *Am J Med.* 1992;93(5):581-582.
430. Shankland KR, Armitage JO, Hancock BW. Non-Hodgkin lymphoma. *Lancet.* 2012;380(9844):848-857.
431. Morschhauser F, Flinn IW, Advani R, et al. Polatuzumab vedotin or pinatuzumab vedotin plus rituximab in patients with relapsed or refractory non-Hodgkin lymphoma: final results from a phase 2 randomised study (ROMULUS). *Lancet Haematol.* 2019;6(5):e254-e265.
432. Dreyling M, Morschhauser F, Bouabdallah K, et al. Phase II study of copanlisib, a PI3K inhibitor, in relapsed or refractory, indolent or aggressive lymphoma. *Ann Oncol.* 2017;28(9):2169-2178.

433. Flinn IW, Miller CB, Ardeshna KM, et al. DYNAMO: a phase II study of duvelisib (IPI-145) in patients with refractory indolent non-Hodgkin lymphoma. *J Clin Oncol*. 2019;37(11):912.
434. Chadha SA, Shastry J, Sunshine J, Choi J, Guggina L. Cutaneous toxicities of PI3K inhibitors: a series of two cases and review of the literature. *SKIN The Journal of Cutaneous Medicine*. 2020;4(6):585-590.
435. Song Y, Zhou K, Zou D, et al. *Treatment of Patients with Relapsed or Refractory Mantle-Cell Lymphoma with Zanubrutinib, a Selective Inhibitor of Bruton's Tyrosine Kinase A C.* 2020.

CHAPTER 75

Cutaneous adverse reactions to immunotherapy

Kelsey Nusbaum, Abraham Korman, Catherine G. Chung, Benjamin H. Kaffenberger, and Brittany O. Dulmage

INTRODUCTION

The field of immunotherapy continues to rapidly advance, transforming the treatment paradigm for hematologic malignancies. With increasing utilization of immunotherapy, a spectrum of accompanying treatment-related cutaneous reactions has emerged. Recognition of clinical presentation and histopathology for these reactions is essential to facilitate early diagnosis and treatment and to allow for uninterrupted or minimally interrupted oncologic therapy. The most common cutaneous adverse events are discussed for two classes of immunotherapy: immune checkpoint inhibitors and chimeric antigen receptor T-cell (CAR-T) therapy.

IMMUNE CHECKPOINT INHIBITORS

Immune checkpoint inhibitors are a promising class of immunomodulatory agents that enhance the antitumor immune response by selectively targeting inhibitory receptors on T-cells. Cancer cells often upregulate these inhibitory receptors as a means of suppressing the immune system and promoting tumor escape.[1] Blockade of cytotoxic T lymphocyte antigen 4, programmed cell death 1 (PD1), or its ligand, PD1 ligand 1 (PDL1), removes this negative regulation, stimulating the generation of tumor-reactive T-cells to overcome tumor-induced immune evasion.[2,3]

There are two FDA-approved immune checkpoint inhibitors with hematologic indications.

Nivolumab is a PD1-directed immune checkpoint inhibitor indicated for the treatment of adult patients with classical Hodgkin lymphoma that has relapsed or progressed after autologous hematopoietic stem cell transplant and posttransplant brentuximab vedotin or three or more lines of systemic therapy that includes autologous hematopoietic stem cell transplant.[4-6]

Pembrolizumab is a PD1-directed immune checkpoint inhibitor indicated for the treatment of adult patients with relapsed or refractory classical Hodgkin lymphoma, pediatric patients with relapsed or refractory classical Hodgkin lymphoma after two or more lines of therapy, and adult and pediatric patients with primary mediastinal large B-cell lymphoma that has relapsed or progressed after two or more lines of therapy.[1,6]

Immune checkpoint inhibitors share a unique profile of adverse events related to their underlying mechanisms of action. By blocking negative regulators of the immune system, immune-related adverse events occur frequently.[7] Cutaneous toxicities are the most commonly observed adverse events, seen in roughly 50% of patients.[8,9] The presence of certain cutaneous adverse events has been found to be associated with improved cancer outcomes in patients treated with immune checkpoint inhibitors.[10,11]

Maculopapular rash is the most frequently observed cutaneous toxicity in patients treated with immune checkpoint inhibitors. The incidence of this rash is approximately 15% with anti-PD1 therapy and less than 10% with anti-PDL1 therapy.[12,13] It typically appears relatively early in treatment, within the first few treatment cycles.[12,14] Patients present with erythematous macules and papules with or without scale typically involving the trunk and extremities and often associated with pruritus.[13-15] Histopathology may demonstrate a lichenoid reaction pattern with superficial dermal perivascular lymphohistiocytic infiltrates.[13,16] Other histological findings include interstitial eosinophils, papillary dermal edema, and spongiosis.[16,17] Immunotherapy can usually be continued as most cases resolve with topical corticosteroids and emollient creams.[13,17] A morbilliform reaction in this setting that displays facial involvement, palmar involvement, dusky coloration, vesicles, or oral erosions should always necessitate stopping treatment, a skin biopsy, and consultation to dermatology out of concern for Stevens-Johnson syndrome (SJS). Severe cutaneous adverse reactions such as SJS and toxic epidermal necrolysis (TEN) are rare in patients treated with immune checkpoint inhibitors. The majority of cases occur after the first few infusions, but there have been reports occurring after several months of therapy.[18-20] Eruptions resemble classic SJS/TEN consisting of dusky macules or papules rapidly progressing to skin desquamation and sloughing with associated mucosal involvement.[18] Histopathology is typical of SJS/TEN, revealing interface dermatitis with full-thickness epidermal necrosis and an inflammatory infiltrate of lymphocytes, neutrophils, and eosinophils.[21,22] Permanent discontinuation of the offending immune checkpoint inhibitor is indicated.[7,18,22] Treatment requires urgent hospitalization with supportive care and systemic immunosuppression.[7,18,22,23]

Vitiligo-like skin hypopigmentation is often seen in melanoma patients treated with PD1 and PDL1 inhibitors but has rarely been reported when these therapies are used to treat other malignancies.[13,24-26] The morphology is distinct from typical vitiligo, as it presents with multiple flecked depigmented macules evolving toward patches.[8,27] This eruption typically involves photoexposed skin including the face, neck, forearms, and hands and uniquely does not exhibit the Koebner phenomenon.[27] Histopathology demonstrates loss of melanocytes in the basal layer of the epidermis, which may be subtle on hematoxylin-eosin staining but highlighted on Melan-A or SOX10 immunohistochemical staining.[25,28,29] Dermal inflammatory infiltrates of CD8+ T-cells are seen in macroscopically normal perilesional skin, but sparsely in the vitiligo-like lesions themselves.[25,28,29] Vitiligo-like skin hypopigmentation has been found to be associated with improved melanoma outcomes and survival.[24,25,30,31] Immunotherapy can usually be continued, and topical corticosteroids or topical tacrolimus may be used for affected areas.[23]

Lichenoid eruptions are another common skin manifestation in patients treated with immune checkpoint inhibitors. Patients present with discrete erythematous to violaceous papules and plaques with scale involving the trunk and extremities.[8,21,32] Oral involvement may be present, appearing as reticulated white streaks or discrete papules and plaques on the buccal mucosa, tongue, palate, or gingivae.[21,32] Histopathology reveals patchy lichenoid interface dermatitis with band-like lymphocytic infiltrates, vacuolar degeneration, and occasional eosinophils.[15,17,33-35] Parakeratosis, spongiosis, and increased abundance of CD163+ histiocytes are distinguishing features not typically observed with idiopathic lichen planus.[8,17,34] Immunotherapy can usually be continued as most lichenoid mucocutaneous reactions resolve with topical corticosteroids.[17,33,35]

Eczematous eruptions are relatively common, occurring months to years after initiation of immune checkpoint inhibitor therapy.[8] The morphology most often resembles classic eczema with erythematous scaly papules and plaques, but may present as nummular plaques, dyshidrotic vesicles, or asteatotic eczema.[8,21] Eczematous eruptions typically involve the back and extremities, but may be seen less frequently on the face, chest, and abdomen.[8] Lesions are often associated with pruritus.[8,21] Histopathology demonstrates eosinophilic spongiosis, a nonspecific histological feature that is normally seen in eczema.[21] Immunotherapy can usually be continued as most cases resolve with topical corticosteroids.[21]

Psoriasiform eruptions are a relatively common cutaneous toxicity induced or exacerbated by immune checkpoint inhibitors. The majority of cases occur in patients with a personal or family history of psoriasis.[36-39] The morphology resembles typical psoriatic lesions, with plaque psoriasis seen most commonly, but scalp, guttate, plaque palmoplantar, pustular palmoplantar, nail, and inverse subtypes have also been observed.[21,36,38,39] Histopathology demonstrates features of typical psoriasis including epidermal hyperplasia with parakeratosis and neutrophils in the stratum corneum, hypogranulosis, thinning of the suprapapillary plates, and a perivascular lymphocytic infiltrate.[17,40,41] Treatment resembles usual psoriasis management with topical corticosteroids, vitamin D analogues, and UVB phototherapy.[21,37,38] Acitretin, apremilast, and methotrexate have also demonstrated efficacy and safety for immune checkpoint inhibitor–mediated psoriasis[39]; however, certain systemic and biologic agents including TNF-alpha inhibitors may be avoided due to risks associated with underlying malignancy.[38,39]

Granulomatous eruptions are a rare, but increasingly recognized cutaneous reaction associated with immune checkpoint inhibitors including sarcoidosis-like reactions, granulomatous panniculitis, granuloma annulare, and granulomatous dermatitis. Sarcoidosis-like reactions are the most common type of granulomatous eruption presenting with papules, plaques, or nodules involving the head, trunk, or extremities, often with associated pulmonary symptoms.[42] Histopathology resembles typical sarcoidosis with noncaseating granulomatous inflammation.[43,44] Granulomatous panniculitis manifests as tender subcutaneous nodules with lobular and septal noncaseating granulomatous panniculitis seen on histopathology.[42,45] Granuloma annulare typically involves pink papules or annular plaques on the extremities. Necrobiotic and palisading granulomas are seen on histopathology.[42,46] Granulomatous dermatitis presents with red-to-brown coalescing papules and plaques on the trunk and extremities, with a superficial dermal lymphohistiocytic infiltrate seen on histopathology.[16,47,48] Immunotherapy can usually be continued after development of a granulomatous eruption, but withdrawal of the offending agent is occasionally necessary, particularly with sarcoid-like reactions.[42] Treatment consists of systemic and topical corticosteroids.[42]

Immunobullous eruptions are a rare cutaneous toxicity associated with immune checkpoint inhibitors, occurring in approximately 1% of patients.[49] These reactions typically develop a few months after initiation of immunotherapy, but may occur after more than a year of treatment.[50-52] Pruritus with nonspecific cutaneous lesions often precludes development of bullous lesions.[50] Patients present with tense vesicles and bullae with or without urticarial plaques involving the trunk and extremities; oral ulcerations are sometimes observed.[21,49] Histopathology demonstrates subepidermal bullae with an eosinophilic infiltrate; linear IgG and C3 are seen at the dermal-epidermal junction on direct immunofluorescence.[21,49] Temporary discontinuation of the offending immune checkpoint inhibitor is usually merited.[49-52] Treatment consists of systemic and topical corticosteroids, plasma exchange, and rituximab or an alternate CD19/20 antibody.[18,49,50,53] Immunobullous lesions may persist for months after immunotherapy discontinuation in the absence of targeted inhibition such as rituximab.[17,51,52,54,55] After clearing with immunosuppression such as rituximab, bullous pemphigoid antibody levels can be monitored with a restart of PD1 therapy.

Eruptive keratoacanthomas have rarely been observed in patients treated with PD1 inhibitors. These lesions typically appear after several months of immunotherapy, presenting with sudden onset of multiple hyperkeratotic nodules and papules involving photoexposed regions of the extremities and upper chest.[56-60] Histopathology reveals crateriform, keratin-filled lesions composed of large glassy eosinophilic keratinocytes.[56,60] Accompanying lichenoid interface dermatitis consisting of CD3+ T-cells with scattered CD20+ B-cells has been reported in several cases, resembling the histopathological features seen in PD1-associated lichenoid mucocutaneous eruptions.[56,58-60] Immunotherapy can usually be continued with localized treatment of lesions.[56-60] Treatment options include topical and intralesional corticosteroids, imiquimod, cryotherapy, and curettage; systemic retinoids are typically avoided due to risks associated with underlying malignancy.[56-60]

CHIMERIC ANTIGEN RECEPTOR T-CELL THERAPY

Chimeric antigen receptor (CAR) T-cell therapy is a novel oncologic therapy in which T-cells derived from patient blood are engineered in vitro to express artificial receptors targeted to a specific tumor antigen with a high degree of specificity.[61] CAR-T cell–mediated targeting of tumors is neither restricted nor dependent on antigen processing and presentation, and thus CAR-T cells are insensitive to tumor escape mechanisms, leading to high levels of efficacy.[62] The production of CAR-T cells involves cell collection from a patient by leukapheresis, followed by removal of myeloid cells, T lymphocyte enrichment, transgene delivery, ex vivo expansion, and subsequent reinfusion into the patient.[63]

There are three FDA-approved CAR-T cell therapies:

Axicabtagene ciloleucel (YESCARTA) is a CD19-directed T-cell immunotherapy indicated for the treatment of adult patients with relapsed or refractory large B-cell lymphoma after two or more lines of systemic therapy, including diffuse large B-cell lymphoma (DLBCL) not otherwise specified, primary mediastinal large B-cell lymphoma, high-grade B-cell lymphoma, and DLBCL arising from follicular lymphoma.[64]

Tisagenlecleucel (KYMRIAH) is a CD19-directed T-cell immunotherapy indicated for the treatment of patients up to 25 years of age with B-cell precursor acute lymphoblastic leukemia that is refractory or in second or later relapse and adult patients with relapsed or refractory large B-cell lymphoma after two or more lines of systemic therapy including DLBCL not otherwise specified, high-grade B-cell lymphoma, and DLBCL arising from follicular lymphoma.[65]

Brexucabtagene autoleucel (TECARTUS) is a CD19-directed T-cell immunotherapy indicated for the treatment of adult patients with relapsed or refractory mantle cell lymphoma.[66]

Reported cutaneous manifestations of CAR-T cell therapy are scarce. Clinical trials and most oncology publications simply classify cutaneous manifestations as "rash." According to the product package inserts, axicabtagene ciloleucel (YESCARTA), tisagenlecleucel (KYMRIAH), and brexucabtagene autoleucel (TECARTUS) were associated with rash in 9%, 16%, and 22% of cases, respectively.[64-66]

A series of five patients described skin lesions that developed after therapy with tisagenlecleucel.[67] The skin lesions included diffuse morbilliform eruptions in three patients, a pseudovesicular eruption in one patient, and a secondary staphylococcal infection in another. Another morbilliform eruption was described with the use of a CD19/CD22 dual-targeted CAR-T therapy in a middle-aged man with DLBCL as well as acral bullous lesions with cyanosis.[68] Skin biopsy of the rash showed marked papillary edema and subepidermal bullae with a superficial dermal, dense perivascular lymphocytic infiltrate composed of CD8+ T-cells. Fluid in the bullae was analyzed and showed a predominance of CAR-T cells, supporting that the rash was secondary to the therapy.

A series that investigated the use of anti-CD30 CAR-T therapy for relapsed/refractory CD30+ lymphoma patients found that two (out of nine) patients developed a skin rash described as inflammatory purpura.[69]

In summary, the skin lesions included eruptions possibly CAR-T cell therapy–related (morbilliform, pseudovesicular, and purpuric) and a secondary infection. Of the rashes that were possibly related, the histopathology was suggestive of the eruption of lymphocyte recovery with mononuclear cell infiltrates perivascularly and mild interface dermatitis. In these cases, transplantation of autologous T-cells may have induced these eruptions.

CONCLUSION

While cutaneous reactions are common side effects of immune checkpoint inhibitors, less is known regarding the skin toxicities associated with CAR-T therapy. As the use of immunotherapies continues to expand for the treatment of hematologic malignancies, the spectrum of adverse cutaneous reactions will be further defined. Recognition of the unique clinicopathological features associated with these cutaneous reactions is essential for timely management of the adverse event and maintenance of uninterrupted oncologic therapy.

References

1. Hargadon KM, Johnson CE, Williams CJ. Immune checkpoint blockade therapy for cancer: an overview of FDA-approved immune checkpoint inhibitors. *Int Immunopharm.* 2018;62:29-39.
2. Jenkins RW, Barbie DA, Flaherty KT. Mechanisms of resistance to immune checkpoint inhibitors. *Br J Cancer.* 2018;118:9-16.
3. Granier C, De Guillebon E, Blanc C, et al. Mechanisms of action and rationale for the use of checkpoint inhibitors in cancer. *ESMO Open.* 2017;2:e00213.
4. Kasamon YL, de Claro RA, Wang Y, Shen YL, Farrell AT, Pazdur R. FDA approval summary: nivolumab for the treatment of relapsed or progressive classical Hodgkin lymphoma. *The oncologist* 2017;22:585.
5. Armand P, Engert A, Younes A, et al. Nivolumab for relapsed/refractory classic Hodgkin lymphoma after failure of autologous hematopoietic cell transplantation: extended follow-up of the multicohort single-arm phase II CheckMate 205 trial. *J Clin Oncol.* 2018;36:1428.
6. Vaddepally RK, Kharel P, Pandey R, Garje R, Chandra AB. Review of indications of FDA-approved immune checkpoint inhibitors per NCCN guidelines with the level of evidence. *Cancers.* 2020;12:738.
7. Brahmer JR, Lacchetti C, Schneider BJ, et al. Management of immune-related adverse events in patients treated with immune checkpoint inhibitor therapy: American Society of Clinical Oncology Clinical Practice Guideline. *J Clin Oncol.* 2018;36:1714.

8. Hwang SJE, Carlos G, Wakade D et al. Cutaneous adverse events (AEs) of anti-programmed cell death (PD)-1 therapy in patients with metastatic melanoma: a single-institution cohort. *J Am Acad Dermatol*. 2016;74:455-461. e1.
9. Ji HH, Tang XW, Dong Z, Song L, Jia YT. Adverse event profiles of anti-CTLA-4 and anti-PD-1 monoclonal antibodies alone or in combination: analysis of spontaneous reports submitted to FAERS. *Clin Drug Invest* 2019;39:319-330.
10. Lee CKM, Li S, Tran DC, et al. Characterization of dermatitis after PD-1/PD-L1 inhibitor therapy and association with multiple oncologic outcomes: a retrospective case-control study. *J Am Acad Dermatol*. 2018;79:1047-1052.
11. Sanlorenzo M, Vujic I, Daud A, et al. Pembrolizumab cutaneous adverse events and their association with disease progression. *JAMA Dermatol*. 2015;151:1206-1212.
12. Sibaud V. Dermatologic reactions to immune checkpoint inhibitors. *Am J Clin Dermatol*. 2018;19:345-361.
13. Belum V, Benhuri B, Postow M, et al. Characterisation and management of dermatologic adverse events to agents targeting the PD-1 receptor. *Eur J Cancer*. 2016;60:12-25.
14. Shi VJ, Rodic N, Gettinger S, et al. Clinical and histologic features of lichenoid mucocutaneous eruptions due to anti–programmed cell death 1 and anti–programmed cell death ligand 1 immunotherapy. *JAMA Dermatol*. 2016;152:1128-1136.
15. Sibaud V, Meyer N, Lamant L, Vigarios E, Mazieres J, Delord JP. Dermatologic complications of anti-PD-1/PD-L1 immune checkpoint antibodies. *Curr Opin Oncol*. 2016;28:254-263.
16. Perret RE, Josselin N, Knol AC, et al. Histopathological aspects of cutaneous erythematous-papular eruptions induced by immune checkpoint inhibitors for the treatment of metastatic melanoma. *Int J Dermatol*. 2017;56:527-533.
17. Geisler AN, Phillips GS, Barrios DM, et al. Immune checkpoint inhibitor–related dermatologic adverse events. *J Am Acad Dermatol*. 2020;83:1255-1268.
18. Coleman EL, Olamiju B, Leventhal JS. The life-threatening eruptions of immune checkpoint inhibitor therapy. *Clin Dermatol*. 2020;38:94-104.
19. Dasanu CA. Late-onset Stevens–Johnson syndrome due to nivolumab use for hepatocellular carcinoma. *J Oncol Pharm Pract*. 2019;25:2052-2055.
20. Hwang A, Iskandar A, Dasanu CA. Stevens-Johnson syndrome manifesting late in the course of pembrolizumab therapy. *J Oncol Pharm Pract*. 2019;25:1520-1522.
21. Coleman E, Ko C, Dai F, Tomayko MM, Kluger H, Leventhal JS. Inflammatory eruptions associated with immune checkpoint inhibitor therapy: a single-institution retrospective analysis with stratification of reactions by toxicity and implications for management. *J Am Acad Dermatol*. 2019;80:990-997.
22. Maloney NJ, Ravi V, Cheng K, Bach DQ, Worswick S. Stevens-Johnson syndrome and toxic epidermal necrolysis-like reactions to checkpoint inhibitors: a systematic review. *Int J Dermatol*. 2020;59:e183-e8.
23. Muntyanu A, Netchiporouk E, Gerstein W, Gniadecki R, Litvinov IV. Cutaneous immune-related adverse events (irAEs) to immune checkpoint inhibitors: a dermatology perspective on management. *J Cutan Med Surg*. 2021;25:59-76.
24. Nakamura Y, Tanaka R, Asami Y, et al. Correlation between vitiligo occurrence and clinical benefit in advanced melanoma patients treated with nivolumab: a multi-institutional retrospective study. *J Dermatol*. 2017;44:117-122.
25. Hua C, Boussemart L, Mateus C, et al. Association of vitiligo with tumor response in patients with metastatic melanoma treated with pembrolizumab. *JAMA Dermatol*. 2016;152:45-51.
26. Liu R, Consuegra G, Chou S, Fernandez Peñas P. Vitiligo-like depigmentation in oncology patients treated with immunotherapies for nonmelanoma metastatic cancers. *Clin Exp Dermatol*. 2019;44:643-646.
27. Larsabal M, Marti A, Jacquemin C, et al. Vitiligo-like lesions occurring in patients receiving anti-programmed cell death–1 therapies are clinically and biologically distinct from vitiligo. *J Am Acad Dermatol*. 2017;76:863-870.
28. Bulat V, Likic R, Bradic L, Speeckaert R, Azdajic MD. Pembrolizumab-induced vitiligo in a patient with lung adenocarcinoma: a case report. *Br J Clin Pharmacol*. 2021;87:2614-2618.
29. Nishino K, Ohe S, Kitamura M, et al. Nivolumab induced vitiligo-like lesions in a patient with metastatic squamous cell carcinoma of the lung. *J Thorac Dis*. 2018;10:E481-E484.
30. Nardin C, Jeand'Heur A, Bouiller K, et al. Vitiligo under anti–programmed cell death-1 therapy is associated with increased survival in melanoma patients. *J Am Acad Dermatol*. 2020;82:770-772.
31. Matsuya T, Nakamura Y, Matsushita S, et al. Vitiligo expansion and extent correlate with durable response in anti-programmed death 1 antibody treatment for advanced melanoma: a multi-institutional retrospective study. *J Dermatol*. 2020;47(6):629-635.
32. Curry JL, Tetzlaff MT, Nagarajan P, et al. Diverse types of dermatologic toxicities from immune checkpoint blockade therapy. *J Cutan Pathol*. 2017;44:158-176.
33. Tetzlaff MT, Nagarajan P, Chon S, et al. Lichenoid dermatologic toxicity from immune checkpoint blockade therapy: a detailed examination of the clinicopathologic features. *Am J Dermatopathol*. 2017;39:121-129.
34. Schaberg KB, Novoa RA, Wakelee HA, et al. Immunohistochemical analysis of lichenoid reactions in patients treated with anti-PD-L1 and anti-PD-1 therapy. *J Cutan Pathol*. 2016;43:339-346.
35. Sibaud V, Eid C, Belum V, et al. Oral lichenoid reactions associated with anti-PD-1/PD-L1 therapies: clinicopathological findings. *J Eur Acad Dermatol Venereol*. 2017;31:e464.
36. Voudouri D, Nikolaou V, Laschos K, et al. Anti-PD1/PDL1 induced psoriasis. *Curr Probl Cancer*. 2017;41:407-412.
37. De Bock M, Hulstaert E, Kruse V, Brochez L. Psoriasis vulgaris exacerbation during treatment with a PD-1 checkpoint inhibitor: case report and literature review. *Case Rep Dermatol*. 2018;10:190-197.
38. Bonigen J, Raynaud-Donzel C, Hureaux J, et al. Anti-PD1-induced psoriasis: a study of 21 patients. *J Eur Acad Dermatol Venereol*. 2017;31:e254.
39. Nikolaou V, Sibaud V, Fattore D, et al. Immune checkpoint-mediated psoriasis: a multicentric European study of 115 patients from European Network for Cutaneous Adverse Event to Oncologic drugs (ENCADO) group. *J Am Acad Dermatol*. 2020.
40. Law-Ping-Man S, Martin A, Briens E, Tisseau L, Safa G. Psoriasis and psoriatic arthritis induced by nivolumab in a patient with advanced lung cancer. *Rheumatology*. 2016;55:2087-2089.
41. Elosua-González M, Pampín-Franco A, Mazzucchelli-Esteban R, et al. A case of de novo palmoplantar psoriasis with psoriatic arthritis and autoimmune hypothyroidism after receiving nivolumab therapy. *Dermatol Online J*. 2017;23:13030/qt12n4m6pm.
42. Cornejo CM, Haun P, English J, Rosenbach M. Immune checkpoint inhibitors and the development of granulomatous reactions. *J Am Acad Dermatol* 2019;81:1165-1175.

43. Lomax AJ, McGuire HM, McNeil C, et al. Immunotherapy-induced sarcoidosis in patients with melanoma treated with PD-1 checkpoint inhibitors: case series and immunophenotypic analysis. *Int J Rheum Dis.* 2017;20:1277-1285.
44. Danlos F-X, Pagès C, Baroudjian B, et al. Nivolumab-induced sarcoid-like granulomatous reaction in a patient with advanced melanoma. *Chest.* 2016;149:e133-e6.
45. Burillo-Martinez S, Morales-Raya C, Prieto-Barrios M, Rodriguez-Peralto JL, Ortiz-Romero PL. Pembrolizumab-induced extensive panniculitis and nevus regression: two novel cutaneous manifestations of the post-immunotherapy granulomatous reactions spectrum. *JAMA Dermatol.* 2017;153:721-722.
46. Wu J, Kwong B, Martires K, et al. Granuloma annulare associated with immune checkpoint inhibitors. *J Eur Acad Dermatol Venereol.* 2018;32:e124.
47. Trinidad C, Nelson KC, Glitza Oliva IC, et al. Dermatologic toxicity from immune checkpoint blockade therapy with an interstitial granulomatous pattern. *J Cutan Pathol.* 2018;45:504-507.
48. Diaz-Perez JA, Beveridge MG, Victor TA, Cibull TL. Granulomatous and lichenoid dermatitis after IgG4 anti-PD-1 monoclonal antibody therapy for advanced cancer. *J Cutan Pathol.* 2018;45:434-438.
49. Siegel J, Totonchy M, Damsky W, et al. Bullous disorders associated with anti–PD-1 and anti–PD-L1 therapy: a retrospective analysis evaluating the clinical and histopathologic features, frequency, and impact on cancer therapy. *J Am Acad Dermatol.* 2018;79:1081-1088.
50. Lopez AT, Khanna T, Antonov N, Audrey-Bayan C, Geskin L. A review of bullous pemphigoid associated with PD-1 and PD-L1 inhibitors. *Int J Dermatol* 2018;57:664-669.
51. Naidoo J, Schindler K, Querfeld C, et al. Autoimmune bullous skin disorders with immune checkpoint inhibitors targeting PD-1 and PD-L1. *Cancer Immunol Res.* 2016;4:383-389.
52. Anastasopoulou A, Papaxoinis G, Diamantopoulos P, et al. Bullous Pemphigoid–like skin lesions and overt eosinophilia in a patient with melanoma treated with nivolumab: case report and review of the literature. *J Immunother.* 2018;41:164-167.
53. Lopez AT, Geskin L. A case of nivolumab-induced bullous pemphigoid: review of dermatologic toxicity associated with programmed cell death protein-1/programmed death ligand-1 inhibitors and recommendations for diagnosis and management. *Oncologist.* 2018;23:1119.
54. Sowerby L, Dewan AK, Granter S, Gandhi L, LeBoeuf NR. Rituximab treatment of nivolumab-induced bullous pemphigoid. *JAMA Dermatol.* 2017;153:603-605.
55. Ridpath AV, Rzepka PV, Shearer SM, Scrape SR, Olencki TE, Kaffenberger BH. Novel use of combination therapeutic plasma exchange and rituximab in the treatment of nivolumab-induced bullous pemphigoid. *Int J Dermatol.* 2018;57:1372-1374.
56. Freites-Martinez A, Kwong BY, Rieger KE, Coit DG, Colevas AD, Lacouture ME. Eruptive keratoacanthomas associated with pembrolizumab therapy. *JAMA Dermatol.* 2017;153:694-697.
57. Antonov NK, Nair KG, Halasz CL. Transient eruptive keratoacanthomas associated with nivolumab. *JAAD Case Rep.* 2019;5:342-345.
58. Fradet M, Sibaud V, Tournier E, et al. Multiple Keratoacanthoma-like lesions in a patient treated with pembrolizumab. *Acta Derm Venereol.* 2019;99:1301-1302.
59. Bednarek R, Marks K, Lin G. Eruptive keratoacanthomas secondary to nivolumab immunotherapy. *Int J Dermatol.* 2018;57:e28-e29.
60. Feldstein SI, Patel F, Larsen L, Kim E, Hwang S, Fung MA. Eruptive keratoacanthomas arising in the setting of lichenoid toxicity after programmed cell death 1 inhibition with nivolumab. *J Eur Acad Dermatol Venereol.* 2018;32:e58-e59.
61. Mohanty R, Chowdhury CR, Arega S, Sen P, Ganguly P, Ganguly N. CAR T cell therapy: a new era for cancer treatment. *Oncol Rep.* 2019;42:2183-2195.
62. Feins S, Kong W, Williams EF, Milone MC, Fraietta JA. An introduction to chimeric antigen receptor (CAR) T-cell immunotherapy for human cancer. *Am J Hematol.* 2019;94:S3-S9.
63. Stroncek DF, Ren J, Lee DW, et al. Myeloid cells in peripheral blood mononuclear cell concentrates inhibit the expansion of chimeric antigen receptor T cells. *Cytotherapy.* 2016;18:893-901.
64. *YESCARTA (Axicabtagene Ciloleucel) [package insert].* Kite Pharma, Inc; 2020.
65. *KYMRIAH (Tisagenlecleucel) [package insert].* Novartis Pharmaceuticals Corporation; 2020.
66. *TECARTUS (Brexucabtagene Autoleucel) [package insert].* Kite Pharma, Inc.; 2020.
67. Rubin CB, Elenitsas R, Taylor L, et al. Evaluating the skin in patients undergoing chimeric antigen receptor modified T-cell therapy. *J Am Acad Dermatol.* 2016;75:1054-1057.
68. Hu Y, Zheng W, Qiao J, et al. Bullous and exanthematous lesions associated with chimeric antigen receptor T-cell therapy in a patient with diffuse large B-cell lymphoma. *JAMA Dermatol.* 2020;156:1026-1028.
69. Wang D, Xiao Y, Li C et al. Anti-CD30 chimeric antigen receptor T cell therapy for CD30+ relapsed/refractory Hodgkin lymphoma and anaplastic large cell lymphoma patients. *Blood.* 2018;132:1660.

PART XIII CUTANEOUS MANIFESTATIONS ASSOCIATED WITH HEMATOLOGIC MALIGNANCY

CHAPTER 76

Sweet and histiocytoid sweet syndrome

Jacqueline M. Junkins-Hopkins and Viktoryia Kazlouskaya

DEFINITION

Sweet syndrome (SS) is a disorder characterized by neutrophil-predominant skin lesions, also known as acute neutrophilic dermatosis, which is frequently associated with systemic involvement. A diagnosis of SS requires the presence of two major criteria: (1) rapid onset of typical skin lesions (tender erythematous plaques, nodules, papules, or rarely blisters) and (2) histopathologic features of an inflammatory infiltrate rich in neutrophils demonstrating leukocytoclasia without evident leukocytoclastic vasculitis, and at least three minor criteria: fever >38 °C; associated malignancy, pregnancy, infection, or inflammatory disease; abnormal laboratory findings—neutrophil count more than 70%, elevated erythrocyte sedimentation rate, C-reactive protein, and/or white blood count; and prompt response to corticosteroids.[1,2] The major criteria are consistently present, but many cases of SS are potentially missed due to failing to fulfill minor criteria, in part due to numerous subtypes that have been described since the initial criteria were put forth. For this reason, a revised set of criteria have been proposed,[3] requiring *constant* clinical and histopathologic features: abrupt onset of painful or tender erythematous papules, plaques, or nodules and histology showing dense dermal neutrophilic infiltrate. In this construct, the term *minor criteria* has been replaced by *variable features*, the absence of which does not exclude SS,[3] and include fever >38 °C, atypical skin lesions (including hemorrhagic blisters, pustular lesions, cellulitis-like lesions), histopathologic variants (subcutaneous, histiocytoid, xanthomatoid, cryptococcoid), and laboratory (elevated erythrocyte sedimentation rate and/or C-reactive protein levels, leukocytosis, neutrophilia, anemia). In this new proposal, the absence of vasculitis is a feature, but it also allows for the presence of vasculitis as a variable feature. However, it is our opinion that the absence of vasculitis be emphasized and the presence of SS with secondary vasculitis be recognized as a separate histopathologic presentation.

EPIDEMIOLOGY AND ETIOLOGY

SS usually manifests in adults, ages 50 to 60 years, but may rarely occur in the pediatric population,[4-6] with a rate of approximately 5% to 8%. Some reports suggest a female predominance, although other studies fail to confirm this.[7] In fact, in kids of ages 3 to 18 years, the male:female ratio is equal, while in kids aged <3 years, male patients predominate.[5] Atypical SS variants have been reported in kids, and there is a difference in associated conditions, depending on the age of the patient. For instance, in kids <3 years old, malignancy is not typically seen, while in ages 3 to 18 years, the risk of malignancy is similar to that of adults, around 44%. Thus, to assist with management, SS in the pediatric population has been designated as neonatal SS (birth to <3 months old), infantile SS (3 month to <3 years), and junior SS (3 to 18 years).[5]

Six main types of SS are known: classic/idiopathic, autoimmune disease–associated, postinfectious, malignancy-associated (MA-SS), pregnancy-associated (PA-SS), and drug-associated (DA-SS). Some consolidate idiopathic, inflammatory, infectious, autoimmune, and pregnancy-related SS under the classic SS subtype.[8]

Autoimmune-associated disorders include systemic lupus erythematosus, dermatomyositis, Hashimoto thyroiditis, Crohn disease, ulcerative colitis, Behçet disease, pemphigus vulgaris, rheumatoid arthritis, and Sjögren syndrome.[7] Other inflammatory conditions such as sarcoidosis and relapsing polychondritis may also present with SS.[9]

Infections have been documented in about 25% of SS cases.[7] Respiratory viral infections are more common, except for the pediatric population prior to 2 months of life, when bacterial infections predominate.[4] Other associated infections include tuberculosis, parvovirus B19, sporotrichosis, tularemia, hepatitis B and C,[10-12] Legionella,[13] lymphogranuloma venereum,[14] and COVID-19.[15]

Adult-onset immunodeficiency (AOID) due to anti–interferon gamma autoantibody is an entity reported primarily in Asian countries, especially Thailand and Taiwan, which is associated with opportunistic infections (OIs), most typically nodal nontuberculous mycobacterium infection that often disseminates, as well as other OIs, and neutrophilic dermatoses, including SS, generalized pustular eruption, and panniculitis. HIV testing is negative, but neutralizing anti–interferon gamma autoantibodies are present in the plasma and serum.[16,17] Cutaneous lesions are reported in up to 80% of cases, up to 82% of which are inflammatory, representing neutrophilic dermatosis.[17] The presence of neutrophilic dermatosis in this group of patients with AIOD is strongly associated with infection; thus, a diagnosis of SS may help diagnose OIs. Other immunodeficiency states associated with SS include common variable immunodeficiency, chronic granulomatous disease, hypogammaglobulinemia, and T-cell lymphopenia.[18]

MA-SS comprises 21% to 51.9% of patients with SS.[19-21] SS lesions may herald the initial onset of the malignancy or may precede the cancer diagnosis for many years. Patients should be monitored for malignancy for a minimum of 16 months.[21] Histiocytoid or subcutaneous SS,[9] absence of arthralgias, anemia, thrombocytopenia, and leukopenia[9,20,21] are seen more in the MA-SS in contrast to the non-MA-SS group and could serve as guidance in the malignancy workup. SS may be a sign of recurrence, but chemotherapy-induced SS should be excluded. Hematologic malignancies represent 85% of all MA-SS cases, with myeloid malignancies leading the list. Acute myelogenous leukemia (AML) is considered to be the most common, but others have found myelodysplastic syndrome (MDS) to occur more often,[20] perhaps due to the close relationship between these entities. SS is seen in about 1% of patients with AML either before or after the diagnosis is made.[22] In over 50% of patients with AML-associated SS, MDS precedes AML. Patients with MA-SS with MDS progressing to AML may have a poor prognosis.[20] Complex cytogenetics (mutations in -5/del(5q) and *FLT3*) and therapy-related AML are among the other AML associations.[22,23] Other hematologic disorders, such as chronic myelogenous leukemia, essential thrombocythemia, and polycythemia vera (PV); paraproteinemias (multiple myeloma and monoclonal gammopathy of undetermined significance [MGUS]); chronic lymphocytic leukemia, some anemias (Fanconi anemia, aplastic anemia, and other refractory anemias), hairy cell leukemia, Hodgkin disease, and diffuse large B-cell lymphoma, are less frequent.[24-28] SS in patients with Fanconi anemia and PV may indicate progression of the disease with evolution to MDS and AML.[29,30] The relationship between SS and cancer is further manifested by the observation that SS refractory to therapy may clear with treatment of the malignancy.[20] Solid tumors associated with SS include gastrointestinal malignancies (esophageal, stomach, colorectal),[20] genitourinary malignancies (ovarian, bladder, prostate, cervical cancers), breast carcinoma, and, less frequently, papillary thyroid carcinoma and lung cancer.[12]

PA-SS comprises less than 2% of SS cases. It may appear in any stage of pregnancy and often recurs during the same or subsequent pregnancies.[31] A normal delivery is expected, although early miscarriage may rarely occur in fulminant SS.[32-34] A case of subcutaneous SS mimicking cellulitis at 12 weeks' gestation has been reported.[35]

Criteria for drug-induced SS include (1) abrupt onset of typical SS lesions, (2) biopsy findings consistent with SS, (3) fever, (4) temporal relationship with drug and lesions or rechallenge confirmation, and (5) temporal relationship after discontinuation of the drug or corticosteroid use.[36-50]

Multiple drugs may cause SS,[51] with granulocyte colony-stimulating factor (G-CSF), vaccines (smallpox, BCG, influenza, pneumococcal), and all-trans-retinoid acid being some of the most common.[52] In one tertiary center, 24% of SS had the drug-induced form in the setting of malignancy, with the most common culprit being Filgrastim. The non-malignancy-associated SS cases with DA-SS was 2%.[9] There have been several reports of SS induced by several vaccines to the SARS CoV2 virus,[41-44] including neuro-SS characterized by acute encephalitis and myoclonus triggered by the mRNA-1273 COVID-19 vaccine.[42] There is a long list of drugs that have been reported to cause SS, some of which include antivirals (acyclovir, abacavir) and antimicrobials (trimethoprim-sulfasalazine, minocycline, nitrofurantoin, ketoconazole, and fluoroquinolones [norfloxacin, ofloxacin, levofloxacin]), which includes the histiocytoid SS variant triggered by levofloxacin and amoxicillin-clavulanate.[51,53] Numerous antineoplastic agents have been associated with the onset of SS (ipilimumab, lenalidomide, ixazomib,[39] letrozole,[48] Palbociclib,[40] midostaurin,[46] and topotecan), including several reports of SS associated with tyrosine kinase inhibitors (TKI)[47] (imatinib, bortezomib, dasatinib, ruxolitinib, nilotinib, ibrutinib, dabrafenib, quizartinib, gilteritinib, vemurafenib). A long latency may be seen. The median time from TKI exposure to SS is around 2 months, but latency may range from 6 months to 6 years. Other miscellaneous medicines that may cause DA-SS include antiseizure medicines (carbamazepine, diazepam, clonazepam), lorazepam, amoxapine, pegfilgrastim,[45] hydralazine, furosemide, gliflozins (dapagliflozin), azathioprine, celecoxib, oral contraceptives, hydroxychloroquine,[50] clopidogrel,[37] tocilizumab,[49] allopurinol.[47] Paradoxical drug reactions have been reported with medications such as azathioprine, ipilimumab, adalimumab, nivolumab, abatacept, and tocilizumab.[54] The lesions resolved after drug discontinuation in 2 to 90 days (median 14 days), at times also requiring concomitant steroid therapy. Cautious rechallenge at a lower dose without recurrence may be attempted.

The incidence of idiopathic SS is ~11%; however, as this group often includes parainflammatory and postinfectious cases, the true incidence of idiopathic SS is not known. Longer follow-up may be needed to reveal an underlying condition.[55]

The pathogenesis of SS[56-60] remains elusive, and the pathogenesis is likely heterogeneous, determined in part by the subtype of SS. Mounting evidence suggests a role for abnormal neutrophilic function, autoinflammation and inflammasomes, genetic predisposition, and/or clonal neutrophils in MA-SS. Abnormal neutrophil function as a cause of SS is supported by documentation of numerous cytokines that have been overexpressed in neutrophilic dermatoses, including G-CSF, interferon-γ, interleukin (IL)-1 (α and β), IL-2, IL-6, IL-8, IL-17, and TNF-α.[8,61,62] Observations that may have etiologic implications include the findings of elevated levels of G-CSF in patients with active SS (compared with inactive disease); IL-1, IL-2, and interferon-γ stimulation of G-CSF production by macrophages; and decreased apoptosis of neutrophils in women, aggravated by progesterone.[61-63] HLA typing has shown

HLA-B54 and Cw1 to be associated with SS. Documenting this HLA phenotype allowed differentiation of neuro-SS from neuro-Behçet in a patient who also was found on a 27-cytokine assay to have an increase in numerous inflammatory cytokines, growth factors, and chemoattractants during the active phase of SS, further supporting a role for a variety of bioactive substances in the pathogenesis of SS.[60] Mouse models with defects in protein tyrosine phosphatases nonreceptor type 6 (PTPN6), which is important in the regulation of the myelopoietic system, have developed neutrophilic dermatosis, and genetic alterations on PTPN6 have been documented in patients with subtypes of neutrophilic dermatoses. CARD9,[57] a myeloid cell–specific signaling protein involved in innate and adaptive immunity, may also play a role in a subset of neutrophilic dermatoses.[58] Some patients with MDS have been shown to have the same clonal mutation in the neutrophilic dermal infiltrates as found in the marrow.[59]

CLINICAL PRESENTATION

Clinically, SS lesions have a predilection for the head, extremities (upper > lower), and dorsal hands but may occur anywhere.[12] Photodistribution may occur (Fig. 76-1). Oral, ocular, and/or genital[64] mucosal involvement may occur, especially in MA-SS, in which widespread involvement is frequent.[65] Morphologically, SS lesions are tender erythematous-violaceous papules, nodules, or plaques (Fig. 76-1B–E). The lesions are often pseudovesicular, and vesicopustular or bullous lesions may be seen in up to 30% of cases.[9] Some lesions may be targetoid.[66] Annular or figurate morphology may be seen (Fig. 76-1F), which some have considered a separate neutrophilic dermatosis, termed chronic annular neutrophilic dermatosis due to the absence of systemic associations. However, it may represent a morphologic variant of SS, since several systemic disorders have since been reported with the condition.[66] SS may mimic various causes of panniculitis (Fig. 76-1G), and clinically it may look nearly identical to erythema nodosum if on the lower extremities. SS may also mimic cellulitis. Giant-cellulitis-like SS presents with large asymmetric erythematous patches and plaques, without lymphadenopathy. Suspicion should arise if there are negative cultures/stains and no response to antimicrobials. Necrotizing neutrophilic dermatosis (NND) may mimic necrotizing fasciitis or pyoderma gangrenosum.[64,67-69] In one study, 94% of NND were misdiagnosed as necrotizing fasciitis, some of which resulted in debridement or amputation; thus, criteria for a diagnosis of NND have been proposed[69] and include pyoderma gangrenosum-like ulcers often with skin breakdown and/or satellite lesions, purulence, purpura, edema, fever >40 °C, shock, leukemoid reaction (≥30,000/μL), leukocytosis (≥11,000/μL), no sign of organisms on histopathologic stains and negative tissue culture, diffuse dermal and subcutaneous neutrophils with leukocytoclasis and edema, dramatic response to corticosteroids, lack of response or worsening with antibiotics, debridement, amputation, and incision and draining. Minor criteria include triggers for SS and history of pathergy. The subtype of SS, termed "neutrophilic dermatosis of the dorsal hands (NDDH)," is usually localized to the area of dorsal hands and fingers, where it presents as tender hemorrhagic, bullous, ulcerated, pseudopustular, or pseudovesicular plaques (Fig. 76-1H), and is frequently biopsied with a suspicion of infection.[70] In a large review of reported cases of NDDH, the palm and other sites were involved as well.[71] Patients with AOID-SS tend to have acral pustular lesions similar to NDDH. In addition to pustular morphology, other clues to the diagnosis include lymphadenopathy and leukocytosis, and this triad should prompt a workup for OI, especially nontuberculous mycobacterium infection in an adult Asian patient.

Patients with SS frequently present concomitantly with fever and arthralgias. Additional extracutaneous symptoms

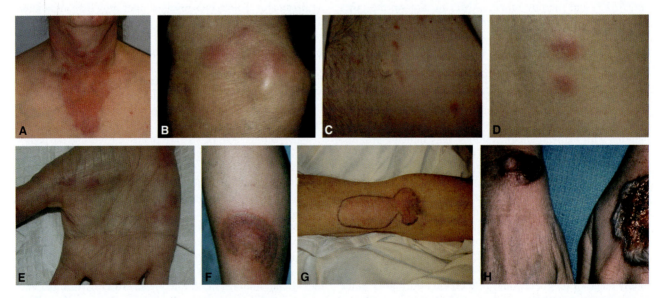

FIGURE 76-1. Clinical lesions of Sweet neutrophilic dermatosis. A. Photodistributed violaceous dermal plaques of SS. Note submental sparing. **B.** Erythematous nonscaly dermal plaques and nodules on the extremity. **C.** Erythematous papules. **D.** Violaceous, juicy papulonodules. **E.** Acral involvement by erythematous papules, nodules, and plaques. **F.** Violaceous and dusky figurate plaque on the leg, exhibiting a targetoid appearance and pseudobullous features, owing to prominent dermal edema. **G.** SS presenting as a panniculitic plaque on the arm. **H.** NDDH—a subtype of SS. Hemorrhagic eroded bullous plaques that simulate infection.

are common, because virtually any organ may be affected by the neutrophilic infiltration. Pulmonary SS may simulate pneumonia with cough and dyspnea, abnormal chest imaging, and neutrophils on bronchioalveolar lavage.[72] Neuro-Sweet may present as meningitis, encephalitis, headaches, epilepsy, hemiparesis, psychiatric disorders, and/or dyskinesias.[73,74] Ocular involvement can be seen in around a third of patients with SS, including blepharitis, conjunctivitis, episcleritis, scleritis, ulcerative keratitis, iritis, panuveitis, glaucoma, retinal vasculitis, and periorbital inflammation[75] and central retinal artery occlusion.[76] Lymph nodes and spleen may also be involved.

HISTOLOGY

Histopathologically, SS lesions, or acute neutrophilic dermatosis, are characterized by the presence of a diffuse pandermal infiltrate that typically includes interstitial neutrophils demonstrating prominent leukocytoclasis (Fig. 76-2A–E) and variable perivascular lymphocytes, which may be prominent (Fig. 76-3). Papillary dermal edema is a classic SS feature (Figs. 76-1A,D and 76-3) but is not always present. The infiltrate may include eosinophils, which may be quite prominent (Fig. 76-2B,C).[77] Histiocytes may be prominent (Fig. 76-4A–C),

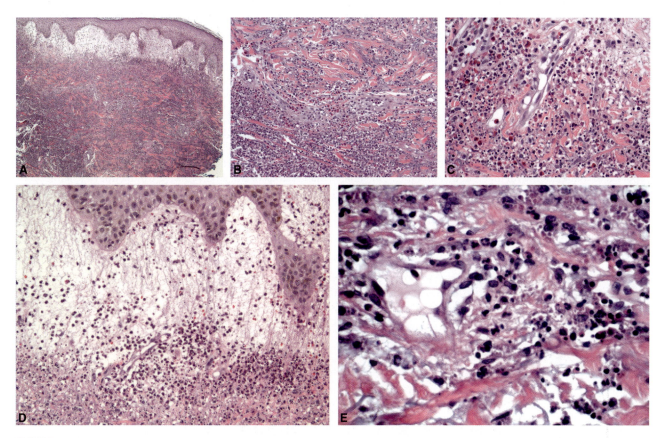

FIGURE 76-2. Histology of Sweet neutrophilic dermatosis. There is a dense, diffuse, pandermal infiltrate of neutrophils (**A–D**) demonstrating prominent leukocytoclasis without vasculitis (**C** and **E**). There is an admixture of eosinophils (**B** and **C**), with marked papillary dermal edema (**D**).

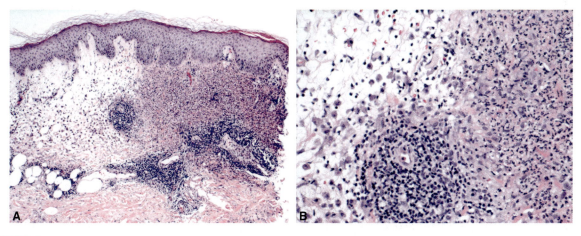

FIGURE 76-3. A. SS with marked edema and a prominent perivascular lymphocytic component. **B.** High-power view demonstrating perivascular lymphocytes and interstitial neutrophils with leukocytoclasis and edema.

possibly reflecting the age of the lesion.[78,79] This should be distinguished from the histiocytoid presentation of immature myeloid cells seen in histiocytoid SS. The neutrophilic component may be difficult to identify due to prominent leukocytoclasis, at times requiring myeloperoxidase stains to confirm that the nuclear fragments are myeloid cells (Fig. 76-5). The lymphocytic component may be inconspicuous, owing to the overwhelming number of neutrophils. A predominance of lymphocytes has been reported in patients with MDS.[78,80,81] In exuberant infiltrates, fibrin leakage and erythrocyte extravasation suggesting an element of vascular damage may be found, especially in long-standing lesions or in NDDH (also known as pustular vasculitis).[82] However, fibrinoid necrosis of vessels typical of a primary leukocytoclastic vasculitis is absent in SS. Intense neutrophilic infiltration may extend into the epidermis, resulting in a pustular lesion. *Subcutaneous SS* is a less common but distinct variant that may or may not arise in conjunction with typical dermal SS changes. There is infiltration of the fat lobules, often without significant destruction of the adipocytes (Fig. 76-6A,B). There may be extension into and widening of the septae, but a granulomatous infiltrate typical of infection is not typically seen. Neutrophils demonstrating leukocytoclasis may be admixed with histiocytoid cells. The subcutaneous variant has been reported in association with myeloid disorders.[9,28,83] In some cases of SS, the neutrophilic component may manifest as immature-appearing myeloid cells with pseudo–Pelger-Huët-type nuclei, termed "*histiocytoid SS*" (*HSS*).[84] This histopathologic subtype exhibits a similar pattern of pandermal infiltration, edema, and leukocytoclasis but is characterized by the presence of non- or hyposegmented myeloid cells, simulating histiocytes, with elongate or large kidney-shaped vesicular nuclei and an inconspicuous nucleolus, admixed with band-like cells, and less conspicuous mature neutrophils.[84] The infiltrate may be dermal and/or subcutaneous.[85] A histopathologic clue to this diagnosis is that of leukocytoclasia, typical of SS (Fig. 76-7A,B). The histiocytoid cells in HSS usually express markers of myeloid origin: myeloperoxidase, CD68, CD43, CD45, and lysozyme.[84,86] While it has been reported that the infiltrate is positive for PG-M1/M2-like macrophage markers,[84,87] histiocytes, as highlighted by CD163, make up only a small component of the infiltrate (usually at the periphery). Instead, the HSS histiocytoid cells primarily coexpress MPO and MDNA, confirming a myelomonocytic and not a histiocytic lineage. CD68+ lesional cells are also present.[86] If in fact there are numerous histiocytes, this could represent a later-stage lesion of SS. HSS diagnosis should prompt a systemic workup, because similar to classic SS there is an association of HSS with malignancy in approximately 30% of cases, with 80% of these representing to hematologic malignancy, especially MDS. Autoimmune diseases, infectious diseases, solid neoplasms,[86,87] and drug-induced cases may be seen.[53,86,88,89] Histiocytes are present in later lesions of SS, so the presence of histiocytes, alone, does not constitute a diagnosis of HSS. Close inspection of the cytomorphology of the MPO-positive cells for nonsegmented nuclei will help confirm the diagnosis of HSS, in conjunction with documenting that these band-like histiocytoid cells

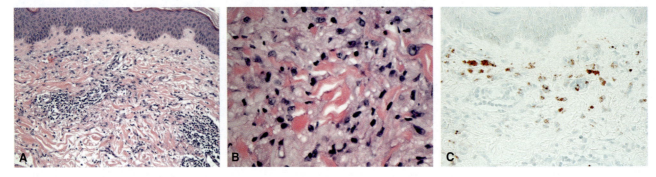

FIGURE 76-4. Histiocyte-rich SS. An older lesion of SS, demonstrating histiocytes, lymphocytes, and nuclear dust of neutrophils (**A** and **B**), confirmed with myeloperoxidase staining (**C**).

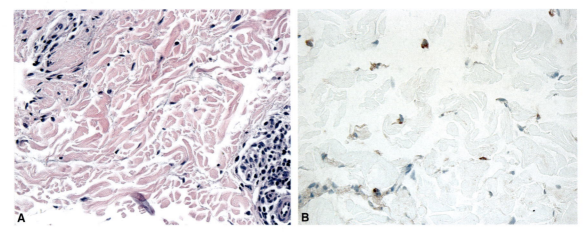

FIGURE 76-5. Subtle SS. A. Fragmentation of neutrophils with perivascular lymphocytes. **B.** Neutrophilic component is highlighted with a myeloperoxidase stain.

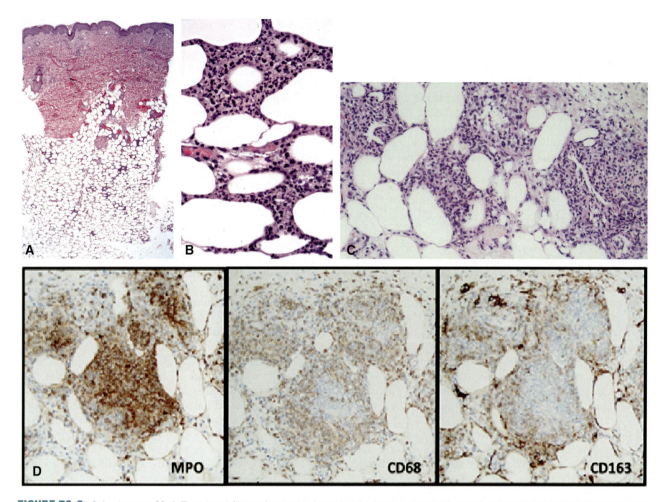

FIGURE 76-6. Subcutaneous SS. A. There is an infiltrate of neutrophils located predominantly in the subcutaneous fat, within the fat lobules. **B.** High-power view demonstrating delicate lacing of the periadipocyte tissue, without destruction. There is leukocytoclasis without vasculitis. **C.** Aggregates of histiocytoid cells surround a jagged cleft, consistent with a Miescher radial granuloma. **D.** The myeloid cells are positive for MPO, partially positive for CD68, and essentially negative for CD163 (stains macrophages).

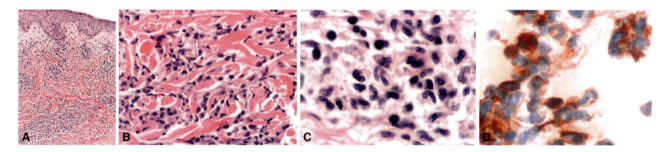

FIGURE 76-7. Histiocytoid SS associated with MDS. A. There is a pandermal infiltrate with papillary dermal edema and leukocytoclasis. **B.** Medium power demonstrating the leukocytoclasis and morphology of the neutrophils to be hyposegmented, band-like and histiocyte-like. **C.** High-power view demonstrating the histiocytoid morphology and abnormal segmentation of the neutrophils. **D.** These cells are confirmed to be neutrophilic with myeloperoxidase staining.

are positive for MPO. The presence of elastolysis associated with neutrophil elastase has been described with histiocytoid SS. This may clinically be associated with acquired cutis laxa (Marshall syndrome).[90] *Cryptoccoid SS* is a recently described histopathologic subtype that is characterized by neutrophils surrounding vacuolated spaces containing basophilic fragmented neutrophils simulating budding yeasts surrounded by capsule-like haloes, mimicking gelatinous cryptococcosis.[91-94] This can be seen in the setting of HSS.[92]

In cases of cryptococcoid SS triggered by infection, hemorrhagic bullous lesions may be seen in conjunction with ANCA positivity, without evidence of systemic ANCA vasculitis.[93] *Xanthomatized neutrophilic dermatosis* is a recently described variant in which there are yellowish papules and plaques on the skin and often oral mucosal tissue with histology showing a dermal infiltrate of neutrophils and xanthomatous histiocytes with foamy cytoplasm.[95,96] The xanthomatous component has been shown to stain positive for MPO and

CD68 (PGM1), with numerous CD163+ histiocytes.[96] Other reports describe the neutrophilic component juxtaposed to the xanthomatous component.[96] The xanthomatous component has been theorized to be a localized response and not systemically derived lipid, but only a handful of cases currently have been reported. Hyperlipidemia has not been documented with this variant, but associated MDS has been documented in reported cases. A case of papular neutrophilic xanthoma of the oral commissure may be a localized form of xanthomatized neutrophilic dermatosis,[97] as it has also been associated with MDS.

DIFFERENTIAL DIAGNOSIS

The differential diagnosis of SS, which is broad and determined by the subtype and stage of evolution, includes urticarial vasculitis, adult Still disease, erythema multiforme, granuloma annulare, insect bite reaction, pyoderma gangrenosum, infection, acute tick bite reaction, cellulitis, necrotizing fasciitis, small vessel neutrophil-rich vasculitis (leukocytoclastic vasculitis), panniculitis, leukemia cutis, Schnitzler syndrome, Wells syndrome, neutrophilic dermatosis of systemic lupus erythematosus, and other neutrophilic dermatoses.

A biopsy will exclude the nonneutrophilic conditions. Fibrin leakage and/or erythrocyte extravasation may make it difficult to differentiate SS from leukocytoclastic vasculitis. In SS, the neutrophils are prominent in the interstitium, with mononuclear cells around the vessels, in contrast to leukocytoclastic vasculitis, in which neutrophils concentrate around and infiltrate the vessel walls, resulting in prominent fibrinoid necrosis. Neutrophilic urticaria and cellulitis are differentiated by the absence of significant leukocytoclasis and a sparser infiltrate. Denser infiltrates will show histopathologic overlap with conditions such as pyoderma gangrenosum, bowel bypass syndrome, and Behçet disease, all of which have distinctive differentiating clinical presentations.[98] Of note, early stages of pyoderma gangrenosum may have indistinguishable histopathologic features. The main clinicopathologic differential will include the other systemic-related aseptic neutrophilic dermatoses, especially "neutrophilic urticarial dermatosis" (NUD), which histologically demonstrates a neutrophilic infiltrate and leukocytoclasis, similar to SS, and is associated with systemic conditions such as cryopirin-associated periodic syndromes (familial cold anti-inflammatory syndrome, Muckle-Wells syndrome, and neonatal-onset multisystem inflammatory disease), adult-onset Still disease, Schnitzler syndrome, and lupus erythematosus (although some consider this latter as a separate condition of neutrophilic cutaneous lupus erythematosus[99]). The absence of dermal edema, presence of necrobiotic collagen alteration, diapedesis of neutrophils, a less dense infiltrate, and sparse-to-absent mononuclear cells favor NUD. Epitheliotropism of neutrophils into eccrine and pilosebaceous epithelium is a unique feature that favors NUD. This is more easily identified with a myeloperoxidase stain.[100] However, an adnexal structure may not be present in the biopsy and some SSs may lack edema; therefore, one should rely on the clinical presentation. NUD lesions are flatter and urticarial, but burn, instead of itch, and are unresponsive to antihistamines, clear spontaneously within 48 hours, and are not triggered as with SS.[101] Early lesions of palisaded neutrophilic and granulomatous dermatosis are neutrophil-rich with leukocytoclasis but are distinguished from SS by the presence of strands of basophilic necrobiotic collagen alteration and vasculitis. Dermal abscess formation due to ruptured folliculitis may show SS-like changes but are frequently accompanied by a granulomatous component and granulation tissue formation. Mycobacterial/atypical mycobacterial and fungal infections may simulate SS, especially in the immunocompromised host, but may present with more basophilic tissue necrosis and/or multinucleated giant cells. Discretion is required to determine the need for special stains prior to diagnosing SS, especially in the NDDH subtype, which clinically shows overlap with local infection. Caution should especially be taken when diagnosing SS in hospitalized neutropenic patients, due to the potential for fusarium or bacterial infection in the lesions, noted in 12.9% of neutropenic patients being evaluated for SS.[102] In these instances, the biopsy may yield a positive culture within a few days, allowing a short delay in instituting a diagnostic/therapeutic trial for SS.

HSS may be difficult to distinguish from a histiocytic infiltrate, such as granuloma annulare. Mucinous collagen degeneration and multinucleated histiocytes favor the latter. Recognizing an admixture of band-like cells, mature neutrophils, and nuclear dust, in addition to the histiocyte-like mononuclear cells, will allow one to consider the possibility of HSS. To confirm the diagnosis, the workup should include myeloperoxidase, to mark the myeloid cells (see Fig. 76-7), because standard histiocyte markers, such as CD68, lysozyme, and MAC 387, will stain both myeloid cells and histiocytes. HSS may be indistinguishable from leukemia cutis, by histopathologic, immunophenotypic, and clinical morphologic parameters, requiring follow-up and correlation with the clinical course.[103] Although a prompt response to oral prednisone helps to confirm a diagnosis of SS, such rare cases have been reported to progress to a clinical picture more typical of leukemia cutis.[103] In some cases of hematologic MA-SS, the same cytogenetic abnormality was seen in the bone marrow and skin, suggesting that HSS may lie on a spectrum with leukemia cutis.[104]

The differential diagnosis of subcutaneous SS includes other neutrophilic panniculitides, including infection, early erythema nodosum, and α1-antitrypsin deficiency.[83] Early erythema nodosum may be indistinguishable and/or may coexist with subcutaneous SS. In subcutaneous SS, the neutrophils delicately infiltrate around the adipocytes, without significant destruction or necrosis, as is typically seen in α1-antitrypsin deficiency, and often in infection. BRAF inhibitor–associated neutrophilic panniculitis is in the differential diagnosis of subcutaneous SS. There are similar histologic features, but it is reported as a distinct entity.[105] Associated arthralgias have been reported, and foci of vasculitis may be seen, differentiating this from SS. Histiocytes may be present in SS, but a significant granulomatous component, especially if accompanied by necrosis or basophilic debris, is more typical of fungal or atypical mycobacterial infectious panniculitis. HSS may present as a panniculitis, requiring myeloperoxidase to confirm. Fixed drug eruption may rarely show histopathologic features of a neutrophilic dermatosis,[106] especially in early lesions,[107] but the clinical presentation of a circular circumscribed lesion arising in the exact same location with a drug trigger distinguishes this from SS.

SS lies on the spectrum of other neutrophilic dermatoses with similar histology but with distinct clinical and/or syndromic presentations, specific disease associations, and management approaches. These include conditions such as pyoderma gangrenosum, Behçet disease, rheumatoid neutrophilic dermatosis, and bowel-associated dermatosis-arthritis syndrome (BADAS). BADAS presents with episodic flu-like symptoms and arthralgias, followed by an eruption of vesicopapules, and subcutaneous nodules. The lesions may be histopathologically identical to SS, but these patients have gastrointestinal conditions such as inflammatory bowel disease, bowel bypass/bariatric surgery, diverticulitis, and appendicitis, which predisposes them to bacterial overgrowth and subsequent immune-complex formation and deposition in the skin.[108,109]

An SS-like neutrophilic dermatosis may present with a distinct constellation of conditions in adult older men (and very rarely in women) with a severe autoinflammatory syndrome due to a somatic mutation in the ubiquitin activating enzyme (UBA1) gene, termed VEXAS (vacuoles, E1 enzyme, X-linked, autoinflammatory, somatic) syndrome. Skin involvement is reportedly seen in 83% to 89% of cases.[59,110-112] Systemic conditions commonly seen include fever, weight loss, MDS, and other hematologic conditions (macrocytic anemia, thrombocytopenia, MGUS, and bone marrow biopsies showing vacuolization of erythroid and myeloid precursors [all patients]), ocular inflammation, relapsing polychondritis, arthralgias, and lymphadenopathy. Cutaneous findings include Sweet-like urticarial papules and nodules, chondritis, periorbital nummular, violaceous lesions or angioedema, vasculitis (small vessel > medium or large vessel), injection site reactions (neutrophilic dermatosis or vasculitis on the biopsy), and erythema nodosum–like lesions. Violaceous variably edematous or umbilicated papules, purpuric infiltrated plaques and nodules, and livedo racemosa have also been described.[59] The neutrophilic infiltrate in VEXSAS has been described as histiocytoid, similar to HSS. The myeloid cells in the skin harbor the same UBA1 mutated myeloid clone found in the marrow.[59] In contrast to SS, vasculitis is often seen on biopsy but may not always be present. In a middle-aged to older male patient with a Sweet-like or histiocytoid neutrophilic dermatosis and any one of the above systemic findings, VEXAS syndrome should be considered and genetic evaluation for UBA1 mutation should be considered.

The prognosis of SS is very good. There is dramatic and prompt response to corticosteroids, which serves as a diagnostic feature. Dapsone, colchicine, potassium iodide, and cyclosporine are additional treatment options. If not ulcerated, lesions of SS resolve without scarring. SS panniculitis may lead to hyperpigmentation and scarring. In children, postinflammatory elastolysis (acquired cutis laxa) follows resolution of SS lesions in 30% of cases.[113] In some severe cases, treatment of the tumor in MA-SS may be required to resolve the SS.[23] Rare fatal cases of SS complicated with inflammatory syndrome have been reported.[114]

References

1. Su WP, Liu HN. Diagnostic criteria for Sweet's syndrome. *Cutis*. 1986;37:167-174.
2. von den Driesch P. Sweet's syndrome (acute febrile neutrophilic dermatosis). *J Am Acad Dermatol*. 1994;31:535-556; quiz 557–560.
3. Nofal A, Abdelmaksoud A, Amer H, et al. Sweet's syndrome: diagnostic criteria revisited. *J Dtsch Dermatol Ges*. 2017;15(11):1081-1088. doi:10.1111/ddg.13350
4. Uihlein LC, Brandling-Bennett HA, Lio PA, et al. Sweet syndrome in children. *Pediatr Dermatol*. 2012;29:38-44.
5. McClanahan D, Funk T, Small A. Sweet syndrome in the pediatric population. *Dermatol Clin*. 2022;40(2):179-190. doi:10.1016/j.det.2021.12.005
6. Bucchia M, Barbarot S, Reumaux H, et al. Age-specific characteristics of neutrophilic dermatoses and neutrophilic diseases in children. *J Eur Acad Dermatol Venereol*. 2019;33(11):2179-2187. doi:10.1111/jdv.15730
7. Rochet NM, Chavan RN, Cappel MA, et al. Sweet syndrome: clinical presentation, associations, and response to treatment in 77 patients. *J Am Acad Dermatol*. 2013;69:557-564.
8. Weiss EH, Ko CJ, Leung TH, et al. Neutrophilic dermatoses: a clinical update. *Curr Dermatol Rep*. 2022;11(2):1-14. doi:10.1007/s13671-022-00355-8
9. Nelson CA, Noe MH, McMahon CM, et al. Sweet syndrome in patients with and without malignancy: a retrospective analysis of 83 patients from a tertiary academic referral center. *J Am Acad Dermatol*. 2018;78(2):303-309.e4. doi:10.1016/j.jaad.2017.09.013
10. Freitas DF, Valle AC, Cuzzi T, et al. Sweet syndrome associated with sporotrichosis. *Br J Dermatol*. 2012;166:212-213.
11. Guo D, Parsons LM. Sweet syndrome in a patient with chronic hepatitis C. *J Cutan Med Surg*. 2014;18:436-438.
12. Cohen PR. Sweet's syndrome—a comprehensive review of an acute febrile neutrophilic dermatosis. *Orphanet J Rare Dis*. 2007;2:34.
13. Jaka A, Tuneu A, Ormaechea N, Zubizarreta J, del Alcazar E. Photodistributed neutrophilic dermatosis in a woman with Legionella pneumonitis. *Int J Dermatol*. 2014;53(3):e209-210. doi:10.1111/j.1365-4632.2012.005824.x
14. Al-Hayani AWM, Alemany IM, Santonja C, et al. Histiocytoid Sweet syndrome associated with anorectal lymphogranuloma venereum in a patient with HIV infection. *Int J Infect Dis*. 2022;115:106-108. doi:10.1016/j.ijid.2021.11.030
15. Taşkın B, Vural S, Altuğ E, et al. COVID-19 presenting with atypical Sweet's syndrome. *J Eur Acad Dermatol Venereol*. 2020;34:e534-e535.
16. Kiratikanon S, Phinyo P, Rujiwetpongstorn R, et al. Adult-onset immunodeficiency due to anti-interferon-gamma autoantibody-associated Sweet syndrome: a distinctive entity. *J Dermatol*. 2022;49(1):133-141. doi:10.1111/1346-8138.16202
17. Jutivorakool K, Sittiwattanawong P, Kantikosum K, et al. Skin manifestations in patients with adult-onset immunodeficiency due to anti-interferon-gamma autoantibody: a relationship with systemic infections. *Acta Derm Venereol*. 2018;98(8):742-747. doi:10.2340/00015555-2959
18. Cook QS, Zdanski CJ, Burkhart CN, Googe PB, Thompson P, Wu EY. Idiopathic, refractory Sweet's syndrome associated with common variable immunodeficiency: a case report and literature review. *Curr Allergy Asthma Rep*. 2019;19(6):32. doi:10.1007/s11882-019-0864-4
19. Wojcik AS, Nishimori FS, Santamaria JR. Sweet's syndrome: a study of 23 cases. *An Bras Dermatol*. 2011;86:265-271.
20. Jung EH, Park JH, Hwan Kim K, et al. Characteristics of Sweet syndrome in patients with or without malignancy. *Ann Hematol*. 2022;101(7):1499-1508. doi:10.1007/s00277-022-04850-7
21. Marcoval J, Martín-Callizo C, Valentí-Medina F, Bonfill-Ortí M, Martínez-Molina L. Sweet syndrome: long-term follow-up of 138 patients. *Clin Exp Dermatol*. 2016;41(7):741-746. doi:10.1111/ced.12899
22. Kazmi SM, Pemmaraju N, Patel KP, et al. Characteristics of Sweet syndrome in patients with acute myeloid leukemia. *Clin Lymphoma Myeloma Leuk*. 2015;15(6):358-363.

23. Roche FC, Paul D, Plovanich M, Mannava KA. Corticosteroid-resistant Sweet syndrome in the setting of acute myeloid leukemia with monosomy 7 and 5q deletion. *JAAD Case Rep*. 2020;6(12):1231-1233. doi:10.1016/j.jdcr.2020.08.039
24. Buck T, Gonzalez LM, Lambert WC, et al. Sweet's syndrome with hematologic disorders: a review and reappraisal. *Int J Dermatol*. 2008;47:775-782.
25. Alkayem M, Cheng W. A case report of hairy cell leukemia presenting concomitantly with Sweet syndrome. *Case Rep Med*. 2014;2014:823286.
26. Miranda CV, Filgueiras Fde M, Obadia DL, et al. Sweet's syndrome associated with Hodgkin's disease: case report. *An Bras Dermatol*. 2011;86:1016-1018.
27. Gille J, Spieth K, Kaufmann R. Sweet's syndrome as initial presentation of diffuse large B-cell lymphoma. *J Am Acad Dermatol*. 2002;46:S11-S13.
28. Levy RM, Junkins-Hopkins JM, Turchi JJ, et al. Sweet syndrome as the presenting symptom of relapsed hairy cell leukemia. *Arch Dermatol*. 2002;138:1551-1554.
29. Gomez Vazquez M, Sanchez-Aguilar D, Peteiro C, et al. Sweet's syndrome and polycythaemia vera. *J Eur Acad Dermatol Venereol*. 2005;19:382-383.
30. Horan MP, Redmond J, Gehle D, et al. Postpolycythemic myeloid metaplasia, Sweet's syndrome, and acute myeloid leukemia. *J Am Acad Dermatol*. 1987;16:458-462.
31. Serrano-Falcon C, Serrano-Falcon MM. Sweet syndrome in a pregnant woman. [Article in Spanish]. *Actas Dermosifiliogr*. 2010;101:558-559.
32. Lopez-Sanchez M, Garcia-Sanchez Y, Marin AP. An unusual evolution of a pregnancy-associated Sweet's syndrome. *Eur J Obstet Gynecol Reprod Biol*. 2008;140:283-285.
33. Pagliarello C, Pepe CA, Lombardi M, et al. Early miscarriage during Sweet's syndrome: uncommon, but probably not coincidental. *Eur J Dermatol*. 2013;23:707-708.
34. Satra K, Zalka A, Cohen PR, et al. Sweet's syndrome and pregnancy. *J Am Acad Dermatol*. 1994;30:297-300.
35. Turner M, Chauhan K. Subcutaneous Sweet syndrome presenting as cellulitis in a pregnant female. *Cureus*. 2021;13(9):e17999. doi:10.7759/cureus.17999
36. Walker DC, Cohen PR. Trimethoprim-sulfamethoxazole-associated acute febrile neutrophilic dermatosis: case report and review of drug-induced Sweet's syndrome. *J Am Acad Dermatol*. 1996;34:918-923.
37. Walterscheid B, Nguyen J, Tarbox M, Eshak N. Clopidogrel-induced Sweet syndrome: severe dermatological complication after percutaneous coronary intervention. *Eur Heart J*. 2021;42(26):2610. doi:10.1093/eurheartj/ehaa656
38. Mattis DM, Limova M, Mully T. Dapagliflozin-induced Sweet syndrome. *Cutis*. 2019;104(2):E22-E24.
39. Yavaşoğlu İ, Bolaman Z. Sweet syndrome associated with ixazomib. *Turk J Haematol*. 2021;38(3):234-235. doi:10.4274/tjh.galenos.2021.2021.0210
40. Fustà-Novell X, Morgado-Carrasco D, García-Herrera A, Bosch-Amate X, Martí-Martí I, Carrera C. Palbociclib-induced histiocytoid Sweet syndrome. *Clin Exp Dermatol*. 2021;46(2):348-350. doi:10.1111/ced.14361
41. Darrigade AS, Théophile H, Sanchez-Pena P, et al. Sweet syndrome induced by SARS-CoV-2 Pfizer-BioNTech mRNA vaccine. *Allergy*. 2021;76(10):3194-3196. doi:10.1111/all.14981
42. Torrealba-Acosta G, Martin JC, Huttenbach Y, et al. Acute encephalitis, myoclonus and Sweet syndrome after mRNA-1273 vaccine. *BMJ Case Rep*. July 26, 2021;14(7):e243173. doi:10.1136/bcr-2021-243173
43. Majid I, Mearaj S. Sweet syndrome after Oxford-AstraZeneca COVID-19 vaccine (AZD1222) in an elderly female. *Dermatol Ther*. 2021;34(6):e15146. doi:10.1111/dth.15146
44. Kinariwalla N, London AO, Soliman YS, Niedt GW, Husain S, Gallitano SM. A case of generalized Sweet syndrome with vasculitis triggered by recent COVID-19 vaccination. *JAAD Case Rep*. 2022;19:64-67. doi:10.1016/j.jdcr.2021.11.010
45. Clarey D, DiMaio D, Trowbridge R. Deep Sweet syndrome secondary to pegfilgrastim. *J Drugs Dermatol JDD*. 2022;21(4):422-424. doi:10.36849/JDD.4794
46. Alkassis S, Rizwan A, Daoud L, Chi J. Midostaurin-induced Sweet syndrome in a patient with FLT3-ITD-positive AML. *BMJ Case Rep*. 2021;14(8):e243615. doi:10.1136/bcr-2021-243615
47. Yang JJ, Maloney NJ, Nguyen KA, Worswick S, Smogorzewski J, Bach DQ. Sweet syndrome as an adverse reaction to tyrosine kinase inhibitors: a review. *Dermatol Ther*. 2021;34(1):e14461. doi:10.1111/dth.14461
48. Cardoso D, Coelho A, Fernandes L, et al. Sweet's syndrome induced by aromatase inhibitor in the treatment of early breast cancer. *Eur J Case Rep Intern Med*. 2020;7(3):001435. doi:10.12890/2020_001435
49. Filippi F, Chessa MA, Patrizi A, Baraldi C, Ferrara F, Bardazzi F. Tocilizumab-induced Sweet syndrome in a patient with polymyalgia rheumatica. *Dermatol Pract Concept*. 2019;10(1):e2020019. doi:10.5826/dpc.1001a19
50. Manzo C, Pollio N, Natale M. Sweet's syndrome following therapy with hydroxychloroquine in a patient affected with elderly-onset primary sjogren's syndrome. *Medicines (Basel)*. 2019;6(4):111. doi:10.3390/medicines6040111
51. Coromilas AJ, Gallitano SM. Neutrophilic drug reactions. *Clin Dermatol*. 2020;38(6):648-659. doi:10.1016/j.clindermatol.2020.06.012
52. Thompson DF, Montarella KE. Drug-induced Sweet's syndrome. *Ann Pharmacother*. 2007;41:802-811.
53. Yuksek T, Gönül M, Gökçe A. Drug-induced histiocytoid Sweet syndrome: two cases with levofloxacin and amoxicillin-clavulanate. *Am J Dermatopathol*. 2022;44(5):380-383. doi:10.1097/DAD.0000000000002131
54. Haber R, Dib N, El Gemayel M, Makhlouf M. Paradoxical neutrophilic dermatosis induced by biologics and immunosuppressive drugs: a systematic review. *J Am Acad Dermatol*. 2021;85(4):1048-1049. doi:10.1016/j.jaad.2021.02.035
55. Abbas O, Kibbi AG, Rubeiz N. Sweet's syndrome: retrospective study of clinical and histologic features of 44 cases from a tertiary care center. *Int J Dermatol*. 2010;49:1244-1249.
56. Satoh TK, Mellett M, Contassot E, French LE. Are neutrophilic dermatoses autoinflammatory disorders? *Br J Dermatol*. 2018;178(3):603-613. doi:10.1111/bjd.15105
57. Nesterovitch AB, Gyorfy Z, Hoffman MD, et al. Alteration in the gene encoding protein tyrosine phosphatase nonreceptor type 6 (PTPN6/SHP1) may contribute to neutrophilic dermatoses. *Am J Pathol*. 2011;178(4):1434-1441. doi:10.1016/j.ajpath.2010.12.035
58. Sheng R, Zhong X, Yang Z, Wang X. The role of CARD9 deficiency in neutrophils. *Mediators Inflamm*. 2021;2021:6643603. doi:10.1155/2021/6643603
59. Zakine E, Schell B, Battistella M, et al. UBA1 variations in neutrophilic dermatosis skin lesions of patients with VEXAS syndrome. *JAMA Dermatol*. 2021;157(11):1349-1354. doi:10.1001/jamadermatol.2021.3344
60. Kusaka H, Nagatani K, Sato T, Minota S. Increase of a wide range of bioactive substances in an active phase of neuro-Sweet disease. *BMJ Case Rep*. 2020;13(4):e233457. doi:10.1136/bcr-2019-233457

61. Kawakami T, Ohashi S, Kawa Y, et al. Elevated serum granulocyte colony-stimulating factor levels in patients with active phase of Sweet syndrome and patients with active Behçet disease: implication in neutrophil apoptosis dysfunction. *Arch Dermatol.* 2004;140:570-574.
62. Giasuddin AS, El-Orfi AH, Ziu MM, et al. Sweet's syndrome: is the pathogenesis mediated by helper T cell type 1 cytokines? *J Am Acad Dermatol.* 1998;39:940-943.
63. Bouman A, Heineman MJ, Faas MM. Sex hormones and the immune response in humans. *Hum Reprod Update.* 2005;11:411-423.
64. Akagi Y, Yamagiwa Y, Shirai H, et al. Aseptic cavernosal abscess: an unrecognized feature of neutrophilic dermatosis. *Intern Med.* 2022;61(6):917-921. doi:10.2169/internalmedicine.7994-21
65. Lobo AM, Stacy R, Cestari D, et al. Optic nerve involvement with panuveitis in Sweet syndrome. *Ocul Immunol Inflamm.* 2011;19:167-170.
66. Philibert F Lombart F, Denamps J, Chatelain D, Lok C, Chaby G. Chronic recurrent annular neutrophilic dermatosis revealing sarcoidosis *JAAD Case Rep.* 2020;6:285-288 doi:10.1016/j.jdcr.2020.02.012
67. Kroshinsky D, Alloo A, Rothschild B, et al. Necrotizing Sweet syndrome: a new variant of neutrophilic dermatosis mimicking necrotizing fasciitis. *J Am Acad Dermatol.* 2012;67:945-954.
68. Paul S, Jammal N, Akhave N, et al. Atypical cases of necrotizing Sweet syndrome in patients with myelodysplastic syndrome and acute myeloid leukaemia. *Br J Haematol.* 2020;191(1):e10-e13. doi:10.1111/bjh.16937
69. Sanchez IM, Lowenstein S, Johnson KA, et al. Clinical features of neutrophilic dermatosis variants resembling necrotizing fasciitis. *JAMA Dermatol.* 2019;155(1):79-84. doi:10.1001/jamadermatol.2018.3890
70. Galaria NA, Junkins-Hopkins JM, Kligman D, et al. Neutrophilic dermatosis of the dorsal hands: pustular vasculitis revisited. *J Am Acad Dermatol.* 2000;43:870-874.
71. Micallef D, Bonnici M, Pisani D, Boffa MJ. Neutrophilic dermatosis of the dorsal hands: a review of 123 cases. *J Am Acad Dermatol.* Published online 2019;S0190-9622(19)32678-7. doi:10.1016/j.jaad.2019.08.070
72. Mizes A, Khosravi H, Bordelon J, et al. Sweet syndrome with pulmonary involvement in a patient with myelodysplastic syndrome. *Dermatol Online J.* 2020;26(3):13030/qt1n73f6k5. PMID: 32609450.
73. Drago F, Ribizzi G, Ciccarese G, et al. Recurrent episodes of neuro-Sweet syndrome in a Caucasian patient. *J Am Acad Dermatol.* 2014;71:192-193.
74. Fortna RR, Toporcer M, Elder DE, et al. A case of Sweet syndrome with spleen and lymph node involvement preceded by parvovirus B19 infection, and a review of the literature on extracutaneous Sweet syndrome. *Am J Dermatopathol.* 2010;32:621-627.
75. Gottlieb CC, Mishra A, Belliveau D, Green P, Heathcote JG. Ocular involvement in acute febrile neutrophilic dermatosis (Sweet syndrome): new cases and review of the literature. *Surv Ophthalmol.* 2008;53(3):219-226.
76. Aghazadeh H, Sia D, Ehmann D. Central retinal artery occlusion associated with Sweet syndrome. *Can J Ophthalmol.* 2021;56(3):e103-e105. doi:10.1016/j.jcjo.2020.12.017
77. Rochael MC, Pantaleao L, Vilar EA, et al. Sweet's syndrome: study of 73 cases, emphasizing histopathological findings. *An Bras Dermatol.* 2011;86:702-707.
78. Jordaan HF. Acute febrile neutrophilic dermatosis: a histopathological study of 37 patients and a review of the literature. *Am J Dermatopathol.* 1989;11:99-111.
79. Going JJ, Going SM, Myskow MW, et al. Sweet's syndrome: histological and immunohistochemical study of 15 cases. *J Clin Pathol.* 1987;40:175-179.
80. Evans AV, Sabroe RA, Liddell K, et al. Lymphocytic infiltrates as a presenting feature of Sweet's syndrome with myelodysplasia and response to cyclophosphamide. *Br J Dermatol.* 2002;146:1087-1090.
81. Kakaletsis N, Kaiafa G, Savopoulos C, et al. Initially lymphocytic Sweet's syndrome in male patients with myelodysplasia: a distinguished clinicopathological entity? case report and systematic review of the literature. *Acta Haematol.* 2014;132:220-225.
82. Malone JC, Slone SP, Wills-Frank LA, et al. Vascular inflammation (vasculitis) in Sweet syndrome: a clinicopathologic study of 28 biopsy specimens from 21 patients. *Arch Dermatol.* 2002;138:345-349.
83. Chan MP, Duncan LM, Nazarian RM. Subcutaneous Sweet syndrome in the setting of myeloid disorders: a case series and review of the literature. *J Am Acad Dermatol.* 2013;68:1006-1015.
84. Requena L, Kutzner H, Palmedo G, et al. Histiocytoid Sweet syndrome: a dermal infiltration of immature neutrophilic granulocytes. *Arch Dermatol.* 2005;141:834-842.
85. Srisuttiyakorn C, Reeve J, Reddy S, et al. Subcutaneous histiocytoid Sweet's syndrome in a patient with myelodysplastic syndrome and acute myeloblastic leukemia. *J Cutan Pathol.* 2014;41:475-479.
86. Alegría-Landa V, Rodríguez-Pinilla SM, Santos-Briz A, et al. Clinicopathologic, immunohistochemical, and molecular features of histiocytoid Sweet syndrome. *JAMA Dermatol.* 2017;153(7):651-659. doi:10.1001/jamadermatol.2016.6092
87. Peroni A, Colato C, Schena D, et al. Histiocytoid Sweet syndrome is infiltrated predominantly by M2-like macrophages. *J Am Acad Dermatol.* 2015;72:131-139.
88. Murase JE, Wu JJ, Theate I, et al. Bortezomib-induced histiocytoid Sweet syndrome. *J Am Acad Dermatol.* 2009;60:496-497.
89. Wu AJ, Rodgers T, Fullen DR. Drug-associated histiocytoid Sweet's syndrome: a true neutrophilic maturation arrest variant. *J Cutan Pathol.* 2008;35:220-224.
90. Jagati A, Shrivastava S, Baghela B, Agarwal P, Saikia S. Acquired cutis laxa secondary to Sweet syndrome in a child (Marshall syndrome): a rare case report. *J Cutan Pathol.* 2020;47(2):146-149. doi:10.1111/cup.13567
91. Ko JS, Fernandez AP, Anderson KA, et al. Morphologic mimickers of cryptococcus occurring within inflammatory infiltrates in the setting of neutrophilic dermatitis: a series of three cases highlighting clinical dilemmas associated with a novel histopathologic pitfall. *J Cutan Pathol.* 2013;40(1):38-45. doi:10.1111/cup.12019
92. Wilson TC, Stone MS, Swick BL. Histiocytoid Sweet syndrome with haloed myeloid cells masquerading as a cryptococcal infection. *Am J Dermatopathol.* 2014;36(3):264-269. doi:10.1097/DAD.0b013e31828b811b
93. Sherban A, Fuller C, Sethi M, et al. Bullous hemorrhagic Sweet syndrome with cryptococcoid neutrophils in patients positive for antineutrophil cytoplasmic antibody without primary vasculitis. *JAAD Case Rep.* 2020;6(12):1196-1200. doi:10.1016/j.jdcr.2020.10.006
94. Wilson J, Gleghorn K, Kelly B. Cryptococcoid Sweet's syndrome: two reports of Sweet's syndrome mimicking cutaneous cryptococcosis. *J Cutan Pathol.* 2017;44(5):413-419. doi:10.1111/cup.12921

95. Ferris GJ, Fabbro S, Gru A, Kaffenberger J. Xanthomatized neutrophilic dermatosis in a patient with myelodysplastic syndrome. *Am J Dermatopathol*. 2017;39(5):384-387. doi:10.1097/DAD.0000000000000774
96. Kamimura A, Yanagisawa H, Tsunemi Y, et al. Normolipemic xanthomatized Sweet's syndrome: a variant of Sweet's syndrome with myelodysplastic syndrome. *J Dermatol*. 2021;48(5):695-698. doi:10.1111/1346-8138.15781
97. Somerset NM, Wolfe CM, Soni BP. Paraproteinemia-associated papular neutrophilic xanthoma of the oral commissure in a patient with myelodysplastic syndrome. *Am J Dermatopathol*. 2014;36(1):103-104. doi:10.1097/DAD.0b013e318288cd8d
98. Dabade TS, Davis MD. Diagnosis and treatment of the neutrophilic dermatoses (pyoderma gangrenosum, Sweet's syndrome). *Dermatol Ther*. 2011;24:273-284.
99. Gusdorf L, Lipsker D. Neutrophilic urticarial dermatosis: a review. *Ann Dermatol Venereol*. 2018;145(12):735-740. doi:10.1016/j.annder.2018.06.010
100. Broekaert SM, Böer-Auer A, Kerl K, et al. Neutrophilic epitheliotropism is a histopathological clue to neutrophilic urticarial dermatosis. *Am J Dermatopathol*. 2016;38(1):39-49. doi:10.1097/DAD.0000000000000390
101. Kieffer C, Cribier B, Lipsker D. Neutrophilic urticarial dermatosis: a variant of neutrophilic urticaria strongly associated with systemic disease. Report of 9 new cases and review of the literature. *Medicine (Baltimore)*. 2009;88(1):23-31. doi:10.1097/MD.0b013e3181943f5e
102. Ravi M, Waters M, Trinidad J, Chung CG, Kaffenberger BH. A retrospective cohort study of infection risk in hospitalized patients evaluated for Sweet syndrome. *Arch Dermatol Res*. 2022. doi:10.1007/s00403-021-02318-8
103. Chow S, Pasternak S, Green P, et al. Histiocytoid neutrophilic dermatoses and panniculitides: variations on a theme. *Am J Dermatopathol*. 2007;29:334-341.
104. Chavan RN, Cappel MA, Ketterling RP, et al. Histiocytoid Sweet syndrome may indicate leukemia cutis: a novel application of fluorescence in situ hybridization. *J Am Acad Dermatol*. 2014;70:1021-1027.
105. Monfort JB, Pages C, Schneider P, et al. Vemurafenib-induced neutrophilic panniculitis. *Melanoma Res*. 2012;22:399-401.
106. Suzuki S, Ho J, Rosenbaum M, Bhawan J. Neutrophilic fixed drug eruption: a mimic of neutrophilic dermatoses. *Clin Exp Dermatol*. 2019;44(2):236-238. doi:10.1111/ced.13740
107. Li A, Kazlouskaya V. Neutrophils in fixed drug eruptions: correction of a mistaken hypothesis. *Am J Dermatopathol*. 2022;44(2):106-110.
108. Johns HR, Shetty N, Cash J, Patel T, Pourciau C. Bowel-Associated-Dermatosis-Arthritis Syndrome (BADAS) as early presentation of ulcerative colitis in an adolescent girl. *Pediatr Dermatol*. Published online 2022. doi:10.1111/pde.14954
109. Havele SA, Clark AK, Oboite M, et al. Bowel-associated dermatosis-arthritis syndrome in a child with very early onset inflammatory bowel disease. *Pediatr Dermatol*. 2021;38(3):697-698. doi:10.1111/pde.14544
110. Georgin-Lavialle S, Terrier B, Guedon AF, et al. Further characterization of clinical and laboratory features in VEXAS syndrome: large-scale analysis of a multicentre case series of 116 French patients. *Br J Dermatol*. 2022;186(3):564-574. doi:10.1111/bjd.20805
111. Sterling D, Duncan ME, Philippidou M, Salisbury JR, Kulasekararaj AG, Basu TN. VEXAS syndrome (vacuoles, E1 enzyme, X-linked, autoinflammatory, somatic) for the dermatologist. *J Am Acad Dermatol*. 2022;S0190-9622(22)00181-5. doi:10.1016/j.jaad.2022.01.042
112. Koster MJ, Kourelis T, Reichard KK, et al. Clinical heterogeneity of the VEXAS syndrome: a case series. *Mayo Clin Proc*. 2021;96(10):2653-2659. doi:10.1016/j.mayocp.2021.06.006
113. Gray PE, Bock V, Ziegler DS, et al. Neonatal Sweet syndrome: a potential marker of serious systemic illness. *Pediatrics*. 2012;129:e1353-e1359.
114. Sawicki J, Morton RA, Ellis AK. Sweet syndrome with associated systemic inflammatory response syndrome: an ultimately fatal case. *Ann Allergy Asthma Immunol*. 2010;105:321-323.

Wells syndrome (eosinophilic cellulitis)

Melinda Jen and Adam I. Rubin

INTRODUCTION

First described in 1971 by George Wells, Wells syndrome (or eosinophilic cellulitis) is an uncommon, recurrent inflammatory dermatosis of unknown etiology. Clinically, individual lesions resemble cellulitis, and "flame figures" with a diffuse eosinophilic infiltrate are seen histologically.

PATHOGENESIS

Wells syndrome appears to be a hypersensitivity reaction to a variety of triggers. Myeloproliferative disorders including chronic myeloid leukemia,[1,2] chronic eosinophilic leukemia,[3] and mantle zone lymphoma[4] have been associated with Wells syndrome. Other associated malignancies, such as gastric cancer,[5] adenocarcinoma of the lung,[6] renal cell carcinoma,[7] and colon carcinoma,[8] have also been reported. A variety of other inciting agents have been associated with Wells syndrome, including infections, infestations, arthropod bites, and medications. Reported inciting medications include etanercept,[9] adalimumab,[10,11] vaccines,[12-15] and hydrochlorothiazide.[16]

The exact pathogenesis of Wells syndrome is unclear, but there is evidence that cytokines such as interleukin 2 (IL-2) and interleukin 5 (IL-5) expressed by T cells prime eosinophils for degranulation.[17-19] T-cell sensitivity to mosquito salivary gland extract has been shown in some patients with Wells syndrome.[20]

CLINICAL MANIFESTATIONS

Wells syndrome classically presents with sudden onset of pruritic, erythematous, edematous papules and plaques that rapidly evolve over days (Figs. 77-1 and 77-2). Seven clinical variants have been described: plaque-type, annular granuloma-like, urticaria-like, papulovesicular, bullous, papulonodular, and fixed drug eruption-like.[21] Children most commonly present with the classic plaque-like lesions, while adults more commonly present with annular granuloma-like lesions.[21] Itching or burning can precede the appearance of lesions. The extremities are more commonly affected, although the trunk and face can also be involved. Lesions resolve within weeks, leaving hyperpigmentation and atrophy. Recurrence is common. The disease tends to wax and wane over years before resolving. Systemic findings, such as fever, malaise, lymphadenopathy, and arthralgias, can be seen.

An elevated white blood cell count with peripheral eosinophilia is frequently seen, especially during the active phases of the disease, but can be normal during quiescent periods. An elevated erythrocyte sedimentation rate can be seen with acute flares.

PATHOLOGY

The histopathology of Wells syndrome will vary by the stage of the lesion. A constant feature over the acute and subacute stages is the presence of eosinophils. There is generally an intense infiltrate of eosinophils that are present in the superficial and deep dermis. Extension of eosinophils into the subcutaneous fat is possible, as well as the fascia and skeletal muscle.[22] The eosinophils are often placed in a perivascular distribution, with involvement of the interstitial dermis as well. The eosinophils can form a band in the upper dermis or be focused in the deeper dermis.[22] In addition to eosinophils, other mixed inflammation including histocytes and lymphocytes can also be present. The epidermis can show variable changes, ranging from minimal change to the development of intraepidermal spongiotic vesicles (Figs. 77-3 and 77-4).

Early acute lesions demonstrate dermal edema in addition to the presence of eosinophils. The dermal edema may be in the papillary dermis, and subepidermal blisters may develop. The subacute stage demonstrates eosinophils that adhere to collagen bundles and show widespread degranulation of eosinophils. It is in the subacute stage that flame figures develop. The resolving state of Wells syndrome includes foreign body–type giant cells, histocytes, and fewer eosinophils.[23,24] Older lesions will resolve without fibrosis and may demonstrate collections of macrophages.[22]

As a lesion becomes more established, flame figures will develop. A flame figure is an area of altered collagen that is eosinophilic in appearance. The contents of degranulating

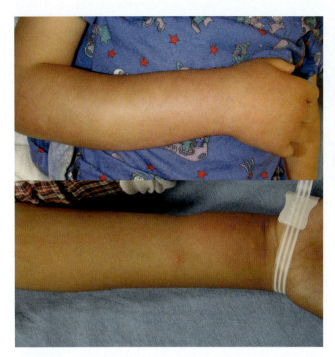

FIGURE 77-1. Characteristic erythematous, edematous plaques seen in Wells syndrome.

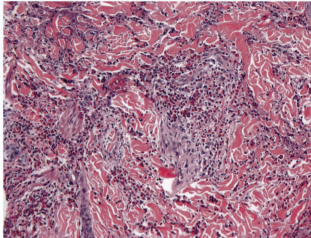

FIGURE 77-3. Numerous eosinophils can be seen in the dermis (H&E 100×).

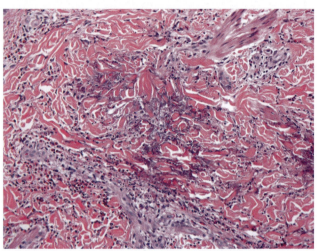

FIGURE 77-4. This flame figure shows characteristic features with necrobiosis of collagen and associated eosinophilic inflammation (H&E 200×).

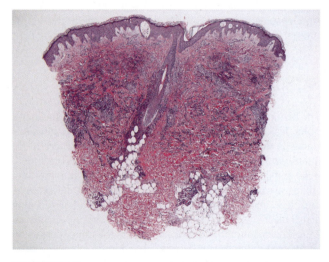

FIGURE 77-2. Low-power view shows an intense inflammatory infiltrate in the upper and mid dermis with multiple flame figures present. Spongiotic vesicles are present in the epidermis (H&E 40×).

eosinophils are deposited on the collagen in the focused areas of the flame figures. Eosinophil major basic protein, which is a component of the eosinophil granule, has been demonstrated in flame figures by immunofluorescence.[25] Established flame figures can show necrobiosis of collagen and show palisading arrangements of eosinophils around the collagen. Older lesions of Wells syndrome can show a granulomatous reaction associated with the flame figures, with histiocytes and multinucleated giant cells around them. Early or resolving lesions of Wells syndrome may not demonstrate flame figures (Fig. 77-5). Luna staining has been reported to be helpful in confirming the presence of flame figures.[26]

Although flame figure is helpful in establishing a diagnosis of Wells syndrome, it is important to note that the flame figure itself is a nonspecific histologic sign that may be present in a variety of other dermatoses. A flame figure can develop in any dermatosis that includes a prominent component of eosinophils. Flame figures have been seen in pathology specimens of bullous pemphigoid, insect bite reactions, follicular mucinosis, urticaria, eczema, prurigo, mastocytoma, scabies, eosinophilic granulomatosis with polyangiitis (EGPA), as well as tinea infections.[27,28] The histologic differential diagnosis for a flame figure could include the Splendore-Hoeppli phenomenon, which can be seen surrounding infectious agents. The Splendore-Hoeppli phenomenon is distinguished from a flame figure by the presence of a PAS-positive rim of eosinophilic material surrounding a central area.[29]

In order to make a specific diagnosis of Wells syndrome, good clinicopathologic correlation is required. If the characteristic skin findings are seen with the histology described above, the specific diagnosis can be established. However, as noted above, similar histology can be seen with

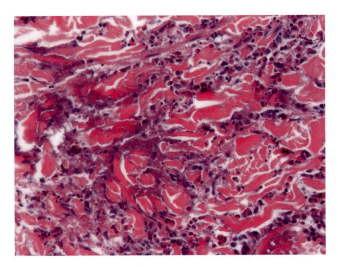

FIGURE 77-5. This high-power view of a flame figure shows the necrobiosis of collagen, deposition of eosinophil granules on altered collagen fibers, and the associated infiltrate of eosinophils (H&E 400×).

other dermatoses, so assessment of the clinical features is essential. Other important histologic features seen in Wells syndrome are the absence of vasculitis and negative direct immunofluorescence testing.

The most common histologic differential diagnosis would be an insect bite reaction. When compared with Wells syndrome, an insect bite reaction generally would have a less intense inflammatory infiltrate of eosinophils and would be localized more to the perivascular areas. More prominent epidermal features such as spongiosis and spongiotic vesicles may be more common in an insect bite reaction as opposed to Wells syndrome. As mentioned above, flame figures may be seen in arthropod bite reactions and may not be used as a distinguishing feature from Wells syndrome. More intense eosinophilic infiltrates and persistence of lesions may be seen with tick bites. Hemorrhagic areas and a central coagulative area may be seen with some tick and spider bites, which could be features that help differentiate from Wells syndrome.[29]

Another consideration in the differential diagnosis would be EGPA, as it also can present with eosinophilic granulomatous inflammation. EGPA can be differentiated from Wells syndrome by the presence of vasculitis, as well as features associated with vasculitis, including leukocytoclasis. EGPA can also demonstrate periarteritis of the deep dermal vasculature as well as the vessels of the subcutaneous fat. Direct immunofluorescence of EGPA can demonstrate IgM and C3 deposition in the dermal blood vessels.[22]

Other dermatoses that may demonstrate flame figures, as mentioned above, could have other distinctive features that would point to the alternative diagnosis. In such instances, these histologic features and clinical correlation would help guide the histologic interpretation.

DIFFERENTIAL DIAGNOSIS

The clinical differential diagnosis for Wells syndrome is cellulitis, urticaria, and arthropod bites. Although individual lesions of Wells syndrome can mimic cellulitis, multifocal cellulitis is exceedingly rare. The presence of multiple lesions would make Wells syndrome more likely. The individual lesions of urticaria last for hours and are more transient than the lesions of Wells syndrome. Arthropod bites are frequently grouped or in a linear configuration. A central punctum can often be seen where the bite occurred. The histologic differential diagnosis is discussed in the pathology section.

TREATMENT

Initial management of Wells syndrome is determined by the severity of disease. Topical steroids can be used alone or in combination with oral steroids. With treatment, skin lesions should resolve within days, and treatment should be slowly tapered over several weeks. Recurrences can be treated with additional courses of oral steroids, but if recurrences are frequent or flares are inadequately controlled, then alternative therapies should be considered. No large-scale therapeutic trials have evaluated systemic treatment for Wells syndrome. A variety of systemic treatments have been reported, including cyclosporine,[30,31] griseofulvin,[32] minocycline,[33] dapsone,[34,35] and adalimumab.[36]

References

1. Nakazato S, Fujita Y, Hamade Y, et al. Wells' syndrome associated with chronic myeloid leukaemia. *Acta Derm Venereol*. 2013;93(3):375-376.
2. Shin D, Kim DY. Chronic relapsing eosinophilic cellulitis associated, although independent in severity, with chronic lymphocytic leukemia. *J Eur Acad Dermatol Venereol JEADV*. 2014;30:159-161.
3. Davis RF, Dusanjh P, Majid A, et al. Eosinophilic cellulitis as a presenting feature of chronic eosinophilic leukaemia, secondary to a deletion on chromosome 4q12 creating the FIP1L1-PDGFRA fusion gene. *Br J Dermatol*. 2006;155(5):1087-1089.
4. Zeeli T, Feinmesser M, Segal R, David M. Insect-bite-like Wells' syndrome in association with mantle-zone lymphoma. *Br J Dermatol*. 2006;155(3):614-616.
5. Kim HS, Kang MJ, Kim H-O, Park YM. Eosinophilic cellulitis in a patient with gastric cancer. *Acta Derm Venereol*. 2009;89(6):644-645.
6. Skellett A, McCann B, Levell N. Eosinophilic cellulitis caused by adenocarcinoma of the lung. *Int J Dermatol*. 2009;48(12):1402-1403.
7. Rajpara A, Liolios A, Fraga G, Blackmon J. Recurrent paraneoplastic wells syndrome in a patient with metastatic renal cell cancer. *Dermatol Online J*. 2014;20(6):13030/qt35w8r1g3.
8. Hirsch K, Ludwig RJ, Wolter M, et al. Eosinophilic cellulitis (Wells' syndrome) associated with colon carcinoma. *J Dtsch Dermatol Ges J Ger Soc Dermatol JDDG*. 2005;3(7):530-531.
9. Winfield H, Lain E, Horn T, Hoskyn J. Eosinophilic cellulitislike reaction to subcutaneous etanercept injection. *Arch Dermatol*. 2006;142(2):218-220.
10. Boura P, Sarantopoulos A, Lefaki I, Skendros P, Papadopoulos P. Eosinophilic cellulitis (Wells' syndrome) as a cutaneous reaction to the administration of adalimumab. *Ann Rheum Dis*. 2006;65(6):839-840.
11. Dabas G, De D, Handa S, Chatterjee D, Radotra BD. Wells syndrome in a patient receiving adalimumab biosimilar: a case report and review of literature. *Indian J Dermatol Venereol Leprol*. 2018;84:594-599.

12. Moreno M, Luelmo J, Monteagudo M, Bella R, Casanovas A. Wells' syndrome related to tetanus vaccine. *Int J Dermatol.* 1997;36(7):524-525.
13. Koh KJ, Warren L, Moore L, James C, Thompson GN. Wells' syndrome following thiomersal-containing vaccinations. *Australas J Dermatol.* 2003;44(3):199-202.
14. Calvert J, Shors AR, Hornung RL, Poorsattar SP, Sidbury R. Relapse of Wells' syndrome in a child after tetanus-diphtheria immunization. *J Am Acad Dermatol.* 2006;54(5 suppl):S232-S233.
15. Yu AM, Ito S, Leibson T, et al. Pediatric Wells syndrome (eosinophilic cellulitis) after vaccination: a case report and review of the literature. *Pediatr Dermatol.* 2018;35(5):e262-e264.
16. Heelan K, Ryan JF, Shear NH, Egan CA. Wells syndrome (eosinophilic cellulitis): proposed diagnostic criteria and a literature review of the drug-induced variant. *J Dermatol Case Rep.* 2013;7(4):113-120.
17. Simon H-U, Plötz S, Simon D, et al. Interleukin-2 primes eosinophil degranulation in hypereosinophilia and Wells' syndrome. *Eur J Immunol.* 2003;33(4):834-839.
18. Yagi H, Tokura Y, Matsushita K, Hanaoka K, Furukawa F, Takigawa M. Wells' syndrome: a pathogenic role for circulating CD4+CD7− T cells expressing interleukin-5 mRNA. *Br J Dermatol.* 1997;136(6):918-923.
19. España A, Sanz ML, Sola J, Gil P. Wells' syndrome (eosinophilic cellulitis): correlation between clinical activity, eosinophil levels, eosinophil cation protein and interleukin-5. *Br J Dermatol.* 1999;140(1):127-130.
20. Koga C, Sugita K, Kabashima K, Matsuoka H, Nakamura M, Tokura Y. High responses of peripheral lymphocytes to mosquito salivary gland extracts in patients with Wells syndrome. *J Am Acad Dermatol.* 2010;63(1):160-161.
21. Caputo R, Marzano AV, Vezzoli P, Lunardon L. Wells syndrome in adults and children: a report of 19 cases. *Arch Dermatol.* 2006;142(9):1157-1161.
22. Lynch JM, Barrett TL. Collagenolytic (necrobiotic) granulomas: part II--the "red" granulomas. *J Cutan Pathol.* 2004;31(6):409-418.
23. Spigel GT, Winkelmann RK. Wells' syndrome. Recurrent granulomatous dermatitis with eosinophilia. *Arch Dermatol.* 1979;115(5):611-613.
24. Mitchell AJ, Anderson TF, Headington JT, Rasmussen JE. Recurrent granulomatous dermatitis with eosinophilia. Wells' syndrome. *Int J Dermatol.* 1984;23(3):198-202.
25. Peters MS, Schroeter AL, Gleich GJ. Immunofluorescence identification of eosinophil granule major basic protein in the flame figures of Wells' syndrome. *Br J Dermatol.* 1983;109(2):141-148.
26. Mejbel HA, Preiszner J, Shurbaji MS, Leicht SS, Youngberg GA. Luna stain: a simple and cost-effective diagnostic tool helps in detecting eosinophilic granules deposition of flame figures and aids in diagnosing eosinophilic cellulitis "Wells Syndrome." *J Histotechnol.* 2020;43(4):196-199.
27. Ferreli C, Pinna AL, Atzori L, Aste N. Eosinophilic cellulitis (Well's syndrome): a new case description. *J Eur Acad Dermatol Venereol JEADV.* 1999;13(1):41-45.
28. Kuwahara RT, Randall MB, Eisner MG. Eosinophilic cellulitis in a newborn. *Pediatr Dermatol.* 2001;18(1):89-90.
29. Wood C, Miller AC, Jacobs A, Hart R, Nickoloff BJ. Eosinophilic infiltration with flame figures. A distinctive tissue reaction seen in Wells' syndrome and other diseases. *Am J Dermatopathol.* 1986;8(3):186-193.
30. Herr H, Koh JK. Eosinophilic cellulitis (Wells' syndrome) successfully treated with low-dose cyclosporine. *J Kor Med Sci.* 2001;16(5):664-668.
31. Kim SH, Kwon JE, Kim H-B. Successful treatment of steroid-dependent eosinophilic cellulitis with cyclosporine. *Allergy Asthma Immunol Res.* 2013;5(1):62-64.
32. Sharma PK, Gautam RK, Sharma AK. Eosinophilic cellulitis - a case study and management with griseofulvin. *Indian J Dermatol Venereol Leprol.* 1995;61(3):163-164.
33. Stam-Westerveld EB, Daenen S, Van der Meer JB, Jonkman MF. Eosinophilic cellulitis (Wells' syndrome): treatment with minocycline. *Acta Derm Venereol.* 1998;78(2):157.
34. Bokotas C, Kouris A, Stefanaki C, Sgotzou T, Christofidou E, Kontochristopoulos G. Wells syndrome: response to dapsone therapy. *Ann Dermatol.* 2014;26(4):541-542.
35. Moon S-H, Shin M-K. Bullous eosinophilic cellulitis in a child treated with dapsone. *Pediatr Dermatol.* 2013;30(4):e46-47.
36. Sarin KY, Fiorentino D. Treatment of recalcitrant eosinophilic cellulitis with adalimumab. *Arch Dermatol.* 2012;148(9):990-992.

CHAPTER 78

Vasculitis

Alejandro A. Gru

INTRODUCTION

Vasculitis refers to a heterogeneous group of disorders characterized by vascular inflammation.[1] The clinical manifestations range from locoregional ischemic and purpuric injuries to systemic disease. The classification of vasculitides takes into account the anatomical site, the size, and type of involved vessels, as well as the type of inflammatory cells and immune complexes mediating the vascular injury.[2] In this chapter, we will focus on the discussion of acute and chronic vasculitides that are associated with lymphoproliferative disorders (Table 78-1). The vascular pathology associated with cryoglobulinemia will be discussed in a separate chapter (Chapter 62).

LEUKOCYTOCLASTIC VASCULITIS

Definition

Leukocytoclastic vasculitis (LCV [hypersensitivity vasculitis, allergic angiitis, necrotizing vasculitis]) is a histopathologic term to denote a small-vessel vasculitis associated with neutrophil fragmentation and nuclear dust formation around inflamed vessels.[1,3,4]

Clinical

Patients present with palpable purpura in dependent areas, typically in the bilateral lower legs. Other clinical presentations include vesicles, papules, nodules, crusted ulcers, and, less commonly, livedo reticularis or annular lesions.[5,6] Extracutaneous manifestations are seen in about 20% of cases and include arthralgias, myositis, low-grade fever, and malaise.

Etiology

There is no discernible etiologic agent in approximately 40% of cases. The most common known etiologic factors include drugs, infections, food or food additives, collagen-vascular diseases, and malignancies. Paraneoplastic (lymphoproliferative-, myeloproliferative-, or carcinoma-induced) vasculitis represents less than 5% of all cases of cutaneous vasculitis.[7] Most paraneoplastic cases are the result of a paraproteinemia secondary to a lymphoproliferative disorder, typically cryoglobulins. In a study of vasculitis associated with hematologic malignancies, 22% of the patients with either lymphoma or leukemia developed cutaneous vasculitis before (26%), concomitantly (39%), or after (35%) the diagnosis of cancer. In 61% of these cases, malignancy was the suspected cause, whereas in the remainder, infections, medication, and mixed cryoglobulinemia were the suspected triggers.[8]

Hematologic dyscrasias associated with LCV include angioimmunoblastic T-cell lymphoma,[9] diffuse large B-cell lymphoma,[10] myelodysplastic syndromes,[11] mycosis fungoides,[12] hairy cell leukemia,[13] acute myeloid leukemia,[14] chronic lymphocytic leukemia,[15] and multiple myeloma.[14,16,17] Medication-induced LCV has been reported with bortezomib,[18] etoposide,[19] interferon-α,[20] methotrexate,[21] sorafenib,[22] lenalidomide,[23] and sunitinib.[24] Patients with type II cryoglobulinemia also present with LCV (usually associated with autoimmune disorders, hepatitis C virus [HCV] infection, and hematologic malignancies).

Histology

The histopathologic features of LCV vary with the age of the lesion (Fig. 78-1).[25] For best histologic findings, biopsy should be taken from lesions of 18 to 24 hours duration.[4] The affected vessels in LCV are the small venules (postcapillary venules), and sometimes the small arterioles. The histopathology reveals infiltration of the vessel walls by neutrophils, which often show cellular disruption with nuclear fragmentation ("leukocytoclasis"). The vessel walls are thickened by edema and fibrinous exudate. Swollen endothelial cells and thrombosis can sometimes be present. The dermis reveals variable edema and extravasation of red blood cells (RBCs).[26] Other inflammatory cells such as eosinophils can also be present and are more common in drug-induced LCV.[27] As the lesions evolve in time, vessel wall changes become less prominent and neutrophils are replaced by lymphocytes and histiocytes. Sometimes, dermal edema evolves into a subepidermal vesicle. Direct immunofluorescence[28] shows variable deposits of fibrinogen, C3, IgM, and IgG within the vessel wall, typically in acute lesions (6-24 hours).[1,4]

Henoch-Schönlein purpura (HSP) is a subtype of superficial dermal LCV characterized by IgA deposits in inflamed postcapillary venules.[29,30] Patients with HSP present with, besides vasculitis, arthralgias, abdominal pain, and renal involvement. More than 90% of HSP cases occur in pediatric

TABLE 78-1 Cutaneous Vasculitis in Hematologic Dyscrasias

Leukocytoclastic vasculitis

Urticarial vasculitis

Henoch-Schönlein purpura

Eosinophilic vasculitis

Erythema elevatum diutinum

Polyarteritis nodosa

Leukemic vasculitis

patients (<10 years old). The clinical signs in childhood HSP resolve within few weeks, whereas in adults the symptoms endure longer with the potential for permanent kidney damage. While most HSP cases are precipitated by upper respiratory infection, the etiology of HSP is unknown. A minority of adult cases is associated with hematologic malignancies including myelodysplastic syndrome, follicular lymphoma, and diffuse large B-cell lymphoma.[31-34]

Wegener granulomatosis (WG), recently renamed as granulomatosis with polyangiitis, presents with superficial and deep LCV.[8] Cases of WG can occur in association with solid tumors as well as lymphomas, leukemias, and myelodysplastic syndromes.[35-38] The incidence of cancers is also increased after therapy for WG.[36] Eosinophilic vasculitis is a recently described entity characterized by a predominantly eosinophilic-rich infiltrate producing a necrotizing vasculitis.[39,40] It presents as pruritic, erythematous, and purpuric papules and plaques. Association with connective tissue disorders,[8] HIV,[41] and hypereosinophilic syndrome[42] had been described.

Urticarial vasculitis (UV) is a form of lymphocytic LCV with urticarial-like clinical findings that last for more than 48 hours. Besides the typical wheals, and angioedema, there is variable purpura. Rarely, hematologic conditions can be associated with UV, including IgA myeloma,[43] IgM disease (Schnitzler syndrome, discussed separately), Castleman disease,[44] and polycythemia vera.[45] It has also been shown

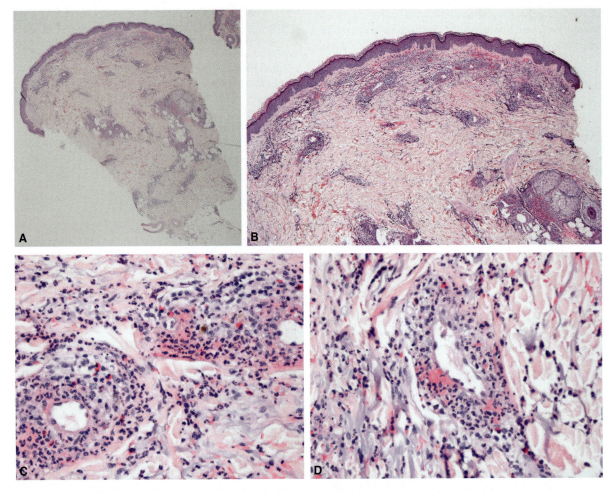

FIGURE 78-1. Leukocytoclastic vasculitis (LCV) **A** and **B.** Busy dermis with associated RBC extravasation in the superficial dermis (hematoxylin and eosin [H&E], 20× and 100×). **C** and **D.** Fibrinoid changes of the vessel walls and prominent leukocytoclasis (H&E, 400×). **E** and **F.** Urticarial vasculitis. Very similar changes to those seen in LCV. Eosinophils are typically more prominent (H&E, 100× and 400×). **G** and **H.** Henoch-Schönlein purpura. Deposits of IgA are present by direct immunofluorescence in the vascular walls.

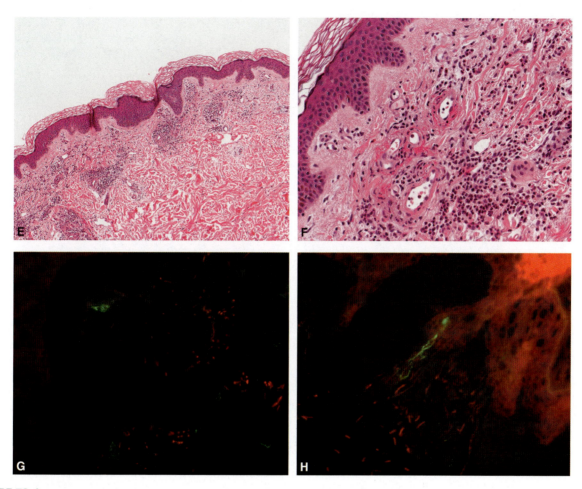

FIGURE 78-1. Cont'd

in association with intravenous Ig and methotrexate administration.

Leukemic vasculitis (LV) is an infrequent histopathological pattern of LC where the vascular injury is caused directly by neoplastic cells.[46-48] This differs from the reactive vascular damage, more frequently observed as a leukocytoclastic vasculitis where benign inflammatory cells mediate the vascular damage. Two types of LV have been reported in the literature: a low grade, with prominent endothelial cells as well as focal deposits of fibrin in small-diameter vessels, and a high grade, with necrotizing vasculitis with thrombosis, extensive fibrin deposition, and leukocytoclasia. Less than 40 cases of LV have been reported in the literature. Papules, nodules, and purpura are the most common clinical manifestations (Fig. 78-2). Most cases of LV are associated with acute myeloid leukemia (with less frequent associations to myelodysplastic syndromes, non-Hodgkin lymphomas, and lymphoblastic leukemias). Figures 78-3 and 78-4 highlight the typical histopathologic features of LV.

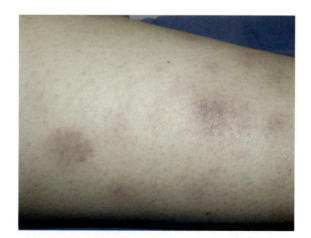

FIGURE 78-2. Leukemic vasculitis. Detail of nodular erythematopurpuric lesions at the lower limbs. (From Kunc K, Biernat W. Carcinoma cuniculatum of the lower leg: A case report and proposed diagnostic criteria. *Am J Dermatopathol.* 2019;41(11):826-831.)

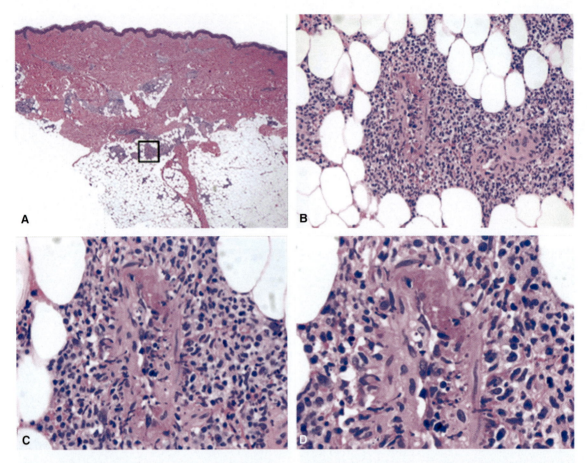

FIGURE 78-3. Leukemic vasculitis. A. H&E ×2. Superficial and deep perivascular nodular infiltration mostly involving dermohipodermal junction and hypodermis. **B.** H&E ×10. Dense perivascular infiltration surrounding an involved muscular vessel. **C.** H&E ×20. Vessel wall with several foci of fibrinoid necrosis as well as obliterated lumen with prominent endothelial cells and cells within the wall. Mostly neutrophilic infiltrates surrounding the affected vessel and red cell extravasation. **D.** H&E ×40. Closer view of the affected arterial wall with presence of monocytoid-like cells showing elongated and reniform nuclei. (From Kunc K, Biernat W. Carcinoma cuniculatum of the lower leg: A case report and proposed diagnostic criteria. *Am J Dermatopathol.* 2019;41(11):826-831.)

ERYTHEMA ELEVATUM DIUTINUM

Definition

Erythema elevatum diutinum (EED) is a rare form of LCV characterized by red, purple, brown, or yellow papules, plaques, or nodules on extensor surfaces. EED and its localized form, granuloma faciale, are chronic vasculitides that could be associated with perivascular fibrosis.[8]

Etiology

EED occurs in patients with connective tissue disorders,[49,50] infection, acquired immune deficiency,[51,52] and hematologic abnormalities, often with an IgA gammopathy.[53-62] Other associations include lymphomas,[63] chronic myeloid leukemia,[64] myelodysplastic syndromes,[65,66] and cryoglobulinemia.[67] Albeit of unknown clinical and pathologic significance, IgA class of antineutrophil cytoplasmic antibodies (IgA ANCAs) have been detected in most patients with EED.[68,69]

Clinical

The clinical lesions of EED are characterized by the presence of symmetric, violaceous, deep red, or brown papules, plaques, or nodules located over the extensor surfaces of the extremities.

Histology

The microscopic features of EED are variable and dependent on the age of the lesion and the presence or absence of recurrent bouts of active vasculitis (Fig. 78-5).[70,71] Early lesions show perivascular neutrophilic infiltrates, with marked fibrinoid changes of the vessel walls, endothelial swelling, and leukocytoclasis. RBC extravasation is not very common. As the lesions evolve, there is a very dense neutrophilic infiltrate in the dermis, a vascular reactive proliferation, and sometimes subepidermal vesicle formation. The epidermis is typically spared (grenz zone). Chronic lesions reveal perivascular fibrosis with an associated spindled fibroblast proliferation, which in some cases might resemble dermatofibroma. Foci of active vasculitis can be frequently noted in chronic lesions.

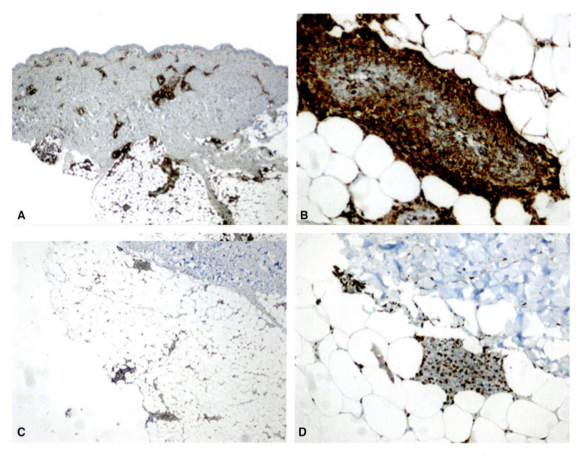

FIGURE 78-4. Leukemic vasculitis. A. Immunostaining with CD43, original magnification ×2. Mostly perivascular and papillary dermis infiltrates of CD43-positive cells. **B.** Original magnification ×20. Detail of the infiltrates surrounding an involved vessel showing CD43-positive cells within the wall and as the main component of the infiltrates. **C.** Immunostaining with myeloperoxidase (MPO), original magnification ×2. MPO-positive cells surrounding hypodermal vessels. **D.** Detail showing up to 40% of MPO-positive cells surrounding vessels as well as isolated positive cells within the dermis and between the adipocytes. (From Kunc K, Biernat W. Carcinoma cuniculatum of the lower leg: A case report and proposed diagnostic criteria. *Am J Dermatopathol.* 2019;41(11):826-831.)

POLYARTERITIS NODOSA

Definition

Polyarteritis nodosa (PAN) is a vasculitis of small to medium-sized muscular arteries with involvement of multiple organs, including kidneys, liver, gastrointestinal tract, and central nervous system.[72,73]

Clinical

Skin findings are present in 10% to 15% of cases[74] (Fig. 78-6). There are usually constitutional symptoms such as fever, weight loss, fatigue, arthralgia, and myalgia. There is a slight predilection for adult males. A cutaneous form of PAN, with a chronic relapsing course but usually no evidence of systemic disease, has been reported.[75-77] Immune complexes appear to plan an important role in the pathogenesis of this disorder. Angiogenic cytokines are also increased (basic fibroblast growth factor and vascular endothelial growth factor). The hepatitis B surface antigen (HbsAg) can be detected in up to 50% of the systemic cases, including those isolated to the skin. HCV has also been detected in some cases.[78]

Association With Hematologic Malignancies

PAN has been shown in association with Hodgkin and non-Hodgkin lymphomas.[31,79] The risk of Hodgkin lymphoma is also increased after the diagnosis of PAN.[80] Specific types of hematologic conditions associated with PAN included angioimmunoblastic T-cell lymphoma,[81,82] lymphoplasmacytic lymphoma,[83,84] marginal zone lymphoma, cutaneous T-cell lymphomas,[85] diffuse large B-cell lymphoma,[86] primary myelofibrosis,[87] myelodysplastic syndromes,[88,89] acute leukemias,[90,91] chronic myelomonocytic leukemia,[92-94] chronic myeloid leukemia,[95] and sickle cell anemia.[96]

Histology

PAN shows different microscopic findings depending on the age of the lesion[97,98] (Fig. 78-6). The biopsies showing different stages of inflammation are not uncommon.[99] Up to a third of the biopsies can be nondiagnostic.[100] In the early stages, thickening of the vessel wall is present, as a result of edema and fibrinous and cellular exudate. The inflammatory infiltrate is typically composed of neutrophils, with scattered eosinophils and lymphocytes. In older lesions,

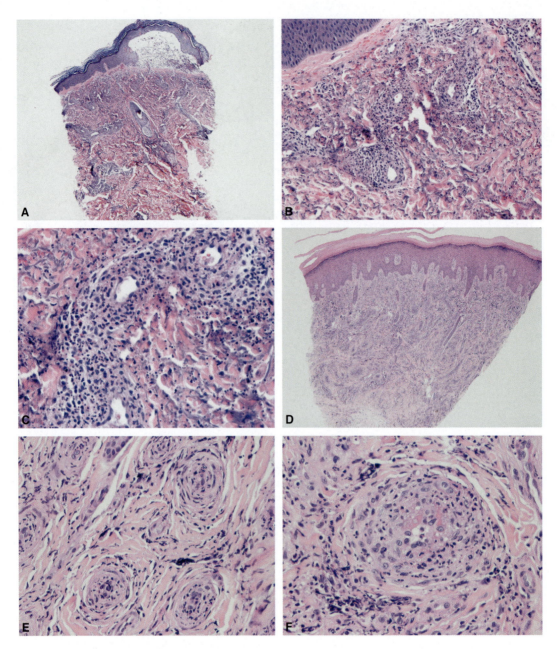

FIGURE 78-5. Erythema elevatum diutinum **A** and **B.** Dermal infiltrate with subepidermal vesicle formation. Leukocytoclasis is prominent (20× and 200×). **C.** Fibrinoid necrosis and neutrophilic infiltrate (400×). **D** and **E.** Chronic phase EED with perivascular dermal fibrosis (40× and 200×). **F.** Focal active vasculitis in chronic EED (400×).

the lymphocytes are the predominant inflammatory cells. Leukocytoclasis can be seen. The lesions can be segmental or involve the entire circumference of the vessel wall and typically affect the small and medium-sized arteries. The pathology is typically centered at the bifurcation of the vessels. Older lesions show intimal and mural fibrosis leading to obliteration of the vessels. In the skin, obtaining significant subcutaneous fat is important for establishing a diagnosis of PAN.

Macular lymphocytic arteritis is regarded by some as a variant of PAN with a predominantly lymphocytic infiltrate and absent or sparse neutrophils.[101-104] A surrounding panniculitis is often present. Many patients have an underlying coagulopathy, such as antiphospholipid antibodies (Fig. 78-7).

KAWASAKI DISEASE AND TAKAYASU ARTERITIS

Kawasaki disease (KD), or mucocutaneous lymph node syndrome, is an acute, multisystemic disease of unknown cause that presents during infancy and early childhood. KD presents with prolonged fever, nonexudative conjunctivitis, cervical lymphadenopathy, pharyngitis, thrombocytosis, and a vasculitis of large-caliber vessels. The coronary arteries are typically affected and, as a result, aneurysms and ectasias develop in 20% of cases. Lymphoid malignancies have been associated with KD in a significant proportion of cases.[105,106]

Takayasu arteritis (TA) is a chronic idiopathic and granulomatous vasculitis, manifesting mainly as a panaortitis.

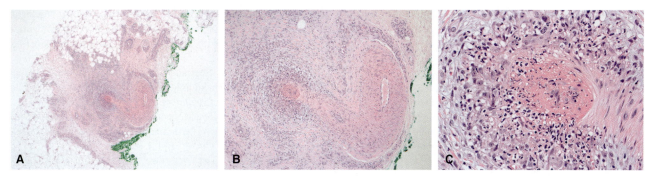

FIGURE 78-6. Polyarteritis nodosa. A. Deep subcutaneous vessel with marked inflammation on the wall. **B.** The inflammation on the wall shows a distinctive localized distribution. **C.** The inflammatory cells include neutrophils and foci of fibrinoid necrosis are seen. (From Hall LD, Dalton SR, Fillman EP, Dohse L, Elston DM. Re-examination of features to distinguish polyarteritis nodosa from superficial thrombophlebitis. *Am J Dermatopathol.* 2013;35:463-471.)

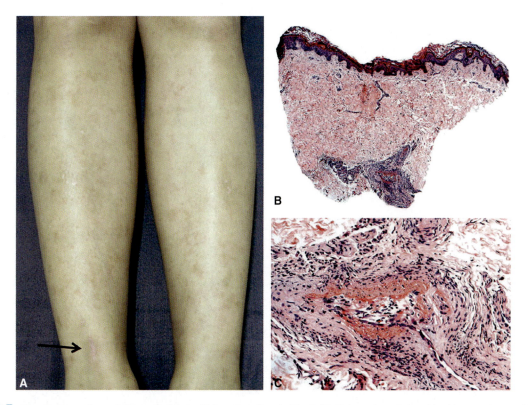

FIGURE 78-7. Macular hyperpigmentation associated with lymphocytic arteritis. A. Mostly hyperpigmented, nonblanching macules are widely scattered over the lower legs associated with vague regions of livedo racemosa and scattered central white stellate scars (atrophie blanche, *arrow*). **B.** Arteritis: a bifurcated artery located at the dermal-hypodermic junction is disrupted by inflammatory infiltrate and intramural fibrin deposits (hematoxylin and eosin, 20×). **C.** Arteritis, subacute-reparative stage. Intimal fibroblastic proliferation partially occludes the lumen, and fibrin deposits are found in the disrupted media. Inflammatory cells are few, mostly lymphocytes in the adventitia or outer media. Nuclear debris, presumptively from neutrophils, is found in the luminal and mural fibrin deposits (hematoxylin and eosin, 200×). (From Macarenco RS, Galan A, Simoni PM, et al. Cutaneous lymphocytic thrombophilic (macular) arteritis: a distinct entity or an indolent (reparative) stage of cutaneous polyarteritis nodosa? Report of 2 cases of cutaneous arteritis and review of the literature. *Am J Dermatopathol.* 2013;35:213-219.)

Autoimmune cell-mediated immunity is probably responsible for the disease. The inflammation commences from the adventitia and progresses to the intima and leads to, both in adults and children, segmental stenosis, occlusion, dilatation, and/or aneurysm formation.[107] Some cases of TA have been seen in the setting of myelodysplastic syndrome.[108,109]

References

1. Sams WM Jr. Necrotizing vasculitis. *J Am Acad Dermatol.* 1980;3:1-13.
2. Magro CM, Crowson AN. The cutaneous neutrophilic vascular injury syndromes: a review. *Semin Diagn Pathol.* 2001;18:47-58.

3. Ramsay C, Fry L. Allergic vasculitis: clinical and histological features and incidence of renal involvement. *Br J Dermatol.* 1969;81:96-102.
4. Sams WM Jr. Hypersensitivity angiitis. *J Invest Dermatol.* 1989;93:78S-81S.
5. Ekenstam E, Callen JP. Cutaneous leukocytoclastic vasculitis. Clinical and laboratory features of 82 patients seen in private practice. *Arch Dermatol.* 1984;120:484-489.
6. Ratnam KV, Boon YH, Pang BK. Idiopathic hypersensitivity vasculitis: clinicopathologic correlation of 61 cases. *Int J Dermatol.* 1995;34:786-789.
7. Loricera J, Calvo-Rio V, Ortiz-Sanjuan F, et al. The spectrum of paraneoplastic cutaneous vasculitis in a defined population: incidence and clinical features. *Medicine (Baltimore).* 2013;92:331-343.
8. Carlson JA, Chen KR. Cutaneous vasculitis update: neutrophilic muscular vessel and eosinophilic, granulomatous, and lymphocytic vasculitis syndromes. *Am J Dermatopathol.* 2007;29:32-43.
9. Endo Y, Tsuji M, Shirase T, et al. Angioimmunoblastic T-cell lymphoma presenting with both IgA-related leukocytoclastic vasculitis and mucous membrane pemphigoid. *Eur J Dermatol.* 2011;21:274-276.
10. Zoroquiain P, Gonzalez S, Molgo M, et al. Leukocytoclastic vasculitis as early manifestation of Epstein–Barr virus-positive diffuse large B-cell lymphoma of the elderly. *Am J Dermatopathol.* 2012;34:330-334.
11. Agha A, Bateman H, Sterrett A, et al. Myelodysplasia and malignancy-associated vasculitis. *Curr Rheumatol Rep.* 2012;14:526-531.
12. Granstein RD, Soter NA, Haynes HA. Necrotizing vasculitis within cutaneous lesions of mycosis fungoides. *J Am Acad Dermatol.* 1983;9:128-133.
13. Spann CR, Callen JP, Yam LT, et al. Cutaneous leukocytoclastic vasculitis complicating hairy cell leukemia (leukemic reticuloendotheliosis). *Arch Dermatol.* 1986;122:1057-1059.
14. Jayachandran NV, Thomas J, Chandrasekhara PK, et al. Cutaneous vasculitis as a presenting manifestation of acute myeloid leukemia. *Int J Rheum Dis.* 2009;12:70-73.
15. Lulla P, Bandeali S, Baker K. Fatal paraneoplastic systemic leukocytoclastic vasculitis as a presenting feature of chronic lymphocytic leukemia. *Clin Lymphoma Myeloma Leuk.* 2011;11(suppl 1):S14-S16.
16. Abouzaid C, Zahlane M, Benjilali L, et al. Paraneoplastic cutaneous leukocytoclastic vasculitis disclosing IgA multiple myeloma [in French]. *Presse Med.* 2013;42:482-484.
17. Carlesimo M, Narcisi A, Orsini D, et al. Angiomatoid lesions (leukocytoclastic vasculitis) as paraneoplastic manifestations of multiple myeloma IgA lambda. *Eur J Dermatol.* 2011;21:260-261.
18. Garcia-Navarro X, Puig L, Fernandez-Figueras MT, et al. Bortezomib-associated cutaneous vasculitis. *Br J Dermatol.* 2007;157:799-801.
19. Turken O, Karagoz B, Bilgi O, et al. Oral etoposide-induced leucocytoclastic vasculitis in a patient with lung carcinoma. *J Eur Acad Dermatol Venereol.* 2007;21:1297-1298.
20. Christian MM, Diven DG, Sanchez RL, et al. Injection site vasculitis in a patient receiving interferon alfa for chronic hepatitis C. *J Am Acad Dermatol.* 1997;37:118-120.
21. Dewan P, Gomber S, Trivedi M, Diwaker P, Madan U. Methotrexate-induced leukocytoclastic vasculitis. *Cureus.* 2021;13(7):e16519.
22. Chung NM, Gutierrez M, Turner ML. Leukocytoclastic vasculitis masquerading as hand-foot syndrome in a patient treated with sorafenib. *Arch Dermatol.* 2006;142:1510-1511.
23. Loree JM, Cai E, Sheffield BS, et al. Leukocytoclastic vasculitis following lenalidomide during the treatment of follicular lymphoma. *Leuk Lymphoma.* 2017;58(3):711-714.
24. Karadimou A, Migou M, Economidi A, et al. Leukocytoclastic vasculitis after long-term treatment with sunitinib: a case report. *Case Rep Oncol.* 2011;4:385-391.
25. LeBoit PE. Dust to dust. *Am J Dermatopathol.* 2005;27:277-278.
26. Bielsa I, Carrascosa JM, Hausmann G, et al. An immunohistopathologic study in cutaneous necrotizing vasculitis. *J Cutan Pathol.* 2000;27:130-135.
27. Bahrami S, Malone JC, Webb KG, et al. Tissue eosinophilia as an indicator of drug-induced cutaneous small-vessel vasculitis. *Arch Dermatol.* 2006;142:155-161.
28. Grunwald MH, Avinoach I, Amichai B, et al. Leukocytoclastic vasculitis—correlation between different histologic stages and direct immunofluorescence results. *Int J Dermatol.* 1997;36:349-352.
29. Heng MC. Henoch–schönlein purpura. *Br J Dermatol.* 1985;112:235-240.
30. Raimer SS, Sanchez RL. Vasculitis in children. *Semin Dermatol.* 1992;11:48-56.
31. Fain O, Hamidou M, Cacoub P, et al. Vasculitides associated with malignancies: analysis of sixty patients. *Arthritis Rheum.* 2007;57:1473-1480.
32. Fox MC, Carter S, Khouri IF, et al. Adult Henoch–Schönlein purpura in a patient with myelodysplastic syndrome and a history of follicular lymphoma. *Cutis.* 2008;81:131-137.
33. Hou JY, Liu HC, Liang DC, et al. Henoch–Schönlein purpura and elevated hepatitis C virus antibody in a girl with nasopharyngeal diffuse large B-cell lymphoma. *Pediatr Neonatol.* 2011;52:349-352.
34. Schena FP, Soerjadi N, Zwi J, et al. Lymphoma presenting as Henoch–Schönlein purpura. *Clin Kidney J.* 2012;5:600-602.
35. Cheon YH, Kim MG, Kim JE, et al. Multiple malignancies in a patient with limited granulomatosis with polyangiitis without immunosuppressive therapy. *Mod Rheumatol.* Published online March 19, 2014.
36. Faurschou M, Sorensen IJ, Mellemkjaer L, et al. Malignancies in Wegener's granulomatosis: incidence and relation to cyclophosphamide therapy in a cohort of 293 patients. *J Rheumatol.* 2008;35:100-105.
37. Shirai T, Takahashi R, Tajima Y, et al. Peripheral T cell lymphoma with a high titer of proteinase-3-antineutrophil cytoplasmic antibodies that resembled Wegener's granulomatosis. *Intern Med.* 2009;48:2041-2045.
38. Sokolowska-Wojdylo M, Florek A, Baranska-Rybak W, et al. Natural killer/T-cell lymphoma, nasal type, masquerading as recalcitrant periodontitis in a patient with a diagnosis of Wegener's granulomatosis. *Am J Med Sci.* 2013;345:163-167.
39. Chen KR, Pittelkow MR, Su D, et al. Recurrent cutaneous necrotizing eosinophilic vasculitis. A novel eosinophil-mediated syndrome. *Arch Dermatol.* 1994;130:1159-1166.
40. Jang KA, Lim YS, Choi JH, et al. Hypereosinophilic syndrome presenting as cutaneous necrotizing eosinophilic vasculitis and Raynaud's phenomenon complicated by digital gangrene. *Br J Dermatol.* 2000;143:641-644.

41. Matsumoto R, Nakamizo S, Tanioka M, et al. Leukocytoclastic vasculitis with eosinophilic infiltration in an HIV-positive patient. *Eur J Dermatol*. 2011;21:103-104.
42. Law AD, Varma S, Varma N, et al. Eosinophilic vasculitis: time for recognition of a new entity? *Indian J Hematol Blood Transfus*. 2014;30:325-330.
43. Borradori L, Rybojad M, Puissant A, et al. Urticarial vasculitis associated with a monoclonal IgM gammopathy: Schnitzler's syndrome. *Br J Dermatol*. 1990;123:113-118.
44. Alizadeh H, Kristenssen J, El Teraifi H, et al. Urticarial vasculitis and Castleman's disease. *J Eur Acad Dermatol Venereol*. 2007;21:541-542.
45. Farell AM, Sabroe RA, Bunker CB. Urticarial vasculitis associated with polycythaemia rubra vera. *Clin Exp Dermatol*. 1996;21:302-304.
46. Reolid A, Rodríguez-Jiménez P, Llamas-Velasco M, Chicharro P, Fraga J, Aragüés M. Leukemic vasculitis: case report and review of the literature. *Am J Dermatopathol*. 2019;41(11):826-831. doi:10.1097/DAD.0000000000001438
47. Nambudiri VE, Aboutalebi A, Granter SR, Saavedra A. Recurrent ALK-negative anaplastic large T-cell lymphoma presenting as necrotizing vasculitis. *Am J Dermatopathol*. 2013;35(4):512-516.
48. Cañueto J, Meseguer-Yebra C, Román-Curto C, et al. Leukemic vasculitis: a rare pattern of leukemia cutis. *J Cutan Pathol*. 2011;38(4):360-364.
49. Chan Y, Mok CC, Tang WY. Erythema elevatum diutinum in systemic lupus erythematosus. *Rheumatol Int*. 2011;31:259-262.
50. Muscardin LM, Cota C, Amorosi B, et al. Erythema elevatum diutinum in the spectrum of palisaded neutrophilic granulomatous dermatitis: description of a case with rheumatoid arthritis. *J Eur Acad Dermatol Venereol*. 2007;21:104-105.
51. Drago F, Semino M, Rampini P, et al. Erythema elevatum diutinum in a patient with human herpesvirus 6 infection. *Acta Derm Venereol*. 1999;79:91-92.
52. Requena L, Sanchez Yus E, Martin L, et al. Erythema elevatum diutinum in a patient with acquired immunodeficiency syndrome. Another clinical simulator of Kaposi's sarcoma. *Arch Dermatol*. 1991;127:1819-1822.
53. Chow RK, Benny WB, Coupe RL, et al. Erythema elevatum diutinum associated with IgA paraproteinemia successfully controlled with intermittent plasma exchange. *Arch Dermatol*. 1996;132:1360-1364.
54. Yiannias JA, El-Azhary RA, Gibson LE. Erythema elevatum diutinum: a clinical and histopathologic study of 13 patients. *J Am Acad Dermatol*. 1992;26:38-44.
55. Sandhu JK, Albrecht J, Agnihotri G, Tsoukas MM. Erythema elevatum et diutinum as a systemic disease. *Clin Dermatol*. 2019;37(6):679-683.
56. Collier PM, Neill SM, Branfoot AC, et al. Erythema elevatum diutinum—a solitary lesion in a patient with rheumatoid arthritis. *Clin Exp Dermatol*. 1990;15:394-395.
57. Hancox JG, Wallace CA, Sangueza OP, et al. Erythema elevatum diutinum associated with lupus panniculitis in a patient with discoid lesions of chronic cutaneous lupus erythematosus. *J Am Acad Dermatol*. 2004;50:652-653.
58. LeBoit PE, Cockerell CJ. Nodular lesions of erythema elevatum diutinum in patients infected with the human immunodeficiency virus. *J Am Acad Dermatol*. 1993;28:919-922.
59. Martin JI, Dronda F, Chaves F. Erythema elevatum diutinum, a clinical entity to be considered in patients infected with HIV-1. *Clin Exp Dermatol*. 2001;26:725-726.
60. Chowdhury MM, Inaloz HS, Motley RJ, et al. Erythema elevatum diutinum and IgA paraproteinaemia: "a preclinical iceberg." *Int J Dermatol*. 2002;41:368-370.
61. Kavanagh GM, Colaco CB, Bradfield JW, et al. Erythema elevatum diutinum associated with Wegener's granulomatosis and IgA paraproteinemia. *J Am Acad Dermatol*. 1993;28:846-849.
62. Wayte JA, Rogers S, Powell FC. Pyoderma gangrenosum, erythema elevatum diutinum and IgA monoclonal gammopathy. *Australas J Dermatol*. 1995;36:21-23.
63. Hatzitolios A, Tzellos TG, Savopoulos C, et al. Erythema elevatum diutinum with rare distribution as a first clinical sign of non-Hodgkin's lymphoma: a novel association? *J Dermatol*. 2008;35:297-300.
64. Atallah J, Garces JC, Loayza E, Carlson JA. Chronic localized fibrosing leukocytoclastic vasculitis associated with lymphedema, intralymphatic and intravascular lymphocytosis, and chronic myelogenous leukemia: a case report of unilateral erythema elevatum diutinum. *Am J Dermatopathol*. 2017;39(6):479-484. doi:10.1097/DAD.0000000000000802
65. Choi JH, Ahn MJ, Park YW, et al. A case of erythema nodosum and serositis associated with myelodysplastic syndrome. *Korean J Intern Med*. 2005;20:177-179.
66. Gubinelli E, Cocuroccia B, Fazio M, et al. Papular neutrophilic dermatosis and erythema elevatum diutinum following erythropoietin therapy in a patient with myelodysplastic syndrome. *Acta Derm Venereol*. 2003;83:358-361.
67. Morrison JG, Hull PR, Fourie E. Erythema elevatum diutinum, cryoglobulinaemia, and fixed urticaria on cooling. *Br J Dermatol*. 1977;97:99-104.
68. Ayoub N, Charuel JL, Diemert MC, et al. Antineutrophil cytoplasmic antibodies of IgA class in neutrophilic dermatoses with emphasis on erythema elevatum diutinum. *Arch Dermatol*. 2004;140:931-936.
69. Shimizu S, Nakamura Y, Togawa Y, et al. Erythema elevatum diutinum with primary Sjögren syndrome associated with IgA antineutrophil cytoplasmic antibody. *Br J Dermatol*. 2008;159:733-735.
70. Katz SI, Gallin JI, Hertz KC, et al. Erythema elevatum diutinum: skin and systemic manifestations, immunologic studies, and successful treatment with dapsone. *Medicine (Baltimore)*. 1977;56:443-455.
71. LeBoit PE, Yen TS, Wintroub B. The evolution of lesions in erythema elevatum diutinum. *Am J Dermatopathol*. 1986;8:392-402.
72. Cohen RD, Conn DL, Ilstrup DM. Clinical features, prognosis, and response to treatment in polyarteritis. *Mayo Clin Proc*. 1980;55:146-155.
73. Goodless DR, Dhawan SS, Alexis J, et al. Cutaneous periarteritis nodosa. *Int J Dermatol*. 1990;29:611-615.
74. Paradela S, Sacristan F, Almagro M, et al. Necrotizing vasculitis with a polyarteritis nodosa-like pattern and selective immunoglobulin A deficiency: case report and review of the literature. *J Cutan Pathol*. 2008;35:871-875.
75. Bauza A, Espana A, Idoate M. Cutaneous polyarteritis nodosa. *Br J Dermatol*. 2002;146:694-699.
76. Cvancara JL, Meffert JJ, Elston DM. Estrogen-sensitive cutaneous polyarteritis nodosa: response to tamoxifen. *J Am Acad Dermatol*. 1998;39:643-646.
77. Ginarte M, Pereiro M, Toribio J. Cutaneous polyarteritis nodosa in a child. *Pediatr Dermatol*. 1998;15:103-107.

78. Crowson AN, Nuovo G, Ferri C, et al. The dermatopathologic manifestations of hepatitis C infection: a clinical, histological, and molecular assessment of 35 cases. *Hum Pathol.* 2003;34:573-579.
79. Fallah M, Liu X, Ji J, et al. Autoimmune diseases associated with non-Hodgkin lymphoma: a nationwide cohort study. *Ann Oncol.* 2014;25:2025-2030.
80. Fallah M, Liu X, Ji J, et al. Hodgkin lymphoma after autoimmune diseases by age at diagnosis and histological subtype. *Ann Oncol.* 2014;25:1397-1404.
81. Ambrosio MR, Rocca BJ, Ginori A, et al. Renal infarction due to polyarteritis nodosa in a patient with angioimmunoblastic T-cell lymphoma: a case report and a brief review of the literature. *Diagn Pathol.* 2012;7:50.
82. Nakashima M, Suzuki K, Okada M, et al. Successful coil embolization of a ruptured hepatic aneurysm in a patient with polyarteritis nodosa accompanied by angioimmunoblastic T cell lymphoma. *Clin Rheumatol.* 2007;26:1362-1364.
83. Mouthon L, Guilpain P, Martin A, et al. Lymphoplasmacytic lymphoma associated with polyradiculoneuritis and cryoglobulinemia mimicking polyarteritis nodosa. *Presse Med.* 2007;36:623-626.
84. Herreman G, Ferme I, Diebold J, et al. Gougerot-Sjögren syndrome, periarteritis nodosa, non-Hodgkin's lymphoplasmocytic lymphoma and acquired C4 deficiency. [Article in French]. *Ann Med Interne (Paris).* 1983;134:19-25.
85. Chircop I, Boespflug A, Antoine C, Lega JC, Dalle S. Paraneoplastic polyarteritis nodosa in a patient with cutaneous T-cell lymphoma. *Lancet Haematol.* 2021;8(3):e240. doi:10.1016/S2352-3026(20)30393-8
86. Ramos-Casals M, Trejo O, Garcia-Carrasco M, et al. Triple association between hepatitis C virus infection, systemic autoimmune diseases, and B cell lymphoma. *J Rheumatol.* 2004;31:495-499.
87. Camos M, Arellano-Rodrigo E, Abello D, et al. Idiopathic myelofibrosis associated with classic polyarteritis nodosa. *Leuk Lymphoma.* 2003;44:539-541.
88. Fernandez-Miranda C, Garcia-Marcilla A, Martin M, et al. Vasculitis associated with a myelodysplastic syndrome: a report of 5 cases. [Article in Spanish]. *Med Clin (Barc).* 1994;103:539-542.
89. Pinal-Fernandez I, Ferrer Fabrega B, Ramentol Sintas M, et al. Histiocytoid Sweet syndrome and cutaneous polyarteritis nodosa secondary to myelodysplastic syndrome. *Int J Rheum Dis.* 2013;16:777-779.
90. Srisuttiyakorn C, Reeve J, Reddy S, et al. Subcutaneous histiocytoid Sweet's syndrome in a patient with myelodysplastic syndrome and acute myeloblastic leukemia. *J Cutan Pathol.* 2014;41:475-479.
91. Leung AC, McLay A, Boulton-Jones JM. Polyarteritis nodosa and monocytic leukaemia. *Postgrad Med J.* 1986;62:35-37.
92. Hamidou MA, Boumalassa A, Larroche C, et al. Systemic medium-sized vessel vasculitis associated with chronic myelomonocytic leukemia. *Semin Arthritis Rheum.* 2001;31:119-126.
93. Roupie AL, Guedon A, Terrier B, et al. Vasculitis associated with myelodysplastic syndrome and chronic myelomonocytic leukemia: French multicenter case-control study. On behalf MINHEMON (French Network of dysimmune disorders associated with hemopathies) and SNFMI. *Semin Arthritis Rheum.* 2020;50(5):879-884.
94. Jacobse J, Sijpkens YWJ, van 't Wout JW, Peters EEM, Vlasveld LT. Vasculitis in myelodysplastic syndrome and chronic myelomonocytic leukemia: a report of two cases. *J Hematol.* 2018;7(4):158-162.
95. Kolodziejczyk TC, Houston N, Davis BC, Wallace EB. Cutaneous polyarteritis nodosa presenting as a paraneoplastic phenomenon in chronic myelogenous leukemia. *JAAD Case Rep.* 2021;12:25-28.
96. Dawe SA, Powell SE, Short KA, et al. Microscopic polyarteritis presenting with skin necrosis in a patient with sickle-cell disease. *Clin Exp Dermatol.* 2006;31:60-62.
97. Rose GA. The natural history of polyarteritis. *Br Med J.* 1957;2:1148-1152.
98. Rose GA, Spencer H. Polyarteritis nodosa. *Q J Med.* 1957;26:43-81.
99. Ishibashi M, Chen KR. A morphological study of evolution of cutaneous polyarteritis nodosa. *Am J Dermatopathol.* 2008;30:319-326.
100. Daoud MS, Hutton KP, Gibson LE. Cutaneous periarteritis nodosa: a clinicopathological study of 79 cases. *Br J Dermatol.* 1997;136:706-713.
101. Buffiere-Morgado A, Battistella M, Vignon-Pennamen MD, et al. Relationship between cutaneous polyarteritis nodosa (cPAN) and macular lymphocytic arteritis (MLA): blinded histologic assessment of 35 cPAN cases. *J Am Acad Dermatol.* 2015;73:1013-1020.
102. Kolivras A, Thompson C, Metz T, et al. Macular arteritis associated with concurrent HIV and hepatitis B infections: a case report and evidence for a disease spectrum association with cutaneous polyarteritis nodosa. *J Cutan Pathol.* 2015;42:416-419.
103. Lee JS, Kossard S, McGrath MA. Lymphocytic thrombophilic arteritis: a newly described medium-sized vessel arteritis of the skin. *Arch Dermatol.* 2008;144:1175-1182.
104. Saleh Z, Mutasim DF. Macular lymphocytic arteritis: a unique benign cutaneous arteritis, mediated by lymphocytes and appearing as macules. *J Cutan Pathol.* 2009;36:1269-1274.
105. Murray JC, Bomgaars LR, Carcamo B, et al. Lymphoid malignancies following Kawasaki disease. *Am J Hematol.* 1995;50:299-300.
106. Suzuki H, Takeuchi T, Minami T, et al. Neoplasms in three patients following Kawasaki disease. *Pediatr Int.* 2005;47:217-219.
107. Vaideeswar P, Deshpande JR. Pathology of Takayasu arteritis: a brief review. *Ann Pediatr Cardiol.* 2013;6:52-58.
108. Cohen MJ, Shyman A, Klein M, et al. Large vessel (Takayasu's) arteritis in a patient with myelodysplastic syndrome: is there a common pathogenesis? *Clin Lymphoma Myeloma Leuk.* 2011;11:60-63.
109. Kato H, Onishi Y, Nakajima S, et al. Significant improvement of Takayasu arteritis after cord blood transplantation in a patient with myelodysplastic syndrome. *Bone Marrow Transpl.* 2014;49:458-459.

CHAPTER 79

Paraneoplastic pemphigus

Katherine France, Milda Chmieliauskaite, and Faizan Alawi

INTRODUCTION

Paraneoplastic pemphigus (PNP) is an autoimmune vesiculobullous disorder.[1] PNP was first described in 1990 as a distinct clinical entity different from pemphigus vulgaris (PV).[1] PNP is most commonly associated with an underlying hematologic neoplasm such as non-Hodgkin lymphoma, chronic lymphocytic leukemia (CLL), or Castleman disease.[2] The heterogeneous clinical presentation often delays diagnosis, and bronchiolitis obliterans, a pulmonary manifestation of this disease, is the primary cause of morbidity and leading cause of mortality in patients with PNP.[3,4] To more appropriately reflect the diverse clinical findings, including organ involvement, it has been proposed that the more inclusive term "paraneoplastic autoimmune multiorgan syndrome" be used and that PNP be employed for those cases in which the manifestations most closely resemble other forms of pemphigus.[5,6]

EPIDEMIOLOGY

The worldwide incidence of PNP is unknown but may represent 1% to 3% of all patients with vesiculobullous disease.[7] It has a bimodal distribution, affecting primarily adults between the ages of 45 and 70 years and children between 7 and 18 years of age.[8] Overall, there is a male predominance.

Approximately 80% of PNP cases are associated with an underlying lymphoproliferative disease.[2,3] Two-thirds of cases are associated with non-Hodgkin lymphomas (38.6%), CLL (18.4%), and Castleman disaese (18.4%).[2,3] PNP has also been reported, albeit less commonly, with thymoma, sarcomas, desmoid tumors, and Waldenstrom macroglobulinemia.[2,3,5,8,9] Various solid malignancies are also reported and include breast cancer, gastric signet cell ring carcinoma and other gastric cancers, and malignant melanoma.[10-13] In pediatric patients, Castleman disease is the most common underlying neoplasm, accounting for some 80% to 90% of cases.[8,14] In addition to underlying neoplasms, HLA-DRB1*03 has been found in up to 61% of cases, and HLA-Cw*14 has also been associated with development of PNP.[15,16] In certain cases, no underlying malignancy is discernible, although an eventual cancer may be diagnosed in some individuals.[17] When not associated with an underlying neoplasm, the trigger of PNP may be idiopathic, a medication, or radiotherapy.[13]

PATHOGENESIS

PNP and PV may appear clinically similar but are distinct regarding immunology and pathogenesis. Both humoral and cell-mediated immunity are involved in the pathogenesis of PNP.[3] Of the humoral effectors, IgG antibodies are most common, with IgA antibodies occasionally observed. IgG1 and IgG2 subclasses predominate in PNP sera, whereas IgG3 and IgG4 have been found less commonly.[18]

Cadherins and plakins, responsible for keratinocyte cell adhesion, are the protein families targeted in PNP.[19,20] From the cadherin family of proteins, autoantibodies are primarily found against the desmosomal proteins desmoglein 3 (Dsg3) and, less commonly, desmoglein 1 (Dsg1).[19] Anti-Dsg3 autoantibodies disrupt desmosomes, thus resulting in acantholysis, suprabasilar clefting, and blistering seen clinically in both PNP and PV.[20] In rare cases of PNP, Dsg1 autoantibodies alone are made, and in some cases of PNP, no circulating autoantibodies are detected, possibly due to progression of cell-mediated immunity without a humoral component.[11,21]

The plakin autoantigens more reliably differentiate PNP from PV. Three Plakin proteins are found in desmosomes and hemidesmosomes and mediate attachments between intermediate filaments and transmembrane adhesion molecules.[3] The entire plakin family constitutes antigens targeted in PNP, including desmoplakin I (250 kDa), desmoplakin II (210 kDa), bullous pemphigoid antigen I (230 kDa), bullous pemphigoid antigen II (180 kDa), envoplakin (210 kDa), epiplakin (>700 kDa), periplakin (190 kDa), plakophilin III (87 kDa), plectin (500 kDa), and desmocollins I, II, and III (each 100 kDa).[13,19,22] α2-Macroglobulin-like 1 A2ML1, a protease inhibitor (170 kDa), is an additional antigen found in the upper layers of the epidermis uniquely targeted in PNP and is used to distinguish it from other forms of pemphigus.[23-25] Compared with PV, there are a greater number of autoantigens recognized in PNP and a broader distribution of epitopes targeted within select autoantigens.[3,18] For example, in PNP, IgG recognizes a wide distribution of epitopes in the Dsg3 extracellular domain, while in PV, autoantibodies primarily target the N terminus.[18]

Cell-mediated immunity is also implicated in PNP pathogenesis and likely plays a central role in the immunophenotype observed.[3,24,26] Mononuclear cell inflammatory infiltrates have been observed at the dermoepidermal junction of histologic specimens in PNP tissue samples and may contain CD8+ cytotoxic T lymphocytes, CD56+ natural killer cells, and CD68+ monocytes/macrophages.[26] Cell-mediated immunity may help explain the various clinical and histologic presentations possible in PNP including the lichenoid-like or erythema multiforme (EM)-like features.[3,26] Furthermore, as demonstrated in neonatal mice, autoantibodies of patients with PNP injected into mice produce the acantholytic skin lesions that are classic of PNP but do not reproduce other internal organ involvement seen in patients with PNP, suggesting that humoral immunity is a necessary but not sufficient component of pathogenesis.[20]

The mechanisms by which neoplasms induce autoimmunity are not well understood; however, a few hypotheses have been proposed. One suggests that the underlying tumor produces autoantibodies targeting the skin and oral mucosa.[3] However, this may not be a universal mechanism because PNP triggered by Waldenstrom macroglobulinemia would be unlikely to produce the IgG-class pathogenic autoantibodies commonly observed in PNP.[3] In addition, there has been no evidence to suggest that the various associated tumors express epithelial proteins that could conceivably initiate autoantibody formation.[3] Other theories suggest that unrelated antigens expressed by an underlying tumor may react with epithelial substrates or that cross-reactivity could develop as a result of epitope spreading.[27] The favored hypothesis, however, is that the malignancy induces dysregulation of cytokines, which may drive the development of autoimmunity.[3]

Serum interleukin 6 (IL-6) may be elevated in hematologic neoplasms associated with PNP including CLL and Castleman disease.[28] Furthermore, increased production of IL-6 has been associated with multiple clinical disorders including other autoimmune diseases and is increasingly shown to be central to the development of PNP.[16,29] In murine models, increased IL-6 promoted B-lymphocyte hyperproliferation, resulting in hypergammaglobulinemia of the IgG1 subclass.[29] Thus, targeted therapies against IL-6 or, more specifically, its receptor may be considered in cases where IL-6 is upregulated.[29] PNP has been suggested to be more common in patients formerly treated with rituximab, an anti-CD20 agent for other causes, presumably as a result of B-cell depletion from treatment.[17] However, this therapy is also thought to have reduced the overall incidence and possibly severity of PNP when used as a treatment for susceptible malignancies.[30]

CLINICAL PRESENTATION AND DIFFERENTIAL DIAGNOSIS

The oral mucosa is invariably affected in patients with PNP. In most cases, the oral ulcerations manifest before any other mucosal or skin sites are affected and, in up to one-third of patients, early signs of PNP may manifest before the underlying associated disease.[13] Indeed, one of the earliest manifestations of PNP is severe and painful, diffuse ulcerative stomatitis refractory to treatment.[3,5,6] These lesions may be deep and indurated and appear red to black with necrosis and crusting.[31] The ulcerations may develop on any oral surface, but there is a tendency for tongue and labial mucosal involvement, starting on the lateral borders of the tongue and labial mucosa and spreading over time to often involve the entire tongue and lip vermillion.[3,12] Patients who initially present with skin lesions will eventually develop mucositis during the course of their disease. In addition to the oral cavity, the mucosal ulcerations may be diffuse and involve the oropharynx, hypopharynx, esophagus, nasal cavity, conjunctiva, and/or genitalia.[3,5] The involvement of conjunctival mucosa may include conjunctivitis, erosions, shortening of the fornix, and more. This ocular component differentiates PNP from PV and may lead to visual loss.[16] However, mucous membrane pemphigoid (MMP) would still be included in the clinical differential diagnosis. To that end, ocular complications typical of MMP, including symblepharon and corneal scarring, may also be evident in PNP.[3,5]

Cutaneous manifestations are polymorphous and may have at least five distinct morphologic appearances: (a) vesiculobullous lesions reminiscent of either PV or (b) MMP/bullous pemphigoid, (c) pruritic papules and plaques with variable erythema resembling lichen planus or lichen planus pemphigoides, (d) erythematous papules and plaques that can appear targetoid as in EM, or become confluent as is seen in Steven-Johnson syndrome, and/or toxic epidermal necrolysis (TEN), and (e) lesions reminiscent of graft-versus-host disease.[3,5,6,16,32] More rarely, the disease may appear more similar to pemphigus foliaceus or pemphigus vegetans.[7,13]

Morphologically distinct skin lesions may be present concomitantly at multiple sites in the same patient, or a single lesional site may experience morphologic change throughout the course of the disease, including evolving from lichen planus-like and other less severe lesions to more widespread, vesiculobullous, or life-threatening presentations.[2,3,33] Lichenoid lesions are also seen more frequently in younger patients and on the torso and limbs, although some lichenoid lesions of the oral cavity are thought to go undiagnosed.[13] Involvement of the palmar and plantar surfaces may help differentiate PNP from PV; these surfaces are very rarely affected in PV, while the scalp is rarely affected in PNP.[2,6,32] Unlike the self-limited course of EM and TEN, which usually resolve over several weeks, PNP persists and is progressive.[3]

PNP is the only form of pemphigus in which internal organs may be affected.[5] Respiratory involvement manifests as a range of signs and symptoms and can progress to bronchiolitis obliterans in approximately 30% to 40% of PNP cases.[3,5,13] In these cases, the development of fibrosis may be connected to anti-epiplakin antibodies, as epiplakin is expressed in the bronchiolar epithelium, although this does not explain why patients with PNP so rarely exhibit fibrosis at other sites.[6,24] Clinically, patients present with progressive dyspnea as a result of irreversible airway obstruction.[4,34] Pulmonary function tests, blood-gas tests, chest radiographs, computed tomography (CT) scans, and endoscopic lung biopsies can aid in the detection of lung involvement in patients with PNP and respiratory symptoms.[4,34] In some patients, gastrointestinal involvement including lesions affecting the esophagus, stomach, duodenum, and colon have been reported and rectal bleeding may be evident.[5] Rare examples of PNP manifesting with glomerulonephritis and neurologic complications have also been described.[35] Myasthenia gravis, which may develop due to cross-reactivity of autoantibodies, is also known to manifest in some cases of PNP with a particular connection to cases arising secondary to thymoma.[16,36] Sepsis may also be a cause of mortality in some patients.[3] In general, patients with PNP present with systemic signs that may be due to either the lesions, underlying malignancy, or both, including fatigue, malaise, weakness, and weight loss.[27]

When PNP develops secondary to Castleman disease, patients present at a mean age of 14 years with mucocutaneous lesions similar to adult forms as well as frequent genital and ocular involvement. These patients most commonly manifest lichenoid appearances and have frequent pulmonary complications that become the primary cause of death. These patients commonly improve after removal of their tumors but generally show little response to other therapies.[37] In fact, this population is overrepresented in cases of PNP that develop bronchiolitis obliterans and demonstrate sloughed epithelial cells in the bronchi and alveolar sacs, possibly as a result of the acantholysis seen in PNP.[24]

Given the clinical variability of the disease and differences in confirmatory test results, major and minor diagnostic criteria have been suggested, but additional studies are needed to validate the criteria.[38]

HISTOPATHOLOGY

PNP has a wide array of histologic presentations, which may correlate with the morphologic pattern of the clinical lesions.[5] These include most commonly acantholysis with suprabasilar clefting and sparse inflammation mimicking PV, and less frequently subepithelial clefting reminiscent of pemphigoid, lichenoid inflammation with or without perivascular involvement thereby resembling either lichen planus or lichenoid mucositis (Fig. 79-1), nonspecific mucositis typical of EM-like eruptions, dyskeratotic keratinocytes, and variable extents of necrosis.[24,39,40] A single biopsy specimen may show multiple histologic features. Direct immunofluorescence (DIF) analyses may also reveal heterogeneous findings including staining patterns that may mimic PV epidermal intercellular deposition of IgG and/or complement, pemphigoid linear basement membrane zone deposition of IgG/C3, a combination of these two patterns, and/or basement membrane zone staining with fibrinogen that is typical of lichenoid reactions (Fig. 79-2). Some samples also elude diagnosis using DIF, both due to the frequency of necrotic tissue from specimens and in cases where cellular immunity predominates.[41] Lesions that exhibit clinical features more similar to lichen planus are likely to appear similarly on histology with lichenoid interface reaction and mononuclear infiltrate at the epidermal junction and are more likely to have negative or unclear DIF results.[16]

As patients with PNP have circulating autoantibodies, indirect immunofluorescence analysis using exogenous tissue substrates may also be used. Monkey esophagus is widely employed as the substrate but may not adequately distinguish PNP from PV, while murine tongue and more reliably bladder are highly specific for PNP due to the prominence of plakin proteins expressed on murine bladder tissue, including more desmoplakin than in human skin.[24,27] Salt split skin has also been proposed as an alternative.[5,39,42]

Enzyme-linked immunosorbent assays (ELISAs), immunoprecipitation, and immunoblotting to identify plakin proteins, specifically envoplakin and periplakin, can also support a diagnosis of PNP.[41] Immunoprecipitation is currently thought to be the most sensitive test for PNP.[24] Although ELISA testing may also reveal Dsg3, Dsg1, BP180, and/or BP230 reactivity, identification of these autoantibodies is not sufficiently diagnostic for PNP. The specialized envoplakin

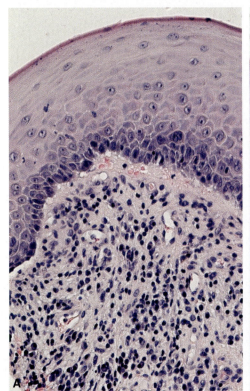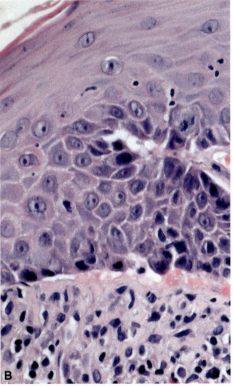

FIGURE 79-1. Lichenoid-type inflammation in oral mucosal tissue from a patient with PNP. **A.** A lymphoplasmacytic infiltrate is noted at the mucosal-submucosal interface; hematoxylin and eosin (H&E), 200×. **B.** Degeneration of the basal cells is seen H&E, 400×.

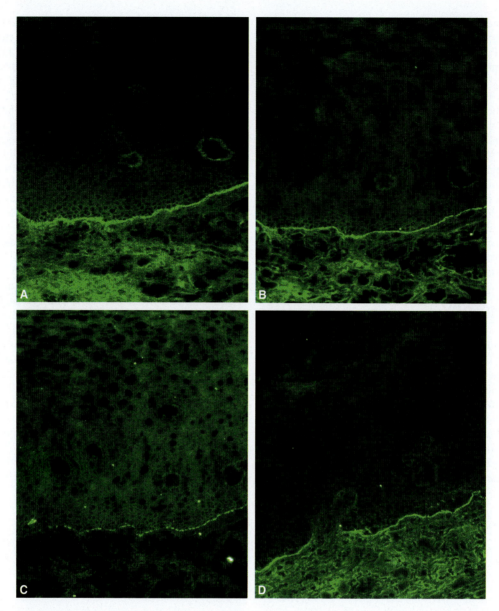

FIGURE 79-2. Direct immunofluorescence analysis of an oral mucosal PNP tissue sample reveals basement membrane zone deposition of **(A)** IgG, **(B)** IgA, **(C)** complement C3, and **(D)** fibrinogen.

and periplakin protein ELISA assays are currently only available through a subset of national and institutional diagnostic laboratories.

TREATMENT AND PROGNOSIS

There are currently no evidence-based guidelines for management of PNP. Treatment approaches have been gathered from case reports, case series, and expert recommendations.[43] The best therapeutic approach for PNP is treatment of the underlying neoplasm.[3,5,43,44] Patients with resectable benign and localized tumors have the best outcomes with resolution of PNP subsequent to complete surgical excision.[3,5,43-46] Patients who had surgical resection of their Castleman tumor exhibited decreased levels of circulating autoantibodies by 5 to 9 weeks following removal, resolving skin lesions by 6 to 11 weeks, and mucosal lesions resolving 5 to 10 months after surgery.[45] Pulmonary damage does not resolve after surgical resection of the tumor and is the most common cause of mortality in patients with PNP.[3,5,43] For patients with ocular involvement, regular ophthalmologic evaluations are recommended to evaluate the extent of disease and monitor damage.[27]

In addition to treating the underlying neoplasm, patients may need further therapy including immunosuppression, immunomodulation, or plasmapheresis.[45,47] High-dose corticosteroids are considered the first-line approach to mucocutaneous lesions; however, oral lesions are often refractory to steroids, resulting in minimal resolution, and are a challenge to manage.[13,47] Increasingly, the anti-CD20 agent rituximab has been used both alone and in combination with other anticancer treatments for treatment of PNP. These additional agents include ibrutinib, bendamustine, and the combination of cyclophosphamide, vincristine sulfate, hydroxydanorubicin, and prednisone (R-CHOP therapy), each of which has been used separately from as well as together with rituximab.[48-51]

These medications may spur continued improvement to PNP lesions when treatment is prolonged after the directed oncologic regimen or may be effective when started separately from treatment of the underlying disease. Additional biologic agents including alemtuzumab and tocilizumab have been proposed for similar reasons.[16] Case reports have also described the use of a wide variety of immunosuppressant medications such as cyclosporine, cyclophosphamide, azathioprine, dapsone, and intravenous immunoglobulin. However, patient outcomes have been varied and inconsistent, and success with these treatment strategies remains anecdotal.[15,43-47] These agents are often used concurrent with corticosteroids to improve response and to decrease steroid burden.[14] While cutaneous lesions often decrease or resolve on the above regimens, mucositis is more resistant to management.[16]

Patients with PNP have a poor prognosis, and cohort studies reported an approximately 38% 5-year survival rate.[5,52] However, the mortality rate has been reported to be as high as 90% in other studies.[5] Unfortunately, prognosis and survival data for PNP are derived from case reports and cohort studies, and the true rates are unknown. Prognosis for patients with PNP depends on the underlying neoplasm, extent of lung damage, and predisposing risk for infection.[52] It has been noted that patients with EM-like lesions and presence of bronchiolitis obliterans may have a worse prognosis compared with other presentations of PNP.[5,50,52] In addition, anti-envoplakin and anti-epiplakin antibodies and clinical manifestations mimicking both TEN and bullous pemphigoid were connected to higher mortality rates in these patients.[22,40] Patients with Castleman disease and thymoma may experience a better overall prognosis.[27]

PNP remains a poorly understood, debilitating disease with a heterogeneous clinical presentation and disease course. Treatment strategies should be tailored to meet the needs of each individual patient. Treating the underlying neoplasm, preventing infection and lung damage, and improving mucosal lesions should be prioritized in patients with PNP, and these require a multidisciplinary approach.

References

1. Anhalt GJ, Kim SC, Stanley JR, et al. Paraneoplastic pemphigus: an autoimmune mucocutaneous disease associated with neoplasia. *N Engl J Med*. 1990;323:1729-1735.
2. Kaplan I, Hodak E, Ackerman L, et al. Neoplasms associated with paraneoplastic pemphigus: a review with emphasis on non-hematologic malignancy and oral mucosal manifestations. *Oral Oncol*. 2004;40:553-562.
3. Anhalt GJ. Paraneoplastic pemphigus. *J Invest Dermatol Symp Proc*. 2004;9:29-33.
4. Maldonado F, Pittelkow MR, Ryu JH. Constrictive bronchiolitis associated with paraneoplastic autoimmune multi-organ syndrome. *Respirology*. 2009;14:129-133.
5. Czernik A, Camilleri M, Pittelkow MR, et al. Paraneoplastic autoimmune multiorgan syndrome: 20 years after. *Int J Dermatol*. 2011;50:905-914.
6. Amber KT. Paraneoplastic autoimmune multi-organ syndrome is a distinct entity from traditional pemphigus subtypes. *Nat Rev Dis Prim*. 2018;4:18012.
7. Calabria E, Fortuna G, Aria M, Mignogna MD. Autoimmune mucocutaneous blistering diseases in the south of Italy: a 25-year retrospective study on 169 patients. *J Oral Pathol Med*. 2020;49:672-680.
8. Mimouni D, Anhalt GJ, Lazarova Z, et al. Paraneoplastic pemphigus in children and adolescents. *Br J Dermatol*. 2002;147:725-732.
9. Sehgal VN, Srivastava G. Paraneoplastic pemphigus/paraneoplastic autoimmune multiorgan syndrome. *Int J Dermatol*. 2009;48:162-169.
10. Lepekhova A, Olisova O, Teplyuk N, Zolotenkov D, Allenova A. A rare association of paraneoplastic pemphigus with gastric signet cell ring carcinoma. *Australas J Dermatol*. 2019;60:e169-e171.
11. Ferguson L, Fearfield L. Paraneoplastic pemphigus foliaceus related to underlying breast cancer. *Clin Exp Dermatol*. 2018;43:817-818.
12. Melnick LE, Beasley JM, Kim R, et al. Paraneoplastic pemphigus in a 34-year-old. *Dermatol Online J*. 2017;23:13.
13. Paolino G, Didona D, Magliulo G, et al. Paraneoplastic pemphigus: insight into the autoimmune pathogenesis, clinical features and therapy. *Int J Mol Sci*. 2017;18:2532.
14. Decaux J, Ferreira I, Van Eeckhout P, Dachelet C, Magremanne M. Buccal paraneoplastic pemphigus multi-resistant: case report and review of diagnostic and therapeutic strategies. *J Stomatol Oral Maxillofac Surg*. 2018;119:506-509.
15. Kranzelbinder B, Hashimoto T, Joch M, et al. Paraneoplastic pemphigus in two pairs of brothers. *J Eur Acad Dermatol Venereol*. 2017;31:e552-e553.
16. Kim JH, Kim S-C. Paraneoplastic pemphigus: paraneoplastic autoimmune disease of the skin and mucosa. *Front Immunol*. 2019;10:1259.
17. Baykal C, Kilic S, Kucukoglu R. Paraneoplastic pemphigus seen in four patients with haematological malignancies formerly treated with rituximab. *J Eur Acad Dermatol Venereol*. 2018;32:e50-e52.
18. Futei Y, Amagai M, Hashimoto T, et al. Conformational epitope mapping and IgG subclass distribution of desmoglein 3 in paraneoplastic pemphigus. *J Am Acad Dermatol*. 2003;49:1023-1028.
19. Maverakis E, Goodarzi H, Wehrli LN, et al. The etiology of paraneoplastic autoimmunity. *Clin Rev Allergy Immunol*. 2012;42:135-144.
20. Amagai M, Nishikawa T, Nousari HC, et al. Antibodies against desmoglein 3 pemphigus vulgaris antigen are present in sera from patients with paraneoplastic pemphigus and cause acantholysis in vivo in neonatal mice. *J Clin Invest*. 1998;102:775-782.
21. Lim JM, Kim JH, Hashimoto T, Kim S-C. Lichenoid paraneoplastic pemphigus associated with follicular lymphoma without detectable autoantibodies. *Clin Exp Dermatol*. 2018;43:592-616.
22. Tsuchisaka A, Numata S, Teye K, et al. Epiplakin is a paraneoplastic pemphigus autoantigen and related to bronchiolitis obliterans in Japanese patients. *J Invest Dermatol*. 2016;139:399-408.
23. Numata S, Teye K, Tsuruta D, et al. Anti-alpha-2-macroglobulin-like-1 autoantibodies are detected frequently and may be pathogenic in paraneoplastic pemphigus. *J Invest Dermatol*. 2013;133:1785-1793.
24. Amber KT, Valdebran M, Grando SA. Paraneoplastic autoimmune multiorgan syndrome PAMS: beyond the single phenotype of paraneoplastic pemphigus. *Autoimmun Rev*. 2018;17:1002-1010.
25. Schepens I, Jaunin F, Begre N, et al. The protease inhibitor alpha-2-macroglobuline-like-1 is the p170 antigen recognized by paraneoplastic pemphigus autoantibodies in human. *PLoS One*. 2010;5:e122250.

26. Nguyen VT, Ndoye A, Bassler KD, et al. Classification, clinical manifestations, and immunopathological mechanisms of the epithelial variant of paraneoplastic autoimmune multiorgan syndrome: a reappraisal of paraneoplastic pemphigus. *Arch Dermatol.* 2001;137:193-206.
27. Maruta CW, Miyamoto D, Aoki V, de Carvalho RGR, Cunha BM, Santi CG. Paraneoplastic pemphigus: a clinical, laboratorial, and therapeutic overview. *An Bras Dermatol.* 2019;94:388-398.
28. Nousari HC, Kimyai-Asadi A, Anhalt GJ. Elevated serum levels of interleukin-6 in paraneoplastic pemphigus. *J Invest Dermatol.* 1999;112:396-398.
29. Calabrese LH, Rose-John S. IL-6 biology: implications for clinical targeting in rheumatic disease. *Nat Rev Rheumatol.* 2014;10:720-727.
30. Kwatra SG, Boozalis E, Pasieka H, Anhalt GJ. Decreased recognition of paraneoplastic pemphigus in patients previously treated with anti-CD 20 monoclonal antibodies. *Br J Dermatol.* 2019;180:1238-1239.
31. Siddiqui S, Bilal M, Otaibi, Bilimoria F, Patel N, Rossetti J. Paraneoplastic pemphigus as a presentation of acute myeloid leukemia: early diagnosis and remission. *Hematol Oncol Stem Cell Ther.* 2017;10:155-160.
32. Vassileva S, Drenovska K, Manuelyan K. Autoimmune blistering dermatoses as systemic diseases. *Clin Dermatol.* 2014;32:364-375.
33. Okahashi L, Oiso N, Ishii N, et al. Paraneoplastic pemphigus presenting lichen planus-like lesions. *J Dermatol.* 2019;46:e140-e142.
34. Nousari HC, Deterding R, Wojtczack H, et al. The mechanism of respiratory failure in paraneoplastic pemphigus. *N Engl J Med.* 1999;340:1406-1410.
35. Qian SX, Li JY, Hong M, et al. Nonhematological autoimmunity glomerulosclerosis, paraneoplastic pemphigus and paraneoplastic neurological syndrome in a patient with chronic lymphocytic leukemia: diagnosis, prognosis and management. *Leuk Res.* 2009;33:500-505.
36. Tu L, Song B, Pu H, Li X, Chen Q, Yang C. Paraneoplastic pemphigus and myasthenia gravis as the first manifestations of a rare case of pancreatic follicular dendritic cell sarcoma: CT findings and review of literature. *BMC Gastroenterol.* 2019;19:92.
37. Han SP, Fu LS, Chen LJ. Masked pemphigus among pediatric patietns with Castleman's disease. *Int J Rheum Dis.* 2019;22:121-131.
38. Camisa C, Helm TN. Paraneoplastic pemphigus is a distinct neoplasia-induced autoimmune disease. *Arch Dermatol.* 1993;129:883-886.
39. Poot AM, Diercks GF, Kramer D, et al. Laboratory diagnosis of paraneoplastic pemphigus. *Br J Dermatol.* 2013;169:1016-1024.
40. Ouedraogo E, Gottlieb J, de Masson A, et al. Risk factors for death and survival in paraneoplastic pemphigus associated with hematologic malignancies in adults. *J Am Acad Dermatol.* 2019;80:1544-1549.
41. Tirado-Sanchez A, Bonifaz A. Paraneoplastic pemphigus. A life-threatening autoimmune blistering disease. *Actas Dermosifiliogr.* 2017;108:902-910.
42. Poot AM, Siland J, Jonkman MF, Pas HH, Diercks GFH. Direct and indirect immunofluorescence staining patterns in the diagnosis of paraneoplastic pemphigus. *Br J Dermatol.* 2016;174:912-915.
43. Frew JW, Murrell DF. Current management strategies in paraneoplastic pemphigus paraneoplastic autoimmune multiorgan syndrome. *Dermatol Clin.* 2011;29:607-612.
44. Zhang J, Qiao Q, Chen X, et al. Improved outcomes after complete resection of underlying tumors for patients with paraneoplastic pemphigus: a single-center experience of 22 cases. *J Cancer Res Clin Oncol.* 2011;137:229-234.
45. Jing L, Shan Z, Yongchu H, et al. Successful treatment of a paraneoplastic pemphigus in a teenager using plasmapheresis, corticosteroids and tumour resection. *Clin Exp Dermatol.* 2011;36:752-754.
46. Fang Y, Zhao L, Yan F, et al. A critical role of surgery in the treatment for paraneoplastic pemphigus caused by localized Castleman's disease. *Med Oncol.* 2010;27:907-911.
47. Nousari HC, Brodsky RA, Jones RJ, et al. Immunoablative high-dose cyclophosphamide without stem cell rescue in paraneoplastic pemphigus: report of a case and review of this new therapy for severe autoimmune disease. *J Am Acad Dermatol.* 1999;40:750-754.
48. Kikuchi T, Mori T, Shimizu T, et al. Successful treatment with bendamustine and rituximab for paraneoplastic pemphigus. *Ann Hematol.* 2017;96:1221-1222.
49. Lee A, Sandhu S, Imlay-Gillespie L, Mulligan S, Shumack S. Successful use of Bruton's kinase inhibitor, ibrutinib, to control paraneoplastic pemphigus in a patient with paraneoplastic autoimmune multiorgan syndrome and chronic lymphocytic leukaemia. *Australas J Dermatol.* 2017;58:e240-e242.
50. Lee S, Yamauchi T, Ishii N, et al. Achievement of the longest survival of paraneoplastic pemphigus with bronchiolitis obliterans associated with follicular lymphoma using R-CHOP chemotherapy. *Int J Hematol.* 2017;106:852-859.
51. Ito Y, Makita S, Maeshima AM, et al. Paraneoplastic pemphigus associated with B-cell chronic lymphocytic leukemia treated with ibrutinib and rituximab. *Intern Med.* 2018;57:2395-2398.
52. Leger S, Picard D, Ingen-Housz-Oro S, et al. Prognostic factors of paraneoplastic pemphigus. *Arch Dermatol.* 2012;148:1165-1172.

CHAPTER 80

Cryoglobulinemia
Alejandro A. Gru

DEFINITION

Cryoglobulins are abnormal serum immunoglobulins that reversibly precipitate at low temperature. Two forms of cryoglobulinemias (CGs) are distinguished based on the composition of the cryoglobulins and associated vascular pathology. In simple CG, type I cryoglobulins are composed of monoclonal immunoglobulins, which result in dermal vasculopathy (thrombosis) as they precipitate in vessels. In mixed CG, cryoglobulins are immune complexes made up of either monoclonal (type II) or polyclonal (type III) rheumatoid factor (RF) bound to the Fc portion of polyclonal IgG. Mixed CG induces leukocytoclastic vasculitis (LCV), typically involving both superficial and deep dermal vessels.[1,2]

LABORATORY FINDINGS

Type I CG represents approximately 25% of all cases of cryoglobulins. The associated monoclonal immunoglobulin is most frequently IgG or IgM and less frequently IgA or light chains.[1,3] Types II and III CG (mixed CG) contain RFs, which are usually IgM and, rarely, IgG or IgA. These RFs form complexes with the fragment, crystallizable (Fc) portion of polyclonal IgG. The actual RF may be monoclonal (in type II CG) or polyclonal (in type III CG) immunoglobulin. Types II and III CG represent 80% of all cryoglobulins.[4,5] Mixed CG takes the form of immune complexes that bind complement and ultimately lead to an inflammatory response.

ETIOLOGY

Type I CG caused by monoclonal IgG is associated with monoclonal gammopathy of undetermined significance (MGUS),[6] multiple myeloma,[7,8] chronic lymphocytic leukemia, marginal zone lymphoma,[9] and lymphoplasmacytic lymphoma (LPL).[3,10-13] Type I CG containing monoclonal IgM is typically linked to MGUS and LPL (Waldenström macroglobulinemia). Cases without associated hematologic dyscrasias are referred to as essential simple CG.[14]

Mixed CG (types II and III) is most frequently associated with hepatitis C virus (HCV) infection. More than 50% of HCV patients have mixed cryoglobulins. Other frequent associations include connective tissue disease (lupus, Sjögren syndrome) and hematologic malignancies.[15] Rare occurrences with EBV,[16] HIV,[17] parvovirus B19,[23] syphilis,[18] and leprosy[19] have been described. An underlying disease cannot be identified in about one-third of mixed CG cases (essential mixed CG).

CLINICAL FINDINGS

Approximately half of patients with type I CG have cutaneous manifestations on presentation.[10] The cutaneous symptoms include Raynaud phenomenon, livedo reticularis,[20,21] and recurrent episodes of cold-induced necrotic purpura of the extremities and urticaria, either cold related or not (Fig. 80-1). Leg ulcers are also a frequent clinical manifestation. Systemic manifestations also include high-grade proteinuria (nephrotic range), nephritic syndrome, acute renal failure, and severe hypertension. Neurologic findings are also seen in 25% of cases, usually in the form of predominantly sensitive polyneuropathy with associated axonal loss. Type I CG is associated with an approximately 10% mortality, related to the hemopathy. Rare cases of multiple myeloma presenting with follicular hyperkeratotic papules in association with CG have also been reported.[22-24]

The symptoms of mixed CG are a consequence of cryoglobulinemic vasculitis. They are characterized by the clinical triad of purpura, arthralgias, and weakness (asthenia). Many other organs may also be involved, particularly the peripheral nervous system and the kidneys.[21] In these patients, high titers of RF and low C4 levels are often observed.

Vasculitis in the skin manifests as nonblanchable palpable purpura in the form of purple, red purpuric lower-extremity macules and papules often triggered by cold exposure or prolonged standing. Palpable purpura can be accompanied by systemic symptoms (70%), arthralgias (60%-70%), glomerulonephritis (55%), neuropathy (40%), and/or pulmonary symptoms of hemoptysis and dyspnea (5%). HCV-related mixed CG is more often associated with arthralgias (61% vs 20%) than mixed CG patients without HCV etiology.[2,25] Koebnerization can rarely occur.[26] Cryoglobulinemia accounts for less than 1% of cases of cutaneous vasculitis in patients hospitalized with complex purpura.[27]

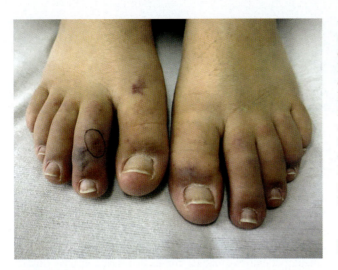

FIGURE 80-1. Purpuric macular lesions on the feet. (From Gammon B, Longmire M, DeClerck B. Intravascular crystal deposition: an early clue to the diagnosis of type 1 cryoglobulinemic vasculitis. *Am J Dermatopathol.* 2014;36:751-755, with permission.)

HISTOPATHOLOGY

Type I CG

Type I CG manifests as thrombo-occlusive vasculopathy (Fig. 80-2). Superficial dermal vessels are occluded by periodic acid Schiff (PAS)-positive homogeneous eosinophilic material. There is no vasculitis, but a scant perivascular lymphocytic infiltrate can be present.[10,14] Rare findings such as LCV, reactive glomeruloid angioendotheliomatosis, and intravascular crystal deposits (Fig. 80-3) have been reported.[10,28,29] Vacuole-like cytoplasmic inclusions were identified in peripheral blood neutrophils, monocytes, lymphocytes, and platelets in CG-associated IgG-κ monoclonal gammopathy.[30] Depending on the patient's hematologic dyscrasia, intravascular thrombi positively stain for either IgG or IgM by direct immunofluorescence (DIF).

Cryocrystalglobulins (CCG) results from the supersaturation of serum paraproteinemic immunoglobulins and is characterized by the deposition of crystallized monoclonal paraprotein within vessels. It is termed CCG if the crystals are cryoprecipitating. CCG is considered a severe variant of CG because it causes more pronounced and rapid end-organ damage than other forms of type 1 CG. CCG aggregate as extracellular crystals; thus, serum cryoglobulins may not be readily detectable in cases of CCG. Clinically, the occlusive vasculopathy resulting in ischemic hypoperfusion manifests as fulminant acute kidney failure, cutaneous necrosis, polyarthralgia, peripheral neuropathy, and gastrointestinal ulceration (Fig. 80-4). The CCG precipitates are visible on light microscopy and are characterized by extracellular oblong, angulated crystals that are eosinophilic, PAS-positive, and exhibit nonbirefringence under polarized light (Fig. 80-5).[31]

Mixed CG

Mixed CG manifests as acute vasculitis, typically in the form of LCV that involves both the superficial and deep dermal vessels. Endothelial swelling, fibrinoid changes of the vessel walls, and leukocytoclasis are the main microscopic findings (Fig. 80-6). The intensity of the inflammatory infiltrate and degree of leukocytoclasis vary and depend on the age of the lesion.[2,25] RBC[32] extravasation and hemosiderin deposits can sometimes be present in chronic lesions. Intravascular hyaline deposits are not typical, but if present, they are seen in the areas of ulceration. Septal panniculitis is another rare association.[33] In a minority of cases, neutrophilic muscular vessel vasculitis (PAN-like) that can coexist with small vessel disease or a lymphocytic small vessel vasculitis is noted.[2] By DIF, the majority of patients will have intravascular immunoglobulins, mostly IgM and/or complement deposits, with less frequent basement membrane zone immunoreactants.

DIFFERENTIAL DIAGNOSIS

Clinically, lesions of CG can resemble perniosis. However, in perniosis, no hyaline vascular thrombi or LCV is noted. A diagnosis of CG is usually based on the presence of the cryoglobulins in the patient's serum. Therefore, when CG is present in the blood and the appropriate clinical and histopathologic findings are noted, a diagnosis of CG can be easily established. Other differential diagnostic considerations include LCV not related to cryoglobulins, where typically a serologic lack of cryoglobulins can help in such distinction. Livedoid vasculopathy (LV) can also histologically mimic CG. In LV, patients often have an underlying vasculopathic disorder, and fibrinoid changes of the vessel walls are characteristically present. The PAS deposits in the lumen of the vessels present in CG are not seen in LV. Drug-induced vasculitis can also be considered in the differential diagnosis. Particularly, levamisole-induced LCV can histologically and clinically mimic CG. A prior history of drug abuse can sometimes be difficult to obtain. Certain connective tissue disorders can also be associated with vasculitis. In particular, many biopsies of lupus erythematosus might display vasculitis. However, the presence of interface changes in such biopsies makes the distinction easier. Churg–Strauss and Wegener granulomatosis are examples of antineutrophil cytoplasmic antibody-positive vasculitis, which can be associated with LCV. However, other accompanying clinical manifestations, such as asthma and tissue eosinophilia (in Churg–Strauss) and lung parenchymal and kidney involvement (in Wegener granulomatosis), can help in the differential diagnosis.

TREATMENT

The treatment in type I CG is aimed toward the underlying hematologic malignancy. Rituximab is often useful in the setting of B-cell lymphoproliferative disorders, but is only of limited value in plasma cell neoplasms. Type II CG therapy targets the use of appropriate antivirals (HCV, HIV), chemotherapy (hematologic dyscrasias), and immune-suppressants (connective tissue disorders).[2,10,25]

CAPSULE SUMMARY

- Cryoglobulins are abnormal immunoglobulins that reversibly precipitate at low temperature.

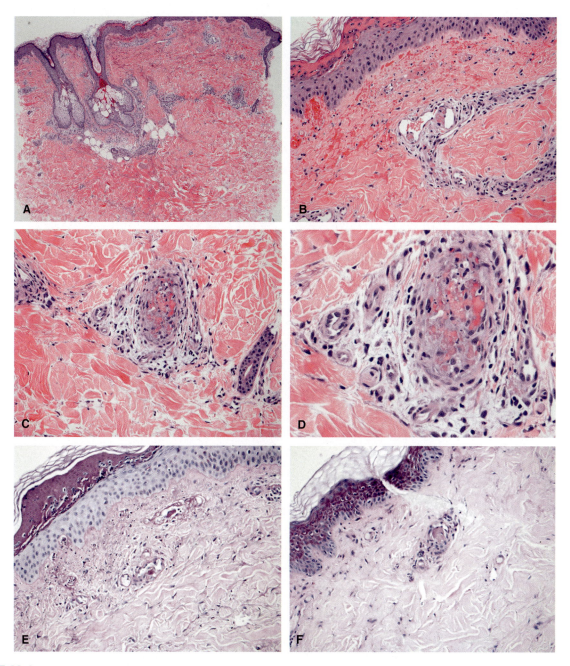

FIGURE 80-2. **Type I CG—Histopathology. A** and **B.** Thrombotic vasculopathy is present with extravasated RBC in the superficial dermis. **C** and **D.** Vessels are filled with hypereosinophilic material. There is minimal perivascular lymphocytic inflammation. **E** and **F.** PAS is positive in the eosinophilic thrombi.

- Two distinct types of cryoglobulins are recognized: monoclonal (type I) and mixed (types II and III).
- Type I CG shows vasculopathy with intravascular immunoglobulin thrombi.
- Type II and III CG manifest as superficial and deep dermal LCV.
- Clinically, the lesions present as purpura, ulcers, and livedo reticularis that are exacerbated with cold.
- Type I CG is associated with hematolymphoid malignancies, whereas type II is most frequently linked to HCV infection and chronic inflammation (autoimmune and connective tissue disorders), and less frequently to hematologic malignancies.

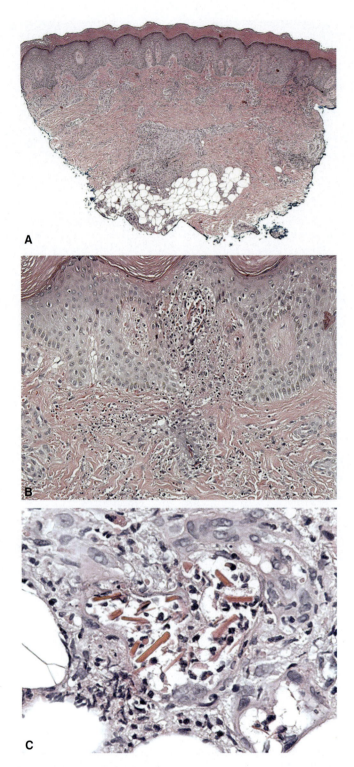

FIGURE 80-3. **Type I CG with intravascular crystals. A–C.** Intravascular rhomboid and rectangular hypereosinophilic crystals. (From Gammon B, Longmire M, DeClerck B. Intravascular crystal deposition: an early clue to the diagnosis of type 1 cryoglobulinemic vasculitis. *Am J Dermatopathol.* 2014;36:751-755, with permission.)

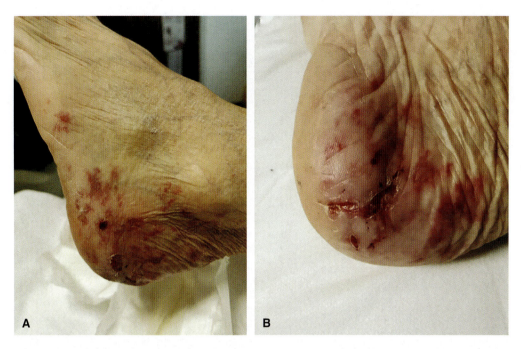

FIGURE 80-4. Crystalcryoglobulinemia. A. Two superficial noninflammatory ulcers with overlying eschar on a background of retiform purpura over the left lateral heel. **B.** Ulcerated fixed retiform purpura over the right medial calcaneus. (From Wee CLP, Lim JHL, Lee JSS. Cryocrystalglobulinemia—an uncommon cutaneous presentation of multiple myeloma and novel finding of transepidermal elimination of crystals. *Am J Dermatopathol*. 2021;43(12):e241-e244. doi:10.1097/DAD.0000000000001944)

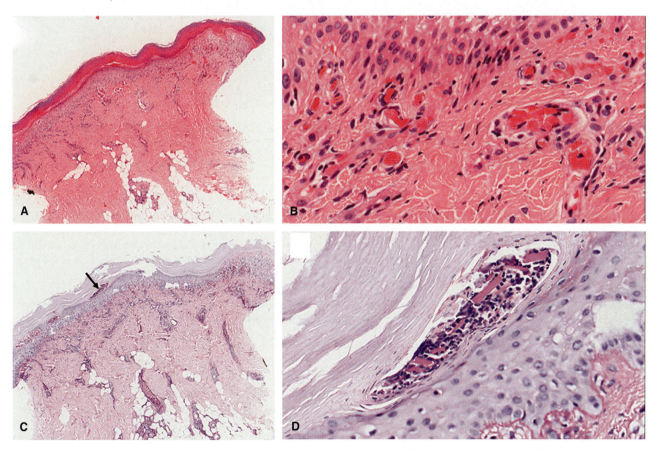

FIGURE 80-5. Crystalcryoglobulinemia. A. Punch biopsy of skin showing occluded superficial dermal blood vessels without significant inflammation (H&E, magnification ×20). **B.** Oblong eosinophilic crystalline structures occluding the lumens of some upper dermal vessels (H&E, magnification ×400). **C.** Scanning magnification showing PAS-positive, diastase-resistant cryocrystalline structures (black arrow) within the stratum corneum following transepidermal elimination (H&E, magnification ×20). **D.** Close-up of the intracorneal cryocrystalline precipitates on PAS-D (H&E, magnification ×400). H&E, hematoxylin and eosin stain. (From Wee CLP, Lim JHL, Lee JSS. Cryocrystalglobulinemia—an uncommon cutaneous presentation of multiple myeloma and novel finding of transepidermal elimination of crystals. *Am J Dermatopathol*. 2021;43(12):e241-e244. doi:10.1097/DAD.0000000000001944)

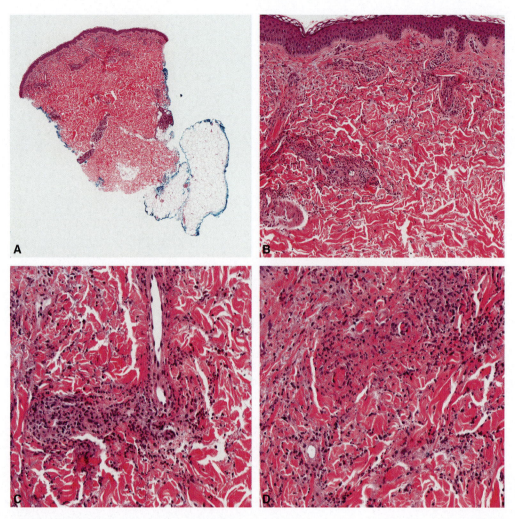

FIGURE 80-6. Type II CG–Histopathology. **A** and **B.** Superficial and perivascular neutrophilic infiltrates are present with associated RBC extravasation. **C** and **D.** Fibrinoid necrosis of dermal vessels and neutrophil fragmentation (leukocytoclasia).

References

1. Bachmeyer C, Wetterwald E, Aractingi S. Cutaneous vasculitis in the course of hematologic malignancies. *Dermatology*. 2005;210:8-14.
2. Carlson JA, Cavaliere LF, Grant-Kels JM. Cutaneous vasculitis: diagnosis and management. *Clin Dermatol*. 2006;24:414-429.
3. Delyon J, Bezier M, Cordoliani F, et al. Cutaneous manifestations revealing cryofibrinogenaemia associated with monoclonal gammopathy. [Article in French]. *Ann Dermatol Venereol*. 2013;140:30-35.
4. Brownell I, Fangman W. Hepatitis C virus infection, type III cryoglobulinemia, and necrotizing vasculitis. *Dermatol Online J*. 2007;13:6.
5. Buob D, Copin MC. Mixed cryoglobulinemia-associated membranoproliferative glomerulonephritis, disclosing gastric MALT lymphoma. [Artice in French]. *Ann Pathol*. 2006;26:267-270.
6. Kagaya M, Takahashi H. A case of type I cryoglobulinemia associated with a monoclonal gammopathy of undetermined significance (MGUS). *J Dermatol*. 2005;32:128-131.
7. Zhang L, Cao XX, Shen KN, et al. Clinical characteristics and treatment outcome of type I cryoglobulinemia in Chinese patients: a single-center study of 45 patients. *Ann Hematol*. 2020;99(8):1735-1740. doi:10.1007/s00277-020-04123-1
8. Payet J, Livartowski J, Kavian N, et al. Type I cryoglobulinemia in multiple myeloma, a rare entity: analysis of clinical and biological characteristics of seven cases and review of the literature. *Leuk Lymphoma*. 2013;54:767-777.
9. Gan C, Howard MD, Mulcahy A, Yazdabadi A. Painful ulcerations: the sole clinical sign of mixed cryoglobulinaemia secondary to marginal zone lymphoma. *BMJ Case Rep*. 2022;15(4):e247780. doi: 10.1136/bcr-2021-247780
10. Harel S, Mohr M, Jahn I, et al. Clinico-biological characteristics and treatment of type I monoclonal cryoglobulinaemia: a study of 64 cases. *Br J Haematol*. 2015;168:671-678.
11. Stone MJ. Waldenstrom's macroglobulinemia: hyperviscosity syndrome and cryoglobulinemia. *Clin Lymphoma Myeloma*. 2009;9:97-99.
12. Zacher NC, Bailey EE, Kwong BY, Rieger KE. Cutaneous reactive angiomatosis associated with intravascular cryoprotein deposition as the presenting finding in a patient with underlying lymphoplasmacytic lymphoma: a case report and review of the literature. *J Cutan Pathol*. 2022;49(2):176-182. doi:10.1111/cup.14144

13. Lacoste C, Duong TA, Dupuis J, et al. Leg ulcer associated with type I cryoglobulinaemia due to incipient B-cell lymphoma. [Article in French]. *Ann Dermatol Venereol.* 2013;140:367-372.
14. den Hollander JG, Swaak AJ. Essential cryoglobulinaemia (type 1) in three patients characterised by Raynaud's phenomenon, arthralgia-arthritis, and skin lesions. *Ann Rheum Dis.* 2002;61:88-89.
15. Perez-Alamino R, Espinoza LR. Non-infectious cryoglobulinemia vasculitis (CryoVas): update on clinical and therapeutic approach. *Curr Rheumatol Rep.* 2014;16:420.
16. Ichinose K, Origuchi T, Tashiro N, et al. An elderly patient with chronic active Epstein–Barr virus infection with mixed cryoglobulinemia and review of the literature. *Mod Rheumatol.* 2013;23:1022-1028.
17. Vitali C. Immunopathologic differences of Sjögren's syndrome versus sicca syndrome in HCV and HIV infection. *Arthritis Res Ther.* 2011;13:233.
18. Shinskii GE, Korobeinikova EA, Kostyreva NI, et al. Cryoglobulinemia in patients with infectious forms of syphilis. [Article in Russian]. *Vestn Dermatol Venerol.* 1973;47:31-34.
19. Thappa DM, Karthikeyan K, Vijaikumar M, et al. Leg ulcers in active lepromatous leprosy associated with cryoglobulinaemia. *Clin Exp Dermatol.* 2002;27:451-453.
20. Relia N, Gokden N, Kulshrestha S, et al. Monoclonal cryoglobulinemia, livedo reticularis, and renal failure. *Kidney Int.* 2012;82:118.
21. Requena L, Kutzner H, Angulo J, et al. Generalized livedo reticularis associated with monoclonal cryoglobulinemia and multiple myeloma. *J Cutan Pathol.* 2007;34:198-202.
22. Tomasini C, Michelerio A, Brazzelli V. Eruptive ulcerative follicular spicules heralding progression of smoldering multiple myeloma. *J Cutan Pathol.* 2019;46(11):844-851. doi:10.1111/cup.13523
23. Lukitsch O, Gebhardt KP, Kövary PM. Follicular hyperkeratosis and cryocrystalglobulinemia syndrome. Occurrence in a patient with multiple myeloma. *Arch Dermatol.* 1985;121(6):795-798.
24. Bork K, Böckers M, Pfeifle J. Pathogenesis of paraneoplastic follicular hyperkeratotic spicules in multiple myeloma. Follicular and epidermal accumulation of IgG dysprotein and cryoglobulin. *Arch Dermatol.* 1990;126(4):509-513.
25. Carlson JA, Chen KR. Cutaneous vasculitis update: small vessel neutrophilic vasculitis syndromes. *Am J Dermatopathol.* 2006;28:486-506.
26. Puerta-Peña M, Agud de Dios M, Fulgencio-Barbarin J, et al. Koebner phenomenon in cryoglobulinemia. *Rheumatology (Oxford).* 2021;60(4):2027-2028. doi:10.1093/rheumatology/keaa528
27. Gehlhausen JR, Wetter DA, Nelson C, et al. A detailed analysis of the distribution, morphology, and histopathology of complex purpura in hospitalized patients: a case series of 68 patients. *J Am Acad Dermatol.* 2021;84(4):1188-1196. doi:10.1016/j.jaad.2020.04.149
28. Liu PY, Prete PE, Kukes G. Leukocytoclastic vasculitis in a patient with type 1 cryoglobulinemia. *Case Rep Rheumatol.* 2011;2011:124940.
29. Gammon B, Longmire M, DeClerck B. Intravascular crystal deposition: an early clue to the diagnosis of type 1 cryoglobulinemic vasculitis. *Am J Dermatopathol.* 2014;36:751-755.
30. Maitra A, Ward PC, Kroft SH, et al. Cytoplasmic inclusions in leukocytes. An unusual manifestation of cryoglobulinemia. *Am J Clin Pathol.* 2000;113:107-112.
31. Wee CLP, Lim JHL, Lee JSS. Cryocrystalglobulinemia—an Uncommon cutaneous presentation of multiple myeloma and Novel finding of transepidermal elimination of crystals. *Am J Dermatopathol.* 2021;43(12):e241-e244. doi:10.1097/DAD.0000000000001944
32. Kolopp-Sarda MN, Miossec P. Cryoglobulinemic vasculitis: pathophysiological mechanisms and diagnosis. *Curr Opin Rheumatol.* 2021;33(1):1-7. doi:10.1097/BOR.0000000000000757
33. Atzeni F, Carrabba M, Davin JC, et al. Skin manifestations in vasculitis and erythema nodosum. *Clin Exp Rheumatol.* 2006;24:S60-S66.

CHAPTER 81

Granulomatous reactions

Zoe O. Brown-Joel and Karolyn A. Wanat

INTRODUCTION

Cutaneous granulomatous inflammation has been reported in association with underlying lymphoproliferative disorders in primarily two patterns: granulomas within or surrounding the cutaneous lymphoma itself and a nonspecific reactive pattern to an underlying systemic or cutaneous lymphoproliferative disease.[1] Similar inflammatory patterns of granulomas have also been described in Hodgkin lymphoma within other organ systems, including lymph nodes, spleen, liver, and bone marrow, and in forms of granulomatous mycosis fungoides.[2,3] The granulomatous response to a cutaneous lymphoma can be prominent, even potentially obscuring the underlying lymphoma.[1] This is hypothesized to be the host defense response to the tumor, but the exact mechanism is unknown. The nonspecific granulomatous inflammation in association with underlying systemic and cutaneous lymphomas could result from a similar immune response.

Granuloma annulare (GA) is a benign, idiopathic, often self-limited granulomatous dermatitis characterized by red, brown, or violaceous papules or plaques that can be annular or polycyclic or more solitary in appearance (Fig. 81-1). GA is most commonly located on the dorsal hands and feet. The eruption may consist of solitary or locally grouped lesions, or it may be a more generalized eruption with lesions on the trunk as well as the extremities. Histopathologic features can comprise a palisaded granulomatous reaction composed of mononuclear histiocytes and multinucleated giant cells surrounding altered collagen, which often has mucinous change, or a diffuse interstitial histiocytic eruption with prominent mucin deposition (Fig. 81-2). The exact, underlying etiology is unknown, but it is thought to be a potentially reactive process to underlying, often unidentified triggers, including diabetes, infections, and malignancies.

Reactive granulomatous dermatitis (RGD) is a recently coined term that encompasses the clinical and histopathologic patterns including palisaded neutrophilic and granulomatous dermatitis (PNGD) and interstitial granulomatous dermatitis (IGD) due to overlapping features. They are also benign, idiopathic granulomatous dermatitides. Clinically PNGD presents with skin-tone to red papules, often distributed symmetrically on the extremities. Histopathological features of PNGD include neutrophilic inflammation, leukocytoclastic vasculitis, karyorrhexis, palisading histiocytes, granulomas, and foci of degenerated collagen. Mucin deposition is not prominent. IGD presents with red to violaceous patches and plaques to linear subcutaneous cords, which are typically found on the upper body or proximal extremities. Histopathologically, IGD displays histiocytes clustered around foci of degenerating collagen. Vasculitis and mucin deposition are not common. The RGD disorders generally develop in the setting of systemic disease and are associated with connective tissue diseases, inflammatory arthritides, and malignancies.[4]

Although evidence for causation is lacking, GA and other granulomatous disorders have been reported in association with neoplasms, including solid organ and visceral cancers.[5-7] Granulomatous dermatitis has also been reported in association with hematolymphoproliferative malignancies, which will be the focus of the remainder of this chapter.

Although GA is a relatively common disease, affecting up to 0.4% of patients who present to dermatology,[8] only a small number of these patients have been reported to develop an underlying hematologic malignancy, and the exact incidence is difficult to calculate secondary to the rarity. GA-like eruptions have been in association with several types of underlying lymphoproliferative disorders, both at the primary site of the malignancy and with the GA occurring at sites distant from the malignancy itself. The largest report by Barksdale et al[9] reported 13 cases of GA with lymphoma. In this report, GA-like lesions occurred in association with Hodgkin disease in three cases. Other than Hodgkin disease, there were three cases of follicular lymphoma, three cases of small lymphocytic lymphoma/chronic lymphocytic lymphoma, three cases of diffuse lymphoma, and one case of Sézary syndrome.[9] The GA eruptions were reported over a wide range of time in association with the malignancy, ranging from 5 years before the diagnosis to 27 years after the diagnosis. The histopathologic features of GA were typical in nature and indistinguishable from other lesions of GA; however, painful lesions and lesions in unusual locations such as the palms, soles, and face were frequently reported in this series.[9] A variety of GA lesions have been reported in association with Hodgkin disease with different morphologies including widespread near-erythrodermic disease, subcutaneous GA, and GA occurring within scars from prior herpes zoster infection, which can occur in nonmalignancy-associated GA as well.[3,10-16]

Cutaneous granulomatous reactions have also been reported in association with several other types of lymphoproliferative diseases. Some of the most commonly reported

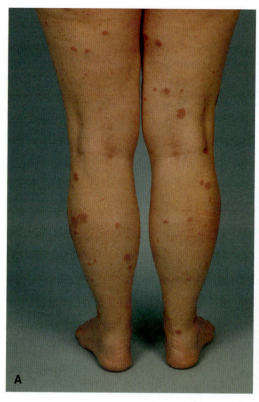
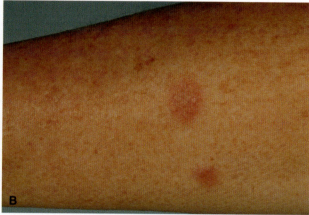

FIGURE 81-1. Clinical appearance of GA in a patient with underlying chronic lymphocytic leukemia. **A** and **B.** The clinical appearance can be indistinguishable from GA with reddish-violaceous plaques. Atypical presentations that include pain; involvement of the face, palms, and soles; and widespread lesions should prompt clinicians to consider an underlying malignancy.

malignancies include acute myelocytic leukemia (AML), myelodysplastic syndrome (in some cases, progressing to AML), chronic myelomonocytic leukemia, and adult T-cell lymphoma.[17-25] Recent reports have also described granulomatous reactions in the setting of polycythemia vera and essential thrombocythemia.[26,27] The histopathologic features of these granulomatous reaction patterns include pathology suggestive of GA, PNGD, granulomatous panniculitis, annular elastolytic giant cell granuloma, nonspecific granulomatous dermatitis, interstitial granulomatous dermatitis, erythema nodosum, and papular sarcoidosis, demonstrating the histopathologic variation that can occur and suggesting that the range of cutaneous granulomatous responses seen is nonspecific and the entities may have significant overlap.[18,19,21,24,25,28-32]

Although the association of granulomatous disease with Hodgkin lymphoma and T-cell lymphomas has been more widely reported, its presentation with other B-cell lymphomas has also occurred. Granulomatous lesions in association with B-cell marginal zone lymphoma, non-Hodgkin lymphoma, diffuse large B-cell lymphoma, chronic lymphocytic leukemia, and mucosal-associated lymphoid tissue lymphoma have also been reported both within the same lesion and at distant sites.[33-39] Granulomatous disorders in association with extracutaneous lymphoma was thought to be the most common presentation,[38,39] but there are more recent reports of coexistent cutaneous granulomatous lesions and lymphoma.[33,34,36,37,40,41] In some cases, the PET-CT imaging highlighted both the cutaneous granulomatous lesions as well as underlying malignancies.[10,35,37] Several authors question whether the cutaneous manifestations represent a primary form of lymphoma/leukemia cutis because atypical cells can appear within the lesion or whether the cutaneous manifestations merely represent a secondary reaction to the underlying lymphoma.

Granulomatous dermatitis and lesions can occur before, after, or concomitantly with the lymphoproliferative disorder.[9,21,28,29,40,42-45] Because of this and occasional lack of response of the granulomatous inflammation when the lymphoma is treated, several authors speculate that the association between these diseases may be random. A recent case control study assessing malignancy prevalence in generalized GA did not find an association and felt development of both conditions may rather be a factor of the patient's age.[46] Given the lack of understanding of the etiopathogenesis of most of these granulomatous reactions when they occur de novo, the strength of the association between these reactions and the underlying malignancies is unclear. Other granulomatous reactions have stronger associations with underlying malignancies, such as necrobiotic xanthogranuloma, in which case the absence of a lymphoproliferative disorder often is atypical. Whether there is prognostic significance to the presence of granulomatous disease is also unclear. In some cases of myelodysplastic syndrome, leukemic transformation was preceded by new development or worsening of granulomatous disease.[17,21,23,26,47]

Even though the association between GA and underlying malignancies has not been shown to be causative, clinicians should consider evaluating patients for potential underlying malignancies in patients presenting with atypical features of GA or other unusual granulomatous dermatitis. Elderly patients with new-onset GA-like lesions or granulomatous dermatitis, painful lesions, atypical-appearing lesions, and

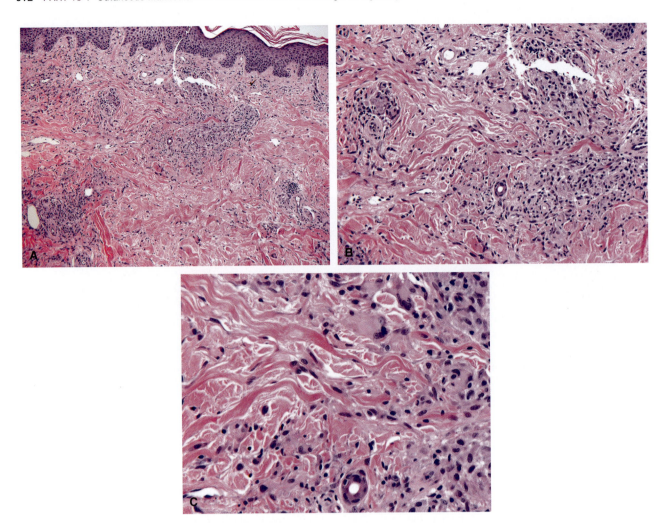

FIGURE 81-2. Histopathologic appearance of GA. **A** and **B** (H&E, 10× and 20×, respectively). Palisaded granulomas composed of histiocytes surrounding mucinous degeneration of collagen are typical of GA. **C.** (H&E, 40×). Higher magnification highlights both mononuclear histiocytes and occasional multinucleated giant cells.

extensive involvement including involvement of the face, palms, or soles should prompt further evaluation.[9,17] In addition, when the disease is explosive in onset or particularly recalcitrant to treatment with continued extensive involvement, clinicians should consider evaluation for underlying malignancy.[9,17]

References

1. Gallardo F, García-Muret MP, Servitje O, et al. Cutaneous lymphomas showing prominent granulomatous component: clinicopathological features in a series of 16 cases. *J Eur Acad Dermatol Venereol*. 2009;23(6):639-647.
2. Choe JK, Hyun BH, Salazar GH, Ashton JK, Sung CY. Epithelioid granulomas of the bone marrow in non-Hodgkin's lymphoproliferative malignancies. *Am J Clin Pathol*. 1984;81(1):19-24.
3. Sacks EL, Donaldson SS, Gordon J, Dorfman RF. Epithelioid granulomas associated with Hodgkin's disease: clinical correlations in 55 previously untreated patients. *Cancer*. 1978;41(2):562-567.
4. Rosenbach M, English JCIIIrd. Reactive granulomatous dermatitis: a review of palisaded neutrophilic and granulomatous dermatitis, interstitial granulomatous dermatitis, interstitial granulomatous drug reaction, and a proposed reclassification. *Dermatol Clin*. 2015;33(3):373-387.
5. Shimizu S, Yasui C, Tsuchiya K. Atypical generalized granuloma annulare associated with two visceral cancers. *J Am Acad Dermatol*. 2006;54(5 suppl):S236-S238.
6. Thomas DJ, Rademaker M, Munro DD, Levison DA, Besser GM. Visceral and skin granuloma annulare, diabetes, and polyendocrine disease. *Br Med J*. 1986;293(6553):977-978.
7. Li JY, Pulitzer MP, Myskowski PL, et al. A case-control study of clinicopathologic features, prognosis, and therapeutic responses in patients with granulomatous mycosis fungoides. *J Am Acad Dermatol*. 2013;69(3):366-374.
8. Muhlbauer JE. Granuloma annulare. *J Am Acad Dermatol*. 1980;3(3):217-230.
9. Barksdale SK, Perniciaro C, Halling KC, Strickler JG. Granuloma annulare in patients with malignant lymphoma: clinicopathologic study of thirteen new cases. *J Am Acad Dermatol*. 1994;31(1):42-48.
10. Dadban A, Slama B, Azzedine A, Lepeu G. Widespread granuloma annulare and Hodgkin's disease. *Clin Exp Dermatol*. 2008;33(4):465-468.
11. Harman RR. Hodgkin's disease, seminoma of testicle and widespread granuloma annulare. *Br J Dermatol*. 1977;97(suppl 15):50-51.
12. Miyamoto T, Mihara M. Subcutaneous granuloma annulare with Hodgkin's disease. *J Dermatol*. 1996;23(6):405-407.

13. Nevo S, Drakos P, Goldenhersh MA, et al. Generalized granuloma annulare post autologous bone marrow transplantation in a Hodgkin's disease patient. *Bone Marrow Transplant.* 1994;14(4):631-633.
14. Sanli HE, Koçyiğit P, Arica E, Kurtyüksel M, Heper AO, Ozcan M. Granuloma annulare on herpes zoster scars in a Hodgkin's disease patient following autologous peripheral stem cell transplantation. *J Eur Acad Dermatol Venereol.* 2006;20(3):314-317.
15. Schwartz RA, Hansen RC, Lynch PJ. Hodgkin's disease and granuloma annulare. *Arch Dermatol.* 1981;117(3):185-186.
16. Setoyama M, Kerdel FA, Byrnes JJ, Kanzaki T. Granuloma annulare associated with Hodgkin's disease. *Int J Dermatol.* 1997;36(6):445-448.
17. Balin SJ, Wetter DA, Kurtin PJ, Letendre L, Pittelkow MR. Myelodysplastic syndrome presenting as generalized granulomatous dermatitis. *Arch Dermatol.* 2011;147(3):331-335.
18. Hinckley MR, Walsh SN, Molnár I, Sheehan DJ, Sangueza OP, Yosipovitch G. Generalized granuloma annulare as an initial manifestation of chronic myelomonocytic leukemia: a report of 2 cases. *Am J Dermatopathol.* 2008;30(3):274-277.
19. Horiuchi Y, Masuzawa M, Nozaki O, Shibahara N, Shiga T, Yoshida M. Unusual cutaneous lesions associated with chronic myelomonocytic leukaemia. *Clin Exp Dermatol.* 1992;17(2):121-124.
20. Bolla G, Lambert M, Boscagli A, et al. Erythema nodosum revealing chronic myelomonocytic leukemia: two cases. [Article in French]. *Rev Med Interne.* 1998;19(11):838-839.
21. Cornejo KM, Lum CA, Izumi AK. A cutaneous interstitial granulomatous dermatitis-like eruption arising in myelodysplasia with leukemic progression. *Am J Dermatopathol.* 2013;35(2):e26-29.
22. Jee MS, Kim ES, Chang SE, Lee MW, Koh JK. Disseminated granuloma annulare associated with chronic myelogenous leukemia. *J Dermatol.* 2003;30(8):631-633.
23. Katz KA. Disseminated cutaneous granulomatous eruption occurring in the setting of myelodysplasia. *Dermatol Online J.* 2003;9(4):22.
24. Vestey JP, Turner M, Biddlestone L, McLaren K, Goulden N, Hunter JA. Disseminated cutaneous granulomatous eruptions associated with myelodysplastic syndrome and acute myeloid leukaemia. *Clin Exp Dermatol.* 1993;18(6):559-563.
25. Kawakami T, Kawanabe T, Soma Y. Granuloma annulare-like skin lesions as an initial manifestation in a Japanese patient with adult T-cell leukemia/lymphoma. *J Am Acad Dermatol.* 2009;60(5):848-852.
26. Lozano-Masdemont B, Baniandrés-Rodríguez O, Parra-Blanco V, Suárez-Fernández R. Granulomatous dermatitis as a cutaneous manifestation of hematologic disorders: the first case associated with polycythemia vera and a new case associated with myelodysplasia. *Actas Dermosifiliogr.* 2016;107(5):e27-32.
27. Polineni SP, Lawyer S. Generalized granuloma annulare associated with essential thrombocythemia. *Clin Case Rep.* 2020;8(6):1065-1068.
28. Pei S, Hinshaw MA. Palisaded neutrophilic granulomatous dermatitis leading to diagnosis of Hodgkin lymphoma: report of rare case and literature review of paraneoplastic granulomatous dermatitides. *Am J Dermatopathol.* 2019;41(11):835-845.
29. Deen J, Banney L, Perry-Keene J. Palisading neutrophilic and granulomatous dermatitis as a presentation of Hodgkin lymphoma: a case and review. *J Cutan Pathol.* 2018;45(2):167-170.
30. Lee C, Hsi A, Lazova R. Subcutaneous panniculitis-like T-cell lymphoma with granulomas as the predominant feature. *Am J Dermatopathol.* 2019;41(9):667-670.
31. Anan T, Imamura T, Yokoyama S, Fujiwara S. Erythema nodosum and granulomatous lesions preceding acute myelomonocytic leukemia. *J Dermatol.* 2004;31(9):741-747.
32. Garg A, Kundu RV, Plotkin O, Aronson IK. Annular elastolytic giant cell granuloma heralding onset and recurrence of acute myelogenous leukemia. *Arch Dermatol.* 2006;142(4):532-533.
33. Fukumoto T, Nagai H, Ichikawa H, Yakusijin K, Nishigori C. Cutaneous granulomatous lesions in a patient with mucosa-associated lymphoid tissue (MALT) lymphoma. *Australas J Dermatol.* 2019;60(3):e240-e242.
34. Fullen DR, Jacobson SN, Valdez R, Novice FM, Lowe L. Granuloma annulare-like infiltrates with concomitant cutaneous involvement by B-cell non-Hodgkin's lymphoma: report of a case. *Am J Dermatopathol.* 2003;25(1):57-61.
35. Shindo M, Yoshida Y, Yamamoto O. Granuloma annulare detected by positron emission tomography with computed tomography in a diffuse large B cell lymphoma. *Eur J Dermatol.* 2009;19(2):174-175.
36. Sokumbi O, Gibson LE, Comfere NI, Peters MS. Granuloma annulare-like eruption associated with B-cell chronic lymphocytic leukemia. *J Cutan Pathol.* 2012;39(11):996-1003.
37. Wanat KA, Elenitsas R, Kim EJ, Rosenbach M. Granuloma annulare associated with cutaneous marginal zone lymphoma: a case linking a hematologic malignancy with granulomatous dermatitis. *Am J Dermatopathol.* 2012;34(8):844-846.
38. Duparc A, Canonne-Courivaud D, Rose C, Creusy C, Modiano P. A pseudotumoral cutaneous form of sarcoidosis associated with non-Hodgkin lymphoma. [Article in French]. *Ann Dermatol Venereol.* 2009;136(6-7):518-521.
39. Randle HW, Banks PM, Winkelmann RK. Cutaneous granulomas in malignant lymphoma. *Arch Dermatol.* 1980;116(4):441-443.
40. Riaz IB, Kamal MU, Segal RJ, Anwer F. First reported association of chronic lymphocytic leukaemia and interstitial granulomatous dermatitis. *BMJ Case Rep.* 2016;2016:bcr2016215108.
41. Fujimoto N, Takahashi T, Yamashita M, Nakanishi G, Okabe H, Tanaka T. Extranodal natural killer/T-cell lymphoma, nasal type, with prominent granulomatous reaction. *J Dermatol.* 2014;41(1):68-69.
42. Choi MJ, Shin D, Kim YC, Oh SH, Kim M. Interstitial granulomatous dermatitis with arthritis accompanied by anaplastic large cell lymphoma. *J Dermatol.* 2014;41(4):363-364.
43. Federmann B, Bonzheim I, Yazdi AS, Schmidt J, Fend F, Metzler G. Generalized palisaded neutrophilic and granulomatous dermatitis—a cutaneous manifestation of chronic myelomonocytic leukemia? A clinical, histopathological, and molecular study of 3 cases. *Hum Pathol.* 2017;64:198-206.
44. Kohlmann J, Schüürmann M, Simon JC, Treudler R. Palisaded neutrophilic and granulomatous dermatitis in a patient with chronic myelomonocytic leukaemia. *J Eur Acad Dermatol Venereol.* 2019;33(6):e241-e242.
45. Patsinakidis N, Susok L, Hessam S, et al. Interstitial granulomatous dermatitis associated with myelodysplastic syndrome—complete clearance under therapy with 5-azacytidine. *Acta Derm Venereol.* 2014;94(6):725-726.
46. Gabaldón VH, Haro-González-Vico V. Lack of an association between generalized granuloma annulare and malignancy: a case-control study. *J Am Acad Dermatol.* 2019;80(6):1799-1800.
47. Aung PP, Bowker B, Masterpol KS, Mahalingam M. Disseminated noninterstitial granulomatous dermatitis as a cutaneous manifestation of the preleukemic state in a patient with myelodysplasia and ulcerative colitis—apropos a case and review of the literature. *Am J Dermatopathol.* 2014;36(7):e117-120.

Pyoderma gangrenosum

Campbell L. Stewart and Roberto Novoa

DEFINITION

Pyoderma gangrenosum (PG) is a rare, ulcerative cutaneous disease of unknown etiology. Its diagnosis critically relies upon the exclusion of other causes of cutaneous ulcers, including infection, malignancy, vasculitis, connective tissue disease, diabetes, and trauma. A third of patients with PG develop new cutaneous ulcers secondary to external trauma to the skin (pathergy). Besides the skin, other organ systems might be also involved, including the lungs, central nervous system, heart, gastrointestinal system, liver, spleen, and lymph nodes. About 50% of the patients have an associated condition such as inflammatory bowel disease, rheumatoid arthritis, or hematologic malignancy.

CLINICAL FEATURES

PG is characterized by the rapid appearance of sterile pustules, tender erythematous nodules, or, rarely, bullae. These primary lesions degrade into a markedly painful ulcer with characteristic undermined, violaceous borders (Fig. 82-1), which may heal with cribriform scarring.[1,2] Multiple ulcers can occur, especially in chronic cases.[3] It most commonly occurs on the lower extremities or trunk, but involvement of the hands, feet, genitalia, and peristomal skin has been reported.[3,4] Adults are much more commonly affected than children, and in certain studies, females are more commonly affected than males.[3] PG is clinically classified into four different subtypes, including ulcerative, pustular, bullous, and vegetative.[5]

EPIDEMIOLOGY

Approximately 1 in 100,000 persons are affected with PG each year in the United States. All ages and both sexes can be affected, but the peak disease incidence occurs in the fourth and fifth decades of life, with a slight female predominance. Only 3% to 4% of cases occur in children.

ETIOLOGY

The exact cause of PG has not been determined. It is likely that PG results from a dysregulation of the immune system and an abnormal wound healing response. In contrast to normal healing wounds, matrix metalloproteinases (MMPs)-9 and -10 as well as tumor necrosis factor-alpha (TNF-α) are upregulated in the stroma of PG lesions. In addition, MMP-1 and -26, which are present in normal healing epithelium, are greatly diminished in PG.[6] Interleukin-8 (IL-8), a chemotactic and activating agent for neutrophils, is also produced at abnormal levels by lesional fibroblasts in patients with PG, who also have elevated levels of serum IL-8. It has been proposed that PG is a clinical reaction to excess, inappropriately secreted circulating IL-8, particularly in the setting of hematologic malignancy.[7] However, abnormalities in chemokines such as TNF-α and IL-8 are not specific to PG.[8,9] In rare heritable autoinflammatory diseases such as pyogenic sterile arthritis, pyoderma gangrenosum, and acne (PAPA) syndrome, defects in PSTPIP-1 appear to increase phosphorylation and pyrin binding, leading to increased activation of the inflammasome.[10]

HISTOLOGIC FEATURES

The histopathologic features of PG are nonspecific and can vary depending on the stage of the lesion as well as the clinical subtype. In ulcerative PG, there is typically central neutrophilic abscess formation (Fig. 82-2A) as well as a variable distal angiocentric lymphocytic inflammatory infiltrate. Pustular PG is characterized by a subcorneal pustule, with a perifollicular neutrophilic infiltrate or a dense dermal neutrophilic infiltrate with subepidermal edema. In bullous lesions, there is subepidermal bulla formation, intraepidermal vesiculation, and a variable dermal neutrophilic infiltrate. The vegetative form of PG demonstrates pseudoepitheliomatous hyperplasia, dermal neutrophilic abscess formation, sinus tracts, and a palisading granulomatous reaction.[5] Varying degrees of leukocytoclastic vasculitis may be seen (Fig. 82-2B).[11] While a biopsy of a PG lesion cannot give a definitive diagnosis, inspection for features consistent with PG, as well as negative stains for microorganisms, can help lead to the diagnosis. Generally, in spite of the risk of pathergy, a skin biopsy for histology and a tissue culture are recommended to diagnose PG.[5]

ASSOCIATED CONDITIONS

PG is not related to a single disease, and in approximately 50% of cases, it is idiopathic. The remaining 50% of cases are mostly associated with inflammatory bowel diseases (30%),

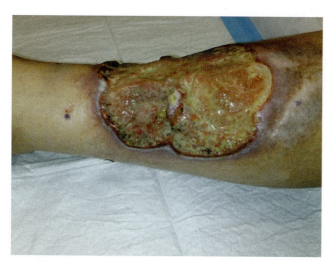

FIGURE 82-1. Pyoderma gangrenosum in a patient with myelodysplastic syndrome. Rapidly evolving, sharply demarcated ulcer on the lower leg with undermined, violaceous border.

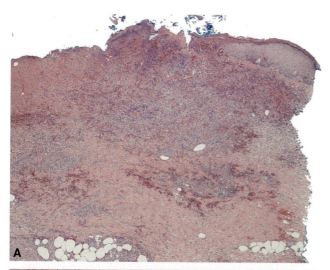

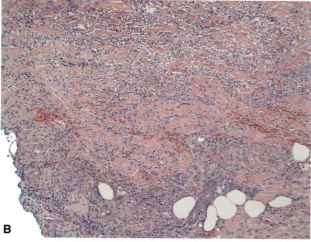

FIGURE 82-2. Histopathology of pyoderma gangrenosum. A. A fibrin-covered ulcer overlies a dense interstitial and perivascular neutrophilic infiltrate (40×). **B.** Leukocytoclastic vasculitis can be seen (100×).

rheumatoid arthritis (10%), and hematologic malignancy (10%).[3,5] Some cases of PG have been associated with more common conditions such as anemia, diabetes mellitus, and metabolic syndrome, as well as thyroid disorders.[1] The most commonly associated hematologic malignancies include acute myelogenous leukemia (AML), chronic myelogenous leukemia, and myeloma.[12,13] PG is also frequently associated with hematologic abnormalities such as myelodysplastic syndrome, monoclonal gammopathies (most commonly IgA), and polycythemia vera.[2] Other reported conditions include Waldenstrom macroglobulinemia, Hodgkin and non-Hodgkin lymphomas, solid malignancies such as carcinoid, as well as colon, breast, and bladder.[2,5,14]

The bullous form of PG is commonly linked with hematologic malignancies, most often a leukemic or preleukemic state.[15] Roughly half to two-thirds of patients with malignancy-associated PG develop the bullous form. Nearly 70% of all bullous PG are related to AML (FAB M2 subtype).[16] Bullous PG can share clinical features with bullous Sweet syndrome, and these two neutrophilic dermatoses may represent different points on a spectrum of disease. Generally, bullous PG portends a poor prognosis for patients with hematologic malignancy, and the development of the bullous lesions often correlates with disease progression or malignant transformation of indolent disease. Patients with bullous PG may also develop neutrophilic infiltrates of their internal organs including the heart and lungs.[17-19] Leukemic cells have rarely been reported in bullous PG lesions; however, their presence may be incidental and not causative.[16]

DIFFERENTIAL DIAGNOSIS

Since the clinical and histologic presentations are nonspecific, the differential diagnosis for PG is extensive and includes halogenodermas, systemic vasculitides, factitial disease, antiphospholipid syndrome, spider bites, cutaneous involvement of malignancy, drug-induced ulcers, and infections related to bacteria, mycobacteria, viruses, or invasive fungi.[5,20] Given the immunosuppressive agents required to treat PG, infectious causes must be excluded before making this diagnosis.

Diagnostic criteria have been proposed and include major and minor criteria. To make a confident diagnosis of PG, both major and at least two minor criteria are required. The major criteria are (1) a rapid progression of a painful, necrolytic cutaneous ulcer with an irregular, violaceous, and undermined border and (2) the exclusion of other potential causes of cutaneous ulceration. The minor criteria are (1) history suggestive of pathergy or clinical finding of cribriform scarring, (2) systemic diseases associated with PG, (3) histopathologic findings compatible with PG (sterile dermal neutrophilia, ± mixed inflammation, ± lymphocytic vasculitis), and (4) treatment response (rapid response to systemic corticosteroids).[11]

PG can easily be mistaken for necrotizing fasciitis and is often debrided if not properly diagnosed. This potential for misdiagnosis is a serious issue, as approximately 30% of PG cases exhibit pathergy. Debridement of a PG lesion can therefore result in large tissue defects, including loss of digits and/or limbs.[3,4] The course of PG can be acute, chronic, or relapsing. If PG is relapsing or chronic, workup for an associated condition should be performed.[21]

TREATMENT

Treatment for PG is challenging. For limited disease, treatment with dapsone or sulfapyridine can be effective.[11] For extensive disease, immunosuppressive agents are the most effective form of therapy. Corticosteroids and cyclosporine are the most common treatments. Other immunosuppressive agents include tacrolimus, azathioprine, and the antimetabolites.[11] Biologic agents, including TNF-α inhibitors, anti-IL-17 antibodies, and anti-IL-12/23 antibodies, have been used with some efficacy.[22-25] Intravenous immunoglobulin has also found recent success.[26] Patients with worsening disease in spite of immunosuppression may need repeat biopsies and wound cultures, as life-threatening superinfections of PG ulcers can occur. Patients with PG requiring inpatient admission generally have poorer outcomes, with long hospital stays, high rate of mortality, and high recurrence rates.[23]

References

1. Al Ghazal P, Herberger K, Schaller J, et al. Associated factors and comorbidities in patients with pyoderma gangrenosum in Germany: a retrospective multicentric analysis in 259 patients. *Orphanet J Rare Dis*. 2013;8:136.
2. Powell FC, Schroeter AL, Su WP, et al. Pyoderma gangrenosum and monoclonal gammopathy. *Arch Dermatol*. 1983;119(6):468-472.
3. Binus AM, Qureshi AA, Li VW, et al. Pyoderma gangrenosum: a retrospective review of patient characteristics, comorbidities and therapy in 103 patients. *Br J Dermatol*. 2011;165(6):1244-1250.
4. Barr KL, Chhatwal HK, Wesson SK, et al. Pyoderma gangrenosum masquerading as necrotizing fasciitis. *Am J Otolaryngol*. 2009;30(4):273-276.
5. Powell FC, Su WP, Perry HO, et al. Pyoderma gangrenosum: classification and management. *J Am Acad Dermatol*. 1996;34(3):395-409; quiz 410-412.
6. Bister V, Mäkitalo L, Jeskanen L, et al. Expression of MMP-9, MMP-10 and TNF-alpha and lack of epithelial MMP-1 and MMP-26 characterize pyoderma gangrenosum. *J Cutan Pathol*. 2007;34(12):889-898.
7. Saito S, Yasui K, Hosoda W, et al. CD30+ anaplastic large cell lymphoma complicated by pyoderma gangrenosum with increased levels of serum cytokines. *Eur J Haematol*. 2006;77(3):251-254.
8. Oka M. Pyoderma gangrenosum and interleukin 8. *Br J Dermatol*. 2007;157(6):1279-1281.
9. Oka M, Berking C, Nesbit M, et al. Interleukin-8 overexpression is present in pyoderma gangrenosum ulcers and leads to ulcer formation in human skin xenografts. *Lab Invest*. 2000;80(4):595-604.
10. Boursier G, Piram M, Rittore C, Sarrabay G, Touitou I. Phenotypic associations of PSTPIP1 sequence variants in PSTPIP1-associated autoinflammatory diseases. *J Invest Dermatol*. 2021;141(5):1141-1147. doi:10.1016/j.jid.2020.08.028
11. Su WP, Davis MD, Weenig RH, et al. Pyoderma gangrenosum: clinicopathologic correlation and proposed diagnostic criteria. *Int J Dermatol*. 2004;43(11):790-800.
12. Sakiyama M, Kobayashi T, Nagata Y, et al. Bullous pyoderma gangrenosum: a case report and review of the published work. *J Dermatol*. 2012;39(12):1010-1015.
13. Jacobs P, Palmer S, Gordon-Smith EC. Pyoderma gangrenosum in myelodysplasia and acute leukaemia. *Postgrad Med J*. 1985;61(718):689-694.
14. Bennett ML, Jackson JM, Jorizzo JL, et al. Pyoderma gangrenosum. A comparison of typical and atypical forms with an emphasis on time to remission. Case review of 86 patients from 2 institutions. *Medicine (Baltimore)*. 2000;79(1):37-46.
15. Perry HO, Winkelmann RK. Bullous pyoderma gangrenosum and leukemia. *Arch Dermatol*. 1972;106(6):901-905.
16. Rafael MR, Fernandes CM, Machado JM, et al. Pyoderma gangrenosum or leukaemia cutis? *J Eur Acad Dermatol Venereol*. 2003;17(4):449-451.
17. Caughman W, Stern R, Haynes H. Neutrophilic dermatosis of myeloproliferative disorders. Atypical forms of pyoderma gangrenosum and Sweet's syndrome associated with myeloproliferative disorders. *J Am Acad Dermatol*. 1983;9(5):751-758.
18. Koester G, Tarnower A, Levisohn D, et al. Bullous pyoderma gangrenosum. *J Am Acad Dermatol*. 1993;29(5, pt. 2):875-878.
19. Fox LP, Geyer AS, Husain S, et al. Bullous pyoderma gangrenosum as the presenting sign of fatal acute myelogenous leukemia. *Leuk Lymphoma*. 2006;47(1):147-150.
20. Weenig RH, Davis MD, Dahl PR, et al. Skin ulcers misdiagnosed as pyoderma gangrenosum. *N Engl J Med*. 2002;347(18):1412-1418.
21. Callen JP, Jackson JM. Pyoderma gangrenosum: an update. *Rheum Dis Clin North Am*. 2007;33(4):787-802, (vi).
22. Brooklyn TN, Dunnill MG, Shetty A, et al. Infliximab for the treatment of pyoderma gangrenosum: a randomised, double blind, placebo controlled trial. *Gut*. 2006;55(4):505-509.
23. Ye MJ, Ye JM. Pyoderma gangrenosum: a review of clinical features and outcomes of 23 cases requiring inpatient management. *Dermatol Res Pract*. 2014;2014:461467.
24. Westerdahl JS, Nusbaum KB, Chung CG, Kaffenberger BH, Ortega-Loayza AG. Ustekinumab as adjuvant treatment for all pyoderma gangrenosum subtypes. *J Dermatol Treat*. Published online June 14, 2021;1-5. doi:10.1080/09546634.2021.1937475
25. Molinelli E, Brisigotti V, Paolinelli M, Offidani A. Novel therapeutic approaches and targets for the treatment of neutrophilic dermatoses, management of patients with neutrophilic dermatoses and future directions in the era of biologic treatment. *Curr Pharmaceut Biotechnol*. 2021;22(1):46-58. doi:10.2174/1389201021666200503050803
26. Song H, Lahood N, Mostaghimi A. Intravenous immunoglobulin as adjunct therapy for refractory pyoderma gangrenosum: systematic review of cases and case series. *Br J Dermatol*. 2018;178(2):363-368. doi:10.1111/bjd.15850

CHAPTER 83

Schnitzler syndrome

Viktoryia Kazlouskaya and Jacqueline M. Junkins-Hopkins

INTRODUCTION

Schnitzler syndrome (SchS) is a rare chronic autoinflammatory multisystem disorder characterized, at least, by a chronic urticarial eruption and a monoclonal gammopathy. The diagnosis is often delayed and may require up to 5 years of follow-up.[1] Other multisystem disorders must also be excluded, such as hematologic, infectious, and similar inflammatory/autoinflammatory disorders. Diagnostic criteria developed by Lipsker et al are most often used to establish the diagnosis of SchS and have recently been validated and found to have a sensitivity and specificity of 100% and 97%, respectively.[1,2] The two major criteria, chronic/recurrent urticarial rash and monoclonal IgM gammopathy, are nearly always present, and the gammopathy helps discriminate this from similar inflammatory conditions, such as cryopyrin-associated periodic syndrome (CAPS).[2] More detailed criteria, developed by an expert group and known as Strasbourg criteria, allow a monoclonal IgG component and include biopsy criteria of neutrophilic urticarial dermatosis (NUD) (Table 83-1).[3] Rare cases of alleged SchS without monoclonal gammopathy have been reported.[4,5] In such instances, one must exclude other anti-IL therapy responsive autoinflammatory syndromes with similar symptoms but lacking gammopathy. Owing to a delay in the monoclonal gammopathy that can span many years, as well as, at times, trace monoclonal components that may escape detection without immunofixation, it is conceivable that other criteria for SchS may be fulfilled prior to a diagnosis of monoclonal gammopathy.[2,6] Biclonal gammopathies with IgM and IgA are also known.[7]

The male-to-female ratio is around 3:1, and mean age of onset of approximately 51 to 57 years.[2,3] Inflammation in SchS is mediated by interleukin (IL)-1β, tumor necrosis factor alfa (TNFα), and IL-6, as highlighted by a dramatic response to treatment with human interleukin-1 receptor antagonist (IL-1Ra) (anakinra), anti-Ilβ (canakinumab), and in some instances anti-IL6 antibody (tocilizumab).[8-10] Circulating mononuclear cells release increased amounts of IL-1β, even in the absence of elevated levels of IL-1.[9,11] IL-18 may participate in regulating IL-1 activity.[12,13] T-cell cytokine dysfunction representing a unique SchS cytokine signature has been described, with decreased levels of Th1, Th2, and Th17 cytokines and diminished IL10 cytokine levels.[9] Levels of CCL2 cytokine are elevated in SchS and correlate with the disease activity.[14] Hypotheses regarding possible genetic mutations have also been put forth.[15,16] Although mutation of *leucin-rich family (NLR), pyrin containing 3 gene (NLRP3)* V198M variant may be found in some SchS patients, similar to patients with CAPS, next-generation sequencing failed to show significant NLRP3 mutations in a series of patients with SchS.[17-19] Instead, activating *MYD88 L265P* mutations were detected in one-third patients with SchS, suggesting a pathogenic as well as possible diagnostic role.[19] The NF-κβ pathway can be activated by gain-of-function mutation in *MYD88*, thus providing a potential connection to the NLRP3 inflammasome pathway.[15] MYD88 induction also occurs in Waldenström macroglobulinemia explaining a possible link between these conditions.[15,16,19]

SchS is characterized by a course of recurrences and spontaneous remissions. Fever is a cardinal feature, and may reach 40°C, but is well tolerated. It may lag the rash by 1 to 14 years, but more often occurs concomitantly. An urticaria-like rash is the most specific and constant symptom in patients with SchS.[3] Lesions are faintly erythematous patches, plaques, or papules, located predominantly on the trunk and extremities, sparing the head and neck and usually palms/soles. Although the rash resembles urticaria in duration (<24 hours) and appearance, the lesions tend to burn instead of itch, edema is not common, and the duration may extend to 48 hours. The rash is characteristically recalcitrant to treatment with antihistamines. Nonpruritic dermographism, angioedema, and mucosal swelling have been reported.[20] The rash may precede the other diagnostic signs and symptoms by years.[6,7]

Biopsies typically reveal NUD. There is a predominantly neutrophilic perivascular and interstitial infiltrate, demonstrating leukocytoclasia without vasculitis, with variable foci of basophilic necrobiotic collagen alteration.[3,21] The infiltrate may concentrate around eccrine glands and in the subcutis (Fig. 83-1A). Epitheliotropism of neutrophils into pilosebaceous and eccrine epithelium is a histopathologic clue, which can be better observed with a myeloperoxidase (MPO) stain.[22] Dermal edema is not typical, and this, along with a less dense infiltrate and absence of perivascular lymphocytes, helps differentiate NUD from lesions of Sweet syndrome (Fig. 83-1B,C). Direct immunofluorescence may reveal IgM and C3 in the vessels or granular deposits of IgM along the basement membrane.[20,23] IL-1b, IL-6, IL-18, MPO, apoptosis-associated speck-like protein containing a CARD (ASC), and caspase-1 biomarkers were reported to be higher in SchS compared with chronic urticaria.[24]

Bone abnormalities with or without joint pain or bone pain are seen in 64% to 80% of patients with SchS.[25,26] They usually affect large bones (femur, tibia, ilium) and present

TABLE 83-1 Lipsker et al and Strasbourg Diagnostic Criteria of Schnitzler Syndrome

Lipsker Criteria[1]	Strasbourg Diagnostic Criteria[2]
Urticarial skin rash, monoclonal IgM component, and at least 2 of the following criteria:	**Definite diagnosis if 2 obligate criteria AND at least 2 minor criteria if IgM, and three minor criteria if IgG** **Probable diagnosis if 2 obligate criteria AND at least 1 minor criterion if IgM, and 2 minor criteria if IgG**
• Fever • Arthralgia or arthritis • Bone pain • Palpable lymph nodes • Liver or spleen enlargement • Elevated erythrocyte sedimentation rate • Leukocytosis • Abnormal findings on bone morphologic investigations	**Obligate criteria** • Chronic urticarial rash • Monoclonal IgM or IgG **Minor criteria** • Recurrent otherwise unexplained fever >38°C, usually occurring with the rash (not obligatory) • Objective findings of abnormal bone remodeling with or without bone pain (assessed by bone scintigraphy, MRI, or elevation of bone alkaline phosphatase) • A neutrophilic dermal infiltrate on skin biopsy (neutrophilic urticarial dermatosis) • Leukocytosis (neutrophils >10,000/mm^3) and/or elevated CRP 30 mg/L

with sclerotic or lytic lesions and rarely periosteal apposition.[26] Bone involvement should be confirmed by imaging or elevated alkaline phosphatase levels. Osteosclerosis can be seen on conventional radiography, but many patients will have a normal X-ray. Increased uptake in the distal femur and proximal tibia ("hot knees sign") on bone technetium scanning is considered to be one of the most sensitive methods to reveal bone abnormalities in patients with SchS.[23] Destructive arthritis has not been reported. Marked elevation of erythrocyte sedimentation rate, complement levels, and neutrophil count is frequently seen. Some patients may have symptomatic anemia of inflammation and chronic disease. Lymph node, splenic, and/or liver enlargement may be seen in a third of patients. Peripheral neuropathy is rare but may be underreported.[27] Other reported symptoms and associations in patients with SchS include cold-induced urticaria, neuropsychological findings (headache, vertigo, depression), pancreatitis, pseudoxanthoma elasticum, membranous nephropathy, hearing loss, thrombophilia with antiphospholipid syndrome, and hyperhomocysteinemia.[7] Aortitis has recently been reported and was documented with a 18F-FDG positron emission tomography/computed tomography scan in a patient with abdominal pain.[28]

SchS is difficult to diagnose in the early stages, resulting in a delayed diagnosis (average time before diagnosis is established is 5 years, range 0-20 years).[27] In patients >40 years old with recurrent fever, neutrophilic infiltrates on biopsy of a chronic urticarial rash, and any of the inflammatory clinical and laboratory presentations listed above, one should exclude a monoclonal gammopathy with serum/urine electrophoresis and immunofixation.[3] Spontaneous remission without treatment is extremely rare.[25] Prognosis is favorable with 91% survival during 15 years after the onset.[7] The median overall survival was reported to be 12.8 years; patients with hemoglobin levels <12 g/dL may have decreased median survival of 8.2 years.[27] Development of lymphoproliferative disorders is the main concern in patients with SchS, with an incidence of about 20%.[27] Some have reported the incidence to be up to 45%.[20] Reported malignancies in patients with SchS include Waldenström macroglobulinemia/lymphoplasmacytic lymphoma, IgM myeloma, chronic lymphocytic leukemia, splenic marginal zone lymphoma, hairy cell leukemia, and marginal zone B-cell lymphoma.[1,20,29,30] Waldenström macroglobulinemia is the most frequently described malignancy associated with SchS.[25,31] It usually develops 10 to 20 years after the first symptoms of SchS appear. Patients with SchS are also at risk of developing systemic AA (serum amyloid A protein) amyloidosis.[32,33]

SchS is differentiated from idiopathic chronic urticaria by the absence of pruritus and the typical systemic involvement, although, because the urticarial rash may be present long before some of the systemic symptoms, continued monitoring for other signs and symptoms of SchS is warranted. Characteristic SchS histopathology showing a neutrophilic infiltrate with leukocytoclasia without vasculitis (NUD) may be seen in other conditions, including Sweet syndrome, systemic lupus erythematosus (SLE), CAPS (familial cold anti-inflammatory syndrome, Muckle-Wells syndrome, and neonatal-onset multisystem inflammatory disease), and adult-onset Still disease (AOSD).[21] SLE typically will have a significantly high positive ANA and photosensitivity. CAPS usually is autosomal-dominantly inherited, with childhood onset, while SchS is not familial and arises in adults, usually around 50 years old. AOSD is differentiated mainly by associated pharyngitis, increased transaminases, and elevated ferritin levels. Elevation of monoclonal paraproteins is not seen in CAPS and AOSD. Normal complement analysis/absence of vasculitis and negative cryoglobulins help to exclude hypocomplementemic urticarial vasculitis and cryoglobulinemia, respectively.[3] Histopathologically, lesions in Sweet syndrome may be indistinguishable from SchS, but Sweet syndrome will have juicy erythematous lesions that persist for more than 24 hours and typically respond promptly to corticosteroids. In addition, Sweet syndrome often has perivascular lymphocytes and dermal edema, in contrast to SchS.

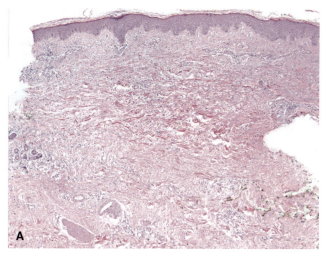
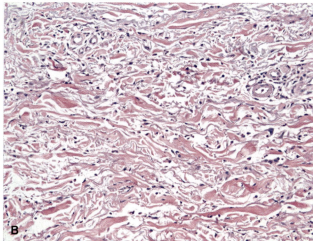
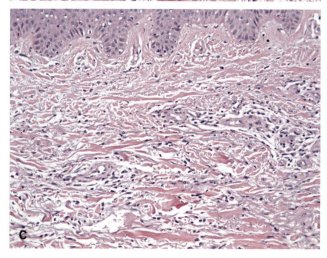

FIGURE 83-1. A. Sparse mixed perivascular and interstitial dermatitis with neutrophils. The infiltrate surrounds eccrine glands. **B.** Interstitial infiltrate, containing neutrophils and eosinophils. **C.** High-power view of neutrophilic infiltrate with leukocytoclasia, without vascular damage or fibrin deposition.

Palisaded neutrophilic granulomatous dermatitis may enter the differential due to leukocytoclasia of neutrophils and basophilic collagen alteration, but the latter is more prominent and consistent and is often accompanied by histiocytes and vasculitis.

Resistance of the rash to antihistamines and corticosteroids, or poor response of systemic manifestations to immunosuppressive agents, may be a clue to the diagnosis. In contrast to urticaria, SchS has a dramatic response (within hours of first injection) to anti-IL-1 agents such as anakinra or canakinumab, which help to confirm the diagnosis, as well as manage the symptoms.[2,4,10]

References

1. Lipsker D, Veran Y, Grunenberger F, Cribier B, Heid E, Grosshans E. The Schnitzler syndrome. Four new cases and review of the literature. *Medicine (Baltimore)*. 2001; 80(1):37-44.
2. Gusdorf L, Asli B, Barbarot S, et al. Schnitzler syndrome: validation and applicability of diagnostic criteria in real-life patients. *Allergy*. 2017;72(2):177-182.
3. Simon A, Asli B, Braun-Falco M, et al. Schnitzler's syndrome: diagnosis, treatment, and follow-up. *Allergy*. 2013;68(5):562-568.
4. Fujita Y, Asano T, Sakai A, et al. A case of Schnitzler's syndrome without monoclonal gammopathy successfully treated with canakinumab. *BMC Musculoskelet Disord*. 2021;22(1):257.
5. Ahn MJ, Yu JE, Jeong J, Sim DW, Koh YI. A case of Schnitzler's syndrome without monoclonal gammopathy-associated chronic urticaria treated with anakinra. *Yonsei Med J*. 2018;59(1):154-157.
6. Darrieutort-Laffite C, Ansquer C, Aubert H, et al. Rheumatic involvement and bone scan features in Schnitzler syndrome: initial and follow-up data from a single-center cohort of 25 patients. *Arthritis Res Ther*. 2020;22(1):272.
7. de Koning HD, Bordar EJ, van der Meer JWM, Simon A; Schnitzler Syndrome Study Group. Schnitzler syndrome: beyond the case reports—review and follow-up of 94 patients with an emphasis on prognosis and treatment. *Semin Arthritis Rheum*. 2007;37(3):137-148.
8. Bonnekoh H, Frischbutter S, Roll S, Maurer M, Krause K. Tocilizumab treatment in patients with Schnitzler syndrome: an open-label study. *J Allergy Clin Immunol Pract*. 2021;9(6):2486-2489.e4.
9. Masson Regnault M, Frouin E, JéruI, et al. Cytokine signature in Schnitzler syndrome: proinflammatory cytokine production associated to Th suppression. *Front Immunol*. 2020;11:588322.
10. Krause K, Bonnekoh H, Ellrich A, et al. Long-term efficacy of canakinumab in the treatment of Schnitzler syndrome. *J Allergy Clin Immunol*. 2020;145(6):1681-1686.e5.
11. Pizzirani C, Falzoni S, Govoni M, et al. Dysfunctional inflammasome in Schnitzler's syndrome. *Rheumatology (Oxford)*. 2009;48(10):1304-1308.
12. Krause K, Feist E, Fiene M, et al. Complete remission in 3 of 3 anti-IL-6-treated patients with Schnitzler syndrome. *J Allergy Clin Immunol*. 2012;129(3):848-850.
13. Bhattacharyya J, Mihara K, Morimoto J, Takihara Y, Hide M. Elevated interleukin-18 secretion from monoclonal IgM+ B cells in a patient with Schnitzler syndrome. *J Am Acad Dermatol*. 2012;67(3):e118-120.
14. Krause K, Sabat R, Wtte-Händel E, et al. Association of CCL2 with systemic inflammation in Schnitzler syndrome. *Br J Dermatol*. 2019;180(4):859-868.
15. van Leersum FS, Potjewijd J, van Geel M, Steijlen PM, Vreeburg M. Schnitzler's syndrome—a novel hypothesis of a

shared pathophysiologic mechanism with Waldenström's disease. *Orphanet J Rare Dis.* 2019;14(1):151.
16. Goodman AM, Cohen PR, Li A, Hinds B, Kurzrock R. Schnitzler syndrome associated with MYD88 L265P mutation. *JAAD Case Rep.* 2019;5(4):312-316.
17. Rowczenio DM, Trojer H, Russell T, et al. Clinical characteristics in subjects with NLRP3 V198M diagnosed at a single UK center and a review of the literature. *Arthritis Res Ther.* 2013;15(1):R30.
18. Loock J, Lamprecht P, Timmann C, Mrowietz U, Csernok E, Gross WL. Genetic predisposition (NLRP3 V198M mutation) for IL-1-mediated inflammation in a patient with Schnitzler syndrome. *J Allergy Clin Immunol.* 2010;125(2):500-502.
19. Pathak S, Rowczenio DM, Owen RG, et al. Exploratory study of MYD88 L265P, rare NLRP3 variants, and clonal hematopoiesis prevalence in patients with Schnitzler syndrome. *Arthritis Rheumatol.* 2019;71(12):2121-2125.
20. Sokumbi O, Drage LA, Peters MS. Clinical and histopathologic review of Schnitzler syndrome: the Mayo Clinic experience (1972-2011). *J Am Acad Dermatol.* 2012;67(6):1289-1295.
21. Kieffer C, Cribier B, Lipsker D. Neutrophilic urticarial dermatosis: a variant of neutrophilic urticaria strongly associated with systemic disease. Report of 9 new cases and review of the literature. *Medicine (Baltim).* 2009;88(1):23-31.
22. Broekaert SM, Böer-Auer A, Kerl K, et al. Neutrophilic epitheliotropism is a histopathological clue to neutrophilic urticarial dermatosis. *Am J Dermatopathol.* 2016;38(1):39-49.
23. Janier M, Bonvalet D, Blanc MF, et al. Chronic urticaria and macroglobulinemia (Schnitzler's syndrome): report of two cases. *J Am Acad Dermatol.* 1989;20(2 pt 1):206-211.
24. Bonnekoh H, Scheffel J, Maurer M, Krause K. Use of skin biomarker profiles to distinguish Schnitzler syndrome from chronic spontaneous urticaria: results of a pilot study. *Br J Dermatol.* 2018;178(2):561-562.
25. Lipsker D. The Schnitzler syndrome. *Orphanet J Rare Dis.* 2010;5:38.
26. Niederhauser BD, Dingli D, Kyle RA, Ringler MD. Imaging findings in 22 cases of Schnitzler syndrome: characteristic para-articular osteosclerosis, and the "hot knees" sign differential diagnosis. *Skeletal Radiol.* 2014;43(7):905-915.
27. Jain T, Offord CP, Kyle RA, Dingli D. Schnitzler syndrome: an under-diagnosed clinical entity. *Haematologica.* 2013;98(10):1581-1585.
28. Bursztejn AC, Imperiale A, Lipsker D. Aortitis: a new feature of Schnitzler syndrome. *JAAD Case Rep.* 2017;3(5):454-456.
29. Dalle S, Dalle S, Dalle S, Dalle S, Dalle S, Dalle S. Schnitzler syndrome associated with systemic marginal zone B-cell lymphoma. *Br J Dermatol.* 2006;155(4):827-829.
30. Fank H, Caers J, Lambert M, et al. Schnitzler syndrome associated with hairy cell leukemia presenting with chronic urticaria and arthralgias. *JAAD Case Rep.* 2018;4(4):386-389.
31. Welsh B, Tate B. Schnitzler's syndrome: report of a case with progression to Waldenström's macroglobulinaemia. *Australas J Dermatol.* 1999;40(4):201-203.
32. Mittal N, Renaut P, Sharma R, Robbie M. Gastrointestinal amyloidosis associated with Schnitzler's syndrome. *Pathology.* 2013;45(4):424-426.
33. Claes K, Bammens B, Delforge M, Evenepoel P, Kuypers D, Vanrenterghem Y. Another devastating complication of the Schnitzler syndrome: AA amyloidosis. *Br J Dermatol.* 2008;158(1):182-184.

INDEX

Note: Page numbers followed by f indicate figures and t indicate tables.

A

ACLH. *See* Atypical cutaneous lymphoid hyperplasia (ACLH)
Acral pseudolymphomatous angiokeratoma of children (APACHE)
    clinical features, 532
    differential diagnosis, 533
    histopathological features, 532–533, 533f
    treatment, 533–534
Actinic reticuloid. *See* Chronic actinic dermatitis (CAD)
Acute leukemias
    anthracyclines, 834–836, 835f–836f
    antimetabolites, 836–838
    enzymes and enzyme inhibitors, 838–841
    multi-targeted protein kinase inhibitors, 841
    small molecule tyrosine kinase inhibitors, 841
    targeted inhibitors, 841
Acute lymphoblastic leukemia/lymphomas (ALLs), 797
    clinical presentation and prognosis, 598–599, 599f
    differential diagnosis, 605
    epidemiology, 598
    etiology, 598
    genetic and molecular findings, 601, 604–605
    histopathology, 599, 600f–603f
    immunophenotype, 599
    postulated cell of origin, 605
Acute myeloid leukemia, 67
AD. *See* Atopic dermatitis (AD)
Adult-onset immunodeficiency (AOID), 873
Adult T-cell leukemia/lymphoma (ATLL), 826
    chronic infection, 311
    classic flower cell of, 312, 312f
    clinical lesion stratification for, 312, 313t
    clinical presentation and prognosis, 312–314, 312f–314f, 313t
    differential diagnosis, 317, 318f, 318t
    epidemiology, 311
    etiology, 311–312, 312t
    follicular papules, 312, 314f
    genetic and molecular findings, 316–317, 317t
    histology, 314, 314t, 315f–316f
    immunophenotype, 314–315, 316f
    plaques and tumors, 312, 343f
    Shimoyama classification of, 312, 313t
Adult xanthogranuloma (AXG), 690–694
AFH. *See* Angiomatoid fibrous histiocytoma (AFH)
Aggressive epidermotropic CD8+ cytotoxic cutaneous t-cell lymphoma, 211
    clinical presentation, 211–212, 211f–212f
    differential diagnosis, 213–215
    epidemiology, 211
    etiology, 211
    genetic and molecular findings, 213
    histology, 212
    immunophenotype, 212–213
    postulated cell of origin, 213
Aggressive natural killer leukemia (ANKL)
    clinical presentation and prognosis, 274
    differential diagnosis, 276
    epidemiology, 274
    etiology, 274
    genetic and molecular findings, 275–276
    histology, 274
    immunophenotype, 275
    skin involvement, 276
ALCL. *See* Anaplastic large cell lymphoma
ALDY. *See* Annular lichenoid dermatosis of youth (ALDY)
Aleukemic leukemia cutis. *See* Leukemia cutis (LC)
ALHE. *See* Angiolymphoid hyperplasia with eosinophilia (ALHE)
Alkylating agents
    chronic leukemias, 843–845
    cutaneous T-cell lymphoma (CTCL), 846–847
    Hodgkin lymphoma (HL), 852
Allergy, 36
All-trans retinoic acid (ATRA), 839–841, 840f
Alopecia
    in B-cell lymphoma
        cutaneous, 826–827
        systemic, 827
    in cutaneous T-cell lymphomas, 820
        adult T-cell leukemia/lymphoma, 826
        CD30+ lymphoproliferative disorders, 825–826
        hepatosplenic T-cell lymphoma, 826
        mycosis fungoides and variants, 820–825
        primary cutaneous CD4+ small to medium T-cell lymphoproliferative disorder, 826, 826f
        subcutaneous panniculitis–like T-cell lymphoma (SPLTCL), 825
    in leukemia, 827
    secondary causes, 827–829
Amplification phase, 79
Amyloidosis, 742
AMZH. *See* Atypical marginal zone hyperplasia (AMZH)
Anagen effluvium, 835
Anaplastic large-cell lymphoma (ALCL), 733–734, 733f
    ALK+
        clinical findings, 781
        differential diagnosis, 782–783
        epidemiology, 781
        etiology, 781
        histologic features, 781–782, 782f–783f
    ALK−
        clinical findings, 770, 771f
        differential diagnosis, 771
        epidemiology, 770
        histologic features, 771, 772f–774f
Angioimmunoblastic T-cell lymphoma (AITL)
    clinical features of, 299t
    clinical presentation/prognosis, 298–299
    dermatological manifestations of, 300f
    differential diagnosis, 306, 307t
    genetics and molecular findings, 303–305, 306f
    histology, 299
    immunophenotype, 300–303, 301t, 304f–305f
    postulated cell of origin, 298
    treatment, 306
Angiolymphoid hyperplasia with eosinophilia (ALHE), 322, 324f, 399
Angiomatoid fibrous histiocytoma (AFH), 536–537, 536f–537f
Angioplasmacellular hyperplasia, 534
Angiosarcoma, 534–536, 535f
Annular lichenoid dermatosis of youth (ALDY)
    clinical presentation, 588, 589f
    differential diagnosis, 589–590
    epidemiology, 588
    etiology and pathogenesis, 588
    genetics/molecular findings, 589
    histology, 588–589, 589f
    immunohistochemistry, 589, 590f
    treatment, 588
Anthracyclines
    acute leukemias, 834–836, 835f–836f
    Hodgkin lymphoma (HL), 852
Antigen-presenting cell (APC), 26
Antimicrotubules, 852
APACHE. *See* Acral pseudolymphomatous angiokeratoma of children (APACHE)
L-Asparaginase, 838
ATLL. *See* Adult T-cell leukemia/lymphoma (ATLL)
Atopic dermatitis (AD), 517–518
Atypical cutaneous lymphoid hyperplasia (ACLH), 552, 553f–555f
Atypical marginal zone hyperplasia (AMZH), 554–555
Autoimmune disease, 37
Axicabtagene ciloleucel (YESCARTA), 869
Azacitidine, 639, 838

B

B-cell differentiation, 12
    memory B-cells, 16
    naïve B-cells, 12
    plasma cells, 16
    precursor B cells, 12
    T-cell–dependent germinal center reaction, 13–16, 14f–15f
    T-cell–independent B-cell differentiation, 12–13
B-cell lineage-acute lymphoblastic leukemia/lymphoma (B-ALL), 598–605
B-cell lymphomas
    Burkitt lymphoma (BL), 729–733
    cutaneous, 826–827
    diffuse large B-cell lymphoma (DLBCL), 724–726, 724f–726f
    extranodal marginal zone B-cell lymphoma, 729, 729f–731f
    follicular lymphoma (FL), 726–728
    mantle cell lymphoma (MCL), 729
    plasmablastic lymphoma (PBL), 726, 726f–728f
    small lymphocytic lymphoma (SLL), 729
    systemic, 827
B-cell malignancies, 66
Bence Jones proteins, 741
Bendamustine, 843–845
Benign cephalic histiocytosis (BCH), 694–695
Benign lymphoid proliferations, 743–746
Benign reactive lymphoid hyperplasia (BLRH), 753
Bexarotene, 849
BIOMED-2, 74–75
    IGH clonality assay, 75, 75f–76f
BL. *See* Burkitt lymphoma (BL)

Blastic indeterminate dendritic cell tumor, 626, 630f
Blastic plasmacytoid dendritic cell neoplasm (BPDCN), 67, 93, 615, 626, 629f
 clinical findings, 803, 803f
 clinical presentation and prognosis, 638–639, 639f
 differential diagnosis, 644–646, 804
 epidemiology, 638, 802
 genetic and molecular findings, 642
 histologic features, 803–804
 histology, 639–640, 640f–645f
 immunophenotype, 642, 645f–647f
 postulated cell of origin, 643
Bleomycin, 852
Blueberry muffin appearance, 608, 609f
Borrelia burgdorferi–associated lymphocytoma cutis, 550–552, 551f–553f
Borrelial lymphocytoma, 569
Bortezomib, 639, 850
BPDCN. *See* Blastic plasmacytoid dendritic cell neoplasm (BPDCN)
BRAF inhibitors, 845–846, 847f
BRAF-V600E mutation, 664
 clinical implications, 667–668
 pathogenesis, 664–667
 pathology, 664–667
Brentuximab vedotin, 244
Brexucabtagene autoleucel (TECARTUS), 869
Burkitt lymphoma (BL), 447–449, 729–733, 853–854
Busulfan, 845

C

CAD. *See* Chronic actinic dermatitis (CAD)
Castleman disease (CD), 477–478
 clinical characteristics, 396
 clinical presentation, 397–398
 differential diagnosis, 399–400
 epidemiology, 397
 histology, 398, 398f–399f
 immunophenotype, 398
 pathogenesis, 398–399, 400f
 subtypes, 397
CBCLs. *See* Cutaneous B-cell lymphomas (CBCLs)
CD. *See* Castleman disease (CD)
CD1C$^+$ DCS (CDC2), 28
CD14$^+$ DCS, 28
CD141$^+$ DCS (CDC1), 28
CD30$^+$ lymphoproliferative disorders, 825–826, 826f
 CD30 antigen, 244
 coexistent C-ALCL/MF *versus* CD30$^+$ large-cell transformation, 248–249, 249f
 lymphomatoid papulosis (LyP), 244–245
  chemotherapy, 246
  expectant management, 245–246
  other treatment options, 246
  phototherapy, 246
  topical agents, 246
 primary cutaneous anaplastic large-cell lymphoma (C-ALCL), 247
  brentuximab vedotin, 248
  chemotherapy, 247–248
  radiotherapy, 247
  surgical excision, 247
  treatment, 247–248, 250
 treatment, 246–247
CD30$^+$ lymphoproliferative disorders (LPDs), 481
CD30 pseudolymphomas. *See* Cutaneous pseudolymphomas (CPLs)
CD8$^+$ aggressive epidermotropic cutaneous T-cell lymphoma, 235
CD8$^+$ cutaneous pseudolymphoma, 235–236
CD8$^+$ resident memory T cells, 6
CD4$^+$ T cells, 2–3
Check-point inhibitors, 829
Chemotherapy
 acute leukemias
  anthracyclines, 834–836, 835f–836f
  antimetabolites, 836–838
  enzymes and enzyme inhibitors, 838–841
  multi-targeted protein kinase inhibitors, 841
  small molecule tyrosine kinase inhibitors, 841
  targeted inhibitors, 841
 alopecia, 827–828
 chronic leukemias, 841
  alkylating agents, 843–845
  antimetabolites, 845
  BRAF inhibitors (BRAFi), 845–846
  monoclonal antibodies (MAbs), 842
  purine analogs, 842
  tyrosine kinase inhibitors (TKIs), 843
 cutaneous T-cell lymphoma (CTCL)
  alkylating agents, 846–847
  corticosteroids, 846
  fusion proteins, 848
  histone deacetylase (HDAC) inhibitors, 847
  interferon-α, 850
  nucleoside analogs, 848–849
  photochemotherapies, 849
  radiotherapy, 849
  retinoids, 849
 Hodgkin lymphoma (HL)
  alkylating agents, 852
  anthracyclines, 852
  antimicrotubules, 852
  glycopeptide antibiotics, 852–853
 multiple myeloma (MM)
  antiangiogenic agents, 851
  cyclophosphamide and melphalan, 851
  monoclonal antibodies (MAbs), 851–852
  proteasome inhibitors, 850–851
 non-Hodgkin lymphoma (NHL)
  Burkitt lymphoma, 853–854
  diffuse large B-cell lymphoma (DLBCL), 853
  follicular lymphoma, 853
  mantle-cell lymphoma (MCL), 853
  marginal-zone lymphoma, 853
  small-cell lymphocytic lymphoma (SCLL), 853
  T-cell lymphomas, 854–855
Chimeric antigen receptor (CAR) T-cell therapy, 869
Chlorambucil, 845
Chromonychia, 836
Chronic actinic dermatitis (CAD)
 clinical presentation and prognosis, 506–507, 507f
 epidemiology, 506
 etiology, 506
 genetics, 507
 histology, 507, 508f
 immunophenotype, 507
Chronic leukemias, 841
 alkylating agents, 843–845
 antimetabolites, 845
 BRAF inhibitors (BRAFi), 845–846
 monoclonal antibodies (MAbs), 842
 purine analogs, 842
 tyrosine kinase inhibitors (TKIs), 843
Chronic lymphocytic leukemia (CLL), 718, 718f
 cutaneous infections, 471
 cutaneous lesions, 463, 464f–465f
 cutaneous nonneoplastic immune infiltrates, 468–469
 differential diagnosis
  primary cutaneous follicle center lymphoma (PCFCL), 464
  primary cutaneous marginal zone B-cell lymphoma (PCMZL), 464
  Richter transformation (RS), 464–467, 469f
 histopathology, 463–464
 immunophenotype, 463–464, 466f–468f
 prevalence, 463
 prognosis, 471
Chronic lymphoproliferative disorders of natural killer (CLPD-NK) cells
 clinical presentation and prognosis, 276
 differential diagnosis, 277
 epidemiology, 276
 etiology, 276
 genetic and molecular findings, 276
 immunophenotype, 276
 morphology, 276
 skin involvement, 276
Chronic myeloid leukemia (CML), 624–626
Chronic myelomonocytic leukemia (CMML), 626, 627f–630f
Cladribine, 842
Classic HL (CHL). *See* Hodgkin lymphoma (HL)
Classic Hodgkin lymphoma (CHL), 171, 723–724
CLH. *See* Cutaneous lymphoid hyperplasia (CLH)
CLL. *See* Chronic lymphocytic leukemia (CLL)
Clonality testing
 basic principle, 74
 BIOMED-2, 74–75
  IGH clonality assay, 75, 75f–76f
 clonal lymphoid process, ascertainment of, 73–74
 EuroClonality consensus primer sets, 74–75
 IGHV hypermutation testing, 74
 lineage determination, 74
 methodology for, 74
 monoclonal/biclonal, 76–77, 77f
 oligoclonal, 77–78
 polyclonal, 78
 residual/recurrent disease, monitoring for, 74
 suitable sample types, 74
 TCRG, 76
 turnaround time, 76
Clonal lymphoid process, ascertainment of, 73–74
Comparative genomic hybridization, 82
Conjunctival lymphomas (CLs), 752, 755–756, 756f–759f
Conventional karyotype, 82–85
Corticosteroids, 846
CPLs. *See* Cutaneous pseudolymphomas (CPLs)
Cryocrystalglobulins (CCG), 904
Cryoglobulinemias (CGs)
 clinical findings, 903, 904f
 differential diagnosis, 904
 etiology, 903
 histopathology, 904, 905f–908f
 laboratory findings, 903
 treatment, 904
Cutaneous anaplastic large cell lymphoma, 87–88
Cutaneous and systemic plasmacytosis (C/SP), 478
 clinical presentation and prognosis, 572–573, 573f
 differential diagnosis, 575
 epidemiology, 572
 etiology, 572
 histology, 573–574, 574f–575f
 treatment, 574–575
Cutaneous B-cell hyperplasia (B-CLH), 542–543, 546f–547f
Cutaneous B-cell immunobiology
 B-cell differentiation, 12
  memory B-cells, 16
  naïve B-cells, 12
  plasma cells, 16
  precursor B cells, 12
  T-cell-dependent germinal center reaction, 13–16, 14f–15f
  T-cell–independent B-cell differentiation, 12–13
 normal skin homeostasis, B-cells in recruitment of, 16
 skin disease, 16–18, 18f

Cutaneous B-cell lymphomas (CBCLs), 336, 361, 794–805, 826–827
  classification, 405
  diagnosis of
    anatomic location, 323
    growth patterns, 323, 327f–332f, 329
    histology, 322, 324f
    molecular approach in skin, 329, 332
    primary, 322, 323t, 325f, 325t–326t, 336, 337t
    systemic, 322, 323t, 326t–327t
    T-cell lymphoproliferative disorder, 322, 325f
  diffuse large B-cell lymphoma, leg type (DLBCL-LT), 54–55, 55f
  disease-specific survival of, 405, 405t
  primary, 405–410
  primary cutaneous follicle center lymphoma (PCFCL), 50–51
    clinical features, 407
    diagnostic workup, 407
    prevalence, 407
    prognosis, 408
    treatment, 408
  primary cutaneous marginal zone lymphoma (PCMZL), 51–54, 52f–53f
    clinical features, 405–406
    diagnostic workup, 406
    prevalence, 405
    prognosis, 406–407
    treatment, 407
  staging, 405, 406t
Cutaneous hematolymphoid proliferations, in children, 770
  aggressive CD8-positive epidermotropic T-cell lymphoma, 786
  cutaneous B-cell lymphomas/leukemias, 794–805
  mature T-cell and NK-cell lymphomas, 770–786
  primary cutaneous CD4+ small to medium T-cell lymphoproliferative disorder, 786
  primary cutaneous γδ T-cell lymphoma, 786–788
  severe mosquito bite allergy, 788–794
Cutaneous hematopathology
  cancer gene set testing, 101
  cancer predisposition testing, 101
  clonality testing, 101–102
Cutaneous low-grade B-cell lymphomas, 323, 327f–328f
Cutaneous lymphadenoma
  clinical features, 525
  differential diagnosis, 526
  histologic features, 525–526, 526f
  treatment, 526
Cutaneous lymphoid hyperplasia (CLH), 354, 542, 543t
  arthropod-bite reaction, 542, 544f
  atypical cutaneous lymphoid hyperplasia (ACLH), 552, 553f–555f
  atypical marginal zone hyperplasia (AMZH), 554–555
  Borrelia burgdorferi–associated lymphocytoma cutis, 550–552, 551f–553f
  causes of, 542, 543t, 545f
  cutaneous B-cell hyperplasia (B-CLH), 542–543, 546f–547f
  cutaneous T-cell hyperplasia (T-CLH), 543–545, 548f–550f
  differential diagnosis, 547–548, 550
  flow cytometry, 546
  immunohistochemistry, 546
  lymphomatoid keratosis (LyK), 555
  mixed T- and B-cell hyperplasia, 542
  molecular findings, 547
  syringolymphoid hyperplasia with alopecia (SLHA), 555
Cutaneous mastocytosis (CM)
  histopathology, 650–651
  subtypes of, 650

Cutaneous myelofibrosis (CMF), 623
Cutaneous myeloid neoplasms
  clinical findings, 800, 801f
  differential diagnosis, 800–801
  epidemiology, 800
  histologic features, 800, 802f–803f
Cutaneous pseudolymphomas (CPLs), 511f
  CD30 expression, 522
  cell of origin, 512
  clinical presentation of, 511
  differential diagnosis, 522–523
  epidemiology, 510
  etiology, 510–511, 511t–512t
  histology, 512, 513f
  immunophenotype, 512, 513f–514f
  infection-associated CD30, 512
  inflammatory dermatoses
    arthropod assault, 517, 518f
    atopic dermatitis (AD), 517–518
    chronic ulceration, 519–521, 520f
    drug-induced, 521–522, 522f
    eruption of lymphocyte recovery (ELR), 519
    pernio, 518
    pityriasis lichenoides et varioliformis acuta (PLEVA), 517
    postscabetic nodules, 517, 518f
    tattoo, 518, 519f
  molecular findings, 512
  prognosis, 511–512
  pseudolymphoma
    Epstein-Barr virus (EBV), 516, 516f
    herpes simplex virus (HSV), 513–515, 514f
    Milker nodules, 516
    molluscum contagiosum (MC), 515–516, 515f
    mycobacteria, 517
    mycotic infections, 516–517
    verruca vulgaris, 516
Cutaneous Rosai–Dorfman disease (CRDD), 684
Cutaneous T-cell hyperplasia (T-CLH), 543–545, 548f–550f
Cutaneous T-cell immunobiology
  CD8+ resident memory T cells, 6
  CD4+ T cells, 2–3
  coreceptors, 1
  follicular T helper cells, 5
  natural killer T cells, 6
  regulatory T cells, 5
  skin, 1–2, 2f
  γδT cells, 6
  T helper 1 (T_H1) cells, 3–4
  T helper 2 (T_H2) cells, 3–4
  T helper 9 (T_H9) cells, 5
  T helper 17 (T_H17) cells, 4
  T helper 22 (T_H22) cells, 4–5
Cutaneous T-cell lymphomas (CTCLs), 820
  adult T-cell leukemia/lymphoma, 826
  alkylating agents, 846–847
  causation, 44
  CD30+ lymphoproliferative disorders, 825–826
  clinical features, 103–104
  corticosteroids, 846
  diagnosis, molecular analyses in, 105–106, 106f
  evolution, 44
  fusion proteins, 848
  histological pattern, 104–105, 105f
  histone deacetylase (HDAC) inhibitors, 847
  immunophenotypic profile, 105
  interferon-α, 850
  mycosis fungoides (MF), 40–41
    variants, 820–825
  nucleoside analogs, 848–849
  photochemotherapies, 849
  primary cutaneous CD30+ lymphoproliferative disorders (ALCL/LYP), 44–46
  primary cutaneous CD4+ small to medium T-cell lymphoproliferative disorder, 826, 826f

  primary cutaneous T-cell lymphomas, 46
  prognostic biomarkers, 47
  radiotherapy, 849
  retinoids, 849
  Sézary syndrome (SS), 40–41
  sources of difficulty, 103
  subcutaneous panniculitis–like T-cell lymphoma (SPLTCL), 46, 825
  systemic T-cell lymphomas, 46–47
  T-cell signaling and differentiation, 41, 41f–43f
    DNA damage response pathways, 44
    epigenetic modification, 43–44
  therapeutic implications, 47
  variants, 46
Cyclophosphamide, 851
Cytarabine, 836–837, 837f
Cytokine production, 22
Cytotoxic cutaneous T-cell lymphomas (CTCLs)
  aggressive epidermotropic CD8+ cytotoxic cutaneous t-cell lymphoma, 211
    clinical presentation, 211–212, 211f–212f
    differential diagnosis, 213–215
    epidemiology, 211
    etiology, 211
    genetic and molecular findings, 213
    histology, 212
    immunophenotype, 212–213
    postulated cell of origin, 213
  primary cutaneous gamma-delta T-cell lymphoma
    clinical presentation, 204
    differential diagnosis, 208–210
    epidemiology, 203
    etiology, 203–204
    genetic and molecular findings, 206–208
    histology, 204–205, 205f
    immunophenotype, 205–206
    postulated cell of origin, 208
    prognosis, 204
Cytotoxicity, 21

D

Dacarbazine, 852
Daratumumab, 851
Dasatinib, 843
Dendritic cell sarcoma (DCS), 702, 703t
  differential diagnosis, 705, 705t
  histopathology, 704–705, 705f
  molecular alterations, 705–706
  subtypes, 703
Dermal fibrosis, 623
Dermatofibroma, 693, 693f
Destombes–Rosai–Dorfman syndrome. *See* Rosai–Dorfman disease (RDD)
Diffuse cutaneous mastocytosis (DCM)
  clinical presentation/prognosis, 656
  differential diagnosis, 657
  epidemiology, 656
  etiology, 656
  treatment, 656
Diffuse large B-cell lymphoma, leg type (DLBCL-LT), 54–55, 55f
Diffuse large B-cell lymphomas (DLBCLs), 724–726, 724f–726f, 853
  Burkitt lymphoma (BL), 447–449
  cell of origin (COO) classification, 431
  de novo CD5-positive, 432, 433f
  EBV+, 434–435, 437–438, 439f–443f
  germinal center types (GCTs), 431
  Hans algorithm for, 432, 432f
  high-grade B-cell lymphoma (HGBCL)
    gray zone lymphomas, 434, 435f–438f
    with 11q aberrations, 432
  plasmablastic lymphoma (PBL), 439–446, 445f
  primary effusion lymphoma (PEL), 446–447, 447f–448f
  T-cell histiocyte-rich large B-cell lymphoma (THRBCL), 449

DLBCLs. *See* Diffuse large B-cell lymphomas (DLBCLs)
DNA sequencing
  emergence of, 97–98
  illumina sequencing, 98
  ion torrent sequencing, 98
  Maxam–Gilbert sequencing, 97
  Sanger sequencing, 97
Doxorubicin, 835
Duvelisib, 841

E

EBV. *See* Epstein–Barr virus (EBV)
EBV+ chronic mucocutaneous ulcer (EBVMCU)
  clinical characteristics, 391
  clinical features, 410
  clinical presentation, 391, 392f
  differential diagnosis, 392
  epidemiology, 391
  genetics, 392
  histology, 391–392, 393f
  immunohistochemistry, 392, 394f–395f
  prognosis, 410
  treatment, 410
EBV+ lymphoproliferative disorders, 329, 331f
EBVMCU. *See* EBV+ chronic mucocutaneous ulcer (EBVMCU)
EBV+ mucocutaneous ulcer (EBV MCU), 384
Eczematous eruptions, 868
EDHM. *See* Eosinophilic dermatosis of hematologic malignancy (EDHM)
EED. *See* Erythema elevatum diutinum (EED)
Elotuzumab, 851
ELR. *See* Eruption of lymphocyte recovery (ELR)
EMH. *See* Extramedullary hematopoiesis (EMH)
Enasidenib, 841
Eosinophilic angiocentric fibrosis, 579–580
Eosinophilic cellulitis. *See* Wells syndrome
Eosinophilic dermatosis of hematologic malignancy (EDHM)
  differential diagnosis, 593–594
  epidemiology, 592, 593f
  histology, 592–593, 593f–594f
  insect bite–like reaction, 592
  pathogenesis, 595, 595f
  prognosis, 595
  treatment, 594–595
  workup, 594
Epidermotropic B-cell lymphomas, 323, 328f
Epithelial tumors
  cutaneous lymphadenoma
    clinical features, 525
    differential diagnosis, 526
    histologic features, 525–526, 526f
    treatment, 526
  lymphoepithelioma-like carcinoma (LELC)
    clinical features, 527
    differential diagnosis, 528
    histologic features, 527–528, 527f–528f
    treatment, 528
  spiradenoma
    clinical features, 526
    differential diagnosis, 526–527, 527f
    histologic features, 526, 527f
    treatment, 527
Epithelioid hemangioma
  clinical features, 530
  differential diagnosis, 532
  histologic features, 530–531, 531f–532f
  treatment, 532
Epstein–Barr virus (EBV), 516, 516f
  Castleman disease (CD), 396–400, 398f–400f
  EBV+ chronic mucocutaneous ulcer (EBVMCU), 391–392, 392f–395f
  lymphoid proliferations, 734–739, 737f–741f
  methotrexate-associated B-cell lymphoproliferative disorders (MTX-LPDs), 392–396, 397f

posttransplant lymphoproliferative disorders (PTLDs), 388–391, 389f–391f
Erdheim–Chester disease (ECD), 680
Eruption of lymphocyte recovery (ELR), 519
Eruptive keratoacanthomas, 868
Eruptive xanthomas, 694, 694f
Erythema elevatum diutinum (EED), 580
  clinical, 890
  etiology, 890
  histology, 890, 891f
Erythrodermic cutaneous T-cell lymphoma, 824, 824f
Erythromelalgia, 621
Essential thrombocythemia (ET), 622–623
Etoposide (topoisomerase II inhibitor), 838–839
EuroClonality consensus primer sets, 74–75
Extracorporeal photopheresis (ECP), 849
Extramedullary hematopoiesis (EMH), 623, 635
  clinical presentation/prognosis/treatment, 635–636, 636f
  differential diagnosis, 636, 805
  epidemiology, 635, 804
  etiology, 635, 804–805
  histologic features, 805, 806f
  histopathology, 636
  immunophenotype, 636
Extranodal marginal zone B-cell lymphoma, 729, 729f–731f
Extranodal marginal zone lymphomas (EMZLs), 752
Extranodal natural killer (NK)/T-cell lymphoma, nasal type (ENKTL), 270, 734, 736f
  clinical findings, 792
  clinical presentation and prognosis, 256–257, 257f, 271
  differential diagnosis, 258–259, 271–273, 273f, 793–794
  epidemiology, 256, 270, 791
  etiology, 256, 270, 792
  genetic and molecular findings, 257–258, 271
  histologic features, 792–793, 793f
  histology, 257, 271
  immunophenotype, 257, 271
  postulated cell of origin, 258
  skin involvement, 271, 272f
Extrinsic cell properties, 62
Eye-associated lymphoid tissue (EALT), 751–752
Eyelid lymphomas, 759–760, 760f, 760t

F

Fibroblastic reticular cell tumor, 671
FL. *See* Follicular lymphoma (FL)
Flow cytometric (FC) analysis, hematopathology diagnosis
  acute myeloid leukemia, 67
  B-cell malignancies, 66
  blastic plasmacytoid dendritic cell neoplasm (BPDCN), 67
  cell characteristics measured by
    extrinsic cell properties, 62
    forward scatter, 62
    immunophenotype characterization, 62–64, 63f–64f
    intrinsic cell properties, 62
    side scatter, 62
  computer system, 61–62
    new-generation advanced flow cytometers, 62
  fluidics, 59
  granulocytic sarcoma, 67
  immunophenotypic profiles, 66
  instrumentation, 59–62
  interpretation of results, 65
  light handling system, 60, 61f
  light sources, 59
  liquid samples processing, 65
  lymph node and skin samples, processing of, 65
  mature T-cell lymphoma

    α/β chain type, 67–68
    clonality studies, 68
    γ/δ type, 68
  natural killer (NK)-cell neoplasms, 67
  optics, 59
  plasma cell neoplasms (PCN), 66–67
  primary cutaneous lymphomas (PCLs), 68–69
  sample collection, 64–65
  T-lymphoblastic lymphoma, 68
Fludarabine, 842
Fluorescent in situ hybridization (FISH), 615
  blastic plasmacytoid dendritic cell neoplasm (BPDCN), 93
  comparative genomic hybridization, 82
  conventional karyotype, 82–85
  cutaneous anaplastic large cell lymphoma, 87–88
  G-banding, 82–85
  lymphomatoid papulosis, 87–88
  mycosis fungoides (MF), 85–87
  nonlymphoid cutaneous hematologic neoplasms, 93
  oncoscan SNP array, 82
  primary cutaneous follicle center lymphoma (PCFCL), 88–91
  primary cutaneous large B-cell lymphoma, leg type (PCLBCL-LT), 91–93
  primary cutaneous marginal zone lymphoma (PCMZL), 93
  Sézary syndrome (SS), 85–87, 86t
Follicular dendritic cell sarcomas (FDCS), 671
Follicular lymphoma (FL), 853
  cutaneous involvement by, 413, 414t
  genetics, 414
  histopathology, 413, 415f
  immunophenotype, 413–414, 416f
  prevalence, 413
Follicular mucinosis (FM), 824–825
Follicular T helper cells, 5
Folliculotropic mycosis fungoides (FMF), 820, 821f–822f
Folliculotropic mycosis fungoides (FTMF), 124–125, 124f–125f
Forward scatter, 62

G

G-banding, 82–85
Generalized eruptive histiocytosis (GEH), 695
GF. *See* Granuloma faciale (GF)
Gilteritinib, 841
Glasdegib, 841
Glycopeptide antibiotics, 852–853
Gout, 621
Granulocyte colony-stimulating factor (G-CSF), 624
Granulocytic sarcoma, 67
Granuloma annulare (GA), 910, 911f–912f
Granuloma faciale (GF), 580
Granulomatous CD8-positive lymphoproliferative disorder
  clinical presentation and prognosis, 233
  diagnosis, 236
  epidemiology, 233
  histology, 233, 234f
  immunophenotype, 234, 235f
Granulomatous dermatitis, 911
Granulomatous eruptions, 868
Granulomatous mycosis fungoides (MF), 107–109, 235
Granulomatous slack skin (GSS), 127–129, 129f–130f

H

HAART. *See* Highly active antiretroviral therapy (HAART)
Halo nevus, melanocytic tumors
  clinical features, 528–529
  differential diagnosis, 530, 530f
  histologic features, 529–530, 529f
  treatment, 530, 530f

Hand–Schüller–Christian disease, 721
Hematopoietic stem cells (HSCs), 635
Henoch–Schönlein purpura (HSP), 887
Hepatosplenic T-cell lymphoma, 826
Herpes simplex virus (HSV), 513–515, 514f
Herpetic viral infections, 567–568, 568f
HGBCL. *See* High-grade B-cell lymphoma (HGBCL)
High-grade B-cell lymphoma (HGBCL)
 gray zone lymphomas, 434, 435f–438f
 with 11q aberrations, 432
Highly active antiretroviral therapy (HAART), 444
Histiocytic neoplasms
 dendritic cell sarcomas (DCS), 702–706, 703t, 705f, 705t
 histiocytic sarcoma (HS), 702–706, 703t, 704f
 histiocytoses, molecular classification of, 664–671
 intralymphatic histiocytosis (ILH), 708–711, 709f–710f
 langerhans cell proliferations and related disorders ("L" group), 674–680
 Melkersson–Rosenthal syndrome 708, 711–712, 711f–712f
 non-Langerhans cell histiocytoses (NLCH), 690–699
 Rosai–Dorfman disease (RDD) 684–688, 685f–686f
Histiocytic sarcoma (HS), 616, 702, 703t
 differential diagnosis, 705, 705t
 histopathology, 702–703, 704f
 molecular alterations, 705–706
 therapy/prognosis, and outcome, 706
Histiocytoses, molecular classification of
 fibroblastic reticular cell tumor, 671
 follicular dendritic cell sarcomas, 671
 histiocytic neoplasms
  BRAF insertion/deletions in, 668
  RAF mutations, 668–669
 mutations, 664–668, 665f–667f
 structural gene rearrangements, 669–671
Histone deacetylase (HDAC) inhibitors, 847
HIV infections. *See* Human immunodeficiency virus (HIV) infections
HL. *See* Hodgkin lymphoma (HL)
Hodgkin and Reed–Sternberg (HRS) cells, 723
Hodgkin-like cells, 339
Hodgkin lymphoma (HL)
 alkylating agents, 852
 anthracyclines, 852
 antimicrotubules, 852
 CD30+ lymphoproliferative disorders (LPDs), 481
 clinical presentation, 481
 cutaneous dissemination, 480–481
 differential diagnosis, 484–488, 486f–487f
 epidemiology, 480
 etiology, 480
 genetics and molecular findings, 481–483
 glycopeptide antibiotics, 852–853
 histopathology, 481, 482f–484f
 immunohistochemistry, 481, 485f
 postulated cell of origin, 484
 prevalence, 480
HS. *See* Histiocytic sarcoma (HS)
HSV. *See* Herpes simplex virus (HSV)
HTLV-1. *See* Human T-lymphotropic virus-1 (HTLV-1)
Human herpes virus 6 (HHV-6), 684
Human immunodeficiency virus (HIV) infections, 569
Human T-lymphotropic virus-1 (HTLV-1), 311–312
Hydroa vacciniforme lymphoproliferative disease
 clinical findings, 790
 differential diagnosis, 791
 epidemiology, 788–790
 etiology, 790
 histologic features, 790–791, 791f
Hydroa vacciniforme lymphoproliferative disorder (HV-LPD)

clinical features, 263–265, 263f–265f
differential diagnosis, 267
epidemiology, 262
etiology, 262
genetic and molecular findings, 266
histopathology, 265–266, 265f–266f
immunophenotype, 266, 268f
postulated cell of origin, 266
Hydroxyurea (HU), 630–631, 631t, 845
Hypereosinophilic syndrome (HES), 626
Hyperpigmentation, 836
Hypopigmented mycosis fungoides (MF), 824, 824f–825f

I

Iatrogenic lymphoproliferative diseases (LPDs), 735
Ibrutinib, 843
Ichthyosiform mycosis fungoides (MF), 824
Ichthyosis, 621
Idiopathic hypereosinophilic syndrome, 626–629
Idiopathic lymphoid hyperplasia, 745, 746f–747f
IgG4-related disease (IgG4-RD)
 clinical presentation and prognosis, 577, 578f
 differential diagnosis, 579–580
 epidemiology, 577
 etiology, 577
 genetic and molecular findings, 578–579
 histology, 577–578, 578f–580f
 immunophenotype, 577–578
 pathogenesis, 578–579
IGH hypermutation testing
 amplification phase, 79
 sequencing phase, 79
IGHV hypermutation testing, 74
ILH. *See* Intralymphatic histiocytosis (ILH)
Imatinib, 631, 843
Immune checkpoint inhibitors, 867–869
Immunobullous eruptions, 868
Immunoglobulin-initiated mast cell activation, 36
Immunoglobulin rearrangement, 73
Immunophenotypic profiles, 66
Indeterminate cell histiocytosis (ICH), 680
Inflammatory dermatoses
 arthropod assault, 517, 518f
 atopic dermatitis (AD), 517–518
 chronic ulceration, 519–521, 520f
 drug-induced, 521–522, 522f
 eruption of lymphocyte recovery (ELR), 519
 pernio, 518
 pityriasis lichenoides et varioliformis acuta (PLEVA), 517
 postscabetic nodules, 517, 518f
 tattoo, 518, 519f
Interferon-α, 850
Interobserver reproducibility, 78–79
Intralymphatic histiocytosis (ILH)
 clinical features, 709
 differential diagnosis, 710–711
 epidemiology, 709
 histopathology, 709, 709f–710f
 immunophenotype, 710, 710f
 management and prognosis, 711
 pathogenesis, 708
Intraocular lymphomas, 760–761, 761f–762f
Intravascular large B-cell lymphoma, 329, 329f
 classification, 410
 clinical features, 410
 diagnostic workup, 410
 prevalence, 409–410
 prognosis, 410
 treatment, 410
Intravascular large B-cell lymphoma (IVLBCL)
 clinical presentation/prognosis, 423–424
 differential diagnosis, 425, 427
 epidemiology, 423
 etiology of, 423
 genetic and molecular findings, 425
 histology, 424, 425f–426f
 immunophenotype, 424, 427f
 postulated cell of origin, 425

treatment, 424
variants, 423
Intravascular lymphoma (IVL), 710
Intrinsic cell properties, 62
Invisible dermatosis, 622
IVLBCL. *See* Intravascular large B-cell lymphoma (IVLBCL)
Ivosidenib, 841
Ixazomib, 850–851

J

Janus kinase inhibitors, 631
Juvenile myelomonocytic leukemia (JMML), 629–630
Juvenile xanthogranuloma (JXG)
 clinical features, 690–691, 691f
 differential diagnosis, 693–694, 693f–694f
 epidemiology, 690
 histopathology, 691–692, 692f
 immunophenotype, 692
 pathogenesis, 691
 xanthomatous granuloma family, 694

K

Kawasaki disease (KD), 892–893
Kimura disease (KD), 399

L

Lacrimal gland lymphomas, 756–758
Langerhans cell histiocytosis (LCH), 653, 664, 721–723, 721f–722f
 clinical presentation, 675, 675f
 differential diagnosis, 678–679, 679f
 epidemiology, 674
 genetics, 677
 histopathology, 675–676, 676f
 immunohistochemistry and ancillary studies, 676–677, 677f–678f
 pathogenesis, 674
 prognosis and therapy, 679–680
Langerhans cell proliferations and related disorders ("L" group)
 Erdheim–Chester disease, 680
 indeterminate cell histiocytosis, 680
 langerhans cell histiocytosis (LCH), 674–680
LC. *See* Leukemia cutis (LC)
LCD. *See* Lymphomatoid contact dermatitis (LCD)
LCH. *See* Langerhans cell histiocytosis (LCH)
LELC. *See* Lymphoepithelioma-like carcinoma (LELC)
Lenalidomide, 639
Letterer–Siwe disease, 721
Leukemia. *See also specific leukemias*
 alopecia in, 827
 etiology, 717
 incidence, 717
 subtypes of, 609, 610t
Leukemia cutis (LC), 624
 clinical presentation and prognosis, 608, 609f
 differential diagnosis, 611–612
 epidemiology, 608
 etiology, 608
 genetic and molecular findings, 611
 histology, 609, 609f–610f, 610t
 immunophenotype, 609–611, 611f–613f
 postulated cell of origin, 611
Leukemic vasculitis (LV), 889
Leukocytoclastic vasculitis (LCV)
 clinical, 887
 etiology, 887
 histology, 887–889, 888f–890f, 888t
Lichenoid
 amalgam reaction, 745, 746f
 eruptions, 868
Lineage determination, 74
Liposomal doxorubicin, 834
Liquid samples processing, 65
LIS. *See* Lymphocytic infiltrate of the skin (LIS)

Livedo reticularis, 850
LPL. *See* Lymphoplasmacytic lymphoma (LPL)
Lupus panniculitis, 579
LyG. *See* Lymphomatoid granulomatosis (LyG)
LyK. *See* Lymphomatoid keratosis (LyK)
Lymph node and skin samples, processing of, 65
Lymphocyte development, gene rearrangement in
    immunoglobulin rearrangement, 73
    T-cell receptor (TCR), 73
Lymphocytic infiltrate of the skin (LIS)
    clinical features, 498, 499
    differential diagnosis, 499–501, 501t
    epidemiology, 498
    etiology, 498–499
    histopathological features, 498
    histopathology, 499, 499f–501f
    immunophenotype, 499
Lymphoepithelial lesions, 729
Lymphoepithelioma-like carcinoma (LELC)
    clinical features, 527
    differential diagnosis, 528
    histologic features, 527–528, 527f–528f
    treatment, 528
Lymphoid hyperplasia, 743, 745f
Lymphoid proliferations
    with bacterial infections, 569–570
    with viral infections, 567–569
Lymphomatoid contact dermatitis (LCD)
    clinical presentation and prognosis, 582, 582f, 583t
    differential diagnosis, 583, 586
    epidemiology, 582
    genetic and molecular findings, 583
    histology, 582–583, 584f–586f
    immunophenotype, 583
Lymphomatoid granulomatosis (LyG), 739
    clinical presentation and prognosis, 378–379, 379f
    differential diagnosis, 382–385
    epidemiology, 378
    etiology, 378
    genetic and molecular findings, 381–382
    grading, 380–381
    histology, 379–380, 380f–384f
    immunophenotype, 380
Lymphomatoid keratosis (LyK), 555
Lymphomatoid papulosis (LyP), 87–88
    clinical findings, 780
    differential diagnosis, 780–781
    epidemiology, 780
    etiology, 780
    expectant management, 245–246
    histologic features, 780–781, 781f
    treatment, 246
Lymphoplasmacytic lymphoma (LPL)
    clinical findings, 418–419
    cutaneous findings, 419, 419f
    epidemiology, 418–419
    histopathology, 419
    immunophenotype, 420, 420t
    laboratory findings, 420
Lymphoproliferative diseases (LPDs), 118, 717

M

Macrophage subsets and function, 29–30, 30f
Maculopapular cutaneous mastocytosis (MPCM), 653–656, 654f–655f
Maculopapular rash, 867
Malignant histiocytosis, 702
Mantle cell lymphoma (MCL), 729, 853
    cutaneous disease, 455–456, 458f
    differential diagnosis, 457–458
    growth pattern, 455
    histopathologic changes, 457, 459f–460f
    immunophenotype, 455, 456f–457f
    prognosis, 458
    treatment, 458
MAP2K1, 668
MAP3K1, 668

Marginal zone lymphoma (MZL), 853
    cutaneous involvement in, 415, 417f
    genetics, 418
    histopathology, 416
    immunophenotype, 417–418, 417f–419f
    prevalence, 414
Mast cell neoplasms, 650–651
    diffuse cutaneous mastocytosis, 656–657
    maculopapular cutaneous mastocytosis, 653–656
    mast cell sarcomas (MCSs), 660
    mastocytoma, 651–653
    systemic mastocytosis with cutaneous involvement (SM+), 657–660
Mast cells (MCs)
    activation, 34–36
    classification, 34
    disease
        allergy, 36
        autoimmune disease, 37
        cancer, 37
    FcεRI, 36
    FcγR, 36
    hematopoietic origins, 34
    identification, 34
    immunoglobulin-initiated mast cell activation, 36
    localization, 34
Mast cell sarcomas (MCSs)
    histology, 660, 660f
    immunophenotype, 660, 661f
    treatment, 660
Mastocytoma, 651–653, 652f
Mature T-cell lymphoma
    α/β chain type, 67–68
    clonality studies, 68
    γ/δ type, 68
MC. *See* Molluscum contagiosum (MC)
Melanocytic tumors
    halo nevus
        clinical features, 528–529
        differential diagnosis, 530, 530f
        histologic features, 529–530, 529f
        treatment, 530, 530f
    regressing melanoma, 528–530
Melkersson–Rosenthal syndrome (MRS)
    differential diagnosis, 712
    etiology, 711
    immunophenotype, 711–712
    pathologic features, 711, 711f–712f
    therapy, 711
Melphalan, 851
Memory B-cells, 16
6-Mercaptopurine, 837–838
Mesenchymal tumors
    acral pseudolymphomatous angiokeratoma of children (APACHE)
        clinical features, 532
        differential diagnosis, 533
        histopathological features, 532–533, 533f
        treatment, 533–534
    angiomatoid fibrous histiocytoma (AFH), 536–537, 536f–537f
    angioplasmacellular hyperplasia, 534
    angiosarcoma, 534–536, 535f
    epithelioid hemangioma
        clinical features, 530
        differential diagnosis, 532
        histologic features, 530–531, 531f–532f
        treatment, 532
    myxoinflammatory fibroblastic sarcoma, 537–539, 538f
Methotrexate (MTX), 837–838, 838, 839f
Methotrexate-associated B-cell lymphoproliferative disorders (MTX-LPDs)
    clinical presentation, 393
    differential diagnosis, 396
    epidemiology, 393
    genetics, 396
    histology, 394, 397f
    immunohistochemistry, 394–395

subcutaneous panniculitis-like T-cell lymphoma (SPTCL), 392
    treatment, 396
Midostaurin, 841
Milker nodules, 516
Mogamulizumab, 244, 848
Molluscum contagiosum (MC), 515–516, 515f, 568–569
Monoclonal antibodies (MAbs)
    chronic leukemias, 842
    multiple myeloma (MM), 851–852
    nucleoside analogs, 848–849
Mononuclear phagocytic system, 702
    antigen-presenting cells
        inflamed skin, 28–29
        normal skin, 26
    CD1C+ DCS (CDC2), 28
    CD14+ DCS, 28
    CD141+ DCS (CDC1), 28
    dermis, 28
    epidermis, 26–28, 27f
    macrophage subsets and function, 29–30, 30f
    plasmacytoid dendritic cells (pDCs), 29
Morbihan disease (MD), 712
MPNs. *See* Myeloproliferative neoplasms (MPNs)
MTX-LPDs. *See* Methotrexate-associated B-cell lymphoproliferative disorders (MTX-LPDs)
Mucosa-associated lymphoid tissue (MALT), 729, 751
Multicentric reticulohistiocytosis (MRH)
    clinical features, 696
    histopathology, 696–697, 697f–698f
    immunophenotype, 698
Multiple myeloma-1 (MUM-1), 340–341
Multiple myeloma (MM), 739–743
    antiangiogenic agents, 851
    cyclophosphamide and melphalan, 851
    diagnosis, 742
    monoclonal antibodies (MAbs), 851–852
    proteasome inhibitors, 850–851
    signs and symptoms, 741
    treatment, 743
Multi-targeted protein kinase inhibitors, 841
MUM-1. *See* Multiple myeloma-1 (MUM-1)
Mycobacteria, 517
Mycosis fungoides (MF), 85–87, 171–172
    alopecia, lymphoproliferative disorders
        erythrodermic cutaneous T-cell lymphoma, 824, 824f
        follicular mucinosis (FM), 824–825
        folliculotropic, 820, 821f–822f
        hypopigmented, 824, 824f–825f
        ichthyosiform, 824
        patch, plaque, and tumor stage, 821f–822f, 823f
        syringotropic mycosis fungoides (SMF), 820–821, 822f–823f
    clinical presentation and prognosis, 110
        patch stage, 110
        plaque stage, 110
        tumor stage, 110–111
    epidemiology, 109
    erythrodermic mycosis fungoides, 130, 131f
    etiology, 109–110
    folliculotropic mycosis fungoides (FTMF), 124–125, 124f–125f
    genetic and molecular findings, 121–123
    granulomatous mycosis fungoides, 127, 129, 134
    granulomatous slack skin (GSS), 127–129, 129f–130f
    histologic differential diagnosis, 134
    histology
        patch stage mycosis fungoides, 111–114, 113f–115f, 113t
        plaque stage mycosis fungoides, 114–115, 115f–116f
        staging and extracutaneous spread, 116–117, 117t–118t
        tumor stage mycosis fungoides, 115–116, 116f

histopathological variants of, 123–124, 123t
hypopigmented, 104, 109, 130, 131f, 132
ichthyosiform, 132
interstitial mycosis fungoides, 132–133
immunophenotype, 118–121, 120f–122f
postulated cell of origin, 123
syringotropic mycosis fungoides (SMF), 125, 127f
variants, 129–134, 131f, 133f
Mycotic infections, 516–517
Myelodysplastic syndrome, 717
Myeloid sarcoma (MS), 718, 718f–720f
clinical presentation and prognosis, 614
differential diagnosis, 615–618, 618f
epidemiology, 613–614
etiology, 614
histology, 614–615, 614f
immunophenotype, 615, 616f–617f
postulated cell of origin, 615
Myelomonocytic cell tumors, 626, 627f
Myeloperoxidase (MPO), 615
Myelophthisic anemia, 717
Myeloproliferative disorders (MPDs), 622, 622t
Myeloproliferative neoplasms (MPNs), 621
disease-related cutaneous manifestations
chronic myeloid leukemia (CML), 624–626
chronic myelomonocytic leukemia (CMML), 626, 627f–630f
essential thrombocythemia (ET), 622–623
idiopathic hypereosinophilic syndrome, 626–629
juvenile myelomonocytic leukemia (JMML), 629–630
polycythemia rubra vera (PRV), 621–622
primary myelofibrosis (PMF), 623–624, 624f–625f
treatment-related cutaneous manifestations
hydroxyurea (HU), 630–631, 631t
Janus kinase inhibitors, 631
tyrosine kinase inhibitors (TKIs), 631, 631t
Myxoinflammatory fibroblastic sarcoma, 537–539, 538f
MZL. *See* Marginal zone lymphoma (MZL)

N

Naïve B-cells, 12
Natural killer (NK)–cell enteropathy (NKE), 277, 277f–278f
Natural killer (NK)–cell leukemias/lymphomas
aggressive natural killer leukemia (ANKL)
clinical presentation and prognosis, 274
differential diagnosis, 276
epidemiology, 274
etiology, 274
genetic and molecular findings, 275–276
histology, 274
immunophenotype, 275
skin involvement, 276
chronic lymphoproliferative disorders of natural killer (CLPD-NK) cells
clinical presentation and prognosis, 276
differential diagnosis, 277
epidemiology, 276
etiology, 276
genetic and molecular findings, 276
immunophenotype, 276
morphology, 276
skin involvement, 276
extranodal natural killer (NK)/T-cell lymphoma, nasal type, 270
clinical presentation and prognosis, 271
differential diagnosis, 271–273, 273f
epidemiology, 270
etiology, 270
genetic and molecular findings, 271
histology, 271
immunophenotype, 271
skin involvement, 271, 272f
natural killer (NK)–cell enteropathy (NKE), 277, 277f–278f

Natural killer (NK) cells, 6
biology, 21
cytokine production, 22
cytotoxicity, 21
development, 21
functions, 21
origins, 21
tissue distribution, 22
tissue frequency
liver, 23
lymph nodes, 22
mucosa-associated lymphoid tissue, 23
peripheral blood and bone marrow, 22
salivary gland, 23
skin, 22
spleen, 22
tissues, immunophenotypic identification, 23
Necrobiotic xanthogranuloma (NXG)
clinical features, 695–696
histopathology, 696
Necrosis, 639
Necrotizing neutrophilic dermatosis (NND), 874
Neutrophilic dermatoses (NDs), 621
Neutrophilic eccrine hidradenitis (NEH), 836
New-generation advanced flow cytometers, 62
Next-generation sequencing (NGS)
bioinformatic aspects
initial processing, 99
reporting, 100
variant annotation, 99–100
cutaneous hematopathology
cancer gene set testing, 101
cancer predisposition testing, 101
clonality testing, 101–102
DNA sequencing
emergence of, 97–98
illumina sequencing, 98
ion torrent sequencing, 98
Maxam–Gilbert sequencing, 97
Sanger sequencing, 97
operational and regulatory considerations
assay validation, 101
professional societies, guidance from, 100–101
turnaround time, 101
third-generation methods, 98–99
NHL. *See* Non-Hodgkin lymphoma (NHL)
Nilotinib, 843
Nivolumab, 867
Non-Hodgkin lymphoma (NHL), 455, 724
B-cell lymphomas, 724–733
Burkitt lymphoma, 853–854
diffuse large B-cell lymphoma (DLBCL), 853
follicular lymphoma, 853
mantle-cell lymphoma (MCL), 853
marginal-zone lymphoma, 853
small-cell lymphocytic lymphoma (SCLL), 853
T-cell lymphomas, 733–734, 854–855
Non-Langerhans cell histiocytosis (NLCH)
ALK-positive histiocytosis, 696
benign cephalic histiocytosis (BCH), 694–695
generalized eruptive histiocytosis (GEH), 695
juvenile and adult xanthogranuloma (JXG-AXG), 690–694
multicentric reticulohistiocytosis (MRH), 696–698
necrobiotic xanthogranuloma (NXG), 695–696
progressive nodular histiocytosis (PNH), 695
solitary reticulohistiocytoma, 698–699
xanthoma disseminatum, 695
Nonlymphoid cutaneous hematologic neoplasms, 93
Normal skin homeostasis, B-cells in
recruitment of, 16
skin disease, 16–18, 18f
Nucleoside analogs, 848–849

O

Ocular adnexa, 751
hematopoietic neoplasms, 763t–765t
lymphoma types, 753t
Ocular adnexal lymphomas (OALs), 751

Ocular lymphoproliferative disorders
anatomical basis, 751
clinical presentation and prognosis, 754
conjunctival lymphomas, 755–756, 756f–759f
epidemiology, 752–753, 753t
etiology, 752
eye-associated lymphoid tissue (EALT), 751–752
eyelid lymphomas, 759–760, 760f, 760t
genetics, 753
immunophenotype of, 753–754
intraocular lymphomas, 760–761, 761f–762f
lacrimal gland lymphomas, 756–758
orbital lymphomas, 754–755, 754f–755f
therapy and management, 761–765, 763t–765t
Optics, 59
Oral lymphoproliferative disorders, 717
benign lymphoid proliferations, 743–746
classic Hodgkin lymphoma (HL), 723–724
EBV-associated lymphoid proliferations, 734–739
Langerhans cell histiocytosis (LCH), 721–723
leukemia, 717–721
multiple myeloma (MM), 739–743
non-Hodgkin lymphoma (NHL), 724–734
plasmacytoma, 743
Oral mucositis, 718
Orbital lymphomas, 754–755, 754f–755f
Osteosclerotic myeloma, 399

P

Paraneoplastic pemphigus (PNP)
clinical presentation, 898–899
differential diagnosis, 898–899
epidemiology, 897
histopathology, 899–900, 899f–900f
pathogenesis, 897–898
treatment and prognosis, 900–901
Patch stage mycosis fungoides, 110, 111–114, 113f–115f, 113t
PBL. *See* Plasmablastic lymphoma (PBL)
PCDLBCL. *See* Primary cutaneous diffuse large B-cell lymphoma, leg type (PCDLBCL)
PCDLBCL-LT. *See* Primary cutaneous diffuse large B-cell lymphoma, leg type (PCDLBCL-LT)
PD-1. *See* Programmed death-1 (PD-1)
PEL. *See* Primary effusion lymphoma (PEL)
Pembrolizumab, 867
Pentostatin, 842
Peripheral T-cell lymphoma, not otherwise specified (PTCL-NOS)
clinical presentation/prognosis/treatment, 220
differential diagnosis, 223
epidemiology, 220
etiology, 220
genetic and molecular findings, 221–223, 223f
histology, 220–221, 222f
immunophenotype, 221
postulated cell of origin, 223
primary cutaneous T-cell lymphomas, 223
Permanent chemotherapy-induced alopecia (PCIA), 828
Persistent pigmented purpuric dermatoses (PPPDs), 503
Photochemotherapies, 849
Pigmented purpuric dermatoses (PPDs)
clinical presentation, 503, 504f
differential diagnosis, 503–504, 504f
epidemiology, 503
histopathology, 503, 504f
Pityriasis lichenoides chronica (PLC)
clinical presentation, 492, 493f
differential diagnosis, 495–496
genetic and molecular findings, 495
histopathology, 493, 494f
immunophenotype, 493, 495f–496f
prognosis, 492, 493f
Pityriasis lichenoides et varioliformis acuta (PLEVA), 172–173, 517
Plaque stage mycosis fungoides, 110, 114–115, 115f–116f

Plasmablastic lymphoma (PBL), 438, 439–446, 445f, 477, 726, 726f–728f
Plasma cell neoplasms (PCN), 66–67
  clinical features, 474, 475f, 475t
  cytogenetic studies, 475–476
  differential diagnosis, 476–478
  epidemiology, 474
  histology, 474, 476f–477f
  immunophenotype, 474–475, 478f
Plasma cells, 16
Plasmacytoid dendritic cells (pDCs), 29, 626, 628f
Plasmacytomas, 743, 744f
PLC. See Pityriasis lichenoides chronica (PLC)
PLEVA. See Pityriasis lichenoides et varioliformis acuta (PLEVA)
Polyarteritis nodosa (PAN)
  clinical, 891, 893f
  with hematologic malignancies, 891
  histology, 891–892, 893f
Polycythemia rubra vera (PRV), 621–622
Polymerase chain reaction (PCR)
  clonality testing, clinical utility of
    basic principle, 74
    BIOMED-2, 74–75
    BIOMED-2 IGH clonality assay, 75, 75f–76f
    clonal lymphoid process, ascertainment of, 73–74
    EuroClonality consensus primer sets, 74–75
    IGHV hypermutation testing, 74
    lineage determination, 74
    methodology for, 74
    residual/recurrent disease, monitoring for, 74
    suitable sample types, 74
    TCRG, 76
    turnaround time, 76
  clonality testing data
    monoclonal/biclonal, 76–77, 77f
    oligoclonal, 77–78
    polyclonal, 78
  IGH hypermutation testing
    amplification phase, 79
    sequencing phase, 79
    interobserver reproducibility, 78–79
    lymphocyte development, gene rearrangement in
      immunoglobulin rearrangement, 73
      T-cell receptor (TCR), 73
Posttransplant lymphoproliferative disorders (PTLDs)
  clinical presentation, 388–389, 389f
  epidemiology, 388
  genetics, 389
  histology, 389, 390f–391f
  immunophenotype, 389
  therapy, 389, 391
Postulated cell of origin, 168
PPDs. See Pigmented purpuric dermatoses (PPDs)
PPPDs. See Persistent pigmented purpuric dermatoses (PPPDs)
Precursor B cells, 12
Precursor T-/B-cell lymphoblastic leukemias/lymphomas
  clinical findings, 797, 799f
  differential diagnosis, 799
  epidemiology, 797
  histologic features, 797–799
Pretibial lymphoplasmacytic plaque (PLP), 477
Primary cutaneous anaplastic large-cell lymphoma (C-ALCL), 247
  brentuximab vedotin, 248
  chemotherapy, 247–248
  radiotherapy, 247
  surgical excision, 247
  treatment, 247–248, 250
Primary cutaneous CD8+ acral lymphoproliferative disorder (CD8+ acral LPD), 234–235
  clinical presentation and prognosis, 225–226, 226f
  differential diagnosis, 228–230, 230t
  epidemiology, 225
  etiology, 225
  genetic and molecular findings, 228
  histology, 226–228, 226f–227f
  immunophenotype, 228, 228f–229f
Primary cutaneous CD30-positive T-cell lymphoproliferative disorders (TLPDs)
  classic Hodgkin lymphoma (CHL), 171
  clinical presentation, 159–161
    lymphomatoid papulosis (LyP), 160–161, 160f–161f
    primary cutaneous anaplastic large cell lymphoma (pcALCL), 159–160, 160f
  differential diagnosis, 169–173
  epidemiology
    lymphomatoid papulosis (LyP), 159
    primary cutaneous anaplastic large cell lymphoma (pcALCL), 158–159
  etiology, 159
  genetic and molecular findings, 166–168
  histology
    lymphomatoid papulosis (LyP), 162–165, 163f–166f
    primary cutaneous anaplastic large cell lymphoma (pcALCL), 161–162, 162f
  immunophenotype
    lymphomatoid papulosis (LyP), 165–166, 170f
    primary cutaneous anaplastic large cell lymphoma (pcALCL), 165, 168f–169f
  mycosis fungoides (MF), 171–172
  other reactive conditions, 173
  other T-cell lymphomas, 172
  pityriasis lichenoides et varioliformis acuta (PLEVA), 172–173
  postulated cell of origin, 168
  prognosis, 159–161
  systemic anaplastic large cell lymphoma (ALCL), 168–171, 173f
Primary cutaneous CD4+ small to medium T-cell lymphoproliferative disorder (SMPTCL), 786
Primary cutaneous diffuse large B-cell lymphoma, leg type (PCDLBCL)
  classification, 408
  clinical features, 408
  diagnostic workup, 408
  prevalence, 408
  prognosis, 408
  treatment, 408–409, 409f
Primary cutaneous diffuse large B-cell lymphoma, leg type (PCDLBCL-LT)
  clinical presentation/prognosis, 360–362, 361f–362f
  differential diagnosis, 367–372, 368f–372f
  epidemiology, 360
  etiology, 360
  genetic and molecular findings, 365–367
  histology, 362, 363f–365f
  immunophenotype, 362–365, 366f
  postulated cell of origin, 367
  treatment, 372
Primary cutaneous follicle center lymphoma (PC-FCL), 50–51, 88–91, 322–323, 332, 464
  clinical and histologic findings, 796, 797f–798f
  clinical presentation and prognosis, 336, 337f–338f
  differential diagnosis, 342–344, 343f, 344t, 796–797
  diffuse-type, 339, 339f–340f, 343f
  epidemiology, 336, 795–796
  etiology, 336
  follicular-type, 338, 338f–339f
  genetic and molecular findings, 342
  histology, 337–339, 338f–340f
  immunophenotype, 340–342, 341f–342f
  postulated cell of, 342

spindle cell, 339, 340f
Primary cutaneous gamma-delta T-cell lymphoma, 786–788, 789f
  clinical presentation, 204
  differential diagnosis, 208–210
  epidemiology, 203
  etiology, 203–204
  genetic and molecular findings, 206–208
  histology, 204–205, 205f
  immunophenotype, 205–206
  postulated cell of origin, 208
  prognosis, 204
Primary cutaneous large B-cell lymphoma, leg type (PCLBCL-LT), 91–93
Primary cutaneous lymphomas (PCLs), 68–69
Primary cutaneous marginal zone lymphoma (PCMZL), 51–54, 52f–53f, 93, 322–323, 332, 464, 476–477
  clinical presentation and prognosis, 348, 348f
  differential diagnosis, 354–355, 355f–356f
  epidemiology, 347
  etiology, 347–348
  genetic and molecular findings, 352, 354
  histology, 348–350, 349f–351f
  immunophenotype, 350–352, 351f, 352t, 353f–354f
  MALT lymphoma, 347
  postulated cell of origin, 354
Primary cutaneous marginal zone lymphoma/lymphoproliferative disorder
  clinical findings, 794, 795f
  differential diagnosis, 795
  epidemiology, 794
  etiology, 794
  histologic features, 794–795, 795f–796f
Primary cutaneous small/medium CD4-positive T-cell lymphoproliferative disorder (LPD)
  clinical features, 193
  differential diagnoses, 197–200
  general features, 193
  genetic and molecular findings, 197
  histopathologic findings, 193–194, 194f–196f
  immunophenotype, 194–197, 197f–199f
  prognosis and therapy, 200
Primary cutaneous T-cell lymphomas (CTCLs)
  allogeneic transplantation, 242
  basic principles, 238–239
  chemotherapy, 241–242
  extracorporeal photochemotherapy (ECP), 242
  phototherapy, 240
    total skin electron beam therapy (TSEBT), 240–241
  Sézary syndrome (SS), 243
  skin-directed therapies
    topical corticosteroids, 239–240
  systemic therapies, 241
    interferon, 241
    retinoids (including bexarotene), 241
Primary effusion lymphoma (PEL), 446–447, 447f–448f
Primary intraocular lymphomas (PIOLs), 760
Primary myelofibrosis (PMF), 623–624, 624f–625f, 635. See also Extramedullary hematopoiesis (EMH)
Progressive nodular histiocytosis (PNH), 695
Proteasome inhibitors, 850
Pseudolymphoma
  Epstein-Barr virus (EBV), 516, 516f
  herpes simplex virus (HSV), 513–515, 514f
  Milker nodules, 516
  molluscum contagiosum (MC), 515–516, 515f
  mycobacteria, 517
  mycotic infections, 516–517
  verruca vulgaris, 516
  with tattoos, 563–565, 564f
  with vaccination, 562–563, 563f
Psoriasiform eruptions, 868
PTLDs. See Posttransplant lymphoproliferative disorders (PTLDs)

Purine analogs, 842
Pyoderma gangrenosum (PG), 914
    associated conditions, 914–915
    clinical features, 914, 915f
    differential diagnosis, 915–916
    epidemiology, 914
    etiology, 914
    histologic features, 914, 915f
    treatment, 916

R

Radiation therapy, 828
Raynaud phenomenon, 850
RDD. *See* Rosai–Dorfman–disease (RDD)
Reactive angioendotheliomatosis (RAE), 710
Reactive granulomatous dermatitis (RGD), 910
Reactive lymphoid hyperplasia (RLH), 752
Reed–Sternberg cells, 339, 380
Regulatory T cells, 5
Residual/recurrent disease, monitoring for, 74
Reticulohistiocytoma (RH), 693, 696
Retinoids, 849
Richter syndrome (RS), 464–467, 469f
Rituximab, 842
Rosai–Dorfman disease (RDD), 684
    clinical presentation and prognosis, 684–685, 685f
    differential diagnosis, 688
    epidemiology, 684
    etiology, 684
    genetic and molecular findings, 687–688
    histology, 685–687, 686f
    immunophenotype, 687
    postulated cell of origin, 688
    treatment, 688

S

Sarcoidosis, 236
Schnitzler syndrome (SchS)
    diagnosis, 918
    Lipsker and Strasbourg diagnostic criteria, 917, 918t
    male-to-female ratio, 917
Severe mosquito bite allergy (SMBA), 788
    extranodal NK/T-cell lymphoma (ENKTL), 791–794
    hydroa vacciniforme lymphoproliferative disease, 788–791
Sézary syndrome (SS), 85–87, 86t
    candidate tumor markers, 152
    clinical presentation, 143–146, 144f–146f
    differential diagnosis, 152–153, 153f
    epidemiology, 143
    etiology, 143
    genetic and molecular findings, 149–150
    histopathology, 147–148, 147f
    immune dysregulation, 150–152, 151f–153f
    immunohistochemistry (IHC), 148
    peripheral blood findings, 148–149, 149f
    postulated cell of origin, 150
    prognosis, 146
    staging, 146
    treatment, 146–147
sFL. *See* Systemic follicular lymphoma (sFL)
Side scatter, 62
SLHA. *See* Syringolymphoid hyperplasia with alopecia (SLHA)
Small-cell lymphocytic lymphoma (SCLL), 853
Small lymphocytic lymphoma (SLL), 718, 718f, 729
Small molecule tyrosine kinase inhibitors, 841
Solitary pagetoid reticulosis (PR) - Woringer-Kolopp disease, 125–127, 128f
Solitary reticulohistiocytoma, 697f
    clinical features, 698
    differential diagnosis, 698
    pathogenesis, 699
    prognosis, 699
Spiradenoma
    clinical features, 526

    differential diagnosis, 526–527, 527f
    histologic features, 526, 527f
    treatment, 527
Subcutaneous panniculitis–like T-cell lymphoma (SPLTCL), 392, 825
    clinical findings, 784
    clinical presentation/prognosis, 179, 179f
    differential diagnosis, 183–184, 184f–188f, 784–786
    epidemiology, 178, 783
    etiology, 178, 783–784
    genetic and molecular findings, 181–183
    histologic features, 784, 785f
    histopathology, 180, 180f–182f
    immunophenotype, 180–181, 183f
    postulated cell of origin, 183
    treatment, 179–180
Sweet syndrome (SS), 872
    clinical presentation, 874–875, 874f–875f
    differential diagnosis, 878–879
    epidemiology, 872–874
    etiology, 872–874
    histology, 875–878
Syringolymphoid hyperplasia with alopecia (SLHA), 555
Syringotropic mycosis fungoides (SMF), 125, 127f, 820–821, 822f–823f
Systemic anaplastic large cell lymphoma
    clinical presentation and prognosis, 280
    differential diagnosis, 286–288, 287f
    epidemiology, 280
    genetic and molecular findings, 284–286
    histology, 280–281
    immunophenotype, 281–282, 282f–285f
    postulated cell of origin, 283
Systemic anaplastic large cell lymphoma (ALCL), 168–171, 173f
Systemic B-cell lymphoma, 827
Systemic chronic active Epstein–Barr virus (EBV) disease
    clinical and histologic findings, 786–788
    epidemiology, 786
Systemic follicular lymphoma (sFL)
    cutaneous involvement by, 413, 414t
    genetics, 414
    histopathology, 413, 415f
    immunophenotype, 413–414, 416f
    prevalence, 413
Systemic marginal zone lymphomas, 414–418
Systemic mastocytosis (SM), 650
    with cutaneous involvement, 657
        clinical presentation, 657–658, 657f–658f
        differential diagnosis, 660
        epidemiology, 657
        etiology, 657
        histopathology, 659, 659f
        prognosis, 658
        treatment, 659–660
Systemic/nodal follicular Lymphoma, 344, 344t

T

Takayasu arteritis (TA), 892–893
T-cell-dependent germinal center reaction, 13–16, 14f–15f
T-cell histiocyte-rich large B-cell lymphoma (THRBCL), 449
T-cell–independent B-cell differentiation, 12–13
T-cell lineage-acute lymphoblastic leukemia/lymphoma (T-ALL), 598–605
T-cell lymphomas
    anaplastic large-cell lymphoma (ALCL), 733–734, 733f
    extranodal NK/T-cell lymphoma, nasal type (ENKTCL), 734, 736f
    mycosis fungoides (MF), 734, 734f–735f
T-cell lymphoproliferative disorder, 322, 325f
T-cell prolymphocytic leukemia (T-PLL)
    clinical presentation and prognosis, 291, 291f–293f

    differential diagnosis, 295
    epidemiology, 291
    etiology, 291
    genetic and molecular findings, 292–295
    histology, 291–292, 293f–294f
    immunophenotype, 292, 294f
    postulated cell of origin, 292
T-cell receptor (TCR), 73
T-cell-rich angiomatoid polypoid pseudolymphoma (TRAPP), 533
γδT cells, 6
TCRG, 76
T helper 1 (T_H1) cells, 3–4
T helper 2 (T_H2) cells, 3–4
T helper 9 (T_H9) cells, 5
T helper 17 (T_H17) cells, 4
T helper 22 (T_H22) cells, 4–5
Third-generation methods, 98–99
THRBCL. *See* T-cell histiocyte-rich large B-cell lymphoma (THRBCL)
Thrombocytopenia, 638
Tibial lymphoplasmacytic plaque (TLP), 533
Tisagenlecleucel (KYMRIAH), 869
TLE. *See* Tumid lupus erythematosus (TLE)
TLP. *See* Tibial lymphoplasmacytic plaque (TLP)
T-lymphoblastic lymphoma, 68
Topical mechlorethamine, 244
Total skin electron beam therapy (TSEBT), 849
TRAPP. *See* T-cell-rich angiomatoid polypoid pseudolymphoma (TRAPP)
Traumatic ulcerative granuloma with stromal eosinophilia (TUGSE), 520–521, 520f
Treponemal infections, 569–570
Tumid lupus erythematosus (TLE)
    clinical features, 498, 499
    differential diagnosis, 499–501, 501t
    epidemiology, 498
    etiology, 498–499
    histopathological features, 498
    histopathology, 499, 499f–501f
    immunophenotype, 499
Type I interferons (IFNs), 498
Tyrosine kinase inhibitors (TKIs), 631, 631t
    chronic leukemias, 843, 843f–844f

U

Urticarial vasculitis (UV), 888

V

Vasculitis, 887
    erythema elevatum diutinum (EED)
        clinical, 890
        etiology, 890
        histology, 890, 891f
    Kawasaki disease (KD), 892–893
    leukocytoclastic vasculitis (LCV)
        clinical, 887
        etiology, 887
        histology, 887–889, 888f–890f, 888t
    polyarteritis nodosa (PAN), 891–892
    Takayasu arteritis (TA), 892–893
Venetoclax, 841
Vinblastine, 852
Vincristine, 839, 852
Vitiligo-like skin hypopigmentation, 868

W

Wegener granulomatosis (WG), 888
Wells syndrome
    clinical manifestations, 883, 884f
    differential diagnosis, 885
    pathogenesis, 883
    pathology, 883–885, 884f
    treatment, 885

X

Xanthoma disseminatum (XD), 695